Kelley's

TEXTBOOK OF Rheumatology

Section 6. Diagnostic Tests and Procedures in Rheumatic Diseases

Section 7. Modalities of Therapy in Rheumatic Diseases: Nonpharmacologic Interventions and Drug Therapy

Section 8. Rheumatoid Arthritis

Section 9. Spondyloarthropathies

Section 10. Systemic Lupus Erythematosus and Related Syndromes

Section 11. Mixed Connective Tissue Disease, Scleroderma, and Inflammatory Myopathies

Section 12. Vasculitis

Section 13. Crystal-induced Inflammation

Section 14. Bone, Cartilage, and Heritable Connective Tissue Disorders

Section 15. Rheumatic Diseases of Childhood

Section 16. Infection and Arthritis

Section 17. Arthritis Accompanying Systemic Diseases

Section 18. The Common Ground of Rheumatology and Orthopaedic Surgery

****SPECIAL FEATURE****
****ON ENCLOSED****
****DVD****

THE GENERAL AND SCREENING MUSCULOSKELETAL EXAMINATION
BY GEORGE LAWRY

V O L U M E 1

Kelley's TEXTBOOK OF Rheumatology

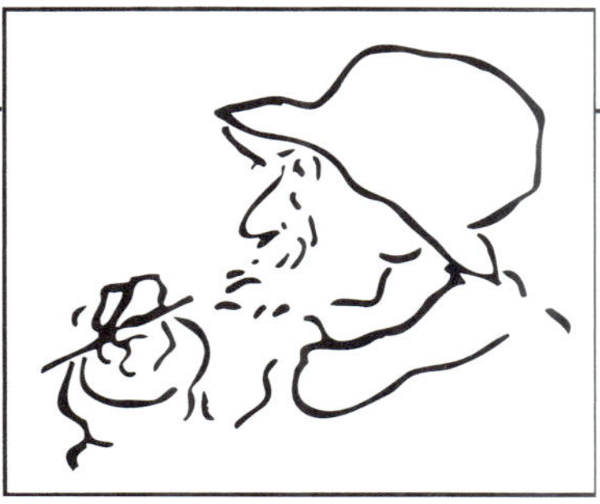

EDITORS

Edward D. Harris, Jr., MD
George DeForest Barnett Professor of Medicine, Emeritus
Stanford University School of Medicine
Academic Secretary to Stanford University
Stanford, California

Ralph C. Budd, MD
Professor of Medicine
Chief of Clinical Services
Division of Immunology and Rheumatology
University of Vermont College of Medicine
Burlington, Vermont

Mark C. Genovese, MD
Associate Professor of Medicine
Chief of Clinical Services
Division of Immunology and Rheumatology
Stanford University
Stanford, California

Gary S. Firestein, MD
Professor of Medicine
Chief, Division of Rheumatology, Allergy and Immunology
University of California, San Diego School of Medicine
La Jolla, California

John S. Sargent, MD
Professor of Medicine and Senior Associate Dean for Clinical Affairs
Vanderbilt University School of Medicine
Chief Medical Officer
Vanderbilt University Medical Center
Nashville, Tennessee

Clement B. Sledge, MD
John B. and Buckminster Brown Professor Emeritus of Orthopedic Surgery
Harvard Medical School
Chairman Emeritus, Department of Orthopedic Surgery
Brigham and Women's Hospital
Boston, Massachusetts

ELECRONIC EDITOR

Shaun Ruddy, MD
Elam C. Toone Professor Emeritus of Internal Medicine, Microbiology and Immunology
Chairman Emeritus, Division of Rheumatology, Allergy, and Immunology
Department of Internal Medicine
Virgina Commonwealth University School of Medicine
Richmond, Virginia

ELSEVIER
SAUNDERS

ELSEVIER
SAUNDERS
The Curtis Center
170 S Independence Mall W 300 E
Philadelphia, Pennsylvania 19106

Kelley's Textbook of Rheumatology, Seventh Edition
ISBN: 0-7216-0141-3

Notice

Surgery is an ever-changing field. Standard safety precautions must be followed, but as new research and clinical experience broaden our knowledge, changes in treatment and drug therapy may become necessary or appropriate. Readers are advised to check the most current product information provided by the manufacturer of each drug to be administered to verify the recommended dose, the method and duration of administration, and contraindications. It is the responsibility of the licensed prescriber, relying on experience and knowledge of the patient, to determine dosages and the best treatment for each individual patient. Neither the publisher nor the author assumes any liability for any injury and/or damage to persons or property arising from this publication.

International Standard Book Number: 0-7216-0141-3

Library of Congress Cataloging-in-Publication Data

Kelley's textbook of rheumatology / edited by Edward D. Harris, Jr. ...[et al.].–7th ed.
p.; cm.
Includes bibliographical references and index.
ISBN 0-7216-0141-3
1. Rheumatism. 2. Arthritis. I. Title: Textbook of rheumatology. II. Harris, Edward D., 1937-III. Kelley, William N., 1939-
[DNLM: 1. Rheumatic Diseases. 2. Arthritis. WE 544 K29 2005]
RC927.T49 2005
616.7′23—dc22 2004052586

Printed in the United States

Last digit is the print number: 9 8 7 6 5 4 3 2 1

The editors are proud to dedicate this seventh edition of Textbook of Rheumatology to our mentors, colleagues in research and the clinics, and family and loved ones. Our mentors showed us the way, giving us focus and a sense of what questions were truly important to answer. Our colleagues amplified our work, gave us course correction, and through their own hard efforts and successes, invigorated our own efforts. To our wives and loved ones (including those dear children and grandkids) we owe deep and abundant thanks for nurture and sustenance in good times and, especially, on those days when all seems bleak. We all agree that we would choose the paths we have taken once again, so long as those mentioned above would be there to join us.

Ted Harris: Many thanks to my mentor, Steve Krane, and for the support of the Harris boys and Eileen...and for the happy smiles of the grandkids—Andrew, Eliza, Maeve, and Liam.

Ralph C. Budd: Sincere thanks to the kind mentoring from Edward D. Harris, Jr., H. Robson MacDonald, and C. Garrison Fathman, as well as to the support of my wife, Lenore, and my children, Graham and Laura.

Gary S. Firestein: Thanks to Linda and our children, David and Cathy, for their patience and support, as well as to Nathan Zvaifler for his guidance for over two decades.

Mark C. Genovese: To my wife Nancy and our daughters, Alexandra, Danielle, and Lauren, for their patience and support, and to Ted Harris for his guidance and mentorship.

Shaun Ruddy: To my wife, Millie; our children, Christi and Candace; and our grandchildren, Kevin, Matthew and Katharine.

John S. Sergent: To Carole and our children, Ellen and Katie, and to our grandchildren, Kathryn, Henry, and Emmaline.

Clement Sledge: To my wife, Georgia; our children, Mego, John, Matthew, and Claire; and our grandchildren, Matthew, Kaitlyn, Kevin, and Brian Tracy; Alexa and Jake Sledge; and Mollie, Reid, and Elsa Smith.

Contributors

Anthony J. Abene, M.D., M.B.A.
Fellow
Sports, Orthopaedics and Rehabilitation
Redwood City, California
Hip and Knee Pain

Steven B. Abramson, M.D.
Professor of Medicine and Pathology
New York University School of Medicine
Division of Rheumatology
New York, New York
Neutrophils and Eosinophils; Pathogenesis of Osteoarthritis

Leena Ala-Kokko
Professor, Department of Medicine
Center for Gene Therapy
Tulane University Health Sciences Center
New Orleans, Louisiana
Collagen and Elastin

Roy D. Altman, M.D.
Professor of Medicine
Division of Rheumatology
David Geffen School of Medicine at the University of California at Los Angeles
Los Angeles, California
Hypertrophic Osteoarthropathy

William P. Arend, M.D.
Scoville Professor of Rheumatology Medicine
University of Colorado School of Medicine
Denver, Colorado
Antigen-Presenting Cells

Erin L. Arnold, M.D.
Rheumatologist
Center for Arthritis and Osteoporosis
Illinois Bone and Joint Institute, LTD
Morton Grove, Illinois
Arthroscopy

William J. Arnold, M.D., F.A.C.P., F.A.C.R.
Rheumatologist
Center for Arthritis and Osteoporosis
Illinois Bone and Joint Institute, LTD
Morton Grove, Illinois
Arthroscopy

Leyla Alparslan, M.D.
Associate Professor
Department of Radiology
Florence Nightingale Hospital
Kadir Has University School of Medicine
Istanbul, Turkey
Imaging

John P. Atkinson, M.D.
Samuel B. Grant Professor of Medicine
Professor of Molecular Microbiology
Department of Medicine/Rheumatology Division
Washington University School of Medicine
Physician
Internal Medicine
Barnes-Jewish Hospital
St. Louis, Missouri
Complement System

Stanley P. Ballou, M.D.
Associate Professor of Medicine
Case Western Reserve University
Director of Rheumatology
Metro Health Medical Center
Cleveland, Ohio
Laboratory Evaluation of Inflammation

N. Nichole Barry, M.D.
Sports Medicine
Stanford University
Palo Alto, California
Hip and Knee Pain

Robert M. Bennett, M.D., FRCP, FACP
Professor of Medicine
Oregon Health and Science University
and Portland, Oregon
Mixed Connective Tissue Disease and Other Overlap Syndromes

Johannes W.J. Bijlsma, M.D., Ph.D.
Professor and Head
Department of Rheumatology and Clinical Immunology
University Medical Center Utrecht
Utrecht, The Netherlands
Glucocorticoid Therapy

Joseph J. Biundo, Jr., M.D.
Emeritus Professor of Medicine
Louisiana State University Health Science Center
New Orleans, Louisiana
Medical Director of Rehabilitation
Kenner Regional Medical Center
Kenner, Louisiana
Rehabilitation of Patients with Rheumatic Diseases

Juergen Braun, M.D., Ph.D.
Medical Director
Professor of Rheumatology
Rheumazentrum Ruhrgebiet
Herne, Germany
Ankylosing Spondylitis

Michael B. Brenner, M.D.
Theodore B. Bayles Professor of Medicine
Harvard Medical School
Chief, Division of Rheumatology, Immunology and Allergy
Brigham and Women's Hospital
Boston, Massachusetts
Synoviocytes

Doreen B. Brettler, M.D.
Professor of Medicine
University of Massachusetts Medical School
Director
New England Hemophilia Center/Staff Hematologist
Hematology/Oncology
University of Massachusetts Memorial Healthcare
Worcester, Massachusetts
Hemophilic Arthropathy

Lenore M. Buckley, M.D., M.P.H.
Professor of Internal Medicine and Pediatrics
Virginia Commonwealth University School of Medicine
Attending Physician
Internal Medicine and Pediatrics
Medical College of Virginia Hospitals
Richmond, Virginia
Development, Execution, and Analysis of Clinical Trials

Ralph C. Budd, M.D.
Professor of Medicine
Director, Immunobiology Program
The University of Vermont College of Medicine
Burlington, Vermont
T Lymphocytes

Nathalie D. Burg, M.D.
Postdoctoral Fellow
Coller Lab
Rockefeller University
Clinical Instructor
Department of Medicine
New York University School of Medicine
New York, New York
Neutrophils and Eosinophils

Jennifer Burkham, M.D., Ph.D.
Department of Rheumatology
University of California, San Francisco
San Francisco, California
Fibromyalgia: A Chronic Pain Syndrome

Leonard H. Calabrese, B.S., D.O.
Department of Rheumatic and Immunologic Disease
Head, Section of Clinical Immunology
R.J. Fasenmyer Chair of Clinical Immunology
Cleveland Clinic Foundation
Cleveland, Ohio
Antineutrophil Cytoplasmic Antibody–Associated Vasculitis

Dennis A. Carson, M.D.
Professor of Medicine
University of California San Diego
La Jolla, California
Rheumatoid Factor

Steve Carsons, M.D.
Professor of Medicine
SUNY Health Science Center at Stony Brook
Stony Brook, New York
Chief, Division of Rheumatology, Allergy and Immunology
Winthrop University Hospital
Meneola, New York
Sjögren's Syndrome

James T. Cassidy, M.D.
Professor and Chief of Pediatric Rheumatology
Department of Child Health
University of Missouri Health Sciences
Columbia, Missouri
Juvenile Rheumatoid Arthritis; Systemic Lupus Erythematosus, Juvenile Dermatomyositis, Scleroderma, and Vasculitis

Eliza F. Chakravarty, M.D.
Assistant Professor
Division of Immunology and Rheumatology
Stanford University School of Medicine
Palo Alto, California
Musculoskeletal Syndromes in Malignancy

Doyt L. Conn, M.D.
Professor of Medicine
Director Division of Rheumatology
Department of Medicine
Emory University School of Medicine
Grady Health System
The Emory Clinic
Atlanta, Georgia
Alternative Care for Arthritis and Related Musculoskeletal Diseases; Cutaneous Small-Vessel Vasculitis

Paul P. Cook, M.D.
Associate Professor of Medicine
Division of Infectious Diseases
Department of Infectious Diseases
Department of Internal Medicine
Brody School of Medicine at East Carolina University
Greenville, North Carolina
Arthritis Caused by Bacteria or Their Components

Joseph E. Craft, M.D.M.D.
Professor of Medicine and Immunobiology
Chief, Section of Rheumatology
Department of Medicine
Yale School of Medicine
Attending and Chief of Rheumatology
Yale-New Haven Hospital
New Haven, Connecticut
Antinuclear Antibodies

Leslie J. Crofford, M.D.
Associate Professor
Internal Medicine, Division of Rheumatology
University of Michigan
Ann Arbor, Michigan
Nonsteroidal Anti-Inflammatory Drugs

Jody A. Dantzig, Ph.D.
Senior Research Investigator
Physiology/Pennsylvania Muscle Institute
School of Medicine
University of Pennsylvania
Philadelphia, Pennsylvania
Muscle: Anatomy, Physiology, and Biochemistry

Devin K. Datta, M.D.
Brevard Orthopaedic Clinic
Melbourne, Florida
Low Back Pain

Jeroen DeGroot, Ph.D.
Head
Matrix Biology Research Group
Division of Biomedical Research
TNO Prevention and Health
Netherlands Organization for Applied Scientific Research
Leiden, the Netherlands
Biological Markers

Betty Diamond, M.D.
Professor of Microbiology and Immunology, Medicine
Albert Einstein College of Medicine
Bronx, New York
B Cells

Federico Díaz-González, M.D.
Staff of Rheumatology
Rheumatology Service
Hospital Universitario de Canarias
La Laguna, Spain
Platelets and Rheumatic Diseases

Paul E. DiCesare, M.D.
Associate Professor of Orthopaedic Surgery and Cell Biology
New York University School of Medicine
Director, Musculoskeletal Research Center
Chief, Adult Reconstructive Surgery
Hospital for Joint Disease
New York, New York
Pathogenesis of Osteoarthritis

Michael F. Dillingham, M.D.
Adjunct Clinical Professor
Division of Orthopedic Surgery
Stanford University School of Medicine
Director and Team Physician
Orthopedics
Stanford University Medical Center
San Francisco, California
Hip and Knee Pain

Maxime Dougados, M.D.
Professor of Rheumatology
Rene(') Descartes University
Chief and Professor
Department of Rheumatology
Hospital Cochin
Paris, France
Clinical Features of Osteoarthritis

Joost P.H. Drenth, M.D., Ph.D.
Research Fellow
Department of Medicine
Division of Gastroenterology and Hepatology
University Medical Center St. Radboud
Nijmegen, The Netherlands
Familial Autoinflammatory Syndromes

George F. Duna, M.D., F.A.C.P.
Associate Professor of Medicine
Baylor College of Medicine
Chief of Rheumatology
St. Luke's Episcopal Hospital
Houston, Texas
Antineutrophil Cytoplasmic Antibody–Associated Vasculitis

Steven M. Edworthy, B.Sc., M.D., F.R.C.P.C.
Associate Professor of Medicine and Community Health Sciences
Department of Medicine
University of Calgary
Associate Professor of Medicine
Foothills Hospital
Calgary, Alberta, Canada
Clinical Manifestations of Systemic Lupus Erythematosus

Keith B. Elkon, M.D.
Professor of Medicine
Division of Rheumatology
University of Washington
Seattle, Washington
Apoptosis

Peng Thim Fan, M.D.
Clinical Professor of Medicine
David Geffen School of Medicine
University of California at Los Angeles
Los Angles, California
Reiter's Syndrome, Undifferentiated Spondyloarthropathy, and Reactive Arthritis

Barbara K. Finck, M.D.
Vice President
Clinical Development
Eos Biotechnology, Inc.
San Francisco, California
Development, Execution, and Analysis of Clinical Trials

Gary S. Firestein, M.D.
Professor of Medicine and Chief
Division of Rheumatology, Allergy and Immunology
University of California San Diego School of Medicine
Director
University of California San Diego Clinical Investigation Institute
La Jolla, California
Etiology and Pathogenesis of Rheumatoid Arthritis

Karen A. Fortner, Ph.D.
Research Associate
Immunobiology Program, Department of Medicine
The University of Vermont College of Medicine
Burlington, Vermont
T Lymphocytes

Andrew G. Franks, Jr., M.D.
Clinical Professor of Dermatology
New York University School of Medicine
Attending Physician in Rheumatology
Hospital for Joint Diseases
New York University Medical Center
New York, New York
The Skin and Rheumatic Diseases

Sherine E. Gabriel, M.D., M.Sc.
Professor of Medicine Rheumatology and Epidemiology
Mayo Clinic
Chair, Department of Health Sciences Research
Mayo Clinic College of Medicine
Rochester, Minnesota
Epidemiology of the Rheumatic Diseases

Rachel A. Garton, M.D.
Chief Resident in Dermatology
Department of Dermatology
Wake Forest School of Medicine
Winston-Salem, North Carolina
Behcet's Disease

Mark C. Genovese, M.D.
Associate Professor of Medicine
Chief of Clinical Services
Division of immunology and Rheumatology
Stanford University
Palo Alto, California
Treatment of Rheumatoid Arthritis; Musculoskeletal Syndromes in Malignancy

Danielle M. Gerlag, M.D.
Assistant Professor of Medicine
Division of Clinical Immunology and Rheumatology
Academic Medical Center
University of Amsterdam
Amsterdam, The Netherlands
Synovial Fluid Analyses, Synovial Biopsy, and Synovial Pathology

Jayashri V. Ghate, M.D.
Department of Dermatology
Wake Forest University School of Medicine
Winston-Salem, North Carolina
Behcet's Disease

Allan Gibofsky, M.D., J.D., F.A.C.P., F.C.L.M.
Professor
Medicine and Public Health
Weill Medical College of Cornell University
Attending Rheumatologist
Hospital for Special Surgery
New York, New York
Acute Rheumatic Fever and Poststreptoccocal Arthritis

Mark H. Ginsberg, M.D.
Professor of Cell Biology
The Scripps Research Institute
La Jolla, California
Adjunct Professor
University of California School of Medicine
San Diego, California
Platelets and Rheumatic Diseases

Dafna O. Gladman, M.D., F.R.C.P.C.
Professor of Medicine/Rheumatology
University of Toronto
Senior Rheumatologist
University Health Network, Toronto Western Hospital
Toronto, Ontario, Canada
Psoriatic Arthritis

Joseph Golbus, M.D.
Associate Professor
Department of Medicine
Northwestern University Medical School
Chicago, Illinois
Head, Division of Rheumatology
Evanston Northwestern Healthcare
Evanston, Illinois
Monarticular Arthritis

Yale E. Goldman, M.D., Ph.D.
Professor, Institute Director
Physiology/Pennsylvania Muscle Institute
School of Medicine, University of Pennsylvania
Philadelphia, Pennsylvania
Muscle: Anatomy, Physiology, and Biochemistry

Mary B. Goldring, Ph.D.
Associate Professor of Medicine (Cell Biology)
Division of Medical Sciences
Harvard Medical School
Associate Professor of Medicine
Department of Medicine/Division of Rheumatology
Beth Israel Deaconess Medical Center
Boston, Massachusetts
Biology of the Normal Joint; Chondrocytes

Steven R. Goldring, M.D.
Professor of Medicine
Harvard Medical School
Chief of Rheumatology
Department of Medicine/Division of Rheumatology
Beth Israel Deaconess Medical Center
Boston, Massachusetts
Biology of the Normal Joint

Emilio B. Gonzalez, M.D.
Clinical Associate Professor
Internal Medicine
Emory University School of Medicine
Chief, Rheumatology Section
Atlanta Medical Center
Atlanta, Georgia
Cutaneous Small-Vessel Vasculitis

Duncan A. Gordon, M.D., M.A.C.R.
Professor
Department of Medicine
University of Toronto
Senior Rheumatologist
Division of Rheumatology
University Health Network, Toronto Western Hospital
Toronto, Ontario, Canada
Second Line Agents

Peter K. Gregersen
Professor of Medicine and Pathology
Department of Medicine and Pathology
New York University School of Medicine
New York, New York
Director
Robert S. Boas Center for Genomics and Human Genetics
North Shore Long Island Jewish Research Institute
Manhasset, New York
Genetics of Rheumatic Diseases

Christine Grimaldi, Ph.D.
Instructor, Microbiology and Immunology
Albert Einstein College of Medicine
Bronx, New York
B Cells

Bevra Hannahs Hahn, M.D.
Chief of Rheumatology and Professor of Medicine
Department of Medicine
David Geffen School of Medicine
University of California, Los Angeles
Los Angeles, California
Pathogenesis of Systemic Lupus Erythematosus; Management of Systemic Lupus Erythematosus

J. Timothy Harrington, M.D.
Associate Professor
Rheumatology Section, Department of Medicine
University of Wisconsin Medical School
Madison, Wisconsin
Mycobacterial and Fungal Infections

Edward D. Harris, M.D.
George DeForest Barnett Professor of Medicine, Emeritus
Stanford University School of Medicine
Academic Secretary to Stanford University
Stanford, California
Biological Markers; Fibromyalgia: A Chronic Pain Syndrome; Clinical Features of Rheumatoid Arthritis; Treatment of Rheumatoid Arthritis

Dick Heinegärd, M.D., Ph.D.
Professor
Department of Cell and Molecular Biology
Lund University
Lund, Sweden
Matrix Glycoproteins and Proteoglycans in Cartilage

David B. Hellman, M.D.
Mary Betty Stevens Professor of Medicine
Johns Hopkins University School of Medicine
Chairman and Physician-in-Chief, Department of Medicine
Johns Hopkins Bayview Medical Center
Baltimore, Maryland
Giant Cell Arteritis and Polymyalgia Rheumatica

George Ho, Jr., M.D.
Professor of Medicine
Division of Allergy, Immunology, and Rheumatology
Department of Internal Medicine
Brody School of Medicine at East Carolina University
Greenville, North Carolina
Arthritis Caused by Bacteria or Their Components

Jeffrey D. Horn, M.D.
Assistant Professor of Ophthalmology
Department of Ophthalmology and Visual Services
Vanderbilt University Medical Center
Nashville, Tennessee
The Eye and Rheumatic Disease

Gene G. Hunder, M.D.
Professor Emeritus
Department of Medicine
Mayo Medical School
Rochester, Minnesota
History and Physical Examination of the Musculoskeletal System; Giant Cell Arteritis and Polymyalgia Rheumatica

Johannes W.G. Jacobs, M.D., Ph.D.
Associate Professor
Department of Rheumatology and Clinical Immunology
University Medical Center Utrecht
Utrecht, The Netherlands
Glucocorticoid Therapy

Charles A. Janeway, Jr., M.D. (Deceased)
Professor
Section of Immunobiology and Howard Hughes Medical Institute
Yale University School of Medicine
New Haven, Connecticut
Innate Immunity

Joseph L. Jorizzo, M.D.
Professor and Former (Founding) Chair
Department of Dermatology
Wake Forest University School of Medicine
Winston-Salem, North Carolina
Behcet's Disease

Sue Joan Jue, M.D.
Associate Professor of Pediatrics
Section of Infectious Diseases
Greenville Hospital Systems
Greenville, South Carolina
Arthritis Caused by Bacteria or Their Components

George A. Karpouzas, M.D.
Clinical Instructor, Assistant Researcher
Department of Medicine
David Geffen School of Medicine
University of California, Los Angeles
Los Angeles, California
Pathogenesis of Systemic Lupus Erythematosus

Arthur Kavanaugh, M.D.
Professor of Medicine
Director of the Center for Innovative Therapy
Division of Rheumatology, Allergy and Immunology
University of California, San Diego
San Diego, California
Anticytokine Therapies

William N. Kelley, M.D.
Professor
Department of Medicine
University of Pennsylvania
Philadelphia, Pennsylvania
Gout and Hyperuricemia

Edward Keystone, M.D., F.R.C.P.(C).
Professor of Medicine
Department of Medicine
University of Toronto
Rheumatologist
Mount Sanai Hospital
Toronto, Ontario, Canada
Emerging Therapies in Rheumatoid Arthritis

Hans P. Kiener, M.D.
Research Fellow
Harvard Medical School
Research Fellow
Brigham and Women's Hospital
Boston, Massachusetts
Synoviocytes

Alice V. Klinkhoff, M.D., F.R.C.P.
Clinical Associate Professor
Department of Medicine
University of British Columbia
Medical Director
Mary Pack Arthritis Program
Vancouver General Hospital
Vancouver, British Columbia, Canada
Second Line Agents

Alisa E. Koch, M.D.
William D. Robinson and Frederick Huetwell Endowed Professor
University of Michigan
Ann Arbor, Michigan
Endothelial Cell Biology, Angiogenesis, and Recruitment of Cells

Joseph H. Korn, M.D.
Alan S. Cohen Professor of Medicine in Rheumatology
Director, Arthritis Center
Boston University School of Medicine
Boston, Massachusetts
Fibroblast Function and Fibrosis

Brian L. Kotzin, M.D.
Professor of Medicine and Immunology
Co-Head, Division of Clinical Immunology
University of Colorado Health Sciences Center
Denver, Colorado
Autoimmunity

Joel M. Kremer, M.D.
Clinical Professor of Medicine
Department of Medicine, Division of Rheumatology
Albany Medical College
Albany, New York
Nutrition and Rheumatic Diseases

Hilal Maradit Kremers, M.D., M.Sc.
Assistant Professor of Epidemiology
Mayo Medical School
Rochester, Minnesota
Research Associate, Department of Health Sciences Research
Mayo Clinic College of Medicine
Rochester, Minnesota
Epidemiology of the Rheumatic Diseases

Irving Kushner, M.D.
Professor of Medicine and Pathology
Case-Western Reserve University
Attending Physician
MetroHealth Medical Center
Cleveland, Ohio
Laboratory Evaluation of Inflammation

Robert Lafyatis, M.D.
Associate Professor of Medicine
Rheumatology Section
Boston University School of Medicine
Associate Professor of Medicine
Department of Rheumatology
Boston University Medical Center
Boston, Massachusetts
Fibroblast Function and Fibrosis

R. Elaine Lambert, M.D.
Adjunct Clinical Associate Professor
Department of Internal Medicine
Stanford School of Medicine
Palo Alto, California
Iron Storage Disease

Nancy E. Lane, M.D.
Associate Professor of Medicine in Residence
Department of Medicine
University of California at San Francisco
Department of Medicine and Division of Rheumatology
San Francisco General Hospital
San Francisco, California
Metabolic Bone Disease

Daniel M. Laskin, DDS, MS
Professor and Chairman Emeritus
Department of Oral and Maxillofacial Surgery
Virginia Commonwealth University School of Dentistry
Attending Oral and Maxillofacial Surgeon
Medical College of Virginia/Virginia Commonwealth University Hospital
Richmond, Virgina
Temporomandibular Joint Pain

Meryl S. LeBoff
Associate Professor
Department of Internal Medicine
Harvard Medical School
Director
Skeletal Health and Osteoporosis
Division of Endocrine, Diabetes and Hypertension
Brigham and Women's Hospital
Boston, Massachusetts
Metabolic Bone Disease

David M. Lee, M.D., Ph.D.
Instructor of Medicine
Harvard Medical School
Division of Rheumatology, Immunology and Allergy
Department of Medicine
Brigham and Women's Hospital
Boston, Massachusetts
Synoviocytes

Michael D. Lockshin, M.D.
Professor of Medicine and Obstetrics and Gynecology
Joan and Sanford Weill Medical College of Cornell University
Attending Physician
Hospital for Special Surgery
New York, New York
Antiphospholipid Antibody Syndrome

Pilar Lorenzo, Ph.D.
Cell and Molecular Biology
Lund University
Rheumatology
Lund University Hospital
Lund, Sweden
Matrix Glycoproteins and Proteoglycans in Cartilage

Kate R. Lorig, RN, DrPH
Professor
Department of Medicine
Stanford University
Palo Alto, California
Education of Patients

Carlos J. Lozada, M.D.
Associate Professor of Medicine
Director, Rheumatology Fellowship Program
Division of Rheumatology and Immunology
University of Miami School of Medicine
Director
Rheumatology Fellowship Training Program and Rheumatology Clinical Services
Jackson Memorial Hospital
Miami, Florida
Management of Osteoarthritis

Maren Lawson Mahowald, M.D.
Professor of Medicine
University of Minnesota
Rheumatology Section Chief
Minneapolis VA Medical Center
Minneapolis, Minnesota
Chronic Musculoskeletal Pain

Scott David Martin, M.D.
Assistant Professor of Orthopedics
Harvard Medical School
Brigham and Women's Hospital
Boston, Massachusetts
Shoulder Pain

W. Joseph McCune, M.D.
Professor of Medicine
Department of Internal Medicine/Rheumatology
University of Michigan Medical Center
Ann Arbor, Michigan
Monarticular Arthritis

Iain B. McInnes, MRCP, Ph.D.
Professor
Division of Immunology, Infection and Inflammation
University of Glasgow
Consultant Rheumatologist
Centre for Rheumatic Diseases
Glasgow Royal Infirmary
Glasgow, Scotland, United Kingdom
Cytokines

Richard T. Meehan, M.D., FACP, FACR
Chief of Rheumatology
Associate Professor of Medicine
National Jewish Medical and Research Center
Associate Clinical Professor of Medicine
Rheumatology, Department of Medicine
University of Colorado Health Sciences Center
Denver, Colorado
Sarcoidosis

Sohail K. Mirza, M.D.
Associate Professor
Department of Orthopaedics and Sports Medicine
Harborview Medical Center
University of Washington
Seattle, Washington
Low Back Pain

Kevin G. Moder, M.D.
Assistant Professor
Division of Rheumatology
Department of Internal Medicine
Mayo Clinic
Rochester, Minnesota
History and Physical Examination of the Musculoskeletal System

Stanley J. Naides, M.D.
Thomas B. Hallowell Professor of Medicine
Chief, Division of Rheumatology
Medicine, Microbiology and Immunology and Pharmacology
Pennsylvania State University College of Medicine
Professor and Chief
Division of Rheumatology
The Milton S. Hershey Medical Center
Hershey Pennsylvania
Viral Arthritis

Kenneth K. Nakano, M.D.
Clinical Professor of Medicine
Albany Medical College
Director of Research
The Center for Rheumatology
Attending Physician
Albany Medical Center Hospital
Albany, New York
Neck Pain

Lee S. Newman, M.D., MA, FCCP
Professor of Medicine
Professor of Preventive Medicine and Biometrics
University of Colorado Health Sciences Center
Professor of Medicine
Head, Division of Environmental and Occupational Health Sciences
National Jewish Medical and Research Center
Denver, Colorado
Sarcoidosis

Urs E. Nydegger, M.D.
Titularprofessor
Faculty of Medicine
University of Bern
Leitender Arzt
University Clinic for Cardiovascular Surgery
Universitätsklinik für Herzund Gefässchirurgie Inselspital
Bern, Switzerland
Immune Complexes

Denis M. O'Day, M.D., F.A.C.S.
Professor of Ophthalmology
Department of Ophthalmology and Visual Sciences
Vanderbilt University School of Medicine
Nashville, Tennessee
The Eye and Rheumatic Disease

James R. O'Dell, BS, M.D.
Professor of Medicine
Chief, Section of Rheumatology and Immunology
Vice-Chairman, Department of Internal Medicine
University of Nebraska Medical Center
Omaha, Nebraska
Methotrexate, Leflunomide, and Combination Therapies

Yasunori Okada, M.D., Ph.D.
Professor and Chairman
Department of Pathology
School of Medicine
Keio University
Tokyo, Japan
Proteinases and Matrix Degradation

Richard S. Panush, M.D.
Clinical Professor
Department of Medicine
Mount Sinai School of Medicine
Chair
Department of Medicine
Saint Barnabas Medical Center
Livingston, New Jersey
Occupational and Recreational Musculoskeletal Disorders

Stanford L. Peng, M.D., Ph.D.
Assistant Professor
Department of Internal Medicine, Division of Rheumatology
Washington University School of Medicine
Assistant Professor
Department of Internal Medicine, Division of Rheumatology
Barnes-Jewish Hospital
St. Louis, Missouri
Antinuclear Antibodies

Jean-Charles Piette, M.D.
Medecine Interne 2
Hospital Pitie-Salpetriere
Paris, France
Relapsing Polychondritis

Lorenzo Pilar, Ph.D.
Department of Cell and Molecular Biology
Lund University
Lund, Sweden
Matrix Glycoproteins and Proteoglycans in Cartilage

Michael H. Pillinger, M.D.
Assistant Professor
Department of Medicine and Pharmacology
New York University School of Medicine
Section Chief, Rheumatology
New York Harbor Veterans Health Care System, Manhattan Campus
New York, New York
Neutrophils and Eosinophils

Robert S. Pinals, M.D.
Professor and Vice-Chairman
Department of Medicine
University of Medicine and Dentistry of New Jersey
Robert Wood Johnson Medical School
Chief, Rheumatology Service
Robert Wood Johnson University Hospital
New Brunswick, New Jersey
Felty's Syndrome

Steven A. Porcelli, M.D.
Associate Professor
Department of Microbiology and Immunology
Department of Medicine
Albert Einstein College of Medicine
Bronx, New York
Innate Immunity

Darwin J. Prockop, M.D., Ph.D.
Director and Chairman
Center for Gene Therapy
Tulane University Health Sciences Center
New Orleans, Louisiana
Collagen and Elastin

Eric L. Radin, M.D.
Adjunct Professor
Orthopaedic Surgery
Tufts University School of Medicine
Boston, Massachusetts
Biomechanics of Joints

Jaya K. Rao, M.D., MHS
Medical Epidemiologist
Health Care and Aging Studies Branch
Centers for Disease Control and Prevention
Adjunct Clinical Associate Professor
Division of Rheumatology
Department of Medicine
Emory University School of Medicine
Atlanta, Georgia
Alternative Care for Arthritis and Related Musculoskeletal Diseases

John D. Reveille, M.D.
George S. Bruce Professor in Arthritis and Other Rheumatic Diseases
Rheumatology, Internal Medicine
The University of Texas Health Science Center at Houston
Director, Division of Rheumatology
Hermann Hospital
Houston, Texas
Rheumatic Manifestations of Human Immunodeficiency Virus Infection

Marco Rizzo, M.D.
Assistant Professor
Division of Orthopaedic Surgery
Duke University Medical Center
Durham, North Carolina
Osteonecrosis

W. Neal Roberts, Jr., M.D.
Director
Rheumatology Training Program
C.W. Thomas Associate Professor of Medicine
Virginia Commonwealth University
Medical College of Virginia
Richmond, Virginia
Psychosocial Management of the Rheumatic Diseases

Andrew E. Rosenberg, M.D.
Associate Professor
Department of Pathology
Harvard Medical School;
Associate Pathologist
Department of Pathology
Massachusetts General Hospital
Boston, Massachusetts
Tumors and Tumor-like Lesions of Joints

Keith T. Rott, M.D., Ph.D.
Assistant Professor
Division of Rheumatology and Immunology
Department of Medicine
Emory University School of Medicine
Atlanta, Georgia
Cutaneous Small-Vessel Vasculitis

David Rowe, M.D.
University of Connecticut Health Science Center
Heritable Disorders of Structural Proteins

Clinton T. Rubin, Ph.D.
Professor and Chair
Department of Biomedical Engineering
Director, Center for Biotechnology
State University of New York
Stony Brook, New York
Biology, Physiology, and Morphology of Bone

Janet E. Rubin, M.D.
Professor of Medicine
Division of Endocrinology and Metabolism
Emory University School of Medicine
Physician
Endocrinology and Metabolism
Atlanta Veterans Affairs Medical Center
Atlanta, Georgia
Biology, Physiology, and Morphology of Bone

Perry J. Rush, M.D.
Assistant Professor
Department of Medicine
University of Toronto
Chief Physiatrist
Department of Medicine
St. John's Rehabilitation Hospital
Toronto Ontario Canada
Rehabilitation of Patients with Rheumatic Diseases

Tore Saxne, M.D., Ph.D.
Professor
Department of Rheumatology
Lund University
Lund, Sweden
Matrix Glycoproteins and Proteoglycans in Cartilage

H. Ralph Schumacher, Jr., M.D.
Professor of Medicine
University of Pennsylvania School of Medicine
Chief of Rheumatology
VA Medical Center
Philadelphia, PA
Hemoglobinopathies and Arthritis

Edward M. Schwarz, Ph.D.
Associate Professor
Department of Orthopaedics
University of Rochester School of Medicine and Dentistry
Rochester, New York
Signal Transduction in Rheumatic Diseases

James R. Seibold, M.D.
Professor of Medicine
Director, Scleroderma Program
University of Medicine and Dentistry of New Jersey
Robert Wood Johnson Medical School Attending Physician
Internal Medicine andand Rheumatology
Robert Wood Johnson University Hospital
New Brunswick, New Jersey
Scleroderma

David C. Seldin, M.D., Ph.D.
Associate Professor of Medicine and Microbiology
Boston University School of Medicine
Attending Physician, Section of Hematology-Oncology
Department of Medicine
Boston Medical Center
Boston, Massachusetts
Amyloidosis

John S. Sergent, M.D.
Professor of Medicine
Vanderbilt University School of Medicine
Vice Chairman for Education
Department of Medicine
Vanderbilt Medical Center
Nashville, Tennessee
Polyarticular Arthritis; Polyarteritis and Related Disorders; Arthritis Accompanying Endocrine and Metabolic Disorders

Jay R. Shapiro, M.D.
Professor
Department of Medicine
Uniformed Services University
Bethesda, Maryland
Director
Osteogenesis Imperfecta Program
Kennedy Krieger Institute
Baltimore, Maryland
Heritable Disorders of Structural Proteins

Leonard H. Sigal, M.D., FACP, FACR
Clinical Professor
Departments of Medicine
Department of Pediatrics
Department of Molecular Genetics and Microbiology
University of Medicine and Dentistry of New Jersey
Robert Wood Johnson Medical School
Attending, Rheumatology Service
Robert Wood Johnson University Hospital
New Brunswick, New Jersey
Lyme Disease

Anna Simon, M.D.
Resident
Department of Medicine
Division of General Internal Medicine
University Medical Center St. Radboud
Nijmegen, The Netherlands
Familial Autoinflammatory Syndromes

Sheldon R. Simon, M.D.
Professor of Clinical Orthopaedics
Albert Einstein School of Medicine
Bronx, New York
Chief Division of Pediatric Orthopaedics
Department of Orthopaedics
Beth Israel Medical Center
New York, New York
Biomechanics of Joints

Martha Skinner, M.D.
Professor
Department of Medicine
Boston University School of Medicine
Director, Amyloid Program
Boston Medical Center
Boston, Massachusetts
Amyloidosis

Clement B. Sledge, M.D.
John B. and Buckminster Brown
Professor of Orthopedic Surgery, Emeritus
Harvard Medical School
Chairman, Department of Orthopedic Surgery, Emeritus
Brigham and Women's Hospital
Boston, Massachusetts
Introduction to Surgical Management of Patients with Arthritis
Principles of Reconstructive Surgery for Arthritis

Nicholas A. Soter, M.D.
Professor of Dermatology
The Ronald O. Perelman Department of Dermatology
New York University School of Medicine
Attending Physician
Tisch Hospital
The University Hospital of NYU
New York, New York
The Skin and Rheumatic Diseases

Timothy M. Spiegel, M.D., MPH
Department of Medicine/Rheumatology
Cottage Hospital
Santa Barbara, California
Ankle and Foot Pain

Paul A. Sponseller, M.D.
Professor and Vice-Chair
Department of Orthopaedics
Head, Pediatric Orthopaedics
Johns Hopkins University
Boston, Massachusetts
Heritable Disorders of Structural Proteins

C. Michael Stein, M.D.
Associate Professor of Medicine
Associate Professor of Pharmacology
Vanderbilt University School of Medicine
Nashville, Tennessee
Immunoregulatory Drugs

John H. Stone, M.D., MPH
Associate Professor of Medicine
Division of Rheumatology
Johns Hopkins University
Director
The Johns Hopkins Vasculitis Center
Baltimore, Maryland
The Classification and Epidemiology of Systemic Vasculitis

Vibeke Strand, M.D.
Adjunct Clinical Professor
Division of Immunology and Rheumatology
Stanford University School of Medicine
Palo Alto, California
Emerging Therapies in Rheumatoid Arthritis

Stephanie Studenski, M.D., MPH
Professor
Department of Medicine
University of Pittsburgh
Staff Physician
Geriatric Research Education and Clinical Center
Virgina Pittsburgh Healthcare System
Pittsburgh, Pennsylvania
Pharmacology and the Elderly

Carrie R. Swigart, M.D.
Assistant Clinical Professor
Department of Orthopaedics and Rehabilitation
Yale University School of Medicine
Associate
Yale–New Haven Hospital
New Haven, Connecticut
Hand and Wrist Pain

Zoltan Szekanecz, M.D., Ph.D., DSC
Associate Professor of Medicine, Rheumatology and Immunology
Head of Rheumatology Division
Third Department of Medicine
Rheumatology Division
Debrecen, Hungary
Endothelial Cell Biology, Angiogenesis, and Recruitment Cells

Paul P. Tak, M.D., Ph.D.
Professor of Medicine
Director, Division of Clinical Immunology and Rheumatology
Academic Medical Center
University of Amsterdam
The Netherlands
Synovial Fluid Analyses, Synovial Biopsy, and Synovial Pathology; Biological Markers

Johan M. TeKoppele, Ph.D.
Head, Division of Biomedical Research
TNO Prevention and Health
Netherlands Organization for Applied Scientific Research
Leiden, The Netherlands
Biological Markers

Jerry Tenenbaum, M.D., FRCPC
Professor of Medicine
University of Toronto;
Director
Ontario International Medical Graduate Program
Mount Sinai Hospital
Toronto, Ontario, Canada
Hypertrophic Osteoarthropathy

Robert Terkeltaub, M.D.
Professor of Medicine in Residence
Director, Rheumatology Training Program
University of California at San Diego
Chief, Rheumatology Section
VA Medical Center
San Diego, California
Diseases Associated with Articular Deposition of Calcium Pyrophosphate Dihydrate and Basic Calcium Phosphate Crystals

Ranjeny Thomas, M.D.
Associate Professor
Centre for Immunology and Cancer Research
University of Queensland
Consultant Rheumatologist
Princess Alexandra Hospital
Brisbane, Australia
Antigen-Presenting Cells

Thomas S. Thornhill, M.D.
John B. and Buckminster Brown
Professor of Orthopaedics
Harvard Medical School
Orthopaedist-in-Chief
Brigham and Women's Hospital
Boston, Massachusetts
Shoulder Pain

Helen Tighe, Ph.D.
Associate Professor of Medicine
University of California San Diego
La Jolla, California
Rheumatoid Factor

Betty P. Tsao, Ph.D.
Professor of Medicine
David Geffen School of Medicine University of California at Los Angeles
Los Angeles, California
Pathogenesis of SLE

Zuhre Tutuncu, M.D.
Assistant Clinical Professor of Medicine
Center for Innovative Therapy
Division of Rheumatology
University of California at San Diego
San Diego, California
Anticytokine Therapies

Katherine S. Upchurch, M.D.
Associate Professor of Medicine
University of Massachusetts Medical School
Associate Chief, Division of Rheumatology
University of Massachusetts Memorial Medical Center
Worcester, Massachusetts
Hemophilic Arthropathy

James R. Urbaniak, M.D.
Virginia Flowers Baker Professor of Orthopedic Surgery
Duke University Medical Center
Durham, North Carolina
Osteonecrosis

Désirée van der Heijde, M.D., Ph.D.
Professor of Rheumatology
Department of Internal Medicine
Division of Rheumatology
University Hospital Maastvicht
Maastvicht, The Netherlands
Ankylosing Spondylitis

Sjef van der Linden, M.D., Ph.D.
Professor of Rheumatology
Department of Internal Medicine
Division of Rheumatology
University Hospital Maastvicht
Maastvicht, The Netherlands
Ankylosing Spondylitis

Jos W.M. van der Meer, M.D., Ph.D., FRCP
Professor of Internal Medicine
Department of Medicine
Division of General Internal Medicine
University Medical Center St. Radboud
Nijmegen, The Netherlands
Familial Autoinflammatory Syndromes

Philippe Vinceneux, M.D.
Medecine Interne 2
Hospital Pitie-Salpetriere
Paris, France
Relapsing Polychondritis

Michael M. Ward, M.D., MPH
Senior Investigator, Intramural Research Program
National Institute of Arthritis and Musculoskeletal and Skin Diseases
National Institutes of Health
U. S. Department of Health and Human Services
Bethesda, Maryland
Assessment of Health Outcomes; Pharmacology and the Elderly

Yasmine Wasfi, M.D.
Instructor, Parker B. Francis Fellow
Department of Medicine
National Jewish Medical and Research Center
Instructor, Division of Pulmonary Sciences and Critical Care Medicine
University of Colorado Health Sciences Center
Denver, Colorado
Sarcoidosis

Barbara N. Weissman, M.D.
Professor
Harvard Medical School
Radiology
Brigham and Women's Hospital
Boston, Massachusetts
Imaging

Augustus A. White, III, M.D., Ph.D.
Ellen and Melvin Gordon Professor of Medical Education
Professor of Orthopaedic Surgery
Harvard Medical School
Orthopedic Surgeon-In-Chief, Emeritus
Beth Israel Deaconess Medical Center
Boston, Massachusetts
Low Back Pain

Christopher M. Wise, M.D.
W. Robert Irby Professor, Internal Medicine
Division of Rheumatology, Allergy, and Immunology
Virginia Commonwealth University Health System
Medical College of Virginia
Richmond, Virginia
Arthrocentesis and Injection of Joints and Soft Tissues

Scott W. Wolfe, M.D.
Professor of Orthopedic Surgery
Weill Medical College of Cornell University
Chief of Hand Surgery
Hospital for Special Surgery
New York, New York
Hand and Wrist Pain

Frank A. Wollheim, M.D., Ph.D., FRCP
Professor of Rheumatology
Department of Rheumatology
University of Lund
Lund University Hospital
Lund, Sweden
Enteropathic Arthritis

Anthony D. Woolf, BSc, MB, BS, FRCP
Honorary Professor of Rheumatology
Institute of Health and Social Care Research
Peninsula Medical School
Universities of Exeter and Plymouth
Consultant Rheumatologist
Department of Rheumatology
Royal Cornwall Hospital
Truro, United Kingdom
Economic Burden of Rheumatic Diseases

Robert L. Wortmann, M.D.
Professor and Chair
Department of Internal Medicine
The University of Oklahoma College of Medicine
Tulsa, Oklahoma
Inflammatory Diseases of Muscle and Other Myopathies; Gout and Hyperuricemia

David Tak Tan Yu, M.D., B.S.
Professor of Medicine
David Geffen School of Medicine
University of California at Los Angeles
Los Angeles, California
Reiter's Syndrome, Undifferentiated Spondyloarthropathy, and Reactive Arthritis

Joseph S. Yu, M.D.
Chief of Musculoskeletal Division
Department of Radiology
Ohio State University Medical Center
Columbus, Ohio
Imaging

John B. Zabriskie, M.D.
Professor Emeritus
Laboratory of Clinical Microbiology/Immunology
Rockefeller University
Senior Scientist, Research Division
Hospital for Special Surgery
New York, New York
Acute Rheumatic Fever and Poststreptoccocal Arthritis

Robert B. Zurier, M.D.
Professor of Medicine
Chief of the Division of Rheumatology
University of Massachusetts Memorial Health Care
Worcester, Massachusetts
Prostaglandins, Leukotrienes, and Related Compounds

International Reviewers

The Publisher wishes to acknowledge the following individuals, who previewed advance materials from Kelley's Textbook of Rheumatology, 7th Edition

Sang-Cheol Bae, MD, PhD, MPH
Professor and Head,
Division of Rheumatology,
Department of Internal Medicine,
The Hospital for Rheumatic Diseases, Hanyang University,
Seoul, Korea

Pradeep Bambery, MD
Professor,
Department of Internal Medicine/Rheumatology,
Postgraduate Institute of Medical Education and Research,
Chandigarh, India

Prof. Em. Dr. Jan Dequeker
Department of Rheumatology,
University Hospital of Leuven,
Leuven, Belgium

Katsuyuki Fujii, MD, PhD
Professor,
Department of Orthopaedic Surgery,
The Jikei University School of Medicine,
Tokyo, Japan

Rajiva Gupta, MD, DNB, MRCP
Assistant Professor of Medicine,
All India Institute of Medical Sciences,
New Delhi, India

Soo-Kon Lee, MD, PhD
Division of Rheumatology,
Department of Internal Medicine,
Yonsei University College of Medicine,
Seoul, Korea

Caio Moreira
Rheumatologist,
Hospital das Clínicas,
Federal University of Minas Gerais,
Brazil. President,
Brasilian Society of Rheumatology 2002/2004

Prakash K. Pispati, MD, FRSM (Lon.)
Consultant Rheumatologist,
Jaslok Hospital & Research Centre,
Bombay, India.
President,
Asia Pacific League of Associations for Rheumatology.
Past President, Indian Rheumatology Association

C. Panchapakesa Rajendran, MBBS, DCH, MD, DM
Professor and Head,
Department of Rheumatology,
Madras Medical College and Government General Hospital,
Chennai, India

Morton Scheinberg, MD, PhD, FACP
Physician and Research Associate,
Hospital Israelita Albert Einstein,
Sao Paulo, Brazil

Yeong-Wook Song, MD, PhD
Professor and Chief,
Division of Rheumatology,
Department of Internal Medicine,
Seoul National University Hospital,
Seoul, Korea

Preface

Twenty-three years have passed since Bill Kelley, Clem Sledge, Shaun Ruddy, and I met with Jack Hanley at W.B. Saunders to plan production of *The Textbook of Rheumatology*. Our goal was to equal or better any current text that described clinical entities and their treatment, but to exceed by far the depth and breadth of existing text in the detail and explication of basic sciences that provide the infrastructure of rheumatology and orthopedic surgery. That first edition, thanks to the diligent writing of many contributors, exceeded our expectations. It became the best-seller of rheumatology texts.

The template for that first edition proved successful, and there has been no reason to change it for subsequent editions. When Bill Kelley stepped down as an active editor, we recognized the importance of "name recognition" and kept the title as *Kelley's Textbook of Rheumatology* while adding John Sergent and Ralph Budd as associate editors in the sixth edition published in 2001. Recognizing as well the reality that new and younger minds should be involved for the present as well as future editions, this seventh edition has seven editors. We added Gary Firestein and Mark Genovese to the group, and the result is highly amplified brain power. Supplementing Shaun, and Ted, and Clem is the basic science knowledge of Gary and Ralph and the clinical science backgrounds of John and Mark. The future of *Kelley's Textbook of Rheumatology* is secure.

This seventh edition was planned with full awareness that we are in the midst of remarkable change in the sciences that form the base of rheumatology. Over the past 70 years we have seen the birth and growth of immunology, biochemistry, cell biology, and genetics. Each of these specialties grew with remarkable independence from the others until recent years. The future of our specialty is now intimately associated with integrative science. Recombinant technology now links genetics with biochemistry, and more important, the translational science that has evolved often enables us to leapfrog directly over traditional basic science to understanding of clinical disease states. Just as in neurobiology, where studies of the basis of consciousness involve psychology, philosophy, mathematics, and computer science, the unraveling of complex diseases such as systemic lupus erythematosus will require collaborative ventures by immunologists, immunogeneticists, biochemists, and cell biologists. Ironically, each of these specialists is using the same molecular tools, and so added to the team must be those who are developing the next methods that will supplant the micro-arrays, Western and Southern blots, and knock-out mice.

It is with the likelihood that this integrative collaboration that can bring true synergism to the understanding of rheumatic disease that this edition of *Kelley's Textbook of Rheumatology* has been planned. Each of the chapters in the section on the basic sciences describes well both the present and future opportunities for application of these specialized data to specific diseases, and each chapter on pathogenesis of specific diseases refers frequently to the advances that science brings to clinical science.

In this seventh edition an accompanying DVD, organized and edited by Shaun Ruddy, provides expansion of clinical photographs, histopathology, and detailed videos of the musculoskeletal system and arthroscopic views of diseased joints.

The corollary of this burst of basic science that can be clearly integrated with clinical science is the need for frequent updates for our readers, updates that fill the gaps between subsequent editions. In response, we are providing "e-ditions" in the format of a web site that will provide every reader with the latest data and their interpretations that will enable basic scientists to plan new experiments, and clinicians to better diagnose and treat their patients.

While we recognize that the future of paper texts is indeterminate amidst the electronic revolution, we are satisfied that this seventh edition of *Kelley's Textbook of Rheumatology* will serve readers better than any other source of information about rheumatology, orthopedic approaches to rheumatic diseases, and the science that drives understanding of the pathogenesis and treatment of the afflictions that our patients suffer from.

Contents

VOLUME I

SECTION XVIII
The Common Ground of Rheumatology and Orthopaedic Surgery

Color Plates

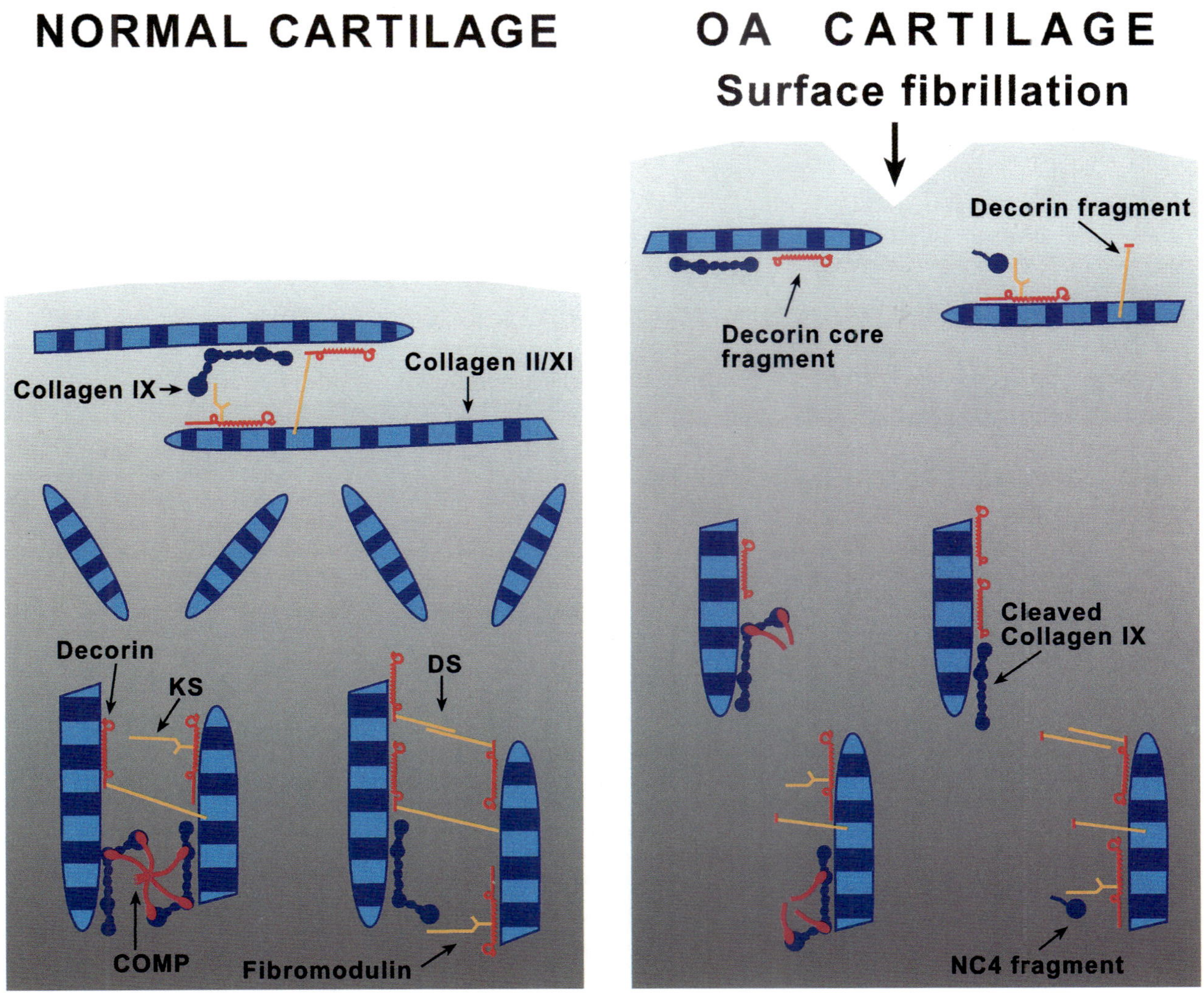

COLOR PLATE 1 • Schematic depiction of the collagen network in articular cartilage and the swelling and surface disruption following disturbance of the collagen network. In osteoarthritis. The dimensions and orientation of the collagen fibers surface by proteolysis will lead to impaired tensile properties of the network and swelling to the tissue on osteoarthritis.

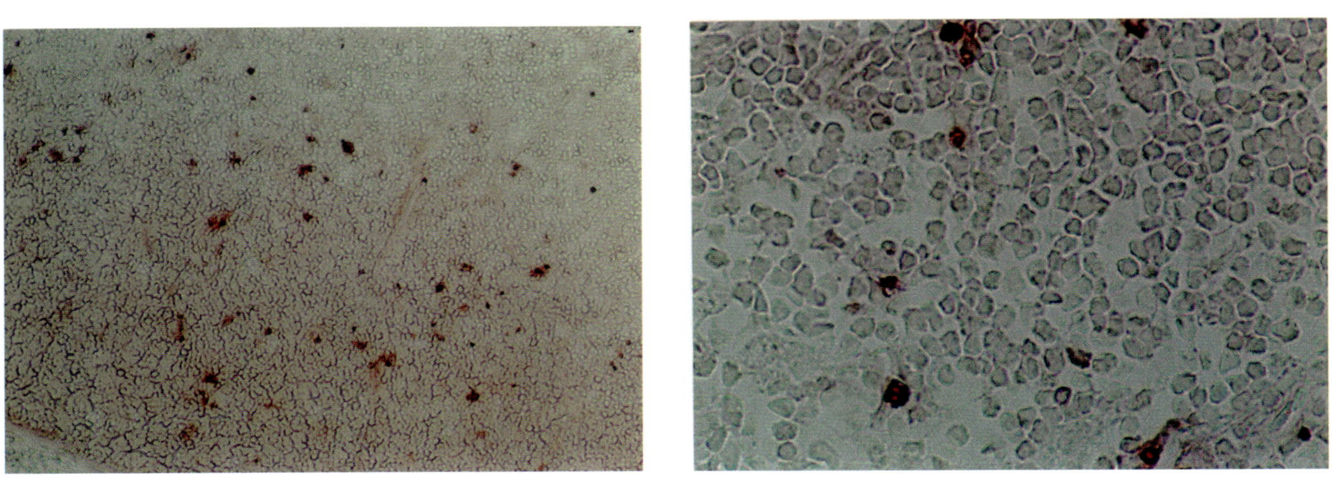

COLOR PLATE 2 • TUNEL assay for nicked DNA in thymocytes undergoing apoptosis. Thymus sections were made from wild-type mice, fixed, and stained by the TUNEL assay. The DNA repair enzyme, TdT, inserts biotinylated dUTP residues at sites of double-stranded breaks, and it is then revealed by avidin horeseradish peroxidase. Shown are sections at 100× and 400×. Apoptotic thymocytes are those undergoing negative selection from either too intense or too weak a T cell receptor (TCR) signal.

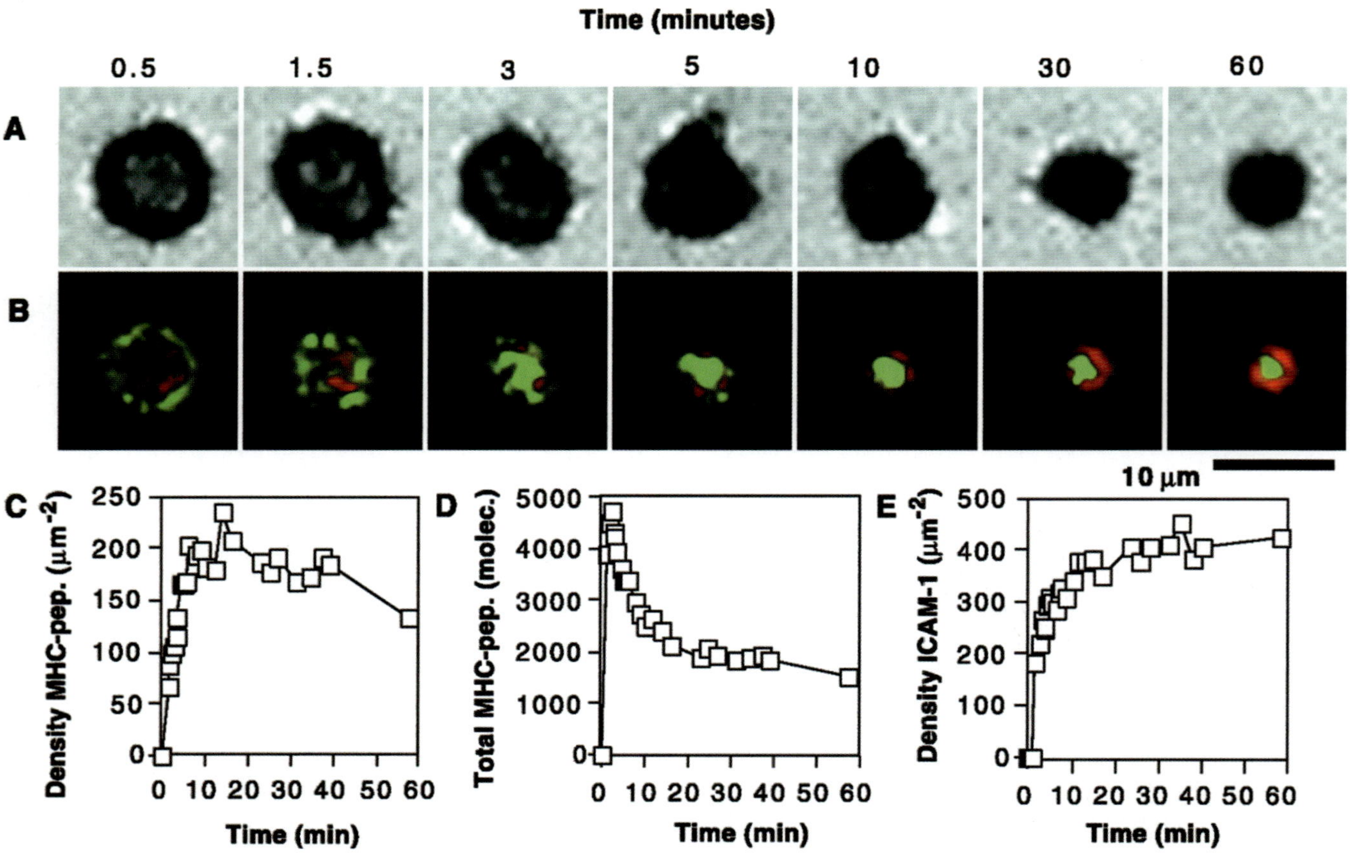

COLOR PLATE 3 • Formation of the Immunologic Synapse. T cells in contact with planar bilayer containing Oregon green E^k-antigen mouse cytochrome peptide 88-103 and Cy5 ICAM-1. Shown is the sequential formation of the immunologic synapse over the time period indicated. (From Grakoui et al: Science 285:221-227, 1999.)

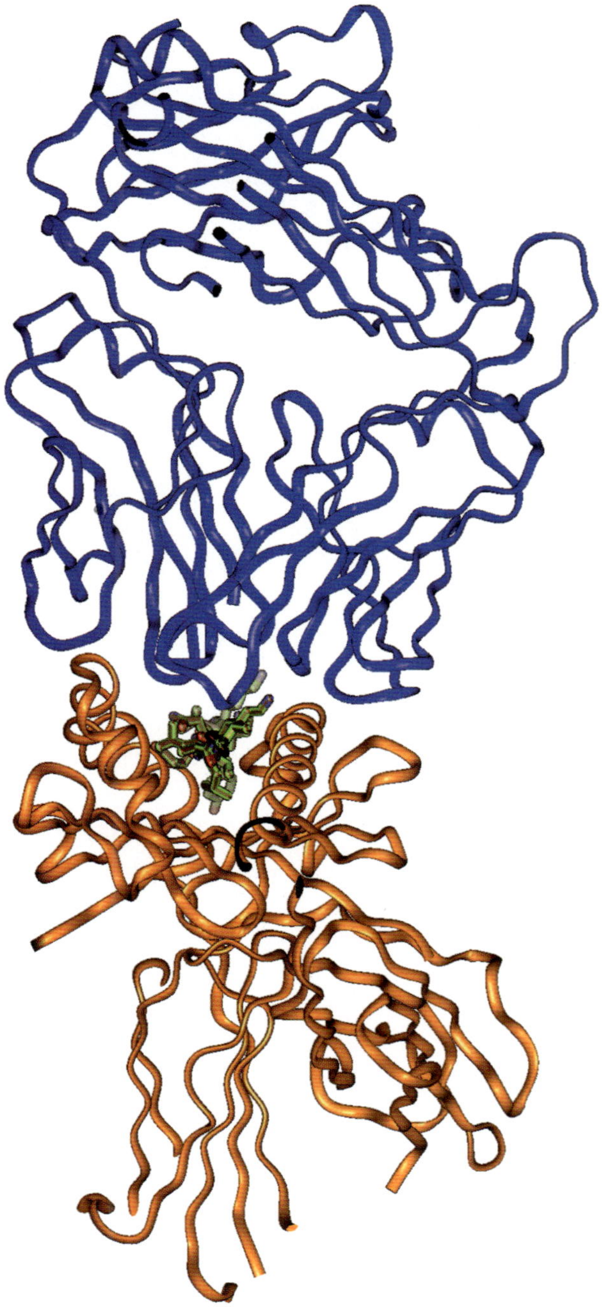

COLOR PLATE 4 • Ribbon diagram derived from the three-dimensional crystal structure of the trimolecular complex of a human a/b-T cell receptor (top, green), influenza hemaglutinin (Ha) antigen peptide, and the MHC class II molecule, DRB1*0401.24 Note that the peptide is contained with the peptide binding cleft of the HLA-DR molecule. The polymorphisms associated with the "shared epitope" are located on a-helical rim (DRB1 chain) of the peptide-binding cleft where they may interact with either the bound peptide antigen or the T cell receptor.

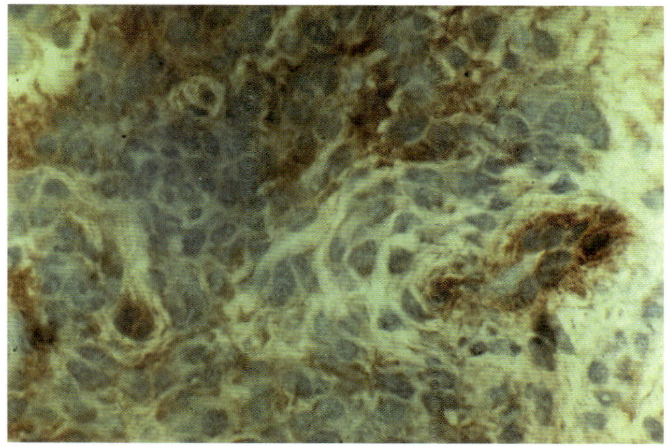

COLOR PLATE 5 • Indirect immunoperoxidase staining of frozen rheumatoid synovial tissue showing endothelial intercellular adhesion molecule-1 (ICAM-1) expression as indicated by the brown color. (×696).

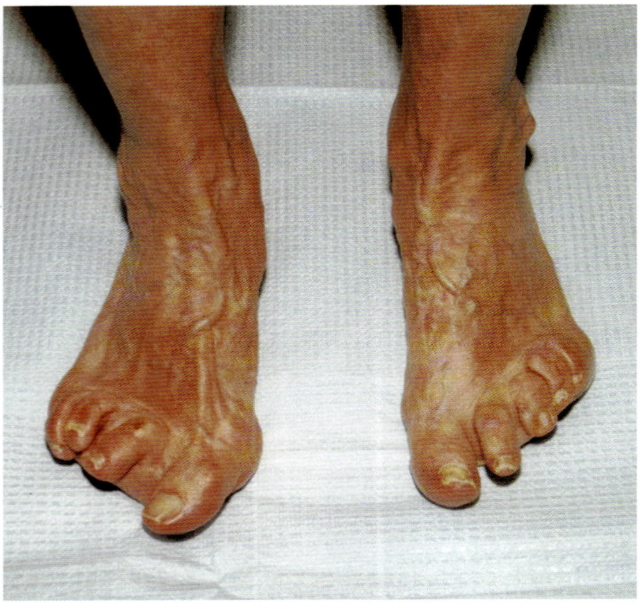

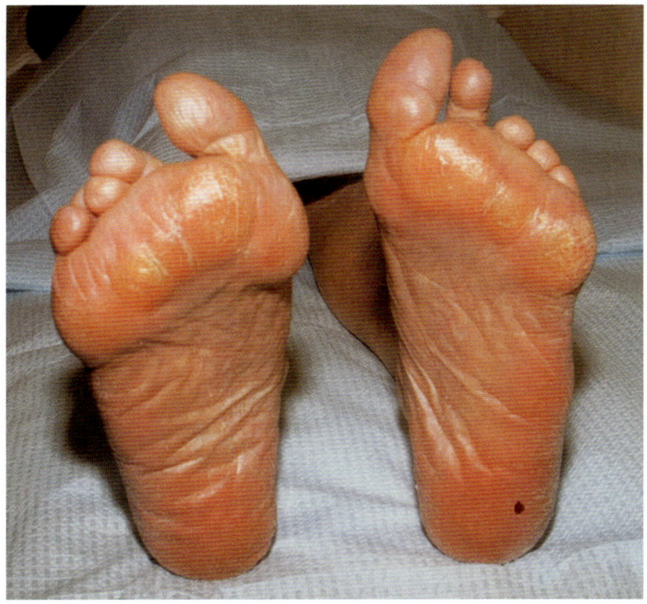

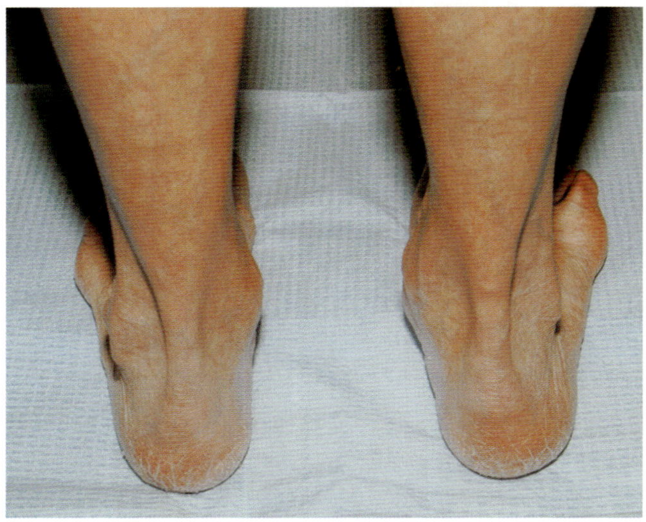

COLOR PLATE 6 • Inflammation of the metatarsals with pronation.

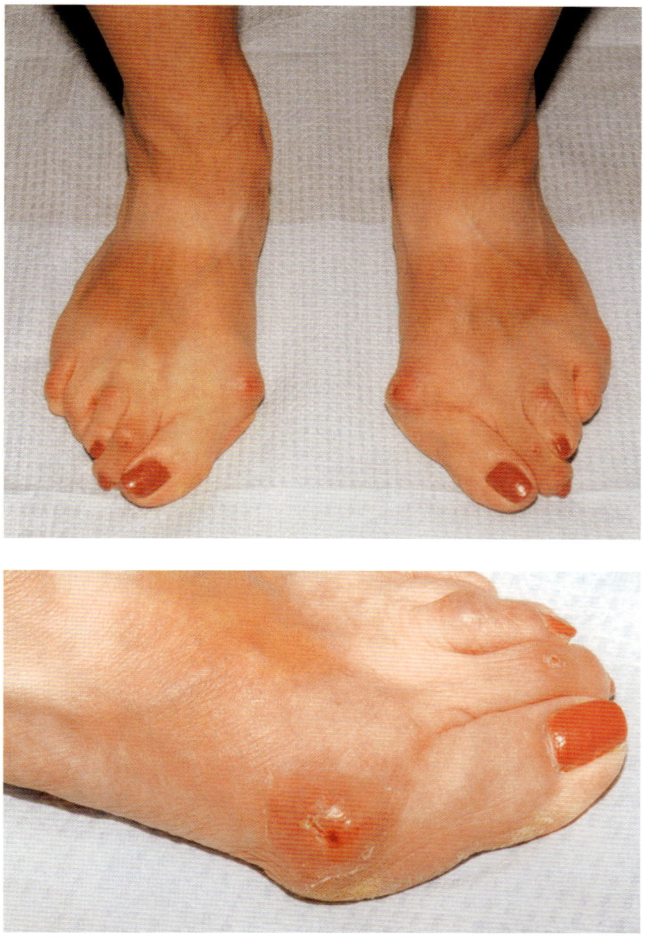

COLOR PLATE 7 • Alignment changes with nodules.

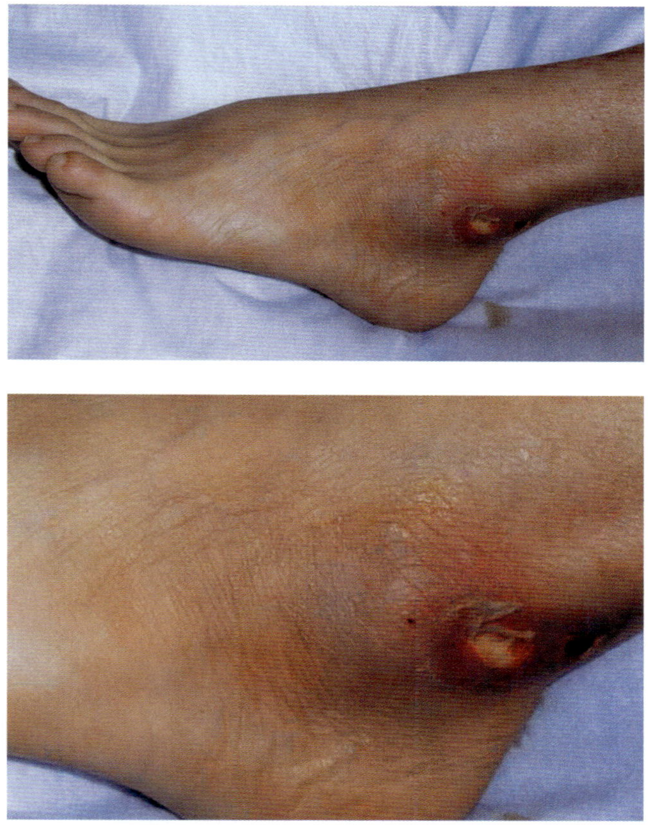

COLOR PLATE 8 • Photographs demonstrating small vasculitis on lateral ankle.

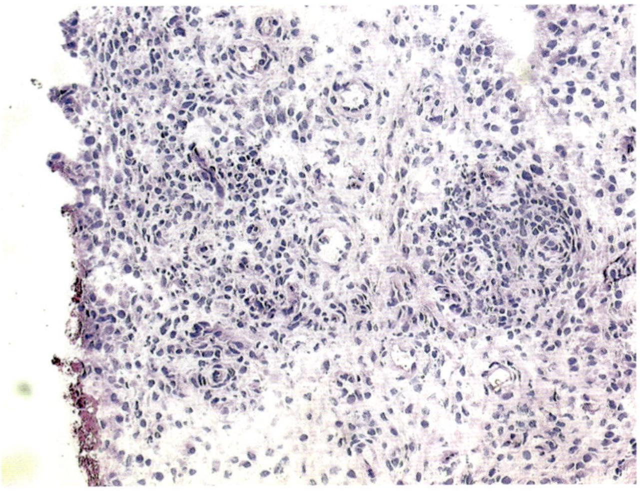

COLOR PLATE 9 • Rheumatoid synovial tissue, showing hyperplasia of the intimal lining layer and infiltration of mononuclear cells in the sublining layer. (H&E, ×200.)

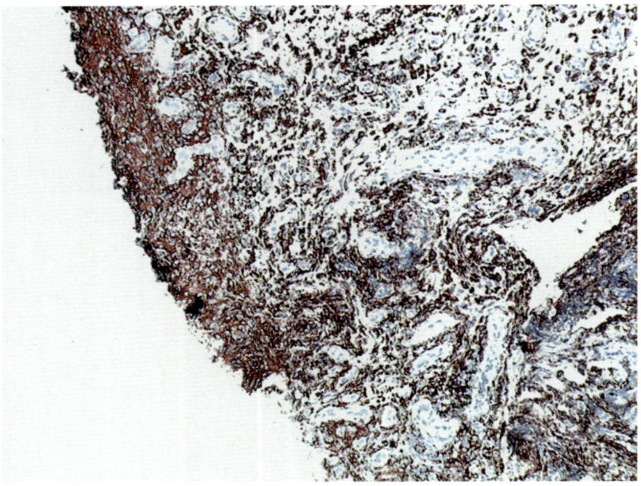

COLOR PLATE 10 • Activated macrophages expressing CD68 (red-brown) in the intimal lining layer and in the sublining layer of rheumatoid synovial tissue. (×100.)

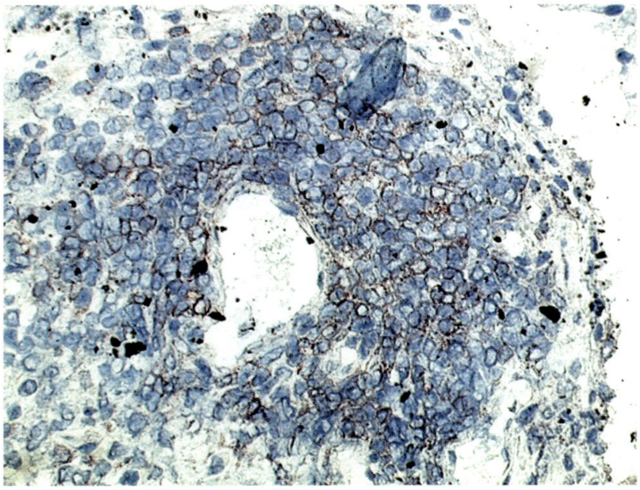

COLOR PLATE 11 • CD4+ T cells in a lymphocytic aggregate in the sublining layer of rheumatoid synovial tissue. (×400.)

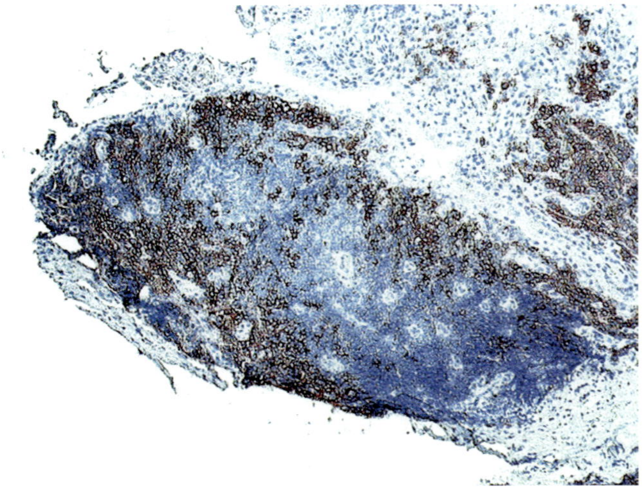

COLOR PLATE 12 • Plasma cells, expressing CD38 (red-brown), surrounding a lymphocyte aggregate in the sublining layer of rheumatoid synovial tissue. This architecture is also called corona. (×100.)

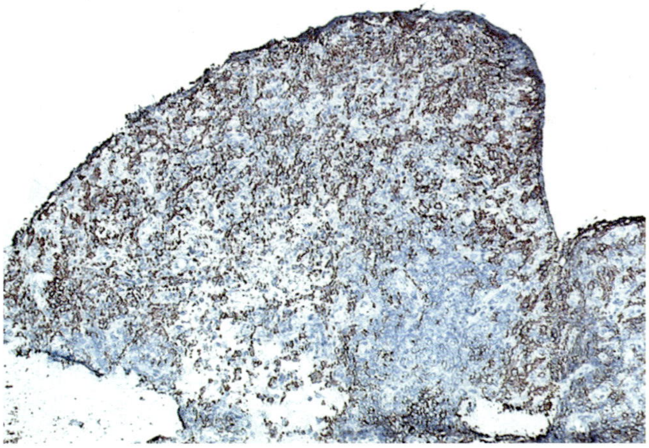

COLOR PLATE 13 • CD163+ macrophages in the intimal lining and sublining layer of rheumatoid synovial tissue. (×100.)

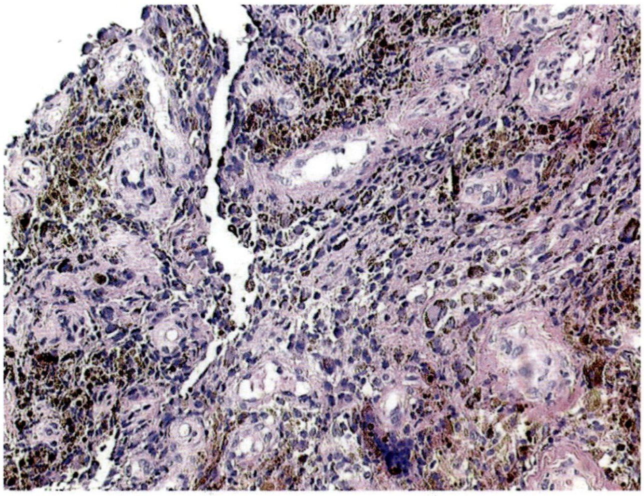

COLOR PLATE 14 • Synovial tissue showing pigmented villonodularis synovitis. (H&E, ×200.)

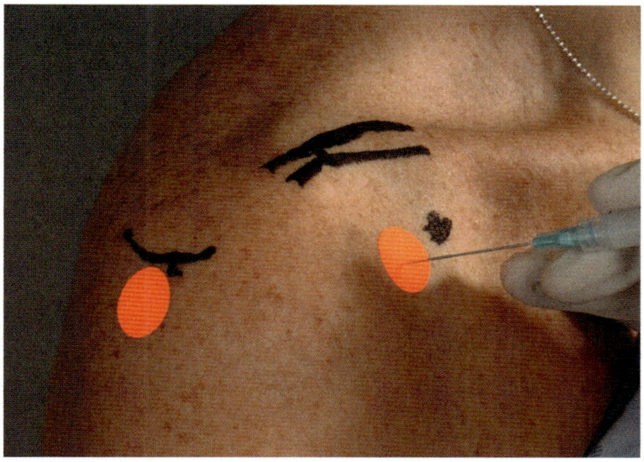

COLOR PLATE 15 • Shoulder (Glenohumeral) Joint Arthrocentesis: Anterior Approach. With the shoulder externally rotated, the needle is inserted at a point just medial to the head of the humerus, slightly inferior and lateral to the coracoid process (marked in black), which is just inferior to the lateral aspect of the clavicle (marked in black above).

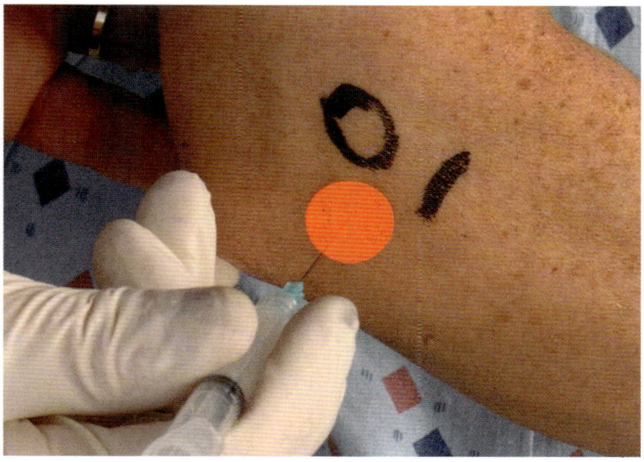

COLOR PLATE 17 • Elbow Arthrocentesis. With the elbow flexed 90 degrees, the needle is inserted into the recess just below the lateral epicondyle (black circle) and radial head (black line) and is directed parallel to the shaft of the radius.

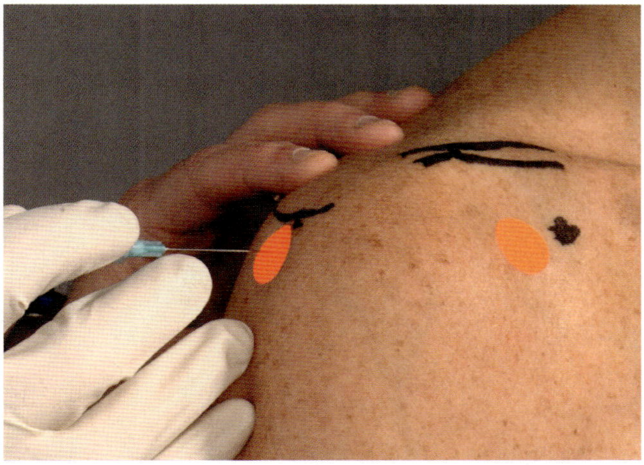

COLOR PLATE 16 • Rotator Cuff Tendon/Subacromial Bursa Injection: Lateral Approach. Over the lateral aspect of the shoulder, the groove between the acromion (marked in black) and humerus is palpated and marked (spot). The needle is inserted at this point and advanced in a horizontal plane medially.

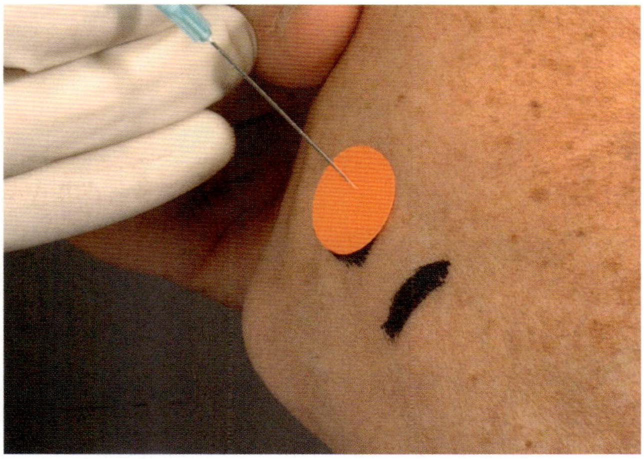

COLOR PLATE 18 • Lateral Epicondyle (Tennis Elbow) Injection. With the elbow flexed and pronated, the needle is inserted at the most tender area over the bony prominence on the anterolateral aspect of the lateral humerus, which is proximal to radial head (black line). A combination of steroid and local anesthetic is then injected into the subcutaneous tissues at the attachment of the extensor muscles to the epicondyle.

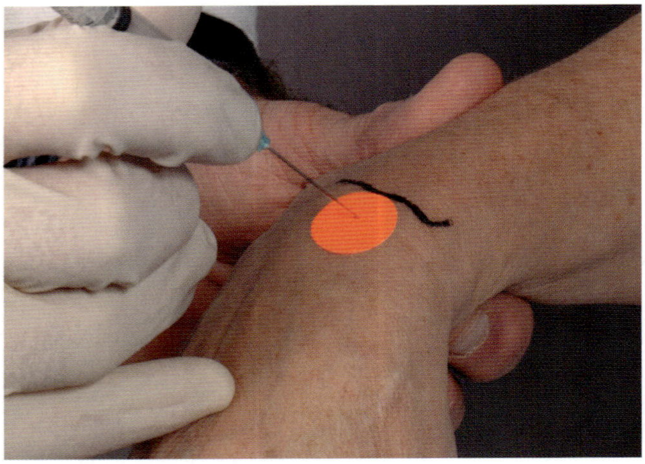

COLOR PLATE 19 • Wrist (Radiocarpal) Arthrocentesis. The needle is inserted just distal to the radius (marked in black) at a point just ulnar to the anatomic snuffbox. It is directed perpendicular to the skin and advanced until fluid is obtained or the needle is advanced 1 to 1.5 inches.

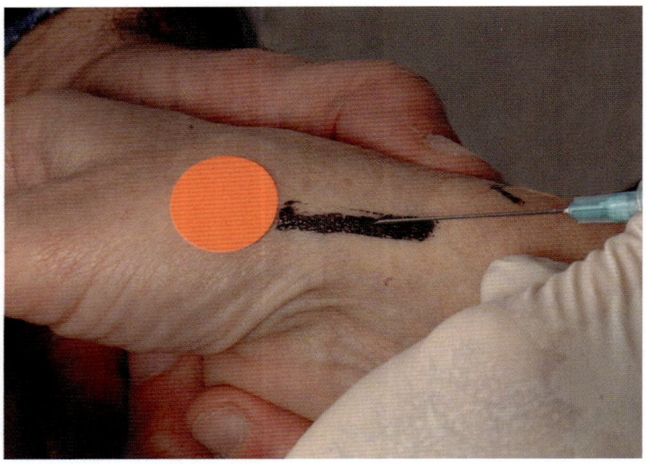

COLOR PLATE 20 • Injection for de Quervain's Tenosynovitis. The needle is inserted along the course of the tendons (black line), proximal to the thumb carpometacarpal joint (spot), at the radial aspect of the anatomic snuffbox. The needle is directed almost parallel to the skin either proximally or distally. As the needle is advanced, a mixture of steroid and anesthetic is injected along the sheath of the tendon, and a palpable bulge is usually felt along the tendon. Care should be taken to avoid injection of steroid into the body of the tendon.

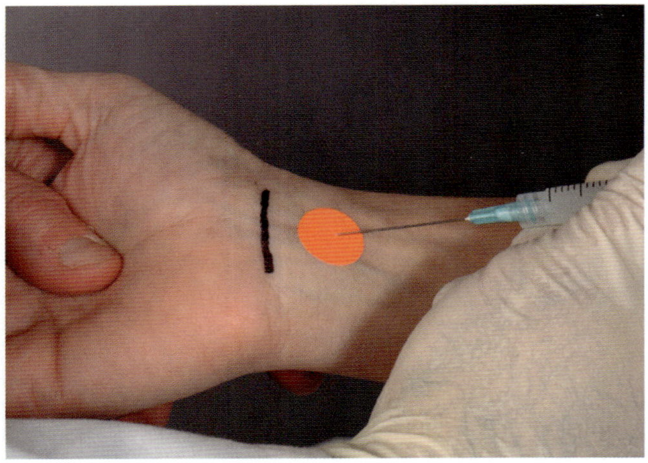

COLOR PLATE 21 • Injection for Carpal Tunnel Syndrome. To begin an injection in this area, the clinician should make a mark on the volar aspect of the wrist along the flexor tendons, on the ulnar side of the long palmar tendon, and approximately 1 inch proximal to the distal volar skin crease at the wrist (black). A 22- to 26-gauge needle is introduced at a 30- to 45-degree angle and is directed proximally or distally along the course of the tendon. The needle should be introduced about Z\x to 1 inch. If the needle meets obstruction, or if the patient experiences paresthesias, the needle should be withdrawn and redirected slightly to avoid injecting into the body of a tendon or into the median nerve itself.

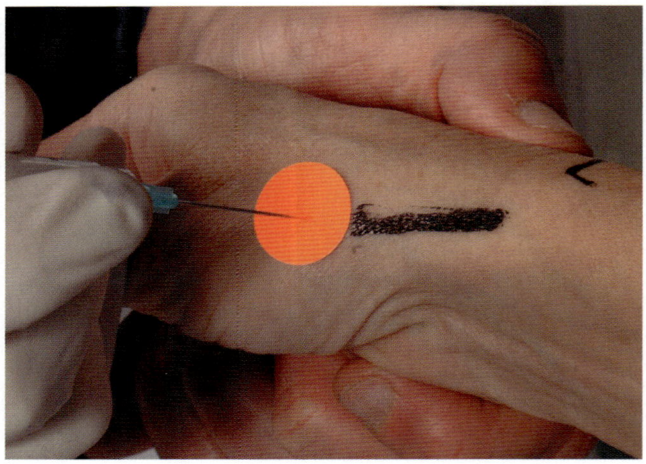

COLOR PLATE 22 • Injection of the Thumb Carpometacarpal Joint. The procedure begins by flexing the thumb across the palm and making a mark at the base of the thumb metacarpal distal to the radial tendons of the snuffbox (black). A 22- to 25-gauge needle is inserted Z\x to 1 inch at this mark and directed away from the radial artery; 0.2 to 0.5 cc of steroid may then be injected.

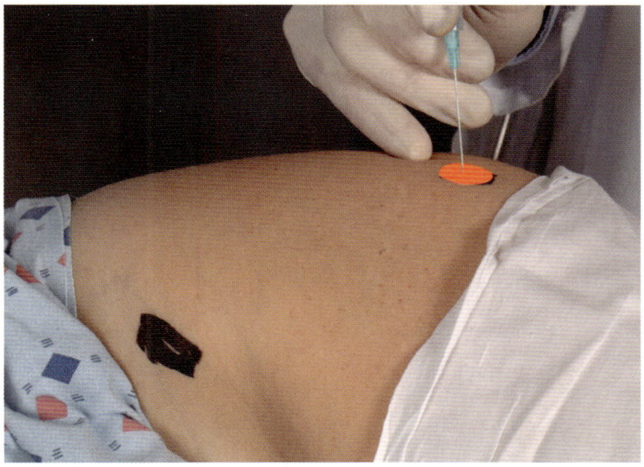

COLOR PLATE 23 • Injection for Trochanteric Pain Syndrome. This area is easily injected after marking the area of tenderness over bony prominence of the lateral hip with the patient lying on the opposite side. A 1- to 3-inch needle is inserted perpendicular to the skin over the bony prominence, and 1 cc of steroid with 2 to 4 cc of local anesthetic are injected into the area. (Anterior superior iliac spine is marked for reference.)

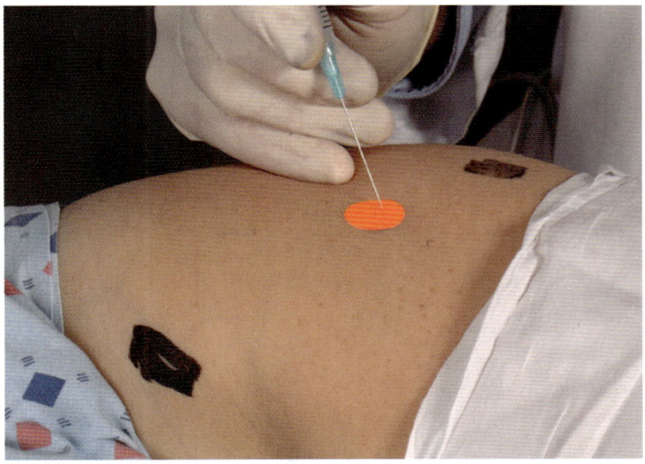

COLOR PLATE 24 • Hip Arthrocentesis: Lateral Approach. With the hip internally rotated, the needle is inserted just anterior to the greater trochanter (black) and directed toward a point slightly below the inguinal ligament (anterior superior iliac spine is marked for reference). As noted in the text, accuracy of any approach to the hip joint is limited, and radiographic guidance should be considered unless synovial fluid is easily obtained using this approach.

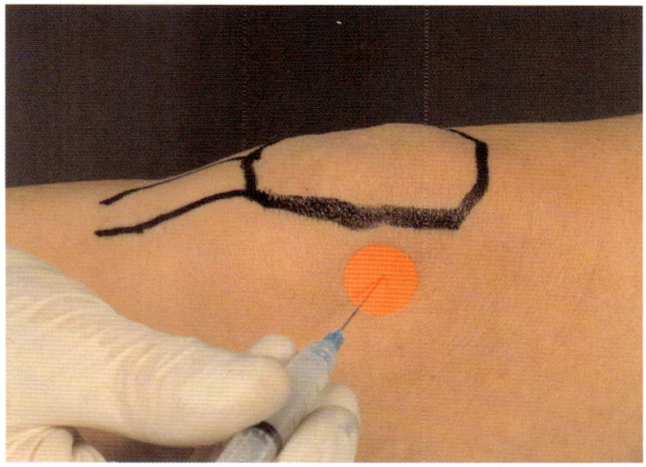

COLOR PLATE 25 • Knee Arthrocentesis: Medial Approach. With the patient supine, a mark is made in the recess (or where there is a fluid bulge) behind the medial portion of the patella (black), approximately at the midline. The needle should be advanced 1.5 inches or more until fluid is obtained (patellar tendon marked for reference).

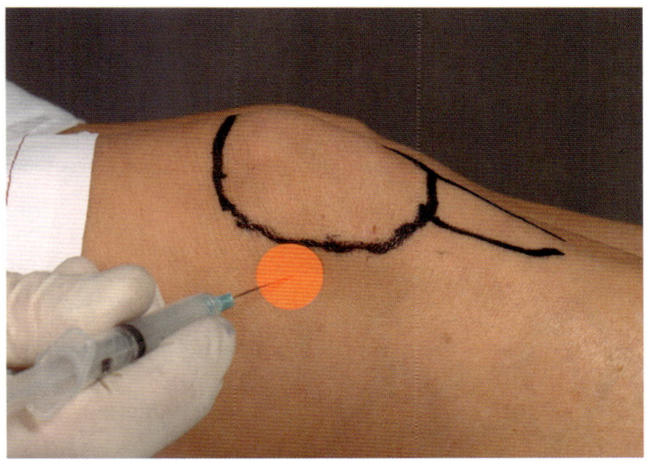

COLOR PLATE 26 • Knee Arthrocentesis: Lateral Approach. With the patient supine, a mark is made in the recess (or where there is a fluid bulge) behind the lateral portion of the patella (black), approximately at the midline. The needle should be advanced 1.5 inches or more until fluid is obtained (patellar tendon marked for reference).

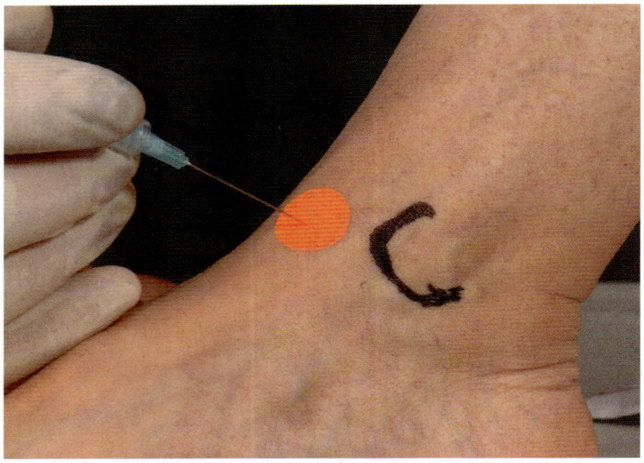

COLOR PLATE 27 • Ankle Arthrocentesis: Anterior Approach (Tibiotalar Joint). With ankle at a 90-degree angle to the lower leg, the needle is inserted at a point just lateral to the medial malleolus (black) and just medial to the tibialis anterior tendon. The needle is then directed posteriorly, perpendicular to the shaft of the tibia.

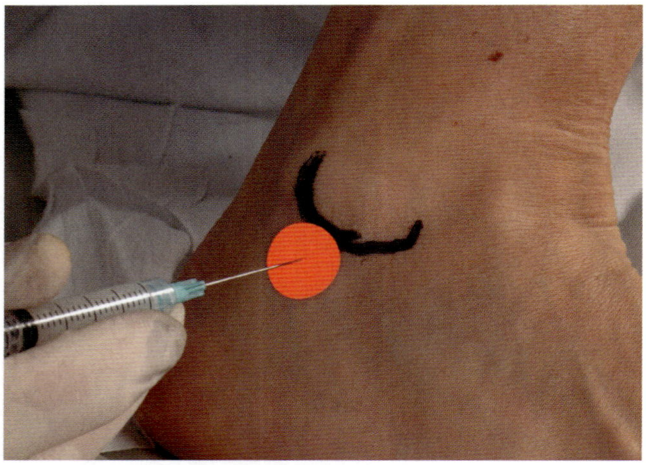

COLOR PLATE 28 • Subtalar (Lateral) Ankle Arthrocentesis. The needle is inserted into the recess just inferior to the tip of the lateral malleolus (black) and directed perpendicularly. A bulge is often easily palpated here if fluid is present in this joint.

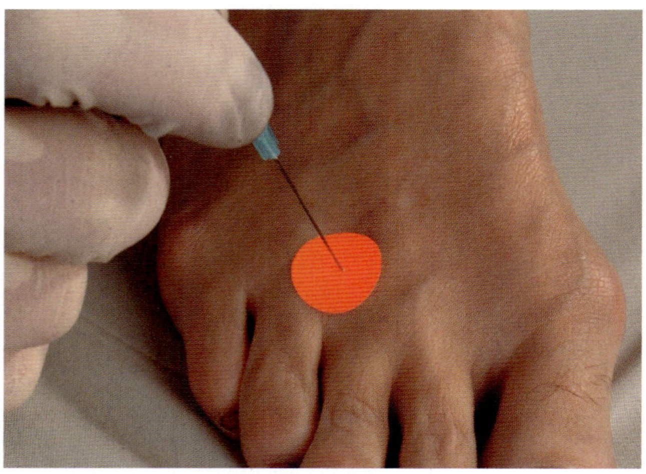

COLOR PLATE 29 • Injection for Interdigital (Morton's) Neuroma. The area is most easily injected from the dorsal aspect, usually between the metarsal heads of the third and fourth toes. The area of tenderness is marked, the needle is inserted 0.5 to 1 inch, and steroid with anesthetic is injected.

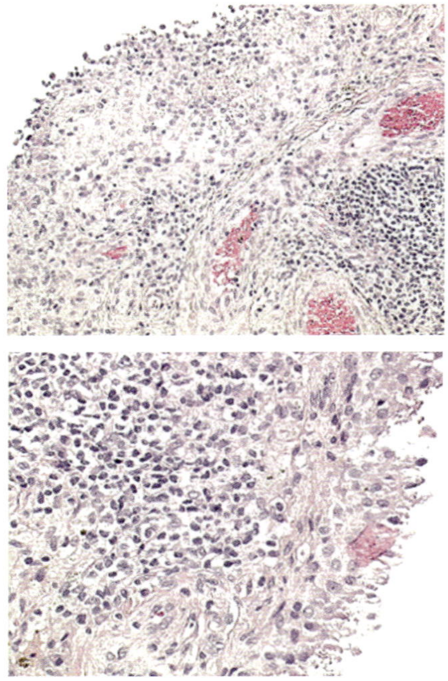

COLOR PLATE 30 • Histopathologic Appearance of Rheumatoid Arthritis (RA) Synovium. Intimal lining hyperplasia, angiogenesis, and a prominent mononuclear cell infiltrate are present. Top panel is magnified ×200 and the bottom panel is ×400. (Courtesy of Dr. Paul-Peter Tak.)

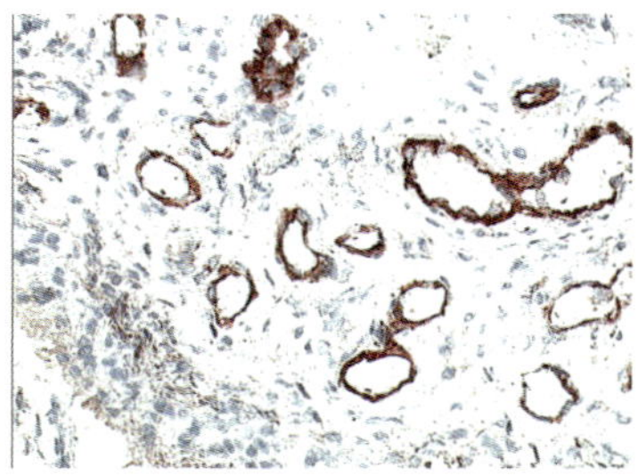

COLOR PLATE 31 • Human Rheumatoid Synovial Membrane Stained with Antibody to Von Willebrand Factor to Delineate Blood Vessels. Virtually all of these blood vessels have formed in response to angiogenic stimuli after the rheumatoid process had been initiated. (Courtesy of Dr. Paul-Peter Tak.)

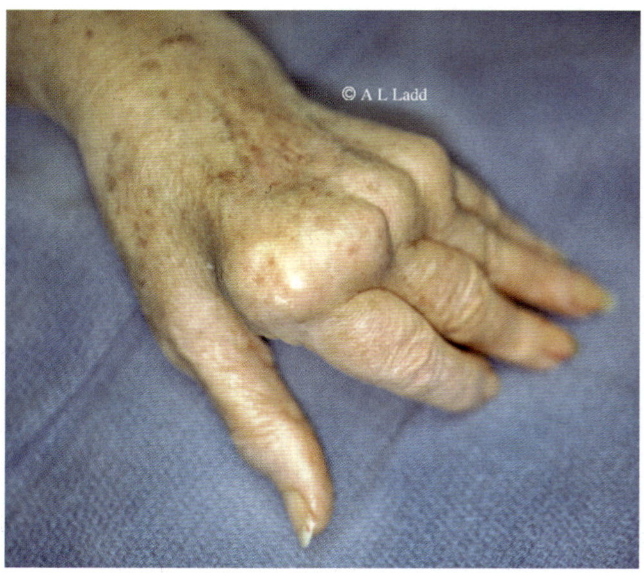

COLOR PLATE 32 • Ulnar Deviation and Subluxation. This left hand shows typical manifestations of end-stage erosive changes about the metacarpophalangeal (MP) joints, with volar dislocation and ulnar drift of the fingers. (Copyright A.L. Ladd)

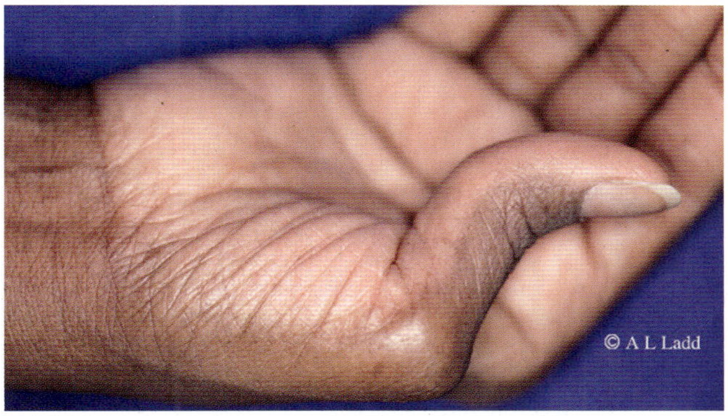

COLOR PLATE 33 • Boutonniére Deformity. This is a right thumb demonstrating typical soft tissue imbalance found in rheumatoid arthritis (RA). The metacarpophalangeal (MP) joint is hyperflexed, and the interphalangeal (IP) joint is hyperextended. (Copyright A.L. Ladd)

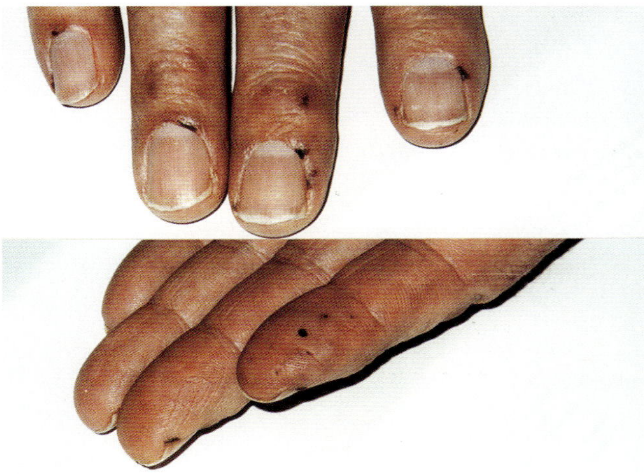

COLOR PLATE 34 • Digital Vasculitis in a 65-year-old man with Seropositive Rheumatoid Arthritis (RA). (Courtesy of Eileen Moynihan, M.D.)

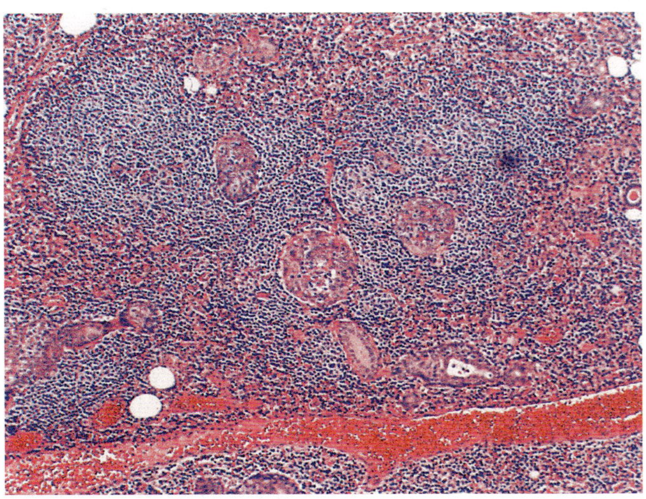

COLOR PLATE 35 • Histopathologic Section of a Salivary Gland from a Patient with Sjögren's Syndrome. Normal glandular architecture is replaced by a sea of mononuclear cells. Remnants of acinar and ductal structures can be seen. Formation of a germinal center-like cluster can be noted. (Courtesy of Dr. John Fantasia, Long Island Jewish Medical Center.)

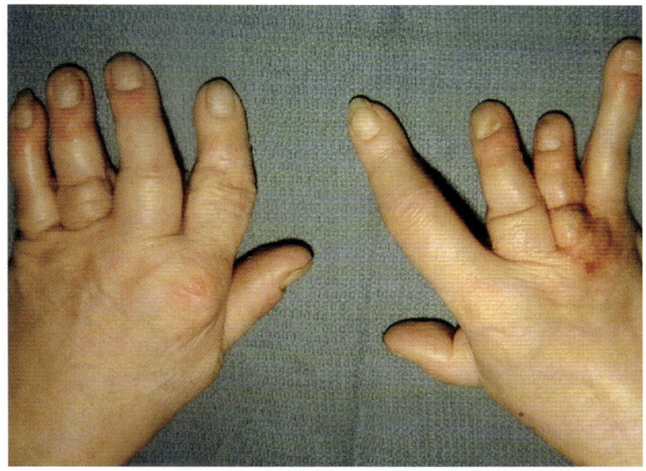

COLOR PLATE 36 • Destructive arthritis (arthritis mutilans) involving all digits, some with shortening, others with ankylosis.

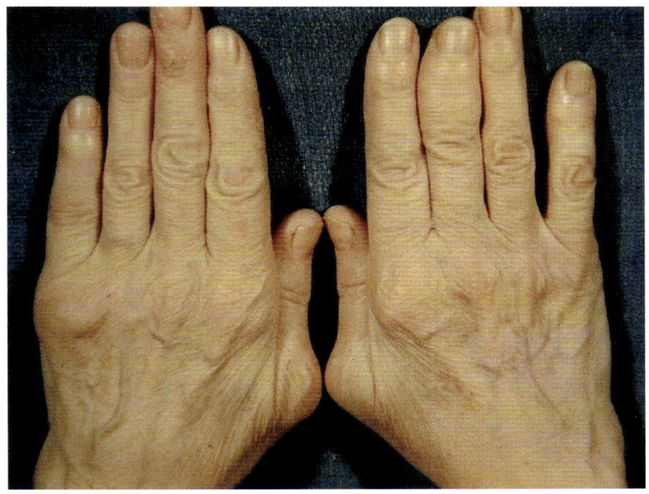

COLOR PLATE 37 • Symmetric polyarthritis indistinguishable from rheumatoid arthritis (RA).

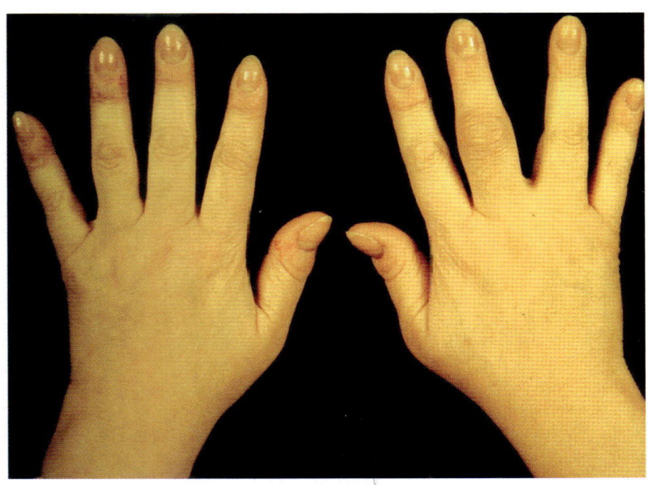

COLOR PLATE 38 • Asymmetric oligoarthritis involving the third proximal interphalangeal joint; the other hand is normal.

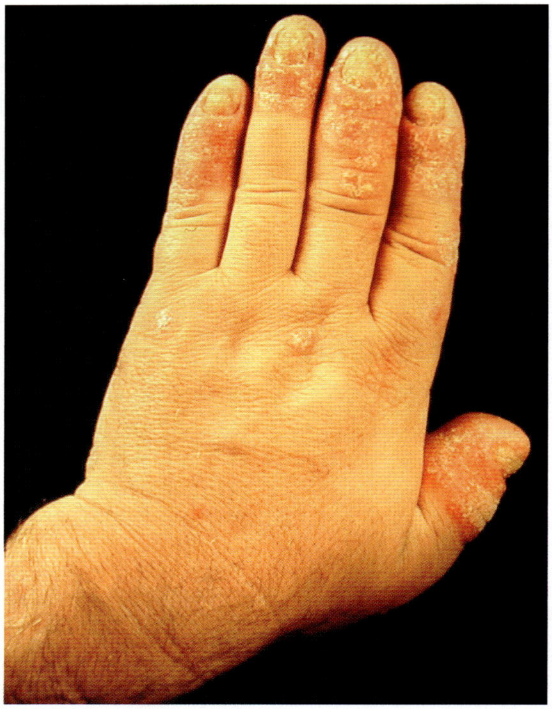

COLOR PLATE 39 • Dactylitis in the third digit and thumb in a patient with psoriatic arthritis (PsA).

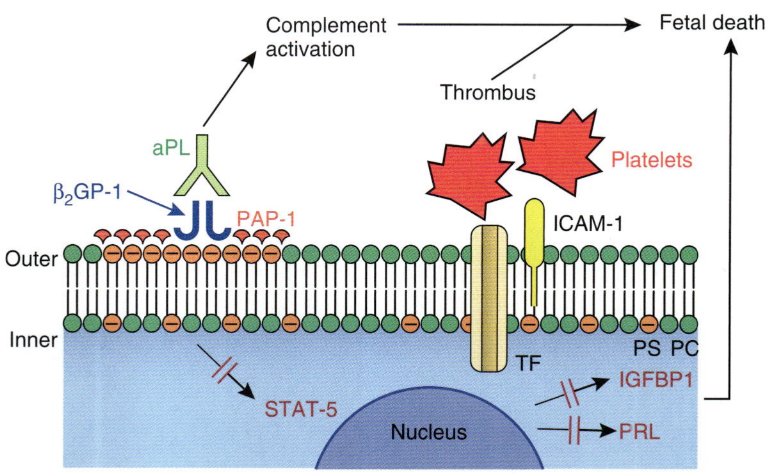

COLOR PLATE 40 • Proposed Mechanism of Throm-bosis and Placental Injury. The negatively charged phospholipid, phosphatidylserine (PS, orange circles), migrates from the inner to the outer cell membrane during activation or apoptosis of platelets and endothelial cells, and it is normally present on trophoblasts. (The neutral phospholipid, phosphatidylcholine [PC, green circles], is the major constituent of the outer layer of unactivated cells.) Dimeric b_2 glycoprotein-I (b_2GPI) then binds to PS and antiphospholipid antibody (aPL) binds to b_2GPI, activating complement and triggering several signals, leading to expression of adhesion molecules (e.g., ICAM-1) and tissue factor (TF), platelet aggregation, and thrombosis. Placental effects of aPL are indicated in red. Placental anticoagulant protein I (PAP-1, annexin V) normally provides a shield on trophoblast PS, protecting the fetus against activation of maternal prothrombotic processes. This shield is broken by b_2GPI-APS complex. It is likely that complement activation, recruiting and stimulating inflammatory cells, is a critical downstream element of fetal injury. APLs also downregulate expression of trophoblast signal transducer and activator of transcription 5 (STAT-5), reducing endometrial stromal cell production of prolactin (PRL) and insulin growth factor binding protein-1 (IGFBP-1). (Adapted from Rai R, Roubey R, Rand J, et al. Presented at the 10th International Antiphospholipid Antibody Conference, Taormina, Sicily, October, 2002.)

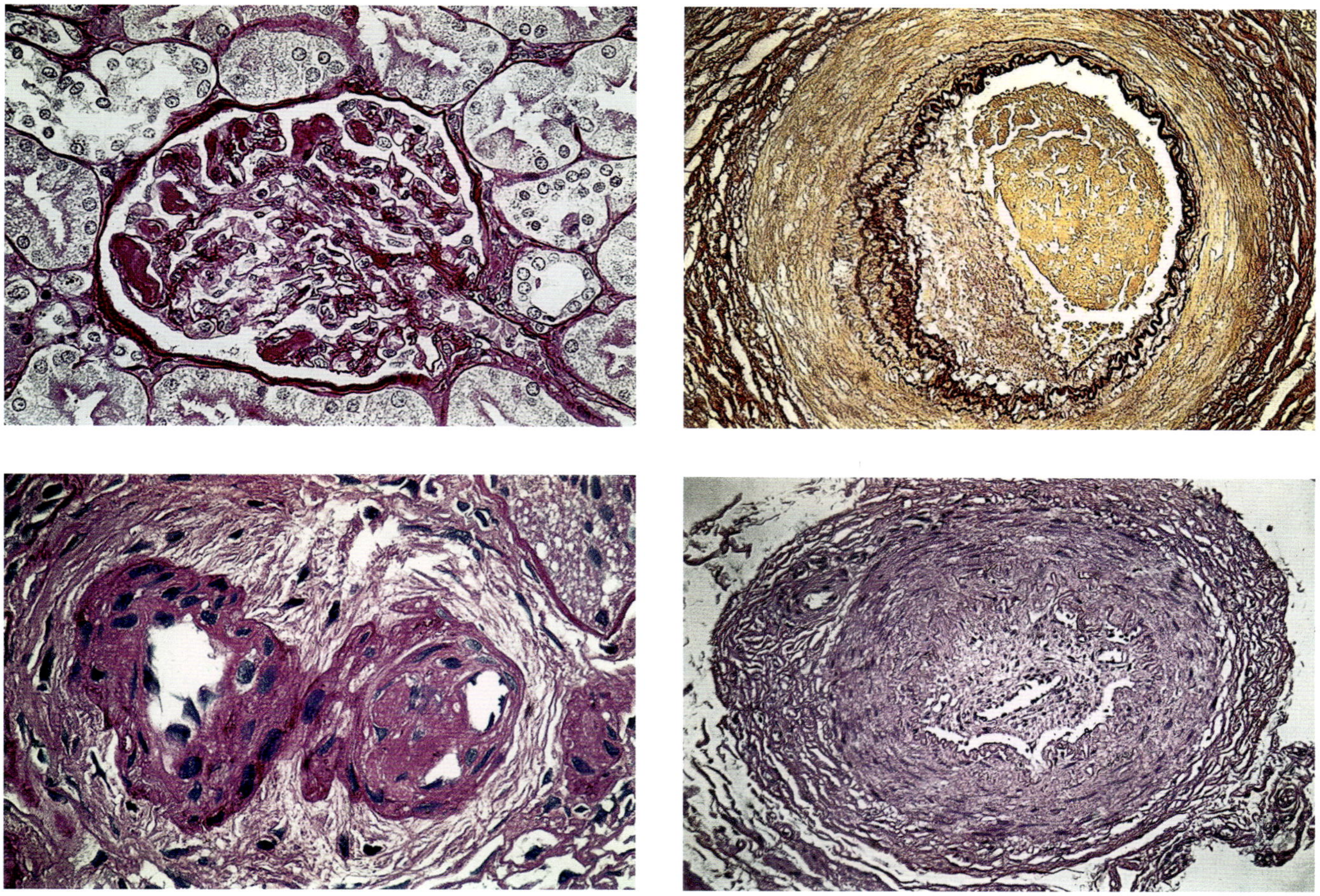

COLOR PLATE 41 • Thrombotic Microangiopathy in the Antiphospholipid Antibody Syndrome (APS). A, Kidney biopsy from a 35-year-old woman with primary antiphospholipid syndrome (PAPS), microhematuria, and non-nephrotic proteinuria. Note the glomerulus containing microthrombi occluding capillary lumina, with endothelial swelling. B, Same patient's small renal artery containing organized thrombus with recanalization and arteriosclerosis (periodic acid-Schiff, ×100). C, Autopsy specimen from a 45-year-old man with PAPS. Note the thrombus in various stages of organization, intact elastic lamina with focal reduplication, and medial thickening (elastic Verhoff's stain, ×100). D, Same patient's medium-sized peripheral artery. Note the organized thrombus with recanalization, severe fibrointimal thickening, medial hypertrophy, and extreme stenosis of lumen (H&E, ×75). (Slides and caption provided by Dr. Surya V. Seshan.)

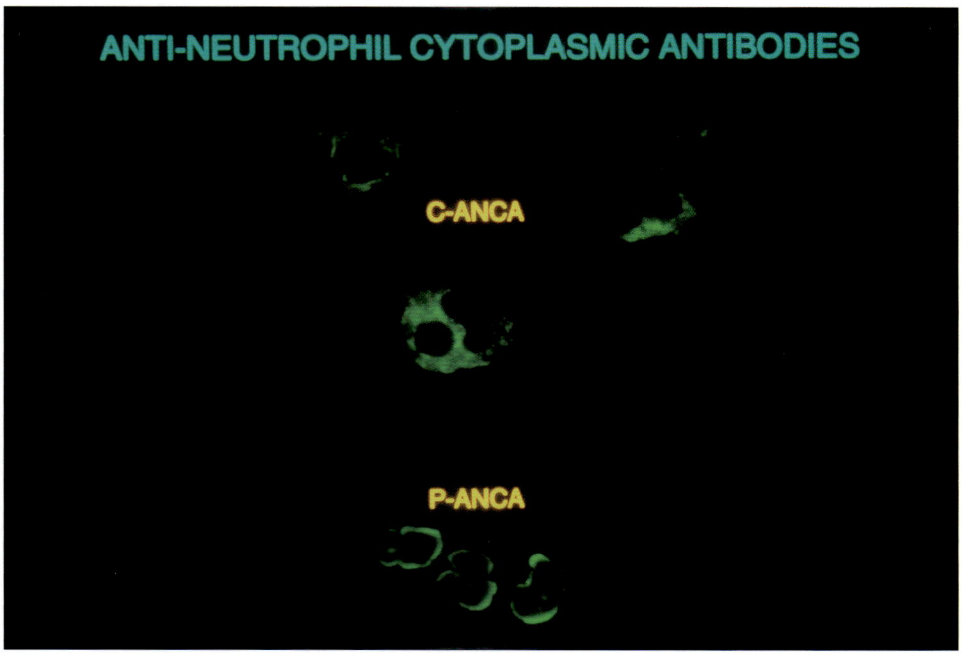

COLOR PLATE 42 • Immunofloure-scence of diffuse or cytoplasmic antineutrophil cytoplasmic antibody (c-ANCA), which is highly correlated with antibodies to proteinase 3 (PR-3) and the less-specific perinuclear pattern (p-ANCA), which is at times indicative of antibodies to myeloperoxidase (MPO). Although immuno-flourescence was historically the standard for ANCA testing, current standards require confirmatory antigen-specific testing for PR 3 and MPO.

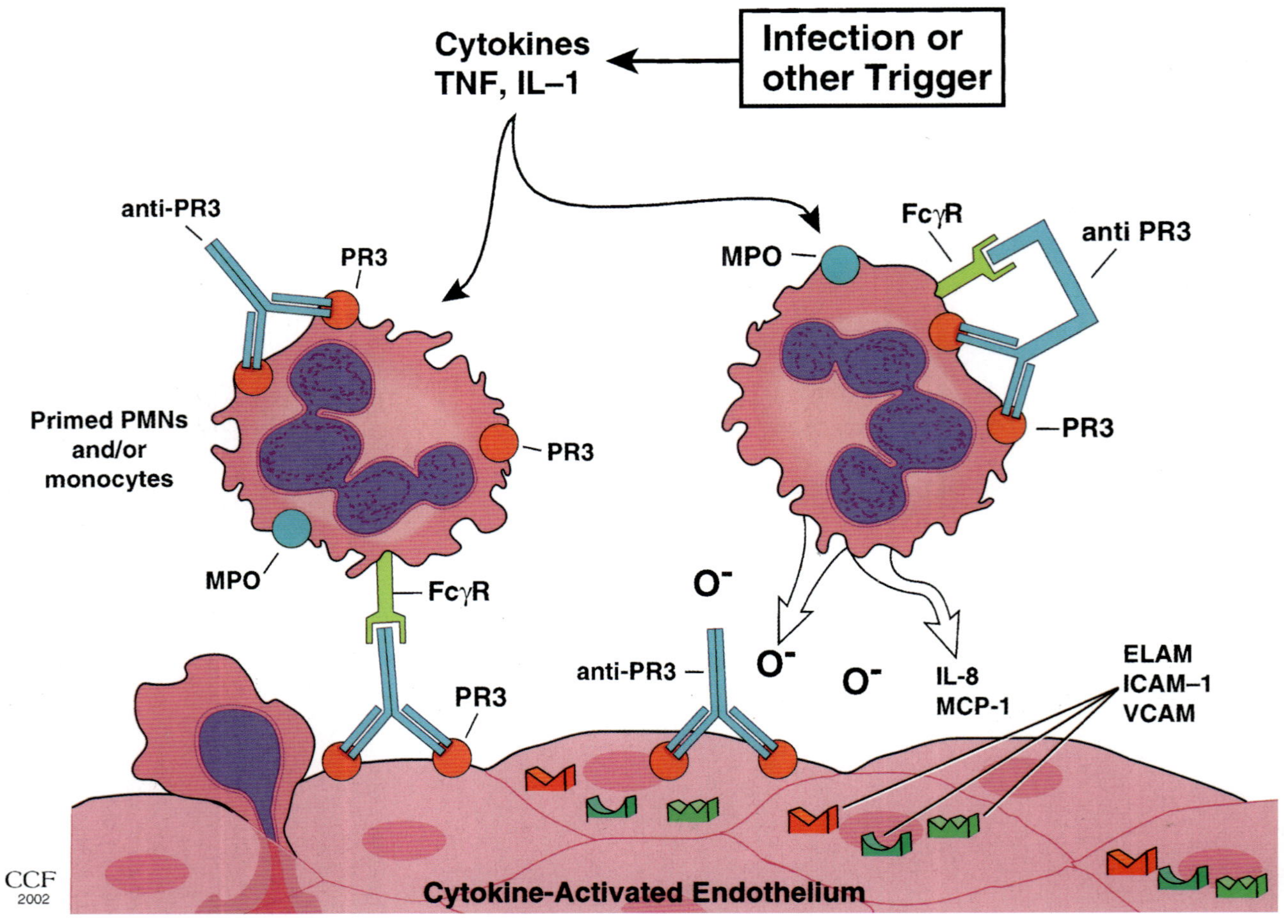

COLOR PLATE 43 • Schematic representation of the immune mechanisms hypothetically involved with antineutrophil cytoplasmic antibody (ANCA) enhancement of vascular injury. In this scheme an infectious trigger or other environmental stimuli leads to a burst of cytokines that serve to prime neutrophils or monocytes and may lead to local upregulation of adhesion molecules on endothelium. The priming process within the inflammatory cells leads to enhanced expression of ANCA antigens on the cell surface. Activated neutrophils or monocytes may degranulate and release reactive oxygen species and lysosomal enzymes, leading to endothelial injury and further activation of the endothelial cell surface. The magnitude of this effect is influenced by the specificity of ANCA for proteinase 3 (PR3) or myeloperoxidase (MPO), as well as different epitopes of these respective antigens. The reaction may also be further influenced by immunoglobulin G (IgG) and the fragment crystallizable gamma (FCg) receptor phenotype engaged. Release of products from degranulated inflammatory cells become bound to endothelial cells and further service targets of ANCA. Release of chemotactic chemokines such as interleukin-8 (IL8) and macrophage chemoattractant protein-1 (MCP-1) serve to augment chemotaxis and inflammatory cell transmigration in conjunction with other adhesion molecules. Thus, the scheme provides the prerequisites for endothelial and vascular injury induced by ANCA namely, 1) the presence of ANCA, b) the expression of target antigens for ANCA on prime neutrophils and monocytes, c) the interaction between prime neutrophils and endothelium via adhesion molecules and finally d) the activation of endothelial cells and ultimate efflux of inflammatory cells to the extra vascular and perivascular tissues.

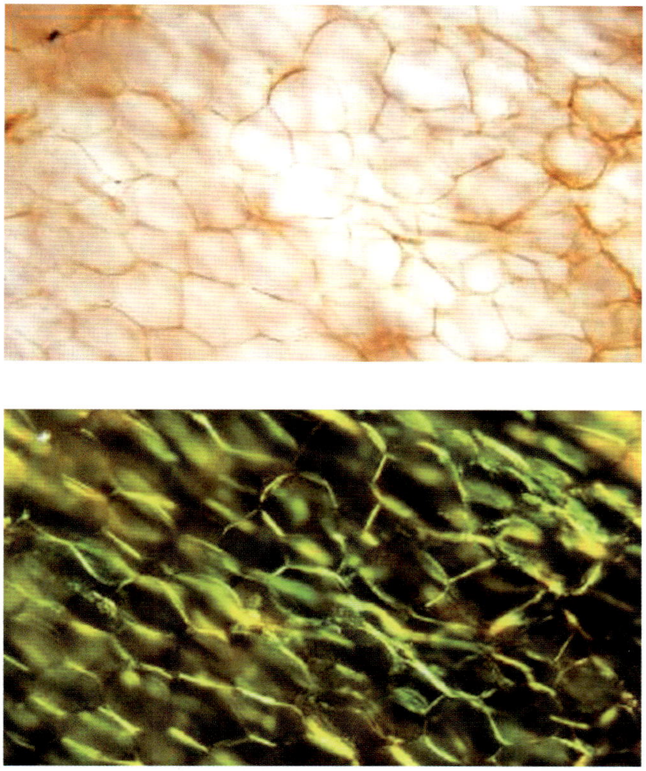

COLOR PLATE 44 • Subcutaneous fat aspirate stained with Congo red. *A,* Sample viewed by light microscopy. *B,* Sample viewed under polarized light (×200). The staining and birefringence is evident in the walls and connective tissue surrounding the adipose

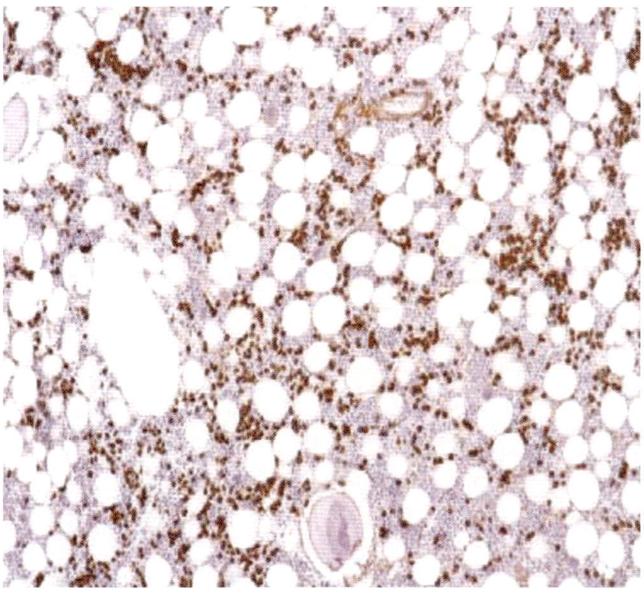

COLOR PLATE 45 • Bone marrow biopsy specimen stained with antibody to δ light chain shows preferential staining of plasma cells as well as staining of amyloid deposit around a blood vessel *(arrow)* (×400).

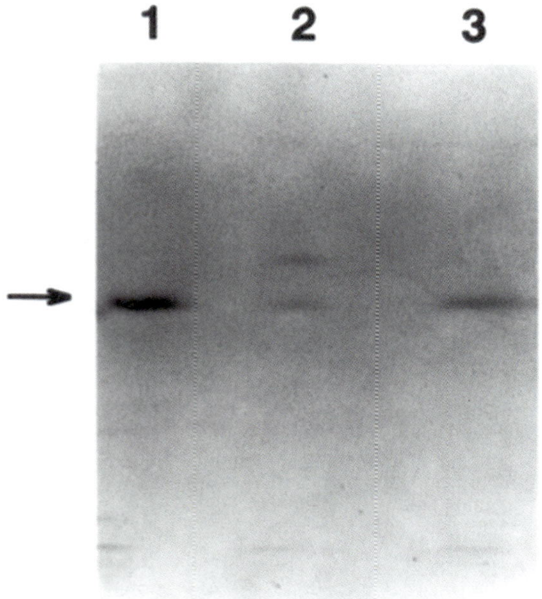

COLOR PLATE 46 • Isoelectric focusing of serum samples shows bands of both variant and wild-type transthyretin (TTR) protein *(arrow)* from a patient with ATTR *(lane 2)* and a single band of wild-type TTR in normal subjects *(lanes 1 and 3).*

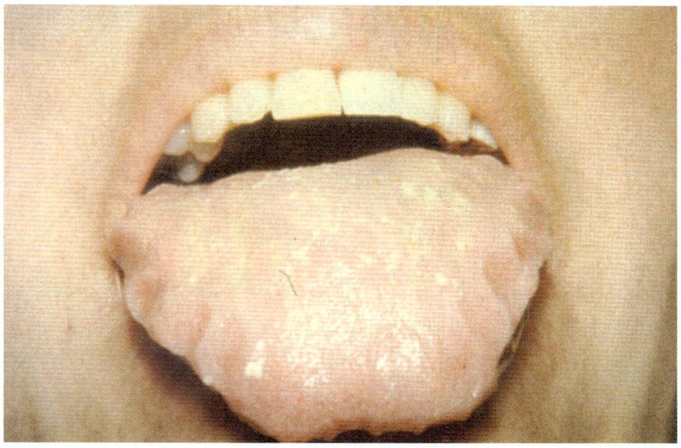

COLOR PLATE 47 • Enlarged tongue of a patient with AL amyloidosis.

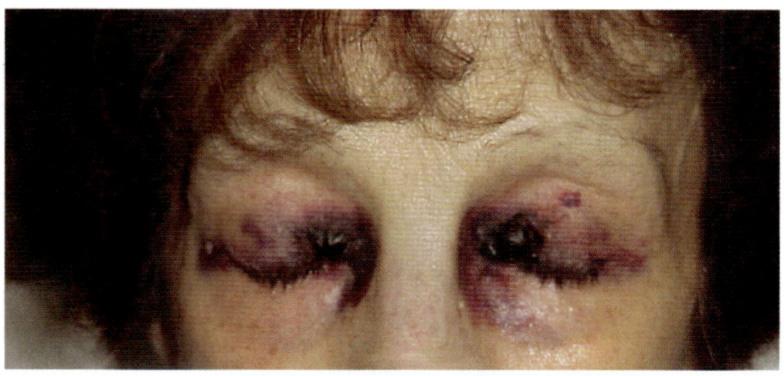

COLOR PLATE 48 • Periorbital ecchymoses and total alopecia of the scalp in a patient with AL amyloidosis.

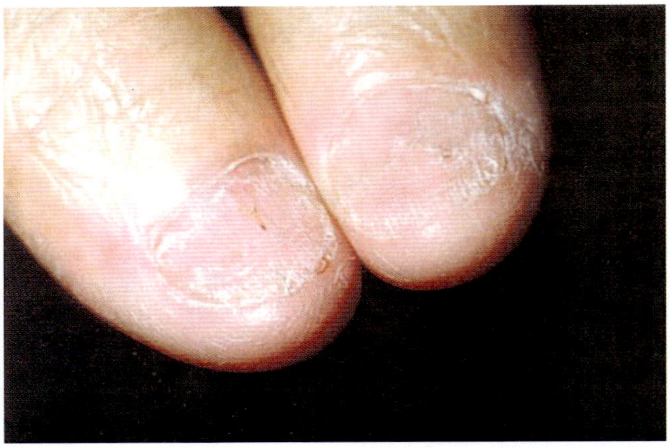

COLOR PLATE 49 • Fingernail dystrophy in a patient with AL amyloidosis.

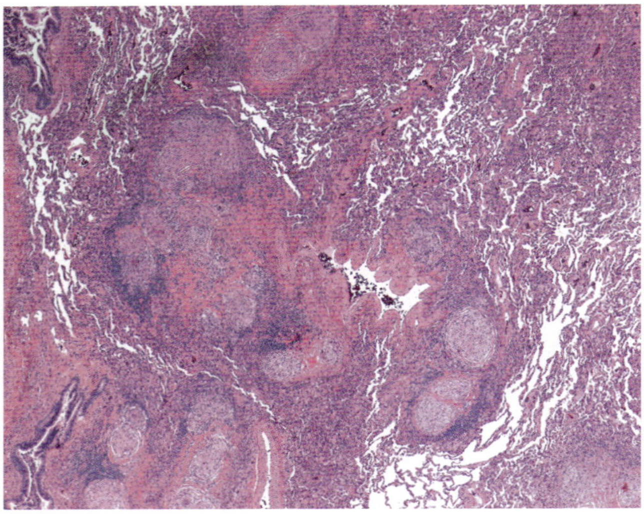

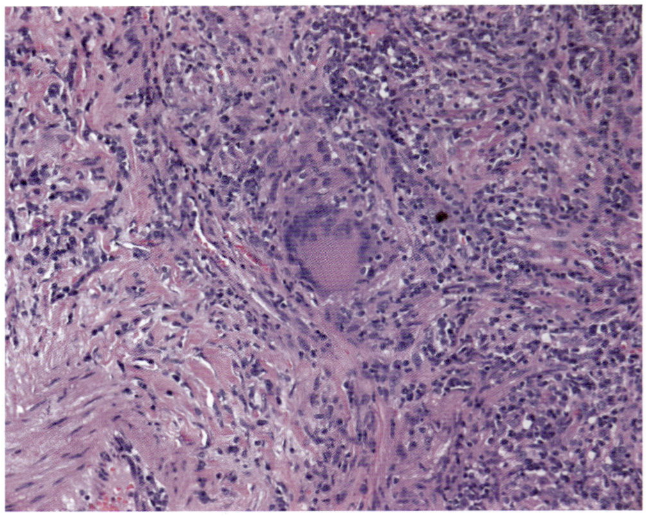

COLOR PLATE 50 • A, The typical pathologic appearance of sarcoidosis consists of non-necrotizing granulomas, which are mononuclear cell infiltrates with varying degrees of adjacent collagen deposition. Shown here is lung tissue (×100, H&E), the most commonly affected organ, infiltrated by multiple noncaseating granulomas adjacent to vessels and bronchioles. B, This ×400 photomicrograph demonstrates the classic, but not pathognomonic, features of the noncaseating granuloma, including multinucleated giant cell (at center), abundant lymphocytes, macrophages, epithelioid cells, mast cells, plasma cells, and fibroblasts. C, Although uncommon, sarcoidosis can cause a non-necrotizing granulomatous vasculitis in virtually any organ. Shown is a ×200 view of a pulmonary artery using an elastic tissue (VVG) stain. The elastic lamina (dark stain) is intact. Within the intima is a large area of non-necrotizing granulomatous inflammation producing a narrowing of the vessel lumen. Efforts must be made to exclude other causes of vasculitis, as discussed in the text. Prognosis is generally poor for this form of sarcoidosis.

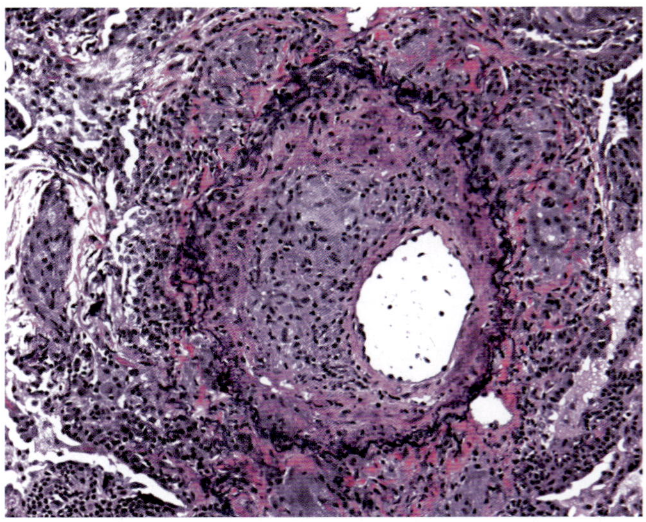

SECTION I

Structure and Function of Bone, Joints, and Connective Tissue

1 Biology of the Normal Joint

STEVEN R. GOLDRING · MARY B. GOLDRING

The normal joint is a specialized, integrated structure consisting of multiple connective tissue elements, including muscles, tendons, ligaments, synovium and capsule, cartilage, and bone, organized in a manner that permits stability and movement of the human skeleton. The joint structures are positioned to distribute normal mechanical stresses optimally and are organized for low-friction load bearing. Deviations from normal structure and physiology of joint tissues have been implicated in the pathogenesis of various forms of arthritis. The differentiation of articular tissues during embryonic development dictates their capacity to respond to insults in later life. Physiologic cellular processes involved in normal joint development, such as differentiation, angiogenesis, macrophage recruitment, and fibroblast proliferation, may reappear in the mature joint and contribute to the pathogenesis of joint disease. Thus, knowledge of the development, structure, and function of normal joint tissues is essential for understanding the underlying mechanisms involved in the pathogenesis of human joint diseases.

Classification of Joints

Human joints provide the structures by which bones join with one another and may be classified according to the histologic features of the union and the range of joint motion. There are three classes of joint design: (1) *synovial* or *diarthrodial* joints (Fig. 1–1), which articulate with free movement, have a synovial membrane lining the joint cavity, and contain synovial fluid; (2) *amphiarthroses*, in which adjacent bones are separated by articular cartilage or a fibrocartilage disk and are bound by firm ligaments permitting limited motion (e.g., pubic symphysis, intervertebral disks of vertebral bodies, the distal tibiofibular articulation, and the sacroiliac joint articulation with pelvic bones); and (3) *synarthroses*, which are found only in the skull (suture lines) where thin, fibrous tissue separates adjoining cranial plates, which interlock to prevent detectable motion prior to the end of normal growth, yet permit growth in childhood and adolescence.[1]

Joints can also be classified according to the connective tissues present. *Symphyses* have a fibrocartilaginous disk separating bone ends that are jointed by firm ligaments (e.g., symphysis pubis and intervertebral joints). In *synchondroses*, the bone ends are covered with articular cartilage, but there is no synovium or significant joint cavity (e.g., sternomanubrial joint). In *syndesmoses*, the bones are joined directly by fibrous ligaments without a cartilaginous interface (the distal tibiofibular articulation is the only joint of this type outside the cranial vault). In *synostoses*, bone bridges are formed between bones, producing ankylosis.

The synovial joints are further classified according to their shapes, which include ball and socket (hip), hinge (interphalangeal), saddle (first carpometacarpal), and plane (patellofemoral) joints. These configurations reflect the varying functions, as the shapes and sizes of the opposing surfaces determine the direction and extent of motion. The various designs permit flexion, extension, abduction, adduction, or rotation. Certain joints can act in one (humero-ulnar), two (wrist), or three (shoulder) axes of motion.

This chapter concentrates on the developmental biology and relationship between structure and function of a "typical," normal human diarthrodial joint—the joint most likely to develop arthritis. Most research has been performed on the knee because of its accessibility, but other joints are described when appropriate.

Developmental Biology of the Diarthrodial Joint

The appendicular skeleton develops in the human embryo from limb buds, which are first visible at around 4 weeks of gestation. Structures resembling adult joints are generated between approximately 4 and 7 weeks of gestation.[2-4] This is followed by many

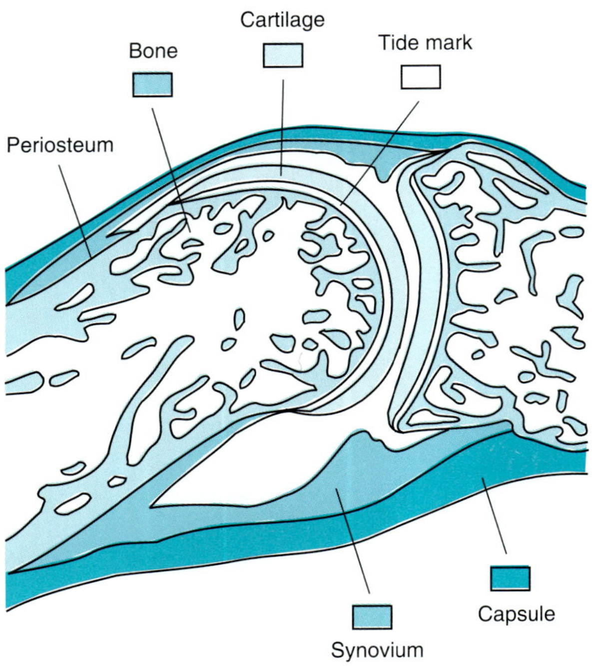

FIGURE 1–1 · A normal human interphalangeal joint, in sagittal section, as an example of a synovial, or diarthrodial, joint. The "tidemark" represents the calcified cartilage that bonds articular cartilage to the subchondral bone plate. (From Sokoloff L, Bland JH: The Musculoskeletal System. Baltimore, Williams & Wilkins, 1975. © 1975, the Williams & Wilkins Co, Baltimore.)

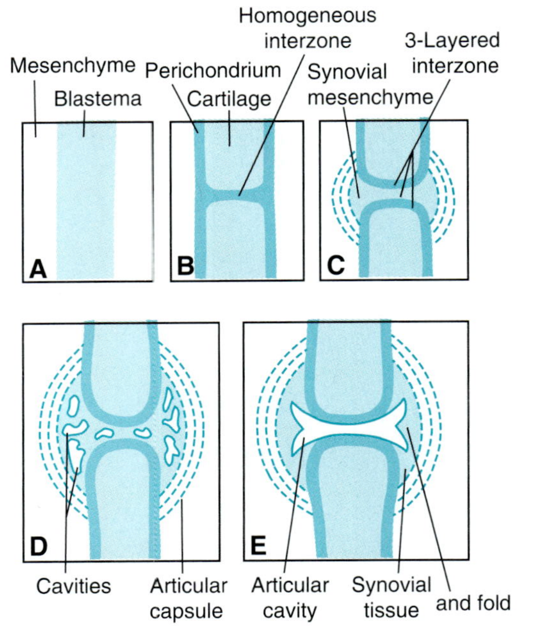

FIGURE 1–2 · The Development of a Synovial Joint. *A*, Condensation. Joints develop from the blastema, not the surrounding mesenchyme. *B*, Chondrification and formation of the interzone. The interzone remains avascular and highly cellular. *C*, Formation of synovial mesenchyme. Synovial mesenchyme forms from the periphery of the interzone and is invaded by blood vessels. *D*, Cavitation. Cavities are formed in the central and peripheral interzone and merge to form the joint cavity. *E*, The mature joint. (From O'Rahilly R, Gardner E: The embryology of movable joints. *In* Sokoloff L (ed): The Joints and Synovial Fluid, Vol 1. New York, Academic Press, 1978.)

other crucial phases of musculoskeletal development, including vascularization of epiphyseal cartilage (8 to 12 weeks), appearance of villous folds in synovium (10 to 12 weeks), evolution of bursae (3 to 4 months), and appearance of periarticular fat pads (4 to 5 months). The upper limbs develop approximately 24 hours earlier than the analogous portions of the lower limbs. Proximal structures, such as the glenohumeral joint, develop before more distal ones, such as the wrist and hand. As a consequence, insults to embryonic development during the period of limb formation affect a more distal portion of the upper limb than of the lower limb. Long bones form as a result of replacement of the cartilage template by endochondral ossification. The stages of limb development are well described by O'Rahilly and Gardner[2,5] and are shown in Fig. 1–2.

CARTILAGE CONDENSATION, INTERZONE FORMATION, AND JOINT CAVITATION

The morphology of the developing synovial joint and the process of joint cavitation have been described in many classic studies carried out on the limbs of mammalian and avian embryos. The developmental sequence of the events occurring during synovial joint formation, and some of the regulatory factors and extracellular matrix components involved, are summarized in Figs. 1–3 and 1–4. The development of the joint is divided into two morphologic events: formation of the cartilaginous anlagen that model skeletal elements and subsequent joint formation. The joint develops from the primitive, avascular, densely packed cellular mesenchyme, termed the *skeletal blastema.* Common precursor mesenchymal cells divide into both chondrogenic and myogenic lineages that determine the differentiation of cartilage, centrally, and muscle, peripherally. The cartilaginous nodules appear in the middle of the blastema, and, simultaneously, cells at the periphery become flattened and elongated to form the perichondrium. The surrounding tissues, particularly epithelium, influence the differentiation of mesenchymal progenitor cells to chondrocytes such that cartilage disks in the vertebral column arise from portions of the somites surrounding the notochord, and nasal and auricular cartilage and the embryonic epiphysis form from the perichondrium. In some cases, the cartilage is replaced by bone (endochondral ossification) or becomes calcified (growth-plate formation). Common arrays of growth factors, signaling molecules, and transcription factors mediate chondrocyte differentiation, although spatial and temporal relationships may vary from one site to the other.

Condensation and Limb-Bud Formation

Formation of the cartilage anlage occurs in four stages: (1) cell migration, (2) aggregation regulated by mesenchymal–epithelial cell interactions, (3) condensation, and (4) overt chondrocyte differentiation, or chondrification.[2,5,6] The aggregation of chondroprogenitor mesenchymal cells into precartilage condensations was first

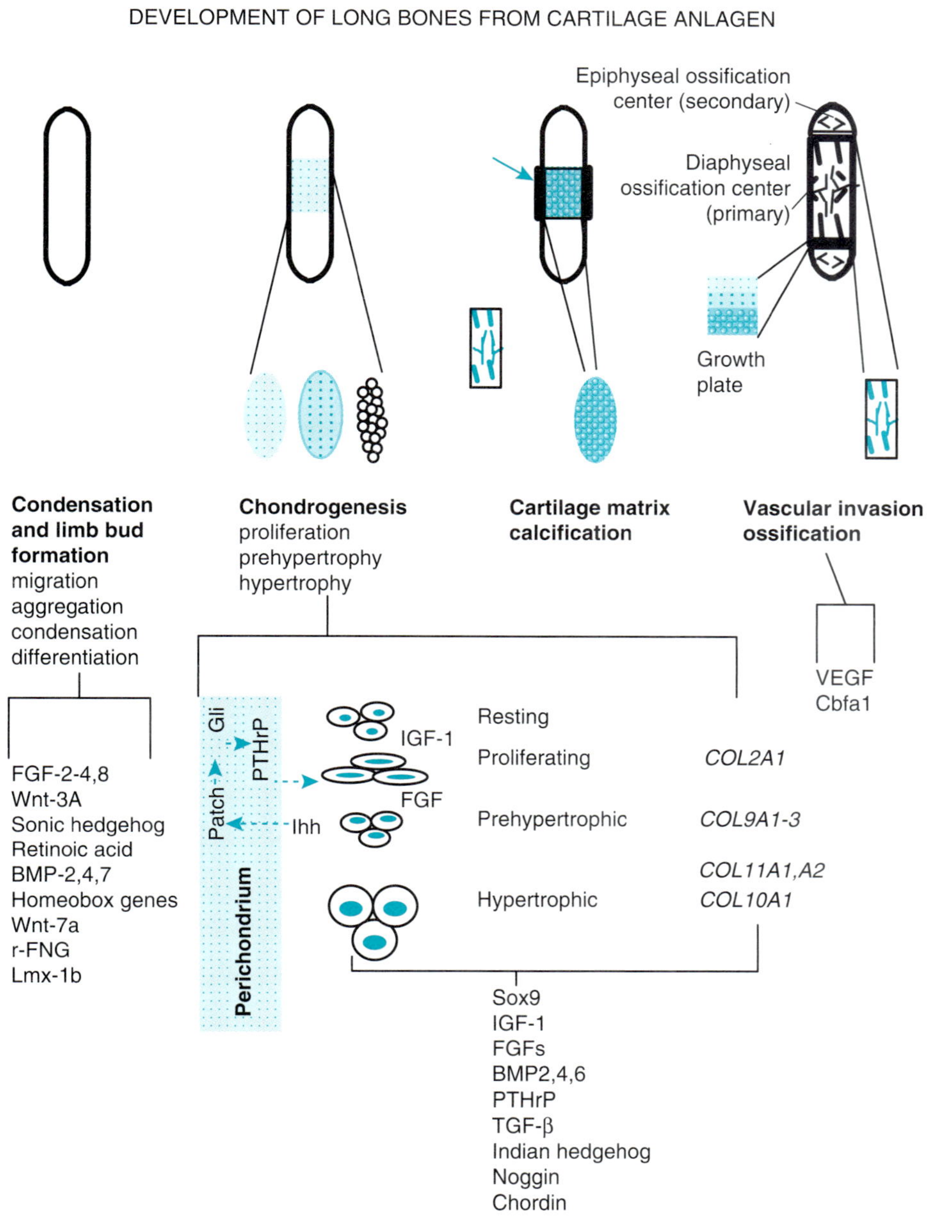

FIGURE 1–3 · The stages of diarthrodial joint formation, and the temporal pattern of expression of the genes involved in regulation at different stages.

described by Fell[7] and represents one of the earliest events in chondrogenesis. This process depends on signals initiated by cell–cell and cell–matrix interactions and is associated with increased cell adhesion, the formation of gap junctions, and changes in the cytoskeletal architecture. Prior to condensation, the prechondrocytic mesenchymal cells produce extracellular matrix that is rich in hyaluronan and collagen type I, as well as type IIA collagen, which contains the exon-2–encoded aminopropeptide found in noncartilage collagens. The initiation of condensation is associated with increased hyaluronidase activity and the appearance of cell adhesion molecules, neural cadherin (N-cadherin), and the neural cell adhesion molecule (N-CAM). Transforming growth factor (TGF-β), which is among the earliest signals of chondrogenic condensation, stimulates the synthesis of fibronectin, which in turn regulates N-CAM. Syndecan, by binding fibronectin, then down-regulates N-CAM and sets condensation boundaries. The extracellular matrix molecules, which also include tenascins and thrombospondins, interact with the cell adhesion molecules to activate intracellular signaling pathways, involving focal adhesion kinase and paxillin, to initiate the transition from chondroprogenitor cells to a fully committed chondrocyte.[8] N-Cadherin and N-CAM disappear in differentiating chondrocytes and are detectable later only in perichondrial cells.

Zwilling[9] proposed that positional information for organization of the limb bud was imparted by diffusible agents generated at the tip of the limb bud and along its posterior margin, promoting the development of a cartilaginous anlage along proximal-distal and anterior-posterior axes, respectively. Limb buds develop from the lateral plate mesoderm.[10] The patterning of

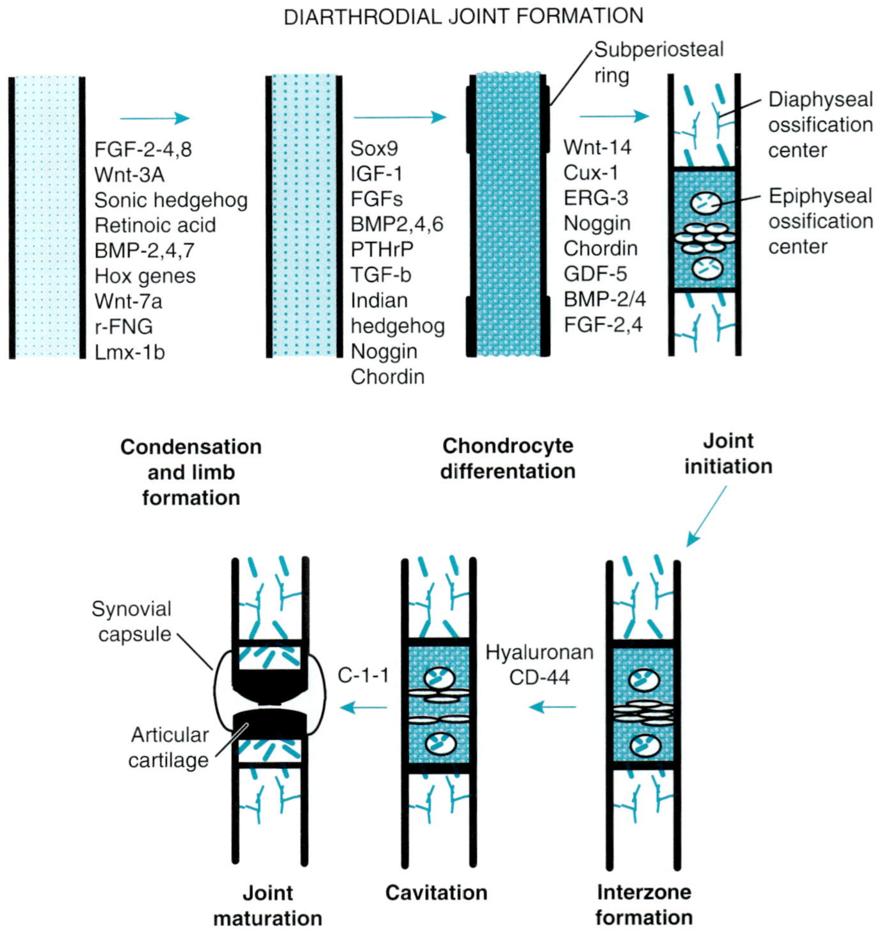

FIGURE 1–4 · Development of long bones from cartilage anlagen.

limb mesenchyme is caused by interactions between the mesenchyme and the overlying epithelium.[11] The embryonic limb possesses two signaling centers, the apical ectodermal ridge (AER) and the zone of polarizing activity (ZPA), which produce signals responsible for directing the proximal-distal outgrowth and anterior-posterior patterning, respectively.[8] Signals from the apical ectoderm of the limb bud probably initiate formation of the anlage by activating expression of the homeobox (Hox) transcription factors in the undifferentiated mesenchyme.[12]

Many of the genes that pattern the distribution and proliferation of mesenchymal condensations at sites of future skeletal elements and control subsequent limb development have been elucidated, but the complexity of their interactions remains to be fully understood.[13] Fig. 1–3 shows a scheme of the different stages of joint development and lists the factors associated with each stage. The Hox genes play an important role in the early events of limb patterning. Fibroblast growth factors (FGF)-2, -4, and -8 (induced by Wnt-3A[14]), from the specialized epithelial cells in the AER that are covering the limb-bud tip, control proximal-distal (shoulder/finger) outgrowth.[15] Sonic hedgehog produced by a small group of cells in the posterior zone of the ZPA (in response to retinoic acid in the mesoderm[16] and FGF-4 in the AER[17]) play a key role in both directing anterior-posterior (little finger/thumb) patterning[16,18] and stimulating expression of bone morphogenetic proteins (BMPs)-2, -4, and -7, and Hox genes.[13,19,20] Dorsal-ventral (knuckles/palm) patterning depends on the secretion of Wnt-7A[21] and expression of the following transcription factors: radical fringe (r-Fng) by the dorsal ectoderm, and homeobox-containing engrailed (En-1) and the LIM-homeodomain protein Lmx1b (which is induced by Wnt-7A) by the ventral endoderm.[22,23] Hoxd11 and -13, and other transcription factors, modulate proliferation of cells within the condensations. BMP-2, -4, and -7 regulate the subsequent growth of the condensations by activating Pax-2, Hoxa2, and Hoxd11 transcription factors.[6] Growth of the condensation ceases when Noggin inhibits BMP signaling and permits overt differentiation to chondrocytes, which are often designated as "chondroblasts." The cartilage thus formed then serves as a template for formation of cartilage elements in the vertebrae, sternum, rib, etc. and for limb elongation or endochondral bone formation. The cellular interactions and signals involved in condensation and the initiation of skeletal development have been reviewed recently.[6,8,24]

Molecular Signals in Cartilage Morphogenesis and the Development of Long Bones: Recent Understanding

The cartilage anlagen grow by cell division and deposition of the extracellular matrix and by apposition of chondroblasts proliferating from the inner chondrogenic layer of the perichondrium. The nuclear transcription factor, Sox9, is one of earliest markers expressed in cells undergoing condensation and is required for the expression of type II collagen and certain other cartilage-specific matrix proteins prior to matrix deposition in the cartilage anlage.[25-27] In addition to type II collagen, the cells in the initial condensations express another member of the hedgehog family, Indian hedgehog (Ihh),[20] and the adjacent, surrounding perichondrial cells express the hedgehog receptor, patched (Ptc), and the Ihh-inducible transcription factor, Gli.[28-31] Homozygous null Ihh mice show severe dwarfism in axial and appendicular skeletal elements and no endochondral bone formation.[32] The runt-domain transcription factor, Core binding factor a1 (Cbfa1; also known as Osf2 and Runx2), is also expressed in all condensations, including those that are destined to form bone.[33-35]

Although these cellular events associated with joint formation have been recognized for many years, only recently have the genes regulating these processes been elucidated. These genes include growth differentiation factor (GDF)-5, Wnt-14, BMP-2, -4, -6, and -7, and the GDF-BMP antagonists, Noggin and Chordin.[36-39] In addition, joint formation is accompanied by the expression of several FGF family members, including FGF-2 and -4.[40] The balance of signaling between BMP and FGF determines the rate of proliferation, thereby adjusting the pace of the differentiation.[41] Two transcription factors, Cux-1, a Hox-containing gene, and C-1-1, an alternatively spliced form of the Ets factor Erg-3,[42,43] are also upregulated and contribute to joint formation, in particular by affecting chondrogenesis, although their specific roles await further evaluation. Hartmann and Tabin[44] have proposed two major roles for Wnt-14. First, it acts at the onset of joint formation as a nega-tive regulator of chondrogenesis. Second, it facilitates interzone formation and cavitation by inducing the expression of GDF-5 (also termed *cartilage-derived morphogenetic protein-1*, or CDMP-1),[45] Wnt-4, Chordin, and the hyaluronan receptor, CD44[44]). Paradoxically, application of GDF-5 to developing joints in mouse-embryo limbs in organ culture causes joint fusion,[46] suggesting that tempero-spatial interactions among distinct cell populations are important for the correct response.

Endochondral Ossification

The development of long bones from the cartilage anlagen occurs by a process termed *endochondral ossification*, which involves chondrocyte hypertrophy, cartilage matrix calcification, vascular invasion, and ossification (Fig. 1–4). This process is initiated when the cells in the central region of the anlage begin hypertrophy, increasing cellular fluid volume by almost 20 times. These cells express the hypertrophic chondrocyte marker, type X collagen. Ihh is expressed in cells as they exit the proliferative phase and enter the hypertrophic phase,[20,47] and Cbfa1 is expressed in the adjacent perichondrium and in the central cartilage anlage, overlapping with Ihh and type X collagen.[47] Ihh signaling is transduced through Ptc and Gli, thereby inducing expression of PTHrP in the perichondrium.[30] PTHrP signaling then stimulates cell proliferation via its receptor expressed in the proliferating chondrocytes.[48] PTHrP also represses chondrocyte maturation by suppressing expression of Ihh, BMP-6, and type X collagen by hypertrophic chondrocytes.[31] Thus, Ihh and PTHrP, by transiently inducing proliferation markers and repressing differentiation markers, function in a tempero-spatial manner to determine the number of cells that remain in the chondrogenic lineage, versus those that enter the endochondral ossification pathway.[24,47]

Angiogenesis in the hypertrophic zone is required for the replacement of cartilage by bone. The angiogenic factor, vascular endothelial growth factor (VEGF), deposited previously in the matrix, promotes vascular invasion by specifically activating localized receptors, including Flk, expressed in endothelial cells in the perichondrium or surrounding soft tissues; neuropilin (Npn) 1, expressed in late hypertrophic chondrocytes; or Npn 2, expressed exclusively in the perichondrium.[49] VEGF is released from the ECM by metalloproteinases (MMPs), such as MMP-9, which is expressed by endothelial cells that migrate into the central region of the hypertrophic cartilage coincident with Flk-positive cells. The membrane (MT)1-MMP (MMP-14) has a broader range of expression than MMP-9; whereas MMP-13, whose expression is regulated by Cbfa1,[50] is found exclusively in late hypertrophic chondrocytes.[51] These events of cartilage matrix remodeling and vascular invasion are prerequisite to migration of osteoclasts and osteoblasts, which begin removing mineralized cartilage matrix and replacing it with bone.

Interzone Formation and Joint Cavitation

In the human embryo, cartilage condensations, or chondrifications, can be detected as early as stage 17, when the embryo is small, approximately 11.7 mm long (Fig. 1–5*A*). In the region of the future joint, following formation of the homogeneous chondrogenic interzone at 6 weeks (stages 18 and 19), a three-layered interzone is formed at approximately 7 weeks (stage 21), which consists of two chondrogenic, perichondrium-like layers that cover the opposing surfaces of the cartilage anlagen and are separated by a narrow band of densely packed cellular blastema that remains and forms the interzone (Fig. 1–5*B*). Cavitation begins in the central interzone at about 8 weeks (stage 23) (Fig. 1–5*C*).

The distribution of collagen types and keratan sulfate in developing avian and rodent joints has been characterized by immunohistochemistry.[52-57] Collagen types I and III characterize the matrix produced by mesenchymal cells, which switch to the production of types II, IX, and XI collagens that typify the cartilaginous matrix at the time of condensation.[58] The mRNAs encoding the small proteoglycans, biglycan and decorin, may be expressed at this time, but the proteins do not appear until after cavitation in the regions destined to become articular cartilage.[59] The interzone regions are marked

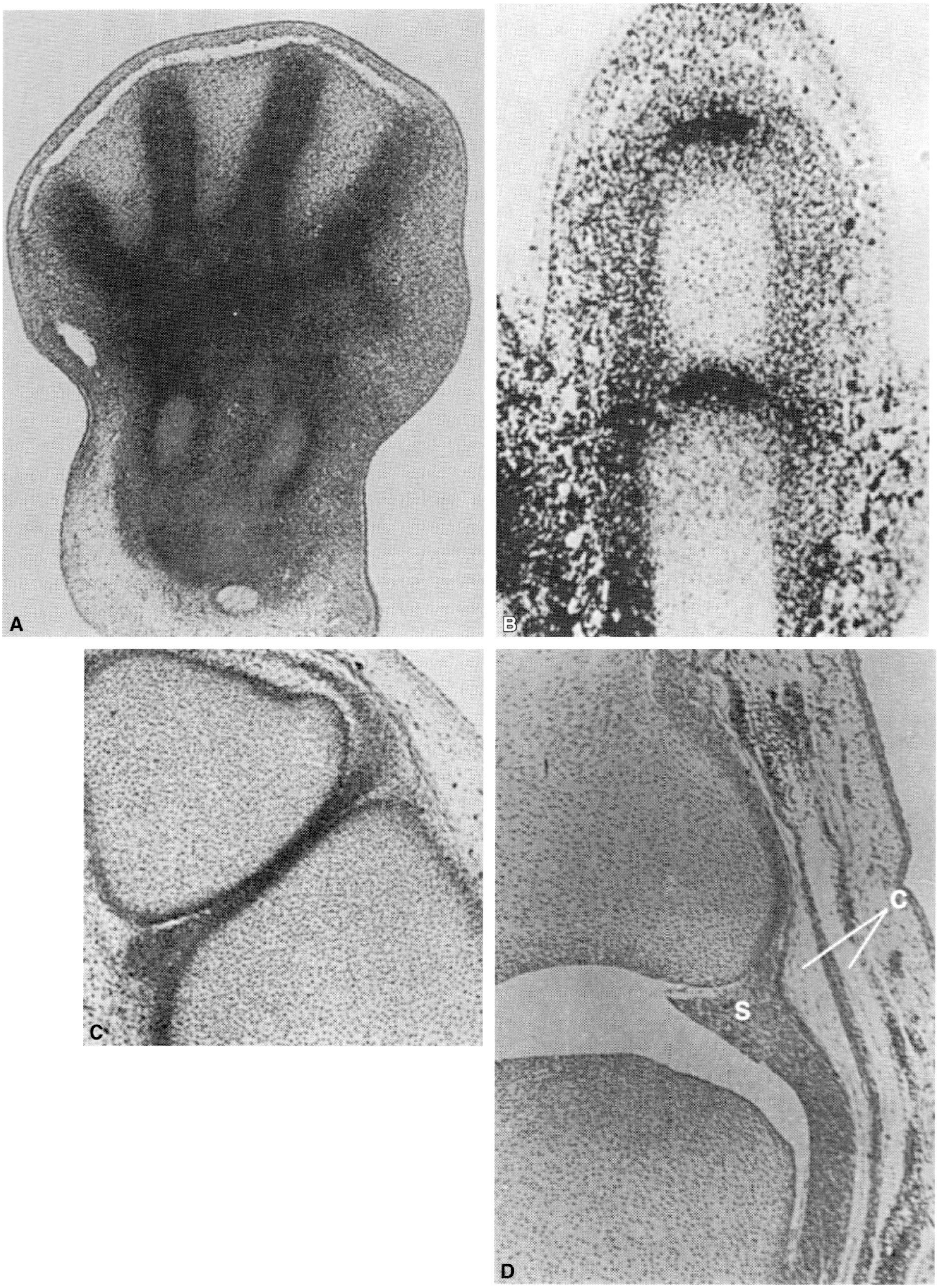
A
B
C
D
S
C

FIGURE 1–5 · *A*, Coronal section of the hand at 11.7 mm (stage 17). The blastema, with its increased cellularity, serves to outline the form of the hand. Faint lightening in the regions of the third and fourth metacarpals indicates very early cartilage condensation. Formation of cartilage anlagen in the radius and ulna is more advanced. (From O'Rahilly R: The development of joints. Ir J Med Sci 6:456, 1957) *B*, Histochemical preparation demonstrating intense localization of acid phosphatase (representing lysosomal activity) in the zone of presumptive joint formation in a mouse embryo. This enzymatic removal of matrix allows cavitation to occur, separating the limb elements.
(From [Milaire J: Enzymatic processes in joint cavitation. *In* Frantz CH (ed): Normal and Abnormal Embryological Development. Washington, DC, National Research Council, 1947, p 61].)
C, The embryonic joint developing between the femur and tibia at stage 23. The lateral meniscus is outlined by cavitation on the femoral side. Cavitation will subsequently spread in a medial direction and develop spontaneously at other foci. (From Gardner E, O'Rahilly R: The early development of the knee joint in staged human embryos. J Anat 102:289, 1968. Used by permission of Cambridge University Press.) *D*, Adjacent phalanges in a human embryonic hand are separated by a clearly demarcated joint space containing early synovial tissue. The dense collagenous joint capsule (C) lying exterior to the synovium (S) is clearly demonstrated. (From Sledge CB: Developmental anatomy of joints. *In* Resnick D, Niwayana G (eds): Diagnosis of Bone and Joint Disorders, 2nd ed. Philadelphia, WB Saunders, 1988, p 618.)

by the expression of type IIA collagen by chondrocyte progenitors in the perichondrial layers, type IIB and XI collagens by overt chondrocytes in the cartilage anlagen, and type I collagen in the interzone as well as in the developing capsule and perichondrium (Fig. 1–6).[60]

The interzone region contains cells that are programmed to undergo joint cavitation. Fluid and macromolecules accumulate in this space and create a nascent synovial cavity. Blood vessels appear in the surrounding capsulo-synovial blastemal mesenchyme before separation of the adjacent articulating surfaces.[61,62] Although it was first assumed that these interzone cells should undergo necrosis or programmed cell death (apoptosis),[61,63] some investigators have found no evidence of DNA fragmentation preceding cavitation.[49,60,64] There is also no evidence that metalloproteinases are involved in loss of tissue strength in the region undergoing cavitation.[65] Instead, the actual joint cavity appears to be formed by mechanospatial changes induced by the synthesis of hyaluronan via uridine diphosphoglucose dehydrogenase (UDPGD) and hyaluronan synthase. Interaction of hyaluronan with its cell surface receptor, CD44, modulates cell migration, but it is thought that the accumulation of hyaluronan and the associated mechanical influences play the major role in forcing the cells apart and inducing rupture of the intervening extracellular matrix by tensile forces.[55,66-69] This mechanism accounts for the observation that joint cavitation is incomplete in the absence of movement.[70] In chick embryos, it has been shown that movement of the limb is essential for normal cavitation,[71] but equivalent data from human embryonic joints are difficult to obtain.[72] In all large joints in the human, complete joint cavities are apparent at the beginning of the fetal period.

DEVELOPMENT OF THE JOINT CAPSULE AND SYNOVIUM

The interzone and the contiguous perichondrial envelope, of which the interzone is a part, contain the mesenchymal cell precursors that give rise to other joint components, including the joint capsule, synovial lining, menisci, intracapsular ligaments, and tendons.[2,4,73-75] The external mesenchymal tissue condenses as a fibrous capsule. The peripheral mesenchyme becomes vascularized and is incorporated as the synovial mesenchyme, which differentiates into a pseudomembrane at about the same time as cavitation begins in the central interzone (stage 23, approximately 8 weeks) (Fig. 1–5*D*). The menisci arise from the eccentric portions of the articular interzone (Fig. 1–5*C*). In common usage, the term *synovium* refers to both the true synovial lining and the subjacent vascular and areolar tissue, up to—but excluding—the capsule. Synovial lining cells can be distinguished as soon as the multiple cavities within the interzone begin to coalesce. At first, these are exclusively fibroblast-like (type B) cells.

As the joint cavity increases in size, synovial-lining cell layers expand by proliferation of fibroblast-like cells and recruitment of macrophage-like (type A) cells from the circulation.[76] The synovial lining cells express the hyaluronan receptor, CD44, and the elevated UDPGD activity persists after cavitation. This increased activity likely contributes to the high concentration of hyaluronan in joint fluids.[68,77,78] Further synovial expansion results in the appearance of synovial villi at the end of the second month, early in the fetal period, which greatly increases the surface area available for exchange between the joint cavity and the vascular space.

The role of innervation in the developing joint is not well understood. A dense capillary network develops in the subsynovial tissue, with numerous capillary loops that penetrate into the true synovial lining layer. The human synovial microvasculature is already innervated by 8 weeks (stage 23) of gestation, around the time of joint cavitation,[73] as is demonstrated by immunoreactivity for the neuronal "housekeeping" enzyme subiquitin C-terminal hydrolase (PGP 9.5).[79,80] However, evidence of neurotransmitter function is not found until much later, with the appearance of the sensory neuropeptide, substance P, at 11 weeks. The putative sympathetic neurotransmitter, neuropeptide Y, appears at 13 weeks of gestation, along with the catecholamine-synthesizing enzyme tyrosine hydroxylase.[79] In developing avian limbs,

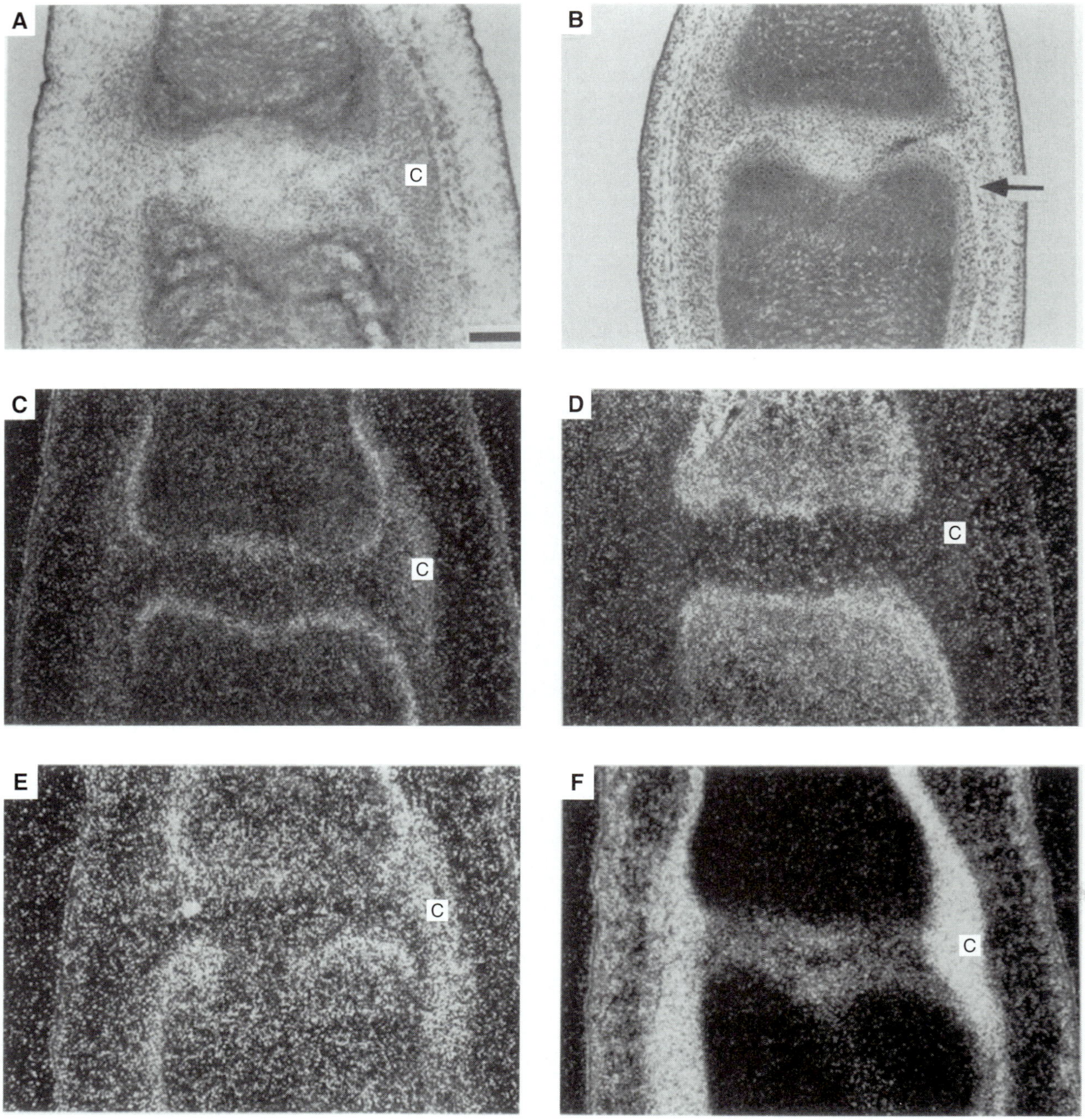

FIGURE 1–6 • In situ hybridization of 13-day-old (stage 39) chicken embryo middle digit, proximal interphalangeal joint, mid-frontal sections. *A*, Bright-field image showing developing joint and capsule (C). *B*, Equivalent paraffin section of opposite limb of same animal, clearly showing onset of cavitation laterally (arrow). *C*, Expression of type II A collagen mRNA in articular surface cells, perichondrium, and capsule. *D*, Type IIB collagen mRNA is expressed only in chondrocytes of the anlagen. *E*, Type XI collagen mRNA is expressed in the surface cells, perichondrium, and capsule, with lower levels in chondrocytes. *F*, Type I collagen mRNA is present in cells of the interzone and capsule. *C* through *F* are dark field. Calibration bar = 1 μm.(From Nalin, AM, Greenlee TK, Jr. Sandell LJ: Collagen gene expression during development of avian synovial joints: transient expression of types II and XI collagen genes in the joint capsule. Develop Dyn 203:352-362, 1995]. With permission.)

tenascin is expressed in the satellite cells that accompany in-growing nerves between stages 24 and 28, but it disappears thereafter.[81] The recent finding that the *slit*-2 gene, which functions for the guidance of neuronal axons and neurons, is expressed in the mesenchyme adjacent to the AER (stages 20 to 22) and in peripheral mesenchyme of the limb bud (stages 23 to 28) suggests that innervation is an integral part of synovial joint development.[82]

DEVELOPMENT OF NONARTICULAR JOINTS

In contrast to articular joints, the temporomandibular joint develops slowly, with cavitation at a crown-rump length of 57 to 75 mm (i.e., well into the fetal stage).[83-85] This may be because this joint develops in the absence of a continuous blastema and involves the insertion between bone ends of a fibrocartilaginous disk that arises from muscular and mesenchymal derivatives of the first pharyngeal arch.

The development of other types of joints, such as synarthroses, is similar to that of diarthrodial joints, except that cavitation does not occur, and synovial mesenchyme is not formed. In these respects, synarthroses and amphiarthroses resemble the "fused" peripheral joints induced by paralyzing chicken embryos,[86] and they may develop as they do because there is relatively little motion during their formation.

Human vertebrae and intervertebral disks develop as units, each derived from a homogeneous blastema arising from a somite. Each embryonic intervertebral disk serves as a rostral and caudal chondrogenic zone for the two adjacent evolving vertebral bodies. The periphery of the embryonic "disk" is replaced by the annulus fibrosus.[87-89] The intervertebral disk bears many similarities to the joint; the annulus is the joint capsule, the nucleus pulposus is the joint cavity, and the vertebral end plates are the cartilage-covered bone ends composing the articulation. The proteoglycans and collagens expressed during development of the intervertebral disc have been mapped[90-92] and reflect the complex structure-function relationships that allow flexibility and resistance to compression in the spine.

DEVELOPMENT OF ARTICULAR CARTILAGE

In the vertebrate skeleton, cartilage is the product of cells from three distinct embryonic lineages. Craniofacial cartilage is formed from cranial neural crest cells,[93,94] the cartilage of the axial skeleton (intervertebral disks, ribs, and sternum) forms from paraxial mesoderm (somites),[95] and the articular cartilage of the limbs is derived from the lateral plate mesoderm.[10] In the developing limb bud, mesenchymal condensations, followed by chondrocyte differentiation and maturation, occur in digital zones, whereas undifferentiated mesenchymal cells in the interdigital web zones undergo apoptotic elimination.[96] Embryonic cartilage is destined for one of several fates: It can remain as permanent cartilage, as on the articular surfaces of bones, or it can provide a template for the formation of bones by endochondral ossification. During development, chondrocyte maturation expands from the central site of the original condensation, which forms the cartilage anlage resembling the shape of the future bone, toward the ends of the forming bones. During joint cavitation, the peripheral interzone is absorbed into each adjacent cartilaginous zone, evolving into the articular surface. The articular surface is destined to become a specialized cartilaginous structure that does not normally undergo vascularization and ossification.

Recent evidence indicates that postnatal maturation of the articular cartilage involves an appositional growth mechanism originating from progenitor cells at the articular surface, rather than by an interstitial mechanism.[97] The chondrocytes of mature articular cartilage are terminally differentiated cells that continue to express cartilage-specific matrix molecules, such as type II collagen and aggrecan.[54,56,60] (see following section). Through the processes described previously, the articular joint spaces are developed and lined on all surfaces either by cartilage or by synovial lining cells. These two different tissues merge at the enthesis, the region at the periphery of the joint where the cartilage melds into bone and where ligaments and the capsule are attached. In the postnatal growth plate, the differentiation of the perichondrium is also linked to the differentiation of the chondrocytes in the epiphysis into different zones of the growth plate, which contributes to longitudinal bone growth[47,49] (Fig. 1–6).

Organization and Physiology of the Mature Joint

The unique structural properties and biochemic components of diarthrodial joints make them extraordinarily durable load-bearing devices.[98] The mature diarthrodial joint is a complex structure, influenced by its environment and mechanical demands (see Chapter 6). There are structural differences between joints determined by their different functions. For example, the shoulder joint, which demands an enormous range of motion, is stabilized primarily by muscles, whereas the hip, requiring both motion and antigravity stability, has an intrinsically stable ball-and-socket configuration. The components of the "typical" synovial joint are the synovium, muscles, tendons, ligaments, bursae, menisci, articular cartilage, and subchondral bone. The anatomy and physiology of muscles are described in detail in Chapter 5.

SYNOVIUM

The synovium, the tissue between the fibrous joint capsule and fluid-filled synovial cavity, is a thin membrane that attaches to skeletal tissues at the bone-cartilage interface and does not encroach upon the surface of the articular cartilage. It is divided into functional compartments: the lining region (synovial intima), the subintimal stroma, and the vasculature (Fig. 1–7). The synovial intima, also termed *synovial lining*, is the superficial layer of the normal synovium that is in contact with the intra-articular cavity.[78,99] The synovial lining is loosely attached to the subintima, which contains blood vessels, lymphatics, and nerves. Capillaries and arterioles are generally located directly underneath the synovial intima, whereas venules are located closer to the joint capsule.

A transition from loose to dense connective tissue occurs from the joint cavity to the capsule. Most cells in the normal subintimal stroma are fibroblasts and macrophages, although adipocytes and occasional mast cells are present.[100] These compartments are not circumscribed by basement membranes but nonetheless have distinct functions; they are separated from each other by chemical barriers, such as membrane peptidases, which limit the diffusion of regulatory factors between compartments.[101] Furthermore, synovial compartments are unevenly distributed within a single joint. Vascularity, for example, is high at the enthesis where synovium, ligament, and cartilage coalesce. Far from being a homogeneous tissue in continuity with the

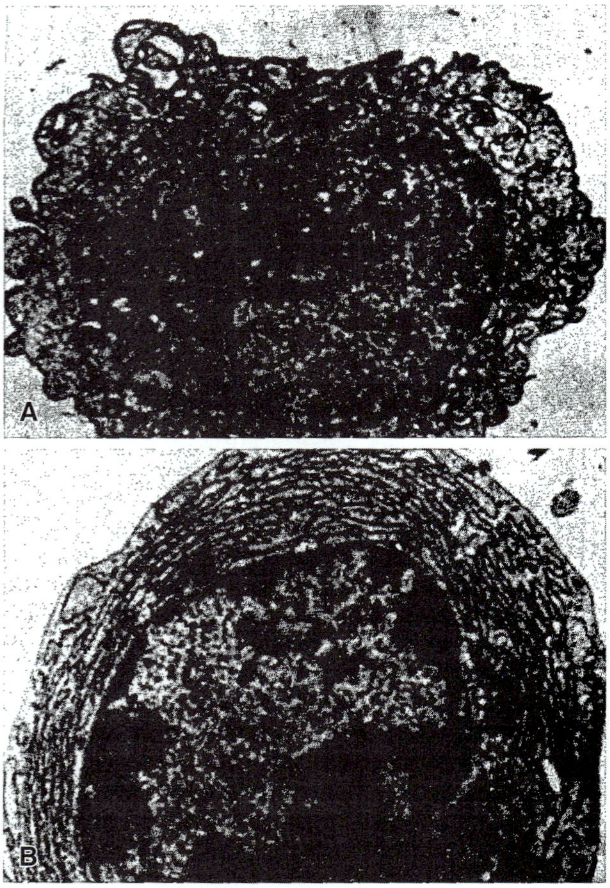

FIGURE 1–7 · *A*, Human synovial intimal macrophage (type A synoviocyte) with many undulations, a prominent Golgi complex, many microvesicles, various and heterogeneous inclusions (residual bodies), and lysosomes. The nucleus contains dense chromatin. Microfilaments are abundant, lying in the long axis of the cell. This cell type has phagocytic capabilities and antigenically resembles mature macrophages. (×11,200) *B*, Human synovial intimal fibroblasts (type B synoviocyte) with a very well-developed rough endoplasmic reticulum and few cell processes and vacuoles. Nuclear chromatin is less dense, and nucleoli are more developed. Cytoplasmic vacuoles and vesicles are rare. These features are consistent with a synthetic function. Type B synovial cells contain the enzyme prolyl hydroxylase, important in collagen synthesis, and so they resemble mature fibroblasts. (×17,500)
(*A* and *B* courtesy of Donald Gates.)

synovial cavity, synovium is highly heterogeneous, and synovial fluid may be poorly representative of the tissue-fluid composition of any synovial tissue compartment.

Synovial Lining

The synovial lining, a specialized condensation of mesenchymal cells and extracellular matrix, is localized between the synovial cavity and stroma. In normal synovium, the lining layer is two to three cells deep, although intra-articular fat pads are usually covered by only a single layer of synovial cells, and ligaments and tendons are covered by synovial cells that are widely separated. At some sites, lining cells are absent, and the extracellular connective tissue constitutes the lining layer.[102] Such "bare areas" become increasingly frequent with advancing age.[103] Although the synovial lining is often referred to as the synovial membrane, the term *membrane* is more correctly reserved for epithelia that have basement membranes, tight intercellular junctions, and desmosomes. Instead, synovial lining cells lie loosely in a bed of hyaluronate interspersed with collagen fibrils. This is the macromolecular sieve that imparts the semipermeable nature of the synovium. The absence of any true epithelial tissue is a major determinant of joint physiology. Please refer to Chapter 11 for more details.

Electron-microscopic studies have characterized lining cells as macrophage-derived type A synoviocytes and fibroblast-derived type B synoviocytes.[104,105] High UDPGD activity is used as a cytochemical marker to distinguish type B synovial cells, whereas nonspecific esterase (NSE) typifies type A cells (Fig. 1–7). Transitional forms, sometimes referred to as type C cells, have been described but may represent type A or B cells at different stages of activation. For example, fibroblast-like synovial cells under certain conditions may express low levels of CD68, a lysosome marker associated with macrophages.[106] Normal synovium is lined predominantly by fibroblast-like cells, whereas macrophage-like cells compose only 10 to 20 percent of lining cells (Fig. 1–8A). Like other fibroblasts, lining cells express the collagen synthesis enzyme prolyl hydroxylase,[107] synthesize extracellular matrix, and have the potential to proliferate, although proliferation markers are rarely seen in normal synovium.[108]

Despite not being a true epithelium, and despite being a boundary to a cavity with no communication to the exterior, synovial lining cells bear abundant membrane peptidases on their surface, capable of degrading a wide range of regulatory peptides, such as substance P and angiotensin II.[101] These enzymes may be important in limiting the diffusion of these potent peptide mediators away from the immediate vicinity of their site of release and action. Synovial lining cells also synthesize non–membrane-bound proteinases and proteinase inhibitors[109] and may regulate matrix turnover, not only in the synovium but also, through the synovial fluid, in articular cartilage.

Type A, macrophage-like synovial cells contain vacuoles, a prominent Golgi apparatus, and filopodia, but they have little rough endoplasmic reticulum. These cells express numerous cell surface markers of the monocyte-macrophage lineage, including CD11b, CD68, CD14, CD163, and the IgG Fc receptor, FcγRIIIa.[78,110,111] Synovial intimal macrophages are phagocytic and may provide a mechanism by which particulate matter can be cleared from the normal joint cavity. Like other tissue macrophages, these cells have little capacity to proliferate and are likely localized to the joint during development. Interestingly, the *op/op* osteopetrotic mouse that is deficient in macrophages due to an absence of macrophage-colony stimulating factor also lacks synovial macrophages.[112] This provides further evidence that type A synovial cells are of a common lineage with other tissue macrophages. Although they rep-

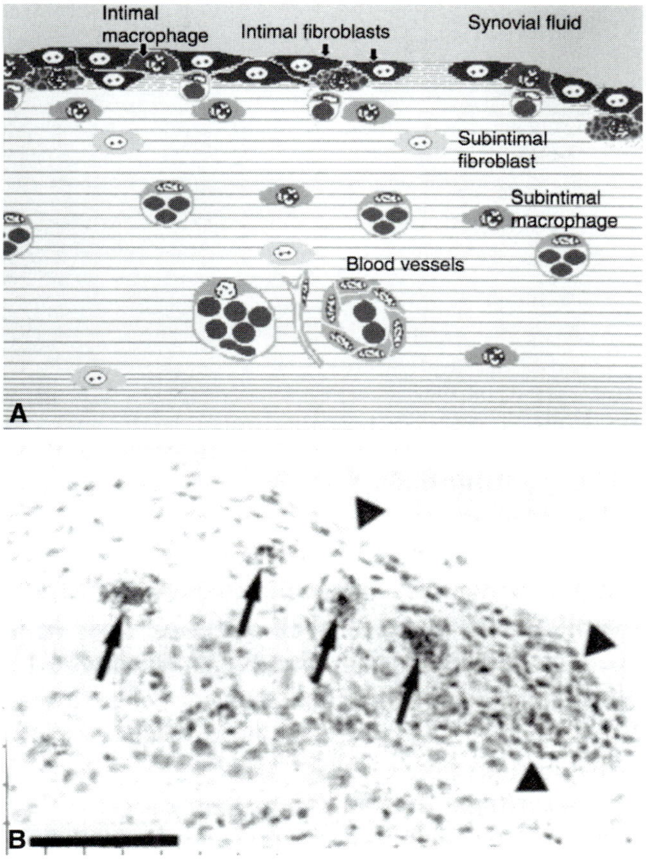

FIGURE 1–8 · *A*, Schematic representation of normal human synovium. The intima contains specialized fibroblasts expressing VCAM-1 and UDPG and specialized macrophages expressing FcγRIIIa. The deeper subintima contains relatively unspecialized counterparts. *B*, Microvascular endothelium in human synovium contains receptors for the vasodilator/growth factor substance P. Silver grains represents specific binding of $[^{125}I]$Bolton Hunter-labeled substance P to synovial microvessels *(arrows)*. Arrowheads indicate the synovial surface. Emulsion-dipped in vitro receptor autoradiography preparations with H&E counterstain. Calibration bar = 1 μm. (A, From Edwards JCW: Fibroblast biology. Development and differentiation of synovial fibroblasts in arthritis. Arthritis Res 2:344-347, 2000. With permission B, From Kelley's Textbook of Rheumatology, 6th edition.)

resent only a small percentage of the cells in the normal synovium, the macrophages are recruited from the circulation during synovial inflammation, in part from subchondral bone marrow through vascular channels near the enthesis.

The type B, fibroblast-like synovial cell contains fewer vacuoles and filopodia than type A cells and has abundant protein-synthetic organelles. Unlike stromal fibroblasts, synovial intimal fibroblasts express UDPGD and synthesize hyaluronan, an important constituent of synovial fluid.[106,113,114] Furthermore, they express CD44, the principal receptor for hyaluronan, and the vascular cell adhesion molecule-1 (VCAM-1).[115-117] The extent to which these specific features of type B synoviocytes contribute to the predisposition of synovium to chronic inflammation awaits further investigation. Hyaluronan, in particular, has many biologic functions, including roles in joint cavitation in the embryo (see previous discussion), regulation of cell–cell and cell–matrix interactions, and lubrication (see following discussion) in the mature joint. Hyaluronan is structurally modified in rheumatoid synovial fluids and may be directly involved in the pathogenesis of synovitis through its angiogenic potential.[118]

Type B cells are responsible for the synthesis of extracellular-matrix proteins of the synovial intimal layer, including collagens, sulfated proteoglycans, fibronectin, and fibrillin-1.[99,119-122] They also synthesize lubricin, which, together with hyaluronan, is necessary for the low-friction interaction of cartilage surfaces in the diarthrodial joint.[123] These cells also synthesize plasminogen activator, which may be involved in both the degradation of fibrinogen and the activation of MMPs that have been implicated in joint destruction.[109]

Although these two types of synoviocytes can be broadly defined morphologically and appear to have distinct ontogenies, some overlap may exist among their functions. It would be overly simplistic to regard type A and type B synoviocytes as purely phagocytic and synthetic, respectively. Type B cells may display phagocytic activity,[124] whereas type A cells synthesize a wide variety of regulatory factors and can contribute matrix components.[125] Furthermore, direct interaction may occur between type A and type B cells in the synovial lining, as suggested by the presence of ligands and receptors expressed by the respective cell types. For example, lining macrophage-like cells express CD97, a member of the secretin superfamily of transmembrane receptors, and lining fibroblast-like cells express CD55, or decay accelerating factor, a specific ligand for CD97.[126] Although the functional consequences of this ligand-receptor interaction is not known, it is possible that CD55 protects cells from complement-mediated damaged and that CD97 transduces signals in the macrophage.

Components of the intercellular matrix of the synovial lining region distinguish it from the underlying stroma, reflecting the specific synthetic activity of lining cells. Hyaluronan, type VI collagen, and chondroitin 6-sulfate are localized to the lining region, with tenascin localized immediately beneath the lining cells.[113,120-122,127] Normal synovial lining cells also express a rich array of adhesion molecules.[117,128,129] These are probably essential for cellular attachment to specific matrix components in the synovial lining region, preventing loss into the synovial cavity of cells subjected to deformation and shear stresses during joint movement. Adhesion molecules such as VCAM-1 are potentially also involved in the recruitment of inflammatory cells during the evolution of arthritis. VCAM-1 expression in intimal and subintimal fibroblasts facilitates binding of α4β1 integrin, which is expressed on mononuclear cells but not on granulocytes.[116] Edwards[78] has speculated that this, in part, accounts for the passage of granulocytes into synovial fluid with retention of mononuclear macrophages in inflamed synovium.

Synovial Stroma

A variable depth of heterogeneous mesenchymal tissue is interposed between the synovial lining region and the joint capsule. At the lateral joint margin of the knee, this synovial stroma is well vascularized and cellular, but it becomes increasingly fibrous with increasing depth until it blends with the joint capsule. The synovial lining of cruciate ligaments is in direct continuity with the underlying hypocellular collagenous fibers; in the suprapatellar pouch, the synovial stroma is composed primarily of adipose tissue. This synovial heterogeneity can make assessment by synovial biopsy material difficult.

Stroma cells in normal synovium are predominantly fibroblasts. Fibroblasts accumulate immediately beneath the lining region and around blood vessels; they bear surface peptidases, such as angiotensin-converting enzyme, dipeptidyl peptidase IV, aminopeptidase M, and—in inflamed synovium—neutral endopeptidase. These enzymes contribute to the functional compartmentalization of peptide regulatory systems within the tissue.[130] The synovial stroma plays an important role in the response of synovium to arthritis because it is host to inflammatory cell infiltrates and lymphoid follicles.

SYNOVIAL VASCULATURE

Normal synovium is richly vascularized,[131,132] providing the high blood flow that is required for solute and gas exchange in the synovium itself and for the generation of synovial fluid (Fig. 1–8B). The avascular articular cartilage also depends on nutrition in the synovial fluid, derived from the synovial vasculature.[133] Thus, the vascularized synovium behaves somewhat like an endocrine organ, generating factors that regulate synoviocyte function and serving as a selective gateway that recruits cells from the circulation during stress and inflammation.[134] Finally, synovial blood flow plays an important role in regulating intra-articular temperature.

Structure-Function Relationships of Synovial Vasculature

The synovial vasculature can be divided, on morphologic and functional grounds, into arterioles, capillaries, and venules. In addition, lymphatics accompany arterioles and larger venules.[135] Arterial and venous networks of the joint are complex and are characterized by arteriovenous anastomoses that communicate freely with blood vessels in periosteum and periarticular bone.[136] As large synovial arteries enter the deep layers of the synovium near the capsule, they give off branches, which bifurcate again to form "microvascular units" in the subsynovial layers. The synovial lining region, the surfaces of intra-articular ligaments, and the entheses (in the angle of ligamentous insertions into bone) are particularly well vascularized.[137] The distribution of synovial vessels, which were formed largely as a result of vasculogenesis during development of the joint, displays considerable plasticity. Vasculogenesis is a dynamic process that depends on the cellular interactions with regulatory factors and the extracellular matrix that are also important in angiogenesis, which is the formation of new vessels from preexisting vasculature. Immobilization in experimental animals actually decreases the number of capillary plexuses, as well as blood flow in joints.[138] Angiogenesis is characteristic of inflammatory arthritis, in which the density of blood vessels decreases relative to the growing synovial mass, thereby creating a hypoxic and acidotic environment.[139,140] Angiogenic factors such as VEGF, via VEGF receptors-1 and -2 (Flt-1 and Flk-1) and bFGF, promote proliferation and migration of endothelial cells, a process that is facilitated by matrix-degrading enzymes and adhesion molecules such as integrin $\alpha v\beta 3$ and E-selectin, expressed by activated endothelial cells.[141-143] Vessel maturation is facilitated by the angiopoietin (Ang)-1 via the Tie-2 receptor, molecules that are restricted to the capillary epithelium in normal synovium but that are elevated in inflamed synovium in both perivascular sites and areas remote from vessels.[144,145]

Regulation of Synovial Blood Flow

Synovial blood flow is regulated by both intrinsic (autocrine and paracrine) and extrinsic (neural and humoral) systems. Locally generated factors, such as the peptide vasoconstrictors angiotensin II and endothelin-1, act on adjacent arteriolar smooth muscle to regulate regional vascular tone.[146,147] Normal synovial arterioles are richly innervated by sympathetic nerves containing vasoconstrictors, such as norepinephrine and neuropeptide Y, and by "sensory" nerves, which also play an efferent vasodilatory role by releasing the neuropeptides substance P and calcitonin gene-related peptide (CGRP).[148] Arterioles regulate regional blood flow. Capillaries and postcapillary venules are sites of fluid and cellular exchange. Correspondingly, regulatory systems are differentially distributed along the vascular axis. For example, angiotensin-converting enzyme, which generates angiotensin II, is localized predominantly in arteriolar and capillary endothelia[101] and decreases during inflammation.[149] Specific receptors for angiotensin II and for substance P are abundant on synovial capillaries, with lower densities on adjacent arterioles.[146,150] Dipeptidyl peptidase IV, a peptide-degrading enzyme, is specifically localized to the cell membranes of venular endothelium.[101] The synovial vasculature, therefore, is not only functionally compartmentalized from the surrounding stroma but also highly specialized along its arteriovenous axis. Other unique characteristics of the normal synovial vasculature include the presence of inducible nitric oxidase synthase (iNOS)-independent 3-nitrotyrosine, a reaction product of peroxynitrite,[151] and the localization of the synoviocyte-derived CXCL12 chemokine on heparan sulfate receptors on endothelial cells,[152] suggesting physiologic roles for these molecules in normal vascular function.

Synovial Fluid Generation and Maintenance of Intra-articular Pressure

The synovial microvasculature is essential for the generation of synovial fluid, formed by admixture of a protein-rich filtrate of blood with synoviocyte-derived hyaluronate. Capillary depth is proposed as the major factor governing fluid exchange in joints.[153] Synovial capillaries are fenestrated; they contain small pores covered by a thin membrane[154] (Fig. 1–9). These fenestrations may facilitate rapid exchange of small molecules, such as glucose and lactate.[155] In normal joints, intra-articular pressures are slightly subatmospheric at rest (0 to –5 mm Hg).[156,157] During exercise, hydrostatic pressure in the normal joint may decrease further.[158] Chronic arthritis leads to increased intra-articular pressures because of the increased volume of synovial fluid and decreased compliance of the joint capsule.[159] Resting intra-articular pressures in rheumatoid joints are around 20 mm Hg, whereas during isometric exercise, they may rise above 100 mm Hg, well above capillary perfusion pressure and, at times, above arterial pressure.[157] Repeated mechanical stresses can interrupt synovial perfusion during joint movement, particularly in the presence of a synovial effusion.

Elevation of intra-articular pressure interrupts not only synovial blood flow but also blood flow in the subchondral bone plate.[160] Massive elevation of intra-articular pressure during exercise is a feature of the chronic synovial inflammation of rheumatoid arthritis, but not of acute traumatic effusions.[156] High resting intra-articular pressures may contribute to resting synovial hypoxia in rheumatoid arthritis and, therefore, contribute to further damage to the joint. The potential volume, and thus the pressure of the synovial cavity, varies according to the degree to which the joint is flexed.[161] During exercise, such as walking, synovial blood flow in the chronically inflamed knee is cyclically occluded, with intermittent reperfusion. Reactive oxygen species generated during these hypoxia-reperfusion cycles may further injure synovial cells.[162] The coordinated interplay of vasodilator and vasocon-strictor regulatory systems may be designed normally to relieve synovial hypoxia while limiting transient reperfusion.

Maintenance of Joint Temperature

The vascular system of the extremities acts as a countercurrent distribution system for tissue temperature, and peripheral joints normally function with intra-articular temperatures well below the core body temperature of 37°C. Intra-articular temperatures may vary widely according to ambient room temperature. In small, peripheral joints with little overlying insulation of fat or muscle, such as the metacarpophalangeal joint, intra-articular temperatures closely parallel those of skin between resting temperatures and 40°C.[163] By contrast, in larger joints, such as the knee, wide variations between joint and skin temperature have been reported.[164,165] Non–weight-bearing active movements increase intra-articular temperature by as much as 1°C, probably by increasing subsynovial tissue blood

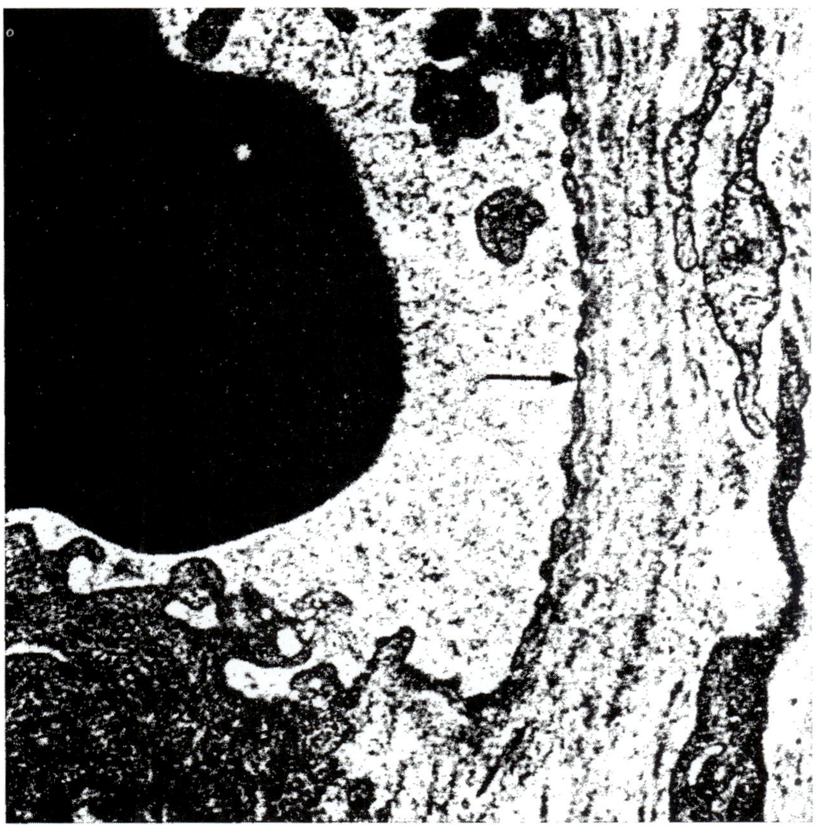

FIGURE 1–9 · Fenestrated Blood Capillary in Human Synovium. The capillary is situated just beneath the lining layer. Pores in the endothelium are indicated by the *arrow*. A red blood cell lies in the lumen of the capillary. (×11,000) (From Bassleer R, Lhosest-Gauthier M-P, Renard A-M, et al: Histological structure and functions of synovium. *In* Franchimont P (ed): Articular Synovium: Anatomy, Physiology, Pathology, Pharmacology, and Therapy. Basel, Karger, 1982, pp 1–26.)

flow, although normal intra-articular temperatures in the knee are always below 36°C at ambient temperatures of around 20°C. In the knee, cold applied to the skin lowers intra-articular temperatures, whereas the application of heat raises it.[166] A painful stimulus, such as apprehension, alarm, or smoking, lowers the skin temperature and elevates intra-articular temperature, presumably by shunting blood from the skin to the synovium. These disparities between skin and intra-articular temperatures complicate the interpretation of thermographic data derived from large joints. Low intra-articular temperatures are important because enzymatic reactions observed in vitro at 37°C may proceed only slowly in the normal joint but may be enhanced during synovial inflammation. At 37°C, for instance, destruction of articular cartilage collagen fibers by synovial collagenase is substantial; at 32°C, it is imperceptible.[167] This suggests that the common practice of applying hot packs to inflamed joints may actually be harmful, due to the subsequent increase in collagenolytic activity.[167]

JOINT INNERVATION

Dissection studies have shown that each joint has a dual nerve supply, consisting of specific articular nerves that penetrate the capsule as independent branches of adjacent peripheral nerves and articular branches that arise from related muscle nerves. The definition of joint position and the detection of joint motion are monitored separately and by a combination of multiple inputs from different receptors in varied systems. Nerve endings in muscle and skin, as well as in the joint capsule, mediate sensation of joint position[168] and movement.[169] Normal joints have both afferent (sensory) and efferent (motor) innervations. Fast-conducting, myelinated A fibers innervating the joint capsule are important for proprioception and detection of joint movement; slow-conducting, unmyelinated C fibers transmit diffuse pain sensation and regulate synovial microvascular function.

Normal synovium is richly innervated by fine, unmyelinated nerve fibers that follow the courses of blood vessels and extend into the synovial lining layers.[170] They do not have specialized endings and are slow-conducting fibers; they may transmit diffuse, burning, or aching pain sensation. Sympathetic nerve fibers surround blood vessels, particularly in the deeper regions of normal synovium.[148] They contain and release both classic neurotransmitters, such as norepinephrine, and neuropeptides that constrict synovial blood vessels. Neuropeptides that are markers of sensory nerves include substance P, CGRP, and neuropeptide Y.[148,171,172] Afferent nerves containing substance P also have an efferent role in the synovium. Substance P is released from peripheral nerve terminals into the joint, and specific, G protein–coupled receptors for substance P are localized to microvascular endothelium in normal synovium.[150,173] Abnormalities of articular innervation that are associated with inflammatory arthritis may contribute to the failure of synovial inflammation to resolve.[148,174] Excessive local neuropeptide release may result in the loss of nerve fibers due to neuropeptide depletion. Furthermore, synovial tissue proliferation without concomitant growth of new nerve fibers may lead to an apparent partial denervation of synovium.[148,174] Studies in patients suggest that free nerve endings containing substance P may modulate inflammation and the pain pathway in osteoarthritis.[175]

Afferent nerve fibers from the joint play an important role in the reflex inhibition of muscle contraction. Trophic factors generated by motor neurons, such as the neuropeptide CGRP, are important in maintaining muscle bulk and a functional neuromuscular junction.[176] Decreases in motor-neuron trophic support during articular inflammation probably contribute to muscle wasting.

Mechanisms of joint pain have been reviewed in detail.[177] In the noninflamed joint, most sensory nerve fibers do not respond to movement within the normal range; these are referred to as silent nociceptors. In the acutely inflamed joint, however, these nerve fibers become sensitized by mediators, such as bradykinin, neurokinin 1, and prostaglandins (peripheral sensitization), such that normal movements induce pain. Pain sensation is further upregulated or downregulated in the central nervous system, both at the level of the spinal cord and in the brain, by central sensitization and "gating" of nociceptive input. Thus, although the normal joint may respond predictably to painful stimuli, there is often a poor correlation between apparent joint disease and perceived pain in chronic arthritis. Pain associated with joint movements within the normal range is a characteristic symptom described by patients with chronically inflamed joints caused by rheumatoid arthritis. Chronically inflamed joints, however, may not be painful at rest, unless exposed to acute inflammation, such as infection.

TENDONS

Tendons are functional and anatomic bridges between muscle and bone.[178,179] They focus the force of a large mass of muscle into a localized area on bone and, by splitting to form numerous insertions, may distribute the force of a single muscle to different bones.[180] Tendons are formed of longitudinally arranged collagen fibrils embedded in an organized, hydrated proteoglycan matrix with blood vessels, lymphatics, and fibroblasts.[178,181] Aldehyde-derived cross-links between adjacent collagen chains or molecules contribute to the tensile strength of the tendon.[182] Tendon collagen fibrillogenesis is initiated during the early development by fibroblasts.[183] Many tendons, particularly those with a large range of motion, run through vascularized, discontinuous sheaths of collagen lined with mesenchymal cells resembling synovium. Gliding of tendons through their sheaths is enhanced by hyaluronic acid produced by the lining cells. Tendon movement is essential for the embryogenesis and maintenance of tendons and their sheaths.[184,185] Degenerative changes appear in tendons, and fibrous adhesions form between tendons and sheaths when inflammation or surgical incision is followed by long periods of immobilization.[185] At the myotendinous junction, recesses between muscle cell processes are filled with collagen fibrils, which blend into the tendon. At its other end, collagen fibers of the tendon typically blend into fibrocartilage, mineralize, and then merge into bone.[184] At some tendon insertions, such as the insertion of the pectoralis major tendon into the humerus, there are no intervening tiers of fibrocartilage.[186] Instead, tendon fibrils run through the periosteum and become continuous with outer bone lamellae, where they are called Sharpey's fibers.

Tendon fibroblasts synthesize and secrete collagens, proteoglycans, and other matrix components, such as fibronectin, as well as MMPs and their inhibitors that can contribute to the breakdown and repair of tendon components.[187-192] Collagen fibrils in tendon are composed primarily of type I collagen with some type III, but there are regional differences in the distribution of other matrix components.[193-195] The compressed region contains the small proteoglycans, biglycan, decorin, fibromodulin, and lumican, and the large proteoglycan versican.[193,195,196] The major components in the tensile region of the tendon are decorin, microfibrillar type VI collagen, fibromodulin, and proline and arginine-rich end teucine-rich repeat protein (PRELP). The presence of collagen oligomeric matrix protein (COMP), aggrecan, and biglycan also are indicative of cells with chondrocyte phenotype[189] (see following discussion).

Failure of the muscle-tendon apparatus is rare, but when it does occur, it is secondary to enormous, quickly generated forces across a joint and usually occurs near the tendon insertion into bone. Factors that may predispose to tendon failure are aging processes, including loss of extracellular water and an increase in intermolecular cross-links of collagen; tendon ischemia; iatrogenic factors, including injection of glucocorticoids; and deposition of calcium hydroxyapatite crystals within the collagen bundles. Alterations in collagen fibril composition and structure are associated with tendon degeneration during aging and may predispose to osteoarthritis.[197,198]

LIGAMENTS

Ligaments provide a stabilizing bridge between bones, permitting a limited range of movements.[199] The ligaments are often recognized only as hypertrophied components of the fibrous joint capsule and are structurally similar to tendons. Although the fibers are oriented parallel to the longitudinal axis of both tissues,[178] the collagen fibrils in ligaments are nonparallel and arranged in fibers that are oriented roughly along the long axis in a wavy, undulating pattern, or "crimp," which can straighten in response to load.[200] Some ligaments have a higher ratio of elastin to collagen (1:4) than tendons (1:50),[180] which permits a greater degree of stretch. For example, the high elastin content of the ligamentum flavum between adjacent vertebral laminae allows stretch during spinal flexion. Ligaments also have larger amounts of reducible cross-links, more type III collagen, slightly less total collagen, and more glycosaminoglycans, compared to tendons.[178] The cells in ligaments appear to be more metabolically active than those in tendons because they have more plump cellular nuclei and higher DNA content.[178] During postnatal growth, the development of ligament attachment zones involves changes in the ratios and distribution of collagen types I, III, and V and the synthesis of type II collagen and proteoglycans by fibrochondrocytes that develop from ligament cells at the attachment zone.[201,202] Attachment zones are believed to permit gradual transmission of the tensile force between ligament and bone.[186,203]

Ligaments play a major role in the passive stabilization of joints, aided by the capsule and, when present, menisci. In the knee, the collateral and cruciate ligaments provide stability when there is little or no load on the joint. As compressive load increases, there is an increasing contribution to stability from the joint surfaces themselves and the surrounding musculature. Injured ligaments generally heal, and structural integrity is restored by contracture of the healing ligament so that it can act again as a stabilizer of the joint.[204,205]

BURSAE

The many bursae in the human body facilitate gliding of one tissue over another, much as a tendon sheath facilitates movement of its tendon. Bursae are closed sacs, lined sparsely with mesenchymal cells similar to synovial cells, but they are generally less well vascularized than synovium. Most bursae differentiate concurrently with synovial joints during embryogenesis. During life, however, trauma or inflammation may lead to the development of new bursae, hypertrophy of previously existing ones,[206] or communication between deep bursae and joints.[180] In patients with rheumatoid arthritis, for example, communications may exist between the subacromial bursae and the glenohumeral joint, between the gastrocnemius or semimembranosus bursae and the knee joint, and between the iliopsoas bursa and the hip joint. It is unusual, however, for subcutaneous bursae, such as the prepatellar bursa or olecranon bursa, to develop communication with the underlying joint.

MENISCI

The meniscus, a fibrocartilaginous, wedge-shaped structure, is best developed in the knee but is also found in the acromioclavicular and sternoclavicular joints, the ulnocarpal joint, and the temporomandibular joint.[207] Until recently, menisci were thought to have little function and a quiescent metabolism with no capability of repair. However, it had been observed that removal of menisci from the knee may lead to premature arthritic changes in the joint.[208] Recent evidence from an arthroscopic study of patients with anterior cruciate ligament (ACL) insufficiency indicates that the pathology of the medial meniscus correlates with that of the medial femoral cartilage.[209] The meniscus is now considered to be an integral component of the knee joint that has important functions in joint stability, load distribution, shock absorption, and lubrication.[210]

The microanatomy of the meniscus is complex and age dependent.[211] The characteristic shape of both the lateral and medial meniscus is achieved early in prenatal development. At that time, the menisci are cellular and highly vascularized; with maturation, however, vascularity decreases progressively from the central margin to the peripheral margin. After skeletal maturity, the peripheral 10 to 30 percent of the meniscus remains highly vascularized by a circumferential capillary plexus and is well innervated. Tears in this vascularized peripheral zone may undergo repair and remodeling.[212] The central portion of the mature meniscus, however, is an avascular fibrocartilage without nerves or lymphatics, consisting of cells surrounded by an abundant extracellular matrix of collagens, chondroitin sulfates, dermatan sulfates, and hyaluronic acid. Tears in this central zone heal poorly, if at all. Collagen constitutes 60 to 70 percent of the dry weight of the meniscus and is mostly type I collagen, with lesser amounts of types III, V, and VI. A small quantity of cartilage-specific type II collagen is localized to the inner, avascular portion of the meniscus. Collagen fibers in the periphery are mostly circumferentially oriented, with radial fibers extending toward the central portion.[213,214] Aggrecan and decorin are the major proteoglycans in the adult meniscus.[215,216] Decorin is the predominant proteoglycan synthesized in the meniscus from young donors, whereas the relative proportion of aggrecan synthesis increases with age. Although the capacity of the meniscus to synthesize sulfated proteoglycans decreases after the teenage years, the age-related increases in expression of decorin and aggrecan mRNAs suggest that the resident cells are able to respond quickly to alterations in the biomechanic environment.[217]

The meniscus was defined originally as a fibrocartilage, based on the rounded or oval shape of most of the cells and the fibrous microscopic appearance of the extracellular matrix.[218] Based on molecular and spatial criteria, three distinct populations of cells are recognized in the meniscus of the knee joint[214,219]: (1) The *fibrochondrocyte* is the most abundant cell in the middle and inner meniscus, synthesizing primarily type I collagen and relatively small amounts of type II and III collagens. It is round or oval in shape and has a pericellular filamentous matrix containing type VI collagen. (2) The *fibroblast-like cells* lack a pericellular matrix and are located in the outer portion of the meniscus. They are distinguished by long, thin, branching cytoplasmic projections that stain for vimentin. They make contact with other cells in different regions via connexin 43-containing gap junctions. The presence of two centrosomes, one associated with a primary celium, suggests a sensory, rather than motile, function that could enable the cells to respond to circumferential tensile loads, rather than compressive loads.[220] (3) The *superficial zone cells* have a characteristic fusiform shape with no cytoplasmic projections. The occasional staining of these cells in the uninjured meniscus with α-actin and their migration into surrounding wound sites suggest that they are specialized progenitor cells that may participate in a remodeling response in the meniscus and surrounding tissues.[221,222] It has also been suggested that the superficial zone cells originate in the synovium and move to the superficial zone through canal-like openings on the surface of the meniscus.[223]

Mature Articular Cartilage

Articular cartilage is a specialized connective tissue that covers the weight-bearing surfaces of diarthrodial joints.[98,224] The principal functions of cartilage layers covering bone ends are to permit low-friction, high velocity movement between bones, to absorb the transmitted forces associated with locomotion, and to contribute to joint stability. Lubrication by synovial fluid provides frictionless movement of the articulating cartilage surfaces. Chondrocytes (see Chapter 13) are the single cellular component of adult hyaline articular cartilage and are responsible for synthesizing and maintaining the highly specialized cartilage matrix macromolecules. The cartilage extracellular matrix is composed of an extensive network of collagen fibrils, which confers tensile strength, and an interlocking mesh of proteoglycans, which provides compressive stiffness through the ability to absorb and extrude water. A brief description of the organization of articular cartilage and structure-function relationships of cartilage matrix components follows. Detailed descriptions of these components can be found in Chapter 2 (collagen) and Chapter 3 (proteoglycans).

CARTILAGE STRUCTURE

Normal articular cartilage is a special type of hyaline cartilage characterized by its translucent (hyaline) appearance. It is an avascular tissue nourished by diffusion from the vasculature of the subchondral bone, as well as from the synovial fluid. Articular cartilage is more than 70 percent water, and it is rather hypocellular compared with other tissues; chondrocytes comprise only 1 to 2 percent of its total volume.[225] More than 90 percent of the dry weight of cartilage consists of two components: type II collagen and the large aggregating proteoglycan, aggrecan. However, several "minor" collagens and small proteoglycans also appear to play a role in cartilage-matrix organization.[226,227] These organic constituents represent only about 20 percent of the wet weight. Collagen, primarily type II, accounts for approximately 15 to 25 percent of the wet weight and about half of the dry weight, except in the superficial zone where it represents most of the dry weight. Proteoglycans, primarily aggrecan, account for up to 10 percent of the wet weight and about 25 percent of the dry weight. The highly cross-linked type II collagen-containing fibrils are thinner than type I collagen fibrils in skin and form a systematically oriented network that traps the highly negatively charged proteoglycan aggregates.[228]

Despite its thinness (7 mm or less) and apparent homogeneity, mature articular cartilage is a heterogeneous tissue with four distinct regions: the superficial tangential (or gliding) zone, the middle (or transitional) zone, the deep (or radial) zone, and the calcified cartilage zone, which is located immediately below the tidemark and above the subchondral bone[225,228-230] (Fig. 1–10). In the superficial zone, the chondrocytes are flattened, and the matrix is composed of thin collagen fibrils in tangential array, associated with a high concentration of the small proteoglycan decorin and a low concentration of aggrecan. The middle zone,

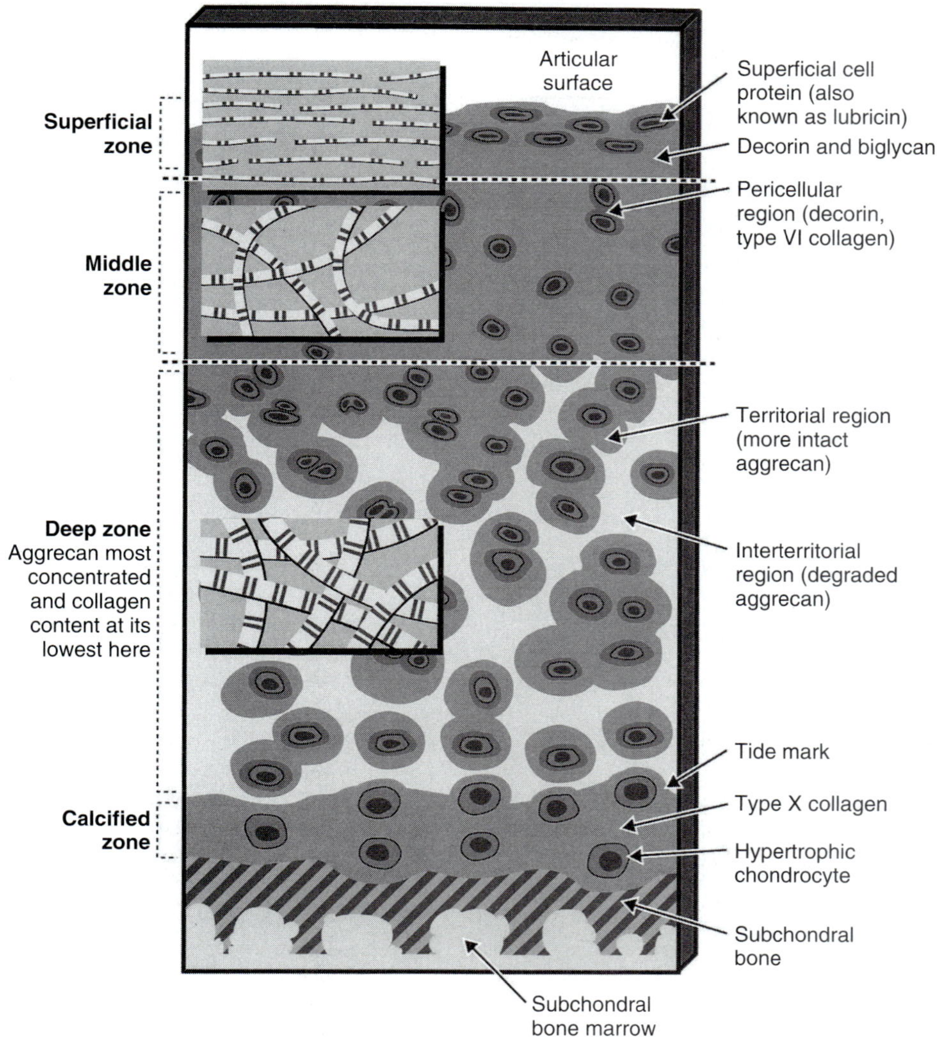

FIGURE 1–10 · The structure of human adult articular cartilage, showing the zones of cellular distribution and the pericellular, territorial, and interterritorial regions of matrix organization. The insets show the relative diameters and orientations of collagen fibrils in the different zones. The positions of the tidemark and subchondral bone and other special features of matrix composition are also noted. (From Poole AR, Kojima T, Yasuda T, et al: Composition and structure of articular cartilage. A template for tissue repair. Clin Ortho-paed Rel Res 391S:S26-S33, 2001. By copyright permission of Lippincott Williams & Wilkins.)

comprising 40 to 60 percent of the cartilage weight, consists of rounded chondrocytes surrounded by radial bundles of thick collagen fibrils. In the deep zone, the chondrocytes are frequently grouped in columns or clusters and resemble the hypertrophic chondrocytes of the growth plate (Fig. 1–11). In this region, the collagen bundles are the thickest and are arranged in a radial fashion. The cell density progressively decreases from the surface to the deep zone, where it is one half to one third of the density in the superficial zone[231]; the chondrocytes in the deep and middle zones have a cell volume that is twice that of the superficial chondrocytes.[232] Water is 75 to 80 percent of the wet weight in the superficial zone and progressively decreases to between 65 and 70 percent with increasing depth. Higher amounts of collagen relative to proteoglycans are present in the superficial zone, compared with the middle and deep zones, and type I collagen may be synthesized in addition to type II collagen.[233,234] With increasing depth, the proportion of proteoglycan increases to 50 percent of the dry weight in the deep zone.[232,235-237] The calcified zone is formed as a result of endochondral ossification and persists as the growth plate is resorbed. The calcified zone serves as an important mechanical buffer between the uncalcified articular cartilage and the subchondral bone.

The physical properties of articular cartilage are determined by the unique fibrillar collagen network, which provides tensile strength, interspersed with proteoglycan aggregates that bestow compressive resilience.[238-240] The proteoglycans are associated with large quantities of water bound to the hydrophilic glycosaminoglycan chains. This cartilaginous extracellular matrix, with its tightly bound water, provides a high degree of resistance to deformation by compressive forces. The capacity to resist compressive forces is associated with the ability to extrude water as the cartilage compresses. Once the compression is released, the proteoglycans (now depleted of balancing counter-ions that were removed with the water) contain sufficient fixed charge to osmotically reabsorb the water and small solutes into the matrix, which then rebounds to its original dimensions.[241,242]

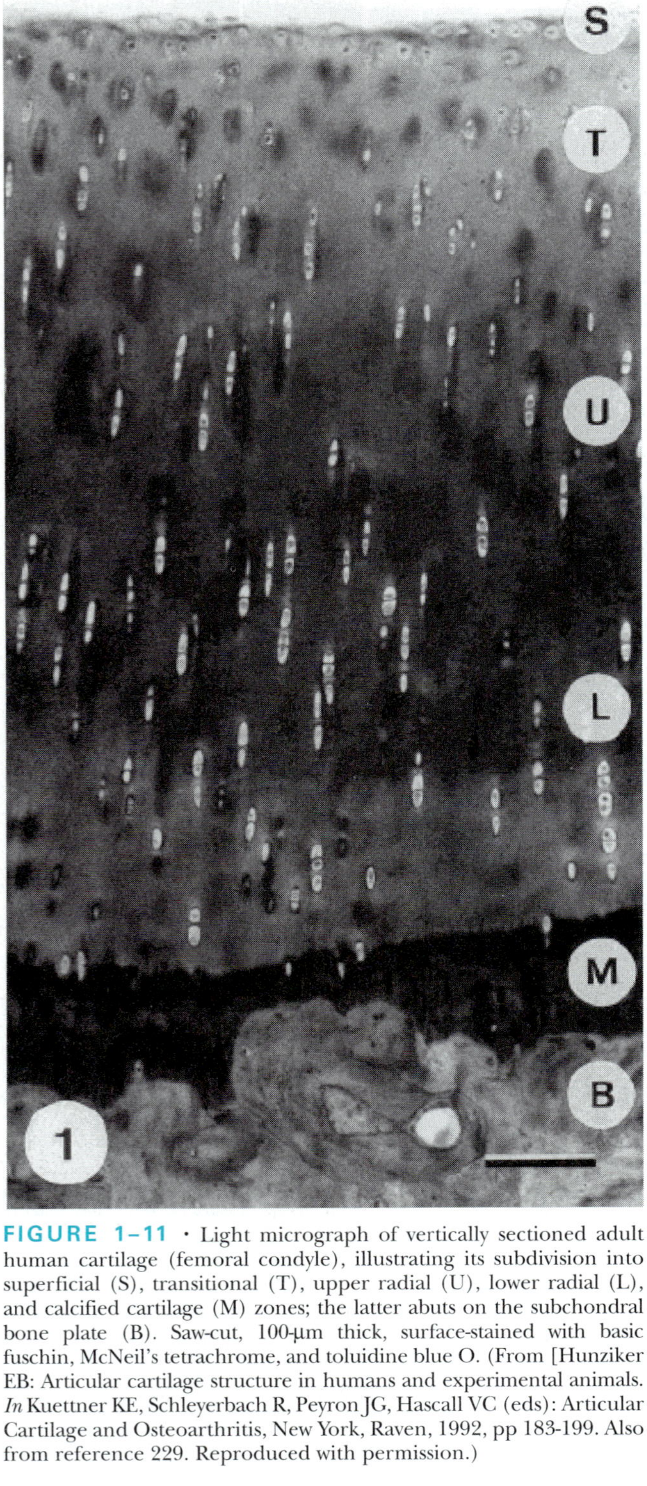

FIGURE 1–11 • Light micrograph of vertically sectioned adult human cartilage (femoral condyle), illustrating its subdivision into superficial (S), transitional (T), upper radial (U), lower radial (L), and calcified cartilage (M) zones; the latter abuts on the subchondral bone plate (B). Saw-cut, 100-μm thick, surface-stained with basic fuschin, McNeil's tetrachrome, and toluidine blue O. (From [Hunziker EB: Articular cartilage structure in humans and experimental animals. *In* Kuettner KE, Schleyerbach R, Peyron JG, Hascall VC (eds): Articular Cartilage and Osteoarthritis, New York, Raven, 1992, pp 183-199. Also from reference 229. Reproduced with permission.)

STRUCTURE-FUNCTION RELATIONSHIPS OF CARTILAGE MATRIX COMPONENTS

The extracellular matrix components synthesized by chondrocytes include highly cross-linked fibrils of triple-helical type II collagen molecules that interact with other collagens, aggrecan, small proteoglycans, and other cartilage-specific specific and nonspecific matrix proteins (Table 1).[98,226,227,230,243,244] The importance of these structural proteins may be observed in heritable disorders, such as chondrodysplasias, or in transgenic animals in which mutations in cartilage-specific collagen genes or in genes that affect sulfation of aggrecan result in cartilage abnormalities.[245,246] Furthermore, knowledge of the composition of the cartilage matrix has permitted the development of methods for identifying molecular markers in serum and synovial fluid that can be used to monitor changes in cartilage metabolism and to assess cartilage damage in osteoarthritis or rheumatoid arthritis.[247-251] Changes in the structural composition of cartilage can markedly affect its biomechanical properties, as is discussed in Chapter 6.

Cartilage Collagens

The major component of the collagen network in adult articular cartilage is the triple-helical type II collagen molecule, which is composed of three identical alpha chains, $[\alpha 1(II)]_3$. These molecules are assembled in fibrils in a quarter-stagger array that can be observed by electron microscopy.[244,252] These fibrils are thinner than the type I collagen-containing fibrils in skin because of the higher number of hydroxylysines that can form cross-links and the presence of other collagen and noncollagen components in the fibril. The type IIB collagen in articular cartilage is a product of alternative splicing and lacks a 69-amino acid, cysteine-rich domain of the amino-terminal propeptide, which is encoded by exon 2 in the human type II collagen gene *(COL2A1)*[253] (see Fig. 1–6). This domain is found in the amino propeptides of other interstitial collagen types and is speculated to play a feedback-inhibitory role in collagen biosynthesis. The type IIA procollagen that contains this domain is expressed normally by chondroprogenitor cells during development, but it may reappear in the middle zone of osteoarthritic cartilage in the pericellular matrix.[254] The reexpression of type X collagen, the hypertrophic chondrocyte marker, in the deep zone of osteoarthritic cartilage also suggests reversion to a developmental phenotype as an attempt to repair the damaged matrix.[255]

Although collagen types VI, IX, XI, XII, and XIV are quantitatively minor components, they may have important structural and functional properties.[252,256] Types IX and XI are relatively specific to cartilage, whereas types VI, XII, and XIV are widely distributed in other connective tissues. Type VI collagen, which is present in cartilage as microfibrils in very small quantities localized around the chondrocytes, may play a role in cell attachment and interacts with other matrix proteins, such as hyaluronan, decorin, and biglycan. Type IX collagen is both a proteoglycan and a collagen, as it contains a chondroitin sulfate chain attachment site in one of the noncollagen domains. The helical domains of the type IX collagen molecule form covalent cross-links with type II collagen telopeptides and are attached to the fibrillar surface, as observed in the electron microscope. It has been suggested that type IX collagen functions as a structural intermediate between type II collagen fibers and the pro-

TABLE 1–1 • EXTRACELLULAR MATRIX COMPONENTS OF CARTILAGE

Molecule	Structure and size	Function and location
Collagens		
Type II	$[\alpha1(II)]_3$; fibril-forming	Tensile strength; major component of collagen fibrils
Type IX	[α1(IX)α2(IX)α3(IX)]; single CS or DS chain; α1(II) gene encodes α3(IX); FACIT	Tensile properties, interfibrillar connections; cross-links to surface of collagen fibril, NC4 domain projects into matrix
Type XI	[α1(XI)α2(XI)α3(XI)]; fibril-forming	Nucleation/control of fibril formation; within collagen fibril
Type VI	[α1(VI)α2(VI)α3(VI)]; microfibrils	Forms microfibrillar network, binds hyaluronan, biglycan, decorin; pericellular
Type X	[α1(X)]3; hexagonal network	Support for endochondral ossification; hypertrophic zone and calcified cartilage
Type XII	$[\alpha1(XII)]_3$; FACIT large cruciform NC3 domain	Associated with collagen I fibrils in perichondrium and articular surface
Type XIV	$[\alpha1(XIV)]_3$; FACIT	Associated with collagen fibrils throughout articular cartilage
Proteoglycans		
Aggrecan	255-kD core protein; CS/KS side chains; C-terminal EGF and lectin-like domains	Compressive stiffness through hydration of fixed charge density; binding through G1 domain to HA stabilized by link protein
Versican	265–370 kD-core protein; CS/DS side chains; C-terminal EGF, C-type lectin, and CRP-like domains	Low levels in articular cartilage throughout life; calcium-binding and selectin-like properties
Perlecan	400–467-kD core protein; HS/CS side chains; no HA-binding	Cell-matrix adhesion; pericellular
Biglycan	38 kD; LRR core protein with two DS chains (76 kD)	Binds collagen VI and TGF-β; pericellular
Decorin	36.5 kD; LRR core protein with one CS or DS side chain (100 kD)	Controls size/shape of collagen fibrils, binds collagen II and TGF-β; interterritorial
Fibromodulin	58 kD; contains KS chains in central LRR region and N-terminal tyrosine sulfate domains	Same as decorin
Lumican	58 kD; structure similar to fibromodulin	Same as decorin
PRELP	58 kD; LRR core protein; proline and arginine-rich N-terminal binding domain for heparin and HS	Mediates cell binding through HS sulfate in syndecan
Chondroadherin	LRR core protein without N-terminal extension	Binding to cells via α2β1 integrin
Other Molecules		
Hyaluronic acid (HA; hyaluronan)	1000–3000 kD	Retention of aggrecan within matrix
Link protein	38.6 kD	Stabilizes attachment of aggrecan G1 domain to HA
Cartilage oligomeric matrix protein (COMP)	550 kD; five 110-kD subunits; thrombospondin-like	Interterritorial in articular cartilage; stabilizes collagen network or promotes collagen fibril assembly; calcium binding
Cartilage matrix protein (CMP, or matrilin-1); matrilin-3	Three 50-kD subunits with vWFA and EGF domains	Tightly bound to aggrecan in immature cartilage
Cartilage intermediate layer protein (CILP)	92 kD; homology with nucleotide pyrophosphohydrolase without active site	Restricted to middle/deep zones of cartilage; increase in early and late OA
Glycoprotein (gp)-39, or YKL-40	39 kD; chitinase homology	Marker of cartilage turnover; chondrocyte proliferation; superficial zone of cartilage
Fibronectin	Dimer of 220-kD subunits	Cell attachment and binding to collagen and proteoglycans; increased In OA cartilage
Tenascin-c	Six 200-kD subunits forming hexabrachion structure	Binds syndecan-3 during chondrogenesis; angiogenesis
Superficial zone protein (SZP), or lubricin	225 kD, 200 nm length	Joint lubrication; superficial zone only
Membrane Proteins		
CD44	Integral membrane protein with extracellular HS/CS side chains	Cell-matrix interactions; binds HA
Syndecan-3	N-terminal HS attachment site; cytoplasmic tyrosine residues	Receptor for tenascin-c during cartilage development; cell-matrix interactions
Anchorin CII (or annexin V)	34 kD; homology to calcium-binding proteins calpactin and lipocortin	Cell surface attachment to type II collagen; calcium binding
Integrins (α1, 2, 3, 5, 6, 10; β1, 3, 5)	Two noncovalently linked transmembrane glycoproteins (α and β subunits)	Cell-matrix binding: α1β1/collagen 1 or VI, α2β1 or α3β1/collagen II, α5β1/ FN; intracellular signaling

Abbreviations: CRP = complement regulatory protein; CS = chondroitin sulfate; DS = dermatan sulfate; EGF = epidermal growth factor; FACIT = fibril-associated collagens with interrupted triple helices; FN, fibronectin; HA, hyaluronic acid; HS = heparan sulfate; KS = keratan sulfate; LRR = leucine-rich repeat; NC, noncollagen; OA, osteoarthritis; PRELP = proline- and arginine-rich end leucine-rich repeat protein; TGF-β, transforming growth factor-β; vWFA = von Willebrand factor.

teoglycan aggregates, thereby serving to enhance the mechanical stability of the fibril network and resist the swelling pressure of the trapped proteoglycans. Destruction of type IX collagen accelerates cartilage degradation and loss of function.

The α3 chain of type XI collagen has the same primary sequence as the α1(II) chain, and the heterotrimeric type XI collagen molecule is buried in the same fibril as type II collagen. Thus, type XI collagen may have a role in regulating fibril diameter. The more recently discovered nonfibrillar fibril-associated collagens with interrupted triple helices (FACIT), XII and XIV, which are structurally related to type IX collagen, do not form fibrils by themselves, but coaggregate with fibril-forming collagens and modulate the packing of collagen fibers by domains projecting from their surfaces.[256,257] Expression of type III and type VI collagens may also be induced or increased in osteoarthritic cartilage.[258]

Deficiencies or disruptions in genes that encode many of these collagens (see Chapter 2) result in decreased cartilage integrity and, in some cases, in premature osteoarthritis.[58,259] Genetic mutations in the type II collagen gene (*COL2A1*) result in chondrodysplasias, characterized by cartilage malformation.[260-263] Targeted expression of SV40 T antigen, directed by the *COL2A1* promoter, results in abnormal cartilage development, presumably because the differentiating chondrocytes are maintained in a proliferative state.[264] Mutations or deficiencies in genes encoding the different chains of the collagens type IX,[265-269] type XI,[270] or type X[271,272] also result in abnormal skeletal development and subsequent loss of cartilage matrix integrity. Defects in type X collagen result in abnormalities in endochondral ossification and growth plate formation associated with defective hematopoiesis.[273,274]

Cartilage Proteoglycans

The major proteoglycan in articular cartilage is the large aggregating proteoglycan, or aggrecan, which consists of a core protein of 225 to 250 kD with covalently attached side chains of glycosaminoglycans (GAGs), including approximately 100 chondroitin sulfate (CS) chains, 30 keratan sulfate (KS) chains, and shorter N- and O-linked oligosaccharides[98,226,275,276] (see also Chapter 3). Link protein, a small glycoprotein, stabilizes the noncovalent linkage between aggrecan and hyaluronic acid (HA; also called hyaluronan) to form the proteoglycan aggregate that may contain as many as 100 aggrecan monomers. The G1 and G2 N-terminal globular domains of aggrecan and its C-terminal G3 domain have distinct structural properties that function as integral parts of the aggrecan core protein and as cleavage products that accumulate with age or in osteoarthritis. The G2 domain is separated from G1 by a linear interglobular domain and has two proteoglycan tandem repeats, but it does not bind to HA. The G3 domain contains sequence homologies to epidermal growth factor, lectin, and complement regulatory protein, and it participates in growth regulation, cell recognition, intracellular trafficking, and the recognition, assembly, and stabilization of the extracellular matrix. About half of the aggrecan molecules in adult cartilage lack the G3 domain, probably due to proteolytic cleavage during matrix turnover. Small amounts of other large proteoglycans are found in cartilage, including versican, which forms aggregates with HA, and perlecan, which is nonaggregating; however, these proteoglycans function primarily during skeletal development, where versican is expressed in prechondrogenic condensations and perlecan in the cartilage anlagen following expression of type II collagen and aggrecan.[276]

The nonaggregating small proteoglycans are not specific to cartilage, but in cartilage, they are thought to serve important roles in matrix structure and function, primarily by modulating collagen-fibril formation.[226,227,257] Of the more than 10 leucine-rich repeat (LRR) proteoglycans discovered thus far, only osteoadherin is not present in cartilage. The 24-amino acid central LRR domain is conserved, but the N- and C-terminal domains have patterns of cysteine residues involved in intrachain disulfide bonds that distin-guish the four subfamilies: (1) biglycan, decorin, fibromodulin, and lumican; (2) keratocan and PRELP; (3) chondroadherin; and (4) epiphycan/PG-Lb and mimecan/osteoglycin. Biglycan has two GAG chains, either CS or dermatan sulfate (DS), or both, attached near the N-terminus through two closely spaced serine-glycine dipeptides. Decorin contains only one CS or DS chain. Fibromodulin and lumican contain KS chains linked to the central domain of the core protein and several sulfated tyrosine residues in the N-terminus. The negatively charged GAG side chains contribute to fixed charge density of the matrix and, together with the highly anionic tyrosine-sulfation sites, permit multiple-site linkage between adjacent collagen fibrils, thereby stabilizing the network. Decorin, the most extensively studied LRR proteoglycan, binds to several collagens present in cartilage, including types II, VI, XII, and XIV, as well as to fibronectin and thrombospondin. Biglycan, decorin, and fibromodulin bind TGF-β and the epidermal growth factor receptor, and may thereby modulate growth, remodeling, and repair. PRELP[277] and chondroadherin[278] may regulate cell–matrix interactions through binding to syndecan and α2β1 integrin, respectively.

Other Extracellular Matrix and Cell-Surface Proteins

Several other noncollagenous matrix proteins may play important roles in determining cartilage matrix integrity.[227,257] COMP, a member of the thrombospondin family, is a disulfide-bonded, pentameric, 550-kD, calcium-binding protein that constitutes approximately 10 percent of the noncollagenous, nonproteoglycan protein in normal adult cartilage.[279] COMP is localized in the interterritorial matrix of adult articular cartilage where it binds to types II and IX collagens, thereby stabilizing the collagen network; however, it is pericellular in the proliferating region of the growth plate, where it may have a role in cell-matrix interactions.[280] The cartilage matrix protein (CMP, or matrilin-1) and matrilin-3 are expressed in cartilage at certain stages of development and are present in tracheal cartilage, but not in mechanically loaded adult articular or intervertebral disk cartilage.[281,282] Tenascin-c, a glycoprotein that is regulated in development, is characteristic of nonossifying cartilage.[283] A splice variant of tenascin-c mRNA is found in chondrosarcomas.[284] The cartilage intermediate layer protein (CILP) is expressed in the middle to deep zones of articular cartilage as a precursor protein that, when cleaved in conjunction with secretion, has structural similarities with nucleotide pyrophosphohydrolase (although it lacks the catalytic site) and may play a role in pyrophosphate metabolism and calcification.[285,286] Asporin is a recently identified LRR protein related to decorin and biglycan whose function in cartilage is as yet unknown.[287] Glycoprotein-39 (gp39, or YKL-40) is found only in the superficial zone of normal cartilage and stimulates proliferation of chondrocytes and synovial cells.[288] Synthesis or release of these proteins or fragments is often increased in cartilage that is undergoing repair or remodeling. COMP and gp39 have been investigated as markers of cartilage damage in arthritis.[248,289,290]

Other matrix proteins, including fibronectin and tenascin-c, may mediate cell-matrix interactions in cartilage by binding to cell-surface integrins or other membrane proteins.[256] Alternative splicing of fibronectin and tenascin-c mRNAs gives rise to different protein products at different stages of chondrocyte differentiation. Both proteins are increased in osteoarthritic cartilage and may thus serve specific functions in remodeling and repair. Fibronectin fragments that are present in osteoarthritic joints have been shown to stimulate chondrocytes to synthesize cartilage-degrading proteinases.[291] Chondrocytes interact with matrix proteins in the pericellular matrix via specific integrins on the cell surface, including $\alpha5\beta1$, $\alpha2\beta1$ and $\alpha3\beta1$ and $\alpha1\beta1$, which bind fibrorectin, type II collagen, and types I and VI collagens respectively. Other integral membrane proteins found in chondrocytes include the cell-surface proteoglycans CD44 and syndecan-3. CD44 is a receptor for hyaluronan and also binds collagen and fibronectin.[292] Syndecan-3 links to the cell surface via glycosyl phosphatidylinositol and binds tenascin-c, as well as growth factors, proteases and inhibitors, and other matrix molecules, through heparan sulfate side chains on the extracellular domain. Anchorin CII, also known as annexin V, is a 34-kD integral membrane protein that binds type II collagen and shares extensive homology with the calcium-binding proteins calpactin and lipocortin.[293]

AGING, DEGENERATION, AND REPAIR OF ARTICULAR CARTILAGE

Zonal differences in tensile strength and compressive resistance are related to differences in matrix composition and can be observed to change during the aging of adult articular cartilage and in response to traumatic damage.[98] There are also differences in composition of the territorial, or pericellular, matrix and the interterritorial matrix that may change with aging. The chondrocytes are normally surrounded by a 2-µm pericellular matrix, composed of a highly branched filamentous network of collagen VI tetramers, that serves as a scaffold for decorin, biglycan, perlecan, and chondroadherin, which predominate in this region, as well as hyaluronan, fibrilin-1, and PRELP. The interterritorial region, in contrast, contains primarily a collagen II/XI fibril network, which binds decorin, fibromodulin, collagen IX, and COMP, and large numbers of intact aggrecan molecules bound via link protein to long chains of hyaluronic acid. In the deep zone, the interterritorial region most remote from the cells contains a larger number of degraded aggrecan molecules that lack the G3 domain. The turnover of type II collagen in adult articular cartilage is extremely low with a half-life of more than 100 years. Although aggrecan and other proteoglycans continue to be synthesized, the complex interrelationships among all of the matrix components may not be replicated precisely with time or after damage.

THE AGING OF ARTICULAR CARTILAGE

It is important, but often difficult, to distinguish between the effects of aging itself and diseases, such as osteoarthritis, that become more common with increasing age. In both cases, biochemic alterations in matrix composition are reflected in changes in cartilage tructure. The thickness of articular cartilage, as demonstrated by magnetic resonance imaging (MRI), decreases with increasing age.[294] Fatigue fracture of superficial collagen bundles and a heterogeneous depletion of glycosaminoglycans at the periphery of joint surfaces may contribute to the mild splitting and fraying of superficial cartilage, which is termed *fibrillation.* If fibrillation progresses into deeper layers of cartilage, abnormal multicellular clusters of chondrocytes that stain intensely for glycosaminoglycans are found at the base of clefts.[295] Fibrillation, by itself, need not necessarily lead to osteoarthritis.[296] In addition to fibrillation of the articular surface, changes in cartilage matrix proteins that accompany aging increase the risk of degeneration. These changes include decreased size and aggregation of aggrecan and increased collagen denaturation, resulting in the loss of compressive stiffness and tensile strength.[297-300] These alterations are probably the result of age-related changes in chondrocyte function that decrease the ability of the cells to maintain the tissue, including decreased synthetic activity, synthesis of smaller and less-uniform aggrecan molecules and less-functional link proteins, and decreased responsiveness to anabolic growth factors.[301,302] Because the proliferative potential of adult articular chondrocytes decreases with age, replicative senescence associated with erosion of telomere length has been proposed to contribute to the age-related changes in normal chondrocyte function.[303,304]

Proteoglycans in aged cartilage have a wide range of sizes, with small forms resulting from low substitution of glycosaminoglycan residues and shorter lengths compared with glycosaminoglycans in young articular cartilage.[301,305,306] Unsubstituted proteoglycan core proteins of aggrecan and biglycan are detectable in articular cartilage from elderly subjects.[307,308] Hyaluronan content increases in aged cartilage, but with a reduced mean chain length, and link protein also appears to be fragmented.[309,310] Collagen fibrils become thinner with age and are less densely packed.[311] During aging, nonenzymatic glycation results in the formation and accumulation of the advanced-glycation endproduct pentosidine in long-lived proteins, including cartilage collagen[312,313] and aggrecan.[314] Such biochemical changes may result in part from changes in chondrocyte synthetic function with age and also from changes in matrix degradation.[315] Increased and more extensive collagen degradation can be observed in cartilage from older, healthy individuals, and similar to cartilage in early osteoarthritis, the damage is concentrated closer to the articular surface and colocalizes with MMP-13 activity.[316] The relevance of age-related changes in the predisposition to osteoarthritis requires further research. (See Chapter 91 for a detailed discussion of osteoarthritis.)

Markers of Cartilage Matrix Degradation and Turnover

With increasing knowledge of the composition of the cartilage matrix, molecular markers in body fluids have been identified for monitoring changes in cartilage metabolism and for assessing joint damage in arthritis.[247-250] Monoclonal antibodies have been developed that recognize products of proteoglycan or collagen degradation (catabolic epitopes) or synthesis of newly synthesized matrix components (anabolic neo-epitopes), which represent attempts to repair the damaged matrix.[251,317,318] For example, different monoclonal antibodies can distinguish subtle biochemical differences in CS or KS chains that result from degraded versus newly synthesized proteoglycans. Such epitopes can be detected in the synovial fluids and sera of patients with osteoarthritis and rheumatoid arthritis, and the synovial fluid-to-serum ratio can be useful as a diagnostic indicator. Antibodies against synthetic epitopes on aggrecan include 846, 3B3(−), and 7D4.[319,320] Other antibodies recognize specific aggrecanase or MMP cleavage sites in the aggrecan core protein.[321,322] (See Chapter 4.)

Similarly, the synthesis of type II collagen can be monitored by measuring serum and synovial fluid levels of the carboxyl-terminal propeptide, and urinary excretion of hydroxylysyl pyridinoline cross-links may indicate collagen degradation.[318,323] Specific antibodies that recognize epitopes on denatured type II collagen at the collagenase cleavage site (for example, N-terminus of the three-quarter fragment) are promising diagnostic reagents.[323,324] These biomarker assays have been used as research tools and are currently being developed and validated as diagnostic tools for monitoring cartilage degradation or repair in osteoarthritis and rheumatoid arthritis patient populations and for assessment of treatment (see Chapter 50). Although a single marker may not be sufficient, a combination may discriminate between different stages of osteoarthritis in different populations. For example, serum levels of COMP, together with expression of the epitope on aggrecan and increased levels of tumor necrosis factor receptor type II (TNFRII), can discriminate between osteoarthritis patients and normal individuals.[325]

REPAIR OF ARTICULAR CARTILAGE

Articular cartilage has a poor capacity for regeneration, and pharmacologic enhancement of cartilage repair would have considerable potential in the treatment of arthritides and intra-articular fractures.[326] The extent of intrinsic repair of a cartilage defect depends on the depth of the lesion and whether the defect penetrates the subchondral bone plate.[327,328] Repair of superficial defects occurs if the chondrocytes remain viable,[327,329,330] and the synthesis of cartilage-specific matrix components may be enhanced by growth and differentiation factors, such as FGF-2 and the BMPs.[331,332] Due to the avascularity of cartilage, it differs from most other tissues in its response to injury; the vascular-dependent inflammatory and reparative phases of the classic healing response are not available. Thus, partial defects generally do not regenerate because resident chondrocytes cannot migrate into the defect, and there is no vascular access for progenitor cells.[327,328] However, deep cartilage defects with disruption of the subchondral bone plate initiate vascular responses—including bleeding, fibrin clot formation, and inflammation—that permit cell invasion from the blood or underlying bone marrow.[333] The lesion becomes filled by granulation tissue, which is eventually replaced by fibrocartilage but rarely by true hyaline cartilage.[328,333-335] Transplantation of cultured autologous chondrocytes has been used somewhat successfully to repair small, full-thickness lesions in knee cartilage in young adults with sports injuries.[336] Evidence of successful repair has been demonstrated by turnover and remodeling of the initial fibrocartilaginous matrix formed by the transplanted chondrocytes due to enzyme degradation and new synthesis of type II collagen.[337] Major challenges are the restoration of the three-dimensional collagen structure and integration of the newly synthesized matrix with the resident tissue. Transfer of genes encoding insulin-like growth factor (IGF)-I, TGF-β, and BMP-2 to chondrocytes prior to transplantation has been proposed as a strategy to promote cartilage-specific matrix synthesis.[338-342] The capacity of the transplanted chondrocytes to express FGFR3, BMP-2, and type II collagen is predictive of successful repair and regeneration.[343] Additional cartilage-engineering approaches include the use of biocompatible scaffolding materials and bone marrow–derived chondroprogenitor stem cells as gene-delivery vehicles.[344,345]

SUBCHONDRAL BONE INTERACTIONS WITH ARTICULAR CARTILAGE

The subchondral bone plate beneath the calcified base of articular cartilage may have many effects on the cartilage above it. Its stiffness modifies the compressive forces to which articular cartilage is subjected, its blood supply may be important in cartilage nutrition (see following section), and its cells may produce peptides that regulate chondrocyte function.[346,347] Several studies have suggested that the responses of the subchondral bone to mechanical stimulation may transmit signals into the articular cartilage.[348-350] Tidemark advancement with thickening of the calcified cartilage and thinning of articular cartilage is associated with fibrillation of the cartilage surface during aging.[351] An increase in subchondral bone density is an early feature of osteoarthritis.[352] Radin and Rose[353] proposed that the initiation of fibrillation is caused by an increase in subchondral bone stiffness. Recent evidence suggests that these changes in subchondral bone stiffness are secondary to cartilage deterioration, but necessary for progression of osteoarthritic lesions, and involve only bone and calcified cartilage close to the joint.[354]

Synovial Fluid and Nutrition of Joint Structures

The volume and composition of synovial fluid is determined by the properties of the synovium and its vasculature. Fluid in normal joints is present in small quantities (2.5 ml in the normal knee) sufficient to coat the synovial surface but not to separate one surface from the other. Tendon sheath fluid and synovial fluid are biochemically similar. [355] Both are essential for the nutrition and lubrication of adjacent avascular structures, including tendon and articular cartilage, and for limiting adhesion formation, thereby maintaining movement. Characterization and measurement of synovial fluid constituents have proven useful for the identification of locally generated regulatory factors, markers of cartilage turnover, and the metabolic status of the joint, as well as for the assessment of the effects of therapy on cartilage homeostasis. However, interpretation of such data requires an understanding of the generation and clearance of synovial fluid and its various components.

GENERATION AND CLEARANCE OF SYNOVIAL FLUID

Synovial fluid concentrations of a protein represent the net contributions of synovial blood flow, plasma concentration, microvascular permeability, and lymphatic removal, as well as its production and consumption within the joint space. Synovial fluid is an ultrafiltrate of plasma, which contains locally generated factors. Generation of this ultrafiltrate depends on the difference between intracapillary and intra-articular hydrostatic pressures and between colloid osmotic pressures of capillary plasma and synovial tissue fluid. Fenestrations in synovial endothelium (see Fig. 1–9) and the macromolecular sieve of hyaluronic acid[356] permit the selective entry of water and low-molecular-weight solutes into the synovium, assisted—in the case of glucose—by an active transport system.[357,358] Proteins are present in synovial fluid at concentrations inversely proportional to molecular size, with synovial fluid albumin concentrations being about 45 percent of those in plasma[359] (Fig. 1–12). Concentrations of electrolytes and small molecules are equivalent to those in plasma.[360,361]

Synovial fluid is cleared through lymphatics in the synovium, assisted by joint movement. Unlike ultrafiltration, lymphatic clearance of solutes is independent of molecular size. In addition, constituents of synovial fluid, such as regulatory peptides, may be degraded locally by enzymes, and low-molecular-weight metabolites may diffuse along concentration gradients into plasma. Thus, the kinetics of delivery and removal of a

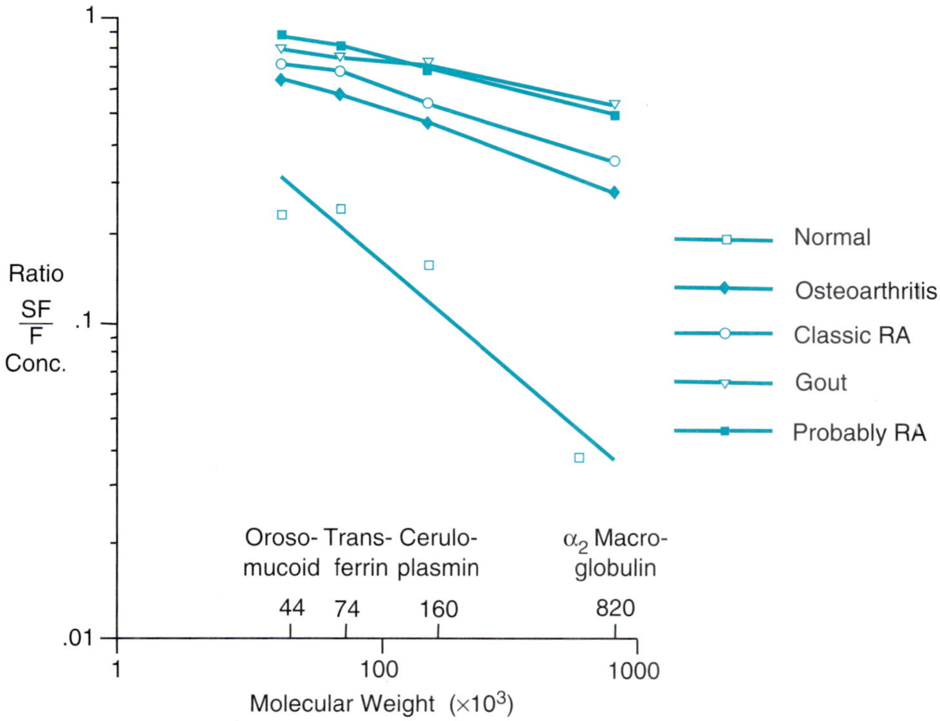

FIGURE 1–12 · Ratio of the concentration of proteins in synovial fluid to that found in serum, plotted as a function of molecular weight. Larger proteins are selectively excluded from normal synovial fluid, but this macromolecular sieve is less effective in diseased synovium. Conc., concentration; RA, rheumatoid arthritis; SF, synovial fluid; S, serum. (From Kushner I, Somerville JA: Permeability of human synovial membrane to plasma proteins. Arthritis Rheum 14;560, 1971. Reprinted with permission of the American College of Rheumatology.)

protein must be determined, using albumin as a reference solute, for example, to assess the significance of its concentration in the joint.[362]

Hyaluronic acid is synthesized by fibroblast-like synovial lining cells, and it appears in high concentrations in synovial fluid at around 3 g/liter, compared to a plasma concentration of 30 μg/liter. Lubricin, a glycoprotein that assists articular lubrication, is another constituent of synovial fluid that is generated by the lining cells.[363] It is now believed that hyaluronan functions in fluid-film lubrication, whereas lubricin is the true boundary lubricant in synovial fluid (see following). Because the volume of synovial fluid is determined by the amount of hyaluronan, water retention appears to be the major function of this large molecule.[364,365]

Despite the absence of a basement membrane, synovial fluid does not mix freely with synovial-tissue fluid. Hyaluronan may trap molecules within the synovial cavity by acting as a filtration screen on the surface of the synovial lining, thereby resisting the movement of synovial fluid out from the joint space.[364] Synovial fluid and its constituent proteins have a rapid turnover time (around 1 hour in normal knees), and equilibrium is not usually reached among all parts of the joint. Tissue fluid around fenestrated endothelium, therefore, is likely to reflect plasma ultrafiltrate most closely, with a low content of hyaluronate compared to synovial fluid. Alternately, locally generated or released peptides, such as endothelin and substance P, may attain much higher perivascular concentrations than those measured in synovial fluid. However, the turnover time for hyaluronan in the normal joint (13 hours) is an order of magnitude slower than that of small solutes and proteins. Thus, association with hyaluronan may result in trapping of solutes within synovial fluid.[366]

SYNOVIAL FLUID AS AN INDICATOR OF JOINT FUNCTION

In the absence of a basement membrane separating synovium or cartilage from synovial fluid, measurements made on synovial fluid may reflect the activity of these structures. A wide range of regulatory factors may be generated locally within the joint, as well as products of synoviocyte metabolism and cartilage breakdown, resulting in marked differences between the composition of synovial fluid and plasma ultrafiltrate.[317,367] Because there is little capacity for the selective concentration of solutes in synovial fluid, those present at higher concentrations than in plasma are probably synthesized locally. However, the local clearance rate must be known to determine whether the solutes present in synovial fluid at lower concentrations than in plasma are generated locally.[361] Although microvascular permeability to protein in highly inflamed rheumatoid joints is more than twice that in osteoarthritic joints, synovial-fluid protein concentrations vary little between the two joint diseases.[368] This is because the enhanced entry of proteins through the microvasculature is largely offset by the increased lymphatic clearance.[369,370] However, because clearance rates from synovial fluid may be slower than those from plasma, synovial fluid levels of drugs or urate, for example, may remain elevated after plasma levels have declined.[358]

Comparisons of synovial fluid constituents between disease groups are often limited by the sparsity of data on normal synovial fluid as a result of difficulties in its collection.[360] Extrapolation from synovial fluid concentrations to local synthetic rates is further complicated because of variations in clearance rates and in synovial fluid volume. Plasma proteins are less effectively filtered in inflamed synovium, perhaps because of increased size of endothelial cell fenestrations or because interstitial hyaluronate-protein complexes are fragmented by enzymes associated with the inflammatory process.[359] Concentrations of proteins, such as α_2 macroglobulin (the principal proteinase inhibitor of plasma), fibrinogen, and immunoglobulin M, therefore, are elevated in inflammatory synovial fluids (see Fig. 1–12), as are associated protein-bound cations. Membrane peptidases may limit the diffusion of regulatory peptides from their sites of release into synovial fluid. In inflammatory arthritis, fibrin deposits may retard flow between the tissue and the liquid phase.

Clearance of synovial fluid and its constituents may be increased in inflamed joints as a result of increased lymphatic drainage,[368] upregulation of membrane peptidases,[101,130] or increased synovial blood flow. Lymphatics, however, appear damaged or depleted in rheumatoid synovium,[135] and there is indirect evidence to suggest that clearance of some synovial fluid components is inadequate in severe inflammation. For instance, complement components and leukocyte-derived proteinases accumulate in synovial fluid in rheumatoid arthritis and may contribute to joint damage.[371,372] Despite these reservations, however, cautious interpretation of synovial-fluid analysis will, no doubt, continue to provide useful information about synovial function (see Chapter 46).

LUBRICATION AND NUTRITION OF THE ARTICULAR CARTILAGE

Lubrication

Synovial fluid serves as a lubricant for articular cartilage, as well as a source of nutrition for the chondrocytes within. Lubrication is essential for protecting cartilage and other joint structures from friction and shear stresses associated with movement under loading.[373] There are two basic categories of joint lubrication. In *fluid-film lubrication*, cartilage surfaces are separated by an incompressible fluid film; hyaluronan functions as the lubricant. In *boundary lubrication*, specialized molecules attached to the cartilage surface permit surface-to-surface contact while decreasing the coefficient of friction.

During loading, a film of fluid is trapped between opposing cartilage surfaces, and because the fluid film is noncompressible, it prevents the surfaces from touching, resulting in so-called "squeeze-film" lubrication.[374] Irregularities in the cartilage surface and its deformation during compression may augment this trapping of fluid. Fluid and low-molecular-weight solutes are forced into articular cartilage from the synovial cavity, thereby concentrating a hyaluronic acid–protein macromolecular gel between cartilage surfaces, preventing cartilage-cartilage contact and "boosting" lubrication.[375] This stable gel layer is approximately 0.1 μm thick in the normal human hip joint, but it can be much thinner in the presence of inflammatory synovial fluids or with increased cartilage porosity.[376,377]

Lubricin is the major boundary lubricant in the human joint.[363] It is a glycoprotein, also called bovine synovial lubricating factor and superficial zone protein (SZP),[123,378] that is synthesized by synovial cells. It has a molecular weight of 225,000, is 200 nm in length, and is 1 to 2 nm in diameter.[123] Dipalmitoyl phosphatidylcholine, which constitutes 45 percent of the lipid in normal synovial fluid, may act together with lubricin as a boundary lubricant.[379] Recent work indicates that lubricin functions as a phospholipid carrier via a mechanism that is common to all tissues.[380,381] Lipid composes 1 to 2 percent of dry weight of cartilage,[382] and experimental treatment of cartilage surfaces with fat solvents impairs lubrication qualities.[383]

Nutrition

As demonstrated by William Hunter[384] in 1743, normal adult articular cartilage contains no blood vessels. Vascularization of cartilage would be expected to alter its mechanical properties. Furthermore, blood flow would be repeatedly occluded during weight bearing and exercise, with reactive oxygen species generated during reperfusion, resulting in repeated damage to both cartilage matrix and chondrocytes. Chondrocytes synthesize specific inhibitors of angiogenesis that maintain articular cartilage as an avascular tissue.[385-387] As a result of the lack of adjacent blood vessels, the chondrocyte normally lives in a hypoxic and acidotic environment, with extracellular fluid pH values around 7.1 to 7.2,[388] and it uses anaerobic glycolysis for energy production.[389] High lactate levels in normal synovial fluid, compared to paired plasma measurements, partly reflect this anaerobic metabolism.[390] There are two sources of nutrients for articular cartilage: (1) the synovial fluid and (2) subchondral blood vessels.

The synovial fluid and, indirectly, the synovial lining, through which synovial fluid is generated, are the major sources of nutrients for articular cartilage. The extracellular fluid of articular cartilage is continuous with synovial fluid, with no intervening basement membrane, and solutes pass easily from the synovial fluid into cartilage. Articular cartilage cannot survive without contact with synovial fluid in vivo; indeed, loose bodies of cartilage in joints actually grow in size.[391] In experimental systems, simple agitation of synovial fluid results in nourishment of even the deepest layers of articular cartilage.[392] Nutrients may enter cartilage from synovial fluid either by diffusion or by mass transport of fluid during compression-relaxation cycles. Molecules as large as hemoglobin (65 kD) can diffuse through normal articular cartilage,[392] and the solutes needed for cellular metabolism are much smaller. It is of interest that diffusion of uncharged small solutes, such as glucose, is not impaired in matrices containing large amounts of glycosaminoglycans, and diffusivity of small molecules through hyaluronate is actually enhanced.[393,394]

Intermittent compression may serve as a pump mechanism for solute exchange in cartilage. The concept has arisen from observations that joint immobilization[395] or dislocation[396] leads to degenerative changes. Exercise, in contrast, increases solute penetration into cartilage in experimental systems.[392] Pressing filter paper against cartilage squeezes out liquid that has the ionic composition of extracellular fluid.[397] McCutchen[398] suggested that during weight bearing, fluid escapes from the load-bearing region by flow to other cartilage sites. When the load is removed, cartilage reexpands and draws back fluid, thereby exchanging nutrients with waste materials.

In the growing child, the deeper layers of cartilage are vascularized, such that blood vessels penetrate between columns of chondrocytes in the hypertrophic zone of the growth plate. It is likely that nutrients diffuse from these tiny end capillaries through the matrix to chondrocytes. Diffusion from subchondral blood vessels is not considered a major route for the nutrition of normal adult articular cartilage because of the barrier provided by its densely calcified lower layer, the "tidemark."[347] Nonetheless, partial defects may normally exist in this barrier,[399] and in pathologic states such as rheumatoid arthritis, neovascularization of the deeper layers of articular cartilage may contribute to cartilage nutrition, as well as to entry of inflammatory cells and cytokines.[400] Furthermore, experimental studies have indicated that cartilage lesions of chondromalacia may develop if the subchondral blood supply of the patella is compromised.[401]

Summary and Conclusion

Normal human synovial joints are complex structures comprised of interacting connective tissue elements that permit constrained and low-friction movement of adjacent bones. The development of synovial joints in the embryo represents a highly ordered process involving complex cell–cell and cell–matrix interactions that lead to the formation of the cartilage anlage and interzone and joint cavitation. Recent understanding of the cellular interactions and molecular factors involved in cartilage morphogenesis and limb development has provided clues to understanding the functions of the synovium, articular cartilage, and associated structures in the mature joint.

The synovial joint is uniquely adapted to responding to environmental and mechanical demands. The synovial lining is composed of two to three cell layers, and there is no basement membrane separating the lining cells from the underlying connective tissue. The synovium produces synovial fluid, which provides nutrition and lubrication to the avascular articular cartilage. Normal articular cartilage contains a single cell type, the articular chondrocyte, which is responsible for maintaining the integrity of the extracellular cartilage matrix. This matrix consists of a complex network of collagens, proteoglycans, and other noncollagenous proteins, which provide tensile strength and compressive resistance. These proteins are distributed differentially within the pericellular, territorial, and interterritorial regions from the superficial to deep zones.

Maintenance of the composition and organization of matrix components is crucial for normal joint function, which is compromised in response to inflammation, biomechanic injury, and aging. Knowledge of the normal structure-function relationships within joint tissues is essential for understanding the pathogenesis and consequences of joint diseases.

REFERENCES

1. Simkin PA: The muskuloskeletal system. A. joints. *In* Klippel JH, Crofford LJ, Stone JH, Weyand CM (eds): Primer on the Rheumatic Diseases. Atlanta, Arthritis Foundation, 2001, pp 5-9.
2. O'Rahilly R, Gardner E: The timing and sequence of events in the development of the limbs in the human embryo. Anat Embryol (Berl) 148:1-23, 1975.
3. Sledge C, Zaleske D: Developmental anatomy of joints. *In* Resnick D, Niwayama G (eds): Diagnosis of Bone and Joint Disorders. Philadelphia, WB Saunders, 1988, pp 2-20.
4. O'Rahilly R, Muller F: Human Embryology and Teratology. New York, Wiley-Liss, 1996.
5. O'Rahilly R, Gardner E: The embryology of movable joints. *In* Sokoloff L (ed): The Joints and Synovial Fluid. New York, Academic Press, 1978, pp 49.
6. Hall BK, Miyake T: All for one and one for all: Condensations and the initiation of skeletal development. Bioessays 22:138-147, 2000.
7. Fell HB: The histogenesis of cartilage and bone in the long bones of the embryonic fowl. J Morphol Physiol 40:417-459, 1925.
8. DeLise AM, Fischer L, Tuan RS: Cellular interactions and signaling in cartilage development. Osteoarthritis Cartilage 8:309-334, 2000.
9. Zwilling E: Limb morphogenesis. Dev Biol 28:12-17, 1972.
10. Cohn MJ, Tickle C: Limbs: A model for pattern formation within the vertebrate body plan. Trends Genet 12:253-257, 1996.
11. Ng JK, Tamura K, Buscher D, Izpisua-Belmonte JC: Molecular and cellular basis of pattern formation during vertebrate limb development. Curr Top Dev Biol 41:37-66, 1999.
12. Davidson DR, Crawley A, Hill RE, Tickle C: Position-dependent expression of two related homeobox genes in developing vertebrate limbs. Nature 352:429-431, 1991.
13. Riddle RD, Tabin C: How limbs develop. Sci Am 280:74-79, 1999.
14. Kengaku M, Capdevila J, Rodriguez-Esteban C, et al: Distinct WNT pathways regulating AER formation and dorsoventral polarity in the chick limb bud. Science 280:1274-1277, 1998.
15. Johnson RL, Riddle RD, Tabin CJ: Mechanisms of limb patterning. Curr Opin Genet Dev 4:535-542, 1994.
16. Riddle RD, Johnson RL, Laufer E, Tabin C: Sonic hedgehog mediates the polarizing activity of the ZPA. Cell 75:1401-1416, 1993.
17. Yang Y, Niswander L: Interaction between the signaling molecules WNT7a and SHH during vertebrate limb development: dorsal signals regulate anteroposterior patterning. Cell 80:939-947, 1995.
18. Laufer E, Nelson CE, Johnson RL, et al: Sonic hedgehog and Fgf-4 act through a signaling cascade and feedback loop to integrate growth and patterning of the developing limb bud. Cell 79:993-1003, 1994.
19. Roberts DJ, Johnson RL, Burke AC, et al: Sonic hedgehog is an endodermal signal inducing Bmp-4 and Hox genes during induction and regionalization of the chick hindgut. Development 121:3163-3174, 1995.
20. Bitgood MJ, McMahon AP: Hedgehog and Bmp genes are coexpressed at many diverse sites of cell-cell interaction in the mouse embryo. Dev Biol 172:126-138, 1995.
21. Parr BA, McMahon AP: Dorsalizing signal Wnt-7a required for normal polarity of D-V and A-P axes of mouse limb. Nature 374:350-353, 1995.
22. Niswander L: Limb mutants: What can they tell us about normal limb development? Curr Opin Genet Dev 7:530-536, 1997.
23. Irvine KD, Vogt TF: Dorsal-ventral signalling in limb development. Curr Opin Cell Biol 8:867-876, 1997.
24. Olsen BR, Reginato AM, Wang W: Bone development. Annu Rev Cell Dev Biol 16:191-220, 2000.
25. Wright E, Hargrave MR, Christiansen J, et al: The Sry-related gene Sox9 is expressed during chondrogenesis in mouse embryos. Nat Genet 9:15-20, 1995.
26. Bell DM, Leung KK, Wheatley SC, et al: SOX9 directly regulates the type-II collagen gene. Nat Genet 16:174-178, 1997.
27. Ng LJ, Wheatley S, Muscat GE, et al: SOX9 binds DNA, activates transcription, and coexpresses with type II collagen during chondrogenesis in the mouse. Dev Biol 183:108-121, 1997.
28. Hui CC, Slusarski D, Platt KA, et al: Expression of three mouse homologs of the Drosophila segment polarity gene cubitus interruptus, Gli, Gli-2, and Gli-3, in ectoderm- and mesoderm-derived tissues suggests multiple roles during postimplantation development. Dev Biol 162:402-413, 1994.
29. Marigo V, Davey RA, Zuo Y, et al: Biochemical evidence that patched is the Hedgehog receptor. Nature 384:176-179, 1996.
30. Vortkamp A, Lee K, Lanske B, et al: Regulation of rate of cartilage differentiation by Indian hedgehog and PTH-related protein. Science 273:613-622, 1996.
31. Iwasaki M, Le AX, Helms JA: Expression of indian hedgehog, bone morphogenetic protein 6 and gli during skeletal morphogenesis. Mech Dev 69:197-202, 1997.
32. St-Jacques B, Hammerschmidt M, McMahon AP: Indian hedgehog signaling regulates proliferation and differentiation of chondrocytes and is essential for bone formation. Genes Dev 13:2072-2086, 1999.
33. Ducy P, Zhang R, Geoffroy V, et al: Osf2/Cbfa1: A transcriptional activator of osteoblast differentiation. Cell 89:747-754, 1997.
34. Komori T, Yagi H, Nomura S, et al: Targeted disruption of Cbfa1 results in a complete lack of bone formation owing to maturational arrest of osteoblasts. Cell 89:755-764, 1997.
35. Otto F, Thornell AP, Crompton T, et al: Cbfa1, a candidate gene for cleidocranial dysplasia syndrome, is essential for osteoblast differentiation and bone development. Cell 89:765-771, 1997.
36. Pacifici M, Liu M, Koyama E: Joint formation: New findings shed more light on this critical process in skeletogenesis. Curr Opin Orthop 13:339-344, 2002.
37. Church VL, Francis-West P: Wnt signalling during limb development. Int J Dev Biol 46:927-936, 2002.
38. Francis-West PH, Abdelfattah A, Chen P, et al: Mechanisms of GDF-5 action during skeletal development. Development 126:1305-1315, 1999.
39. Edwards CJ, Francis-West PH: Bone morphogenetic proteins in the development and healing of synovial joints. Semin Arthritis Rheum 31:33-42, 2001.
40. Xu X, Weinstein M, Li C, Deng C-X: Fibroblast growth factor receptors (FGFRs) and their roles in limb development. Cell Tissue Res 296:33-43, 1999.
41. Minina E, Kreschel C, Naski MC, et al: Interaction of FGF, Ihh/Pthlh, and BMP signaling integrates chondrocyte proliferation and hypertrophic differentiation. Dev Cell 3:439-449, 2002.
42. Iwamoto M, Higuchi Y, Koyama E, et al: Transcription factor ERG variants and functional diversification of chondrocytes during limb long bone development. J Cell Biol 150:27-40, 2000.
43. Lizarraga G, Lichtler A, Upholt WB, Kosher RA: Studies on the role of Cux1 in regulation of the onset of joint formation in the developing limb. Dev Biol 243:44-54, 2002.
44. Hartmann C, Tabin CJ: Wnt-14 plays a pivotal role in inducing synovial joint formation in the developing appendicular skeleton. Cell 104:341-351, 2001.
45. Tsumaki N, Tanaka K, Arikawa-Hirasawa E, et al: Role of CDMP-1 in skeletal morphogenesis: promotion of mesenchymal cell recruitment and chondrocyte differentiation. J Cell Biol 144:161-173, 1999.
46. Storm EE, Kingsley DM: GDF5 coordinates bone and joint formation during digit development. Dev Biol 209:11-27, 1999.

47. Ferguson CM, Miclau T, Hu D, et al: Common molecular pathways in skeletal morphogenesis and repair. Ann N Y Acad Sci 857:33-42, 1998.
48. Lanske B, Karaplis AC, Lee K, et al: PTH/PTHrP receptor in early development and Indian hedgehog-regulated bone growth. Science 273:663-666, 1996.
49. Colnot CI, Helms JA: A molecular analysis of matrix remodeling and angiogenesis during long bone development. Mech Dev 100:245-250, 2001.
50. Jimenez MJ, Balbin M, Lopez JM, et al: Collagenase 3 is a target of Cbfa1, a transcription factor of the runt gene family involved in bone formation. Mol Cell Biol 19:4431-4442, 1999.
51. Kim IS, Otto F, Zabel B, Mundlos S: Regulation of chondrocyte differentiation by Cbfa1. Mech Dev 80:159-170, 1999.
52. von der Mark H, von der Mark K, Gay S: Study of differential collagen synthesis during development of the chick embryo by immunofluorescence. I. Preparation of collagen type I and type II specific antibodies and their application to early stages of the chick embryo. Dev Biol 48:237-249, 1976.
53. Craig FM, Bentley G, Archer CW: The spatial and temporal pattern of collagens I and II and keratan sulphate in the developing chick metatarsophalangeal joint. Development 99:383-391, 1987.
54. Morrison EH, Ferguson MW, Bayliss MT, Archer CW: The development of articular cartilage: I. The spatial and temporal patterns of collagen types. J Anat 189(Pt 1):9-22, 1996.
55. Pitsillides AA, Archer CW, Prehm P, et al: Alterations in hyaluronan synthesis during developing joint cavitation. J Histochem Cytochem 43:263-273, 1995.
56. Murphy JM, Heinegard R, McIntosh A, et al: Distribution of cartilage molecules in the developing mouse joint. Matrix Biol 18:487-497, 1999.
57. Kavanagh E, Osborne AC, Ashhurst DE, Pitsillides AA: Keratan sulfate epitopes exhibit a conserved distribution during joint development that remains undisclosed on the basis of glycosaminoglycan charge density. J Histochem Cytochem 50:1039-1047, 2002.
58. Mundlos S, Olsen BR: Heritable diseases of the skeleton. Part II: Molecular insights into skeletal development-matrix components and their homeostasis. FASEB J 11:227-233, 1997.
59. Kavanagh E, Ashhurst DE: Development and aging of the articular cartilage of the rabbit knee joint: Distribution of biglycan, decorin, and matrilin-1. J Histochem Cytochem 47:1603-1616, 1999.
60. Nalin AM, Greenlee TK, Jr, Sandell LJ: Collagen gene expression during development of avian synovial joints: Transient expression of types II and XI collagen genes in the joint capsule. Dev Dyn 203:352-362, 1995.
61. Mitrovic DR: Development of the metatarsophalangeal joint of the chick embryo: Morphological, ultrastructural and histochemical studies. Am J Anat 150:333-347, 1977.
62. Mitrovic D: Development of the diarthrodial joints in the rat embryo. Am J Anat 151:475-485, 1978.
63. Kimura S, Shiota K: Sequential changes of programmed cell death in developing fetal mouse limbs and its possible roles in limb morphogenesis. J Morphol 229:337-346, 1996.
64. Roach HI, Clarke NM: Physiological cell death of chondrocytes in vivo is not confined to apoptosis. New observations on the mammalian growth plate. J Bone Joint Surg Br 82:601-613, 2000.
65. Edwards JCW, Wilkinson LS, Soothill P, et al: Matrix metalloproteinases in the formation of human synovial joint cavities. J Anat 188(Pt 2):355-360, 1996.
66. Craig FM, Bayliss MT, Bentley G, Archer CW: A role for hyaluronan in joint development. J Anat 171:17-23, 1990.
67. Archer CW, Morrison H, Pitsillides AA: Cellular aspects of the development of diarthrodial joints and articular cartilage. J Anat 184 (Pt 3):447-456, 1994.
68. Edwards JCW, Wilkinson LS, Jones HM, et al: The formation of human synovial joint cavities: A possible role for hyaluronan and CD44 in altered interzone cohesion. J Anat 185(Pt 2):355-367, 1994.
69. Dowthwaite GP, Edwards JC, Pitsillides AA: An essential role for the interaction between hyaluronan and hyaluronan binding proteins during joint development. J Histochem Cytochem 46:641-651, 1998.
70. Persson M: The role of movements in the development of sutural and diarthrodial joints tested by long-term paralysis of chick embryos. J Anat 137(Pt 3):591-599, 1983.
71. Drachman DB, Sokoloff L: The role of movement in embryonic joint development. Dev Biol 14:401, 1966.
72. Yasuda Y: Differentiation of human limb buds in vitro. Anat Rec 175:561, 1973.
73. Merida-Velasco JA, Sanchez-Montesinos I, Espin-Ferra J, et al: Development of the human knee joint. Anat Rec 248:269-278, 1997.
74. Merida-Velasco JA, Sanchez-Montesinos I, Espin-Ferra J, et al: Development of the human elbow joint. Anat Rec 258:166-175, 2000.
75. Merida-Velasco JA, Sanchez-Montesinos I, Espin-Ferra J, et al: Develop- ment of the human knee joint ligaments. Anat Rec 248:259-268, 1997.
76. Izumi S, Takeya M, Takagi K, Takahashi K: Ontogenetic development of synovial A cells in fetal and neonatal rat knee joints. Cell Tissue Res 262:1-8, 1990.
77. Edwards JC: The nature and origins of synovium: Experimental approaches to the study of synoviocyte differentiation. J Anat 184(Pt 3):493-501, 1994.
78. Edwards JCW: Fibroblast biology. Development and differentiation of synovial fibroblasts in arthritis. Arthritis Res 2:344-347, 2000.
79. Hukkanen MV, Mapp PI, Moscoso G, et al: Innervation of the human knee joint, a study in foetal material. Br J Rheumatol 29:32, 1990.
80. Hukkanen M, Konttinen YT, Rees RG, et al: Distribution of nerve endings and sensory neuropeptides in rat synovium, meniscus and bone. Int J Tissue React 14:1-10, 1992.
81. Kardon G: Muscle and tendon morphogenesis in the avian hind limb. Development 125:4019-4032, 1998.
82. Holmes G, Niswander L: Expression of slit-2 and slit-3 during chick development. Dev Dyn 222:301-307, 2001.
83. Simons N: The development of the temperomandibular joint. J Anat 86:326, 1952.
84. Morimoto K, Hashimoto N, Suetsugu T: Prenatal developmental process of human temporomandibular joint. J Prosthet Dent 57:723-730, 1987.
85. Merida-Velasco JR, Rodriguez-Vazquez JF, Merida-Velasco JA, et al: Development of the human temporomandibular joint. Anat Rec 255:20-33, 1999.
86. Bradley SJ: An analysis of self-differentiation of chick limb buds in chorio-allantoic grafts. J Anat 107:479-490, 1970.
87. Walmsley R: The development and growth of the intervertebral disc. Edinburgh Med J 60:341, 1983.
88. Christ B, Wilting J: From somites to vertebral column. Anat Anz 174:23-32, 1992.
89. Bareggi R, Grill V, Sandrucci MA, et al: Developmental pathways of vertebral centra and neural arches in human embryos and fetuses. Anat Embryol (Berl) 187:139-144, 1993.
90. Eyre DR, Matsui Y, Wu JJ: Collagen polymorphisms of the intervertebral disc. Biochem Soc Trans 30:844-848, 2001.
91. Hayes AJ, Benjamin M, Ralphs JR: Extracellular matrix in development of the intervertebral disc. Matrix Biol 20:107-121, 2001.
92. Zhu Y, McAlinden A, Sandell LJ: Type IIA procollagen in development of the human intervertebral disc: Regulated expression of the NH(2)-propeptide by enzymic processing reveals a unique developmental pathway. Dev Dyn 220:350-362, 2001.
93. Bronner-Fraser M: Neural crest cell formation and migration in the developing embryo. FASEB J 8:699-706, 1994.
94. Noden DM: Cell movements and control of patterned tissue assembly during craniofacial development. J Craniofac Genet Dev Biol 11:192-213, 1992.
95. Tam PP, Trainor PA: Specification and segmentation of the paraxial mesoderm. Anat Embryol 189:275-305, 1994.
96. Pizette S, Niswander L: Early steps in limb patterning and chondrogenesis. Novartis Found Symp 232:23-36; discussion 36-46, 2001.
97. Hayes AJ, MacPherson S, Morrison H, et al: The development of articular cartilage: Evidence for an appositional growth mechanism. Anat Embryol (Berl) 203:469-479, 2001.
98. Poole AR: Cartilage in health and disease. *In* Koopman WJ (ed): Arthritis and Allied Conditions: A Textbook of Rheumatology,

14th ed. Philadelphia, Lippincott, Williams & Wilkins, 2001, pp 226-284.
99. Henderson B, Pettipher ER: The synovial lining cell: biology and pathobiology. Semin Arthritis Rheum 15:1-32, 1985.
100. Lydyard PM, Edwards JC: The pathophysiology of rheumatoid arthritis. Clin Exp Rheumatol 12(Suppl 11):S55-58, 1994.
101. Walsh DA, Mapp PI, Wharton J, et al: Neuropeptide degrading enzymes in normal and inflamed human synovium. Am J Pathol 142:1610-1621, 1993.
102. Bassleer R, Lhosest-Gauthier M-P, Renard A-M, et al: Histological structure and functions of synovium. *In* Franchimont P (ed): Articular Synovium. Basel, Karger, 1982, pp 1-26.
103. Pasquali-Ronchetti I, Frizziero L, Guerra D, et al: Aging of the human synovium: an in vivo and ex vivo morphological study. Semin Arthritis Rheum 21:400-414, 1992.
104. Barland P, Novikoff AB, Hamerman D: Electron microscopy of the human synovial membrane. J Cell Biol 14:207-220, 1962.
105. Ghadially F, Roy S: Ultrastructure of Synovial Joints in Health and Disease. London, Butterworths, 1969.
106. Wilkinson LS, Pitsillides AA, Worrall JG, Edwards JC: Light microscopic characterization of the fibroblast-like synovial intimal cell (synoviocyte). Arthritis Rheum 35:1179-1184, 1992.
107. Smith SC, Folefac VA, Osei DK, Revell PA: An immunocytochemical study of the distribution of proline-4-hydroxylase in normal, osteoarthritic and rheumatoid arthritic synovium at both the light and electron microscopic level. Br J Rheumatol 37:287-291, 1998.
108. Qu Z, Garcia CH, O'Rourke LM, et al: Local proliferation of fibroblast-like synoviocytes contributes to synovial hyperplasia. Results of proliferating cell nuclear antigen/cyclin, c-myc, and nucleolar organizer region staining. Arthritis Rheum 37:212-220, 1994.
109. Andersen RB, Gormsen J: Fibrinolytic and fibrin stabilizing activity of synovial membranes. Ann Rheum Dis 29:287-293, 1970.
110. Athanasou NA, Quinn J: Immunocytochemical analysis of human synovial lining cells: Phenotypic relation to other marrow derived cells. Ann Rheum Dis 50:311-315, 1991.
111. Edwards JCW: The muskuloskeletal system. A. synovium. *In* Klippel JH, Crofford LJ, Stone JH, Weyand CM (eds): Primer on the Rheumatic Diseases. Atlanta, Arthritis Foundation, 2001, pp 22-26.
112. Naito M, Umeda S, Takahashi K, Shul z LD: Macrophage differentiation and granulomatous inflammation in osteopetrotic mice (op/op) defective in the production of CSF-1. Mol Reprod Dev 46:85-91, 1997.
113. Yielding KL, Tomkins GM, Bunim JJ: Synthesis of hyaluronic acid by human synovial tissue slices. Science 125:1300-1306, 1957.
114. Worrall JG, Bayliss MT, Edwards JC: Morphological localization of hyaluronan in normal and diseased synovium. J Rheumatol 18:1466-1472, 1991.
115. Henderson KJ, Edwards JC, Worrall JG: Expression of CD44 in normal and rheumatoid synovium and cultured synovial fibroblasts. Ann Rheum Dis 53:729-734, 1994.
116. Wilkinson LS, Edwards JC, Poston RN, Haskard DO: Expression of vascular cell adhesion molecule-1 in normal and inflamed synovium. Lab Invest 68:82-88, 1993.
117. Morales-Ducret J, Wayner E, Elices MJ, et al: Alpha 4/beta 1 integrin (VLA-4) ligands in arthritis. Vascular cell adhesion molecule-1 expression in synovium and on fibroblast-like synoviocytes. J Immunol 149:1424-1431, 1992.
118. Henderson EB, Grootveld M, Farrell A, Smith EC, Thompson PW, Blake DR: A pathological role for damaged hyaluronan in synovitis. Ann Rheum Dis 50:196-200, 1991.
119. Waller HA, Butler MG, McClean JG, et al: Localisation of fibronectin mRNA in the rheumatoid synovium by in situ hybridisation. Ann Rheum Dis 51:735-740, 1992.
120. Waggett AD, Kielty CM, Shuttleworth CA: Microfibrillar elements in the synovial joint: Presence of type VI collagen and fibrillin-containing microfibrils. Ann Rheum Dis 52:449-453, 1993.
121. Worrall JG, Wilkinson LS, Bayliss MT, Edwards JC: Zonal distribution of chondroitin-4-sulphate/dermatan sulphate and chondroitin-6-sulphate in normal and diseased human synovium. Ann Rheum Dis 53:35-38, 1994.
122. Revell PA, al-Saffar N, Fish S, Osei D: Extracellular matrix of the synovial intimal cell layer. Ann Rheum Dis 54:404-407, 1995.
123. Jay GD, Lane BP, Sokoloff L: Characterization of a bovine synovial fluid lubricating factor. III. The interaction with hyaluronic acid. Connect Tissue Res 28:245-255, 1992.
124. Norton WL, Lewis DC, Ziff M: Electron-dense deposits following injection of gold sodium thiomalate and thiomalic acid. Arthritis Rheum 11:436-443, 1968.
125. Roy S, Ghadially FN: Synthesis of hyaluronic acid by synovial cells. J Pathol Bacteriol 93:555-557, 1967.
126. Hamann J, Wishaupt JO, van Lier RA, et al: Expression of the activation antigen CD97 and its ligand CD55 in rheumatoid synovial tissue. Arthritis Rheum 42:650-658, 1999.
127. Cutolo M, Picasso M, Ponassi M, et al: Tenascin and fibronectin distribution in human normal and pathological synovium. J Rheumatol 19:1439-1447, 1992.
128. Demaziere A, Athanasou NA: Adhesion receptors of intimal and subintimal cells of the normal synovial membrane. J Pathol 168:209-215, 1992.
129. Johnson BA, Haines GK, Harlow LA, Koch AE: Adhesion molecule expression in human synovial tissue. Arthritis Rheum 36:137-146, 1993.
130. Mapp PI, Walsh DA, Kidd BL, et al: Localization of the enzyme neutral endopeptidase to the human synovium. J Rheumatol 19:1838-1844, 1992.
131. Stevens CR, Blake DR, Merry P, et al: A comparative study by morphometry of the microvasculature in normal and rheumatoid synovium. Arthritis Rheum 34:1508-1513, 1991.
132. Castor CW: The microscopic structure of normal human synovial tissue. Arthritis Rheum 3:140-151, 1960.
133. Simkin PA: Physiology of normal and abnormal synovium. Semin Arthritis Rheum 21:179-183, 1991.
134. Wilkinson LS, Edwards JC: Microvascular distribution in normal human synovium. J Anat 167:129-136, 1989.
135. Wilkinson LS, Edwards JC: Demonstration of lymphatics in human synovial tissue. Rheumatol Int 11:151-155, 1991.
136. Liew M, Dick WC: The anatomy and physiology of blood flow in a diarthrodial joint. Clin Rheum Dis 7:131-148, 1981.
137. Haywood L, Walsh DA: Vasculature of the normal and arthritic synovial joint. Histol Histopathol 16:277-284, 2001.
138. Lindstrom J: Microvascular anatomy of synovial tissue. Acta Rheum Scand 7:1, 1963.
139. Firestein GS: Starving the synovium: Angiogenesis and inflammation in rheumatoid arthritis. J Clin Invest 103:3-4, 1999.
140. Walsh DA: Angiogenesis and arthritis. Rheumatology (Oxford) 38:103-112, 1999.
141. Koch AE: Review: angiogenesis: implications for rheumatoid arthritis. Arthritis Rheum 41:951-962, 1998.
142. Walsh DA, Wade M, Mapp PI, Blake DR: Focally regulated endothelial proliferation and cell death in human synovium. Am J Pathol 152:691-702, 1998.
143. Storgard CM, Stupack DG, Jonczyk A, et al: Decreased angiogenesis and arthritic disease in rabbits treated with an alphavbeta3 antagonist. J Clin Invest 103:47-54, 1999.
144. Uchida T, Nakashima M, Hirota Y, et al: Immunohistochemical localisation of protein tyrosine kinase receptors Tie-1 and Tie-2 in synovial tissue of rheumatoid arthritis: Correlation with angiogenesis and synovial proliferation. Ann Rheum Dis 59:607-614, 2000.
145. Gravallese EM, Pettit AR, Lee R, et al: Angiopoietin-1 is expressed in the synovium of patients with rheumatoid arthritis and is induced by tumour necrosis factor alpha. Ann Rheum Dis 62:100-107, 2003.
146. Walsh DA, Suzuki T, Knock GA, et al: AT1 receptor characteristics of angiotensin analogue binding in human synovium. Br J Pharmacol 112:435-442, 1994.
147. Wharton J, Rutherford RA, Walsh DA, et al: Autoradiographic localization and analysis of endothelin-1 binding sites in human synovial tissue. Arthritis Rheum 35:894-899, 1992.
148. Mapp PI, Kidd BL, Gibson SJ, et al: Substance P-, calcitonin gene-related peptide- and C-flanking peptide of neuropeptide Y-immunoreactive fibres are present in normal synovium but depleted in patients with rheumatoid arthritis. Neuroscience 37:143-153, 1990.
149. Walsh DA, Catravas J, Wharton J: Angiotensin converting enzyme in human synovium: Increased stromal [(125)I]351A binding in rheumatoid arthritis. Ann Rheum Dis 59:125-131, 2000.

150. Walsh DA, Mapp PI, Wharton J, et al: Localisation and characterisation of substance P binding to human synovial tissue in rheumatoid arthritis. Ann Rheum Dis 51:313-317, 1992.
151. Mapp PI, Klocke R, Walsh DA, Chana JK, et al: Localization of 3-nitrotyrosine to rheumatoid and normal synovium. Arthritis Rheum 44:1534-1539, 2001.
152. Pablos JL, Santiago B, Galindo M, et al: Synoviocyte-derived CXCL12 is displayed on endothelium and induces angiogenesis in rheumatoid arthritis. J Immunol 170:2147-2152, 2003.
153. McDonald JN, Levick JR: Pressure induced deformation of the interstitial route across synovium and its relation to hydraulic conductance. J Rheumatol 17:341-348, 1990.
154. Schumacher HR: The microvasculature of the synovial membrane of the monkey: Ultrastructural studies. Arthritis Rheum 12:387-404, 1969.
155. Levick JR: Microvascular architecture and exchange in synovial joints. Microcirculation 2:217-233, 1995.
156. Merry P, Williams R, Cox N, et al: Comparative study of intra-articular pressure dynamics in joints with acute traumatic and chronic inflammatory effusions: Potential implications for hypoxic-reperfusion injury. Ann Rheum Dis 50:917-920, 1991.
157. Gaffney K, Williams RB, Jolliffe VA, Blake DR: Intra-articular pressure changes in rheumatoid and normal peripheral joints. Ann Rheum Dis 54:670-673, 1995.
158. Gaffney K, Edmonds SE, Stevens CR, Blake DR: Pressure and vascular changes in mobile joints: Implications for inflammatory joint disease. Scand J Rheumatol Suppl 101:21-26, 1995.
159. Myers DB, Palmer DG: Capsular compliance and pressure-volume relationships in normal and arthritic knees. J Bone Joint Surg Br 54:710-716, 1972.
160. Gronlund J, Kofoed H, Svalastoga E: Effect of increased knee joint pressure on oxygen tension and blood flow in subchondral bone. Acta Physiol Scand 121:127-131, 1984.
161. Jayson MI, Dixon AS: Intra-articular pressure in rheumatoid arthritis of the knee. 3. Pressure changes during joint use. Ann Rheum Dis 29:401-408, 1970.
162. Blake DR, Winyard PG, Marok R: The contribution of hypoxia-reperfusion injury to inflammatory synovitis: The influence of reactive oxygen intermediates on the transcriptional control of inflammation. Ann N Y Acad Sci 723:308-317, 1994.
163. Mainardi CL, Walter JM, Spiegel PK, et al: Rheumatoid arthritis: Failure of daily heat therapy to affect its progression. Arch Phys Med Rehabil 60:390-393, 1979.
164. Hollander JL, Horvath SM: The influence of physical therapy procedures on the intra-articular temperature of normal and arthritic subjects. Am J Med Sci 218:543, 1949.
165. Horvath SM, Hollander JL: Intra-articular temperature as a measure of joint reaction. J Clin Invest 28:469, 1949.
166. Oosterveld FG, Rasker JJ: Effects of local heat and cold treatment on surface and articular temperature of arthritic knees. Arthritis Rheum 37:1578-1582, 1994.
167. Harris ED Jr, McCroskery PA: The influence of temperature and fibril stability on degradation of cartilage collagen by rheumatoid synovial collagenase. N Engl J Med 290:1-6, 1974.
168. Ferrell WR, Crighton A, Sturrock RD: Position sense at the proximal interphalangeal joint is distorted in patients with rheumatoid arthritis of finger joints. Exp Physiol 77:675-680, 1992.
169. Dee R: Structure and function of hip joint innervation. Ann R Coll Surg Engl 45:357-374, 1969.
170. Mapp PI: Innervation of the synovium. Ann Rheum Dis 54:398-403, 1995.
171. Buma P, Verschuren C, Versleyen D, et al: Calcitonin gene-related peptide, substance P and GAP-43/B-50 immunoreactivity in the normal and arthrotic knee joint of the mouse. Histochemistry 98:327-339, 1992.
172. Hukkanen M, Platts LA, Corbett SA, et al: Reciprocal age-related changes in GAP-43/B-50, substance P and calcitonin gene-related peptide (CGRP) expression in rat primary sensory neurones and their terminals in the dorsal horn of the spinal cord and subintima of the knee synovium. Neurosci Res 42:251-260, 2002.
173. Yaksh TL: Substance P release from knee joint afferent terminals: modulation by opioids. Brain Res 458:319-324, 1988.
174. Niissalo S, Hukkanen M, Imai S, et al: Neuropeptides in experimental and degenerative arthritis. Ann N Y Acad Sci 966:384-399, 2002.
175. Saito T, Koshino T: Distribution of neuropeptides in synovium of the knee with osteoarthritis. Clin Orthop 172-182, 2000.
176. New HV, Mudge AW: Calcitonin gene-related peptide regulates muscle acetylcholine receptor synthesis. Nature 323:809-811, 1986.
177. Schaible HG, Ebersberger A, Von Banchet GS: Mechanisms of pain in arthritis. Ann N Y Acad Sci 966:343-354, 2002.
178. Amiel D, Frank C, Harwood F, et al: Tendons and ligaments: A morphological and biochemical comparison. J Orthop Res 1:257-265, 1984.
179. Gelberman RH, Goldberg V, An K-N, et al: Tendon. *In* Woo SL-Y, Buckwalter JL (eds): Injury and Repair of the Musculoskeletal Soft Tissues. Park Ridge, Ill., American Academy of Orthopaedic Surgeons, 1988, p 5.
180. Canoso JJ: Bursae, tendons and ligaments. Clin Rheum Dis 7:189, 1981.
181. Clark J, Stechschulte DJ Jr: The interface between bone and tendon at an insertion site: A study of the quadriceps tendon insertion. J Anat 192 (Pt 4):605-616, 1998.
182. Davison PF: The contribution of labile crosslinks to the tensile behavior of tendons. Connect Tissue Res 18:293-305, 1989.
183. Trelstad RL, Hayashi K: Tedon collagen fibrillogenesis: Intracellular sub-assemblies and cell surface changes associated with fibril growth. Dev Biol 71:228-242, 1979.
184. Kieny M, Chevallier A: Autonomy of tendon development in the embryonic chick wing. J Embryol Exp Morphol 49:153-165, 1979.
185. Kannus P, Jozsa L, Kvist M, et al: The effect of immobilization on myotendinous junction: An ultrastructural, histochemical and immunohistochemical study. Acta Physiol Scand 144:387-394, 1992.
186. Cooper RR, Misol S: Tendon and ligament insertion. A light and electron microscopic study. J Bone Joint Surg Am 52:1-20, 1970.
187. Dalton S, Cawston TE, Riley GP, et al: Human shoulder tendon biopsy samples in organ culture produce procollagenase and tissue inhibitor of metalloproteinases. Ann Rheum Dis 54:571-577., 1995.
188. Blevins FT, Djurasovic M, Flatow EL, Vogel KG: Biology of the rotator cuff tendon. Orthop Clin North Am 28:1-16, 1997.
189. Vogel KG, Meyers AB: Proteins in the tensile region of adult bovine deep flexor tendon. Clin Orthop S344-355, 1999.
190. Jain A, Nanchahal J, Troeberg L, et al: Production of cytokines, vascular endothelial growth factor, matrix metalloproteinases, and tissue inhibitor of metalloproteinases 1 by tenosynovium demonstrates its potential for tendon destruction in rheumatoid arthritis. Arthritis Rheum 44:1754-1760, 2001.
191. Tillander B, Franzen L, Norlin R: Fibronectin, MMP-1 and histologic changes in rotator cuff disease. J Orthop Res 20:1358-1364, 2002.
192. Jarvinen TA, Jozsa L, Kannus P, et al: Mechanical loading regulates the expression of tenascin-C in the myotendinous junction and tendon but does not induce de novo synthesis in the skeletal muscle. J Cell Sci 116:857-866, 2003.
193. Vogel KG, Ordog A, Pogany G, Olah J: Proteoglycans in the compressed region of human tibialis posterior tendon and in ligaments. J Orthop Res 11:68-77, 1993.
194. Robbins JR, Vogel KG: Regional expression of mRNA for proteoglycans and collagen in tendon. Eur J Cell Biol 64:264-270, 1994.
195. Berenson MC, Blevins FT, Plaas AH, Vogel KG: Proteoglycans of human rotator cuff tendons. J Orthop Res 14:518-525, 1996.
196. Waggett AD, Ralphs JR, Kwan AP, et al: Characterization of collagens and proteoglycans at the insertion of the human Achilles tendon. Matrix Biol 16:457-470, 1998.
197. Kumagai J, Sarkar K, Uhthoff HK: The collagen types in the attachment zone of rotator cuff tendons in the elderly: an immunohistochemical study. J Rheumatol 21:2096-2100, 1994.
198. Ameye L, Aria D, Jepsen K, et al: Abnormal collagen fibrils in tendons of biglycan/fibromodulin-deficient mice lead to gait impairment, ectopic ossification, and osteoarthritis. FASEB J 16:673-680, 2002.
199. Frank C, Woo S, Andriacchi T, et al: Normal ligament. *In* Woo SL-Y, Buckwalter JL (eds): Injury and Repair of the Musculoskeletal Soft Tissues. Park Ridge, Ill, American Academy of Orthopaedic Surgeons, 1988, p 45.
200. Bessette GC, Hunter RE: The anterior cruciate ligament. Orthopedics 13:551-562, 1990.

201. Nawata K, Minamizaki T, Yamashita Y, Teshima R: Development of the attachment zones in the rat anterior cruciate ligament: changes in the distributions of proliferating cells and fibrillar collagens during postnatal growth. J Orthop Res 20:1339-1344, 2002.
202. Bland YS, Ashhurst DE: Changes in the distribution of fibrillar collagens in the collateral and cruciate ligaments of the rabbit knee joint during fetal and postnatal development. Histochem J 28:325-334, 1996.
203. Gao J, Messner K: Quantitative comparison of soft tissue-bone interface at chondral ligament insertions in the rabbit knee joint. J Anat 188(Pt 2):367-373, 1996.
204. Faryniarz DA, Chaponnier C, Gabbiani G, et al: Myofibroblasts in the healing lapine medial collateral ligament: possible mechanisms of contraction. J Orthop Res 14:228-237, 1996.
205. Frank CB, Hart DA, Shrive NG: Molecular biology and biomechanics of normal and healing ligaments—a review. Osteoarthritis Cartilage 7:130-140, 1999.
206. Kuhns J: Adventitious bursa. Arch Surg 46:687, 1943.
207. Arnoczky SP, Adams M, DeHaven KE, et al: Meniscus. *In* Woo SL-Y, Buckwalter JL (eds): Injury and Repair of the Musculoskeletal Soft Tissues. Park Ridge, Ill, American Academy of Orthopaedic Surgeons, 1988, p 487.
208. Fairbank T: Knee joint changes after meniscectomy. J Bone Joint Surg Br 30:664, 1948.
209. Murrell GA, Maddali S, Horovitz L, et al: The effects of time course after anterior cruciate ligament injury in correlation with meniscal and cartilage loss. Am J Sports Med 29:9-14, 2001.
210. Arnoczky SP, McDevitt CA: The meniscus: structure, function repair, and replacement. *In* Buckwalter JL, Einhorn TA, Simon SR (eds): Orthopaedic Basic Science: Biology and Biomechanics of the Muskuloskeletal System. Park Ridge, Ill, American Academy of Orthopaedic Surgeons, 2000, pp 531-546.
211. Messner K, Gao J: The menisci of the knee joint. Anatomical and functional characteristics, and a rationale for clinical treatment. J Anat 193 (Pt 2):161-178, 1998.
212. Arnoczky SP, Warren RF: The microvasculature of the meniscus and its response to injury. An experimental study in the dog. Am J Sports Med 11:131-141, 1983.
213. Eyre DR, Muir H: The distribution of different molecular species of collagen in fibrous, elastic and hyaline cartilages of the pig. Biochem J 151:595-602, 1975.
214. McDevitt CA, Webber RJ: The ultrastructure and biochemistry of meniscal cartilage. Clin Orthop 8-18, 1990.
215. Roughley PJ, McNicol D, Santer V, Buckwalter J: The presence of a cartilage-like proteoglycan in the adult human meniscus. Biochem J 197:77-83, 1981.
216. Roughley PJ, White RJ: The dermatan sulfate proteoglycans of the adult human meniscus. J Orthop Res 10:631-637, 1992.
217. McAlinden A, Dudhia J, Bolton MC, et al: Age-related changes in the synthesis and mRNA expression of decorin and aggrecan in human meniscus and articular cartilage. Osteoarthritis Cartilage 9:33-41, 2001.
218. Ghadially FN, Lalonde JM, Wedge JH: Ultrastructure of normal and torn menisci of the human knee joint. J Anat 136(Pt 4):773-791, 1983.
219. McDevitt CA, Mukherjee S, Kambic H, Parker R: Emerging concepts of the cell biology of the meniscus. Curr Opin Orthop 13:345-350, 2002.
220. Hellio Le Graverand MP, Ou Y, Schield-Yee T, et al: The cells of the rabbit meniscus: their arrangement, interrelationship, morphological variations and cytoarchitecture. J Anat 198:525-535, 2001.
221. Kambic HE, Futani H, McDevitt CA: Cell, matrix changes and alpha-smooth muscle actin expression in repair of the canine meniscus. Wound Repair Regen 8:554-561, 2000.
222. Ahluwalia S, Fehm M, Murray MM, et al: Distribution of smooth muscle actin-containing cells in the human meniscus. J Orthop Res 19:659-664, 2001.
223. Hu SY, Wang S, Zuo RT, et al: Meniscus and synovial membrane: an electronmicroscopic study on rabbits. Can J Appl Physiol 26:254-260, 2001.
224. Goldring MB: The muskuloskeletal system. B. articular cartilage. *In* Klippel JH, Crofford LJ, Stone JH, Weyand CM (eds): Primer on the Rheumatic Diseases. Atlanta, Arthritis Foundation, 2001, pp 10-16.
225. Stockwell RA, Meachim G: The chondrocytes. *In* Freeman MAR (ed): Adult Articular Cartilage. Tunbridge Wells, England, Pitman Medical, 1979, pp 69-144.
226. Hardingham T: Proteoglycans and glycoaminoglycans. *In* Seibel MJ, Robins SP, Bilezekian JP (eds): Dynamics of Bone and Cartilage Metabolism. New York, Academic Press, 1999, pp 71-81.
227. Heinegard D, Lorenzo P, Saxne T: Noncollagenous proteins: glycoproteins and related proteins. *In* Seibel MJ, Robins SP, Bilezekian JP (eds): Dynamics of Bone and Cartilage Metabolism. New York, Academic Press, 1999, pp 59-69.
228. Poole AR, Pidoux I, Reiner A, Rosenberg L: An immunoelectron microscope study of the organization of proteoglycan monomer, link protein, and collagen in the matrix of articular cartilage. J Cell Biol 93:921-937, 1982.
229. Hunziker EB, Michel M, Studer D: Ultrastructure of adult human articular cartilage matrix after cryotechnical processing. Microsc Res Tech 37:271-284, 1997.
230. Poole AR, Kojima T, Yasuda T, et al: Composition and structure of articular cartilage: A template for tissue repair. Clin Orthop S26-33, 2001.
231. Stockwell RA: Inter-relationship of articular cartilage thickness and cellularity. Ann Rheum Dis 31:424, 1972.
232. Wong M, Wuethrich P, Buschmann MD, et al: Chondrocyte biosynthesis correlates with local tissue strain in statically compressed adult articular cartilage. J Orthop Res 15:189-196, 1997.
233. Muir H, Bullough P, Maroudas A: The distribution of collagen in human articular cartilage with some of its physiological implications. J Bone Joint Surg Br 52:554-563, 1970.
234. Stanescu V, Stanescu R, Maroteaux P: Differences in distribution of type I and type II collagens in the superficial and intermediary zones of articular cartilage. C R Acad Sci Hebd Seances Acad Sci D 283:279-282, 1976.
235. Maroudas A, Muir H, Wingham J: The correlation of fixed negative charge with glycosaminoglycan content of human articular cartilage. Biochim Biophys Acta 177:492-500, 1969.
236. Franzen A, Inerot S, Hejderup SO, Heinegard D: Variations in the composition of bovine hip articular cartilage with distance from the articular surface. Biochem J 195:535-543, 1981.
237. Ratcliffe A, Fryer PR, Hardingham TE: The distribution of aggregating proteoglycans in articular cartilage: Comparison of quantitative immunoelectron microscopy with radioimmunoassay and biochemical analysis. J Histochem Cytochem 32:193-201, 1984.
238. Kempson GE, Muir H, Swanson SA, Freeman MA: Correlations between stiffness and the chemical constituents of cartilage on the human femoral head. Biochim Biophys Acta 215:70-77, 1970.
239. Kempson GE, Muir H, Pollard C, Tuke M: The tensile properties of the cartilage of human femoral condyles related to the content of collagen and glycosaminoglycans. Biochim Biophys Acta 297:456-472, 1973.
240. Schmidt MB, Mow VC, Chun LE, Eyre DR: Effects of proteoglycan extraction on the tensile behavior of articular cartilage. J Orthop Res 8:353-363, 1990.
241. Urban JP, Maroudas A, Bayliss MT, Dillon J: Swelling pressures of proteoglycans at the concentrations found in cartilaginous tissues. Biorheology 16:447-464, 1979.
242. Lai WM, Hou JS, Mow VC: A triphasic theory for the swelling and deformation behaviors of articular cartilage. J Biomech Eng 113:245-258, 1991.
243. von der Mark K: Structure, biosynthesis, and gene regulation of collagens in cartilage and bone. *In* Seibel MJ, Robins SP, Bilezekian JP (eds): Dynamics of Bone and Cartilage Metabolism. New York, Academic Press, 1999, pp 3-29.
244. Eikenberry EF, Bruckner P: Supramolecular structure of cartilage matrix. *In* Seibel MJ, Robins SP, Bilezekian JP (eds): Dynamics of Bone and Cartilage Metabolism. New York, Academic Press, 1999, pp 289-300.
245. Mundlos S, Olsen BR: Heritable diseases of the skeleton. Part II: Molecular insights into skeletal development-matrix components and their homeostasis. FASEB J 11:227-233, 1997.
246. Goldring MB: The role of cytokines as inflammatory mediators in osteoarthritis: Lessons from animal models. Connec Tiss Res 40:1-11, 1999.

247. Thonar EJ-M, Lenz ME, Masuda K, Manicourt D-H: Body fluid markers of cartilage metabolism. *In* Seibel MJ, Robins SP, Bilezekian JP (eds): Dynamics of Bone and Cartilage Metabolism. New York, Academic Press, 1999, pp 453-464.
248. Garnero P, Rousseau J-C, Delmas PD: Molecular basis and clinical use of biochemical markers of bone, cartilage and synovium in joint diseases. Arthritis Rheum 43:953-968, 2000.
249. Goldring SR, Goldring MB: Rheumatoid arthritis and other inflammatory joint pathologies. *In* Seibel MJ, Robins SP, Bilezekian JP (eds): Dynamics of Bone and Cartilage Metabolism. New York, Academic Press, 1999, pp 623-636.
250. Akesson K: Osteoarthritis and degenerative spine pathologies. *In* Seibel MJ, Robins SP, Bilezekian JP (eds): Dynamics of Bone and Cartilage Metabolism. New York, Academic Press, 1999, pp 637-648.
251. Poole AR: Can serum biomarker assays measure the progression of cartilage degeneration in osteoarthritis? Arthritis Rheum 46:2549-2552, 2002.
252. Mayne R: Structure and function of collagen. *In* Koopman WJ (eds): Arthritis and Allied Conditions: A Textbook of Rheumatology. Baltimore, Williams and Wilkins, 1997, pp 207-227.
253. Sandell LJ, Morris N, Robbins JR, Goldring MB: Alternatively spliced type II procollagen mRNAs define distinct populations of cells during vertebral development: Differential expression of the amino-propeptide. J Cell Biol 114:1307-1319, 1991.
254. Aigner T, Zhu Y, Chansky HH, et al: Reexpression of type IIA procollagen by adult articular chondrocytes in osteoarthritic cartilage. Arthritis Rheum 42:1443-1450, 1999.
255. Sandell LJ, Aigner T: Articular cartilage and changes in arthritis. An introduction: cell biology of osteoarthritis. Arthritis Res 3:107-113, 2001.
256. Olsen BR: Matrix molecules and their ligands. *In* Lanza R, Langer R, Chick W (eds): Principles in Tissue Engineering. Austin, Tex., R.G. Landes Company, 1997, pp 47-65.
257. Svensson L, Oldberg A, Heinegard D: Collagen binding proteins. Osteoarthritis Cartilage 9(Suppl A):S23-28, 2001.
258. Aigner T, Dudhia J: Phenotypic modulation of chondrocytes as a potential therapeutic target in osteoarthritis: a hypothesis. Ann Rheum Dis 56:287-291, 1997.
259. Aszodi A, Hunziker EB, Olsen BR, Fassler R: The role of collagen II and cartilage fibril-associated molecules in skeletal development. Osteoarthritis Cartilage 9 (Suppl A):S150-159, 2001.
260. Vikkula M, Metsaranta M, Ala-Kokko L: Type II collagen mutations in rare and common cartilage diseases. Ann Med 26:107-114, 1994.
261. Ritvaniemi P, Korkko J, Bonaventure J, et al: Identification of COL2A1 gene mutations in patients with chondrodysplasias and familial osteoarthritis. Arthritis Rheum 38:999-1004, 1995.
262. Freisinger P, Ala-Kokko L, LeGuellec D, et al: Mutation in the COL2A1 gene in a patient with hypochondrogenesis. Expression of mutated COL2A1 gene is accompanied by expression of genes for type I procollagen in chondrocytes. J Biol Chem 269:13663-13669, 1994.
263. Chan D, Cole WG, Chow CW, et al: A COL2A1 mutation in achondrogenesis type II results in the replacement of type II collagen by type I and III collagens in cartilage. J Biol Chem 270:1747-1753, 1995.
264. Cheah KS, Levy A, Trainor PA, et al: Human COL2A1-directed SV40 T antigen expression in transgenic and chimeric mice results in abnormal skeletal development. J Cell Biol 128:223-237, 1995.
265. Nakata K, Ono K, Miyazaki J, et al: Osteoarthritis associated with mild chondrodysplasia in transgenic mice expressing alpha 1(IX) collagen chains with a central deletion. Proc Natl Acad Sci U S A 90:2870-2874, 1993.
266. Fassler R, Schnegelsberg PN, Dausman J, et al: Mice lacking alpha 1 (IX) collagen develop noninflammatory degenerative joint disease. Proc Natl Acad Sci U S A 91:5070-5074, 1994.
267. Muragaki Y, Mariman EC, van Beersum SE, et al: A mutation in the gene encoding the alpha 2 chain of the fibril-associated collagen IX, COL9A2, causes multiple epiphyseal dysplasia (EDM2). Nat Genet 12:103-105, 1996.
268. Annunen S, Paassilta P, Lohiniva J, et al: An allele of COL9A2 associated with intervertebral disc disease. Science 285:409-412, 1999.
269. Paassilta P, Lohiniva J, Annunen S, et al: COLL9A3 A third locus for multiple epiphyseal dysplasia. Am J Hum Genet 64:1036-1044, 1999.
270. Vikkula M, Mariman EC, Lui VC, et al: Autosomal dominant and recessive osteochondrodysplasias associated with the COL11A2 locus. Cell 80:431-437, 1995.
271. Warman ML, Abbott M, Apte SS, et al: A type X collagen mutation causes Schmid metaphyseal chondrodysplasia. Nat Genet 5:79-82, 1993.
272. Chan D, Jacenko O: Phenotypic and biochemical consequences of collagen X mutations in mice and humans. Matrix Biol 17:169-184, 1998.
273. Jacenko O, Roberts DW, Campbell MR, et al: Linking hematopoiesis to endochondral skeletogenesis through analysis of mice transgenic for collagen X. Am J Pathol 160:2019-2034, 2002.
274. Gress CJ, Jacenko O: Growth plate compressions and altered hematopoiesis in collagen X null mice. J Cell Biol 149:983-993, 2000.
275. Vertel BM: The ins and outs of aggrecan Trends Cell Biol 5:458-464, 1995.
276. Knudson CB, Knudson W: Cartilage proteoglycans. Semin Cell Dev Biol 12:69-78, 2001.
277. Bengtsson E, Neame PJ, Heinegard D, Sommarin Y: The primary structure of a basic leucine-rich repeat protein, PRELP, found in connective tissues. J Biol Chem 270:25639-25644, 1995.
278. Camper L, Heinegard D, Lundgren-Akerlund E: Integrin alpha2beta1 is a receptor for the cartilage matrix protein chondroadherin. J Cell Biol 138:1159-1167, 1997.
279. Hedbom E, Antonsson P, Hjerpe A, et al: Cartilage matrix proteins. An acidic oligomeric protein (COMP) detected only in cartilage. J Biol Chem 267:6132-6136, 1992.
280. Thur J, Rosenberg K, Nitsche DP, et al: Mutations in cartilage oligomeric matrix protein causing pseudoachondroplasia and multiple epiphyseal dysplasia affect binding of calcium and collagen I, II, and IX. J Biol Chem 276:6083-6092, 2001.
281. Zhang Y, Chen Q: Changes of matrilin forms during endochondral ossification. Molecular basis of oligomeric assembly. J Biol Chem 275:32628-32634, 2000.
282. Segat D, Paulsson M, Smyth N: Matrilins: Structure, expression and function. Osteoarthritis Cartilage 9 (Suppl A):S29-35, 2001.
283. Pacifici M: Tenascin-C and the development of articular cartilage. Matrix Biol 14:689-698, 1995.
284. Ghert MA, Qi WN, Erickson HP, et al: Tenascin-C expression and distribution in cultured human chondrocytes and chondrosarcoma cells. J Orthop Res 20:834-841, 2002.
285. Lorenzo P, Bayliss MT, Heinegard D: A novel cartilage protein (CILP) present in the mid-zone of human articular cartilage increases with age. J Biol Chem 273:23463-23468, 1998.
286. Hirose J, Ryan LM, Masuda I: Up-regulated expression of cartilage intermediate-layer protein and ANK in articular hyaline cartilage from patients with calcium pyrophosphate dihydrate crystal deposition disease. Arthritis Rheum 46:3218-3229, 2002.
287. Lorenzo P, Aspberg A, Onnerfjord P, et al: Identification and characterization of asporin. A novel member of the leucine-rich repeat protein family closely related to decorin and biglycan. J Biol Chem 276:12201-12211, 2001.
288. Recklies AD, White C, Ling H: The chitinase 3-like protein human cartilage glycoprotein 39 (HC-gp39) stimulates proliferation of human connective-tissue cells and activates both extracellular signal-regulated kinase- and protein kinase B-mediated signalling pathways. Biochem J 365:119-126, 2002.
289. Sharif M, Saxne T, Shepstone L, et al: Relationship between serum cartilage oligomeric matrix protein levels and disease progression in osteoarthritis of the knee joint. Br J Rheumatol 34:306-310, 1995.
290. Bleasel JF, Poole AR, Heinegard D, et al: Changes in serum cartilage marker levels indicate altered cartilage metabolism in families with the osteoarthritis-related type II collagen gene COL2A1 mutation. Arthritis Rheum 42:39-45, 1999.
291. Homandberg GA: Cartilage damage by matrix degradation products: fibronectin fragments. Clin Orthop S100-107, 2001.
292. Kurtis MS, Tu BP, Gaya OA, et al: Mechanisms of chondrocyte adhesion to cartilage: role of beta1-integrins, CD44, and annexin V. J Orthop Res 19:1122-1130, 2001.

293. von der Mark K, Mollenhauer J: Annexin V interactions with collagen. Cell Mol Life Sci 53:539-545, 1997.
294. Karvonen RL, Negendank WG, Teitge RA, et al: Factors affecting articular cartilage thickness in osteoarthritis and aging. J Rheumatol 21:1310-1318, 1994.
295. Collins DH: Sulphate ($^{35}SO_4$) fixation by human articular cartialge compared in the knee and should joints. Ann Rheum Dis 20:1961, 1961.
296. Byers PD, Contepomi CA, Farkas TA: Post-mortem study of the hip joint. II. Histological basis for limited and progressive cartilage alterations. Ann Rheum Dis 35:114-121, 1976.
297. Bader DL, Kempson GE: The short-term compressive properties of adult human articular cartilage. Biomed Mater Eng 4:245-256, 1994.
298. Kempson GE: Age-related changes in the tensile properties of human articular cartilage: A comparative study between the femoral head of the hip joint and the talus of the ankle joint. Biochim Biophys Acta 1075:223-230, 1991.
299. Aurich M, Poole AR, Reiner A, et al: Matrix homeostasis in aging normal human ankle cartilage. Arthritis Rheum 46:2903-2910, 2002.
300. Martin JA, Buckwalter JA: Aging, articular cartilage chondrocyte senescence and osteoarthritis. Biogerontology 3:257-264, 2002.
301. Bayliss MT, Ali SY: Age-related changes in the composition and structure of human articular-cartilage proteoglycans. Biochem J 176:683-693, 1978.
302. Guerne PA, Blanco F, Kaelin A, et al: Growth factor responsiveness of human articular chondrocytes in aging and development. Arthritis Rheum 38:960-968, 1995.
303. Martin JA, Buckwalter JA: Human chondrocyte senescence and osteoarthritis. Biorheology 39:145-152, 2002.
304. Price JS, Waters JG, Darrah C, Pennington C, Edwards DR, Donell ST, Clark IM: The role of chondrocyte senescence in osteoarthritis. Aging Cell 1:57-65, 2002.
305. Buckwalter JA, Roughley PJ, Rosenberg LC: Age-related changes in cartilage proteoglycans: Quantitative electron microscopic studies. Microsc Res Tech 28:398-408, 1994.
306. Wells T, Davidson C, Morgelin M, et al: Age-related changes in the composition, the molecular stoichiometry and the stability of proteoglycan aggregates extracted from human articular cartilage. Biochem J 370:69-79, 2003.
307. Roughley PJ, White RJ, Magny MC, et al: Non-proteoglycan forms of biglycan increase with age in human articular cartilage. Biochem J 295(Pt 2):421-426, 1993.
308. Vilim V, Fosang AJ: Characterization of proteoglycans isolated from associative extracts of human articular cartilage. Biochem J 293(Pt 1):165-172, 1993.
309. Holmes MW, Bayliss MT, Muir H: Hyaluronic acid in human articular cartilage. Age-related changes in content and size. Biochem J 250:435-441, 1988.
310. Mort JS, Caterson B, Poole AR, Roughley PJ: The origin of human cartilage proteoglycan link-protein heterogeneity and fragmentation during aging. Biochem J 232:805-812, 1985.
311. Wachtel E, Maroudas A, Schneiderman R: Age-related changes in collagen packing of human articular cartilage. Biochim Biophys Acta 1243:239-243, 1995.
312. Uchiyama A, Ohishi T, Takahashi M, et al: Fluorophores from aging human articular cartilage. J Biochem (Tokyo) 110:714-718, 1991.
313. Verzijl N, DeGroot J, Ben ZC, et al: Crosslinking by advanced glycation end products increases the stiffness of the collagen network in human articular cartilage: A possible mechanism through which age is a risk factor for osteoarthritis. Arthritis Rheum 46:114-123, 2002.
314. Verzijl N, DeGroot J, Bank RA, et al: Age-related accumulation of the advanced glycation endproduct pentosidine in human articular cartilage aggrecan: The use of pentosidine levels as a quantitative measure of protein turnover. Matrix Biol 20:409-417, 2001.
315. Hollander AP, Pidoux I, Reiner A, et al: Damage to type II collagen in aging and osteoarthritis starts at the articular surface, originates around chondrocytes, and extends into the cartilage with progressive degeneration. J Clin Invest 96:2859-2869, 1995.
316. Wu W, Billinghurst RC, Pidoux I, et al: Sites of collagenase cleavage and denaturation of type II collagen in aging and osteoarthritic articular cartilage and their relationship to the distribution of matrix metalloproteinase 1 and matrix metalloproteinase 13. Arthritis Rheum 46:2087-2094, 2002.
317. Poole AR: NIH White Paper: Biomarkers, the osteoarthritis initiative. *In* NIAMS News and Events: Bethesda, National Institutes of Health, 2000, *http://www.niams.nih.gov/ne/oi/oabiomarwhipap.htm*
318. Garnero P, Ayral X, Rousseau JC, et al: Uncoupling of type II collagen synthesis and degradation predicts progression of joint damage in patients with knee osteoarthritis. Arthritis Rheum 46:2613-2624, 2002.
319. Visco DM, Johnstone B, Hill MA, et al: Immunohistochemical analysis of 3-B-(-) and 7-D-4 epitope expression in canine osteoarthritis. Arthritis & Rheumatism 36:1718-1725, 1993.
320. Poole AR, Ionescu M, Swan A, Dieppe PA: Changes in cartilage metabolism in arthritis are reflected by altered serum and synovial fluid levels of the cartilage proteoglycan aggrecan. Implications for pathogenesis. J Clin Invest 94:25-33, 1994.
321. Lark MW, Bayne EK, Flanagan J, et al: Aggrecan degradation in human cartilage. Evidence for both matrix metalloproteinase and aggrecanase activity in normal, osteoarthritic, and rheumatoid joints. J Clin Invest 100:93-106, 1997.
322. Hughes CE, Caterson B, Fosang AJ, et al: Monoclonal antibodies that specifically recognize neoepitope sequences generated by 'aggrecanase' and matrix metalloproteinase cleavage of aggrecan: application to catabolism in situ and in vitro. Biochem J 305:799-804, 1995.
323. Nelson F, Dahlberg L, Laverty S, et al: Evidence for altered synthesis of type II collagen in patients with osteoarthritis. J Clin Invest 102:2115-2125, 1998.
324. Dahlberg L, Billinghurst RC, Manner P, et al: Selective enhancement of collagenase-mediated cleavage of resident type II collagen in cultured osteoarthritic cartilage and arrest with a synthetic inhibitor that spares collagenase 1 (matrix metalloproteinase 1). Arthritis Rheum 43:673-682, 2000.
325. Otterness IG, Swindell AC, Zimmerer RO, et al: An analysis of 14 molecular markers for monitoring osteoarthritis: segregation of the markers into clusters and distinguishing osteoarthritis at baseline. Osteoarthritis Cartilage 8:180-185., 2000.
326. Buckwalter JA, Mankin HJ: Articular cartilage repair and transplantation. Arthritis Rheum 41:1331-1342, 1998.
327. Buckwalter JA: Cartilage repair in osteoarthritis. *In* Moskowitz RW, Howell DS, Goldberg VM, Mankin HJ (eds): Osteoarthritis: Diagnosis and Surgical Management. Philadelphia, W.B. Saunders, 1992, pp 71-108.
328. Hunziker EB: Articular cartilage repair: Are the intrinsic biological constraints undermining this process insuperable? Osteoarthritis Cartilage 7:15-28, 1999.
329. Palmoski M, Perricone E, Brandt KD: Development and reversal of a proteoglycan aggregation defect in normal canine knee cartilage after immobilization. Arthritis Rheum 22:508-517, 1979.
330. Reimann I, Christensen SB, Diemer NH: Observations of reversibility of glycosaminoglycan depletion in articular cartilage. Clin Orthop 258-264, 1982.
331. Cuevas P, Burgos J, Baird A: Basic fibroblast growth factor (FGF) promotes cartilage repair in vivo. Biochem Biophys Res Commun 156:611-618, 1988.
332. Nishida Y, Knudson CB, Eger W, et al: Osteogenic protein 1 stimulates cells-associated matrix assembly by normal human articular chondrocytes: Up-regulation of hyaluronan synthase, CD44, and aggrecan. Arthritis Rheum 43:206-214, 2000.
333. Shapiro F, Koide S, Glimcher MJ: Cell origin and differentiation in the repair of full-thickness defects of articular cartilage. J Bone Joint Surg Am 75:532-553, 1993.
334. Landells J: The reactions of injured human articular cartilage. J Bone Joint Surg -Br 39:548, 1957.
335. Meachim G, Osborne G: Repair at the femoral articular cartilage surface in osteoarthritis of the hip. J Pathol 102:1, 1970.
336. Brittberg M, Lindahl A, Nilsson A, et al: Treatment of deep cartilage defects in the knee with autologous chondrocyte transplantation. N Engl J Med 331:889-895, 1994.
337. Roberts S, Hollander AP, Caterson B, et al: Matrix turnover in human cartilage repair tissue in autologous chondrocyte implantation. Arthritis Rheum 44:2586-2598, 2001.
338. Evans CH, Ghivizzani SC, Oligino TA, Robbins PD: Future of adenoviruses in the gene therapy of arthritis. Arthritis Res 3:142-146, 2001.

339. Smith P, Shuler FD, Georgescu HI, et al: Genetic enhancement of matrix synthesis by articular chondrocytes: Comparison of different growth factor genes in the presence and absence of interleukin-1. Arthritis Rheum 43:1156-1164, 2000.
340. S ellers RS, Zhang R, Glasson SS, et al: Repair of articular cartilage defects one year after treatment with recombinant human bone morphogenetic protein-2 (rhBMP-2). J Bone Joint Surg Am 82:151-160, 2000.
341. Hunziker EB: Growth-factor-induced healing of partial-thickness defects in adult articular cartilage. Osteoarthritis Cartilage 9:22-32, 2001.
342. Blunk T, Sieminski AL, Gooch KJ, et al: Differential effects of growth factors on tissue-engineered cartilage. Tissue Eng 8:73-84, 2002.
343. Dell'Accio F, De Bari C, Luyten FP: Molecular markers predictive of the capacity of expanded human articular chondrocytes to form stable cartilage in vivo. Arthritis Rheum 44:1608-1619, 2001.
344. Solchaga LA, Dennis JE, Goldberg VM, Caplan AI: Hyaluronic acid-based polymers as cell carriers for tissue-engineered repair of bone and cartilage. J Orthop Res 17:205-213, 1999.
345. Yoo JU, Barthel TS, Nishimura K, et al: The chondrogenic potential of human bone-marrow-derived mesenchymal progenitor cells. J Bone Joint Surg Am 80:1745-1757, 1998.
346. Burr DB, Radin EL: Trauma as a factor in the initiation of osteoarthritis. *In* Brandt KD (ed): Cartilage Changes in Osteoarthritis. Indianapolis, Indiana University School of Medicine, 1990, pp 73-80.
347. Oegema TR: Cartilage-bone interface (Tidemark). *In* Brandt KD (ed): Cartilage Changes in Osteoarthritis. Indianapolis, Indiana University School of Medicine, 1990, pp 43-52.
348. Radin EL, Burr DB, Caterson B, Fyhrie D, et al: Mechanical determinants of osteoarthrosis. Sem Arthritis Rheum 21:12-21, 1991.
349. Moskowitz RW: Bone remodeling in osteoarthritis: subchondral and osteophytic responses. Osteoarthritis Cartilage 7:323-324, 1999.
350. Westacott CI, Webb GR, Warnock MG, et al: Alteration of cartilage metabolism by cells from osteoarthritic bone. Arthritis Rheum 40:1282-1291, 1997.
351. Green WT Jr, Martin GN, Eanes ED, Sokoloff L: Microradiographic study of the calcified layer of articular cartilage. Arch Pathol 90:151-158, 1970.
352. Reimann I, Mankin HJ, Trahan C: Quantitative histologic analyses of articular cartilage and subchondral bone from osteoarthritic and normal human hips. Acta Orthop Scand 48:63-73, 1977.
353. Radin EL, Rose RM: Role of subchondral bone in the initiation and progression of cartilage damage. Clin Orthop 213:34-40, 1986.
354. Burr DB, Schaffler MB: The involvement of subchondral mineralized tissues in osteoarthrosis: Quantitative microscopic evidence. Microsc Res Tech 37:343-357, 1997.
355. Hagberg L, Heinegard D, Ohlsson K: The contents of macromolecule solutes in flexor tendon sheath fluid and their relation to synovial fluid. A quantitative analysis. J Hand Surg Br 17:167-171, 1992.
356. Nettelbladt E, Sundblad L, Jonsson E: Permeability of the synovial membrane to proteins. Acta Rheum Scand 9:28, 1963.
357. Simkin PA, Pizzorno JE: Transynovial exchange of small molecules in normal human subjects. J Appl Physiol 36:581-587, 1974.
358. Simkin PA: Synovial perfusion and synovial fluid solutes. Ann Rheum Dis 54:424-428, 1995.
359. Kushner I, Somerville JA: Permeability of human synovial membrane to plasma proteins. Relationship to molecular size and inflammation. Arthritis Rheum 14:560-570, 1971.
360. Ropes MW, Bauer EA: Synovial Fluid Changes in Joint Diseases. Cambridge, Mass, Harvard University Press, 1953.
361. Simkin PA: Fluid dynamics of the joint space and trafficking of matrix products. *In* Seibel MJ, Robins SP, Bilezekian JP (eds): Dynamics of Bone and Cartilage Metabolism. New York, Academic Press, 1999, pp 319-324.
362. Levick JR: A method for estimating macromolecular reflection by human synovium, using measurements of intra-articular half lives. Ann Rheum Dis 57:339-344, 1998.
363. Swann DA, Silver FH, Slayter HS, et al: The molecular structure and lubricating activity of lubricin isolated from bovine and human synovial fluids. Biochem J 225:195-201, 1985.
364. Levick JR, McDonald JN: Fluid movement across synovium in healthy joints: Role of synovial fluid macromolecules. Ann Rheum Dis 54:417-423, 1995.
365. Simkin PA, Bassett JE, Koh EM: Synovial perfusion in the human knee: A methodologic analysis. Semin Arthritis Rheum 25:56-66, 1995.
366. Myers SL, Brandt KD: Effects of synovial fluid hyaluronan concentration and molecular size on clearance of protein from the canine knee. J Rheumatol 22:1732-1739, 1995.
367. Simkin PA, Bassett JE: Cartilage matrix molecules in serum and synovial fluid. Curr Opin Rheumatol 7:346-351, 1995.
368. Wallis WJ, Simkin PA, Nelp WB: Protein traffic in human synovial effusions. Arthritis Rheum 30:57-63, 1987.
369. Myers SL, Brandt KD, Eilam O: Even low-grade synovitis significantly accelerates the clearance of protein from the canine knee. Implications for measurement of synovial fluid "markers" of osteoarthritis. Arthritis Rheum 38:1085-1091, 1995.
370. Myers SL, O'Connor BL, Brandt KD: Accelerated clearance of albumin from the osteoarthritic knee: Implications for interpretation of concentrations of "cartilage markers" in synovial fluid. J Rheumatol 23:1744-1748, 1996.
371. Ruddy S, Austen KF: Activation of the complement and properdin systems in rheumatoid arthritis. Ann N Y Acad Sci 256:96-104, 1975.
372. Opdenakker G, Masure S, Grillet B, Van Damme J: Cytokine-mediated regulation of human leukocyte gelatinases and role in arthritis. Lymphokine Cytokine Res 10:317-324, 1991.
373. McCutchen CW: Lubrication of joints. *In* Sokoloff L (ed): The Joints and Synovial Fluid. New York, Academic Press, 1978, p 437.
374. Fein R: Are synovial joints squeeze-film lubricated? Proc Inst Mech Eng 181:125, 1967.
375. Walker PS, Dowson D, Longfield MD, Wright V: "Boosted lubrication" in synovial joints by fluid entrapment and enrichment. Ann Rheum Dis 27:512-520, 1968.
376. Hlavacek M: The role of synovial fluid filtration by cartilage in lubrication of synovial joints—II. Squeeze-film lubrication: homogeneous filtration. J Biomech 26:1151-1160, 1993.
377. Jin ZM, Dowson D, Fisher J: The effect of porosity of articular cartilage on the lubrication of a normal human hip joint. Proc Inst Mech Eng [H] 206:117-124, 1992.
378. Jay GD, Tantravahi U, Britt DE, et al: Homology of lubricin and superficial zone protein (SZP): Products of megakaryocyte stimulating factor (MSF) gene expression by human synovial fibroblasts and articular chondrocytes localized to chromosome 1q25. J Orthop Res 19:677-687, 2001.
379. Williams PF 3rd, Powell GL, LaBerge M: Sliding friction analysis of phosphatidylcholine as a boundary lubricant for articular cartilage. Proc Inst Mech Eng [H] 207:59-66, 1993.
380. Hills BA: Boundary lubrication in vivo. Proc Inst Mech Eng 214:83-94, 2000.
381. Jay GD, Harris DA, Cha CJ: Boundary lubrication by lubricin is mediated by O-linked beta(1-3)Gal-GalNAc oligosaccharides. Glycoconj J 18:807-815, 2001.
382. Stockwell RA: Lipid content of human costal and articular cartilage. Ann Rheum Dis 26:481-486, 1967.
383. Pickard JE, Fisher J, Ingham E, Egan J: Investigation into the effects of proteins and lipids on the frictional properties of articular cartilage. Biomaterials 19:1807-1812, 1998.
384. Hunter W: On the structure and diseases of articulating cartilage. Philos Trans R Soc Lond Biol 42:514, 1743.
385. Brem H, Folkman J: Inhibition of tumor angiogenesis mediated by cartilage. J Exp Med 141:427-439, 1975.
386. Kuettner KE, Pauli BU: Inhibition of neovascularization by a cartilage factor. Ciba Found Symp 100:163-173, 1983.
387. Moses MA, Sudhalter J, Langer R: Identification of an inhibitor of neovascularization from cartilage. Science 248:1408-1410, 1990.
388. Pita JC, Howell DS: Micro-biochemical studies of cartilage. *In* Sokoloff L (ed) The Joints and Synovial Fluid. New York, Academic Press, 1978, p 273.
389. Bywaters E: The metabolism of joint tissues. J Pathol Bacteriol 44:247, 1937.
390. Naughton DP, Haywood R, Blake DR, et al: A comparative evaluation of the metabolic profiles of normal and inflammatory knee-joint synovial fluids by high resolution proton NMR spectroscopy. FEBS Lett 332:221-225, 1993.

391. Strangeways T: The nutrition of the articular cartilage. Br Med J 1:661, 1920.
392. Maroudas A, Bullough P, Swanson SA, Freeman MA: The permeability of articular cartilage. J Bone Joint Surg Br 50:166-177, 1968.
393. Hadler NM: Synovial fluids facilitate small solute diffusivity. Ann Rheum Dis 39:580-585, 1980.
394. O'Hara BP, Urban JP, Maroudas A: Influence of cyclic loading on the nutrition of articular cartilage. Ann Rheum Dis 49:536-539, 1990.
395. Sood SC: A study of the effects of experimental immobilisation on rabbit articular cartilage. J Anat 108:497-507, 1971.
396. Bennett G, Bauer W, Lewis P: Joint changes resulting from patellar displacement and their relation degenerative hip disease. J Bone Joint Surg Am 19:667, 1959.
397. Lewis P, McCutchen CW: Experimental evidence for weeping lubrication in mammalian joints. Nature 184:1285, 1959.
398. McCutchen CW: An approximate equation for weeping lubrication, solved with an electrical analogue. Ann Rheum Dis 34:1975.
399. Mital MA, Millington PF: Osseous pathway of nutrition to articular cartilage of the human femoral head. Lancet 1:842, 1970.
400. Bromley M, Bertfield H, Evanson JM, Woolley DE: Bidirectional erosion of cartilage in the rheumatoid knee joint. Ann Rheum Dis 44:676-681, 1985.
401. Neusel E, Graf J: The influence of subchondral vascularisation on chondromalacia patellae. Arch Orthop Trauma Surg 115:313-315, 1996.

2 Collagen and Elastin

LEENA ALA-KOKKO • DARWIN J. PROCKOP

Connective tissue, or extracellular matrix, is loosely defined as the compartments and components that provide structural support for the body and bind together its cells, organs, and tissues. The major connective tissues are bone, skin, tendons, ligaments, and cartilage. Connective tissue is also a term applied to blood vessels and to synovial spaces and fluids. In effect, however, all organs and tissues contain connective tissue in the form of membranes and septa.

All connective tissues contain large amounts of water, salt, albumin, and other components of plasma. The characteristic feature of connective tissues, however, is that they contain a series of specific macromolecules assembled into large, complex structures that define the size and shape of most organs. Two of the most characteristic macromolecules of connective tissue are the fibrous proteins *collagen* and *elastin*. Connective tissues also contain a series of proteoglycans and related molecules.

The differences among connective tissues such as bone, skin, and cartilage are, in part, attributable to differences in their content of specific macromolecules, such as collagens. Tendons and ligaments, for example, consist primarily of fibrils of type I collagen bound together into large fibers. They also contain small amounts of other types of collagen that bind to, and probably help organize, the fibrils of type I collagen. Cartilage contains large amounts of type II collagen, a protein similar to type I collagen. The fibrils of type II collagen in cartilage form an arcade-like network that is distended by the presence of highly charged proteoglycans that trap large amounts of water and salts. Blood vessels such as the aorta contain large amounts of another fibrillar collagen, known as type III, and large amounts of elastin. The differences among connective tissues also depend on variations in the size, orientation, and packing of collagen fibrils. Fibrils and fibers of type I collagen in tendons are in a parallel orientation; the type I collagen fibrils of skin are randomly oriented in the plane of the skin; and the type I collagen fibrils in cortical bone are deposited in complex helical H arrays around haversian canals. Accordingly, the differences in the morphology and function of connective tissues are based in part on their content of specific macromolecules and in part on the organization of these macromolecules within the extracellular spaces.

Collagen and elastin, the subjects of this chapter, are similar in that they are both tough, fibrous proteins. At the same time, they are dramatically different; the monomers of most collagens spontaneously self-assemble into highly ordered structures, whereas elastin forms amorphous fibrils in which it is difficult to find any evidence of an ordered structure.

Collagens

More than 20 different types of collagens have now been identified in different tissues of vertebrates.[1–3] The family of collagens can be divided into seven subclasses (Table 2–1).

All the fibrillar collagens form fibrils that appear similar when viewed by electron microscopy. They vary in diameter and probably length, but they have a characteristic cross-striated pattern that reflects the gaps between the ends of the molecules found on the surface of the fibrils[4] (Fig. 2–1*A*). The major fibrillar proteins (types I, II, and III) are among the most abundant proteins in the body. Fibrils and fibril bundles or fibers of type I collagen account for 60 to 90 percent of the dry weight of skin, ligaments, and bone (demineralized).

Type I collagen is also found in many other tissues, including the lungs, dentin, and the sclerae of the eyes. In addition, it is the major constituent of mature scars.

Type II collagen accounts for more than half the dry weight of cartilage, and it is found in the vitreous gel of the eye. It is also transiently present in many tissues during embryonic development.

Type III collagen is abundant in large blood vessels and is found in small amounts in most tissues that contain type I collagen, but it is not present in bone. Of special interest is a large percentage of the type III collagen found in some tissues, particularly skin: It is found in a partially processed precursor form that retains the N propeptides (see discussion later in chapter). The partially processed form, defined as type III pNcollagen, binds to the surface of type I collagen fibrils and thereby limits their lateral growth.[5] The less abundant fibrillar collagen, known as *type V* collagen, is found as thin fibrils in the synovial membranes, lung, skin, and a few other tissues.

Type XI collagen, another fibril-forming collagen, is uniformly distributed in articular cartilage, where it accounts for about 5 percent of the total collagen. The fibrils formed by type V and type XI collagens appear to be similar to those of the major fibrillar collagens, but they have not been studied as extensively.[3]

A second class of collagens (types IV, VIII and X)is defined as network-forming collagens. Type IV collagen is an example of a large, network-forming collagen and is a major constituent of all major membranes.

TABLE 2–1 • MAJOR TYPES OF COLLAGEN AND THEIR α-CHAINS AND TISSUE DISTRIBUTION

Classes	α-Chains	Tissue Distribution
Fibril-Forming Collagens		
Type I	α1(I), α2(I)	Most connective tissues; abundant in bone, skin, and tendon
Type II	α1(II)	Cartilage, intervertebral disk, vitreous humor
Type III	α1(III)	Most connective tissues, particularly skin, lung, blood vessels
Type V	α1(V), α2(V), α3(V)	Tissues containing type I collagen, quantitatively minor component
Type XI	α1(XI), α2(XI), α3(XI)	Cartilage, intervertebral disk, vitreous humor
Network-Forming Collagens		
Type IV	α1(IV), α2(IV), α3(IV), α4(IV), α5(IV), α6(IV)	Basement membranes
Type VIII	α1(VIII), α2(VIII)	Several tissues, especially endothelium
Type X	α1(X)	Hypertrophic cartilage
FACIT Collagens		
Type IX	α1(IX), α2(IX), α3(IX)	Cartilage, intervertebral disk, vitreous humor
Type XII	α1(XII)	Tissues containing type I collagen
Type XIV	α1(XIV)	Tissues containing type I collagen
Type XVI	α1(XVI)	Several tissues
Type XIX	α1(XIX)	Rhabdomyosarcoma cells
Beaded Filament-Forming Collagen		
Type VI	α1(VI), α2(VI), α3(VI)	Most connective tissues
Collagen of Anchoring Fibrils		
Type VII	α1(VII)	Skin, oral mucosa, cervix, cornea
Collagens with a Transmembrane Domain		
Type XIII	α1(XIII)	Endomysium, perichondrium, placenta, mucosa of the intestine, meninges
Type XVII	α1(XVII)	Skin, cornea
Collagen Types XV and XVIII		
Type XV	α1(XV)	Many tissues, especially skeletal and heart muscle, placenta
Type XVIII	α1(XVIII)	Many tissues, especially kidney, liver, lung

Monomers of the protein bind to one another through globular extensions found at both ends of the molecule to form large structures resembling a wire network (Fig. 2–2). The network formed by type IV collagen serves as a scaffold for the binding of other membrane constituents, such as laminin, nidogen, and large heparan sulfate proteoglycans. The decorated scaffold then serves as an important barrier to fluids and solids and as an important surface for the attachment and movement of cells.

The two other network-forming collagens, type VIII and type X, have a structure different from that of type IV but similar to each other. The α1(VIII), α2(VIII), and α1(X) chains all contain a collagenous sequence of almost the same size and with eight imperfections in similar positions in the -Gly-X-Y-sequences. Descemet's membrane, which separates the corneal endothelial cells from the stromal, consists of stacks of hexagonal lattices made of type VIII collagen.[3] Type X collagen is among the most specialized of the collagens and is synthesized primarily by hypertrophic chondrocytes in the deep calcifying zone of cartilage. The assembled form of type X collagen resembles the hexagonal lattice of type VIII in Descemet's membrane.

The **f**ibril-**a**ssociated **c**ollagens with **i**nterrupted **t**riple helices (FACIT collagens, types IX, XII, XIV, XVI, XIX) do not form fibrils themselves but are found attached to the surfaces of preexisting fibrils of the fibril-forming collagens. All these collagens are characterized by short triple-helical domains, interrupted by short noncollagenous sequences.

The type IX collagen molecule consists of three triple-helical domains and four noncollagenous domains. The protein is commonly found on the surface of fibrils of type II collagen, covalently bound to molecules of type II collagen in antiparallel orientation. One unusual feature of collagen IX is that a side chain of glycosaminoglycans is covalently attached to the third noncollagenous domain of the α2(IX)-chain.

Type VI collagen is referred to as a beaded filament-forming collagen because of structures it forms in a variety of connective tissues. Each of the three different chains of protein contains a short triple-helical domain; the remainder consists of large N-terminal and C-terminal globular domains.

Type VII is the collagen of the anchoring fibrils that link basement membranes to the plaques of type IV collagen and laminin in the underlying matrix of structures such as skin. The triple-helical domain of type VII collagen is longer than the triple-helical domain of any other known collagen. The protein is first assembled into antiparallel dimers, formed by a small overlap at the C-terminal globular domains. The dimers then associate laterally and, in register, become the main constituents of anchoring fibrils.

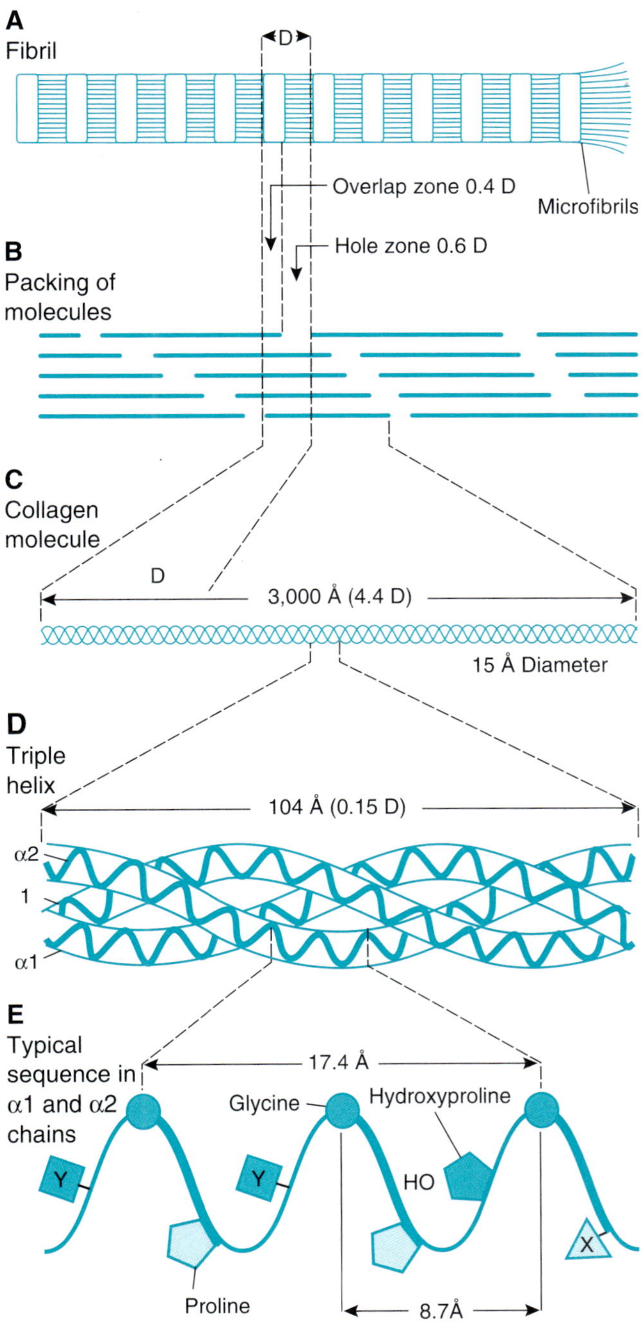

FIGURE 2–1 · A–E, Schematic Representation of the Structure of a Fibril of Type I Collagen. (From Prockop DJ, Guzman NA: Collagen diseases and the biosynthesis of collagen. Hosp Pract 12:61-68, 1977. © 1977, The McGraw-Hill Companies, Inc. Illustration by Bunji Tagawa.)

Two recently discovered collagens contain a transmembrane domain and, therefore, are not secreted in the extracellular matrix. Type XIII collagen is found in many tissues. In contrast, type XVII collagen is found primarily in the hemidesmosomes of the skin and is one of the two antigens that produce the autoimmune disease bullous pemphigoid. These two collagens are not homologous in structure, but they contain a single transmembrane domain and an N-terminal domain that is apparently cytoplasmic. The remainder of the molecule is extracellular.

Two other recently discovered collagens, type XV and type XVIII, apparently constitute a separate class. They have a large N-terminal globular domain, a highly interrupted triple helix, and a large C-terminal globular domain. Both collagens contain several potential attachment sites for serine-linked glycosaminoglycans and asparagine-linked oligosaccharides, which suggests that these collagens may be extensively glycosylated. A fragment of 20 kD from the C terminus of type XVIII collagen was shown to be identical to an antiangiogenic factor called endostatin.[6] Both type XV and type XVIII collagen are found in many tissues, but type XVIII collagen is expressed at much higher levels in liver.[7]

STRUCTURE OF COLLAGEN FIBRILS

The fibrils formed by the fibrillar collagens consist almost entirely of monomers of the protein tightly packed in a quarter-stagger array (see Fig. 2–1). The molecular structure of type I collagen is composed of two identical polypeptide chains, called α1(I), and one slightly different polypeptide chain, called α2(I) (see Table 2–1). Type II collagen is a homotrimer made of three identical α1(II)-chains, and type III collagen is a homotrimer composed of three α1(III)-chains. The structure of each α-chain of the fibrillar collagens is highly repetitive. Glycine is every third amino acid, and each α-chain has about 1000 amino acids. Therefore, the sequence of each α-chain can be defined as $(Gly\text{-}X\text{-}Y)_{333}$. The X position in the sequence is frequently occupied by proline, and the Y position is frequently occupied by hydroxyproline, an unusual amino acid that is abundant in collagen but rare in any other protein. An important feature of the triple helix of collagen is that the glycine residues are packed into a restricted space near the center of the triple helix, which can accommodate only glycine, the smallest amino acid residue.[1] Because proline and hydroxyproline are saturated-ring amino acids, they keep the α-chains in an extended configuration that stabilizes the structure of the triple helix. Some of the X and Y positions in each α-chain contain hydrophobic or charged amino acids, which appear in clusters. The clusters of hydrophobic and charged amino acids are on the surface of the triple helix, and direct binding of one molecule to another so that each is quarter-staggered relative to its nearest neighbor in a fibril (see Fig. 2–1). Each of the α-chains of a fibrillar collagen also contains short sequences of about 25 amino acids at each end (known as telopeptides) that do not have a triple-helical structure and that play an important, but incompletely defined, role in assembly of the proteins into fibrils.

All collagens have at least one triple-helical domain similar to the large triple-helical domain that accounts for most of the structure of a fibrillar collagen. In the nonfibrillar collagens, however, the repetitive Gly-X-Y sequences are frequently interrupted by short regions of other amino acid sequences that introduce more flexible hinge regions into the proteins. Type IV collagen, for

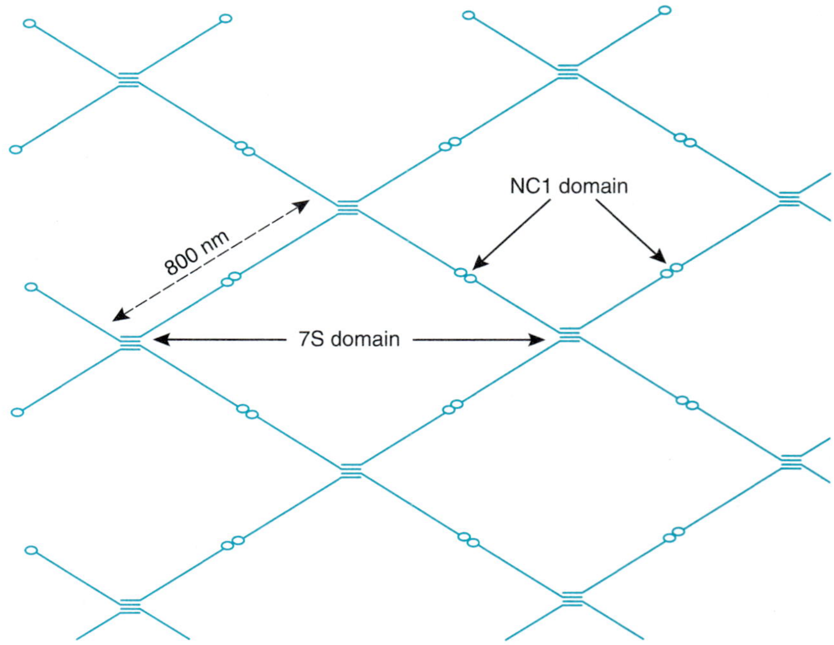

FIGURE 2–2 · Schematic Representation of the Network-like Structures formed by the Assembly of type IV Collagen in Basement Membranes. The NC1 domains are the globular extensions at the C-terminus of the molecule. The 7S domains are noncollagenous domains at the N-terminus of the protein.

example, has numerous short interruptions of its large triple-helical domain that are probably important for its assembly into network-like structures (see Fig. 2–2) or binding of other basement-membrane constituents. One of the hinge regions of type IX collagen is an attachment site for chondroitin sulfate.

STRUCTURE OF COLLAGEN GENES

The genes for collagens have several unusual features. Each of the genes for the major fibrillar collagens (types I, II, and III) has over 40 exons that code for the large triple-helical domain of the protein.[1–3,8] The most common exon size is 54 base pairs (bp); some exons are 108 bp (twice 54), and one is 162 (three times 54). Still other exons are variations on the 54-bp theme in that they are 99 bp (54 plus 45). With one exception, the sizes of specific exons are identical in the two genes for type I procollagen (*COL1A1* and *COL1A2*), the gene for type II procollagen (*COL2A1*), and the gene for type III procollagen (*COL3A1*). In addition, the same exons have the same sizes in genes from humans, rodents, and chickens. The unusual 54-bp motif of the genes for fibrillar collagens may indicate either that the genes arose by duplication of a 54-bp exon or that the molecular mechanisms for replication of the genes specifically perpetuate a 54-bp motif.

The same 54-bp motif is seen in parts of the structures for nonfibrillar collagens. However, some of the exons of the genes for these other collagens have varying structures, and many of the exons begin with the second base for a glycine codon rather than a complete codon for glycine, as seen in the exons for fibrillar collagens.

BIOSYNTHESIS

The biosynthesis of collagen involves a large number of post-translational processing steps.[1]

The major fibrillar collagens (types I, II, and III) are first assembled as large precursor procollagens that have additional N-terminal and C-terminal propeptides not found in the nonfibrillar collagens (Fig. 2–3). The three proα-chains of a procollagen are initially synthesized with N-terminal signal sequences that direct their binding to the ribosomes of the cisternae of the rough endoplasmic reticulum. As the proα-chains pass into the cisternae, the signal peptides are cleaved, and the proα-chains undergo a series of hydroxylations and glycosylations. About 100 prolyl residues in the Y positions are hydroxylated to hydroxy-4-proline, and about 10 lysyl residues in the Y positions are hydroxylated to hydroxylysine. Some of the hydroxylysyl residues are subsequently modified by the addition of galactose, or both galactose and glucose, to the epsilon-hydroxyl (ε-hydroxyl) group. The hydroxylation of proline and that of lysine require ascorbic acid. Of the two hydroxylations, the hydroxylation of proline to hydroxyproline is more critical because a stable collagen triple helix cannot be formed at body temperature unless each α-chain contains about 100 hydroxyprolyl residues. The requirement for ascorbic acid in the enzymatic hydroxylation of proline probably explains the failure of wounds to heal in cases of scurvy. In addition to the modifications of the prolyl and lysyl residues, a mannose-rich carbohydrate is added to the C-terminal propeptide of each proα-chain. As these modifications of the proα-chains are occurring, the three chains come together through their globular C propeptides and become disulfide linked. After the three chains associate and acquire the necessary content of hydroxyproline, a nucleus of triple helix forms near the C-terminus of the α-chain domains. The triple-helical conformation is then propagated from the C- to the N-terminus of the molecule.

An usual relationship exists between the folding of procollagen into a triple-helical conformation and

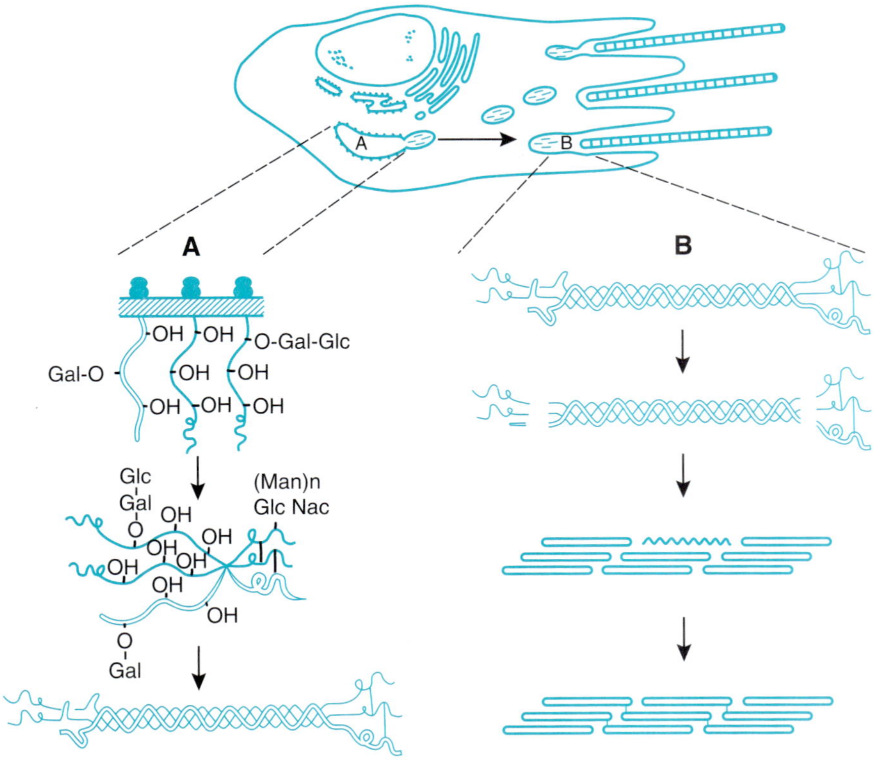

FIGURE 2–3 · A, B, Schematic Representations of how a Fibroblast Assembles Collagen Fibrils. *A,* Intracellular post-translational modifications of proα-chains, association of C propeptide domains, and folding into the triple-helical conformation. *B,* Enzymatic cleavage of procollagen to collagen, self-assembly of collagen monomers into fibrils, and cross-linking of fibrils into fibers. (From Prockop DJ, Kivirikko KI: Heritable diseases of collagen. N Engl J Med 311:376-386, 1984. Reprinted with permission from the New England Journal of Medicine.)

the post-translational modifications that introduce hydroxyproline, hydroxylysine, and glycosylated hydroxylysine.[1-3] The two hydroxylases and the two glycosyltransferases involved in the reactions can modify only proα-chains or α-chains that are in a random coil conformation. As soon as the protein folds into a triple helix, the enzymes no longer interact with the proα-chains. Because the protein cannot fold into a triple helix until most of the Y-position prolyl residues are hydroxylated to hydroxyproline, the content of hydroxyproline in most fibrillar collagens is essentially the same. The contents of hydroxylysine and glycosylated hydroxylysine vary, however, and depend on several poorly controlled factors, such as the relative concentrations of the proα-chain substrates, the enzymes, and the cofactors for the enzymes in the cisternae of the rough endoplasmic reticulum. The lack of precise control of these factors probably explains why the contents of hydroxylysine and glycosylated hydroxylysine are higher in embryonic tissues than in adult tissues. The content of glycosylated hydroxylysine in collagen affects its biologic function because the glycosylated hydroxylysyl residues project from the surface of the triple helix and interfere with lateral packing of the molecule into fibrils. Therefore, an increase in glycosylated hydroxylysine decreases the diameter of the fibrils formed. Any condition that delays folding of the proα-chains into a triple helix increases the contents of hydroxylysine and glycosylated hydroxylysine. As a result, most mutations that change the amino acid sequences of proα-chains increase the content of hydroxylysine and glycosylated hydroxylysine in procollagen and collagen (see discussion later in chapter).

The folding of procollagen into a triple-helical conformation is also intimately related to its secretion from cells. Under normal conditions, secretion begins only after the protein is correctly folded. In a condition such as ascorbate deficiency, the rate of hydroxylation of prolyl residues (and hence the rate of protein folding) is decreased. Consequently, there is an accumulation of nonhelical proα-chains in the rough endoplasmic reticulum and an overall decrease in the secretion of helical procollagen molecules. Accumulation of nonhelical proα-chains is also seen with agents that inhibit prolyl hydroxylase and with mutations in the structure of the proα-chains that delay folding (see discussion later in chapter).

As soon as the protein folds into a triple-helical conformation, it is transported from the rough endoplasmic reticulum to Golgi vesicles, from which it is secreted. The protein is then further processed extracellularly by a specific procollagen N-proteinase that cleaves the N propeptides and a separate procollagen C-proteinase that cleaves the C propeptides. After the propeptides are cleaved, the solubility of the protein decreases more than 1000-fold to less than 1 μg/ml at 37°C, and it spontaneously self-assembles into fibrils.[1,9] The fibers initially assembled have the same morphology as mature fibers of collagen, but they do not achieve their optimal tensile strength until some of the lysyl and glycosylated hydroxylysyl residues are enzymatically deaminated by the enzyme-lysyl oxidase to generate aldehydes that project from the surfaces of the molecules. The aldehydes then spontaneously form covalent cross-links among adjacent molecules in the fibril. The formation of the cross-links stabilizes the fibril structure so that it acquires a tensile strength approximately that of a steel wire.

Two observations about procollagen C-proteinase have illuminated unexpected features of the collagen biosynthetic pathway. First, the enzyme can process an inactive precursor form of lysyl oxidase to the active enzyme in vitro.[10] Therefore, it may play a role in the synthesis of the covalent cross-links that are essential for the normal tensile strength of fibers of both collagen and elastin (see discussion later in chapter). Second, C-proteinase is a product of the same gene that synthesizes bone morphogenic protein 1 (BMP-1).[11,12] BMP-1, in turn, was shown to be similar in structure to a large family of proteins that play critical roles in the development of organisms that include *Drosophila*, hydra, sea urchin, frogs, fish, and mammals. The homologous enzymes C-proteinase/BMP-1/tolloid cleave complexes containing inhibitory proteins (chordin/sog) and thereby release active forms of *Drosophila* decapentaplegic (dpp)/BMP-2/BMP-4 at the margin of dorsoventral development in embryos.[13-16] Therefore, the enzyme essential to assembling the collagen fibrils that largely define the size, shape, and strength of most complex organisms plays additional roles in embryonic development.

The biosynthetic pathways for nonfibrillar collagens are similar to those for the fibrillar collagens, but they have not been studied as extensively. Most of the nonfibrillar collagens have globular extensions at both ends, but there is no evidence that the globular ends of the proteins are cleaved in a manner comparable to that of the globular ends of fibrillar procollagens. Instead, the globular ends persist in tissues and appear to be involved in the assembly of matrix structures (see Fig. 2–2).

METABOLIC TURNOVER

The collagens in adult tissues are highly stable structures. However, dramatic degradation and resynthesis of collagen fibrils occur during embryonic development as tissues change their shape and increase in size.[1] Considerable metabolic turnover of collagens continues throughout the growth of the organism. After maturity of the skeleton, the collagen fibrils and fibers in most tissues become stable metabolically so that they have half-lives of many weeks or months. In bone, however, collagen continues to be degraded and resynthesized as remodeling continues throughout life. In addition, large amounts of collagen can be lost from the skin and other connective tissues during periods of malnutrition or starvation.

The collagen in many tissues, therefore, is a replenishable source of amino acids for gluconeogenesis. Also, diseases of connective tissue produce marked increases in collagen turnover. For example, there are marked increases in the metabolic turnover of collagen in bone in Paget's disease, hyperparathyroidism, and metastatic diseases. There are large increases in the turnover of collagen, as well as most other proteins, in hyperthyroidism. Increases in collagen turnover are accompanied by increases in the excretion of peptide-bound hydroxyproline and hydroxylysine in urine, because some of the peptide bonds in collagen resist cleavage. Assays of the urinary excretion of hydroxyproline and glycosylated hydroxylysine have, therefore, been used clinically to measure turnover of collagen. Immunoassays of serum levels of procollagen propeptides have been used to follow changes in rates of collagen biosynthesis. Assays of the serum levels of the N propeptide of type III procollagen and the 7S fragment of type IV collagen have been particularly useful in following liver fibrosis.[17,18]

The degradation of the collagen in tissues is initiated by cleavage of the molecule by one of several specific collagenases. The collagenases cleave the molecule at a site that is about three quarters of the distance from the N- to the C-terminus. The resulting 3/4 and 1/4 fragments then partially unfold so that they are further degraded by nonspecific proteases, such as gelatinases and stromelysin. In addition to the extracellular degradation of collagen fibrils, part of the newly synthesized proα-chains in cells appears to be degraded before being incorporated into functional procollagen or collagen molecules. The intracellular degradation of the newly synthesized chains may represent a mechanism for correcting errors in biosynthesis.

PRINCIPLE OF NUCLEATED GROWTH IN COLLAGEN BIOSYNTHESIS

One of the unusual features of collagen biosynthesis is that it employs a principle of nucleated growth whereby a few molecules first assemble into a structure defined as a nucleus, and the structure of the nucleus is then propagated by the orderly and rapid addition of thousands of the same molecules.[9] The principle of nucleated growth is used extensively in nature in the formation of crystals by many inorganic materials, including the formation of snowflakes by water. In collagen biosynthesis, the principle of nucleated growth is used in folding the protein, in that a nucleus of triple helix is formed near the C-terminus of the procollagen molecule and is then rapidly propagated to the N-terminus (see Fig. 2–3). In addition, the principle of nucleated growth is employed in the assembly of fibrils; a few molecules of the protein first form a nucleus of a fibril, then the nucleus grows by the orderly and rapid addition of many collagen molecules.

Nucleated growth is a highly efficient mechanism for assembly of large structures with a precisely defined architecture; however, it requires that all the molecules or subunits in the system have the same structure. As illustrated by the growth of inorganic crystals, a few molecules with a defective structure prevent propagation of the nucleus and "poison" the system. Because collagen biosynthesis extensively employs the principle of nucleated growth, it is markedly disturbed by mutations that change the amino acid sequence of the protein. In particular, a single-base mutation that converts a glycine codon to a codon for an amino acid with a bulkier side residue can prevent propagation of the triple helix so the molecule cannot form a functional protein. The presence of one proα-chain with a single glycine substitution can prevent folding and cause degradation of both the abnormal proα-chain and two normal proα-chains in a process referred to as procollagen suicide (Fig. 2–4). Surprisingly, however, some mutations that substitute bulkier amino acids for glycine residues have little effect on the folding of the protein but produce subtle changes in conformation, such as a flexible "kink" in the triple helix that is visible by electron microscopy (Fig. 2–5).[19] The presence of conformational kinks in the molecule can poison fibril assembly, generating fibrils with highly distorted morphology (Fig. 2–6)[20] or markedly decreasing the amount of collagen incorporated in the fibrils.

MUTATIONS IN COLLAGEN GENES THAT PRODUCE HUMAN DISEASES

Mutations in collagen genes produce a variety of disease phenotypes (Table 2–2). Mutations in collagen genes were first encountered in studies on osteogenesis imperfecta, a heritable disorder, characterized by brittleness of bones, that is frequently associated with changes in other tissues rich in collagen. More than 90 percent of patients with osteogenesis imperfecta have a mutation in the gene for the proα1(I)-chain (COL1A1) or the gene for the proα2(I)-chain (COL1A2) of type I procollagen.[3,21,22] Mild forms of osteogenesis imperfecta are caused primarily by mutations that decrease the synthesis of proα1(I)-chains. However, more severe variants of osteogenesis imperfecta are caused by mutations that produce synthesis of abnormal, but partially functional, proα1(I)- or proα2(I)-chains of type I procollagen. Unrelated patients and families rarely have the same mutation, and hundreds of different mutations have now been defined.

The devastating effects of mutations that change the structure of a proα1(I)-chain or proα2(I)-chain are explained by the extensive use of nucleated growth in collagen biosynthesis.[9] Of special interest has been a large number of single-base mutations that convert a codon for glycine to a codon for a bulkier amino acid. The glycine substitutions are highly position specific in that a substitution of one glycine position can produce procollagen suicide, whereas a substitution of the same or a similar amino acid for a nearby glycine position has essentially no effect on the folding of the triple helix but can markedly alter fibril assembly (Fig. 2–7 and Table 2–3). Also, the glycine substitutions are position specific in the sense that substitutions for some glycine residues produce severe osteogenesis imperfecta that is lethal in utero or shortly after birth, whereas others cause only mild forms of the disease. The results suggest that some regions of the α-chains may be more critical than others to the stability of the triple helix. Some regions of the molecule may be important for its normal function in tissues such as bone, whereas other regions are more important for its function elsewhere. Such generalizations probably explain why some patients with moderately severe osteogenesis imperfecta have fragile bones together with evidence of decreased collagen in other tissues, such as blue sclerae, severe dentinogenesis imperfecta,

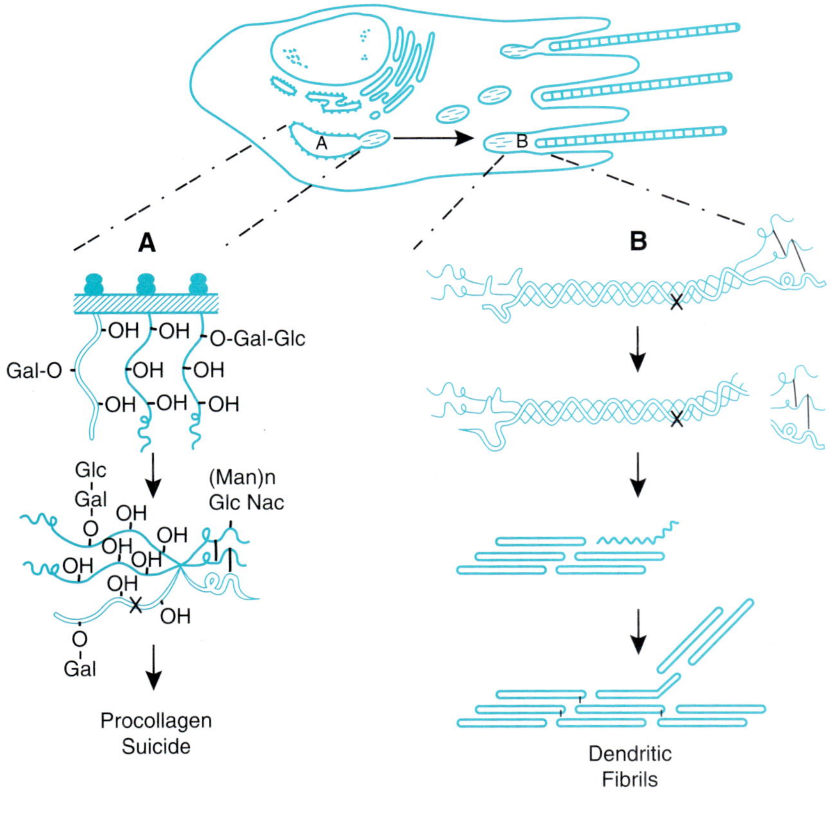

FIGURE 2–4 · A, B, Schematic Representations of how Mutations that Change the Structure of type I Collagen can Interfere with either the Intracellular Assembly of the Protein or the Subsequent Assembly of Collagen Fibrils. As discussed in the text, a mutation that converts a codon for a glycine residue to a codon for a bulkier amino acid can prevent the folding of the protein into a triple-helical conformation. If folding is prevented, both the normal proα-chains and the mutated proα-chains are degraded through a process referred to as "procollagen suicide". Alternatively, a glycine substitution or other mutation can allow folding into a triple-helical conformation but introduces a subtle change in conformation of the protein, such as a kink. Monomers with an altered conformation can interfere with fibril assembly so that highly abnormal fibrils are generated. (From Prockop DJ, Kivirikko KI: Heritable diseases of collagen. N Engl J Med 311:376-386, 1984. Reprinted with permission from the New England Journal of Medicine.)

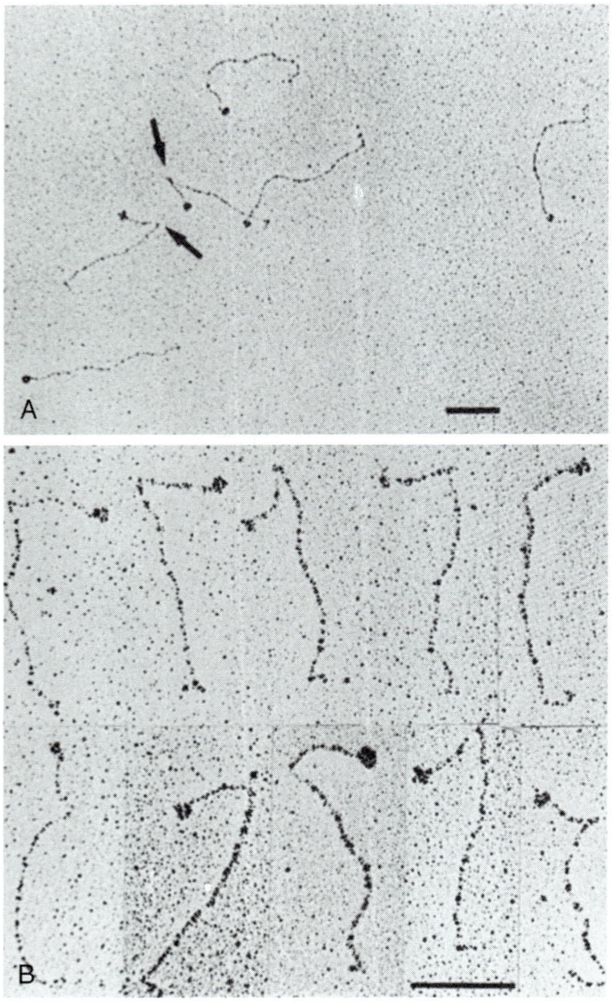

FIGURE 2–5 · **Rotary Shadowing Electron Microscopy of Mutated Type I Procollagen Molecules.** A panel of individual molecules is presented. The C-terminus of the protein can be identified because the globular C propeptide is larger than the globular N propeptide. The molecules demonstrate the presence of a flexible kink at the site of a mutation that has converted the codon for glycine at position α1-748 to a codon for cysteine. (From Vogel BE, Doelz R, Kadler KE, et al: A substitution of cysteine for glycine 748 of the α1 chain produces a kink at this site in the procollagen I molecule and an altered N-proteinase cleavage site over 225 nm away. J Biol Chem 263:19249-19255, 1988.)

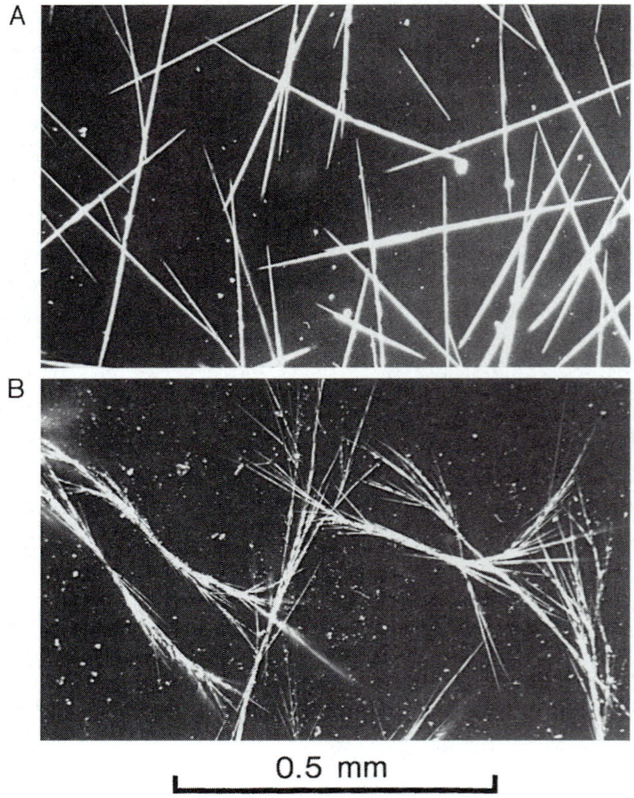

FIGURE 2–6 · **Collagen Fibrils Assembled from Normal Human Type I Collagen (A) and Collagen from a Proband with a Heterozygous Mutation that Converted the Codon for Glycine at Position α1-748 to a Codon for Cysteine (B).** About 10% of the protein in the fibrils is the mutated type I collagen, and 90% is normal type I collagen. As indicated, the presence of the mutated protein generates fibrils that are abnormally branched. (From Kadler KE, Torre-Blanco A, Adachi E, et al: A type I collagen with substitution of a cysteine for glycine-748 in the α1[I] chain copolymerizes with normal type I collagen and can generate fractal-like structures. Biochemistry 30:5081-5088, 1991. Reproduced by permission from Biochemistry. Copyright 1991, American Chemical Society.)

and strikingly thin skin, whereas other patients with equally fragile bones have apparently normal sclerae, teeth, and skin.

The large number of mutations in the type I procollagen genes causing osteogenesis imperfecta prompted a search for mutations in other procollagen genes that might cause other heritable disorders of connective tissue. A series of mutations in five genes for four different collagens produce cartilage phenotypes (Table 2–4). Similarly, mutations in the gene for type III procollagen (*COL3A1*) have been shown to cause the potentially lethal form of Ehlers-Danlos syndrome, known as type IV, which produces marked changes in tissues rich in type III collagen, such as thinness and scarring of skin and rupture of large arteries and other whole organs. Mutations in four genes for type IV collagen (*COL4A3, COL4A4, COL4A5,* and *COL4A6*) have been shown to cause Alport's syndrome,[3] a hereditary disorder characterized by hematuria and nephritis and frequently associated with deafness. Mutations in the genes for type V collagen (*COL5A1* and *COL5A2*) cause type I and type II Ehlers-Danlos syndrome, with hyperextensible skin and lax joints.[23,24] Mutations in the three genes for type VI collagen (*COL6A1, COL6A2,* and *COL6A3*) cause an early-onset myopathy and joint contractures.[25-28] Mutations in the gene for type VII collagen *(COL7A1)* may cause the dystrophic form of epidermolysis bullosa, in which blistering occurs below the basement membrane of the skin and is associated with a decrease in the anchoring fibrils[3] formed by type VII collagen. Mutations in the gene for type XVII *(COL17A1)* cause a variant of epidermolysis bullosa with tissue separation of hemidesmosomes.[29]

In addition, mutations in collagen genes can cause common diseases. There are two reported examples of glycine substitutions in type I collagen that cause either postmenopausal osteoporosis or juvenile osteoporosis in patients who may show some phenotypic overlap with osteogenesis imperfecta.[30,31] In addition, there are con-

TABLE 2–2 • TYPES OF COLLAGENS AND DISEASES CAUSED BY MUTATIONS IN COLLAGEN GENES

Collagen	Human Disease
Type I	Osteogenesis imperfecta, Ehlers-Danlos syndrome, osteoporosis
Type II	Several chondrodysplasias, osteoarthritis
Type III	Ehlers-Danlos syndrome type IV, aortic aneurysms
Type IV	Alport's syndrome
Type V	Ehlers-Danlos syndrome types I and II
Type VI	Bethlem myopathy
Type VII	Epidermolysis bullosa
Type IX	Multiple epiphyseal dysplasia, intervertebral disk disease
Type X	Schmid type metaphyseal dysplasia
Type XI	Otospondylomegaepiphyseal dysplasia, Marshall's syndrome, Stickler's syndrome (nonsyndromic hearing loss)
Type XVII	Epidermolysis bullosa

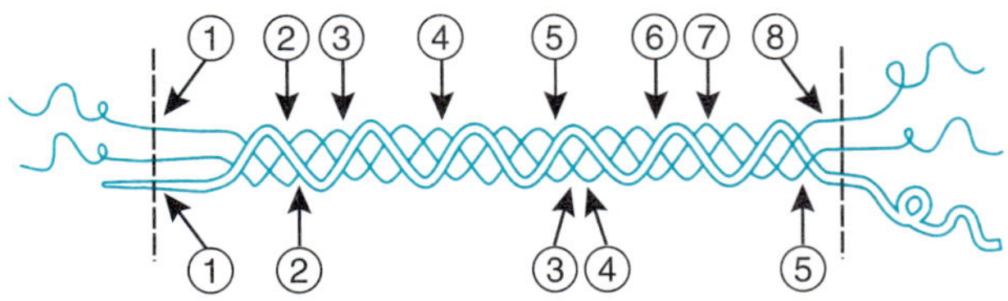

FIGURE 2–7 • Approximate Sites of Mutations that Alter the Primary Structure of Type I Procollagen. *Numbers above the molecule:* approximate sites of mutations in the proα1(I)-chain. *Numbers below the molecule:* approximate sites of mutations in the proα2(I)-chain. Effects of the mutations are summarized in Table 2–3.

flicting reports as to whether a polymorphism in the gene for the α1(I)-chain of type I collagen is associated with reduced bone density and osteoporotic fractures.[32,33] A glycine substitution in type III procollagen was shown to cause aortic aneurysms in a family without any of the characteristic features of Ehlers-Danlos syndrome type IV or Marfan syndrome.[34] Linkage studies suggested that a mutation in the gene for type II procollagen was a cause of osteoarthritis in two large Finnish families.[35] In addition, a mutation that converted an arginine codon to a codon for cysteine[36] was shown to cause osteoarthritis associated with a mild chondrodysplasia in one family (Fig. 2–8). Subsequently, four additional families with the same mutation and a similar phenotype were described.[37,38] The presence of several rare polymorphisms in the same allele indicates that three of the families are probably descendants of the same Icelandic founder. Also, three families with similar syndromes had similar mutations in the gene for type II collagen that converted the codon for Arg-75 to a codon for Cys.[38] Mutations that introduced a tryptophan codon into the α2(IX)-chain of type IX collagen cause dominantly inherited vertebral disk disease.[39] A similar tryptophan mutation in the α3(IX)-chain of type IX collagen is associated with the same phenotype and increases the risk for the disease three-fold.[40]

Elastin

The elastic properties of tissues such as skin, large blood vessels, lung, and large ligaments depend on the presence of rubber-like elastic fibers.[41-43] In contrast to collagen fibrils and fibers, elastic fibers are amorphous structures; their molecular components are not assembled in a regular pattern that can be detected by electron microscopy or x-ray diffraction. The major constituent of elastic fibers is elastin, an unusual protein composed of a single polypeptide chain of 72 kD. The protein has large domains of hydrophobic amino acids joined by shorter sequences that are rich in alanine and lysine. The amino acid sequences of the hydrophobic domains are similar to the α-chains of collagen in that they frequently have sequences of Gly-X-Y. A few of the prolines in the Y position of the sequences are hydroxylated to hydroxyproline, but the presence of hydroxyproline in elastin appears to have no functional significance. The regions rich in alanine and lysine are sites for covalent cross-links among different regions of the same chain and among different chains of the protein. The elastic properties of the protein

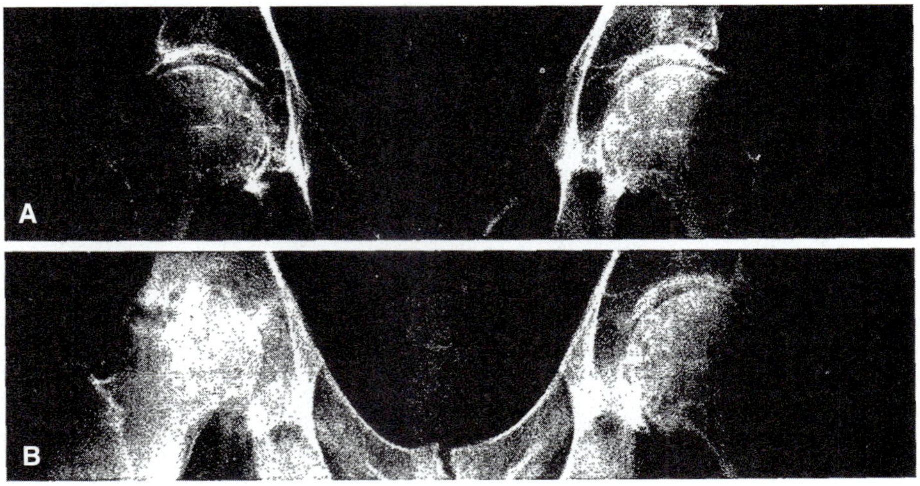

FIGURE 2–8 • Radiographs from an affected Member of the Family with Primary Generalized Osteoarthritis Associated with Mild Chondrodysplasia. *A*, Radiograph showing osteoarthritis in both hips, but no apparent dysplasia. *B*, Radiograph of same patient 3 years later. There is a progressive increase in osteoarthritis-induced changes that are more pronounced on the right. (From Knowlton RG, Katzenstein PL, Moskowitz RW, et al: Genetic linkage of a polymorphism in the type II procollagen gene *[COL2A1]* to primary osteoarthritis associated with mild chondrodysplasia. N Engl J Med 322:526, 1990. Reprinted with permission from the New England Journal of Medicine.)

TABLE 2–3 • EXAMPLES OF MUTATIONS IN TYPE I PROCOLLAGENS, THEIR EFFECTS ON THE PROTEIN, AND THE PHENOTYPES THEY PRODUCE*

	Molecular Mechanism		
Mutation	Procollagen Suicide	Abnormal Fibrils	Disease Phenotype
Proα1-chain			
Splicing of exon 6		+	Loose joints (EDS VIIA)†
Gly^{175}→Cys	±	+	Moderate OI
Gly^{244}→Cys	0	(+)	Lethal OI
Gly^{391}→Arg	±	(+)	Lethal OI
Gly^{598}→Ser	+		Lethal OI
Gly^{748}→Cys	+	+	Moderate OI
Gly^{832}→Cys	±	(+)	Moderate OI
Gly^{988}→Cys	+	+	Lethal OI
Proα2-chain			
Splicing of exon 6		+	Loose joints (EDS VIIA)†
Partial deletion of IVS10/exon 11	+	+	Loose joints or fragile bones
Gly^{646}→Cys	±	(+)	Mild OI
Gly^{661}→Ser	0	(+)	Osteoporosis
Gly^{907}→Asp	+	(?)	Lethal OI

*For summaries of mutations and their effects, see Kuivaniemi et al[22] and Byers.[21]

†Mutations that prevent cleavage of the N propeptide.

Key: +, proven mechanism; ±, secondary mechanism; (+), probable mechanism. Superscript numbers indicate amino acid position in the α1(I)-chain or α2(I)-chain.

Abbreviations: EDS, Ehlers-Danlos syndrome; OI, osteogenesis imperfecta.

TABLE 2–4 • EXAMPLES OF MUTATIONS IN COLLAGEN GENES THAT PRODUCE CARTILAGE PHENOTYPES

Mutation	Disease Phenotype
Type II collagen, proα1(II)-chain	
Gly^{943}→Ser	Lethal (achondrogenesis II)
Gly^{997}→Ser	Moderate (spondyloepiphyseal dysplasia)
Skipping of exon 12	Moderate (Kniest dysplasia)
Premature STOP	Mild (Stickler's syndrome)
Gly^{519}→Cys	Mild (osteoarthritis with mild chondrodysplasia)
Type IX collagen, α2(IX)-chain	
Skipping of exon 3	Mild (multiple epiphyseal dysplasia)
Gln^{326}→Trp	Mild (intervertebral disk disease)
Type IX collagen, α3(IX)-chain	
Skipping of exon 3	Mild (multiple epiphyseal dysplasia)
Arg^{103}→Trp	Mild (intervertebral disk disease)
Type XI collagen, α1(XI)-chain	
Skipping of exon 50	Mild (Marshall's syndrome)
Gly^{148}→Arg	Mild (Stickler's syndrome)
Type XI collagen, α2(XI)-chain	
Premature STOP (recessive)	Moderate (otospondylomegaepiphyseal dysplasia)
Skipping of exon 60	Mild (nonocular Stickler's syndrome)

derive from the marked tendency of the hydrophobic domains to fold in on themselves and form coil-like compartments within the fibers. Stretching the fibers unfolds the hydrophobic domains and extends the polypeptide chains so they are held together primarily by the cross-links. As soon as the stretching force is released, the hydrophobic domains spontaneously refold. Detailed studies on elastin, however, are hampered by the fact that the protein is among the most insoluble proteins in nature and cannot be extracted from tissues with solvents as harsh as 8 M urea or hot alkali.

In addition to elastin, elastic fibers in tissues contain poorly defined microfibrillar structures. The microfibrillar structures are seen early in embryonic development as elastic fibers are first formed. They are also seen at the edges of elastic fibrils in mature tissues. The composition of the microfibrillar structures has not been fully defined, but a major component has been identified as *fibrillin*, a large glycoprotein of about 300 kD that appears to be associated with most elastin fibrils.[44]

THE GENE FOR ELASTIN AND FIBRILLIN

The human gene for elastin contains 34 exons that range in size from 27 to 186 bp and code for a polypeptide chain of 786 amino acids.[45] The hydrophobic and the cross-linking domains of the protein are coded by separate exons. The introns of the gene are relatively large compared to genes for collagens and other proteins, and they contain a large number of *Alu* repetitive sequences, particularly at the 3′ end of the gene.

One of the most interesting features of the elastin gene is that RNA transcripts are spliced by a number of alternative pathways to generate a large series of messenger RNAs that differ because they lack the codons from one or more exons of the gene.[45,46] As a result, cells synthesizing elastin produce a variety of polypeptide chains of different sizes and amino acid compositions. The reasons for these variations are not known.

The microfibrils associated with elastin have diameters of 10 to 12 nm. Ten or more gene products are found in microfibrils, but the best characterized are two similar 350-kD glycoproteins known as fibrillin-1 and fibrillin-2.[44,47–50] Both have complex repetitive structures that include 43 domains, similar to the precursor of epidermal growth factor, which has a consensus sequence for calcium binding. The isolated proteins are found as long strands of globular structures joined by thin fibrils.[47] The proteins are encoded by multiexonic genes; the gene for fibrillin-1 is on chromosome 15, and the similar gene for fibrillin-2 is on chromosome 5.[48]

BIOSYNTHESIS AND METABOLIC TURNOVER

Elastin is synthesized by smooth muscle cells and, to a lesser extent, by fibroblasts. Initial studies suggested that the protein was first synthesized as a larger and more soluble precursor protein, but this possibility was subsequently excluded by more detailed biosynthetic studies.[49–51] Therefore, it is not apparent how this highly insoluble protein is synthesized without premature aggregation in cells. Also, little information is available about the biosynthesis of fibrillin.

After elastin is secreted, it undergoes extensive cross-linking reactions.[52] The cross-linking reactions (Fig. 2–9) begin with removal of the ε-amino group of lysine by lysyl oxidase, the same enzyme involved in collagen cross-linking. About 40 lysine residues in elastin are deaminated to generate aldehydes that undergo a series of apparently spontaneous interactions to form

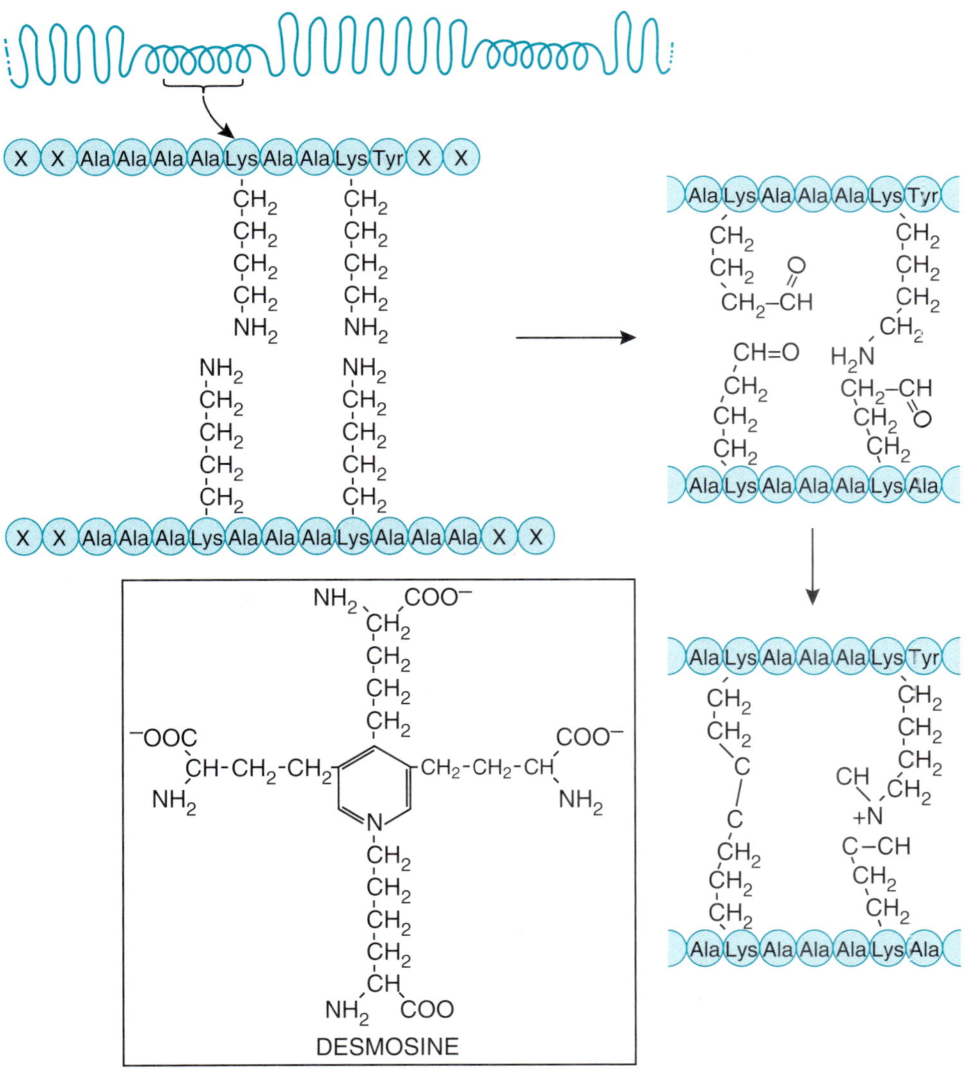

FIGURE 2–9 · Formation of Peptidyl Cross-links in the Conversion of Soluble Elastin to Insoluble Elastin. The large loop of the tropoelastin structure represents hydrophilic stretchable areas composed primarily of the amino acids glycine, proline, valine, pheylalanine, isoleucine, and leucine. The small coiled areas represent the alanmerich areas that surround the lysine residues involved in cross-link formation. This is an α-helical region containing two lysine residues separated by two and three alanine residues. Two peptide chains are parallel such that the side chains of lysine or allysine after oxidative deamidation can spontaneously condense to form the stable peritoneum ring structure with three double bonds (as depicted). The desmosine molecule, therefore, is composed of three allysine residues and one lysine residue in a peritoneum ring structure to form the tetrafunctional amino acid that participates in both interchain and intrachain cross-linking.

complex aromatic structures. The parent compound is desmosine, but a number of variations on the structure are also found, including reduced aldehyde-condensation products.

Elastases that degrade elastin are present in polymorphonuclear leukocytes and in the pancreas.[53,54] Because desmosine is metabolized poorly, if at all, the urinary excretion of desmosine has been used to assay metabolic turnover of elastin. The results suggest that only about 1 percent of total body elastin is degraded per year in a normal adult.[55]

DISEASES RELATED TO ELASTIN AND FIBRILLIN

As may be expected from the role of elastin in maintaining the elasticity of skin, mutations in the elastin gene cause cutis laxa, a rare and heterogeneous group of disorders characterized by skin that is both lax and inelastic.[56,57] Three different frame-shift mutations were found in three unrelated families with dominant forms of the disease. Surprisingly, other mutations in the elastin gene produce phenotypes that primarily involve the aorta, whose elasticity again depends on the presence of elastin. Mutations in the elastin gene, which include chromosome translocations, intragenic deletions, and point mutations, cause supravalvular aortic stenosis, a congenital narrowing of the ascending aorta.[58-60] As with other mutations in genes for structural protein, such as collagens, it is not clear at the moment why some mutations in the elastin gene primarily affect the skin and others affect the aorta. A more complex situation arises in Williams' syndrome.[58-60] In this case, a large deletion that encompasses the elastin gene together with additional genes in the same locus produces a phenotype that includes supravalvular aortic stenosis, growth retardation, characteristic facies, and an unusual mental phenotype of low intelligence quotient and a high degree of sociability.

Mutations in the gene for fibrillin-1 are a primary cause of Marfan's syndrome.[47,48,61-63] The mutations that produce Marfan's syndrome include premature termination codons, partial gene deletions, and single-base substitutions, including those that probably alter the binding of calcium to the epidermal growth factor–like domains. Mutations in the fibrillin-2 gene cause a rarer form of Marfan's syndrome that is characterized by contractural arachnodactyly.[61] Other mutations in the fibrillin-1 gene produce a range of clinical phenotypes.[63] Marfan's syndrome was initially defined on the basis of a triad of symptoms: ectopia lentis; aneurysms of the ascending thoracic aorta; and skeletal changes that include long extremities, loose jointedness, and arachnodactyly. However, it was apparent that some affected members of selected families had a phenotype involving only one of these tissues. Accordingly, some mutations in the fibrillin-1 gene cause isolated ectopia lentis.[63] Others cause isolated aneurysms of the descending aorta, and still others cause isolated skeletal defects. A rare mutation also produces aortic dilatation and arachnodactyly with craniosynostosis and mental retardation (Shprintzen-Goldberg syndrome). A DNA test is now available that identifies mutations in the fibrillin-1 gene causing Marfan's syndrome.[64]

REFERENCES

1. Prockop DJ, Kivirikko KI: Heritable diseases of collagen. N Engl J Med 311:376, 1984.
2. Myllyharju J, Kivirikko KI: Collagens and collagen-related diseases. Ann Med 33:7, 2001.
3. Prockop DJ, Kivirikko KI: Collagen: molecular biology, diseases and potentials for therapy. Annu Rev Biochem 64:403–434, 1995.
4. Prockop DJ, Guzman NA: Collagen diseases and the biosynthesis of collagen. Hosp Pract 12:61, 1977.
5. Romanic AM, Adachi E, Kadler KE, et al: Copolymerization of pNcollagen III and collagen I: pNcollagen III decreases the rate of incorporation of collagen I into fibrils, the amount of collagen incorporated, and the diameter of fibrils formed. J Biol Chem 266:12703, 1991.
6. O'Reilly MS, Boehm T, Shing Y, et al: Endostatin: an endogenous inhibitor of angiogenesis and tumor growth. Cell 88:277, 1997.
7. Pihlajaniemi T, Rehn M: Two new collagen subgroups: membrane associated collagens and types XV and XVIII. Prog Nucleic Acid Res Mol Biol 50:255, 1995.
8. Chu ML, Prockop DJ: Collagen: Gene structure. *In* Royce PM, Steinmann B (eds): Connective Tissue and Its Heritable Disorders. New York, Wiley-Liss, 1993, p 149.
9. Engel J, Prockop DJ: The zipper-like folding of collagen triple helices and the effects of mutations that disrupt the zipper. Annu Rev Biophys Biophys Chem 20:137, 1991.
10. Panchenko MV, Stetler-Stevenson WG, Trubetskoy OV, et al: Metalloproteinase activity secreted by fibrogenic cells in the processing of prolysyl oxidase: potential role of procollagen C-proteinase. J Biol Chem 271:7113, 1996.
11. Li SW, Sieron AL, Fertala A, et al: The C-proteinase that processes procollagens to fibrillar collagens is identical to the protein previously identified as bone morphogenic protein-1. Proc Natl Acad Sci U S A 93:5127, 1996.
12. Kessler E, Takahara K, Biniaminov L, et al: Bone morphogenetic protein-1: the type I procollagen C-proteinase. Science 271:360, 1996.
13. Padgett RW, Wozney JM, Gelbart WM: Human BMP sequences can confer normal dorsal-ventral patterning in the *Drosophila* embryo. Proc Natl Acad Sci U S A 90:2905, 1993.
14. Shimell MJ, Ferguson EL, Childs SR, O'Connor MB: The *Drosophila* dorsal-ventral patterning gene *tolloid* is related to human bone morphogenic protein 1. Cell 67:469, 1991.
15. Marques G, Musacchio M, Shimell MJ, et al: Production of a DPP activity gradient in the early *Drosophila* embryo through the opposing actions of the SOG and TLD proteins. Cell 91:417, 1997.
16. Piccolo S, Agius E, Lu B, et al: Cleavage of Chordin by xolloid metalloprotease suggests a role for proteolytic processing in the regulation of Spemann organizer activity. Cell 91:407, 1997.
17. Rohde H, Vargas L, Hahn E, et al: Radioimmunoassay for type III procollagen peptide and its application to human liver disease. Eur J Clin Invest 9:451, 1979.
18. Ala-Kokko L, Günzler V, Hoek JB, et al: Hepatic fibrosis in rats produced by carbon tetrachloride and dimethyl-nitrosamine: observations suggesting immunoassays of serum for the 7S fragment of type IV collagen are a more sensitive index of liver damage than immunoassays for the NH_2-terminal propeptide of type III procollagen. Hepatology 16:167, 1992.
19. Vogel BE, Doelz R, Kadler KE, et al: A substitution of cysteine for glycine-748 of the α1 chain produces a kink at this site in the procollagen I molecule and an altered N-proteinase cleavage site over 225 nm away. J Biol Chem 263:19249, 1988.
20. Kadler KE, Torre-Blanco A, Adachi E, et al: A type I collagen with substitution of a cysteine for glycine-748 in the α1(I) chain copolymerizes with normal type I collagen and can generate fractal-like structures. Biochemistry 30:5081, 1991.

21. Byers PH: Osteogenesis imperfecta. *In* Royce PM, Steinmann B (eds): Connective Tissue and Its Heritable Disorders. New York, Wiley-Liss, 1993, p 317.
22. Kuivaniemi H, Tromp G, Prockop DJ: Mutations in collagens type I, II, III, X and XI cause a spectrum of diseases of bone, cartilage and blood vessels. Hum Mutat 9:300, 1997.
23. Toriello HV, Glover TW, Takahara K, et al: A translocation interrupts the *COL5A1* gene in a patient with Ehlers-Danlos syndrome and hypomelanosis of Ito. Nat Genet 13:361, 1996.
24. Michalickova K, Susic M, Willing MC, et al: Mutations of the α2(V) chain of type V collagen impair matrix assembly and produce Ehlers-Danlos syndrome type I. Hum Mol Genet 7:249, 1998.
25. Jobsis GJ, Keizers H, Vreijling JP, et al: Type VI collagen mutations in Bethlem myopathy, an autosomal dominant myopathy with contractures. Nat Genet 14:113, 1996.
26. Lamande SR, Bateman JF, Hutchison W, et al: Reduced collagen VI causes Bethlem myopathy: a heterozygous *COL6A1* nonsense mutation results in mRNA decay and functional haploinsufficiency. Hum Mol Genet 7:981, 1998.
27. Pan TC, Zhang RZ, Pericak-Vance MA, et al: Missense mutation in a von Willebrand factor type A domain of the α3(VI) collagen gene (*COL6A3*) in a family with Bethlem myopathy. Hum Mol Genet 7:807, 1998.
28. Demir E, Sabatelli P, Allamand V, et al: Mutations in COL6A3 cause severe and mild phenotypes of Ullrich congenital muscular dystrophy. Am J Hum Genet 70:1446, 2002.
29. Pulkkinen L, Uitto J: Hemidesmosomal variants of epidermolysis bullosa: mutations in the α6β4 integrin and the 180-kD bullous pemphigoid antigen/type XVII collagen genes. Exp Dermatol 7:46–64, 1998.
30. Spotila LD, Constantinou CD, Sereda L, et al: Mutation in a gene for type I procollagen (*COL1A2*) in a woman with postmenopausal osteoporosis: evidence for phenotypic and genotypic overlap with mild OI. Proc Natl Acad Sci U S A 88:6624, 1991.
31. Dawson PA, Kelly TE, Marini JC: Extension of phenotype associated with structural mutations in type I collagen: siblings with juvenile osteoporosis have an α2(I)Gly436 → Arg substitution. J Bone Miner Res 14:449, 1999.
32. Grant SF, Reid DM, Blake G, et al: Reduced bone density and osteoporosis associated with a polymorphic Sp1 binding site in the collagen type I α1 gene. Nat Genet 14:203, 1996.
33. Han KO, Moon IG, Hwang CS, et al: Lack of an intronic Sp1 binding-site polymorphism at the collagen type I α1 gene in healthy Korean women. Bone 24:135, 1999.
34. Kontusaari S, Tromp G, Kuivaniemi H, et al: A mutation in the gene for type III procollagen (*COL3A1*) in a family with aortic aneurysms. J Clin Invest 86:1465, 1990.
35. Palotie A, Vaisanen P, Ott J, et al: Predisoposition to familial osteoarthrosis linked to type II collagen gene. Lancet 1:924, 1989.
36. Ala-Kokko L, Baldwin CT, Moskowitz RW, Prockop DJ: Single base mutation in the type II procollagen gene (*COL2A1*) as a cause of primary osteoarthritis associated with a mild chondrodysplasia. Proc Natl Acad Sci U S A 87:6565, 1990.
37. Williams CJ, Rock M, Considine E, et al: Three new point mutations in type II procollagen (COL2A1) and identification of a fourth family with the COL2A1 ARG519 → CYS base substitution using conformation sensitive gel electrophoresis. Hum Mol Genet 4:309–312, 1995.
38. Prockop DJ, Ala-Kokko, L, McLain DA, et al: Can mutated genes cause common osteoarthritis? Br J Rheumatol 36:827, 1997.
39. Annunen S, Paassilta P, Lohiniva J, et al: An allele of COL9A2 associated with intervertebral disc disease. Science 285:409, 1999.
40. Paassilta P, Lohiniva, J, Göring HH, et al: Identification of a novel common risk factor for lumbar disk disease. JAMA 285:1843, 2001.
41. Sandberg LB, Soskel NJ, Solt MS: Structure of the elastin fiber: an overview. J Invest Dermatol 79:128, 1982.
42. Vrhovski B, Weiss AS: Biochemistry of tropoelastin. Eur J Biochem 15:1, 1998.
43. Rosenbloom J, Abrams WR, Mecham R: Extracellular matrix 4: the elastic fiber. FASEB J 7:1208, 1993.
44. Sakai LY, Keene DR, Glanville RW, Bachinger HP: Purification and partial characterization of fibrillin, a cysteine-rich structural component of connective tissue microfibrils. J Biol Chem 266:14763, 1991.
45. Rosenbloom J, Abrams WR, Indik Z, et al: Structure of the elastin gene. Ciba Found Symp 192:59, 1995.
46. Indik Z, Yeh H, Ornstein-Goldstein N, et al: Alternate splicing of human elastin mRNA indicated by sequence analysis of cloned genomic and complementary DNA. Proc Natl Acad Sci USA 84:5680, 1987.
47. Raghunath M, Kielty CM, Kainulainen K, et al: Analyses of truncated fibrillin caused by a 336 bp deletion in the *FBN1* gene resulting in Marfan syndrome. Biochem J 302:889–896, 1994.
48. Dietz HC, Ramirez F, Sakai LY: Marfan's syndrome and other microfibrillar diseases Adv Hum Genet 22:153–186, 1994.
49. Brown-Augsburger P, Broekelmann T, Rosenbloom J, Mechan RP: Functional domains on elastin and microfibril-associated glycoprotein involved in elastic fibre assembly. Biochem J 318:149, 1996.
50. Kielty CM, Shuttleworth CA: Microfibrillar elements of the dermal matrix. Microsc Res Tech 38:413, 1997.
51. Bressan GM, Prockop DJ: Synthesis of elastin in aortas from chick embryos: conversion of newly secreted elastin to cross-linked elastin without apparent proteolysis of the molecule. Biochemistry 16:1406, 1977.
52. Smith-Mungo LI, Kagan HM: Lysyl oxidase: properties, regulation and multiple functions in biology. Matrix Biol 16:387, 1998.
53. Shapiro SD, Campbell EJ, Welgus HG, Senior RM: Elastin degradation by mononuclear phagocytes. Ann N Y Acad Sci 624:69, 1991.
54. Snider GL, Ciccolella DE, Morris SM, et al: Putative role of neutrophil elastase in the pathogenesis of emphysema. Ann N Y Acad Sci 624:45, 1991.
55. Partridge SM, Elsden DF, Thomas J: Biosynthesis of the desmosine and isodesmosine cross-bridges in elastin. Biochem J 93:30, 1964.
56. Tassabehji M, Metcalfe K, Hurst J, et al: An elastin gene mutation producing abnormal tropoelastin and abnormal elastic fibres in a patient with autosomal dominant cutis laxa. Hum Mol Genet 7:1021, 1998.
57. Zhang M-C, He L, Giro MG, et al: Cutis laxa arising from frameshift mutations in exon 30 of the elastin gene *(ELN)*. J Biol Chem 274:981, 1999.
58. Morris CA: Genetic aspects of supravalvular aortic stenosis. Curr Opin Cardiol 13:215, 1998.
59. Chowdhury T, Reardon W: Elastin mutation and cardiac disease. Pediatr Cardiol 20:183, 1999.
60. Ewart AK, Morris CA, Atkinson D, et al: Hemizygosity at the elastin locus in a developmental disorder, Williams syndrome. Nat Genet 5:11, 1993.
61. Ramirez F: Fibrillin mutations in Marfan syndrome and related phenotypes. Curr Opin Genet Dev 6:309, 1996.
62. Dietz HC, Pyeritz RE: Mutations in the human gene for fibrillin-1 (*FBN1*) in the Marfan syndrome and related disorders. Hum Mol Genet 4:1799, 1995.
63. Hayward C, Brock DJ: Fibrillin-1 mutations in Marfan syndrome and other type-1 fibrillinopathies. Hum Mutat 10:415, 1997.
64. Körkkö J, Kaitila I, Lönnqvist L, et al: Sensitivity of conformational sensitive gel electrophoresis in detecting mutations in Marfan syndrome and related conditions. J Med Genet 39:34, 2002.

3 Matrix Glycoproteins and Proteoglycans in Cartilage

DICK HEINEGÅRD • PILAR LORENZO • TORE SAXNE

In joint diseases such as osteoarthritis (OA) and rheumatoid arthritis (RA), cartilage, bone, tendons, and ligaments are affected. It is not clear which of these tissues is the primary target and to what extent alterations in the various tissues are secondary to an altered function of the initial target. It is important to bear in mind that the tissues are in close proximity such that factors (i.e., cytokines) released from one affected tissue will have an opportunity to affect also the other connective-tissue components. Furthermore, the close mechanical relationship among joint structures is such that any alterations in one of the tissues will result in compensatory changes in the others. The end stage of chronic disease affecting the joints is often total erosion of the cartilage and very extensive remodeling of the underlying bone, which changes considerably, indicating the dynamic behavior of the tissue.

The most common joint disease is OA, primarily a disease of older age. Among those over 60 years of age, 25 percent suffer from pain and disability due to OA. The same age-group also suffers from osteoporosis, with much less mechanically stable bone-enabling fractures. In these patients, OA appears to be rare, perhaps indicating that bone with less rigidity may not support the osteoarthritic process.

In RA, the process affecting the cartilage may result in its total degradation at the same time as bone is undergoing extensive alterations and periarticular osteoporosis. One of the problems in depicting the sequence of events in joint structures during disease progression is that traditional diagnostic methods are rather insensitive. In most cases, alterations in the joint structure are detected only when they become morphologically apparent. At the same time, it is apparent that the earliest alteration in tissue structure will occur at the molecular level, combining effects of cells degrading matrix constituents, or trying to repair damage by a synthetic response, or both. Loss of proteoglycans from the tissue is an example of such an early response. Why the cells initiate this response is not clear, but it is likely to include triggering by cytokines from an inflammatory response.

Research, particularly during recent decades, has increased our understanding of some functional elements of cartilage and bone. We now view the tissues as composite structures containing a variety of elements. Cartilage has collagen networks composed of collagen fibrils that provide tensile strength. Glycoproteins and proteoglycans bound at the surface of these fibrils modify their properties and provide opportunities for interactions with other tissue structural elements. This includes cross-linking of one collagen fibril to neighboring ones in ways that enhance the mechanical stability of the collagen network. Other proteins bound at the collagen-fibril surface appear to have roles in preventing neighboring fibrils from fusing as a complementary factor in regulating the properties of the collagen.

Another major component of articular cartilage are the large, highly negatively charged proteoglycan complexes that provide a "swelling pressure" that is counteracted by the collagen fibrillar network (see Chapter 5). Together, these components form a tissue extremely well adapted to take up and distribute load with minimal deformation. These complex organizations are assembled outside the chondrocytes in the extracellular environment, but their assembly and properties are tightly controlled by the cells. These regulate assembly of the matrix to be different in their close environment (i.e., the pericellular and territorial area) compared to the matrix more distant to the cell (i.e., the interterritorial matrix) (Fig. 3–1).

The biology of cartilage is influenced by the underlying bone. The bone, whose major functions depend on a rigid structure, contains a major organic component of collagen and a dominant inorganic matrix of hydroxyapatite. The crystals of the mineral are deposited using the collagen fibers as a scaffold. The interface between cartilage and bone provides a tight anchor and sequesters processes to either of these two very different tissues. Little is known about this interface, but several proteins are particularly enriched at this site, indicating specific roles. These proteins include Bone Sialoprotein (BSP) and osteoadherin.[1,2]

Cartilage can be viewed as a composite containing aggrecan and having more than 100 chondroitin sulfate side chains, each with about 50 carboxyl and 50 sulfate groups. The other major component is the fibrillar network, consisting of collagen linked to noncollagenous and collagenous matrix proteins. A number of proteins have roles in cell binding combined with binding back to elements in the matrix. They are capable of eliciting signals in response to altered conditions in the matrix. Mechanical insults or inflammation can lead to degradation of one or more components of this highly specialized tissue. The character of the ensuing repair response ranges from successful repair to inadequate restoration leading to tissue failure. This chapter describes a number of noncollagenous molecular constituents of cartilage and iterates how information about them can be used in understanding normal and pathologic tissue biology.

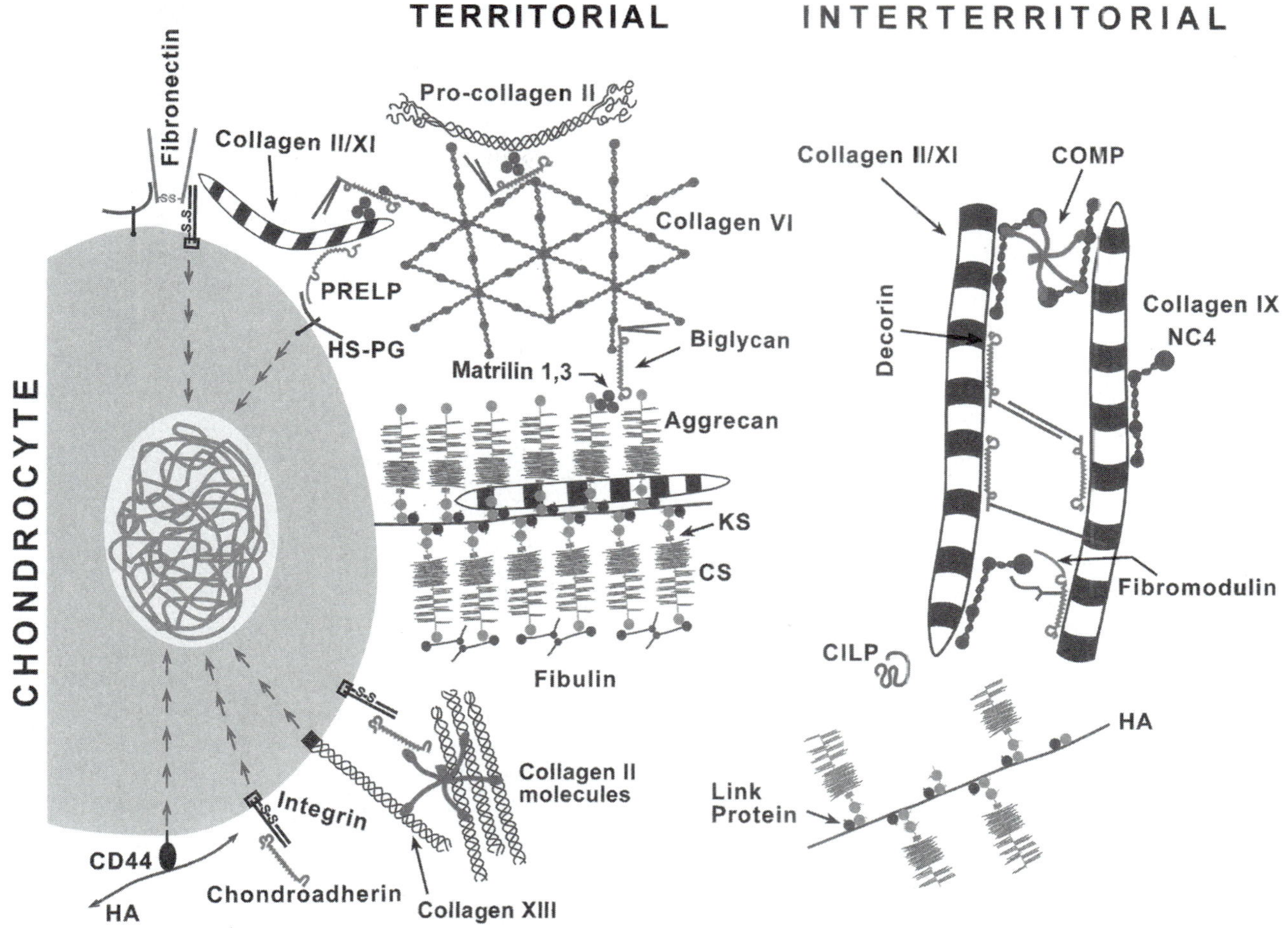

FIGURE 3–1 · Schematic Illustration of Molecular Assemblies of Cartilage Matrix. Note the different macromolecular composition and organization of the territorial (close to cells) and the interterritorial (at distance) matrix. Also indicated are a number of putative and verified interactions between matrix constituents and cells, as well as between various matrix constituents. These interactions are important for the mechanisms of assembly and maintenance of networks. Note the two networks of collagen VI and II and how they are cross-linked to other matrix constituents by cross-bridging molecules with at least two functional domains. *Abbreviations:* CHAD, chondroadherin; CILP, cartilage intermediate layer protein; COMP, cartilage oligomeric matrix protein (thrombospondin-5); CS, chondroitin sulfate; DS, dermatan sulfate; KS, keratan sulfate; HA, hyaluronan; HS-PG, heparan sulfate proteoglycan (e.g., syndecan); PRELP, proline- and arginine-rich end leucine rich repeat protein; NC-4, the noncollagenous N-terminal globular domain of collagen IX.

Aggregating Proteoglycans

CHARACTERIZATION OF AGGRECAN

Aggrecan, the large aggregating proteoglycan in cartilage, has a major role in providing fixed charge groups that attract ions of opposite charge, which creates an osmotic pressure in the cartilage, retaining water and restricting water flow.[3-6] The proteoglycan exerts a "swelling pressure" within the cartilage, which is resisted by the network of fibrillar collagens modulated in properties by noncollagenous and collagenous matrix proteins. One consequence of this water retention is that deformation is counteracted and limited when the tissue is loaded. When load on normal cartilage is released, the tissue rebounds quickly to its original volume. This is an essential function of aggrecan in taking up and distributing load over the cartilage tissue and onto the underlying bone.[6]

Considerable information on the detailed structure of the aggrecan, including its interactions and its turnover has been gathered.[7,8] This molecule contains several structural domains. The N-terminal domain, G1, binds specifically (dissociation constant 10^{-9}) to hyaluronan through a decasaccharide sequence.[9,10] This binding permits more than 100 aggrecan molecules to bind to a very long filament of hyaluronan, forming complexes that are micrometers in size.[11] This binding is stabilized by the link protein, which binds with the same specificity and affinity to hyaluronan[10] and at the same time to the G1 domain.[12,13] This ternary complex is very stable, functionally approaching a covalent bond.

A second globular domain, G2, shares similarities with the G1 domain, but it lacks the ability to bind to hyaluronan.[11,14] Following G2, there is a stretched domain carrying the major part of approximately 30 keratan sulfate chains with one to two bound to a polypeptide stretch of six amino acid residues repeated

23 times in bovine aggrecan.[15,16] The next major part of the core protein contains the chondroitin sulfate chains attached, through their reducing terminus, to serine residues. This domain bears the major part of the charged groups, and one important function of this part of the proteoglycan is to fix these charged groups in the matrix.[17] The distribution of the approximately 100 chondroitin sulfate chains is variable along this part of the core protein, such that two subdomains with somewhat different clustering of these chains are observed.[14,16] Overall, there is a high degree of packing of the charged chondroitin sulfate chains. In the C-terminal part there is a variably spliced Epidermal Growth Factor (EGF) homology domain,[18] a lectin homology domain, and a complement regulatory-like protein domain.[14] Early data indicate that the lectin may bind monosaccharides,[19] but best characterized are a number of protein-protein interactions. One of these targets tenascin,[20] a molecule that is not present in normal adult cartilage. Another interaction of the C-terminal lectin homology domain is to a fibrillar matrix protein, Fibulin-1 (see Fig. 3–1), which is present in developing cartilage, as well as Fibulin-2, which is found also in adult cartilage. These protein-to-protein interactions do not involve carbohydrate; they are directed to EGF-like calcium binding motifs in the proteins.[21,22] Similarly this domain of the related proteoglycan versican has been shown to bind to the EGF-domain rich protein fibrillin-1, which also is expressed in cartilage.[23] These interactions of aggrecan, via its C-terminus, with other molecules that themselves have the capacity to form complexes probably are important for matrix assembly. It is of interest to note that in adult cartilage the major proportion of the aggrecan molecules have been proteolytically modified such that they lack the C-terminal lectin domain. Although this is true in the interterritorial matrix at a distance from the cells, the aggrecan molecules in the territorial matrix close to the cells (where there is active turnover of the molecule) still contains the C-terminal domain (Aspberg and Heinegård, unpublished) (see Fig. 3–1).

A very large complex of many aggrecan molecules bound to hyaluronan present in cartilage is likely to have the important functions of sequestering molecules in the matrix and regulating diffusion of nutrients and other molecules participating in the assembly of the matrix (see Fig. 3–1). Aggregates are apparently formed at the cell surface, with aggrecan bound to the hyaluronan present there.[24,25] As a consequence, the pericellular environment probably is organized in a way that is important for promoting matrix assembly.

Aggrecan in Disease

A prominent feature of joint disease is the considerably reduced levels of aggrecan. Loss of this results from proteolytic degradation of the aggrecan molecules. At least two distinct enzymes appear to be involved. Major breakdown and release seems to be caused by the so-called aggrecanases, two members (4 and 5) of the a disintegrin and metalloproteinase with thrombospondin motif (ADAMTS) family of zinc-binding metalloproteinases (MMPs).[26-28] These enzymes appear to be responsible for normal aggrecan turnover, increased turnover upon immobilization of the joint, and the increased release in many inflammatory processes, such as reactive arthritis.[29] Even though the loss of aggrecan from the tissue may be extensive, the process apparently can be reversed if the collagen network is not damaged. Aggrecanases can cleave the aggrecan at four sites, with cleavage starting at the most C-terminal site in the domain carrying the chondroitin sulfate chains and the last at the most N-terminal site in the interglobular domain adjacent to the G1, hyaluronan-binding structure.[30,31]

Other MMPs that may cause release of aggrecan produce a different pattern of cleavage. Stromelysin (MMP-3), for example, cleaves between a glutamine and a phenylalanine in the interglobular domain between G1 and G2 (-DIPEN_FFG-).[32,33] In contrast, aggrecanases cleave between a glutamic acid and an alanine residue (-NITEGE_ARG-) in this interglobular domain.[29,34] The relative activities of these MMPs, stromelysin and aggrecanase, are not clear, although most of the aggrecan release appears to be caused by aggrecanases. There may be different relative activities of the enzymes and a different sequence of events in aggrecan degradation in different pathologic joint conditions.

One consequence of the loss of aggrecan from tissue and the associated loss of fixed charged groups is that the osmotic environment is altered and the ability to retain water impaired. The distribution of load over the tissue is less efficient and the process may perpetuate itself with impaired ability of the cells to accomplish repair.

A typical finding in both OA and RA is loss of aggrecan. However, very early in the process of OA, the level of aggrecan appears conserved in the cartilage. At the same time, the correlation of the tissue content of aggrecan to the staining of fixed charged groups by alcian blue, ruthenium red, or toluidine blue may be impaired, possibly because the polyanionic groups are blocked by other, newly synthesized proteins laid down in the matrix (P. Lorenzo, M. Bayliss and D. Heinegård, unpublished).

One known function of the aggrecan molecule is to form a compartment with an extremely high density of fixed charged groups that are part of polysaccharide chains covalently bound to protein, resulting in supramolecular aggregates linked to hyaluronan. This network creates the osmotic environment and "swelling pressure." In this manner, the proteoglycan has a major function in retaining tissue shape, resisting compression, and distributing load over a large volume of the tissue.

Collagen-Binding Glycoproteins

COLLAGEN NETWORKS

Other major functional units in cartilage are the collagen networks. One such network contains fibrils with collagen II as the major constituent. These fibrils are linked together by a number of noncollagenous proteins bound on their surface. The fibrils are made up of more than one type of collagen. Thus, in addition to collagen II, the complex contains a small percentage of collagen XI,[35] which may have a role in regulating the dimensions of the collagen II fibril,[36] analogous to the situation between collagen I and V in other tissues.[37] At the surface of the collagen fibrils is found collagen IX,[35] which is often covalently linked to collagen II.[38] In diseases such as OA, collagen X, normally found primarily in hypertrophic cartilage, is expressed by some articular cartilage chondrocytes.[39] This collagen may form its own network around the cells.

Collagen VI, present in many tissues, forms beaded fibrils close to the cell surface (see Fig. 3–1).[40,41] The role of these fibers is not well known, but this collagen interacts with other matrix constituents. Collagen VI filaments can be extracted from cartilaginous tissues with a linker module attached at their N-terminal structures.[42] This module is made up of a small leucine-rich-region proteoglycan (further discussed in following paragraphs), such as biglycan alternating with decorin linked to the collagen VI or to a matrilin (matrilin-1, -2, or -3)[42] (see Fig. 3–1). The matrilin, in turn, links to a set of collagen structures ranging from procollagen II to completed collagen II fibers.[42] It is possible that the collagen VI functions as a scaffold important in organizing the collagen II fibril formation. The matrilin is alternatively found linking to aggrecan molecules. Collagen VI, therefore, appears to have a central role in connecting and organizing the matrix in the territorial compartment of cartilage.

Other major components in the matrix include several noncollagenous proteins that bind to the surface of the collagen fibrils. These proteins appear to have major roles in regulating the assembly of the fibrils and in modulating the collagen-fibril surface properties and thereby the interactions with other matrix constituents, including other collagen fibrils.

The collagen networks are assembled outside the cells. The collagen fibrillar dimensions vary between different parts of the tissue, as is indicated in Figures 3–1 and 3–2. In the deeper layers, the collagen fibers are generally thicker than in the superficial layers, with a predominant arrangement perpendicular to the cartilage surface. In the superficial layer, the arrangement of the thinner collagen fibers is largely parallel to the surface[43-45] (see Fig. 3–2) There is a gradient such that the fibril dimensions

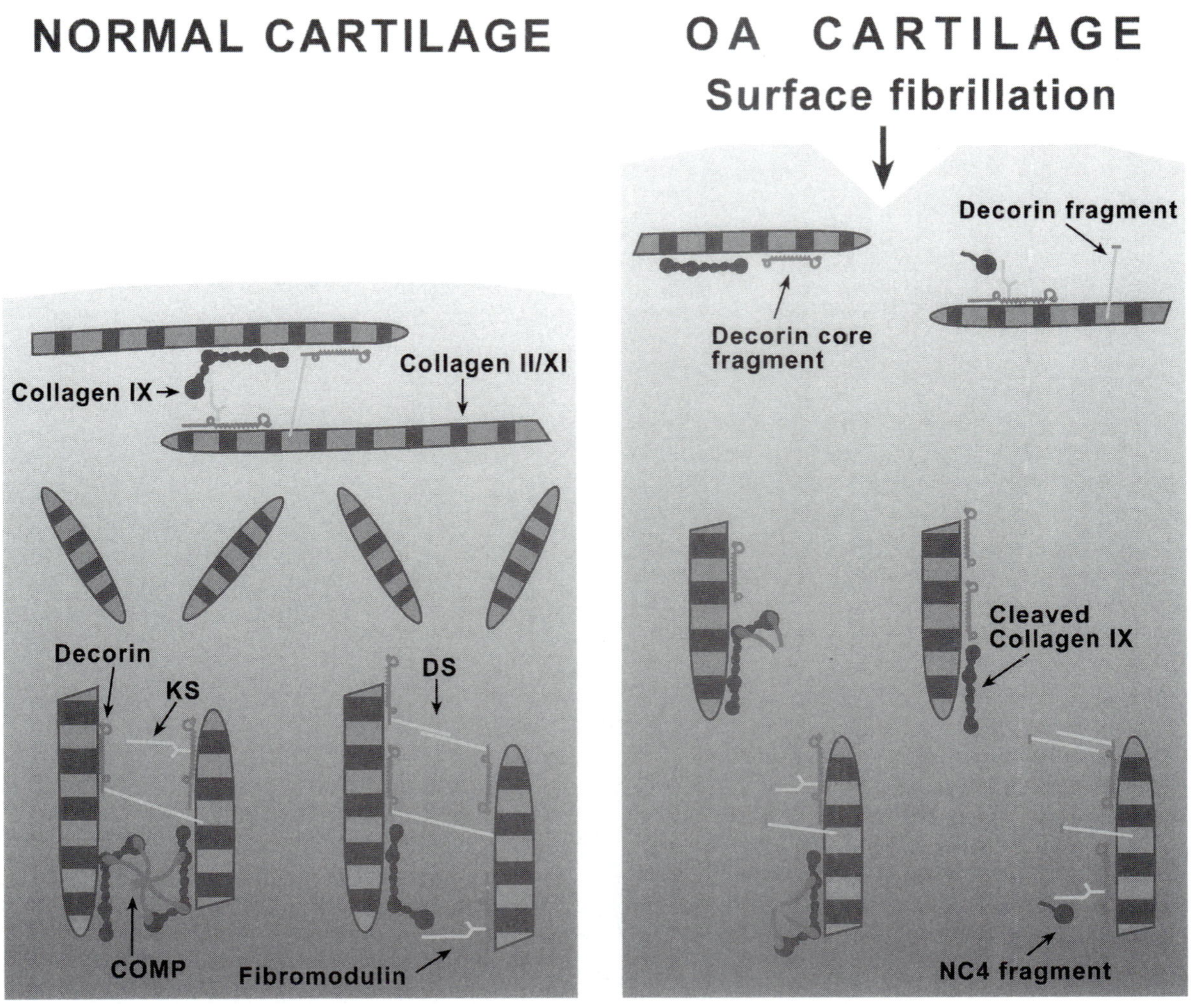

FIGURE 3–2 · Schematic Depiction of the Collagen Network in Articular Cartilage and the Swelling and Surface Disruption Following Disturbance of the Collagen Network in Osteoarthritis. The dimensions and orientation of the collagen fibers surface by proteolysis will lead to impaired tensile properties of the network and swelling to the tissue in osteoarthritis. (See color plate 1.)

close to the cells are thinner than those farther away from the cells in the so-called interterritorial matrix[45] (see Fig. 3–1 and Chapter 13).

Control of the collagen-fibril assembly appears to be a highly regulated process in which several other molecules (including the Leucine Rich Repeat [LRR] proteins to be discussed later) participate. These molecules bind to the surface of collagen molecules, as well as to the surface of the forming fiber, thereby regulating accretion of new collagen molecules. By regulating the relative abundance of the various collagen-binding molecules between them and relative to collagen itself, the cells have the capacity to modulate the orientation and dimensions of the collagen fibrils.

Assembly of the collagen fibrils also depends on the exclusion properties of the network of aggrecan molecules that regulate the diffusion of collagen precursors. In a matrix, such as articular cartilage, this consists of a gel of aggrecan, facilitating translational diffusion along the long axis of the extremely asymmetric collagen fiber.[46] At the same time, diffusion in other directions is extremely hampered. One possibility in the assembly of the collagen fibrils is diffusion through regions in the matrix that are less occupied by other constituents. One such potential "hole" region (see Fig. 3–1) is formed by the central domain of the aggrecan, where there is a more open structure, devoid of large glycosaminoglycan chains. This keratan sulfate domain can bind to collagen.[47] It is possible that one template for collagen-fibril assembly is provided by the proteoglycan aggregates and their central domain, particularly in the area close to the cells. However, further work is needed to establish this hypothesis, although available data show that in the pericellular territorial environment, a large proportion of the collagen fibrils appear to pass through the center of the aggrecan.[47]

COLLAGEN-ASSOCIATED MOLECULES

An important functional component of the collagen network appears to be the set of small collagen-binding molecules (see Figs. 3–1 and 3–3). These include decorin,[48] biglycan,[49] fibromodulin,[50] lumican,[51] proline, arginine-rich end leucine-rich repeat protein (PRELP),[52] chondroadherin,[53] and probably asporin.[54] They are members of a family of proteins containing several repeats of about 25 amino acids, with leucine residues in conserved locations. There are many similar intracellular proteins with variable numbers of these repeat sequences, whereas those in the extracellular matrix primarily contain 10 to 11 such repeats. There is also a family of these extracellular proteins with only six repeats (see Fig. 3–3). The repeat region is flanked by disulfide-loop structures, and in the N-terminus, most of the molecules carry a peptide

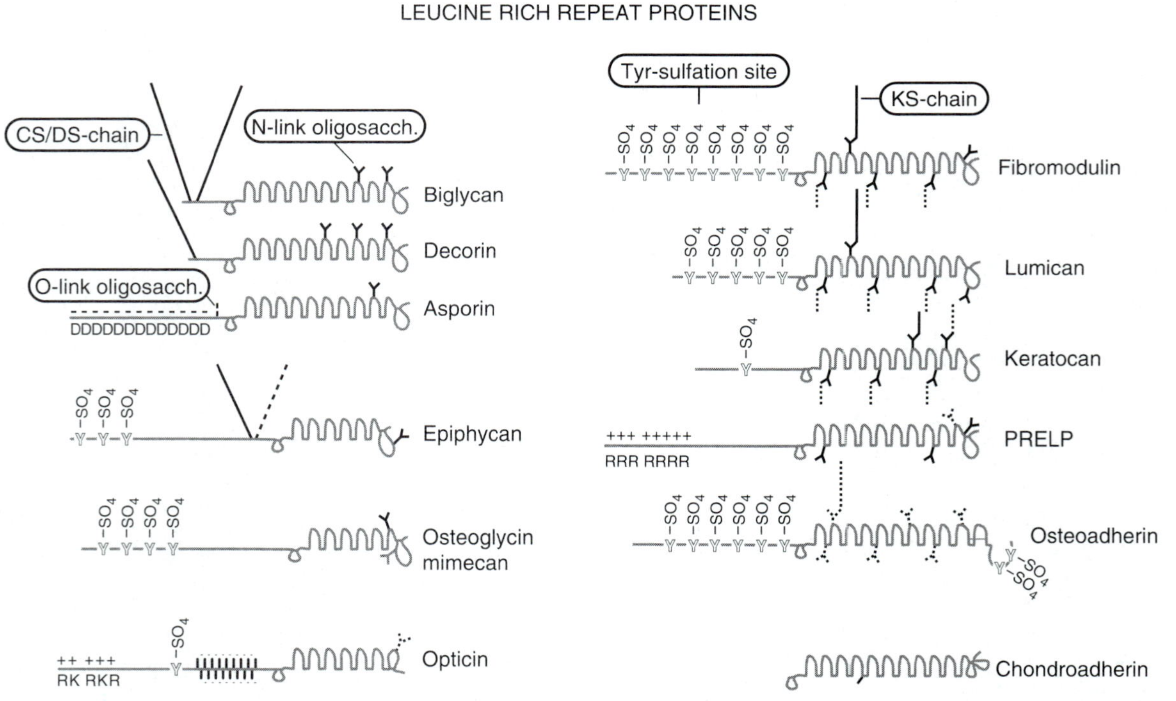

FIGURE 3–3 · Schematic Illustration of Leucine Rich Repeat Proteins in Extracellular Matrices. Each repeat is indicated, as well as the disulfide loops surrounding the repeat region. This repeat-containing domain is a key element in many interactions, including those with collagen. Note that the N- and C-terminal domains are variable with different functional implications. Biglycan and decorin bind tightly to collagen VI, as well as to matrilins, providing a cross-link. Decorin, fibromodulin, and probably lumican are bound at the collagen II fiber surface and provide interactions with other matrix constituents including collagens. Proline- and arginine-rich end leucine rich repeat protein (PRELP) can bind to collagens I and II and concomitantly to heparan sulfate side chains of proteoglycans, such as perlecan. Chondroadherin (CHAD) binds tightly to collagen molecules and can bind to integrin $\alpha2\beta1$ at the cell surface. Osteoadherin can bind to the integrin $\alpha V\beta3$.

domain with substituents of glycosaminoglycan chains (decorin and biglycan) or tyrosine sulfate (fibromodulin, lumican, osteoadherin, and keratocan).[55] Asporin has no substituents in this domain, but it is built from a long, continuous stretch of aspartic acid residues providing an anionic character.[54] PRELP has a basic N-terminal domain with clusters of arginine residues providing for binding to heparan sulfate,[56] whereas chondroadherin completely lacks this extension.[53] The molecules within the family with a shorter repeat structure bear overall similarities to the larger molecules.[55]

It has been shown that many of these molecules bind collagen with high affinity, having dissociation constants in the nanomolar range. These proteins include decorin,[57,58] biglycan,[59] fibromodulin,[60] lumican,[61] PRELP,[62] and chondroadherin.[63] It appears that also asporin,[54] and most likely osteoadherin and keratocan, have this ability to bind to collagen.

The most extensively studied collagen-associated molecules are decorin, fibromodulin, lumican, PRELP, and chondroadherin (see Fig. 3–3). They can bind to the collagen II fibrillar surface primarily through their core protein. For decorin, repeats four and five appear to provide the major binding site.[58,64] Overall, the interactions are likely to involve one surface of the molecules where the leucine-rich repeats form a β-sheet structure that is particularly suited for interactions, as has been outlined in studies of the structurally related ribonuclease inhibitor.[65]

There appear to be differences in the specificity of the binding. Biglycan shows particular affinity for collagen VI,[59] whereas it does not appear to bind to collagen I or II in the fiber form.[58] Decorin binds to both types of collagen, and the binding site on collagen VI is identical to the one for biglycan and is found in the globular structure corresponding to the N-terminus of the collagen.[59] Fibromodulin binds to both collagens, but to a different site on collagens I and II than decorin.[57] Chondroadherin also binds to collagens I and II and has been recovered from cartilaginous chondrosarcoma tissue bound to collagen II. The sites appear to be unique for this molecule, as are the sites on collagen VI, where chondroadherin is found in the tissue at the globular structures corresponding to the N-terminus, as well as that corresponding to the C-terminus.[66] PRELP binds to collagens I and II at what appear to be sites unique for this molecule.[62] All these interactions are mediated by the coreprotein and appear to involve some of the repeats in the LRR-structure.[55] Binding is in all cases strong, usually with a dissociation constant of about 10^{-9} M.

Available data indicate that these molecules serve to cross-bridge to surrounding structures, including other collagen molecules, by binding to one collagen fibril through their core protein and using their N-terminal functional domain to bind to other structures. The glycosaminoglycan side chain of decorin has been shown to bind at specific sites along the collagen fiber, but this appears to be other than the one carrying the bound core protein of the same molecule (see Figs. 3–1 and 3–2). The binding sites on the collagen may be represented by cationic domains along the fiber. In addition, dermatan sulfate side chains, exemplified by those on cartilage decorin appear to have the capacity to self interact (see Figs. 3–1 and 3–2).[67] Other putative binding sites are represented by the basic non-collagenous (NC) 4 domain of collagen IX known to extend from the collagen II fiber surface (see Fig. 3–1).[35] Both biglycan and decorin use the core protein to bind to collagen VI and the side chains to organize the further assembly of this collagen.[66] These molecules, at the same time that they bind to collagen VI, can bind to one of several members of the matrilin family of proteins.[42] These are tri- or tetramers and use the other subunits to bind to surrounding matrix structures, including collagen,[42] as discussed previously (see Fig. 3–1).

PRELP can bind via its LRR-region to collagen I, and most likely to collagen II, at the same time as the protein binds via its N-terminal heparan sulfate binding domain to proteoglycans such as Perlecan,[62] which is bound to other structures in tissues, typically basement membranes.

A consequence of the large number of interactions that occur between neighboring fibrils is a knitting together of the various fibrils in a tight network. The collagen-associated molecules may have an important role in maintaining the volume of the tissue by enforcing the ability of the collagen fibrils to resist the swelling pressure exerted by aggrecan.

Collagen Fibrillar Network in Disease

Although little is known about the early changes in the matrix in disease, one of the earliest observations in joint disease (initially observed in animal models of OA) is swelling of the cartilage, along with surface irregularities such as fibrillation. This could arise only if the collagen network has lost its ability to resist the osmotic charge pressure of the aggrecan molecules, which could result from degradation of the collagen-associated molecules, causing separation of their two or more binding sites (see Fig. 3–2). The forces holding the neighboring collagen fibrils together would then be abolished. The collagen fibrils are less likely to be degraded at this early stage because of their relative resistance to nonspecific proteolytic enzymes.[68]

Animal and Tissue Culture Models of Cartilage Degradation

Verification that the collagen-binding molecules are degraded requires studies of events far ahead of the time when clinical symptoms arise. To depict early changes in disease, studies of models of arthritis are important. The relevance of the results to human disease may be substantiated by using molecular-marker technology applied to samples from patients that provide information on the early events of matrix degradation.

An example of such a model is explant cultures of cartilage stimulated by the addition of inflammatory cytokines (e.g., IL-1) to induce tissue breakdown. Characterization of fragmented molecules released into culture medium over time will unravel cleavage sequences to enable the search for enzymes responsible for degradation. Information on cleavage sites may be used to develop assays specific for the responsible proteases.

Loosening of the collagen fibrillar network resulting from degradation of the collagen-binding molecules may represent the first irreversible step in matrix destruction. Indeed, when cartilage fragments are stimulated in vitro by IL-1, there is an initial release of aggrecan followed by molecules such as cartilage oligomeric matrix protein (COMP) and fibromodulin, apparently representing constituents released from the collagen fibril surface. Only later is collagen fragmented and released from the tissue.[68]

Another important role of these collagen-binding molecules is in the regulation of collagen fibril assembly during development and in repair and remodeling. Much information has been obtained by gene-inactivation, or knockout, studies. Mice with an inactivated gene for decorin[69] and lumican,[70] respectively, show increased collagen-fiber dimensions in the skin, and the fibers show irregular morphology. The tensile properties of the skin also is altered.[69] A surprising finding in mice with the fibromodulin gene inactivated was a larger abundance of thinner fibrils in tendons. At the same time, the level of lumican protein was higher. Surprisingly, the mRNA level for lumican was lower.[71] These seemingly contradictory results may be explained by a slower catabolism of the lumican in the absence of fibromodulin. Taken together, the data indicate a sequence of events in which individual molecules have different roles during collagen fibril assembly.

One consequence of the altered collagen stability in the mice with inactivated genes of these collagen-binding molecules is illustrated by those with a knockout of fibromodulin. These mice do develop an early-onset OA at the age of 7 or 8 months.[72] They also show lesions of the cruciate ligaments, and it is possible that the primary cause of the joint problems is defective stability due to insufficiency of the ligaments.

THROMBOSPONDINS

The thrombospondins represent a family of five members.[73,74] COMP (i.e., thrombospondin-5) has a restricted tissue distribution and is found primarily in cartilage, but it also exists in other structures with related morphology, including pressure-loaded parts of tendons.[75,76] Thrombospondin-1 (TSP-1),[77,78] -3,[79] -4,[80] and -5[81] have been found in cartilage. Two distinct subgroups within this family carry three or five subunits. COMP is a representative of the group of TSP-3,[82] - 4,[83] and -5 (COMP)[84,85] with five identical subunits, each with a molecular mass of about 87,000 D.[86] They are linked together close to the N-terminus through a heptad repeat structure, which is further stabilized by disulfide bonds.[87] The subunits contain a number of structurally different motifs also found in other connective tissue proteins, including those that can bind calcium.[84,88] The C-terminal part of each chain forms a globular structure.[85] COMP can bind with other matrix constituents by its five identical putative binding structures in the globular domain.

Thrombospondin-1 contains three subunits that are larger than COMP.[73,74] These are bound together in a heptad repeat, but they leave a free N-terminal domain at the linkage point. These chains have globular domains in their C-terminal ends, very similar to those in COMP.

The functional role of thrombospondins such as COMP in cartilage is unknown, although mutations affecting their calcium-binding ability result in multiple epiphyseal dysplasia or pseudoachondroplasia.[89,90] Despite the presence of the protein, particularly in pressure-loaded parts of normal tendon, an altered phenotype in COMP-deficient mice cannot be detected. Part of the phenotype in human disease may depend on the mutated protein forming large intracellular deposits,[91,92] which possibly interfere with the normal function of the cell. There also are indications that COMP can bind to cells,[78] but the details have not been elucidated. Although the protein is found close to the cell in growing cartilage (as in the growth plate), in adult, normal articular cartilage, the protein is almost exclusively localized at a distance from the cell,[93] which excludes direct interactions.

A clue to the function of COMP is obtained by studies of collagen binding[94] in which the protein binds tightly, with a dissociation constant in the order of 10^{-9} M. This interaction depends on presence of zinc ions, and calcium does not seem to promote the interaction. There are four apparently identical sites with binding properties on the collagen molecule. However, an individual COMP molecule is only capable of interacting with one such site on each collagen.[94] The other four binding sites can bind to other collagen molecules and facilitate more efficient collagen fibril formation. Although COMP binds tightly to collagen molecules, it does not remain bound at the completed fiber.[95] Thus, the molecule acts as a catalyst involved only in the early steps occurring close to the cell surface (see Fig. 3–1).

COMP also binds tightly at the noncollagenous domains of collagen IX. Because this molecule is bound covalently at the surface of the collagen II fibers, COMP has the potential to cross-bridge neighboring fibers[88] (see Fig. 3–1). In adult cartilage, COMP is found primarily in the interterritorial matrix where the collagen fibers are most prominent.[93]

MATRILINS

Matrilins[96] represent a novel family of proteins; cartilage matrix protein (CMP), or matrilin-1, was the first described.[97] Matrilins-1 and -3[98] are particularly prominent in normal cartilage.[99] Matrilin-1 is selectively found only in some cartilages,[100] including tracheal, nasal, ear, and epiphyseal cartilage. The protein is not detected in normal adult articular cartilage or in the intervertebral disk structures. This protein is a trimer with each of three identical subunits having a molecular mass of about 50,000 D.[96,97] The subunits are held together by a coiled-coiled domain, and the interaction is further stabilized by disulfide bonds. A functional structure present in all the matrilins is the von Willebrand factor (vWf) A domain. Matrilin-1 contains two such domains, whereas matrilin-3, also present in cartilage, contains only one.[98] One function of the vWf A domain is to contribute collagen-binding properties to proteins. Matrilin-1 can bind to collagen and appears to colocalize with the fibers in the tissue.[101] In addition to the collagen binding, it appears that the protein may self assemble, forming its own network[102] in a manner that may involve the vWf A domain. In this respect, the increasing levels of the protein in aging are interesting. As is discussed previously matrilins-1, -2, and -3 occur in tissue bound to one of the small LRR-proteoglycans, decorin or biglycan, which in turn bind to the N-terminal globular domain of collagen VI.[42] The matrilin in this complex concomitantly binds to collagen II at various organizational levels from molecule to fiber.[42] The matrilin also binds to specific locations along the aggrecan core protein.[103] Thus, matrilins appear to serve as linkers able to bind to different structures through their identical subunits.

Mutations in the matrilin-3 gene have been found associated with multiple epiphyseal dysplasia,[104] an indication of its role in cartilage matrix assembly. More recently, a mutation in the matrilin-3 gene has been associated with OA in the hands.[105] The protein is increased in OA cartilage.[106]

The detailed function of the several members of this family is only partially understood. A composite protein containing subunits of both matrilin-1 and -3 occurs in cartilage.[107] This further highlights the complexity of the functional aspects of these proteins.

Cell-Binding Glycoproteins

Chondrocytes constantly remodel the cartilage to meet new requirements and to remove old, nonfunctional tissue. In this process, the cells can secrete and activate catabolic enzymes leading to tissue breakdown, followed by secretion of newly synthesized molecules to accomplish repair. Unfortunately, the process may fail and lead to cartilage destruction, as in diseases such as RA and OA. We do not know how catabolism and anabolism are regulated and why the process may fail. However, a key issue in understanding the regulation of this well-coordinated and balanced degradation and repair in the remodeling process includes a better characterization of the roles of the cells, particularly with regard to factors that trigger their responses. It is likely that the interactions of the cell with its environment have crucial roles. These interactions usually involve matrix proteins that bind to specific receptors (e.g., integrins) at the cell surface. Integrins consist of an α-chain in combination with a β-chain. More than 10 α-chains have been identified; α10 is particularly restricted to cartilage. Integrins with other α-chains do not show a restricted distribution to this tissue.

An integrin dimer consists of one of these α-chains combined with a particular β-chain, primarily β1 or β3, such that the total number of integrins exceeds 20. The various combinations of subunits have different specificities for binding to specific ligands. For example, there are integrins primarily binding to collagen and others to fibronectin.

When integrins bind to a specific matrix protein, responses are elicited that may involve signals to the cytoskeleton resulting in cell spreading, movement, or division. Other responses, involving a cascade of tyrosine phosphorylation reactions, result in the activation of transcription factors, with ensuing modulated synthesis of matrix macromolecules, growth factors, and proteinases.

COLLAGEN

Collagen triple-helical domains of, for example, fibril-forming collagens I and II (see Chapter 2) have been shown to bind primarily α1β1, α2β1, α10β1, and α11β1 integrins.[108,109] When the cells bind to collagen in vitro, they respond by spreading and eventually dividing. At the same time, production of matrix constituents is often altered.

FIBRONECTIN

Fibronectin is not a cartilage-specific component, although the variant present in this tissue appears to be specifically spliced.[110,111] The primary ligand is the α5β1 integrin, but the protein may also bind to other integrins.[112] Fibronectin contains the classic cell-binding sequence identified as arginine-glycine-aspartic acid (RGD).[113] Cell binding to immobilized fibronectin can be inhibited by addition of RGD-containing short peptides, which saturate the integrins and do not contain binding sites cross-linking to other matrix structures. Fibronectin is upregulated in OA[114,115] and may have a role in the response to events in the matrix.

Fragments of fibronectin only containing heparin-binding sequence have been shown to change cellular behavior. When such fragments are added to joint structures in vitro and in vivo they can induce catabolic events.[116,117] Although the details of the mechanism are not known, and these fragments do not bind directly to integrins at the cell surface, they may bind to heparan sulfate proteoglycans at the cell surface. It is possible that one mechanism driving cartilage breakdown in joint disease is the formation of fibronectin fragments or, indeed, fragments of other proteins binding to other proteins or receptors at the cell surface.

CHONDROADHERIN

Chondroadherin is a member of the leucine-rich repeat protein family described previously (see Fig. 3–3). The protein is different from the other members of the family in that it contains no N-terminal extension and has a short C-terminal peptide region outside the disulfide loop structures.[53] The protein is somewhat basic and, uniquely for extracellular matrix proteins, appears to contain no carbohydrate structures and has no attachment site for N-glycosidically linked oligosaccharides.

Chondroadherin can promote cell attachment mediated by the α2β1 integrin,[107] which is normally seen as a collagen-binding receptor. However, when cells are plated on chondroadherin, they attach, but fail to spread in contrast to their more common behavior upon integrin binding, including that to collagen through the same receptor.[107] This is of particular interest because cell spreading is an early event in cell division, and chondrocytes normally do not divide. It appears that different matrix proteins, even when involving the same integrin, may elicit different responses. This is possibly a result of a binding by different types of interactions. Whether the cells also respond by activating different repair or catabolic events is not clear.

Chondroadherin, in addition, binds triple-helical collagens II at two distinct sites.[63] This tight binding (dissociation constant ~10^{-9} M) occurs in vivo; extraction of collagen molecules with bound chondroadherin results from using activation of endogenous MMPs in the cartilage.[63] The presence of such a complex between the monomeric collagen molecule and chondroadherin in the tissue indicates a role of the protein in collagen fibrillogenesis. Chondroadherin also occurs in the pressure-loaded part of tendon, which has a cartilage-like structure.[76]

PROLINE- AND ARGININE-RICH END LEUCINE RICH REPEAT PROTEIN

PRELP was originally purified as a prominent component of bovine articular cartilage. It has a molecular mass of around 58 kD.[118] The protein belongs to the leucine-rich repeat protein family[52] (see Fig. 3–3) and has been found in different types of cartilage and in many non-cartilaginous tissues.

At the chondrocyte cell surface, PRELP can interact with heparan sulfate chains. The latter are localized primarily on the proteoglycan syndecan, which is intercalated into the cell membrane by its protein core.[118] Other ligands for heparan sulfate include specific domains of fibronectin and collagen. These domains are different from the integrin-binding domain of these proteins. The concomitant binding of heparan sulfate and integrin appears essential for some of the cellular reactions, particularly spreading.[120] PRELP seems to selectively bind heparan sulfate through its N-terminal extension, which contains proline and clustered arginine residues. This represents a motif typical for binding to this glycosaminoglycan. Cells can attach to surfaces coated with PRELP,[121] a process probably mediated by heparan sulfate. This attachment can be inhibited by digestion of the cells with heparan sulfate–cleaving enzymes (E. Bengtsson, A. Aspberg and D. Heinegård, unpublished observation). Ligands binding to the heparan sulfate chains of the syndecan may elicit intracellular signals.[119] PRELP, in this interaction, may have a role in feedback from matrix to chondrocytes. The molecule may interfere with the binding of growth factors, such as basic fibroblast growth factor (FGF) and platelet-derived growth factor (PDGF) to heparan sulfate.

Another ligand for PRELP is triple-helical collagen.[62] Binding is in the nanomolar range. It leaves the N-terminal domain free to interact with heparan sulfate on other extracellular matrix components. Complexes of perlecan bound to PRELP via one of its heparan sulfate chains, where the PRELP is further bound to collagen molecules in vitro, has been visualized by negative-staining electron microscopy.[62] Whether this interaction is a reason for the severe growth disturbances and altered collagen fibril network observed in mice with the perlecan gene inactivated[122,123] is not known.

Other Matrix Glycoproteins

No function has been identified for several matrix proteins. One such protein, which shows alterations in joint disease such as OA, is cartilage intermediate layer protein (CILP).

CARTILAGE INTERMEDIATE LAYER PROTEIN

CILP was initially isolated from articular cartilage and found to be present in a number of different cartilages, although not in other tissues.[124] Cloning and sequence determination of the protein has revealed an unusual gene[125] that encodes a protein precursor that has, in the N-terminal portion, the approximately 82-kD CILP protein and in its C-terminal part, a nucleotide pyrophosphohydrolase homologue (NTPPHase). The precursor protein is efficiently cleaved at the time of secretion by what appears to be a furin-type protease. Only the two separated proteins are found in the extracellular environment. CILP, although upregulated in early OA, has no known function. Its amino acid sequence presents an entirely novel protein without presenting functional clues.[125] A piece of information of potential importance is that the protein is not distributed throughout the articular cartilage, but is particularly enriched at the middle to lower part of the tissue. This indicates some special function for this part of the tissue, where CILP should fulfill a role. The NTPPHase enzyme homology part of the gene product, if active, may have a role in generating pyrophosphate. This component may be involved in formation of calcium pyrophosphate precipitates, or, on the other hand, it could inhibit hydroxyapatite crystal growth. The upregulation of this molecule in OA may have a particular role in regulating mineral homeostasis and, perhaps, formation of crystal deposits.

There are few examples where one gene encodes two proteins, and the CILP-NTPPHase gene is also rare in that the border between the two proteins occurs within the last exon 9.[126]

Although we currently do not have an understanding of the functional roles of CILP, further studies should reveal more information about its functional implications in disease.

OTHER GLYCOPROTEINS

Glycoprotein-39 (gp39), or YKL-40, is present in cartilage and in a number of other connective tissues, including the synovial capsule. It is predominantly found in the more superficial parts of articular cartilage.[127]

A novel proteoglycan, which has been referred to as the superficial zone protein,[128] contains both keratan sulfate and chondroitin sulfate chains. It was first found in megakaryocytes,[129] and probably corresponds to a previously identified lubricating activity in synovial fluid.[130] In articular cartilage it is present primarily in the superficial part, and it is also produced in the joint capsule.[131] Little is known of its functional properties.

WARP (von Willebrand factor A related protein) is a novel protein that appears unique to cartilage. This protein contains vWf A domains and is, therefore, likely to participate in as-yet-unknown interactions with other matrix proteins. WARP is present in the superficial parts of articular cartilage.[132]

SUMMARY

Thus, cartilage tissue can be viewed as a composite of aggrecan, containing more than 100 negatively charged chondroitin sulfate side chains, each with some 50 carboxyl and 50 sulfate groups. The other major component is the fibrillar network, which consists of collagen and attached cross-bridging and -linking noncollagenous, as well as collagenous, matrix proteins. There are also a number of proteins with roles in cell binding capable of eliciting signals in response to altered conditions in the matrix. Yet other proteins may have primary roles in regulating processes in the tissue.

Applications of Matrix Proteins in Studies of Disease

ALTERED MATRIX PROTEINS AND TISSUE IN DISEASE

The information gained about matrix constituents and some of their functional roles have provided insights into the mechanisms of tissue damage resulting from disease. The early stages of cartilage damage have been defined by a single superficial lesion of fibrillation or surface roughening of the cartilage in the knee joint. Metabolic labeling of samples obtained at surgery involving amputation because of a tumor in the lower limb have provided important information on altered specific cellular activities (P. Lorenzo, M. Bayliss, and D. Heinegård, unpublished information). Studies demonstrated a particularly pronounced increase in the synthesis of COMP, CILP, and fibronectin; the latter observation had been made previously by Lust and collaborators[114] in studies of canine OA. Another 40-kD protein represents a novel member of the leucine-rich repeat protein family, asporin, which has a polyaspartate N-terminal tail[54,133] (see Fig. 3–3). This altered pattern of protein synthesis provides a type of fingerprint, characteristic of early features of OA. In situ hybridization has revealed that the distribution of cells in the cartilage expressing increased amounts of COMP and CILP was different in early tissue damage than in the normal tissue (K. King, P. Lorenzo, M. Bayliss and D. Heinegård, unpublished observation).

A hallmark of early OA is that CILP and COMP, normally deposited in the interterritorial matrix at a distance from the cells, are particularly enriched in deeper regions of the cartilage, where they are laid down in a ring in close proximity to the chondrocyte. At the same time, the proteins have virtually been lost from the interterritorial matrix (K. King, P. Lorenzo, M. Bayliss and D. Heinegård, unpublished observation). This pattern must be a consequence of the increased turnover in combination with a high level of synthesis. The altered location of these two proteins represents the earliest sign of the process that may lead to OA and is corroborated by a similar appearance in late-stage disease. In view of the putative role of COMP in collagen fibrillogenesis, the very high COMP production coupled to a low production of collagen may lead to hampered collagen-fiber formation. This is caused when each binding site on the collagen is occupied by an individual COMP molecule, with the effect that no cross-bridging to other collagen molecules will occur.

Further information that corroborates cartilage alterations in disease can be obtained in studies of synovial fluid. Some of the fragments produced in tissues as a result of the altered turnover of matrix constituents will be released initially to the synovial fluid and later into the systemic circulation. Studies of these molecular fragments are referred to as molecular-marker technology (see Chapter 1).

MOLECULAR-MARKER TECHNOLOGY IN DIAGNOSIS AND MONITORING OF DISEASE

In diseases such as OA and RA, the normal balance between breakdown of cartilage matrix constituents and their replacement by newly synthesized elements is disturbed. It is shifted toward excessive degradation in established disease and eventually leads to disruption of the structural and functional integrity of the cartilage. The macromolecules or their fragments released into the synovial fluid may be used to monitor the intensity and character of the process. These fragments eventually may reach the blood stream, and those representing the peptides containing the cross-links from collagen may be recovered from the urine.[134-137] This sequence of events, depicted in Figure 3–4, is the basis for efforts to identify processes in the tissue by quantifying matrix molecules, or molecular markers, in body fluids. Immunoassays provide noninvasive methods for monitoring pathologic tissue processes.[138]

Molecular markers are analyzed for diagnostic and prognostic purposes and for monitoring the effects of therapy on the joint cartilage. Another approach, which has proven feasible in studies of the pathophysiology of tissue destruction in arthritis, is the concomitant quantification of a number of tissue markers in the same fluid sample to depict different processes. This includes assay for the activity in the inflammatory process which can, for example, be done using a sensitive assay for C-reactive protein[139,140] at the same time as assays are performed for the process in the different structures of the joint, exemplified by COMP for cartilage[140,141] and BSP for bone.[141] The pattern observed represents a "fingerprint" that may be used to distinguish and characterize the process destroying the joint and to assess how far the damage has progressed at the level of the molecular organization. Delineating the fragment pattern will aid in identifying the enzymes responsible for the tissue breakdown. It needs to be stressed that the molecular markers depict the activity of the ongoing process and do not provide any direct information on the extent of tissue loss depicted by imaging methods.

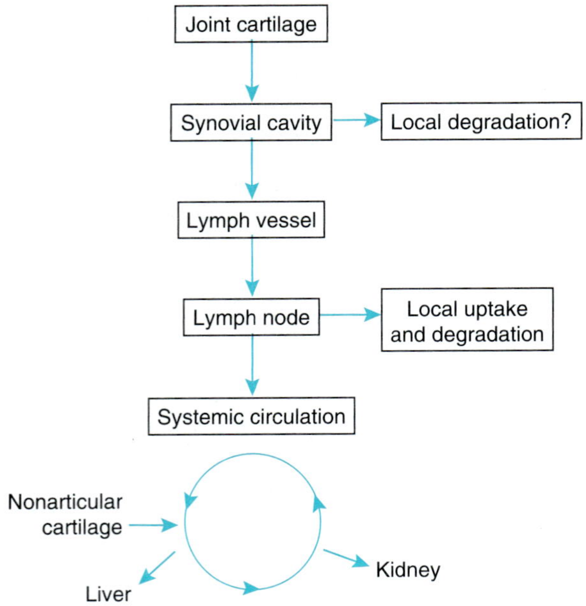

FIGURE 3–4 · **Release from Articular Cartilage and Flux of Fragmented Macromolecules between Body Fluids.** Cartilage macromolecular constituents become fragmented by proteases and are released into the synovial fluid. They are then cleared by lymphatic drainage to the blood and removed by hepatic degradation or renal clearance. Note that some types of fragments, such as aggrecan, are eliminated in the lymph nodes. Also note the influx of fragments from extra-articular cartilage.

Increased release of fragmented tissue molecular elements indicates upregulated tissue turnover, which, if persistent and not compensated by repair, eventually will lead to permanent joint damage. Increased or increasing synovial fluid or serum levels of cartilage macromolecules may foretell cartilage destruction and add prognostic value. The feasibility of this approach has indeed been shown in studies of RA[142-144] and OA[141,145] and has been supported in studies of experimental models of arthritis[145,146,147] (see Chapter 1). Serum levels of these markers do not necessarily correlate with inflammation. For example, in a model of collagen II-induced arthritis, inflammation can be inhibited by tumor necrosis factor-alpha (TNF-α) antagonists without affecting cartilage destruction and levels of markers from cartilage found in the blood.[148]

Marker technology provides a measure of the disease process not accounted for in clinical practice, except when destruction of joint structures can be demonstrated by radiographs or magnetic resonance imaging (MRI) in follow-up studies. Assessment of tissue-protective effects of therapy by analysis of tissue-derived molecular markers has the potential to provide a means of obtaining information on the influence on the tissue, particularly cartilage, at the time when therapy is given, rather than waiting for destruction to progress sufficiently to be detected by imaging techniques. Preliminary results from RA trials are encouraging, but the information obtained in studies of experimental arthritis is more extensive and lays the groundwork for studying human disease.[149,150] For example, serum levels of COMP have convincingly been shown to reflect cartilage involvement in experimental arthritis.[147,148,151] Treatment modalities, which by histopathologic examination were shown to differ in their effects on joint cartilage, were also shown to differ in their effects on serum COMP levels. Prevention of cartilage damage resulted in normalization of serum COMP levels.[148,152]

Because the cartilage structure is very different in various layers and compartments, the consequences of a disease process may vary considerably according to tissue location. For instance, a disturbance close to the chondrocyte is more likely to be corrected than is one occurring in the interterritorial matrix, where the greater distance to the cell is likely to hamper the assembly of structural elements for efficient repair. Aggrecan turnover, normally and in some cases when accelerated, appears to result in the loss of fragments that are replaced without influencing the long-term function or structure. This process is demonstrated by the marked release into the synovial fluid of aggrecan fragments in patients with reactive arthritis.[153] If more widespread structural derangement occurs, progressive joint destruction is likely to gradually involve new matrix structures. The pattern of fragmented macromolecules found in the early stages of disease changes into a different pattern in later stages of disease development.

The concept of assessing the stage and damage at the molecular level has been substantiated in a series of studies of RA and OA. For example, the synovial fluid content of fragments derived from the chondroitin sulfate–rich region of aggrecan is increased early in RA, whereas the aggrecan G1 domain remains in the tissue bound to hyaluronan and protected in the ternary complex with this molecule and with the link protein. This domain is released at later stages, and its release indicates more advanced and perhaps irreversible tissue damage.[154]

Molecular-marker technology offers opportunities to evaluate the different processes that affect the joint in disease. Thus, it has been shown possible to monitor the inflammatory process in OA by a sensitive C-reactive protein (CRP) assay showing elevated levels and indicating that inflammation is a component of late-stage disease.[139] In prospective studies of patients developing OA compared to those not developing the clinical disease over the same extended period, it was shown that the serum CRP levels were elevated only in those that developed clinical disease. This occurred before signs of a process in the cartilage characterized by elevated serum COMP levels were found, which also were found only in the group that developed clinical disease.[140] Thus, it appears that inflammation may be a very early event in the pathogenesis of OA and may actually alter the sensitivity of the cartilage to everyday use, triggering the process leading to disease.

Molecular-marker technology facilitates the identification of pathologic processes in the tissue and aids the design and evaluation of agents that block these destructive pathways in joint diseases. A full understanding of the release or retention of matrix macromolecules requires analyses of the factors governing the flux of fragments from the affected tissue into the synovial fluid and then into the general circulation through the lymphatic system (see Fig. 3–4). For example, fragments of aggrecan (the region rich in chondroitin sulfate) and COMP are cleared differently. Aggrecan fragments are well represented in the synovial fluid, but are largely eliminated in the lymph nodes en route to the circulation (R. Frazer, T. Saxne, and D. Heinegård, unpublished). COMP appears to quantitatively reach the circulation, with no apparent elimination in the lymph nodes (R. Frazer, T. Saxne, and D. Heinegård, unpublished). Consequently, measurements of glycosaminoglycans, such as keratan sulfate and peptide epitopes of the chondroitin sulfate–rich domain, can be informative when synovial fluid is analyzed, but serum samples are not representative. In contrast, measurements of COMP (and probably other proteins) in synovial fluid and serum can provide information on processes in joints.

Despite potential limiting factors, the application of molecular-marker technology in research and clinical practice offers great potential for monitoring the effects of disease on target tissues. Molecular markers represent biologic measures for studies of the mechanisms of tissue destruction and for monitoring the tissue process, which is essential to evaluating the effects of novel forms of therapy.

REFERENCES

1. Hultenby K, Reinholt FP, Norgård M, et al: Distribution and synthesis of bone sialoprotein in metaphyseal bone of young rats show a distinctly different pattern from that of osteopontin. Eur J Cell Biol 63:230-239, 1994.
2. Ramstad V, Franzén A, Heinegård D, et al: Ultrastructural distribution of osteoadherin in rat bone show pattern similar to that of bone sialoprotein. Calcif Tissue Int 72:57-64, 2003.
3. Akizuki S, Mow VC, Müller F, et al: Tensile properties of human knee joint cartilage. I. Influence of ionic conditions, weight bearing, and fibrillation on the tensile modulus. J Orthop Res 4: 379-392, 1986.
4. Akizuki S, Mow VC, Müller F, et al: Tensile properties of human knee joint cartilage. II. Correlations between weight bearing and tissue pathology and the kinetics of swelling. J Orthop Res 5:173-186, 1987.
5. Mow VC, Holmes MH, Lai WM: Fluid transport and mechanical properties of articular cartilage: a review. Biomechanics 17(5): 377-394, 1984.
6. Maroudas A: Physicochemical properties of articular cartilage. *In* Freeman MAR (ed): Adult Articular Cartilage. Turnbridge Wells, Pitman Medical, 1979, pp 215-290.
7. Hardingham TE, Fosang AJ: Proteoglycans: many forms and many functions. FASEB J 6:861-870, 1992.
8. Heinegård D, Oldberg å: Glycosylated matrix proteins. *In* Royce PM, Steinmann B (eds): Connective Tissue and Its Heritable Disorders. New York, Wiley-Liss, 1992, pp 189-209.
9. Hascall VC, Heinegård D: Aggregation of cartilage proteoglycans. II. Oligosaccharide competitors of the proteoglycan-hyaluronic acid interaction. J Biol Chem 249:4242-4249, 1974.
10. Tengblad A: A comparative study of the binding of cartilage link protein and the hyaluronate-binding region of the cartilage proteoglycan to hyaluronate-substituted Sepharose gel. Biochem J 199:297-305, 1981.
11. Mörgelin M, Heinegård D, Engel J, Paulsson M: The cartilage proteoglycan aggregate: assembly through combined protein-carbohydrate and protein-protein interactions. Biophys Chem 50:113-128, 1994.
12. Heinegård D, Hascall VC: The effects of dansylation and acetylation on the interaction between hyaluronic acid and the hyaluronic acid-binding region of cartilage proteoglycans. J Biol Chem 254:921-926, 1979.
13. Yasumoto T, Bird JL, Sugimoto K, et al: The G1 domain of aggrecan released from porcine articular cartilage forms stable complexes with hyaluronan/link protein. Rheumatology (Oxford) 42:336-342, 2003.
14. Doege KJ, Sasaki M, Kimura T, Yamada Y: Complete coding sequence and deduced primary structure of the human cartilage large aggregating proteoglycan, aggrecan. J Biol Chem 266:894-902, 1991.
15. Heinegård D, Axelsson I: Distribution of keratan sulfate in cartilage proteoglycans. J Biol Chem 252:1971-1979, 1977.
16. Antonsson P, Heinegård D, Oldberg Å: The keratan sulfate-enriched region of bovine cartilage proteoglycan consists of a consecutively repeated hexapeptide motif. J Biol Chem 264:16170-16173, 1989.
17. Maroudas A: Physical chemistry and the structure of cartilage. J Physiol (Lond) 223:21P-22P, 1972.
18. Baldwin C, Reginato A, Prockop D: A new epidermal growth factor-like domain in the human core protein for the large cartilage-specific proteoglycans: evidence for alternative splicing of the domain. J Biol Chem 264:15747-15750, 1989.
19. Halberg DF, Proulx G, Doege K, et al: A segment of the cartilage proteoglycan core protein has lectin-like activity. J Biol Chem 263:9486-9490, 1968.
20. Aspberg A, Miura R, Bourdoulous S, et al: The C-type lectin domains of lecticans, a family of aggregating chondroitin sulfate proteoglycans, bind tenascin-R by protein-protein interactions independent of carbohydrate moiety. Proc Natl Acad Sci U S A 94:10116-10121, 1997.
21. Aspberg A, Adam S, Kostka G, et al: Fibulin-1 is a ligand for the C-type lectin domains of aggrecan and versican. J Biol Chem 274:20444-20449, 1999.
22. Olin AI, Mörgelin M, Sasaki T, et al: The proteoglycans aggrecan and versican form networks with fibulin-2 through their lectin domain binding. J Biol Chem 276:1253-1261, 2001.
23. Isogai Z, Aspberg A, Keene DR, et al: Versican interacts with fibrillin-1 and links extracellular microfibrils to other connective tissue networks. J Biol Chem, 277:4565-4572, 2002.
24. Kimura JH, Hardingham TE, Hascall VC: Assembly of newly synthesized proteoglycan and link protein into aggregates in cultures of chondrosarcoma chondrocytes. J Biol Chem 255(15):7134-7143, 1980.
25. Sommarin Y, Heinegård D: Specific interaction between cartilage proteoglycans and hyaluronic acid at the chondrocyte cell surface. Biochem J 214:777-784, 1983.
26. Tortorella MD, Burn TC, Pratta MA, et al: Purification and cloning of aggrecanase-1: a member of the ADAMTS family of proteins [see comments]. Science 284:1664-1666, 1999.
27. Tortorella MD, Liu RQ, Burn T, et al: Characterization of human aggrecanase 2 (ADAM-TS5): substrate specificity studies and comparison with aggrecanase 1 (ADAM-TS4). Matrix Biol 21:499-511, 2002.
28. Tortorella MD, Malfait AM, Deccico C, Arner E: The role of ADAM-TS4 (aggrecanase-1) and ADAM-TS5 (aggrecanase-2) in a model of cartilage degradation. Osteoarthritis Cartilage 9:539-552, 2001.
29. Sandy JD, Flannery CR, Neame PJ, Lohmander LS: The structure of aggrecan fragments in human synovial fluid: evidence for the involvement in osteoarthritis of a novel proteinase which cleaves the Glu 373-Ala 374 bond of the interglobular domain. J Clin Invest 89:1512-1516, 1992.
30. Westling J, Fosang AJ, Last K, et al: ADAMTS4 cleaves at the aggrecanase site (Glu373-Ala374) and secondarily at the matrix metalloproteinase site (Asn341-Phe342) in the aggrecan interglobular domain. J Biol Chem 277:16059-16066, 2002.
31. Sandy JD, Thompson V, Doege K, Verscharen C: The intermediates of aggrecanase-dependent cleavage of aggrecan in rat chondrosarcoma cells treated with interleukin-1. Biochem J 351:161-166, 2000.
32. Hughes CE, Caterson B, Fosang AJ, et al: Monoclonal antibodies that specifically recognize neoepitope sequences generated by 'aggrecanase' and matrix metalloproteinase cleavage of aggrecan: application to catabolism in situ and in vitro. Biochem J 305:799-804, 1995.
33. Fosang AJ, Last K, Knäuper V, et al: Fibroblast and neutrophil collagenases cleave at two sites in the cartilage aggrecan interglobular domain. Biochem J 295:273-276, 1993.
34. Hughes CE, Little CB, Buttner FH, et al: Differential expression of aggrecanase and matrix metalloproteinase activity in chondrocytes isolated from bovine and porcine articular cartilage. J Biol Chem 273:30576-30582, 1998.

35. Mendler M, Eich-Bender SG, Vaughan L, et al: Cartilage contains mixed fibrils of collagen types II, IX, and XI. J Cell Biol 108: 191-197, 1989.
36. Blaschke UK, Eikenberry EF, Hulmes DJ, et al: Collagen XI nucleates self-assembly and limits lateral growth of cartilage fibrils. J Biol Chem 275:10370-10378, 2000.
37. Marchant JK, Hahn RA, Linsenmayer TF, Birk DE: Reduction of type V collagen using a dominant-negative strategy alters the regulation of fibrillogenesis and results in the loss of corneal-specific fibril morphology. J Cell Biol 135:1415-1426, 1996.
38. Wu JJ, Woods PE, Eyre DR: Identification of cross-linking sites in bovine cartilage type IX collagen reveals an antiparallel type II-type IX molecular relationship and type IX to type IX bonding. J Biol Chem 267:23007-23014, 1992.
39. Girkontaite I, Frischholz S, Lammi P,et al: Immunolocalization of type X collagen in normal fetal and adult osteoarthritic cartilage with monoclonal antibodies. Matrix Biology 15:231-238, 1996.
40. Ayad S, Marriott A, Morgan K, Grant ME: Bovine cartilage types VI and IX collagens. Characterization of their forms in vivo. Biochem J 262:753-761, 1989.
41. Kielty CM, Boot-Handford RP, Ayad S, et al: Molecular composition of type VI collagen. Evidence for chain heterogeneity in mammalian tissues and cultured cells. Biochem J 272:787-795, 1990.
42. Wiberg C, Klatt A, Wagener R, et al: Complexes of matrilin-1 and biglycan or decorin connect collagen VI microfibrils to both collagen II and aggrecan. J Biol Chem, in press.
43. Yarker YE, Hukins DW, Nave C: X-ray diffraction studies of tibial plateau cartilage using synchrotron radiation. Connect Tissue Res 12:337-343, 1984.
44. Aspden RM, Hukins DWL: Stress in collagen fibrils of articular cartilage calculated from their measured orientations. Matrix 9:486-488, 1989.
45. Hedlund H, Mengarelli-Widholm S, Reinholt FP, Svensson O: Stereologic studies on collagen in bovine articular cartilage. APMIS 101:133-140, 1993.
46. Laurent TC, Pertoft H, Preston BN, et al: Diffusion of macromolecules through compartments containing polysaccharides. Bibl Anat 15:489-492, 1977.
47. Hedlund H, Hedbom E, Heinegård D, et al: Association of the aggrecan keratan sulfate-rich region with collagen in bovine articular cartilage. J Biol Chem 274:5777-5781, 1999.
48. Krusius T, Ruoslahti E: Primary structure of an extracellular matrix proteoglycan core protein deduced from cloned cDNA. Proc Natl Acad Sci U S A 83:7683-7687, 1986.
49. Fisher LW, Termine JD, Young MF: Deduced protein sequence of bone small proteoglycan I (biglycan) shows homology with proteoglycan II (decorin) and several nonconnective tissue proteins in a variety of species. J Biol Chem 264:4571-4576, 1989.
50. Oldberg Å, Antonsson P, Lindblom K, Heinegård D: A collagen-binding 59-kd protein (fibromodulin) is structurally related to the small interstitial proteoglycans PG-S1 and PG-S2 (decorin). EMBO J 8:2601-2604, 1989.
51. Blochberger T, Vergnes J-P, Hempel J, Hassell J: cDNA to chick lumican (corneal keratan sulfate proteoglycan) reveals homology to the small interstitial proteoglycan gene family and expression in muscle and intestine. J Biol Chem 267:347-352, 1992.
52. Bengtsson E, Neame PJ, Heinegård D, Sommarin Y: The primary structure of a basic leucine-rich repeat protein, PRELP, found in connective tissues. J Biol Chem 270:25639-25644, 1995.
53. Neame PJ, Sommarin Y, Boynton RE, Heinegård D: The structure of a 38-kDa leucine-rich protein (chondroadherin) isolated from bovine cartilage. J Biol Chem 269:21547-21554, 1994.
54. Lorenzo P, Aspberg A, Önnerfjord P, et al: Identification and characterization of asporin-a -novel member of the leucine rich repeat protein family closely related to decorin and biglycan. J Biol Chem 276:12201-12211, 2001.
55. Heinegård D, Aspberg A, Franzén A, Lorenzo P: Non-collagenous glycoproteins in the extracellular matrix, with particular reference to cartilage and bone. *In* Royce P, Steinmann B, (eds): Connective Tissue and Its Heritable Disorders: Molecular, Genetic, and Medical Aspects. New York, Wiley-Liss, 2002, pp 271-291.
56. Bengtsson E, Aspberg A, Heinegård D, et al: The amino-terminal part of PRELP binds to heparin and heparan sulfate. J Biol Chem 270:40696-40702, 2000.
57. Hedbom E, Heinegård D: Binding of fibromodulin and decorin to separate sites on fibrillar collagens. J Biol Chem 268:27307-27312, 1993.
58. Svensson L, Heinegård D, Oldberg Å: Decorin-binding sites for collagen type I are mainly located in leucine-rich repeats 4-5. J Biol Chem 270:20712-20716, 1995.
59. Wiberg C, Hedbom E, Khairullina A, et al: Biglycan and decorin bind close to the n-terminal region of the collagen VI triple helix. J Biol Chem 276:18947-18952, 2001.
60. Hedbom E, Heinegård D: Interaction of a 59-kDa connective tissue matrix protein with collagen I and collagen II. J Biol Chem 264:6898-6905, 1989.
61. Svensson L, Narlid I, Oldberg A: Fibromodulin and lumican bind to the same region on collagen type I fibrils. FEBS Lett 470: 178-182, 2000.
62. Bengtsson E, Mörgelin M, Sasaki T, et al: The leucine rich repeat protein PRELP binds perlecan and collagens and may function as a basement membrane anchor. J Biol Chem 277:15061-15068, 2002.
63. Månsson B, Wenglén C, Mörgelin M, et al: Association of chondroadherin with collagen type II. J Biol Chem 276:32883-32888, 2001.
64. Kresse H, Liszio C, Schönherr E, Fisher L: Critical role of glutamate in a central leucine-rich repeat of decorin for interaction with type I collagen. J Biol Chem 272:18404-18410, 1997.
65. Kobe B, Deisenhofer J: The leucine-rich repeat: a versatile binding motif. Trends Biochem Sci 19:415-421, 1994.
66. Wiberg C, Heinegård D, Wenglén C, et al: Biglycan organizes collagen VI into hexagonal-like networks resembling tissue structures. J Biol Chem 51:49120-49126, 2002.
67. Cöster L, Fransson L-Å: Self-association of dermatan sulphate proteoglycans from bovine sclera. Biochem J 197:483-490, 1981.
68. Goldberg R, Spirito S, Doughty J, et al: Time dependent release of matrix components from bovine cartilage after IL-1 treatment and the relative inhibition by matrix metalloproteinase inhibitors. Trans Orthop Res Soc USA 20:125, 1995.
69. Danielson KG, Baribault H, Holmes DF, et al: Targeted disruption of decorin leads to abnormal collagen fibril morphology and skin fragility. J Cell Biol 136:729-743, 1997.
70. Chakravarti S, Magnuson T, Lass J, et al: Lumican regulates collagen fibril assembly: skin fragility and corneal opacity in the absence of lumican. J Cell Biol 141:1277-1286, 1998.
71. Svensson L, Aszodi A, Reinholt FP, et al: Fibromodulin-null mice have abnormal collagen fibrils, tissue organization, and altered lumican deposition in tendon. J Biol Chem 274:9636-9647, 1999.
72. Gill MR, Oldberg A, Reinholt FP: Fibromodulin-null murine knee joints display increased incidences of osteoarthritis and alterations in tissue biochemistry. Osteoarthritis Cartilage 10:751-757, 2002.
73. Lawler J, Duquette M, Urry L, et al: The evolution of the thrombospondin gene family. J Mol Evol 36:509-516, 1993.
74. Bornstein P, Sage EH: Thrombospondins. Methods in Enzymology: Extracellular Matrix Proteins. Academic Press, 1994, pp 62-85.
75. DiCesare P, Hauser N, Lehman D, et al: Cartilage oligomeric matrix protein (COMP) is an abundant component of tendon. FEBS Lett 354:237-240, 1994.
76. Smith RK, Zunino L, Webbon P, Heinegård D: The distribution of cartilage oligomeric matrix protein (COMP) in tendon and its variation with tendon site, age and load. Matrix Biol 16:255-271, 1997.
77. Tucker RP, Hagios C, Chiquet-Ehrismann R, Lawler J: In situ localization of thrombospondin-1 and thrombospondin-3 transcripts in the avian embryo. Dev Dyn 208:326-337, 1997.
78. DiCesare P, Mörgelin M, Mann K, Paulsson M: Cartilage oligomeric matrix protein and thrombospondin 1. Purification from articular cartilage, electron microscopic structure, and chondrocyte binding. Eur J Biochem 223:927-937, 1994.
79. Qabar AN, Lin Z, Wolf FW, et al: Thrombospondin 3 is a developmentally regulated heparin binding protein. J Biol Chem 269:1262-1269, 1994.
80. Tucker RP, Adams JC, Lawler J: Thrombospondin-4 is expressed by early osteogenic tissues in the chick embryo. Dev Dyn 203: 477-490, 1995.
81. Hedbom E, Antonsson P, Hjerpe A, et al: Cartilage matrix proteins. An acidic oligomeric protein (COMP) detected only in cartilage. J Biol Chem 267:6132-6136, 1992.

82. Vos HL, Devarayalu S, de Vries Y, Bornstein P: Thrombospondin 3 (Thbs3), a new member of the thrombospondin gene family. J Biol Chem 267:12192-12196, 1992.
83. Lawler J, Duquette M, Whittaker CA, et al: Identification and characterization of thrombospondin-4, a new member of the thrombospondin gene family. J Cell Biol 120:1059-1067, 1993.
84. Oldberg Å, Antonsson P, Lindblom K, Heinegård D: COMP (cartilage oligomeric matrix protein) is structurally related to the thrombospondins. J Biol Chem 267:22346-22350, 1992.
85. Mörgelin M, Heinegård D, Engel J, Paulsson M: Electron microscopy of native cartilage oligomeric matrix protein purified from the Swarm rat chondrosarcoma reveals a five-armed structure. J Biol Chem 267:6137-6141, 1992.
86. Zaia J, Boynton RE, McIntosh A, et al: Post-translational modifications in cartilage oligomeric matrix protein: characterization of the N-linked oligosaccharides by matrix-assisted laser desorption ionization time-of-flight mass spectrometry. J Biol Chem 272:14120-14126, 1997.
87. Malashkevich VN, Kammerer RA, Efimov VP, et al: The crystal structure of a five-stranded coiled coil in COMP: a prototype ion channel? Science 274:761-765, 1996.
88. Thur J, Rosenberg K, Nitsche DP, et al: Mutations in cartilage oligomeric matrix protein causing pseudoachondroplasia and multiple epiphyseal dysplasia affect binding of calcium and collagen I, II, and IX. J Biol Chem 276:6083-6092, 2001.
89. Briggs MD, Hoffman SMG, King LM, et al: Pseudoachondroplasia and multiple epiphyseal dysplasia due to mutations in the cartilage oligomeric matrix protein gene. Nature Genetics 10:330-336, 1995.
90. Deere M, Sanford T, Ferguson HL, et al: Identification of twelve mutations in cartilage oligomeric matrix protein (COMP) in patients with pseudoachondroplasia. Am J Med Genetics 80: 510-513, 1998.
91. Maddox BK, Keene DR, Sakai LY, et al: The fate of cartilage oligomeric matrix protein is determined by the cell type in the case of a novel mutation in pseudoachondroplasia. J Biol Chem 272:30993-30997, 1997.
92. Dinser R, Zaucke F, Kreppel F, et al: Pseudoachondroplasia is caused through both intra- and extracellular pathogenic pathways. J Clin Invest 110:505-513, 2002.
93. Shen Z, Heinegård D, Sommarin Y: Distribution and expression of cartilage oligomeric matrix protein and bone sialoprotein show marked changes during rat femoral head development. Matrix Biol 14:773-781, 1995.
94. Rosenberg K, Olsson H, Mörgelin M, Heinegård D: Cartilage oligomeric matrix protein shows high affinity zinc-dependent interaction with triple helical collagen. J Biol Chem 273: 20397-20403, 1998.
95. Rosenberg K, Mörgelin M, Heinegård D: COMP (Cartilage oligomeric matrix protein) as a catalyst in collagen fibrillogenesis. J Biol Chem. Submitted.
96. Deak F, Wagener R, Kiss I, Paulsson M: The matrilins: a novel family of oligomeric extracellular matrix proteins. Matrix Biol 18:55-64, 1999.
97. Paulsson M, Heinegård D: Purification and structural characterization of a cartilage matrix protein. Biochem J 197:367-375, 1981.
98. Wagener R, Kobbe B, Paulsson M: Primary structure of matrilin-3, a new member of a family of extracellular matrix proteins related to cartilage matrix protein (matrilin-1) and von Willebrand factor. FEBS Lett 413:129-134, 1997.
99. Segat D, Frie C, Nitsche PD, et al: Expression of matrilin-1, -2, and -3 in developing mouse limbs and heart. Matrix Biol 19:649-655, 2000.
100. Paulsson M, Heinegård D: Radioimmunoassay of the 148-kilodalton cartilage protein: distribution of the protein among bovine tissues. Biochem J 207:207-213, 1982.
101. Winterbottom N, Tondravi MM, Harrington TL, et al: Cartilage matrix protein is a component of the collagen fibril of cartilage. Dev Dyn 193:266-276, 1992.
102. Chen Q, Johnson D, Haudenschild D, et al: Cartilage matrix protein forms a type II collagen-independent filamentous network: analysis in primary cell cultures with a retrovirus expression system. Mol Biol Cell 6:1743-1753, 1995.
103. Hauser N, Paulsson M, Heinegård D, Mörgelin M: Interaction of cartilage matrix protein with aggrecan: increased covalent cross-linking with tissue maturation. J Biol Chem 271:32247-32252, 1996.
104. Chapman KL, Mortier GR, Chapman K, et al: Mutations in the region encoding the von Willebrand factor A domain of matrilin-3 are associated with multiple epiphyseal dysplasia. Nat Genet 28:393-396, 2001.
105. Stefansson SE, Jonsson H, Ingvarsson T, et al: Genomewide scan for hand osteoarthritis: a novel mutation in matrilin-3. Am J Hum Genet 72:1448-1459, 2003.
106. Pullig O, Weseloh G, Klatt AR, et al: Matrilin-3 in human articular cartilage: increased expression in osteoarthritis. Osteoarthritis Cartilage 10:253-263, 2002.
107. Wu JJ, Eyre DR: Matrilin-3 forms disulfide-linked oligomers with matrilin-1 in bovine epiphyseal cartilage. J Biol Chem 273:17433-17438, 1998.
108. Camper L, Heinegård D, Lundgren-Åkerlund E: Integrin alpha2beta1 is a receptor for the cartilage matrix protein chondroadherin. J Cell Biol 138:1159-1167, 1997.
109. Gullberg DE, Lundgren-Akerlund E: Collagen-binding I domain integrins: What do they do? Prog Histochem Cytochem 37:3-54, 2002.
110. MacLeod JN, Burton-Wurster N, Gu DN, Lust G: Fibronectin mRNA splice variant in articular cartilage lacks bases encoding the V, III-15, and I-10 protein segments. J Biol Chem 271:18954-18960, 1996.
111. Burton-Wurster N, Lust G: Molecular and immunologic differences in canine fibronectins from articular cartilage and plasma. Arch Biochem Biophys 269(1):32-45, 1989.
112. Hynes RO: Integrins: versatility, modulation, and signaling in cell adhesion. Cell 69:11-25, 1992.
113. Pierschbacher MD, Ruoslahti E: Influence of stereochemistry of the sequence Arg-Gly-Asp-Xaa on binding specificity in cell adhesion. J Biol Chem 262(36):17294-17298, 1987.
114. Burton-Wurster N, Lust G: Deposition of fibronectin in articular cartilage of canine osteoarthritic joints. Am J Vet Res 46: 2542-2545, 1985.
115. Lust G, Burton-Wurster N, Leipold H: Fibronectin as a marker for osteoarthritis. J Rheumatol 14:28-29, 1987.
116. Homandberg GA, Kang Y, Zhang J, et al: A single injection of fibronectin fragments into rabbit knee joints enhances catabolism in the articular cartilage followed by reparative responses but also induces systemic effects in the non-injected knee joints. Osteoarthritis Cartilage 9:673-683, 2001.
117. Xie DL, Hui F, Meyers R, Homandberg GA: Cartilage chondrolysis by fibronectin fragments is associated with release of several proteinases: stromelysin plays a major role in chondrolysis. Arch Biochem Biophys 311:205-212, 1994.
118. Heinegård D, Larsson T, Sommarin Y, et al: Two novel matrix proteins isolated from articular cartilage show wide distributions among connective tissues. J Biol Chem 261:13866-13872, 1986.
119. Woods A, Couchman JR: Syndecans: synergistic activators of cell adhesion. Trends Cell Biol 8:189-192, 1998.
120. Woods A, Longley RL, Tumova S, Couchman JR: Syndecan-4 binding to the high affinity heparin-binding domain of fibronectin drives focal adhesion formation in fibroblasts. Arch Biochem Biophys 374:66-72, 2000.
121. Sommarin Y, Larsson T, Heinegård D: Chondrocyte-matrix interactions: attachment to proteins isolated from cartilage. Exp Cell Res 184:181-192, 1989.
122. Costell M, Gustafsson E, Aszodi A, et al: Perlecan maintains the integrity of cartilage and some basement membranes. J Cell Biol 147:1109-1122, 1999.
123. Arikawa-Hirasawa E, Watanabe H, Takami H, et al: Perlecan is essential for cartilage and cephalic development. Nat Genet 23:354-358, 1999.
124. Lorenzo P, Bayliss MT, Heinegård D: A novel cartilage protein (CILP) present in the mid-zone of human articular cartilage increases with age. J Biol Chem 273:23463-23468, 1998.
125. Lorenzo P, Neame P, Sommarin Y, Heinegård D: Cloning and deduced amino acid sequence of a novel cartilage protein (CILP) identifies a proform including a nucleotide pyrophosphohydrolase. J Biol Chem 273:23469-23475, 1998.

126. Lorenzo P, Åman P, SommarinY, Heinegård D: The human CILP gene: exon/intron organization and chromosomal mapping. Matrix Biol 18:445-454, 1999.
127. Hakala BE, White C, Recklies AD: Human cartilage gp-39, a major secretory product of articular chondrocytes and synovial cells, is a mammalian member of a chitinase protein family. J Biol Chem 268:25803-25810, 1993.
128. Schumacher BL, Block JA, Schmid TM, et al: A novel proteoglycan synthesized and secreted by chondrocytes of the superficial zone of articular cartilage. Arch Biochem Biophys 311:144-152, 1994.
129. Flannery CR, Hughes CE, Schumacher BL, et al: Articular cartilage superficial zone protein (SZP) is homologous to megakaryocyte stimulating factor precursor and is a multifunctional proteoglycan with potential growth-promoting, cytoprotective and lubricating properties in cartilage metabolism. Biochem Biophys Res Commun 254:535-541, 1999.
130. Swann DA, Silver FH, Slayter HS, et al: The molecular structure and lubricating activity of lubricin isolated from bovine and human synovial fluids. Biochem J 225:195-201, 1985.
131. Jay GD, Tantravahi U, Britt DE, et al: Homology of lubricin and superficial zone protein (SZP): products of megakaryocyte stimulating factor (MSF) gene expression by human synovial fibroblasts and articular chondrocytes localized to chromosome 1q25. J Orthop Res 19:677-687, 2001.
132. Fitzgerald J, Tay TS, Bateman JF: WARP is a new member of the von Willebrand factor A-domain superfamily of extracellular matrix proteins. FEBS Lett 517:61-66, 2002.
133. Henry SP, Takanosu M, Boyd TC, et al: Expression pattern and gene characterization of asporin-a newly discovered member of the leucine repeat protein family. J Biol Chem 276:12212-12221, 2001.
134. Poole AR, Dieppe PA: Biological markers in rheumatoid arthritis. Semin Arthritis Rheum 23:17-31, 1994.
135. Thonar EJ, Shinmei M, Lohmander LS: Body fluid markers of cartilage changes in osteoarthritis. Rheum Dis Clin North Am 19:635-657, 1993.
136. Garnero P, Rousseau JC, Delmas PD: Molecular basis and clinical use of biochemical markers of bone, cartilage, and synovium in joint diseases. Arthritis Rheum 43:953-968, 2000.
137. Saxne T, Månsson B: Molecular markers for assessment of cartilage damage in rheumatoid arthritis. *In* Firestein G, Panai G, Wollheim F (eds): Rheumatoid Arthritis: New Frontiers in Pathogenesis and Treatment. Oxford, Oxford University Press, 2000, pp 291-304.
138. Saxne T, Heinegård D: Matrix proteins: potentials as body fluid markers of changes in the metabolism of cartilage and bone in arthritis. J Rheumatol Suppl 43:71-74, 1995.
139. Spector TD, Hart DJ, Nandra D, et al: Low-level increases in serum C-reactive protein are present in early osteoarthritis of the knee and predict progressive disease. Arthritis Rheum 40:723-727, 1997.
140. Saxne T, Lindell M, Månsson B, et al: Inflammation is a feature of the disease process in early knee joint osteoarthritis. Rheumatology (Oxford), in press.
141. Petersson IF, Boegård T, Svensson B, et al: Changes in cartilage and bone metabolism identified by serum markers in early osteoarthritis of the knee joint. Br J Rheumatol 37:46-50, 1998.
142. Månsson B, Geborek P, Saxne T: Cartilage and bone macromolecules in knee joint synovial fluid in rheumatoid arthritis: relation to development of knee or hip joint destruction. Ann Rheum Dis 56:91-96, 1997.
143. Saxne T, Wollheim F, Pettersson H, Heinegård D: Proteoglycan concentration in synovial fluid: predictor of future cartilage destruction in rheumatoid arthritis? Br Med J (Clin Res Educ) 295:1447-1448, 1987.
144. Månsson B, Carey D, Alini M, et al: Cartilage and bone metabolism in rheumatoid arthritis: differences between rapid and slow progression of disease identified by serum markers of cartilage metabolism. J Clin Invest 95:1071-1077, 1995.
145. Sharif M, Saxne T, Shepstone L, et al: Relationship between serum cartilage oligomeric matrix protein levels and disease progression in osteoarthritis of the knee joint. Br J Rheumatol 34:306-310, 1995.
146. Larsson E, Mussener A, Heinegård D, et al: Increased serum levels of cartilage oligomeric matrix protein and bone sialoprotein in rats with collagen arthritis. Br J Rheumatol 36:1258-1261, 1997.
147. Vingsbo LC, Saxne T, Olsson H, Holmdahl R: Increased serum levels of cartilage oligomeric matrix protein in chronic erosive arthritis in rats. Arthritis Rheum 41:544-550, 1998.
148. Joosten LA, Helsen MM, Saxne T, et al: IL-1 alpha beta blockade prevents cartilage and bone destruction in murine type II collagen-induced arthritis, whereas TNF-alpha blockade only ameliorates joint inflammation. J Immunol 163:5049-5055, 1999.
149. den Broeder AA, Joosten LA, Saxne T, et al: Long term antitumour necrosis factor alpha monotherapy in rheumatoid arthritis: effect on radiological course and prognostic value of markers of cartilage turnover and endothelial activation. Ann Rheum Dis 61:311-318, 2002.
150. Crnkic M, Månsson B, Geborek P, et al: Serum-COMP decreases in rheumatoid arthritis patients treated with infliximab or etanercept. Arthritis Res Ther 5:181-185, 2003.
151. Larsson E, Erlandsson HH, Lorentzen JC, et al: Serum concentrations of cartilage oligomeric matrix protein, fibrinogen and hyaluronan distinguish inflammation and cartilage destruction in experimental arthritis in rats. Rheumatology (Oxford) 41:996-1000, 2002.
152. Joosten LA, Helsen MM, Saxne T, et al: Synergistic protection against cartilage destruction by low dose prednisolone and interleukin-10 in established murine collagen arthritis. Inflamm Res 48:48-55, 1999.
153. Saxne T, Glennas A, Kvien TK, et al: Release of cartilage macromolecules into the synovial fluid in patients with acute and prolonged phases of reactive arthritis. Arthritis Rheum 36:20-25, 1993.
154. Saxne T, Heinegård D: Synovial fluid analysis of two groups of proteoglycan epitopes distinguishes early and late cartilage lesions. Arthritis Rheum 35:385-390, 1992.

4 Proteinases and Matrix Degradation

YASUNORI OKADA

Extracellular matrix (ECM) plays critical roles in the normal development and function of organisms by interacting with cells and supporting tissue structures. The in vivo cellular functions regulated by cell-ECM interaction include proliferation, differentiation, apoptosis, and motility. The proteolytic turnover and remodeling of ECM is transient and highly controlled under physiologic conditions, and excessive degradation of ECM components by proteinases causes tissue destruction in many pathologic conditions. In rheumatoid arthritis and osteoarthritis, ECM-degrading proteinases are elevated without sufficient endogenous inhibitors, and they are believed to play central roles in the destruction of articular cartilage and bone on the basis of a local imbalance between proteinases and inhibitors. This chapter provides recent information about the ECM-degrading proteinases and their inhibitors. The chapter covers developments in the areas of proteinases and matrix degradation that have occurred since the sixth edition of this book was published in 2001. Okada[1] offers more comprehensive coverage of the older literature.

Extracellular Matrix–Degrading Proteinases

ECM is degraded by endopeptidases (i.e., proteinases) that act internally on polypeptide chains; little evidence is present for the roles of exopeptidases that cleave one or a few amino acids from the N- or C-terminus. Proteinases are comprised of aspartic proteinases, cysteine proteinases, serine proteinases, and metalloproteinases, which are classified according to catalytic mechanism. Proteinases from each the four classes are involved in the degradation of ECM macromolecules.

ASPARTIC PROTEINASES

The most aspartic proteinases have two aspartic-acid residues in their catalytic sites, at which the nucleophile that attacks the scissile peptide bond is an activated water molecule. Among the proteinases belonging to this group, cathepsin D is the major aspartic proteinase involved in ECM degradation (Table 4–1). Cathepsin D is a lysosomal proteinase synthesized as a preproenzyme that is processed to procathepsin D, which undergoes autocatalytic cleavage to a mature active enzyme in the lysosomes. It exhibits proteolytic activity against most substrates, such as aggrecan and collagen telopeptides, with pH optima between pH 3.5 and 5.0. Because of the acidic pH optima and intracellular localization within lysosomes, cathepsin D is probably responsible for intracelluar degradation of phagocytozed ECM fragments that perviously were degraded in the extracellular spaces. However, a recent study on cartilage explant cultures using the aspartic proteinase inhibitor suggests the possibility that cathepsin D secreted extracellularly contributes to the degradation of aggrecan in articular cartilage.[2]

CYSTEINE PROTEINASES

Cysteine proteinases are endopeptidases in which the nucleophile of the catalytic site is the sulfhydryl group of a cysteine residue. The ECM-degrading cysteine proteinases include lysosomal cathepsins B, L, S, and K and the calpains (see Table 4–1). Cathepsins B and L digest the telopeptide regions of fibrillar collagen types I and II, the nonhelical regions of collagen types IX and XI, and aggrecan at acidic pH.[1] Cathepsin S has a similar spectrum of substrates within a broad range of pH values. Cathepsin K, also called cathepsin O, O2, or X, is a collagenolytic cathepsin that efficiently cleaves type I collagen at the triple-helical regions at pH values between 4.5 and 6.6.[3] This proteinase also degrades gelatin and osteonectin. Because cathepsins B, L, S, and K are expressed in synovium, articular cartilage, or both in cases of rheumatoid arthritis and osteoarthritis, they may be involved in cartilage destruction through degradation of the ECM macromolecules. Cathepsin K also plays a key role in bone resorption under such joint diseases (see following discussion).

Calpains are Ca^{2+}-dependent, papain-like cysteine proteinases and are ubiquitously distributed among mammalian cells. The best-characterized members of the calpain superfamily are μ-calpain and m-calpain, which are also called conventional and classical calpains, respectively.[4] Calpains are involved in various pathologic conditions such as muscle dystrophy by acting intracellularly. However, they are also present in the extracellular spaces and in osteoarthritic synovial fluid, and they can degrade aggrecan.

SERINE PROTEINASES

Serine proteinases require the hydroxyl group of a serine residue to act as the nucleophile that attacks the peptide bond. They include the largest number of proteinases, classified to about 40 families. Most can degrade ECM macromolecules. The major ECM-degrading serine proteinases in joint tissues are subsequently described (see also Table 4–1).

TABLE 4–1 • PROTEINASES THAT MAY BE INVOLVED IN DEGRADATION OF EXTRACELLULAR MATRIX

Enzyme	Molecular Mass (kD)	Source	Inhibitor
Aspartic Proteinases			
Cathepsin D	34	Lysosome	Pepstatin
Cysteine Proteinases			
Cathepsin B	25	Lysosome	Cystatins
Cathepsin L	24	Lysosome	Cystatins
Cathepsin S	24	Lysosome	Cystatins
Cathepsin K	29	Lysosome	Cystatins
Calpain	110(80+30)	Cytosol	Calpastatin
Serine Proteinases			
Neutrophil elastase	30	Neutrophils	α1-PI
Cathepsin G	30	Neutrophils	α1-Antichymotrypsin
Proteinase 3	29	Neutrophils	α1-PI, elafin
Plasmin	94	Plasma	Aprotinin
Plasma kallikrein	88/85	Plasma	Aprotinin
Tissue kallikrein	46	Glandular tissues	Aprotinin, kallistatin
Tissue-type plasminogen activator (tPA)	67-72	Endothelial cells, chondrocytes	PAI-1, PAI-2
Urokinase-type plasminogen activator (uPA)	54/33	Fibroblasts, chondrocytes	PAI-1, PAI-2, PN-1
Tryptase	30-35	Mast cells	Trypstatin
Chymase	26	Mast cells	α1-PI
Metalloproteinases			
Secreted-type MMPs			
Collagenases			
Interstitial collagenase (MMP-1)	52/56*	Fibroblasts, synovial cells, chondrocytes, macrophages, endothelial cells, cancer cells	TIMPs
Neutrophil collagenase (MMP-8)	75*	Neutrophils	TIMPs
Collagenase-3 (MMP-13)	65	Chondrocytes, breast carcinoma cells	TIMPs
Gelatinases			
Gelatinase A (MMP-2)	72	Fibroblasts, chondrocytes, mesangial cells, macrophages, endothelial cells	TIMPs, RECK
Gelatinase B (MMP-9)	92*	Neutrophils, macrophages, osteoclasts, trophoblasts, T-lymphocytes, cancer cells	TIMPs
Stromelysins			
Stromelysin-1 (MMP-3)	57/59*	Synovial cells, chondrocytes, fibroblasts	TIMPs
Stromelysin-2 (MMP-10)	56	Cancer cells, T-lymphocytes	TIMPs
Matrilysins			
Matrilysin-1 (MMP-7)	28	Cancer cells, chondrocytes, macrophages, mesangial cells, gland cells	TIMPs
Matrilysin-2 (MMP-26)	28	Placenta, endometrium	TIMPs
Furin-activated MMPs			
Stromelysin-3 (MMP-11)	58	Cancer stromal cells	TIMPs
Epilysin (MMP-28)	56	Epidermis, testis, lung, cancer cells	TIMPs
Other secreted-type MMPs			
Metalloelastase (MMP-12)	54	Macrophages	TIMPs
RASI-1 (MMP-19)	57	Synovial cells, ovary	TIMPs
Enamelysin (MMP-20)	54	Enameloblast	TIMPs
MMP-21	Unknown	Unknown	Unknown
MMP-27	Unknown	Unknown	Unknown
Membrane-anchored MMPs			
Type I transmembrane-type MMPs			
MT1-MMP (MMP-14)	66	Cancer cells, glioma cells, chondrocytes, fibroblasts, synovial cells	TIMPs except for TIMP-1, RECK
MT2-MMP (MMP-15)	68	Cancer cells, glioma cells	TIMPs except for TIMP-1
MT3-MMP (MMP-16)	64	Glioma cells	TIMPs except for TIMP-1
MT5-MMP (MMP-24)	63	Brain, glioma cells	Unknown
GPI-linked MMPs			
MT4-MMP (MMP-17)	Unknown	Unknown	Unknown
MT6-MMP (MMP-25)	Unknown	Leukemia cells	Unknown
Type II transmembrane-type MMP			
MMP-23	Unknown	Ovary, endometrium, testis, prostate	Unknown

(Continued)

TABLE 4–1 • PROTEINASES THAT MAY BE INVOLVED IN DEGRADATION OF EXTRACELLULAR MATRIX—cont'd

Enzyme	Molecular Mass (kD)	Source	Inhibitor
ADAMTS			
ADAMTS1	90	Kidney, heart	Unknown
ADAMTS2	135	Skin, tendon	Unknown
ADAMTS3	135	Brain	Unknown
ADAMTS4	69	Brain, heart, chondrocytes, synovial cells	TIMP-3
ADAMTS5	74	Uterus, placenta, chondrocytes	TIMP-3

* Glycosylated form.

MMP-4, MMP-5 and MMP-6 are missing MMPs.

MMP-18 (Xenopus collagenase 4; from Stolow et al: Identification and characterization of a novel collagenase in Xenopus laevis: possible roles during frog development. Mol Biol Cell 7:1471, 1996), and MMP-22 (chick MMP; Yang and Kurkinen: Cloning and characterization of a novel matrix metalloproteinase (MMP), CMP, from chicken embryo fibroblasts. MMP, Xenopus, XMMP, and human MMP19 have a conserved unique cysteine in the catalytic domain. J Biol Chem 273:17893, 1998.) are not mammalian, and thus omitted in this list.

Abbreviations: PI, proteinase inhibitor; PAI, plasminogen activator inhibitor, PN, proteinase nexin; TIMP, tissue inhibitor of metalloproteinases; RECK, reversion-inducing, cysteine-rich protein with Kazal motifs.

Neutrophil Elastase and Cathepsin G

Neutrophil elastase and cathepsin G are serine proteinases synthesized as precursors in promyelocytes within bone marrow and subsequently stored in the azurophil granules of polymorphonuclear leukocytes as active enzymes. Mature leukocytes do not synthesize elastase, but they mobilize azurophil granules to the cell surface and release the proteinases in response to various stimuli. Monocytes have low levels of elastase but lose the enzyme during the differentiation into macrophages. Neutrophil elastase and cathepsin G are basic glycoproteins with isoelectric points somewhat larger than 9 and about 12, respectively. Thus, they can be readily trapped in cartilage matrix that has a negative charge.

Neutrophil elastase and cathepsin G cleave elastin; the telopeptide region of fibrillar collagens I, II, and III; other collagen types IV, VI, VIII, IX, X, and XI; and other ECM components such as fibronectin, laminin, and aggrecan at neutral pH. These serine proteinases can also be involved indirectly in the breakdown of ECM by activating the zymogen of matrix metalloproteinases (proMMPs)[5] and by inactivating endogenous proteinase inhibitors, such as α_2-antiplasmin, α_1-antichymotrypsin, and tissue inhibitor of metalloproteinases.

Mast Cell Chymase and Tryptase

Chymase and tryptase are packaged in secretory granules with histamine and other mediators in mast cells, which are infiltrated in rheumatoid synovium. Chymase is a chymotrypsin-like proteinase with a broad spectrum of activity against ECM components, such as type VI collagen[6] and aggrecan. It also activates proMMPs, such as proMMP-1, proMMP-3, and proMMP-9.[5] Although prochymase is activated intracellularly and stored in the granules, the activity in the granules is limited at low pH and becomes fully active when released extracellularly. Tryptase is a trypsin-like proteinase that degrades collagen type VI[6] and fibronectin; it also activates proMMP-3.[5] Active tryptase exists as a tetramer of approximately 135 kD, which is stabilized by tightly bound heparin proteoglycan. Heparin or heparin proteoglycan is essential to its activity because the tetramer is transposed to inactive monomer in the absence of heparin.

Plasmin and Plasminogen Activators

Plasminogen is synthesized in liver and secreted to plasma. It can bind to fibrin and to cells, and after activation by plasminogen activators, plasmin readily digests fibrin. Membrane-bound plasmin also degrades a number of ECM components, including proteoglycan, fibronectin, type IV collagen, and laminin.[7] Another important function of plasmin is to initiate the activation of proMMPs,[5] activate latent cell-associated transforming growth factor (TGF) β1, and act as proenzyme convertase. Plasmin is generated through activation of plasminogen mainly by plasminogen activators, principally two serine proteinases: tissue-type plasminogen activator (tPA) and urinary- or urokinase-type plasminogen activator (uPA).

The tPA is synthesized as a proenzyme of 70 kD and is secreted into the circulating blood primarily by endothelial cells and others such as fibroblasts, chondrocytes, and tumor cells.[7] In addition to being a major activator of plasminogen for fibrinolysis, tPA plays a key role in the clearance of fibrin from circulation.

The uPA molecule was first purified from urine as a proenzyme of 54 kD.[7] It is converted to the active form of two chains, 30 kD and 24 kD, linked by a disulfide bond. Another fully active form of 33 kD is generated by plasmin. Although the expression of uPA is limited to some cells, such as renal tubules and bladder urothelium, under the physiologic conditions, it is more widely expressed in various cells, including invasive cancer cells, migrating keratinocytes, and activated leukocytes, in pathologic situations. Pro-uPA and two-chain uPA bind to a specific uPA receptor, a single-chain glycoprotein with a glycosylphosphatidylinositol (GPI) moiety expressed on fibroblasts, macrophages, and tumor cells. Receptor-bound uPA preferentially activates cell membrane–bound plasminogen into plasmin. Cell membrane–bound plasmin can activate receptor-bound pro-uPA. Among its specificities, uPA has a limited action on fibronectin.

Kallikreins

Two types of kallikreins, plasma and tissue kallikreins, are known. Plasma kallikrein, with two disulfide-linked chains (36 kD and 52 kD), is generated from prokallikrein of 88 kD by coagulation factor XIIa or by kallikrein itself. It activates kininogens to bradykinin and activates proMMP-1 and proMMP-3.[5] Tissue kallikrein is synthesized in glandular tissues. It releases Lys-bradykinin from kininogen and activates proMMP-8.[5]

METALLOPROTEINASES

Like aspartic proteinases, metalloproteinases are endopeptidases in which the nucleophilic attack on a peptide bond is mediated by a water molecule. A divalent metal cation, usually zinc, activates the water molecule. Among the metalloproteinase groups, matrix metalloproteinases (MMPs), which are also designated matrixins (a subfamily of the metzincin superfamily), are key ECM-degrading zinc-dependent endopeptidases (see Table 4–1). However, recently accumulated evidence indicates that some members of the a disintegrin and metalloproteinase (ADAM) family, which is an MMP-related gene family, are also involved in ECM degradation (Table 4–1).

Matrix Metalloproteinases

The human MMP family contains 23 members that have both MMP designation (numbered according to a sequential numbering system) and common names coined by the authors of the reported papers (see Table 4–1 and Table 4–2). The MMP family members were originally classified into several groups based on their substrate specificity for ECM components, such as collagenases, gelatinases, and stromelysins. However, as data on the biochemical properties provided by the domain structures and on their substrate specificity are accumulated, these family members now can be classified into two major subgroups: secreted-type MMPs and membrane-anchored MMPs. MMP-4, MMP-5, and MMP-6 are excluded from the list because they are identical to other known MMPs (i.e., MMP-3 and MMP-2). MMP-18 and MMP-22 are also missing in Tables 4–1 and 4–2 because they are assigned to xenopus collagenase-4 and chicken MMP, respectively.

Most secreted-type MMPs, including collagenases, stromelysins, and other MMPs, are composed of three basic domains—the propeptide, catalytic, and hemopexin-like domains—that are preceded by hydrophobic signal peptides (Fig. 4–1). The N-terminal propeptide domain has one unpaired cysteine in the conserved sequence of PRCGXPD. The cysteine residue in the sequence interacts with the essential zinc atom in the catalytic domain to prevent it from binding the catalytic water molecule, maintaining the proenzyme in an inactive state. The catalytic domain has the zinc-binding motif HEXGHXXGXXH, in which three histidines bind to the catalytic zinc atom. The four-blade C-terminal hemopexin-like domain, which is connected to the catalytic domain by a proline-rich hinge region, interacts with ECM components and can play a role in determining the substrate specificity in some MMPs. Gelatinases have these domains with additional insertions of collagen-binding type II repeats of fibronectin in the catalytic domain (see Fig. 4–1); this provides them with collagen-binding properties. On the other hand, matrilysins are the shortest, lacking the hemopexin-like domains. Furin-activated MMPs contain insertions of a basic motif with a cleavage site by proprotein convertases, including furin, at the end of the propeptide domains (see Fig. 4–1).

Membrane-anchored MMPs include three types: type I transmembrane-type MMPs, GPI-linked MMPs, and type II transmembrane-type MMP. MT1, 2, 3, 5-MMPs have type I transmembrane domains in the C-terminal region, but MT4, 6-MMPs contain GPI anchors in the C-terminal region without transmembrane domains (see Fig. 4–1). On the other hand, MMP-23 is unique in that it has type II transmembrane domain, a cysteine array, and an immunoglobulin-like domain instead of hemopexin-like domain (see Fig. 4–1).

Secreted-type MMPs

Collagenases (MMP-1, -8, and -13)

The collagenases include MMP-1 (interstitial collagenase, collagenase-1), MMP-8 (neutrophil collagenase, collagenase-2), and MMP-13 (collagenase-3). These MMPs attack triple-helical regions of interstitial collagen types I, II, and III at a specific single site following a glycine residue Gly (Ile or Leu)-(Ala or Leu), located about three quarters of the distance from the N-terminus. Thus, this cleavage generates fragments approximately three-fourths and one-fourth the size of the collagen molecules. MMP-13 is unique in that it cleaves α-chains of type II collagen at two sites of the Gly^{906}-Leu^{907} and Gly^{909}-Gln^{910} bonds.[8] All these collagenases degrade the interstitial collagens, but their specific activities against the collagens are different; MMP-1, MMP-8, and MMP-13 preferentially digest collagen types III, I, and II, respectively.[8,9] Although rodents, such as mice, were originally thought to have only two collagenases (MMP-8 and MMP-13) and lack the MMP-1 gene, rodent homologues of human MMP-1 gene were recently cloned and named mouse collagenase A and B (Mcol-A and Mcol-B).[10]

In addition to the interstitial fibrillar collagens, MMP-1, MMP-8, and MMP-13 degrade a number of other ECM macromolecules. MMP-1 digests entactin, collagen X, gelatins, perlecan, aggrecan, and cartilage link protein (see Table 4–2). MMP-8 digests aggrecan, gelatins, and cartilage link protein (see Table 4–2). MMP-13 hydrolyzes aggrecan; type IV, IX, X, and XIV collagens; fibronectin; and tenascin.[1] Non-ECM substrates of MMP-1, MMP-8, and MMP-13 include α_2-macroglobulin, α1-antiproteinase inhibitor, α1-antichymotrypsin, and insulin-like growth factor binding proteins-2, -3 (IGF-BP-2, -3) (see Table 4–2).

Gelatinases (MMP-2 and -9)

MMP-2 (gelatinase A) and MMP-9 (gelatinase B) belong to the gelatinase subgroup. Both MMPs readily digest

TABLE 4–2 • SUBSTRATES OF HUMAN MATRIX METALLOPROTEINASES

Enzymes	ECM Substrates	Non-ECM Substrates
Secreted-type MMPs		
Collagenases		
Interstitial collagenase (MMP-1)	Collagens I, II, III, VII and X; gelatins; aggrecan; link protein; entactin; tenascin; perlecan	α2-M; α1-PI; α1-antichymotrypsin; IGF-BP-2,3,5; pro-IL-1β; CTGF
Neutrophil collagenase (MMP-8)	Collagens I, II and III; gelatins; aggrecan; link protein	α1-PI
Collagenase-3 (MMP-13)	Collagens I, II, III, IV, IX, X and XIV; aggrecan; Fn; tenascin	CTGF; Pro-TGF-β; α1-antichymotrypsin
Gelatinases		
Gelatinase A (MMP-2)	Gelatins; collagens IV, V, VII and XI; Ln; Fn; elastin; aggrecan; link protein	Pro-TGF-β; FGF receptor I; MCP-3; IGF-BP-5; pro-IL-1β; galectin-3; plasminogen
Gelatinase B (MMP-9)	Gelatins; collagens III, IV and V; aggrecan; elastin; entactin; link protein	Pro-TGF-β; IL-2 receptor α; Kit-L; IGF-BP-3; pro-IL-1β; α1-PI; galectin-3
Stromelysins		
Stromelysin-1 (MMP-3)	Aggrecan; decorin; gelatins; Fn; Ln; collagens III, IV, IX and X; tenascin; link protein; perlecan	IGF-BP-3; pro-IL-1β; HB-EGF; CTGF; E-cadherin; α1-antichymotrypsin; α1-PI; α2-M; plasminogen; uPA
Stromelysin-2 (MMP-10)	Aggrecan; Fn; Ln; collagens III, IV and V; link protein	Unknown
Matrilysins		
Matrilysin-1 (MMP-7)	Aggrecan; gelatins; Fn; Ln; elastin; entactin; collagen IV; tenascin; link protein	Pro-α-defensin; Fas-L; β4 integrin; E-cadherin; pro-TNFα; CTGF; HB-EGF
Matrilysin-2 (MMP-26)	Gelatin; collagen IV; Fn; fibrinogen	α1-PI
Furin-activated MMPs		
Stromelysin-3 (MMP-11)	Fn; Ln; aggrecan; gelatins	α1-PI; α2-M; IGF-BP-1
Epilysin (MMP-28)	Unknown	Unknown
Other secreted-type MMPs		
Metalloelastase (MMP-12)	Elastin; Fn; collagen V; osteonectin	Plasminogen; apolipoprotein-a
RASI-1 (MMP-19)	Collagen IV; gelatin; Fn; Tenascin; aggrecan; COMP; Ln; nidogen	Unknown
Enamelysin (MMP-20)	Amelogenin; aggrecan; gelatin; COMP	Unknown
MMP-21	Unknown	Unknown
MMP-27	Unknown	Unknown
Membrane-anchored MMPs		
Type I transmembrane-type MMPs		
MT1-MMP (MMP-14)	Collagens I, II and III; gelatins; aggrecan; Fn; Ln; fibrin; Ln-5	CD44; tissue transglutaminase
MT2-MMP (MMP-15)	Fn; tenascin; nidogen; aggrecan; perlecan; Ln	Tissue transglutaminase
MT3-MMP (MMP-16)	Collagen III; Fn; gelatin	Tissue transglutaminase
MT5-MMP (MMP-24)	PG	Unknown
GPI-linked MMPs		
MT4-MMP (MMP-17)	Gelatin; fibrinogen	Unknown
MT6-MMP (MMP-25)	Gelatin; collagen IV; fibrin; Fn; Ln	Unknown
Type II transmembrane-type MMP		
MMP-23	Gelatin	Unknown

Abbreviations: Fn, fibronectin; Ln, laminin; COMP, cartilage oligomeric matrix protein; PG, proteoglycan; α2-M, α2-macroglobulin; α1-PI, α1-proteinase inhibitor, IGF-BP, insulin-like growth factor binding protein; CTGF, connective tissue growth factor; IL-1, interleukin-1; TGF, transforming growth factor.; MCP-3, monocyte chemoattractant protein; HB-EGF, heparin-binding epidermal growth factor.; uPA, urokinase-type plasminogen activator.

gelatins and also cleave collagen types IV and V.[11,12] Elastin, aggrecan, and cartilage link protein are also substrates of the gelatinases.[1] Although MMP-2 and MMP-9 share such substrates, they have different activities on several ECM macromolecules. For example, MMP-2, but not MMP-9, digests fibronectin and laminin,[11] and type III collagen and α_2-chains of type I collagen are degraded only by MMP-9.[12] The gelatinases also process directly TGF-β into an active ligand (see Table 4–2). MMP-2 and MMP-9 cleave fibroblast growth factor (FGF) receptor type I and interleukin (IL)-2 receptor type-α, respectively (see Table 4–2). MMP-9 also releases soluble kit ligand.[13] MMP-2 processes monocyte chemoattractant protein (MCP)-3 into an MCP-3 fragment, deleting the N-terminal four amino acids, which can bind to CC-chemokine receptors and act as a general chemokine antagonist.[14]

Stromelysins (MMP-3 and -10)

The subgroup of stromelysins consists of MMP-3 (stromelysin-1) and MMP-10 (stromelysin-2). They share 78 percent of their amino acid sequences and have similar enzymatic properties.[15] The enzymes hydrolyze a number of ECM macromolecules, including aggrecan, fibronectin, laminin, and collagen IV (see Table 4–2).[16] Collagen III, IX, and X and telopeptides of collagens I, II, and XI are also digested by MMP-3.[17] In addition to the ECM components, MMP-3 is also active on IGF-BP-3,

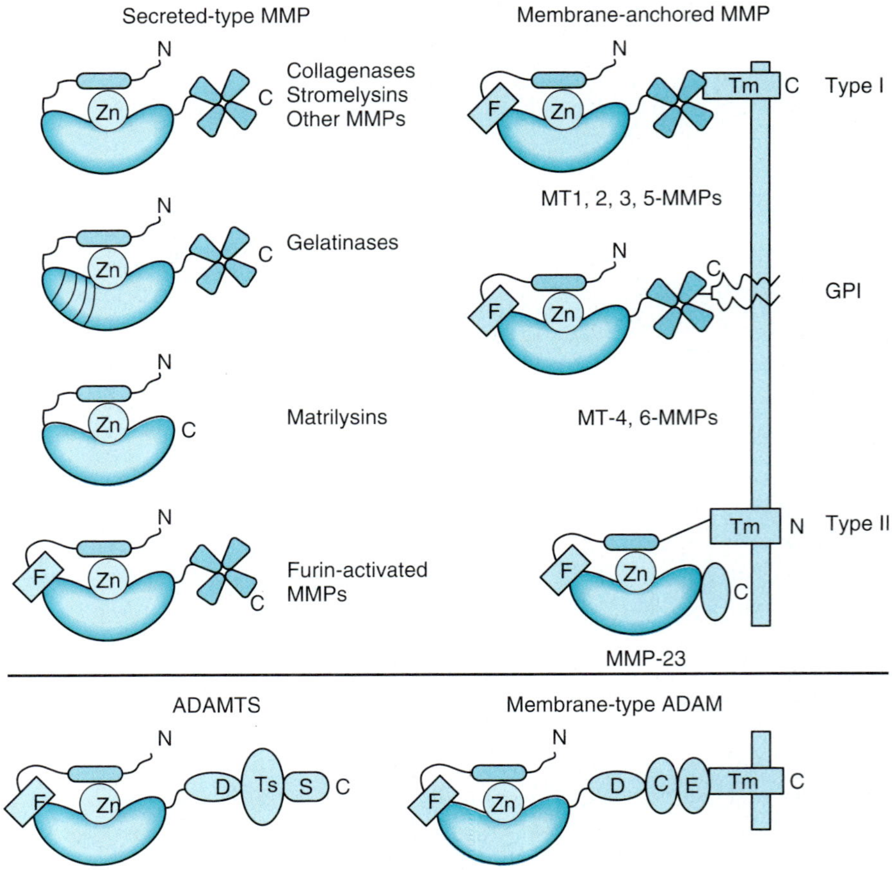

FIGURE 4–1 · The Domain Structures of Two Types of MMPs (Secreted-type MMP and Membrane-anchored MMP) and Two Types of ADAMs (ADAMTS and Membrane-type ADAM). Typical domain structure of most secreted-type MMPs (collagenases, stromely-sins, and other MMPs) is composed of a prodomain, a catalytic domain, a hinge, and hemopexin-like domain. Gelatinases (MMP-2 and MMP-9) have additional insertions of collagen-binding type II repeats of fibronectin in the catalytic domain, while matrilysins (MMP-7 and MMP-26) lack a hemopexin-like domain. Furin-activated MMPs (MMP-11 and MMP-28) contain an RKRR sequence (furin recognition site = F) at the end of the propeptide. Membrane-anchored MMPs are composed of type I transmembrane-type MMPs (MT1-, 2-, 3-, 5-MMPs), GPI-linked MMPs (MT4-, 6-MMPs) and type II transmembrane-type MMP (MMP-23). All of them have furin-recognition sites. ADAMTS has a prodomain, a furin recognition site (F), a catalytic domain, a hinge, a disintegrin domain (D), thrombospondin motifs (Ts), and a spacer domain (S). Membrane-type ADAM is composed of a prodomain, a furin-recognition site (F), a catalytic domain, a hinge, a disintegrin domain (D), a cysteine-rich domain (C), an EGF-like domain (E), and a transmembrane domain (Tm).

IL-1β, heparin-binding epidermal growth factor (HB-EGF), connective tissue growth factor (CTGF), E-cadherin, α_1-antichymotrypsin, and α_1-proteinase inhibitor (see Table 4–2). MMP-3 also activates many proMMPs.[5] A similar activator function has been identified for MMP-10.[18]

Matrilysins (MMP-7 and -26)

Matrilysins include MMP-7 (matrilysin-1) and MMP-26 (matrilysin-2), which are the smallest of the MMPs, having only the propeptide and catalytic domains. The substrate specificity of MMP-7 is similar to that of stromelysins; it digests numerous ECM components, including aggrecan; gelatins; fibronectin; laminin; elastin; entactin; collagen types III, IV, V, IX, X, and XI; fibrin/fibrinogen; vitronectin; tenascin; and link protein (see Table 4–2). Although these substrates overlap with those of other MMPs, the specific activity of MMP-7 for most substrates is the highest among the MMPs.[19,20] Non-ECM molecules such as α-defensin, Fas ligand, β4 integrin, E-cadherin, plasminogen, tumor necrosis factor (TNF)-α, and CTGF are also substrates for MMP-7 (see Table 4–2). MMP-26 degrades gelatin, collagen IV, fibronectin, fibrinogen, and α1-proteinase inhibitor,[21-23] but information about other substrates is still limited.

Furin-activated MMPs (MMP-11 and 28)

MMP-11 (stromelysins-3) and MMP-28 (epilysin) contain an RKRR sequence at the end of the propeptide, which is a unique motif for intracellular processing of proproteins to mature molecules by furin and other proprotein convertases. ProMMP-11 is indeed activated intracellularly by the action of furin.[24] MMP-11 shows only weak proteolytic activity against gelatin, laminin, fibronectin, and aggrecan,[25] but it has respectable catalytic action in digesting α1-proteinase inhibitor, α2-macroglobulin, and IGF-BP-1[26,27] (see Table 4–2). MMP-28 can degrade casein, but its natural substrates are not known.[28]

Other Secreted-Type MMPs (MMP-12, -19, -20, -21, and -27)

MMP-12 (metalloelastase),[29] MMP-19 (RASI-1),[30] MMP-20 (enamelysin),[31] MMP-21,[23] and MMP-27 have structural characteristics similar to those of collagenases and stromlysins. However, these MMPs are not classified into the previously mentioned subgroups because their substrates and other biochemical characters have not been fully examined at present. Overall information on the substrate specificity of MMP-12,[29] MMP-19,[32,33] and MMP-20,[31,33] however, suggests that they are stromelysin-like proteinases. MMP-12[29] digests elastin, fibronectin, collagen V, osteonectin, and plasminogen (see Table 4–2). MMP-19, which was originally reported as MMP-18 but renamed as MMP-19, cleaves type IV collagen, laminin, fibronectin, gelatin, tenascin, entactin, fibrin/fibrinogen, aggrecan, and cartilage oligomeric matrix protein (COMP)[32,33] (see Table 4–2). MMP-20 also digests amelogenin, aggrecan, and COMP.[33] However, substrates of MMP-21 and MMP-27 are not known.

Membrane-Anchored MMPs

Type I transmembrane-type MMPs include MT1-MMP (MMP-14),[34] MT2-MMP (MMP-15),[35] MT3-MMP (MMP-16),[36] and MT5-MMP (MMP-24).[37] All these MT-MMPs can activate proMMP-2, but MT1-MMP may play a major role in the activation of proMMP-2 in various tissues (see following discussion). Besides the activator function, however, MT1-MMP digests the triple-helical portions of interstitial collagen types I, II, and III and other ECM components, including fibronectin, laminin, aggrecan, and gelatin[38] (see Table 4–2). MT2-MMP also digests fibronectin, tenascin, nidogen, aggrecan, perlecan, and laminin.[39] MT3-MMP cleaves collagen type III, fibronectin, and gelatins.[40] MT4-MMP (MMP-17)[41] and MT6-MMP (MMP-25)[42] are GPI-linked MMPs. Both MT4-MMP and MT6-MMP have ability to digest gelatin and fibrin/fibrinogen[42,43,44](see Table 4–2). MMP-23 (cysteine array-MMP, MIFR) is type II transmembane-type MMP,[45] and two almost-identical genes are cloned; therefore, they are called MMP-23A and MMP-23B. MMP-23 digests gelatin,[46] but no information about other substrates is available (see Table 4–2). A unique aspect of MMP-23 is that this MMP is expressed in only female and male reproductive organs, such as endometrium, ovary, testis, and prostate,[46] but its functions are not well established.

ADAM Family

The disintegrin and metalloproteinase (ADAM) family members, which are also called mammalian reprolysins, comprise the common domains, including propeptide, metalloproteinase, and disintegrin, and are classified into two groups—ADAM metalloproteinases and catalytically inactive nonproteolytic homologues—according to the difference in the active-site sequence of the metalloproteinase domain. Based on the C-terminal strucutural differences of the molecules, ADAM metalloproteinases are divided into two subgroups (see Fig. 4–1): membrane-type ADAM with transmembrane domain (ADAM1, 8, 9, 10, 12, 13, 15, 17, 19, 20, 21, 24, 25, 26, 28, 30, 33, and 34) and secreted-type ADAMTS with thrombospondin motifs (ADAMTS1, 2, 3, 4, 5, 6, 7, 8, 9, 10, 12, 13, 14, 15, 16, 17, 18, and 19). The active sites in the catalytic domains of both subgroups' members contain a common sequence of HEXGHXXGXXHD with "Met-turn," which is also present in MMP members. Among the membrane-type ADAMs, ADAM8, ADAM9, ADAM10, ADAM12, ADAM17, and ADAM19 are demonstrated to have proteinase activity. Although ADAM10 degrades type IV collagen and myelin basic protein, the main substrates of these ADAMs are various membrane proteins, which include precursors of cytokines and growth factors such as TNF-α, HB-EGF, and neureglin; receptors such as p75 TNF receptor and IL-1 receptor II; and other membrane proteins related to development such as Notch ligand and ephrin.[47-51] According to these data, one of the major functions of the membrane-type ADAMs is shedding of the membrane proteins. ADAM17 cleaves proform of TNF-α at the physiological processing site into the soluble form of TNF-α and is called TNFα-converting enzyme (TACE). ADAM17 is also involved in release of L-selectin, TGF-α, and p75 TNF receptor.[47]

ADAMTS subgroup includes 18 members. Although information about substrates and biological functions is still limited, ADAMTS1, 2, 3, 4, and 5 are all ECM-degrading proteinases. ADAMTS1,[52] ADAMTS4,[53] and ADAMTS5[54] can preferentially cleave aggrecan at the five Glu-X bonds, including the Glu^{373}-Ala^{374} bond (the aggrecanase site). Because of aggrecan-degrading activity, ADAMTS4 and ADAMTS5 are named as aggrecanase-1 and aggrecanase-2, respectively,[53,54] but versican is also digested by these proteinases,[55] and brevican is cleaved by ADAMTS4.[56] ADAMTS2 and ADAMTS3 process the N-terminal propeptides of type I and II collagens, and thus are named procollagen N-proteinase. On the other hand, ADAMTS13 is a von Willebrand factor-cleaving proteinase, and its mutation causes thrombotic thrombocytopenic purpura. Proteinase activities of other ADAMTS species are still unknown.

Endogenous Proteinase Inhibitors

Endogenous proteinase inhibitors control the activities of proteinases in vivo. The inhibitors are derived from plasma or cells in the local tissues. Plasma contains several proteinase inhibitors, and about 10 percent of all the plasma proteins are proteinase inhibitors. Most are proteinase class specific, but α_2-macroglobulin inhibits the activities of proteinases from all four groups. Major endogenous inhibitors of the ECM-degrading proteinases are listed in Table 4–3.

α_2-MACROGLOBULIN

The α_2-macroglobulin molecule is a large plasma glycoprotein of 725 kD, which consists of four identical subunits of 185 kD that are linked in pairs by disulfide bonds. The pairs assemble noncovalently. Almost all active proteinases, regardless of the proteinase classes, bind and attack the so-called bait region, located near the center of the subunit. After cleaving within the bait region, the proteinase is physically trapped within the molecule by inducing a conformational change of the inhibitor, resulting in a proteinase/α2-macroglobulin complex. Although the proteinase in the complex remains active against very small substrates, it is trapped by the arms of the α_2-macroglobulin and prevented from degrading larger, extracellular proteins. Besides the function as a proteinase inhibitor, α_2-macroglobulin may act as a carrier protein because it also binds to a number of growth factors and cytokines, such as platelet-derived growth factor (PDGF), bFGF, TGF-β, insulin, and IL-1β.

The α_2-macroglobulin molecule is synthesized mainly in liver but also locally by macrophages, fibroblasts, and adrenocortical cells. Concentration of the inhibitor in plasma is 250 mg/dl. Because of its large molecular weight, it is not present in noninflammatory synovial fluid. During synovial inflammation, α_2-macroglobulin penetrates into the joint cavity. Rheumatoid synovial fluid, for example, has about the same concentration of the inhibitor as plasma.

TABLE 4–3 • ENDOGENOUS INHIBITORS OF EXTRACELLULAR MATRIX-DEGRADING PROTEINASES

Inhibitor	Molecular Mass (kD)	Source	Target Enzyme
α2-Macroglobulin	725	Plasma (liver), macrophages, fibroblasts	Most proteinases from all classes
Inhibitors of Serine Proteinase			
Serpins			
α1-Proteinase inhibitor	52	Plasma, macrophages	Neutrophil elastase, cathepsin G, proteinase 3
α1-Antichymotrypsin	58	Plasma	Cathepsin G, chymotrypsin, chymase, tissue kallikrein
α2-Antiplasmin	67	Plasma	Plasmin
Proteinase nexin-1	45	Fibroblasts	Thrombin, uPA, tPA, plasmin, trypsin, trypsin-like serine proteinase
PAI-1	45	Endothelial cells, fibroblasts, platelets, plasma	tPA, uPA
PAI-2	47	Plasma, macrophages	uPA, tPA
Protein C inhibitor	57	Plasma, urine	Active protein C, tPA, uPA, tissue kallikrein
C1-inhibitor	96	Plasma	Plasma kallikrein, C1 esterase
Kallistatin	92	Plasma, liver, stomach, kidney, pancreas	Tissue kallikrein
Kunins			
Aprotinin	7	Mast cells	Plasmin, kallikrein
Trypstatin	6	Mast cells	Tryptase
Proteinase nexin-2 (β-amyloid protein precursor)	100	Fibroblasts	EGF binding protein, NGF-γ, trypsin, chymotrypsin, factor XIa
Others			
Secretory leukocyte proteinase inhibitor (SLPI)	15	Bronchial secretions, seminal plasma, cartilage	Neutrophil elastase, cathepsin G, chymotrypsin, trypsin
Elafin	7	Horny layers of skin	Neutrophil elastase, proteinase 3
Inhibitors of Cysteine Proteinase			
Stefin A	11	Cytosol	Cysteine proteinases
Stefin B	11	Cytosol	Cysteine proteinases
Cystatin C	13	Body fluids	Cysteine proteinases
Cystatin S	13	Seminal plasma, tears, saliva	Cysteine proteinases
Kininogens	50-78/108-120	Plasma	Cysteine proteinases
Calpastatin	120	Cytosol	Calpains
Metalloproteinase Inhibitors			
TIMP-1	28	Connective tissue cells, macrophages	MMPs
TIMP-2	22	Connective tissue cells, macrophages	MMPs
TIMP-3	21/24*	Fibroblasts, synovial cells	MMPs, ADAMs, ADAMTS
TIMP-4	21	Heart, brain, testis	MMPs
RECK	Unknown	Many tissue cells, fibroblasts	MMP-2, MT1-MMP

* Glycosylated form.

Abbreviations: PA, plasminogen activator, PAI, plasminogen activator inhibitor; EGF, epidermal growth factor; NGF, nerve growth factor; TIMP, tissue inhibitor of metalloproteinases; RECK, reversion-inducing, cysteine-rich protein with Kazal motifs.

INHIBITORS OF SERINE PROTEINASES

The primary inhibitors of serine proteinases include the members of the serpin (serine proteinase inhibitor) gene family, Kunitz-type inhibitors, and others (see Table 4–3). The serpins are glycoproteins of 50 to 100 kD and share homology with human α_1-proteinase inhibitor.[57] α_1-Proteinase inhibitor, α_1-antichymotrypsin, α_2-antiplasmin, plasminogen activator inhibitors (PAI-1 and PAI-2), protein C inhibitor (PAI-3), C1-inhibitor, kallistatin, and proteinase nexin-1 (PN-1) are the major serpins involved in the regulation of ECM-degrading serine proteinases. The main proteinases inhibited by these molecules are listed in Table 4–3. Although PAI-1 and PAI-2 inhibit both tPA and uPA, inhibition by PAI-1 and PAI-2 is more effective on tPA and uPA, respectively.

Kunitz-type inhibitors include aprotinin, trypstatin, and proteinase nexin-2, which is identical to a β-amyloid protein precursor. Secretory leukocyte proteinase inhibitor, which inhibits neutrophil elastase and cathepsin G, is present in many secretory and inflammatory fluids and also in cartilage. Elafin is a serine proteinase inhibitor that has 38 percent identity with the second domain of secretory leukocyte proteinase inhibitor; it inhibits neutrophil elastase and proteinase 3.

INHIBITORS OF CYSTEINE PROTEINASES

The members of the cystatin superfamily and calpastatin belong to the family of inhibitors of ECM-degrading cysteine proteinases (see Table 4–3). Cystatins capable of inhibiting lysosomal cysteine proteinases consist of three groups. Subgroup 1 includes stefins A and B. Each has a molecular mass of 11 kD, and the stefins reside within cells. Subgroup 2 includes cystatin C and S, each with a molecular mass of 13 kD. They occur at relatively high concentrations in cerebrospinal fluid and saliva. Subgroup 3 is the kininogens. Kininogens that participate in blood coagulation and inflammation are also inhibitors of cysteine proteinases. Calpains are not inhibited by cystatins but are inhibited by calpastatin (120 kD), which is a cytosolic-specific inhibitor of calpain.

TISSUE INHIBITORS OF METALLOPROTEINASES

Tissue inhibitors of metalloproteinases (TIMPs) are a gene family consisting of four different members with approximately 40 to 50 percent sequence identity (i.e., TIMP-1, TIMP-2, TIMP-3, and TIMP-4), which have molecular masses ranging from 21 to 28 kD in humans.[58-61] Virtually all TIMPs inhibit the activities of MMPs by binding in a 1:1 molar ratio to form tight, noncovalent complexes,[58] except that TIMP-1 does not efficiently inhibit MT-MMPs.[39,40,62] TIMPs contain 12 highly conserved cysteine residues that form six intrachain disulfide bonds, which are essential for maintaining the correct ternary structure of the molecule[60,63] and stable inhibitor activity.[58] The TIMP molecules have two structurally distinct subdomains: an N-terminal subdomain (loops 1 through 3) and a C-terminal subdomain (loops 4 through 6). The N-terminal subdomain of each TIMP molecule contains the inhibitory activity for MMPs.[58] Studies on the crystal structures of the MMP/TIMP complexes demonstrate that the wedge-shaped TIMPs bind with their edge into the entire length of the active-site cleft of their cognate MMPs[60] (Fig. 4–2). In an MMP-3/TIMP-1 complex, six sequentially separate polypeptide segments of TIMP-1 (four in the N-terminal and two in the C-terminal subdomains) interact with the catalytic domain of MMP-3.[63] Among them, two central disulfide-linked segments (Cys^1-Thr^2-Cys^3-Val^4-Pro^5 and Ser^{68}-Val^{69}-Ala^{70}) play an essential role in the inhibition of the activity by binding to either side of the catalytic zinc; the other four segments have direct, but weaker, contacts with MMP-3.[63] High affinity and efficient inhibitor activity of TIMP-2 to MT1-MMP are explained by the additional interaction between a quite long hairpin loop of TIMP-2 with a loop over the rim of the active-site cleft of MT1-MMP[64] (see Fig. 4–2).

TIMP-1 and TIMP-2 are unique in that they form the complexes with proMMP-9 and proMMP-2, respectively (i.e., the proMMP-9/TIMP-1 and proMMP-2/TIMP-2 complexes). Similar complex formation is also known between TIMP-4 and proMMP-2. Because the complexes are made through the interation between their C-termini,[58] TIMPs in the complexes retain inhibitor activity against MMPs. The activation of proMMP-9 and proMMP-2 is suppressed in the complex forms; the complex formation may be a safety device for these gelatinases.[12] On the other hand, the proMMP-2/TIMP-2 complex is useful for the efficient activation of proMMP-2 by MT1-MMP on the cell membranes because MT1-MMP captures proMMP-2 at the cell membranes through the trimolecular complex formation between the catalytic domain of MT1-MMP and the N-terminal domain of TIMP-2[65] (see following).

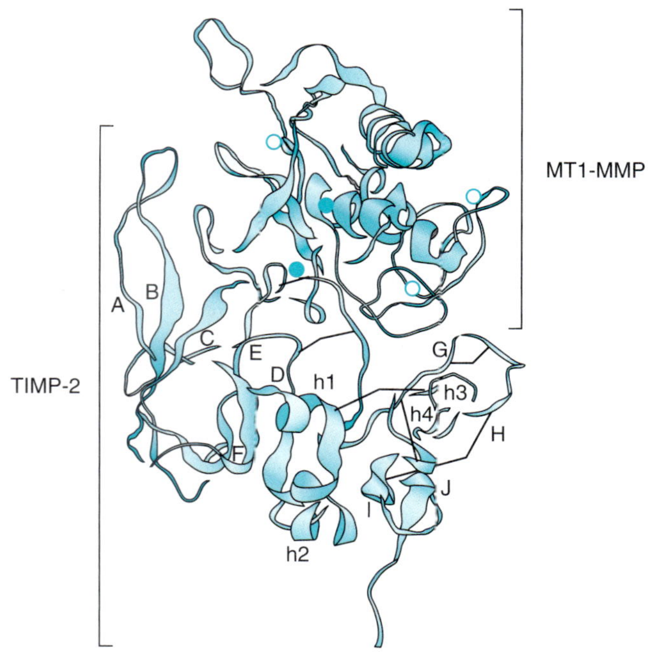

FIGURE 4–2 · **Diagram of the Complex of TIMP-2 and the Catalytic Domain of MT1-MMP.** The catalytic and structural zinc ions and the three calcium ions are shown as closed and open spheres, respectively. Strands and helices in TIMP-2 are labeled as A-J and h1-h4, respectively. Disulfide bonds in TIMP-2 are also shown. The wedge-shaped TIMP-2 binds with its edge made by six segments into the active site cleft of the MT1-MMP. Interaction between a long, hairpin loop of TIMP-2 made by segments *A* and *B* and a loop over the rim of the active-site cleft of MT1-MMP is seen. The image was prepared from the Brookhaven Protein Data Bank entry using Ras Mol V. 2.6.

Besides the inhibition and interations of TIMPs to MMPs, TIMP-3, among the TIMPs, specifically inhibits the activities of ADAM10, ADAM12, and ADAM17, although ADAM8 and ADAM9 are not inhibited by TIMPs. Because TIMP-3 also efficiently inhibits the aggrecan-degrading activity of ADAMTS4,[66] TIMP-3 may be a common tissue inhibitor of the ADAM members. Some structural elements of TIMP-3 are suspected to be critical to the inhibition of the activities of ADAM members.

TIMPs are multifunctional proteins with diverse actions beyond being MMP/ADAM inhibitors. These other actions include growth factor activity, antiangiogenic activity, and regulatory activity of apoptosis. TIMP-1, -2, and -3 have growth fatocr activity to various cell lines. Although the activity is present in the N-terminal domains of the TIMPs independently of MMP inhibitor activity, the precise mechanism is not known. It is also reported that

TIMP-2 and TIMP-3, but not TIMP-1, are antiangiogenic. The effects are explained in several ways, such as by preventing degradation of the ECM, inhibiting endothelial cell migration, and blocking the release of ECM-bound angiogenic factors. TIMP-1 and TIMP-2 are known to inhibit apoptosis, but TIMP-3 promotes apoptosis.[67] Antiapoptotic activity of TIMP-1 and TIMP-2 may be related to their MMP inhibitory and growth promoting activities,[1] and apoptosis-promoting activity of TIMP-3 can be explained by the stabilization of the TNF receptor through the prevention of its shedding by ADAM members.

A new MMP inhibitor, reversion-inducing, cysteine-rich protein with Kazal motifs (RECK), was recently discovered.[68] RECK is a GPI-linked glycoprotein harboring three inhibitor-like domains, and it inhibits the activities of at least MMP-2 and MT1-MMP. Although this inhibitor seems to play a key role in the angiogenic processes in vivo, biochemical mechanism as an MMP inhibitor and functions in pathologic conditions such as arthritides remain unknown.

Regulation of Proteinase Activity

The activities of ECM-degrading proteinases in tissues are regulated by the balance between the proteianses and their inhibitors. The balance at the local tissues depends on several factors, including production rates of proteinases and inhibitors, their secretion, activation of proenzymes, and anchoring systems of the activated proteinases to cell surfaces. Production levels of the proteinases and inhibitors within the cells are controlled mainly by their gene expression. Activation processes of proMMPs and membrane anchoring of their activities have been recently established by extensive experimental work.

GENE EXPRESSION OF PROTEINASES AND INHIBITORS

Matrix Metalloproteinases and Tissue Inhibitors of Metalloproteinases

Normal cells, except for inflammatroy cells, do not produce MMPs or TIMPs in the tissues under physiologic conditions, but instead, they start their expression by stimulation with many factors under pathologic conditions. Neutrophils and macrophages synthesize MMP-8 and MMP-9 during the differentiation and store them within the granules of the differentiated cells. Tumor cells express many MMPs, such as MMP-1, MMP-7, MMP-9, MMP-10, and MT1-MMP, and TIMP-1 predominantly by oncogenic transformation, although their expression is also modulated by cytokines and growth factors. However, the gene expression of MMPs and TIMPs in the tissue cells, other than inflammatory cells and tumor cells, is regulated by numerous factors, including cytokines, growth factors, and chemical and physical stimuli.

Much information is available for regulators of MMP-1 and MMP-3, which are coordinately expressed in many cell types after stimulation with cytokines and growth factors, factors acting at cell surface, chemical agents, and so on (Table 4–4). The induced production of MMP-1 and MMP-3 is suppressed by retinoic acid, TGF-β, and glucocorticoid. The gene expression of MMP-7 and MMP-9 is also regulated by the similar factors, but the regulation is more strict and fewer factors modulate the expression (see Table 4–4). MT1-MMP expression is upregulated by phorbormyristate acetate (TPA), concanavalin A, basic FGF, and TNF-α, and it is downregulated by glucocorticoids in various cells. TNF-α and IL-1α stimulate osteoarthritic chondrocytes to express the MT1-MMP gene.[69] In contrast to these MMPs, MMP-2 and TIMP-2 are unique in that factors capable of enhancing the production of MMP-1, MMP-3, and TIMP-1 are inactive.

The 5′-flanking regions of the genes encoding MMP-1, MMP-3, MMP-7, MMP-9, and MMP-10 have a TATA box and a TPA-responsive element (TRE)—a TGAGTCA sequence—that binds to AP-1 proteins (Fos and Jun). The enhanced expression of these MMPs by TPA, IL-1, or TNF-α is considered to be mediated by TRE in the promoter. The promoter regions of these MMPs (except for MMP-9) also contain Ets binding sites ([A/C]GGAA). The MMP-9 gene lacks the Ets binding site, but it contains the SP-1 and NF-κB binding sites and the GT box, the latter of which is involved during the activation with v-Src. TGF-β inhibitor element (TIE) is identified in the promoter regions of MMP-1, MMP-3, and MMP-7, and involvement of TIE in the suppression of the gene expression is demonstrated with MMP-3. The suppression of MMP-1 transcripts by glucocorticoid results from the binding of the hormone receptor with c-Jun, which prevents interaction between AP-1 and TRE. The retinoic acid/retinoic acid receptor complex binds to the promoter of MMP-3, which also prevents the interaction of AP-1 and TRE. The promoter region of MMP-2 is different from those of these MMPs in that it lacks a TATA box and a TRE element, but it has an adenovirus E1A-responsive element and two regions that function as a silencer. The 5′-flanking region of the MT1-MMP gene lacks TATA box, but it contains putative regulatory elements, including Sp-1 sites, CCAAT boxes, a binding site for the β-catenin/Tcf4 complex,[70] and an Egr-1 site that partially overlaps with the Sp1 sites. Increased binding of Egr-1 to the MT1-MMP promoter correlates with enhanced transcriptional activity.[71]

TIMP-1 expression is enhanced or suppressed in response to many factors, including cytokines, growth factors, and oncogenic transformation (see Table 4–4). Effects of these stimulatory factors are common to the gene expression of MMPs, but they are regulated independently. For example, TGF-β, retinoic acid, progesterone, and estrogen enhance TIMP-1 expression in fibroblasts, but they suppress the expression of MMP-1 and MMP-3. The human TIMP-1 gene has 10 consensus sequences for Sp1, 6 for AP-1, 6 for polyoma enhancer A3 (PEA3), 12 for AP-2, and 5 CCAAT boxes.[72] In addition, upstream TIMP-1 element-1, where unknown cellular proteins bind, is identified as a novel regulatory element to control TIMP-1 expression in normal and pathologic states.[73] The regulation of TIMP-3 gene expression appears similar to that of TIMP-1 because TIMP-3 gene

TABLE 4–4 • FACTORS THAT MODULATE SYNTHESIS OF MMPS AND TIMPS

Enzyme or TIMP	Stimulating Factor*	Suppressive Factor
MMP-1	**Cytokines and growth factors:** IL-1, TNF-α, EGF, PDGF, bFGF, VEGF, NGF, TGF-α, IFN-α, INF-β and IFN-γ, leukoregulin, relaxin **Factors acting at cell surface:** Calcium ionophore A23187, cell fusion, collagen, concanavalin A, integrin receptor antibody, crystals of urate, hydroxyapatite and calcium pyrophosphate, SPARC (osteonectin/BM 40), iron, extracellular matrix metalloproteinase inducer (EMMPRIN/CD147/basigin/M6 antigen), phagocytosis **Chemical agents:** cAMP, colchicine, cytochalasins B and D, LPS, pentoxifylline, TPA, calmodulin inhibitors, serotonin, 1,25-$(OH)_2$ vitamin D3, platelet-activating factor, serum amyloid A, β-microglobulin **Physical factors:** heat shock, ultraviolet irradiation **Others:** viral transformation, oncogenes, autocrine agents, aging of fibroblasts	Retinoic acids, glucocorticoids, estrogen, progesterone, TGF-β, transmembrane neural cell adhesion molecule, cAMP, INF-γ, adenovirus E1A
MMP-2	TGF-β, concanavalin A, H-ras transformation, extracellular matrix metalloproteinase inducer (EMMPRIN/CD147/basigin/M6 antigen)	Adenovirus E1A
MMP-3	IL-1, TNF-α, EGF, concanavalin A, SPARC (osteonectin/BM 40), LPS, TPA, extracellular matrix metalloproteinase inducer (EMMPRIN/CD147/basigin/M6 antigen), viral transformation, oncogenes, integrin receptor antibody, heat shock, calcium ionophore A23187, cytochalasin B	Retinoic acids, glucocorticoids, estrogen, progesterone, TGF-β, adenovirus E1A
MMP-7	IL-1, TNF-α, EGF, TPA, LPS	Unknown
MMP-8	TNF-α, TPA, IL-1	Unknown
MMP-9	IL-1, TNF-α, EGF, TGF-β, TPA, H-ras, v-Src, SPARC (osteonectin/BM40)	Retinoic acids, adenovirus E1A
MMP-10	TPA, A23187, TGF-α, EGF	Unknown
MMP-11	Retinoic acids	bFGF
MMP-13	bFGF, TNF-α, TGF-β	Unknown
MT1-MMP	Concanavalin A, TPA, bFGF, TNF-α, IL-1α	Glucocorticoids
TIMP-1	IL-1, IL-6, IL-11, TPA, TGF-β, TNF-β, retinoic acids, LPS, progesterone, estrogen, oncogenic transformation, viral infection	Extracellular matrix, cytochalasins
TIMP-2	Progesterone	TGF-β, LPS
TIMP-3	EGF, TGF-β, TPA, TNF-α, glucocorticoids, oncostatin M	Unknown

* Factors regulating gene expression of other MMPs are excluded from this table, and those for TIMP-4 are not known.

Abbreviations: AMP, adenosine 5′-monophosphate; EGF, epidermal growth factor; FGF, fibroblast growth factor; INF, interferon; IL, interleukin; LPS, lipopolysaccharide; NGF, nerve growth factor; PDGF, platelet-derived growth factor; TGF, transforming growth factor; TNF, tumor necrosis factor; TPA, 12-*O*-teradecanoylphorbol 13-acetate; VEGF, vascular endothelial growth factor.

expression is inducible by AP-1 and NF-κB activators, TPA, and TNF-α(see Table 4–4). TIMP-3 is a TATA-less gene, and its promoter has six AP-1 binding sites, two NF-κB sites, a c-Myc site, and two copies of a p53 binding motif,[74] the last of which is, however, not reactive with p53 protein. One of the unique characters of TIMP-3 is that the gene expression is silenced by hypermethylation (or hypomethylation) of the promoter in non–small cell lung carcinomas and other tumor cell lines,[75] although it is not known whether this is special to tumor cells. On the other hand, TIMP-2 gene, which is constitutively expressed by many cells, has several features observed in housekeeping genes and differs significantly from TIMP-1 and TIMP-3 genes. The TIMP-2 promoter has a TATA-like element, several SP-1 binding sites, an AP-1 site, two AP-2 sites, and three PEA-3 sites.[76] Despite the presence of a complete AP-1 consensus and a typical CpG island, the promoter does not respond to TPA treatment or methylation of this island. TIMP-4 is the TATA-less gene and contains consensus motifs for Sp1 and an inverted CCAAT box, both of which are implicated in the gene expression.[77] Factors controlling the gene expression of TIMP-4 are not well known.

Serine Proteinases and Their Inhibitors

Neutrophil elastase, cathepsin G, chymase, and tryptase are stored within the secretory granules and secreted into the extracellular milieu after activation of neutrophils and mast cells. The expression of these serine proteinases is controlled mainly by the cellular differentiation. Precursors of plasmin and plasma kallikrein are constitutively synthesized predominantly in the liver.

They circulate in blood as zymogen forms (i.e., plasminogen and prekallikrein) and reach the inflammed tissues by being released from blood vessels. Thus, the proteinase activities in the tissues are controlled mainly through activation of the proenzymes by activators. The uPA and tPA molecules (activators of plasminogen) are synthesized by tissue cells, and their gene expression is regulated by many factors (Table 4–5). The uPA synthesis is upregulated in a number of normal cell types and in transformed cells by agents that increase intracellular cyclic adenosine monophosphate (cAMP) levels (e.g., calcitonin, vasopressin, cholera toxin, cAMP analogues); growth factors (e.g., EGF, PDGE, VEGF); cytokines (IL-1, TNF-α); and phorbol esters, whereas glucocorticoid decreases the expression.[7] The expression of tPA is also regulated by the similar factors (see Table 4–5). In endothelial cells, proteinases are enhancers; thrombin and plasmin stimulate the production of tPA.[7] PAI-1 and PAI-2 are also regulated by common factors, many of which also enhance the production of uPA and tPA (see Table 4–5). On the other hand, most serpins are constitutively produced in the liver and secreted to plasma.

Lysosomal Cysteine and Aspartic Proteinases

The expression of lysosomal cysteine proteinases—cathepsins B, L, and K—is generally constitutive, but cellular transformation is often associated with increased synthesis of cathepsins B and L. Cathepsin B transcription varies with cell type and the state of differentiation of tumor cells; it is increased in chondrocytes by IL-1. The synthesis of cathepsin L is stimulated by malignant transformation, tumor promoters, and growth factors. Cathepsin K gene expression in monocyte-macrophage lineage depends on the cellular differentiation to osteoclasts, but all-*trans* retinoic acid upregulates the expression in rabbit osteoclasts. Lysosomal aspartic proteinase, cathepsin D, is constitutively expressed in almost all cells, although estradiol, calcitriol, and retinoic acid can regulate the expression.

ACTIVATION MECHANISMS OF THE ZYMOGENS OF METALLOPROTEINASES

All the MMPs are synthesized as inactive zymogens (proMMPs), and thus activation of proMMPs is prerequisite to their functioning in vivo. ProMMPs are kept inactive by an interaction between a cysteine-sulfhydryl group in the conserved propeptide sequence PRCGXPD and the zinc ion bound to the catalytic domain, preventing the formation of a water-zinc complex that is essential to the enzymatic reaction. Activation requires proteolytic removal of the propeptide domain. There are three pathways of the proMMP activation: extracellular, intracellular, and pericellular (Fig. 4–3).

Extracellular Activation

The extracellular activation, which is applicable to many secreted MMPs (i.e., proMMP-1, proMMP-3, proMMP-7, proMMP-8, proMMP-9, proMMP-10, proMMP-12, and proMMP-13), is initiated through the disruption of the Cys-Zn^{2+} interaction by treatment with nonproteolytic agents or proteinases and completed by autocatalytic processing.[5] Nonproteolytic activators used in vitro include thiol-modifying reagents (e.g., mercurial compounds, iodoacetamide, *N*-ethylmaleimide, oxidized glutathione), hypochlorous acid, sodium dodecyl sulfate, chaotropic agents, and physical factors (heat and acid exposure).[5] Most of these factors, especially 4-aminophenylmercuric acetate (APMA), enable proMMP molecules to generate a short-lived intermediate that is formed by removal of part of a propeptide by an intramolecular reaction.[5] The fully activated form is made by an intermolecular autocatalysis that cleaves three amino acids downstream from the conserved sequence PRCGXPD and leads to generation of active MMPs, starting with Tyr or Phe at the N-terminus. However, such a process may not be essential for proMMP-9 activation by APMA because a fully active form, retaining the PRCGVPD sequence, is generated by the cleavage of the Ala^{74}-Met^{75} bond upstream of the conserved sequence.[12]

A similar stepwise activation is also proposed for the proteolytic activation of proMMPs. Proteinases initially attack the proteinase-susceptible bait regions in the propeptides and generate proteolytically active intermediates through destabilization of the Cys-Zn^{2+} interaction.[5] In the second step, the final activation site is autolytically catalyzed by the active intermediate instead of the trigger proteinases, and active MMPs without propeptides are made. In many cases, the bait-region sequences in the propeptide dictate which proteinases can become an activator of a particu-

TABLE 4–5 • FACTORS THAT REGULATE EXPRESSION OF PLASMINOGEN ACTIVATORS AND THEIR INHIBITORS

Enzyme or Inhibitor	Stimulatory Factor	Suppressive Factor
uPA	TPA, IL-1, INF-γ, EGF, PDGF, bFGF, VEGF, TGF-β, cholera toxin, cAMP, estrogen, calcitonin, vasopressin, disruption of E-cadherin–dependent cell-cell adhesion	Glucocorticoids, TGF-β
tPA	TPA, EGF, bFGF, VEGF, retinoic acids, glucocorticoids, cAMP, thrombin, plasmin, follicle-stimulating hormone, luteinizing hormone, gonadotropin-releasing hormone	TNF-α
PAI-1	IL-1, TNF-α, TGF-β, bFGF, VEGF, TPA, glucocorticoids	cAMP
PAI-2	TPA, LPS, TNF-α, colony-stimulating factor, cholera toxin, dengue virus	Glucocorticoids
PN-1	TPA, EGF, thrombin	Unknown

Abbreviations: AMP, adenosine 5′-monophosphate; EGF, epidermal growth factor; FGF, fibroblast growth factor; IL, interleukin; INF, interferon; LPS, lipopolysaccharide; PAI, plasminogen activator inhibitor; PDGF, platelet derived growth factor; PN, proteinase nexin; TGF, transforming growth factor; TNF, tumor necrosis factor; TPA, 12-*O*-teradecanoylphorbol 13-acetate; tPA, tissue-type plasminogen activator; uPA, urokinase-type plasminogen activator; VEGF, vascular endothelial growth factor.

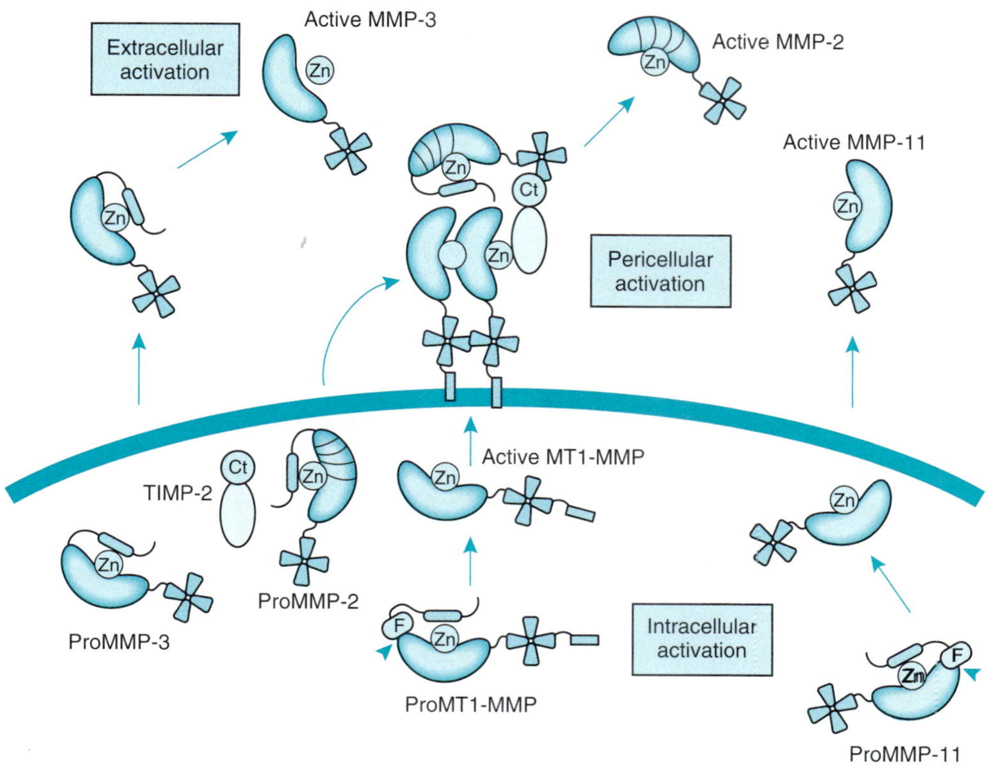

FIGURE 4–3 · **Activation Mechanisms of proMMPs.** Most secreted-type proMMPs, such as proMMP-3, are activated extracellularly by many proteinases (extracellular activation). Furin-activated secreted proMMPs, including proMMP-11, and proMT-MMPs such as proMT1-MMP are intracellularly activated through removal of the propeptides *(arrowheads)* by the action of proprotein convertases such as furin (intracellular activation). ProMMP-2 is activated on the cell membrane by MT1-MMP; this activation requires trimolecular complex of MT1-MMP/TIMP-2/proMMP-2 and dimerization of MT1-MMP (pericellular activation). Ct, C-terminal domain of TIMP-2; F, furin-recognition site.

lar MMP.[5] Potential activators of proMMPs are listed in Table 4–6. Plasmin may play a major role in the activation of proMMP-3 and proMMP-10 in vivo because treatment of these proMMPs with plasmin leads to full activation in vitro.[78] However, proMMP-1 activation by plasmin alone results in only about 25 percent of the potential MMP-1 activity, and full activation requires the subsequent cleavage of the Gln[80]-Phe[81] bond by active MMP-3, MMP-7, or MMP-10.[5,20] On the other hand, MMP-3 and MMP-10 can directly activate proMMP-7,[20] proMMP-8, proMMP-9,[12,18] and proMMP-13[9] into fully active forms. This intermolecular activation cascade of MMPs may be important to in vivo activation of proMMPs.

Intracellular Activation

Because proMT-MMPs, proMMP-23, proMMP-11, and proMMP-28 have basic motifs containing a RXKR sequence at the end of the propeptide domains, proprotein convertases such as furin, a processing enzyme in the *trans* Golgi apparatus, are considered to intracellularly activate these proMMPs (see Fig. 4–3). Actually, intracellular activation of proMMP-11 and proMT1-MMP by

TABLE 4–6 · ACTIVATORS OF PROMATRIX METALLOPROTEINASES

ProMMP	Activator
ProMMP-1	Trypsin (partial), plasmin (partial), plasma kallikrein (partial), chymase (partial), MMP-3, MMP-7, MMP-10, MMP-11
ProMMP-2	MT1-MMP, MT2-MMP, MT3-MMP, MT5-MMP
ProMMP-3	Plasmin, plasma kallikrein, trypsin, tryptase, chymase, cathepsin G, chymotrypsin, neutrophil elastase, thermolysin
ProMMP-7	MMP-3, MMP-10 (partial), trypsin, plasmin (partial), neutrophil elastase (partial)
ProMMP-8	MMP-3, MMP-10, tissue kallikrein, neutrophil elastase, cathepsin G, trypsin
ProMMP-9	MMP-3, MMP-2, MMP-7, MMP-10 (partial), MMP-13, trypsin, chymotrypsin, cathepsin G, tissue kallikrein
ProMMP-10	Plasmin, trypsin, chymotrypsin
ProMMP-11	Furin
ProMMP-13	MMP-2, MMP-3, MT1-MMP, plasmin
ProMT1-MMP	Furin

furin has been demonstrated.[24,79] After the activation, MMP-11 is secreted from the cells, and MT1-MMP is expressed on the cell membranes. Because other proMT-MMPs, such as proMMP-23 and proMMP-28, also have the motif, furin is presumably responsible for the intracellular activation of these proMMPs.

Pericellular Activation

ProMMP-2 is unique in that it is activated pericellularly by type I transmembrane-type MMPs, including MT1-MMP, MT2-MMP, MT3-MMP, and MT5-MMP, but not by ordinary MMP-activatable endopeptidases.[11] This pericellular activation has been extensively studied with MT1-MMP and found to occur in a two-step manner. MT1-MMP cleaves the Asn^{37}-Leu^{38} bond in the propeptide of proMMP-2, generating an intermediate form that is converted to a fully activated enzyme by an intermolecular autocatalytic mechanism.[62] TIMP-2 is essential to the efficient pericellular activation of proMMP-2 by MT1-MMP. The N-terminal inhibitor and C-terminal tail domains of TIMP-2 bind to the catalytic domain of MT1-MMP and the C-terminal hemopexin-like domain of proMMP-2, respectively, forming a trimolecular complex of MT1-MMP/TIMP-2/proMMP-2 on the cell membranes (see Fig. 4–3). Capturing proMMP-2 by the trimolecular complex formation on the cell membranes facilitates proMMP-2 activation by increasing a local concentration of proMMP-2 and presenting it to the near, noninhibited MT1-MMP.[65] Dimerization of MT1-MMP through an interaction of the C-terminal hemopexin-like domain is required for the efficient activation of proMMP-2 by MT1-MMP.[80] MT1-MMP initiates proMMP-2 activation by attacking a part of the proMMP-2 propeptide, and another already activated MMP-2 finally activates proMMP-2 by removing a residual portion of the propeptide. Integrins such as $\alpha_v\beta_3$ may be involved in the process as an additional receptor for transferring activated MMP-2 to the integrin.[81] MT2-MMP, MT3-MMP, or MT5-MMP can activate proMMP-2 in the transfected cells,[35-37] but the activation mechanisms for these MT-MMPs are not well understood. MT1-MMP also activates proMMP-13,[82] and this activation appears not to require TIMP-2.[83]

PERICELLULAR DOCKING OF MMPS

Discovery of membrane-anchored MMPs (i.e., MT1, 2-, 3-, 4-, 5-, 6-MMPs and MMP-23) and subsequent studies on proMMP-2 activation by MT1-MMP have established pericellular actions of these MMPs, including MMP-2. Secreted MMPs were originally thought to extracellularly digest ECM macromolecules after the activation, but recent studies have indicated that they may also function on the cell membranes through their cell-surface docking.[84-86] Besides the proMMP-2/TIMP-2/MT1-MMP system, several secreted MMPs are reported to interact with cell membrane proteins, which include α2-chains of integrin α2β1 and CD147 (EMMPRIN) for MMP-1,[87] αvβ3 integrin and caveolin-1 for MMP-2,[81,88] CD44 heparan sulfate proteoglycan for MMP-7,[89] and CD44 for MMP-9.[90] Because all these cell membrane proteins bind to active forms of the MMPs, their proteolytic activities can be used on the cell surfaces to digest ECM and non-ECM molecules located close to the cell membranes. The importance of pericellular docking of secreted MMPs in arthritic tissues, however, should be demonstrated by further work.

Joint Destruction and Proteinases

DEGRADATION OF ECM IN ARTICULAR CARTILAGE

In most joint diseases, such as rheumatoid arthritis and osteoarthritis, articular cartilage is the major target tissue for destruction, and excessive degradation of cartilage ECM by proteinases is a key process in the destruction. Histologically, depletion of proteoglycans from articular cartilage (degradation of proteoglycans) is a common initial change in these joint diseases, and subsequently, collagen fibrils are degraded, which leads to fibrillation and laceration because of destruction of the arcade structures of collagen fibrils in the articular cartilage. Articular cartilage is composed of the superficial (I), transitional (II), radial (III), and calcified zones (IV) (Fig. 4–4).

Aggrecan, a major proteoglycan in cartilage, is susceptible to degradation by a number of proteinases, including MMPs, ADAMTS species, neutrophil elastase, cathepsin G, and cathepsin B. Because most of these proteinases mainly cleave the peptide bonds located in the interglobular G1-G2 domain, the major glycosaminoglycan-bearing aggrecan fragments are detached from the hyaluronan attachment site (G1 domain) after the cleavage and released from the cartilage matrix. The two major aggrecan fragments with the N-terminal sequences starting from Phe^{342} or Ala^{374} of the core protein are detected in joint fluids from patients with various inflammatory arthritides and osteoarthritis.[91] Many MMPs, including MMP-1, MMP-2, MMP-3, MMP-7, MMP-8, MMP-9, MMP-13, and MT1-MMP, preferentially cleave the Asn^{341}-Phe^{342} bond (the MMP site).[19] On the other hand, ADAMTS1,[52] ADAMTS4,[53] and ADAMTS5[54] clip the Glu^{373}-Ala^{374} bond (the aggrecanase site) in addition to other sites in the G2-G3 domains. Thus, members of both the MMP and ADAMTS families may play central roles in the aggrecan degradation in arthritides. Decorin, a leucine-rich repeat proteoglycan, is also digested by MMP-2, MMP-3, and MMP-7.[92] However, information about proteinases responsible for the degradation of other proteoglycans, including fibromodulin, lumican, biglycan, proline- and arginine-rich end leucine repeat protein (PRELP), chondroadherin, and syndecan present in articular cartilage, is limited.

Fibrillar interstitial collagens (i.e., type I, II, and III collagens) are extremely resistant to most proteinases because of their triple-helical structures. In general, classic collagenases, including MMP-1, MMP-8, and MMP-13, are responsible for degradation of these collagens. Among them, MMP-13 may be most important for the degradation of cartilage collagen because it preferentially digests type II collagen.[9] MT1-MMP degrades type I, II, and III collagens.[38] Type III collagen is also

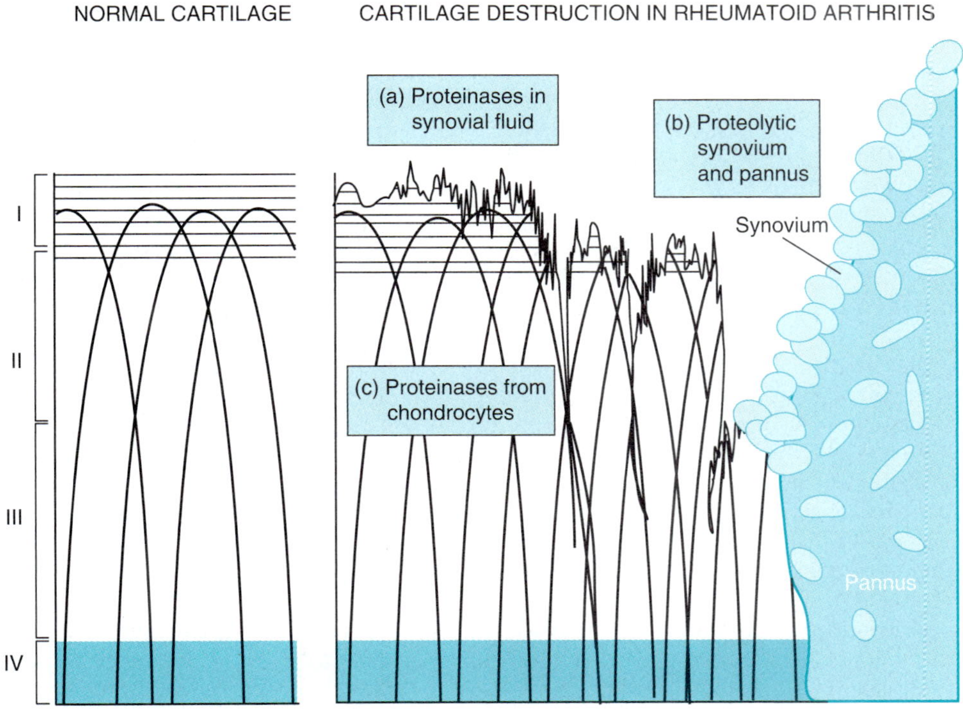

FIGURE 4–4 · **Structure of Normal Articular Cartilage and its Destruction by Proteinases in Rheumatoid Arthritis.** Normal articular cartilage is divided into four zones (I, II, III, and IV). Collagen fibrils are aligned parallel to the articular surface in the superficial zone, and they blend with radial fibers and form plates or sheets sweeping vertically through the middle zone, showing arcade structures that originate from the calcified zone (IV). In rheumatoid arthritis, synovial tissue cells and inflammatory cells produce various proteinases, most of which are secreted into synovial fluid. These proteinases in synovial fluid attack the surface of the articular cartilage from the synovial fluid (a). At the periphery of the articular surface, proteolytic synovium degrades cartilage by direct contact, and pannus tissue covers and invades cartilage (b). Chondrocytes, which secrete proteinases by stimulation with various cytokines and growth factors, also are implicated in cartilage destruction (c).

susceptible to degradation by MMP-3,[78] MMP-9,[12] MT3-MMP,[40] and neutrophil elastase. Cleavage of the telopeptides by the telopeptidase activity of MMP-3,[17] MMP-9,[12] neutrophil elastase, cathepsin G, and cysteine proteinase cathepsins is important for depolymerization of the cross-linked collagens.[1] Once the collagen molecules are cleaved, the helical structures are unwound at 37°C (i.e., body temperature) and become denatured into gelatins, which are digested into smaller peptides by gelatinases (MMP-2 and MMP-9).[11,12] Collagen V is readily digested by MMP-2[11] and MMP-9.[12] In contrast, type VI collagen is resistant to most MMPs, including MMP-1, MMP-2, MMP-3, MMP-7, MMP-9, MMP-10, and MT1-MMP, but it is susceptible to neutrophil elastase, cathepsin G, chymase, and tryptase.[6] Type IX collagen is degraded by MMP-3.[17] Type X collagen is susceptible to MMP-1 and MMP-2, and collagen XI is degraded by MMP-2.

Fibronectin is degraded by many MMPs including MMP-2, MMP-3, MMP-7, MMP-10, MMP-11, MMP-13, MMP-19, MT1-MMP, MT2-MMP, MT3-MMP, and other serine proteinases. Link protein is also susceptible to many proteinases, such as MMP-1, MMP-2, MMP-3, MMP-7, MMP-8, MMP-9, MMP-10, neutrophil elastase, and cathepsin G. Cartilage oligomeric matrix protein (COMP) is digested by MMP-19 and MMP-20.[33] However, proteinases capable of digesting cartilage matrix protein (CMP) and cartilage intermediate layer protein (CILP) are not known.

CARTILAGE DESTRUCTION BY PROTEINASES IN RHEUMATOID ARTHRITIS

Articular cartilage in rheumatoid arthritis is destroyed by proteinases in three pathways: (1) destruction from surfaces of articular cartilage by proteinases present in synovial fluid; (2) destruction through direct contact of proteolytic synovium, pannus tissue, or both to articular cartilage; (3) intrinsic destruction pathway by proteinases derived from chondrocytes (see Fig. 4–4).

Rheumatoid arthritis is characterized by chronic proliferative synovitis, which shows hyperplasia of the synovial lining cells, inflammatory cell infiltration, and angiogenesis in the sublining cell layer (see Chapter 65). Hyperplastic synovial lining cells overproduce MMP-1, MMP-3, MMP-9, and MT1-MMP, as well as TIMP-1 and TIMP-3.[1,93,94] Sublining fibroblasts produce MMP-2 and TIMP-2.[1] Polymorphonuclear leukocytes infiltrated in the synovium and joint cavity contain MMP-8 in the specific granules and MMP-9, as well as neutrophil elastase, cathepsin G, and proteinase 3, in the azurophil granules. These substances are released from cells during phagocytosis of tissue debris and immune complexes. Other inflammatory cells in the synovium include macrophages, lymphocytes, and mast cells. Macrophages produce MMP-1, MMP-9, TIMP-1, and TIMP-2. uPA and cathepsins B, L, and D are also secreted from activated macrophages. T-lymphocytes in the synovium synthesize MMP-9. Chymase and tryptase are degranulated from mast cells in response to activation by immune complexes. Endothelial cells express many MMPs, including MMP-1, MMP-2, MMP-3, MMP-9, and MT1-MMP, as well as tPA and their inhibitors. These proteinases may be involved in tissue remodeling during angiogenesis in the synovium, instead of cartilage destruction.

All these proteinases and inhibitors produced by synovial tissue cells and inflammatory cells seem to be secreted into the synovial fluid, and they attack the surfaces of articular cartilage when active proteinases overwhelm inhibitors. Actually, MMP-1, MMP-2, MMP-3,

MMP-8, MMP-9, TIMP-1, and TIMP-2 are detectable in rheumatoid synovial fluids, and the molar ratios of MMPs to TIMPs correlate with MMP activity, which is detectable in rheumatoid synovial fluids.[95] Thus, MMPs are thought to be in favor of proteinase in rheumatoid synovial fluids. The cartilage in the central part of the articular surface shows surface irregularity (fibrillation) and proteoglycan depletion without being covered by pannus tissue, even in the early stage of rheumatoid arthritis. This cartilage degradation may be ascribed to proteolytic damage by the action of the proteinases present in synovial fluid (see Fig. 4–4).

Articular cartilage at the margins of the articular surface, to which synovial tissue can directly attach, is progressively degraded even in the disease's early stage. Because rheumatoid synovial lining cells exhibit strong gelatinolytic activity, which is probably generated through activation of proMMP-2 by the action of MT1-MMP,[93] direct contact of the proteolytically active synovial tissue to articular cartilage is a destruction pathway (see Fig. 4–4). Although rheumatoid synovium contains high concentrations of active proteinases, the synovium can avoid the attack by MMPs because type VI collagen, a major component in the lining cell layer,[96] is resistant to the activities of MMP-1, MMP-2, MMP-3, and MT1-MMP.[38,96] Pannus tissue is proliferative, and vascular tissue growing from the marginal transitional zone onto the surface of the partially degraded articular cartilage.[1] It is unknown whether pannus tissue formation is a sign of active destruction or repair of the articular cartilage, but the balance of data favors the former. Immunolocalization of MMP-1 and phagocytosis of collagen fibrils by pannus cells at sites of pannus-cartilage junction may suggest a role of the tissue in the cartilage destruction.

In addition to the extrinsic pathway for the cartilage damage, cartilage may be destroyed by proteinases derived from chondrocytes (see Fig. 4–4), which are activated to produce proteinases by cytokines. Chondrocytes, under stimulation, are capable of expressing various proteinases including MMP-1, MMP-2, MMP-3, MMP-7, MMP-9, MMP-13, MT1-MMP, MT3-MMP, ADAM9, ADAM10, ADAM17, ADAMTS4, and other classes of proteinases. In rheumatoid arthritic cartilage, MMP-1, MMP-2, MMP-3, MMP-7, MMP-9, MMP-13, and MT1-MMP are expressed in the chondrocytes located in the proteoglycan-depleted zone. Once large areas of the cartilage surface are ulcerated, after degradation of cartilage ECM, death of chondrocytes occurs, leading to further progressive cartilage destruction.

BONE RESORPTION IN RHEUMATOID ARTHRITIS

Bone is resorbed by osteoclasts even in the early stage of rheumatoid arthritis. This is commonly observed at the bare zone, where pannus-like granulation tissue invades the bone marrow and destroys subchondral bone. Activated osteoclasts attach only to mineralized bone matrix, and this cell-matrix contact is carried out between $\alpha v\beta 3$ integrin of osteoclasts and Arg-Gly-Asp (RGD) sequence of osteopontin in the matrix. ECM degradation of the mineralized bone is possible only after demineralization of the bone matrix by protons secreted by osteoclasts because proteinases cannot permeate the matrix components in the mineralized tissues. Thus, matrix degradation by osteoclasts is performed in the subosteoclastic compartments, which have acidic (pH 4 to 5) and hypercalcemic (40 to 50 mM Ca^{++}) conditions.[97]

The major component of the ECM proteins in mature bone is insoluble highly cross-linked type I collagen, although type III and V collagens are also present. Other minor components in bone matrix are leucine-rich repeat proteoglycans (decorin and biglycan) and glycoproteins such as osteopontin, osteonectin (SPARC), osteocalcin (bone Gla-protein), and thrombospondin. Among collagenolytic cysteine proteinases, including cathepsins B, K, L, and S, cathepsin K is considered most important for bone resorption because of its collagenolytic activity with a broad pH optimum and selective expression in osteoclasts and giant cells of giant-cell tumors.[1] Mutations of human cathepsin K are responsible for pycnodysostosis, an autosomal recessive osteochondrodysplasia characterized by osteopetrosis and short stature.[98] Moreover, cathepsin K–deficient mice have a similar phenotype. Despite the importance of cathepsin K in bone resorption, osteoclastic bone resorption cannot be completely inhibited by cysteine proteinase inhibitors; it is inhibited to a similar degree by MMP inhibitors.[97] MMP-9 is highly expressed in osteoclasts in normal and rheumatoid bones[99] and in giant cells of giant-cell tumors. MMP-9 has telopeptidase activity against soluble and insoluble type I collagen and also strong gelatinolytic activity.[12,99] ProMMP-9 is activated by acid exposure, and once activated, it is proteolytically active under acidic and hypercalcemic conditions.[99] MMP-9–deficient mice show a transient disturbance of growth plate development. Accordingly, both cathepsin K and MMP-9 may be involved in bone resorption in rheumatoid arthritis. Although MT1-MMP is reportedly expressed in osteoclasts in rheumatoid arthritis,[100] evidence of the direct involvement in osteoclastic bone resorption is limited.

CARTILAGE DESTRUCTION BY PROTEINASES IN OSTEOARTHRITIS

In osteoarthritis, no prominent inflammatory changes occur in the synovium during early stages of the disease, but elevated production of enzymes by the chondrocytes themselves contributes to the breakdown of cartilage. Many MMPs, including MMP-1,[101] MMP-2,[69,102] MMP-3,[103] MMP-7,[104] MMP-8,[101] MMP-9,[102] MMP-13,[8,101] and MT1-MMP,[69] are expressed in osteoarthritic cartilage. MMP-3, MMP-7, and MT1-MMP are immunolocalized to chondrocytes in the proteoglycan-depleted zone of osteoarthritic cartilage, and the levels of their staining correlate directly with the histologic Mankin score.[69,103,104] Among the classic collagenolytic MMPs (i.e., MMP-1, MMP-8, and MMP-13), MMP-13 may be most important for degradation of the cartilage collagen because of its preferential digestion of type II collagen over type I and III collagens.[8,9] Because MT1-MMP efficiently activates proMMP-2 within the osteoarthritic cartilage,[69] and it can also activate proMMP-13.[83] MT1-MMP may play a key role in cartilage degradation through activation of proMMP-2 and proMMP-13 and its own proteolytic activity against cartilage ECM. Considering intermolecular activation cascade for proMMPs by active MMPs, another key MMP in osteoarthritic cartilage tissue is MMP-3, which can activate proMMP-1, proMMP-7, proMMP-8, proMMP-9, and proMMP-13. MMP-3 not only digests many cartilage ECM components such as aggrecan, type IX collagen, and link protein, but it also activates those proMMPs.

Other proteinases implicated for cartilage destruction in osteoarthritis are members of the ADAMTS family. Chondrocytes are known to express ADAMTS1, ADAMTS4, and ADAMTS5. However, information about their expression and regulation of the activities in osteoarthritic cartilage is still limited. Members of the membrane-type ADAM family (i.e., ADAM10, ADAM12, ADAM15, and ADAM17) are expressed in osteoarthritic cartilage, but the functions of these ADAMs in osteoarthritic cartilage are unknown.

REFERENCES

1. Okada Y: Proteinases and matrix degradation. Philadelphia, W.B. Saunders, 2001, pp 55-72.
2. Handley CJ, Mok MT, Ilic MZ, et al: Cathepsin D cleaves aggrecan at unique sites within the interglobular domain and chondroitin sulfate attachment regions that are also cleaved when cartilage is maintained at acid pH. Matrix Biol 20:543-553, 2001.
3. Bromme D, Okamoto K, Wang BB, et al: Human cathepsin O2, a matrix protein-degrading cysteine protease expressed in osteoclasts: functional expression of human cathepsin O2 in *Spodoptera frugiperda* and characterization of the enzyme. J Biol Chem 271:2126-2132, 1996.
4. Sorimachi H, Suzuki K: The structure of calpain. J Biochem (Tokyo) 129:653-664, 2001.
5. Nagase H: Activation mechanisms of matrix metalloproteinases. Biol Chem 378:151-160, 1997.
6. Kielty CM, Lees M, Shuttleworth CA, et al: Catabolism of intact type VI collagen microfibrils: susceptibility to degradation by serine proteinases. Biochem Biophys Res Commun 191:1230-1236, 1993.
7. Saksela O, Rifkin DB: Cell-associated plasminogen activation: regulation and physiological functions. Annu Rev Cell Biol 4:93-126, 1988.
8. Mitchell PG, Magna HA, Reeves LM, et al: Cloning, expression, and type II collagenolytic activity of matrix metalloproteinase-13 from human osteoarthritic cartilage. J Clin Invest 97:761-768, 1996.
9. Knauper V, Lopez-Otin C, Smith B, et al: Biochemical characterization of human collagenase-3. J Biol Chem 271:1544-1550, 1996.
10. Balbin M, Fueyo A, Knauper V, et al: Identification and enzymatic characterization of two diverging murine counterparts of human interstitial collagenase (MMP-1) expressed at sites of embryo implantation. J Biol Chem 276:10253-10262, 2001.
11. Okada Y, Morodomi T, Enghild JJ, et al: Matrix metalloproteinase 2 from human rheumatoid synovial fibroblasts: purification and activation of the precursor and enzymic properties. Eur J Biochem 194:721-730, 1990.
12. Okada Y, Gonoji Y, Naka K, et al: Matrix metalloproteinase 9 (92-kDa gelatinase/type IV collagenase) from HT 1080 human fibrosarcoma cells. Purification and activation of the precursor and enzymic properties. J Biol Chem 267:21712-21719, 1992.
13. Heissig B, Hattori K, Dias S, et al: Recruitment of stem and progenitor cells from the bone marrow niche requires MMP-9 mediated release of kit-ligand. Cell 109:625-637, 2002.
14. McQuibban GA, Gong JH, Tam EM, et al: Inflammation dampened by gelatinase A cleavage of monocyte chemoattractant protein-3. Science 289:1202-1206, 2000.
15. Nagase H, Ogata Y, Suzuki K, et al: Substrate specificities and activation mechanisms of matrix metalloproteinases. Biochem Soc Trans 19:715-718, 1991.
16. Okada Y, Nagase H, Harris ED Jr: A metalloproteinase from human rheumatoid synovial fibroblasts that digests connective tissue matrix components: purification and characterization. J Biol Chem 261:14245-14255, 1986.
17. Wu JJ, Lark MW, Chun LE, et al: Sites of stromelysin cleavage in collagen types II, IX, X, and XI of cartilage. J Biol Chem 266:5625-5628, 1991.
18. Nakamura H, Fujii Y, Ohuchi E, et al: Activation of the precursor of human stromelysin 2 and its interactions with other matrix metalloproteinases. Eur J Biochem 253:67-75, 1998.
19. Fosang AJ, Neame PJ, Last K, et al: The interglobular domain of cartilage aggrecan is cleaved by PUMP, gelatinases, and cathepsin B. J Biol Chem 267:19470-19474, 1992.
20. Imai K, Yokohama Y, Nakanishi I, et al: Matrix metalloproteinase 7 (matrilysin) from human rectal carcinoma cells: activation of the precursor, interaction with other matrix metalloproteinases and enzymic properties. J Biol Chem 270:6691-6697, 1995.
21. Uria JA, Lopez-Otin C: Matrilysin-2, a new matrix metalloproteinase expressed in human tumors and showing the minimal domain organization required for secretion, latency, and activity. Cancer Res 60:4745-4751, 2000.
22. Park HI, Ni J, Gerkema FE, et al: Identification and characterization of human endometase (matrix metalloproteinase-26) from endometrial tumor. J Biol Chem 275:20540-20544, 2000.
23. Marchenko GN, Ratnikov BI, Rozanov DV, et al: Characterization of matrix metalloproteinase-26, a novel metalloproteinase widely expressed in cancer cells of epithelial origin. Biochem J 356: 705-718, 2001.
24. Pei D, Weiss SJ: Furin-dependent intracellular activation of the human stromelysin-3 zymogen. Nature 375:244-247, 1995.
25. Noel A, Santavicca M, Stoll I, et al: Identification of structural determinants controlling human and mouse stromelysin-3 proteolytic activities. J Biol Chem 270:22866-22872, 1995.
26. Pei D, Majmudar G, Weiss SJ: Hydrolytic inactivation of a breast carcinoma cell-derived serpin by human stromelysin-3. J Biol Chem 269:25849-25855, 1994.
27. Manes S, Mira E, Barbacid MM, et al: Identification of insulin-like growth factor-binding protein-1 as a potential physiological substrate for human stromelysin-3. J Biol Chem 272:25706-25712, 1997.
28. Lohi J, Wilson CL, Roby JD, et al: Epilysin, a novel human matrix metalloproteinase (MMP-28) expressed in testis and keratinocytes and in response to injury. J Biol Chem 276: 10134-10144, 2001.
29. Shapiro SD, Kobayashi DK, Ley TJ: Cloning and characterization of a unique elastolytic metalloproteinase produced by human alveolar macrophages. J Biol Chem 268:23824-23829, 1993.
30. Pendas AM, Knauper V, Puente XS, et al: Identification and characterization of a novel human matrix metalloproteinase with unique structural characteristics, chromosomal location, and tissue distribution. J Biol Chem 272:4281-4286, 1997.
31. Llano E, Pendas AM, Knauper V, et al: Identification and structural and functional characterization of human enamelysin (MMP-20). Biochemistry 36:15101-15108, 1997.
32. Stracke JO, Hutton M, Stewart M, et al: Biochemical characterization of the catalytic domain of human matrix metalloproteinase 19: evidence for a role as a potent basement membrane degrading enzyme. J Biol Chem 275:14809-14816, 2000.
33. Stracke JO, Fosang AJ, Last K, et al: Matrix metalloproteinases 19 and 20 cleave aggrecan and cartilage oligomeric matrix protein (COMP). FEBS Lett 478:52-56, 2000.
34. Sato H, Takino T, Okada Y, et al: A matrix metalloproteinase expressed on the surface of invasive tumour cells. Nature 370: 61-65, 1994.
35. Will H, Hinzmann B: cDNA sequence and mRNA tissue distribution of a novel human matrix metalloproteinase with a potential transmembrane segment. Eur J Biochem 231:602-608, 1995.
36. Takino T, Sato H, Shinagawa A, et al: Identification of the second membrane-type matrix metalloproteinase (MT-MMP-2) gene from a human placenta cDNA library. MT-MMPs form a unique

membrane-type subclass in the MMP family. J Biol Chem 270:23013-23020, 1995.
37. Pei D: Identification and characterization of the fifth membrane-type matrix metalloproteinase MT5-MMP. J Biol Chem 274:8925-8932, 1999.
38. Ohuchi E, Imai K, Fujii Y, et al: Membrane type 1 matrix metalloproteinase digests interstitial collagens and other extracellular matrix macromolecules. J Biol Chem 272:2446-2451, 1997.
39. d'Ortho MP, Will H, Atkinson S, et al: Membrane-type matrix metalloproteinases 1 and 2 exhibit broad-spectrum proteolytic capacities comparable to many matrix metalloproteinases. Eur J Biochem 250:751-757, 1997.
40. Shimada T, Nakamura H, Ohuchi E, et al: Characterization of a truncated recombinant form of human membrane type 3 matrix metalloproteinase. Eur J Biochem 262:907-914, 1999.
41. Itoh Y, Kajita M, Kinoh H, et al: Membrane type 4 matrix metalloproteinase (MT4-MMP, MMP-17) is a glycosylphosphatidylinositol-anchored proteinase. J Biol Chem 274:34260-34266, 1999.
42. Pei D: Leukolysin/MMP25/MT6-MMP: a novel matrix metalloproteinase specifically expressed in the leukocyte lineage. Cell Res 9:291-303, 1999.
43. Wang Y, Johnson AR, Ye QZ, et al: Catalytic activities and substrate specificity of the human membrane type 4 matrix metalloproteinase catalytic domain. J Biol Chem 274:33043-33049, 1999.
44. English WR, Puente XS, Freije JM, et al: Membrane type 4 matrix metalloproteinase (MMP17) has tumor necrosis factor-alpha convertase activity but does not activate pro-MMP2. J Biol Chem 275:14046-14055, 2000.
45. Pei D, Kang T, Qi H: Cysteine array matrix metalloproteinase (CA-MMP)/MMP-23 is a type II transmembrane matrix metalloproteinase regulated by a single cleavage for both secretion and activation. J Biol Chem 275:33988-33997, 2000.
46. Velasco G, Pendas AM, Fueyo A, et al: Cloning and characterization of human MMP-23, a new matrix metalloproteinase predominantly expressed in reproductive tissues and lacking conserved domains in other family members. J Biol Chem 274:4570-4576, 1999.
47. Peschon JJ, Slack JL, Reddy P, et al: An essential role for ectodomain shedding in mammalian development. Science 282: 1281-1284, 1998.
48. Sunnarborg SW, Hinkle CL, Stevenson M, et al: Tumor necrosis factor-alpha converting enzyme (TACE) regulates epidermal growth factor receptor ligand availability. J Biol Chem 277:12838-12845, 2002.
49. Black RA: Tumor necrosis factor-alpha converting enzyme. Int J Biochem Cell Biol 34:1-5, 2002.
50. Yan Y, Shirakabe K, Werb Z: The metalloprotease Kuzbanian (ADAM10) mediates the transactivation of EGF receptor by G protein-coupled receptors. J Cell Biol 158:221-226, 2002.
51. Asakura M, Kitakaze M, Takashima S, et al: Cardiac hypertrophy is inhibited by antagonism of ADAM12 processing of HB-EGF: metalloproteinase inhibitors as a new therapy. Nat Med 8:35-40, 2002.
52. Rodriguez-Manzaneque JC, Westling J, Thai SN, et al: ADAMTS1 cleaves aggrecan at multiple sites and is differentially inhibited by metalloproteinase inhibitors. Biochem Biophys Res Commun 293:501-508, 2002.
53. Tortorella MD, Burn TC, Pratta MA, et al: Purification and cloning of aggrecanase-1: a member of the ADAMTS family of proteins. Science 284:1664-1666, 1999.
54. Abbaszade I, Liu RQ, Yang F, et al: Cloning and characterization of ADAMTS11, an aggrecanase from the ADAMTS family. J Biol Chem 274:23443-23450, 1999.
55. Sandy JD, Westling J, Kenagy RD, et al: Versican V1 proteolysis in human aorta in vivo occurs at the Glu441-Ala442 bond, a site that is cleaved by recombinant ADAMTS-1 and ADAMTS-4. J Biol Chem 276:13372-13378, 2001.
56. Nakamura H, Fujii Y, Inoki I, et al: Brevican is degraded by matrix metalloproteinases and aggrecanase-1 (ADAMTS4) at different sites. J Biol Chem 275:38885-38890, 2000.
57. Potempa J, Korzus E, Travis J: The serpin superfamily of proteinase inhibitors: structure, function, and regulation. J Biol Chem 269:15957-15960, 1994.
58. Murphy G, Willenbrock F: Tissue inhibitors of matrix metalloendopeptidases. Methods Enzymol 248:496-510, 1995.
59. Gomez DE, Alonso DF, Yoshiji H, et al: Tissue inhibitors of metalloproteinases: structure, regulation and biological functions. Eur J Cell Biol 74:111-122, 1997.
60. Bode W, Fernandez-Catalan C, Tschesche H, et al: Structural properties of matrix metalloproteinases. Cell Mol Life Sci 55:639-652, 1999.
61. Brew K, Dinakarpandian D, Nagase H: Tissue inhibitors of metalloproteinases: evolution, structure and function. Biochim Biophys Acta 1477:267-283, 2000.
62. Will H, Atkinson SJ, Butler GS, et al: The soluble catalytic domain of membrane type 1 matrix metalloproteinase cleaves the propeptide of progelatinase A and initiates autoproteolytic activation: regulation by TIMP-2 and TIMP-3. J Biol Chem 271:17119-17123, 1996.
63. Gomis-Ruth FX, Maskos K, Betz M, et al: Mechanism of inhibition of the human matrix metalloproteinase stromelysin-1 by TIMP-1. Nature 389:77-81, 1997.
64. Fernandez-Catalan C, Bode W, Huber R, et al: Crystal structure of the complex formed by the membrane type 1-matrix metalloproteinase with the tissue inhibitor of metalloproteinases-2, the soluble progelatinase A receptor. EMBO J 17:5238-5248, 1998.
65. Kinoshita T, Sato H, Okada A, et al: TIMP-2 promotes activation of progelatinase A by membrane-type 1 matrix metalloproteinase immobilized on agarose beads. J Biol Chem 273:16098-16103, 1998.
66. Kashiwagi M, Tortorella M, Nagase H, et al: TIMP-3 is a potent inhibitor of aggrecanase 1 (ADAM-TS4) and aggrecanase 2 (ADAM-TS5). J Biol Chem 276:12501-12504, 2001.
67. Baker AH, Zaltsman AB, George SJ, et al: Divergent effects of tissue inhibitor of metalloproteinase-1, -2, or -3 overexpression on rat vascular smooth muscle cell invasion, proliferation, and death in vitro: TIMP-3 promotes apoptosis. J Clin Invest 101:1478-1487, 1998.
68. Oh J, Takahashi R, Kondo S, et al: The membrane-anchored MMP inhibitor RECK is a key regulator of extracellular matrix integrity and angiogenesis. Cell 107:789-800, 2001.
69. Imai K, Ohta S, Matsumoto T, et al: Expression of membrane-type 1 matrix metalloproteinase and activation of progelatinase A in human osteoarthritic cartilage. Am J Pathol 151:245-256, 1997.
70. Lohi J, Lehti K, Valtanen H, et al: Structural analysis and promoter characterization of the human membrane-type matrix metalloproteinase-1 (MT1-MMP) gene. Gene 242:75-86, 2000.
71. Haas TL, Stitelman D, Davis SJ, et al: Egr-1 mediates extracellular matrix-driven transcription of membrane type 1 matrix metalloproteinase in endothelium. J Biol Chem 274:22679-22685, 1999.
72. Clark IM, Rowan AD, Edwards DR, et al: Transcriptional activity of the human tissue inhibitor of metalloproteinases 1 (TIMP-1) gene in fibroblasts involves elements in the promoter, exon 1 and intron 1. Biochem J 324:611-617, 1997.
73. Trim JE, Samra SK, Arthur MJ, et al: Upstream tissue inhibitor of metalloproteinases-1 (TIMP-1) element-1, a novel and essential regulatory DNA motif in the human TIMP-1 gene promoter, directly interacts with a 30-kDa nuclear protein. J Biol Chem 275:6657-6663, 2000.
74. Sun Y, Hegamyer G, Kim H, et al: Molecular cloning of mouse tissue inhibitor of metalloproteinases-3 and its promoter: specific lack of expression in neoplastic JB6 cells may reflect altered gene methylation. J Biol Chem 270:19312-19319, 1995.
75. Zochbauer-Muller S, Fong KM, Virmani AK, et al: Aberrant promoter methylation of multiple genes in non-small cell lung cancers. Cancer Res 61:249-255, 2001.
76. Hammani K, Blakis A, Morsette D, et al: Structure and characterization of the human tissue inhibitor of metalloproteinases-2 gene. J Biol Chem 271:25498-25505, 1996.
77. Young DA, Phillips BW, Lundy C, et al: Identification of an initiator-like element essential for the expression of the tissue inhibitor of metalloproteinases-4 (Timp-4) gene. Biochem J 364:89-99, 2002.
78. Nagase H: Human stromelysins 1 and 2. Methods Enzymol 248:449-470, 1995.
79. Sato H, Kinoshita T, Takino T, et al: Activation of a recombinant membrane type 1-matrix metalloproteinase (MT1-MMP) by furin and its interaction with tissue inhibitor of metalloproteinases (TIMP)-2. FEBS Lett 393:101-104, 1996.
80. Itoh Y, Takamura A, Ito N, et al: Homophilic complex formation of MT1-MMP facilitates proMMP-2 activation on the cell surface and promotes tumor cell invasion. EMBO J 20:4782-4793, 2001.

81. Brooks PC, Stromblad S, Sanders LC, et al: Localization of matrix metalloproteinase MMP-2 to the surface of invasive cells by interaction with integrin alpha v beta 3. Cell 85:683-693, 1996.
82. Cowell S, Knauper V, Stewart ML, et al: Induction of matrix metalloproteinase activation cascades based on membrane-type 1 matrix metalloproteinase: associated activation of gelatinase A, gelatinase B and collagenase 3. Biochem J 331:453-458, 1998.
83. Knauper V, Bailey L, Worley JR, et al: Cellular activation of proMMP-13 by MT1-MMP depends on the C-terminal domain of MMP-13. FEBS Lett 532:127-130, 2002.
84. Sternlicht MD, Werb Z: How matrix metalloproteinases regulate cell behavior. Annu Rev Cell Dev Biol 17:463-516, 2001.
85. Egeblad M, Werb Z: New functions for the matrix metalloproteinases in cancer progression. Nat Rev Cancer 2:161-174, 2002.
86. Seiki M: The cell surface: the stage for matrix metalloproteinase regulation of migration. Curr Opin Cell Biol 14:624-632, 2002.
87. Guo H, Li R, Zucker S, et al: EMMPRIN (CD147), an inducer of matrix metalloproteinase synthesis, also binds interstitial collagenase to the tumor cell surface. Cancer Res 60:888-891, 2000.
88. Puyraimond A, Fridman R, Lemesle M, et al: MMP-2 colocalizes with caveolae on the surface of endothelial cells. Exp Cell Res 262:28-36, 2001.
89. Yu WH, Woessner JF, Jr., McNeish JD, et al: CD44 anchors the assembly of matrilysin/MMP-7 with heparin-binding epidermal growth factor precursor and ErbB4 and regulates female reproductive organ remodeling. Genes Dev 16:307-323, 2002.
90. Yu Q, Stamenkovic I: Cell surface-localized matrix metalloproteinase-9 proteolytically activates TGF-beta and promotes tumor invasion and angiogenesis. Genes Dev 14:163-176, 2000.
91. Fosang AJ, Last K, Maciewicz RA: Aggrecan is degraded by matrix metalloproteinases in human arthritis: evidence that matrix metalloproteinase and aggrecanase activities can be independent. J Clin Invest 98:2292-2299, 1996.
92. Imai K, Hiramatsu A, Fukushima D, et al: Degradation of decorin by matrix metalloproteinases: identification of the cleavage sites, kinetic analyses and transforming growth factor-beta1 release. Biochem J 322:809-814, 1997.
93. Yamanaka H, Makino K, Takizawa M, et al: Expression and tissue localization of membrane-types 1, 2, and 3 matrix metalloproteinases in rheumatoid synovium. Lab Invest 80:677-687, 2000.
94. Takizawa M, Ohuchi E, Yamanaka H, et al: Production of tissue inhibitor of metalloproteinases 3 is selectively enhanced by calcium pentosan polysulfate in human rheumatoid synovial fibroblasts. Arthritis Rheum 43:812-820, 2000.
95. Yoshihara Y, Nakamura H, Obata K, et al: Matrix metalloproteinases and tissue inhibitors of metalloproteinases in synovial fluids from patients with rheumatoid arthritis or osteoarthritis. Ann Rheum Dis 59:455-461, 2000.
96. Okada Y, Naka K, Minamoto T, et al: localization of type VI collagen in the lining cell layer of normal and rheumatoid synovium. Lab Invest 63:647-656, 1990.
97. Delaisse J, Vaes G: Mechanism of mineral solubilization and matrix degradation in osteoclastic bone resorption. In Biology and Physiology of the Osteoclast. Edited by Riflein BR and Gay CV, Boca Raton, Fla., CRC Press, 1992, pp 289-314.
98. Gelb BD, Shi GP, Chapman HA, et al: Pycnodysostosis, a lysosomal disease caused by cathepsin K deficiency. Science 273: 1236-1238, 1996.
99. Okada Y, Naka K, Kawamura K, et al: Localization of matrix metalloproteinase 9 (92-kilodalton gelatinase/type IV collagenase = gelatinase B) in osteoclasts: implications for bone resorption. Lab Invest 72:311-322, 1995.
100. Pap T, Shigeyama Y, Kuchen S, et al: Differential expression pattern of membrane-type matrix metalloproteinases in rheumatoid arthritis. Arthritis Rheum 43:1226-1232, 2000.
101. Shlopov BV, Lie WR, Mainardi CL, et al: Osteoarthritic lesions: involvement of three different collagenases. Arthritis Rheum 40:2065-2074, 1997.
102. Mohtai M, Smith RL, Schurman DJ, et al: Expression of 92-kD type IV collagenase/gelatinase (gelatinase B) in osteoarthritic cartilage and its induction in normal human articular cartilage by interleukin 1. J Clin Invest 92:179-185, 1993.
103. Okada Y, Shinmei M, Tanaka O, et al: Localization of matrix metalloproteinase 3 (stromelysin) in osteoarthritic cartilage and synovium. Lab Invest 66:680-690, 1992.
104. Ohta S, Imai K, Yamashita K, et al: Expression of matrix metalloproteinase 7 (matrilysin) in human osteoarthritic cartilage. Lab Invest 78:79-87, 1998.

5 Muscle: Anatomy, Physiology, and Biochemistry

YALE E. GOLDMAN • JODY A. DANTZIG

Approximately 660 skeletal muscles support and move the body under the control of the central nervous system. They constitute up to 40 percent of the adult human body mass. Most skeletal muscles are fastened by collagenous tendons across joints in the skeleton. The transduction of chemical energy into mechanical work by the muscle cells leads to muscle shortening and consequent movement. A high degree of specialization in this tissue is evident from the intricate architecture and kinetics of intracellular membrane systems, the contractile proteins, and the molecular components that transmit force extracellularly to the basement membrane and tendons. Muscle cells normally exhibit wide variations in activity level and are able to adapt in size, isoenzyme composition, membrane organization, and energetics. In pathologic states, they often become deconditioned. These examples of plasticity can be surprisingly swift and extensive. This chapter outlines the structure and function of muscle and its relationship to the associated connective tissue. It also introduces the basis for the highly adaptive response to altered functional demands and diseases. Two excellent Web sites can be accessed for further information in these areas[1,2]

Muscle Development

EMBRYOGENESIS

During embryogenesis, connective tissue, bone, and skeletal muscle are derived from mesodermal cells of the somites. The mechanisms that control the expression of skeletal muscle–specific genes and regulate skeletal muscle cell differentiation and maturation are emerging from developmental biologic studies and serve as a paradigm for developmental regulation in many tissues. Sequentially expressed transcriptional regulators, such as the myocyte-enhancer factors[3] and the myogenic basic helix-loop-helix proteins (MyoD, Myf-5, Mrf-4, and myogenin),[4-8] initiate the transcription of skeletal muscle–specific genes in myoblasts (precursors of muscle cells). MyoD and Myf-5 regulate cell lineage commitment, whereas Mrf-4 and myogenin control differentiation. Although the "master switch" for myogenesis remains to be determined, the detailed relationships of these myogenic regulatory factors (Mrfs) with other ubiquitous regulatory factors[9,10] and their roles in specification, differentiation, and repair are emerging.[11]

MYOFIBRILLOGENESIS

When mesenchymal cells from the myotome of the somites commit to the myogenic cell line, the presumptive myoblasts proliferate and migrate to sites of muscle development within the embryo. This induction and patterning is controlled by diffusible messengers, such as sonic hedgehog, bone morphogenetic proteins (BMPs), and Wnt proteins, that are secreted from nearby structures, including the neural tube, notochord, dorsal ectoderm, and lateral mesoderm.[12] The presumptive myoblasts withdraw from the cell cycle, differentiate into spindle-shaped myoblasts, and begin to synthesize embryonic isoforms of muscle-specific proteins.[13] Myoblasts align in columns and fuse to produce multinucleated primary myotubes (Fig. 5–1). The contractile organelle, the myofibril, which is comprised of long columns of sarcomeres (see Fig. 5–4), self-assembles on cytoskeletal scaffolding. The sequence of molecular events in the assembly mechanism of these elaborate structures has been described.[14,15] Myofibrils first appear near the periphery of the myotubes and fill in toward the center of the newly formed muscle fibers (skeletal muscle cells). Myofibrillogenesis continues until the cytoplasm is packed with parallel, laterally aligned sarcomeres. The nuclei then migrate from the center to the periphery, where they remain, even in mature, multinucleated muscle fibers. Central nuclei in adult muscle biopsies are thus diagnostic of abnormal muscle-cell turnover (see also Chapter 80).

An extracellular matrix (see Chapters 2 and 3) of type IV collagen, proteoglycans, fibronectin, and laminin is secreted by the myotubes to form the basal lamina, which fully ensheathes the fiber membrane (sarcolemma) except at the neuromuscular junction.[16] Myoblasts continue to proliferate, and later generations elongate, fuse, and differentiate within the basal laminae of the primary myotubes, forming independent secondary myotubes.[17] Both sets of myotubes develop into phenotypically distinct muscle fiber types by sequentially expressing a series of embryonic, neonatal, and mature isoforms of the contractile proteins.[18] Some of the developmental and mature isoforms of the contractile proteins, (Table 5–1) appearing in fast, slow, and cardiac muscle, are encoded by multigene families, whereas others are differentially expressed by alternative splicing of messenger RNA.

Under normal conditions, the number of muscle fibers within a skeletal muscle is virtually constant throughout life. Myogenic stem cells (satellite cells) remain situated in mature muscles between the sarcolemmas and basal laminae, providing a reservoir for muscle repair and

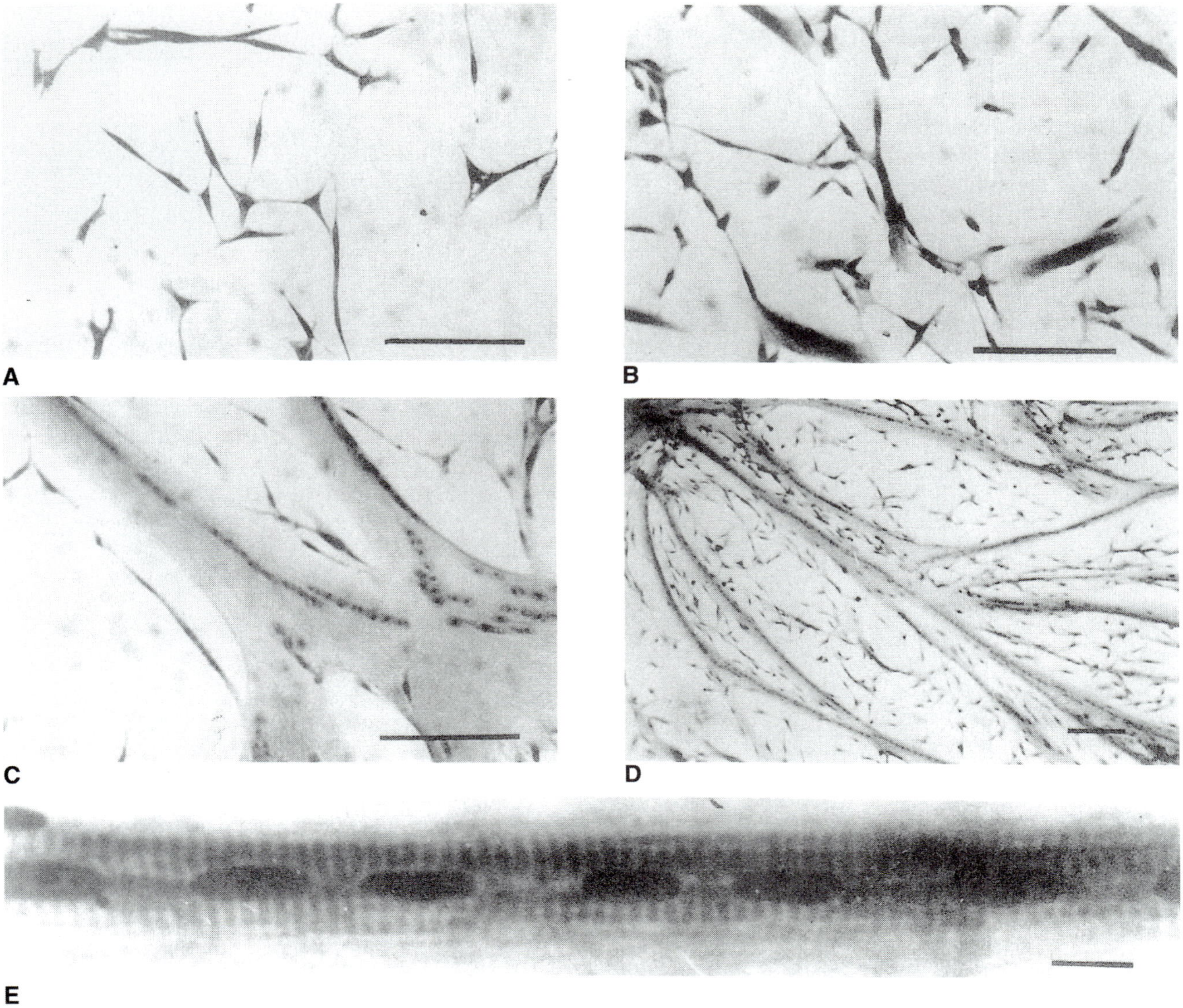

FIGURE 5–1 · Developmental Progression of Myoblasts During Fusion into Myotubes. *A*, Unicellular myoblasts. *B*, Initial fusion of myoblasts. *C*, Multinucleated myotubes. *D*, Lower-magnification micrograph of multinucleated myotubes showing the extent of cell fusion. *E*, Multinucleated myotube with cross-striations. *A–D*, Calibration bar = 100 μm; *E*, calibration bar = 10 μm.
(*A–E* From Buckley PA, Konigsberg IR: myogenic fusion and the duration of the post-mitotic gap (G_1). Dev Biol 37:198, 1974.)

growth.[19,20] When a muscle fiber is damaged or necrosed, mitogenic factors and peptide regulators released from the damaged cells[18,20,21] trigger satellite cells to proliferate and migrate into the affected area, guided by the basal lamina. Satellite cells differentiate into myoblasts, fuse, and form new muscle fibers. The supply of these stem cells is limited, however, which affects the potential for repair in severe degenerative conditions.

Structure

MUSCLE TISSUE

Parallel, aligned bundles of skeletal muscle fibers make up approximately 85 percent of muscle tissue. Nerves, blood supply, and connective tissue structures that provide support, elasticity, and force transmission to the skeleton (see later discussion) constitute the remaining volume. Muscle fibers range in length from a few millimeters to many centimeters and in diameter from 10 to 150 μm. This elongated shape is determined by the organization of the contractile proteins that occupy the majority of the sarcoplasm. Each muscle has a limited range of shortening that is amplified into large motions by lever systems of the skeleton, which is usually operating at a mechanical disadvantage. Variations in geometric arrangements of the fibers—parallel, fan-shaped, fusiform (spindle-like), or pennate (feather-like)—determine some of the mechanical properties. For example, the slant of the fibers in a pennate muscle increases the magnitude of force generation at the expense of speed and range of movement, compared to a similarly sized muscle with fibers aligned parallel to the

TABLE 5–1 • SIGNALING AND CONTRACTILE PROTEINS OF SKELETAL MUSCLE

Protein	Molecular Weight (kDa)	Subunits (kDa)	Location	Function
Acetylcholine receptor	~250	5 × ~50	Postsynaptic membrane of neuromuscular junction	Neuromuscular signal transmission
Dihydropyridine receptor	~380	1 × ~160 1 × ~130 1 × ~60 1 × ~30	T tubule membrane	Voltage sensor
Ryanodine receptor	1800	4 × 450	Terminal cisternae of SR	SR Ca^{2+} release channel
Ca^{2+} ATPase	110	—	Longitudinal SR	Uptake of Ca^{2+} into the SR
Calsequestrin	63	—	SR terminal cisternae lumen	Binding and storage of Ca^{2+}
Troponin	78	1 × 18 1 × 21 1 × 31	Thin filament	Regulation of contraction
Tropomyosin	70	2 × 35	Thin filament	Regulation of contraction
Myosin tion	500	2 × 220 2 × 15 2 × 20	Thick filament	Chemomechanical energy transduc-
Actin tion	42	—	Thin filament	Chemomechanical energy transduc-
MM creatine phosphokinase	40	—	M line	ATP buffer, structural protein
α-Actinin	190	2 × 95	Z line	Structural protein
Titin	3000	—	From Z line to M line	Structural protein
Nebulin	600	—	Thin filaments, in the I band	Structural protein
Dystrophin	400	—	Subsarcolemma	Structural integrity of sarcolemma

Abbreviations: ATP, adenosine triphosphate; SR, sarcoplasmic reticulum.

tendons.[22] Muscles designed for strength (e.g., gastrocnemius) are typically pennate, whereas those designed for speed (e.g., biceps) tend to have parallel fibers. Muscles are commonly arranged around joints as antagonistic pairs facilitating bidirectional motion. When one muscle (the *agonist*) contracts, another (its *antagonist*) is relaxed and passively extended. Their roles reverse to actively generate the opposite motion, unless it occurs passively by the force of gravity.

An extensive network of connective tissue, forming the endomysium, surrounds each muscle fiber. Fine nerve branches and the small capillaries, necessary for the metabolic exchange of nutrients and waste products, penetrate this layer. The endomysium is continuous with the perimysium, a connective tissue network that ensheathes small parallel bundles of muscle fibers known as *fasciculi*, intrafusal fibers, larger nerves, and blood vessels. The epimysium encompasses the whole muscle. All three layers of connective tissue contain collagen, mostly types I, III, IV, and V, with types IV and V predominating in the basement membranes surrounding each skeletal muscle fiber. The $\alpha 1_2 \alpha 2$-chain composition of the collagen IV isoform is the most prevalent and provides the mechanical stability and flexibility of the basil lamina[23,24] (see Chapter 2). The perimysium and endomysium merge at the junction between the muscle fibers and the tendons, aponeuroses, and fasciae. These layers give the attachment sites great tensile strength and distribute axial force into shear forces over a larger surface area.

FIBER TYPES

Muscles adapt to their specific functions. Fibers can be classified according to their size, twitch duration, speed of contraction, balance between aerobic and glycolytic metabolism, and resistance to fatigue (Table 5–2). In addition, isoenzymes of the signaling, regulatory, and contractile proteins and the surface area of the sarcoplasmic reticulum membranes are key features that distinguish functional properties of fiber types. For instance, the duration of the twitch is influenced by the rates of the sarcoplasmic reticulum Ca^{2+} release and reuptake. The velocity of shortening is determined by myosin isoenzyme composition. Type IIB (fast) fibers are less "red" than the other fiber types because they contain less of the iron-heme–containing proteins, myoglobin and mitochondrial cytochromes. Classification schemes are not, however, absolute because some groups of fibers have composite or intermediate functional, ultrastructural, and histochemical characteristics.

During development, fiber-type specificity may be partly determined before innervation.[25] Although the biologic events and signals responsible for designating functional specialization in muscle fibers are not fully understood, classic cross-innervation experiments demonstrate that innervation can dynamically specify and modify the muscle fiber type.[26] After cross-innervation, the functional and histologic properties listed in Table 5–2 shift toward the target fiber type over a few weeks' time, indicating the ability of muscles to adapt and remodel in accordance with the pattern of neuronal activity.

TABLE 5–2 • CLASSIFICATION OF MUSCLE FIBER TYPES

	I	IIA	IIB	IIC
General Features				
Size	Moderate	Small	Large	Small
Mitochondria	Many	Intermediate	Few	Intermediate
Capillary blood supply	Extensive	Sparse	Sparse	Sparse
SR membrane	Sparse	Extensive	Extensive	Extensive
Z line	Wide	Wide	Narrow	Narrow
Protein Isoforms				
Myosin heavy chain	MHCI	MHCIIA	MHCIIB	MHCI and MHCIIA
Myosin essential light chain	ELC1s	ELC1f, ELC3f	ELC1f, ELC3f	ELC1f, ELC3f, and ELC1s
Myosin regulatory light chain	RLC2s	RLC2f	RLC2f	RLC2f and RLC2s
Regulatory proteins	Slow	Fast	Fast	Fast
Mechanic Properties				
Contraction time	Slow and sustained	Fast twitch	Fast twitch	Moderate twitch
SR calcium ATPase rate	Low	High	High	High
Actomyosin ATPase rate	Low	High	High	Moderate
Shortening velocity	Slow	Fast	Fast	Moderate
Resistance to fatigue	High	Moderate	Low	Moderate
Metabolic Profile				
Oxidative capacity	High	Intermediate	Low	High
Glycolytic capacity	Moderate	High	High	High
NADH-TR/SDH/MDH	High	Moderate	Low	Moderate
LDH and phosphorylase	Low	Medium	High	Moderate
Glycogen	Low	High	High	Variable
Myoglobin	High	Medium	Low	High

Abbreviations: ELC, Myosin essential light chain; f, fast; LDH, lactate dehydrogenase; MDH, malate dehydrogenase; MHC, myosin heavy chain; NADH-TR, nicotinamide adenine dinucleotide tetrazolium reductase; RLC, myosin regulatory light chain; s, slow; SDH, succinate dehydrogenase; SR, sarcoplasmic reticulum.

Events During Muscle Contraction

NEURAL CONTROL

Normally, a skeletal muscle fiber is activated briefly and then relaxes. This *twitch,* which is 5 to 40 msec long, is initiated by an action potential propagated from the central nervous system along an α-motoneuron, synaptic transmission across the neuromuscular junction, and an action potential in the muscle sarcolemma. Muscle fibers are typically innervated at one or two sites along their length by branches of an α-motoneuron axon arising from the ventral horn of the spinal column. A motoneuron and the approximately 5 to 1600 homogeneous muscle fibers it innervates constitute a motor unit. Although the spatial domains of different units are intermingled, when an α-motoneuron is excited, all fibers in the motor unit are triggered to contract together. Functional properties, such as speed and susceptibility to fatigue, vary with the dynamic requirements set by the neuronal firing pattern and the mechanical load, but they are homogeneous within a motor unit. The level of muscle activity is dynamically controlled by varying the firing rate of twitches and the number of active motor units. As activity increases, more and larger units are recruited.

A second class of fibers, the *intrafusal fibers,* are innervated by γ-motoneurons and control the sensitivity of the Golgi tendon organs and spindle receptors that provide local feedback to the spinal cord regarding muscle length and force. Afferent feedback pathways modulate activity to control the desired movement. The same feedback system generates the monosynaptic stretch reflex.

NEUROMUSCULAR TRANSMISSION

At the neuromuscular junction, the axon tapers and loses its myelin sheath. The postsynaptic sarcolemmal membrane (the motor end plate) is indented into folds that increase its surface area (Fig. 5–2). Mitochondria and nuclei are concentrated in this region. The junctional cleft is a 50-nm-wide space between the presynaptic axonal membrane and the sarcolemma.

When the nerve action potential reaches the presynaptic terminal, local Ca^{2+} channels are gated open for the influx of Ca^{2+}, which triggers fusion of acetylcholine-loaded membrane vesicles with the neuronal presynaptic membrane.[27] Exocytosed acetylcholine rapidly diffuses across the junctional cleft and binds to nicotinic acetylcholine-gated ion channels in the crests of the postsynaptic membrane folds. Ligand gating of the acetylcholine receptors increases their cation permeability, locally depolarizing the muscle cell. This change of membrane potential initiates a regenerative action potential, mediated by voltage-gated Na^+ and K^+ channels. The action potential propagates at velocities up to 5 m/sec from the motor end plate throughout the sarcolemma.

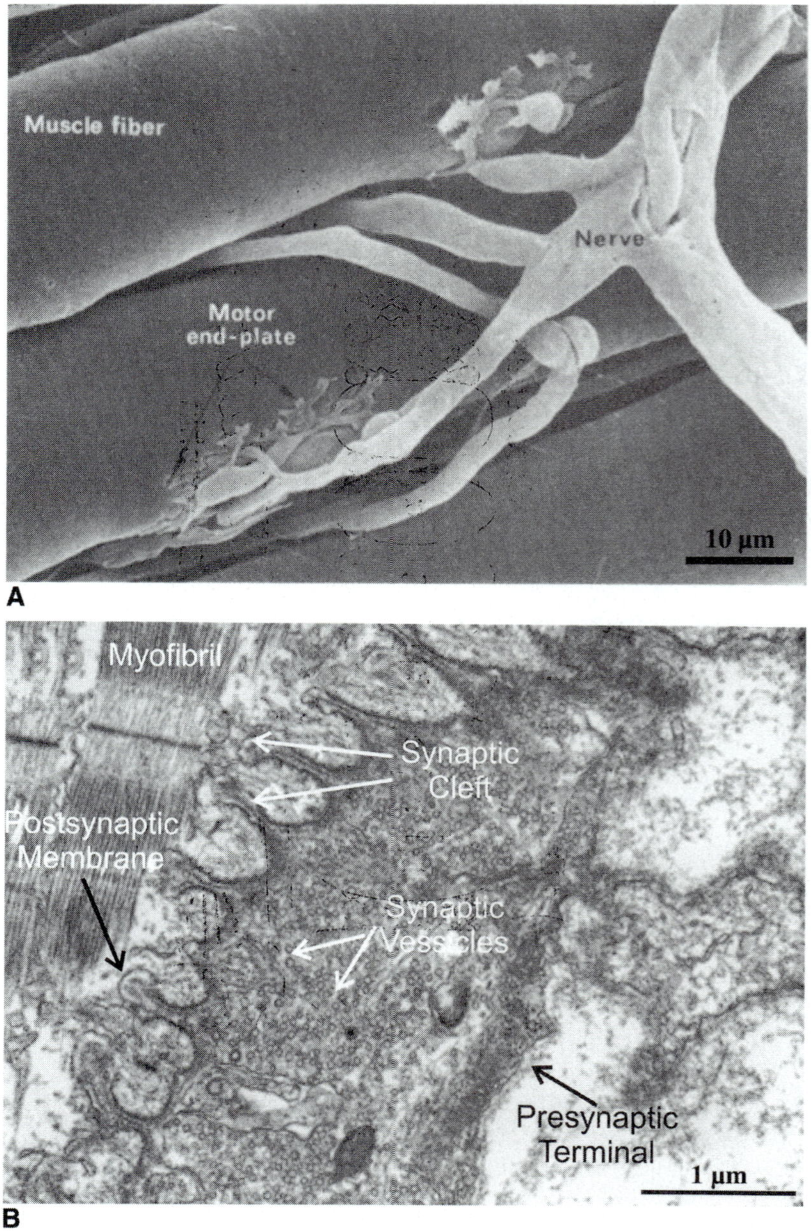

FIGURE 5–2 · Neuromuscular Junction. *A*, Scanning electron micrograph of an α-motoneuron innervating several muscle fibers in its motor unit. Calibration bar = 10 μm. (From Bloom W, Fawcett DW: A Textbook of Histology, 10th ed. Philadelphia, WB Saunders, 1975.) *B*, Transmission electron micrograph. Calibration bar = 1 μm. (Courtesy of Dr. Clara Franzini-Armstrong, University of Pennsylvania, Philadelphia.)

EXCITATION-CONTRACTION COUPLING

Invaginations of the sarcolemma at regular intervals constitute the transverse tubule (T tubule) network, which pervades the fiber and surrounds the contractile apparatus with connected longitudinal and lateral segments (Fig. 5–3). The lumen of this network is open to the extracellular space, and it contains the high Na^+ and low K^+ concentrations of interstitial fluid.[28] Action potentials at the surface membrane invade the entire T tubular system. A specialized type of endoplasmic reticulum forms an entirely intracellular membrane system termed the *sarcoplasmic reticulum* (SR). Prevalent structures containing a T tubule flanked by two terminal cisternae of the SR to form junctional complexes are termed triads. Terminal cisternae contain the oligomers of the Ca^{2+}-binding protein calsequestrin, which provides the fiber with an internal reservoir of calcium ions. The Ca^{2+} channels, termed *dihydropyridine receptors* (DHPRs), are localized in the T tubule membranes juxtaposed to a cytoplasmic domain of SR Ca^{2+}-release channels (the *ryanodine receptors* [RyRs], or foot proteins) in the terminal cisternae membranes.[29] These membrane proteins are further characterized in Table 5–1.

When an action potential depolarizes the T tubular membrane, the DHPRs, primarily voltage sensors in skeletal muscle (but not in myocardium), transfer a signal from the T tubules to the RyRs by direct interprotein coupling. Ca^{2+} is then released cooperatively through the RyRs from the SR into the myoplasm, where it activates the contractile machinery.[30] This sequence of events is termed *excitation-contraction coupling*.

Mutations in the α-subunit of the DHPR in dysgenic mice lead to paralysis because in these mutants membrane depolarization in skeletal muscle does not initiate the release of Ca^{2+} from the SR. Excitation-

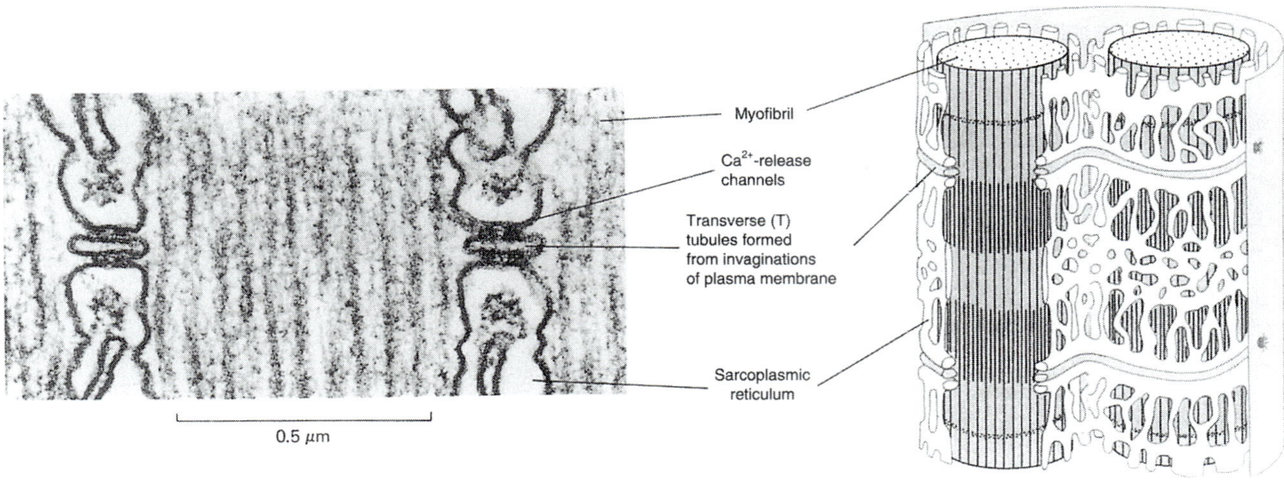

FIGURE 5–3 · Membrane Systems That Relay the Excitation Signal from the Sarcolemma to the Cell Interior. In the electron micrograph, two T tubules are cut in cross-section. The electron densities spanning the gap between the T tubules and sarcoplasmic reticulum membranes are the ryanodine receptors, channels that release calcium into the myoplasm. (From Alberts B, Bray D, Lewish J, et al: Molecular Biology of the Cell, 2nd ed. New York, Garland Publishers, 1989. Micrograph courtesy of Dr. Clara Franzini-Armstrong, University of Pennsylvania, Philadelphia.)

contraction coupling can be restored in cultured cells from these mice by transfection with the complementary DNA encoding for the DHPR,[31] and transfections using chimeric constructs[32] have pinpointed the domain within the DHPR that specifies skeletal- or cardiac-type excitation-contraction coupling.[33] Isoforms of the RyRs also help determine the characteristics of the coupling between T tubules and the SR.[34] Channelopathies in human skeletal and heart muscle have been linked to DHPR mutations.[35,36] Human malignant hyperthermia occurs in individuals with mutant RyRs that become trapped in the open state after exposure to halothane anesthetic agents.[37]

CONTRACTILE APPARATUS

The specific locations and functions of the contractile proteins are listed in Table 5–1. *Myofibrils* (Fig. 5–4*D*) are long, 1-μm-diameter cylindrical organelles that contain the contractile protein arrays responsible for work production, force generation, and shortening. Each myofibril is a column of sarcomeres, the basic contractile units, which are approximately 2.5 μm in length and delimited by Z lines (see Fig. 5–4*D* and *E*) containing the densely packed structural protein α-actinin. The contractile and structural proteins within each sarcomere form a highly ordered, nearly crystalline lattice of interdigitating thick and thin myofilaments[38] (see Fig. 5–4*E, I,* and *J*). Myofilaments are remarkably uniform in both length and lateral registration, even during contraction,[39] resulting in the cross-striated histologic appearance of skeletal and cardiac muscles. This highly periodic organization has facilitated biophysic studies of muscle by sophisticated structural[38] and spectroscopic techniques.[40,41]

Thick filaments (1.6-μm long) containing the motor protein myosin are located in the center of the sarcomere in the optically anisotropic A band (see Fig. 5–4*D*). The thick filaments are organized into a hexagonal lattice stabilized by M protein[42] and muscle-specific creatine phosphokinase[43] in the M line (see Fig. 5–4*D* and *E*). Myosin (see Fig. 5–4*K*) is a highly asymmetric 470-kD protein containing two 120-kDa globular NH_2-terminal heads, termed the *cross-bridge* or *subfragment-1*(S1) (see Fig. 5–4*L*), and an α-helical coiled-coil rod. Two light chains, essential and regulatory, ranging from 15 to 22 kDa, are associated with the heavy chain in each S1 (see Fig. 5–4*L*). The rod portions of approximately 300 myosin molecules polymerize in a three-stranded helix to form the backbone of each thick filament (see Fig. 5–4*K*). The cross-bridges, protruding from these backbones, contain adenosine triphosphatase (ATPase) and actin-binding sites responsible for the conversion of chemical energy into mechanical work. Besides their role in muscle contraction, at least 15 classes of myosins accomplish diverse tasks in cell motility such as chemotaxis, cytokinesis, pinocytosis, targeted vesicle transport, and signal transduction.[44] Thus, myosin is the target for mutations leading to a number of inherited muscle and neurologic diseases.[45,46]

Thin filaments (see Fig. 5–4*I*) are double-stranded helical polymers of actin that extend 1.1 μm from each side of the Z line and occupy the optically isotropic I band (see Fig. 5–4*D* and *E*). A regulatory complex containing one tropomyosin molecule and three troponin subunits (TnC, TnT, and TnI) is associated with each successive group of seven actin monomers along the thin filament (see Fig. 5–4*J*).[38] In the region where the thick and thin filaments overlap, the thin filaments are positioned within the hexagonal lattice equidistant from three thick filaments (see Fig. 5–4*F*). Both sets of filaments are polarized. In an active muscle, an interaction between the two filaments causes a concerted translation of the thin filaments toward the M line that shortens the sarcomere, and thus the whole muscle. Actin is ubiquitous in the cytoskeleton of eukaryotic cells and, like myosin, fulfills many roles in determining cell shapes and motions.[47,48] Control of the actin cytoskeleton and diseases due to mutations in actin-binding proteins are being intensively investigated.[49]

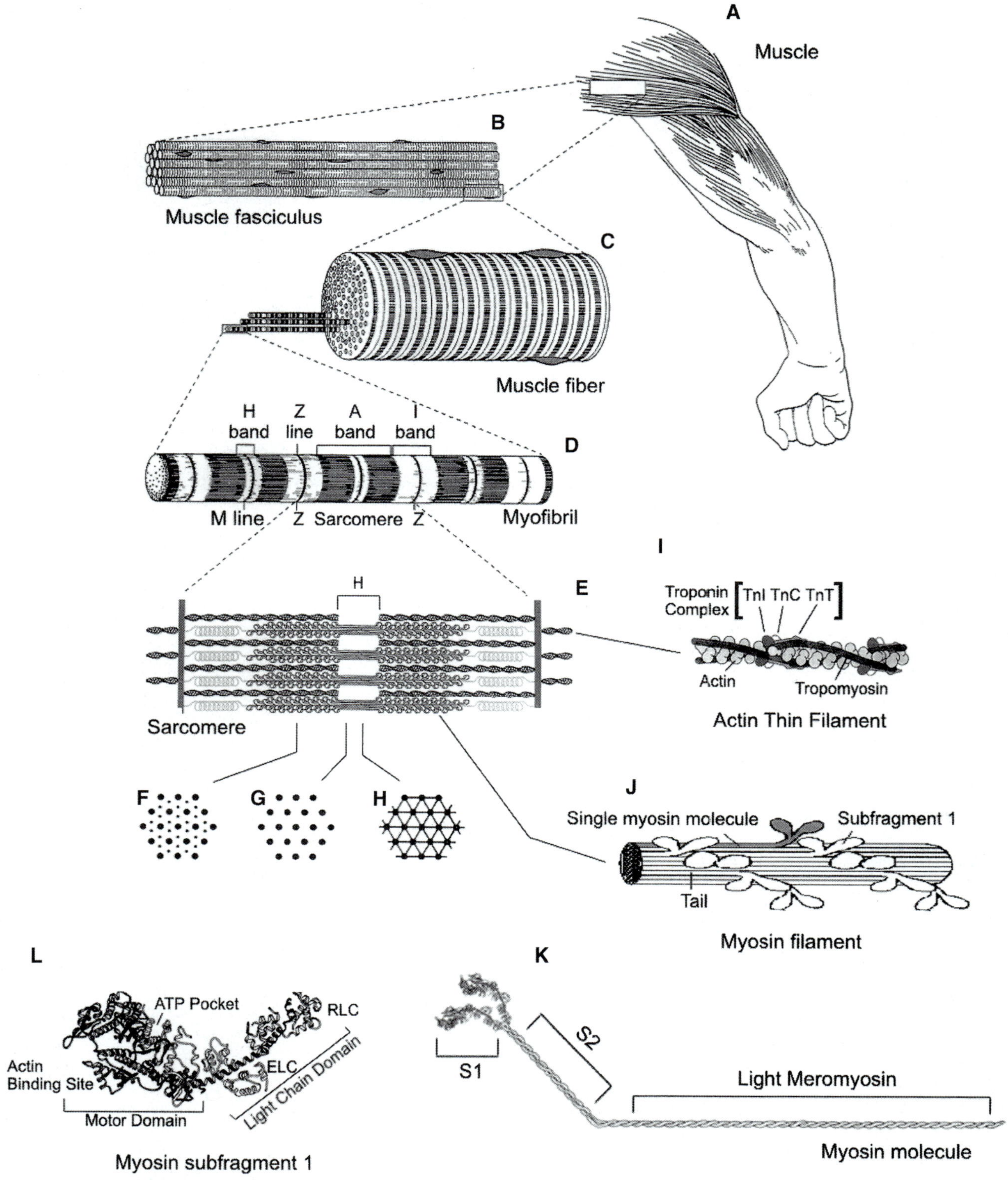

FIGURE 5–4 • Components of the contractile apparatus at successively increasing magnifications from the whole muscle *(A)* to the molecular level *(I–L)*. The myofibril *(D)* shows the banding pattern created by the lateral alignment of the myofilaments *(I, J)* in the sarcomeres *(D,E)*. Diagrams *F* to *H* show the cross-sectional structure of the filament lattice at various points within the sarcomere. Myosin is shown at the single two-headed molecule level *(K)*, and the crystal structure of the globular motor domain is shown *(L, S-1)* with the essential and regulatory light chains. (From Juanqueira LC, Carneiro J, Long JA: Basic Histology, 5th ed. Norwalk, Conn, Appleton-Lange, 1986. Modified from Bloom W, Fawcett DW: A Textbook of Histology, 10th ed. Philadelphia, WB Saunders, 1975 and Rayment I, Rypniewski WR, Schmidt-Base K, et al: Three-dimensional structure of myosin subfragment-1: a molecular motor. Science 261:50, 1993.)

Two of the largest identified proteins, titin and nebulin, function in the assembly and maintenance of the sarcomeric structure. Individual titin molecules (~3000 kDa) are associated with the thick filament and extend from the M line to the Z line.[50] Titin contains repeating fibronectin-like immunoglobulin and unusual proline-rich domains that confer molecular elasticity on the resting sarcomere.[51] Nebulin (~800 kDa) is associated with the Z line and thin filaments.[50] Protein connections from the contractile apparatus through the sarcolemma to the extracellular matrix are described later in this chapter. The cytoskeleton of muscle fibers also contains cytoplasmic actin, microtubules, and intermediate filaments.[52]

FORCE GENERATION AND SHORTENING

At rest, the thin filament–regulatory proteins, troponin and tropomyosin, inhibit contraction (see Fig. 5-4*I*). During a twitch, Ca^{2+} released from the SR binds to TnC, relieving this inhibition and thus allowing cross-bridges to attach to actin. A contraction results from a cyclic interaction between actin and myosin (the cross-bridge cycle) that produces a relative sliding force between the thin and thick filaments.[53] The energy source is the hydrolysis of adenosine triphosphate (ATP) to adenosine diphosphate (ADP) and orthophosphate (P_i).

A simplified model of the chemomechanical events in the cross-bridge cycle is illustrated in Figure 5–5. Motor proteins, including myosin, can now be studied by single-molecule biophysic techniques, which provide unprecedented detail on their dynamics.[54] When Ca^{2+} is present, a complex of myosin, ADP, and P_i attaches to the thin filament (step a) and a structural change associated with P_i release (b) generates the sliding force.[55,56] The conformational change in the cross-bridge that leads to force generation is apparently a tilting motion of the light chain region.[41,57,58] After ADP is released (c), ATP binds to the active site and dissociates myosin from actin (d). Myosin then hydrolyzes ATP (e) to form the ternary myosin-ADP-P_i complex, which can reattach to actin for the next cycle.

If the mechanic load on the muscle is high, the contractile apparatus produces a mechanic force without changing length (an isometric contraction). If the load is moderate, the thin filaments slide actively toward the M line of the sarcomere, resulting in shortening of the whole muscle. The width of the muscle increases during shortening, so the volume stays constant. Work production (concomitant force and sliding) is associated with an increase of the ATPase rate. The thermodynamic efficiency (mechanical power divided by energy liberated by ATPase activity) approaches 50 percent, a remarkable figure considering that manufactured combustion engines seldom achieve efficiencies greater than 20 percent.

RELAXATION

The twitch is terminated by reversal of all the steps in activation. Ca^{2+} released from the SR is taken up again by Ca^{2+}-ATPase pumps located in longitudinal membranes of the SR. The myoplasmic Ca^{2+} concentration then decreases and Ca^{2+} dissociates from TnC, deactivating the thin filament. When the number of attached cross-bridges declines below a certain threshold, tropomyosin inhibits further cross-bridge attachment and tension declines to the resting level. Ca^{2+} diffuses within the longitudinal SR to the calsequestrin sites in terminal cisternae in preparation for the next twitch. Myosin continues to hydrolyze ATP at a low rate in relaxed muscle, accounting for a sizable proportion of basal metabolism.

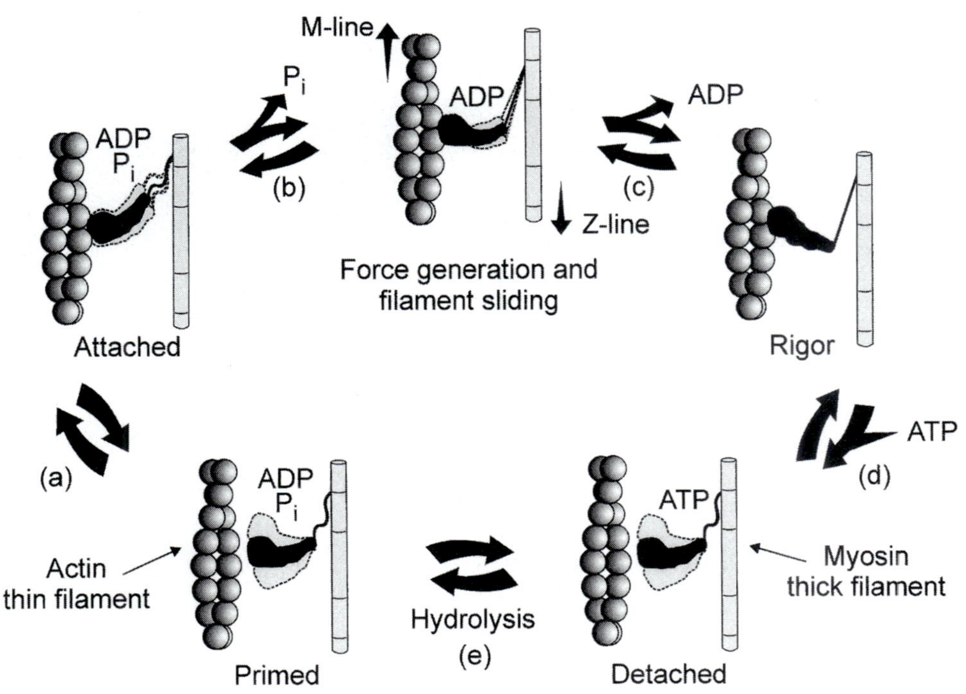

FIGURE 5–5 · The Actomyosin Cross-Bridge Cycle. Myosin molecules normally have two globular head regions (cross-bridges), but for clarity only one is shown. Each head binds with two actin monomers. The sequence of reactions is attachment *(A)*; P_i release and the force-generating transition *(B)*; ADP release *(C)*; ATP binding and detachment *(D)*; and ATP hydrolysis *(E)*. The heads near the detached and force-generating myosin heads indicate high mobility of the cross-bridges in these states. ADP, adenosine diphosphate; P_i, inorganic phosphate.

Transmission of Force to the Exterior

CELL-MATRIX ADHESIONS

The muscle cell is closely connected to the basal lamina along its entire surface. Several transmembrane macromolecular complexes link the myofibrils and actin cytoskeleton to laminins and collagen in the extracellular matrix. Attachment complexes for muscle, analogous to the focal adhesions of motile and epithelial cells and to adhesion plaques and intercalated disks in cardiac muscle, contain filamentous actin, vinculin, talin, and the transmembrane protein integrin (primarily the α7β1 isoform), which is the laminin receptor (Fig. 5–6). In muscle, the main laminin isoforms are laminin-2 (α2β1γ1) and laminin-4 (α2β2γ1), which are collectively termed *merosin.* In addition to providing mechanical coupling between the cytoskeleton and the extracellular matrix, the laminin-integrin system may provide a signaling pathway to regulate localized protein expression.[59] Defects of integrin and laminin expression lead to various forms of muscular dystrophy.[60]

A specialized linkage between the cytoskeleton and basal lamina in muscle, complementary to the integrin focal adhesion system, is the dystrophin-glycoprotein complex (see Fig. 5–6). Dystrophin, a 427-kDa peripheral cytoskeletal protein, has been postulated to function as a mechanical link between the cytoskeleton and the cell membrane, as a shock absorber, or to contribute mechanical strength to the membrane. Its absence or truncation causes Duchenne and Becker muscular dystrophies.[61] The unusual intricacy of muscle cell–matrix connection systems may relate to the high forces generated during contraction.

The NH_2-terminus of dystrophin binds to actin via a region with sequence homology to the actin-binding domain of α-actinin. This end of the dystrophin molecule may be linked to the basal lamina via the same proteins described previously for the focal adhesion-like complexes (see Fig. 5–6). The COOH-terminus binds to a transmembrane dystroglycan-sarcoglycan complex, which in turn binds to the laminins. Muscular dystrophies of varied severity are associated with a loss of these components.[62] Dystroglycans are also required for early embryonic development of muscle, possibly organizing laminin localization and assembly.[63,64] Utrophin, a smaller protein (395 kDa) related to dystrophin, may also link the actin cytoskeleton to the dystroglycans, especially near the neuromuscular junction

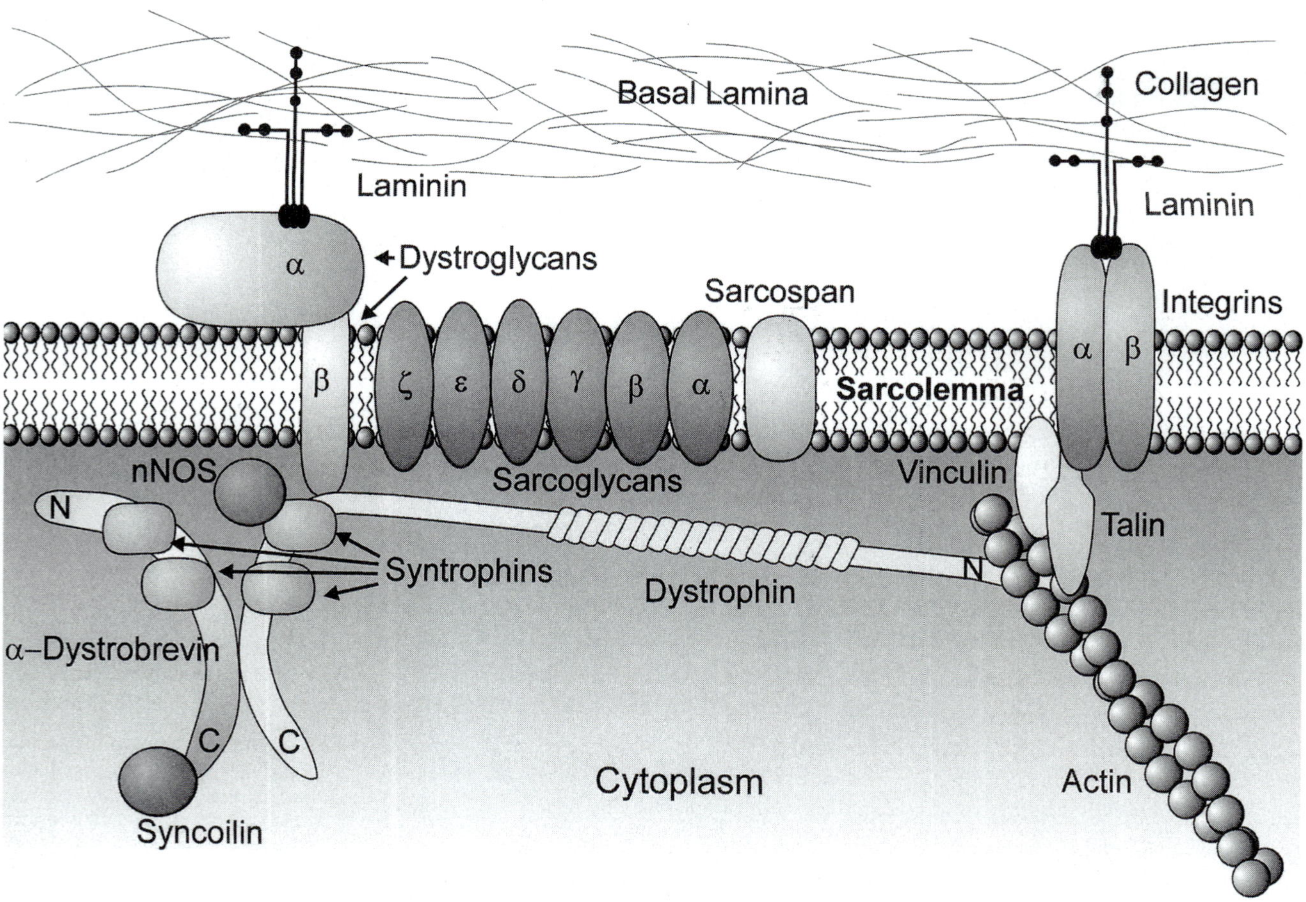

FIGURE 5–6 • Connections Between the Muscle Cytoskeleton and Extracellular Matrix. Actin is linked through integrins to the matrix, as in many cell types. Dystrophin forms an extra link through the dystroglycan-sarcoglycan complex of glycosylated proteins. The helical section of dystrophin is homologous to spectrin and may form homodimers or oligomers. Diagram was prepared following consultation with Thomas Krag and Tejvir Khurana, University of Pennsylvania, Philadelphia.

and in nonmuscle cells. Overexpression of this protein or truncated dystrophin constructs are promising avenues for gene therapy in Duchenne muscular dystrophy.[65]

MYOTENDINOUS JUNCTION

The force of muscle contraction is transmitted to the skeleton via the tendons, which are composed of collagens type I and III, blood vessels, lymphatic ducts, and fibroblasts. At the ends of the muscle fibers, myofibrils are separated by invaginations of sarcolemma filled with long bundles of collagen arising from the tendon. The membrane folds increase the surface area for bearing the mechanical load by approximately 30-fold. Instead of terminating in the Z disks, actin filaments insert into a subsarcolemmal matrix containing α-actinin, vinculin, talin, and integrin. The force is transmitted through laminin to the collagen of the tendon.

Energetics

Metabolic pathways in muscle cells are specialized for the variable, and at times extreme, rates of ATP splitting by the contractile apparatus and the membrane pumps. Because the muscle tissue compartment is large and specific protein isoforms are expressed, circulating levels of some metabolic enzymes (e.g., lactate dehydrogenase and creatine phosphokinase) are useful in the diagnosis of sarcolemmal disruption. Only the most important enzymes are mentioned here in regard to the function of normal muscle.

BUFFERING OF ADENOSINE TRIPHOSPHATE CONCENTRATION

The ATP content (~5 mM) is sufficient for only a few seconds of contraction, so rapid and effective buffering of ATP during contraction is essential for the maintenance of activity. ADP formed by the hydrolysis of ATP is rephosphorylated by transfer of a phosphate group from creatine phosphate (20 mM in a resting cell) by creatine phosphokinase located within the M line of the sarcomere, in the myoplasm, and between the inner and outer membranes of the mitochondria. Adenylate kinase, known as myokinase in muscle, catalyzes the transfer of a phosphate group between two ADP molecules, forming ATP and adenosine monophosphate (AMP). The by-products of the rapid enzymatic reactions that maintain ATP concentration are, therefore, creatine, P_i, and AMP. Some of the AMP is converted to inosine monophosphate by adenylate deaminase. A creatine phosphate shuttle has been proposed to enhance energy flux.[66] According to this hypothesis, creatine phosphate is split within the contractile apparatus and creatine is predominantly rephosphorylated in the mitochondria.

GLYCOLYSIS

Muscles use glucose as fuel when possible, otherwise they use fatty acids and ketone bodies (acetoacetate and 3-hydroxybutyrate). Most of the body storage of glycogen, which is converted to glucose 6-phosphate for local use, is in the muscle compartment. Muscle fibers lack glucose 6-phosphatase and thus do not export glucose. During intense activity, especially in anaerobic conditions, the rate of glycolysis and the production of pyruvate exceed the rate of pyruvate consumption by the citric acid cycle. The excess pyruvate is reduced to lactate by lactate dehydrogenase, which has tissue-specific isoforms. The lactate-dehydrogenase reaction also produces nicotinamide adenine dinucleotide (NAD^+), which is necessary for glycolysis, but otherwise lactate is not useful within the muscle. Lactate is freely permeable through the sarcolemma, and local increase in the extracellular lactate concentration or acidification produces exertional pain ("the burn"). Lactate is transported through the blood to the liver where it is converted back to pyruvate and then glucose, which is excreted into the blood for use by other tissues, such as muscle and brain. This sequence of steps, termed the *Cori cycle,* transfers some of the high metabolic load to the liver and "buys time" until oxidative metabolism is available.

OXIDATIVE PHOSPHORYLATION

In aerobic conditions, pyruvate enters the mitochondria, where it is oxidized to CO_2 and H_2O, generating reduced NAD (NADH). An H^+ gradient across the mitochondrial membrane is produced by the electron transport chain and, finally, ADP is phosphorylated to ATP by the mitochondrial ATP synthase. This remarkable rotary motor-generator has been studied extensively using single-molecule biophysic techniques.[67] Combining glycolysis and oxidative phosphorylation, up to 38 ATP molecules can be generated by the oxidation of each molecule of glucose. This process is energetically much more favorable than the production of lactate, but it can only occur when molecular oxygen is available. Myoglobin is an iron–heme complex protein that facilitates oxygen transport within the muscle cells. The tissue pressure in a contracting muscle often exceeds arterial perfusion pressure, so the strongest contractions are anaerobic. The content of oxidative enzymes, myoglobin, and mitochondria determines the predominant type of energy metabolism and varies in different muscle types, as discussed previously (see Table 5–2).

FATIGUE AND RECOVERY

During intense or prolonged activity, muscle fatigue is caused by alterations of metabolite levels that suppress force generation at the contractile apparatus,[68] in excitation-contraction coupling, or both.[69] Markedly increased myoplasmic P_i and H^+ concentrations and decreased creatine phosphate levels have been detected by magnetic resonance spectroscopy.[70] When the creatine phosphate level declines, maintained activity depends on glycogenolysis until glycogen stores are depleted. During prolonged intense activity, the respiratory and circulatory systems are unable to meet the oxygen demands of the tissue. Force production declines well before the ATP concentration is compromised.

The chemomechanical link between P_i release and force generation (see Fig. 5–5) implies that the increase of myoplasmic P_i in fatigued muscle reduces the magnitude of force simply by mass action.[56] Decreased pH in the muscle, partly from lactate accumulation, and insufficient availability of acetylcholine at the neuromuscular junction, leading to failure of synaptic transmission, also contribute to decreased work production. Because the respiratory and circulatory systems do not supply sufficient oxygen to support the metabolism during intense activity, an oxygen debt is incurred. Blood flow and oxygen uptake continue at an enhanced level after the period of exercise to reclaim this energy. Rephosphorylation of creatine can take place within a few minutes, but glycogen resynthesis requires several hours. Recovery processes also involve restoration of ionic gradients across the membrane-bound compartments and require consumption of further energy.

Plasticity

The strength and endurance of a muscle are altered dramatically within weeks after changes in the demands for its use, its mobility, or its hormonal or metabolic environment. The effects of this adaptive response should be considered in any clinic situation that causes a substantial shift in these factors and in regard to the long-term lifestyle, satisfaction, and independence of the patient.

ADAPTATION TO EXERCISE

Exercise leads to adaptations in the muscle fibers that include alterations in specific contractile, regulatory, structural, and metabolic proteins, as well as optimization of motor-unit recruitment. The frequency, intensity, and duration of a training stimulus and the external load influence the adaptive response.[71] Trophic factors liberated from the nerve play a minor role, if any. Strength training causes cross-sectional hypertrophy of fast type IIB fibers (see Table 5–2), the expression of fast myosin isoforms, an increase in amino acid uptake, and decreased synthesis of mitochondrial proteins. Endurance training enhances the oxidative capacity and volume density of mitochondria in oxidative type I and IIA fibers, redistributes blood flow to these motor units, and increases the synthesis of contractile proteins. Long-term hyperplasia does not usually occur after training in humans. Although hypertrophy of preexisting fiber types is observed, training also induces changes in myosin isoform distribution, especially in fibers already containing more than one isoform. There is little evidence that voluntary training regimens can switch fibers between the major categories.

When physical activity is reduced, for instance in limb immobilization, the cross-section of the fibers decreases and endurance is reduced as a result of a decreased metabolic reserve. Acute exercise hypertrophy and disuse atrophy are both reversible, but after extensive alterations, the restoration may be incomplete.[72]

ENDOCRINE CONTROL

The endocrine system also participates in adaptation. For example, normal circulating levels of thyroid hormones are required during muscle development and differentiation.[73] Experimental alterations of thyroid hormone concentrations promote changes in the relative levels of myosin and regulatory protein isoforms, as well as changes in the activity of some metabolic enzymes.[74] An intact nerve supply is required for these thyroid effects. Myogenesis is partly controlled by growth hormone release from the pituitary via the production of insulin-like growth factor I (IGF-I) in the liver. IGF-I activates satellite cells for muscle regeneration and stimulates the hypertrophy of mature muscle cells.[75,76] Abuse of growth factors, such as IGF-I, drugs, steroids, and metabolites, by athletes (primarily young men) to increase muscle mass and strength is a medical and societal problem.[77,78]

As in other tissues, insulin regulates the entry of glucose through the cell membrane. In muscle, it also promotes the uptake of branched-chain amino acids (valine, leucine, and isoleucine), which are necessary for rapid protein synthesis, and inhibits protein degradation.

AGING

Normal individuals exhibit an approximately 30 percent decrease in total muscle mass between the ages of 30 and 80. The cross-sectional area of the fibers decreases, leading to a significant loss of strength. Gradual decreases in muscle activity, as well as neuronal changes, contribute to this muscle atrophy, which can exacerbate age-related joint degeneration, making joints less stable and more prone to injury.

A decline in estrogen and testosterone levels in aging individuals has been hypothesized to affect muscle strength. Aging also produces a marked decrease in the level of IGF-I and the subsequent ability to repair or build new muscle. Recombinant IGF-I delivered via virus-mediated gene transfer has been shown to increase the muscle mass and strength of the aged mouse.[79] Further manipulations of specific growth factors may ameliorate muscle loss due to muscular dystrophies, other chronic illnesses, and aging.[80] Muscle mass, strength, and flexibility are major factors in the maintenance of independent and productive lifestyles among the elderly.

Summary

The complex functional capacity of muscle to produce finely tuned and coordinated movements is ultimately expressed as the transduction of chemical to mechanical energy by actomyosin. A twitch is initiated by an action potential propagated from the central nervous system along an α-motoneuron, neuromuscular chemical transmission, direct protein–protein communication at the T tubule–sarcoplasmic reticulum junction, Ca^{2+} diffusion in the myoplasm, and Ca^{2+} binding to thin filament regulatory proteins. Because the central nervous system controls activity through the recruitment of motor units, the gradation and coordination of movement depend critically on the pattern of connections between the α-motoneurons and the muscle fibers and on variations of properties among motor units. The development, maintenance, and aging of the muscular system involve a complex series of genetic programs and cellular interactions that are just beginning to be understood at the molecular level. Adaptation of motor unit properties is evident not only in training regimens but also in reduced activity caused by pain or joint immobilization and in compromised metabolic, hormonal, or nutritional conditions. Hence, the plasticity of muscle impacts on the clinical course of many diseases. In addition to its importance in pathophysiology, muscle serves as an excellent substrate for understanding the molecular basis of cell development, protein structure-function relationships, cell signaling, and energy transduction processes.

REFERENCES

1. The Myosin Home Page. Hosted by the Myosin Group at the MRC Laboratory of Molecular Biology and the Cambridge Institute for Medical Research, http://www.mrc-lmb.cam.ac.uk/myosin/myosin.html
2. Illingworth JA: Muscle structure and function. Leeds, School of Biochemistry and Molecular Biology, University of Leeds, XXXX, http://www.bmb.leeds.ac.uk/illingworth/muscle/
3. Kaushal S, Schneider JW, Nadal-Ginard B, Mahdavi V: Activation of the myogenic lineage by MEF2A, a factor that induces and cooperates with MyoD. Science 266:1236, 1994.
4. Emerson CP: Myogenesis and developmental control genes. Curr Opin Cell Biol 2:1065, 1990.
5. Weintraub H, Davis R, Tapscott S, et al: The *myoD* gene family: Nodal point during specification of the muscle cell lineage. Science 251:761, 1991.
6. Edmondson DG, Olson EN: Helix-loop-helix proteins as regulators of muscle-specific transcription. J Biol Chem 268:755, 1993.
7. Olson EN: Signal transduction pathways that regulate skeletal muscle gene expression. Mol Endocrinol 7:1369, 1993.
8. Molkentin JD, Olson EN: Combinatorial control of muscle development by basic helix-loop-helix and MADS-box transcription factors. Proc Natl Acad Sci U S A 93:9366, 1996.
9. Lassar AB, Davis RL, Wright WE, et al: Functional activity of myogenic HLH proteins requires hetero-oligomerization with E12/E47-like proteins in vivo. Cell 66:305, 1991.
10. Blackwell TK, Weintraub H: Differences and similarities in DNA-binding preferences of MyoD and E2A protein complexes revealed by binding site selection. Science 250:1104, 1990.
11. Sabourin LA, Rudnicki MA: The molecular regulation of myogenesis. Clin Genet 57:16, 2000.
12. Cossu G, Tajbakhsh S, Buckingham M: How is myogenesis initiated in the embryo? Trends Genet 12:218, 1996.
13. Buckley PA, Konigsberg IR: Myogenic fusion and the duration of the post-mitotic gap (G_1). Dev Biol 37:193, 1974.
14. Holtzer H, Hijikata T, Lin ZX, et al: Independent assembly of 1.6 μm long bipolar MHC filaments and I-Z-I bodies. Cell Struct Funct 22:83, 1997.
15. Sanger JW, Chowrashi P, Shaner NC, et al: Myofibrillogenesis in skeletal muscle cells. Clin Orthop 403S:S153, 2002.
16. Kühl U, Öcalan M, Timpl R, et al: Role of muscle fibroblasts in the deposition of type-IV collagen in the basal lamina of myotubes. Differentiation 28:164, 1984.
17. Kelly AM, Rubinstein NA: Development of neuromuscular specialization. Med Sci Sports Exerc 18:292, 1986.
18. Buckingham M: Skeletal muscle formation in vertebrates. Curr Opin Genet Dev 11:440, 2001.
19. Bischoff R: Interaction between satellite cells and skeletal muscle fibers. Development 109:943, 1990.
20. Hawke TJ, Garry DJ: Myogenic satellite cells: Physiology to molecular biology. J Appl Physiol 91:534, 2001.
21. Florini JR: Hormonal control of muscle growth. Muscle Nerve 10:577, 1987.
22. Gowitzke BA, Milner M: Scientific Bases of Human Movement, 3rd ed. Baltimore, Williams & Wilkins, 1988, pp 144–145.
23. Hudson BG, Reeders ST, Tryggvason K: Type IV collagen: Structure, gene organization, and role in human diseases. Molecular basis of Goodpasture and Alport syndromes and diffuse leiomyomatosis. J Biol Chem 268:26033, 1993.
24. Kühn K: Basement membrane (type IV) collagen. Matrix Biol 14:439 1994.
25. Miller JB, Stockdale FE: What muscle cells know that nerves don't tell them. Trends Neurosci 10:325, 1987.
26. Buller AJ, Eccles JC, Eccles RM: Differentiation of fast and slow muscles in the cat hind limb. J Physiol 150:399, 1960.
27. Südhof TC: The synaptic vesicle cycle: A cascade of protein-protein interactions. Nature 375:645, 1995.
28. Somlyo AV, Gonzalez-Serratos H, Shuman H, et al: Calcium release and ionic changes in the sarcoplasmic reticulum of tetanized muscle: An electron-probe study. J Cell Biol 90:577, 1981.
29. Franzini-Armstrong C, Protasi F: Ryanodine receptors of striated muscles: A complex channel capable of multiple interactions. Physiol Rev 77: 699, 1997.
30. Rios E, Brum G: Involvement of dihydropyridine receptors in excitation-contraction coupling in skeletal muscle. Nature 325:717, 1987.
31. Tanabe T, Beam KG, Powell JA, Numa S: Restoration of excitation-contraction coupling and slow calcium current in dysgenic muscle by dihydropyridine receptor complementary DNA. Nature 336:134, 1988.
32. Tanabe T, Beam KG, Adams BA, et al: Regions of the skeletal muscle dihydropyridine receptor critical for excitation-contraction coupling. Nature 346:567, 1990.
33. Nakai J, Ogura T, Protasi F, et al: Functional nonequality of the cardiac and skeletal ryanodine receptors. Proc Natl Acad Sci U S A 94:1019, 1997.
34. Murayama T, Ogawa Y: Roles of two ryanodine receptor isoforms coexisting in skeletal muscle. Trends Cardiovasc Med 12:305, 2002.
35. Barchi RL: Ion channel mutations and diseases of skeletal muscle. Neurobiol Dis 4:254, 1997.
36. Ptácek LJ: Channelopathies: Ion channel disorders of muscle as a paradigm for paroxysmal disorders of the nervous system. Neuromuscul Disord 7:250, 1997.
37. Gillard EF, Otsu K, Fujii J, et al: A substitution of cysteine for arginine 614 in the ryanodine receptor is potentially causative of human malignant hyperthermia. Genomics 11:751, 1991.
38. Squire J: The Structural Basis of Muscular Contraction. New York, Plenum Press, 1981.
39. Sosa H, Popp D, Ouyang G, Huxley HE Ultrastructure of skeletal muscle fibers studied by a plunge quick freezing method: myofilament lengths. Biophys J 67:283, 1994.
40. Thomas DD: Spectroscopic probes of muscle cross-bridge rotation. Ann Rev Physiol 49:691, 1987.
41. Irving M, Allen TStC, Sabido-David C, et al: Tilting of the light-chain region of myosin during step length changes and active force generation in skeletal muscle. Nature 375:688, 1995.
42. Chowrashi PK, Pepe FA: M-band proteins: Evidence for more than one component. *In* Pepe FA, Sanger JW, Nachmias VT (eds): Motility in Cell Function. New York, Academic Press, 1979.
43. Walliman T, Pelloni G, Turner DC, Eppenberger HM: Removal of the M-line by treatment with Fab′ fragments of antibodies against MM-creatine kinase. *In* Pepe FA, Sanger JW, Nachmias VT (eds): Motility in Cell Function. New York, Academic Press, 1979.
44. Mermall V, Post PL, Mooseker MS: Unconventional myosins in cell movement, membrane traffic, and signal transduction. Science 279:527, 1998.
45. Hasson T: Unconventional myosins, the basis for deafness in mouse and man. Am J Hum Genet 61:801, 1997.
46. Redowicz MJ: Myosins and deafness. J Muscle Res Cell Motil 20:241, 1999.
47. Small JV, Rottner K, Kaverina I, Anderson KI: Assembling an actin cytoskeleton for cell attachment and movement. Biochim Biophys Acta 1404:271, 1998.

48. Sheterline P, Clayton J, Sparrow JC (eds): Actin, 4th ed. New York, Oxford University Press, 1998.
49. Janmey PA, Chaponnier C: Medical aspects of the actin cytoskeleton. Curr Opin Cell Biol 7:111, 1995.
50. Wang K: Sarcomere-associated cytoskeletal lattices in striated muscle. *In* Shay JW (ed): Cell and Muscle Motility. Vol 6. New York, Plenum Press, 1985.
51. Labeit S, Kolmerer B: Titins: Giant proteins in charge of muscle ultrastructure and elasticity. Science 270:293, 1995.
52. Toyama Y, Forry-Schaudies S, Hoffman B, Holtzer H: Effects of taxol and Colcemid on myofibrillogenesis. Proc Natl Acad Sci U S A 79:6556, 1982.
53. Goldman YE: Wag the tail: Structural dynamics of actomyosin. Cell 93:1, 1998.
54. Leuba SH, Zlatanova J (eds): Biology at the Single Molecule Level. England, Pergamon Press, 2001.
55. Goldman YE: Kinetics of the actomyosin ATPase in muscle fibers. Annu Rev Physiol 49:637, 1987.
56. Dantzig JA, Goldman YE, Millar NC, et al: Reversal of the cross-bridge force-generating transition by photogeneration of phosphate in rabbit psoas muscle fibres. J Physiol 451:247, 1992.
57. Dobbie I, Linari M, Piazzesi G, et al: Elastic bending and active tilting of myosin heads during muscle contraction. Nature 396:383, 1998.
58. Forkey JN, Quinlan ME, Shaw MA, et al: Three-dimensional structural dynamics of myosin V by single-molecule fluorescence polarization. Nature 422:399, 2003.
59. Chicurel ME, Singer RH, Meyer CJ, Ingber DE: Integrin binding and mechanical tension induce movement of mRNA and ribosomes to focal adhesions. Nature 392:730, 1998.
60. Vachon PH, Xu H, Liu L, et al: Integrins ($\alpha7\beta1$) in muscle function and survival. Disrupted expression in merosin-deficient congenital muscular dystrophy. J Clin Invest 100:1870, 1997.
61. Durbeej M, Campbell KP: Muscular dystrophies involving the dystrophin-glycoprotein complex: An overview of current mouse models. Curr Opin Genet Dev 12:349, 2002.
62. Matsumura K, Ohlendieck K, Ionasescu VV, et al: The role of the dystrophin-glycoprotein complex in the molecular pathogenesis of muscular dystrophies. Neuromuscul Disord 3:533, 1993.
63. Henry MD, Campbell KP: A role for dystroglycan in basement membrane assembly. Cell 95:859, 1998.
64. Campbell KP, Stull JT: Skeletal muscle basement membrane-sarcolemma-cytoskeleton interactions minireview series. J Biol Chem 278:12599, 2003.
65. Wells DJ, Wells KE: Gene transfer studies in animals: what do they really tell us about the prospects for gene therapy in DMD? Neuromuscul Disord 12:S11, 2002.
66. Bessman SP, Carpenter CL: The creatine-creatine phosphate energy shuttle. Ann Rev Biochem 54:831, 1985.
67. Kinosita K Jr, Yasuda R, Noji H: F1-ATPase: A highly efficient rotary ATP machine. Essays Biochem 35:3, 2000.
68. Dawson MJ, Gadian DG, Wilkie DR: Muscular fatigue investigated by phosphorus nuclear magnetic resonance. Nature 274:861, 1978.
69. Lännergren J, Westerblad H: Force and membrane potential during and after fatiguing, continuous high-frequency stimulation of single *Xenopus* muscle fibres. Acta Physiol Scand 128:359, 1986.
70. Meyer RA, Brown TR, Kushmerick MJ: Phosphorus nuclear magnetic resonance of fast- and slow-twitch muscle. Am J Physiol 248:C279, 1985.
71. Faulkner JA, White TP: Adaptations of skeletal muscle to physical activity. *In* Bouchard C, Shephard RJ, Stephens T, et al (eds): Exercise, Fitness, and Health. Champaign, Ill, Human Kinetics, 1990, pp 265–279.
72. Appell HJ: Muscular atrophy following immobilisation. A review. Sports Med 10:42, 1990.
73. Rubinstein NA, Lyons GE, Kelly AM: Hormonal control of myosin heavy chain genes during development of skeletal muscles. Ciba Found Symp 138:35, 1988.
74. Nwoye L, Mommaerts WFHM: The effects of thyroid status on some properties of rat fast-twitch muscle. J Musc Res Cell Motil 2:307, 1981.
75. Florini JR, Ewton DZ, Coolican SA: Growth hormone and the insulin-like growth factor system in myogenesis. Endocrine Rev 17:481, 1996.
76. Lamberts SW, van den Beld AW, van der Lely A-J: The endocrinology of aging. Science 278:419, 1997.
77. Bower KJ: Anabolic steroid abuse and dependence. Curr Psych Reports 4:377, 2002.
78. Bowers LD: Abuse of performance-enhancing drugs in sport. Therap Drug Monitor 24:178, 2002.
79. Barton-Davis ER, Shoturma DI, Musaro A, et al: Viral mediated expression of insulin-like growth factor I blocks the aging-related loss of skeletal muscle function. Proc Natl Acad Sci U S A 95:15603, 1998.
80. Bogdanovich S, Krag TOB, Barton ER, et al: Functional improvement of dystrophic muscle by myostatin blockade. Nature 420:418, 2002.

6 Biomechanics of Joints

SHELDON R. SIMON • ERIC L. RADIN

Joint physiology depends on the interaction of tissue biology and biomechanics. This chapter reviews the biomechanics of normal joints, including structure, motion, forces, stability, and control. Selected aspects of the biomechanics of joint degeneration are addressed briefly throughout.

Joint Structure

Normal functioning of any joint requires that all structures (i.e., cartilage, bone, ligaments, synovium, capsule, muscle, nerves, and higher control centers) act in combination to allow smooth, steady motion while maintaining stability. During performance of the activities of daily living, it is estimated that the joints of a person's lower extremities undergo at least 2 million oscillatory cycles each year. Even under these extreme loading conditions, most of our joints do not wear out for up to 80 years.[1] The joint lubricant (i.e., synovial fluid), bearing surfaces, and articular cartilage are built to withstand the range of intra-articular frictional forces created. The biochemical composition and geometric distribution of water and organic matrix within the articular cartilage provide some conformational load bearing. Although cartilage is flexible, the subchondral trabecular bony bed on which the cartilage sits is also flexible, and by conforming under load, it absorbs some of the shock of impulsive loading.[2] Ligaments passively restrict and muscles (in concert with the central nervous system [CNS]) actively control the movement of joints. Cartilage interstitial fluid circulation and the blood supply to bone are enhanced by intermittent tissue motion. Each aspect of the joint structure is optimized to allow joint movement to occur, reduce the mechanical forces it must withstand, and provide nourishment and protection. Alteration of any individual component affects the delicate balance and can lead to mechanical breakdown of the joint. Although many factors may initiate cartilage damage, mechanical factors lead to the progressive joint dysfunction known as osteoarthrosis (see chapters 91 and 92).

Joint Motions

The types of motions and the degree to which each motion is allowed are distinct for each joint. In humans, the primary function of the upper extremities is to carry and manipulate objects, and the primary function of the lower extremities is locomotion.

To provide for the wide extent of function that an extremity can encompass, the most proximal joints must have the widest range of motion. The joint configuration established to suit these demands at the shoulder is a ball (the humeral head) on a relatively flat surface (the glenoid).[3] A large range of motion linked with a minimum of bony and ligament constraint requires significant muscular stability. The hip, utilizing only a slightly smaller range of rotational motion, functions to balance body mass and has a need for greater stability. It derives much of its stability from encapsulating bony contours; the femoral head and neck "like a lollipop" in the socket of the acetabulum can still achieve large rotational motions. Muscles still play an important stabilizing role,[4] as noted by the fact that paralyzed individuals are more likely to dislocate their hips than individuals with functional hip musculature.

For an extremity to function at all points within its range, a means is provided to alter the length of the limb. Bending the elbow and knee joints with rotation of the limb segments, primarily in a single plane, allows effective limb-length changes[5,6] (Fig. 6–1).

Environmental interactions primarily occur at the end of an extremity. Whether it is a hand or a foot and the need is prehension, grasp, or movement on irregular ground, requirements are multiple and vary in nature and magnitude. These demands are met with sets of multiple small joints providing movements in many directions.

Joint Forces

The force causing joint rotation about an axis is a *torque*. It is not merely the magnitude of the force but the product of this force multiplied by the distance between the joint's center of rotation and the point of application of the force. Most external forces acting on an extremity are exerted at a distance from a joint, causing large destabilizing rotational torques. These external rotational torques are resisted by muscular contraction (Fig. 6–2). The tendons placed at the periphery of the joint give the muscle a mechanical advantage, and this leverage creates the greatest torque with the least effort. The distances over which the muscles act, however, are far below those of the external forces; muscle forces created to balance or overcome external torques must be several times higher. Thus, during normal walking, in most of the weight-bearing joints in the lower extremities, intra-articular forces are in the range of three to four times body weight

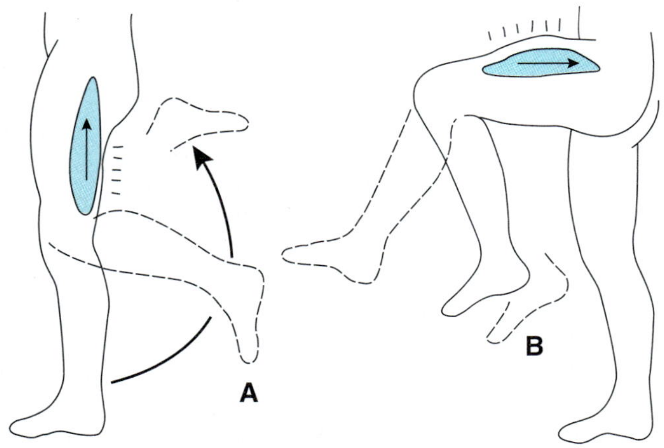

FIGURE 6–1 • *A*, If the femur is stationary, knee motions alone are not an effective means of producing limb shortening. Under such circumstances, the foot can move only in a single prescribed 180-degree arc behind the knee. *B*, However, if at the same time the thigh is allowed to move by rotatory motions produced about the hip, the limb can be shortened or placed within a wide, spheric volume.

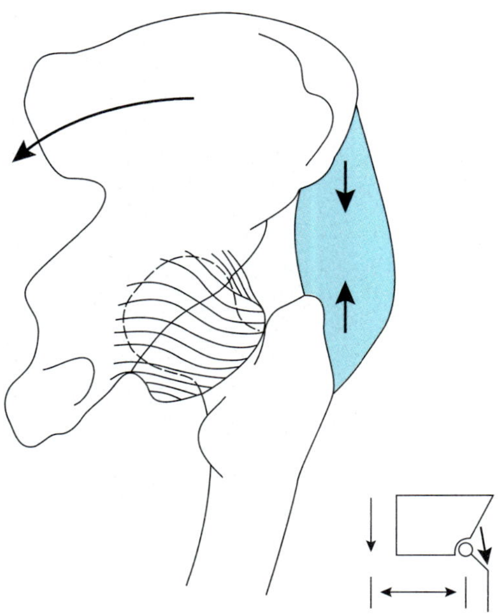

FIGURE 6–2 • When one-legged support is required, the abductor muscles contract to produce a rotational force about the hip joint opposite to that produced by body weight. The farther away the muscle-tendon complex is from the center of the joint, the lower the muscle force needs to be to create the same rotational force. In most cases the distance of the muscle-tendon complex from the center of the joint is less than that of the weight it is trying to counteract. This produces a larger force from the muscles than the weight it balances. As a consequence, during the functional activities of daily living, the major muscles about the hip typically produce forces two to four times those of body weight.

because of the muscle forces produced to counteract body weight.

JOINT MINIMIZATION OF FRICTIONAL FORCES

Flexion-extension movements of a joint create sliding or rolling motions of one articular surface on another. Such motions should create shear or frictional forces between the two surfaces, causing joint breakdown. However, joints do not wear down by pure rubbing because their lubrication is effective.[7] There is essentially no shear force on normal joint surfaces.

Frictional force is defined as the resistance a moving surface exerts to impede its progress. Such resistance depends on the compression load, the composition of the interface materials, and the characteristics of the lubricant interposed between the two surfaces (Fig. 6–3). The resistance to movement may be quantified by a dimensionless number called the *coefficient of friction*. The lower this number is, the more slippery the movement and the lower the shear forces created between the moving surfaces. Well-manufactured joints, such as steel-on-steel lubricated by oil, operate at coefficients of friction between 0.1 and 0.5. Biologic diarthrodial joints, in contrast, operate at coefficients of friction of approximately 0.002, nearly one-hundredth that of machine-made bearings. If a walking man weighing 70 kg creates a 200-kg compressive force across a lower-extremity joint, the shear, or frictional, force at the joint would be less than 0.4 kg.

Articular cartilage, with an intact surface layer but without any fluid imbibed within it, has a coefficient of friction of 0.3. If saline is added, the cartilage imbibes and releases the fluid like a sponge. As the wet cartilage surfaces slide against each other, the coefficient of friction is reduced to as little as 0.010. If glycoprotein molecules (e.g., lubricin), which naturally occur in synovial fluid and adhere to the cartilage surfaces, are added to the saline, the coefficient of friction is further reduced to 0.002. The self-pressurized fluid squeezed out of the fluid-soaked cartilage and the lubricating molecules in the synovial fluid are the major features that reduce the frictional force so effectively that articular surfaces see little shear stress at their surfaces.[8]

How the various lubricating mechanisms interact to produce low levels of frictional resistance is controversial. Many theories have been proposed; common to

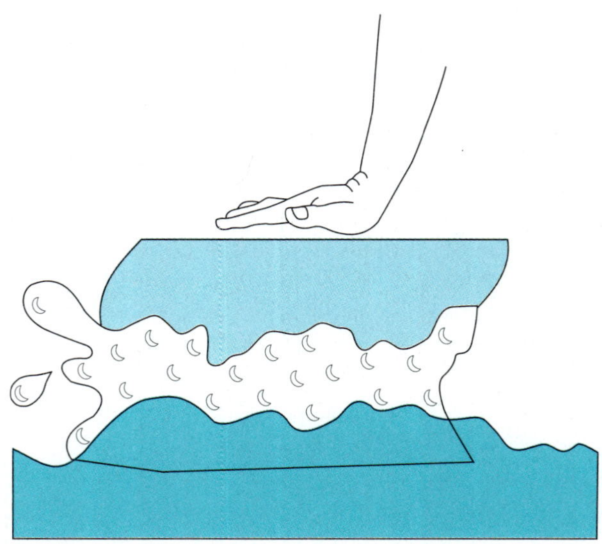

FIGURE 6–3 • The ease with which one surface may slide over another is dependent on the compressive load, the characteristics of the two opposing materials and their surfaces, and the nature of the material interposed between the two surfaces.

each is the movement of fluid in and out of the porous cartilage. McCutchen[9] postulated that, as the cartilage is compressed, the fluid from within seeps out and forms a self-pressurized layer separating the two surfaces. Theoretical evidence and in vitro test results[10] suggest that fluid is imbibed into articular surfaces in the trailing area of compression, whereas at the leading edge, where compression is developing, fluid is expressed (Fig. 6–4). The lubrication mechanisms in joints are so efficient that the joint's frictional forces do not appear to be a cause of articular-cartilage breakdown.

JOINT RESISTANCE TO COMPRESSIVE AND TENSILE FORCES

Cartilage is constructed in an ideal way to also withstand compressive forces or stresses. It has two components: a liquid and a solid. The liquid is a dialysate of synovial fluid; it is incompressible, but it can flow. However, for this fluid to withstand the compressive loads that joints sustain, the fluid must be contained, and its flow must be minimized. The cartilage matrix resembles a sponge with directional pores. The small diameter of these functional pores and their arrangement in circuitous "tunnels," created by the hydrophilic collagen and highly charged proteoglycan matrix components, prevent large molecules from entering the cartilage and offer considerable resistance to interstitial fluid flow. These characteristics provide adequate containment and flow to enable the fluid to support load.[11]

At any instant, only a part of the joint is bearing a load (i.e., in compression). If one part is in compression, the adjacent area is being stretched and pulled apart. This places high compressive and tensile stresses on the matrix of cartilage in its deeper layers.

Although there is agreement about the tangential parallel arrangement of the collagen fibers on the surface of articular cartilage and the perpendicular arrangement at their base, controversy about the arrangement of the collagen in the middle zone of articular cartilage persists.[12] Some authorities believe the midzone fibers alter their alignment under compression to provide maximal resistance against load. Such changes allow the matrix to accommodate the imposed loads, decrease the pore size, and increase resistance to fluid flow through the cartilage, with permeability of the tissue (ease of flow) decreasing exponentially. The mechanical strength of cartilage increases as greater loads are imposed. The greater the depth of the cartilage layer examined, the more important these relationships are.[13]

The electrical properties of proteoglycans and their interaction with the surrounding matrix constituents contribute to the material properties of the articular cartilage. The carboxyl and sulfate groups of the glycosaminoglycans are endowed with highly negative charges. The large, fixed proteoglycan molecules are highly charged and attract a large volume of water, which tends to neutralize the fixed negative charge. Under compressive loads, water is pushed out of the zone of highest pressure, allowing the cartilage to compress and to increase its fixed-charge density. This increases the resistance to the flow of such fluid away from it, increasing the mechanical strength of the cartilage. When the pressure is removed, the fixed negative charge osmotically attracts water, and the cartilage regains its precompressed thickness. In most circumstances, this fluid flow under pressure allows articular cartilage to compress under a load without permanent damage to its matrix.[11]

In light of the preceding discussion, it is easy to understand how enzymatic destruction of cartilage matrix in arthritic (primarily inflammatory) joint conditions can lead to cartilage destruction. In arthrotic (primarily mechanical) joint deterioration, it is believed that repetitive, impulsive loading damages the matrix. In this circumstance, the compressive load is applied too rapidly for the interstitial cartilage water to have the time to flow, and the cartilage matrix can be subjected to microdamage.[8]

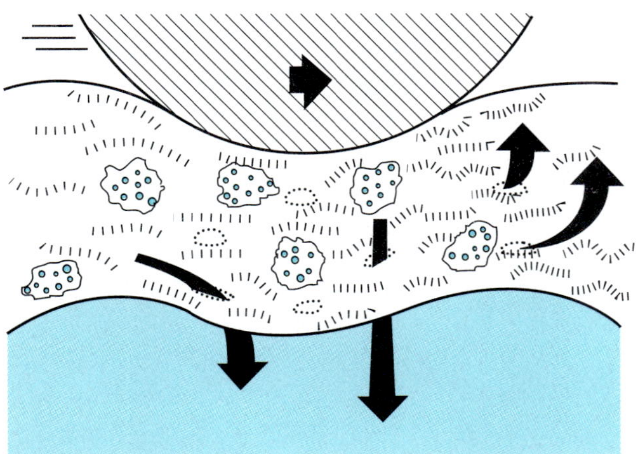

FIGURE 6–4 • To minimize the resistance of moving one cartilage surface over another, the porous cartilaginous surface is layered with viscous macromolecules and weeps synovial fluid dialysate at the leading edge; it then absorbs this fluid in the trailing area, and deforms in the "area of contact," allowing the two cartilaginous surfaces to be kept apart.

MAXIMIZATION OF CONTACT AREA

The breakdown of any mechanical structure depends on the total force and the area over which it is loaded (i.e., contact pressure). For example, if a tack is pressed into a person's finger, the person's reaction depends on whether the point or the flat part of the tack is being pushed into the skin. Joint structures are designed to provide an increasing contact surface with increasing forces to keep articular-compressive stress minimal.

The articular cartilage rests on a layer of calcified cartilage, which is supported by a subchondral bone plate. This plate is supported by subchondral trabecular bone, whose lattice arrangement follows the major stress trajectories of the transmitted load (Fig. 6–5). The trabecular bone density is related to the quantity of the habitually transmitted load. The articular ends of the joints are expanded under load to increase their potential contact area and diminish the articular stress. Trabecular bone is 10 times more compliant than cortical bone; micromotion of the subchondral plate and

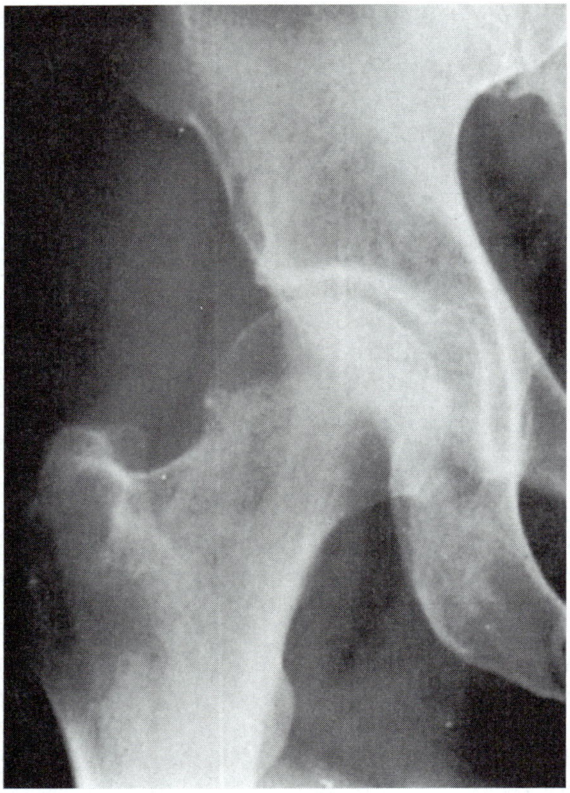

FIGURE 6–5 · At the hip, trabecular bone in the femoral head is concentrated along an axis 160 degrees to the vertical, where the greatest concentration of forces occurs. In contrast, the trabecular bone on the acetabular side flares out to occupy an area greater than the joint's contacting surface, distributing the same forces over a wide area, thereby reducing the stresses and allowing some of the stresses to be absorbed by bone deformation.

trabecular bone aids in joint conformation under load[14] and can probably help absorb impulsive loads if they are not applied too quickly.[12]

At the hip, the concave acetabulum under low loads contacts the head of the femur about its periphery. As the load increases, the surface tends to flare out for maximum joint confinement under load.[14] Movement of the marrow and slight bending of the acetabular and femoral head trabeculae allow subchondral deformation without matrix damage. Under load, the acetabular socket spreads, and the femoral head flattens to increase hip contact area.[14]

Cartilage compression under load increases surface area, and joints conform better under load because of subchondral bone deformation. In the knee joints, the load-bearing contact area of the knee becomes greater with increasing loads because the menisci increase the contact area. The contact area of the tibiotalar joint increases with load sharing of the fibulotalar joint. Physiologic joint pressure approximates 5.0 meganewtons (MN)/m, and pressures in all joints are equivalent. The joints in the upper extremities are smaller than those in the lower extremities, but so are their loads.[15]

The ability of the subchondral bone to diffuse compressive loads provides added protection for the cartilage in most circumstances. Although cartilage is compliant, even in its normal state it is not thick enough to deform sufficiently to absorb impulsive loads. At very high rates of loading, there is insufficient time for marrow flow, and the trabecular bone can be subjected to microdamage. The microdamage resulting from repetitive, impulsive loading can accumulate and lead to fatigue failure.[16] The repair of the subchondral bone damage stiffens the trabecular structure. This process advances the tidemark on which the articular cartilage rests. The enchondral ossification front advances at the expense of its overlying articular cartilage, which is thinned. This process increases the shear stress on the articular cartilage, particularly in its depths, which can lead to fragmentation.[17] It has been suggested that chronic, mechanically induced, progressive articular cartilage loss requires subchondral plate thickening and cartilage thinning as prerequisites.[18]

Joint Stability

Joints need to maintain their integrity; if dislocation or subluxation occurs, joint efficiency is lost and early arthritis results.[19] To maintain joint stability, joint motion must be primarily rotational (i.e., flexing and extending) and minimally translational (i.e., sliding side to side). Joint stability is created by bony configurations, ligaments, and muscles. Different joint anatomies emphasize different combinations of these constructs.[3] Although each joint is characterized by its unique contour, one side is usually concave, and the other is convex.[20] Because bone is the most rigid anatomic structure, the greater the arc of motion enclosed by the bone, the greater the amount of inherent stability but the less the motion. As mentioned previously, the shoulder, with a small, relatively flat socket and minimally enclosed humeral head, is easier to dislocate or subluxate than the hip, where the spherical femoral head is almost enclosed by a hemispheric arc of bony acetabulum[21,22] (Fig. 6–6).

Ligaments are passive elements with fixed properties to resist tensile forces. Situated across joints to resist rotational or translational forces, they restrict joint motions. They provide some stability; however, they provide it only in circumstances of modest loading, because ligaments can easily tear.[23,24]

Muscle action is the primary stabilizer of joints. Because muscle actions are dynamic, the forces they produce to resist or create motions can change. Where

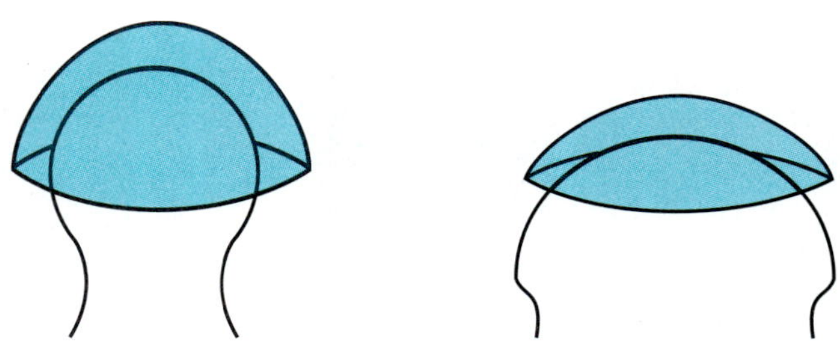

FIGURE 6–6 · Neither the hip nor the shoulder joints have rotational restrictions, and each has a similar ball-socket shape. The glenoid socket does not stabilize the humeral head as well as the acetabulum stabilizes the femoral head.

considerable motion is intrinsic to a joint, muscles can act without the presence of ligaments, allowing motion but controlling the magnitude of torque and the speed at which the motion is produced (e.g., quadriceps action during knee flexion and extension). The shear force or rotational torque parallel to the joint line caused by muscle action can help to stabilize the joint against inertial or weight-bearing forces.[25,26] In other cases in which motion is restricted or limited, muscles act in concert with ligaments (e.g., the hamstrings and tensor fascia lata spare pulling on the medial and lateral knee collateral ligaments; similarly, peroneal muscles spare lateral collateral ankle ligaments).[23,25] Muscle action can generate greater restraining forces than ligaments, a fact that protects the latter from tearing. Ligaments tear only when appropriate muscle action fails to occur in time or the damaging force is overwhelming.[23]

The spine illustrates the intricate balance between all the existing structural stabilizers. To protect the spinal cord while allowing rotatory motions of the trunk, a sophisticated stabilizing arrangement has evolved. The intervertebral "unit" (i.e., vertebra–intervertebral disk–vertebra) is composed of several elements, as follows:[27,28]

1. A bony articulation composed of one amphiarthrodial joint (the intervertebral disk and the vertebral bony end plates) and two diarthrodial intervertebral facet joints
2. Ligaments on all sides (anterior and posterior longitudinal, ligamentum flavum, and interspinous)
3. A multitude of paraspinal muscles

The disk is a major supporting unit between the vertebral bony units and helps to maintain the vertical rigidity of the system. Although the disk stabilizes vertical loads and prevents vertical translation, it does not stabilize horizontal translation. Bending puts the body's weight anterior to the spine. This configuration compresses the disk and tends to collapse the spine by creating forces that tilt and slide one vertebral unit over the one below it. The posterolateral intervertebral facet joints prevent sliding and rotation. The ligaments and muscles limit the extent of motion within the constraints of the disk and body fit, control the degree of and speed with which motions occur, and act as the major source of stability in rotation (Fig. 6–7). Control of the position of the loaded spine ultimately depends on the paraspinal muscles.[29]

Disks are ruptured by a combination of compression and rotation. Heavy compressive loads, in the absence of rotation, do not rupture disks. Disk rupture is more likely while bending to tie a shoelace than from lifting a heavy object kept in front of the person. Mechanically induced disk rupture may be related to an internal weakness of the intervertebral interspace, such as an anatomic asymmetry or remodeling changes.[29] Many disks appear to rupture from the outside in, rather than from the inside out.[30]

Joint Control

Because ligaments and bone are only passive stabilizers, the activity of muscles controls joint motion. For example, during walking, the knee flexes only 15 to 20 degrees as the heel strikes the ground (i.e., at the onset of the stance phase). The quadriceps muscle attempts to prevent collapse of the leg under the body's weight as the leg is decelerating at the end of the swing phase. At this time, most of the force exerted on the joints is compressive. If an individual walks faster, greater muscle activity is needed for deceleration, creating higher compressive loads across the joint. Quadriceps activity increases even further during running, when muscle action is needed for acceleration as well. In contrast, during the swing phase of slow walking, in which momentum and gravity are the major contributors to leg motions, no significant muscle activity is needed, and knee joint forces are minimal. It is most efficient to provide such control with a single muscle that spans two joints (Fig. 6–8). The hamstrings crossing the hip and knee joints and active at the end of swing exemplify this point. At this time, the knee is extending but the hip is flexing. As one joint (the knee) moves in a direction to stretch the muscle, the other (the hip) rotates in an

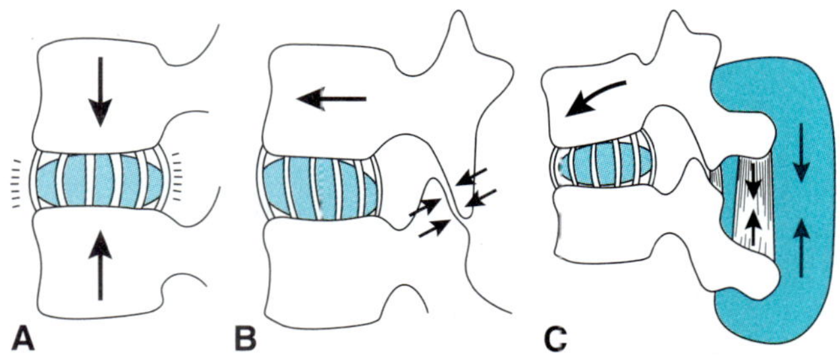

FIGURE 6–7 · The Intervertebral Unit of the Spine has Multiple Structures Contributing to Its Stability. *A*, The disk prevents vertical translational motions, as would a balloon placed in a coffee can. *B*, The facet joints prevent forward translation, permitting the more proximal vertebrae only to rotate about the more distal one in a prescribed arc. *C*, Multiple ligaments and paraspinal muscles control the speed and extent of motion within this arc of movement through their "clamping" effect on the posterior elements.

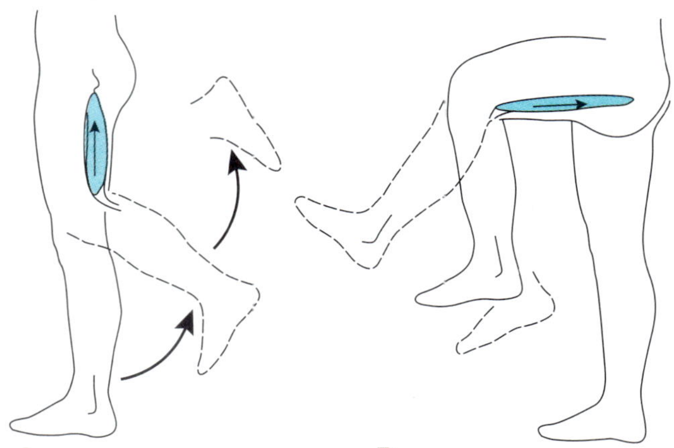

FIGURE 6–8 · *A*, The hamstring muscles originate above the hip and insert below the knee. With the hip straight, considerable contraction of the hamstrings is necessary to bend the knee. *B*, With the hip flexed, however, the hamstrings are stretched behind the hip, and a relatively modest contraction is all that is necessary to bend the knee in that circumstance.

opposite direction, lessening the degree of active contraction necessary.

Quadriceps and other muscle activity at all joints during common activities appears to be dictated by fixed, preprogrammed neurologic responses (i.e., locomotion or pattern "generators") located in the brain stem. There are separate generators for the upper and lower extremities.[31] Activities requiring involvement of the low back usually involve the participation of one or more joints of the upper and lower extremities.

The speed at which an activity is carried out can be controlled voluntarily by the higher cortical centers. The locomotion generators and cerebellum coordinate these motions during common activities of daily living, such as walking and writing. Changes in the performance of activities of daily living may have important implications with regard to the progression of osteoarthrosis. Bone and articular cartilage are viscoelastic; when they are compressed slowly, their interstitial water flows and protects the matrix. Rapidly compressed interstitial water has no time to flow, and matrix can be damaged. It is advantageous to avoid rapid (i.e., impulsive) loading of joints during the activities of daily living. Normally, a person automatically accomplishes this primarily by decelerating the limb just before it is about to hit an object. This momentary deceleration may be important in avoiding the matrix damage that is found in osteoarthrotic tissues.

The magnitude of the intra-articular forces depend on muscle action as it relates to what the functional activity is, how the activity is performed, and how fast it is carried out. About one third of normal adults lack protective, timely limb deceleration. As a result, these people impulsively load their joints during the activities of daily living. Such individuals have been referred to as *microklutzes*, and the repetitive, impulsive loading can be deleterious to their joints over time.[32]

The ability of an individual to perform a task in a chosen manner depends on the strength of the relevant muscle groups. For example, if a person has strong-enough back muscles, he or she may pick something up by keeping the legs straight and bending only the spine, or the person may bend at the hips, knees, and ankles, keeping the back straight, and lift the object mainly with the leg muscles. A person may choose to use a combination of these two methods, employing back and lower-extremity muscles. Using a combination of upper- and lower-extremity efforts, plus the paraspinal muscles, places less stress on the lumbar joints.

REFERENCES

1. Sokoloff L: The Biology of Degenerative Joint Disease. Chicago, University of Chicago Press, 1969.
2. Radin EL: The physiology and degeneration of joints. Semin Arthritis Rheum 2:245, 1973.
3. Kumar VP: Biomechanics of the shoulder. Ann Acad Med Singapore 31(5):590-592, 2002.
4. Kapandji IA: The Physiology of Joints, 2nd ed. Edinburgh, Scotland, ERS Livingstone, 1970.
5. Bernstein AD, Jazrawi LM, Rokito AS, et al: Elbow joint biomechanics: basic science and clinical applications. Orthopedics 23(12):1293-1301, 2000.
6. Zimmerman NB: Clinical application of advances in elbow and forearm anatomy and biomechanics. Hand Clin 18(1):1-19, 2002.
7. Radin EL, Paul IL: A consolidated concept of joint lubrication. J Bone Joint Surg Am 54:607, 1972.
8. Radin EL, Paul IL, Rose RM, et al: The mechanics of joints as it relates to their degeneration. American Academy of Orthopaedic Surgeons Symposium on Osteoarthritis. St. Louis, Mosby, 1976, p 34.
9. McCutchen CW: Mechanism of animal joints: sponge-hydrostatic and weeping bearings. Nature 184:1284, 1959.
10. Torzilli PA, Mow VC: On the fundamental fluid transport mechanisms through normal and pathological articular cartilage during function. II. The analysis, solution and conclusions. J Biomech 9:587, 1976.
11. Maroudas A: Physico-chemical properties of articular cartilage. *In* Freeman MAR (ed): Adult Articular Cartilage. New York, Grune & Stratton, 1974, p 215.
12. Clark JR: Variation of collagen fiber alignment in a joint surface: a scanning electron microscope study of total plateau in dog, rabbit, and man. J Orthop Res 9:246, 1991.
13. Mansour JM, Mow VC: The permeability of articular cartilage under compressive strain and at high pressures. J Bone Joint Surg Am 58:509, 1976.
14. Bullough PG, Goodfellow JB, Greenwald AS, et al: Incongruent surfaces in the human joint. Nature 217:1290, 1968.
15. Radin EL, Fyhrie D: Joint physiology and biomechanics. *In* Mow VC, Woo SYL, Ratcliffe T (eds): Symposium on Biomechanics of Diarthrodial Joints. Vol II. New York, Springer-Verlag, 1990.
16. Radin EL, Parker HG, Pugh JW, et al: response of joints to impact loading. III. Relationship between trabecular microfractures and cartilage degeneration. J Biomech 6:61, 1973.
17. O'Conner JJ, Johnston I: Transmission of rapidly applied load through articular cartilage: the mechanics of osteoarthrosis. *In* Turner-Smith AR (ed): Micromovement in Orthopaedics. Oxford, Clarendon Press, 1993, p 244.
18. Radin EL, Burr DB, Fyhrie D, et al: Characteristics of joint loading as it applies to osteoarthrosis. *In* Mow VC, Woo SYL, Ratcliffe T (eds): Symposium on Biomechanics of Diarthrodial Joints. Vol I. New York, Springer-Verlag, 1990, p 437.
19. Berdia S, Wolfe SW: Effects of scaphoid fractures on the biomechanics of the wrist. Hand Clin 17(4):533-540, 2001.
20. Simkin PA, Graney DO, Fiechtner JJ: Roman arches, human joint, and disease: differences between convex and concave sides of joints. Arthritis Rheum 23:1308, 1980.
21. Halder AM, Itoi E, An K: Anatomy and biomechanics of the shoulder. Orthop Clin North Am 31(2):159-176, 2000.
22. Doukas WC, Speer KP: Anatomy, pathophysiology, and biomechanics of shoulder instability. Orthop Clin North Am 32(3):381-391, vii, 2001.
23. O'Conner J, Biden E, Bradley J, et al: The muscle-stabilized knee. *In* Daniel DD, Akeson WH, O, Connor JJ (eds): Knee Ligaments: Structure, Function, Injury, and Repair. New York, Raven Press, 1990.
24. Woo SL, Debski RE, et al: Biomechanics of knee ligaments. Am J Sports Med 27(4):533-543, 1999.
25. Hintermann B: Biomechanics of the unstable ankle joint and clinical implications. Med Sci Sports Exerc 31(7 Suppl):S459-S469, 1999.
26. Denham RA: Hip mechanics. J Bone Joint Surg Br 41:550, 1959.
27. Bogduk N, Mercer S: Biomechanics of the cervical spine. I. Normal kinematics. Clin Biomech (Bristol, Avon) 15(9):633-648, 2000.
28. Davis KG, Marras WS: The effects of motion on trunk biomechanics. Clin Biomech (Bristol, Avon) 15(10):703-717, 2000.
29. Farfan HF: Mechanical Disorders of the Low Back: The Effects of Torsion on the Lumbar Intervertebral Joints. Philadelphia, Lea & Febiger, 1973.
30. Gordon SJ, Yang KY, Mater PJ, et al: Mechanism of disc rupture. Spine 16:450, 1991.
31. Grillner S: Locomotion in vertebrates: Central mechanisms and reflex interactions. Physiol Rev 55:247, 1975.
32. Radin EL, Yang KH, O'Connor JJ, et al: Relationship between lower limb dynamics and knee joint pain. J Orthop Res 9:398, 1991.

SECTION II

Cells Involved in Autoimmune Diseases and Inflammation

7 Antigen-Presenting Cells

RANJENY THOMAS • WILLIAM P. AREND

Antigen-presenting cells (APC) are of prime importance in the innate immune response and are instrumental in the initiation of adaptive immune responses to exogenous and endogenous antigens. A discussion of innate immunity is presented in Chapter 8 of this text, and adaptive immunity is covered in chapters 9 and 10. Innate immunity represents a phylogenetically older host defense mechanism against primarily infectious agents and does not depend on previous exposure to these agents or to material derived from them. Cells of the innate immune system recognize specific and fixed pathogen-associated molecular patterns (PAMPs) through sets of pattern-recognition receptors (PRRs). The adaptive immune system evolved later, possibly because of the inability of innate responses to protect against new and different microbial agents and noninfectious materials. Adaptive immune responses use selection and mutation of the somatically generated immune repertoire to develop protection against foreign substances. These responses endow the organism with the ability to respond to repeated contact with specific antigens in a highly targeted manner.

The principal cells of the innate immune system include dendritic cells (DC) and macrophages, which recognize specific sets of microbial surface structures in an antigen-nonspecific fashion. However, these same cells are the major APCs, initiating antigen-specific adaptive immune responses in B and T lymphocytes. Thus, the innate immune system stimulates and shapes adaptive immune responses.

This chapter will summarize the major phenotypic and functional characteristics of DC and macrophages, both as integral cells in innate immunity and as APCs for adaptive immunity. Other cells that can function as APCs, such as follicular dendritic cells (FDC) and B lymphocytes, also will be briefly discussed. An antigen is defined as any molecule capable of being recognized by antibodies or T cell receptors (TCR). In contrast, immunogens are antigens capable of inducing antibody formation. Antigens are processed by proteolysis in APCs into short peptides and are presented by major histocompatability complex (MHC) class I and II molecules to specific TCR, a function known as antigen presentation. APCs must either synthesize (endogenous) or acquire by phagocytosis (exogenous) antigenic material, process it, and specifically present it to T cells. Antigen presentation by APCs leading to a primary immune response requires MHC-TCR interactions, as well as the collaboration of a variety of costimulatory molecules. The development of specific immunity in response to an immunogenic antigen leads to the generation of memory T or B cells, capable of rapidly responding to subsequent contact with the antigen.

In addition to their role as APCs, macrophages carry out many important efferent functions in host defense and in maintenance of homeostasis, such as removal of senescent cells, killing of microbial agents, mediating inflammation and wound healing, and killing malignant cells. APCs also may play key roles in mechanisms of disease if their normally protective functions are not properly regulated or become inappropriately directed against self-determinants. The involvement of APCs in rheumatic diseases will be discussed briefly in this chapter and in more detail in other chapters on specific diseases.

The Mononuclear Phagocyte System

ORIGIN AND DIFFERENTIATION

In Messina, Sicily, in 1882, Metchnikoff performed a historic experiment by placing a thorn under the skin of a starfish larva. On the following morning, he observed that wandering cells had gathered at the tip of the thorn at the point of injury.[1] His experiment may have represented the first observation of an inflammatory response, with mobilization and chemotaxis of protective cells after tissue injury. Metchnikoff and other scientists had earlier observed the ingestion of particulate matter by cells in invertebrates, leading, in 1884, to a definition of phagocytosis and to a comprehensive theory of cellular protection against infection. Metchnikoff later described cells that primarily ingested bacteria, called microphages (polymorphonuclear leukocytes), and larger cells that scavenged materials throughout the body, now known as macrophages. In the 1920s, Aschoff coined the term *reticuloendothelial system* based on observations that similar large phagocytic cells were present in lymphatic tissues and lining sinusoids of the liver and spleen. Further findings by electron microscopy, surface labeling studies, and cell trafficking experiments led van Furth, in 1970, to introduce the term *mononuclear phagocyte system.*[2]

The mononuclear phagocyte system includes promonocytes in the bone marrow (BM), circulating monocytes, and tissue macrophages.[3] Pluripotential hematopoietic stem cells, either $CD34^+$ or $CD34^-$, comprise 1 to 2 percent of mononuclear cells in the BM. Under the influence of a variety of cytokines, including interleukin (IL)-1, IL-3, and stem cell factor (SCF), $CD34^+$ stem cells differentiate into myeloid cells that express CD33, CD34, and HLA-DR. Further differentiation into colony-forming unit granulocyte-monocyte (CFU-GM) progenitors is stimulated by granulocyte-monocyte colony-stimulating factor (GM-CSF), monocyte colony-stimulating factor (M-CSF), and IL-3, with eventual development into monoblasts, promonocytes, and monocytes. Mature monocytes then enter the blood where they circulate for 1 to 2 days before entering tissues where they differentiate into macro-phages. Blood monocytes lose the expression of CD34, but they do express CD33, HLA-DR, CD14 (a component of the receptor for lipopolysaccharide [LPS]), and Fc receptors, including Fc-gamma receptor I (FcγRI) (or CD64), FcγRII (or CD32), FcγRIII (or CD16), and CD89, the receptor for IgA. These cells contain a large, pale nucleus; azurophilic granules; and intracytoplasmic lysosomes.

TISSUE MACROPHAGES

Tissue macrophages are particularly prominent in the lung (alveolar macrophages), liver (Kupffer cells), spleen, and BM and may divide several times over a life span of more than 60 days.[4] The characteristics of more differentiated tissue macrophages vary with the organ of residence, and they are influenced by local environments, including activation by T cells. Macrophages express a variety of cell surface–adhesion molecules and receptors, and they secrete a large number of products involved in carrying out heterogeneous functions.

ADHESION MOLECULES AND CHEMOKINE RECEPTORS

A full discussion of adhesion molecules on phagocytic cells, and their roles in cell function, can be found in Chapter 24. The principle adhesion molecules on cells of the mononuclear phagocyte system are summarized in Table 7–1.[5,6] These molecules, in general, mediate monocyte migration into inflammatory tissues and may initiate the process of cell activation. L-selectin (CD62-L) is present on all circulating leukocytes and binds to endothelial cells, initiating cell rolling prior to migration into inflammatory tissues. The variety of integrins found on monocytes and macrophages is important in mediating firm adhesion to endothelial cells and transmigration through the vessel wall. Integrins also bind to various components of the connective-tissue matrix, including fibronectin, vitronectin, fibrinogen, thrombospondin, osteopontin, collagen, and laminin, to enhance cell migration into tissues. Furthermore, cell activation results from interaction with integrins manifested by initiation of transcription factor pathways and production of inflammatory cytokines and metalloproteinases (MMP). The presence of adhesion molecules of the Ig superfamily on monocytes and macrophages may be constitutive or inducible and may primarily mediate interaction with endothelial cells and lymphocytes.

Chemokines play an important role in mediating the migration of leukocytes into inflammatory tissues, and receptors for many chemokines are present on monocytes and macrophages.[7] The described chemokines and their receptors present on these cells are summarized in Table 7–2. Chemokines are secreted by resident tissue cells, resident and recruited inflammatory cells, and endothelial cells, primarily after stimulation by IL-1, tumor necrosis factor (TNF)α, LPS, and viruses. These potent molecules are retained in tissues by binding to heparin sulfate proteoglycans on endothelial cells and in connective-tissue matrix. A chemokine gradient is established with stimulation of integrins on leukocytes converting rolling to firm arrest and adherence to endothelial cells with subsequent migration into tissues. In addition to chemokines, transforming growth factor (TGF)-β is chemotactic to monocytes and helps recruit them into inflammatory tissues.

RECEPTORS ON MONOCYTES AND MACROPHAGES

In addition to chemokine receptors, a variety of other receptors are present on the surface of monocytes and macrophages (Table 7–3). Receptors for immunoglobulins and their complement components are very important in recognition of opsonized soluble or particulate material in phagocytosis and in cell stimulation. The activating multichain Fcγ receptors FcγRI and FcγRIIIa bind Fc through single α-chains that possess immunoreceptor tyrosine-based activation motifs (ITAMs) in their intracellular domains[8] (Fig. 7–1). These ITAMs interact with homodimeric γ-chains to transduce signals. FcγRIIa also possess ITAMs in their intracellular domains, but these do not interact with γ-chains. FcγRIIIb does not contain an ITAM, or even an intracellular domain, but is anchored in the outer part of the plasma membrane by a glycosylphosphatidylinositol (GPI) anchor; this receptor is found only on neutrophils and can mediate phagocytosis.

Stimulatory responses by cells depend more on the cell itself than on the type of FcγR present. On macrophages, FcγRI, FcγRIIa, and FcγRIIIa all initiate the same group of responses, which includes internalization of bound soluble or particulate materials, stimulation of a respiratory burst, and secretion of inflammatory cytokines and other molecules. In contrast, ITAM-containing FcγR on DC

TABLE 7–1 • ADHESION MOLECULES ON MONONUCLEAR PHAGOCYTES

Adhesion molecule	Function
Selectin	
L-selectin (LAM-1, Mel-14, CD62L)	Binds to counter receptors on endothelial cells
Integrins	
α4β1 (VLA-4, CD49a/CD29)	Binds to fibronectin and VCAM-1
α5β1 (VLA-5, CD49e/CD29)	Binds to fibronectin
αLβ2 (LFA-1, CD11a/CD18)	Binds to ICAM-1, ICAM-2, and ICAM-3
αXβ2 (p150/95, CD11c/CD18)	Binds to C3bi and fibrinogen
αvβ3 (VNR, CD51/CD61)	Binds to a variety of connective tissue components
αvβ5	Binds to vitronectin and fibronectin
Immunoglobulin-like	
ICAM-1 (CD54)	Binds to αLβ2, αMβ2, and CD43
ICAM-2 (CD102)	Binds to αLβ2
ICAM-3 (CD50)	Binds to αLβ2
VCAM-1 (CD106)	Binds to α4β1 and α4β7
PECAM-1 (CD31)	Binds to CD31 and αvβ3
LFA-3 (CD58)	Binds to CD2
Other	
CD34	Present on immature myeloid cells only
CD44	Binds to fibronectin, collagen, hyaluronic acid, and glycosaminoglycans

Abbreviations: LFA-1, laurocyte formation-associated antigen, Type 1; LAM-1, leurocyte adhesion-molecule, Type 1; ICAM, intercellular adhesion molecule; PECAM, plately/endolthelial cell adhesion molecule; VCAM, vascular cell adhesion molecule; VLA, very late activation antigen; VNR, vitranectin receptor.

mediate internalization and endocytic transport of immune complexes leading to processing and presentation of antigens. The inhibitory FcγRIIb, when coaggregated with ITAM-expressing receptors by a multivalent ligand, leads to blockade of phagocytosis and other cell responses. Cross-linking of stimulatory FcγR leads to phosphorylation of tyrosines in the ITAM by Src kinases, recruitment of the SH2-domain tyrosine kinase Syk, and activation of the phosphatidylinositol-3 kinase (PI3K) signal transduction pathway with an influx of Ca^{++} (see Fig. 7–1). In contrast, coaggregation of inhibitory FcγRIIb leads to phosphorylation of tyrosines in inhibitory motifs in the intracellular domain, recruitment of SH2-containing inositol 5′-phosphatase (SHIP), and hydrolysis of phosphatidylinositol (3,4,5)-diphosphate (PIP_3) into phosphatidylinositol (4,5)-triphosphate (PIP_2). This response blocks Ca^{++} flux with inhibition of subsequent events in the stimulatory PI3k pathway. In cells that possess both stimulatory and inhibitory FcγRII, the ultimate cell response is dependent on the balance between the two types of FcγR.

TABLE 7–2 • CHEMOKINE RECEPTORS PRESENT ON MONOCYTES AND MACROPHAGES

Receptor	Chemokine ligands
CCR1	CCL3, 5, 7, 14-16, 23 (MCP-3, MCP-4, MIP-1α, RANTES, and MPIF-1)
CCR2	CCL 2, 7, 8, 13, CCL12 (MCP-1, -2, -3, -4, and -5)
CCR5	CCL2-4, 5, 7, 8, 13 (MIP-1α, MIP-1β, RANTES, and MCP-1 through –4)
CCR7	CCL19, 21 (MIP-3β and SLC)
CCR8	CCL1, 4, 17 (I-309, TARC, and MIP-1β)
CXCR1	CXCL6, 8 (IL-8 and GCP-2)
CXCR2	CXCL1-3, 5-8 (IL-8, GCP-2, GRO-α, -β, and -γ, ENA-78, and NAP-2)
CXCR4	CXCL12 (SDF-1α/β)
CX3CR1	CX3CL1 (Fractalkine)
XCR1	XCL1 (Lymphotactin)

Abbreviations: ENA, epithelial cell-derived neutrophil attractant; GCP-2, granulocyte chemoattractant protein-2; GRO, growth-related oncogene; MCP, monocyte chemoattractant protein; MPIF-1, myeloid progenitor inhibitory factor-1; MIP, macrophage inflammatory protein; NAP, neutrophil activating peptide; RANTES, regulated upon activation normal T cell expressed and secreted; SDF, stromal–cell-derived factor; SLC, secondary lymphoid tissue chemokine; and TARC, thymus and activation-regulated chemokine.

From [Hoczarenko M, Campbell JJ, Silberstein LE: Chemokines and Chemokine Receptors. *In* Rich R, Fleisher T, Kotzin B, Schroeder Jr H (eds): Clinical Immunology: Principles and Practice, 2nd ed., St. Louis, Mosby, 2001, 13.1].

Allelic polymorphisms are present in FcγRIIa, and FcγRIIIa and may be predisposing factors for immune-complex diseases.[8] FcγRIIa has two codominantly expressed alleles: H131, which binds IgG2 avidly, and R131, which binds IgG2 weakly. An individual who carries the H131 allele may not clear IgG2-containing immune complexes well and also may be prone to infections with encapsulated bacteria such as *Neisseria, Haemophilus,* and *Streptococcus.* FcγRIIIa also has two codominantly expressed alleles: V176, which binds IgG1 and IgG3 avidly, and F176, which binds these IgG subclasses weakly. Carrying FcγRIIa-R131 is associated with systemic lupus erythematosus (SLE) in African Americans, and FcγRIIIa-F176 is associated with SLE in Causcasians and other ethnic groups. The observation that IgG2 and IgG3 subclasses may predominate in immune deposits in lupus kidneys supports the hypothesis that FcγRIIa and FcγRIIIa genes may play a predisposing role. Two allelic variants

TABLE 7–3 • RECEPTORS ON MONOCYTES, MACROPHAGES, AND DENDRITIC CELLS

Receptor	Function
Immunoglobulin	
FcγRI (CD64)	High-affinity receptor for monomeric IgG
FcγRIIa (CD32)	Low-affinity activating receptor (absent in mouse)
FcγRIIb2 (CD32)	Inhibitory receptor when coligated with FcγRI, IIa, or IIIa
FcγRIIIa (CD16)	Intermediate affinity receptor that binds immune complexes
FcγRIIIb (CD16)	Lacks an intracellular domain
FcεRIIa and b (CD23)	Low-affinity receptor for IgE
FcαR (CD89)	Low-affinity receptor for IgA
Complement	
CR1 (CD35)	Binds C3b and C4b
CR2 (CD21)	Binds C3bi, C3dg, and C3d
CR3 (CD11b and CD18)	Binds C3bi, LPS, and fibrinogen
C1q receptors	Bind immune complexes containing C1q, producing cell activation
C3a and C5a	Bind these complement fragments with subsequent cell activat on
Leucine-rich proteins	
CD14	Binds bacterial LPS
Toll-like receptors (TLR)	Binds bacterial, viral, and fungal products, DNA, etc.
Scavenger	
SR-A, B, C, D, and E	Bind polyanionic ligands, lipoteichoic acid, phosphatidylserine, modified LDL, and apoptotic cell structures
C-type lectins	
Mannose receptor	Binds mannose or frucose
Cytokines	Bind specific cytokines and stimulate signal transduction pathways

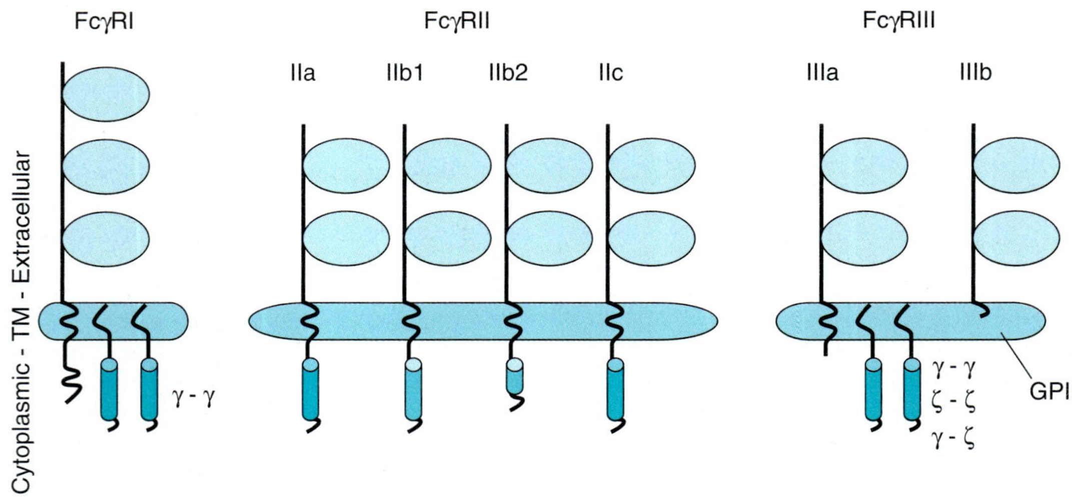

FIGURE 7–1 • Human Fcγ Receptor (FcγR) Family Members. FcγR α-chains contain two or three disulfide-linked immunoglobulin-like extracellular domains that mediate binding to IgG. The cytoplasmic domains of FcγR or their associated subunits are responsible for signal transduction. FcγRIIIb is the only FcγR that lacks a cytoplasmic tail. FcγRI and FcγRIIIa are multichain receptors that associate with immunoreceptor tyrosine-based activation motif (ITAM; black cylinders) bearing γ-or ξ-chain dimers to mediate positive signaling. FcγRIIa and FcγRIIc are single-chain stimulatory receptors containing ITAMs in their cytoplasmic tails. FcγRIIb1 and FcγRIIb2 are single-chain inhibitory receptors containing immunoreceptor tyrosine-based inhibitory motifs (ITIMs; white cylinders) in their cytoplasmic tails. TM, transmembrane; GPI, glycosyl phosphatidylinositol. (From [Salmon JE, Pricop L: Human receptors for immunoglobulin G: Key elements in the pathogenesis of rheumatic disease. Arthritis Rheum 44:739, 2001].)

of FcγRIIIb have been described, NA1 and NA2, with NA1 stimulating more vigorous responses in neutrophils.

C-reactive protein (CRP) is a major acute-phase protein that is produced in large amounts by the liver in response to IL-1 and IL-6 during the innate immune response to infection and tissue injury. CRP binds to encapsulated bacteria and enhances their clearance. FcγRIIa is the primary receptor for CRP on monocytes, and this receptor demonstrates reciprocal binding affinities for IgG2a and CRP.[9] FcγRIIa allele R131, which binds IgG2 weakly, binds CRP strongly and vice versa, thus endowing individuals who carry R131 with some resistance to bacterial infection.[10] In addition, CRP binds nucleosomes and apoptotic cells, clearing them through FcγRIIa.[11] Thus, a deficiency in this clearance mechanism may lead to prolonged exposure of the adaptive immune system to altered self with enhanced possibility for the development of autoimmunity.[12] CRP also stimulates production of both IL-1β and IL-1Ra in human monocytes, but it inhibits LPS-induced production of these two cytokines in alveolar macrophages.[13]

Complement receptors (CR) on monocytes and macrophages mediate a variety of functions[14] (see Table 7–3). C1qR may promote opsonizatation of immune complexes, followed by enhanced antibody-dependent cellular cytotoxicity (ADCC) and cytokine release. The major role of CR1 on tissue macrophages is to mediate the removal from circulation of C3-coated erythrocytes. CR1 cooperates with FcγR to mediate phagocytosis in resting macrophages, but CR1 alone can mediate phagocytosis only in activated macrophages. CR1 also exhibits an additional function as a regulator of complement activity. CR2 is expressed primarily on B cells, where it acts as a costimulator after binding of antigens coated with IgM and C3. CR2 also may be involved in binding of antigens by FDC. CR3 (CD11b, CD18) is a heterodimer that belongs to the β_2-integrin family and binds both C3 and C3 fragments. It may be involved in organization of cytoskeletal events during phagocytosis. Receptors for C3a and C5a respond to binding of these potent anaphylatoxins by releasing a variety of inflammatory molecules. Macrophage stimulation by C5a is particularly important in acute and chronic inflammatory diseases. C5a binding to alveolar macrophages induces the expression of stimulatory FcγRIII and suppresses expression of inhibitory FcγRIIb, enhancing the ability of these cells to respond to immune complexes.[15] Furthermore, mice rendered genetically deficient in expression of C5a receptors do not develop experimental inflammatory joint disease, indicating the importance of this receptor in inflammatory diseases.[16]

Other receptors on mononuclear phagocytes carry out important roles in the housekeeping functions of these cells and in mediation of inflammatory diseases.[17] The Toll-like receptors (TLR) are discussed extensively in Chapter 8. As an example of TLR function in macrophages, LPS binds to TL4 on macrophages in close contact with CD14, leading to activation of the NF-κB signal transduction pathway and enhanced transcription of inflammatory cytokines and other molecules. Scavenger receptors are instrumental in removal of senescent and apoptotic cells from the body. However, macrophage scavenger receptors also mediate uptake of acetylated low-density lipoproteins (LDL), possibly contributing to the development of atherosclerotic lesions in vessel walls.[18] The mannose receptor binds pathogens expressing that sugar, thereby mediating uptake and possibly processing for antigen presentation by MHC class II molecules. Lastly, monocytes and macrophages express receptors for a large number of cytokines, including IL-8 and other chemokines; IL-1, -2, -4, -6, -10, and -13; TNF-α; interferon (IFN)γ; TGF-β; and platelet-derived growth factor (PDGF). These receptors mediate chemotactic responses, production of inflammatory cytokines and other molecules, and production of anti-inflammatory proteins such as (IL-1 receptor antagonist, IL-1Ra).

PHAGOCYTOSIS

The surfaces of microbial agents express specific repeating molecular structures (PAMPs) that are recognized by receptors (PRRs) on DC and macrophages, leading to phagocytosis of the pathogen and initiation of the innate immune response.[19] Coating of foreign material with complement components and antibodies facilitates phagocytosis. Fc and C receptors enhance binding of coated particles and induce rearrange-ments in actin filaments, which leads to internalization and formation of cytoplasmic vacuoles. In addition, mononuclear phagocytes may ingest material through other mechanisms, such as pinocytosis and receptor-mediated endocytosis.

The mechanisms of internalization and intracellular responses differ between Fc and C receptors. FcγR are constitutively active and employ a zipper mechanism during phagocytosis with pseudopodia enveloping IgG-coated particles and drawing them into the body of the macrophage with actin microfilaments.[20] In contrast, C receptors on macrophages bind, but do not internalize, coated particles in the absence of additional stimulation provided by cytokines or attachment to matrix molecules such as laminin or fibronectin. Complement-coated particles are not surrounded by pseudopodia but appear to gently sink into the cell via microtubules. Phagocytosis induced by FcγR is tightly coupled to stimulation of transcription and release of proinflammatory mediators, whereas C-mediated internalization is not accompanied by these responses. Phagocytosis by the mannose receptor also leads to the production of proinflammatory cytokines and other molecules. Following internalization mediated by FcγR, the phagosome gradually fuses with late endosomes and lysosomes, forming a phagolysosome that moves through the cell on microtubules. Acid hydrolyases are present in these vacuoles, leading to enzymatic degradation of the ingested particle.

Many bacteria are internalized through a different process, called macropinocytosis, which differs from phagocytosis mediated by FcγR or CR. Addition of growth factors or some bacteria to macrophages results in extensive surface ruffling with random extension of pseudopods. Actin-mediated engulfment is then triggered, leading to formation of large macropinosomes that may contain other bystander materials present around the cell. These vesicles may not fuse with lysosomes, but bacteria may multiply inside the vacuole.

Other bacteria, such as *Mycobacteria*, are ingested using a variety of receptors, but the phagosomes resist fusion with lysosomes unless the cell is activated, leading to persistence of bacteria-laden vacuoles in the cell.

Apoptic cells acquire new surface determinants, such as phosphatidylserine, and are phagocytosed by macrophages using scavenger receptors, CR, and CD14. When apoptotic cells are recognized and engulfed by macrophages, production of proinflammatory molecules is downregulated by the release of TGF-β, prostaglandin (PG)E_2, and other anti-inflammatory mediators.[21] However, ingestion of microbial agents not expressing phosphatidlyserine on their cell surface results in the rapid production and release of proinflammatory molecules such as IL-1, TNF-α, GM-CSF, and leukotriene C_4. Deficiency of C1q predisposes to SLE, possibly because of a delay in the clearance of apoptotic cells by macrophages and a resultant increase in DC phagocytosis of nuclear debris and stimulation of autoimmune responses.[22] However, the predominant receptors expressed by macrophages vary with the state of cell differentiation and activation, influencing whether phagocytosis of apoptic cells leads to the release of proinflammatory or anti-inflammatory products.

SECRETORY PRODUCTS

Cells of the mononuclear phagocytic system participate in complex functions of inflammatory and immune responses primarily through secretion of a large number of products. Secretory responses of macrophages are stimulated by engagement of specific cell surface receptors. Some of the major categories of secretory products of macrophages are summarized in Table 7–4.[23,24] A detailed list of these secretory products can be found in review articles and further information about their relevance for rheumatic diseases can be found in other chapters in this text. Among the secretory products important for rheumatic diseases are proinflammatory and anti-inflammatory cytokines, matrix metallo-protensis (MMPs) responsible for tissue turnover and degradation, components of the classic and alternative complement pathways, prostaglandins and leukotrienes, and reactive oxygen and nitrogen intermediates. As innate immune cells, monocytes and macrophages release substances that both incite acute inflammation and nonspecifically stimulate cells of the adaptive immune system. As effector cells, macrophages secrete a variety of products that induce chronic inflammation and tissue repair, in large part through the stimulation of other nearby cells. Thus, these multifaceted cells play important roles in maintaining internal homeostasis but may contribute to diseases when they are inappropriately and chronically stimulated.

TABLE 7–4 • SECRETORY PRODUCTS OF MONONUCLEAR PHAGOCYTES*

Polypeptide hormones and cytokines
Complement components
Coagulation factors
Proteolytic enzymes
Lipases and other enzymes
Inhibitors of enzymes
Proteins of extracellular matrix or cell adhesion
Binding proteins for metals, vitamins, lipids, etc.
Bioactive lipids, including cyclooxygenase and lipoxygenase products
Reactive oxygen and nitrogen intermediates
Nucleosides and metabolites

*For a detailed listing of compounds in each category, see references 23,24.

ANTIGEN PROCESSING AND PRESENTATION IN MACROPHAGES

DC are the most potent APCs in the body because of their expression of MHC class I and class II molecules and costimulatory molecules such as CD80 and CD86. However, macrophages may also function as efficient APCs, particularly when stimulated to express higher levels of costimulatory molecules and, as discussed later in this chapter, they may differentiate into DC. Macrophages use the same mechanisms as DC to process and present antigenic material. In general, MHC class I molecules were thought to present endogenous antigens and MHC class II molecules to present peptides derived from exogenous materials.[25] However, it now appears that the major determinants of the presentation pathway used for exogenous material reside with the APC and the antigen. Macrophages and DC process endocytosed antigens for presentation by both MHC class I and class II molecules, whereas B cells present endocytosed antigens primarily by the class II pathway. Particulate antigens, lipoproteins and lipopeptides, and immune complex antigens are particularly likely to be processed by the endogenous pathway after endocytosis. Endocytosed antigens are subjected to the same ultimate processing mechanisms as are endogenous antigens, after transport from endosomal to cytosolic compartments for MHC class I presentation.

Antigen processing for MHC class I presentation involves a different proteolytic pathway for each end of the antigenic protein (Figure 7–2). Proteins are ubiquitinated and enter the 26S proteasome, where processing of the carboxy termini takes place, followed by amino-terminal processing by aminopeptidases in the cytosol and endoplasmic reticulum (ER). The processed peptides then interact with transport associated with antigen processing (TAP) molecules that shuttle the peptide from the cytosol into the ER. Endogenous antigens may also be transported to the ER by TAP molecules, but a TAP-independent pathway exists, which uses signal recognition particles (SRP) as a transport mechanism for endogenous proteins possessing signal peptides. Heavy chains of MHC class I molecules are inserted into the ER membrane, via the protein secretory pathway, where they first associate with the β_2-microglobulin (β_2m) light chain. A class I loading complex containing heavy and light chains and other components is assembled in the ER and binds the processed peptide. MHC class I molecules with bound peptide are released from the loading complex and traffic to the Golgi, then to the cell surface. MHC class I molecules that have not bound peptide are degraded in the ER. The binding cleft of MHC class I molecules

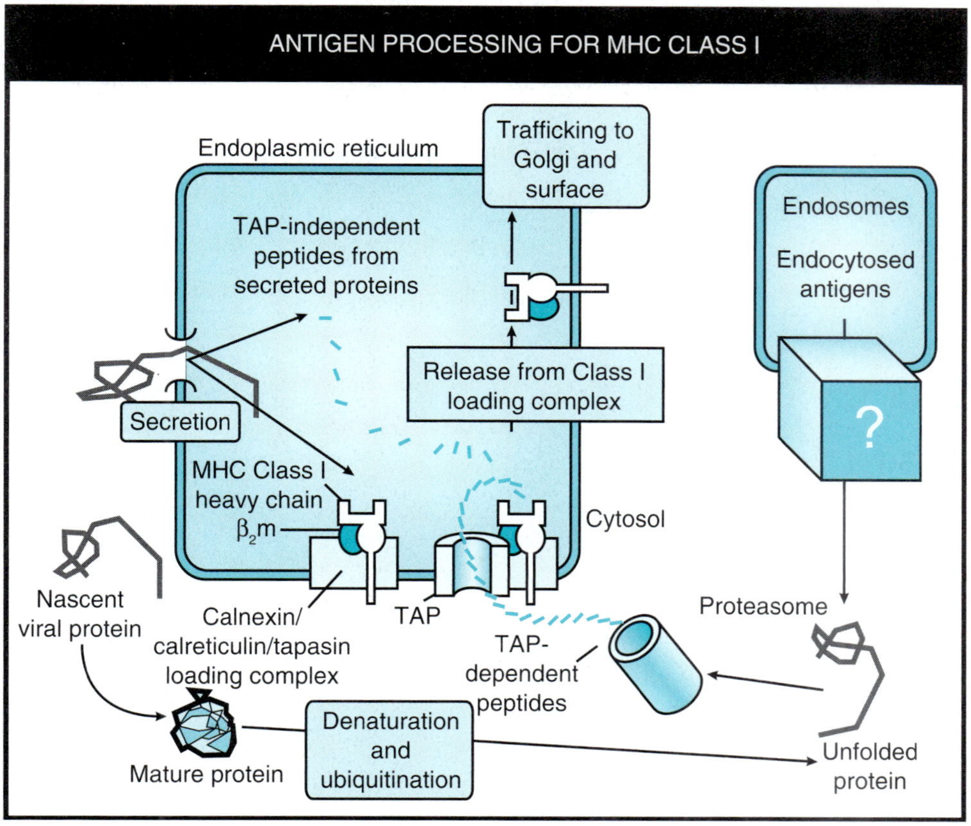

FIGURE 7–2 · **Antigen Processing for MHC Class I Presentation.** Two major pathways for antigen processing interact within the cytosol. *1,* Most endogenous antigens are synthesized on cytosolic ribosomes, processed by proteasomes, and enter the endoplasmic reticulum (ER) through the transport associated with antigen processing (TAP) transporter. A minor set of antigens is processed within the ER from proteins secreted into the ER. *2,* Professional antigen-presenting cells (APCs) transfer endocytosed antigens into the cytosol for processing. Note that peptide may not be available to diffuse freely in the ER, as depicted, but may always be complexed with a peptide carrier protein (not shown). (From [Rodgers JR, Rich R: Antigens and antigen presentation *In* Rich R, Fleisher T, Kotzin B, Schroeder Jr H (eds): Clinical Immunology: Princi-ples andPractice, 2nd ed. St. Louis, Mosby, 2001, 7.1].)

binds peptides containing 8 to 10 amino acid residues with the carboxy and amino termini embedded in the cleft. Anchoring of the peptide in the MHC class I cleft is mediated by the terminal residues, the peptide backbone, and by side chains. Thus, the structural requirements for peptide binding to MHC class I molecules are quite rigid. On the cell surface, peptides bound by MHC class I molecules are recognized by TCR on CD8+ T cells, stimulating the generation of cytotoxic T lymphocytes (CTL).

The mechanism of antigen processing and presentation by MHC class II molecules is quite different (Figure 7–3). The mechanisms of entry into the cell for material destined for the MHC class II pathway include pinocytosis of soluble antigens, receptor-mediated uptake of immune complexes, recycling through clathrin-coated pits, and phagocytosis of microbial agents or apoptotic bodies.[25] The antigenic substances are enzymatically degraded in the endolysosome. The MHC class II molecules assemble in the ER, where an invariant chain occupies the antigen-binding cleft. The assembled αβ dimers of MHC class II with invariant chain move through the Golgi to MHC class II–rich late endosomes (MIIC) containing processed peptides. After subsequent proteolysis, a small peptide of the invariant chain (CLIP, or class II–associated invariant chain peptide) remains in the cleft and HLA-DM molecules catalyze and exchange it for a processed antigenic peptide. The initial binding to MHC class II molecules is by large unfolded proteins or protein fragments that subsequently are trimmed by exopeptidases as the complex is moved to the cell surface. The final peptides present in MHC class II molecules are 15 to 20 amino acids long, with the ends of the antigen-binding cleft open and the peptide hanging out. Thus, the mechanisms of binding and presentation of peptides by MHC class II molecules are not as rigid as by class I. Peptides bound by MHC class II molecules are recognized by TCR on $CD4^+$ T cells, leading to the generation of humoral and cellular immune responses.

It should be noted that most MHC class I and II molecules on the surface of resting APCs contain self peptides. The absence of stimulatory signaling of TCR by these self peptides may be due to the low density of costimulatory molecules. Two important costimulatory molecules on APCs are CD80 (B7.1) and CD86 (B7.2), which interact with CD28 ligand on T cells. Expression of costimulatory molecules on APCs is enhanced by exposure to LPS from microbial agents; by cytokines of the innate immune system, such as IL-1 and TNF-α; and by CD40 ligation as a result of T cell activation. A naïve T cell may be rendered anergic by interaction with MHC molecules containing bound peptide in the absence of accompanying expression of adequate levels of costimulatory molecules. Thus, generation of primary adaptive immune responses is dependent on the level of expression of costimulatory molecules, as well as on presentation of MHC-bound immunogenic peptides. However, the reactivity of memory T cells to an antigen is not so dependent on costimulation.

In addition to presenting immunogens or antigens bound to MHC class I or II and expressing costimulatory molecules, macrophages enhance and shape the immune response through the release of cytokines. The combination of CD80 (B7.1) and IL-12 promote

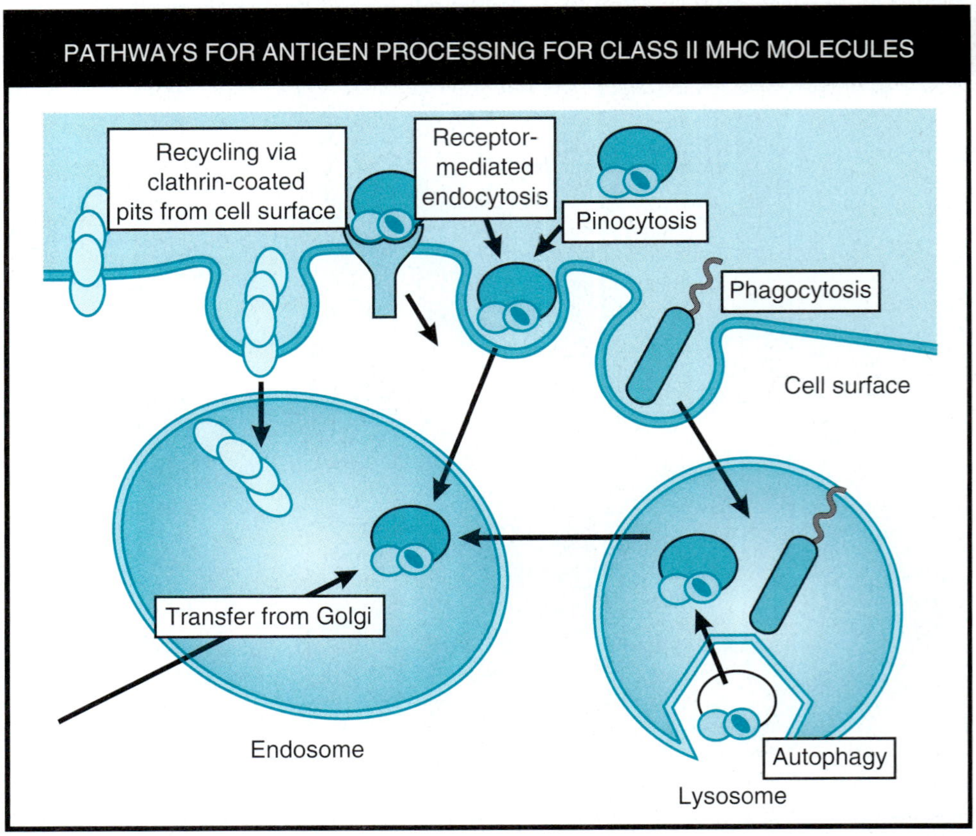

FIGURE 7–3 · **Antigen Processing for MHC Class II Presentation.** The most prominent pathway used by a professional antigen-presenting cell (APC) is endocytosis: pinocytosis of soluble antigens; receptor-mediated endocytosis of ligands (e.g., uptake of antigen-antibody complexes via Fc receptors); recycling through clathrin- coated pits of surface proteins such as human immunodeficiency virus (HIV) gp 120; and phagocytosis of microbes and apoptotic bodies. Minor pathways include transfer from the Golgi to endosomes and autophagy. A few peptides bind to class II molecules in the endoplasmic reticulum (ER) before they are transferred to endosomes from the Golgi (not shown). (From [Rodgers JR, Rich R: Antigens and antigen presentation *In* Rich R, Fleisher T, Kotzin B, Schroeder Jr H (eds): Clinical Immunology. Principles and Practice, 2nd ed. St. Louis, Mosby, 2001, 7.1].)

the differentiation of resting $CD4^+$ T cells into Th1 cells, and CD86 (B7.2) and IL-4 lead to differentiation into Th2 cells. IL-12 interacting with $CD8^+$ T cells enhances the development of CTL. In contrast, T cell proliferation is inhibited by the release of IL-10 and TGF-β from macrophages, in part through the down-regulation of costimulatory molecule expression.

MHC-independent antigen presentation may occur via CD1 molecules that bind lipids and glycolipids. CD1 proteins are similar in structure to MHC class I heavy chains, are noncovalently linked to β_2m on the cell surface, and present antigens to $CD8^+$ or $CD8^-CD4^-$ αβ T cells. CD1 possesses a more narrow and deep antigen-binding cleft than MHC class I, and it may bind hydrophobic peptides in an antigen-nonspecific fashion. The CD1 system is thought to be of primary importance in presentation of antigens from *Mycobacteria* and other microbes.

ANTIGEN PROCESSING AND PRESENTATION BY B CELLS

Any cell that expresses MHC class I or class II molecules has the potential to function as an APC, but most of these cells do not possess the capacity to ingest and process antigens or to express costimulatory molecules. Although not as potent as DC or macrophages, B cells can bind and express antigens for which they possess specific Ig receptors. The induction of costimulatory molecules on these B cells endows them with the capacity to present antigens to T cells. B cells also express FcγRIIb that cannot be endocytosed and thus does not function in antigen capture and processing. However, CR2, when ligated by C3d, serves as a costimulator in antigen-induced B cell activation by amplifying signals initiated through the Ig receptors for antigen.[14] CR2 carries out this function through coassociation with the B cell–specific protein CD19 and with two other proteins. CR2 on B cells is involved in primary and secondary immune responses. Indeed, when given to mice in vivo, a recombinant model antigen fused to several copies of C3d was 1000-fold more immunogenic than antigen alone. In this way, the opsonin C3d functions as a molecular adjuvant of innate immunity that profoundly influences an acquired immune response through the CR2 receptor.[26]

MACROPHAGE EFFECTOR FUNCTIONS

As part of the innate immune system, mononuclear phagocytes exhibit potent antimicrobial properties. After recognition and phagocytosis of nonencapsulated bacteria, killing ensues in the phagolysosomes through the activities of lysosomal enzymes, reactive oxygen and nitrogen intermediates, toxic radicals, and chloramines. Macrophage killing of pathogens is enhanced after IgG and C coating of the particle and after activation by IFN-γ. Anitmicrobial responses of macrophages may also have more broad effects. The toxic radical nitric oxide (NO) is produced by many cells besides macrophages, such as endothelial cells and neurons. NO influences the production of a wide variety of cytokines by other cells and may also inhibit lymphocyte proliferation.

Macrophages also play important roles in the resolution of acute inflammation and in wound repair. The release of TGF-β by tissue macrophages in sites of tissue injury leads to the chemotaxis of monocytes and neutrophils and to the production of IL-1, TNF-α, IL-6, and IL-12. Macrophages engulf tissue debris and also contribute to angiogenesis, formation of granulation tissue, and re-epithelialization of the wound. The release of growth factors, such as PDGF, fibroblast growth factor (FGF), vascular endothelial growth factor (VEGF), and TGF-β, stimulates fibroblast proliferation and production of matrix proteins. The release of anti-inflammatory proteins such as IL-1Ra also enhances tissue repair.

SYNOVIAL MACROPHAGES

Macrophages are present in the normal synovial lining as type A cells and are prominent in the proliferative synovitis of rheumatoid arthritis (RA)[27,28] (see Chapter 65). Blood-borne monocytes enter the normal and inflamed synovium with subsequent differentiation into mature cells influenced by TNF-α and GM-CSF. Macrophage release of multiple cytokines, particularly TNF-α and IL-1, plays a central role in the mechanisms of tissue injury in the rheumatoid synovium. The inflammatory effects of these cytokines include upregulating adhesion-molecule expression on endothelial cells, enhancing migration of more cells into the joint, and stimulating release of MMPs from fibroblasts and chondrocytes. Monocytes and macrophages in the rheumatoid synovium also may be differentiated into DC and osteoclasts, with the latter cells responsible for erosion of marginal bone. The role of macrophages in the initiation of the inflammatory joint pathology of RA and seronegative spondyloarthropathies is not known, but their involvement may include harboring intracellular pathogens or their remnants or involvement in generation of proinflammatory cytokines and other products in response to immune-complex antigen. Macrophages certainly are important in chronic synovitis, where they may be activated both by direct contact with T cells and by T cell–independent mechanisms.[29] Macrophages may acquire relatively autonomous function in this disease process, not requiring continual T cell stimulation. Therapeutic approaches in RA directed at macrophages include blocking their entry into the joint, inhibiting their activation, counteracting their inflammatory products, and killing the cells.

OSTEOCLAST DIFFERENTIATION

Receptor activator of nuclear factor (NF)-κB ligand (RANKL) is essen-tial for osteoclast (OC) differentiation. The cognate RANKL receptor, RANK, is expressed by monocytes, DC, and osteoclasts. RANK expression is critical for later stages of OC differentiation. This process has potential significance for the development of bony erosions in the rheumatoid joint. Monocytes, macrophages, or c-kit$^+$ c-fms$^+$ RANK$^-$ osteoclast precursors can be induced to differentiate into mature osteoclasts, with bone resorptive capacity, in the presence of RANKL and M-CSF.[30] In rheumatoid synvoial tissue, RANKL may be derived from bone stromal cells, synovial fibroblasts, or T cells. In support of this pathway, RANKL-deficient mice are protected from bone erosion in a model of inflammatory arthritis.[31]

Dendritic Cells

Dendritic cells (DC) were discovered by Steinman in 1973 as "large stellate" cells in the mouse spleen.[32] DC are derived from hematopoietic stem cells.[33] They comprise a heterogeneous population of cells with dendritic morphology that express high levels of MHC class II and costimulatory molecules and that possess characteristic endocytic pathways for antigen uptake and processing. In antigen-specific assays or mixed lymphocyte reactions, DC induce higher levels of T cell proliferation than any other APC and are able to prime resting T cells to antigen in vitro. In vivo, DC are specialized in their capacity to prime the immune response to novel antigens.[34]

In the periphery, DC sample antigens, including self antigens, by endocytosis of particulate and soluble antigens. Immature DC possess high levels of ability to capture antigens with moderate levels of costimulatory molecule (CD80/86) expression. In peripheral sites, inflammatory cytokines, bacterial products, or molecules exposed in damaged tissues, such as proteoglycans, induce differentiation or maturation of DC through PRRs, leading to increased costimulatory molecule expression, altered chemokine receptor expression, and IL-12 production.[35-37] As a result, DC migrate to the secondary lymphoid organs, where they complete their maturation through interaction with CD154 (CD40 ligand) expressed by T cells.[37] As a result of these antigen-presenting properties, DC have been termed *nature's adjuvant*—a property applied to clinical protocols for tumor immunotherapy.[38]

ORIGIN OF DC

DC originate from hematopoietic progenitors in the bone marrow and traffic in the blood to peripheral tissues.[39] DC precursors comprise 0.5 to 3 percent of the mononuclear cells in peripheral blood.[40-42] Their numbers may be increased in circulation by granulocyte colony-stimulating factor (G-CSF), exercise, and surgical stress, with kinetics similar to those of granulocytes.[43] In mice and humans, a common myeloid developmental pathway has been demonstrated for monocytes/macrophages, DC, and granulocytes: from an MHC class II progenitor in the bone marrow.[44-46] In support, in mice transgenic for the E-GFP (green fluorescent protein) driven by the M-CSF receptor promoter, common myeloid progenitors as well as the macrophage and DC systems of the mouse are fluorescent.[47] Production of DC from hemopoietic progenitors in vivo can be greatly enhanced by the cytokines Flt-3L and G-CSF.[48] Both human and murine DC express the integrin CD11c. In addition, there is some evidence for a lymphoid DC lineage[33] (Fig. 7–4). Of clinical importance, peripheral blood monocytes can differentiate into DC in the

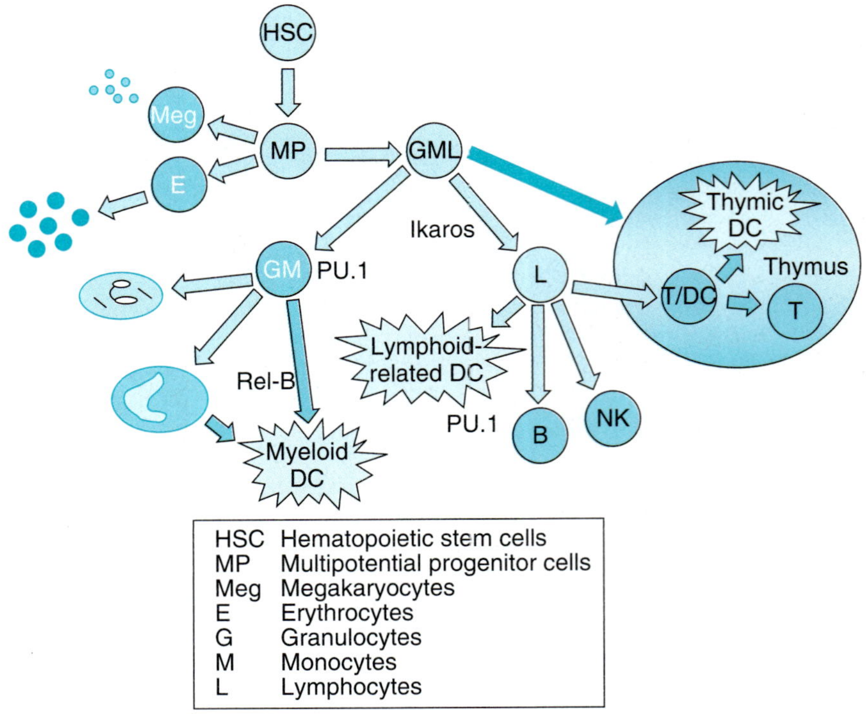

FIGURE 7–4 • Proposed schema for dendritic cell (DC) development from hemopoietic stem cells and the role of transcription factors in the differentiation of subpopulations. Hemopoietic stem cells (HSC) differentiate into multipotential progenitor cells (MP) with the capacity to generate megakaryocytes (Meg), erythrocytes (E), granulocytes (G), monocytes (M), lymphocytes (L) and DC. DC can derive in close association with either myeloid or lymphoid lineages. Ikaros is essential for the formation of lymphocytes and some DC. RelB is essential for development of myeloid-related DC. PU-1 is essential for the development of B cells, monocytes, and putative myeloid DC. (From [Lotze MT, Thomson AW (eds): Dendritic Cells, 2nd ed. London, Academic Press, 2001].)

presence of GM-CSF and IL-4 for 2 to 7 days.[49,50] Immature DC derived from monocytes retain macrophage-development potential[50] (Fig. 7–5).

Accumulating evidence supports the view that DC development and function result from environmental signals ("instruction") rather than from inflexible lineage-restricted traits ("selection"), although arguments have been put forward for the alternative view. Many cells, including monocytes and T, B, and NK cells, retain the ability to differentiate into DC until the point of terminal differentiation.[51]

Subpopulations of DC: Specialized Functions

In the mouse, CD11c expression appears to be restricted to DC. Murine CDllc$^+$ DC populations have been classified according to the surface expression of CD8αα homodimer. Shortman and colleagues have noted three major subsets using this marker, with particular distribution in the lymphoid organs: CD8α$^+$CD4$^-$, CD8α$^-$CD4$^+$, and CD8α$^-$CD4$^-$.[52] A further CD45R$^+$CDllc^{dim} population, known as plasmacytoid DC, has also been identified.[53] CD8α$^+$ and 8α$^-$ DC are found in the spleen, skin-draining lymph nodes (LN), and mesenteric LN. In the spleen, CD8α$^+$ DC are found in the T cell region, whereas the CD8α$^-$ DC are located in the marginal zone and only migrate into the T cell area following microbial challenge[54] (Fig. 7–6). The thymus contains a preponderance of CD8α$^+$ DC.[55] Both CD8α$^+$ and CD8α$^-$ subsets arise from a CDllc$^+$ MHC class II$^-$ precursor, which expresses low cell-surface CD40.[56] The DC precursor can reconstitute B220$^+$ DC, as well as CD8α$^+$ and CD8α$^-$ DC subsets, when transferred into congenic mice. CD40$^-$ DC are also observed in the rat, after cannulation of afferent lymphatics and isolation of DC, migrating constitutively from the periphery to the draining LN in the absence of priming.[57]

In contrast to CD8α$^-$ DC, which produce low levels of IL-12, CD8α$^+$ DC produce high levels of IL-12 in response to microbial and CD154 signals.[58] IL-12 can be induced by microbial stimuli that signal through TLR, or through CD154 signaling of CD40.[59] The microbial

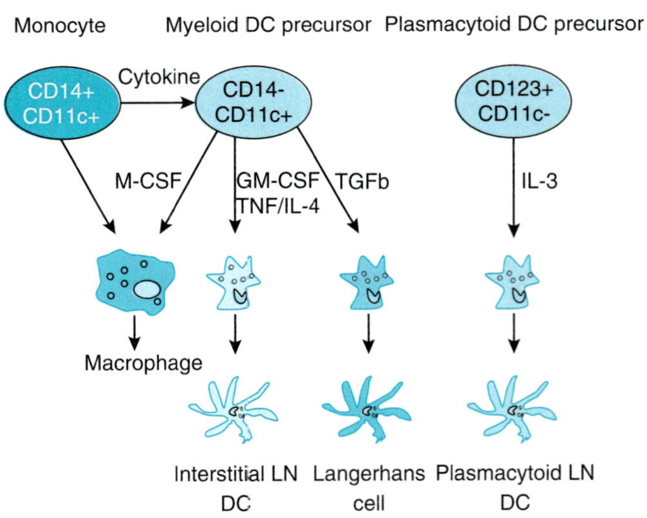

FIGURE 7–5 • Dendritic Cell (DC) Subsets in Humans. Two subsets of dendritic cell precursors circulate in peripheral blood: CD11c$^+$ myeloid DC and CD11c$^-$CD123$^+$ plasmacytoid DC. CD11c$^+$ precursors may originate from monocytes. CD11c$^+$ precursors can give rise to Langerhans cells, interstitial DC (found in T cell area of lymph nodes and spleen), or macrophages. CD11c$^-$CD123$^+$ plasmacytoid DC depend on IL-3 and CD154 for survival and maturation and are also found in the T cell areas of lymphoid organs. (From [Lotze MT, Thomson AW (eds): Dendritic Cells, 2nd ed. London, Academic Press, 2001].)

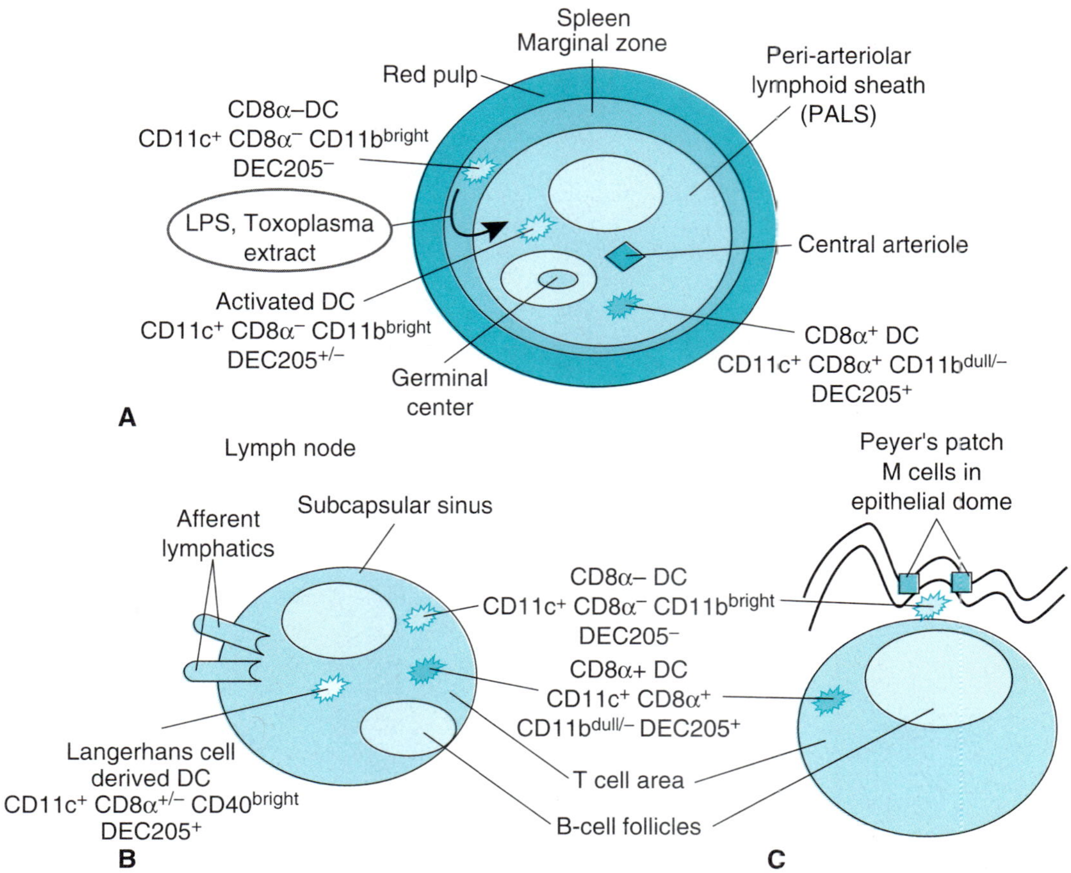

FIGURE 7–6 · Dendritic Cell (DC) Subsets in Lymphoid Organs in Mice. In the spleen, CD8α$^+$ and CD8α$^-$ DC can be identified. CD8α$^+$ DC are located in the periarticular lymphoid sheath (PALS), and CD8α$^-$ subsets are in the marginal zones. Certain microbial products such as LPS can induce rapid migration of CD8α$^-$ marginal zone DC to the PALS. In the lymph nodes, CD8α$^+$ and CD8α$^-$ DC and Langerhans cells are found. These DC express the DEC205 receptor and high levels of CD40. In the Peyer's patches, CD8α$^+$ and CD8α$^-$ DC are found. (From [Lotze MT, Thomson AW (eds): Dendritic Cells, 2nd ed. London, Academic Press, 2001].)

pathway may be important for stimulation of rapid IL-12 production, and the CD40-dependent pathway may increase in importance during the later stages of infection as a result of sustained DC-T cell signaling in the LN. Thus, these two pathways are unlikely to be mutually exclusive.[60] In the human, circulating DC precursors express CD11c and the myeloid lineage markers CD13 and CD33, but they are distinguished from monocytes by their lack of high levels of CD14. They differentiate spontaneously into mature DC in vitro.[40,61]

Plasmacytoid DC

Plasmacytoid DC (PDC) circulate in human peripheral blood as CDllc$^-$ MHC class II$^+$ precursors that uniformly express high levels of IL-3Rα (CD123) and CD62L.[62] IL-3 and CD154 promote their survival and differentiation into APC in vitro.[63] This discrete DC population, present in mice and humans, is believed to play a role linking the innate response against pathogens and the adaptive immune response as APC. PDC are the principal source of type I IFN, and they produce large amounts of IFNα in response to viral infection, including human immunodeficiency virus (HIV).[64]

Langerhans Cells

Epithelial DC or Langerhans cells (LC) were discovered in 1868 by medical student Paul Langerhans. LC can be identified by expression of langerin, possession of specialized intracellular vesicles known as Birbeck granules, and, after migration in peripheral (epithelial-draining) LN, as CDllc$^+$CD40^{high} cells (see Fig. 7–6B). Consistent with the anatomy of priming in LN, CD40^{high} DC are only found in peripheral LN and not in spleen, thymus, Peyer's patches, or mesenteric LN. Monocyte-derived DC develop into LC-like cells in the presence of TGF-β1[65] (see Fig. 7–5). TGF-β is essential for the development of epithelial LC, as is demonstrated by their absence in TGF-β-deficient mice.[66]

DC DIFFERENTIATION AND MATURATION

Morphological changes accompanying DC maturation include a loss of adhesive molecules, cytoskeletal reorganization, and acquisition of high cellular motility.[67] Phenotypically, DC upregulate cell surface expression of MHC class II molecules as they translocate from intracellular compartments to the cell surface; costimulatory molecules, including the B7 family and CD40;

adhesion molecules; DC–lysosome-associated membrane protein (DC-LAMP); and chemokine receptors. Mature DC exhibit a loss of antigen capture capacity and an increase in migratory capacity, thus allowing DC that have been signaled for maturation to migrate to draining LN (Fig. 7–7). Immature DC express functional chemokine receptors for inflammation-induced chemokines, such as CCRl, CCR2, CCR3, CCR5, and CXCR1. However, upon maturation, DC downregulate expression of inflammatory chemokine receptors and upregulate CCR7 expression.[68] This change has significance for attraction of mature DC to the T cell areas of lymphoid organs as the CCR7 ligands CCL19 and 21 are expressed in the T cell areas and, in the case of CCL21, by afferent lymphatic endothelium.[69] Functionally, immature DC are poor allogenic stimulators and can induce T cell anergy, but fully mature DC are strong allogenic stimulators and can induce immunity. Fully mature DC also produce cytokines and chemokines, including IL-12 p40 and p70, TNF-α, IL-l, IL-6, and many others.

At least five types of surface receptors trigger DC maturation:

1. *Toll-like receptors (TLR):* Bacterial wall components such as LPS, unmethylated CpG motifs, and double-stranded RNA are recognized by a large family of surface receptors called TLR. The TLR family consists of phylogenetically conserved transmembrane proteins that are essential for innate immunity. To date, mammals have been found to express more than 10 members of the TLR family. DC express some of these molecules, including TLR2, TLR3, and TLR4.[70] They trigger functional DC maturation in response to bacterial peptidoglycans, lipopeptides, LPS, and mycoplasma lipoproteins. PDC specifically express TLR9 and, therefore, respond to immunostimulatory CpG motifs in unmethylated DNA, typically producing large amounts of IFN-α.
2. *Cytokine receptors:* Pathogens may trigger secretion of inflammatory mediators, such as TNF-α, IL-lβ, IL-12, and PGE_2, which may subsequently activate DC.[38]
3. *Tumor-necrosis factor (TNF)-receptor (TNF-R) superfamily molecules, including CD40:* Activation of the CD40 receptors is a critical signal that triggers full maturation of DC into highly efficient APC.[37] Functional maturation of DC also occurs by ligation of other superfamily members, including Fas and OX40L.[71]
4. *FcγR:* DC may also be activated through receptors for Ig. Engagement of most FcγR by immune complexes or specific antibodies induces DC maturation.[72] This process requires the FcR-associated γ-chain that contains an ITAM. DC may also be downregulated by engagement of inhibitory, ITIM-associated FcR.
5. *Sensors for cell death:* Necrotic, but not apoptotic, cell death induces DC maturation in vitro.[73] Heat-shock proteins (HSP), including gp96, HSP90, and HSP70, released by necrotic cells, provide potent signals for DC maturation, signaling through CD91 or CD40.[74] CD40 has been shown to act as an endocytic receptor for HSP-peptide complexes, potentially playing a critical role in cross-priming.[75] Nucleotides, such as adenosine triphosphate (ATP) and uridine triphosphate (UTP), may also activate DC through purinergic receptors.

DC SURVIVAL

Viability of a DC is inversely related to the level of maturation. Survival can be enhanced by CD154 and RANKL, which are expressed by T cells. Both signals inhibit apoptosis of DC and improve the ability of DC to prime T cells.[76] IFN-α enhances the sensitivity of DC to activation-induced apoptosis.

Pathways Signaling DC Maturation

NF-κB Pathway

The NF-κB family of molecules is essential for cell differentiation, viability, and activation. This pathway is, therefore, of major importance in inflammation. The NF-κB family is a key transducer of inflammatory signals to the DC maturation program. The NF-κB complex comprises homodimers and heterodimers of the structurally related proteins p50, p52, RelA (p65), c-Rel, and RelB. NF-κB proteins are present in an inactive form in the cytosol, bound to inhibitor proteins called IκB. Signaling through NF-κB-inducing kinase and other kinases induces phosphorylation of IκB and nuclear translocation of NF-κB.[77,78] Blockade of all NF-

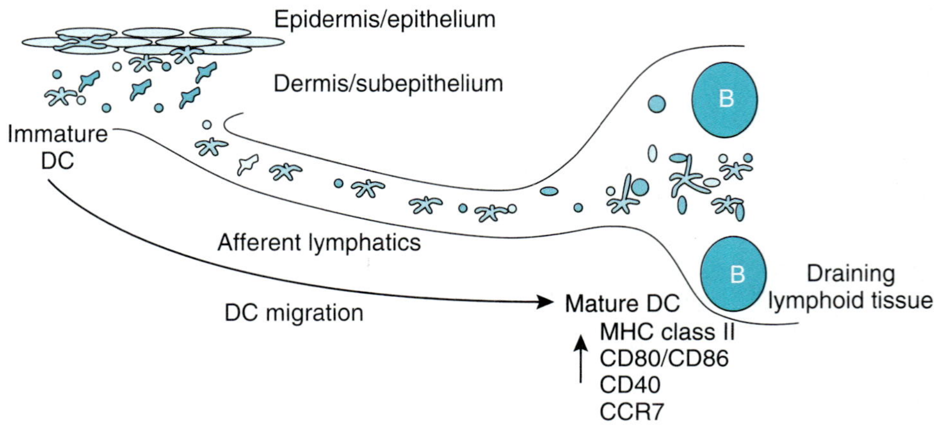

FIGURE 7–7 · Dendritic Cell (DC) Distribution in Epithelium and Migration to Draining Lymph Node. Immature DC within the stratified squamous epithelium and dermis survey and capture antigens and traffic in dermal lymphatics to subcapsular sinus and T cell areas of draining lymph nodes. In the context of inflammatory signals, DC mature and induce antigen-specific immunity in the lymph node. (From [Lotze MT, Thomson AW (eds): Dendritic Cells, 2nd ed. London, Academic Press, 2001].)

κB subunits by a variety of modalities prevents DC maturation and IL-12 secretion.

p38 MAPK Pathway

Similarly to NF-κB, the three mitrogen-activated protein kinase (MAPK) pathways (ERK, JNK, and p38) are activated by CD40 stimulation of DC.[79] However, whereas the p38 MAPK regulates IL-12 production by DC, ERK regulates DC survival.[79,80] In addition to playing an important role in IL-12 production, p38 MAPK is also critical for induction of costimulatory molecule expression by DC following microbial challenge.[81,82] Neither CD86 nor CD40 is upregulated when an inhibitor of the p38 MAPK is added at the time of microbial challenge to DC in vitro.[82] The importance of the p38 MAPK and NF-κB pathways to IL-12 production by DC suggests synergism between the two pathways. p38 MAPK enhances the accessibility of NF-κB binding sites within the IL-12 promoter. In contrast to CD154, TNF-α stimulation of DC only marginally induces p38 MAPK activity, similar to the weak induction of NF-κB in DC in response to TNF-α compared to CD154.[83,84]

The NF-κB pathway in DC is activated by CD40 ligation, and it regulates CD40 expression.[85-87] Although RelA has been shown to bind the CD40 promoter, RelB may also be required for CD40 transcription; DC generated from RelB-deficient mice fail to express CD40. Furthermore, enhanced CD40 expression by activated DC or B cells can be signaled directly as a result of RelB nuclear translocation.[88,89] A second NF-κB-independent pathway of DC activation exists, which involves signaling through triggering receptor expressed on myeloid cells (TREM2)/DAP12. Activation of MDDC by anti-TREM2 mAb also induces CD40 expression by the DC, thereby enhancing susceptibility to the CD40/RelB program of DC activation.[90]

IFN-γ primes DC to produce high levels of IL-12 and also increases expression of CD40 by DC.[91] IL-10 has suppressive functions on DC and can retard the upregulation of CD40 cell-surface expression. When added to DC cultures, IL-10 alters the capacity of the DC to signal T cells such that the population of regulatory T cells is expanded.[92-94] The finding that IL-10 can prevent degradation of IκB explains the potent CD40-suppressive capacity of IL-10.[95]

Antigen-Presenting Function of DC

Several molecules are involved in DC-T cell interactions. Engagement of the T cell receptor with the DC MHC-peptide complex alone is insufficient to trigger T cell proliferation and requires assistance from costimulatory and adhesion molecules to stabilize the bond and enhance further signaling between DC and T cells.[96] Only after 6 to 30 hours of continuous contact are naïve T cells committed to clonal expansion. The type of T cell response is dependent on DC-derived signals, including the type of MHC molecule, antigen density, level of costimulatory molecule expression, and cytokines.[97]

DC are capable of inducing the full repertoire of effector T cell responses, including Th0, Thl, Th2, and regulatory T cells.[95] DC also activate naïve CD8$^+$ CTL through presentation of antigen in the context of MHC class I molecules.[98] Th1 responses following DC stimulation require the cytokine IL-12 p70.[99] The mechanism of Th2 development is less understood, and lack or loss of IL-12, rather than the presence of IL-4, appears to be the predominant mechanism.[100] However CD86 signaling of CD28 may also play a role in Th2 development.

Type 1 CD4$^+$ helper T cells are crucial for the development of CTL.[101] Two mechanisms for this response have been suggested. The three-cell interaction model has now replaced the unspecific cytokine-secretion hypothesis. In this model, DC are partially matured by inflammatory signals in the periphery. However, the level of MHC and costimulatory molecule expression is insufficient for CTL induction, and fully mature ("conditioned") DC can only be obtained through interaction with CD4$^+$ T cells. Of importance, in the secondary lymphoid organs, interaction between CD4$^+$ T cells and DC with exposure to DC-derived IL-12 induces CD154 expression on activated CD4$^+$ T cells.[102,103] CD40 signaling of DC induces higher levels of IL-12 secretion and higher expression of MHC and CD86.[102] Both CD86 and IL-12, following CD40 ligation, are critical factors for CTL induction (Fig. 7–8).

ANTIGEN LOADING

Immature DC take up antigen efficiently through a variety of mechanisms, including receptor-mediated endocytosis, macropinocytosis, and phagocytosis of particles. Antigens can be processed and presented either by MHC class I or class II pathways.[104,105] MHC class I and class II molecules are highly polymorphic membrane proteins that bind and transport peptide fragments of intact proteins to the surface of APC and provide a display of peptide fragments of intracellular and environmental proteins for scrutiny by T cells. Class II molecules predominantly present antigens that are derived by processing soluble exogenous proteins or the extracellular domains of transmembrane proteins.[106,107] In contrast, class I molecules predominantly present antigen derived from endogenous or virally encoded proteins.[108] In certain circumstances, class II molecules present peptides derived from endogenous proteins,[109] and class I molecules present antigens derived from soluble proteins or from the extracellular domains of transmembrane proteins—a phenomenon known as *cross-presentation.*[110]

DC have phagocytic capability, although less than that of a macrophage. Engagement of specific receptors initiates a cascade of signal transduction. In immature DC, macropinocytosis is constitutive, allowing DC to rapidly and nonspecifically sample large amounts of surrounding fluid. Immature DC phagocytose bacteria, as well as *Saccharomyces cerevisae* and *Candida albicans* yeast cells and hyphae, through coiling and zipper types of phagocytosis.[111] DC also internalize parasites such as *Leishmania,* or malaria-parasitized red blood cells (RBC).[112] Apoptotic cells induced by viral infection, γ- or ultraviolet (UV) irradiation, serum starvation, or Fas- or tumor necrosis factor-related apoptosis-inducing ligand (TRAIL) ligation

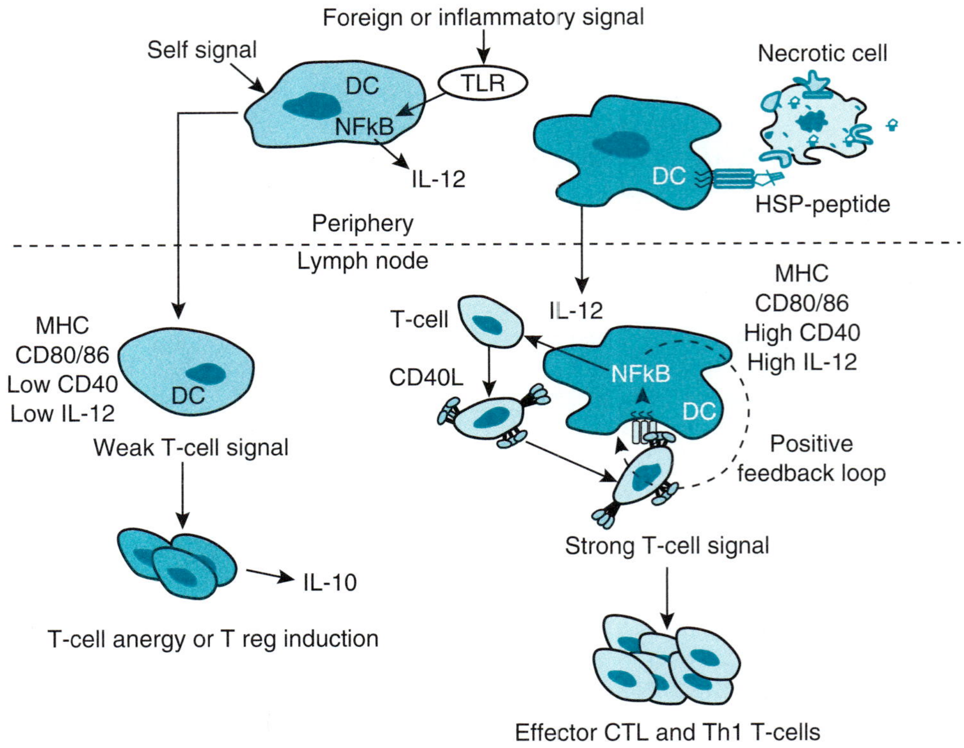

FIGURE 7–8 • T Cell Activation by Dendritic Cells (DC). In the absence of inflammation, DC express low levels of surface CD40 and secrete low level IL-12. These DC anergize T cell or induce IL-10–producing regulatory T cells. Micro-bial signals activate Toll-like receptors (TLR) and induce DC to express high levels of surface CD40 and secrete high levels of IL-12. IL-12 enhances CD40L surface expression by T cells, which signals DC to activate NF-κB. Activated NF-κB leads to enhanced DC differentiation and IL-12 secretion, promoting CTL and Th1 T cells.

are internalized by immature DC. DC similarly internalize necrotic bodies, but these activate DC as a result of HSP-mediated signaling.[113] Phagocytes identify such targets using complement receptors, CD14, integrins (including αvβ3 and αvβ5, which can act in cooperation with CD36 and thrombospondin-l), scavenger receptor family members, or the recently described phosphatidylserine-specific receptor.[114]

DC Sense the Environment Using Receptors

The most abundant antigen receptors expressed by DC are C-type lectin family members that recognize glycosylated antigens. They include proteins expressed specifically by DC, such as DEC-205, and more ubiquitous receptors such as the mannose receptor (MMR). After recognition of oligosaccharides on the bacterial surface by the MMR, the constant domain of Ig and Ig-coated particles by Fc receptors, or the plasma membrane of apoptotic cells by scavenger receptors, phagocytosis is initiated.[115] The MMR mediates antigen capture, transport to endosomes and lysosomes, and efficient antigen presentation.[116] It is expressed by DC but not by LC. DEC-205 belongs to the same receptor family as the MMR. It is involved in antigen uptake as well as post-Ag uptake functions, but its antigen specificity is largely unknown.[117] However, targeting of antigen to the DEC-205 receptor in vivo can induce antigen-specific tolerance.[118]

Immature DC express complement receptors CR3 and CR4, but not CR1 and CR2.[119] Dermal DC, but not LC, express CD88, the C5a receptor, thereby allowing for the uptake of antigen coated with complement. DC-specific ICAM3-grabbing nonintegrin (DC-SIGN) and langerin are two type II lectins with mannose specificity, expressed by interstitial DC and LC, respectively.[120,121] The normal function of DC-SIGN is adhesive, in that it binds to ICAM-2 and 3, which is expressed by T cells or endothelial cells. Therefore, DC-SIGN plays a role in DC-T cell interactions and DC emigration from blood or lymph. Langerin induces the formation of a unique endocytic compartment of LC, the Birbeck granules.[120]

Downmodulation of antigen internalization by mature DC restricts the specificity of T cell stimulation to those antigens encountered in the periphery, where antigen is taken up. There are two mechanisms proposed. First, most antigen receptors, including FcR, MMR, DEC-205, and receptors for HSP and apoptotic bodies, are downregulated after induction of DC maturation. This decreased expression of antigen receptors by mature DC represents a first level of control of antigen uptake. Second, mature DC downregulate the endocytic process itself.

Consequences of DC Regulation for Antigen Presentation

RelB activity is required for myeloid DC differentiation.[122-124] In addition to the contact-dependent interaction between the DC and T cell, the cytokine environment plays a role in determining the outcome of an encounter between DC and T cells. Recent studies suggest a mechanism by which peripheral tolerance might be constitutively maintained by myeloid DC in which RelB activity and CD40 are either suppressed or not induced. Constitutive presentation of self antigen may occur by RelB^{-} DC draining from the periphery to LN in the absence of inflammation. At uninflamed sites of antigen uptake, myeloid immature DC lack RelB activity.[125] Furthermore, a proportion of unmanipulated DC in both the periphery and LN has been shown to express little, if any, CD40 constitutively and to rely upon infectious signals for CD40 induction and concomitant IL-12 production.[126] Therefore, in the absence of proinflammatory signals, myeloid DC may reach LN lacking RelB activity and cell surface CD40.[127] Thus, upstream signaling of DC by microbial antigens through TLR and other pattern recognition receptors, which lead to RelB nuclear translocation and CD40 induction, provides a key pathway for discrimination by the immune system of antigens loaded by myeloid peripheral tissue DC (see Fig. 7–8). DC that are capable of inducing T cell tolerance in LN are characterized by low to absent cell surface CD40-expression and nuclear RelB/p50 expression.[88] When presenting self antigens derived from somatic cells, it is proposed that these DC actively induce self antigen–specific regulatory T cells that contribute to the maintenance of peripheral tolerance.[128]

DC in Rheumatic Disease

Myeloid DC can be identified in freshly purified blood, synovial fluid, or synovial tissue cell suspensions of patients with RA, spondyloarthropathies, and gout.[129] Myeloid DC are three- to four-fold enriched in fresh synovial fluid or synovial tissue compared with the blood and are more differentiated than blood-DC precursors.[130,131] Synovial fluid DC and blood DC stimulate resting allogeneic T cells with equivalent efficacy and more efficiently than synovial fluid monocytes. However, synovial fluid DC are markedly more efficient simulators of autologous T cells in the absence of exogenous antigen.[130] DC-expressing markers of both differentiated and undifferentiated cells have been identified in RA synovial tissue. DC in perivascular, T cell–enriched areas of synovial tissue are characterized by expression of CD86, nuclear RelB, and CCR7 and are associated with cells expressing CCL19 and 21.[132-134] Of interest, ectopic expression of CCL19 is sufficient for formation of lymphoid tissue similar to that seen in rheumatoid synovial tissue.[135] In contrast, immature DC in the synovial lining and sublining layers are characterized by CCR6 expression and are associated with CCL20-expressing cells.[134]

In patients with SLE, PDC are reduced in blood and IFN-α-activated monocytes are effective APC in vitro.[136] It has been proposed that these monocyte-derived DC might efficiently capture apoptotic cells and nucleosomes present in SLE patients' blood and tissues.[137] IFN-α activates not only myeloid cells, including monocytes and myeloid DC, but also PDC themselves, which are enriched in the inflammatory site in SLE skin lesions.[138]

Follicular Dendritic Cells

Follicular dendritic cells (FDC) reside in germinal centers of B cell follicles of lymphoid organs. They have a cell body similar in size to a lymphocyte but are characterized by long, beaded dendritic processes. B cells with high affinity for antigen are formed in germinal centers, resulting in formation of memory B cells. In the follicles, proliferating antigen-specific B cells undergo somatic hypermutation of the variable parts of the Ig genes, giving rise to progeny with varying affinities of the B cell receptor (BcR) for antigen. FDC rescue high-affinity, germinal-center B cells from apoptotic cell death, thus supporting the differentiation of a high-affinity clone of memory B cells (Fig. 7–9). FDC differ from DC in that they neither internalize and process antigens, nor present antigens in the context of MHC class II. Rather, FDC present native antigens in the form of immune complexes on their surface as immune complex–coated bodies or "iccosomes." On the surface of FDC, immune complexes are associated with complement receptors 1 and 2 (CD35, CD21) and FcγRIIb.[139] These molecules are not unique to FDC. However, expression of the long-splice variant of CD21 does appear to be a specific FDC marker.[140] Germinal-center B cells express Fas, and Fas ligation accelerates apoptosis unless the B cells are in contact with FDC. FDC block apoptosis by supporting upregulation of the anti-apoptotic molecule cellular FLICE-like inhibitory protein (cFLIP) by B cells.[141] FDC attract B cells to the follicles through the secretion of the chemokine CXCL-13, which binds to the B cell receptor CXCR5.[12,142] B cells adhere to FDC by means of IgR/CD21, and integrin interactions.[143]

The cellular origin of FDC has not been characterized. There is evidence that this precursor may be BM-derived but also that it may have a mesenchymal origin. These possibilities are not mutually exclusive, especially because mesechymal precursors may have an origin in BM-derived stem cells and can traffic in the peripheral blood of infants and adults. Studies of mice deficient in the TNF and TNF-R families demonstrate the importance of TNF-α, lymphotoxin (LT)α_3, LT$\alpha_2\beta_1$, and TNF-R1 in the interaction between lymphocytes and the FDC precursor for the generation of the FDC network.[144] RelB, the same transcription factor critical for the differentiation of DC, also plays an important transcriptional role in FDC. RelB is present in the nucleus of a proportion of FDC in both normal lymph nodes and ectopic lymphoid tissue, including rheumatoid synovium. Consistent with its central role in the development of the lymph node structure, RelB-deficient mice completely lack lymph nodes. RelB is able to heterodimerize in the nucleus only with p50 or p52. Of interest, both RelB- and p52-deficient mice have impaired follicle formation, and FDC networks are defective after antigen challenge. Although expression of TNF/LT is only mildly affected, expression of CXCL-13 is strongly reduced in RelB-deficient spleen. Thus, activation of p52-RelB heterodimers downstream of TNF/LT is required for normal expression of homing chemokines and proper development of lymphoid organs. Considerable plasticity to the FDC network exists, as FDC networks disappear after administration of soluble LTβR, but reestablish upon cessation of treatment. Similarly, patients undergoing antiretroviral treatment for HIV infection can regenerate their FDC

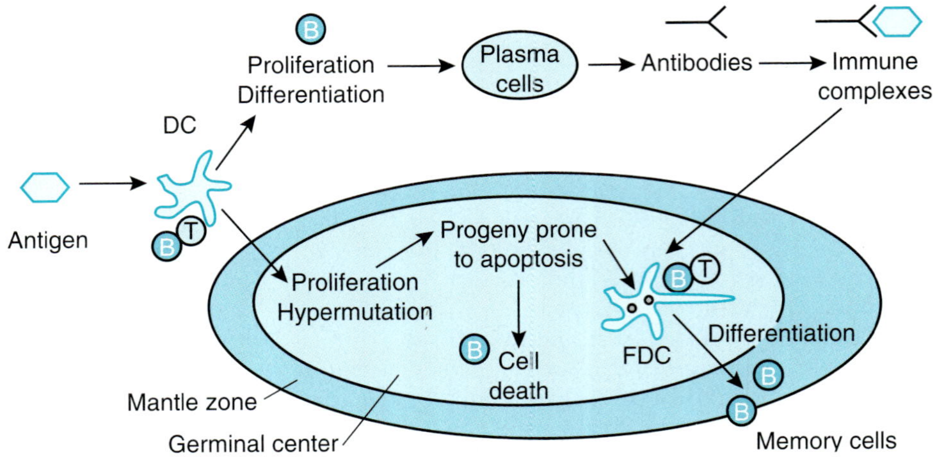

FIGURE 7–9 · **Role of Follicular Dendritic Cells (FDC) in the Germinal Center.** Antigen-specific B cell activation starts in the T cell area, as dendritic cells (DC) present antigen to T cells and interact with B cells. Some B cells differentiate into antibody-producing plasma cells. Resulting immune complexes are either cleared in the liver or trapped on the surface of FDC. In the germinal center, there is proliferation and somatic hypermutation of B cells. Only those B cells with high-affinity IgR bind the Ag presented by FDC, thereby preventing apoptosis.

network even after severe dysfunction and follicular involution in advanced disease.[145]

Human FDC bear similarities to fibroblasts. Furthermore, there is evidence that FDC develop outside secondary lymphoid organs at sites of chronic inflammation, such as in the thyroid in Hashimoto's thyroiditis, in salivary glands in Sjögren's syndrome, and in rheumatoid synovial tissue. In RA, these FDC express the long form of CD21 and chemoattract B cells through secretion of CXCL-13. The likely scenario is that local high levels of TNF-α and LT have contributed to the differentiation of FDC from either fibroblast or blood-borne precursors in situ. Of relevance, synovial fibroblast cell lines can be induced to differentiate into cells with FDC-like characteristics and function, including inhibition of B cell apoptosis.[146-148] Characteristic FDC markers can be induced in some lines in the presence of TNF-α or IL-1 in vitro.[149] Taken together, the data suggest that products and contact mechanisms derived from lymphocytes at inflammatory sites may drive the differentiation of FDC from fibroblasts.

Concluding Remarks

From lymphoid-organ DC to osteoclasts, brain microglia, and Kupffer cells, the evolutionarily ancient mononuclear phagocyte system illustrates the remarkable diversity of phenotype and function resulting from the differentiation of myeloid precursors and monocytes in responses to environmental signals. Not only are these cells key to the maintenance of self-recognition and host defense, but they also play a critical role in the pathology of inflammatory diseases.

REFERENCES

1. Karnovsky ML: Metchnikoff in Messina: a century of studies on phagocytosis. N Engl J Med 304:1178, 1981.
2. van Furth R: A proposed new classification of macrophages, monocytes and their precursor cells. Nat New Biol 240:65, 1972.
3. Lewis D, Harriman GR: Cells and tissues of the immune system *In* Rich R, Fleisher T, Kotzin B, Schroeder Jr H (eds): Clinical Immunology: Principles and Practice, 2nd ed. St. Louis, Mosby, 2001, 2.1.
4. Gordon S, Cohn ZA: The macrophage. Int Rev Cytol 36:171, 1973.
5. Oppenheimer-Marks N, Lipsky PE: Adhesion molecules as targets for the treatment of autoimmune diseases. Clin Immunol Immunopathol 79:203, 1996.
6. Mojcik CF, Shevach EM: Adhesion molecules: a rheumatologic perspective. Arthritis Rheum 40:991, 1997.
7. Hoczarenko M, Campbell JJ, Silberstein LE: Chemokines and Chemokine Receptors. *In* Rich R, Fleisher T, Kotzin B, Schroeder Jr H (eds): Clinical Immunology. Principles and Practice, 2nd ed., St. Louis, Mosby, 2001, 13.1.
8. Salmon JE, Pricop L: Human receptors for immunoglobulin G: key elements in the pathogenesis of rheumatic disease. Arthritis Rheum 44:739, 2001.
9. Bharadwaj D, Stein MP, Volzer M, et al: The major receptor for C-reactive protein on leukocytes is Fcgamma receptor II. J Exp Med 190:585, 1999.
10. Stein MP, Edberg JC, Kimberly RP, et al: C-reactive protein binding to FcgammaRIIa on human monocytes and neutrophils is allele-specific. J Clin Invest 105:369, 2000.
11. Gershov D, Kim S, Brot N, et al: C-Reactive protein binds to apoptotic cells, protects the cells from assembly of the terminal complement components, and sustains an antiinflammatory innate immune response: implications for systemic autoimmunity. J Exp Med 192:1353, 2000.
12. Legler DF, Loetscher M, Roos RS, et al: B cell-attracting chemokine 1, a human CXC chemokine expressed in lymphoid tissues, selectively attracts B lymphocytes via BLR1/CXCR5. J Exp Med 187:655, 1998.
13. Pue CA, Mortensen RF, Marsh CB, et al: Acute phase levels of C-reactive protein enhance IL-1 beta and IL-1ra production by human blood monocytes but inhibit IL-1 beta and IL-1ra production by alveolar macrophages. J Immunol 156:1594, 1996.
14. Holers VM: Complement. *In* Rich R, Fleisher T, Kotzin B, Schroeder Jr H (eds): Clinical Immunology: Principles and Practice, 2nd ed. St. Louis, Mosby, 2001, 21.1.
15. Shushakova N, Skokowa J, Schulman J, et al: C5a anaphylatoxin is a major regulator of activating versus inhibitory FcgammaRs in immune complex-induced lung disease. J Clin Invest 110:1823, 2002.
16. Grant EP, Picarella D, Burwell T, et al: Essential role for the C5a receptor in regulating the effector phase of synovial infiltration and joint destruction in experimental arthritis. J Exp Med 196:1461, 2002.
17. Smith PD, Smythies LE, Wahl SM: Macrophage effector function *In* Rich R, Fleischer B, Kotzin B, Schroeder Jr H (eds): Clinical Immunology: Principles and Practice, 2nd ed. St. Louis, Mosby, 2001, 19.1.
18. Rigotti A, Acton SL, Krieger M: The class B scavenger receptors SR-BI and CD36 are receptors for anionic phospholipids. J Biol Chem 270:16221, 1995.

19. Aderem A, Underhill DM: Mechanisms of phagocytosis in macrophages. Annu Rev Immunol 17:593, 1999.
20. Swanson JA, Baer SC: Phagocytosis by zippers and triggers. Trends Cell Biol 5:89, 1995.
21. Fadok VA, Bratton DL, Konowal A, et al: Macrophages that have ingested apoptotic cells in vitro inhibit proinflammatory cytokine production through autocrine/paracrine mechanisms involving TGF-beta, PGE2, and PAF. J Clin Invest 101:890, 1998.
22. Taylor PR, Carugati A, Fadok VA, et al: A hierarchical role for classical pathway complement proteins in the clearance of apoptotic cells in vivo. J Exp Med 192:359, 2000.
23. Rappolee DA, Werb Z: Secretory products of phagocytes. Curr Opin Immunol 1:47, 1988.
24. Nathan CF, Murray HW, Cohn ZA: The macrophage as an effector cell. N Engl J Med 303:622, 1980.
25. Rodgers JR, Rich R: Antigens and antigen presentation *In* Rich R, Fleisher T, Kotzin B, Schroeder Jr H (eds): Clinical Immunology: Principles and Practice, 2nd ed. St. Louis, Mosby, 2001, 7.1.
26. Dempsey PW, Allison ME, Akkaraju S, et al: C3d of complement as a molecular adjuvant: bridging innate and acquired immunity. Science 271:348, 1996.
27. Burmester GR, Stuhlmuller B, Keyszer G, et al: Mononuclear phagocytes and rheumatoid synovitis: mastermind or workhorse in arthritis? Arthritis Rheum 40:5, 1997.
28. Kinne RW, Brauer R, Stuhlmuller B, et al: Macrophages in rheumatoid arthritis. Arthritis Res 2:189, 2000.
29. Firestein GS, Zvaifler NJ: How important are T cells in chronic rheumatoid synovitis? II. T cell-independent mechanisms from beginning to end. Arthritis Rheum 46:298, 2002.
30. Kotake S, Udagawa N, Hakoda M, et al: Activated human T cells directly induce osteoclastogenesis from human monocytes: possible role of T cells in bone destruction in rheumatoid arthritis patients. Arthritis Rheum 44:1003, 2001.
31. Pettit AR, Ji H, von Stechow D, et al: TRANCE/RANKL knockout mice are protected from bone erosion in a serum transfer model of arthritis. Am J Pathol 159:1689, 2001.
32. Steinman RM, Cohn ZA: Identification of a novel cell type in peripheral lymphoid organs of mice. I. Morphology, quantitation, tissue distribution. J Exp Med 137:1142, 1973.
33. Liu YJ, Kanzler H, Soumelis V, et al: Dendritic cell lineage, plasticity and cross-regulation. Nat Immunol 2:585, 2001.
34. Grabbe S, Kampgen E, Schuler G: Dendritic cells: multi-lineal and multi-functional. Immunol Today 21:431, 2000.
35. Sallusto F, Lanzavecchia A, Mackay CR: Chemokines and chemokine receptors in T-cell priming and Th1/Th2-mediated responses. Immunol Today 19:568, 1998.
36. Banchereau J, Steinman RM: Dendritic cells and the control of immunity. Nature 392:245, 1998.
37. O'Sullivan B, Thomas R: CD40 and dendritic cell function. Crit Rev Immunol 23: 83, 2003.
38. Banchereau J, Briere F, Caux C, et al: Immunobiology of dendritic cells. Annu Rev Immunol 18:767, 2000.
39. Austyn JM: Dendritic cells. Curr Opin Hematol 5:3, 1998.
40. Thomas R, Davis LS, Lipsky PE: Isolation and characterization of human peripheral blood dendritic cells. J Immunol 150:821, 1993.
41. Thomas R, Lipsky PE: Human peripheral blood dendritic cell subsets: isolation and characterization of precursor and mature antigen-presenting cells. J Immunol 153:4016, 1994.
42. O'Doherty U, Peng M, Gezelter S, et al: Human blood contains two subsets of dendritic cells, one immunologically mature and the other immature. Immunology 82:487, 1994.
43. Ho CS, Lopez JA, Vuckovic S, et al: Surgical and physical stress increases circulating blood dendritic cell counts independently of monocyte counts. Blood 98:140, 2001.
44. Reid CD: The dendritic cell lineage in haemopoiesis. Br J Haematol 96:217, 1997.
45. Caux C, Vanbervliet B, Massacrier C, et al: $CD34^+$ hematopoietic progenitors from human cord blood differentiate along two independent dendritic cell pathways in response to GM-CSF and TNFα. J Exp Med 184:695, 1996.
46. Strunk D, Rappersberger E, C., Strobl H, et al: Generation of human dendritic cells/Langerhans cells from circulating $CD34^+$ hematopoietic progenitor cells. Blood 87:1292, 1996.
47. Sasmono RT, Oceandy D, Pollard JW, et al: A macrophage colony-stimulating factor receptor-green fluorescent protein transgene is expressed throughout the mononuclear phagocyte system of the mouse. Blood 101:1155, 2003.
48. O'Keeffe M, Hochrein H, Vremec D, et al: Effects of administration of progenipoietin 1, Flt-3 ligand, granulocyte colony-stimulating factor, and pegylated granulocyte-macrophage colony-stimulating factor on dendritic cell subsets in mice. Blood 99: 2122, 2002.
49. Sallusto F, Lanzavecchia A: Efficient presentation of soluble antigen by cultured human dendritic cells is maintained by granulocyte/macrophage colony-stimulating factor plus interleukin 4 and downregulated by tumor necrosis factor alpha. J Exp Med 179:1109, 1994.
50. Palucka KA, Taquet N, Sanchez-Chapuis F, et al: Dendritic cells as the terminal stage of monocyte differentiation. J Immunol 160:4587, 1998.
51. Izon D, Rudd K, DeMuth W, et al: A common pathway for dendritic cell and early B cell development. J Immunol 167:1387, 2001.
52. Vremec D, Pooley J, Hochrein H, et al: CD4 and CD8 expression by dendritic cell subtypes in mouse thymus and spleen. J Immunol 164:2978, 2000.
53. Nakano H, Yanagita M, Gunn MD: CD11c(+)B220(+)Gr-1(+) cells in mouse lymph nodes and spleen display characteristics of plasmacytoid dendritic cells. J Exp Med 194:1171, 2001.
54. De Smedt T, Pajak B, Muraille E, et al: Regulation of dendritic cell numbers and maturation by lipopolysaccharide in vivo. J Exp Med 184:1413, 1996.
55. Vremec D, Zorbas M, Scollay R, et al: The surface phenotype of dendritic cells purified from mouse thymus and spleen: investigation of the CD8 expression by a subpopulation of dendritic cells. J Exp Med 176:47, 1992.
56. del Hoyo GM, Martin P, Vargas HH, et al: Characterization of a common precursor population for dendritic cells. Nature 415:1043, 2002.
57. Turnbull E, MacPherson G: Immunobiology of dendritic cells in the rat. Immunol Rev 184:58, 2001.
58. Hochrein H, Shortman K, Vremec D, et al: Differential production of IL-12, IFN-alpha, and IFN-gamma by mouse dendritic cell subsets. J Immunol 166:5448, 2001.
59. Mason N, Aliberti J, Caamano JC, et al: Cutting edge: identification of c-Rel-dependent and -independent pathways of IL-12 production during infectious and inflammatory stimuli. J Immunol 168:2590, 2002.
60. Edwards AD, Manickasingham SP, Sporri R, et al: Microbial recognition via Toll-like receptor-dependent and -independent pathways determines the cytokine response of murine dendritic cell subsets to CD40 triggering. J Immunol 169:3652, 2002.
61. O'Doherty U, Steinman RM, Peng M, et al: Dendritic cells freshly isolated from human blood express CD4 and mature into typical immunostimulatory dendritic cells after culture in monocyte-conditioned medium. J Exp Med 178:1067, 1993.
62. Cella M, Jarrossay D, Facchetti F, et al: Plasmacytoid monocytes migrate to inflamed lymph nodes and produce large amounts of type I interferon [see comments]. Nat Med 5:919, 1999.
63. Grouard G, Rissoan MC, Filgueira L, et al: The enigmatic plasmacytoid T cells develop into dendritic cells with interleukin (IL)-3 and CD40-ligand. J Exp Med 185:1101, 1997.
64. Siegal FP, Kadowaki N, Shodell M, et al: The nature of the principal type 1 interferon-producing cells in human blood [see comments]. Science 284:1835, 1999.
65. Rossi G, Heveker N, Thiele B, et al: Development of a Langerhans cell phenotype from peripheral blood monocytes. Immunol Lett 31:189, 1992.
66. Borkowski TA, Letterio JJ, Farr AG, et al: A role for endogenous transforming growth factor β1 in Langerhans cell biology: the skin of transforming growth factor β1 null mice is devoid of epidermal Langerhans cells. J Exp Med 184:2417, 1996.
67. Winzler C, Rovere P, Rescigno M, et al: Maturation stages of mouse dendritic cells in growth factor-dependent long-term cultures. J Exp Med 185:317, 1997.
68. Sozzani S, Allavena P, G DA, et al: Differential regulation of chemokine receptors during dendritic cell maturation: a model for their trafficking properties. J Immunol 161:1083, 1998.

69. Gunn MD, Tangemann K, Tam C, et al: A chemokine expressed in lymphoid high endothelial venules promotes the adhesion and chemotaxis of naive T lymphocytes. Proc Natl Acad Sci U S A 95:258, 1998.
70. Muzio M, Mantovani A: Toll-like receptors (TLRs) signalling and expression pattern. J Endotoxin Res 7:297, 2001.
71. Ohshima Y, Tanaka Y, Tozawa H, et al: Expression and function of OX40 ligand on human dendritic cells. J Immunol 159:3838, 1997.
72. Regnault A, Lankar D, Lacabanne V, et al: Fcγ receptor-mediated induction of dendritic cell maturation and major histocompatibility complex class I-restricted antigen presentation after immune complex internalization. J Exp Med 189:371, 1999.
73. Sauter B, Albert ML, Francisco L, et al: Consequences of cell death: exposure to necrotic tumor cells, but not primary tissue cells or apoptotic cells, induces the maturation of immunostimulatory dendritic cells. J Exp Med 191:423, 2000.
74. Basu S, Binder RJ, Ramalingam T, et al: CD91 is a common receptor for heat shock proteins gp96, hsp90, hsp70, and calreticulin. Immunity 14:303, 2001.
75. Wang Y, Kelly CG, Karttunen JT, et al: CD40 is a cellular receptor mediating mycobacterial heat shock protein 70 stimulation of CC-chemokines. Immunity 15:971, 2001.
76. Josien R, Li HL, Ingulli E, et al: TRANCE, a tumor necrosis factor family member, enhances the longevity and adjuvant properties of dendritic cells in vivo. J Exp Med 191:495, 2000.
77. Ghosh S, May MJ, Kopp EB: NF-kappa B and Rel proteins: evolutionarily conserved mediators of immune responses. Annu Rev Immunol 16:225, 1998.
78. Garceau N, Kosaka Y, Masters S, et al: Lineage-restricted function of nuclear factor kappaB-inducing kinase (NIK) in transducing signals via CD40. J Exp Med 191:381, 2000.
79. Aicher A, Shu GL, Magaletti D, et al: Differential role for p38 mitogen-activated protein kinase in regulating CD40-induced gene expression in dendritic cells and B cells. J Immunol 163:5786, 1999.
80. Rescigno M, Martino M, Sutherland CL, et al: Dendritic cell survival and maturation are regulated by different signaling pathways. J Exp Med 188:2175, 1998.
81. Ardeshna KM, Pizzey AR, Devereux S, et al: The PI3 kinase, p38 SAP kinase, and NF-kappaB signal transduction pathways are involved in the survival and maturation of lipopolysaccharide-stimulated human monocyte-derived dendritic cells. Blood 96:1039, 2000.
82. Arrighi JF, Rebsamen M, Rousset F, et al: A critical role for p38 mitogen-activated protein kinase in the maturation of human blood-derived dendritic cells induced by lipopolysaccharide, TNF-alpha, and contact sensitizers. J Immunol 166:3837, 2001.
83. Saccani S, Pantano S, Natoli G: p38-Dependent marking of inflammatory genes for increased NF-kappa B recruitment. Nat Immunol 3:69, 2002.
84. O'Sullivan BJ, Thomas R: CD40 Ligation conditions dendritic cell antigen-presenting function through sustained activation of NF-kappaB. J Immunol 168:5491, 2002.
85. Tsukamoto N, Kobayashi N, Azuma S, et al: Two differently regulated nuclear factor kappaB activation pathways triggered by the cytoplasmic tail of CD40. Proc Natl Acad Sci U S A 96:1234, 1999.
86. Pullen SS, Dang TT, Crute JJ, et al: CD40 signaling through tumor necrosis factor receptor-associated factors (TRAFs): binding site specificity and activation of downstream pathways by distinct TRAFs. J Biol Chem 274:14246, 1999.
87. Tone M, Tone Y, Babik JM, et al: The role of Sp1 and NF-kappa B in regulating CD40 gene expression. J Biol Chem 277:8890, 2002.
88. Martin E, O'Sullivan BJ, Low P, et al: Antigen-specific suppression of a primed immune response by dendritic cells mediated by regulatory T cells secreting interleukin-10. Immunity 18:155, 2003.
89. O'Sullivan BJ, MacDonald KP, Pettit AR, et al: RelB nuclear translocation regulates B cell MHC molecule, CD40 expression, and antigen-presenting cell function. Proc Natl Acad Sci U S A 97:11421, 2000.
90. Bouchon A, Hernandez-Munain C, Cella M, et al: A DAP12-mediated pathway regulates expression of CC chemokine receptor 7 and maturation of human dendritic cells. J Exp Med 194:1111, 2001.
91. Hilkens CM, Kalinski P, de Boer M, et al: Human dendritic cells require exogenous interleukin-12-inducing factors to direct the development of naive T-helper cells toward the Th1 phenotype. Blood 90:1920, 1997.
92. Buelens C, Willems F, Delvaux A, et al: Interleukin-10 differentially regulates B7-1 (CD80) and B7-2 (CD86) expression on human peripheral blood dendritic cells. Eur J Immunol 25:2668, 1995.
93. Steinbrink K, Jonuleit H, Muller G, et al: Interleukin-10-treated human dendritic cells induce a melanoma-antigen-specific anergy in CD8(+) T cells resulting in a failure to lyse tumor cells. Blood 93:1634, 1999.
94. Steinbrink K, Wolfl M, Jonuleit H, et al: Induction of tolerance by IL-10-treated dendritic cells. J Immunol 159:4772, 1997.
95. Schottelius AJ, Mayo MW, Sartor RB, et al: Interleukin-10 signaling blocks inhibitor of kappaB kinase activity and nuclear factor kappaB DNA binding. J Biol Chem 274:31868, 1999.
96. Lanzavecchia A, Sallusto F: Regulation of T cell immunity by dendritic cells. Cell 106:263, 2001.
97. Kalinski P, Hilkens CM, Wierenga EA, et al: T-cell priming by type-1 and type-2 polarized dendritic cells: the concept of a third signal. Immunol Today 20:561, 1999.
98. Porgador A, Gilboa E: Bone marrow-generated dendritic cells pulsed with a class I-restricted peptide are potent inducers of cytotoxic T lymphocytes. J Exp Med 182:255, 1995.
99. Moser M, Murphy KM: Dendritic cell regulation of TH1-TH2 development. Nat Immunol 1:199, 2000.
100. Langenkamp A, Messi M, Lanzavecchia A, et al: Kinetics of dendritic cell activation: impact on priming of TH1, TH2 and nonpolarized T cells. Nat Immunol 1:311, 2000.
101. Shortman K, Heath WR: Immunity or tolerance? That is the question for dendritic cells. Nat Immunol 2:988, 2001.
102. Cella M, Scheidegger D, Palmer Lehmann K, et al: Ligation of CD40 on dendritic cells triggers production of high levels of interleukin-12 and enhances T cell stimulatory capacity: T-T help via APC activation. J Exp Med 184:747, 1996.
103. Peng X, Remacle JE, Kasran A, et al: IL-12 up-regulates CD40 ligand (CD154) expression on human T cells. J Immunol 160:1166, 1998.
104. Braciale TJ, Morrison LA, Sweetser MT, et al: Antigen presentation pathways to class I and class II MHC-restricted T lymphocytes. Immunological Reviews 98:114, 1987.
105. Germain RN: MHC-dependent antigen processing and peptide presentation: providing ligands for T lymphocyte activation. Cell 76:287, 1994.
106. Chesnut RW, Grey HM: Studies on the capacity of B cells to serve as antigen-presenting cells. J Immunol 126:1075, 1981.
107. Ziegler K, Unanue ER: Identification of a macrophage antigen-processing event required for I-region-restricted antigen presentation to T lymphocytes. J Immunol 127:1869, 1981.
108. Townsend AR, Gotch FM, Davey J: Cytotoxic T cells recognize fragments of the influenza nucleoprotein. Cell 42:457, 1985.
109. Moreno J, Vignali DAA, Nadimi F, et al: Processing of an endogenous protein can generate MHC class II-restricted T cell determinants distinct from those derived from exogenous antigen. J Immunol 147:3306, 1991.
110. Albert ML, Sauter B, Bhardwaj N: Dendritic cells acquire antigen from apoptotic cells and induce class I-restricted CTLs. Nature 392:86, 1998.
111. d'Ostiani CF, Del Sero G, Bacci A, et al: Dendritic cells discriminate between yeasts and hyphae of the fungus *Candida albicans*: Implications for initiation of T helper cell immunity in vitro and in vivo. J Exp Med 191:1661, 2000.
112. Gorak PM, Engwerda CR, Kaye PM: Dendritic cells, but not macrophages, produce IL-12 immediately following *Leishmania donovani* infection. Eur J Immunol 28:687, 1998.
113. Subklewe M, Paludan C, Tsang ML, et al: Dendritic cells cross-present latency gene products from Epstein-Barr virus-transformed B cells and expand tumor-reactive CD8(+) killer T cells. J Exp Med 193:405, 2001.
114. Fadok VA, Chimini G: The phagocytosis of apoptotic cells. Semin Immunol 13:365, 2001.
115. Platt N, da Silva RP, Gordon S: Recognizing death: the phagocytosis of apoptotic cells. Trends Cell Biol 8:365, 1998.

116. Sallusto F, Cella M, Danieli C, et al: Dendritic cells use macropinocytosis and the mannose receptor to concentrate macromolecules in the major histocompatibility complex class II compartment: downregulation by cytokines and bacterial products. J Exp Med 182:389, 1995.
117. Jiang W, Swiggard WJ, Heufler C, et al: The receptor DEC-205 expressed by dendritic cells and thymic epithelial cells is involved in antigen processing. Nature 375:151, 1995.
118. Hawiger D, Inaba K, Dorsett Y, et al: Dendritic cells induce peripheral T cell unresponsiveness under steady state conditions in vivo. J Exp Med 194:769, 2001.
119. Reis E, Sousa C, Stahl PD, Austyn JM: Phagocytosis of antigens by Langerhans cells in vitro. J Exp.Med 178:509, 1993.
120. Valladeau J, Ravel O, Dezutter-Dambuyant C, et al: Langerin, a novel C-type lectin specific to Langerhans cells, is an endocytic receptor that induces the formation of Birbeck granules. Immunity 12:71, 2000.
121. Geijtenbeek TB, Torensma R, van Vliet SJ, et al: Identification of DC-SIGN, a novel dendritic cell-specific ICAM-3 receptor that supports primary immune responses. Cell 100:575, 2000.
122. Burkly L, Hession C, Ogata L, et al: Expression of relB is required for the development of thymic medulla and dendritic cells. Nature 373:531, 1995.
123. Weih F, Carrasco D, Durham SK, et al: Multiorgan inflammation and hematopoietic abnormalities in mice with a targeted disruption of RelB, a member of the NF-kappa B/Rel family. Cell 80:331, 1995.
124. Wu L, D'Amico A, Winkel KD, et al: RelB is essential for the development of myeloid-related CD8alpha-dendritic cells but not of lymphoid-related CD8alpha+ dendritic cells. Immunity 9:839, 1998.
125. Thompson AG, Pettit AR, Padmanabha J, et al: Nuclear RelB+ cells are found in normal lymphoid organs and in peripheral tissue in the context of inflammation, but not under normal resting conditions. Immunol Cell Biol 80:164, 2002.
126. Schulz O, Edwards DA, Schito M, et al: CD40 triggering of heterodimeric IL-12 p70 production by dendritic cells in vivo requires a microbial priming signal. Immunity 13:453, 2000.
127. Huang FP, Platt N, Wykes M, et al: A discrete subpopulation of dendritic cells transports apoptotic intestinal epithelial cells to T cell areas of mesenteric lymph nodes. J Exp Med 191:435, 2000.
128. Thompson AG, Thomas R: Induction of immune tolerance by dendritic cells: implications for preventative and therapeutic immunotherapy of autoimmune disease. Immunol Cell Biol 80:509, 2002.
129. Pettit AR, Ahern M, Zehntner S, et al: Comparison of differentiated dendritic cell infiltration of autoimmune and osteoarthritic synovial tissue. Arthritis Rheum 44:105, 2001.
130. Thomas R, Davis LS, Lipsky PE: Rheumatoid synovium is enriched in mature antigen-presenting dendritic cells. J Immunol 152:2613, 1994.
131. Bergroth V, Tsai V, Zvaifler NJ: Differences in responses of normal and rheumatoid arthritis peripheral blood T cells to synovial fluid and peripheral blood dendritic cells in allogeneic mixed leukocyte reactions. Arthritis Rheum 32:1381, 1989.
132. Thomas R, Quinn C: Functional differentiation of dendritic cells in rheumatoid arthritis: role of CD86 in the synovium. J Immunol 156:3074, 1996.
133. Pettit AR, MacDonald KPA, O'Sullivan B, et al: Differentiated dendritic cells expressing nuclear RelB are predominantly located in rheumatoid synovial tissue perivascular mononuclear cell aggregates. Arthritis Rheum 43:791, 2000.
134. Page G, Lebecque S, Miossec P: Anatomic localization of immature and mature dendritic cells in an ectopic lymphoid organ: correlation with selective chemokine expression in rheumatoid synovium. J Immunol 168:5333, 2002.
135. Fan L, Reilly CR, Luo Y, et al: Cutting edge: ectopic expression of the chemokine TCA4/SLC is sufficient to trigger lymphoid neogenesis. J Immunol 164:3955, 2000.
136. Blanco P, Palucka AK, Gill M, et al: Induction of dendritic cell differentiation by IFN-alpha in systemic lupus erythematosus. Science 294:1540, 2001.
137. Amoura Z, Piette JC, Chabre H, et al: Circulating plasma levels of nucleosomes in patients with systemic lupus erythematosus: correlation with serum antinucleosome antibody titers and absence of clear association with disease activity. Arthritis Rheum 40:2217, 1997.
138. Farkas L, Beiske K, Lund-Johansen F, et al: Plasmacytoid dendritic cells (natural interferon-alpha/beta-producing cells) accumulate in cutaneous lupus erythematosus lesions. Am J Pathol 159:237, 2001.
139. Tew JG, Wu J, Fakher M, et al: Follicular dendritic cells: beyond the necessity of T-cell help. Trends Immunol 22:361, 2001.
140. Liu YJ, Xu J, de Bouteiller O, et al: Follicular dendritic cells specifically express the long CR2/CD21 isoform. J Exp Med 185:165, 1997.
141. van Nierop K, de Groot C: Human follicular dendritic cells: function, origin and development. Semin Immunol 14:251, 2002.
142. Ansel KM, Ngo VN, Hyman PL, et al: A chemokine-driven positive feedback loop organizes lymphoid follicles. Nature 406:309, 2000.
143. Koopman G, Keehnen RM, Lindhout E, et al: Adhesion through the LFA-1 (CD11a/CD18)-ICAM-1 (CD54) and the VLA-4 (CD49d)-VCAM-1 (CD106) pathways prevents apoptosis of germinal center B cells. J Immunol 152:3760, 1994.
144. Futterer A, Mink K, Luz A, et al: The lymphotoxin beta receptor controls organogenesis and affinity maturation in peripheral lymphoid tissues. Immunity 9:59, 1998.
145. Zhang ZQ, Schuler T, Cavert W, et al: Reversibility of the pathological changes in the follicular dendritic cell network with treatment of HIV-1 infection. Proc Natl Acad Sci U S A 96:5169, 1999.
146. Shi K, Hayashida K, Kaneko M, et al: Lymphoid chemokine B cell-attracting chemokine-1 (CXCL13) is expressed in germinal center of ectopic lymphoid follicles within the synovium of chronic arthritis patients. J Immunol 166:650, 2001.
147. Shimaoka Y, Attrep JF, Hirano T, et al: Nurse-like cells from bone marrow and synovium of patients with rheumatoid arthritis promote survival and enhance function of human B cells. J Clin Invest 102:606, 1998.
148. Hayashida K, Shimaoka Y, Ochi T, et al: Rheumatoid arthritis synovial stromal cells inhibit apoptosis and up-regulate Bcl-xL expression by B cells in a CD49/CD29-CD106-dependent mechanism. J Immunol 164:1110, 2000.
149. Lindhout E, van Eijk M, van Pel M, et al: Fibroblast-like synoviocytes from rheumatoid arthritis patients have intrinsic properties of follicular dendritic cells. J Immunol 162:5949, 1999.
150. Cebon J, Davis I, Luft T, et al: Dendritic cells as recipients of cytokine signals. *In* Lotze MT, Thomson AW (eds): Dendritic Cells, 2nd ed. London, Academic Press, 2001.
151. Kalinski P, Lotze MT, Kapsenberg ML: Dendritic cell-related immunoregulation: signals and mediators. *In* Lotze MT, Thomson AW (eds): Dendritic Cells, 2nd ed. London, Academic Press, 2001.

8 Innate Immunity

STEVEN A. PORCELLI • CHARLES A. JANEWAY, JR.

It has become common practice in immunology to divide the mechanisms involved in host defense into adaptive and innate components (Table 8–1). A specific immune response, such as the production of antibodies or T cells against a particular pathogen, is referred to as *adaptive immunity* because it represents an adaptation that occurs during the lifetime of an individual as a result of exposure to that pathogen. Adaptive immune responses involve the clonal expansion of T and B lymphocytes bearing a large repertoire of somatically generated receptors that can be selected to recognize virtually any pathogen. The adaptive immune system of any given individual is profoundly molded by the immunologic challenges encountered by that individual during the course of a lifetime. A hallmark of adaptive immune responses is that they are highly specific for the triggering agent, and they provide the basis for immunologic memory, which allows increased resistance against future infection with the same pathogen.

Adaptive immunity is essential for the survival of all mammals and most other vertebrates, but a wide variety of other mechanisms that do not involve antigen-specific lymphocyte responses also are involved in successful immune protection. These diverse mechanisms are collectively known as *innate immunity* because they are not dependent on prior exposure to specific pathogens for their amplification. Such responses are controlled by the products of germline genes that are inherited and similarly expressed by all normal individuals. Innate immune mechanisms involve both consitutive and inducible components and use a wide variety of recognition and effector mechanisms. Importantly, it has become clear in recent years that innate immune responses have a profound influence on the generation and outcome of adaptive immune responses. This ability of the innate immune system to instruct the responses of the adaptive immune system suggests multiple ways in which innate immunity could influence the development of both long-term specific immunity and autoimmune diseases.

Evolutionary Origins of Innate Immunity

In spite of its obvious importance for most vertebrate organisms, the adaptive immune system is a relatively recent evolutionary development (Fig. 8–1). In fact, all invertebrate animals, and even some lower vertebrates, completely lack the ability to generate lymphocyte populations bearing large families of clonally diverse antigen receptors.[1,2] The ability to construct such receptors required the acquisition of a specialized recombination system that mediates the assembly of gene segments in the T cell and B cell receptor families, which most likely occurred as the result of the invasion of the genome of a primitive vertebrate by a transposable element or virus carrying this machinery.[3,4] This critical step in the evolution of the immune system can be traced back to the emergence of the ancestors of present day jawed fish because these represent the most primitive species on the earth today that are known to possess an adaptive immune response.[5]

In contrast, elements of innate immunity are believed to exist in all animals and plants and must have evolved with the earliest multicellular forms of life. In many cases, components of the innate immune system are significantly conserved in structure and function from the lowliest invertebrates all the way to the most complex vertebrates.[1] This preservation of innate immune mechanisms, with their functions largely intact, through such vast evolutionary distances is a clear indication of their importance, even in animals that have developed sophisticated adaptive immune responses.

Pathogen Recognition by the Innate Immune System

Some mechanisms of innate immunity are constitutive, meaning they are continuously expressed and not significantly modulated by the presence or absence of infection. Examples of this can be found in the barrier functions provided by epithelial surfaces that are continuously exposed to microbial flora, such as those of the skin and intestinal and genital tracts. In contrast, the inducible mechanisms of innate immunity involve the increased production of mediators and upregulation of effector functions that eliminate microorganisms. The induction occurs as a result of exposure to a wide variety of microbes and represents a less-specific form of immune recognition than is associated with specific antibodies and T cells that mediate adaptive immunity. The basic principle underlying this form of response is a process known as *pattern recognition*. This recognition strategy is based on the detection of commonly occurring and conserved molecular patterns that are essential products or structural components of microbes.

TABLE 8–1 • CONTRASTING FEATURES OF THE INNATE AND ADAPTIVE IMMUNE SYSTEMS*

Property	Innate Immune System	Adaptive Immune System
Receptors	Relatively few (~several hundred?) Fixed in genome Gene rearrangement not required	Many (potentially 10^{14} or more) Encoded in gene segments Gene rearrangement required
Distribution	Nonclonal All cells of a class identical	Clonal All cells of a class distinct
Targets	Conserved molecular patterns Lipopolysaccharides Lipoteichoic acids Glycans Others	Details of molecular structure Proteins Peptides Carbohydrates
Self–nonself discrimination	Perfect: selected over evolutionary time	Imperfect: selected in individual somatic cells
Action time	Immediate or rapid (seconds to hours)	Delayed (days to weeks)
Response	Microbicidal effector molecules Antimicrobial peptides Superoxide Nitric oxide Cytokines (IL-1, IL-6, others) Chemokines (IL-8, others)	Clonal expansion or anergy of specific T and B lymphocytes Cytokines (IL-2, IL-4, IFNγ, others) Specific antibody production Specific cytolytic T cell generation

*Adapted with slight modification from Medzhitov R, Janeway, CA Jr: Innate immune recognition. Annu Rev Immunol 20:197-216, 2002.)

PATHOGEN-ASSOCIATED MOLECULAR PATTERNS

The general name given to the targets of innate immune recognition is *pathogen-associated molecular patterns* (PAMPs). These are structural features or components distinctive for microorganisms and are not normally found in the animal host. The best known example of a PAMP is bacterial lipopolysaccharide (LPS), a ubiquitous glycolipid constituent of the outer membranes of gram-negative bacteria. Another important example is the peptidoglycan structure present as the basic cell-wall structure in nearly all bacteria. These structures may vary partially from one bacterium to another, but the basic elements are conserved, thus providing the possibility of recognizing a very broad array of pathogens by sensing a single or relatively small number of PAMPs. Many PAMPs that serve as targets of recognition for the innate immune response are now known to be associated with bacteria, fungi, and viruses.

Pattern-Recognition Receptors

The recognition of PAMPs is mediated by a collection of germline encoded molecules known collectively as *pattern-recognition receptors* (PRRs) (Table 8–2). These receptors are host proteins that have evolved, through many millions of years of natural selection, to have defined specificities for particular PAMPs expressed by microorganisms. The total number of PRRs present in complex vertebrates such as humans is estimated to be several hundred, a number limited by the size of the genome of any animal and the number of genes it can dedicate to immune protection. The human genome, for example, is estimated to contain approximately 30,000 genes, most of which are not related directly to the immune system. This demonstrates one of the strong points of contrast between the innate and adaptive immune systems because the latter can possess in the range of 10^{14} or more different somatically generated receptors for foreign antigens in the form of antibodies and T cell receptors. With its much more limited array of receptors, the innate immune system uses the strategy of targeting highly conserved PAMPs that are shared broadly by large classes of microorganisms. Because most pathogens contain PAMPs, this strategy allows the generation of at least partial immunity against most infections.

PRRs are expressed by many cell types, some of which are specialized effector cells of the immune system (e.g., neutrophils, macrophages, dendritic cells, lymphocytes) and some that are not generally regarded as part of the immune system (e.g., epithelial and endothelial cells). Unlike the T and B cell receptors used for adaptive immune recognition, the expression of PRRs is not clonal, which means all of the receptors displayed by a given cell type (e.g., macrophages) have identical structure and specificity. When PRRs are engaged by recognition of their associated PAMPs, effector cells bearing the PRRs are triggered to perform their immune-effector functions immediately, rather than after undergoing proliferation and expansion, as in the case of adaptive immune responses. This accounts for the much more rapid onset of innate immune responses.

In recent years, considerable progress has been made toward identifying many of the important PRRs involved in the induction of innate immunity. These receptors can be classified into three functional classes: secreted, endocytic, and signaling PRRs (see Table 8–2). In addition, many of the known PRRs can be classified into structurally defined families on the basis of a few characteristic protein domains. Among these, the best known include proteins with calcium-dependent lectin domains, scavenger receptor domains, and leucine-rich repeat domains.

PRRs of the Lectin Family

Calcium-dependent lectin domains are common modules of secreted and membrane-bound proteins involved

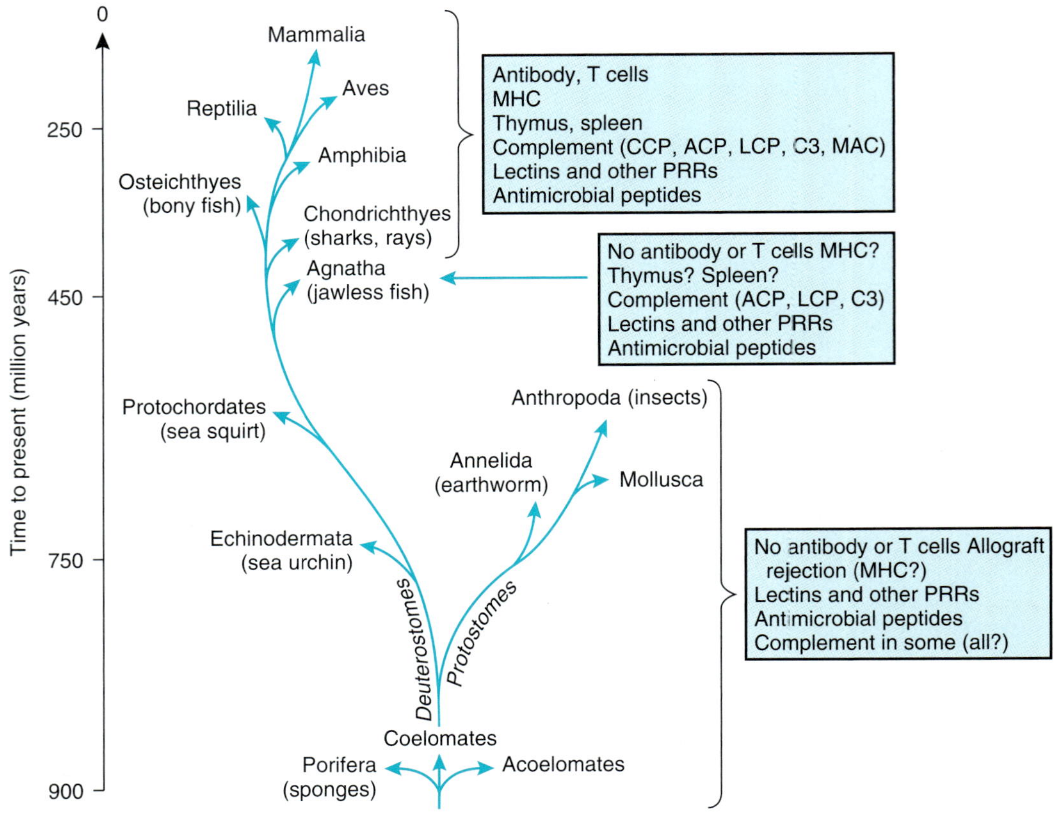

FIGURE 8–1 · **Ancient Evolutionary Origin of the Innate Immune System.** Studies of the immune systems of a wide range of vertebrates and invertebrates have revealed that even the most primitive invertebrates possess many components of innate immunity (e.g., pattern-recognition receptors of the lectin and toll-like families, antimicrobial peptides, and complement proteins). The innate immune system is thus extremely ancient, having arisen early in the evolution of multicellular life. In contrast, the adaptive immune system is a much more recent development, which did not appear until the emergence of the ancestors of present day sharks and rays, approximately 400 million years ago. The first species to acquire an adaptive immune system must have arisen after the appearance of the direct ancestors of present day jawless fish (lampreys and hagfish), which are the most highly evolved living species that seem to lack all elements of adaptive immunity (*arrow*). ACP, alternative complement pathway; CCP, classical complement pathway; MAC, membrane attack complex; MHC, major histocompatibility complex; LCP, lectin-activated complement pathway. (Adapted from Sunyer JO, Zarkadis IK, Lambris JD: Complement diversity: a mechanism for generating immune diversity? Immunol Today 19:519, 1998.)

in the binding of carbohydrate structures. A well-characterized PRR belonging to this class is the mannan-binding lectin (MBL), also known as soluble mannose binding protein, which represents a secreted PRR that functions in the initiation of the complement cascade (Fig. 8–2).[6,7] This protein is synthesized primarily in the liver on a constitutive basis, although its production can be increased as an acute-phase reactant following many types of infections. MBL binds to carbohydrates on the outer membranes and capsules of many bacteria,[8-10] as well as fungi,[11] and some viruses[12,13] and parasites.[14] Although mannose and fucose sugars bound by MBL can also be found on the surfaces of normal mammalian cells, these are present at too low a density or in the wrong orientation to efficiently engage the lectin domains of MBL. In contrast, the coats of many microorganisms contain an array of these sugars that allows strong binding of MBL. Thus, in this case, the spacing and orientation of specific carbohydrate residues comprise the PAMP that triggers activation of innate immunity by MBL. The MBL functions as one of a small number of secreted PRRs that can initiate the lectin pathway of complement activation. At least two other soluble proteins with lectin activity in human plasma, known as ficolins (ficolin/P35 and H-ficolin), can also activate this pathway following their interaction with bacterial polysaccharides.[15]

Several of the soluble lectin-type PRRs are also known to play an important role in opsonization of microbes by binding to their surfaces and directing them to receptors on phagocytic cells. Among these are the pulmonary surfactant proteins (SP), SP-A and SP-D, which similarly recognize and bind to the surface-sugar codes of microbes in the respiratory tract.[16-18] These molecules are similar in structure to MBL, having both collagen-like and lectin domains, and together they comprise a family of soluble PRRs known as collectins.[17] Another family of soluble PRRs that performs a similar function in plasma is the pentraxins, so called because they are formed by association of five identical protein subunits.[19] This family includes the acute-phase reactants C-reactive protein (CRP) and serum amyloid P protein (SAP)[19,20]

TABLE 8–2 • PATTERN RECOGNITION RECEPTORS (PRRS)

Receptor Class	Examples	Prominent Sites of Expression	Major Ligands	Function
Secreted PRRs	Collectins Mannan-binding lectin Ficolins Surfactant proteins (SP-A, SP-B) Short pentraxins (CRP, SAP) Long pentraxins	Plasma	Carbohydrate arrays typical of bacterial capsules, fungi, and other microbes Apoptotic cells and cellular debris including chromatin	Complement activation Opsonization
Endocytic PRRs	Lectin-family receptors Macrophage mannose receptor DEC-205 Dectin-1 Scavenger receptor A MARCO Complement receptors CD11b/CD18 (CR3) CD21/35 (CR2/1)	Macrophages, dendritic cells, some endothelia, epithelia, and smooth muscle cells	Cell-wall polysaccharides (mannans and glucans), LPS, LTA, and opsonized cells and particles	Pathogen uptake by phagocytes Delivery of ligands to antigen-processing compartments Clearance of cellular and extracellular debris
Signaling PRRs	Toll-like receptors NOD proteins	Macrophages, dendritic cells, epithelia	Multiple conserved pathogen-associated molecular patterns (LPS, LTA, dsRNA, lipoproteins, flagellin, bacterial DNA, others)	Activation of inducible innate immunity (antimicrobial peptides, cytokines, reactive oxygen/nitrogen intermediates) Instruction of adaptive immune response

Abbreviations: CR2/1, complement receptors 2 and 1; CR3, complement receptor 3; CRP, C-reactive protein; DEC-205, dendritic and epithelial cells, 205 kDalton; dsRNA, double-stranded RNA; LPS, lipopolysaccharide; LTA, lipoteichoic acid; MARCO, macrophage receptor with collagenous structure; NOD, nucleotide-binding oligomerization domain; SAP, serum amyloid P protein; SP-A, surfactant protein A; SP-B, surfactant protein B.

and also a number of so-called long pentraxins, which have an extended polypeptide structure with homology to the classic short pentraxins (i.e., CRP and SAP) only at their carboxy-terminal domains.[21,22] Long pentraxins are expressed in a variety of different tissues and cells, and their functions are mostly unknown. However, the long pentraxin PTX3 has been shown to play an important nonredundant role in resistance to fungal infections in mice, indicating that at least some of these proteins are involved in innate immunity.[23]

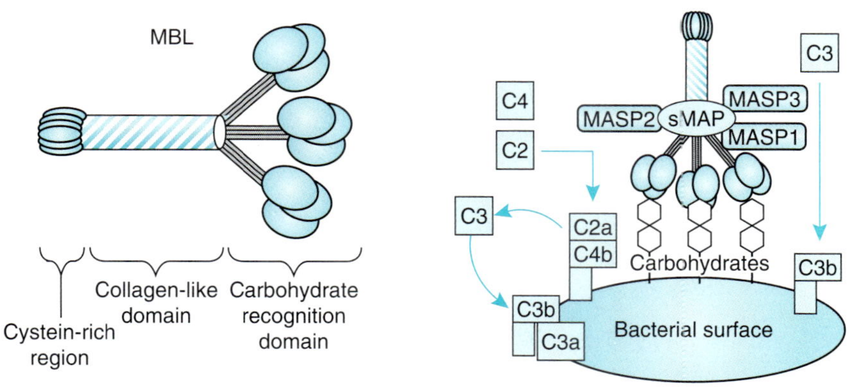

FIGURE 8–2 • **Structure and Function of Mannan-Binding Lectin (MBL), an Example of a Soluble Pattern-Recognition Receptor.** *Left:* MBL is a multimer protein structure with multiple carbohydrate-binding lectin domains. Three identical 32- kDa polypeptides associate to form a subunit, which then oligomerize to form functional complexes (the trimeric form consisting of three subunits is illustrated, which is one of several different oligomer sizes that has been observed for MBL). Each polypeptide in the subunit contains an N-terminal cysteine-rich domain, a collagen-like domain, a neck region, and a C-terminal carbohydrate-recognition domain. *Right:* Initiation of the lectin pathway for complement activation by MBL. The carbohydrate-recognition domains of MBL bind to carbohydrates that are characteristic of bacterial surfaces. This leads to the recruitment of several other serum proteins, including small MBL-associated protein (sMAP), and the three MBL-associated serine proteases (MASP1, MASP2, MASP3). The protease activity of MASP2 cleaves complement C4 and C2 subunits, generating the C3 convertase (C4bC2a). MASP1 is able to cleave C3 directly. The deposit of C3 cleavage products on the bacterial surface results in opsonization and phagocytosis of the bacterial cell.

In addition to these soluble proteins, a large number of membrane-bound glycoproteins with lectin domains are known to exist, and some of these participate in innate immunity by serving as endocytic PRRs for the uptake of microbes or microbial products (Fig. 8–3). One of the most extensively studied of these is the macrophage mannose receptor (MMR).[24] Although originally identified on alveolar macrophages and known to be expressed on macrophage subsets throughout the body, this receptor is also expressed on a variety of other cell types including certain endothelia, epithelia, and smooth muscle cells. The MMR is a membrane-anchored, multilectin domain-containing protein that mediates the binding of a broad range of pathogens, leading to their internalization via endocytosis and phagocytosis.[6,25-27] Although the major function of the MMR appears to be directing uptake of its ligands, there is also evidence that this receptor may be capable of signaling to modify macrophage functions following receptor engagement.[28]

PRRs of the Scavenger Receptor Family

The scavenger receptor family contains a broad range of cell-surface proteins that are expressed most prominently on macrophages, dendritic cells, and endothelial cells[29,30] (see Fig. 8–3). Although they were defined originally by their ability to bind and take up modified serum lipoproteins, they also bind a wide range of other ligands that include bacteria and some of their associated products. Two members of this family that have been implicated as PRRs for innate immunity are

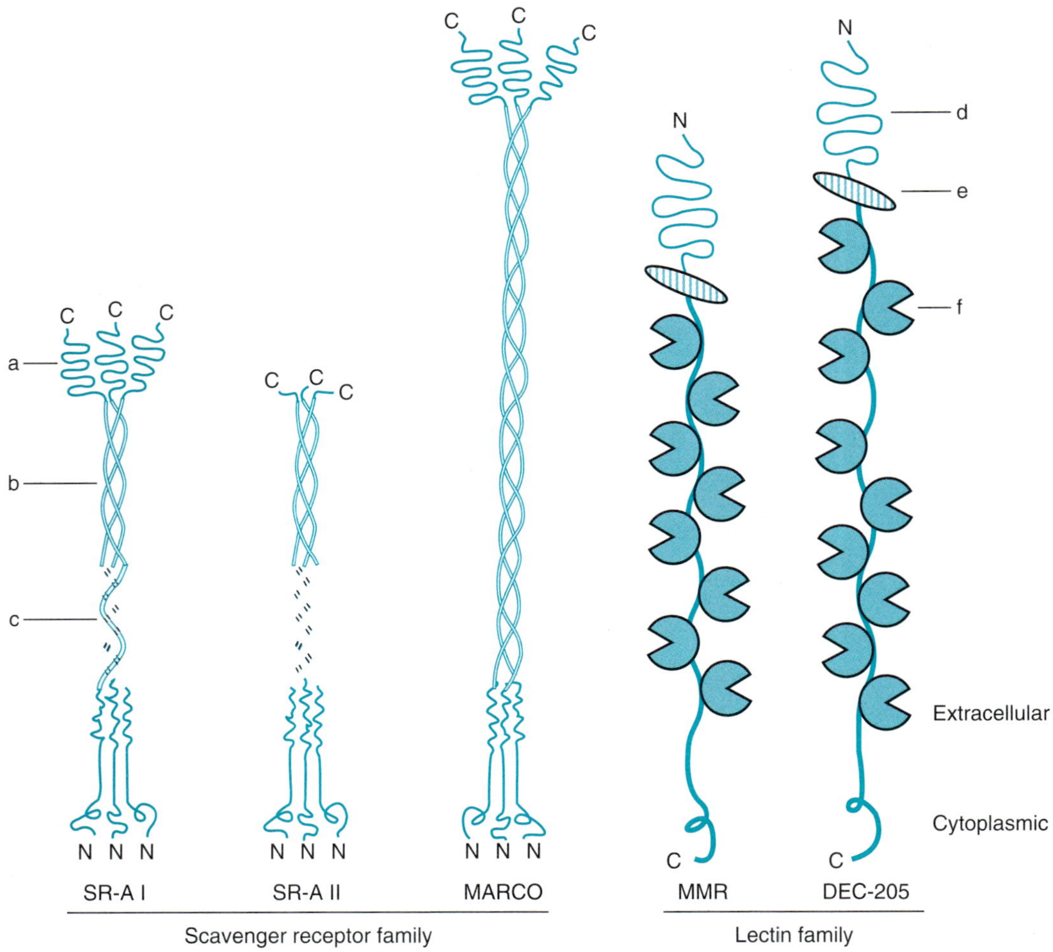

FIGURE 8–3 · **Endocytic Pattern-Recognition Receptors of the Scavenger Receptor and Lectin Families.** On the left are schematic illustrations of three members of the scavenger receptor family. These are trimeric complexes of type II transmembrane polypeptides that have their N-termini positioned in the cytoplasm and their C-termini in the extracellular space. Three distinct extracellular structural domains are indicated: *(a)* the scavenger receptor cysteine-rich (SRCR) domain (absent in SR-A II), which has no currently known function; *(b)* the collagen-like domain that is implicated in the binding of polyanionic ligands; *(c)* the α-helical coiled-coil domain (absent in MARCO) that is believed to assist in receptor trimerization. On the right are two examples of multilectin domain endocytic pattern-recognition receptors, the macrophage mannose receptor (MMR) and DEC-205. Distinct extracellular domains in these receptors include: *(d)* a cysteine-rich N terminal domain; *(e)* a fibronectin-like domain; and *(f)* multiple calcium-dependent (C-type) lectin domains that bind various carbohydrate ligands. (Reproduced in part from Peiser L, Mukhopadhyay S, Gordon S: Scavenger receptors in innate immunity. Curr Op Immunol 14:123-128, 2002.)

the scavenger receptor A (SR-A) and a related molecule called macrophage receptor with collagenous structure (MARCO).[30-33] Both of these molecules contain a scavenger receptor cysteine-rich (SRCR) domain in their membrane distal ends and a collagen-like stalk with a triple-helical structure. Both are known to bind bacteria, and SR-A has been shown to bind well-known PAMPs such as lipoteichoic acids and LPS.[34,35] Mice that have been made deficient in SR-A by targeted gene disruption show increased susceptibility to infections caused by a variety of bacteria, thus providing strong evidence for a role of scavenger receptors in protective immunity, most likely through activation of innate immune mechanisms.[36-38] Although these members of the scavenger receptor family clearly function as endocytic PRRs in the uptake of microbes, their potential to serve as signaling receptors is not yet established.

PRRs with Leucine-Rich Repeat Domains

Leucine-rich repeat domains (LRRs) are structural modules found in many proteins, including PRRs involved in signaling the activation of innate immunity. Molecules in this class include most notably the recently discovered family of mammalian Toll-like receptors (TLRs), which are membrane-bound signal-transducing molecules that play a central role in the recognition of extracellular and vacuolar pathogens. The cytoplasmic nucleotide-binding oligomerization domain (NOD) proteins are another group of LRR-containing receptors that are soluble proteins within the cytosol and most likely are involved in the recognition of PAMPs expressed by intracellular pathogens.[39-42] These molecules are closely related in structure and function to proteins found in invertebrates and plants that are also involved in pathogen resistance, highlighting the ancient evolutionary origin of these pathways for host defense, which appear to have been recognizably conserved through approximately 1 billion years of evolution.[43,44]

Toll-like Receptors

The first member of the Toll family to be discovered was the drosophila Toll protein, which was identified as a component of a signaling pathway controlling dorsoventral polarity during the development of the fly embryo.[45] The sequence of Toll showed it to be a transmembrane protein with a large extracellular domain containing multiple tandemly repeated LRRs at the N-terminal end, followed by a cysteine-rich domain and an intracellular signaling domain (Fig. 8–4). A role for Toll in immune responses was suggested by the observation that its intracellular domain shows homology to the mammalian interleukin-1 receptor (IL-1R) cytoplasmic domain.[46] This association was later confirmed in studies showing that Toll was critical for the antifungal response in the fly, linking this pathway for the first time to innate immunity.[47] The identification of drosophila Toll eventually led to a search for similar proteins in mammals, and this effort has been richly rewarded, yielding at least 10 mammalian Toll-like receptors (TLRs) in both mice and humans.[48,49] All of these molecules contain large extracellular domains with multiple LRRs, as well as intracellular signaling domains known as Toll/IL-1R or TIR domains. Many of these TLRs have now been linked to the innate immune responses against various PAMPs of different microorganisms.

TLR4 and the Response to LPS. The first human TLR to be identified was the molecule now designated as TLR4, which is a major component in the response to one of the most common of all PAMPs, bacterial LPS.[50] Earlier studies on the response to LPS had identified two proteins, CD14 and LPS-binding protein (LBP), as molecules involved in the binding of LPS to the surface of LPS-responsive cells. However, these molecules did not possess any potential for transducing signals into the cell, so it was unclear how LPS binding would lead to activation of cellular responses associated with gram-negative bacterial infection. The answer to this conundrum was provided by positional cloning studies of the *lps* gene in the LPS hyporesponsive C3H/HeJ mouse.[51,52] This revealed a single amino acid substitution in the signaling domain of TLR4. Subsequent specific deletion of the TLR4 gene by targeted gene disruption in mice confirmed the essential role of this molecule in the response to LPS because these TLR4 knockout mice have almost no response to LPS and are highly resistant to endotoxic shock.[53-55] Biochemical studies provide further support for the identification of TLR4 as a component of the LPS receptor. These show that LPS bound to the surface of cells is in close contact with both CD14 and TLR4, as well as another protein called MD-2 that appears to perform an accessory function in the binding of LPS to the receptor complex.[56] Further studies have elucidated many of the downstream elements in the signaling pathways that connect TLR4 to the activation of genes associated with inducible innate immunity[57-61] (see Fig. 8–4). Studies of Toll signaling pathways in drosophila identified the transcription factor nuclear factor κB (NF-κB) as one of the key effectors of gene activation following engagement of Toll, and this basic pathway in the fly appears to be largely conserved in higher animals, including mammals.[62]

Other PAMPs Recognized by TLRS. The search for ligands that lead to signaling through various TLRs has demonstrated that this family of PRRs is collectively responsible for innate immune responses to an extraordinary array of PAMPs. In addition to its central role in the signaling of responses to LPS, TLR4 has been shown to be involved in responses to multiple different self and nonself ligands. The antimitotic agent Taxol has been shown to mimic LPS-induced signaling in mouse cells through a pathway that requires both TLR4 and MD-2.[63-65] Other foreign ligands of TLR4 are the fusion protein (F protein) of respiratory syncytial virus[66,67] and heat-shock protein 60 (HSP60) of chlamydia.[68,69] Interestingly, TLR4 can also signal in response to mammalian HSP60, a protein expressed at increased levels and most likely released by stressed or damaged cells.[70] This represents a variation of the pattern-recognition principle in which the pattern is not a PAMP produced directly by a pathogen, but

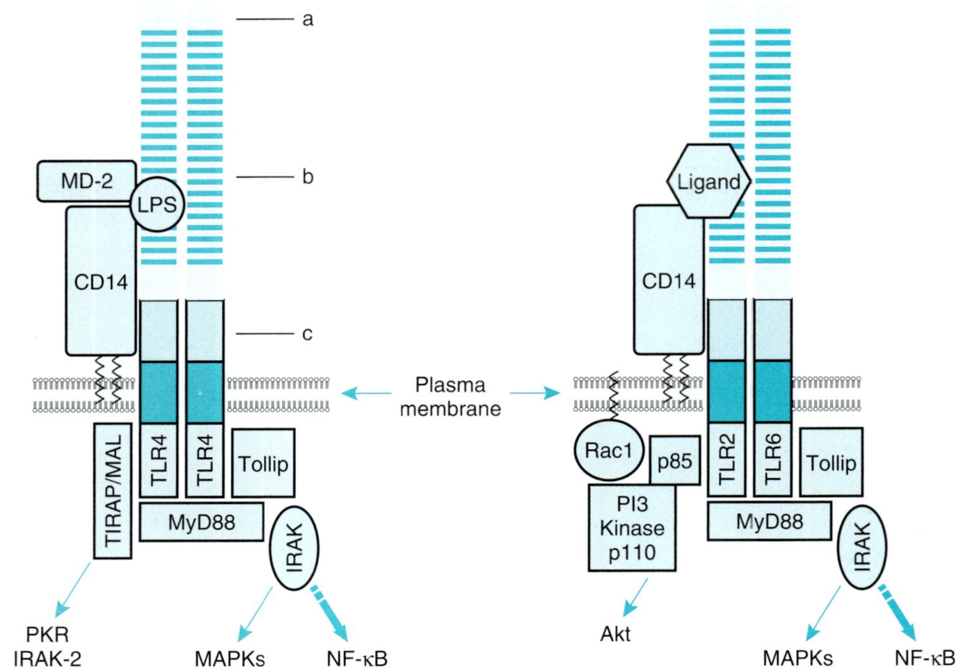

FIGURE 8–4 • **Toll-like Receptors and Associated Proteins.** *Left:* TLR4 is a transmembrane polypeptide present in the plasma membrane as a homodimer. The TLR4 polypeptide has three distinct extracellular regions: *(a)* an N-terminal flanking domain; *(b)* the leucine-rich repeat (LRR) region, which contains 21 leucine-rich motifs and is thought to be directly involved in binding to LPS and other ligands; and *(c)* a C-terminal flanking cysteine-rich domain. The cytoplasmic domains of TLR4 and all other TLRs have homology to the human IL-1 receptor and are designated Toll-IL-1 receptor (TIR) domains. The extracellular portion of TLR4 associates with at least two other proteins, CD14 and MD-2, which are involved in ligand recognition. The intracellular TIR domains associate with multiple adaptor proteins (MyD88, TIRAP/MAL, Tollip), which link the receptor complex to kinases that activate signaling cascades. For TLR4, and probably most other TLRs, activation of the IL-1 receptor-associated kinase (IRAK) is an important step leading to the release of the active form of transcription factor NF-κB. In addition, signaling through TLR4 also leads to signal transduction through activation of mitogen-activated protein kinases (MAPKs), double-stranded RNA-binding protein kinase (PKR), and other members of the IRAK family, such as IRAK-2. *Right:* A different set of ligands is recognized by TLR2, which functions as part of a heterodimeric complex with other TLRs, such as TLR6. The TLR2/6 complex shares many features with the TLR4 complex in terms of its associated proteins. However, the TIR domain of TLR2 also appears to recruit phosphatidyl-3-OH kinase (PI3 kinase, p85 and p110 subunits) and the membrane-associated GTPase Rac1, which allows the activation of other signaling molecules, such as the serine/threonine kinase Akt. Thus, although the major signaling pathways activated by different TLRs are similar or identical (i.e., activation of NF-kB and MAPKs), it appears likely that each TLR complex may show subtle differences in their secondary pathways of signal transduction. These differences may lead to partially overlapping but distinct outcomes in response to ligands recognized by different TLR complexes. (Adapted from Underhill DM, Ozinsky A: Toll-like receptors: key mediators of microbe detection. Curr Op Immunol 14:103-110, 2002.)

rather a structural feature associated with infected or physically damaged cells of the host. Another example of this is provided by the activation of signaling through TLR4 by the extra domain A (EDA) region of fibronectin, which is produced by alternative RNA splicing in response to tissue injury or inflammation.[71]

The range of PAMPs recognized through TLR2 is probably even greater than for TLR4. Currently, TLR2 is known to be involved in signaling in response to multiple PAMPs of gram-negative and gram-positive bacteria, including such structures as LPS, peptidoglycan, bacterial lipoproteins, parasite-derived glycolipids, and fungal cell-wall polysaccharides.[54,72-75] TLR2 does not function independently in responding to these PAMPs but forms heterodimers with either TLR1 or TLR6. This ability to pair with other TLRs appears thus far to be unique to TLR2 because other TLRs that have been studied carefully (e.g., TLR4 and TLR5) most likely function only as homodimers. Other TLRs with currently defined ligands are TLR5 (involved in the response to bacterial flagellin),[76] TLR3 (double-stranded RNA),[77] and TLR9 (unmethylated bacterial DNA).[78] It is apparent that most, if not all, microbes contain multiple PAMPs that are recognized by different TLRs. For example, a typical bacterium expressing LPS will also contain unmethylated DNA and peptidoglycan, and thus will generate signals not only through TLR4, but presumably also through TLR2 and TLR9. Because different TLRs are capable of activating distinct signaling cascades (see Fig. 8–3), the ability of a single cell to detect several different features of a pathogen simultaneously with multiple TLRs may help the innate immune response to be more finely tuned to respond to a particular challenge.[79]

Effector Mechanisms of Innate Immune Responses

The ability to recognize pathogens through PRRs allows numerous antimicrobial effector mechanisms to be activated by the innate immune response. These responses lead to killing of pathogens through the production of effector molecules with direct microbicidal activities, including the membrane attack complex of complement, a variety of antimicrobial peptides and the caustic reactive oxygen and reactive nitrogen intermediates generated within phagocytic cells. In invertebrates, these mechanisms represent virtually the entire protective response against microbial invaders. However, in most vertebrates, including mammals, innate immune recognition also has profound effects on triggering and programming the adaptive immune response that follows somewhat later. This ability of the innate immune system to instruct the adaptive response has major implications for the development of long-term protective immunity to infections, and may also play a critical part in mechanisms leading to autoimmunity.

CELL TYPES MEDIATING INNATE IMMUNITY

Many types of cells have the ability to mount at least a limited response to PAMPs, but the most effective cell types in this regard are probably the specialized phagocytes, such as macrophages, neutrophils, and dendritic cells. Upon recognition of microbial stimuli, these cells have the ability to upregulate the NADPH oxidase by assembling the components of this enzyme complex on phagosomal membranes, leading to an oxidative burst that produces microbicidal superoxide ions.[80] Many phagocytic cells also increase their expression of the inducible nitric oxide synthase (iNOS, or NOS2) upon contact with various PAMPs.[81,82] This leads to the production of reactive nitrogen intermediates, including nitric oxide and peroxynitrite, which have potent direct antimicrobicidal activities. These responses are synergistic because the antimicrobial activity of the phagocyte oxidase system is frequently enhanced by expression of reactive nitrogen intermediates.

INNATE-LIKE LYMPHOCYTES

A number of distinct lymphocyte subsets also play important roles in innate immune responses. One group of such lymphocytes, the natural killer (NK) cells, appear to be true members of the innate immune system. These lymphocytes do not express receptors generated by somatic recombination and thus depend on germline-encoded receptors for signaling their responses against pathogen-infected cells.[83] NK cells are participants in the early innate response against virally, and probably also bacterially, infected cells through the expression of cytotoxic activity and the secretion of cytokines.[84]

Several other subsets of lymphocytes belonging in the T and B cell lineages have been identified as participants in the rapid response against pathogens to which the host has not previously been exposed. Although these cells express clonally variable, somatically rearranged antigen receptors (i.e., T cell antigen receptors or membrane immunoglobulins), and thus could be classified as components of the adaptive immune system, their manner of functioning is much more characteristic of innate than adaptive immunity. These innate-like lymphocytes (ILLs) may represent the remnants of the earliest primitive adaptive immune systems, and they appear to have been conserved to varying degrees because they continue to make specialized contributions to host immunity.[85]

Among the currently recognized ILLs are two B cell populations, known as the B1 and marginal zone (MZ) B cell subsets.[86,87] These are involved in the spontaneous production of natural antibodies, which are largely germline-encoded immunoglobulins that are reactive to commonly expressed microbial determinants. In addition, both of these B cell populations generate rapid T cell–independent responses following bacterial challenges and thus contribute to the first line of immune defense that precedes the delayed onset of adaptive immunity.

Among the T cells, two populations of ILLs have been identified and characterized in detail: γδ T cells and NK T cells. The γδ T cells express somatically rearranging receptors that use a limited number of variable region genes and are thought to recognize a narrow spectrum of foreign or self ligands.[88] In humans, the specificities of two subsets of γδ T cells have been at least partially defined. One of these, the major circulating population expressing the Vδ2 gene product, respond rapidly and without prior immunization to a variety of small alkyl phosphate and alkyl amine compounds that are produced by many bacteria. Another subset, characterized by its expression of the Vδ1 gene product, responds to major histocompatibility complex (MHC) class I–related self molecules of the MHC class I chain-related A and B (MICA/B) and CD1 families.[89,90] These molecules may serve as markers of cellular stress and are upregulated on cells in the context of infection or inflammation, leading to the activation of Vδ1-bearing γδ T cells.

A similar principle appears to be involved in the functioning of NK T cells, which are so named because of their coexpression of an αβ T cell antigen receptor and a variety of receptor molecules that are typically associated with NK cells.[85,91] Like γδ T cells, NK T cells have somatically rearranged antigen receptors that use a limited array of V genes and most likely recognize a narrow range of foreign or self antigens. A major population of NK T cells is reactive with the MHC class I–like CD1d molecule, and these ILLs appear to be activated by recognition of a variety of lipid or glycolipid ligands that can be presented by CD1d. NK T cells make important contributions to a variety of different types of innate and adaptive immune responses[91] and may play a particularly important role in immunoregulation to prevent autoimmunity[92] (see also Chapter 9 on T lymphocytes).

ANTIMICROBIAL PEPTIDES

Antimicrobial peptides are the key effector molecules of inducible innate immunity in many invertebrates and are now being increasingly recognized as important elements of innate immunity in higher animal species, including mammals.[93] They are evolutionarily ancient components of host defense that are widely distributed throughout all multicellular organisms in the animal and plant kingdoms. There are now more than 500 such peptides known (for current list, see *http://www.bbcm.univ.trieste.it/~tossi/antimic.html*), and their diversity is so great that it is difficult to categorize them. However, at a structural and mechanistic level, most of these peptides share several basic features. They are generally composed of amino acids arranged to create an amphipathic structure with hydrophobic and cationic regions. The cationic regions target a fundamental difference in membrane design between microbes and multicellular animals, which is the abundance of negatively charged phospholipid headgroups on the outer leaflet of the lipid bilayer. The preferential association of antimicrobial peptides with microbial membranes leads to a membrane-disrupting activity, most likely involving the interaction of the hydrophobic regions of the peptide with membrane lipids.[94-96]

Antimicrobial peptides produced in response to engagement of various PRRs account for the majority of the inducible immunity against microbes in many invertebrate animals and plants. Although probably less central to host immunity in most vertebrates, there is evidence that they make important contributions to immunity in more highly evolved animals, including mammals.[97] In humans, active antimicrobial peptides, such as the β-defensins, are either constitutively or inducibly produced in skin and in epithelia of the gastrointestinal and respiratory tracts.[98-101] These molecules most likely act as natural preservatives of epithelia that are colonized or frequently exposed to microbial flora. Because the acquisition of resistance against these agents by sensitive microbial strains is extremely unusual, antimicrobial peptides are of great interest currently as templates for the development of new antimicrobial pharmaceuticals.[102]

Influence of Innate Mechanisms on Adaptive Immunity

In addition to functioning as a first line of defense against invading pathogens, another critical feature of the innate immune system in higher animals such as mammals is its effect on activating the adaptive immune system. In fact, it is now clear that in most situations, the adaptive immune system will only mount a response to a pathogen after the pathogen has first generated signals via PRRs of the innate immune system. This principle is the basis for what has been known for many years as the adjuvant effect, which is the observation that antibody and T cell responses are only efficiently generated against protein antigens if these are introduced together with a nonspecific activator of the immune system, which is generically known as an adjuvant. Most adjuvants are in fact extracts or products of bacteria, and it is now clear that adjuvant effects result in most or all cases from the activation of the innate immune response.[103]

There are many ways in which innate immune responses can prime or potentiate the adaptive immune response that follows (Fig. 8–5). In the case of T cell responses, one extremely important and well-recognized mechanism involves the upregulation of costimulatory molecules. T cells require at least two signals to become activated from a naïve, resting state. One signal is provided through the T cell antigen receptor by its binding to a specific peptide ligand presented by a MHC class I or II molecule. The second signal is provided by one of several costimulatory ligands that are expressed by specialized antigen-presenting cells such as dendritic cells. The best studied of these are the molecules of the B7 family, B7-1 (CD80) and B7-2 (CD86), which engage the activating receptor CD28 on the surface of the T cell. The expression of B7 family costimulatory molecules on the surface of antigen-presenting cells is controlled by the innate immune system, such that these molecules are induced to appear at functional levels only after PRRs, such as members of the TLR family, have been activated by recognition of their cognate PAMPs.[50]

Innate immune responses also trigger the production of many cytokines and chemokines that enhance the development of adaptive immune responses and change the nature of the adaptive response generated. For example, the contact of dendritic cells with PAMPs such as LPS or bacterial lipoproteins leads to the production of interleukin-12 as a result of signaling through TLRs.[73,103,104] This cytokine acts on antigen-specific T cells to promote their differentiation into T helper type 1 (Th1) cells, which are associated with strong production of interferon-γ and other effector mechanisms that favor the clearance of bacterial pathogens.[105] In the case of myeloid-lineage dendritic cells, signaling through TLRs, and potentially other PRRs, induces a process known as maturation, which is associated with the increased expression of antigen-presenting and costimulatory molecules that enables the efficient priming of naive antigen-specific T cells.[103,106]

This requirement for the innate immune response to "switch on" the expression of molecules required for the priming and differentiation of T cell responses helps ensure that proinflammatory adaptive immune responses mainly occur in the setting of a relevant infectious challenge. After activation, helper T cells control other components of adaptive immunity, such as the activation of cytotoxic T cells, B cells, and macrophages. Innate immune recognition, therefore, appears to control all the major aspects of the adaptive immune responses through the initial recognition of infectious microbes by PRRs. Recently, this paradigm has been extended and slightly reinterpreted by the observation that certain self molecules upregulated by cellular stress or damage can substitute for PAMPs of infectious microbes in bringing about the subsequent activation of adaptive immune responses.[70,71] This more extended view, sometimes referred to as the "danger model," helps explain why certain self ligands produced or released in the setting of infections or tissue damage can function in essentially the same manner as the PAMPs associated with microorganisms.[107]

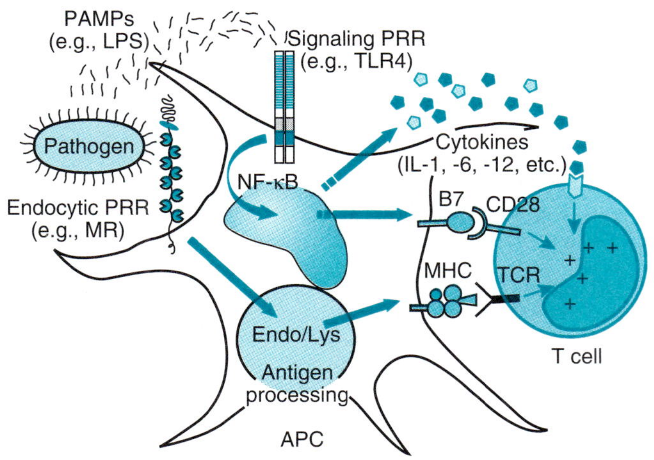

FIGURE 8–5 · **Instruction of the Adaptive Immune Response by the Innate Immune System.** When an antigen-presenting cell (APC) comes into contact with a pathogen bearing pathogen-associated molecular patterns (PAMPs), responses are triggered via innate immune mechanisms that dramatically alter the ability of the APC to stimulate an adaptive (T cell–mediated) immune response. For example, signals generated by contact with PAMPs such as lipopolysaccharide (LPS) with TLR4 lead to the activation of transcription factor NF-κB, which enters the nucleus of the APC and assists in switching on genes for cytokines (e.g., IL-1, -6, -12, and a variety of chemokines) and costimulatory molecules (e.g., the B7 family members CD80 and CD86). In addition, binding of the pathogen to endocytic pattern-recognition receptors (PRRs) such as the mannose receptor leads to the delivery of the pathogen to endosomes (Endo) and lysosomes (Lys). There, the protein antigens of the pathogen are partially degraded to generate antigenic peptides that can be presented by major histocompatibility complex (MHC) class II molecules for recognition by the T cell antigen receptors (TCR) of specific T cells. These effects of pattern recognition by the innate immune system lead to the expression of the signals that are required for the activation of quiescent antigen-specific T cells and the subsequent generation of specific antibodies. (Adapted from Medzhitov R, Janeway C Jr: Innate Immunity. New Eng J Med 343:338-344, 2000.)

Disease Associations Involving Innate Immunity

Given the obvious role of the innate immune response in virtually all types of infectious diseases, one might expect that defects in mechanisms of innate immunity should occur relatively rarely and in association with clinical immunodeficiency. In fact, there is increasing evidence that mutations that inactivate various innate immune pathways can lead to increased pathogen sensitivity in both laboratory mice and in humans.[9,37,97,108] Because many of the pathways leading to innate immunity are amplified during recurrent or prolonged activation of the immune system, these must also participate in mediating tissue damage in chronic inflammatory diseases. In addition, certain self molecules that are produced or released at increased levels as a result of inflammation, such as heat-shock proteins and DNA-nucleoprotein complexes, may act in a manner analogous to PAMPs. These may signal through TLRs or other PRRs to stimulate adjuvant-like effects that increase the potential for autoreactive lymphocytes to be activated.[70,109]

Perhaps a more surprising finding has been that certain defects in innate immunity are associated with a markedly increased predisposition to autoimmune disease. Several different mechanisms have been proposed to explain this paradoxical association. Mechanisms of the innate immune response play an important role in the clearance of self antigens released from necrotic or apoptotic cells, resulting in a noninflammatory clearance of self antigens that tends to favor tolerance rather than the stimulation of immune responses.[110] A failure of such clearance may lead to excessive exposure to self antigens with triggering of normally silent autoreactive lymphocyte clones to expand and differentiate into effector cells. This may account for the development of lupus-like autoimmunity in mice with targeted deletion of the gene for the short pentraxin SAP, which, along with other components of the innate immune system, appears to play a significant role in clearance of DNA-chromatin complexes.[111]

Deficiencies of the early components of the classic pathway of complement activation have been strongly associated with lupus-like autoimmunity in both humans and mouse models.[112-116] This may also be the result of alterations in the clearance of apoptotic cells or other sources of self antigens resulting in increased stimulation of normally silent autoreactive lymphocytes.[117-119] An alternate, but nonexclusive, mechanism relates to the involvement of the complement system, particularly the early components C1 and C4, in facilitating the induction of self-tolerance by the adaptive immune system by increasing the localization of autoantigens such as dsDNA and nucleoproteins within the primary lymphoid compartment.[113,120,121] Thus, a deficiency of C1 or C4 appears to result in a failure to delete or functionally inactivate autoreactive B cell clones as they arise during lymphopoiesis in the bone marrow.[120,122] Studies carried out in mouse models suggest that this tolerance-inducing mechanism is also partially disrupted in animals that are deficient in a variety of other components of innate immunity, including SAP component and the complement receptors CD21/CD35.[111,120]

Other defects in innate immune mechanisms that predispose to autoimmunity have also begun to emerge from recent studies. Deficiencies in at least two populations of innate-like lymphocytes, NK cells and NK T cells, have been associated with multiple autoimmune syndromes in both humans and mice.[91,92,123-126] This is believed to reflect a significant role for these ILLs in regulating adaptive immune responses, although the precise mechanisms by which they act are still not known.[127] Another example of a defect in innate immunity that leads to loss of normal self-tolerance is provided by genetic mapping studies that identified the IBD1 locus conferring susceptibility to Crohn's disease as the gene for NOD2, a member of the nucleotide-binding oligomerization domain (NOD) protein family, which is a cytoplasmic PRR in the LRR family.[128-131] This protein normally signals to induce cytokine production in response to bacterial LPS, but mutant alleles associated with increased risk of Crohn's disease are defective in this function.[128] In this case, it may be a failure of innate immunity to adequately control bacterial colonization or infection in the intestine that leads to the final expression of disease. Given the complex interplay between innate and adaptive immunity, it is extremely likely that further examples of associations between alterations in innate immunity and autoimmune diseases will continue to emerge.

REFERENCES

1. Mushegian A, Medzhitov R: Evolutionary perspective on innate immune recognition. J Cell Biol 155:705, 2001.
2. Hoffmann JA, Reichhart JM: Drosophila innate immunity: An evolutionary perspective. Nat Immunol 3:121, 2002.
3. Agrawal A, Eastman QM, Schatz DG: Transposition mediated by RAG1 and RAG2 and its implications for the evolution of the immune system. Nature 394:744, 1998.
4. Schatz DG: Transposition mediated by RAG1 and RAG2 and the evolution of the adaptive immune system. Immunol Res 19:169, 1999.
5. Flajnik MF: Churchill and the immune system of ectothermic vertebrates. Immunol Rev 166:5, 1998.
6. Fraser IP, Koziel H, Ezekowitz RA: The serum mannose-binding protein and the macrophage mannose receptor are pattern recognition molecules that link innate and adaptive immunity. Semin Immunol 10:363, 1998.
7. Stover C, Endo Y, Takahashi M, et al: The human gene for mannan-binding lectin-associated serine protease-2 (MASP-2), the effector component of the lectin route of complement activation, is part of a tightly linked gene cluster on chromosome 1p36.2-3. Genes Immun 2:119, 2001.
8. Jack DL, Jarvis GA, Booth CL, et al: Mannose-binding lectin accelerates complement activation and increases serum killing of Neisseria meningitidis serogroup C. J Infect Dis 184:836, 2001.
9. Jack DL, Klein NJ, Turner MW: Mannose-binding lectin: Targeting the microbial world for complement attack and opsonophagocytosis. Immunol Rev 180:86, 2001.
10. Polotsky VY, Belisle JT, Mikusova K, et al: Interaction of human mannose-binding protein with Mycobacterium avium. J Infect Dis 175:1159, 1997.
11. Fraser IP, Takahashi K, Koziel H, et al: Pneumocystis carinii enhances soluble mannose receptor production by macrophages. Microbes Infect 2:1305, 2000.
12. Kase T, Suzuki Y, Kawai T, et al: Human mannan-binding lectin inhibits the infection of influenza A virus without complement. Immunology 97:385, 1999.
13. Thielens NM, Tacnet-Delorme P, Arlaud GJ: Interaction of C1q and mannan-binding lectin with viruses. Immunobiology 205:563, 2002.
14. Klabunde J, Uhlemann AC, Tebo AE, et al: Recognition of Plasmodium falciparum proteins by mannan-binding lectin, a component of the human innate immune system. Parasitol Res 88:113, 2002.
15. Matsushita M, Kuraya M, Hamasaki N, et al: Activation of the lectin complement pathway by H-ficolin (Hakata antigen). J Immunol 168:3502, 2002.
16. Lu J, Teh C, Kishore U, et al: Collectins and ficolins: Sugar pattern recognition molecules of the mammalian innate immune system. Biochim Biophys Acta 1572:387, 2002.
17. Reid KB, Colomb M, Petry F, et al: Complement component C1 and the collectins—first-line defense molecules in innate and acquired immunity. Trends Immunol 23:115, 2002.
18. McCormack FX, Whitsett JA: The pulmonary collectins, SP-A and SP-D, orchestrate innate immunity in the lung. J Clin Invest 109:707, 2002.
19. Gewurz H, Zhang XH, Lint TF: Structure and function of the pentraxins. Curr Opin Immunol 7:54, 1995.
20. Szalai AJ, Agrawal A, Greenhough TJ, et al: C-reactive protein: Structural biology, gene expression, and host defense function. Immunol Res 16:127, 1997.
21. Goodman AR, Cardozo T, Abagyan R, et al: Long pentraxins: an emerging group of proteins with diverse functions. Cytokine Growth Factor Rev 7:191, 1996.
22. Bottazzi B, Vouret-Craviari V, Bastone A, et al: Multimer formation and ligand recognition by the long pentraxin PTX3. Similarities and differences with the short pentraxins C-reactive protein and serum amyloid P component. J Biol Chem 272:32817, 1997.
23. Garlanda C, Hirsch E, Bozza S, et al: Non-redundant role of the long pentraxin PTX3 in anti-fungal innate immune response. Nature 420:182, 2002.
24. East L, Isacke CM: The mannose receptor family. Biochim Biophys Acta 1572:364, 2002.
25. Zamze S, Martinez-Pomares L, Jones H, et al: Recognition of bacterial capsular polysaccharides and lipopolysaccharides by the macrophage mannose receptor. J Biol Chem 277:41613, 2002.
26. Apostolopoulos V, McKenzie IF: Role of the mannose receptor in the immune response. Curr Mol Med 1:469, 2001.
27. Martinez-Pomares L, Linehan SA, Taylor PR, et al: Binding properties of the mannose receptor. Immunobiology 204:527, 2001.
28. Nigou J, Zelle-Rieser C, Gilleron M, et al: Mannosylated lipoarabinomannans inhibit IL-12 production by human dendritic cells: Evidence for a negative signal delivered through the mannose receptor. J Immunol 166:7477, 2001.
29. Peiser L, De Winther MP, Makepeace K, et al: The class A macrophage scavenger receptor is a major pattern recognition receptor for Neisseria meningitidis which is independent of lipopolysaccharide and not required for secretory responses. Infect Immun 70:5346, 2002.
30. Krieger M: The other side of scavenger receptors: Pattern recognition for host defense. Curr Opin Lipidol 8:275, 1997.
31. Peiser L, De Winther MP, Makepeace K, et al: The class A macrophage scavenger receptor is a major pattern recognition receptor for Neisseria meningitidis which is independent of lipopolysaccharide and not required for secretory responses. Infect Immun 70:5346, 2002.
32. Kraal G, van der Laan LJ, Elomaa O, et al: The macrophage receptor MARCO. Microbes Infect 2:313, 2000.
33. Elshourbagy NA, Li X, Terrett J, et al: Molecular characterization of a human scavenger receptor, human MARCO. Eur J Biochem 267:919, 2000.
34. Hampton RY, Golenbock DT, Penman M, et al: Recognition and plasma clearance of endotoxin by scavenger receptors. Nature 352:342, 1991.
35. Dunne DW, Resnick D, Greenberg J, et al: The type I macrophage scavenger receptor binds to gram-positive bacteria and recognizes lipoteichoic acid. Proc Natl Acad Sci U S A 91:1863, 1994.
36. Suzuki H, Kurihara Y, Takeya M, et al: A role for macrophage scavenger receptors in atherosclerosis and susceptibility to infection. Nature 386:292, 1997.
37. Thomas CA, Li Y, Kodama T, et al: Protection from lethal gram-positive infection by macrophage scavenger receptor-dependent phagocytosis. J Exp Med 191:147, 2000.
38. Haworth R, Platt N, Keshav S, et al: The macrophage scavenger receptor type A is expressed by activated macrophages and protects the host against lethal endotoxic shock. J Exp Med 186:1431, 1997.
39. Inohara N, Ogura Y, Nunez G: Nods: A family of cytosolic proteins that regulate the host response to pathogens. Curr Opin Microbiol 5:76, 2002.
40. Bertin J, Nir WJ, Fischer CM, et al: Human CARD4 protein is a novel CED-4/Apaf-1 cell death family member that activates NF-kappaB. J Biol Chem 274:12955, 1999.
41. Inohara N, Koseki T, del Peso L, et al: Nod1, an Apaf-1-like activator of caspase-9 and nuclear factor-kappaB. J Biol Chem 274:14560, 1999.
42. Inohara N, Ogura Y, Chen FF, et al: Human Nod1 confers responsiveness to bacterial lipopolysaccharides. J Biol Chem 276:2551, 2001.
43. Dangl JL, Jones JD: Plant pathogens and integrated defence responses to infection. Nature 411:826, 2001.
44. Medzhitov R, Janeway C Jr: Innate immune recognition: mechanisms and pathways. Immunol Rev 173:89, 2000.
45. Hashimoto C, Hudson KL, Anderson KV: The Toll gene of Drosophila, required for dorsal-ventral embryonic polarity, appears to encode a transmembrane protein. Cell 52:269, 1988.
46. Gay NJ, Keith FJ: Drosophila Toll and IL-1 receptor. Nature 351:355, 1991.
47. Lemaitre B, Nicolas E, Michaut L, et al: The dorsoventral regulatory gene cassette spatzle/Toll/cactus controls the potent antifungal response in Drosophila adults. Cell 86:973, 1996.
48. Janeway CA Jr, Medzhitov R: Innate immune recognition. Annu Rev Immunol 20:197, 2002.
49. Kimbrell DA, Beutler B: The evolution and genetics of innate immunity. Nat Rev Genet 2:256, 2001.

50. Medzhitov R, Preston-Hurlburt P, Janeway CA Jr: A human homologue of the Drosophila Toll protein signals activation of adaptive immunity. Nature 388:394, 1997.
51. Poltorak A, He X, Smirnova I, et al: Defective LPS signaling in C3H/HeJ and C57BL/10ScCr mice: Mutations in Tlr4 gene. Science 282:2085, 1998.
52. Qureshi ST, Lariviere L, Leveque G, et al: Endotoxin-tolerant mice have mutations in Toll-like receptor 4 (Tlr4). J Exp Med 189:615, 1999.
53. Hoshino K, Takeuchi O, Kawai T, et al: Cutting edge: Toll-like receptor 4 (TLR4)-deficient mice are hyporesponsive to lipopolysaccharide: evidence for TLR4 as the Lps gene product. J Immunol 162:3749, 1999.
54. Takeuchi O, Hoshino K, Kawai T, et al: Differential roles of TLR2 and TLR4 in recognition of gram-negative and gram-positive bacterial cell wall components. Immunity 11:443, 1999.
55. Takeuchi O, Akira S: Genetic approaches to the study of Toll-like receptor function. Microbes Infect 4:887, 2002.
56. da Silva CJ, Soldau K, Christen U, et al: Lipopolysaccharide is in close proximity to each of the proteins in its membrane receptor complex: transfer from CD14 to TLR4 and MD-2. J Biol Chem 276:21129, 2001.
57. Medzhitov R, Preston-Hurlburt P, Kopp E, et al: MyD88 is an adaptor protein in the hToll/IL-1 receptor family signaling pathways. Mol Cell 2:253, 1998.
58. Horng T, Barton GM, Medzhitov R: TIRAP: An adapter molecule in the Toll signaling pathway. Nat Immunol 2:835, 2001.
59. Horng T, Barton GM, Flavell RA, et al: The adaptor molecule TIRAP provides signaling specificity for Toll-like receptors. Nature 420:329, 2002.
60. Fitzgerald KA, Palsson-McDermott EM, Bowie AG, et al: Mal (MyD88-adapter-like) is required for Toll-like receptor-4 signal transduction. Nature 413:78, 2001.
61. Yamamoto M, Sato S, Hemmi H, et al: Essential role for TIRAP activation of the signalling cascade shared by TLR2 and TLR4. Nature 420:324, 2002.
62. Belvin MP, Anderson KV: A conserved signaling pathway: The Drosophila toll-dorsal pathway. Annu Rev Cell Dev Biol 12:393, 1996.
63. Kawasaki K, Akashi S, Shimazu R, et al: Involvement of TLR4/MD-2 complex in species-specific lipopolysaccharide-mimetic signal transduction by Taxol. J Endotoxin Res 7:232, 2001.
64. Kawasaki K, Gomi K, Nishijima M: Cutting edge: Gln22 of mouse MD-2 is essential for species-specific lipopolysaccharide mimetic action of Taxol. J Immunol 166:11, 2001.
65. Kawasaki K, Akashi S, Shimazu R, et al: Mouse toll-like receptor 4-MD-2 complex mediates lipopolysaccharide-mimetic signal transduction by Taxol. J Biol Chem 275:2251, 2000.
66. Haynes LM, Moore DD, Kurt-Jones EA, et al: Involvement of toll-like receptor 4 in innate immunity to respiratory syncytial virus. J Virol 75:10730, 2001.
67. Kurt-Jones EA, Popova L, Kwinn L, et al: Pattern recognition receptors TLR4 and CD14 mediate response to respiratory syncytial virus. Nat Immunol 1:398, 2000.
68. Sasu S, LaVerda D, Qureshi N, et al: Chlamydia pneumoniae and chlamydial heat shock protein 60 stimulate proliferation of human vascular smooth muscle cells via toll-like receptor 4 and p44/p42 mitogen-activated protein kinase activation. Circ Res 89:244, 2001.
69. Vabulas RM, Ahmad-Nejad P, da Costa C, et al: Endocytosed HSP60s use toll-like receptor 2 (TLR2) and TLR4 to activate the toll/interleukin-1 receptor signaling pathway in innate immune cells. J Biol Chem 276:31332, 2001.
70. Ohashi K, Burkart V, Flohe S, et al: Cutting edge: Heat shock protein 60 is a putative endogenous ligand of the toll-like receptor-4 complex. J Immunol 164:558, 2000.
71. Okamura Y, Watari M, Jerud ES, et al: The extra domain A of fibronectin activates Toll-like receptor 4. J Biol Chem 276:10229, 2001.
72. Aliprantis AO, Yang RB, Mark MR, et al: Cell activation and apoptosis by bacterial lipoproteins through toll-like receptor-2. Science 285:736, 1999.
73. Brightbill HD, Libraty DH, Krutzik SR, et al: Host defense mechanisms triggered by microbial lipoproteins through toll-like receptors. Science 285:732, 1999.
74. Campos MA, Almeida IC, Takeuchi O, et al: Activation of Toll-like receptor-2 by glycosylphosphatidylinositol anchors from a protozoan parasite. J Immunol 167:416, 2001.
75. Akira S, Takeda K, Kaisho T: Toll-like receptors: Critical proteins linking innate and acquired immunity. Nat Immunol 2:675, 2001.
76. Hayashi F, Smith KD, Ozinsky A, et al: The innate immune response to bacterial flagellin is mediated by Toll-like receptor 5. Nature 410:1099, 2001.
77. Alexopoulou L, Holt AC, Medzhitov R, et al: Recognition of double-stranded RNA and activation of NF-kappaB by Toll-like receptor 3. Nature 413:732, 2001.
78. Hemmi H, Takeuchi O, Kawai T, et al: A Toll-like receptor recognizes bacterial DNA. Nature 408:740, 2000.
79. Underhill DM, Ozinsky A: Toll-like receptors: Key mediators of microbe detection. Curr Opin Immunol 14:103, 2002.
80. Babior BM, Lambeth JD, Nauseef W: The neutrophil NADPH oxidase. Arch Biochem Biophys 397:342, 2002.
81. Xie QW, Cho HJ, Calaycay J, et al: Cloning and characterization of inducible nitric oxide synthase from mouse macrophages. Science 256:225, 1992.
82. Nathan C: Inducible nitric oxide synthase in the tuberculous human lung. Am J Respir Crit Care Med 166:130, 2002.
83. Vilches C, Parham P: KIR: Diverse, rapidly evolving receptors of innate and adaptive immunity. Annu Rev Immunol 20:217, 2002.
84. Biron CA, Nguyen KB, Pien GC, et al: Natural killer cells in antiviral defense: Function and regulation by innate cytokines. Annu Rev Immunol 17:189, 1999.
85. Bendelac A, Bonneville M, Kearney JF: Autoreactivity by design: Innate B and T lymphocytes. Nat Rev Immunol 1:177, 2001.
86. Berland R, Wortis HH: Origins and functions of B-1 cells with notes on the role of CD5. Annu Rev Immunol 20:253, 2002.
87. Martin F, Kearney JF: Marginal-zone B cells. Nat Rev Immunol 2:323, 2002.
88. Carding SR, Egan PJ: $\gamma\delta$ T cells: Functional plasticity and heterogeneity. Nat Rev Immunol 2:336, 2002.
89. Wu J, Groh V, Spies T: T cell antigen receptor engagement and specificity in the recognition of stress-inducible MHC class I-related chains by human epithelial $\gamma\delta$ T cells. J Immunol 169:1236, 2002.
90. Dutronc Y, Porcelli SA: The CD1 family and T cell recognition of lipid antigens. Tissue Antigens, 60:337, 2002.
91. Godfrey DI, Hammond KJ, Poulton LD, et al: NKT cells: Facts, functions and fallacies. Immunol Today 21:573, 2000.
92. van der Vliet HJ, von Blomberg BM, Nishi N, et al: Circulating Vα24+ Vβ11+ NKT cell numbers are decreased in a wide variety of diseases that are characterized by autoreactive tissue damage. Clin Immunol 100:144, 2001.
93. Zasloff M: Antimicrobial peptides of multicellular organisms. Nature 415:389, 2002.
94. Shai Y: Mechanism of the binding, insertion and destabilization of phospholipid bilayer membranes by α-helical antimicrobial and cell non-selective membrane-lytic peptides. Biochim Biophys Acta 1462:55, 1999.
95. Yang L, Weiss TM, Lehrer RI, et al: Crystallization of antimicrobial pores in membranes: magainin and protegrin. Biophys J 79:2002, 2000.
96. Matsuzaki K: Why and how are peptide-lipid interactions utilized for self-defense? Magainins and tachyplesins as archetypes. Biochim Biophys Acta 1462:1, 1999.
97. Nizet V, Ohtake T, Lauth X, et al: Innate antimicrobial peptide protects the skin from invasive bacterial infection. Nature 414:454, 2001.
98. Harder J, Bartels J, Christophers E, et al: A peptide antibiotic from human skin. Nature 387:861, 1997.
99. Harder J, Bartels J, Christophers E, et al: Isolation and characterization of human β-defensin-3, a novel human inducible peptide antibiotic. J Biol Chem 276:5707, 2001.
100. Singh PK, Jia HP, Wiles K, et al: Production of β-defensins by human airway epithelia. Proc Natl Acad Sci U S A 95:14961, 1998.
101. O'Neil DA, Porter EM, Elewaut D, et al: Expression and regulation of the human β-defensins hBD-1 and hBD-2 in intestinal epithelium. J Immunol 163:6718, 1999.

102. Shai Y: From innate immunity to de-novo designed antimicrobial peptides. Curr Pharm Des 8:715, 2002.
103. Schnare M, Barton GM, Holt AC, et al: Toll-like receptors control activation of adaptive immune responses. Nat Immunol 2:947, 2001.
104. Barton GM, Medzhitov R: Control of adaptive immune responses by Toll-like receptors. Curr Opin Immunol 14:380, 2002.
105. Constant SL, Bottomly K: Induction of Th1 and Th2 CD4+ T cell responses: the alternative approaches. Annu Rev Immunol 15:297, 1997.
106. Banchereau J, Steinman RM: Dendritic cells and the control of immunity. Nature 392:245, 1998.
107. Matzinger P: The danger model: A renewed sense of self. Science 296:301, 2002.
108. Kuhns DB, Long Priel DA, Gallin JI: Endotoxin and IL-1 hyporesponsiveness in a patient with recurrent bacterial infections. J Immunol 158:3959, 1997.
109. Leadbetter EA, Rifkin IR, Hohlbaum AM, et al: Chromatin-IgG complexes activate B cells by dual engagement of IgM and Toll-like receptors. Nature 416:603, 2002.
110. Gershov D, Kim S, Brot N, et al: C-reactive protein binds to apoptotic cells, protects the cells from assembly of the terminal complement components, and sustains an antiinflammatory innate immune response: Implications for systemic autoimmunity. J Exp Med 192:1353, 2000.
111. Bickerstaff MC, Botto M, Hutchinson WL, et al: Serum amyloid P component controls chromatin degradation and prevents antinuclear autoimmunity. Nat Med 5:694, 1999.
112. Walport MJ: Complement and systemic lupus erythematosus. Arthritis Res 4(Suppl 3):S279-S293, 2002.
113. Einav S, Pozdnyakova OO, Ma M, et al: Complement C4 is protective for lupus disease independent of C3. J Immunol 168:1036, 2002.
114. Paul E, Pozdnyakova OO, Mitchell E, et al: Anti-DNA autoreactivity in C4-deficient mice. Eur J Immunol 32:2672, 2002.
115. Mitchell DA, Pickering MC, Warren J, et al: C1q deficiency and autoimmunity: The effects of genetic background on disease expression. J Immunol 168:2538, 2002.
116. Chen Z, Koralov SB, Kelsoe G: Complement C4 inhibits systemic autoimmunity through a mechanism independent of complement receptors CR1 and CR2. J Exp Med 192:1339, 2000.
117. Korb LC, Ahearn JM: C1q binds directly and specifically to surface blebs of apoptotic human keratinocytes: complement deficiency and systemic lupus erythematosus revisited. J Immunol 158:4525, 1997.
118. Cutler AJ, Botto M, van Essen D, et al: T cell-dependent immune response in C1q-deficient mice: defective interferon-γ production by antigen-specific T cells. J Exp Med 187:1789, 1998.
119. Mitchell DA, Taylor PR, Cook HT, et al: Cutting edge: C1q protects against the development of glomerulonephritis independently of C3 activation. J Immunol 162:5676, 1999.
120. Prodeus AP, Goerg S, Shen LM, et al: A critical role for complement in maintenance of self-tolerance. Immunity 9:721, 1998.
121. Paul E, Carroll MC: SAP-less chromatin triggers systemic lupus erythematosus. Nat Med 5:607, 1999.
122. Goodnow CC, Cyster JG, Hartley SB, et al: Self-tolerance checkpoints in B lymphocyte development. Adv Immunol 59:279, 1995.
123. Fort MM, Leach MW, Rennick DM: A role for NK cells as regulators of CD4+ T cells in a transfer model of colitis. J Immunol 161:3256, 1998.
124. Zhang B, Yamamura T, Kondo T, et al: Regulation of experimental autoimmune encephalomyelitis by natural killer (NK) cells. J Exp Med 186:1677, 1997.
125. Shi FD, Wang HB, Li H, et al: Natural killer cells determine the outcome of B cell-mediated autoimmunity. Nat Immunol 1:245, 2000.
126. Wilson SB, Kent SC, Patton KT, et al: Extreme Th1 bias of invariant Vα24JαQ T cells in type 1 diabetes. Nature 391:177, 1998.
127. Shi F, Ljunggren HG, Sarvetnick N: Innate immunity and autoimmunity: From self-protection to self-destruction. Trends Immunol 22:97, 2001.
128. Ogura Y, Bonen DK, Inohara N, et al: A frameshift mutation in NOD2 associated with susceptibility to Crohn's disease. Nature 411:603, 2001.
129. Hugot JP, Chamaillard M, Zouali H, et al: Association of NOD2 leucine-rich repeat variants with susceptibility to Crohn's disease. Nature 411:599, 2001.
130. Cuthbert AP, Fisher SA, Mirza MM, et al: The contribution of NOD2 gene mutations to the risk and site of disease in inflammatory bowel disease. Gastroenterology 122:867, 2002.
131. Hampe J, Grebe J, Nikolaus S, et al: Association of NOD2 (CARD 15) genotype with clinical course of Crohn's disease: a cohort study. Lancet 359:1661, 2002.

9 T Lymphocytes

RALPH C. BUDD • KAREN A. FORTNER

The immune system is foremost an organ of defense against infection. The evolutionary pressures that have molded the particular structures of the immune response and promoted a highly diverse repertoire clearly derive from infectious agents. Two very different strategies exist. The more primitive innate immune response (see Chapter 8) uses a limited repertoire of nonpolymorphic receptors that recognize structural motifs common to many microorganisms. These include small glycolipids and lipopeptides. The alternative strategy of the evolutionarily newer adaptive immune response relies on generating myriad receptors that might recognize the wide array of foreign compounds from infectious agents. Whereas the innate immune response allows a rapid response, the adaptive one permits a wider array of response, as well as immune memory.

T lymphocyte development constantly confronts the dilemma of combating infection without provoking a response to the host. The price for generating an increasingly varied population of antigen receptors needed to recognize a wide spectrum of pathogens is the progressive risk of producing self-reactive lymphocytes that can provoke an autoimmune diathesis. To minimize the possibility of self-reactive cells, T lymphocytes are subjected to a rigorous selection process during development in the thymus. In addition, premature activation of mature T cells is prevented by requiring two signals for activation. Finally, the tremendous expansion of T cells that occurs during the response to an infection is resolved by the active induction of cell death. In perhaps no other organ are the processes of cell proliferation and death more dynamically displayed than by lymphocytes during an immune response. The consequences of inefficient lymphocyte removal at any one of these junctures can be devastating to the health of the organism. This is vividly displayed in both humans and mice where naturally arising mutations in death receptors, such as Fas, result in massive accumulation of lymphocytes and autoimmune sequelae. These are discussed in more detail in Chapter 26 on apoptosis.

The activation of T lymphocytes yields a variety of effector functions pivotal to arresting infectious processes. Cytolytic T cells can kill infected cells through the expression of perforin, which produces holes in cell membranes, or ligands for death receptors such as Fas or tumor necrosis factor-alpha (TNF-α) receptor. Production of T cell cytokines such as interferon-γ (IFN-γ) can inhibit viral replication, whereas other cytokines such as interleukin-4 (IL-4) and IL-5 are critical for optimal B cell growth and immunoglobulin production.[1,2] However, this same armamentarium can also precipitate damage to host tissues and provoke autoimmune responses. This is most dramatically apparent in situations in which T cell infiltration can be observed histologically, such as in the synovium of inflammatory arthritides, pancreatic islets in type I diabetes, and the central nervous system in multiple sclerosis. Damage in these cases need not be directly the result of recognition of target tissues by the T cells. T cells may be activated elsewhere and then migrate to the tissue and damage innocent bystander cells. T cells may also promote an autoimmune diathesis through the augmentation of B cell responses.

In describing the development and function of T lymphocytes in this chapter, emphasis is placed on highlighting the various junctures at which autoreactive T cells may arise, either through inefficient elimination, accidental clonal expansion through cross-reactivity between infectious and self antigens, or nonspecific activation with resulting bystander injury.

T Cell Development

T cells must traverse two stringent hurdles during their development. First, a T cell must successfully rearrange the genes encoding the two chains of the T cell antigen receptor (TCR). Second, a T cell must survive thymic selection during which self-reactive T cells are eliminated. The survival rate of these two independent selection processes is less than 3 percent, which is in part necessary to minimize the chances of autoreactive T cells escaping to the periphery.

The TCR is an 80- to 90-kD disulfide-linked heterodimer composed of a 48- to 54-kD α-chain and a 37- to 42-kD β-chain. An alternate TCR composed of γ- and δ-chains is expressed on 2 to 3 percent of peripheral blood T cells and is discussed later in the chapter. The TCR has an extracellular ligand-binding pocket and a short cytoplasmic tail that, by itself, cannot signal. Consequently, it is noncovalently associated with as many as five invariant chains of the CD3 complex. The structure of the TCR gene is, not surprisingly, very similar to what was first described for immunoglobulin genes in B cells (see Chapter 10). Each overcame the problem of how to encode approximately 10 million different T or B cell specificities within the human genome, which contains only about 30,000 genes. To economically package this diversity, the process of gene rearrangement and splicing evolved using machinery similar to that which already existed to promote gene translocations. The β- and δ-chain genes of the TCR contain four segments known as the V (variable), D (diversity), J (joining), and C (constant) regions. The α- and γ-chains are similar but lack the J component. Each of the segments has several family members (approximately 50 to 100 V, 15 D, 6 to 60 J, and 1 to 2 C members). An orderly process occurs during TCR gene rearrangement in which a D segment is spliced adjacent to a J segment, which is subsequently spliced to a V segment. Following transcription, the VDJ sequence is spliced to a C segment to produce a mature TCR messenger RNA. Arithmetically, this random rearrangement of a single chain of the TCR locus can give rise to minimally 50V × 15D × 6J × 2C, or about 9000 possible combinations. At each of the splice sites, which must occur in-frame to be functional, additional nucleotides not encoded by the genome (so-called N-region nucleotides) can be incorporated, adding further diversity to the rearranging gene. The combinations from the two TCR chains, plus N-region diversity, yield at least 10^8 theoretic possible combinations. The cutting, rearranging, and splicing are directed by specific enzymes. Mutations in the genes for these processes can result in an arrest in lymphocyte development. For example, mutation in the gene encoding a DNA-dependent protein kinase required for receptor gene recombination results in severe-combined immunodeficiency (SCID).

Thus, TCR gene recombination presents the first of the two major hurdles for developing lymphocytes. Because the developing T cell has two copies of each chromosome, there are two chances to successfully rearrange each of the two TCR chains. As soon as successful rearrangement occurs, further β-chain rearrangements on either the same or the other chromosome are suppressed, a process known as *allelic exclusion.* This limits the chance of dual TCR expression by an individual T cell. The high percentage of T cells that contain rearrangements of both β-chain genes attests to the inefficiency of this complex event. Rearrangement of the α-chain occurs later in thymocyte development in a similar fashion, although without apparent allelic exclusion. This can lead to dual TCR expression by a single T cell.

Development of T cells occurs within a microenvironment provided by the thymic epithelial stroma. The thymic anlage is formed from embryonic ectoderm and endoderm and is then colonized by hematopoietic cells, which give rise to dendritic cells, macrophages, and developing T cells.[2] The hematopoietic and epithelial components combine to form two histologically defined compartments: the cortex, which contains immature thymocytes, and the medulla, which contains mature thymocytes (Fig. 9–1A). As few as 50 to 100 bone marrow–derived stem cells enter the thymus daily.[3]

The stages of thymocyte development can be defined by the status of rearrangement and expression of the two genes that encode the α- and β-chains of the TCR and the expression of CD4 and CD8, proceeding in an orderly fashion from CD4-8– to CD4+8+ to CD4+8– or CD4-8+ (see Fig. 9–1B). CD4 and CD8 define, respectively, the helper and cytolytic subsets of mature T cells.

CD4-8– thymocytes can be further subdivided based on their expression of CD25 (the high affinity IL-2 receptor α-chain) and CD44 (the hyaluronate receptor).[4] Development proceeds in this order:

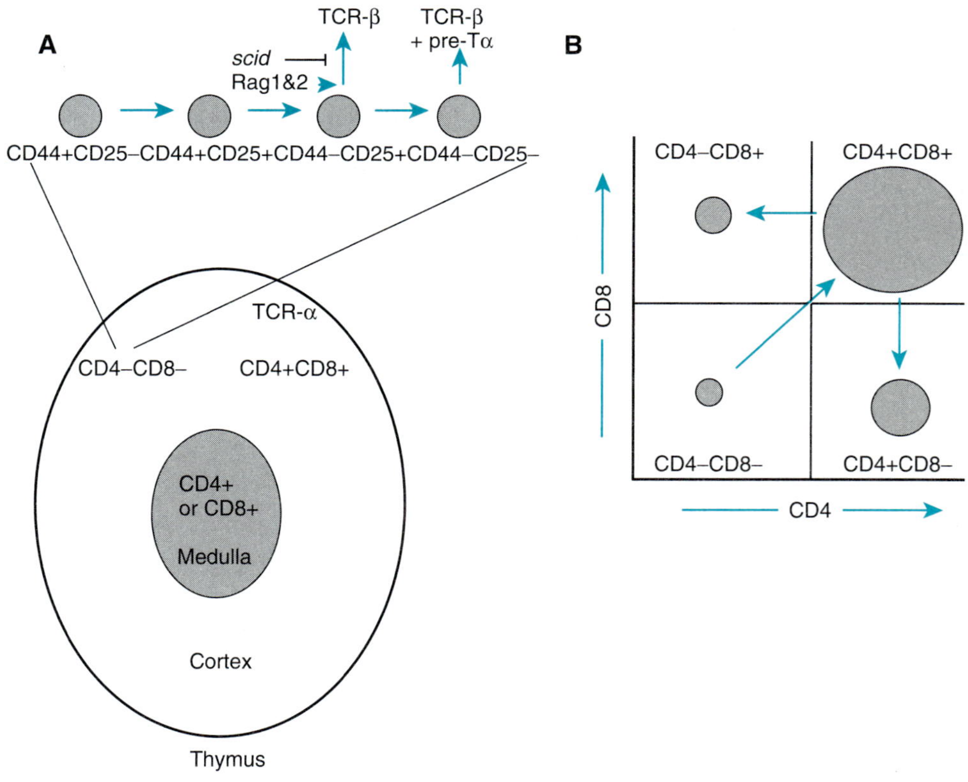

FIGURE 9–1 · Sequence of Thymocyte Development. *A,* The earliest thymocyte precursors lack expression of CD4 and CD8 (CD4–CD8–). These can be further divided into four subpopulations based on the sequential expression of CD44 and CD25. It is at the CD44-CD25+ stage that the T cell receptor (TCR) β-chain rearranges. The severe combined immunodeficiency (SCID) mutation or deficiencies of the recombination activating genes, Rag-1 and Rag-2, result in inability to rearrange the β-chain and maturational arrest at this stage. Those thymocytes that successfully rearrange the β-chain express it associated with a surrogate α-chain known as pre-T α. Concomitant with a proliferative burst, development can then progress to the CD4+CD8+ stage in the cortex in which the TCR α-chain rearranges and pairs with the β-chain to express a mature TCR complex. These cells then undergo thymic positive and negative selection (see Fig. 9–3B). Successful completion of this rigorous selection process results in mature CD4+ or CD8+ T cells in the medulla, which eventually emigrate to peripheral lymphoid sites. *B,* Schematic two-color flow cytometry shows subpopulations of thymocytes defined by CD4 and CD8 expression in their relative proportions.

CD25-CD44+ → CD25+CD44+ → CD25+CD44−→ CD25-CD44−

These subpopulations correspond to discrete stages of thymocyte differentiation. CD25-44+ cells express low levels of CD4, and their TCR genes are in germline configuration. These cells downregulate CD4 and upregulate CD25 to give rise to CD25+CD44+ thymocytes, which now express surface CD2 and low levels of CD3ε. At the next stage (CD25+CD44–), there is a brief burst of proliferation followed by upregulation of the recombination-activating genes, RAG-1 and RAG-2, and the concomitant rearrangement of the genes of the TCR β-chain. A small subpopulation of T cells rearranges and expresses a second pair of TCR genes known as γ and δ. Productive TCR β-chain rearrangement results in downregulation of RAG and a second proliferative burst. Loss of CD25 then yields CD25-CD44– thymocytes.

The TCR β-chain cannot be stably expressed without an α-chain. Because the TCR α-chain has not yet rearranged, a surrogate invariant TCR pre–α-chain is disulfide linked to the β-chain. When associated with components of the CD3 complex, this allows a low-level surface expression of a pre-TCR and progression to the next developmental stage. Failure to successfully rearrange the TCR β-chain results in a developmental arrest at the transition from CD25+CD44− to CD25–CD44−. This occurs in RAG-deficient mice as well as in SCID mice and humans.[5,6]

A number of signaling molecules are required for early T cell development[7] (Fig. 9–2), The IKAROS gene encodes a family of transcription factors required for the development of cells of lymphoid origin. Notch-1, a molecule known to regulate cell-fate decisions, is also required at the earliest stage of T cell lineage development.[8] Cytokines including IL-7 promote the survival and expansion of the earliest thymocytes.[9] In mice deficient for IL-7, its receptor components, IL-7Rα or γ_c, or the cytokine receptor-associated signaling molecule janus-associated kinase (JAK-3), thymocyte development is inhibited at the $CD25^-CD44^+$ stage. In humans, mutations in γ_c or *JAK-3* result in the most frequent form of SCID.[10] Pre-TCR signaling is required for the $CD25^+44^-$ to $CD25^-CD44^-$ transition. Thus, loss of signaling components, including Lck, SLP-76, and *LAT-1*, results in a block at this stage of T cell development.[11] TCR signals are also required for differentiation of CD4+8+ to CD4+ or CD8+ cells. Humans deficient in zeta-associated protein (*ZAP-70*) have CD4+ but not CD8+ T cells in the thymus and periphery.[12]

CD25–CD44– cells upregulate expression of CD4 and CD8 to become CD4+8+. It is as a CD4+CD8+ thymocyte that the α-chain of the TCR rearranges. Unlike the β-chain, allelic exclusion of the α-chain is not apparent. Rearrangement of the α-chain can occur simultaneously on both chromosomes, and if one attempt is unsuccessful, repeat rearrangements to other Vα segments are possible. Reports have been made of dual TCR expression by as many as 30 percent of mature T cells, in which a T cell expresses different α-chains paired with the same β-chain.[13] However, in most cases of dualing TCR α-chains, one is downregulated during positive selection through ubiquitination, endocytosis, and degradation.[14]

Although the structure of immunoglobulin and TCR are quite similar, they recognize fundamentally different antigens. Immunoglobulins recognize intact antigens in isolation, either soluble or membrane bound, and they are often sensitive to the tertiary structure. The TCRαβ recognizes linear stretches of antigen peptide fragments bound within the grooves of either major histocompatability complex (MHC) class I or class II molecules (Fig. 9–3A). Thymic selection molds the repertoire of emerging TCR so that they recognize peptides within the groove of self-MHC molecules,

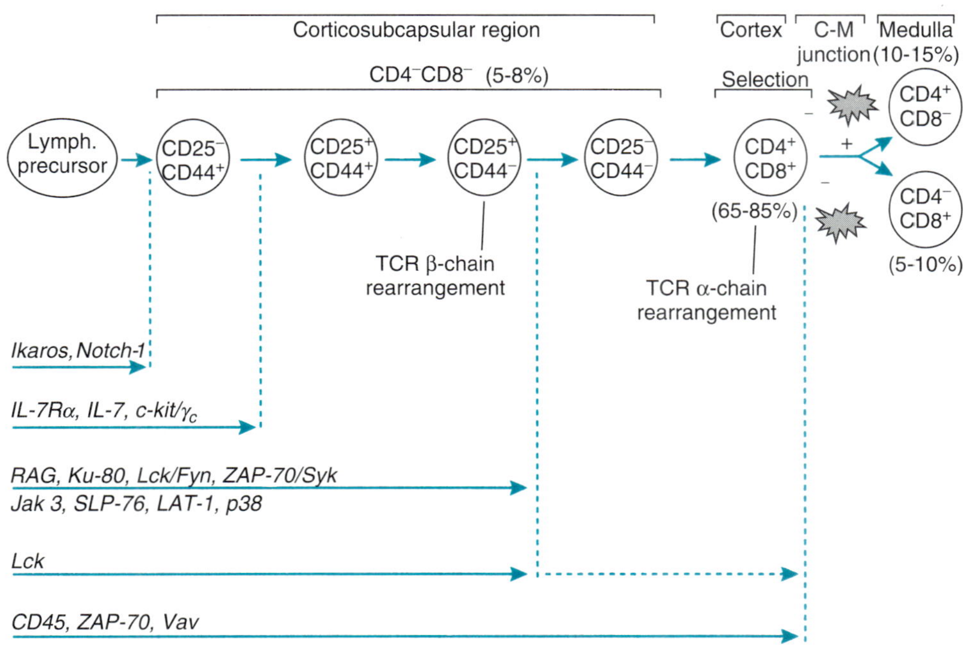

FIGURE 9–2 · Sequence of αβ T Cell Development in the Thymus. The earliest thymocyte precursors lack expression of CD4 and CD8 (CD4–CD8–). These can be further divided into four subpopulations based on the sequential expression of CD25 and CD44. At the CD25+CD44– stage, the T cell receptor (TCR) β-chain rearranges and associates a surrogate α-chain known as pre-T α. Concomitant with a proliferative burst, thymocytes progress to the CD4+CD8+ stage, rearrange the TCR α-chain, and express a mature TCR complex. These cells then undergo thymic positive and negative selection. Those thymocytes that survive this rigorous selection process differentiate into mature CD4+ or CD8+ T cells. Also shown are the various signaling molecules involved at specific stages of thymic development.

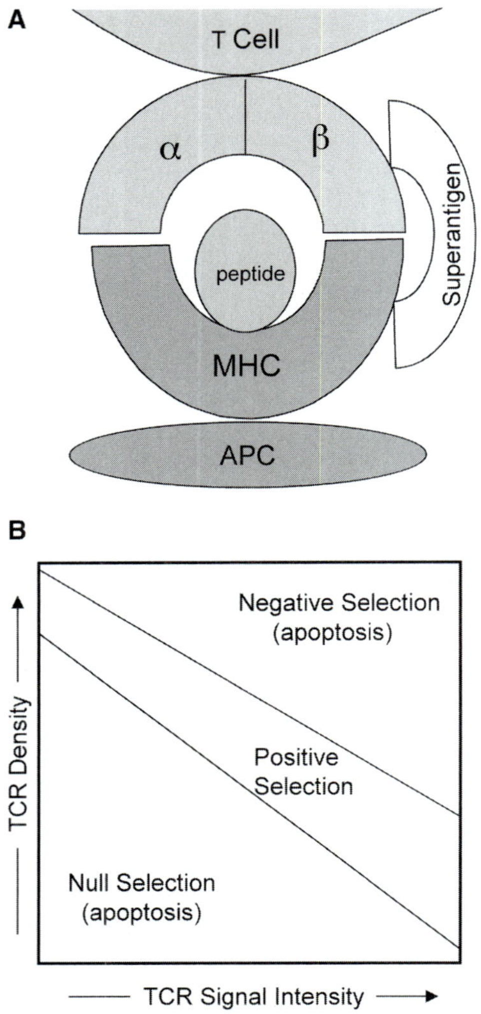

FIGURE 9–3 • *A*, T cell receptor (TCR) interaction with the major histocompatibility complex (MHC)/peptide complex. Polymorphic residues within the variable region of the α- and β-chains of the TCR make contact with determinants on the MHC molecule on an antigen-presenting cell (APC), as well as with the peptide fragment that sits in the MHC binding groove. *B*, Schematic diagram illustrates that during thymocyte development, those TCR conferring either a very low signal intensity, null selection, or high-intensity negative selection each leads to apoptosis. Only those thymocytes whose TCR can engage MHC/peptides and confer moderate intensity survive by positive selection.

ensuring the self-MHC restriction of T cell responses. The MHC structure is described in detail in Chapter 17. Pockets within the MHC groove bind particular residues along the peptide sequence of seven to nine amino acids for MHC class I and nine to 15 amino acids for MHC class II molecules. As a result, depending on the particular MHC molecule, certain amino acids will make strong contact with the MHC groove, whereas others will contact the TCR.

The contact between the TCR and antigen or MHC has been revealed by crystal structure to be remarkably flat, rather than the deep lock-and-key structure one might imagine.[15,16] The TCR axis is tipped about 30 degrees to the long axis of the MHC class I molecule and is slightly more skewed to MHC class II. The affinity of the TCR for antigen or MHC is in the micromolar range.[17] This is less than many antibody-antigen affinities, and several logs less than many enzyme-substrate affinities. This has lead to the notion that TCR interactions with antigen or MHC are brief, and successful activation of the T cell requires multiple interactions, resulting in a cumulative signal.

Once the T cell has successfully rearranged and expressed a TCR in association with the CD3 complex, it encounters the second major hurdle in T cell development, thymic selection. Selection has two phases, positive and negative, and the outcome is based largely upon the intensity of TCR signaling in response to interactions with MHC or self peptides expressed on thymic epithelium and dendritic cells. TCR signals that are either too weak (death by neglect) or too intense (negative selection) result in elimination by apoptosis, whereas those with intermediate signaling intensity survive by positive selection (see Fig. 9–3B). Successful positive selection at the CD4+8+ stage is coincident with upregulation of surface TCR, the activation markers CD5 and CD69, and the survival factor Bcl-2.[18-20] T cells bearing a TCR that recognizes MHC class I maintain CD8 expression, downregulate CD4, and become CD4-8+. T cells expressing a TCR that recognizes MHC class II become CD4+8-.

Not surprisingly, a variety of signaling molecules activated by TCR engagement are important to thymic selection. These include *Lck*, the *Ras* → Raf-1 → MEK1→ ERK kinase cascade, the kinase *ZAP-70*, and the phosphatases CD45 and calcineurin, which are involved with positive selection.[11] Among these, the *Ras* to *ERK* pathway is particularly important, as dominant negative versions of these molecules can disrupt positive selection. Conversely, an activator of *Ras* known as *GRP1* assists the positive selection of thymocytes expressing weakly selecting signals.[21] These molecules are discussed in more detail in the section on TCR signaling. By contrast, although a number of molecules may promote negative selection, including the mitogen-activated protein (MAP) kinases JNK and p38, there appears to be sufficient redundancy so that only rarely does elimination of any one of these molecules affect deletion of thymocytes. The few exceptions include CD40, CD40L, or CD30, where preservation of at least some thymocytes bearing self-reactive TCR could be observed in mice deficient in these molecules.[22-24]

The survivors of these two stringent processes of TCR gene rearrangement and thymic selection represent less than 3 percent of total immature thymocytes. This is reflected by the presence of a high rate of cell death in developing thymocytes. This can be visualized by the measurement of DNA degradation, a hallmark of apoptosis, as shown in Figure 9–4. The survivors become either CD4+ helper or CD8+ cytolytic T cells and reside in the thymic medulla for 12 to 14 days before emigrating to the periphery. The decision to become a CD4+ versus CD8+ T cell involves further developmental signals, including once again *Notch-1*.[25] *Notch-1* signaling is required for progression to CD8+ but not CD4+ thymocytes. This parallels the observation that long TCR interactions are required for CD4 progression, whereas shorter TCR engagement is required for CD8 progression.[26]

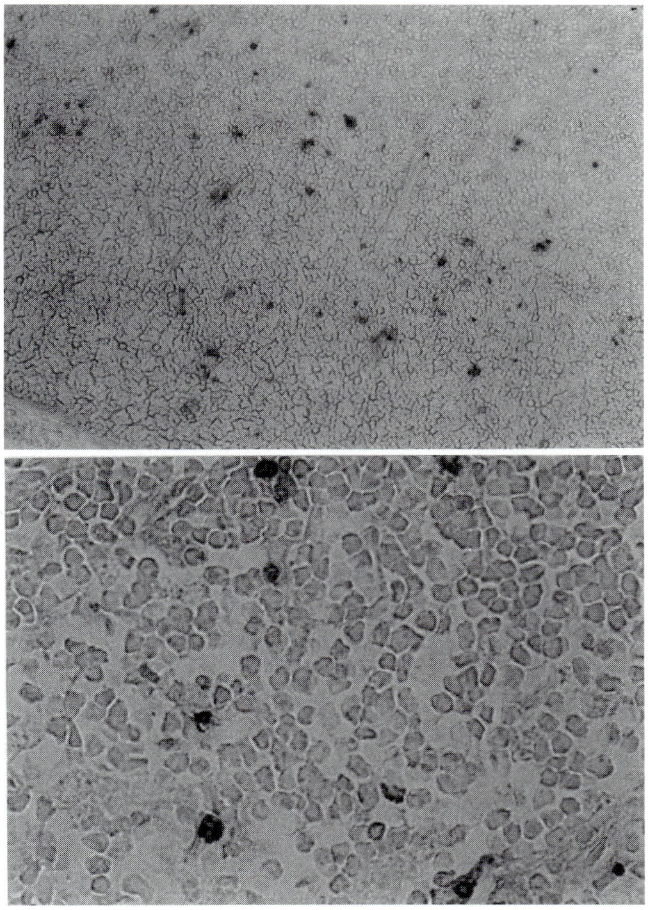

FIGURE 9–4 · Terminated Deoxynucleotidyl Transferase-mediated dUTP Nick End Labeling (TUNEL) Assay for Nicked DNA in Thymocytes Undergoing Apoptosis. Thymus sections were made from wild-type mice, fixed, and stained by the TUNEL assay. The DNA repair enzyme, terminal deoxynucleotidyl transferase (TdT), inserts biotinylated dUTP residues at sites of double-stranded breaks, and it is then revealed by avidin horeseradish peroxidase. Shown are sections at 100 × and 400 ×. Apoptotic thymocytes are those undergoing negative selection from either too intense or too weak a T cell receptor (TCR) signal. (See color plate 2.)

Extrathymic T Cell Development

In the absence of a thymus, as in nude (nu/nu) mice, T cell populations in the lymph nodes and spleen are severely reduced and oligoclonal, but they are not absent. Whereas some of this extrathymic T cell development occurs within the liver, a significant amount also occurs in contact with the intestinal epithelium.

Intestinal intraepithelial lymphocytes (IEL) have a very different phenotype from thymus-derived T cells. In contrast to the predominance of CD4+ T cells over CD8+ T cells in normal lymph nodes, IEL contain large portions of CD8+ and CD4$^-$8– T cells.[27] Many CD8+ IEL express only the CD8α-chain as an αα homodimer. γδ T cells also comprise a significant portion of IEL. The antigens to which IEL respond are not known, although in humans some of the γδ IEL recognize the MHC class Ib molecule MICA.[28] IEL have a memory CD44+ T cell phenotype (see following) and are cytolytic when freshly isolated.

Abnormalities of Human T Cell Development

Given the vast number of developmental events in T cell development, it is not surprising that a multiplicity of causes can underlie human T cell immunodeficiencies.[29,30] The influence of the thymic stroma on thymocyte ontogeny is underscored in the DiGeorge anomaly in which development of the pharyngeal pouches is disrupted and the thymic rudiment fails to form.[31] This results in the failure of normal T cell development. Less severe T cell deficiencies are associated with a failure to express MHC class I, class II, or both (the "bare lymphocyte syndrome"), which are directly involved with interactions required to induce the positive selection of, respectively, CD8+ and CD4+ mature T cells.

Metabolic disorders can affect thymocytes more directly. The absence of functional adenosine deaminase (ADA) and purine nucleoside phosphorylase (PNP) results in the build-up of metabolic by-products that are toxic to developing T and B lymphocytes. This ultimately produces forms of SCID.

The inability to express a number of surface molecules important in TCR and cytokine signaling also has the potential to perturb development. The failure to express TCR-CD3 components (specifically CD3γ and CD3ε), CD18, and IL-2Rγ[32] have all been noted among patients who exhibit varying degrees of T cell deficiency or dysfunction. All of these molecules are involved in signaling of thymocyte development and survival, and their absence clearly has the potential to alter developmental fate.

Peripheral Migration of T Cells

The migration of naïve T cells to peripheral lymphoid structures, or their infiltration into other tissues, requires the coordinate regulation of an array of cell-adhesion molecules. T cell recirculation is essential for host surveillance and is carefully regulated by a specific array of homing receptors. Entry from the circulation to tissues occurs via two main anatomic sites: the flat endothelium of the blood vessels or specialized postcapillary venules, known as high endothelial venules (HEV).[33] A three-step model has been proposed for lymphocyte migration: rolling, adhesion, and migration.[34] L-selectin expressed by naïve T cells binds via lectin domains to carbohydrate moieties of GlyCAM-1 (cell adhesion molecule) and CD34 (collectively known as peripheral node addressin), which are expressed on endothelial cells, particularly HEV. The weak binding of CD62L to its ligand mediates a weak adhesion to the vessel wall, which, combined with the force of blood flow, results in rolling of the T cell along the endothelium. The increased cell contact facilitates the interaction of a second adhesion molecule on lymphocytes, the integrin LFA-1 (CD11a/CD18) with its ligands, intercellular adhesion molecule-1 (ICAM-1) (CD54) and ICAM-2 (CD102). This results in the arrest of rolling and firm attachment. Migration into the extracellular matrix of tissues may involve additional lymphocyte cell surface molecules, such as the hyaluronate receptor

(CD44) or the integrin α4β7 (CD49d/β7), which binds the mucosal addressin cell-adhesion molecule-1 (MAdCAM-1) on endothelium of Peyer's patches and other endothelial cells.

Other cytokines known as chemokines may contribute to lymphocyte homing. Chemokines are structurally and functionally related to proteins bearing an affinity for heparan sulfate proteoglycan and promote migration of various cell types.[35,36] The chemokines "regulated on activation normal T expressed secreted" (RANTES), MIP-1α, MIP-1β, MCP-1, and IL-8 are produced by a number of cell types, including endothelium, activated T cells, and monocytes, and are present at inflammatory sites such as rheumatoid synovium (see Chapter 24).

A more recently recognized capacity of peripheral T cells is homeostatic proliferation.[37,38] This reflects the ability of mature T cells to undergo proliferation in lymphopenic environments. Experimentally this is studied by the adoptive transfer of T cells into RAG-deficient or irradiated mice. However, a similar phenomenon has been shown to occur in normal newborn mice.[39] Newborn mice do not reach the adult levels of T cells until day 7 in lymph nodes and day 15 in the spleen. Because this expansion of T cells requires the presence of MHC or self peptides, this may become an area of considerable interest in future studies of autoimmune mechanisms. In this regard, it is of interest that one of the standard models of autoimmunity is day-3 thymectomy, which results in lymphopenia.[40,41] It will be of interest to learn the possible contribution of homeostatic proliferation to this syndrome.

Activation of T Cells

T cell activation initiates intracellular signaling cascades, which activate transcription factors and induce new gene transcription. This ultimately results in proliferation, effector function, or death, depending on the developmental stage of the cell. To guard against premature or excessive activation, T cells have a requirement of two independent signals for full activation. Signal 1 is an antigen-specific signal provided by the binding of the TCR to antigenic peptide complexed with MHC. Signal 2 is mediated by either cytokines or the engagement of costimulatory molecules such as B7.1 (CD80) and B7.2 (CD86) on the antigen-presenting cell (APC).

T CELL RECEPTORS AND TYROSINE KINASES

TCR αβ and γδ have very short cytoplasmic domains and by themselves are unable to transduce signals.[42,43] The molecules of the noncovalently associated CD3 complex couple the TCR to intracellular signaling machinery (Fig. 9–5). The CD3 complex contains nonpolymorphic members known as CD3ε, CD3γ, CD3δ, as well as ζ- and η-chains that are alternatively spliced forms of the same gene and are not genetically linked to the CD3 complex. Although the functional stoichiometry of the TCR complex is not completely defined, current data indicate that each TCR heterodimer is associated with three dimers: CD3 εγ, CD3εδ, and ζζ or ζη.[44] CD3ε, -γ, and -δ have an immunoglobulin-like extracellular domain, a transmembrane region, and a modest cytoplasmic domain, whereas ζ contains a longer cytoplasmic tail. The transmembrane domains of ζ and the CD3 chains contain a negatively charged residue that interacts with positively charged amino acids in the transmembrane domain of the TCR.

None of the proteins in the TCR complex has intrinsic enzymatic activity. Instead, the cytoplasmic domains of the invariant CD3 chains contain conserved activation domains that are required for coupling the TCR to intracellular signaling molecules. These immunoreceptor tyrosine-based activation motifs (ITAMS) contain a min-

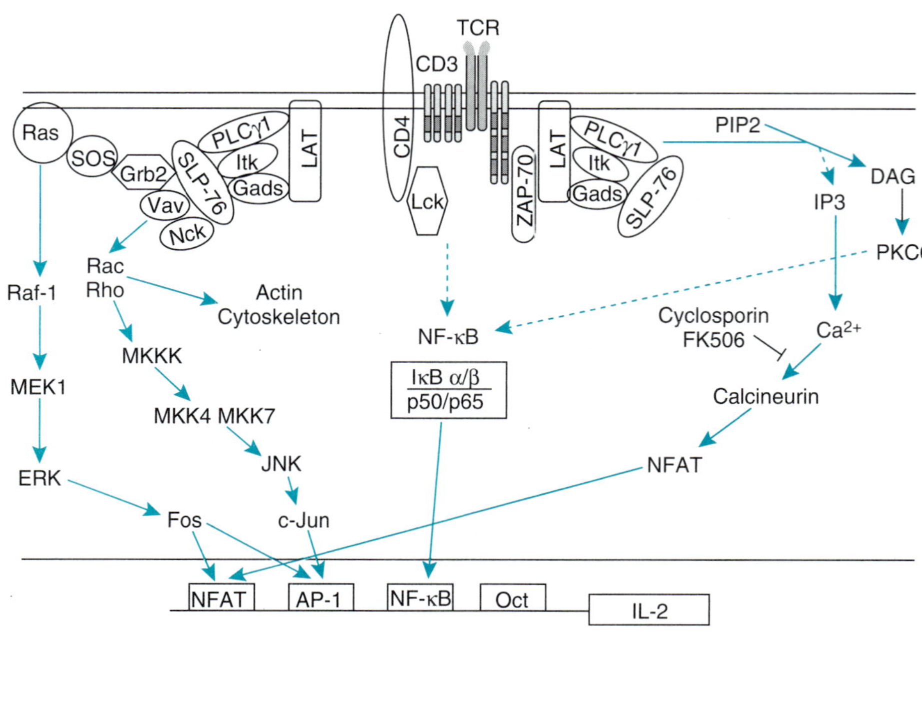

FIGURE 9–5 • T cell Receptor (TCR) Signal Pathways. Schema show the principle signal pathways resulting from TCR activation and how they impinge on the regulatory region of the interleukin-2 (IL-2) gene. See text for details.

imal functional consensus sequence of paired tyrosines (Y) and leucines (L): $(D/E)XXYXXL(X)_{6\text{-}8}YXXL$.[45] ITAMs are substrates for cytoplasmic protein tyrosine kinases (PTKs) and, upon phosphorylation, recruit additional molecules to the TCR complex.[46] Each ζ-chain contains three ITAMs, whereas there is one in each of the CD3ε, -γ, and -δ chains. Thus, each TCR complex can contain 10 total ITAMs.

Activation of PTKs is one of the earliest signaling events following TCR stimulation. Four families of PTKs are known to be involved in TCR signaling: Src, Csk, Tec, and Syk.[47] The Src family members Lck and Fyn[T] have a central role in TCR signaling and are expressed exclusively in lymphoid cells. Src PTKs contain multiple structural domains including: 1) N-terminal myristylation and palmitylation sites which allow association with the plasma membrane; 2) a Src-homology 3 (SH3) domain that associates with proline-rich sequences; 3) an SH2 domain that binds phosphotyrosine-containing proteins; and 4) a carboxy-terminal negative regulatory site. Their catalytic activity is regulated by the balance between the actions of kinases and phosphatases. Activity is repressed by phosphorylation of a conserved carboxy-terminal tyrosine and dephosphorylation by the phosphatase CD45 is critical for the initiation of TCR-mediated signal transduction. In addition, autophosphorylation of other tyrosines within the kinase domain enhances catalytic activity. Lck is physically and functionally associated with CD4 and CD8. Fifty to 90 percent of total Lck molecules are associated with CD4 and and 10 to 25 percent with CD8. CD4 and CD8 physically associate with the TCR/CD3 complex during antigen stimulation as a result of their interaction with MHC class II and class I molecules and thus enhance TCR-mediated signals by recruiting Lck to the TCR complex. Lck phosphorylates the CD3 chains, *TCRζ, ZAP-70,* phospholipase *C-γ1* (PLCγ1), *Vav,* and *Shc.* Fyn binds TCRζ and CD3ε and, although its substrates are less well defined, T cells lacking *Fyn* have diminished response to TCR signals.[48,49] In addition, the SH2 and SH3 domains of Src PTKs can mediate their association with, respectively, phosphotyrosine- and proline-containing molecules.

Somewhat less is known about the Csk and Tec PTKs. Csk negatively regulates TCR signaling by phosphorylating the carboxy-terminal tyrosine of Lck and Fyn. Dephosphorylation of this negative regulatory tyrosine is mediated by the transmembrane tyrosine phosphatase CD45. CD45 activity is essential for TCR signaling as CD45-deficient T cells fail to activate by TCR stimulation.[50] The Tec family member *Itk* is preferentially expressed in T cells. T cells from Itk-deficient mice have diminished response to TCR stimulation.[51] The mechanism by which *Itk* regulates TCR signaling has not been determined, although recent studies have shown that *Itk* is an important component of the pathway leading to increased intracellular Ca^{2+}.

Phosphorylation of the ITAM motifs on the CD3 complex recruits the *Syk* kinase family member *ZAP-70* by its tandem SH2 domains. ZAP-70 is expressed exclusively in T cells and is required for TCR signaling. Like the *Src*-family PTKs, *ZAP-70* is positively and negatively regulated by its phosphorylation. Phosphorylation of tyrosine 493 by *Lck* activates *ZAP-70* kinase activity. In murine thymocytes and ex vivo T cells, inactive nonphosphorylated *ZAP-70* is constitutively associated with the basally phosphorylated *TCRζ*-chain via the *SH2* domain of *ZAP-70.*[52] TCR stimulation is required for *ZAP-70* phosphorylation and activation. The recruitment of ZAP-70 to the TCR complex facilitates the tyrosine phosphorylation and activation of ZAP-70 by Lck. These data suggest that the receptor-signaling complex in these cells is primed, but an initiating event is still required to activate ZAP-70. ZAP-70 can also act as a scaffold, binding to other proteins via its SH2 domain and phosphorylated tyrosines. ZAP-70 interacts with Lck, Ras-GAP, Vav, the phosphatase SHP-1, and Cbl, and these proteins may regulate ZAP-70 activity or serve as substrates. ZAP-70 phosphorylates tyrosine residues in a number of molecules including phospholipase Cγ1 and the adaptor proteins SLP-76 and LAT.

ADAPTOR PROTEINS

Phosphorylation of tyrosine residues in ITAMs and PTKs following TCR stimulation creates docking sites for adaptor proteins. Adaptor proteins contain no known enzymatic or transcriptional activities but instead mediate protein-protein interactions or protein-lipid interactions.[53] They function to bring proteins in proximity to their substrates and regulators, as well as sequester signaling molecules to specific subcellular locations. The protein complexes formed can function as either positive or negative regulators of TCR signaling, depending on the molecules they contain.

Two critical adaptor proteins for linking proximal and distal TCR signaling events are *SH2*-domain-containing leukocyte protein of 76 kD (*SLP-76*) and linker for activation of T cells (LAT) (see Fig. 9–5). Loss of these adaptor proteins has profound consequences for T cell development. Mice deficient for *LAT* or *SLP-76* manifest a block in T cell development at the CD4-8-CD25+44+ stage. LAT is constitutively localized to lipid rafts and, following TCR stimulation, is phosphorylated on tyrosine residues by *ZAP-70.* Phosphorylated *LAT* then recruits *SH2*-domain–containing proteins including *PLCγ1,* the p85 subunit of phosphoinositide-3 kinase, *Itk,* and the adaptors Grb2 and Gads. Because the *SH3* domain of Gads is constitutively associated with *SLP-76,* this brings *SLP-76* to the complex where it is phosphorylated by *ZAP-70. SLP-76* contains three protein-binding motifs: tyrosine phosphorylation sites, a proline-rich region, and an *SH2* domain. The N terminus of *SLP-76* contains tyrosine residues that associate with the SH2 domains of *Vav,* the adaptor *Nck,* and *Itk. Vav* is a 95-kD protein that acts as guanine nucleotide exchange factor for the *Rho/Rac/cdc42* family of small G-proteins. Through its association with *Vav* and *Nck, SLP-76* links TCR signals to *Rac/Rho* guanosine triphosphate-ases (GTPases) and the actin cytoskeleton. The association of phosphorylated *LAT* with *PLCγ1* and Grb2 couples the TCR signaling to both the *Ras* and phosphatidylinositol pathways (see following). *Grb2* contains a central *SH2* domain flanked by two SH3 domains and associates with the proline-rich regions of Sos, a guanine nucleotide exchange factor for Ras. Recruitment of Grb2 to the receptor brings Sos to the plasma membrane where it activates Ras. The complex of LAT, SLP-76/Gads, PLCγ1, and associated molecules results in the full activation of PLCγ1 and activation of Ras.

In addition to acting as positive regulators for TCR signaling, adaptors can also mediate negative regulation. As described previously, the activity of the Src-family kinases is regulated by the interaction of kinases (Csk) and phosphatases (CD45) specific for inhibitory C-terminal phosphotyrosine, and this is determined by the subcellular localization of these regulatory molecules. The interactions that control the localization of CD45 are just now being analyzed. The localization of Csk is dependent on an adaptor known as phosphoprotein associated with glycosphingolipid-enriched microdomains (PAG or Csk binding protein, CBP). Collectively the data suggest the following model. PAG is constitutively associated with membrane lipid rafts. In resting cells, PAG/CBP is tyrosine phosphorylated, which mediates the association with the SH2 domains of Csk. This colocalizes Csk with Src-family kinases in lipid rafts and controls the basal activation of Src-family PTK through phosphorylation of inhibitory C-terminal tyrosine residues. Upon TCR stimulation, PAG becomes dephosphorylated, resulting in the dissociation of Csk. Loss of Csk from the rafts reverses the inhibition of Src PTK activity and permits the initiation of downstream signaling.

A second mechanism by which adaptor proteins can negatively regulate TCR signaling is through regulation of protein stability. c-Cbl and Cbl-b are members of a conserved family of proteins that contains a highly conserved N-terminal region containing a tyrosine kinase-binding and RING-finger domains. c-CBL RING finger domain binds the E2 ubiquitin-conjugating enzymes. Active E2 enzymes are brought into proximity with tyrosine kinase–binding proteins resulting in their ubiquination and degradation by the proteosome complex. Syk and ZAP-70 associate with c-Cbl, whereas Vav, ZAP-70, LCK, PLCγ1, and the p85 subunit of PI3K associate with Cbl-b.

DOWNSTREAM TRANSCRIPTION FACTORS

The previously mentioned signaling events couple TCR stimulation to downstream pathways that culminate in changes in gene transcription that are required for proliferation and effector function (see Fig. 9–4). One of the best-characterized genes induced following T cell activation is the T cell growth factor, IL-2. Transcription of the IL-2 gene is regulated in part by the transcription factors activator protein-1 (AP-1), nuclear factor of activated T cells (NF-AT), and nuclear factor kappa B (NFκB), all of which are activated following TCR stimulation. Proximal signaling events lead to the activation of Ras and PLCγ.[54,55] Ras initiates a cascade of kinases including Raf-1, MEK, and the MAP kinase ERK, which leads to the production of the transcription factor Fos. Ligation of the costimulatory molecule CD28 results in the activation of another member of the MAP kinase family, c-Jun N-terminal kinase (JNK), and phosphorylation of the transcription factor c-Jun. c-Jun and Fos associate to form AP-1. PLCγ hydrolyzes membrane inositol phospholipids to generate phosphoinositide second messengers including inositol 1,4,5 trisphosphate (IP_3) and diacylglycerol. IP_3 stimulates the mobilization of calcium from intracellular stores. Diacylglycerol activates protein kinase C (especially PCKθ in T cells) and, along with CARMA, connects with the NFκB pathway.[56]

Increased intracellular calcium is central to many forms of cellular activation. Calcium activates the calcium/calmodulin-dependent serine phosphatase calcineurin, which dephosphorylates NF-AT.[57] Dephosphorylated NF-AT translocates to the nucleus and, together with AP-1, forms a trimolecular transcription factor for the IL-2 gene. The immunosuppressive agents Cyclosporin-A and FK-506 specifically inhibit the calcium-dependent activation of calcineurin, thereby blocking activation of NF-AT and the transcription of NF-AT–dependent cytokines, such as IL-2, IL-3, IL-4, and granulocyte-macrophage colony-stimulating factor (GM-CSF). Recently, it has been appreciated that differences in the amplitude and duration of calcium signals mediate different functional outcomes. Although high spikes of calcium are easily measured in lymphocytes during the first 10 minutes following antigen stimulation, sustained low-level calcium spikes over a few hours are necessary for full activation.[58] These latter, more-subtle calcium fluxes appear to be controlled by cyclic-adenosine diphosphate (ADP)-ribose and ryanodine receptors.[59] Selective inhibitors exist for these molecules, opening the potential for new specific blockers of T cell activation.

COSTIMULATION

Signal 2 is mediated either by growth-factor cytokines or through a costimulatory molecule, of which the prototype is CD28 interacting with CD80 (B7-1) or CD86 (B7-2). CD28 is a disulfide-linked homodimer constitutively expressed on the surface of T cells.[60] Virtually all murine T cells express CD28, whereas in human T cells, nearly all CD4+ and 50 percent of CD8+ cells express CD28. The cytoplasmic domain of CD28 has no known enzymatic activity but does contain two SH3 and one SH2 binding sites. CD28 interacts with PI_3-kinase and GRB2 and promotes JNK activation, as noted previously. CD28 ligation alone does not transmit a proliferative response to T cells, but in conjunction with TCR engagement it augments IL-2 production at the level of both transcription and translation. It also increases the production of other cytokines including IL-4, IL-5, IL-13, IFN-γ, and TNF-α, as well as the chemokines IL-8 and RANTES.[61]

The ligands for CD28, CD80, and CD86 are expressed in a restricted distribution on B cells, dendritic cells, monocytes, and activated T cells. CD80 and CD86 have similar structures but share only 25 percent amino acid homology. They each contain rather short cytoplasmic tails that may signal directly, and they bind to CD28 with different activities.

IMMUNOLOGIC SYNAPSE

Antigen-specific interaction between the T cell and APCs results in the formation of a specialized contact region called the immunological synapse or supramolecular activation cluster (SMAC)[62] (Fig. 9–6). Synapse formation is an active, dynamic process that requires a specific antigen to drive synapse formation; TCR-MHC interaction alone is not sufficient. The synapse also overcomes the obstacles to close T cell/APC contact involving short molecules (e.g., TCR, MHC, CD4, CD8) caused by interactions recruiting long molecules (ICAM-1, LFA-1, CD45). Two stages of assembly have been described. During the nascent stage, cell adhesion molecules, such as ICAM-1 on APC and LFA-1 on T cells, make contact in a central zone, surrounded by an annulus of close contact between MHC and TCR.[62] Within minutes the engaged TCR migrates to the central area, resulting in a mature synapse in which the initial relationships are reversed: The central area (CSMAC) now contains TCR, CD2, CD28, and CD4 and is enriched for Lck, Fyn, and PKCθ.[63,64] Surrounding the central domain is a peripheral ring (pSMAC) that contains CD45, LFA-1, and associated talin. T cell activation leads to compartmentalization of activated TCR and TCR signaling molecules to plasma-membrane microdomains call "rafts."[65,66] Rafts are composed primarily of glycosphingolipids and cholesterol and are enriched in signaling molecules, actin, and actin-binding proteins.[67,68] Src-family kinases, Ras-like G proteins, LAT, and phosphatidylinositol-anchored membrane proteins have all been shown to localize to raft domains.

During T cell stimulation, activation of many tyrosine kinases precedes formation of the immunologic synapse.[69,70] After TCR ligation, rafts become enriched for Vav, Shc, phosphorylated ζ, PLCγ1, and ZAP-70.[66,71] TCR engagement induces rapid reorganization of the T cell cytoskeleton toward the T cell-APC junction.[72] This results in the redistribution of surface molecules and the release of cytokines and cytotoxic mediators toward the site of the T cell stimulus.[73] Among the known molecules connecting signaling and structural proteins is the Wiskott Aldrich syndrome protein (WASp). WASp contains a GTPase binding domain that mediates binding to activated cdc42.[74] This promotes the coupling of TCR engagement with actin polymerization.

Full T cell activation requires engagement of a minimum of about 100 to 200 MHC/peptide molecules on an APC, which can serially stimulate 2000 to 8000 TCR. It has been estimated that naïve T cells also require a sustained signal for 15 to 20 hours to commit to proliferation.[75] T cells face a number of obstacles to achieving full activation, including the small physical size of the TCR and MHC molecules compared to other cell surface molecules, the low affinity of TCR for MHC-peptide complex, and the low number of MHC molecules present on the APC that contain the antigenic

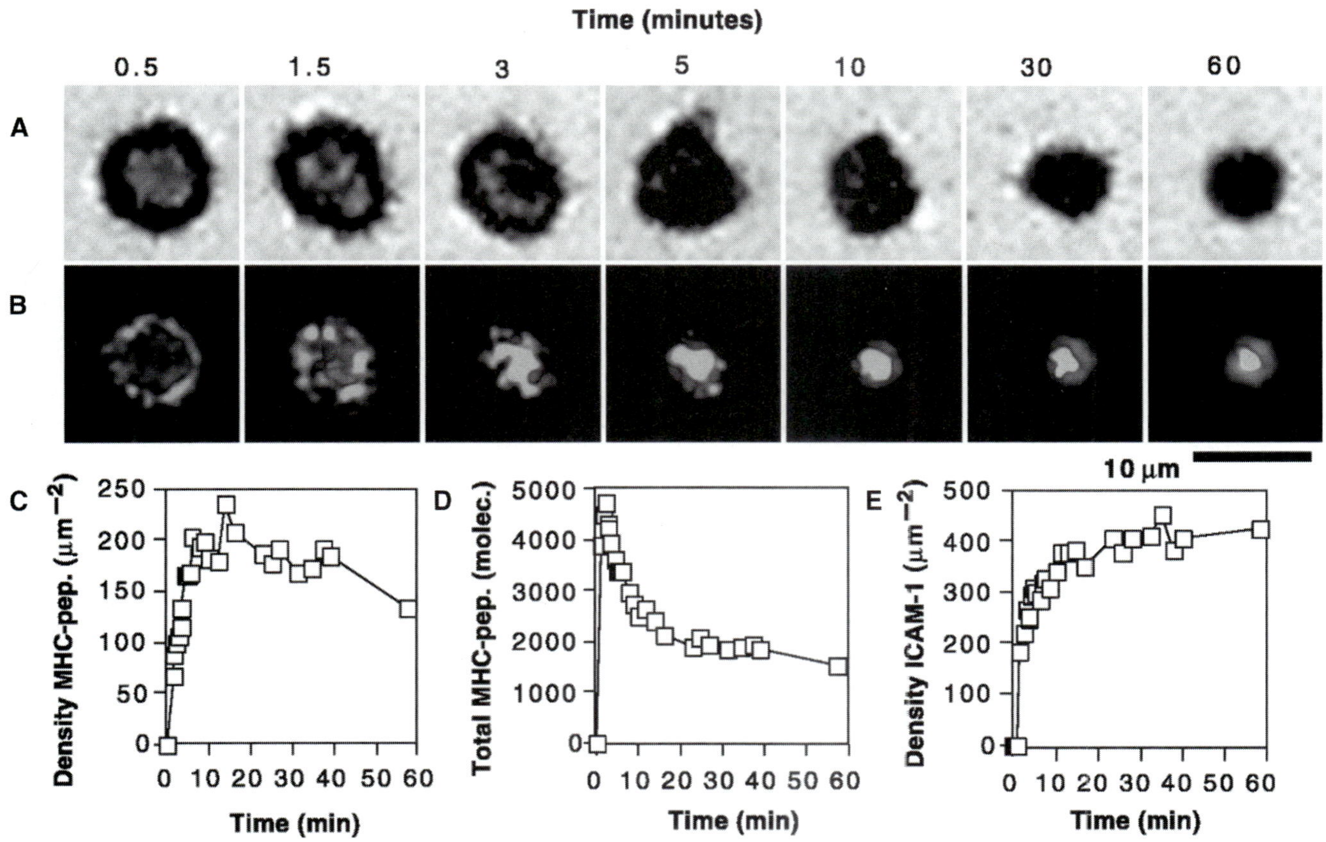

FIGURE 9–6 · Formation of the Immunologic Synapse. T cells in contact with planar bilayer containing Oregon green E^{k}-antigen mouse cytochrome peptide 88-103 and Cy5 ICAM-1. Shown is the sequential formation of the immunologic synapse over the time period indicated. (From Grakoui A, Bromley SK, Sumen C, et al: The immunological synapse: A molecular machine controlling T cell activation. Science 285:221-227, 1999.) (See color plate 3.)

peptide.[76] The immunologic synapse may provide the mechanism for overcoming these barriers and achieving the duration of TCR stimulation necessary to commit the cell to proliferation.[62] The spatial organization of the synapse juxtaposes the membranes of the APC and T cell, facilitating the interaction of the TCR and MHC-peptide complex. The available MHC-peptide complexes and TCR are concentrated at the site of contact via actin cytoskeleton-mediated transport. The multistep process of mature synapse formation may also enable the T cell to discriminate between the potential antigen-containing MHC-peptide complexes it encounters on the APC cell surface. Recently, it has been shown that costimulatory signals may contribute to synapse formation by initiating the transport of membrane rafts containing the kinases and adaptor molecules required for TCR signaling to the site of contact.[77,78]

Tolerance and Control of Autoreactive T Cells

The immune system is constantly confronted by the problem of how to ensure that T cells are activated only under conditions in which there is a true need for a response to a foreign pathogen and not merely a self component. This is not a trivial point as, like all biologic filters, the thymus is not 100-percent efficient and not all self-reactive T cells are eliminated. Hence, a variety of fail-safe mechanisms are engaged to suppress the ability of these errant T cells from premature clonal expansion. Part of nature's solution to this dilemma was the ingenious design of requiring two distinct signals from separate molecules to be coordinately triggered for T cell activation and proliferation to proceed. If only one of the signals is received, the T cell will not proliferate and will actually enter a nonresponsive state known as tolerance or anergy.

The anergy that results from the absence of a CD28 costimulatory signal manifests at a signal level by a failure to fully couple the TCR signal to Ras/MAP kinase pathway and consequent AP-1 transcriptional activity. An additional method of provoking an incomplete TCR signal and unresponsiveness is to make amino acid substitutions in the recognized peptide antigen. These so called "altered peptide ligands" (APL) cause a suboptimal phosphorylation of TCRζ and consequent inefficient recruitment of ZAP-70.[79]

Following the discovery of CD28 as a costimulatory molecule, a related structure known as cytotoxic lymphocyte-associated antigen-4 (CTLA-4) was found to also bind to CD80 and CD86 with 20-fold higher affinity than CD28. Unlike CD28, CTLA-4 is expressed only transiently following T cell activation and confers an inhibitory signal for T cell proliferation.[80] The mechanism by which this occurs is not clearly defined, although two reports have suggested that the phosphatase SHP-2 may associate with the cytoplasmic tail of CTLA-4.[77,81] A more recent report showed that CTLA-4 signaling keeps CD3ζ out of the immunoligic synapse and thus diminished the density of surface TCR and its consequent signaling.[82] In this capacity, CTLA-4 functions to limit T cell clonal expansion induced by CD28. The consequences of the loss of this negative regulation are striking. The genetic deletion of the *CTLA-4* gene in mice results in enormous uncontrolled T cell expansion and an autoimmune diathesis.[83,84]

Chronic exposure to certain inflammatory cytokines, most notably TNF-α, can also induce anergy. It has been appreciated for some time that T cells from rheumatoid synovium manifest profound deficiencies of proliferation and cytokine production.[85,86] Because TNF-α is one of the major cytokines detectable in rheumatoid synovial fluid, it was soon appreciated that chronic exposure of T cell clones to TNF-α for 10 to 12 days suppressed proliferative and cytokine responses to antigen by as much as 70 percent.[87] Furthermore, a single administration of anti–TNF-α receptor monoclonal antibody to patients with rheumatoid arthritis (RA) rapidly restored the response of peripheral T cells to mitogens and recall antigens.[87] Similar observations have been made in TCR transgenic mice following TNF-α exposure.[88] The observation that chronic TNF-α exposure inhibited calcium responses following TCR ligation[88] supports the view that TNF-α may uncouple TCR signaling. Conceivably, other members of the TNF-α family may invoke similar T cell anergy.

Another layer of regulation has been the long-held theoretic concept that a subset of T cells might exist that could actively suppress the immune response. In the past, clear demonstration of these cells was elusive as was their acceptance by the immunology community. However, more recently, a phenotypically defined subpopulation of CD4+CD25+ regulatory T cells has been identified with an ability to inhibit antigen-induced proliferation.[89] This subset is expressed in the periphery at a low frequency and appears to be thymic dependent. The latter point may be of interest as it suggests that the absence of regulatory T cells following day-3 thymectomy may be involved with the subsequent development of autoimmune disease in these animals.[90] Indeed, diminished levels of CD4+CD25+ regulatory T cells have been observed in other autoimmune syndromes, and the transfer of regulatory T cells to autoimmune mice has shown some alleviation of symptoms. At present, the lineage of CD4+CD25+ cells is quite unclear, as is their exact mechanism of suppression. Recently, CD4+CD25+ cells were observed to selectively express Foxp3, a regulatory gene that upon transfection into naïve T cells was able to confer functional characteristics of regulatory T cells.[91] This is a very active area of research because of the potential therapeutic implications for autoimmune diseases.

Subsets and Function of Peripheral T Cells

CD4 HELPER AND CD8 CYTOLYTIC T CELLS

αβ T cells can be subdivided into two main subsets based on their recognition of peptides presented by MHC class I or class II molecules and their respective expression of CD8 or CD4. CD4+ and CD8+ T cells have different functions and recognize antigens derived from different cellular compartments. The peptides presented by MHC class I molecules are produced by the proteasome[92,93] and can be derived from either self proteins or intracellular foreign proteins as might occur during viral infection. MHC class II–bound peptides are derived largely from extracellular infectious agents or self cell-surface proteins that have been engulfed and degraded in the lysosomal complex.

CD4+ T cells express a variety of cytokines and cell surface molecules that are important to B cell proliferation, immunoglobulin production, and CD8+ T cell function. Following antigen stimulation, CD4+ T cells differentiate into two major classes of effector T cells based on their cytokine profiles, which are called T helper type 1 (Th1) and T helper type 2 (Th2)[94] (see following). The CD4 molecule is structurally related to immunoglobulins and has an affinity for nonpolymorphic residues on the MHC class II molecule. In this capacity, CD4 presumably increases the efficiency with which CD4+ T cells recognize antigen in the context of class II molecules, which are restricted in their expression to B cells, macrophages, dendritic cells, and a few other tissues during states of inflammation. In addition, the cytoplasmic tail of CD4 binds to *Lck* and promotes signaling by the TCR, as described earlier. However, ligation of CD4 prior to engagement of the TCR renders the T cell susceptible to apoptosis upon subsequent engagement of the TCR.[95] This is clinically important in human immunodeficiency virus (HIV) infections in which the gp120 molecule of HIV binds to CD4 and primes the T cell to undergo cell death when later triggered by the TCR.[96] Accelerated apoptosis of CD4+ T cells has been demonstrated in acquired immune deficiency syndrome (AIDS) patients.[97]

CD8+ T cells are very efficient killers of pathogen-infected cells. Given the ubiquitous expression of class I molecules, mature cytolytic T cells (CTL) can recognize viral infections in a wide array of cells, in distinction to the more-restricted distribution of class II molecules and their recognition by CD4+ T cells. CTL induce lysis of target cells through the production of perforin, which induces holes in cell membranes, and the expression of Fas ligand (FasL) and TNF-α, which induce apoptosis. In this capacity, CTL kill virally infected target cells in an attempt to restrict the spread of infection. Similar to CD4, CD8 manifests an affinity for MHC class I molecules, enhances the signaling of CTL, and also binds Lck by its cytoplasmic tail.

T CELLS IN THE INNATE IMMUNE RESPONSE

In addition to the broad array of antigens recognized by αβ T cells, there is growing appreciation that the immune system also contains small subpopulations of T cells that may be specialized to recognize conserved structures that are either uniquely expressed by prokaryotic pathogens or on stressed host cells. These are discussed in detail in Chapter 8. Such common antigenic motifs include bacterial lipoproteins recognized by Toll-like receptor (TLR)-2 and TLR-4, double-stranded RNA from RNA viruses that binds TLR-3, and methylated cytosine residues in bacterial CpG sequences that bind to TLR-9.[98] TLR expressed by APC can trigger the release of cytokines and costimulatory molecules for T cells. Another family of molecules that likely binds bacterial components is CD1. CD1 structurally resembles MHC class I but contains a deeper and more hydrophobic binding pocket that can accommodate certain lipopeptides and glycolipids.[99] By using such molecular strategies to focus on common and nonpolymorphic molecules, the immune response may be able to respond quickly during the early phase of infections. This response is part of innate immunity. Although it may represent the remnants of an evolutionarily more-primitive immune response, it nevertheless provides a very vital early defense system. Among T cells this function is provided by γδ and natural killer (NK) T cells.

γδ T CELLS

The γδ T cell is among the oddest of immunology's distinguished oddities. Their study stems from the serendipitous discovery of rearranged genes while searching for the TCR-α–chain gene, rather than a preexisting knowledge of their presence and biologic function.[100] Structurally, the γ-chain locus contains at least 14 Vγ-region genes, of which six are pseudogenes, each capable to rearranging to any of five Jγ regions and two Cγ regions. The δ-chain genes are nested within the α-chain gene locus between Vα and Jα. There are about six Vδ regions, two Dδ, two Jδ regions, and a single Cδ gene. Transcription of rearranged γ and δ genes begins prior to αβ genes and is apparent on days 15 to 17 of mouse-thymus development, after which it declines in the adult thymus. In addition to the ordered appearance of *TCRγδ* before *TCRαβ*, there is also a highly ordered expression of γ and δ V-region genes during early thymic development. This results in successive waves of oligoclonal γδ T cells migrating to the periphery. The reason for this remarkable regimentation remains unclear.

γδ T cells manifest a number of differences from αβ T cells. γδ T cells are often anatomically sequestered to epithelial barriers or sites of inflammation,[101] and they frequently manifest cytotoxicity toward a broad array of targets.[102] In contrast to αβ T cells, γδ cells can respond to antigen directly, without evidence of MHC restriction,[103] or conversely, they can react to MHC molecules without peptide.[104]

Human γδ T cell clones, particularly those expressing the Vδ2 gene and derived from peripheral blood of normal individuals or synovial fluid of RA patients, frequently react to mycobacterial extracts.[105,106] Although a few of these Vδ2 clones respond to a heat-shock protein, the major stimulatory components have recently been identified as phosphate-containing nonpeptide molecules such as nucleotide triphosphates,[107] prenyl pyrophosphates,[108] and alkylamines.[109] These molecules are, respectively, subunits in DNA and RNA, substrates in lipid metabolism for the synthesis of farnesyl pyrophosphate, and products of pathogenic organisms. In mammalian cells, farnesyl addition is a critical modification for targeting certain signaling molecules to the cell membrane, such as Ras. This process appears critical to cell transformation. These phosphate-containing nonpeptides can be found in both microbial and mammalian cells. This suggests that γδ cells may recognize a class of antigens shared by a number of pathogens, as well as by damaged or transformed mammalian cells, and may provide insight into the role of γδ cells in infection and their accumulation at sites of inflammation. Recently a subpopulation of γδ T cells typically found in the intestine and expressing the Vδ1 gene (which is also found in inflamed synovial fluid) was shown to react to newly discovered MHC class I–like molecules known as MICA and MICB.[28] Unlike classic MHC class I molecules that are expressed ubiquitously and continuously, MICA and MICB expression appears to be restricted to gut epithelium and occurs only during times of stress, similar to that of a heat-shock response.

The contribution of γδ T cells to defense against infection has been examined in mice using a number of pathogens including *Listeria*,[110] *Leishmania*,[111] *Mycobacterium*,[112] *Plasmodium*,[113] and *Salmonella*.[57] All of these studies have shown a moderately protective role for γδ T cells. In some cases of rapid bacterial growth, γδ T cells appear to be protective early during infection by reducing bacterial growth,[110] whereas in less-virulent infections such as influenza or Sendai virus, γδ cells appear later in inflammatory lesions.[114] In only a few instances, however, have γδ clones derived from an infected animal been shown to react to the causative organism. In human infections, γδ T cells from cutaneous lesions of leprosy patients respond to *M. leprae*,[115] and γδ cells from Lyme arthritis synovial fluid will respond to the causative spirochete, *Borrelia burgdorferi*.[116] This response by Lyme synovial γδ cells requires lipidated hexapeptides of the outer surface proteins of *B. burgdorferi*, and the tripalmitate lipid moiety is as important for activation of γδ T cells as the hexapeptide portion.

γδ T cells accumulate at inflammatory sites in autoimmune disorders such as RA,[117] coeliac disease,[118] and sarcoidosis.[119] The reason for this remains an enigma. However, there is evidence that γδ cells can be highly cytolytic toward a variety of tissues, including CD4+ T cells,[120] in part due to their high and sustained expression of surface *FasL*.[121] Their presence can strongly bias the cytokine profiles of the infiltrating CD4+ cells, in some instances toward Th1 profiles[122] and in others toward Th2.[123]

NATURAL KILLER T CELLS

A minor subpopulation of T cells bearing the NK determinant manifest perhaps the most restricted of TCR repertoires and determinants of recognition. NK T cells are found within the CD4+ and CD4-8-subsets of T cells and, in both mouse and human, express a very limited number of TCR-V β chains and an invariant α-chain.[124] Furthermore, NK T cells are restricted in their response to a monomorphic MHC class I–like molecule, CD1. Recent crystallographic analysis of CD1 has shown that it contains a deeper groove than traditional MHC molecules and is highly hydrophobic, suggesting it may bind lipid moieties.[99] This may represent another type of innate T cell response whereby bacterial lipids or lipopeptides may be presented to NK T cells to provoke a rapid early immune response.

The potential importance of NK T cells in autoimmune disease stems from their production of high levels of certain cytokines, particularly IL-4 and IFN-γ.[124] In this capacity, the IL-4 response may be important for modulating inflammatory responses dominated by Th1 infiltrates. This has been noted in the nonobese diabetic (NOD) mouse model of diabetes, which lacks NK T cells.[125] Adoptive transfer of NK T cells into NOD mice blocks the onset of diabetes.[126] A recent study extended this observation to human type I diabetes. The NK T cells of diabetic individuals produced more IFN-γ and less IL-4 than their unaffected siblings.[127] Thus, this minor population of T cells may play a pivotal role in early innate responses to certain infections and also in the regulation of inflammatory lesions.

NAÏVE VERSUS MEMORY T CELLS

CD4+ and CD8+ T cells emigrate from the thymus bearing a naïve phenotype. Naïve T cells produce IL-2 but only low levels of other cytokines and, therefore, manifest little B cell helper activity. They express high levels of Bcl-2 and can survive for extended periods without antigen, but they require the presence of MHC molecules. Naïve T cells circulate from the blood to lymphoid tissues of the spleen and lymph nodes, which concentrate antigen, APC, T cells, and B cells. Particularly important in this environment as APC are dendritic cells, which are derived from both lymphoid and myeloid progenitors and are particularly adept at concentrating and presenting antigen. Dendritic cells can migrate from other areas of the body, such as the skin, and thus transport antigen to lymphoid tissues (see Chapter 7). These specialized cells express high and constitutive levels of MHC class II and costimulatory molecules CD80 and CD86 that are critical to promoting proliferation of naïve T cells. In this capacity, dendritic cells are particularly adept at promoting clonal expansion of antigen-specific T cells, which may be present at as low a frequency as 1 in 10^6 prior to immunization, but can increase to 1 in 100 or more within 1 week. The recent development of antigen peptide/MHC tetramer technology has led to a more direct quantification of these values using flow cytometry and suggests their frequency may be considerably higher.[128]

During the process of clonal expansion of naïve T cells and their differentiation into effector and eventually memory T cells, as many as 100 genes are induced. These are manifest primarily as increased expression of certain surface molecules involved with cell adhesion and migration (CD44, ICAM-1, LFA-1, α4β1, and α4β7 integrins), activation (CD45 change from high-molecular-weight CD45RA to lower-molecular-weight CD45RO isotype), cytokine production (increased production of IFN-γ, IL-3, IL-4, and IL-5) and death receptors (e.g., Fas/CD95) (Table 9–1). More transiently induced are CD69, the survival factor *Bcl-xL*, and the high-affinity IL-2 receptor α-chain (CD25), the last being necessary for T cell proliferation.

The concept of immune memory has existed since the first successful vaccinations by Jenner for smallpox. For years memory T cells could only be identified at a

TABLE 9–1 • SURFACE MARKERS ON NAIVE AND MEMORY T CELLS

Molecule	Other Designation	Molecular Weight (kD)	Characteristic	Expression	
				Memory	Naive
CD58	LFA-3	45–66	Ligand for CD2	+ +	+
CD2	T11	50	Alternative activation pathway	+ + +	+ +
CD11a/CD18	LFA-1	180–195	Receptor for ICAM-1, ICAM-2, ICAM-3	+ + +	+ +
CD29		130	β-chain of β_1 (VLA) integrins	+ + + +	+
CD45RO		220	Isoform of CD45	+ + + +	–
CD45RA		80–95	Isoform of CD45	–	+ + + +
CD44	Pgp-1	90	Receptor for hyaluronic acid	+ + +	+ +
CD54	ICAM-1	120	Counter-receptor for LFA-1	+	–
CD26		40	Dipeptidyl peptidase IV	+	–
CD7		Multichain complex	T cell lineage marker	+/–	+ +
CD3			Part of TCR complex	+	+

Abbreviations: CD, Cluster of differentiation, ICAM, intercellular adhesion molecule; LFA, leukocyte function-associated antigen; TCR, T cell antigen receptor, VLA, very late activation antigen.

functional level by demonstrating the presence of an enhanced proliferative response of peripheral blood lymphocytes (PBL) from an individual previously vaccinated against an antigen such as tetanus toxoid. In the late 1980s, a series of cell surface memory T cell markers were identified. The first of these was CD44, the hyaluronate receptor.[129] Surface CD44 is low on mature T cells as they emerge from the thymus, but its expression is upregulated upon the first encounter with antigen stimulation in the periphery. Several other markers have been shown to change upon primary antigenic stimulation. Most notable for human T cells is CD45, in which an isoform known as CD45RA is expressed on naïve T cells, whereas CD45RO expression characterizes memory T cells (see Table 9–1). Using these markers it has been possible to identify a variety of differences between naïve and memory T cells. Activation of memory T cells appears to be more efficient than that of naïve T cells and not absolutely dependent on costimulation. Memory T cells are also able to migrate to nonlymphoid tissues such as lung, skin, liver, and joints.[130]

T HELPER TYPE 1 VERSUS T HELPER TYPE 2 CELLS

Th1 cells participate in cell-mediated inflammatory reactions, activate macrophages, and produce IL-2, TNF-β, and IFN-γ. Th2 cells activate B cells and produce IL-4, IL-5, IL-6, and IL-10. IL-4 and IL-5 are important B cell growth factors, as are surface CD40-ligand and the recently described BAFF.[131] In addition, IL-4 promotes B cell secretion of immunoglobulin (Ig)G_1 and IgE, whereas IFN-γ drives IgG_{2a} production. Because Th1 and Th2 cells mediate different functions, the type of response generated can influence susceptibility to disease.

In response to repetitive antigenic stimulation, responding CD4+ cells can differentiate into effector cells expressing polarized patterns of cytokine production. Th1 cells are characterized by production of IL-2, IFN-γ, TNF-α, and TNF-β, whereas Th2 cells produce IL-4, IL-5, IL-6, IL-10, and IL-13.[94] A list of cytokines and their properties is described in Table 9–2. These patterns have been best characterized during chronic infections. In general, a Th1 response helps eradicate intracellular microorganisms, such as *Leishmania major* and *Brucella abortus*,[94] whereas a Th2 cell response can better control extracellular pathogens, such as the helminth *Nippostrongylus braciliensis*.[132] The cytokine profiles of Th1 and Th2 cells are mutually inhibitory, such that the Th1 cytokine IFN-γ, or IL-12 from APC, suppresses Th2 responses and augments Th1 cytokine gene expression, whereas the Th2 cytokines IL-4, or IL-6 from APC, promote the opposite pattern.[133] Polarization of the cytokine environment also occurs at the sites of inflammation in many autoimmune syndromes. Th2 skewing has been observed in models of systemic lupus erythematosus (SLE) in which increased levels of immunoglobulins and autoantibodies are typical, as well as in chronic allergic conditions such as asthma.[134] Frequently, however, the infiltrating lymphocytes exhibit a bias toward Th1 cytokines. This occurs with brain-infiltrating lymphocytes in multiple sclerosis and in its animal model, experimental allergic encephalomyelitis (EAE)[135]; β islet lymphocytes in diabetes[136]; and synovial lymphocytes in inflammatory arthritides.[137,138] Unlike the beneficial effects of Th1 responses during infections, these same cytokines can be quite deleterious in autoimmune disorders. Thus, therapies based on inhibition of certain Th1 cytokines have been of considerable interest and are often ameliorative, such as anti–TNF-α treatment of EAE[135] and in RA.[139] Several cytokines can have pleotropic effects, and predicting the effects of modulating their levels can be complex. For example, despite the tendency of IL-6 to promote a Th2-cytokine profile, blocking IL-6 has been reported to be extremely beneficial in RA.[140]

Costimulatory molecules and other cytokines produced by APC can also influence cytokine polarization. CD80 and IL-12 promote a Th1 emergence,[141,142] whereas CD86, IL-4, and IL-6 can evoke a Th2 predominance.[133,142,143] Th1 cells are also generally thought to be more easily tolerized and more susceptible to activation-induced cell death (AICD),[144,145] perhaps because they express more *FasL* than Th2 cells.[146,147] Increased

TABLE 9–2 • T CELL–DERIVED CYTOKINES

Cytokine	Abbreviation	Other Names	Mr of Natural Protein (kD)	Amino Acids of Mature Protein	Chromosome	Receptor	Activity
Interleukin-1α	IL-1α	Lymphocyte-activating factor (LAF) Endogenous pyrogen (EP); catabolin Osteoclast activating factor (OAF) Epidermal cell-derived thymocyte-activating factor (ETAF)	17.5	159	2	Single chain; CDw121a; type I receptor; 80 kD or p80; binds IL-1α, IL-1β, and IL-1R antagonist	Costimulates T and B cell activation and the secretion of cytokines (IL-2, IFN-γ) and antibody; increases killing by NK cells; myriad of effects on nonlymphoid cells
Interleukin-2	IL-2	T cell growth factor (TCGF)	15–20	133	4	Low-affinity, CD25, IL-2Rα, p55; CD122, IL-2Rβ, p75; non-IL-2 binding p64 IL-2γ; intermediate affinity IL-2R, IL-2Rα/γ, or IL-2Rβ/γ; high affinity is IL-2Rα/β/γ. γ-chain associated with IL-4R, IL-7R, IL-15R (? IL-13R and IL-9R)	Promotes growth and differentiation of activated T and B cells; activates NK cells, macrophages
Interleukin-3	IL-3	Multipotential colony-stimulating factor (multi-CSF) Mast cell growth factor (MCGF) Erythroid colony-stimulating factor (ECSF) Megakaryocyte colony-stimulating factor (Meg-CSF) Eosinophil colony-stimulating factor (Eo-CSF)	14–30	133	5	α-chain, p70; β-chain, p120; IL-3R associated with tyrosine kinase activity	Stimulates proliferation and differentiation of precursors of all hematopoietic cell lineages
Interleukin-4	IL-4	B cell stimulatory factor I (BSF-1) B cell differentiation factor-γ (BCDF-γ) T cell growth factor-2 (TCGF-2) Mast cell growth factor-2 (MCGF-2)	15–20	129	5	High-affinity, IL-4Rα + IL-2R γ-chain or "common γ-chain," γc; CD124 is IL-4R α-chain, p140; low-affinity IL-4R reported; soluble IL-4Rα is potent IL-4 antagonist	Promotes growth and differentiation of T cells, B cells; enhances tumoricidal activity of macrophages, but inhibits IL-1 and TNF-α production
Interleukin-5	IL-5	B cell growth factor II (BCGF-II) T cell replacing factor Eosinophil differentiation factor (EDF) IgA-enhancing factor (IgA-EF)	45	115	5	Low-affinity, CD125, IL-5α, p60; IL-5R β-chain is nonbinding and shared with IL-3R and GM-CSFR	Promotes growth of cytotoxic cells and differentiation of B cells
Interleukin-6	IL-6	Interferon-β2 (IFN-β2) B cell stimulatory factor-2 (BSF-2) Hepatocyte stimulatory factor II (HSF-II) Hybridoma plasmacytoma growth factor (HPGF, IL-HP1) Myeloma cell growth factor (MCGF)	26	183	7	High-affinity, IL-6R α-chain (p80) + gp130; gp130 is nonbinding and forms homodimer when complexed with IL-6Rα, acts to transduce signal	Enhances IL-2 production from T cells and Ig production by B cells; myriad of effects on nonlymphoid cells
Interleukin-8	IL-8	Neutrophil-activating protein (NAP-1) Granulocyte chemotactic protein (GCP)	6–8	77	4	High-affinity IL-8R, CDw128, p58–67; low affinity IL-8R also binds GRO/MGSA, NAP-2	Produced by many cell types, mainly acts as neutrophil and lymphocyte chemoattractant and activation factor
Interleukin-9	IL-9	P40, mast cell growth-enhancing activity; T cell growth factor III	32–39	126	5	IL-9R is single chain, p64	Produced by activated Th2 cells; enhances T cell proliferation, mast cell lines and erythroid precursors

Interleukin-10	IL-10	Cytokine synthesis inhibition factor (CSIF) B cell-derived T cell growth factor (B-TCGF)	35–40	160	1	IL-10R is single chain, p90–110	Stimulates Th2 cell and thymocyte growth; inhibits Th1 cell proliferation, IL-2 and IFN-γ production; inhibits macrophage cytokine production
Interleukin-12	IL-12	Natural killer cell stimulatory factor (NKSF) Cytotoxic lymphocyte maturation factor (CLMF)	30–33 35–44	196/306	?	High-affinity, IL-12R, type I receptor, p180	Induces Th1 cell differentiation; enhances IFN-γ production by T cells and NK cells; stimulates proliferation of T cells
Interleukin-13	IL-13	Murine P600	10–17	112	5	Unknown; may share nonbinding chain with IL-4	Produced by activated T cells; inhibits production of inflammatory cytokines (IL-1β, IL-6, TNFα, IL8); induces CD23 on B cells, promotes human B cell proliferation and Ig secretion
Interleukin-14	IL-14	High-molecular-weight B cell growth factor (HMW-BCGF)	60	483	?	Unknown; also binds Bb component of complement	Produced by activated T cells; promotes B cell proliferation, inhibits Ig secretion; shares homology with complement factor Bb
Interleukin-15	IL-15	None	14–15	114	?	IL15R binding chain unknown; shares IL-2Rβ and γ-chains (not IL-2Rα)	Produced by many cells; enhances T cell proliferation, cytotoxic activity and LAK activity
Granulocyte-macrophage colony-stimulating factor	GM-CSF	Colony-stimulating factor-α Pluripoietin Colony-stimulating factor 2	22	127	5	Low-affinity, CDw116, α-chain, p80; β-chain, p130, shared with IL-3R and IL-5R; high affinity α-+ β-chains	Activates macrophages
Interferon-γ	IFN-γ	Macrophage-activating factor (MAF)	20–25	143	12	High-affinity, CDw119, binding chain, second chain transduces signal	Enhances differentiation of T and B cells; counteracts effects of IL-4; enhances kiling by NK cells; activates macrophages; induces class II MHC molecules on many nonimmune cells
Lymphotoxin	LT	Tumor necrosis factor-β (TNF-β)	25	171	6	Type I receptor, CD120a, p55; second receptor is type II receptor, CD120b, p75; both members of NGFR/TNFR superfamily	LT and TNF-α have the same activities; enhance T and B cell proliferation; enhance B cell differentiation; increase killing by NK cells
Tumor necrosis factor-α	TNF-α	Cachectin	52	157	6	Same as LT	Same as LT
Transforming growth factor-β	TGFβ	None	25	2 × 112	19/14	Three receptors; high-affinity type I and II, p55 and p80; low-affinity type III, p250–300	Inhibits T cell growth and cytokine secretion; inhibits B cell growth and differentiation; counteracts effects of IFN-γ on nonimmune cells

expression of Fas-associating phosphatase-1 (FAP-1) by Th2 cells may also contribute to their resistance to AICD by inhibiting Fas signaling.[144] However, other investigators have observed that Th1 and Th2 cells are equally sensitive to apoptosis upon Fas ligation.[146]

MOLECULAR MIMICRY

Perhaps the oldest concept in autoimmune mechanisms is that of molecular mimicry: the notion that the response of the immune system to a foreign substance may provoke cross-reactivity to a self protein. This is best established in rheumatic heart disease, where a B cell antibody response to a group A streptococcal cell-wall component can precipitate a cross-reactivity to cardiac myosin. Similarly for T cells, investigators used the peptide sequence of myelin basic protein (MBP) recognized by specific T cell clones from patients with multiple sclerosis to search a database of infectious agents. Some of the candidate sequences obtained were able to stimulate the MBP-reactive T cell clones.[148] This suggested for the first time that T cells responding to an infectious agent might manifest cross-reactivity to self peptides. More recently it was observed that one of the outer surface proteins of *B. burgdorferi*, known as OspA, may trigger a cross-reactive response in Lyme arthritis.[149] Furthermore, a T cell immunodominant peptide of outer surface protein A (OspA) has been identified in a subset of HLA-DR4 patients who are more resistant to antibiotic treatment and manifest an antibody as well as a T cell response to OspA.[150] Using a sequence algorithm to identify homologous peptides that bind the DR4 pocket, a sequence in LFA-1 was identified that bound DR4 and stimulated a T cell response from these OspA-reactive patients.[149] The technology of peptide/ MHC tetramers discussed previously will enable investigators to determine whether a given subpopulation of T cells within an inflammatory synovium might manifest dual specificity for both a foreign pathogen and a cross-reacting self protein.

Death of T Cells

The rapid removal of the effector T cells following clearance of an infection is as important as the initial clonal expansion of responding T cells for the health of the organism. Failure to clear activated lymphocytes increases the risk of cross-reactivity with self antigens and a sustained autoimmune reaction. To ensure that resolution of an immune response occurs rapidly, a number of processes promote active cell death of clonally expanded T cells. One means to control T cell proliferation is through limited availability of growth factors. Upon activation, T cells express receptors for various growth cytokines for approximately 7 to 10 days, but they only produce cytokines during the first 48 hours. This results in an unstable situation in which T cells tend to outgrow the availability of cytokines. T cells expressing IL-2R, for example, in the absence of IL-2 will rapidly undergo programmed cell death. Another method is restimulation of TCR on actively dividing T cells, which triggers the death cascade AICD.

The discovery of a family of death receptors expressed by T cells elucidated an additional regulatory process. These molecules are described more extensively in Chapter 26 and will only be discussed here as they relate to T cell function. The best described of these is Fas (CD95). Both Fas-deficient mice[151] and humans bearing Fas mutations (Canele-Smith Syndrome)[152] manifest a profound lymphadenopathy accompanied by an autoimmune diathesis. This underscores the importance of efficiently removing T cells after their activation. Nearly all cells have some level of surface Fas, whereas expression of its ligand (FasL) is restricted primarily to activated T cells and B cells. Consequently, regulation of Fas-mediated apoptosis is, to a large extent, under the governance of the immune system. FasL expression has also been reported for certain components of the eye, the Sertolli cells of the testis, and perhaps some tumors.[153] Expression of FasL by these nonlymphoid cells is thought to prevent immune responses at sites where such inflammation might cause tissue damage. For years immunologists have been aware of these so-called "immune privileged" sites within which immune responses are difficult to initiate.

During T cell activation, expression of FasL is rapidly induced at the level of RNA, and the ability to kill Fas-sensitive target cells is easily demonstrated. Yet expression of surface FasL protein has been difficult to demonstrate. This may be due to a sensitivity of surface FasL to certain proteinases, which results in its rapid cleavage and release from the cell in a manner similar to the release of another member of the Fas family, TNF-α. Resting T cells are not sensitive to Fas-induced death; they must first enter the cell cycle for approximately 3 days. During this period, the cellular level of an endogenous inhibitor of Fas known as *c-FLIP* (FLICE [caspase-8] inhibatory protein) is downregulated and this presumably allows Fas signaling to progress.[154] Thus, c-FLIP may function to protect resting T cells from unnecessary death and restrict apoptosis to activated T cells to limit their expansion. The importance of *c-FLIP* as an inhibitor of cell death is reinforced by the discovery that certain herpes viruses express a homolog of mammalian FLIP, called E8, that can prevent death of host cells.[155] E8 expression may alter the tumorigenic potential of herpes viruses.[156] Although it is generally well accepted that Fas is a major regulator of AICD in vitro, it is less clear that Fas plays much role in the death and removal of T cells following activation in vivo.

The sequence of T cell activation followed by cell death is graphically displayed following the administration to mice of bacterially or virally derived compounds called superantigens. Superantigens activate T cells by directly cross-linking MHC class II molecules with particular β-chain V families of the TCR (see Fig. 9–3A). The superantigen staphylococcal enterotoxin B (SEB) strongly activates V β8+ T cells.[157] This initiates a rapid expansion of Vβ8+ T cells over 2 to 3 days, followed by an equally rapid loss of these cells, such that by day 7 very few V β8+ T cells remain. A similar process of T cell activation occurs in the human disease toxic shock syndrome in which a related staphylococcal toxin (TSST) stimulates the expansion of Vβ2+ T cells.[158] The devastating illness that results from this profound activation of a large proportion of T cells underscores the need to rapidly eliminate activated T cells. At least some of the damage in toxic shock syndrome likely results from the extensive T cell expression of FasL and TNF-α, particularly in certain tissues such as the liver. Hepatocytes are exquisitely sensitive to damage by these ligands.[159] Activation of T lymphocytes leads to homing to the liver, and administration of antigen to TCR transgenic mice can yield a syndrome resembling autoimmune hepatitis.[160] Thus, certain autoimmune disorders may result from the death or damage of "innocent bystander" cells as a consequence of the migration of activated T cells to an organ and nonspecific damage due to the expression of FasL family members.

Although it was initially assumed that Fas would largely regulate this process, Fas-deficient mice eliminate T cells activated by either traditional antigens or superantigens nearly as efficiently as wild-type mice. Rather, a more recently identified family of compounds known as *Bim, Bad,* and *Bax* appear to regulate AICD in vivo.[161] These molecules are related to the cell-survival molecule, Bcl-2, but are more truncated, containing only the BH3 domain of Bcl-2—hence their designation as the "BH3-only" family. They function as sentinels within the cell in that they are attached to various cytoskeletal proteins and organelles and sense cellular damage. If damage occurs, they are released from these sequestered areas and migrate to the mitochondria to inhibit the survival function of Bcl-2.

T Cells at Sites of Inflammation

The observation that T cells infiltrate target organs in autoimmune diseases such as RA, type I diabetes mellitus, and multiple sclerosis quickly lead to an analysis of T cell subsets and, more recently, to a more detailed study of the T cell repertoire based on TCR expression. In many of these disorders, the known HLA class II association is paralleled by a predominant, though by no means exclusive, infiltration of CD4+ T cells.[162] Many of these CD4+ T cells also manifest a Th1-like cytokine profile as discussed earlier.[135,136,138] Evidence for the importance of these CD4+ cells derives from numerous studies showing the efficacy of CD4 depletion in animal models of these disorders.[163] A parallel situation has often occurred in humans with these autoimmune diseases who concurrently become infected with HIV. The CD4 depletion occurring during AIDS can actually ameliorate RA.[164] However, the resulting CD8 predominance during HIV infection has also frequently resulted in exacerbation of psoriatic arthritis and Sjögren's syndrome, suggesting the CD8+ subset of T cells may be important in these disorders.[164]

The ability to assess the TCR repertoire of infiltrating T cells has added further insight into the degree of clonality present within inflamed tissues. Many studies have examined the TCRβ-chain because of its association with superantigen responses, as well as the TCRα-chain.[165] From the dozens of publications, perhaps most certain is that a very broad array of TCR types is usually observed in most T cell–mediated diseases. In the few studies that have analyzed the earliest lesions, T cell oligoclonality has been observed.[166] However, it is possible that the oligoclonality in these situations may simply reflect the limited number of T cells in early lesions. These are, nonetheless, provocative findings that warrant further analysis.

REFERENCES

1. Pawson T, Scott JD: Signaling through scaffold, anchoring, and adaptor proteins. Science 278: 2075-2080, 1997.
2. Rudd CE: Adaptors and molecular scaffolds in immune cell signaling. Cell 96:5-8, 1999.
3. Scollay R, Smith J, Stauffer V: Dynamics of early T cells: Prothymocyte migration and proliferation in the adult mouse thymus. Immunol Rev 91:129-157, 1986.
4. Godfrey DI, Kennedy J, Suda T, Zlotnik A: A developmental pathway involving four phenotypically and functionally distinct subsets of CD3-CD4-CD8-triple-negative adult mouse thymocytes defined by CD44 and CD25 expression. J Immunol 150:4244-4252, 1993.
5. Bosma GC, Custer RP, Bosma MJ: A severe combined immunodeficiency mutation in the mouse. Nature 301:527-530, 1983.
6. Mombaerts P, et al: RAG-1-deficient mice have no mature B and T lymphocytes. Cell 68:869-877, 1992.
7. Rodewald HR, Fehling HJ: Molecular and cellular events in early thymocyte development. Adv Immunol 69:1-112, 1998.
8. Radtke F, et al: Deficient T cell fate specification in mice with an induced inactivation of Notch1. Immunity 10:547-558, 1999.
9. Peschon JJ, et al: Early lymphocyte expansion is severely impaired in interleukin 7 receptor-deficient mice. J Exp Med 180:1955-1960, 1994.
10. Uribe L, Weinberg KI: X-linked SCID and other defects of cytokine pathways. Semin Hematol 35:299-309, 1998.
11. Farrar MA, Doerfler P, Sauer K: Signal transduction pathways regulating the development of alpha beta T cells. Biochim Biophys Acta 1377:F35-F78, 1998.
12. Elder ME, et al: Human severe combined immunodeficiency due to a defect in ZAP-70, a T cell tyrosine kinase. Science 264: 1596-1599, 1994.
13. Padovan E, et al: Expression of two T cell receptor α chains: Dual receptor T cells. Science 262:422-424, 1993.
14. Niederberger N, et al: Allelic exclusion of the TCR alpha-chain is an active process requiring TCR-mediated signaling and c-Cbl. J Immunol 170:4557-4563, 2003.
15. Garboczi DN, et al: Structure of the complex between human T-cell receptor, viral peptide and HLA-A2. Nature 384:134-141, 1996.
16. Garcia KC, et al: An α β T cell receptor structure at 2.5 A and its orientation in the TCR-MHC complex. Science 274:209-219, 1996.
17. Matsui K, et al: Low affinity interaction of peptide-MHC complexes with T cell receptors. Science 254:1788-1791, 1991.
18. Yamashita I, Nagata T, Tada T, Nakayama T: CD69 cell surface expression identifies developing thymocytes which audition for T cell antigen receptor-mediated positive selection. Int Immunol 5:1139-1150, 1993.
19. Punt JA, Osborne BA, Takahama Y, et al: Negative selection of CD4+CD8+ thymocytes by T cell receptor-induced apoptosis requires a costimulatory signal that can be provided by CD28. J Exp Med 179:709-713, 1994.
20. Linette GP, et al: Bcl-2 is upregulated at the CD4 + CD8 + stage during positive selection and promotes thymocyte differentiation at several control points. Immunity 1:197-205, 1994.
21. Priatel JJ, Teh SJ, Dower NA, et al: RasGRP1 transduces low-grade TCR signals which are critical for T cell development, homeostasis, and differentiation. Immunity 17:617-627, 2002.
22. Amakawa R, et al: Impaired negative selection of T cells in Hodgkin's disease antigen CD30-deficient mice. Cell 84:551-562, 1996.
23. Kawabe T, et al: The immune responses in CD40-deficient mice: Impaired immunoglobulin class switching and germinal center formation. Immunity 1:167-178, 1994.

24. Xu J, et al: Mice deficient for the CD40 ligand. Immunity 1: 423-431, 1994.
25. Deftos ML, He YW, Ojala EW, Bevan MJ: Correlating notch signaling with thymocyte maturation. Immunity 9:777-786, 1998.
26. Yasutomo K, Doyle C, Miele L, et al: The duration of antigen receptor signalling determines CD4 + versus CD8 + T-cell lineage fate. Nature 404:506-510, 2000.
27. Lefrancois L, Puddington L: Extrathymic intestinal T-cell development: Virtual reality? Immunol Today 16:16-21, 1995.
28. Groh V, Steinle A, Bauer S, Spies T: Recognition of stress-induced MHC molecules by intestinal epithelial γδ T cells. Science 279:1737-1740, 1998.
29. Arnaiz-Villena A, et al: Human T-cell activation deficiencies. Immunol Today 13:259-265, 1992.
30. Buckley RH: Primary cellular immunodeficiencies. J Allergy Clin Immunol 109:747-757, 2002.
31. Hong R: The DiGeorge anomaly. Clin Rev Allergy Immunol 20:43-60, 2001.
32. Noguchi M, et al: Interleukin-2 receptor gamma chain mutation results in X-linked severe combined immunodeficiency in humans. Cell 73:147-157, 1993.
33. van Dinther-Janssen AC, Pals ST, Scheper R, et al: Dendritic cells and high endothelial venules in the rheumatoid synovial membrane. J Rheumatol 17:11-17, 1990.
34. Butcher EC, Picker LJ: Lymphocyte homing and homeostasis. Science 272: 60-66, 1996.
35. Bodolay E, Koch AE, Kim J, et al: Angiogenesis and chemokines in rheumatoid arthritis and other systemic inflammatory rheumatic diseases. J Cell Mol Med 6:357-376, 2002.
36. Szekanecz Z, Kim J, Koch AE: Chemokines and chemokine receptors in rheumatoid arthritis. Semin Immunol 15:15-21, 2003.
37. Troy AE, Shen H: Cutting edge: homeostatic proliferation of peripheral T lymphocytes is regulated by clonal competition. J Immunol 170:672-676, 2003.
38. Goldrath AW, Bogatzki LY, Bevan MJ: Naive T cells transiently acquire a memory-like phenotype during homeostasis-driven proliferation. J Exp Med 192:557-564, 2000.
39. Min B, et al: Neonates support lymphopenia-induced proliferation. Immunity 18:131-140, 2003.
40. Miller JF, Osoba D: Current concepts of the immunological function of the thymus. Physiol Rev 47:437-520, 1967.
41. Yunis EJ, et al: Postthymectomy wasting associated with autoimmune phenomena. I. Antiglobulin-positive anemia in A and C57BL-6 Ks mice. J Exp Med 125:947-966, 1967.
42. Weiss A, Littman DR: Signal transduction by lymphocyte antigen receptors. Cell 76:263-274, 1994.
43. Howe LR, Weiss A: Multiple kinases mediate T-cell-receptor signaling. Trends Biochem Sci 20:59-64, 1995.
44. Weissman AM: The T-cell antigen receptor: A multisubunit signaling complex. Chem Immunol 59:1-18, 1994.
45. Cambier JC: Antigen and F_c receptor signaling. The awesome power of the immunoreceptor tyrosine-based activation motif ITAM. J Immunol 155:3281-3285, 1995.
46. Wange RL, Samelson LE: Complex complexes: Signaling at the TCR. Immunity 5:197-205, 1996.
47. Mustelin T, Tasken K: Positive and negative regulation of T-cell activation through kinases and phosphatases. Biochem J 371: 15-27, 2003.
48. Appleby MW, et al: Defective T cell receptor signaling in mice lacking the thymic isoform of $p59^{fyn}$. Cell 70:751-763, 1992.
49. Stein PL, Lee HM, Rich S, Soriano P: $pp59^{fyn}$ mutant mice display differential signaling in thymocytes and peripheral T cells. Cell 70:741-750, 1992.
50. Koretzky GA, Picus J, Thomas ML, Weiss A: Tyrosine phosphatase CD45 is essential for coupling T-cell antigen receptor to the phosphatidyl inositol pathway. Nature 346:66-68, 1990.
51. Liao XC, Littman DR: Altered T cell receptor signaling and disrupted T cell development in mice lacking Itk. Immunity 3:757-769, 1995.
52. van Oers NS, Killeen N, Weiss A: ZAP-70 is constitutively associated with tyrosine-phosphorylated TCR ζ in murine thymocytes and lymph node T cells. Immunity 1:675-685, 1994.
53. Jordan MS, Singer AL, Koretzky GA: Adaptors as central mediators of signal transduction in immune cells. Nat Immunol 4: 110-116, 2003.
54. Alberola-Ila J, Takaki S, Kerner JD, Perlmutter RM: Differential signaling by lymphocyte antigen receptors. Annu Rev Immunol 15:125-154, 1997.
55. Cantrell D: T cell antigen receptor signal transduction pathways. Annu Rev Immunol 14:259-274, 1996.
56. Sun Z, et al: PKC-theta is required for TCR-induced NF-kappaB activation in mature but not immature T lymphocytes. Nature 404:402-407, 2000.
57. Crabtree GR, Olson EN: NFAT signaling: Choreographing the social lives of cells. Cell 109(Suppl):S67-S79, 2002.
58. Dolmetsch RE, Lewis RS, Goodnow CC, Healy JI: Differential activation of transcription factors induced by Ca2+ response amplitude and duration. Nature 386:855-858, 1997.
59. Guse AH, et al: Regulation of calcium signalling in T lymphocytes by the second messenger cyclic ADP-ribose. Nature 398:70-73, 1999.
60. Lenschow DJ, Walunas TL, Bluestone JA: CD28/B7 system of T cell costimulation. Annu Rev Immunol 14:233-258, 1996.
61. Loetscher P, Seitz M, Baggiolini M, Moser B: Interleukin-2 regulates CC chemokine receptor expression and chemotactic responsiveness in T lymphocytes. J Exp Med 184:569-577, 1996.
62. Grakoui A, et al: The immunological synapse: A molecular machine controlling T cell activation. Science 285:221-227, 1999.
63. Monks CR, Freiberg BA, Kupfer H, et al: Three-dimensional segregation of supramolecular activation clusters in T cells. Nature 395:82-86, 1998.
64. Dustin ML, et al: A novel adaptor protein orchestrates receptor patterning and cytoskeletal polarity in T-cell contacts. Cell 94: 667-677, 1998.
65. Montixi C, et al: Engagement of T cell receptor triggers its recruitment to low-density detergent-insoluble membrane domains. EMBO J 17:5334-5348, 1998.
66. Xavier R, Brennan T, Li Q, et al: Membrane compartmentation is required for efficient T cell activation. Immunity 8:723-732, 1998.
67. Simons K, Ikonen E: Functional rafts in cell membranes. Nature 387:569-572, 1997.
68. Harder T, Simons K: Caveolae, DIGs, and the dynamics of sphingolipid-cholesterol microdomains. Curr Opin Cell Biol 9:534-542, 1997.
69. Lee KH, et al: T cell receptor signaling precedes immunological synapse formation. Science 295:1539-1542, 2002.
70. Stoll S, Delon J, Brotz TM, Germain RN: Dynamic imaging of T cell-dendritic cell interactions in lymph nodes. Science 296:1873-1876, 2002.
71. Rozdzial MM, Malissen B, Finkel TH: Tyrosine-phosphorylated T cell receptor ζ chain associates with the actin cytoskeleton upon activation of mature T lymphocytes. Immunity 3:623-633, 1995.
72. Kupfer A, Swain SL, Singer SJ: The specific direct interaction of helper T cells and antigen-presenting B cells. II. Reorientation of the microtubule organizing center and reorganization of the membrane-associated cytoskeleton inside the bound helper T cells. J Exp Med 165:1565-1580, 1987.
73. Kupfer A, Mosmann TR, Kupfer H: Polarized expression of cytokines in cell conjugates of helper T cells and splenic B cells. Proc Natl Acad Sci U S A 88:775-779, 1991.
74. Badour K, et al: The Wiskott-Aldrich syndrome protein acts downstream of CD2 and the CD2AP and PSTPIP1 adaptors to promote formation of the immunological synapse. Immunity 18:141-154, 2003.
75. Iezzi G, Karjalainen K, Lanzavecchia A: The duration of antigenic stimulation determines the fate of naive and effector T cells. Immunity 8:89-95, 1998.
76. Shaw AS, Dustin ML: Making the T cell receptor go the distance: a topological view of T cell activation. Immunity 6:361-369, 1997.
77. Lee K-M, et al: Molecular basis of T cell inactivation by CTLA-4. Science 282:2263-2266, 1998.
78. Viola A, Schroeder S, Sakakibara Y, Lanzavecchia A: T lymphocyte costimulation mediated by reorganization of membrane microdomains. Science 283:680-682, 1999.
79. Sloan-Lancaster J, Shaw AS, Rothbard JB, Allen PM: Partial T cell signaling: altered phospho-ζ and lack of zap70 recruitment in APL-induced T cell anergy. Cell 79:913-922, 1994.
80. Krummel MF, Allison JP: CD28 and CTLA-4 have opposing effects on the response of T cells to stimulation. J Exp Med 182:459-465, 1995.

81. Marengere LE, et al: Regulation of T cell receptor signaling by tyrosine phosphatase SYP association with CTLA-4. Science 272:1170-1173, 1996.
82. Chikuma S, Imboden JB, Bluestone JA: Negative regulation of T cell receptor-lipid raft interaction by cytotoxic T lymphocyte-associated antigen 4. J Exp Med 197:129-135, 2003.
83. Tivol EA, et al: Loss of CTLA-4 leads to massive lymphoproliferation and fatal multiorgan tissue destruction, revealing a critical negative regulatory role of CTLA-4. Immunity 3:541-547, 1995.
84. Waterhouse P, et al: Lymphoproliferative disorders with early lethality in mice deficient in Ctla-4. Science 270:985-988, 1995.
85. Firestein GS, Zvaifler NJ: Peripheral blood and synovial fluid monocyte activation in inflammatory arthritis. I. A cytofluorographic study of monocyte differentiation antigens and class II antigens and their regulation by gamma-interferon. Arthritis Rheum 30:857-863, 1987.
86. Verwilghen J, Vertessen S, Stevens EA, et al: Depressed T-cell reactivity to recall antigens in rheumatoid arthritis. J Clin Immunol 10:90-98, 1990.
87. Cope AP, et al: Chronic exposure to tumor necrosis factor TNF in vitro impairs the activation of T cells through the T cell receptor/CD3 complex; reversal in vivo by anti-TNF antibodies in patients with rheumatoid arthritis. J Clin Invest 94:749-760, 1994.
88. Cope AP, et al: Chronic tumor necrosis factor alters T cell responses by attenuating T cell receptor signaling. J Exp Med 185:1573-1584, 1997.
89. Sakaguchi S, et al: Immunologic tolerance maintained by CD25+ CD4+ regulatory T cells: their common role in controlling autoimmunity, tumor immunity, and transplantation tolerance. Immunol Rev 182:18-32, 2001.
90. Shevach EM, McHugh RS, Piccirillo CA, Thornton AM: Control of T-cell activation by CD4+ CD25 + suppressor T cells. Immunol Rev 182:58-67, 2001.
91. Hori S, Nomura T, Sakaguchi S: Control of regulatory T cell development by the transcription factor Foxp3. Science 299: 1057-1061, 2003.
92. Pamer E, Cresswell P: Mechanisms of MHC class I–restricted antigen processing. Annu Rev Immunol 16:323-358, 1998.
93. Rock KL, Goldberg AL: Degradation of cell proteins and the generation of MHC class I-presenting peptides. Annu Rev Immunol 17:739-777, 1999.
94. Street NE, et al: Heterogeneity of mouse helper T cells: Evidence from bulk cultures and limiting dilution cloning for precursors of Th1 and Th2 cells. J Immunol 144:1629-1639, 1990.
95. Newell MK, Haughn LJ, Maroun CR, Julius MH: Death of mature T cells by separate ligation of CD4 and the T-cell receptor for antigen. Nature 347:286-289, 1990.
96. Fauci AS: Host factors and the pathogenesis of HIV-induced disease. Nature 384:529-534, 1996.
97. Casella CR, Finkel TH: Mechanisms of lymphocyte killing by HIV. Curr Opin Hematol 4:24-31, 1997.
98. Janeway CA Jr, Medzhitov R: Innate immune recognition. Annu Rev Immunol 20:197-216, 2002.
99. Zeng Z, et al: Crystal structure of mouse CD1: An MHC-like fold with a large hydrophobic binding groove. Science 277:339-345, 1997.
100. Saito H, et al: Complete primary structure of a heterodimeric T-cell receptor deduced from cDNA sequences. Nature 309: 757-762, 1984.
101. Itohara S, et al: Homing of a gamma delta thymocyte subset with homogeneous T-cell receptors to mucosal epithelia. Nature 343:754-757, 1990.
102. Wright A, et al: Cytotoxic T lymphocytes specific for self tumor immunoglobulin express T cell receptor delta chain. J Exp Med 169:1557-1564, 1989.
103. Sciammas R, et al: Unique antigen recognition by a herpesvirus-specific TCR-gamma delta cell. J Immunol 152:5392-5397, 1994.
104. Schild H, et al: The nature of major histocompatibility complex recognition by gamma delta T cells. Cell 76:29-37, 1994.
105. Holoshitz J, Koning F, Coligan JE, et al: Isolation of CD4-CD8- mycobacteria-reactive T lymphocyte clones from rheumatoid arthritis synovial fluid. Nature 339:226-229, 1989.
106. Kabelitz D, Bender A, Schondelmaier S, et al: A large fraction of human peripheral blood γ δ+ T cells is activated by Mycobacterium tuberculosis but not by its 65-kD heat shock protein. J Exp Med 171:667-679, 1990.
107. Constant P, et al: Stimulation of human γδ T cells by nonpeptidic mycobacterial ligands. Science 264 267-270, 1994.
108. TanakaY, et al: Natural and synthetic non-peptide antigens recognized by human γ δ T cells. Nature 375:155-158, 1995.
109. Bukowski JF, Morita CT, Brenner MB: Human γδ T cells recognize alkylamines derived from microbes, edible plants, and tea: implications for innate immunity. Immunity 11:57-65, 1999.
110. Hiromatsu K, et al: A protective role of γδ T cells in primary infection with Listeria monocytogenes in mice. J Exp Med 175:49-56, 1992.
111. Rosat JP, MacDonald HR, Louis JA: A role for γδ+ T cells during experimental infection of mice with Leishmania major. J Immunol 150:550-555, 1993.
112. Kaufmann SH, Ladel CH: Role of T cell subsets in immunity against intracellular bacteria: Experimental infections of knock-out mice with Listeria monocytogenes and Mycobacterium bovis BCG. Immunobiology 191:509-519, 1994.
113. Tsuji M, et al: γ δ T cells contribute to immunity against the liver stages of malaria in αβ T-cell-deficient mice. Proc Natl Acad Sci U S A 91:345-349, 1994.
114. Carding SR, et al: Late dominance of the inflammatory process in murine influenza by γ δ+ T cells. J Exp Med 172:1225-1231, 1990.
115. Modlin RL, et al: Lymphocytes bearing antigen-specific γδ T-cell receptors accumulate in human infectious disease lesions. Nature 339:544-548, 1989.
116. Vincent MS, et al: Lyme arthritis synovial gamma delta T cells respond to Borrelia burgdorferi lipoproteins and lipidated hexapeptides. J Immunol 161:5762-5771, 1998.
117. Brennan FM, et al: T cells expressing γδ chain receptors in rheumatoid arthritis. J Autoimmunity 1:319-326, 1988.
118. Rust C, et al: Phenotypical and functional characterization of small intestinal TcR γ δ+ T cells in coeliac disease. Scand J Immunol 35:459-468, 1992.
119. Balbi B, Moller DR, Kirby M, et al: Increased numbers of T lymphocytes with γδ + antigen receptors in a subgroup of individuals with pulmonary sarcoidosis. J Clin Invest 85:1353-1361, 1990.
120. Vincent MS, et al: Apoptosis of Fashigh CD4 + synovial T cells by borrelia-reactive Fas-ligand high gamma delta T cells in Lyme arthritis. J Exp Med 184:2109-2117, 1996.
121. Roessner K, et al: High expression of Fas ligand by synovial fluid-derived gamma delta T cells in Lyme arthritis. J Immunol 170:2702-2710, 2003.
122. Huber S, Shi C, Budd RC: Gammadelta T cells promote a Th1 response during coxsackievirus B3 infection in vivo: Role of Fas and Fas ligand. J Virol 76:6487-6494, 2002.
123. Schramm CM, et al: Proinflammatory roles of T-cell receptor TCRgammadelta and TCRalphabeta lymphocytes in a murine model of asthma. Am J Respir Cell Mol Biol 22:218-225, 2000.
124. Bendelac A, Rivera MN, Park SH, Roark JH: Mouse CD1-specific NK1 T cells: Development, specificity, and function. Annu Rev Immunol 15:535-562, 1997.
125. Lehuen A, et al: Overexpression of natural killer T cells protects V α14-J α281 transgenic nonobese diabetic mice against diabetes. J Exp Med 188:1831-1839, 1998.
126. Baxter AG, Kinder SJ, Hammond KJ, et al: Association between αβTCR+ CD4-CD8-T-cell deficiency and IDDM in NOD/Lt mice. Diabetes 46:572-582, 1997.
127. Wilson SB, et al: Extreme Th1 bias of invariant Vα24J αQ T cells in type 1 diabetes. Nature 391:177-181, 1998.
128. Doherty PC: The new numerology of immunity mediated by virus-specific CD8 + T cells. Curr Opin Microbiol 1:419-422, 1998.
129. Budd RC, Cerottini JC, MacDonald HR: Phenotypic identification of memory cytolytic T lymphocytes in a subset of Lyt-2+ cells. J Immunol 138:1009-1013, 1987.
130. Masopust D, Vezys V, Marzo AL, Lefrancois L: Preferential localization of effector memory cells in nonlymphoid tissue. Science 291:2413-2417, 2001.
131. Schneider P, et al: BAFF, a novel ligand of the tumor necrosis factor family, stimulates B cell growth. J Exp Med 189:1747-1756, 1999.
132. Coffman RL, Seymour BW, Hudak S, et al: Antibody to interleukin-5 inhibits helminth-induced eosinophilia in mice. Science 245:308-310, 1989.

133. Rincon M, Anguita J, Nakamura T, et al: Interleukin IL-6 directs the differentiation of IL-4-producing CD4+ T cells. J Exp Med 185:461-469, 1997.
134. Fuss IJ, et al: Characteristic T helper 2 T cell cytokine abnormalities in autoimmune lymphoproliferative syndrome, a syndrome marked by defective apoptosis and humoral autoimmunity. J Immunol 158:1912-1918, 1997.
135. Ruddle NH, et al: An antibody to lymphotoxin and tumor necrosis factor prevents transfer of experimental allergic encephalomyelitis. J Exp Med 172:1193-1200, 1990.
136. Heath WR, et al: Autoimmune diabetes as a consequence of locally produced interleukin-2. Nature 359:547-549, 1992.
137. Saxne T, Palladino MA Jr, Heinegard D, et al: Detection of tumor necrosis factor a but not tumor necrosis factor β in rheumatoid arthritis synovial fluid and serum. Arthritis Rheum 31:1041-1045, 1988.
138. Yssel H, et al: Borrelia burgdorferi activates a T helper type 1-like T cell subset in Lyme arthritis. J Exp Med 174:593-601, 1991.
139. Elliott MJ, et al: Randomised double-blind comparison of chimeric monoclonal antibody to tumour necrosis factor alpha cA2 versus placebo in rheumatoid arthritis. Lancet 344:1105-1110, 1994.
140. Choy EH, et al: Therapeutic benefit of blocking interleukin-6 activity with an anti-interleukin-6 receptor monoclonal antibody in rheumatoid arthritis: A randomized, double-blind, placebo-controlled, dose-escalation trial. Arthritis Rheum 46:3143-3150, 2002.
141. Hsieh CS, et al: Development of TH1 CD4+ T cells through IL-12 produced by Listeria-induced macrophages. Science 260:547-549, 1993.
142. Kuchroo VK, et al: B7-1 and B7-2 costimulatory molecules activate differentially the Th1/Th2 developmental pathways: application to autoimmune disease therapy. Cell 80:707-718, 1995.
143. Le Gros G, Ben-Sasson SZ, Seder R, et al: Generation of interleukin 4 IL-4-producing cells in vivo and in vitro: IL-2 and IL-4 are required for in vitro generation of IL-4-producing cells. J Exp Med 172:921-929, 1990.
144. Zhang X, et al: Unequal death in T helper cell Th1 and Th2 effectors: Th1, but not Th2, effectors undergo rapid Fas/FasL-mediated apoptosis. J Exp Med 185:1837-1849, 1997.
145. Gilbert KM, Hoang KD, Weigle WO: Th1 and Th2 clones differ in their response to a tolerogenic signal. J Immunol 144: 2063-2071, 1990.
146. Ramsdell F, et al: Differential ability of Th1 and Th2 T cells to express Fas ligand and to undergo activation-induced cell death. Int Immunol 6:1545-1553, 1994.
147. Suda T, et al: Expression of the Fas ligand in cells of T cell lineage. J Immunol 154:3806-3813, 1995.
148. Wucherpfennig KW, Strominger JL: Molecular mimicry in T cell-mediated autoimmunity: viral peptides activate human T cell clones specific for myelin basic protein. Cell 80:695-705, 1995.
149. Gross DM, et al: Identification of LFA-1 as a candidate autoantigen in treatment-resistant Lyme arthritis. Science 281:703-706, 1998.
150. Kalish RA, Leong JM, Steere AC: Association of treatment-resistant chronic Lyme arthritis with HLA-DR4 and antibody reactivity to OspA and OspB of Borrelia burgdorferi. Infect Immunity 61:2774-2779, 1993.
151. Budd RC, Van Houten N, Clements J, Mixter PF: Parallels in T lymphocyte development between lpr and normal mice. Semin Immunol 6:43-48, 1994.
152. Vaishnaw AK, et al: The molecular basis for apoptotic defects in patients with CD95 Fas/Apo-1 mutations. J Clin Invest 103:355-363, 1999.
153. Griffith TS, Brunner T, Fletcher SM, Green DR, Ferguson TA: Fas ligand-induced apoptosis as a mechanism of immune privilege. Science 17:1189-1192, 1995.
154. Irmler M, et al: Inhibition of death receptor signals by cellular FLIP. Nature 388:190-195, 1997.
155. Thome M, et al: Viral FLICE-inhibitory proteins FLIPs prevent apoptosis induced by death receptors. Nature 386:517-521, 1997.
156. Tschopp J, Thome M, Hofmann K, Meinl E: The fight of viruses against apoptosis. Curr Opin Genet Dev 8:82-87, 1998.
157. Kawabe Y, Ochi A: Selective anergy of V beta 8+, CD4+ T cells in Staphylococcus enterotoxin B-primed mice. J Exp Med 172: 1065-1070, 1990.
158. Choi Y, et al: Selective expansion of T cells expressing V beta 2 in toxic shock syndrome. J Exp Med 172:981-984, 1990.
159. Kennedy NJ, Russell JQ, Michail N, Budd RC: Liver damage by infiltrating CD8+ T cells is Fas dependent. J Immunol 167: 6654-6662, 2001.
160. Russell JQ, et al: Liver damage preferentially results from CD8+ T cells triggered by high affinity peptide antigens. J Exp Med 188:1147-1157, 1998.
161. Hildeman DA, et al: Activated T cell death in vivo mediated by proapoptotic bcl-2 family member bim. Immunity 16:759-767, 2002.
162. Steere AC, Duray PH, Butcher EC: Spirochetal antigens and lymphoid cell surface markers in Lyme synovitis: Comparison with rheumatoid synovium and tonsillar lymphoid tissue. Arthritis Rheum 31:487-495, 1988.
163. Ranges GE, Sriram S, Cooper SM: Prevention of type II collagen-induced arthritis by in vivo treatment with anti-L3T4. J Exp Med 162:1105-1110, 1985.
164. Winchester RJ: HIV infection and rheumatic disease. Bull Rheum Dis 43:5-8, 1994.
165. Wucherpfennig KW, et al: T cell receptor V α-V β repertoire and cytokine gene expression in active multiple sclerosis lesions. J Exp Med 175:993-1002, 1992.
166. Yang Y, Charlton B, Shimada A, et al: Monoclonal T cells identified in early NOD islet infiltrates. Immunity 4:189-194, 1996.

10 B Cells

BETTY DIAMOND • CHRISTINE GRIMALDI

Immunoglobulin Structure and Function

The principal role of B lymphocytes in the immune system is the synthesis of immunoglobulins (also referred to as antibodies), which are globular proteins that bind foreign substances known as antigens. Immunoglobulins exist as secreted proteins, which circulate throughout the body, or as cell membrane–associated receptors that help mediate B cell activation and maturation. The tertiary structure of an antibody molecule adopts a Y-shaped form that contains two functional moieties: two identical variable regions and the constant region (Fig. 10–1). Each variable region of an antibody molecule contains an antigen-binding pocket; the constant region directs immunoglobulin-effector functions that mediate the killing and removal of invading organisms. The amino acid composition of the immunoglobulin variable region exhibits great diversity, which facilitates the recognition of a wide array of antigens. As the name implies, the constant region exhibits far less diversity and can be subdivided into a few distinct classes known as isotypes.

The fundamental units of an immunoglobulin are the light (L) chain polypeptide, which has an apparent molecular mass of 25 kD, and the heavy (H) chain polypeptide, which has an apparent molecular mass of 50 to 65 kD. An immunoglobulin monomer consists of two identical L chain molecules covalently linked by disulfide bonds to two identical H chain molecules, which are also linked by disulfide bonds (see Fig. 10–1). Early studies analyzing proteolytic fragments of molecules demonstrated distinct functional components.[1] Cleavage with papain generates the antigen-binding fragment (Fab), either of two identical fragments that retain the ability to recognize antigen. The Fab portion is composed of the variable region domains of the H and L chains, the first H chain constant region domain (C_H1), and the L chain constant region domain (C_L). Cleavage with pepsin occurs below the disulfide linkage of the two H chains and generates a molecule that contains two disulfide-bonded Fab fragments called $F(ab')_2$. The presence of two Fab regions in a single immunoglobulin monomer creates a bivalent binding capacity to interact with repetitive determinants present in multivalent antigens (i.e., polysaccharide) or two separate antigen molecules containing the same antigenic determinant. The remaining component, termed *fragment crystallizable* (Fc) on the basis of its ability to readily undergo crystal formation, is unable to interact with antigen but contains the C_H2 and C_H3 domains of the H chain that mediate immune-effector functions.

Within the variable region of the immunoglobulin molecule are discrete regions, known as complementarity-determining regions, that make direct contact with antigen. The amino acid sequences of the complementarity-determining regions are highly variable and are flanked by more conserved amino acid sequences called framework regions. The H and L chain molecules each contain three complementarity-determining regions and four framework regions (see Fig. 10–1). The minimal antigenic determinant recognized by the H and L complementarity-determining regions is known as an epitope, which may be a continuous or discontinuous region on a protein, carbohydrate, lipid, or nucleic acid.

IMMUNOGLOBULIN CONSTANT REGION

The specific binding interactions that occur between the immunoglobulin variable region and the antigen may be sufficient to block microbial infectivity or neutralize toxins. However, the ability to eliminate pathogens is mediated by the Fc portion of the molecule. The Fc regions of antigen-antibody complexes are made accessible to serum factors or to cytotoxic and phagocytic cells that mediate destruction and removal of the pathogen. The ways in which the Fc region directs the destruction of pathogens are: (1) activation of the complement cascade, and (2) engagement of Fc-specific receptors on effector cells, such as monocytes, macrophages, neutrophils, and natural killer (NK) cells. In mice and humans, there are five different types of H chain constant regions, or isotypes, designated IgM (μ),IgD (δ), IgG (γ), IgA (α), and IgE (ε), each encoded by a distinct constant region gene segment present in the H chain locus. Each immunoglobulin molecule is capable of specific effector functions, depending on its H chain constant region. The number of C_H domains, the presence of a hinge region to increase flexibility of the Fab region, serum half-life, the ability to form polymers, complement activation, and Fc-receptor binding vary among isotypes. Characteristics of the different immunoglobulin H chain isotypes are presented in Table 10–1.[2-4] These isotypes may also differ in the intracellular signaling they initiate when bound by antigen in their membrane-associated form.

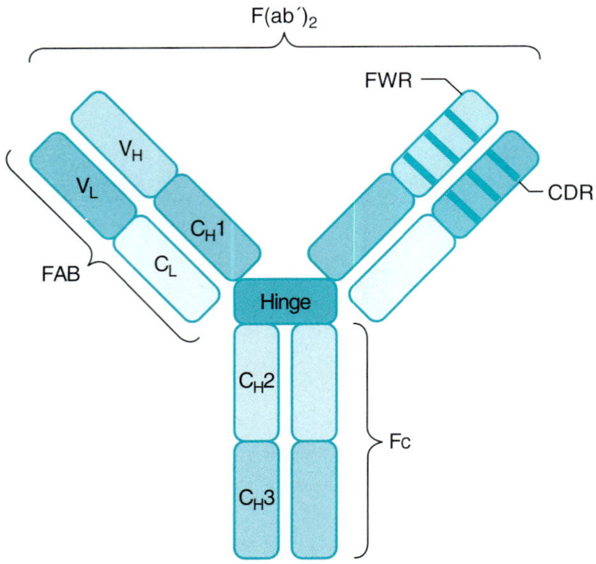

FIGURE 10–1 • Schematic of the Antibody Molecule. An antibody monomer consists of two heavy (H) chain molecules covalently linked to two light (L) chain molecules. The variable region is comprised of the V_H and V_L domains of the H and L chains, respectively. Within the V_H and V_L domains are four framework regions (FWR) and three complementarity-determining regions (CDR), which together make up the antigen-binding pocket. Papain digestion generates the Fab portion, which consists of V_H, C_H1, V_L, and C_L domains, and pepsin digestion generates two covalently linked Fabs, known as the $F(ab')_2$. The Fc region of the H chain constant region, which mediates immune-effector functions, consists of the hinge domain (only in IgG, IgA, and IgD), which promotes flexibility, and C_H2 and C_H3 domains.

H Chains

Immunoglobulin M

IgM is the first isotype generated in developing B cells and the first antibody secreted during a primary immune response. The secreted form of IgM exists mainly as a pentamer. IgM also exists as a hexamer, which represents approximately 5 percent of total serum IgM.[5] Pentameric IgM is linked together by a molecule called the J chain, whereas the hexameric form is not. IgM antibodies usually exhibit low affinity for antigen because the process that increases antibody affinity for a particular antigen (affinity maturation) has not yet been initiated during the early stages of a primary immune response. However, polymeric IgM displays high avidity for antigen. The presence of multiple Fab regions makes the IgM molecule suitable to bind large, multimeric antigens. IgM is found predominantly in serum but is also present in mucosal secretions and breast milk.

The Fc region of IgM (as well as some of the IgG isotypes) is a potent activator of the classic complement pathway.[3] The complement cascade is composed of a series of enzymes that, on activation, mediate the removal and lysis of invading organisms. In general, antibody molecules bound to antigen can activate the classic complement pathway. Deposit of antibody molecules or complement components on the surface of the antigen facilitates phagocytosis. Proteins, such as antibody and complement, that enhance phagocytosis are called opsonins. Once the complement cascade has been activated, monocytes, macrophages, or neutrophils engulf opsonized particles through specific receptors present on phagocytic cells (CD21) that recognize fragments of the C3 complement component. Activation of the complement pathway also results in the generation of the membrane-attack complex, which is composed of late complement components and directly lyses C3-opsonized pathogens.

Immunoglobulin G

IgG is the most common isotype found in serum. IgG antibodies are usually of higher affinity than IgM antibodies and predominate in a secondary, or memory, immune response. There are four subclasses of IgG in humans: IgG1, IgG2, IgG3, and IgG4. All IgG subclasses exist as monomers. Each of the four subclasses appears to predominate in different immune responses. IgG1 and IgG2 antibodies are observed in responses to polysaccharide antigens; IgG1, IgG3, and IgG4 participate in immune responses to viral and protein antigens, and IgG4 participates in responses to nematodes.[6]

IgG1 and IgG3 are more potent activators of the classic complement pathway than are IgG2 and IgG4. Several immunoglobulin isotypes, including IgG1, are

TABLE 10–1 • PROPERTIES OF HUMAN IMMUNOGLOBULIN ISOTYPES

Characteristics	IgM	IgG	IgA	IgE	IgD
Valency	pentamer, hexamer	monomer	dimer (IgA2), monomer (IgA1)	monomer	monomer
C_H domains	4	3	3	4	3
Serum values (mg/ml)	0.7-1.7	9.5-12.5	1.5-2.6	0.0003	0.04
Serum half-life (days)	5	23	6	2.5	3
Complement activation (classic)	yes	yes	no	no	no
Complement activation (alternative)	no	yes	yes	no	yes
FcR binding	no	yes	yes	yes	no
FcR-mediated phagocytosis	no	yes	yes	no	no
ADCC	no	yes	no	no	no
Placental transfer	no	yes	no	no	no
Presence in mucosal secretions	yes	no	yes	no	no

Abbreviations: ADCC, Antibody-dependent cell-mediated cytotoxicity; FcR, F_c receptor.

capable of initiating the alternative complement pathway (see also Chapter 22). The mechanisms by which antibody activates the alternative pathway are poorly understood, but specific binding sites for the C3 complement component have been identified on some immunoglobulin isotypes.[7,8]

All IgG subclasses engage specific Fc gamma receptors (FcγR) present on macrophages, neutrophils, and NK cells to mediate phagocytosis of antibody-coated antigens and to initiate antibody-dependent cell-mediated cytotoxicity. The FcγR on phagocytic cells, such as monocytes, macrophages, and neutrophils, mediate the removal of immune complexes.[4] Engagement of FcγR with immune complexes results in receptor activation. This, in turn, stimulates phagocytic cells to ingest opsonized antigens to destroy them in the phagosome compartment. The FcγR on NK cells mediate killing of antibody-coated cells by the antibody-dependent cell-mediated cytotoxicity pathway, resulting in the release of granules that contain perforin, a pore-forming protein, and enzymes known as granzymes that induce programmed cell death (also known as apoptosis) of target cells.[9]

Another important role of IgG is that it is the only source of maternal antibodies for a developing fetus during pregnancy. The transcytosis of maternal IgG antibodies into the fetal blood supply is mediated by another type of Fc receptor, FcRn.[10] FcRn expressed on endothelial cells regulates the half-life of serum IgG by blocking IgG catabolism.[10]

Immunoglobulin A

There are two subclasses of IgA in humans, designated IgA1 and IgA2.[3] IgA1 exists mainly as a monomer and is present in serum; IgA2 exists as a dimer linked by the J chain and is the predominant isotype in saliva, tears, colostrum, breast milk, and respiratory and vaginal secretions. Secretory IgA (and also IgM) is produced by B cells in the lamina propria, which is beneath the mucosal lining of polarized epithelial cells. Specific receptors for secretory immunoglobulin, termed polymeric immunoglobulin receptors (pIgR), expressed on the basolateral surface of epithelial cells mediate transport of immunoglobulin polymers across the epithelium.[11] The pIgR binds dimeric IgA with higher affinity than IgM. During transport, the pIgR undergoes proteolytic cleavage to generate a fragment called secretory component. Before transcytosis is complete, the IgA dimer associates with secretory component, which renders it resistant to enzymatic degradation.

Secretory IgA may play an important role in the protection against foreign organisms by directly blocking infection and neutralizing toxins in the mucosa. IgA is unable to activate complement through the classic pathway, but IgA1 can activate the alternative complement pathway.[8] Patients with IgA deficiency have reduced levels of both serum and secretory IgA, and at least half of these patients exhibit increases in respiratory and diarrheal infections.[12] An increase in autoimmune disorders has also been observed in patients with IgA deficiency. An IgA-specific FcαR has been identified. The physiologic role of this receptor is not well understood, but there is evidence that FcαR expressed on monocytes, macrophages, neutrophils, and eosinophils mediates the phagocytosis of IgA-coated pathogens.[13]

Immunoglobulin E

IgE exists as a monomer. Only a small amount of IgE is detectable in serum. IgE triggers immune responses associated with allergic reactions.[6] The Fc region of IgE interacts with the high-affinity IgE Fc receptor, FcεR, that is found on the surface of mast cells and basophils.[4] When multimeric antigen cross-links the variable region of IgE molecules bound to FcεR molecules, mast cells and basophils degranulate and release vasoactive molecules associated with anaphylaxis, such as histamine, prostaglandin D_2, and leukotrienes. IgE has been implicated in protection against parasitic infections, because cross-linking of FcεR results in the activation of mast cells, which are involved in immune responses to parasites and help skew the T cell response to parasites to a Th2 cytokine profile (see Chapter 9).

Immunoglobulin D

Little is known about the function of IgD. The membrane form of IgD is coexpressed with the membrane form of IgM. Surface expression of IgD occurs during the later stages of B cell development (see later section "B Cell Development"). The role of IgD in a humoral immune response is unclear. Unlike the other four H chain isotypes, IgD is not secreted from activated B cells, and therefore, it is unlikely to play a protective role against infection. Studies performed with IgD-transgenic mice suggest that surface IgD protects against tolerance induction because autoreactive IgM^+, IgD^+ B cells—but not IgM^+, IgD^- B cells—are resistant to deletion by antigen.[14] Targeted disruption of the IgD gene in mice, however, does not appear to interfere with normal immune functions. Although the total number of B cells is slightly reduced and affinity maturation is delayed, there is no evidence of autoreactivity.[15,16]

L Chains

There are two distinct L chain polypeptides, designated kappa (κ) and lambda (λ). L chains contain a variable region and a single constant region domain. Amino acid residues in the L chain variable region interact with residues in the H chain variable region to create the antigen-binding cleft. Even though there are two L chain isotypes, there is no known function associated with the L chain constant regions. The κ-chain is used more often than the λ-chain in human (65 percent) and mouse (95 percent) immunoglobulin molecules.[17]

IMMUNOGLOBULIN VARIABLE REGION

For the recognition of a virtually unlimited number of antigens to occur, immunoglobulin molecules must be generated that possess different antigenic specificities. The molecular basis of immunoglobulin diversity is now well understood. Immunoglobulin H and L chain genes are encoded by distinct gene segments residing on separate chromosomes; the H chain locus is on human chromosome 14, the κ-chain locus is on chromosome 2, and the λ-chain locus is on chromosome 22. Individual genes encode the variable and constant regions of an immunoglobulin molecule. A limited number of separate H and L chain variable region gene segments undergo somatic rearrangement to generate a multitude of immunoglobulin molecules bearing different antigenic specificities.[18] The H chain variable region is composed of a variable (V_H), a diversity (D_H), and a joining (J_H) gene. The L chain is composed of V_κ and J_κ or V_λ and J_λ genes and does not contain D genes. Immunoglobulin genes can exist as functional gene segments, which are able to be expressed as H or L chain polypeptides, or as pseudogenes, which are unable to be expressed. The human H chain locus contains approximately 51 V_H, 30 D_H, and 6 J_H functional genes. The κ-chain locus contains approximately 32 V_κ genes and 5 J_κ functional genes; the λ-chain locus contains 29 V_λ and 4 J_λ functional genes.[19]

Variable Region Gene Rearrangement

During variable/diversity/joining (VDJ) rearrangement, different V_H, D_H, and J_H, or V_L and J_L gene segments are randomly combined to generate a large number of different immunoglobulin molecules (Fig. 10–2). VDJ recombination occurs in the absence of antigen stimulation. The molecular mechanism that regulates VDJ rearrangement is activated during B cell maturation in primary lymphoid tissue (see later section "B Cell Development"). Specific DNA sequences that flank the V, D, and J gene segments are recognized by components of the recombination machinery. These highly conserved sequences that compose the recombination signal sequences are either seven base pairs (heptamer) or nine base pairs (nonamer) in length, followed by DNA spacers that are 12 or 23 base pairs in length.[20] Specific enzymes termed recombination-activating gene 1 (RAG-1) and recombination-activating gene 2 (RAG-2) initiate VDJ gene rearrangement at the H chain or L chain loci by generating double-stranded DNA breaks at recombination signal sequence sites. The cleaved V, D, and J segments are joined by a complex of several polypeptides that includes Ku70, Ku80, and DNA-dependent protein kinase.[21] The same recombinase machinery also mediates the somatic rearrangement of gene segments for the T cell receptor (see Chapter 9).

Variable Region Diversity

The random recombination that occurs among V, D, and J gene segments can generate a diverse immunoglobulin

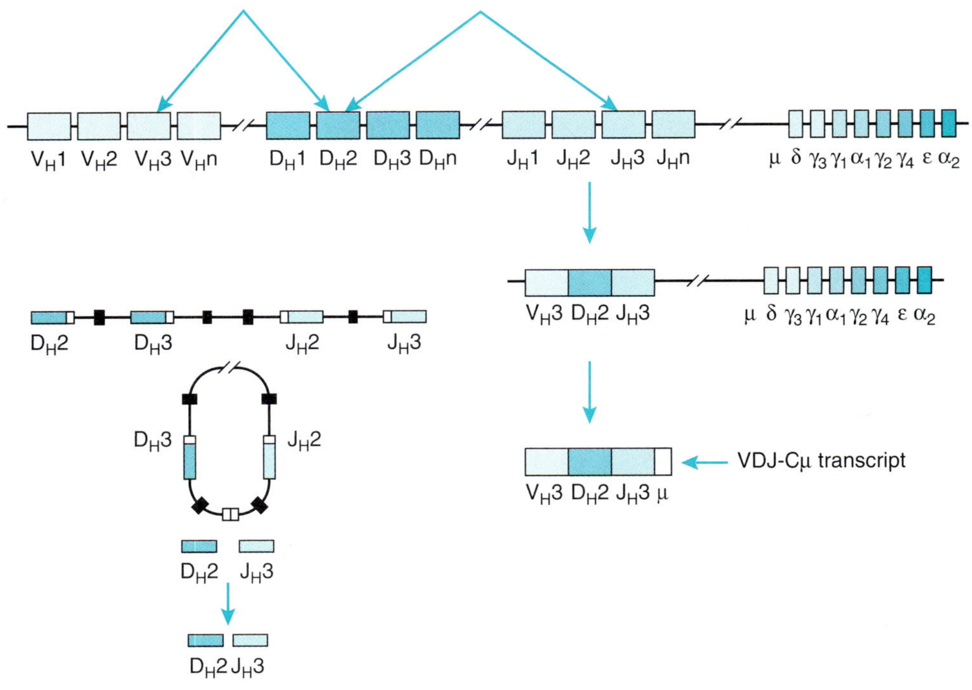

FIGURE 10–2 · V(D)J Recombination at the Immunoglobulin Gene (H Chain) Locus. A single V_H gene segment randomly recombines with a D_H and J_H gene segment residing on the same chromosome. Following $V_HD_HJ_H$ recombination, a transcript containing the IgM H chain constant region gene (Cμ) is generated. The inset represents an example of VDJ recombination occurring between a single D_H and J_H gene segment. The *white squares* represent the heptamer, and the *black squares* represent the nonamer recombination recognition sequences (RSS). Following recognition and cleavage of these sequences, the coding junctions of the rearranged D_H and J_H gene segments are ligated. A V_H gene segments then recombines with the rearranged D_HJ_H segment. L chain rearrangement is mediated by the same mechanism.

repertoire without the need for a large number of germline H and L chain genes. During H chain recombination, nucleotides may be added at V_HD_H and D_HJ_H junctions by the enzyme terminal deoxynucleotidyl transferase. These non–germline-encoded sequences are known as N additions. As long as these nucleotide changes do not disrupt the reading frame or lead to the incorporation of premature stop codons, the random addition of N sequences increases the diversity of the amino acid sequence. Furthermore, imprecise ligation at the coding junctions may result in the loss of nucleotides, thereby altering the amino acid sequence. The expression of different H and L chain combinations also contributes to the creation of diverse binding specificities.[3]

A process known as somatic mutation can further increase variable region diversity.[22] Somatic mutations are point mutations that occur at a high frequency (approximately 10^3 per base pair per cell division) in the variable region of H and L chain genes. Unlike the other genetic events described previously, which increase diversity in developing B cells, somatic mutations occur in mature, antigen-stimulated B cells present in secondary lymphoid tissue in discrete regions called germinal centers (see later section "B Cell Activation"). Nucleotide changes that occur in the complementarity-determining region can increase the affinity of the immunoglobulin variable region for a particular antigen or, in some cases, change the specificity from one antigen to another.[23] Antigen selection results in more replacement mutations in the complementarity-determining regions and fewer in framework regions.

B Cell Development

The development of undifferentiated hematopoietic stem cells into mature B lymphocytes is divided into two phases; the early stages of B cell lymphopoiesis take place in sites known as primary lymphoid tissue, whereas differentiation into B cells that either secrete large quantities of immunoglobulin or persist as long-lived memory cells occurs in secondary or peripheral lymphoid tissue. Primary lymphoid tissue includes the fetal liver and the bone marrow. One of the major events associated with B cell lymphopoiesis in these tissues is immunoglobulin gene rearrangement. Mature naïve B cells exit the primary lymphoid tissue and home to secondary lymphoid tissue, such as the spleen, lymph nodes, tonsils, and Peyer's patches of the intestine. At these sites, B cells interact with foreign antigens and specific humoral immune responses are activated.

B CELL SUBSETS

Two subsets of B lymphocytes exist that are designated B1 B cells and B2 B cells. The B1 subset is produced earlier in ontogeny than are the B2 B cells; the B2 subset includes "conventional" B cells that are replenished from precursor cells in the bone marrow. These subsets are distinguished by surface markers known as clusters of differentiation (CD).

B1 B Cells

B1 B cells can be distinguished from B2 cells on the basis of their expression of specific cell-surface molecules and the types of humoral immune responses in which they participate (Table 10–2). B1 B cells are subdivided into B1a and B1b B cells. One of the characteristic markers expressed on B1a B cells is constitutive expression the CD5 surface molecule, which is absent on B1b and can be induced on B2 B cells. The CD5 molecule is a common marker for chronic lymphocytic leukemia, which is a B cell tumor derived from B1a B cells.[24]

The origin and the maintenance of the B1 B cell populations has yet to be resolved. Two theories exist; one is that B1 B cells are a distinct lineage arising during gestation in the yolk sac and fetal liver and have the unusual property of self-renewal[25]; the other is that B1 B cells derive from a common B cell lineage with B2 B cells and are replenished by bone marrow-derived precursors after birth.[26] Terminal deoxynucleotidyl transferase is

TABLE 10–2 • CHARACTERISTICS OF B CELL SUBSETS

	B 1a	B 1b	Follicular	Marginal Zone
Surface IgM	High	High	Low	High
Surface IgD	Low	Low	High	Low
CD5	+	−	−	−
CD21	−	−	+	++
CD23	−	−	+	−
***CD11b/CD18**	+	+	−	−
Bone marrow progenitors	−	+	+	+
Self-renewal capacity	+	+	−	−
Response to TI antigens	+	+	+/−	+
Response to TD antigens	+/−	+/−	+	+/−
Predominant isotype	IgM	IgM	IgG	IgM
Anatomic locations	Peritoneum, pleura, spleen	Peritoneum, pleura, spleen	Spleen, lymph nodes, Peyer's patches, tonsils, peripheral blood	Spleen and tonsils

*B1 B cells in the spleen do not express CD11b/CD18.

Abbreviations: CD, Clustens of differentiation; TD, T cell dependent; TI, T cell independent.

not expressed during the development of B1 B cells, consistent with the absence of N nucleotide additions at the V_HD_H and J_HD_H junctions observed in H chain genes of these B cells. The role of B1 B cells may be to form a first line of defense against bacteria, producing antibodies that are broadly cross-reactive with bacterial antigens and becoming activated before the adaptive arm of the immune system has time to respond to these antigens.[27]

B2 B Cells and the Bone Marrow Microenvironment

In humans and mice, B2 B cells are produced from hematopoietic stem cells in the bone marrow. Hematopoietic precursor cells are self-renewing, pluripotent stem cells that give rise to all blood-cell types. The environmental cues required for stem cell self-renewal and hematopoiesis are contained within the bone marrow. The microenvironment of the bone marrow stroma consists of several different cell types, including endothelial cells, macrophages, and adipose tissue surrounded by extracellular matrix components.

Hematopoietic stem cells fail to differentiate in vitro in the absence of cultured stromal cells. The reconstitution of B cell differentiation in vitro using stromal cell lines has led to the discovery of a number of cell-surface molecules and soluble factors that are required for B cell lymphopoiesis. During the early stages of lymphopoiesis, B cell precursors are dependent on direct interactions with stromal cells. Some of these cell-surface interactions include vascular adhesion molecule 1 expressed on endothelial cells and macrophages with very late antigen (VLA) 4 expressed on B cell progenitors, intercellular adhesion molecule expressed on stromal cells with VLA 5 expressed on B cell progenitors, hyaluronate present on stromal cells with CD44 expressed on B cell progenitors, and neural cell adhesion molecules expressed on stromal cells with the membrane proteoglycan syndecan expressed on B cell progenitors.[19,28] Although many of the soluble factors important in B cell lymphopoiesis have yet to be definitively identified, there is evidence that interleukin (IL)-4, IL-7, IL-11, insulin-like growth factor, and sex hormones play a role in human B cell development.[29,30] As B cells begin to express surface IgM molecules, they migrate toward the center of the bone marrow cavity and become less dependent on direct interaction with the stroma.

STAGES OF B CELL DEVELOPMENT

The stages of B cell development are defined, in part, by the differential expression of surface markers and genes associated with immunoglobulin gene rearrangement. In the laboratory, these markers are identified by flow cytometry with specific antibodies or by reverse transcription–polymerase chain reaction. Many of the cell surface markers used to define particular B cell subsets mediate important signal-transduction events associated with maturation and activation, whereas others have no known function at present. Because the events associated with B cell development are not strictly linear, the nomenclature and classification of particular stages vary slightly among the different laboratories working in this field. For simplicity, we have divided the stages of B cell lymphopoiesis into pro-B, pre-B, immature, transitional, and mature cell stages (Table 10–3).

The Pro-B Cell Stage

In humans, the earliest hematopoietic stem cells express the CD34 surface marker. The progression from CD34+ cells into B cell progenitors is regulated by specific

TABLE 10–3 • HUMAN B CELL MATURATION MARKERS OF B CELL PROGENITORS

Markers	Stem Cell	Pro-B Cell	Pre-B Cell	Immature B Cell
CD34	+	+	−	−
CD19	−	+	+	+
CD10	−	+	+	−
CD20	−	+	+	+
CD21	−	+	+	+
CD22	−	+	+	+
CD23	−	−	−	−
CD38	−	+	+	+
CD40	−	+	+	+
CD45RB	−	+	+	+
RAG-1	−	+	+	−
RAG-2	−	+	+	−
Tdt	−	+	+	−
Igα	−	+	+	+
Igβ	−	+	+	+
H chain	−	+ (D^H-J^H)	+ (V^H-D^H-J^H)	+
Pre-BCR	−	−	+	−
Surface IgM	−	−	−	+
Surface IgD	−	−	−	−
L chain	−	−	+ ($V^κ$-$J^κ$, $V^λ$-$J^λ$)	+

Abbreviations: BCR, B cell receptor; CD, clusters of differentiation; H, heavy; L, light; RAG, recombination-activating gene; Tdt, terminal deoxynucleotidyl transferase.

transcription factors, including PU.1, Ikaros, E2A, early B cell factor (EBF) and B cell–specific activation protein (BSAP).[31] Pro-B cells continue to express CD34, as well as the surface markers CD19, CD10, CD20, CD21, CD22, CD38, CD40, and CD45RB and the major histocompatibility complex (MHC) class II. The surface immunoglobulin accessory molecules Ig-α and Ig-β are also expressed during the pro-B stage. Pro-B cells are dependent on interactions with endothelial cells present in the stroma. The VLA 4 integrin receptor and the CD44 molecules, which mediate adhesion to stromal cells, are highly expressed at this stage and are believed to be important for development.[19] Pro-B cells also express high levels of Bcl-2. As will be discussed further, this molecule plays a pivotal role in protection against apoptosis.

At the onset of pro-B cell development, the variable gene segments on both H and L chain loci are in the unrearranged germline configuration. Before VDJ rearrangement, the genes required for recombination, such as those encoding RAG-1, RAG-2, terminal deoxynucleotidyl transferase, and the Ku complex, are expressed. After expression of the recombinase machinery, a D_H gene segment on one H chain chromosome rearranges with a J_H gene segment residing on the same chromosome (see Fig. 10–2), often with the inclusion of N nucleotides at the junction.

The Pre-B Cell Stage

During the pre-B cell stage of development, a V_H gene rearranges to the D_HJ_H gene fragment. Completion of $V_HD_HJ_H$ gene rearrangement leads to the generation of an H chain transcript that contains the IgM constant region (C_μ), the constant region gene most proximal to the variable region genes on the chromosome (see Fig. 10–2). The different H chain transcripts each encode either a transmembrane molecule or a secretory molecule determined by alternative splicing. In pre-B cells, however, only transmembrane C_μ is produced.

A critical developmental checkpoint in B cell lymphopoiesis is the cell-surface expression of the pre-B cell receptor (pre-BCR) complex at the pre-B cell stage. Before L chain gene rearrangement, the transmembrane form of the C_μ polypeptide expressed in pre-B cells associates with two other polypeptides, Vpre-B and lambda 5 (λ5), which form the surrogate L chain.[32,33] The genes for these molecules are located on human chromosome 22, which also carries the λ-chain locus. There are three separate genes for λ5, known as 14.1, 16.1, and Fλ1; however, only 14.1 has been shown to encode a protein. A disulfide-linked complex is formed between C_μ and surrogate L chain, which is expressed on the cell surface in association with the accessory molecules Ig-α and Ig-β.

The pre-BCR complex appears to play an important role in B cell maturation. Surface expression of the pre-BCR transduces a signal to the developing pre-B cell that VDJ rearrangement was successful and halts recombination of the second H chain allele. This process of allelic exclusion ensures that all immunoglobulin molecules generated within each B cell are identical and have the same specificity. If rearrangement of the first allele is nonproductive (e.g., genes contain a premature stop codon and cannot be translated into a full-length polypeptide), the absence of pre-BCR signaling permits rearrangement of the second H chain allele. If the second rearrangement also results in a nonproductive H chain molecule, the absence of pre-BCR–mediated signal induces apoptosis. Because it has been estimated that about two thirds of VDJ rearrangements are nonproductive, the inability to express the pre-BCR complex ensures that B cells without a productive H chain will not undergo further differentiation. Targeted disruption of genes encoding the pre-BCR complex, such as the IgM transmembrane constant region domain, λ5, or the Ig-α and Ig-β accessory molecules, results in a profound decrease in developing B cells.

After expression of the H chain polypeptide, L chain rearrangement occurs. Because terminal deoxynucleotidyl transferase expression is reduced at this stage, L chains do not usually contain N sequences at the V_LJ_L junction. Ig-α and Ig-β, CD10, CD19, CD20, CD21, CD22, CD38, CD40, CD45RB, and MHC class II expression continues throughout the pre-B cell stage; the antiapoptotic molecule Bcl-XL is upregulated in pre-B cells, whereas expression of Bcl-2 is downregulated.

The Immature B Cell Stage

L chain gene rearrangement marks the transition from the pre-B cell stage to the immature B cell stage. The rearranged transmembrane C_μ and L chain polypeptides assemble into functional immunoglobulin molecules. At this stage, surface immunoglobulin, which is also known as the B cell receptor (BCR), is expressed. It is believed that surface expression of the BCR on immature B cells transduces signals that enforce allelic exclusion at the L chain locus and downregulate expression of the RAG genes. As discussed in a later section of this chapter, one of the functions of surface immunoglobulin is to mediate negative selection of autoreactive B cells arising in the bone marrow.

Despite the necessity of expressing a single H and L chain molecule in each B cell, circumstances exist that permit the rearrangement of either a second H or L chain allele. Autoreactivity generated during B cell development in the bone marrow can arise by the random expression of different H and L chains. One of the mechanisms that prevents the survival of potentially autoreactive B cells is a process called receptor editing. Reexpression of the RAG genes in immature B cells permits rearrangement and expression of the second H or L chain allele in autoreactive B cells, thus altering antibody specificity. Expression of the antiapoptotic molecule Bcl-XL has been implicated in receptor editing.[34] This molecule may prevent apoptosis of autoreactive B cells by extending the window for receptor editing to occur. The mechanism of receptor editing and its role in the regulation of autoreactivity is discussed later in more detail (see later section "Negative Selection").

Transitional B Cells

There is recent evidence that the later stages of B cell maturation occur outside the bone marrow. Studies in rodents now provide evidence that immature B cells differentiate into a phenotypically distinct population known as transitional type 1 (T1) B cells and localize to the spleen prior to becoming mature B cells.[35] The transitional T1 population is similar to the immature B cell population and appears also to be subject to negative selection following exposure to self antigen (see later section "Negative Selection"). Transitional T1 B cells that survive the selection process differentiate into transitional type2 (T2) B cells, which are the precursors of mature B2 cell subsets. The recently described B cell survival factor, known as B cell activating factor of the tumor necrosis factor family (BAFF; also known as Blys), that is secreted by myeloid cells appears to play an important role in T2 cell development because blockade of BAFF binding leads to arrested development at the T2 stage.[36] During the transitional B cell stage, an IgD (C_δ) H chain is coexpressed along with the C_μ H chain that bears the same variable region and associates with the same L chain. The switch from IgM^+, IgD^- to IgM^+, IgD^+ occurs at the level of transcription during the final phase of maturation in the bone marrow. A long transcript containing both C_μ and C_δ genes undergoes alternative splicing to generate both IgM and IgD H chains.

The Mature B Cell Stage

Transitional T2 B cells give rise to the mature B2 B cell populations, follicular and marginal zone B cells. These mature subsets are both phenotypically and functionally distinct from each other and, thus, respond to different types of antigens (see later section "B Cell Activation"). The Bcl-2 molecule is upregulated in both populations. Follicular B cells are IgM^+, IgD^+, $CD23^+$ and display intermediate expression for CD21, whereas marginal zone B cells are IgM^+, IgD^-, $CD23^-$ and display high expression for CD21. Unlike follicular B cells, marginal zone B cells are absent in humans under the age of 2; children under 2 are, therefore, unable to generate immune responses to certain antigens.

EXIT INTO THE PERIPHERY

Several different types of secondary lymphoid tissue exist. These include the spleen, lymph nodes, and mucosa-associated lymphoid tissue (such as Peyer's patches, appendix, and tonsil). Secondary lymphoid tissues are well adapted to trap circulating antigen. Foreign antigens in lymph are drained into lymph nodes, whereas antigens in the circulation are trapped in the spleen. Peripheral lymphoid tissue contains specialized antigen-presenting cells known as dendritic cells (see also Chapter 7). The Peyer's patches of the intestines collect foreign antigen in specialized epithelial cells known as M cells. Even though peripheral lymphoid tissues vary in structure and cellular organization, they all possess antigen-presenting cells and B cell–containing follicles surrounded by T cell–rich zones. As will become more evident in the following section, antigen, T cells, and dendritic cells are required for B cell activation and differentiation into immunoglobulin-secreting plasma cells or memory B cells.

B1 B cells typically home to the peritoneal and pleural cavities and also to the spleen. Follicular B cells enter the peripheral circulation by passing through the endothelial lining of the sinusoids of secondary lymphoid tissue and recirculate throughout the follicles of secondary lymphoid tissues. Because follicular B cells require antigen-specific T cell help for activation, the localization of this subset at the T cell zone of B cell follicles facilitates the chance encounter between antigen-specific B cells and cognate T cells. Conversely, marginal zone B cells respond to antigen without the need for cognate T cell help. They are found exclusively in the spleen of mice, and in the spleen and tonsils of humans, due to interactions between adhesion molecules and chemokine receptors that sequester marginal zone B cells within the marginal sinuses. The location of marginal zone B cells makes them well suited to capture blood-borne antigens.

B Cell Activation

B cells develop without bias for a particular antigenic specificity, ensuring that a diverse repertoire of different immunoglobulin molecules is produced. Despite the expression of antiapoptotic molecules such as Bcl-2, naïve B cells are short-lived unless they are activated in the presence of antigen and accessory cells, such as dendritic cells and T cells. Antigen-activated B cells undergo clonal expansion; B cells that do not interact with antigen are destined to undergo programmed cell death in a matter of days or weeks. The B1 and B2 B cell subsets are regulated by different activation mechanisms and are involved in different immune responses (see Table 10–2).

B1 B CELL ACTIVATION

B1 B cells respond to T cell–independent antigens. There are two classes of T cell–independent antigens: type I, which includes lipopolysaccharide (LPS); and type II, which includes large, multivalent antigens with repetitive epitopes that are often found on the surface of bacteria. T cell–independent antigens can directly activate B cells, resulting in the secretion of antibody. The B cell coreceptor contains activating molecules such as CD19, CD21, CD81, and Leu-13, which associate with the BCR and may enhance B cell responsiveness to T cell–independent antigens. There is strong evidence that these surface molecules are important for B1 activation because mice deficient in the genes that encode CD19 and CD21 have a reduced number of B1 B cells.[37] Soluble factors, such as IL-5 and IL-10, also appear to be involved in the maintenance and activation of B1 B cells.

B1 B cells do not require activation by antigen-specific T cells. However, $CD4^+$ helper T cells (Th cells) appear to augment B1 B cell activation, enhance immunoglobulin production, and influence isotype class switching, although the mechanisms are unclear.

The main H chain isotypes produced by B1 B cells in response to T cell–independent antigens are IgM, IgA, and IgG.

MARGINAL ZONE B CELL ACTIVATION

Marginal zone B cells are similar to B1 B cells in that they do not require cognate T cell help for activation. Marginal zone B cells respond to T cell–independent type II antigens and play an important role in protection against blood-borne pathogens. Soluble factors derived from dendritic cells, such as BAFF, and T cell–derived cytokines appear to be important for marginal zone B cell activation. Following activation, marginal zone B cells differentiate rapidly into antibody-secreting plasma cells. Marginal zone B cells secrete predominantly IgM antibodies, and to a lesser extent they secrete IgG antibodies.

FOLLICULAR B CELL ACTIVATION

As naïve follicular B cells leave the circulation and contact antigen and antigen-specific Th cells, B cells with BCR specific for antigen will be sequestered and activated. Engagement of the BCR by antigen signals B cells to engulf the antigen, process it intracellularly, and express peptide fragments bound to MHC class II molecules on the B cell surface.

After the expression of peptide fragments bound to MHC class II molecules, antigen-activated B cells present peptide to primed Th cells. B and T cells interact through T cell receptor recognition of a peptide-MHC complex on the B cell and through engagement of costimulatory molecules B7 and CD40 (Fig. 10–3). The B7 molecule, which interacts with CD28 on Th cells, is not constitutively expressed on B cells but is induced after antigen uptake by B cells. Th cells secrete cytokines, such as IL-3, IL-4, IL-5, and IL-10, and provide costimulatory signals that are important for B cell maturation and differentiation.[38] B cell activation during a T cell–dependent immune response also depends on engagement of the CD40 receptor expressed on B cells with the CD40 ligand (CD40L) expressed on T cells.[39] The importance of signal transduction events mediated by CD40-CD40L engagement is evident from studies of patients with a type of X-linked hyper-IgM syndrome, an immunodeficiency disease resulting from a defect in the CD40L. These individuals do not mount strong immune responses to T cell–dependent antigens; they have high concentrations of circulating IgM, but only trace amounts of IgG isotypes, and no affinity maturation of the antibody response.

Activated follicular B cells can have two different fates. Some of the activated B cells begin to proliferate to form primary foci.[40] These B cells can differentiate into short-lived plasma cells that secrete an immediate supply of antigen-specific antibody during a primary immune response (i.e., the first time a particular antigen is encountered by the immune system). The antibodies produced by these short-lived plasma cells are usually of the IgM isotype and are of low affinity because of the absence of somatic mutations. Alternatively, the proliferating B cells, along with the activating antigen-specific Th cells, can migrate to the primary follicles of secondary lymphoid tissue. During a primary immune response, antigen-activated follicular B cells form discrete structures in the primary follicles known as germinal centers. Isotype class switching, affinity maturation, and differentiation into memory B cells or plasma cells occur in germinal centers.

MATURATION IN GERMINAL CENTERS

Germinal centers can be subdivided into separate regions where the different stages of B cell maturation take place (Fig. 10–4). The dark zone is composed of

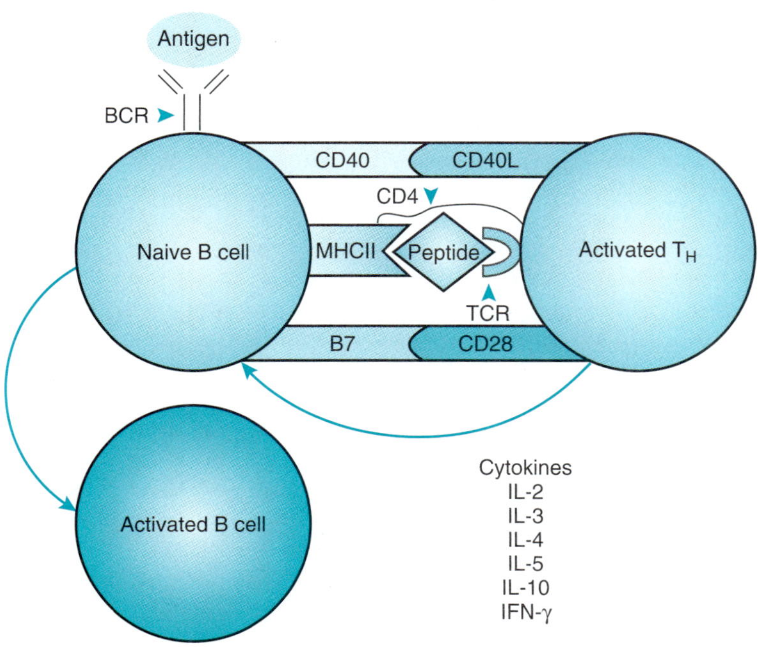

FIGURE 10–3 · B Cells as Antigen-Presenting Cells. Antigen bound to surface immunoglobulin on naïve B cells triggers endocytosis and intracellular processing into peptide fragments. B cells engage antigen-specific T helper (TH) cells though recognition of foreign peptide by the T cell receptor (TCR) and through binding of a conserved region of the major histocompatibility complex (MHC) II molecule by CD4. Coligation of CD40 and B7 expressed on B cells with CD40L and CD28 on T cells provide critical costimulatory signals and secretion of cytokines that are required for B cell activation.

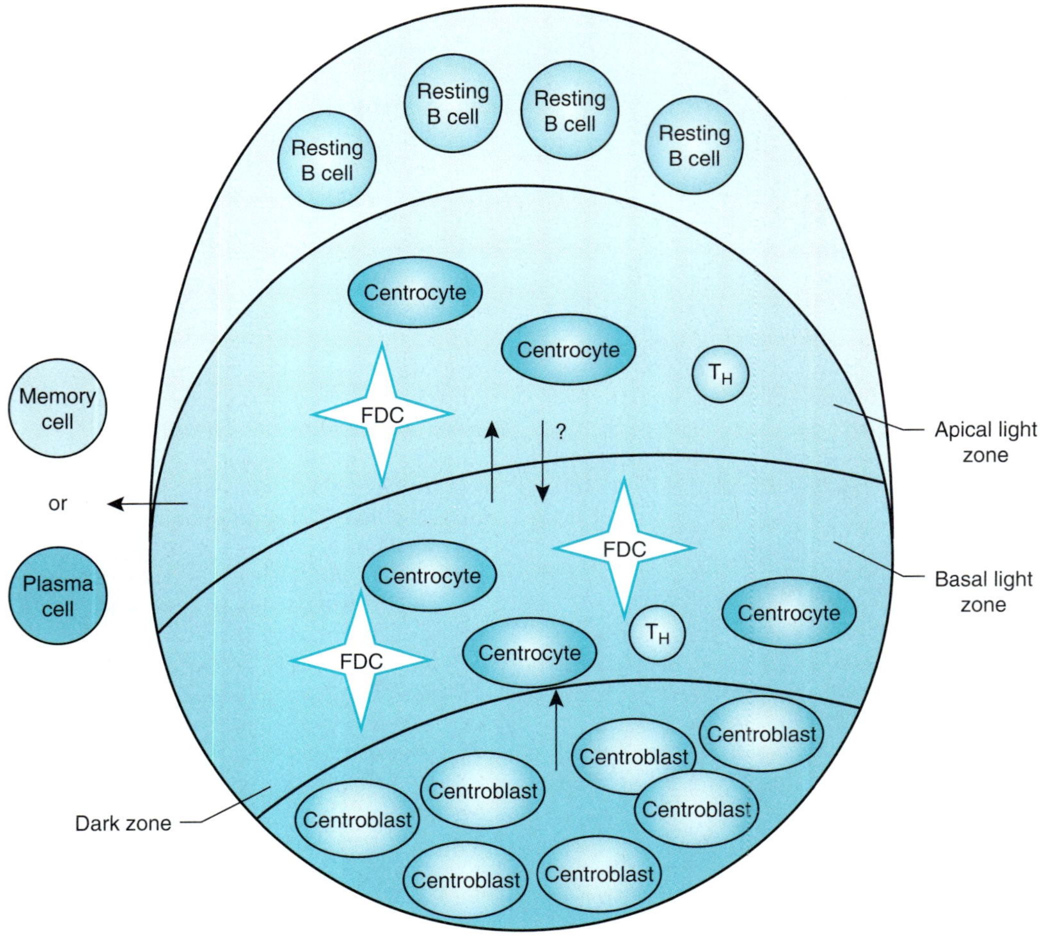

FIGURE 10–4 · **B Cell Maturation in Germinal Centers.** Following exposure to antigen, B cells in the primary follicles form germinal centers or migrate to previously formed germinal centers. Centroblasts located in the dark zone undergo proliferation and acquire somatic mutations. A small number of proliferating centroblasts can give rise to a larger number of centrocytes present in the basal light zone. As these cells pass through a dense network of follicular dendritic cells (FDC) and helper T cells, centrocytes bearing surface immunoglobulin receptors with high affinity for antigen will undergo positive selection. Centrocytes in the apical light zone are nondividing cells that undergo differentiation into memory B cells or plasma cells. It has been suggested that centrocytes may return to the dark zone where additional somatic mutations may be acquired. Resting B cells that are not activated by antigen are pushed aside to form the follicular mantle zone.

rapidly dividing cells called centroblasts, which develop into cells known as centrocytes. Centrocytes migrate to the light zone, where they encounter a dense network of follicular dendritic cells (FDC) and Th cells. B cells that do not express moderate- to high-affinity BCR are excluded from the light zone; B cells that receive vital survival signals differentiate into plasma or memory cells. Each stage of maturation is characterized by the differential expression of B cell surface markers (Table 10–4).

Centroblasts in the dark zone are rapidly proliferating cells derived from a relatively small number of antigen-activated B cells. Expression of the antiapoptotic Bcl-2 protein is low in these cells, whereas expression of the proapoptotic Fas protein is upregulated.[41] Low levels of Bcl-2 expression render developing B cells sensitive to apoptosis, but these cells can be rescued by antigen and CD40-CD40L interactions provided by antigen-specific Th cells.

The process of somatic mutation is activated during the centroblast stage. As discussed previously, somatic mutation is a process that introduces nucleotide base-pair changes in the DNA sequence of immunoglobulin genes, giving rise to antibodies with potentially higher affinity for antigen. The mechanisms that regulate the somatic mutation process are poorly understood. Current data show that: 1) Somatic mutations are introduced only into rearranged immunoglobulin genes; 2) *cis*-acting DNA elements that flank immunoglobulin genes may help target the variable region genes for mutation; and 3) immunoglobulin gene transcription is required.[22] A recently discovered molecule known as activation-induced cytidine deaminase (AID) has been shown to play a critical role in somatic mutation and also isotype class switching (see following) because the immunoglobulin variable regions of humans and mice with genetic lesions in the AID gene are largely unmutated.[42,43] The insertion of somatic mutations

TABLE 10–4 • MARKERS OF ANTIGEN-ACTIVATED B CELLS IN SECONDARY LYMPHOID TISSUE

	Naïve	Centroblast	Centrocyte	Memory	Plasma
Surface IgD	+	–	–	–	–
Surface IgM, IgG, IgA, or IgE	+	–	+	+	–
CD10	–	+	+	–	–
CD20	+	+	+	+	–
CD38	–	+	+	–	+
CD77	–	+	–	–	–
Presence of somatic mutation	–	+	+	+	+
Isotype class switch	–	–	+	+	+
Bcl-2	+	–	*+/–	+	+
Fas	+	+	+	+	–
AID	–	+	–	–	–
BLIMP-1	–	–	–	?	+

*Bcl-2 is only expressed in centrocytes following interaction with follicular dendritic cells.

Abbreviations: AID, Activation-induced cytidine deaminase; BLIMP, B lymphocyte-induced maturation protein; CD, clusters of differentiation.

occurs throughout the coding region of the variable gene segment and within 1 kilobase in each direction of the coding region between the promoter region and constant region of the rearranged immunoglobulin gene. DNA sequences known as "hot spot" motifs have been identified that appear to be targeted by the somatic mutation machinery with a higher frequency than are non–hot spot sequences.[44] B cell clones that express surface immunoglobulin with an increased affinity for antigen will be selectively expanded during the affinity maturation process, whereas B cells that express somatically mutated immunoglobulins with low affinity for antigen or altered affinity for self antigens will be targeted for apoptosis or inactivation. The importance of somatic mutation and affinity maturation during an immune response is underscored by the fact that patients with mutations in the AID gene are severely immunocompromised.

Centroblasts give rise to centrocytes located in the basal region of the germinal center light zone.[41] Because centrocytes are short-lived cells and express high levels of Fas and low levels of Bcl-2, they require survival signals from specialized germinal center cells called FDC. FDC differ from the other types of antigen-presenting cells in that they do not process antigen and present peptide–MHC class II complexes on the cell's surface. Instead, they trap antigen by collecting antigen-antibody complexes known as iccosomes (immune complex–coated bodies) on the cell surface. Iccosomes bind to FcγR present on FDC and deliver an antigen-specific signal to B cells through the BCR (Fig. 10–5). Centrocytes with specificity for antigen on FDC are saved from apoptosis by upregulation of the Bcl-2 molecule. Engagement of the complement receptors CR1 and CR2 (CD21 and CD35, respectively) on B cells by components of the C3 complement protein (iC3b, C3dg, and C3d) bound to FDC may mediate a secondary costimulatory signal.[45] If centrocytes do not receive these positive selection signals, they rapidly die. As antigen-selected centrocytes move into the apic light zone,

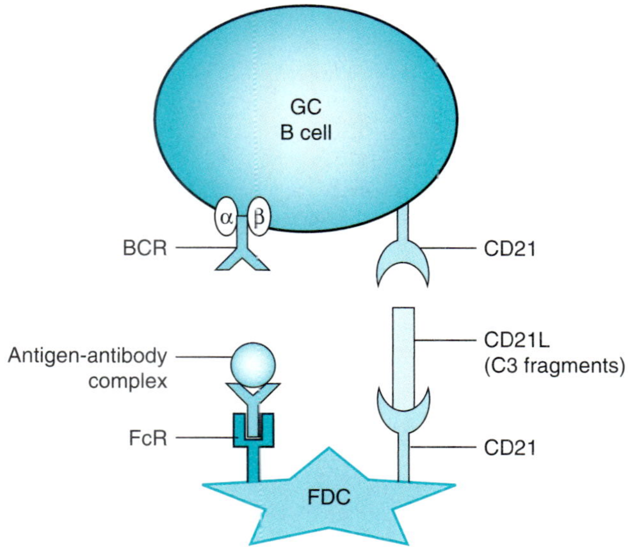

FIGURE 10–5 • **Engagement of B Cells with Follicular Dendritic Cells (FDC).** Interaction between FDC and B cells results in signals that mediate the positive selection of B cells in germinal centers. Antigen-antibody complexes trapped on the FDC surface deliver a signal to the B cell receptor (BCR). A second signal is delivered by the binding of CD21 on B cells to C3 complement components on the surface of FDC.

they no longer divide but continue maturing into memory B cells or plasma cells.

Concurrent with the positive selection of antigen-specific centrocytes in germinal centers, signaling events mediated by CD40L-CD40 and Th-derived cytokines promote isotype class switching in B cells. Th cells secrete IL-4, which mediates class switching to IgG4 and IgE, and IL-10, which mediates class switching to IgG1 and IgG3. Switching occurs by a deletion mechanism that brings a downstream constant region gene into juxtaposition with the VDJ gene segment.[6] Upstream of each constant region gene segment are switch recombination sequences, which contain binding sites for proteins known as switch factors. A putative enzyme known as switch recombinase catalyzes the removal of the upstream constant region gene sequences. The AID molecule, which plays a critical role in somatic mutation, is also required for isotype class switching, and patients and mice with mutations in the AID gene exhibit a hyper-IgM syndrome due to a defect in class switching.[43]

MEMORY B CELLS

During the final stages of B cell development in the germinal center, centrocytes develop into either memory B cells or plasma cells. These B cells typically express immunoglobulin genes that have undergone isotype class switching and possess somatic mutations. It is believed that the CD40-CD40L interaction directs centrocytes to undergo maturation into long-lived memory B cells. The exact life span of memory B cells is unknown, but it has been postulated that these B cells may persist throughout the life span of the host.[46]

Memory B cells circulate throughout the body in a quiescent state until the same antigen is reencountered and triggers a potent secondary immune response. Much less antigen is required to activate a secondary response than a primary response. Furthermore, a secondary immune response is generated more quickly than a primary immune response. Memory B cells ingest antigen and express peptide–MHC class II fragments. After antigen presentation of peptide to Th cells, memory B cells are activated to undergo expansion and maturation, giving rise to a second wave of plasma cells or memory B cells.

PLASMA CELLS

At the end of the B cell maturation cascade is the generation of plasma cells, which are factories for the secretion of soluble antibody molecules. B cells undergoing differentiation into plasma cells exit the lymphoid follicles and migrate to extrafollicular regions of secondary lymphoid tissue or to the bone marrow, where the final stage of plasma cell maturation occurs. There is evidence suggesting that IL-5 and IL-6 help induce plasma-cell differentiation, whereas engagement of CD40-CD40L molecules blocks this differentiation pathway. The transcriptional repressor known as B lymphocyte-induced maturation protein (BLIMP-1) has been shown also to play a critical role in the differentiation into plasma cells.[47] Plasma cells are terminally differentiated and have a finite life span, which can be quite long.[48] Studies performed with immunized mice demonstrate that long-lived plasma cells generated within germinal centers have a half-life of more than 100 days; short-lived plasma cells that arise from extrafollicular B cells have a half-life of less than 10 days.[49]

Regulation of B Cell Activation

Engagement of surface immunoglobulin by antigen triggers a series of cellular events that regulate B cell proliferation and differentiation. Receptor cross-linking leads to the rapid activation of proximal mediators of the BCR signal transduction pathway. This results in the activation of second messengers, such as phospholipase C, phosphatidylinositol 3-kinase, and Ras pathways. Induction of these pathways ultimately transmits signals to the nucleus, initiating new gene expression. Depending on the type of signal that is delivered and the stage of maturation, B cells can either undergo differentiation into memory B cells and plasma cells or undergo apoptosis. Along with surface immunoglobulin, several other receptors modulate antigen-induced signal transduction.

THE B CELL RECEPTOR

The BCR complex is composed of surface immunoglobulin along with the accessory molecules Ig-α and Ig-β. The role of surface immunoglobulin is to recognize foreign antigen; the Ig-α and Ig-β molecules are responsible for the induction of signal-transduction pathways required for B cell activation. The cytoplasmic domains of Ig-α and Ig-β contain a specific signaling motif known as the immunoreceptor tyrosine-based activation motif (ITAM). The ITAM amino acid sequence contains two tyrosine residues that are critical for signaling. After phosphorylation of these tyrosine residues, the ITAM acts as a docking site to recruit other signaling molecules.

The binding of antigen to surface immunoglobulin results in BCR clustering on the cell surface.[50] Once the receptors are cross-linked, the BCR-associated tyrosine kinases, which include the Src family members Blk, Fyn, and Lyn, mediate phosphorylation of the Ig-α and Ig-β ITAM tyrosine residues (Fig. 10–6). Subsequently, the tyrosine kinases Syk and Btk interact with the phosphorylated ITAM and are activated by tyrosine phosphorylation. The phosphorylation of Syk triggers the activation of phospholipase C, phosphatidylinositol 3-kinase, and Ras pathways. The activation of Syk appears to be absolutely critical for BCR-mediated signal transduction, because Syk-deficient cell lines exhibit a loss in BCR-induced signaling. Btk also appears to be required for the activation of second-messenger pathways. In patients with X-linked agammaglobulinemia, a mutation in the Btk gene results in impaired BCR signaling at the pre-B cell stage.[51] As a consequence, these patients have a greatly reduced number of mature B cells and generate poor antibody responses. In mice, however, a mutation in Btk leads to a disease known as X-linked immunodeficiency. B cell development is impaired at the transitional T2 stage, and B cells that do go on to maturity are unable to respond to certain T cell–independent antigens.

Signaling through the BCR leads to numerous events, such as B cell activation and endocytosis of antigen-antibody complexes, B cell proliferation, B cell differentiation, and apoptosis. Many molecules can modulate BCR signal transduction, either enhancing or diminishing the signal derived by antigen. The B cell coreceptor complex (CD19/CD21/CD81/Leu-13), CD45, SHP-1, SHP-2, SHIP, CD22, FcγRIIB1, CD5, CD72, PIR-B,

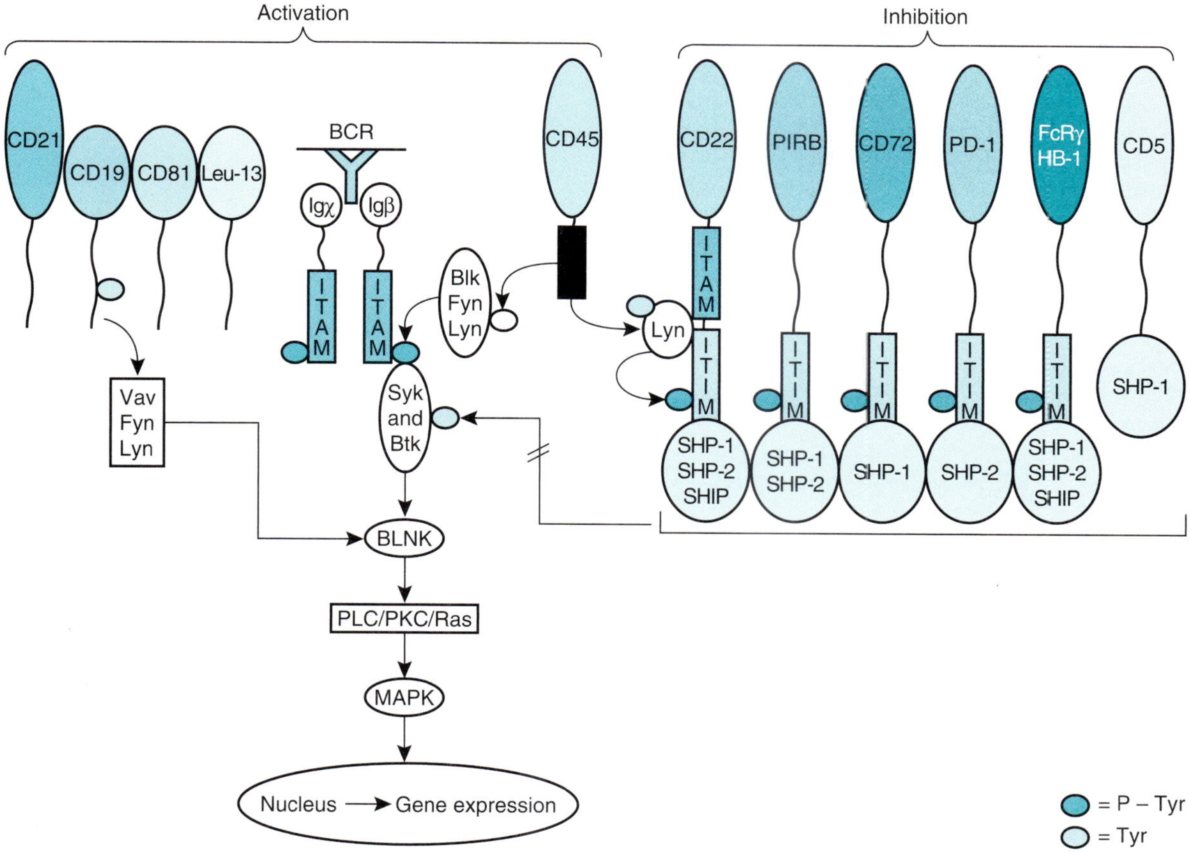

FIGURE 10–6 · **Molecules That Regulate the Activation State of B Cells.** Coligation of surface immunoglobulin results in the tyrosine phosphorylation at specific tyrosine residues present in the immunoreceptor tyrosine activation motif (ITAM) of Igα and Igβ cytoplasmic domains. This occurs following the removal of the inhibitory tyrosine residues of the B cell receptor (BCR)-associated cytoplasmic kinases, such as Blk, Fyn, and Lyn, which are mediated by CD45. The phosphorylated ITAMs recruit and activate the Syk and Btk kinases, which, in turn, activate a series of second messenger pathways (phospholipase C [PLC], protein kinase C [PKC], and Ras) that result in the upregulation of genes required for B cell activation and survival. Coligation of the pre-BCR complex (CD19, CD21, CD81, and Leu-13) results in phosphorylation of tyrosine residues residing in the cytoplasmic domain of CD19. Cytoplasmic kinases, including Vav, Fyn, and Lyn, become activated and enhance the signaling mediated by the BCR. Following the activation of PLC, PKC and Ras, molecules of the mitogen-activated protein kinase (MAPK) pathway become activated and translocate to the nucleus to regulate gene expression. Signals delivered mediated by CD22, paired immunoglobulin-like receptor PIR B), CD72, PD-1, FcγRIIB1, and CD5 deliver negative signals that block BCR activation by the phosphatases SH2 containing tyrosine phosphatase-1 (SHP-1), SH2 containing tyrosine phosphatase-2 (SHP-2), and SH2-containing inositol 5′-phosphatase (SHIP) to immunoreceptor tyrosine inhibitory motif (ITIMs).

and PD-1 (see Fig. 10–6) determine the threshold for activation, as well as the strength of the BCR signal.

THE B CELL CORECEPTOR COMPLEX

The B cell coreceptor complex is composed of CD19, CD21, CD81, and a recently identified interferon-inducible molecule called Leu-13.[5] CD19 has also been shown to associate with surface immunoglobulin.[50] After antigen cross-linking of surface immunoglobulin, specific tyrosine residues contained within the CD19 cytoplasmic domain become rapidly phosphorylated. There is evidence that ligation of CD19 leads to recruitment and activation of Vav, phosphatidylinositol 3-kinase, Fyn, Lyn, and Lck.[52] To date, the natural ligand for CD19 is not known. In vitro studies have demonstrated that ligation of CD19 with anti-CD19 antibody lowers the threshold required for BCR-mediated B cell activation and enhances the proliferative effect of anti-IgM treatment on B cells.[53] A role for CD19 in B cell activation has been clearly defined in mice that either are deficient in or overexpress CD19.[37] The CD19 molecule is required for germinal center formation and humoral responses to T cell–dependent antigens and possibly T cell–independent antigens.

The CD21 molecule serves as a receptor for cleavage fragments of the C3 component of complement, iC3b, C3dg, and C3d. Mice deficient in CD21 also have impaired responses to T cell–dependent and T cell–independent antigens and a defect in germinal-center formation.[37,54]

The functions of the remaining two components of the B cell coreceptor complex, CD81 and Leu-13, have not been characterized, although it has been suggested that these molecules may mediate homotypic cell adhesion.

CD45

Receptor tyrosine kinases require activation by phosphorylation of specific tyrosine residues, and they also require inactivation. Their inactivation in resting B cells is maintained by the phosphorylation of specific inhibitory tyrosine residues. For B cell activation to occur, phosphate groups must first be removed from the inhibitory tyrosine residues of the BCR-associated Src tyrosine kinases by CD45. CD45 has an extensive extracellular domain, with no clearly defined ligand specificity, and a cytoplasmic domain that possesses tyrosine phosphatase activity. One of the targets for CD45 dephosphorylation is Lyn; when activated, Lyn leads to the activation of Syk and Btk.[51] Mice deficient for CD45 display a diminished response to antigen and have a decreased number of mature B cells, indicating that some level of BCR activation is required for the transition of immature to mature B cells during lymphopoiesis.[55] CD45 is generally considered to be a positive regulator of BCR signaling, but it can also act as a negative regulator by initiation of a feedback loop to limit the extent of BCR activation (see following section "CD22").

SHP-1

SHP-1, another tyrosine phosphatase, is a potent negative regulator of BCR signaling. SHP-1 is a cytosolic protein found in association with transmembrane proteins, such as CD22, FcγRIIB1, CD5, CD72, and PIR-B (see following section). SHP-1 antagonizes BCR signaling by inactivating tyrosine kinases associated with signaling. Potential candidates for SHP-1 dephosphorylation include Ig-α and Ig-β, CD19, and Syk.[56] The function of SHP-1 has been extensively studied in mice that bear a naturally occurring mutation in the SHP-1 gene. Mice with this genetic defect are known as moth-eaten mice because of the appearance of their fur. These mice have a decreased number of conventional B cells and an elevation in B1 B cells, accompanied by high titers of autoreactive IgM antibodies.[57] This defect in B cell regulation underscores the importance of SHP-1 in limiting the extent of BCR signaling.

SHP-2

The intracellular tyrosine phosphatase SHP-2 is structurally similar to SHP-1. As with SHP-1, SHP-2 is recruited to the ITIM of inhibitory receptors. Mice deficient in SHP-2 are not viable, suggesting that SHP-2 plays a role in embryonic development.[58] Studies of chimeric mice suggest that SHP-2 plays a role in hematopoiesis and that SHP-1 and SHP-2 act in antagonistic fashion.[59]

SHIP

SHIP is an inositol phosphatase that inhibits B cell activation by hydrolyzing the 5′ phosphate from phosphatidylinositol 3,45-triphosphate, a critical component of numerous signaling pathways. As with SHP-1 and SHP-2, SHIP is recruited to ITIM motifs following BCR cross-linking. The role of SHIP in downregulating BCR-induced signals is demonstrated by its association with FcRγIIB1. Mice deficient in SHIP display splenomegaly and elevated levels of serum antibody.[60]

CD22

The CD22 receptor is a surface molecule that can also associate with the BCR, presumably through interaction with $\alpha_{2,6}$-sialylate sugars present on IgM.[61] Although CD22 contains an ITAM motif and is able to recruit Src tyrosine kinase to its cytoplasmic domain,[62] CD22 is most likely a negative regulator of BCR activation. Within the cytoplasmic domain of CD22 is a specific motif known as the immunoreceptor tyrosine-based inhibition motif (ITIM). As with the ITAM, a critical tyrosine residue resides in the ITIM that mediates signal transduction events. After activation of Lyn by CD45, it is believed that the ITIM of CD22 is phosphorylated by Lyn, leading to the recruitment of intracellular phosphatases, such as SHP-1.[61] B cells of mice deficient for CD22[62] and Lyn[63] have a phenotype similar to the SHP-1–deficient viable moth-eaten mice.

FCγRIIB1

FcγRIIB1 appears to be expressed exclusively on B cells, and unlike other types of FcγR, it is unable to mediate phagocytosis. The simultaneous ligation of both the BCR and FcγRIIB1 sends an inhibitory signal to prevent antigen activation of naïve B cells. In the presence of high levels of circulating immune complexes, this inhibitory signal provides a negative feedback mechanism to attenuate an antigen-induced antibody response. Recruitment and activation of SHIP by the FcγRIIB1 is required for downregulation of BCR signaling.[64] After coligation of the FcγRIIB1 and BCR, it is believed that Lyn phosphorylates the FcγRIIB1.[63] SHIP then associates with the FcγRIIB1 and mediates the dephosphorylation of CD19, thereby terminating BCR signaling.[65] Depending on the genetic background, mice deficient in FcγRIIB1 display a lupus-like phenotype.[66]

CD5

The role of CD5 in B1a B cell function is not well understood. After BCR cross-linking, CD5 is thought to mediate signals that induce apoptosis and block proliferation.[67] Cross-linking of CD5 with an anti-CD5 monoclonal antibody results in apoptosis. There is some evidence that CD5 recruits the inhibitory phosphatase SHP-1 to its cytoplasmic domain. However, unlike CD22 and FcγRIIB1, CD5 does not contain a strong ITIM consensus sequence and may recruit SHP-1 indirectly.[56] The ligand-binding region of CD5 remains to be elucidated, but recent evidence demonstrates that CD5 is a ligand for another negative regulator of BCR signaling, CD72.

CD72

CD72 is a transmembrane receptor that is expressed as a homodimer. The cytoplasmic tail of CD72 contains

ITIMs, and experiments have shown that CD72 recruits SHP-1. Mice with a targeted disruption of the CD72 gene reveal that CD72 plays a negative role in B cell activation. These B cells of CD72-deficient mice are similar to the viable moth-eaten phenotype and have an expansion of B1 B cells, are hyperresponsive to BCR cross-linking, and are more resistant to BCR-mediated apoptosis.[68] There are several putative ligands for CD72, including CD5 and CD100.

PAIRED IMMUNOGLOBULIN-LIKE RECEPTORS

The paired immunoglobulin-like receptors (PIR) A and B are expressed in a paired fashion as their name implies. These receptors are believed to have opposing functions, with PIR-A inducing an activation signal and PIR-B inducing an inhibitory signal. The ligands for PIR-A and PIR-B remain to be elucidated. Although less is known about the role of PIR-A in B cell activation, recent data demonstrate that PIR-B plays a role in downregulating B cell responses. The cytoplasmic tail of PIR-B possesses several ITIMs that recruit inhibitory phosphatases. Mice that harbor a targeted disruption of the PIR-B gene exhibit a phenotype similar to mice that are deficient in the other ITIM-bearing inhibitory receptors, such as an expansion of B1 B cells and B cell hyperresponsiveness.[69]

PD-1

PD-1 is an inhibitory molecule expressed predominantly on activated B and T cells. The ligand-binding domain binds PD-1L, and the cytoplasmic tail of PD-1 contains ITIMs that recruit SHP-2 to attenuate BCR signals. When expressed on certain genetic backgrounds, PD-1–deficient mice display an autoimmune phenotype.[70] The B cells of PD-1–deficient mice are hyperresponsive to BCR signaling, and these mice display an augmented response to T cell–independent type II antigens.

Negative Selection

An important feature of the immune system is the discrimination between foreign and self antigens. Self antigens are molecules derived from intracellular or extracellular components of the host. B cells with surface immunoglobulin receptors that recognize self components are subjected to a process known as negative selection, or tolerance induction, to avoid autoreactivity. The immune system has evolved several mechanisms to selectively inactivate B cells that recognize self antigen, while still permitting activation and expansion of B cells recognizing foreign antigen. In an intact immune system, autoreactive B cells generated in either the bone marrow or the periphery can be regulated by various mechanisms; the choice of which tolerance mechanism is used depends on the strength of the BCR signal delivered by self antigen and the developmental stage of the B cell. The concentration of self antigen and the affinity of the antibody for self antigen determine the degree of receptor occupancy of surface immunoglobulin and the strength of the BCR signal. If there is little receptor cross-linking, either because antigen concentration is low or because the affinity of the antibody is weak, there is no BCR signaling, and the autoreactive B cells are not tolerized. If receptor cross-linking reaches the threshold necessary to trigger a signaling cascade, an autoreactive B cell in the absence of T cell help will undergo tolerance induction. Three mechanisms are currently believed to mediate tolerance induction: receptor editing, anergy, and deletion. When mechanisms that regulate autoreactive B cells fail, the breakdown of self tolerance can lead to the development of autoimmune disease.

CENTRAL AND PERIPHERAL TOLERANCE

There are two stages in B cell development when autoreactive B cells can be generated. The first wave of autoreactivity arises in the bone marrow after VDJ rearrangement and expression of surface immunoglobulin on immature B cells. Because of the vast number of different antibody molecules that can be formed through the random recombination of H and L chain variable region genes, all individuals have the potential to generate autoreactive B cells. The process preventing the exit of autoreactive B cells from the bone marrow is known as central tolerance. Immature B cells are particularly sensitive to tolerance induction, probably owing to the absence of Bcl-2 expression and the lack of costimulation by Th cells. Peripheral tolerance refers to the downregulation of autoreactive B cells in peripheral lymphoid tissue. Transitional B cells may undergo peripheral tolerance if they encounter autoantigen for the first time in the periphery. Antigen-activated B cells that have acquired autoreactivity by somatic mutation in germinal centers may also undergo peripheral tolerance. At this developmental stage, it is crucial that the maturation of autoreactive B cells into memory B cells or plasma cells be blocked.

RECEPTOR EDITING

Cross-linking of the BCR on autoreactive B cells with high affinity for self antigen results in tolerance induction. However, these B cells can be salvaged if the original autospecificity is modified by a process known as receptor editing. In this process, the immunoglobulin surface receptor undergoes revision to acquire a new, nonautoreactive specificity. This occurs by secondary gene rearrangement events, such as intrachromosomal deletion accompanied by V_H or V_L replacement, novel intrachromosomal rearrangement of upstream V_L genes and downstream J_L genes, or rearrangement of H and L chain genes on an unrearranged locus.[71]

Studies from transgenic mice suggest that receptor editing occurs in both immature and transitional B cells and possibly in germinal-center B cells. Autoreactive B cells in transgenic mice expressing self-reactive specificities, such as anti–double-stranded DNA[72] or anti–MHC class I haplotype,[73] encounter self antigen in the bone marrow. They continue to express RAG-1 and

RAG-2 and generate DNA excision products resulting from secondary immunoglobulin gene rearrangement events. In these models, survival of edited B cells depends on the expression of a second L chain molecule that is able to associate with the transgene-encoded H chain and displace the initial L chain. There is evidence that H chain receptor editing can also occur in the bone marrow.[74,75] It still remains to be elucidated whether mature B cells in the periphery can also undergo receptor editing.

ANERGY

Some autoreactive B cells enter a hyporesponsive state known as anergy. Anergy is thought to be induced in immature B cells when they undergo a modest degree of BCR cross-linking. Anergic B cells downregulate surface immunoglobulin receptors and display a desensitization of the BCR, blocking activation of downstream mediators of signaling. Furthermore, anergic B cells are short-lived. Goodnow and colleagues[76] have performed classic studies on B cell tolerance induction in mice engineered to express an anti–hen egg lysozyme (HEL) antibody, along with soluble HEL, which acts as a self antigen. In the anti-HEL transgenic mouse model, B cells that encounter soluble, monovalent HEL are anergized. These B cells populate secondary lymphoid tissue but do not secrete anti-HEL antibody and cannot be recruited into a germinal-center response. This phenomenon is known as follicular exclusion.[77]

It appears that anergy can be reversed under certain conditions. Experimentally, anergy is broken in vitro by treatment with lipopolysaccharide or anti-CD40 antibody and IL-4. Exposure of anergic B cells in vivo to multivalent antigen in the presence of activated Th cells may also lead to their activation.[78] It has been suggested that anergic B cells serve as a potential source of autoantibody and may be activated in inflammatory conditions.[76b]

DELETION

Extensive BCR cross-linking in the absence of Th costimulation leads to a type of tolerance induction called deletion. In the transgenic model described previously, when anti-HEL B cells encounter multivalent membrane-bound HEL autoantigen in the bone marrow, they are deleted.[79] These results suggest that when antigen binding exceeds the threshold for anergy induction, cell death is triggered. Deletion of autoreactive B cells also occurs in the periphery and may be a means to control B cells expressing somatically mutated, high-affinity autoantibodies.

B cells are deleted from the immune system by a process known as apoptosis or programmed cell death. Apoptosis is a highly regulated event that is distinct from necrotic cell death, which results from destruction of the plasma membrane (see Chapter 26). Apoptotic cell death is primarily mediated through the activation of a series of endogenous proteases. Once apoptosis is triggered, characteristic morphologic and cellular changes take place that include a decrease in cell volume, membrane blebbing, movement of phosphatidylserine to the outer leaflet of the plasma membrane, chromatin condensation, and DNA fragmentation. The pathways that regulate apoptosis at the different stages of B cell development are not entirely understood, but at least two pathways have been shown to play an active role in regulating B cell death, the Fas pathway and the Bcl-2 pathway.

Fas (also known as CD95 or Apo-1), a member of the tumor necrosis factor receptor gene family, and Fas ligand (FasL) are transmembrane proteins expressed on a variety of cell types. Because Fas ligand is a homotrimeric molecule, it can bind three Fas molecules. Clustering of Fas on the cell surface, which occurs when Fas molecules bind Fas ligand, activates a cascade of intracellular enzymes, or caspases, that mediate apoptosis.[80]

It appears that when B cells engage CD40L expressed on Th cells in the absence of BCR ligation, Fas signaling induces apoptosis.[81,82] Other triggers for Fas-mediated death have not been clearly identified. Mutations in Fas *(lpr)* or Fas ligand *(gld)* in mice result in a systemic lupus erythematosus–like syndrome characterized by the production of pathogenic autoantibodies and lymphadenopathy. In humans, similar mutations lead to lymphadenopathy and antierythrocyte antibodies, but anti-DNA antibodies and glomerulonephritis are not present in these individuals.[83]

The Bcl-2 gene family is composed of molecules that either protect against or induce apoptosis in many cell types. Relative levels of these molecules dictate cell fate. For example, excess Bcl-2 promotes cell survival, whereas excess Bax induces cell death.[84]

The expression pattern of the antiapoptotic molecules Bcl-2 and Bcl-XL during B cell development suggests that they may play an important role in B cell survival. Levels are low at times of repertoire selection in the bone marrow or germinal centers and increase concomitantly with positive selection. B cells from mice deficient in Bcl-2 undergo spontaneous apoptosis,[85] whereas certain mouse strains that overexpress Bcl-2 in B cells produce autoantibodies.[86]

B Cell Autoimmunity

B cell activation must be tightly regulated at multiple levels to prevent the development of autoantibody-mediated autoimmune diseases. Many autoimmune disorders, including several rheumatologic diseases, involve the production of autoantibodies. The specific autoantigens and the affected organ systems vary among these different disorders. It has been speculated that B cell–associated autoimmune diseases may be linked by a common defect in the machinery that regulates B cell tolerance, but the etiology of most autoimmune diseases remains unsolved.

ORIGIN OF AUTOREACTIVE B CELLS

One of the fundamental questions surrounding B cell autoimmunity is the origin of autoreactive B cells. There is evidence that both B1 and B2 B cell subsets contribute to autoimmunity.[87] B1 B cells have been suggested to be a source of autoantibodies because this subset is known to secrete high levels of polyreactive antibody and can be directly activated by BCR cross-linking with multivalent antigens in the absence of antigen-specific T cell help.[88] Despite the production of autoreactive antibodies by this population, it is not clear whether these antibodies contribute to disease. B1 B cells in nonautoimmune individuals produce low-affinity autoantibodies that are nonpathogenic. It has been proposed that these autoantibodies may actually play a protective role against the tissue damage from more pathogenic autoantibodies.[88b] There is also some evidence that marginal zone B cells can secrete autoantibodies; however, there is also no direct evidence that these antibodies are pathogenic. Furthermore, it is not clear whether B1 and marginal zone B cells can also secrete high-affinity autoantibodies in autoimmune individuals. Yet a number of recently described genetically engineered mice have increased numbers of marginal zone B cells, produce autoantibodies, and exhibit autoantibody-mediated tissue damage.

Antibody production by the follicular subset requires the involvement of T cells. These B cells undergo H chain class switching and somatic mutation in germinal centers. Analysis of autoantibodies produced in both New Zealand black (NZB) and New Zealand white (NZW) F1 mice and MRL/lpr mice that spontaneously develop systemic lupus erythematosus demonstrate extensive somatic mutation and class switching to IgG isotypes, suggesting that they arise from follicular B cells.[89,90] The relative importance of each B cell subset in the generation of autoreactive B cells is still being debated.

INITIATION AND PROPAGATION OF AUTOIMMUNITY

There are several prevailing theories that attempt to explain the activation and expansion of B cells that should normally be silenced. Autoimmunity is thought to arise by a combination of environmental factors, such as infectious agents that initiate an autoimmune response, and genetic defects that alter B cell regulation. Proposed models for autoimmunity include 1) cross-reactivity of foreign antigen with self antigen, 2) inappropriate costimulation, and 3) altered thresholds for BCR signaling.

Much of our understanding of the breakdown of self-tolerance and progression of autoimmunity comes from the examination of mouse models. Autoimmune mouse models can be divided into three broad categories: 1) induced autoimmunity, 2) spontaneously occurring autoimmunity, and 3) genetically manipulated mice. Even though the progression of autoimmunity in humans is thought to be a highly complex process that involves multiple genetic and environmental factors, these animal models have provided much information on the molecular events that maintain self-tolerance.

MOLECULAR MIMICRY

One proposed model for the initiation of autoreactivity is that cross-reactive antiself, antiforeign B cells escape central tolerance because self antigen is present at too low a concentration to trigger tolerance induction or because the affinity of the antibody for autoantigen is below the signaling threshold. These B cells become activated in the periphery by foreign pathogens resembling self antigen and produce antibodies that bind both foreign and self antigen. This cross-reactivity is known as molecular mimicry. Molecular mimicry remains a popular model to explain the induction of many autoimmune disorders.[91] Once the pathogen is cleared, the autoantibody response is terminated because antigen-specific T cell help is no longer present. In the case of autoimmune-prone individuals, it is possible that intrinsic B cell defects prevent the down-regulation of autoantibody production, even after foreign antigen disappears.

The data that support molecular mimicry as a trigger for B cell–mediated autoimmunity are circumstantial; antigens from infectious agents have been identified that cross-react with self molecules associated with specific autoimmune diseases[91-95] (Table 10–5). The strongest evidence for molecular mimicry as a trigger for autoimmune disease is the cross-reactivity observed between the M protein of group A streptococcus and cardiac myosin in rheumatic heart disease. There is also experimental evidence that phosphorylcholine, a

TABLE 10–5 • EVIDENCE FOR ANTIBODY CROSS-REACTIVITY BETWEEN FOREIGN AND SELF ANTIGENS

Foreign Antigen	Self Antigen
Yersinia, *Klebsiella*, and *Streptococcus*[a]	DNA
Epstein Barr virus nuclear antigen 1[a]	ribonucleoprotein SmD
Streptococcus M protein[b]	cardiac myosin
Coxsackie B3 capsid protein[c]	cardiac myosin
Klebsiella nitrogenase[d]	HLA B27
Yersinia lipoprotein[e]	thyrotropin receptor
Mycobacteria heat-shock protein[f]	mitochondrial components
Escherichia, *Klebsiella*, and *Proteus*[g]	acetylchloline receptor
gpD derived from herpes simplex virus[g]	acetylcholine receptor

Autoimmune disorders exhibiting cross-reactive antibodies: [a], systemic lupus erythomatosus (SLE); [b], rheumatic fever; [c], myocarditis; [d], ankylosing spondylitis; [e], Graves' disease; [f], primary biliary cirrhosis; and [g], myasthenia gravis.

component of the cell wall found in many bacterial strains, mimics the structure of double-stranded DNA. Immunization of a nonautoimmune mouse strain with phosphorylcholine coupled to a protein carrier routinely generates anti–double-stranded DNA antibodies in germinal-center B cells.[96] However, these B cells are normally downregulated before contributing to a serum response.

In general, an initial immune response is generated against a dominant set of epitopes, followed by a later response to secondary or "cryptic" epitopes, a process known as epitope spreading.[97] Epitope spreading is an important aspect of a protective immune response because the ability to recognize multiple antigenic determinants increases the efficiency of neutralization and removal of pathogens. When an autoimmune response has been triggered, epitope spreading can lead to the production of additional autoantibodies with specificity for multiple self antigens. There are several proposed mechanisms by which epitope spreading triggers a cascade of T and B cell activation. Antigen-presenting cells present a foreign peptide that mimics a self peptide to T cells (Fig. 10–7*A*). These cross-reactive T cells become activated and provide costimulation to autoreactive B cells that recognize self antigen. This results in the production of autoantibodies specific for the antigen recognized by the T cell. After internalization of the self antigen by the autoreactive B cell, the autoantigen is processed and new cryptic epitopes of the self antigen are presented to T cells. A B cell binding to self antigen will internalize not only that self antigen but any complex of molecules that include the self antigen. The B cell may, therefore, present cryptic epitopes of many self antigens and activate autoreactive T cells with multiple autospecificities. T cells are present in the periphery that have not been tolerized to these epitopes and so are activated by self peptide. These activated T cells in turn help provide costimulation and activate other autoreactive B cells.

Alternatively, cross-reactive B cells may be activated first after exposure to foreign antigen and T cell help (see Fig. 10–7*B*). These B cells will internalize self antigen and present cryptic peptides to T cells that have not been tolerized, as described previously, leading to activation of autoreactive T cells and initiating the cascade. Thus, molecular mimicry and epitope spreading can lead to the activation of T and B cells specific for multiple autoantigens so long as the autoantigens form a complex in vivo.

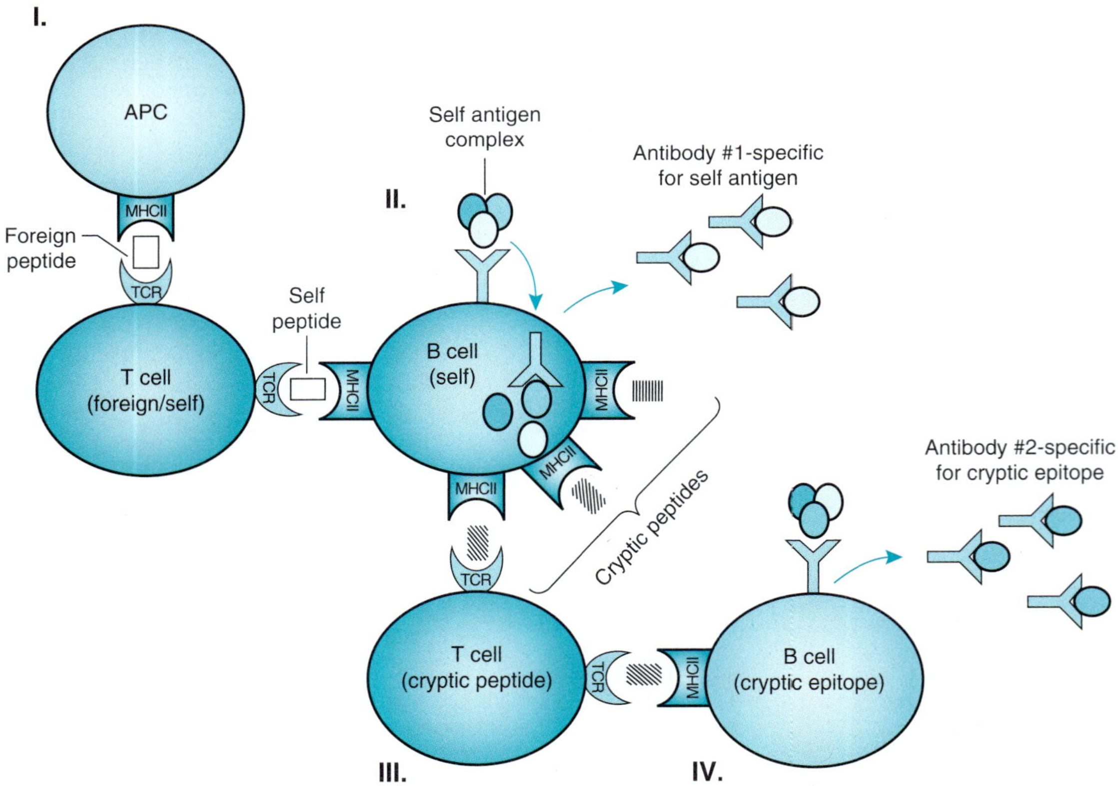

FIGURE 10–7A · Epitope Spreading by Activation of Cross-Reactive T Cells. **I.** Following antigen presentation of a foreign peptide that is recognized by a cross-reactive T cell, costimulatory signals are delivered to B cells with surface immunoglobulin receptors that recognize an epitope that is part of a self antigen complex. **II.** The complex is engulfed by a self-reactive B cell, and antibodies specific for the self antigen are generated. **III.** Self-reactive B cells process the self molecules and present cryptic peptide–major histocompatibility complex (MHC) class II complexes on the cell surface. **IV.** If these cryptic peptides are recognized by nontolerized autoreactive T cells, B cells specific for these cryptic epitopes are activated, and the autoantibody response spreads to other components of the self antigen complex.

Both nonautoimmune and autoimmune-prone individuals have the capacity to generate autoantibodies. Therefore, it is not likely that cross-reactivity between foreign and self antigens is solely responsible for the breakdown of tolerance that leads to autoimmunity. A plausible explanation is that foreign antigen acts as a molecular trigger to initiate an autoimmune response to self molecules, and a defect in the mechanism that regulates B cell activation leads to the propagation of an autoimmune response.

COSTIMULATION

It is evident that costimulatory signals play a critical role in B cell activation. Therefore, it is reasonable to envision that inappropriate costimulation could lead to the propagation of an immune response directed against a self antigen. The interaction between B7 on B cells and CD28 on T cells is crucial for activation of antigen-specific T and B cells. When a genetically engineered protein that inhibits B7/CD28 interactions is administered to NZB/NZW F1 lupus-prone mice, progression of disease is blocked.[98] Reciprocally, autoreactive B cells present in mice that constitutively overexpress B7 are not sensitive to Fas killing and display high serum-autoantibody titers.[99] Overexpression of CD40 or CD40L may also activate autoreactivity. In vitro studies have demonstrated that CD40-CD40L ligation in the presence of IL-4 activates anergic cells. It has been suggested that CD40L may be overexpressed in lymphoid cells of patients with systemic lupus erythematosus.[100,101] Enhanced survival and activation of autoreactive B cells has been demonstrated in mice that overexpress BAFF.[102] An increase in serum levels of BAFF has been observed in some patients with lupus, rheumatoid arthritis, and Sjögrens syndrome.[103] There is also evidence that autoreactive B cell activation is enhanced through the cross-linking of Toll-like receptor 9 (TLR9), which binds unmethylated CpG containing nucleic acid sequences with the BCR.[104] This mechanism could lead to the activation of chromatin-reactive B cells. It seems clear that perturbations in costimulatory pathways alter thresholds for B cell activation and death and could be responsible for the progression of autoimmune disease.

B CELL SIGNALING THRESHOLDS

The effects of altering the threshold for BCR signaling have been demonstrated in several mouse models. In transgenic mice that overexpress the BCR coreceptor complex component CD19, anergic B cells are activated and secrete autoantibody.[105] These results suggest that a decrease in the minimal requirement for antigen activation of the BCR can lead to inappropriate induction of autoreactive B cells. Viable moth-eaten mice also develop an autoimmune syndrome due to a naturally occurring deficiency in the SHP-1 phosphatase, a potent negative regulator of BCR signaling.[57] In these mice, B1 B cells are responsible for the production of IgM anti-DNA antibodies. Transgenic mice deficient in other signaling molecules that alter threshold activation, such as CD22[62] and Lyn,[63] also produce autoantibodies. Thus, changes in thresholds for antigen-induced B cell activation can lead to activation of autoreactive B cells.

Summary

The generation of a diverse repertoire of antibody molecules provides an important line of defense against microbial infections. The immune system is exquisitely controlled at multiple levels to allow the maturation of

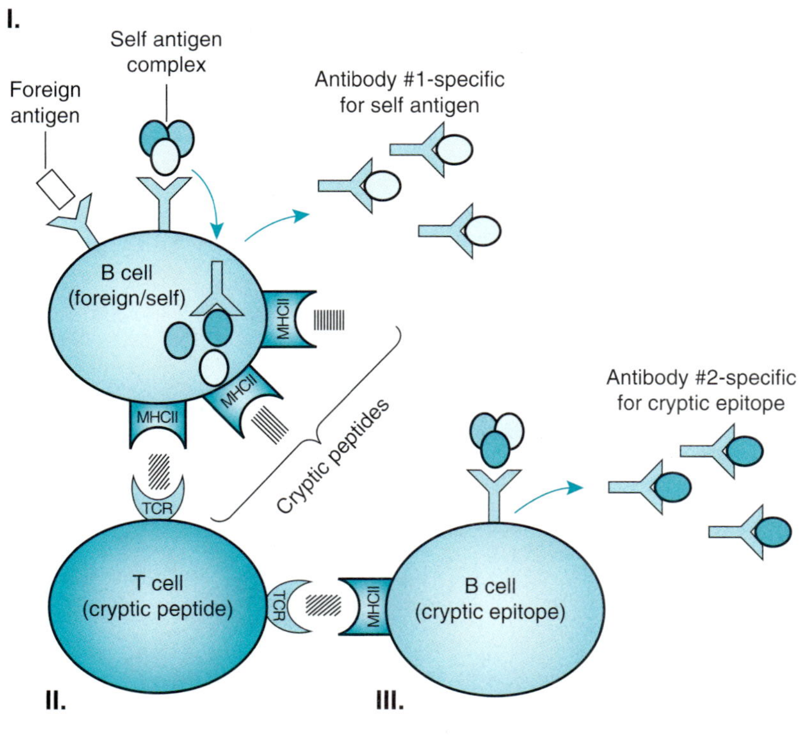

FIGURE 10–7B · Epitope Spreading by Activation of Autoreactive B Cells. **I.** A foreign antigen that mimics a self antigen can mediate the endocytosis of a self antigen complex. The self molecules of the complex are processed and expressed on the cell surface of the B cell as cryptic peptide–MHC class II complexes. **II.** If the cryptic peptides are recognized by nontolerized autoreactive T cells, **III.** These T cells provide costimulation to B cells that recognize cryptic epitopes, resulting in the production of additional self-reactive antibodies.

B cells that produce protective antibodies, while attempting to avoid the production of autoantibodies. Only a small percentage of B cell precursors that are generated complete the maturation scheme. During the pro-B and pre-B cell stages of development, B cells with aberrantly rearranged H or L chain genes are eliminated. As the remaining precursor cells transit into the immature B cell stage, they are subjected to negative selection; immature B cells bearing autospecificity are either deleted or inactivated, and B cells that can potentially bind foreign antigen are released into the periphery. B cells that are stimulated by foreign antigen are selectively expanded and undergo further immunoglobulin gene diversification in peripheral lymphoid tissue. During this stage of development, B cells that express high-affinity immunoglobulin receptors undergo positive selection, whereas B cells with a diminished affinity, or those that have acquired autoreactivity, are eliminated. B cells that pass through these critical developmental checkpoints differentiate into long-lived memory B cells or plasma cells. The underlying causes of B cell–associated autoimmunity are not well understood, but it seems likely that multiple defects in the regulatory mechanisms that control B cell maturation and differentiation contribute to autoimmune disease.

REFERENCES

1. Janeway JA, Travers P, Walport M, et al: The structure of a typical antibody molecule. *In:* Immunobiology, 5th ed. New York and London, Garland, 2001, p 96.
2. Janeway JA, Travers P, Walport M, et al: Structural variation in immunoglobulin constant regions. *In:* Immunobiology, 5th ed. New York and London, Garland, 2001, p 142.
3. Frazer JK, Capra JD: Immunoglobulins: Structure and function. *In* Paul, WE (ed): Fundamental Immunology, 4th ed. Philadelphia, Lippincott-Raven, 1999, p 37.
4. Raghavan M, Bjorkman PJ: Fc receptors and their interactions with immunoglobulins. Annu Rev Cell Dev Biol 12:181, 1996.
5. Bradbury LE, Kansas GS, Levy S, et al: The CD19/CD21 signal transducing complex of human B lymphocytes includes the target of antiproliferative antibody-1 and Leu-13 molecules. J Immunol 149:2841, 1992.
6. Snapper CM, Finkelman FD: Immunoglobulin class switching. *In* Paul, WE (ed): Fundamental Immunology, 4th ed. Philadelphia, Lippincott-Raven, 1999, p 831.
7. Shohet JM, Pemberton P, Carroll MC: Identification of a major binding site for complement C3 on the IgG1 heavy chain. J Biol Chem 268:5866, 1993.
8. Hiemstra PS, Biewenga J, Gorter A, et al: Activation of complement by human serum IgA, secretory IgA and IgA1 fragments. Mol Immunol 25:527, 1988.
9. Froelich CJ, Hanna WL, Poirier GG, et al: Granzyme B/perforin-mediated apoptosis of Jurkat cells results in cleavage of poly(ADP-ribose) polymerase to the 89-kDa apoptotic fragment and less abundant 64-kDa fragment. Biochem Biophys Res Commun 227:658, 1996.
10. Ghetie V, Ward ES: FcRn: The MHC class I-related receptor that is more than an IgG transporter. Immunol Today 18:592, 1997.
11. Aroeti B, Casanova J, Okamoto C, et al: Polymeric immunoglobulin receptor. Int Rev Cytol 137B:157, 1992.
12. Burrows PD, Cooper MD: IgA deficiency. Adv Immunol, 65:245, 1997.
13. Stewart WW, Kerr MA: The specificity of the human neutrophil IgA receptor (Fc alpha R) determined by measurement of chemiluminescence induced by serum or secretory IgA1 or IgA2. Immunology 71:328, 1990.
14. Carsetti R, Kohler G, Lamers MC: A role for immunoglobulin D: interference with tolerance induction. Eur J Immunol 23:168, 1993.
15. Nitschke L, Kosco MH, Kohler G, et al: Immunoglobulin D-deficient mice can mount normal immune responses to thymus-independent and -dependent antigens. Proc Natl Acad Sci U S A 90:1887, 1993.
16. Roes J, Rajewsky K: Immunoglobulin D (IgD)-deficient mice reveal an auxiliary receptor function for IgD in antigen-mediated recruitment of B cells. J Exp Med 177:45, 1993.
17. Janeway JA, Travers P, Walport M, et al: The structure of a typical antibody molecule. *In:* Immunobiology, 5th ed. New York and London, Garland, 2001, p 95.
18. Tonegawa S: Somatic generation of antibody diversity. Nature 302:575, 1983.
19. Duchosal MA: B-cell development and differentiation. Semin Hematol 34:2, 1997.
20. Akira S, Okazaki K, Sakano H: Two pairs of recombination signals are sufficient to cause immunoglobulin V-(D)-J joining. Science 238:1134, 1987.
21. Chu G: Role of the Ku autoantigen in V(D)J recombination and double-strand break repair. Curr Top Microbiol Immunol 217:113, 1996.
22. Wiesendanger M, Scharff MD, Edelmann W: Somatic hypermutation, transcription, and DNA mismatch repair. Cell 94:415, 1998.
23. Diamond B, Scharff MD: Somatic mutation of the T15 heavy chain gives rise to an antibody with autoantibody specificity. Proc Natl Acad Sci U S A 81:5841, 1984.
24. Boumsell L, Bernard A, Lepage V, et al: Some chronic lymphocytic leukemia cells bearing surface immunoglobulins share determinants with T cells. Eur J Immunol 8:900, 1978.
25. Kantor AB, Stall AM, Adams S, et al: Differential development of progenitor activity for three B-cell lineages. Proc Natl Acad Sci U S A 89:3320, 1992.
26. Huang CA, Henry C, Iacomini J, et al: Adult bone marrow contains precursors for CD5+ B cells. Eur J Immunol 26:2537, 1996.
27. Casali P, Schettino EW: Structure and function of natural antibodies. Curr Top Microbiol Immunol 210:167, 1996.
28. Picker LJ, Siegelman MH: Lymphoid tissues and organs. *In* Paul, WE (ed): Fundamental Immunology, 4th ed. Philadelphia, Lippincott-Raven, 1999, p 479.
29. Dorshkind K: Regulation of hemopoiesis by bone marrow stromal cells and their products. Annu Rev Immunol 8:111, 1990.
30. Kincade PW: B lymphopoiesis: global factors, local control. Proc Natl Acad Sci U S A 91:2888, 1994.
31. O'Riordan M, Grosschedl R: Transcriptional regulation of early B-lymphocyte differentiation. Immunol Rev 175:94, 2000.
32. Melchers F, Haasner D, Grawunder U, et al: Roles of IgH and L chains and of surrogate H and L chains in the development of cells of the B lymphocyte lineage. Annu Rev Immunol 12:209, 1994.
33. Papavasiliou F, Jankovic M, Nussenzweig MC: Surrogate or conventional light chains are required for membrane immunoglobulin mu to activate the precursor B cell transition. J Exp Med 184:2025, 1996.
34. Fang W, Weintraub BC, Dunlap B, et al: Self-reactive B lymphocytes overexpressing Bcl-xL escape negative selection and are tolerized by clonal anergy and receptor editing. Immunity 9:35, 1998.
35. Loder F, Mutschler B, Ray RJ, et al: B cell development in the spleen takes place in discrete steps and is determined by the quality of B cell receptor-derived signals. J Exp Med 190:75, 1999.
36. Gross JA, Dillon SR, Mudri S, et al: TACI-Ig neutralizes molecules critical for B cell development and autoimmune disease. impaired B cell maturation in mice lacking BLyS. Immunity 15:289, 2001.
37. Tedder TF, Inaoki M, Sato S: The CD19-CD21 complex regulates signal transduction thresholds governing humoral immunity and autoimmunity. Immunity 6:107, 1997.
38. Abbas AK, Murphy KM, Sher A: Functional diversity of helper T lymphocytes. Nature 383:787, 1996.

39. van Kooten C, Banchereau J: Functions of CD40 on B cells, dendritic cells and other cells. Curr Opin Immunol 9:330, 1997.
40. Smith KG, Hewitson TD, Nossal GJ, et al: The phenotype and fate of the antibody-forming cells of the splenic foci. Eur J Immunol 26:444, 1996.
41. Liu YJ, Arpin C: Germinal center development. Immunol Rev 156:111, 1997.
42. Revy P, Muto T, Levy Y, et al: Activation-induced cytidine deaminase (AID) deficiency causes the autosomal recessive form of the Hyper-IgM syndrome (HIGM2). Cell 102:565, 2000.
43. Muramatsu M, Kinoshita K, Fagarasan S, et al: Class switch recombination and hypermutation require activation-induced cytidine deaminase (AID), a potential RNA editing enzyme. Cell 102:553, 2000.
44. Betz AG, Neuberger MS, Milstein C: Discriminating intrinsic and antigen-selected mutational hotspots in immunoglobulin V genes. Immunol Today 14:405, 1993.
45. Tew JG, Wu J, Qin D, et al: Follicular dendritic cells and presentation of antigen and costimulatory signals to B cells. Immunol Rev 156:39, 1997.
46. Sprent J: Immunological memory. Curr Opin Immunol 9:37, 1997.
47. Shaffer AL, Lin KI, Kuo TC, et al: Blimp-1 orchestrates plasma cell differentiation by extinguishing the mature B cell gene expression program. Immunity 17:51, 2002.
48. Merville P, Dechanet J, Desmouliere A, et al: Bcl-2+ tonsillar plasma cells are rescued from apoptosis by bone marrow fibroblasts. J Exp Med 183:227, 1996.
49. Slifka MK, Ahmed R: Long-lived plasma cells: A mechanism for maintaining persistent antibody production. Curr Opin Immunol 10:252, 1998.
50. Birkeland ML, Monroe JG: Biochemistry of antigen receptor signaling in mature and developing B lymphocytes. Crit Rev Immunol 17:353, 1997.
51. Kurosaki T: Molecular mechanisms in B cell antigen receptor signaling. Curr Opin Immunol 9:309, 1997.
52. Sato S, Jansen PJ, Tedder TF: CD19 and CD22 expression reciprocally regulates tyrosine phosphorylation of Vav protein during B lymphocyte signaling. Proc Natl Acad Sci U S A 94:13158, 1997.
53. Carter RH, Fearon DT: CD19: lowering the threshold for antigen receptor stimulation of B lymphocytes. Science 256:105, 1992.
54. Haas KM, Hasegawa M, Steeber DA, et al: Complement receptors CD21/35 link innate and protective immunity during Streptococcus pneumoniae infection by regulating IgG3 antibody responses. Immunity 17:713, 2002.
55. Kishihara K, Penninger J, Wallace VA, et al: Normal B lymphocyte development but impaired T cell maturation in CD45-exon 6 protein tyrosine phosphatase-deficient mice. Cell 74:143, 1993.
56. Neel BG: Role of phosphatases in lymphocyte activation. Curr Opin Immunol 9:405, 1997.
57. Westhoff CM, Whittier A, Kathol S, et al: DNA-binding antibodies from viable motheaten mutant mice: implications for B cell tolerance. J Immunol 159:3024, 1997.
58. Qu CK, Yu WM, Azzarelli B, et al: Biased suppression of hematopoiesis and multiple developmental defects in chimeric mice containing Shp-2 mutant cells. Mol Cell Biol 18:6075, 1998.
59. Qu CK, Nguyen S, Chen J, et al: Requirement of Shp-2 tyrosine phosphatase in lymphoid and hematopoietic cell development. Blood 97:911, 2001.
60. Helgason CD, Kalberer CP, Damen JE, et al: A dual role for Src homology 2 domain-containing inositol-5-phosphatase (SHIP) in immunity: aberrant development and enhanced function of B lymphocytes in ship −/− mice. J Exp Med 191:781, 2000.
61. Cyster JG, Goodnow CC: Tuning antigen receptor signaling by CD22: integrating cues from antigens and the microenvironment. Immunity 6:509, 1997.
62. Sato S, Miller AS, Inaoki M, et al: CD22 is both a positive and negative regulator of B lymphocyte antigen receptor signal transduction: altered signaling in CD22-deficient mice. Immunity 6:551, 1996.
63. Chan VW, Meng F, Soriano P, et al: Characterization of the B lymphocyte populations in Lyn-deficient mice and the role of Lyn in signal initiation and down-regulation. Immunity 7:69, 1997.
64. Coggeshall KM: Inhibitory signaling by B cell Fc gamma RIIb. Curr Opin Immunol 10:306, 1998.
65. Hippen KL, Buhl AM, D'Ambrosio D, et al: Fc gammaRIIB1 inhibition of BCR-mediated phosphoinositide hydrolysis and Ca2+ mobilization is integrated by CD19 dephosphorylation. Immunity 7:49, 1997.
66. Bolland S, Ravetch JV: Spontaneous autoimmune disease in Fc(gamma)RIIB-deficient mice results from strain-specific epistasis. Immunity 13:277, 2000.
67. Bikah G, Carey J, Ciallella JR, et al: CD5-mediated negative regulation of antigen receptor-induced growth signals in B-1 B cells. Science 274:1906, 1996.
68. Pan C, Baumgarth N, Parnes JR: CD72-deficient mice reveal nonredundant roles of CD72 in B cell development and activation. Immunity 11:495, 1999.
69. Ujike A, Takeda K, Nakamura A, et al: Impaired dendritic cell maturation and increased T(H)2 responses in PIR-B(−/−) mice. Nat Immunol 3:542, 2002.
70. Nishimura H, Nose M, Hiai H, et al: Development of lupus-like autoimmune diseases by disruption of the PD-1 gene encoding an ITIM motif-carrying immunoreceptor. Immunity 11:141, 1999.
71. Radic M, ZZouali M: Receptor editing, immune diversification, and self-tolerance. Immunity 5:505, 1996.
72. Gay D, Saunders T, Camper S, et al: Receptor editing: An approach by autoreactive B cells to escape tolerance. J Exp Med 177:999, 1993.
73. Tiegs SL, Russell DM, Nemazee D: Receptor editing in self-reactive bone marrow B cells. J Exp Med 177:1009, 1993.
74. Chen C, Radic MZ, Erikson J, et al: Deletion and editing of B cells that express antibodies to DNA. J Immunol 152:1970, 1994.
75. Bertrand FE, Golub R, Wu GE: V(H) gene replacement occurs in the spleen and bone marrow of non-autoimmune quasi-monoclonal mice. Eur J Immunol 28:3362, 1998.
76. Goodnow CC, Crosbie J, Adelstein S, et al: Altered immunoglobulin expression and functional silencing of self-reactive B lymphocytes in transgenic mice. Nature 334:676, 1988.
76b. Goodnow CC, Brink R, Adams E: Breakdown of self-tolerance in anergic B lymphocytes. Nature 352:532, 1991.
77. Cyster JG, Hartley SB, Goodnow CC: Competition for follicular niches excludes self-reactive cells from the recirculating B-cell repertoire. Nature 371:389, 1994.
78. Cooke MP, Heath AW, Shokat KM, et al: Immunoglobulin signal transduction guides the specificity of B cell-T cell interactions and is blocked in tolerant self-reactive B cells. J Exp Med 179:425, 1994.
79. Hartley SB, Goodnow CC: Censoring of self-reactive B cells with a range of receptor affinities in transgenic mice expressing heaavy chains for a lysozyme specific antibody. Int Immunol 6:1417, 1994.
80. Ashkenazi A, Dixit VM: Death receptors: signaling and modulation. Science 281:1305, 1998.
81. Schattner EJ, Elkon KB, Yoo DH, et al: CD40 ligation induces Apo-1/Fas expression on human B lymphocytes and facilitates apoptosis through the Apo-1/Fas pathway. J Exp Med 182:1557, 1995.
82. Garrone P, Neidhardt EM, Garcia E, et al: Fas ligation induces apoptosis of CD40-activated human B lymphocytes. J Exp Med 182:1265, 1995.
83. Elkon KB, Marshak-Rothstein A: B cells in systemic autoimmune disease: recent insights from Fas-deficient mice and men. Curr Opin Immunol 8:852, 1996.
84. Knudson CM, Korsmeyer SJ: Bcl-2 and Bax function independently to regulate cell death. Nat Genet 16:358, 1997.
85. Veis DJ, Sorenson CM, Shutter JR, et al: Bcl-2-deficient mice demonstrate fulminant lymphoid apoptosis, polycystic kidneys, and hypopigmented hair. Cells 75:229, 1993.
86. Strasser A, Whittingham S, Vaux DL, et al: Enforced BCL2 expression in B-lymphoid cells prolongs antibody responses and elicits autoimmune disease. Proc Natl Acad Sci U S A 88:8661, 1991.
87. Ye YL, Chuang YH, Chiang BL: In vitro and in vivo functional analysis of CD5+ and CD5− B cells of autoimmune NZB x NZW F1 mice. Clin Exp Immunol 106:253, 1996.
88. Murakami M, Honjo T: Involvement of B-1 cells in mucosal immunity and autoimmunity. Immunol Today 16:534, 1995.
88b. Boes M, Schmidt T, Linkermann K, et al: Accelerated development of IgG autoantibodies and autoimmune disease in the absence of secreted IgM. Proc Natl Acad Sci USA 97:1184.

89. Marion TN, Bothwell AL, Briles DE, et al: IgG anti-DNA autoantibodies within an individual autoimmune mouse are the products of clonal selection. J Immunol 142:4269, 1989.
90. Shlomchik M, Mascelli M, H S, et al: Anti-DNA antibodies from autoimmune mice arise by clonal expansion and somatic mutation. J Exp Med 171:265, 1990.
91. Davies JM: Molecular mimicry: Can epitope mimicry induce autoimmune disease? Immunol Cell Biol 75:113, 1997.
92. Cunningham MW: Bacterial antigen mimicry. *In* Bona C, Siminovitch K, Zanetti M, Theophilopoulos A (eds): Molecular Pathology of Autoimmune Diseases. Chur, Switzerland, Harwood Academic, 1993, p 245.
93. Zhang H, Kaur I, Niesel DW, et al: Lipoprotein from Yersinia enterocolitica contains epitopes that cross-react with the human thyrotropin receptor. J Immunol 158:1976, 1997.
94. El-Roiey A, Sela O, Isenberg DA, et al: The sera of patients with Klebsiella infections contain a common anti-DNA idiotype (16/6) and anti-polynucleotide activity. Clin Exp Immunol 67:507, 1987.
95. Putterman C, Limpanasithikul W, Edelman M, et al: The double edged sword of the immune response; mutational analysis of a murine anti-pneumococcal, anti-DNA antibody. J Clin Invest 97:2251, 1996.
96. Ray SK, Putterman C, Diamond B: Pathogenic autoantibodies are routinely generated during the response to foreign antigen: a paradigm for autoimmune disease. Proc Natl Acad Sci U S A 93:2019, 1996.
97. McCluskey J, Farris AD, Keech CL, et al: Determinant spreading: lessons from animal models and human disease. Immunol Rev 164:209, 1998.
98. Daikh DI, Finck BK, Linsley PS, et al: Long-term inhibition of murine lupus by brief simultaneous blockade of the B7/CD28 and CD40/gp39 costimulation pathways. J Immunol 159:3104, 1997.
99. Rathmell JC, Fournier S, Weintraub BC, et al: Repression of B7.2 on self-reactive B cells is essential to prevent proliferation and allow Fas-mediated deletion by CD4(+) T cells. J Exp Med 188:651, 1998.
100. Koshy M, Berger D, Crow MK: Increased expression of CD40 ligand on systemic lupus erythematosus lymphocytes J Clin Invest 98:826, 1996.
101. Desai-Mehta A, Lu L, Ramsey-Goldman R, et al: Hyperexpression of CD40 ligand by B and T cells in human lupus and its role in pathogenic autoantibody production. J Clin Invest 97:2063, 1996.
102. Mackay F, Woodcock SA, Lawton P, et al: Mice transgenic for BAFF develop lymphocytic disorders along with autoimmune manifestations. J Exp Med 190:1697, 1999.
103. Groom J, Kalled SL, Cutler AH, et al: Association of BAFF/BLyS overexpression and altered B cell differentiation with Sjogren's syndrome. J Clin Invest 109:59, 2002.
104. Leadbetter EA, Rifkin IR, Hohlbaum AM, et al: Chromatin-IgG complexes activate B cells by dual engagement of IgM and Toll-like receptors. Nature 416:603, 2002.
105. Inaoki M, Sato S, Weintraub BC, et al: CD19-regulated signaling thresholds control peripheral tolerance and autoantibody production in B lymphocytes. J Exp Med 186:1923, 1997.

11 Synoviocytes

DAVID M. LEE • HANS P. KIENER • MICHAEL B. BRENNER

Normal Synovium

MICROANATOMY AND TISSUE ORGANIZATION

The biology of synoviocytes is best considered in the context of their microanatomy: the synovium, a complex tissue composed of heterogeneous cellular populations, acellular stroma, nerves, lymphatics, and blood vessels. Normal synovial tissue resides between the fluid-filled joint cavity and the fibrous joint capsule. Histologically, at the light-microscopic level, classic synovial descriptions focus on characterization of discrete anatomic morphologies identifiable in the joint lining[1,2]; differing forms (areolar, adipose, and fibrous) are present to varying degrees interspersed throughout the joint capsule. Their characterization is entirely descriptive; there is no known functional difference between these morphologic types of synovium.

The transition from synovium to periosteum and cartilage is indistinct and gradual.[3] The synovium is thought to overlie the periosteum with little connecting interface, with the exception of the hyaline cartilage boundary where the synovium is tightly bound and has a fibrous appearance. In man, synovial tissue extends onto the cartilage surface for only a short distance and has the appearance of a wedge at the joint margin.[4]

The synovium reveals a condensed accumulation of cells one to four cells thick, which forms an apparent lining layer overlaying a more loosely packed stroma. The upper region has been variably defined as the synovial lining layer (or intima) and the underlying region is called the sublining (or subintima). Unlike endothelium and cuboidal or columnar epithelium whose structures contain a basement membrane, tight junctions, and desmosomes, the synovial lining is porous, with intercellular spaces apparent between some of the lining cells.[5,6]

Cellular Composition

Within the synovial lining, two cell types predominate. In electron microscopic analyses of the human synovium,[5] two discrete cell populations were identified, type A and type B synoviocytes. A large golgi apparatus, numerous large vacuoles, filopodia, vesicles, and mitochondria typify type A synoviocytes, whereas type B synoviocytes feature abundant ergastoplasm (granular endoplasmic reticulum) with narrow cisternae, a well-developed golgi apparatus, and far fewer vacuoles. Scientists accurately hypothesized that these morphologic differences corresponded to discrete functional differences: Type A cells appear phagocytic and type B cells appear to have largely synthetic and secretory function (Fig. 11–1). Immunohistochemical analyses have further delineated the two predominant cellular populations within the synovial lining. Type A synoviocytes (also called macrophage-like synoviocytes) express markers of hematopoietic origin most consistent with the monocyte/macrophage lineage; their surface receptor profile is similar to other tissue resident macrophage populations[7] (see Fig. 11–1). Characteristic expression markers of type A synoviocytes include CD14, CD16, and CD68. In animal models, the bone marrow origin of this lineage postnatally was confirmed in mouse radiation chimera experiments. Bone marrow from beige mice (bg), which contains characteristic large cytoplasmic granules, was transplanted into irradiated recipient mice. Analysis of recipient mouse synovium revealed contribution from the donor bone marrow that was exclusively present in the type A synoviocyte population.[8] These and other studies suggest that type A synoviocytes are tissue macrophages that turn over and are replaced by recruitment and maturation from the peripheral blood monocyte pool.[9,10] Type B synoviocytes express (also called fibroblast like synoviocytes) markers common to mesenchymal (fibroblast) cells in other anatomic sites, including collagen, vimentin, and CD90 (see Fig. 11–1). However, in contrast to many other fibroblast populations, they express uridine diposphoglucose dehydrogenase (UDPDG), CD55 (delay acceleration factor [DAF], mAb67), and CD106 (vascular cell adhesion molecule-1 [VCAM-1]).[11,12] The fibroblast-like populations in the synovium demonstrate marked differences in the lining and sublining layers. Synovial lining layer fibroblasts have increased cellular compaction relative to fibroblasts in the sublining. In addition, fibroblast-like cells in the synovial sublining lack expression of CD55, CD106, and UDPDG. These immunohistologic expression studies imply functional differences between the fibroblast-like synoviocyte (FLS) subpopulations in the synovial lining and sublining.[13-17]

The postnatal maintenance and replenishment of synovial lining FLS may occur by replacement by proliferation of resident cells, recruitment of extrasynovial progenitor cells, or recruitment of FLS from the sublining for continuous repopulation of the lining layer. However, there exists no direct evidence to resolve which of these possibilities predominates. Histologic examination of type B synoviocytes reveals only rare mitotic figures, and DNA-incorporation experiments revealed very low rates of division in human synovial explants.[18,19] In contrast, cells with mesenchymal progenitor features have been isolated from synovial tissues, providing a candidate source for lining layer repopulation.[20]

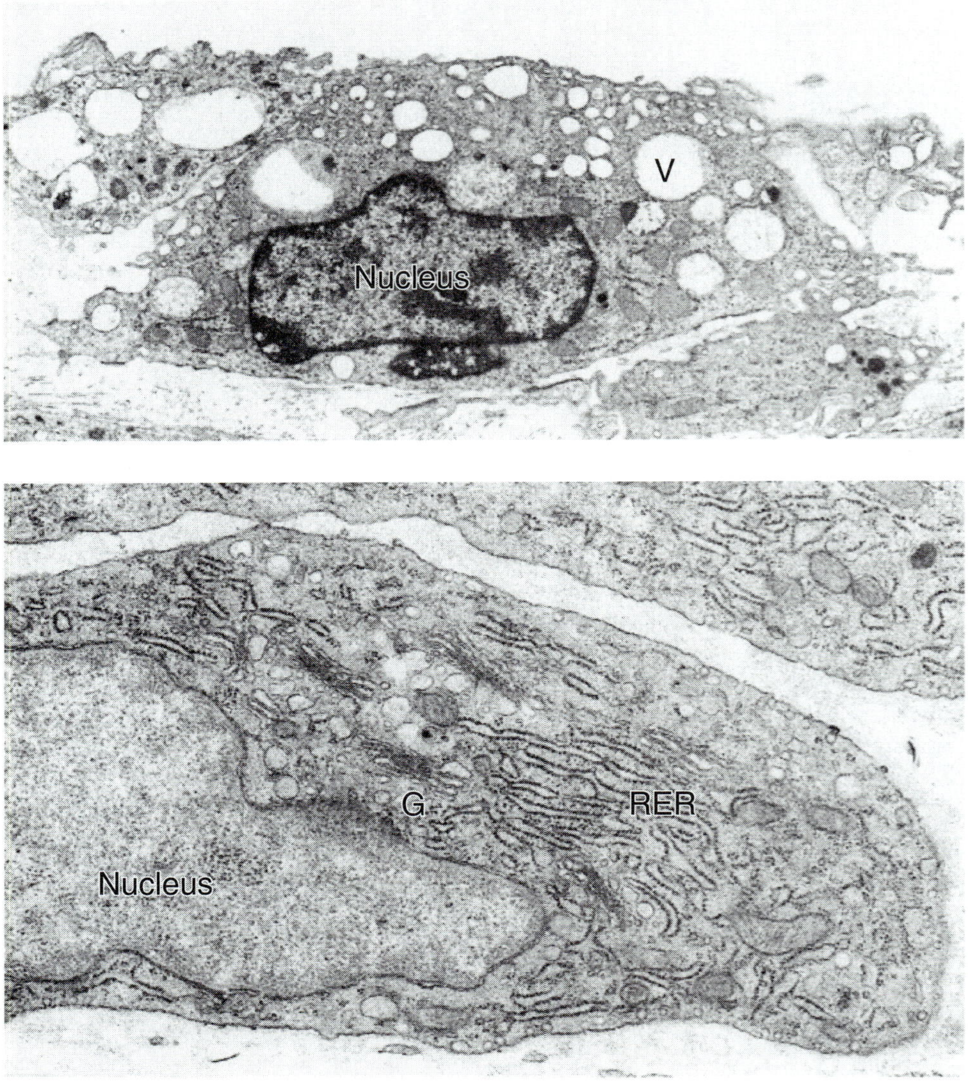

FIGURE 11–1 • Transmission electron micrographs of macrophage-like (Type A) and fibroblast-like (Type B) synoviocytes. Note the characteristic prominent cytoplasmic vacuoles and vesicles (V) characteristic of tissue macrophages evident in the Type A synoviocte. Within the Type B synoviocyte are prominent rough endoplasmic reticulum (RER) and extensive golgi apparatus (G). The nucleus demonstrates an open chromatin pattern. Table 11–1 lists sele-cted markers expressed by macrophage-like and fibroblast-like synoviocytes. (Adapted by Advanced Medical Graphics from Henderson B, Edwards JCW: The Synovial Lining in Health and Disease. London, Chapman and Hall, 1987.)

TABLE 11–1 • N MACROPHAGE-LIKE (TYPE A) SYNOVIOCYTES

Marker	
CD16/CD64	Immunoglobulln G Fc high- and low-affinity receptor
CD45	Leukocyte common antigen, tyrosine phos phatase
CD14	LPS/LBP receptor
CD68	Lysoosomal glycoprotein
CD11b/CD18	Integrin adhesion molecule and complement receptor "Mac-1"
MHC class II	Antigen presenting molecule
Fibroblast-Like (Type B) Synoviocytes	
Marker	
UDPGD	Uridine diphospho-glucose dehydrogenase
VCAM-1	Vascular cell adhesion molecule-1, CD106
DAF	Complement decay–accelerating factor, CD55
Cadherin-11	Homophillic adhesion molecule
Vlmentin	Intermediate filament protein
Thy-1	CD90

In contrast to the ordered and compact layer of synovial lining, the sublining is more amorphous and heterogeneous, yet it plays a critical role in influencing the synovial lining. The sublining consists of loose connective tissue that serves as a microanatomic base upon which the synovial lining attaches and allows the free diffusion of solutes extravasated from the capillary serum ultrafiltrate. Many cellular populations are constituents of the synovial sublining, including vascular cells, nerves, adipocytes, lymphatics, lymphocytes, mast cells, phagocytes, and fibroblast-like cells. Thus, the synovial sublining provides a means for communication of both molecular and cellular elements from circulating blood to the synovial lining and the synovial fluid space. In addition, it provides a resident immunologic cellular population for infectious surveillance and a possible reservoir of FLS for continuous repopulation of the synovial lining.

Synovial Lining

Most body surfaces and organ structures are lined with epithelia or endothelia whose structural integrity is maintained by tight intercellular junctions and further supported structurally by an underlying basement membrane. The junctions that connect cells to other cells are typically multiprotein complexes made of the transmembrane adhesion molecules (classical cadherins) and cytoplasmic proteins (catenins, vinculin, others) that link the surface adhesion molecules to the cytoskeleton (actin filaments). These multiprotein complexes provide both regulated intercellular adhesive function and a mechanism to transduce signals initiated by cellular interactions that regulate cytoskeletal organization, cell migration, cell proliferation, and cell differentiation.[21] The critical importance of cadherin-based intercellular adhesive interactions for the formation of epithelia has been demonstrated in vivo. In chimeric mice, intestinal epithelial cells that lack E-cadherin expression due to a dominant negative cadherin demonstrate aberrations in cell differentiation, epithelial cell polarity, and integrity of the epithelium.[22]

Underlying an epithelial lining, an acellular basement membrane, composed predominantly of the structural extracellular matrix proteins fibronectin, laminins, and collagens, contributes to epithelial structure by providing a durable tissue scaffold as well as a site for attachment of epithelial cells. The basement membrane also contributes to epithelial function by providing a semipermeable barrier for passage of fluid and small solutes.

In contrast to the highly organized epithelia, the synovial lining structure lacks tight junctions, desmosomes, and a discrete basement membrane.[5] Rather, it is composed of a network of cells within a meshwork of extracellular matrix. This combination of cells and matrix components form a functional "cellular basement membrane" between the specialized synovial fluid compartment and the richly enervated and vascularized synovial sublining region (Fig. 11–2).

Mechanisms contributing to the synovial lining structural integrity are beginning to emerge. Although electron microscopic analyses demonstrated synovial lining discontinuity with evidence of significant intercellular matrix space, they also demonstrated a degree of cell–cell contact with interdigitation of cellular processes.[5] The molecular interactions mediating synoviocyte–cellular interactions differ significantly from those in traditional epithelia. Heterophilic adhesion molecule receptor–ligand pairs, including CD55-CD97 and VLA-4–CD106 (VCAM-1) are expressed by FLS and synovial macro-phages,[13,23] providing a means for mediating heterotypic or homotypic cellular interactions. The recent identification of synovial expression of cadherin 11 by Type B FLS[24] provides further insight into mechanisms of synovial lining formation, structural organization, and integrity. The homophilic (like-like) adhesion properties of cadherin 11 provide a means for specifying FLS-FLS adhesion critical for structural integrity of the synovial lining. Furthermore, synovial lining cadherin expression provides a molecular mechanism for regulating shape and function of FLS within this distinct microanatomic compartment.

SYNOVIOCYTE FUNCTIONS

The durable synovial lining provides a deformable tissue architecture to the joint cavity that allows movement. Importantly, the synovial lining is largely responsible

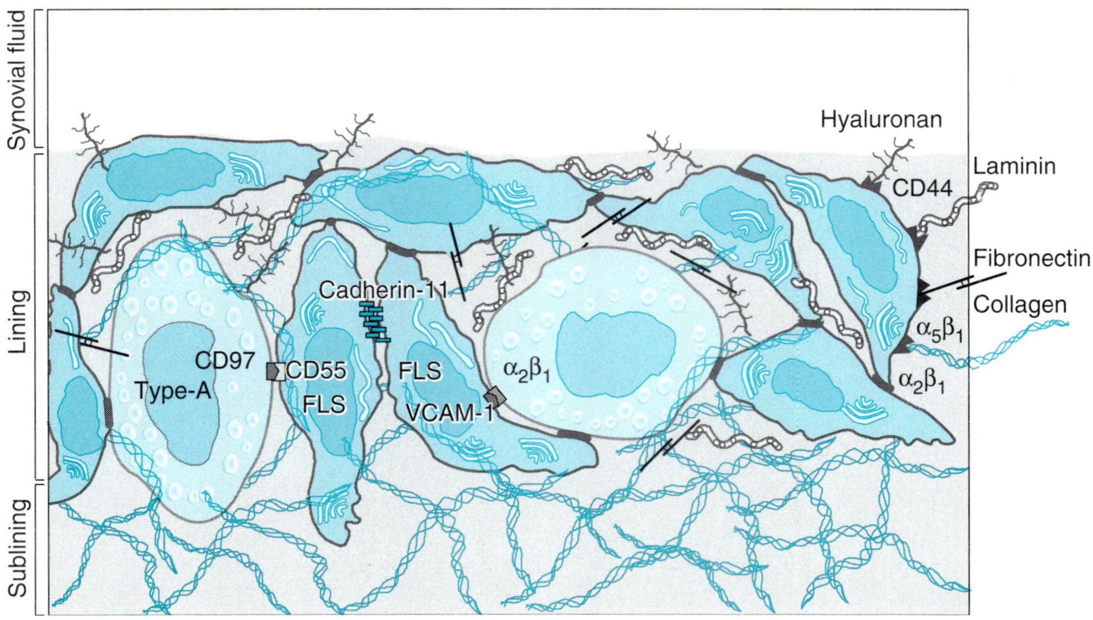

FIGURE 11–2 · Normal Synovial Lining Microenvironment. Synoviocytes form localized contacts between cells (denoted by dark lines) while embedded in a fibrillar extracellular matrix. Cell–cell molecular interactions include homophilic adhesion by cadherin 11 (fibroblast-like synoviocyte [FLS]-FLS) and heterophilic adhesion by vascular cell adhesion molecule [VCAM-1]:$\alpha4\beta_1$ (FLS-FLS and FLS-Type A). Cell-matrix adhesion includes cellular integrin species (e.g., $\alpha2\beta1$,$\alpha3\beta1$,$\alpha6\beta1$,$\alpha4\beta1$,$\alpha5\beta1$) and CD44, which can bind to matrix constituents (e.g., collagens, laminin, fibronectin, chondroitins, and hyaluronan). Other cell-cell interactions include those mediated by receptor-ligand pairs such as CD55-CD97. Together these cell–cell and cell-matrix connections provide for structural integrity and anatomic organization of the lining, as well as allowing for solute permeability. (Advanced Medical Graphics.)

for joint homeostasis. The porous organization of the synovial lining allows passage of small solutes from serum ultrafiltrate in close proximity to the cartilage surface, a process thought to be important for supplying nutrients to the avascular chondrocyte population.[25] Concurrently, by providing a selectively permeable barrier function, the synovial cellular matrix lining mediates production and clearance of the synovial fluid.[26] The synoviocytes themselves also produce and take up synovial fluid components (see following).

Macrophage-Like Synoviocytes (Type A Synoviocytes)

Electron microscopic studies of synovial macrophages (Type A cells) document that they contain numerous vacuoles consistent with active phagocytic activity.[5] Injection of particulate matter into experimental animals results in uptake and clearance by this population.[27] A prevailing hypothesis is that these phagocytic cells participate in particulate clearance from the joint space. In the inflamed state, synovial macrophages become a major substituent of the synovial lining layer and produce a host of inflammatory mediators.

Fibroblast-Like Synoviocytes (Type B Synoviocytes)

Synovial Fluid

Both the extensive network of organelles involved in protein production and assembly (golgi and rough endoplasmic reticulum) seen on electron microscopic ultrastructural analysis and in vitro measurement of synthetic function indicate that the FLS are key producers of the molecular constituents in the synovial fluid and matrix. The need for synthetic activity has been demonstrated by fluid and hyaluronan metabolic studies: The synovial fluid volume is exchanged approximately every 60 minutes, and the hyaluronic acid turns over daily.[26] Hyaluronic acid, present in both synovial fluid and matrix, is manufactured within the synovium.[28] Although FLS production of hyaluronic acid has not been formally demonstrated, FLS—and not other synovial cellular populations—express high levels of UDPGD, an enzyme required for hyaluronan synthesis.[11,29,30] In addition to production of hyaluronic acid, FLS also manufacture the synovial fluid constituent, lubricin, which is critical for lubricating ability of synovial fluid.[31-33]

Extracellular Matrix

The synovial matrix is in contact with the synovial fluid compartment and is present in the intercellular space throughout the synovium. The extracellular matrix (ECM) constituents include collagen species (types I, III, IV, V, and VI), structural glycoproteins (fibronectin, vitronectin, laminin), proteoglycans (hyaluronan, heparan sulfate, keratan sulfate, chondroitin sulfate), and elastin.[3,34-47] These constituents are not present diffusely within the matrix; rather, their inclusion appears to result from an ordered process with subsets of matrix molecules present in discrete regions of the synovium. Collagens are present in relatively low numbers in the lining compared to the sublining matrix, whereas fibronectin, laminin, and hyaluronic acid are relatively enriched in the lining matrix. Type IV collagen, laminin, and fibronectin, prominent constituents of the basement membrane underlying cells at other anatomic sites, are present specifically in the intercellular matrix of the synovial lining region.[17,48,49] The absence of the cross-linking ECM component entactin may explain in part the structural differences between the loosely organized synovial lining matrix and highly organized basement membrane architecture of epithelial tissues.

FLS are major participants in all aspects of the active, continuous process of maintaining the synovial ECM. Histochemical studies show the production of matrix components (fibronectin, collagens, laminin, tenascin, and the proteoglycans) by FLS.[40,43,46,49-52] In addition to producing molecular constituents of the ECM, FLS also direct matrix component assembly via cell surface expression of integrin species, such as $\alpha5\beta1$ and $\alpha V\beta3$, which direct fibrillogenesis of matrix components such as fibronectin.[53] FLS also synthesize degradative enzymes necessary for matrix remodeling and cellular movement. Cathepsins, serine proteases, metalloproteinases (MMPs), and the membrane-type metalloproteinases (MT-MMP) are all expressed by FLS. In combination, these proteases contain activities capable of digesting the protein contents of the synovial matrix.[54-57] These proteases also allow cross-activation of zymogen pro-forms of each other, providing a means for amplification of the matrix degradative process. Furthermore, many of the cleavage products generated by these proteases have biologic activities besides protein cleavage. For example, they can regulate cellular migration, proliferation, apoptosis, and angiogenesis.[58] The activity of MMPs is regulated in part by endogenous inhibitory proteins, many of which are expressed by FLS. These inhibitors include α_2-macroglobulin and a family of proteins called tissue inhibitors of metalloproteinases (TIMPs).[59] The importance of degradative enzymes in normal joint physiology has been underscored in clinical trials of MMP inhibitors. In these oncology trials, a prominent side effect of MMP inhibitors included a progressive polyarthritis with joint pain and stiffness.[57,60-62] Synovial matrix remodeling, therefore, results from a delicate balance between matrix degradation, matrix synthesis, and matrix assembly, all of which are substantially influenced by FLS.

The FLS populations also produce a number of other bioactive factors, including growth factors (fibroblast growth factor [FGF], stem cell factor [SCF], vascular endothelial growth factor [VEGF], granulocyte-macrophage colony-stimulating factor [GM-CSF]), prostaglandins, complement components, and receptor activator of NFκB (RANK) ligand. The role of these mediators in normal joint physiology, including cellular division, cellular maturation, angiogenesis, regulation of blood flow, and other functions, has been hypothesized and remains a matter of investigation.[63-65] Thus, synoviocytes, especially lining layer FLS, actively participate in diarthrodial joint function including manufacture of joint lubrication, synovial fluid maintenance, cartilage nutrition, and synovial lining flexibility and integrity.

Synovitis

In the context of inflammatory arthritis, the synovium undergoes profound changes in cellular content and physiology. Histologically, there is hyperplasia of the synovial lining layer composed of macrophages (Type A) and FLS (Type B), in which the macrophage synoviocyte (Type A) becomes the majority population.[7,31,66,67] Ultrastructurally, consistent with their activated phenotype, these tissue macrophages display increased numbers of lysosomes and cisternal dilatation of the rough endoplasmic reticulum.[31,68] Similarly, the FLS (Type B) population demonstrates expansion, thickening, and dilatation of the rough endoplasmic reticulum with large numbers of associated polyribosomes, numerous vesicles containing granular material, prominent centrioles, and changes in cytoskeletal organization[69] consistent with a stimulated, metabolically active, secretory cellular state.

In addition to the changes observed in the resident cellular synovial lining populations, the normally sparsely populated synovial sublining undergoes massive infiltration with inflammatory cells including T lymphocytes, B lymphocytes, macrophages, plasma cells, mast cells, and neutrophils. Although these inflammatory infiltrates can vary in composition, lymphoid populations generally predominate with lymphoid follicle formation occurring on occasion in chronic synovitis.[70] Vascular changes, including new vessel formation (angiogenesis)[71] and the generation of high endothelial venules,[72] are notable in the sublining, as are changes in ECM content of the connective tissue stroma. FLS both respond to and actively contribute to the alterations seen in synovitis, in particular to the destructive components of rheumatoid synovitis.

MECHANISMS OF SYNOVIOCYTE ACTIVATION AND SYNOVIAL HYPERPLASIA

Synoviocyte Activation

Synovial Macrophages

Type A (macrophage-like) synoviocytes are abundant in the inflamed synovial lining and sublining, as well as in the erosive pannus. Both their high-level major histocompatability complex (MHC) class II expression and prominent cytokine expression demonstrate that these cells are activated in the context of inflammatory arthritis. This activation occurs in response to cell–cell contact as well as to soluble factors.[73-75] Cell contact–mediated macrophage stimulation is mediated in part by lymphocytes and may involve lymphocyte counterreceptors interacting with CD40, lymphocyte function–associated antigen-1 (LFA-1), and CD69 expressed on macrophages.[75-78] Macrophages can also be stimulated via soluble factors including cytokines (e.g., interferon-γ and interleukin-17 [IL-17]), components of infectious organisms (via CD14, Toll-like receptors, and other pattern-recognition receptors) and sex hormones.[79] Synovial macrophages participate in inflammatory arthritis predominantly via secretion of effector molecules, including cytokines, MMPs, and nitric oxide. Indeed, synovial macrophage populations are the major producers of IL-1 and tumor necrosis factor-alpha (TNF-α).[80,81] These mediators in turn increase endothelial adhesion molecule expression and may recruit and stimulate infiltrating leukocytes, induce angiogenesis, and stimulate responses seen in the Type B (fibroblast-like) synoviocytes.

Fibroblast-like Synoviocytes

The inflammatory leukocyte accumulation that occurs in conditions such as rheumatoid arthritis (RA) mainly occurs in the synovial sublining region. WD The major means by which leukocytes infiltrating the synovial sublining influence the synovial lining FLS is via secretion of soluble inflammatory mediators, especially cytokines.[82,83] In the case of FLS, the effects of leukocyte-derived cytokines on their activation are legion. IL-1 and TNF-α can potently stimulate FLS proliferation in vitro[84,85]; FLS remain responsive to these cytokines even after long-term culture. These cytokines stimulate induction of FLS proliferation, which provides a mechanism for the prominent synovial hyperplasia seen in vivo in conditions such as RA. Furthermore IL-1 and TNF-α can induce the expression of degradative enzymes such as collagenase and stromelysin in FLS and thereby contribute to matrix and cartilage destructive processes seen in vivo.[84,86-89] Cytokine stimulation of FLS can also induce FLS to secrete cytokines (e.g., TNF-α can stimulate FLS IL-1 production, TNF-α and IL-1 can stimulate FLS IL-11 expression) as well as prostaglandins (e.g., prostaglandin E2).[84,88-91] This cytokine-stimulated production of inflammatory mediators by FLS provides a means by which the FLS amplify and perpetuate the synovial inflammatory response. A thorough discussion of synovial cytokines in inflammatory arthritis is presented in Chapter 65.

Other soluble mediators found within the inflamed synovium have bioactivity on FLS. Three growth factor species that are present in high concentration in inflamed synovium and that display potent mitogenic activity for FLS are platelet-derived growth factor (PDGF), transforming growth factor-beta (TGF-β), and FGF. FGF appears to operate in an autocrine manner in FLS. TGF-β, produced by synovial macrophages and other cells, is present in both synovial tissue and fluid.[92,93] TGF-β stimulates cellular proliferation and production of collagen by cultured FLS in vitro.[94] In vivo, injection of TGF-β directly into joints of experimental animals induces significant synovial hyperplasia, which far exceeds the degree of concomitant inflammatory infiltration.[95] PDGF, another growth factor found in inflamed synovium, is one of the most potent inducers known of cultured FLS proliferation in vitro.[96] PDGF is produced by inflamed RA synovial macrophages[97] and endothelial cells, whereas synovial fibroblasts express the PDGF receptor,[98] suggesting a paracrine mechanism for regulating synovial fibroblast growth.

Further bioactive mediators in the synovium that activate FLS include mast cell proteases (tryptases) and neuropeptides such as vasoactive intestinal peptide (VIP). Tryptase produced by synovium resident mast cells potently activates fibroblasts to produce collagen and induces fibroblast chemotaxis.[99,100] Synovial production of neuropeptides, such as substance P,[101] and the anti-inflammatory properties of VIP[102] suggest a role for these mediators in regulating FLS function. The specific role of neuropeptides in FLS biology is not well understood.

Together cellular, cytokine, and noncytokine factors stimulate a cycle of Type A and Type B synoviocyte activation, which contributes importantly to the cyclic amplification and perpetuation of synovial activation and hyperplasia that participate in joint damage in inflammatory arthritis such as RA.

Synovial Hyperplasia

Type A Synoviocytes

Both macrophages and FLS populations contribute to synovial lining hyperplasia. The significant increase in synovial macrophages[7] is accomplished by recruitment from circulating monocyte progenitors. In animal studies, macrophage-like synoviocytes are recruited from outside the synovium and accounted for the majority of the hyperplasia within 4 days.[103] In humans, recruitment of peripheral blood monocytes is mediated via synovial production of chemoattractant molecules called chemokines. Synovial production of chemokines known to attract monocytes, including IL-8, monocyte chemoattractant protein-1 (MCP-1), macrophage inflammatory protein-1α (MIP-1α), MIP-1β, regulated on activation normal T expressed secreted (RANTES), and fraktalkine, has been demonstrated. In addition, the chemokine receptors CCR1, CCR2, CCR5, CXCR1, CXCR2, and CX3CR1 are expressed by synovial macro-phages.[104-106] In humans, peripheral blood monocytes demonstrate increased integrin expression (CD11a/ CD18 [lymphocyte function-associated antigen-1 (LFA-1)], CD11b/CD18 [Mac-1]) and increased matrix-binding ability.[107] Furthermore, inflamed RA vascular endothelium demonstrates an induction of functional leukocyte adhesion molecules P-selectin and E-selectin.[108] Thus, chemokine signals coupled with increased monocyte and vascular endothelium adhesion molecule expression facilitate the rapid influx of macrophages into inflammatory synovium.

Fibroblast-like Synoviocytes

Several possible mechanisms can contribute to FLS hyperplasia in the inflamed synovium: increased proliferation, decreased apoptosis, and recruitment of progenitor populations. The relative importance of each remains to be determined, although distinct processes might account for increased numbers of FLS early in inflammatory arthritis compared to late disease.

Proliferation

Under inflammatory conditions, FGF and TGF-β are found in high concentrations in synovial fluid and are produced abundantly by cultured FLS.[109] These cytokines can potently stimulate FLS proliferation and may play a role in FLS hyperplasia.[110,111] Similarly, TNF-α is produced in substantial quantities by cultured FLS[112] and can stimulate FLS proliferation and MMP and prostaglandin production.[88] Chemokines produced spontaneously by FLS are capable of stimulating the production of inflammatory cytokines by cultured FLS.[113] It is likely that these and other autocrine factors contribute to the proliferation and activation of FLS in vivo and to the observed stable "inflammatory" phenotype of FLS obtained from patients with inflammatory arthritis.

However, the means by which synovial lining FLS numbers increase in inflammatory synovial hyperplasia are not fully understood. Histologic analyses have observed only rare mitotic cells. Although other studies have documented a modest increase in proliferating cells, the absolute proliferation rates were very low.[19,114] Immunohistologic stains for cellular proliferation markers noted some reactivity with the proliferating cell nuclear antigen (PcNA) antigen but only rare Ki-67 antigen–positive cells.[115,116] Taken together, these findings suggest that FLS proliferation occurs but that rapid cellular proliferation, by itself, does not account for the impressive synovial hyperplasia seen in inflammatory arthritis.

Apoptosis

Pathways that alter apoptosis in FLS may contribute to hyperplasia. Fas receptor ligation is a potent, but regulated means of inducing apoptosis. FLS express the Fas antigen both in vivo and in vitro. Under specific circumstances, ligation of Fas in vivo in animal models and in vitro on cultured FLS potently induces programmed cell death. However, exposure of FLS to cytokines present in the inflamed synovium, such as IL-1, renders them resistant to death by Fas ligation. Furthermore, FLIP (FLICE inhibitory protein [Fas associated death domain-like Ii-1β converting enzyme]), an inhibitor of Fas-mediated apoptosis, is expressed in both lining and sublining FLS at higher levels in RA than in osteoarthritis (OA) synovium.[117] Similarly, expression of Bcl-2 and sentrin, other inhibitors of Fas-mediated apoptosis, can be demonstrated in synovial FLS.[118,119] Interestingly, demonstration of frequent mutations in the tumor-suppressing gene p53 in inflamed synovial FLS also can affect apoptosis.[120,121] Experimental studies in cultured FLS demonstrated both increased cell division and inhibition of Fas-mediated apoptosis with p53 inhibition in vitro[122] and increased FLS invasiveness in vivo.[123] Morphologic analyses of RA tissues has revealed very few apoptotic cells, suggesting that reduced cell death may contribute to synovial hyperplasia. However, apoptosis as assessed by both terminal dUTP nuclear end labeling (TUNEL) assay and DNA fragmentation are demonstrable in normal, OA, and RA synovial tissue[124,125] with higher rates of DNA damage in RA tissues. This apparent discrepancy may be resolved either by rapid clearance of apoptotic cells by synovial macrophages, making their detection by morphologic criteria difficult,[126] or by increased DNA damage without progression to apoptosis. Overall, the respective contributions of increased proliferation and reduced apoptosis both seem to contribute to hyperplasia of the synovial FLS in RA, yet neither process can be confirmed as dominant in RA pathogenesis.

Recruitment and Maturation

The recruitment and differentiation of mesenchymal progenitor cells into synovial-lining FLS as a mechanism for synovial lining hyperplasia is appealing but remains hypothetical. From a kinetics standpoint, synovial hyperplasia can occur extremely rapidly, with animal models demonstrating substantial hyperplasia within 4 to 5 days after administration of an arthritogenic stimulus.[127,128] This rapid hyperplasia cannot readily be ascribed to proliferation of resident lining cells and is reminiscent of the process of rapid recruitment of infiltrating leukocytes to sites of inflammation. Further, work in experimental models has demonstrated that mesenchymal progenitor cells (or even less-differentiated, multipotent stem cells) are present in the circulatory system and can be recruited for functional contribution to multiple anatomic sites.[129] The presence of mesenchymal progenitors within the inflamed synovium is suggested by the identification of cells expressing mesenchymal progenitor cell surface markers (e.g., bone morphogenetic protein receptor [BMPR], CD44, type I collagen, vimentin) by flow cytometric and immunohistologic analysis of inflammatory synovial fluid and synovial biopsy tissues.[20] These mesenchymal lineage cells with multipotential differentiative capacity can be grown from cultures of synovial fluid and tissue.[20,130] Multipotent mesenchymal progenitor cells that share immunophenotype with synovial populations (BMPR, CD44, Type I collagen, vimentin) have been demonstrated in peripheral blood of normal human volunteers, providing a potential circulating reservoir for cells observed in the inflammatory synovium.[131] Furthermore, it is becoming apparent that many of the molecular and cellular pathways utilized during limb and joint development continue and are relevant in these postnatal processes. In vitro studies of *wnt* family member expression in healthy and diseased synovium have implicated this family in fibronectin, MMP, and inflammatory cytokine production by RA synoviocytes.[132,133] The expression of TGF-β, FGF, BMP, and Hox genes have all been demonstrated in RA synoviocytes.[134-139] Taken together, these findings suggest that the FLS cellular increase noted in the hyperplastic inflamed synovium may also involve recruitment and maturation of tissue resident or circulating mesenchymal progenitor cells.

FIBROBLAST-LIKE SYNOVIOCYTES AS INFLAMMATORY CELLS IN SYNOVITIS

Inflammatory Mediator Production

In addition to responding to inflammatory mediators elaborated by infiltrating leukocytes, there is growing evidence that the FLS cellular population, like fibroblasts from other anatomic sites, plays an active role in the propagation of inflammatory synovitis.[140,141] FLS are capable of substantial primary cytokine production, both constitutively[142] and in response to stimuli. The cytokines produced by FLS include IL-6, which can activate synovial macrophages and lymphocytes, as well as TNF-α and IL-1, which have pleiotropic autocrine and paracrine effects. In addition, the list of other cytokines expressed by FLS continues to expand (IL-8, IL-11, IL-15, IL-16, leukemia inhibitory factor [LIF], TGF-β, PDGF, GM-CSF, granulocyte colony-stimulating factor [G-CSF], FGF, VEGF, epidermal growth factor [EGF]).[143] FLS also elaborate chemokines, including IL-8, GRO-α, MCP-1, MIP-1α, MIP-1β and RANTES, which are potently capable of leukocyte recruitment.[113,144-147] They secrete macrophage colony-stimulating factor (M-CSF) and stem cell factor (SCF), which function in synovial macrophage and mast cell recruitment and maturation, respectively.[148-150] Additionally, FLS express both cyclooxygenases (COX-1 and COX-2)[151,152] and elaborate prostaglandins (most notably prostaglandin E) whose biologic activities include vasodilatation, modulation of vascular permeability, and regulation of bone formation through osteoblast stimulation and bone resorption via osteoclast stimulation and differentiation.[153-155] The in vivo importance of COX-2 has been demonstrated in both the collagen-induced and anti-collagen antibody transfer mouse models of inflammatory arthritis, in which COX-2 deficiency confers resistance to arthritis.[156]

Angiogenesis

FLS can participate in angiogenesis via elaboration of angiogenic factors, such as vascular endothelial growth factor (VEGF), Ang-1, Ang-2, IL-8, PDGF, EGF and basic fibroplast growth factor (bFGF).[135,157-159] Indeed, VEGF production by FLS can be induced by IL-1, a cytokine present in the inflamed synovium.[159] The relative contribution of FLS production of angiogenic factors in vivo has not been determined; however, elaboration of these angiogenic factors by FLS provides a means for establishing a vascular supply to the hyperplastic synovium and correlates with the highly vascular nature of the inflamed synovium.

FIBROBLAST-LIKE SYNOVIOCYTES AS DESTRUCTIVE CELLS IN SYNOVITIS

Pannus Formation

In rheumatoid synovitis a distinct mesenchymal reaction yields the formation of a condensed mass of cells that encroaches on and invades the cartilage from the periphery of the joint. This aggressive tissue resembles a cloth spreading out over the cartilage and has therefore been referred to as *pannus* (Latin for shroud or cloth). The predominant cell type found in pannus exhibits fibroblast-like features and is presumably derived from synovial FLS. Similarly to activated FLS, these pannus cells exhibit rhomboid morphology, express high levels of VCAM-1, produce type-1 collagen, and contain intracellular vimentin. Most direct evidence that FLS contribute to pannus formation comes from in vivo studies. Coimplantation of cultured human rheumatoid FLS and cartilage under the renal capsule of severe combined immunodeficiency (SCID) mice leads to spontaneous pannus formation with FLS invasion and destruction of the adjacent cartilage, even in the absence of an inflammatory infiltrate.[160]

Despite the link to FLS, there remains debate about the origin and complexity of cells within the pannus. Distinct cells in the pannus are morphologically rhomboid and can retain this phenotype for extended periods of time in in vitro culture.[161] Immunohistochemical and cytochemical studies have demonstrated that these distinct pannus cells express high levels of VCAM-1, as well as type I collagen. However, they also share markers associated with chondrocytes, such as inducible lymphocyte antigen (ILA).[161] Of note, these rhomboid-shaped cells in the pannus are prominent, particularly at the eroding interface with cartilage. They have been variably labeled in the medical literature as "pannocytes" or "Type C cells." Whether these terms identify the same population remains a matter of dispute, as does their origin. Perhaps it is surprising that the precise identity of this and other populations of cells in the pannus are still under some speculation.

The pannus is often vascularized and contains laminated fibrous matrix. Unlike other portions of the hyperplastic synovium, no lining cell layer can be distinguished in the pannus. Instead, it is a continuous mass of cells that is attached to and extends onto the articular cartilage. The recent identification of cadherin-11 expression in FLS may provide insight into molecular mechanisms involved in cell adhesion and the formation of pannus tissue. Cadherins comprise a family of calcium-dependent cell-cell adhesion proteins that typically mediate homophilic cellular adhesion through binding the same cadherin species on a cell of the same type. They are responsible for cell sorting during development and for tissue shape and integrity in adults.[21] Cadherins have been implicated in tissue morphogenesis during development, as well as in determining the architecture of tissue projections by directing cells to crawl over one another and thereby altering a tissue to become locally invasive.[46,162] This process may be critical not only during limb development, when N-cadherin mediates the condensation of mesenchymal cells during initial stages of chondrogenesis,[162] but also for pathologic processes evident in pannus formation.

Cartilage Invasion and Destruction

The FLS population in rheumatoid pannus is metabolically active and serves as the major source of MMPs, serine proteases, and cathepsins—factors that can mediate matrix and cartilage turnover, as well as their destruction. FLS also produce physiologic inhibitors of MMPs, TIMPs, suggesting that in vivo, the extent of matrix degradation is determined by the ratio of active proteases to their inhibitors.

Historically, MMPs were thought to predominantly degrade matrix components, thereby facilitating cell invasion. However, recent studies indicate additional and more complex roles for MMPs in modulating cell functions. Cleavage of matrix components can result in the generation of bioactive fragments or in the release of growth factors from extracellular complexes. MMPs exert their effects not only by cleaving matrix components directly but also by the conversion of other substrates that alter their bioactivity, including growth factor receptors, adhesion molecules, growth factor precursors, and other proteinases.[163] For instance, MMP-9 is highly expressed in FLS derived from rheumatoid synovium and has been implicated in the release and activation of TGF-β.[164,165] Notably, proteolytically active MMP-9 was shown to associate with the hyaluronan receptor CD44, and the localization of MMP-9 to the cell surface was required for its ability to promote cell invasion.[165] Consistent with the notion that regulated cell surface localization of soluble proteases is functional in the synovium, FLS express a variety of candidate docking receptors for proteases, such as CD44, urinary-type plasminogen activator receptor (uPAR),[166] and integrin αvβ3.[167] The coordinated function of transmembrane surface proteins, MMPs, and MMP substrates may provide a molecular mechanism for influencing the behavior of the pannus tissue that attaches to and erodes into cartilage and bone.

The cells making up the pannus not only produce matrix-degrading proteases but are manufacturing plants for matrix components such as collagens and fibronectin. Fibronectin synthesis is of particular interest because recent evidence indicates that this matrix glycoprotein can regulate the invasive capacity of FLS. In tumor cells, fibronectin expression is associated with increased malignancy and metastasis.[168] Fibronectin exerts its cellular effects via integrins, the cell surface adhesion receptors that bind it. Formation of adhesive contacts by the engagement of fibronectin-binding integrins (α4β1, α5β1, αvβ3) expressed on the cell surface of FLS initiates the assembly of protein complexes composed of nonreceptor tyrosine kinases, adaptor proteins, and actin-binding proteins at the cytoplasmic face of the adhesion receptors.[169] These multiprotein complexes not only link the adhesive integrins to the cytoskeleton but also transduce signals to the cell that regulate cell functions including cell migration.[169] In the context of destructive synovitis, fibronectin may operate as a haptotactic motility factor, guiding FLS to invade deeper into the cartilage. The formation of cell-matrix adhesive contacts and cell migration are highly regulated processes. Determinants include level of integrin expression, integrin avidity, and ligand-receptor binding affinity (inside out signaling).[170] Additionally, fibronectin-induced upregulation of MMPs may further enhance the invasive capacity of FLS.[171]

Bone Erosions

Although osteoclasts have been primarily implicated in the process of bone erosion in inflammatory arthritis,[172-174] FLS are also found at the sites of bone erosion. FLS produce degradative enzymes, namely the MMPs, which are capable of degrading the organic components of bone.[54] FLS have also been shown to produce M-CSF and RANKL, both of which are potent inducers of osteoclast differentiation and function.[65,149,175,176] It is thought that FLS elaboration of these osteoclastogenic factors[177] is a primary means by which FLS orchestrate bone erosions in inflammatory arthritis. Although FLS have not been shown to possess mechanisms to solubilize the inorganic hydroxyapatite matrix present in bone, recent reports have demonstrated the ability of cultured RA FLS to erode into bone slices in the absence of osteoclasts, suggesting that FLS may contain the ability to degrade bone directly in vivo.[178] Thus, FLS participate in bone destruction via elaboration of proteolytic enzymes and via secretion of stimulators of osteoclast function.

TRANSFORMED-LIKE STATE OF FIBROBLAST-LIKE SYNOVIOCYTES IN SYNOVITIS

Like fibroblasts from other anatomic sites, FLS are easily cultured for many passages in vitro. After several passages, leukocyte populations are lost, yet FLS continue to produce substantial levels of cytokines. However, because senescence is observed after extended culture, FLS are not transformed tumor cells. Rather, they display selected features that occur in transformed cells. In vivo, when implanted near cartilage in SCID mice (which lack lymphocytes), RA FLS proliferate and invade cartilage despite the lack of donor human or murine macrophages or other inflammatory cell populations.[160] Furthermore, in mice bearing a TNF-α transgene, significant FLS hyperplasia and cartilage destruction are seen despite lack of prominent synovial inflammatory infiltrates.[179] Taken together, these findings suggest that FLS exposed to inflammatory and other mitogenic signals may develop a chronic activated phenotype that can perpetuate the inflammatory response after the inciting stimulus is resolved.

The abnormal behavior of FLS in inflammatory arthritis might be the result of spontaneous mutations leading to disregulation of FLS function,[180] or the result of FLS undergoing long-term changes ("imprinting") in the context of stimulation in inflammatory synovitis,[141] or both. As noted previously, somatic mutations of tumor-suppressor genes such as p53 occur in FLS, and experimental interruption of p53 function increases aggressiveness of invading FLS in the SCID mouse model.[123] In addition, there is evidence that FLS from RA patients arise from oligoclonal progenitors, implying somatic mutations within a small number of FLS progenitors, which subsequently populate the synovium.[121,181] However, there is also evidence that FLS are not a homogenous population, but exist as intermingled nonclonal subsets of cells, much like those found

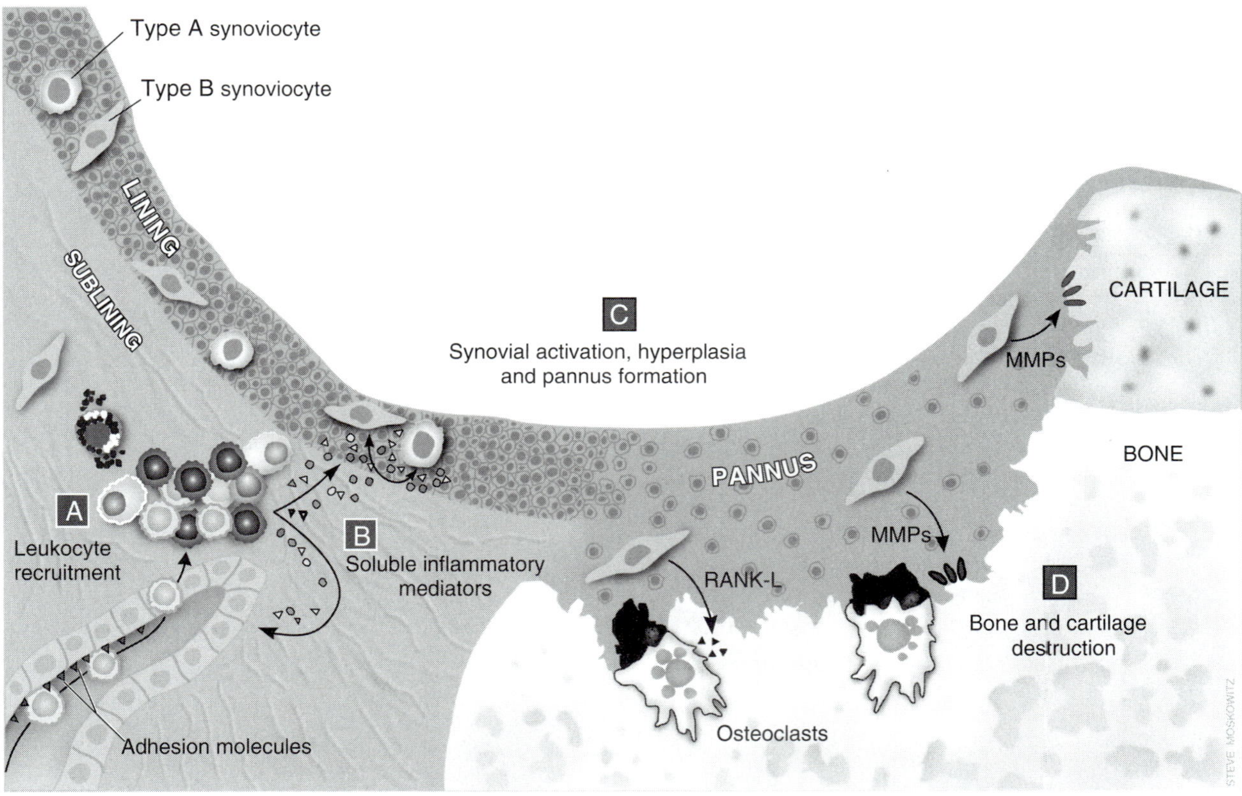

FIGURE 11–3 · Synoviocytes in the Context of Inflammatory Arthritis. The elements of arthritis can be grouped into four broad categories: (1) recruitment and accumulation of leukocytes; (2) soluble mediator production (cytokines, chemokines, angiogenic signals, and other soluble inflammatory molecules); (3) fibroblast-like synoviocyte (FLS) activation, hyperplasia, and pannus formation; and (4) bone and cartilage destruction (digestion, invasion, and erosion). *A*, Initiating signals incite the infiltration of inflammatory leukocytes into the synovial sublining via chemokine-mediated recruitment and coordinate upregulation of adhesion molecules on vascular endothelium. *B*, These infiltrating leukocytes contribute to inflammatory synovitis by generating cytokines and other soluble inflammatory molecules. *C*, A prominent FLS response in inflammatory arthritis includes extensive hyperplasia within the synovial lining and the formation of synovial pannus. *D*, In the hyperplastic synovial lining and pannus, FLS produce tissue-degrading enzymes, inflammatory cytokines, and prostaglandins. This process results in cartilage and bone erosion mediated both by activated FLS and by bone-resorbing osteoclasts responding to RANKL, macrophage colony-stimulating factor (M-CSF), and other stimuli to pathologically destroy bone. (Advanced Medical Graphics.)

among tissue macrophage, mast cell, lymphocyte, and dendritic cell populations.[141] Furthermore, fibroblasts isolated from other anatomic sites of inflammation display stable, discrete phenotypic alterations over long periods of in vitro culture.[140,141,182-184] Thus, the driving force for FLS and pannus behavior in chronic inflammatory arthritis may result from this stimulation by inflammatory mediators, or by their autonomously activated and partially transformed nature.

Summary

Synoviocytes in the normal state enable function of the diarthrodial joint. They maintain a deformable, resilient joint lining composed of a cellular basement membrane capable of withstanding joint motion and synovial fluid hydraulic forces. They synthesize and regulate the highly specialized lubricating synovial fluid and provide phagocytic function for clearance of joint debris. They also allow the transudation of nutritional support for cells in the avascular cartilage.

The major pathologic tissue in inflammatory arthritis is the synovium. Infiltrating leukoctyes including lymphocytes (T and B cells), macrophages, neutrophils, and mast cells, largely in the synovial sublining, are abundant and produce inflammatory mediators that contribute to arthritis. Prominent among these are inflammatory cytokines (e.g., TNF-α, IL-1, and IL-6) and chemokines. However, synovitis is much more than inflammation of the synovium. It is the response of the synovial tissues, including the FLS and the pannus that mediate much of the pathogenesis of tissue damage in inflammatory synovitis. The parallels between the synovial FLS reaction in synovitis and tumor growth are striking; common mechanisms regulating angiogenesis, cellular proliferation, cellular migration, tissue condensation, ECM remodeling, and invasion have been demonstrated. FLS may respond to continuous mitogenic input from hematopoietic lineage cells or undergo fundamental physiologic or genetic change after inflammatory stimulation, allowing autonomous participation in synovial changes. Figure 11–3 summarizes the mechanisms of participation of FLS in inflammatory arthritis.

REFERENCES

1. Key JA: The synovial membrane of joints and bursae. *In* Cowdry, EV (ed): Special Cytology II. New York, Paul B. Hoeber, 1932, p 1055.
2. Castor CW: The microscopic structure of normal human synovial tissue. Arthritis Rheum 3:140, 1960.
3. Henderson B, Edwards JCW: The Synovial Lining in Health and Disease. London, Chapman and Hall, 1987.
4. Allard SA, Bayliss MT, Maini RN: The synovium-cartilage junction of the normal human knee. Implications for joint destruction and repair. Arthritis Rheum 33:1170, 1990.
5. Barland P, Novikoff AB, Hamerman D: Electron microscopy of the human synovial membrane. J Cell Biol 14:207, 1962.
6. Lever JD, Ford HER: Histological, histochemical and electron microscopic observations on synovial membrane. Anat Rec 132:525, 1958.
7. Athanasou NA, Quinn J: Immunocytochemical analysis of human synovial lining cells: phenotypic relation to other marrow derived cells. Ann Rheum Dis 50:311, 1991.
8. Edwards JC, Willoughby DA: Demonstration of bone marrow derived cells in synovial lining by means of giant intracellular granules as genetic markers. Ann Rheum Dis 41:177, 1982.
9. Athanasou NA: Synovial macrophages. Ann Rheum Dis 54:392, 1995.
10. Koch AE, Burrows JC, Skoutelis A, et al: Monoclonal antibodies detect monocyte/macrophage activation and differentiation antigens and identify functionally distinct subpopulations of human rheumatoid synovial tissue macrophages. Am J Pathol 138:165, 1991.
11. Wilkinson LS, Pitsillides AA, Worrall JG, Edwards JC: Light microscopic characterization of the fibroblast-like synovial intimal cell (synoviocyte). Arthritis Rheum 35:1179, 1992.
12. Wilkinson LS, Moore AR, Pitsillides AA, et al: Comparison of surface fibroblastic cells in subcutaneous air pouch and synovial lining: Differences in uridine diphosphoglucose dehydrogenase activity. Int J Exp Pathol 74:113, 1993.
13. Morales-Ducret J, Wayner E, Elices MJ, et al: Alpha 4/beta 1 integrin (VLA-4) ligands in arthritis. Vascular cell adhesion molecule-1 expression in synovium and on fibroblast-like synoviocytes. J Immunol 149:1424, 1992.
14. Stevens CR, Mapp PI, Revell PA: A monoclonal antibody (Mab 67) marks type B synoviocytes. Rheumatol Int 10:103, 1990.
15. Edwards JC, Wilkinson LS: Distribution in human tissues of the synovial lining-associated epitope recognised by monoclonal antibody 67. J Anat 188:119, 1996.
16. Fairburn K, Kunaver M, Wilkinson LS, et al: Intercellular adhesion molecules in normal synovium. Br J Rheumatol 32:302, 1993.
17. Demaziere A, Athanasou NA: Adhesion receptors of intimal and subintimal cells of the normal synovial membrane. J Pathol 168:209, 1992.
18. Mohr W, Beneke G, Mohing W: Proliferation of synovial lining cells and fibroblasts. Ann Rheum Dis 34:219, 1975.
19. Nykanen P, Helve T, Kankaanpaa U, Larsen A: Characterization of the DNA-synthesizing cells in rheumatoid synovial tissue. Scand J Rheumatol 7:118, 1978.
20. Marinova-Mutafchieva L, Taylor P, Funa K, et al: Mesenchymal cells expressing bone morphogenetic protein receptors are present in the rheumatoid arthritis joint. Arthritis Rheum 43:2046, 2000.
21. Gumbiner BM: Cell adhesion: The molecular basis of tissue architecture and morphogenesis. Cell 84:345, 1996.
22. Hermiston ML, Gordon JI: Inflammatory bowel disease and adenomas in mice expressing a dominant negative N-cadherin. Science 270:1203, 1995.
23. Hamann J, Wishaupt JO, van Lier RA, et al: Expression of the activation antigen CD97 and its ligand CD55 in rheumatoid synovial tissue. Arthritis Rheum 42:650, 1999.
24. Valencia X, Higgins JMG, Gravallese EM, et al: Cadherin-11 mediates homophilic adhesion of type-B synoviocytes in rheumatoid arthritis. Arthritis Rheum 42:S111, 1999.
25. Levick JR: Microvascular architecture and exchange in synovial joints. Microcirculation 2:217, 1995.
26. Levick JR, McDonald JN: Fluid movement across synovium in healthy joints: Role of synovial fluid macromolecules. Ann Rheum Dis 54:417, 1995.
27. Adams WS: Fine structure of the synovial membrane: Phagocytosis of colloidal carbon from the joint cavity. Laboratory Investigator 15:680, 1966.
28. Yielding KL, Tomkins GM, Bunim JJ: Synthesis of hyaluronic acid by human synovial tissue slices. Science 125:1300, 1957.
29. Pitsillides AA, Blake SM: Uridine diphosphoglucose dehydrogenase activity in synovial lining cells in the experimental antigen induced model of rheumatoid arthritis: an indication of synovial lining cell function. Ann Rheum Dis 51:992, 1992.
30. Pitsillides AA, Wilkinson LS, Mehdizadeh S, et al: Uridine diphosphoglucose dehydrogenase activity in normal and rheumatoid synovium: The description of a specialized synovial lining cell. Int J Exp Pathol 74:27, 1993.
31. Henderson B, Pettipher ER: The synovial lining cell: Biology and pathobiology. Semin Arthritis Rheum 15:1, 1985.

32. Jay GD, Britt DE, Cha CJ: Lubricin is a product of megakaryocyte stimulating factor gene expression by human synovial fibroblasts. J Rheumatol 27:594, 2000.
33. Swann DA, Silver FH, Slayter HS, et al: The molecular structure and lubricating activity of lubricin isolated from bovine and human synovial fluids. Biochem J 225:195, 1985.
34. Myers DB, Highton TC, Rayns DG: Acid mucopolysaccharides closely associated with collagen fibrils in normal human synovium. J Ultrastruct Res 28:203, 1969.
35. Eyre DR, Muir H: Type III collagen: A major constituent of rheumatoid and normal human synovial membrane. Connect Tissue Res 4:11, 1976.
36. Scott DL, Salmon M, Morris CJ, et al: Laminin and vascular proliferation in rheumatoid arthritis. Ann Rheum Dis 43:551, 1984.
37. Clemmensen I, Holund B, Andersen RB: Fibrin and fibronectin in rheumatoid synovial membrane and rheumatoid synovial fluid. Arthritis Rheum 26:479, 1983.
38. Iwai-Liao Y, Ogita Y, Tsubai T, Higashi Y: Scanning electron microscopy of elastic system fibers in the articular disc of the rat mandibular joint. Okajimas Folia Anat Jpn 71:211, 1994.
39. Konttinen YT, Li TF, Xu JW, et al: Expression of laminins and their integrin receptors in different conditions of synovial membrane and synovial membrane-like interface tissue. Ann Rheum Dis 58:683, 1999.
40. Revell PA, al-Saffar N, Fish S, Osei D: Extracellular matrix of the synovial intimal cell layer. Ann Rheum Dis 54:404, 1995.
41. Waggett AD, Kielty CM, Shuttleworth CA: Microfibrillar elements in the synovial joint: presence of type VI collagen and fibrillin-containing microfibrils. Ann Rheum Dis 52:449, 1993.
42. Worrall JG, Wilkinson LS, Bayliss MT, Edwards JC: Zonal distribution of chondroitin-4-sulphate/dermatan sulphate and chondroitin-6-sulphate in normal and diseased human synovium. Ann Rheum Dis 53:35, 1994.
43. Smith SC, Folefac VA, Osei DK, Revell PA: An immunocytochemical study of the distribution of proline-4-hydroxylase in normal, osteoarthritic and rheumatoid arthritic synovium at both the light and electron microscopic level. Br J Rheumatol 37:287, 1998.
44. Schneider M, Voss B, Rauterberg J, et al: Basement membrane proteins in synovial membrane: distribution in rheumatoid arthritis and synthesis by fibroblast-like cells. Clin Rheumatol 13:90, 1994.
45. Linck G, Stocker S, Grimaud JA, Porte A: Distribution of immunoreactive fibronectin and collagen (type I, III, IV) in mouse joints. Fibronectin, an essential component of the synovial cavity border. Histochemistry 77:323, 1983.
46. Ashhurst DE, Bland YS, Levick JR: An immunohistochemical study of the collagens of rabbit synovial interstitium. J Rheumatol 18:1669, 1991.
47. Marsh JM, Wiebkin OW, Gale S, et al: Synthesis of sulphated proteoglycans by rheumatoid and normal synovial tissue in culture. Ann Rheum Dis 38:166, 1979.
48. Okada Y, Naka K, Minamoto T, et al: Localization of type VI collagen in the lining cell layer of normal and rheumatoid synovium. Lab Invest 63:647, 1990.
49. Pollock LE, Lalor P, Revell PA: Type IV collagen and laminin in the synovial intimal layer: an immunohistochemical study. Rheumatol Int 9:277, 1990.
50. Mapp PI, Revell PA: Fibronectin production by synovial intimal cells. Rheumatol Int 5:229, 1985.
51. Wolf J, Carsons SE: Distribution of type VI collagen expression in synovial tissue and cultured synoviocytes: relation to fibronectin expression. Ann Rheum Dis 50:493, 1991.
52. McCachren SS, Lightner VA: Expression of human tenascin in synovitis and its regulation by interleukin-1. Arthritis Rheum 35:1185, 1992.
53. Danen EH, Sonneveld P, Brakebusch C, et al: The fibronectin-binding integrins alpha5beta1 and alphavbeta3 differentially modulate RhoA-GTP loading, organization of cell matrix adhesions, and fibronectin fibrillogenesis. J Cell Biol 159:1071, 2002.
54. Okada Y, Nagase H, Harris ED Jr: Matrix metalloproteinases 1, 2, and 3 from rheumatoid synovial cells are sufficient to destroy joints. J Rheumatol 14 Spec No:41, 1987.
55. Woessner JF Jr: Matrix metalloproteinases and their inhibitors in connective tissue remodeling. FASEB J 5:2145, 1991.
56. Konttinen YT, Ainola M, Valleala H, et al: Analysis of 16 different matrix metalloproteinases (MMP-1 to MMP-20) in the synovial membrane: different profiles in trauma and rheumatoid arthritis. Ann Rheum Dis 58:691, 1999.
57. Close DR: Matrix metalloproteinase inhibitors in rheumatic diseases. Ann Rheum Dis 60 (Suppl 3):iii62, 2001.
58. Egeblad M, Werb Z: New functions for the matrix metalloproteinases in cancer progression. Nat Rev Cancer 2:161, 2002.
59. Fassina G, Ferrari N, Brigati C, et al: Tissue inhibitors of metalloproteases: Regulation and biological activities. Clin Exp Metastasis 18:111, 2000.
60. Wojtowicz-Praga S, Torri J, Johnson M, et al: Phase I trial of marimastat, a novel matrix metalloproteinase inhibitor, administered orally to patients with advanced lung cancer. J Clin Oncol 16:2150, 1998.
61. Rasmussen HS, McCann PP: Matrix metalloproteinase inhibition as a novel anticancer strategy: A review with special focus on batimastat and marimastat. Pharmacol Ther 75:69, 1997.
62. Nemunaitis J, Poole C, Primrose J, et al: Combined analysis of studies of the effects of the matrix metalloproteinase inhibitor marimastat on serum tumor markers in advanced cancer: Selection of a biologically active and tolerable dose for longer-term studies. Clin Cancer Res 4:1101, 1998.
63. Salmon JA, Higgs GA, Vane JR, et al: Synthesis of arachidonate cyclo-oxygenase products by rheumatoid and nonrheumatoid synovial lining in nonproliferative organ culture. Ann Rheum Dis 42:36, 1983.
64. Crofford LJ: COX-1 and COX-2 tissue expression: Implications and predictions. J Rheumatol 24(Suppl 49):15, 1997.
65. Gravallese EM, Manning C, Tsay A, et al: Synovial tissue in rheumatoid arthritis is a source of osteoclast differentiation factor. Arthritis Rheum 43:250, 2000.
66. Schumacher HR, Kitridou RC: Synovitis of recent onset. A clinicopathologic study during the first month of disease. Arthritis Rheum 15:465, 1972.
67. Kulka JP, Bocking D, Ropes MW, Bauer W: Early joint lesions of rheumatoid arthritis. Arch Pathol 59:129, 1955.
68. Barland P, Novikoff AB, Hamerman D: Lysosomes in the synovial membrane in rheumatoid arthritis: A mechanism for cartilage erosion. Trans Assoc Am Physicians 77:239, 1964.
69. Hollywell C, Morris CJ, Farr M, Walton KW: Ultrastructure of synovial changes in rheumatoid disease and in seronegative inflammatory arthropathies. Virchows Arch A Pathol Anat Histopathol 400:345, 1983.
70. Van Boxel JA, Paget SA: Predominantly T-cell infiltrate in rheumatoid synovial membranes. N Engl J Med 293:517, 1975.
71. Koch AE: Review: Angiogenesis: implications for rheumatoid arthritis. Arthritis Rheum 41:951, 1998.
72. FitzGerald O, Soden M, Yanni G, et al: Morphometric analysis of blood vessels in synovial membranes obtained from clinically affected and unaffected knee joints of patients with rheumatoid arthritis. Ann Rheum Dis 50:792, 1991.
73. Sebbag M, Parry SL, Brennan FM, Feldmann M: Cytokine stimulation of T lymphocytes regulates their capacity to induce monocyte production of tumor necrosis factor-alpha, but not interleukin-10: possible relevance to pathophysiology of rheumatoid arthritis. Eur J Immunol 27:624, 1997.
74. Vey E, Zhang JH, Dayer JM: IFN-gamma and 1,25(OH)2D3 induce on THP-1 cells distinct patterns of cell surface antigen expression, cytokine production, and responsiveness to contact with activated T cells. J Immunol 149:2040, 1992.
75. Malik N, Greenfield BW, Wahl AF, Kiener PA: Activation of human monocytes through CD40 induces matrix metalloproteinases. J Immunol 156:3952, 1996.
76. Wagner DH Jr, Stout RD, Suttles J: Role of the CD40-CD40 ligand interaction in CD4+ T cell contact-dependent activation of monocyte interleukin-1 synthesis. Eur J Immunol 24:3148, 1994.
77. MacDonald KP, Nishioka Y, Lipsky PE, Thomas R: Functional CD40 ligand is expressed by T cells in rheumatoid arthritis. J Clin Invest 100:2404, 1997.
78. McInnes IB, Leung BP, Sturrock RD, et al: Interleukin-15 mediates T cell-dependent regulation of tumor necrosis factor-alpha production in rheumatoid arthritis. [comment]. Nature Medicine. 3:189, 1997.

79. Kinne RW, Brauer R, Stuhlmuller B, et al: Macrophages in rheumatoid arthritis. Arthritis Res 2:189, 2000.
80. Wood NC, Dickens E, Symons JA, Duff GW: In situ hybridization of interleukin-1 in CD14-positive cells in rheumatoid arthritis. Clin Immunol Immunopathol 62:295, 1992.
81. Chu CQ, Field M, Feldmann M, Maini RN: Localization of tumor necrosis factor alpha in synovial tissues and at the cartilage-pannus junction in patients with rheumatoid arthritis. Arthritis Rheum 34:1125, 1991.
82. Arend WP: Physiology of cytokine pathways in rheumatoid arthritis. Arthritis Rheum 45:101, 2001.
83. Feldmann M, Brennan FM, Maini RN: Role of cytokines in rheumatoid arthritis. Ann Rev Immunol 14:397, 1996.
84. Dayer JM, de Rochemonteix B, Burrus B, et al: Human recombinant interleukin 1 stimulates collagenase and prostaglandin E2 production by human synovial cells. J Clin Invest 77:645, 1986.
85. Alvaro-Gracia JM, Zvaifler NJ, Firestein GS: Cytokines in chronic inflammatory arthritis. V. Mutual antagonism between interferon-gamma and tumor necrosis factor-alpha on HLA-DR expression, proliferation, collagenase production, and granulocyte macrophage colony-stimulating factor production by rheumatoid arthritis synoviocytes. J Clin Invest 86:1790, 1990.
86. Ito A, Itoh Y, Sasaguri Y, et al: Effects of interleukin-6 on the metabolism of connective tissue components in rheumatoid synovial fibroblasts. Arthritis Rheum 35:1197, 1992.
87. MacNaul KL, Chartrain N, Lark M, et al: Discoordinate expression of stromelysin, collagenase, and tissue inhibitor of metalloproteinases-1 in rheumatoid human synovial fibroblasts. Synergistic effects of interleukin-1 and tumor necrosis factor-alpha on stromelysin expression. J Biol Chem 265:17238, 1990.
88. Dayer JM, Beutler B, Cerami A: Cachectin/tumor necrosis factor stimulates collagenase and prostaglandin E2 production by human synovial cells and dermal fibroblasts. J Exp Med 162:2163, 1985.
89. Kumkumian GK, Lafyatis R, Remmers EF, et al: Platelet-derived growth factor and IL-1 interactions in rheumatoid arthritis. Regulation of synoviocyte proliferation, prostaglandin production, and collagenase transcription. J Immunol 143:833, 1989.
90. Dinarello CA, Cannon JG, Wolff SM, et al: Tumor necrosis factor (cachectin) is an endogenous pyrogen and induces production of interleukin 1. J Exp Med 163:1433, 1986.
91. Mino T, Sugiyama E, Taki H, et al: Interleukin-1alpha and tumor necrosis factor alpha synergistically stimulate prostaglandin E2-dependent production of interleukin-11 in rheumatoid synovial fibroblasts. Arthritis Rheum 41:2004, 1998.
92. Schlaak JF, Pfers I, Meyer KH, et al: Different cytokine profiles in the synovial fluid of patients with osteoarthritis, rheumatoid arthritis and seronegative spondylarthropathies. Clin Exp Rheumatol 14:155, 1996.
93. Szekanecz Z, Haines GK, Harlow LA, et al: Increased synovial expression of transforming growth factor (TGF)-beta receptor endoglin and TGF-beta 1 in rheumatoid arthritis: possible interactions in the pathogenesis of the disease. Clin Immunol Immunopathol 76:187, 1995.
94. Sarkissian M, Lafyatis R: Transforming growth factor-beta and platelet derived growth factor regulation of fibrillar fibronectin matrix formation by synovial fibroblasts. J Rheumatol 25:613, 1998.
95. Allen JB, Manthey CL, Hand AR, et al: Rapid onset synovial inflammation and hyperplasia induced by transforming growth factor beta. J Exp Med 171:231, 1990.
96. Thornton SC, Por SB, Penny R, et al: Identification of the major fibroblast growth factors released spontaneously in inflammatory arthritis as platelet derived growth factor and tumour necrosis factor-alpha. Clin Exp Immunol 86:79, 1991.
97. Remmers EF, Sano H, Lafyatis R, et al: Production of platelet derived growth factor B chain (PDGF-B/c-sis) mRNA and immunoreactive PDGF B-like polypeptide by rheumatoid synovium: coexpression with heparin binding acidic fibroblast growth factor-1. J Rheumatol 18:7, 1991.
98. Reuterdahl C, Tingstrom A, Terracio L, et al: Characterization of platelet-derived growth factor beta-receptor expressing cells in the vasculature of human rheumatoid synovium. Lab Invest 64:321, 1991.
99. Abe M, Kurosawa M, Ishikawa O, Miyachi Y: Effect of mast cell-derived mediators and mast cell-related neutral proteases on human dermal fibroblast proliferation and type I collagen production. J Allergy Clin Immunol 106:S78, 2000.
100. Gruber BL, Kew RR, Jelaska A, et al: Human mast cells activate fibroblasts: Tryptase is a fibrogenic factor stimulating collagen messenger ribonucleic acid synthesis and fibroblast chemotaxis. J Immunol 158:2310, 1997.
101. Inoue H, Shimoyama Y, Hirabayashi K, et al: Production of neuropeptide substance P by synovial fibroblasts from patients with rheumatoid arthritis and osteoarthritis. Neurosci Lett 303:149, 2001.
102. Delgado M, Abad C, Martinez C, et al: Vasoactive intestinal peptide prevents experimental arthritis by downregulating both autoimmune and inflammatory components of the disease. Nat Med 7:563, 2001.
103. Dreher R: Origin of synovial type A cells during inflammation. An experimental approach. Immunobiology 161:232, 1982.
104. Katschke KJ Jr, Rottman JB, Ruth JH, et al: Differential expression of chemokine receptors on peripheral blood, synovial fluid, and synovial tissue monocytes/macrophages in rheumatoid arthritis. Arthritis Rheum 44:1022, 2001.
105. Ruth JH, Volin MV, Haines GK III, et al: Fractalkine, a novel chemokine in rheumatoid arthritis and in rat adjuvant-induced arthritis. Arthritis Rheum 44:1568, 2001.
106. Patterson AM, Schmutz C, Davis S, et al: Differential binding of chemokines to macrophages and neutrophils in the human inflamed synovium. Arthritis Res 4:209, 2002.
107. Liote F, Boval-Boizard B, Weill D, et al: Blood monocyte activation in rheumatoid arthritis: increased monocyte adhesiveness, integrin expression, and cytokine release. Clin Exper Immunol 106:13, 1996.
108. Grober JS, Bowen BL, Ebling H, et al: Monocyte-endothelial adhesion in chronic rheumatoid arthritis. In situ detection of selectin and integrin-dependent interactions. [comment]. J Clin Invest 91:2609, 1993.
109. Goddard DH, Grossman SL, Williams WV, et al: Regulation of synovial cell growth. Coexpression of transforming growth factor beta and basic fibroblast growth factor by cultured synovial cells. Arthritis Rheum 35:1296, 1992.
110. Hamilton JA, Butler DM, Stanton H: Cytokine interactions promoting DNA synthesis in human synovial fibroblasts. J Rheumatol 21:797, 1994.
111. Gitter BD, Koehneke EM: Retinoic acid potentiates interleukin-1– and fibroblast growth factor–induced human synovial fibroblast proliferation. Clin Immunol Immunopathol 61:191, 1991.
112. Brennan FM, Chantry D, Jackson AM, et al: Cytokine production in culture by cells isolated from the synovial membrane. J Autoimmun 2(Suppl):177, 1989.
113. Nanki T, Nagasaka K, Hayashida K, et al: Chemokines regulate IL-6 and IL-8 production by fibroblast-like synoviocytes from patients with rheumatoid arthritis. J Immunol 167:5381, 2001.
114. Nykanen P, Bergroth V, Raunio P, et al: Phenotypic characterization of 3H-thymidine incorporating cells in rheumatoid arthritis synovial membrane. Rheumatol Int 6:269, 1986.
115. Qu Z, Garcia CH, O'Rourke LM, et al: Local proliferation of fibroblast-like synoviocytes contributes to synovial hyperplasia. Results of proliferating cell nuclear antigen/cyclin, c-myc, and nucleolar organizer region staining. Arthritis Rheum 37:212, 1994.
116. Lalor PA, Mapp PI, Hall PA, Revell. PA: Proliferative activity of cells in the synovium as demonstrated by a monoclonal antibody, Ki67. Rheumatol Int 7:183, 1987.
117. Schedel J, Gay RE, Kuenzler P, et al: FLICE-inhibitory protein expression in synovial fibroblasts and at sites of cartilage and bone erosion in rheumatoid arthritis. Arthritis Rheum 46:1512, 2002.
118. Matsumoto S, Muller-Ladner U, Gay RE, et al: Ultrastructural demonstration of apoptosis, Fas and Bcl-2 expression of rheumatoid synovial fibroblasts. J Rheumatol 23:1345, 1996.
119. Franz JK, Pap T, Hummel KM, et al: Expression of sentrin, a novel antiapoptotic molecule, at sites of synovial invasion in rheumatoid arthritis. Arthritis Rheum 43:599, 2000.

120. Inazuka M, Tahira T, Horiuchi T, et al: Analysis of p53 tumour suppressor gene somatic mutations in rheumatoid arthritis synovium. Rheumatology (Oxford) 39:262, 2000.
121. Yamanishi Y, Boyle DL, Rosengren S, et al: Regional analysis of p53 mutations in rheumatoid arthritis synovium. Proc Natl Acad Sci U S A 99:10025, 2002.
122. Aupperle KR, Boyle DL, Hendrix M, et al: Regulation of synoviocyte proliferation, apoptosis, and invasion by the p53 tumor suppressor gene. Am J Pathol 152:1091, 1998.
123. Pap T, Aupperle KR, Gay S, et al: Invasiveness of synovial fibroblasts is regulated by p53 in the SCID mouse in vivo model of cartilage invasion. Arthritis Rheum 44:676, 2001.
124. Nakajima T, Aono H, Hasunuma T, et al: Apoptosis and functional Fas antigen in rheumatoid arthritis synoviocytes. Arthritis Rheum 38:485, 1995.
125. Firestein GS, Yeo M, Zvaifler NJ: Apoptosis in rheumatoid arthritis synovium. J Clin Invest 96:1631, 1995.
126. Nishioka K, Hasunuma T, Kato T, et al: Apoptosis in rheumatoid arthritis: a novel pathway in the regulation of synovial tissue. Arthritis Rheum 41:1, 1998.
127. Korganow AS, Ji H, Mangialaio S, et al: From systemic T cell self-reactivity to organ-specific autoimmune disease via immunoglobulins. Immunity 10:451, 1999.
128. Terato K, Hasty KA, Reife RA, et al: Induction of arthritis with monoclonal antibodies to collagen. J Immunol 148:2103, 1992.
129. Blau HM, Brazelton TR, Weimann JM: The evolving concept of a stem cell: Entity or function? Cell 105:829, 2001.
130. De Bari C, Dell'Accio F, Tylzanowski P, Luyten FP: Multipotent mesenchymal stem cells from adult human synovial membrane. Arthritis Rheum 44:1928, 2001.
131. Zvaifler NJ, Marinova-Mutafchieva L, Adams G, et al: Mesenchymal precursor cells in the blood of normal individuals. Arthritis Res 2:477, 2000.
132. Sen M, Lauterbach K, El-Gabalawy H, et al: Expression and function of wingless and frizzled homologs in rheumatoid arthritis. Proc Natl Acad Sci U S A 97:2791, 2000.
133. Sen M, Reifert J, Lauterbach K, et al: Regulation of fibronectin and metalloproteinase expression by Wnt signaling in rheumatoid arthritis synoviocytes. Arthritis Rheum 46:2867, 2002.
134. Miossec P, Naviliat M, Dupuy d'Angeac A, et al: Low levels of interleukin-4 and high levels of transforming growth factor beta in rheumatoid synovitis. Arthritis Rheum 33:1180, 1990.
135. Melnyk VO, Shipley GD, Sternfeld MD, et al: Synoviocytes synthesize, bind, and respond to basic fibroblast growth factor. Arthritis Rheum 33:493, 1990.
136. Sano H, Forough R, Maier JA, et al: Detection of high levels of heparin binding growth factor-1 (acidic fibroblast growth factor) in inflammatory arthritic joints. J Cell Biol 110:1417, 1990.
137. Fowler MJ Jr, Neff MS, Borghaei RC, et al: Induction of bone morphogenetic protein-2 by interleukin-1 in human fibroblasts. Biochem Biophys Res Commun 248:450, 1998.
138. Nguyen NC, Nakazawa M, Nakamura H, et al: Synovial fibroblasts with HoxD9 protein escape from apoptosis in vivo. Arthritis Rheum 43S:S161, 2000.
139. Jorgensen C, Noel D, Gross G: Could inflammatory arthritis be triggered by progenitor cells in the joints? Ann Rheum Dis 61:6, 2002.
140. Smith RS, Smith TJ, Blieden TM, Phipps RP: Fibroblasts as sentinel cells. Synthesis of chemokines and regulation of inflammation. Am J Pathol 151:317, 1997.
141. Buckley CD, Pilling D, Lord JM, et al: Fibroblasts regulate the switch from acute resolving to chronic persistent inflammation. Trends Immunol 22:199, 2001.
142. Bucala R, Ritchlin C, Winchester R, Cerami A: Constitutive production of inflammatory and mitogenic cytokines by rheumatoid synovial fibroblasts. J Exp Med 173:569, 1991.
143. Ritchlin C: Fibroblast biology. Effector signals released by the synovial fibroblast in arthritis. Arthritis Res 2:356, 2000.
144. Hayashida K, Nanki T, Girschick H, et al: Synovial stromal cells from rheumatoid arthritis patients attract monocytes by producing MCP-1 and IL-8. Arthritis Res 3:118, 2001.
145. Szekanecz Z, Strieter RM, Kunkel SL, Koch AE: Chemokines in rheumatoid arthritis. Springer Semin Immunopathol 20:115, 1998.
146. Konig A, Krenn V, Toksoy A, et al: Mig, GRO alpha and RANTES messenger RNA expression in lining layer, infiltrates and different leucocyte populations of synovial tissue from patients with rheumatoid arthritis, psoriatic arthritis and osteoarthritis. Virchows Arch 436:449, 2000.
147. Rathanaswami P, Hachicha M, Sadick M, et al: Expression of the cytokine RANTES in human rheumatoid synovial fibroblasts. Differential regulation of RANTES and interleukin-8 genes by inflammatory cytokines. J Biol Chem 268:5834, 1993.
148. Seitz M, Loetscher P, Fey MF, Tobler A: Constitutive mRNA and protein production of macrophage colony-stimulating factor but not of other cytokines by synovial fibroblasts from rheumatoid arthritis and osteoarthritis patients. Br J Rheumatol 33:613, 1994.
149. Hamilton JA, Filonzi EL, Ianches G: Regulation of macrophage colony-stimulating factor (M-CSF) production in cultured human synovial fibroblasts. Growth Factors 9:157, 1993.
150. Kiener HP, Hofbauer R, Tohidast-Akrad M, et al: Tumor necrosis factor alpha promotes the expression of stem cell factor in synovial fibroblasts and their capacity to induce mast cell chemotaxis. Arthritis Rheum 43:164, 2000.
151. Siegle I, Klein T, Backman JT, et al: Expression of cyclooxygenase 1 and cyclooxygenase 2 in human synovial tissue: differential elevation of cyclooxygenase 2 in inflammatory joint diseases. Arthritis Rheum 41:122, 1998.
152. Crofford LJ, Wilder RL, Ristimaki AP, et al: Cyclooxygenase-1 and -2 expression in rheumatoid synovial tissues. Effects of interleukin-1 beta, phorbol ester, and corticosteroids. J Clin Invest 93:1095, 1994.
153. Sato T, Morita I, Sakaguchi K, et al: Involvement of prostaglandin endoperoxide H synthase-2 in osteoclast-like cell formation induced by interleukin-1 beta. J Bone Miner Res 11:392, 1996.
154. Nefussi JR, Baron R: PGE2 stimulates both resorption and formation of bone in vitro: differential responses of the periosteum and the endosteum in fetal rat long bone cultures. Anat Rec 211:9, 1985.
155. Zhang X, Schwarz EM, Young DA, et al: Cyclooxygenase-2 regulates mesenchymal cell differentiation into the osteoblast lineage and is critically involved in bone repair. J Clin Invest 109:1405, 2002.
156. Myers LK, Kang AH, Postlethwaite AE, et al: The genetic ablation of cyclooxygenase 2 prevents the development of autoimmune arthritis. Arthritis Rheum 43:2687, 2000.
157. Scott BB, Zaratin PF, Colombo A, et al: Constitutive expression of angiopoietin-1 and -2 and modulation of their expression by inflammatory cytokines in rheumatoid arthritis synovial fibroblasts. J Rheumatol 29:230, 2002.
158. Fava RA, Olsen NJ, Spencer-Green G, et al: Vascular permeability factor/endothelial growth factor (VPF/VEGF): Accumulation and expression in human synovial fluids and rheumatoid synovial tissue. J Exp Med 180:341, 1994.
159. Jackson JR, Minton JA, Ho ML, et al: Expression of vascular endothelial growth factor in synovial fibroblasts is induced by hypoxia and interleukin 1beta. J Rheumatol 24:1253, 1997.
160. Muller-Ladner U, Kriegsmann J, Franklin BN, et al: Synovial fibroblasts of patients with rheumatoid arthritis attach to and invade normal human cartilage when engrafted into SCID mice. Am J Pathol 149:1607, 1996.
161. Zvaifler NJ, Tsai V, Alsalameh S,et al: Pannocytes: Distinctive cells found in rheumatoid arthritis articular cartilage erosions. Am J Pathol 150:1125, 1997.
162. Oberlender SA, Tuan RS: Expression and functional involvement of N-cadherin in embryonic limb chondrogenesis. Development 120:177, 1994.
163. McCawley LJ, Matrisian LM: Matrix metalloproteinases: They're not just for matrix anymore! Curr Opin Cell Biol 13:534, 2001.
164. Unemori EN, Hibbs MS, Amento EP Constitutive expression of a 92-kD gelatinase (type V collagenase) by rheumatoid synovial fibroblasts and its induction in normal human fibroblasts by inflammatory cytokines. J Clin Invest 88:1656, 1991.
165. Yu Q, Stamenkovic I: Cell surface-localized matrix metalloproteinase-9 proteolytically activates TGF-beta and promotes tumor invasion and angiogenesis. Genes Dev 14:163, 2000.
166. Gonzalez-Gronow M, Gawdi G, Pizzo SV: Characterization of the plasminogen receptors of normal and rheumatoid arthritis human synovial fibroblasts. J Biol Chem 269:4360, 1994.

167. Brooks PC, Stromblad S, Sanders LC, et al: Localization of matrix metalloproteinase MMP-2 to the surface of invasive cells by interaction with integrin alpha v beta 3. Cell 85:683, 1996.
168. Clark EA, Golub TR, Lander ES, Hynes RO: Genomic analysis of metastasis reveals an essential role for RhoC. Nature 406:532, 2000.
169. Hynes RO: Integrins: Bidirectional, allosteric signaling machines. Cell 110:673, 2002.
170. Liddington RC, Ginsberg MH: Integrin activation takes shape. J Cell Biol 158:833, 2002.
171. Tremble P, Damsky CH, Werb Z: Components of the nuclear signaling cascade that regulate collagenase gene expression in response to integrin-derived signals. J Cell Biol 129:1707, 1995.
172. Kong YY, Feige U, Sarosi I, et al: Activated T cells regulate bone loss and joint destruction in adjuvant arthritis through osteoprotegerin ligand. Nature 402:304, 1999.
173. Pettit AR, Ji H, von Stechow D, et al: TRANCE/RANKL knockout mice are protected from bone erosion in a serum transfer model of arthritis. Am J Pathol 159:1689, 2001.
174. Gravallese EM, Harada Y, Wang JT, et al: Identification of cell types responsible for bone resorption in rheumatoid arthritis and juvenile rheumatoid arthritis. Am J Pathol 152:943, 1998.
175. Takayanagi H, Iizuka H, Juji T, et al: Involvement of receptor activator of nuclear factor kappaB ligand/osteoclast differentiation factor in osteoclastogenesis from synoviocytes in rheumatoid arthritis. Arthritis Rheum 43:259, 2000.
176. Shigeyama Y, Pap T, Kunzler P, et al: Expression of osteoclast differentiation factor in rheumatoid arthritis. Arthritis Rheum 43:2523, 2000.
177. Takayanagi H, Oda H, Yamamoto S, et al: A new mechanism of bone destruction in rheumatoid arthritis: synovial fibroblasts induce osteoclastogenesis. Biochem Biophys Res Commun 240:279, 1997.
178. Hummel KM, Claus A, Blaschke S, et al: Osteoclast-independent bone resorption in synovial fibroblasts (RASF) from patients with RA. Arthritis Rheum 46:S569, 2002.
179. Keffer J, Probert L, Cazlaris H, et al: Transgenic mice expressing human tumour necrosis factor: a predictive genetic model of arthritis. EMBO J 10:4025, 1991.
180. Firestein GS: Invasive fibroblast-like synoviocytes in rheumatoid arthritis. Passive responders or transformed aggressors? Arthritis Rheum 39:1781, 1996.
181. Imamura F, Aono H, Hasunuma T, et al: Monoclonal expansion of synoviocytes in rheumatoid arthritis. Arthritis Rheum 41:1979, 1998.
182. Brouty-Boye D, Pottin-Clemenceau C, Doucet C, et al: Chemokines and CD40 expression in human fibroblasts. Eur J Immunol 30:914, 2000.
183. Hogaboam CM, Steinhauser ML, Chensue SW, Kunkel SL: Novel roles for chemokines and fibroblasts in interstitial fibrosis. Kidney Int 54:2152, 1998.
184. Ritchlin C, Dwyer E, Bucala R, Winchester R: Sustained and distinctive patterns of gene activation in synovial fibroblasts and whole synovial tissue obtained from inflammatory synovitis. Scand J Immunol 40:292, 1994.

12 Fibroblast Function and Fibrosis

JOSEPH H. KORN • ROBERT LAFYATIS

The fibroblast plays a critical role in tissue repair, that is, in laying down collagen and other matrix proteins in response to injury. This reparative function may be a response to physical injury—a surgical incision, for example—or to tissue destruction from other causes. In both instances, the fibroblast responds to sets of signals from its microenvironment (Fig. 12–1). These signals include mediators, cytokines, and growth factors released by immune and inflammatory cells, platelets, endothelial cells, and smooth muscle cells, as well as signals from the noncellular environment. The noncellular signals include plasma and serum factors, oxygen tension, pH, and matrix proteins.

Excessive stimulation of the fibroblast may lead to persistent activation, with resulting fibrosis.[1,2] This can result from increased matrix deposition, especially collagen, with or without an increase in fibroblast numbers. The process of repair also involves tissue remodeling, necessitating degradation of matrix proteins. Fibroblasts release a variety of enzymes that can degrade collagen proteoglycans and other matrix components. In some instances, such as in rheumatoid synovitis, net matrix destruction, rather than fibrosis, may result owing to activation of synovial fibroblasts with release of matrix-degrading enzymes (Fig. 12–2).

Several areas of fibroblast biology have received increasing attention in recent years and have significant bearing on the processes of inflammation and repair. A large repertoire of cytokines has been defined that influence fibroblast function.[3-5] The delineation of these and their mechanisms of action has shed considerable light on the fibrotic process. It has also become clear that the fibroblast is a cell involved in inflammation by actions other than synthesis and degradation of matrix. The original concept was that the fibroblast was only a responder to environmental signals that governed its level of metabolic activity. However, the fibroblast is capable of interacting with the immune system, with hematopoietic cell precursors, and with other cell types in more complex and interdependent ways (Fig. 12–3). This can occur through release from the fibroblast of soluble mediators, including cytokines thought originally to derive only from immune cells, or through direct cell–cell interactions mediated by adhesion ligands. These interactions can result in profound alterations of immune-cell localization and function, which in turn may alter fibroblast metabolism.

Another area in which the view of fibroblast biology has expanded is in the appreciation of differences among and within fibroblast populations. Fibroblasts are mesenchyme-derived cells that have a widespread tissue distribution. Fibroblasts from a variety of sites can be morphologically similar; indeed, fibroblasts have been "identified" by their spindle-shaped morphology in culture. It is clear, however, that there are differences among fibroblasts from skin, lung, synovium, periosteum, gingiva, cornea, bone marrow, and the interstitium of various organs. Furthermore, evidence has accumulated that even among fibroblasts derived from a single site, there are substantial differences in proliferation and in biosynthetic activity.[6] Characterization of fibroblast heterogeneity and specialized activities is incomplete but is discussed further later (see "Fibroblast Heterogeneity").

Normal Fibroblast Function

Fibroblasts are ubiquitous in the body and perform a variety of functions, many specialized to the resident tissue or organ. However, certain capabilities are common to all fibroblasts. These are consistent with their role as the primary resident cell type in connective tissues. Connective tissues provide structural support, form barriers to infections, anchor white blood cells during inflammation, and repair damaged tissue. Orchestrating these normal and physiologic functions requires several distinctive fibroblast capabilities. In normal connective tissue, the relatively sparse population of fibroblasts must monitor and maintain the extracellular matrix (ECM). During injury, fibroblasts must move to damaged regions and synthesize or degrade appropriate ECM molecules. Interacting with the ECM is central to these fibroblast roles.

FIBROBLAST RESPONSE TO INJURY

In the unperturbed state, in vivo, fibroblasts are relatively quiescent with little cell turnover and low levels of matrix synthesis. In response to injury, an increase in fibroblast numbers and an increase in metabolic activity are seen. Fibroblasts synthesize collagens, fibronectin, proteoglycans, elastin, and a variety of other glycoproteins. In addition to types I and III collagen, the predominant types synthesized by skin and interstitial fibroblasts, fibroblasts synthesize several other collagens that are important in collagen-fibril organization. These include types V, VI, and VII (see Chapter 2).

Surgical Wound

The most straightforward type of injury is a surgical wound of either the skin or another site. Normal wound

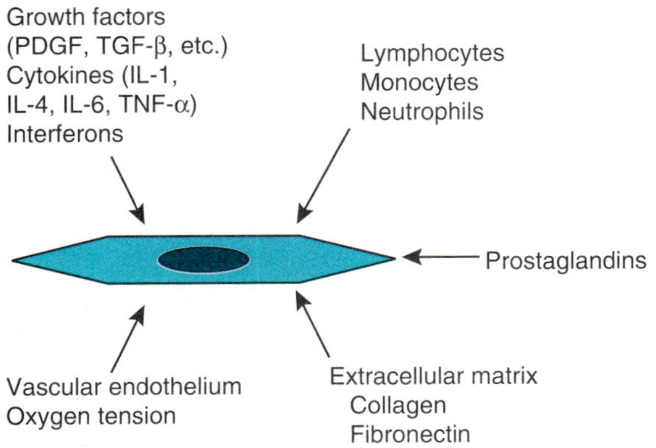

FIGURE 12–1 · **Features of the Microenvironment That Influence Fibroblast Growth and Metabolism.** Cells, matrix, nutritive factors, and spatial orientation provide signals that regulate fibroblast activity. These factors may individually, or in combination, relay signals through intracellular messengers, initiating or inhibiting gene transcription.

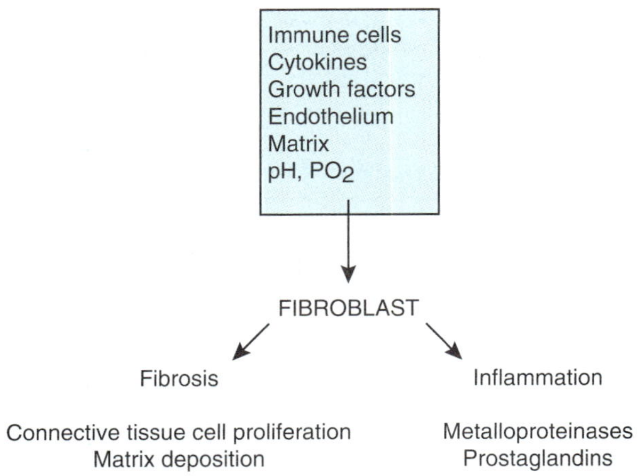

FIGURE 12–2 · **Fibroblast Products That Alter the Microenvironment.** Fibroblast responses to signals in the microenvironment include not only proliferation but also expression of new surface proteins, matrix proteins, matrix-degrading enzymes, and soluble molecules that can influence the metabolic activity of other cells.

healing involves several phases. During each phase, the ECM, integrin expression, and cytokines coordinately determine fibroblast movement, proliferation, and gene expression. Immediately after wounding, the blood clot forms a provisional fibrin-fibronectin matrix, and degranulating platelets release an array of growth factors, including transforming growth factor-β (TGF-β) and platelet-derived growth factor (PDGF). In this type of injury, it is clear that PDGF plays a central role in the reparative response.[7] PDGF can also be released by other cell types including endothelial cells, smooth muscle cells, macrophages, renal mesangial cells, and Langerhans cells. It, thus, can play a role in fibroproliferative events not only after mechanical injury to the skin but also after damage at other tissue sites.

The accumulated fibroblasts are activated by these and other stimuli to initiate repair. TGF-β and PDGF stimulate increased synthesis of matrix proteins that form the granulation tissue of the wound.[8] As scar tissue is formed, increasing amounts of type I collagen are incorporated into the matrix, and fibronectin levels

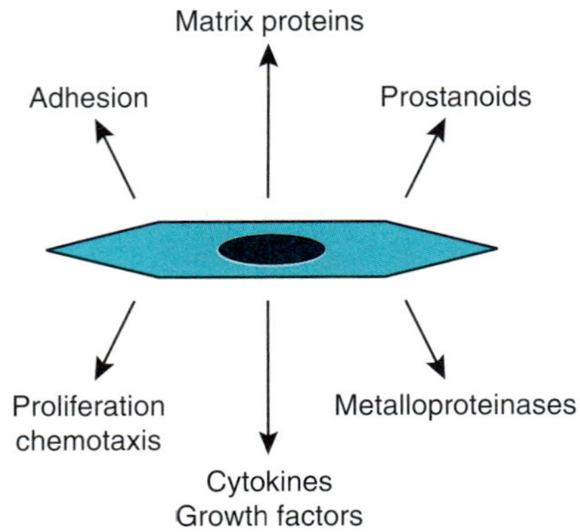

FIGURE 12–3 · **Alternative Pathways of Fibroblast Activation.** The mix of signals to which the fibroblast is exposed and the type of responding fibroblast determine whether responses are primarily fibrotic and reparative or degrading and inflammatory in nature. Both types of processes coexist in most situations, and inflammation followed by repair is a common and "normal" sequence.

decrease. Fibroblasts produce high levels of $\alpha_2\beta_1$-integrin, which binds collagen and promotes contraction of matrix; PDGF stimulates $\alpha_2\beta_1$ expression, and PDGF and TGF-β stimulate collagen expression.[9-11] In later stages of wound healing, there is decreased mechanical stress on the ECM, and collagen synthesis is downregulated.[12] These processes of sequential collagen synthesis, matrix contraction, and then relaxation with quiescence of collagen synthesis can be modeled by growing fibroblasts in vitro in stressed and relaxed collagen gels.[11,12]

Matrix Deposition

Fibroblasts regulate matrix macromolecule deposition at multiple steps, including production, processing, and cross-linking. Collagen is secreted as soluble procollagen.[13] Procollagen must be processed at both amino- and carboxy-termini by C- and N-procollagen proteinases after which it can spontaneously assemble into collagen fibrils.[13] Collagen deposition is stabilized by cross-linking through the action of lysyl oxidase.

Assembly of fibronectin into fibrillar polymers requires more active involvement of the fibroblast. Fibroblasts assemble secreted fibronectin into a fibrillar matrix after dimeric fibronectin binds to cell-surface integrin receptors (Fig. 12–4). For fibrillar-matrix assembly to proceed, the integrin receptor must be in a high-affinity conformation. Integrin affinity can be modulated by intracellular signals impacting integrin α- and β-subunit cytoplasmic domains.[14] The cell cytoskeleton also contributes to fibronectin-matrix assembly.[15] Stress fibers exert tension on the fibronectin molecule, exposing a site required for sequential binding of fibronectin dimers.[16] Thus, fibroblasts control matrix composition in response to multiple intracellular cues.

FIBROBLAST ADHESION TO EXTRACELLULAR MATRIX DIRECTS FIBROBLAST MIGRATION INTO THE WOUND

Fibroblasts migrate into the wound from adjacent sites in response to chemotactic stimuli, including PDGF and

TGF-β from platelets, thrombin, and peptides of collagen, fibronectin, and elastin, that may be released in the course of injury.[17-22] Cells move by binding to ECM proteins, including collagen, fibronectin, laminins, and vitronectin. Cell surface receptors known collectively as integrins mediate cell binding to the ECM. Intracellular cytoskeletal structures also attach to integrins, forming focal adhesion complexes. Thus, integrins serve as the focus point on the cell membrane between the intracellular cytoskeleton and the ECM.

Integrin Receptors

Integrin receptors include an array of protein dimers formed by combination in pairs of several different α-and β-subunits.[23] Most integrins mediating fibroblast adhesion to ECM components contain either an α_v- or a β_1-subunit (Table 12–1). Integrins containing α_v-subunits are best characterized for interacting with vitronectin ($\alpha_v\beta_1$, $\alpha_v\beta_3$, $\alpha_v\beta_5$), whereas those containing β_1-subunits interact with collagen ($\alpha_1\beta_1$ and $\alpha_2\beta_1$), laminin ($\alpha_3\beta_1$), or fibronectin ($\alpha_4\beta_1$ and $\alpha_5\beta_1$). Other β_1-integrin receptors have been described, and, depending on the cell type, ligand specificity of each of these receptor dimers can vary. Various cytokines, principally PDGF and TGF-β, regulate levels of integrin-receptor expression.[11]

Integrin engagement leads to formation of an actin-based cytoskeleton, regulates gene expression and provides a second signal required for fibroblast proliferation[24] (see Fig. 12–4). Actin-based stress fibers terminate at the plasma membrane in focal adhesions composed of both structural and signaling proteins, including α-actinin, talin, vinculin, paxillin, tensin, and integrin-linked kinase (ILK) and focal adhesion kinase (FAK).[25] A variety of protein kinases mediate integrin signals intracellularly, including focal adhesion–associated kinases, FAK and ILK, and soluble Rho and mitogen-activated protein (MAP) family kinases.[26,27] FAK, a tyrosine kinase, is phosphorylated on receptor cross-linking by any of the β_1- or α_v-integrin receptors.[28] It mediates integrin signals for both cell survival and growth.[29,30] FAK stimulates several intracellular signaling

TABLE 12–1 • PRIMARY INTEGRINS RELEVANT FOR FIBROBLAST-MEDIATED INTERACTIONS WITH EXTRACELLULAR MATRIX COMPONENTS

Integrin Family	Associated Subunit	Extracellular Matrix Ligand
β_1	α_1	Collagens, laminins
	α_2	Collagens, laminins
	α_3	Collagens, fibronectin, epiligrin (laminin 5)
	α_4	Fibronectin (CS-1)
	α_5	Fibronectin (RGD)
α_v	β_1	Vitronectin, fibronectin
	β_3	Vitronectin, fibronectin, collagen (others)
	β_5	Vitronectin
	β_6	Fibronectin

pathways, including the MAP kinase, extracellular signal-regulated kinase (ERK).[27,29] FAK-independent signaling of MAP kinase has been also described through Shc, an adaptor protein.[31] ILK is a serine-threonine kinase activated by integrins. It binds to integrin β-chains, promotes cell survival, anchors actin filaments to integrins, and activates Akt.[32-34] The roles of these and other signaling molecules in the diverse biologic functions of integrins remain under intense investigation.

Fibroblast Movement

Fibroblast movement requires several distinctive cellular appendages, including filopodia, lamellipodia, and stress fibers.[35,36] Different cytoskeletal formations support each of these appendages. Filopodia are elongated extensions from the cell that may mediate the first step in directed cell movement. Actin fibers run parallel to the extensions. Lamellipodia are broad-based projections from the cell membrane that may represent the second step in cell locomotion. Lamellipodia form after filopodia at the leading edge, extending the cell forward. Circumferential actin fibers support lamellipodia, and PDGF can stimulate their formation. Stress-fiber contraction in the lagging cell edge may serve to complete cell movement forward. Stress fibers are linear actin arrays that radiate from focal adhesions to the cell interior. They form during cell spreading and are required for wound contraction. Stress fibers form on stimulation with lysophosphatidic acid or serum. Thus, factors released during clot formation provide stimuli for cell movement as well as for proliferation.

Intracellular Signaling for Cell Movement Through Ras Family Guanosine Triphosphatases

Cell movement may be coordinated intracellularly by sequential activation of Ras family guanosine triphosphatases (GTPases): Cdc42 activates Rac, which activates Rho[35] (Fig. 12–5). This activation cascade causes extension of filopodia mediated by Cdc42, followed by formation of lamellipodia mediated by Rac, followed by stress-fiber formation mediated by Rho. Integrin engagement by ECM is also required for stress-fiber formation and stimulates retrograde movement of the receptor cytoskeletal-ECM complex.[37] Ras is also required for cell movement, possibly by regulating turnover of focal adhesions.[38,39]

CYTOKINES REGULATE FIBROBLAST PROLIFERATION, METABOLISM, AND APOPTOSIS

PDGF Stimulates Fibroblast Proliferation

PDGF may exist as either a homodimer or a heterodimer of PDGF-A and PDGF-B chains.[40] Some cells release one isoform of PDGF preferentially; others, such as platelets, release multiple isoforms. The PDGF receptor also functions optimally as a dimer, constituted as either a homodimer or heterodimer of α- and β-chains, with different cells having different receptor

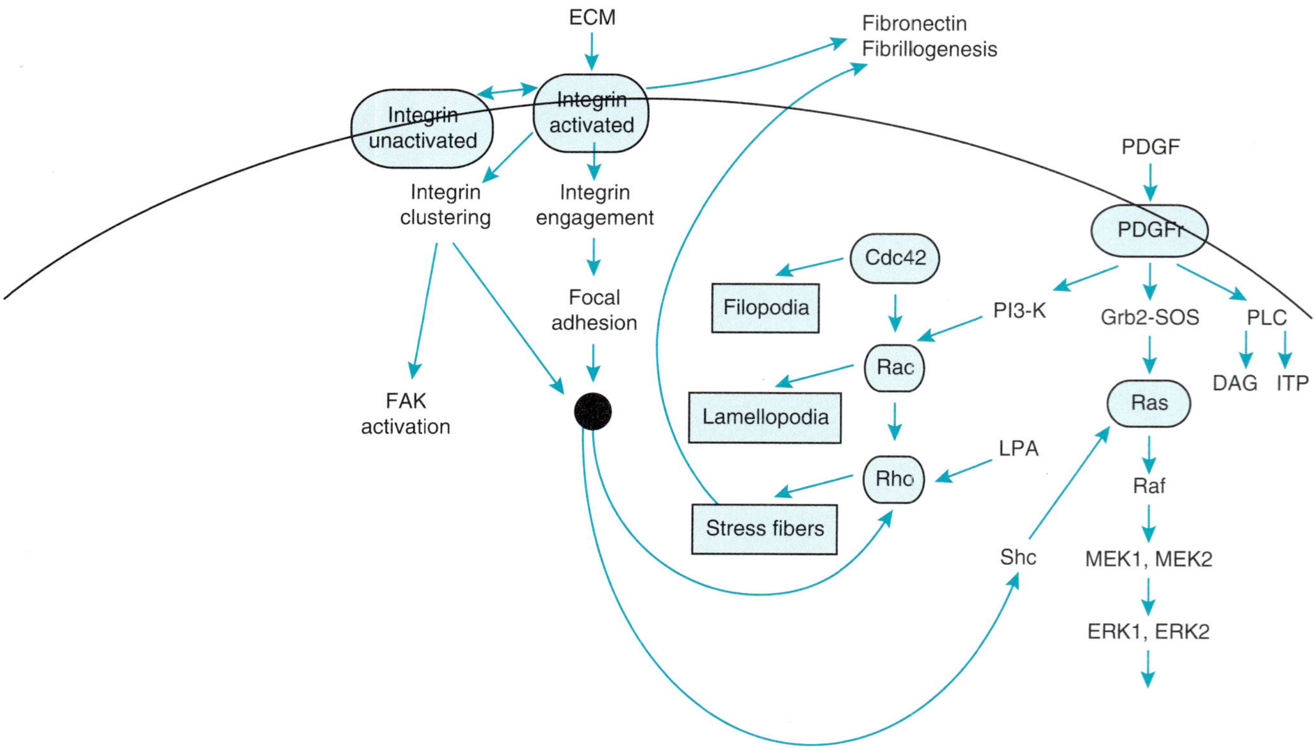

FIGURE 12–4 · Intracellular Signals Mediating Growth Factor–Induced Cellular Proliferation. Platelet-derived growth factor (PDGF) and other growth factors (fibroblast growth factor [FGF] and epidermal growth factor [EGF]) stimulate receptor autophosphorylation. Phosphorylated tyrosine on these receptors binds and activates downstream signaling proteins (Grb2-SOS, phosphatidylinositol 3-kinase, and phospholipase C). Guinine exchange factors (such as SOS) activate Ras and Ras family members, stimulating downstream mitogen-activated protein (MAP) kinase cascades.

forms.[41] The BB PDGF isoform binds to all possible receptor dimers (αα, αβ, and ββ) with high affinity, whereas PDGF-AA binds with high affinity only to the αα receptor.[42] The binding of PDGF to specific fibroblast cell surface αα-receptors is followed by receptor activation, autophosphorylation, and initiation of fibroblast proliferation.[43]

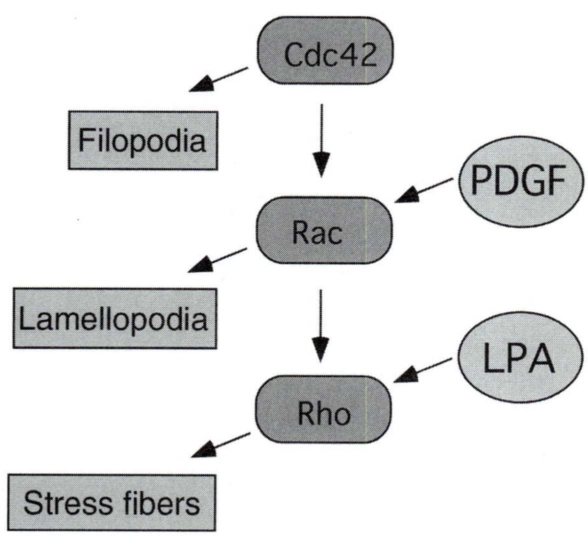

FIGURE 12–5 · Ras family guanosine triphosphatase (GTPase) activation of intracellular cytoskeletal structures. The Cdc42 to Rac to Rho cascade of GTPase activation contributes to cell movement.

Intracellular Signaling

Dimeric PDGF binds to PDGF receptor monomers, inducing receptor dimerization and autophosphorylation or transphosphorylation on intracellular tyrosine residues through the receptor's tyrosine kinase activity[44] (Fig. 12–6). Signaling through cell surface receptors is often dependent on kinase activity: Kinases phosphorylate proteins at specific amino acid residues, leading to their activation. These phosphorylated, activated proteins can also have kinase activity and can phosphorylate and activate additional proteins. The membrane tyrosine kinase receptors for fibroblast growth factor (FGF) and epidermal growth factor (EGF), although not dimerized, are activated similarly to PDGF.[45] Phosphorylated tyrosine residues serve as docking sites for proteins with Src homology 2 (SH2) domains, including Src, GTPase-activating protein, Grb2, phospholipase C, and phosphatidylinositol 3-kinase. Binding of each SH2 domain–containing protein spawns secondary signals, at least some of which are critical to cell proliferation. Amino acids surrounding phosphorylated tyrosines determine SH2 domain–binding specificity, permitting different responses to different growth factors.

Receptor tyrosine kinases control Ras and Ras family GTPases through SH2 domain signaling proteins (see Fig. 12–6). Ras family GTPases are active when bound to GTP and inactive when bound to guanosine diphosphate (GDP). Guanine exchange factors activate Ras family members by catalyzing the release of GDP from

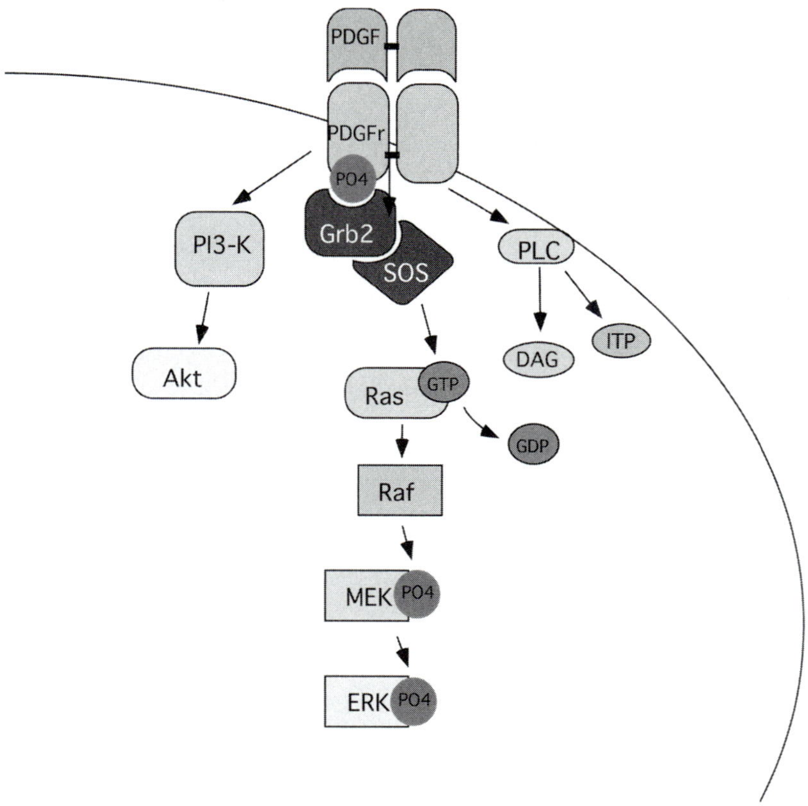

FIGURE 12–6 · Extracellular matrix (ECM) proteins signal through both integrin-receptor engagement and clustering. Integrins stimulate focal adhesion kinase (FAK) phosphorylation. Lysophosphatidic acid (LPA) and integrin engagement activates Rho, leading to stress-fiber formation. Fibronectin polymerization requires integrin-receptor activation and stress-fiber formation.

Ras, which then binds intracellular GTP. PDGF activates Ras by binding to Grb2, an SH2 domain adaptor protein, that is constitutively bound to SOS, a guanine exchange factor. SOS thus activates Ras.[44] Other guanine exchange factors with overlapping specificities can activate Ras and related GTPases. Ras activation stimulates cell proliferation through MAP kinases.[46]

Mitogen-Activated Protein Kinases in Proliferation and the Stress Response

Many signal pathways mediating proliferative and stress responses are transmitted by MAP kinase cascades[45,47] (see Fig. 12–6). The most important of these cascades for cell proliferation is initiated by Ras activation of Raf, an MAP kinase kinase kinase. Raf is a serine-threonine kinase recruited to the membrane by binding to activated Ras, where it is activated by phosphorylation. Raf, in turn, phosphorylates the MAP kinase kinases MEK1 and MEK2, which are ERK kinases. MAP kinase kinases are dual-specificity kinases that, on activation, phosphorylate MAP kinases. MEK1 and MEK2 phosphorylate the MAP kinases ERK1 and ERK2. MAP kinases are serine-threonine kinases that, on phosphorylation, enter the nucleus, where they activate specific transcription factors or other mediators. Activated ERK1 and ERK2 phosphorylate a wide variety of cytoplasmic and nuclear proteins but most importantly Elk-1 and Myc, proteins critical in cellular growth and transformation. Other parallel MAP kinase cascades have been described. Jun kinase is another MAP kinase activated through a parallel pathway of MEK kinase (the MAP kinase kinase kinase), stress-activated protein kinase (SAPK, or SEK) or Jun N-terminal kinase kinase (the MAP kinase kinases), and Jun kinase. Jun kinase phosphorylates and activates Jun; Jun activation has been implicated in regulation of metalloproteinases (MMPs). This pathway may play an important, incompletely defined role in inflammation and tissue remodeling.

Fibroblast Apoptosis

During the last several years, we have learned that not only is proliferation carefully regulated, but cell death as well. Studies done on fibroblasts have shown that normal cells have a finite life span, then are "programmed" to die.[48] The process of programmed cell death, or apoptosis, is universal, and its molecular regulation was first appreciated in studies of specific death genes in the worm *Caenornabditis elegans*. In apoptosis, there is fragmentation of DNA, nuclear condensation and blebbing, and then cell death, a process different from cell necrosis or injury to cell membranes. In humans, as in *C. elegans*, a specific set of cell surface and intracellular proteins are important in the apoptotic pathway (see Chapter 26). Fas is a cell surface protein, part of the tumor necrosis factor receptor (TNF-R) family, whose ligation triggers apoptosis in lymphocytes and fibroblasts.[49] There are a number of other cell death genes and proteins, including c-Myc and p53, whose action eventually leads to activation of cellular caspases (enzymes related to interleukin-1 [IL-1]–converting enzyme) that initiate DNA cleavage and cell death. c-Myc is also key in cell proliferation, and it is clear that proliferation and apoptosis are alternative branch points after cellular activation.[50]

In addition to proapoptotic molecules, there are also molecules such as Bcl-2 that suppress apoptosis. Another TNF-R family member, CD40, mediates an antiapoptotic signal. The natural counter-receptors for Fas and CD40, Fas ligand and CD40 ligand, are expressed on activated lymphocytes.[51] Antiapoptotic signals could be mediated by CD40. In lymphocytes, in which the term *activation-induced cell death* is used, apoptosis is an important event in regulating the immune response and eliminating autoreactive cells. Other than serving as a mechanism for elimination of senescent cells, the role of apoptosis in fibroblasts is less clear. However, apoptosis may lead to elimination of particular fibroblast subpopulations and alterations of phenotypic expression.

Other Intracellular Signaling Pathways Regulating Fibroblast Metabolism

Growth factors and cytokines activate other intracellular signaling pathways that may affect a variety of metabolic processes in addition to cell proliferation and death. For example, phospholipase C is another SH2 domain–containing protein activated on growth factor receptor phosphorylation (see Fig. 12–6). It cleaves membrane components into two "second messengers": inositol 1,4,5-triphosphate and diacylglycerol. Inositol 1,4,5-triphosphate stimulates increased Ca^{2+}, and diacylglycerol activates protein kinase C. Other important second messengers include cyclic nucleotides (cyclic adenosinemonophosphate), G proteins, and phosphatidylinositol 3-kinase. The level of fibroblast proliferation may be due not only to the absence of "on" signals (e.g., growth factors) but also to the presence of "off" signals. Generation of arachidonic acid metabolites such as prostaglandin E_2 by IL-1 or TNF-α leads to cyclic adenosine monophosphate generation that suppresses cellular proliferation.[52-54]

TRANSFORMING GROWTH FACTOR-β FAMILY MEMBERS REGULATE MATRIX PRODUCTION AND DEPOSITION

TGF-βs, TGF-β1, TGF-β2, and TGF-β3, are part of a larger family of growth and morphogenic factors that include the bone morphogenic proteins (BMPs), activins and inhibins (discussed in Chapters 1 and 89). TGF-β stimulates extracellular deposition of multiple matrix proteins, including collagen, fibronectin, and fibrillin. TGF-β coordinately simulates multiple steps in the process of collagen synthesis and deposition. It promotes synthesis of procollagen by stimulating transcription of collagen genes. It markedly stimulates collagen matrix deposition by activating BMP-1/procollagen C-proteinase and procollagen N-proteinase–mediated processing.[55] Finally, TGF-β increases collagen cross-linking by activating lysyl oxidase.[56]

Multiple cell types produce TGF-βs in vivo. Platelets provide a rich source of TGF-β for healing wounds. Fibroblasts also secrete TGF-β, providing potential autoregulation of fibroblast function. However, secreted TGF-β is inactive. The aminoterminus of the TGF-β propeptide, known as the latency-associated peptide (LAP), maintains the active carboxyterminus of TGF-β in a latent state through a noncovalent interaction.[57] Further, latent TGF-β can be stored in connective tissues by covalent binding to latent TGF-β binding proteins (LTBPs).[58,59] Several factors can activate TGF-β, including proteases, the αvβ6 integrin receptor, and thrombospondin.[60-62] The relative importance of these activation mechanisms is unclear in the various roles TGF-β plays in vivo.[57]

Receptors and Intracellular Signaling

TGF-β interacts with receptor serine-threonine kinases[63] (Fig. 12–7). TGF-β binding to TGF-βRII stimulates autophosphorylation, binding of the complex to TGF-βRI, and phosphorylation of TGF-βRI. Smad family proteins mediate TGF-β effects on gene transcription. Phosphorylated TGF-βI receptor recruits and phosphorylates Smad2 and Smad3. These Smads then complex with Smad4 and translocate into the nucleus. Smad complexes can bind DNA directly or enhance binding of other proteins to DNA, regulating promoter activity of target genes. Smad6 and Smad7 inhibit TGF-β signaling by blocking phosphorylation of Smad2 and Smad3. Although Smads play a primary role in TGF-β signaling, other transcription factors, such as activator protein-1 (AP-1) and SP1, interact directly with Smads or modify their effect on target promoters. Connective tissue growth factor, a cytokine strongly induced by TGF-β, may also mediate certain effects of TGF-β.[64]

Immune Modulation of Fibroblast Function

LYMPHOCYTE RECRUITMENT AND LOCALIZATION

Lymphocytes normally reside in specialized lymphoid tissues (e.g., lymph nodes and spleen) and in the circulation. Lymphocytes may gain entry to the circulation from lymphoid organs or other tissues, and they may leave to recirculate through the lymphatic system. Establishment of a chronic inflammatory focus is characterized by both increased lymphocyte and monocyte emigration from the vasculature and localization of these cells to tissue (Fig. 12–8). Recirculation, homing, and localization of immune cells are rigorously controlled by the expression and engagement of cell surface receptors.[65]

Mononuclear Cells Express Adhesion Molecules That Bind to Fibroblasts

Lymphocytes and monocytes express cell surface molecules that interact with ligands on endothelial cells, fibroblasts, and ECM to promote cell adhesion (see Chapter 24). As an initial event, immune-cell activation leads to increased expression and function of adhesion ligands. Endothelial cells at sites of inflammation are

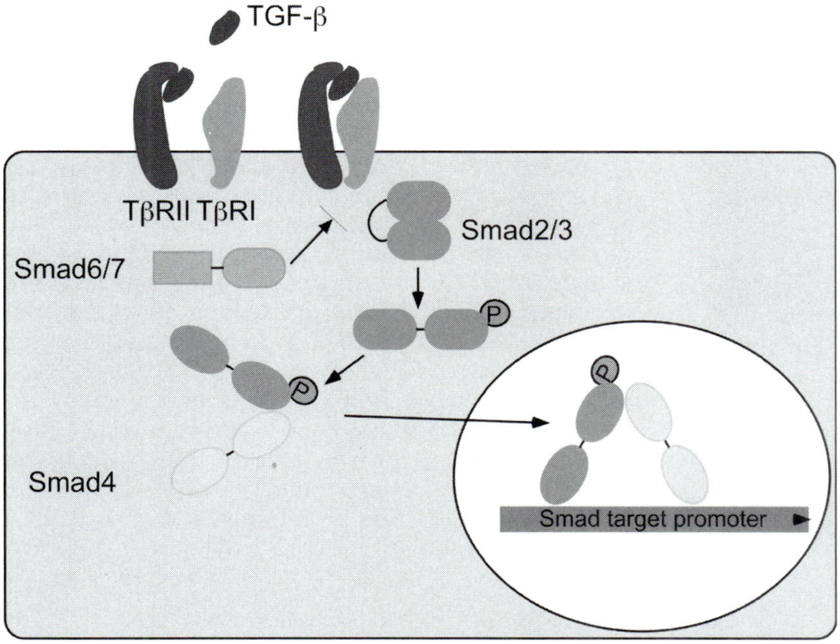

FIGURE 12–7 · **Transforming Growth Factor-β (TGF-β) Intracellular Signaling.** TGF-β binds to the type II TGF-β receptor. This complex then associates with the type I TGF-β receptor. These receptor serine-threonine kinases phosphorylate Smad2 and Smad3, which bind to Smad4, regulating the promoter activity of target genes.

activated by immune cell cytokines, particularly IL-1 and TNF-α from monocytes, or by other stimuli (e.g., endotoxin) to increase expression of counter-receptors, or ligands, for lymphocyte and monocyte receptors. The endothelial cell ligands include vascular cell adhesion molecule-1 (VCAM-1), endothelial leukocyte adhesion molecule-1 (E-selectin), mucosal addressin cell adhesion molecule-1, CD34 (CD, or cell determinant, designations are catalog numbers for identified proteins), and P-selectin, as well as intercellular adhesion molecule (ICAM)-1, -2, and -3. Lymphocyte and monocyte ligands, including L-selectin, sialated glycoproteins, the β_2-integrin, leukocyte function–associated antigen 1 (CD11a, CD18, or $\alpha_1\beta_2$), very late antigen-4 (VLA-4) (CD49d, CD29, or $\alpha_4\beta_1$), and Mac-1 ($\alpha_M\beta_2$ or CD11b, CD18), bind to these endothelial cell receptors and modulate the egress of lymphocytes and monocytes from the vasculature (Fig. 12–9). This can be facilitated by chemotactic stimuli such as the chemokines IL-8, "regulated on activation normal T expressed secreted" (RANTES), monocyte inflammatory protein-1α, and monocyte chemotactic protein-1, -2, and -3, as well as by other chemotactic stimuli including collagen peptides.[66-69]

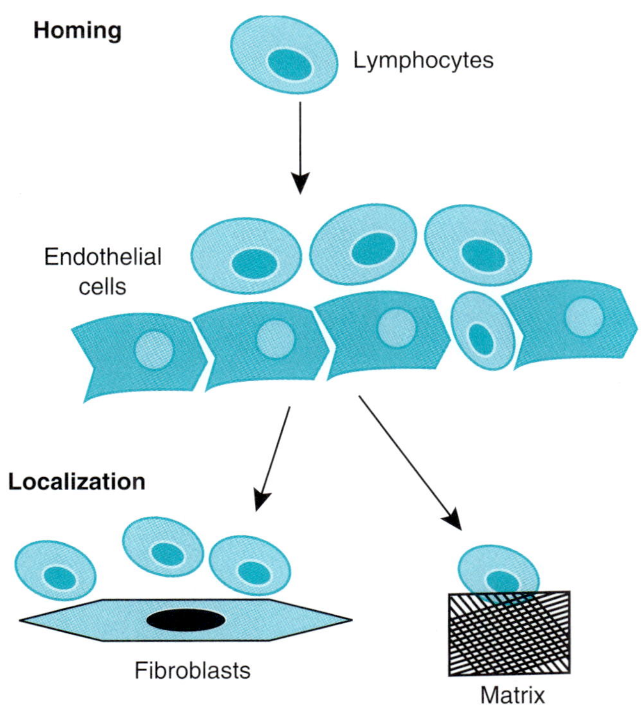

FIGURE 12–8 · **Homing and Localization of Mononuclear Cells to Connective Tissue.** The localization of lymphocytes and monocytes requires cellular activation, egress from the vasculature, and binding to cellular and matrix elements of the connective tissue. These processes are tightly regulated by the expression of specific adhesion ligands.

Fibroblasts and Matrix Bind Mononuclear Cells

Lymphocyte localization requires activation of and adhesion molecule expression by fibroblasts. ICAM-1 and leukocyte function-associated antigen-3 (LFA-3) mediate lymphocyte-fibroblast attachment[70-72] (see Fig. 12–9). ICAM-1 on fibroblasts is induced by interferon-γ (IFN-γ), TNF-α, IL-1, and IL-4.[71,73,74] In addition, lymphocytes may bind to noncellular ligands expressed on collagen and fibronectin through surface integrins, which include VLA-1 ($\alpha_1\beta_1$) and VLA-4 ($\alpha_4\beta_1$).[75-77] Lymphocytes that initially leave the vasculature and bind to connective tissue are presumably activated; however, there is further recruitment of monocytes and lymphocytes in response to immune cell and connective tissue signals, including the chemotactic factors noted before. Cellular binding, per se, may result in activation of immune cells and connective tissue cells as a result of receptor activation.[78]

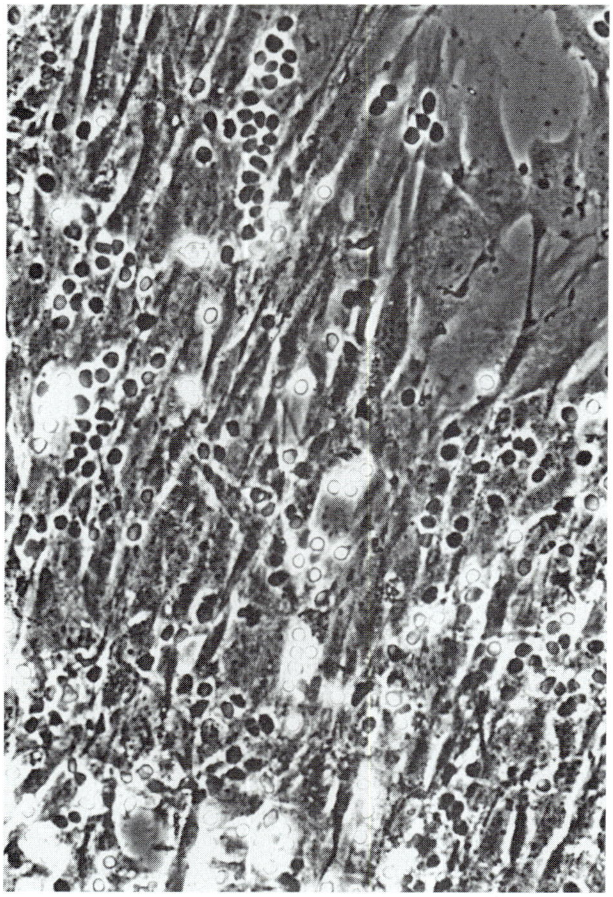

FIGURE 12–9 • Purified Human T Lymphocytes Are Bound to Human Dermal Fibroblasts Grown in Culture. Fibroblasts were activated by interferon-γ (IFN-γ) before the binding process. Fibroblasts appear spindle shaped. Lymphocytes are small, round, dark cells, tightly adherent and flattened, or bright, round cells more loosely adherent and rounded. (Viewed under phase-contrast microscopy; original magnification ×400.)

FIBROBLAST ENVIRONMENT, CYTOKINE NETWORKS, AND MATRIX METABOLISM

Fibroblasts In Vivo

Fibroblasts in vivo exist under environmental conditions markedly different from those used to study growth factors in vitro. Such conditions, including the presence of a surrounding ECM and different oxygen tension, profoundly influence fibroblast behavior in general, as well as responses to growth factors. For example, in vitro responses to PDGF, as well as to EGF, are altered by the presence of an ECM[79-81]; PDGF signaling is decreased when cells are grown in an in vitro matrix.[82] There is evidence that other cytokines and growth factors stimulating fibroblast proliferation may mediate their effect through PDGF action. IL-1 and TNF-α stimulate synthesis and release of endogenous fibroblast PDGF-AA.[83] TGF-β_1 appears to increase expression of fibroblast PDGF-αα receptors.[84] Some growth factors, such as insulin-like growth factor,[85] are not mitogenic by themselves but potentiate the mitogenic action of other substances. At low oxygen tension, which may occur after vascular injury, there is decreased binding of TGF-β and EGF, whereas proliferative responses to EGF may be augmented.[86]

Immune Cell Cytokines Regulate Fibroblast Functions

Although direct cell contact between fibroblast and immune cells may have reciprocal effects on cell metabolism, the preponderant regulation of fibroblast metabolism occurs through release from immune cells of soluble cytokines and growth factors (Table 12–2). These are often active at nanomolar concentrations, a range readily achieved in the confines of the interstitial space. Cytokines and growth factors released by lymphocytes and monocytes that regulate fibroblast metabolism include IL-1, IL-4, IL-6, IL-10, IL-13, TNF-α, IFN-γ, TGF-β, PDGF, and endothelins. As already noted, IL-1, TGF-α, and PDGF stimulate both proliferation and collagen synthesis by fibroblasts; IL-4 stimulates fibroblast chemotaxis, proliferation, and matrix synthesis.[87-89] IL-6 stimulates synthesis of collagen and glycosaminoglycans.[90] IL-13 is a member of the profibrotic family of cytokines. It stimulates matrix gene expression in fibroblasts, as well as adhesion molecule expression.[91,92] TNF-α increases fibroblast proliferation by stimulating endogenous fibroblast PDGF-AA. It has variable effects on collagen synthesis, stimulates proteoglycans, and suppresses fibronectin production.[93-95] IFN-γ, IFN-α, and

TABLE 12–2 • CYTOKINES STIMULATING FIBROBLAST FUNCTION

Proliferation	Matrix Biosynthesis	Metalloproteinases	Adhesion-Molecule Expression	Chemotaxis
PDGF	TGF-β	TNF-α	IFN-γ	TGF-β
FGF	IL-1	IL-1	TNF-α	PDGF
IL-1 via PDGF	IL-4	IL-10	IL-1	IL-4
IL-4	PDGF		IL-4	IFN-γ
CTAPs	FGF			TNF-α
Endothelin	Endothelin			Fibronectin
TNF-α	IL-6 (proteoglycan)			Collagen peptides
	IL-13			EGF
				C3a/C5
				Endothelin
				Leukotriene B_4

Abbreviations: C3a/C5, Complement components C3a, C5; CTAPs, connective tissue activating peptides; EGF, epidermal growth factor; FGF, fibroblast growth factor; IFN-γ, interferon γ; IL, interleukin; PDGF, platelet-derived growth factor; TGF-β, transforming growth factor β; TNFα, tumor necrosis factor α.

IL-10 suppress collagen synthesis.[96] Endothelins are a family of polypeptides with potent effects on endothelial cells, smooth muscle cells, and fibroblast metabolism.[97] In fibroblasts they stimulate proliferation and matrix biosynthesis.[98] The overall effect on collagen synthesis thus depends on the balance of cytokines and growth factors, the type of responding fibroblast, and other environmental factors.

Fibroblasts Elaborate Matrix-Degrading Enzymes and Enzyme Inhibitors

The net amount of accumulated collagen and other matrix components depends not only on synthesis, but on degradation. Fibroblasts, as well as other cell types, elaborate connective tissue matrix-degrading enzymes, termed *matrix MMPs* because of their dependence on metal ions for activity. Seven of these enzymes are related structurally and genetically, the prototype being interstitial collagenase[99] (see Chapter 4). These enzymes are secreted as latent enzymes and are activated extracellularly. Fibroblast (also called interstitial) collagenase (MMP-1) and neutrophil collagenase (MMP-8) can cleave native (nondenatured) collagen.[100] Once cleaved, collagen becomes denatured (gelatin = denatured collagen) and is susceptible to further degradation by gelatinases. MMP-2 (also called 72-kD gelatinase because of its molecular weight) and MMP-3 (stromelysin) are gelatinases produced constitutively by fibroblasts; MMP-9, stromelysin-2, and pump-1 (uterine MMP) are inducible gelatinases. MMP-3, or stromelysin, also degrades proteoglycans, fibronectin, laminin, and cartilage link protein and activates latent procollagenase (see Chapter 4). Fibroblasts also make elastases, cathepsins, and other enzymes, some of which are membrane-bound enzymes.[101,102] Elastases not only are important in degradation of vascular, skin, and lung elastin, but they also have the capability of degrading matrix proteins and causing significant tissue injury.

Cytokine Regulation of Matrix Degradation

Cytokines may have concordant or discordant effects on synthesis of collagen and the enzymes that degrade collagen and other matrix macromolecules. IL-1, which stimulates production of collagen, also stimulates production of collagenase (MMP-1) and stromelysin.[103-105] TNF-α is a potent stimulator of MMP-9 and also stimulates production of collagenase and stromelysin.[106] Both IL-1 and TNF-α induce the transcription factor c-*jun* in fibroblasts, and the increase in c-*jun* probably plays a direct role in activating collagenase gene transcription.[107,108] IL-1 and TNF-α also individually and synergistically stimulate fibroblast prostaglandin E_2 synthesis, and prostaglandin E_2 suppresses collagenase production.[52,109-111] In direct contrast to IL-1, IFN-γ suppresses both collagen synthesis and synthesis of collagenase and stromelysin.[112,113] TGF-β, perhaps the most potent stimulus for collagen synthesis, also suppresses synthesis of collagenase and stromelysin.[112,113] Glucocorticoids, in general, suppress production of MMPs. Finally, fibroblasts synthesize autokines (self-stimulating cytokines), which augment collagenase production.[114]

In addition to elaborating matrix and matrix-degrading enzymes, fibroblasts synthesize inhibitors of MMPs. Tissue inhibitor of MMPs (TIMP) inhibits the action of the entire family of mammalian MMPs.[99] TIMP is induced in fibroblasts by IL-1, IL-6, and IL-11.[115-117] Both IL-6 and IL-11 are fibroblast products, or autokines, whose production in fibroblasts is, in turn, stimulated by IL-1 and TNF-α.[118,119] IL-11 production can also be stimulated by TGF-β.[120] Thus, TGF-β has an overall matrix-promoting effect, augmenting production of collagen and collagenase inhibitor, suppressing collagenase production, and potentially playing a critical role in the development of fibrotic disease.

The Balance of Forces on the Fibroblast Determines Tissue Repair or Degradation

The balance of forces on the fibroblast, as well as the particular tissue involved, determines whether inflammatory stimuli lead to net proliferation and repair or to tissue degradation and destruction. The skin fibroblast is normally a relatively quiescent cell that divides slowly and, in the absence of injury, elaborates little matrix. Inflammation in the skin tends to lead to net increases in matrix (e.g., wound healing). In contrast, synovial tissue responds to inflammation, predominantly with increased MMP production and destruction of subadjacent cartilage and bone. Within the synovium per se, however, there is increased synovial fibroblast proliferation and matrix deposition. A similar situation exists for the gingival fibroblast; proliferation and matrix deposition in the gingiva are accompanied by destruction and resorption of adjacent bony tissues.

Fibroblast Cytokines

CHEMOKINES AND OTHER LEUKOCYTE CHEMOTACTIC FACTORS

As just noted, the stimulation of fibroblasts by IL-1, TNF-α, and other cytokines leads to fibroblast proinflammatory activities by stimulating matrix degradation. Peptides of degraded collagen and fibronectin may further stimulate lymphocyte and monocyte recruitment by their chemotactic properties. Fibroblasts may also have more direct effects on leukocyte recruitment and activation. Stimulation of fibroblasts by TNF-α leads to synthesis of the chemotaxin IL-8 and leukemia-inhibitory factor, which are chemotactic for and activate leukocytes.[78,121] Fibroblasts also elaborate the lymphocyte chemotactic factors monocyte chemotactic protein-1, -2, and -3 and monocyte inflammatory protein-1α.[66,122] IL-16 is made by fibroblasts and acts as a lymphocyte chemoattractant.[123] TNF-α also stimulates production of membrane-associated IL-1α in fibroblasts; IL-1 has multiple stimulatory influences on lymphocytes and monocytes. Both IL-1 and TNF-α stimulate production of IL-6 by fibroblasts[118,119]; IL-6 is a major inducer of acute-phase proteins in hepatocytes and is an important promoter of plasma cell proliferation.[124-126]

BONE MARROW FIBROBLASTS PRODUCE CYTOKINES LEADING TO HEMATOPOIETIC CELL DIFFERENTIATION

Fibroblasts are also an important source of cytokines that regulate development of hematopoietic precursors. In this respect, bone-marrow fibroblasts serve key nutritive and differentiating functions; fibroblasts make granulocyte colony-stimulating factor (G-CSF), granulocyte-monocyte colony-stimulating factor (GM-CSF), and IL-11, the last in response to IL-1, TNF-α, and TGF-β.[120,127,128] Finally, fibroblasts make growth factors including TGF-β and PDGF, which can not only serve as autokines but act on other cells as well.[83,129] Thus, fibroblast-derived cytokines affect a variety of cells including immune cells, mesenchymal cells, and bone-marrow stem cells.

Fibroblast Heterogeneity

DERMAL FIBROBLAST HETEROGENEITY

In addition to the obvious differences in functional expression among dermal, synovial, lung, and other fibroblast populations, it has become apparent that even fibroblasts derived from a single source are heterogeneous. Thus, among fibroblasts derived from human skin, there are marked differences in proliferation and in the synthesis of collagen, glycosaminoglycans, prostaglandins, and MMPs.[130-133] Furthermore, there are differences in responses to growth-regulatory cytokines and in adhesion-molecule expression.[129,134] The heterogeneity among fibroblasts has been ascertained both by study of cloned dermal fibroblast populations and by study of whole populations by flow cytometry, immunohistochemistry, and in situ hybridization. Similar heterogeneity has been seen in populations of fibroblasts derived from lung and other tissues.[135]

The importance of this heterogeneity is sometimes difficult to assess. One possibility is that it represents a continuum of states of fibroblast differentiation. Alternatively, there may be discrete subtypes of fibroblast lineage, each with somewhat different metabolic capabilities. Because subtypes may have differential responses to environmental factors, including growth-modulatory cytokines, it is possible that subpopulations of fibroblasts may become selectively increased. This process of "clonal selection" may explain some abnormalities of fibroblast metabolism seen in fibrotic states. Scleroderma fibroblasts, for example, maintain increased collagen synthesis in vitro in the absence of continued stimulation by immune-derived cytokines that might have stimulated collagen synthesis in vivo.[136] In cultured scleroderma fibroblasts, compared to normal, there is overrepresentation of the subpopulations of cells with high collagen synthesis.[137] One possibility that could explain this finding is that in vivo processes have "selected" for high collagen–producing cells or clones. Indeed, it has been shown that the fibroblast subpopulation with high levels of receptors for C1q (first complement component) also maintains high levels of collagen synthesis.[138]

Several new techniques, including differential display and, more recently, gene array, promise to highlight further the differences between fibroblast populations, as well as the effects of cytokines on gene expression. Genes overexpressed by scleroderma fibroblasts and novel genes regulated by TGF-β have been identified using these techniques.[139,140]

MYOFIBROBLASTS

Myofibroblasts represent a subtype of fibroblasts that stain for a specific isoform of actin generally associated with smooth muscle cells: alpha-smooth muscle actin. In some cases, myofibroblasts may represent a distinct fibroblast cell lineage, but alpha-smooth muscle actin can also be induced from resting fibroblasts by TGF-β.[141] Myofibroblasts are present when there is active matrix deposition or connective tissue repair; increased numbers of myofibroblasts are present in granulation tissue and in scleroderma.[142]

Alpha-smooth muscle actin is not only a marker for myofibroblasts, but also plays a critical role in the special function of these cells. Fibers containing alpha-smooth muscle actin colocalize with beta-actin containing stress fibers and mediate the contractile force generated by these cells[143] (Fig. 12–10). This fibroblast "muscle" is important in generating the contractile force across healing wounds. It may also lead to pathologic contractile forces in fibrotic disease such as scleroderma. Myofibroblasts may also contribute to pathologic fibrosis through increased expression of collagen. Disruption of alpha-smooth muscle actin–containing fibers inhibits collagen expression by myofibroblasts. Thus, the formation of alpha-smooth muscle actin

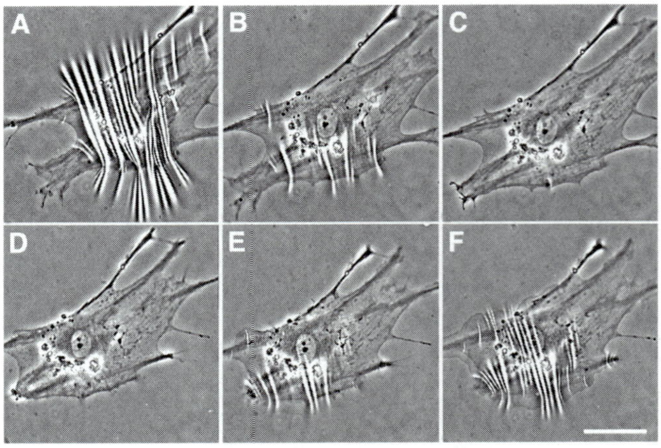

FIGURE 12-10 · Time-lapse photomicrographs of the effect of a specific inhibitor of alpha-smooth muscle actin on myofibroblast contraction of a silicone substrate. *A*, Myofibroblasts wrinkle the substrate. *B*, Inhibition of alpha-smooth muscle actin fibers for 15 minutes decreased wrinkling. *C*, Inhibition of alpha-smooth muscle actin fibers for 30 minutes also decreased wrinkling. *D*, Removal of the inhibitor leads to a gradual reoccurrence of wrinkling after 10 minutes. *E*, After 30 minutes. *F*, After 60 minutes. (Reproduced with permission from Hinz B, Gabbiani G, Chaponnier C: The NH2-terminal peptide of alpha-smooth muscle actin inhibits force generation by the myofibroblast in vitro and in vivo. J Cell Biol 157: 657-663, 2002.)

fibers mediates the contractile and fibrotic phenotype of these cells.

SYNOVIAL FIBROBLAST HETEROGENEITY

Fibroblast heterogeneity in normal synovial tissues has been shown by the characterization of markers present on synovial lining and sublining fibroblasts. Lining-layer fibroblasts express uridine diphosphoglucose dehydrogenase activity, an enzyme required for hyaluronan synthesis, indicating the specialized function of these cells in synovial fluid production. Both lining and sublining fibroblasts express VCAM-1. Neither of these markers is found on other fibroblast populations. Further uncharacterized heterogeneity may also exist as in the skin. Similar to dermal fibroblasts in scleroderma, abnormalities displayed by rheumatoid synovial cells in vitro may reflect overgrowth of particular synovial cell subpopulations.

Summary

The fibroblast is the foremost cell involved in reparative functions both in skin and visceral tissues. Reparative processes are initiated in response to injury or inflammatory stimuli. The fibroblast responds to cytokines and growth factors released in these circumstances by initiating cellular proliferation and matrix biosynthesis. In addition, the fibroblast is capable of matrix degradation and remodeling, a process that normally accompanies repair. With excessive activity of the immune system, reparative processes may not cease, because of either persistent stimulatory signals or the failure of inhibitory signals to retard fibroblast activity. In the latter instance, excessive and pathologic fibrosis may result. In addition, the fibroblast elaborates a variety of regulatory cytokines that modulate the proliferation and biosynthetic activity of other cell types.

REFERENCES

1. Agelli M, Wahl SM: Cytokines and fibrosis. Clin Exp Rheumatol 4:379-388, 1986.
2. Kovacs EJ: Fibrogenic cytokines: The role of immune mediators in the development of scar tissue. Immunol Today 12:17-23, 1991.
3. Korn JH, Piela-Smith T: Interaction of immune and connective tissue cells. *In* Nickoloff BJ (ed): Dermal Immune System. Vol. 1. Boca Raton, Fla., CRC Press, 1993, pp 185-208.
4. Piela TH, Korn JH: Lymphokines and cytokines in the reparative process. *In* Cohen S (ed): The Role of Lymphokines in the Immune Response. Boca Raton, Fla., CRC Press, 1990, pp 255-273.
5. Postlethwaite AE: Dermal fibroblast function. *In* Nickoloff BJ (ed): Dermal Immune System. Vol. 1. Boca Raton, Fla., CRC Press, 1993, pp 163-184.
6. Fries KM, Blieden T, Looney RJ, et al: Evidence of fibroblast heterogeneity and the role of fibroblast subpopulations in fibrosis. Clin Immunol Immunopathol 72:283-292, 1994.
7. Pierce GF, Mustoe TA, Altrock BW, et al: Role of platelet-derived growth factor in wound healing. J Cell Biochem 45: 319-326, 1991.
8. Pierce GF, Vande Berg J, Rudolph R, et al: Platelet-derived growth factor-BB and transforming growth factor beta1 selectively modulate glycosaminoglycans, collagen, and myofibroblasts in excisional wounds. Am J Pathol 138:629-646, 1991.
9. Klein CE, Dressel T, Steinmayer C, et al: Integrin alpha2beta1 is upregulated in fibroblasts and highly aggressive melanoma cells in three-dimensional collagen lattices and mediates the reorganization of collagen I fibrils. J Cell Biol 115:1427, 1991.
10. Nusgens B, Merrill C, Lapiere C, et al: Collagen biosynthesis by cells in a tissue equivalent matrix in vitro. Collagen Relat Res 4:351, 1984.
11. Xu J, Clark RF: Extracellular matrix alters PDGF regulation of fibroblast integrins. J Cell Biol 132:239, 1996.
12. Mochitate K, Pawelek P, Grinnell F: Stress relaxation of contracted collagen gels: Disruption of actin filament bundles, release of cell surface fibronectin, and downregulation of DNA and protein synthesis. Exp Cell Res 193:198, 1991.
13. Kadler KE, Holmes DF, Trotter JA, et al: Collagen fibril formation. Biochem J 316:1-11, 1996.
14. Hughes PE, Pfaff M: Integrin affinity modulation. Trends Cell Biol 8:359-364, 1998.
15. Wu C, Keivens VM, O'Toole TE, et al: Integrin activation and cytoskeletal interaction are essential for the assembly of a fibronectin matrix. Cell 83:715-724, 1995.
16. Zhong C, Chrzanowska-Wodnicka M, Brown J, et al: Rho-mediated contractility exposes a cryptic site in fibronectin and induces fibronectin matrix assembly. J Cell Biol 141:539-551, 1998.
17. Dawes KE, Gray AJ, Laurent GJ: Thrombin stimulates fibroblast chemotaxis and replication. Eur J Cell Biol 61:126-130, 1993.
18. Fukai F, Suzuki H, Suzuki K, et al: Rat plasma fibronectin contains two distinct chemotactic domains for fibroblastic cells. J Biol Chem 266:8807-8813, 1991.
19. Gu X-F, Raynaud F, Evain-Brion D: Increased chemotactic and mitogenic response of psoriatic fibroblasts to platelet-derived growth factor. J Invest Dermatol 91:599-602, 1988.
20. Postlethwaite AE, Seyer JM, Kang AH: Chemotactic attraction of human fibroblasts to type I, II, and III collagens and collagen-derived peptodes. Proc Natl Acad Sci U S A 75:871-875, 1978.
21. Postlethwaite AE, Keski-Oja J, Moses HL, et al: Stimulation of the chemotactic migration of human fibroblasts by transforming growth factor β. J Exp Med 165:251-256, 1987.
22. Senior RM, Griffin GL, Mecham RP: Chemotactic responses of fibroblasts to tropoelastin and elastin-derived peptides. J Clin Invest 70:614-618, 1982.
23. Hynes RO: Integrins: Versatility, modulation, and signaling in cell adhesion [Review]. Cell 69:11-25, 1992.
24. Assoian RK, Marcantonio EE: The extracellular matrix as a cell cycle control element in atherosclerosis and restenosis. J Clin Invest 98:2436-2439, 1996.
25. Yamada KM, Miyamoto S: Integrin transmembrane signaling and cytoskeletal control. Curr Opin Biol 7:681-689, 1995.
26. Chen Q, Kinch MS, Lin TH, et al: Integrin-mediated cell adhesion activates Mitogen-activated protein kinases. J Biol Chem 269:26602-26605, 1994.
27. Clark EA, Hynes RO: Ras activation is necessary for integrin-mediated activation of extracellular signal-regulated kinase 2 and cytosolic phospholipase A2 but not for cytoskeletal organization. J Biol Chem 271:14814-14818, 1996.
28. Hanks SK, Calalb MB, Harper MC, et al: Focal adhesion protein-tyrosine kinase phosphorylated in response to cell attachment to fibronectin. Proc Natl Acad Sci U S A 89:8487-8491, 1992.
29. Renshaw MW, Price LS, Schwartz MA: Focal adhesion kinase mediates the integrin signaling requirement for growth factor activation of MAP kinase. J Cell Biol 147:611-618, 1999.
30. Almeida EA, Ilic D, Han Q, et al: Matrix survival signaling: from fibronectin via focal adhesion kinase to c-Jun NH(2)-terminal kinase. J Cell Biol 149:741-754, 2000.
31. Wary KK, Mainiero F, Isakoff SJ, et al: The adaptor protein Shc couples a class of integrins to the control of cell cycle progression. Cell 87:733-743, 1996.
32. Persad S, Attwell S, Gray V, et al: Inhibition of integrin-linked kinase (ILK) suppresses activation of protein kinase B/Akt and induces cell cycle arrest and apoptosis of PTEN-mutant prostate cancer cells. Proc Natl Acad Sci U S A 97:3207-3212, 2000.
33. Hannigan GE, Leung-Hagesteijn C, Fitz-Gibbon L, et al: Regulation of cell adhesion and anchorage-dependent growth by a new beta 1-integrin-linked protein kinase. Nature 379:91-96, 1996.
34. Wu C, Dedhar S: Integrin-linked kinase (ILK) and its interactors: A new paradigm for the coupling of extracellular matrix to actin

cytoskeleton and signaling complexes. J Cell Biol 155:505-510, 2001.
35. Nobes CD, Hall A: Rho, Rac, and Cdc42 GTPases regulate the assembly of multimolecular focal complexes associated with actin stress fibers, lamellipodia and filopodia. Cell 81:53-62, 1995.
36. Tapon N, Hall A: Rho, Rac and Cdc42 GTPases regulate the organization of the actin cytoskeleton. Curr Opin Cell Biol 9: 86-92, 1997.
37. Felsenfeld DP, Choquet D, Sheetz MP: Ligand binding regulates the directed movement of z1 integins on fibroblasts. Nature 383:438-440, 1996.
38. Bar-Sagi D, Hall A: Ras and Rho GTPases: a family reunion. Cell 103:227-238, 2000.
39. Nobes CD, Hall A: Rho GTPases control polarity, protrusion, and adhesion during cell movement. J Cell Biol 144:1235-1244, 1999.
40. Beckmann MP, Betsholtz C, Heldin C-H, et al: Comparison of biological properties and transforming potential of human PDGF-A and PDGF-B chains. Science 241:1346-1349, 1988.
41. Seifert RA, Hart CE, Phillips PE, et al: Two different subunits associate to create isoform-specific platelet-derived growth factor receptors. J Biol Chem 264:8771-8778, 1989.
42. Hart CE, Forstrom JW, Kelly JD, et al: Two classes of PDGF receptor recognize different isoforms of PDGF. Science 240:1529-1531, 1988.
43. Heldin C-H, Ernlund A, Rorsman C, et al.: Dimerization of B-type platelet-derived growth factor receptors occurs after ligand binding and is closely associated with receptor kinase activation. J Biol Chem 264:8905-8912, 1989.
44. Heldin CH, Ostman A, Ronnstrand L: Signal transduction via platelet-derived growth factor receptors. Biochim Biophys Acta 1378:79-113, 1998.
45. Denhardt DT: Signal-transducing protein phosphorylation cascades mediated by Ras/Rho proteins in the mammalian cell: The potential for multiplex signalling. Biochem J 318:729-747, 1996.
46. Vojtek AB, Cooper JA: Rho family members: Activators of MAP kinase cascades. Cell 82:527-529, 1995.
47. Marshall CJ: Specificity of receptor tyrosine kinase signaling: Transient versus sustained extracellular signal-regulated kinase activation. Cell 80:179-185, 1995.
48. Hayflick L: The limited in-vitro lifetime of human diploid cell strains. Exp Cell Res 37:614-636, 1965.
49. Jelaska A, Korn JH: Anti-Fas induces apoptosis and proliferation in human dermal fibroblasts: Differences between foreskin and adult fibroblasts. J Cell Physiol 175:19-29, 1998.
50. Evan GI, Wyllie AH, Gilbert CS, et al: Induction of apoptosis in fibroblasts by c-myc protein. Cell 69:119-128, 1992.
51. Laytragoon LN: Programmed cell death: The influence of CD40, CD95 (Fas or Apo-I) and their ligands. Med Oncol 15:15-19, 1998.
52. Dayer J-M, Breard J, Chess L, et al: Participation of monocytes-macrophages and lymphocytes in the production of a factor that stimulates collagenase and prostaglandin release by rheumatoid synovial cells. J Clin Invest 64:1386-1392, 1979.
53. Korn JH, Halushka PV, LeRoy EC: Mononuclear cell modulation of connective tissue function: suppression of fibroblast growth by stimulation of endogenous prostaglandin production. J Clin Invest 65:543-554, 1980.
54. Magnaldo I, PouyssÇgur J, Paris S: Cyclic AMP inhibits mitogen-induced DNA synthesis in hamster fibroblasts, regardless of the signalling pathway involved. FEBS Lett 245:65-69, 1989.
55. Lee S, Solow-Cordero DE, Kessler E, et al: Transforming growth factor-beta regulation of bone morphogenetic protein-1/procollagen C-proteinase and related proteins in fibrogenic cells and keratinocytes. J Biol Chem 272:19059-19066, 1997.
56. Uzel MI, Scott IC, Babakhanlou-Chase H, et al: Multiple bone morphogenetic protein 1-related mammalian metalloproteinases process pro-lysyl oxidase at the correct physiological site and control lysyl oxidase activation in mouse embryo fibroblast cultures. J Biol Chem 276:22537-22543, 2001.
57. Munger JS, Harpel JG, Gleizes PE, et al: Latent transforming growth factor-beta: Structural features and mechanisms of activation. Kidney Int 51:1376-1382, 1997.
58. Kanzaki T, Olofsson A, Moren A, et al: TGF-beta 1 binding protein: a component of the large latent complex of TGF-beta 1 with multiple repeat sequences. Cell 61:1051-1061, 1990.
59. Saharinen J, Hyytiainen M, Taipale J, et al: Latent transforming growth factor-beta binding proteins (LTBPs)– structural extracellular matrix proteins for targeting TGF-beta action. Cytokine Growth Factor Rev 10:99-117, 1999.
60. Lyons RM, Keski-Oja J, Moses HL: Proteolytic activation of latent transforming growth factor-beta from fibroblast-conditioned medium. J Cell Biol 106:1659-1665, 1988.
61. Munger JS, Huang X, Kawakatsu H, et al: The integrin alpha v beta 6 binds and activates latent TGF beta 1: A mechanism for regulating pulmonary inflammation and fibrosis. Cell 96:319-328, 1999.
62. Ribeiro SM, Poczatek M, Schultz-Cherry S, et al: The activation sequence of thrombospondin-1 interacts with the latency-associated peptide to regulate activation of latent transforming growth factor-beta. J Biol Chem 274:13586-13593, 1999.
63. Verrecchia F, Mauviel A: Transforming growth factor-beta signaling through the Smad pathway: Role in extracellular matrix gene expression and regulation. J Invest Dermatol 118:211-215, 2002.
64. Leask A, Holmes A, Abraham DJ: Connective tissue growth factor: A new and important player in the pathogenesis of fibrosis. Curr Rheumatol Rep 4:136-142, 2002.
65. Springer TA: Traffic signals for lymphocyte recirculation and leukocyte emigration: The multistep paradigm [Review]. Cell 76:301-314, 1994.
66. Carr MW, Roth SJ, Luther E, et al: Monocyte chemoattractant protein 1 acts as a T-lymphocyte chemoattractant. Proc Natl Acad Sci U S A 91:3652-3656, 1994.
67. Cruikshank WW, Center DM, Nisar N, et al: Molecular and functional analysis of a lymphocyte chemoattractant factor: Association of biologic function with CD4 expression. Proc Natl Acad Sci U S A 91:5109-5113, 1994.
68. Korn JH, Downie E: Clonal interactions in fibroblast proliferation: recognition of self vs. non-self. J Cell Physiol 141:437-440, 1989.
69. Taub DD, Lloyd AR, Wang JM, et al: The effects of human recombinant MIP-1 alpha, MIP-1 beta, and RANTES on the chemotaxis and adhesion of T cell subsets. Adv Exp Med Biol 351:139-146, 1993.
70. Piela TH, Korn JH: Lymphocyte-fibroblast adhesion induced by interferon-gamma. Cell Immunol 114:149-160, 1988.
71. Rothlein R, Czajkowski M, O'Neill MM, et al: Induction of intercellular adhesion molecule 1 on primary and continuous cell lines by pro-inflammatory cytokines: Regulation by pharmacologic agents and neutralizing antibodies. J Immunol 141:1665-1669, 1988.
72. Abraham D, Lupoli S, McWhirter A, et al: Expression and function of surface antigens on scleroderma fibroblasts. Arthritis Rheum 34:1164-1172, 1991.
73. Piela TH, Korn JH: ICAM-1 dependent fibroblast-lymphocyte adhesion: discordance between expression and function of ICAM-1. Cell Immunol 129:125-137, 1990.
74. Piela-Smith TH, Broketa G, Hand A, et al: Regulation of ICAM-1 expression and function in human dermal fibroblasts by IL-4. J Immunol 148:1375-1381, 1992.
75. Gullberg D, Gehlsen KR, Turner DC, et al: Analysis of alpha 1 beta 1, alpha 2 beta 1 and alpha 3 beta 1 integrins in cell–collagen interactions: identification of conformation dependent alpha 1 beta 1 binding sites in collagen type I. EMBO J 11:3865-3873, 1992.
76. Liao N-S, St. John J, McCarthy JB, et al: Adhesion of lymphoid cells to the carboxyl-terminal heparin-binding domains of fibronectin. Exp Cell Res 181:348-361, 1989.
77. Takada Y, Elices MJ, Crouse C, et al: The primary structure of the alpha 4 subunit of VLA-4: Homology to other integrins and a possible cell-cell adhesion function. EMBO J 8:1361-1368, 1989.
78. Lorenzo JA, Jastrzebski SL, Kalinowski JF, et al: Tumor necrosis factor alpha stimulates production of leukemia inhibitory factor in human dermal fibroblast cultures. Clin Immunol Immunopathol 70:260-265, 1994.
79. Nakagawa S, Pawelek P, Grinnell F: Extracellular matrix organization modulates fibroblast growth and growth factor responsiveness. Exp Cell Res 182:572-582, 1989.
80. Nishiyama T, Akutsu N, Horii I, et al: Response to growth factors of human dermal fibroblasts in a quiescent state owing to cell-matrix contact inhibition. Matrix 11:71-75, 1991.

81. Rhudy RW, McPherson JM: Influence of the extracellular matrix on the proliferative response of human skin fibroblasts to serum and purified platelet-derived growth factor. J Cell Physiol 137:185-191, 1988.
82. Lin YC, Grinnell F: Decreased level of PDGF-stimulated receptor autophosphorylation by fibroblasts in mechanically relaxed collagen matrices. J Cell Biol 122:663-672, 1993.
83. Raines EW, Dower SK, Ross R: Interleukin 1 mitogenic activity for fibroblasts and smooth muscle cells is due to PDGF-AA. Science 243:393-396, 1989.
84. Ishikawa O, LeRoy EC, Trojanowska M: Mitogenic effect of transforming growth factor beta 1 on human fibroblasts involves the induction of platelet-derived growth factor alpha receptors. J Cell Physiol 145:181-186, 1990.
85. Phillips PD, Pignolo RJ, Cristofalo VJ: Insulin-like growth factor-I: Specific binding to high and low affinity sites and mitogenic action throughout the life span of WI-38 cells. J Cell Physiol 133:135-143, 1987.
86. Storch TG, Talley GD: Oxygen concentration regulates the proliferative response of human fibroblasts to serum and growth factors. Exp Cell Res 175:317-325, 1988.
87. Monroe JG, Haldar S, Prystowsky MB, et al: Lymphokine regulation of inflammatory processes: Interleukin-4 stimulates fibroblast proliferation. Clin Immunol Immunopathol 49:292-298, 1988.
88. Postlethwaite AE, Seyer JM: Fibroblast chemotaxis induction by human recombinant interleukin-4. Identification by synthetic peptide analysis of two chemotactic domains residing in amino acid sequences 70-88 and 89-122. J Clin Invest 87:2147-2152, 1991.
89. Postlethwaite AE, Katai H, Raghow R: Human fibroblasts synthesize elevated levels of extracellular matrix in response to interleukin 4. J Clin Invest 90:1479-1485, 1992.
90. Duncan MR, Berman B: Stimulation of collagen and glycosaminoglycan production in cultured human adult dermal fibroblasts by recombinant human interleukin 6. J Invest Dermatol 97:686-692, 1991.
91. Doucet C, Brouty-Boye D, Pottin-Clemenceau C, et al: IL-4 and IL-13 specifically increase adhesion molecule and inflammatory cytokine expression in human lung fibroblasts. Int Immunol 10:1421-1433, 1998.
92. Oriente A, Fedarko NS, Pacocha SE, et al: Interleukin-13 modulates collagen homeostasis in human skin and keloid fibroblasts. J Pharmacol Exp Ther 292:988-994, 2000.
93. Duncan MR, Berman B: Differential regulation of collagen, glycosaminoglycan, fibronectin, and collagenase activity production in cultured human adult dermal fibroblasts by interleukin 1-alpha and beta and tumor necrosis factor-alpha and beta. J Invest Dermatol 92:699-706, 1989.
94. Mauviel A, Daireaux M, RÇdini F, et al: Tumor necrosis factor inhibits collagen and fibronectin synthesis in human dermal fibroblasts. FEBS Lett 236:47-52, 1988.
95. Paulsson Y, Austgulen R, Hofsli E, et al: Tumor necrosis factor-induced expression of platelet-derived growth factor A-chain messenger RNA in fibroblasts. Exp Cell Res 180:490-496, 1989.
96. Reitamo S, Remitz A, Tamai K, et al: Interleukin-10 modulates type I collagen and matrix metalloproteaseX gene expression in cultured human skin fibroblasts. J Clin Invest 94:2489-2492, 1994.
97. Inoue A, Yanagisawa M, Kimura S, et al: The human endothelin family: Three structurally and pharmacologically distinct isopeptides predicted by three separate genes. Proc Natl Acad Sci U S A 86:2863-2867, 1989.
98. Xu S, Denton CP, Holmes A, et al: Endothelins: Effect on matrix biosynthesis and proliferation in normal and scleroderma fibroblasts. J Cardiovasc Pharmacol 31:360-363, 1998.
99. Woessner JF Jr: Matrix metalloproteinases and their inhibitors in connective tissue remodeling. FASEB J 543:2145-2154, 1991.
100. Harris ED J, DiBona DR, Krane SM: Collagenase in human synovial fluid. J Clin Invest 48:2104-2113, 1969.
101. Redini F, Lafuma C, Pujol JP, et al: Effect of cytokines and growth factors on the expression of elastase activity by human synoviocytes, dermal fibroblasts and rabbit articular chondrocytes. Biochem Biophys Res Commun 155:786-793, 1988.
102. Smith TH, Korn JH: Aminopeptidase N: A constitutive cell surface protein on human dermal fibroblasts. Cell Immunol 162:42-48, 1995.
103. Dayer JM, Russell RGG, Krane SM: Collagenase production by rheumatoid synovial cells: stimulation by a human lymphocyte factor. Science 195:181-183, 1977.
104. Postlethwaite AE, Lachman LB, Mainardi CL, et al: Interleukin 1 stimulation of collagenase production of cultured fibroblasts. J Exp Med 157:801-806, 1983.
105. Sirum-Connolly K, Brinckerhoff CE: Interleukin-1 or phorbol induction of the stromelysin promoter requires an element that cooperates with AP-1. Nucleic Acids Res 19:335-341, 1991.
106. Dayer JM, Beutler B, Cerami A: Cachectin/tumor necrosis factor stimulates collagenase and prostaglandin E2 production by human synovial cells and dermal fibroblasts. J Exp Med 162:2163-2168, 1985.
107. Brenner DA, O'Hara M, Angel P, et al: Prolonged activation of jun and collagenase genes by tumour necrosis factor-alpha. Nature 337:661-663, 1989.
108. Conca W, Kaplan PB, Krane SM: Increases in levels of procollagenase messenger RNA in cultured fibroblasts induced by human recombinant interleukin 1z or serum follow c-jun expression and are dependent on new protein synthesis. J Clin Invest 83:1753-1757, 1989.
109. Elias JA, Gustilo K, Baeder W, et al: Synergistic stimulation of fibroblast prostaglandin production by recombinant interleukin-1 and tumor necrosis factor. J Immunol 138:3812-3816, 1987.
110. Krane SM, Dayer J-M, Simon LS, et al: Mononuclear cell-conditioned medium containing mononuclear cell factor (MCF), homologous with interleukin 1, stimulates collagen and fibronectin synthesis by adherent rheumatoid synovial cells: Effects of prostaglandin E_2 and indomethacin. Collagen Related Res 5:99-117, 1985.
111. Mizel SB, Dayer JM, Krane SM, et al: Stimulation of rheumatoid synovial cell collagenase and prostaglandin by partially purified lymphocyte-activating factor (interleukin-1). Proc Natl Acad Sci U S A 78:2474-2477, 1981.
112. Overall CM, Wrana JL, Sodek J: Independent regulation of collagenase, 72-kDa progelatinase, and metalloendoproteinase inhibitor expression in human fibroblasts by transforming growth factor-bz. J Biol Chem 264:1860-1869, 1989.
113. Varga J, Jimenez SA: Stimulation of normal human fibroblast collagen production and processing by transforming growth factor-beta. Biochem Biophys Res Commun 138:974-980, 1986.
114. Brinckerhoff CE, Mitchell TI, Karmilowicz MJ, et al: Autocrine induction of collagenase by serum amyloid A-like and beta 2-microglobulin-like proteins. Science 243:655-657, 1989.
115. Lotz M, Guerne P-A: Interleukin-6 induces the synthesis of tissue inhibitor of metalloproteinases-1/erythroid potentiating activity (TIMP-1/EPA). J Biol Chem 266:2017-2020, 1991.
116. Maier R, Ganu V, Lotz M: Interleukin-11, an inducible cytokine in human articular chondrocytes and synoviocytes, stimulates the production of the tissue inhibitor of metalloproteinases. J Biol Chem 268:21527-21532, 1993.
117. Murphy G, Reynolds JJ, Werb Z: Biosynthesis of tissue inhibitor of metalloproteinases by human fibroblast cultures: Stimulation by 12-0-tetradecanoylphorbol 13-acetate and interleukin-1 in parallel with collagenases. J Biol Chem 260:3079-3083, 1985.
118. Walther Z, May LT, Sehgal PB: Transcriptional regulation of the interferon-beta 2/B cell differentiation factor BSF-2/hepatocyte-stimulating factor gene in human fibroblasts by other cytokines. J Immunol 140:974-977, 1988.
119. Zilberstein A, Ruggieri R, Korn JH, et al: Structure and expression of cDNA and genes for human interferon-beta-2, a distinct species inducible by growth-stimulatory cytokines. EMBO J 5:2529-2538, 1986.
120. Elias JA, Zheng T, Whiting NL, et al: IL-1 and transforming growth factor-beta regulation of fibroblast-derived IL-11. J Immunol 152:2421-2429, 1994.
121. DeMarco D, Kunkel SL, Strieter RM, et al: Interleukin-1 induced gene expression of neutrophil activating protein (interleukin-8) and monocyte chemotactic peptide in human synovial cells. Biochem Biophys Res Commun 174:411-416, 1991.

122. Taub DD, Conlon K, Lloyd AR, et al: Preferential migration of activated CD4+ and CD8+ T cells in response to MIP-1 alpha and MIP-1z. Science 260:355-358, 1993.
123. Franz JK, Kolb SA, Hummel KM, et al: Interleukin-16, produced by synovial fibroblasts, mediates chemoattraction for CD4+ T lymphocytes in rheumatoid arthritis. Eur J Immunol 28: 2661-2671, 1998.
124. Gauldie J, Richards C, Harnish D, et al: Interferon beta 2/B-cell stimulatory factor type 2 shares identity with monocyte-derived hepatocyte-stimulating factor and regulates the major acute phase protein response in liver cells. Proc Natl Acad Sci U S A 84:7251-7255, 1987.
125. Geiger T, Andus T, Bauer J, et al: Cell-free-synthesized interleukin-6 (BSF-2/IFN-z2) exhibits hepatocyte-stimulating activity. Eur J Biochem 175:181-186, 1988.
126. Marinkovic S, Jahreis GP, Wong GG, et al: IL-6 modulates the synthesis of a specific set of acute phase plasma proteins in vivo. J Immunol 142:808-812, 1989.
127. Fibbe WE, Van Damme J, Billiau A, et al: Human fibroblasts produce granulocyte-CSF, macrophage-CSF, and granulocyte-macrophage-CSF following stimulation by interleukin-1 and poly(rI).poly(rC). Blood 72:860-866, 1988.
128. Mantovani L, Henschler R, Brach MA, et al: Regulation of gene expression of macrophage-colony stimulating factor in human fibroblasts by the acute phase response mediators interleukin (IL)-1z, tumor necrosis factor-‡ and IL-6. FEBS Lett 280:97-102, 1991.
129. Needleman BW, Choi J, Burrows-Mezu A, et al: Secretion and binding of transforming growth factor beta by scleroderma and normal dermal fibroblasts. Arthritis Rheum 33:650-656, 1990.
130. Goldring SR, Stephenson ML, Downie E, et al: Heterogeneity in hormone responses and patterns of collagen synthesis in cloned dermal fibroblasts. J Clin Invest 85:798-803, 1990.
131. Korn JH: Substrain heterogeneity in prostaglandin E2 synthesis of human dermal fibroblasts: differences in prostaglandin E2 synthetic capacity of substrains are not stimulus restricted. Arthritis Rheum 28:315-322, 1985.
132. Korn JH, Brinckerhoff CE, Edwards RL: Synthesis of PGE2, collagenase and tissue factor by fibroblast substrains: substrains are differentially activated for different metabolic products. Collagen Relat Res 5:437-447, 1985.
133. Whiteside TL, Ferrarini M, Hebda P, et al: Heterogeneous synthetic phenotype of cloned scleroderma fibroblasts may be due to aberrant regulation in the synthesis of connective tissues. Arthritis Rheum 31:1221-1229, 1988.
134. Korn JH, Torres D, Downie E: Clonal heterogeneity in the fibroblast response to mononuclear cell derived mediators. Arthritis Rheum 27:174-179, 1984.
135. Jordana M, Schulman J, McSharry C, et al: Heterogeneous proliferative characteristics of human adult lung fibroblast lines and clonally derived fibroblasts from control and fibrotic tissue. Am Rev Respir Dis 137:579-584, 1988.
136. LeRoy EC: Increased collagen synthesis by scleroderma skin fibroblasts in vitro: a possible defect in the regulation or activation of the scleroderma fibroblast. J Clin Invest 54:880-889, 1974.
137. Jelaska A, Arakawa M, Broketa G, et al: Heterogeneity of collagen synthesis in normal and systemic sclerosis skin fibroblasts.Increased proportion of high collagen-producing cells in systemic sclerosis fibroblasts. Arthritis Rheum 39:1338-1346, 1996.
138. Bordin S, Page RC, Narayanan AS: Heterogeneity of normal human diploid fibroblasts: isolation and characterization of one phenotype. Science 223:171-173, 1984.
139. Strehlow D, Jelaska A, Strehlow K, et al: A potential role for protease nexin 1 overexpression in the pathogenesis of scleroderma. J Clin Invest 103:1179-1190, 1999.
140. Verrecchia F, Chu ML, Mauviel A: Identification of novel TGF-beta /Smad gene targets in dermal fibroblasts using a combined cDNA microarray/promoter transactivation approach. J Biol Chem 276:17058-17062, 2001.
141. Desmouliere A, Geinoz A, Gabbiani F, et al: Transforming growth factor-beta 1 induces alpha-smooth muscle actin expression in granulation tissue myofibroblasts and in quiescent and growing cultured fibroblasts. J Cell Biol 122:103-111, 1993.
142. Kissin E, Korn JH: Apoptosis and myofibroblasts in the pathogenesis of systemic sclerosis. Curr Rheumatol Rep 4:129-135, 2002.
143. Hinz B, Gabbiani G, Chaponnier C: The NH2-terminal peptide of alpha-smooth muscle actin inhibits force generation by the myofibroblast in vitro and in vivo. J Cell Biol 157:657-663, 2002.

WEBSITES

Fibroblast contractility and α-smooth muscle actin:
http://www.jcb.org/cgi/content/full/jcb.200201049/DC1
Scleroderma foundation:
www.scleroderma.org

13 Chondrocytes

MARY B. GOLDRING

Chondrocytes are the single cellular component of hyaline cartilage. Articular chondrocytes are considered to be fully differentiated cells that reside in cartilage once it is formed. Their apparent role is to maintain matrix constituents in a low turnover state of equilibrium. Chondrocytes serve diverse functions during development and postnatal life. In the embryo, they provide the templates, or cartilage anlagen, for the developing skeletal elements. Chondrocytes also represent the major cellular element in the growth plate, where the process of endochondral ossification leads to rapid postnatal growth of the skeleton. During development, the chondrocyte arises from mesenchymal progenitors from diverse sources, including the cranial neural crest of the neural ectoderm, cephalic mesoderm, sclerotome of the paraxial mesoderm, and the somatopleure of the lateral plate mesoderm. Temporal and spatial signals determine the stages of differentiation, which include proliferation, differentiation, maturation, and apoptosis and result in the formation of hyaline, elastic, and fibrous cartilage. Within the epiphyseal growth plate, the chondrocyte is responsible for longitudinal growth of the skeleton. The processes that control the different stages of skeletal development are described in Chapter 1.

In the adult, the anatomic distribution of cartilage is restricted primarily to the joints, trachea, and nasal septum, where the major function is anatomic support. In joints, cartilage has the additional function of providing low-friction articulation (see Chapter 6). In adult articular cartilage, chondrocytes comprise 2 to 5 percent of the tissue volume; the remainder is composed of a specialized matrix of collagens, proteoglycans, and other cartilage-specific and nonspecific proteins (see Chapter 1). Adult articular chondrocytes are relatively inactive metabolically due, in part, to the absence of a vascular supply and innervation in the tissue. Mature chondrocytes are remnants of the resting, proliferating, and prehypertrophic chondrocytes that laid down the original cartilage matrix during chondrogenesis and growth plate formation. The adult chondrocyte cannot recapitulate precisely the zonal variations in the cartilage matrix network that was formed originally, but it can respond to mechanic stimuli, growth factors, and cytokines that influence normal homeostasis in a positive or negative manner. Thus, it is within the articular cartilage that the chondrocyte has clinical importance. This chapter will focus on the articular chondrocyte, its normal functions, and its responses to adverse environmental insults that may modify its function.

Morphology, Classification, and Normal Function of Chondrocytes

MORPHOLOGY

The characteristic feature of the chondrocyte embedded in cartilage matrix is its rounded or polygonal morphology. The exception occurs at tissue boundaries, such as the articular surface of joints, where chondrocytes may be flattened or discoid. Intracellular features, including a rough endoplasmic reticulum, a juxtanuclear Golgi apparatus, and deposition of glycogen, are characteristic of a synthetically active cell. Stockwell[1] calculated that the cell density of full-thickness, human, adult, femoral condyle cartilage is maintained at 14.5 (± 3.0) × 10^3 cells per mm^3 from age 20 to 30 years. Because senescence of chondrocytes is known to occur with aging, it is logical to suppose that dead chondrocytes are replaced by mitosis. Mitotic figures, however, are not observed in normal adult articular cartilage.[2]

The morphology, density, and synthetic activity of an adult chondrocyte varies according to its position within the different zones of articular cartilage.[3,4] In the region of highest cell density, the superficial zone, the cells are flattened and oriented parallel to the surface along with the collagen fibers. Chondrocytes within the middle zone appear larger and more rounded and display a random distribution within the matrix, where the collagen fibers are also more randomly arranged. The chondrocytes in the deeper zones form columns that, along with the collagen fibers, are oriented perpendicular to the cartilage surface. The chondrocytes may exhibit different behaviors depending on their position within the different layers, and these zonal differences in synthetic properties may persist in primary chondrocyte cultures.[5,6] Chondrocyte volume in situ increases from the superficial through the deep zones and with the degree of cartilage degeneration.[7] A recent study, using confocal scanning laser microscopy (CSLM) of live, unfixed cartilage, has revealed fine cytoplasmic processes extending from the cell bodies of up to 40 percent of chondrocytes of all cartilage grades.[8] These processes are proposed to permit interactions among the chondrocytes and the cartilage matrix at near and remote sites. They are distinct from the cilia, which are observed by electron microscopy,[9] but not by CSLM.[8]

One of the challenges to researchers in the field of cartilage biology is the maintenance of morphology as a marker of chondrocyte phenotype for in vitro studies. When chondrocytes are isolated from their matrix and cultured in monolayer, they adhere to the culture dish and readily respond to serum growth factors, which stimulate proliferation of the normally quiescent cells. When plated at high density they maintain a polygonal, though flattened, morphology. However, at low plating densities, with prolonged culture, and upon expansion in serial subculture, they gradually assume a more elongated, "fibroblast-like" morphology. Early work suggested that this change in morphology is associated with a loss of phenotype, whereby the synthesis of cartilage-specific matrix molecules such as type II collagen and aggrecan decreases or disappears.[10] This "dedifferentiated phenotype," which has been described thus far only in vitro, is marked by the appearance of synthesis of type I and type III collagens, although type I collagen mRNA can be detected in normal articular cartilage, particularly in the superficial zone. A lack of correlation between cell shape and chondrocyte phenotype has been reported.[11,12] However, dedifferentiation of chondrocytes in monolayer culture appears to be associated with increased expression of genes involved in cell proliferation, such as cyclin D1.[13]

CLASSIFICATION: CELL ORIGIN AND DIFFERENTIATION

The chondrocyte arises in the embryo from mesenchymal origin. As described in detail in Chapter 1, chondrogenesis occurs as a result of cellular condensations at sites where skeletal elements will form.[14,15] The prechondrocytic mesenchymal cells produce extracellular matrix (ECM) rich in hyaluronan and collagen type I, as well as type IIA collagen containing the exon 2–encoded aminopropeptide found in noncartilage collagens. They initiate condensation by increasing hyaluronidase activity and the synthesis of the cell adhesion molecules, N-cadherin and neural cell adhesion molecule (N-CAM), which disappear in differentiating chondrocytes and are detectable later only in perichondrial cells. Fibronectin, syndecan, tenascin, and thrombospondin, as well as the intracellular signaling molecules, focal adhesion kinase and paxillin, are also expressed in the transition from chondroprogenitor cells to a fully committed chondrocyte. The transcription factor, Sox9, together with two other members of the Sry-type high mobility group box (SOX) family, L-Sox5 and Sox6, are early markers of the differentiating chondrocyte and are required for the onset of expression of type II (B) collagen, aggrecan, and other cartilage-specific matrix proteins such as type IX collagen. Common arrays of growth factors, signaling molecules, and transcription factors mediate responses at different stages of chondrocyte differentiation, although spatial and temporal relationships may vary from one stage to the other. Thus, the fate of a chondrocyte is dependent upon origin and location (Fig. 13–1).

The articular cartilage persists after joint cavitation. The chondrocytes that comprise the epiphyseal growth plates proceed through a differentiation program that leads to chondrocyte hypertrophy—a terminally differentiated state marked by type X collagen and chondrocyte apoptosis that facilitates endochondral ossification whereby bone replaces the calcified cartilaginous matrix of the hypertrophic chondrocyte (see Chapter 1). Thus, one major function of the chondrocyte is growth of the skeleton through proliferation and production of more cells, ECM production, and increased cell volume through hypertrophy. Following cessation of growth, the resting chondrocyte remains as part of the supporting structures in articular, tracheal, and nasal cartilages.

NORMAL FUNCTION OF THE ADULT ARTICULAR CHONDROCYTE

The mature articular chondrocyte embedded in its ECM is a resting cell with no detectable mitotic activity and a very low rate of synthetic activity. Because articular cartilage is not vascularized, the chondrocyte must rely upon diffusion from the articular surface for the exchange of nutrients and metabolites. As a consequence, the chondrocyte metabolism operates at low oxygen tension within the cartilage matrix, ranging from 10 percent at the surface to less than 1 percent in the deep zone. The majority of the energy requirements are fulfilled by glycolysis and, thus, the chondrocytes do not normally contain abundant mitochondria. Nevertheless, when cultured in a range of oxygen tensions between 0.1-percent O_2 and 20-percent O_2, the lower oxygen tensions upregulate the levels of anabolic genes, such as transforming growth factor-β (TGF-β) and connective tissue growth factor.[16] Chondrocytes are able to adapt to low oxygen tension, in part by changes in transcription factors such as hypoxia inducible factor-1 (HIF-1) and activator protein-1 (AP-1).[17] However, hyperoxic (55% O_2) conditions may increase the breakdown of cartilage collagens in articular cartilage in the presence of vascularized rheumatoid synovium.[18] Chondrocytes also maintain active membrane transport systems for exchange of cations, including Na^+, K^+, $Ca2^+$, and H^+, whose intracellular concentrations fluctuate with load and changes in the composition of the cartilage matrix.[19]

The consumption of oxygen by cartilage on a per-cell basis is only 2 to 5 percent of that in liver or kidney, although the amounts of lactate produced are comparable. Thus, energy metabolism in chondrocytes depends strongly on the glucose supply, and the requirements may be modulated by mechanical stress.[20] Glucose serves as the major energy source for the chondrocytes and as an essential precursor for glycosaminoglycan synthesis.[21-23] Facilitated glucose transport in chondrocytes is mediated by several distinct glucose transporter proteins (GLUTs) that are either constitutively expressed (GLUT3 and GLUT8) or cytokine-inducible (GLUT1 and GLUT6).[24,25] The relative expression of these proteins may determine the capacity of chondrocytes to survive in cartilage matrix and to modulate metabolic activity in response to the environmental changes.

CHONDROCYTE SYNTHETIC PRODUCTS

The expression patterns of matrix proteins by chondrocytes within cartilage from human and animal sources have been mapped by immunohistochemistry and in situ hybridization to localize protein and mRNA levels, respectively (see Chapter 1, Table 1-1 for complete listing

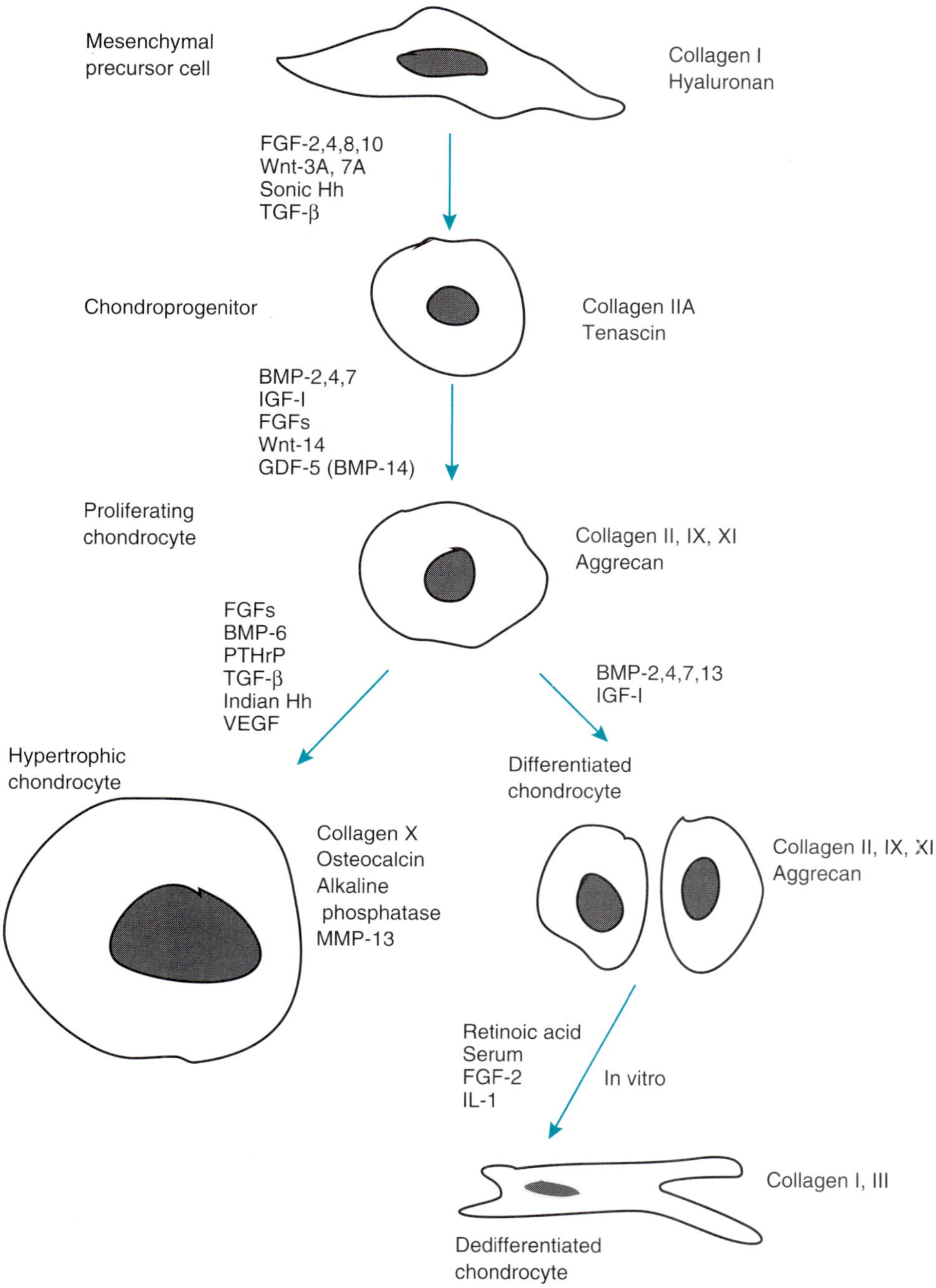

FIGURE 13–1 · Schematic representation of cellular phenotypes associated with developmental fates during chondrocyte differentiation. Some of the regulatory factors active at different stages are listed adjacent to the arrows. The major extracellular matrix genes are listed to the right of each cell type in which they are differentially expressed.

of cartilage matrix constituents). The markers of mature articular chondrocytes are type II collagen (COL2A1) other cartilage-specific collagens, such as IX (COL9) and XI (COL11), the large aggregating proteoglycan aggrecan, and link protein (Table 13–1). The synthesis of small proteoglycans such as biglycan and decorin and other specific and nonspecific matrix proteins has been examined both in vivo and in vitro. In normal adult articular cartilage, the chondrocytes synthesize matrix components very slowly. The turnover of collagen has been estimated to occur with a half-life of more than 100 years,[26,27] whereas the glycosaminoglycan constituents on the aggrecan core protein are more readily replaced, and the half-life of aggrecan subfractions has been estimated in the range of 3 to 24 years.[28] The chondrocyte maintains a steady-state metabolism resulting from equilibrium between anabolic processes and catabolic processes that result in the normal turnover of matrix molecules. The complex composition of the articular cartilage matrix is more difficult for the chondrocyte to replicate if severe damage to the collagen network occurs. Nevertheless, chondrocytes in vivo respond to structural changes in the surrounding cartilage matrix as occurs during the initial stages of osteoarthritis (OA), in which increased chondrocyte proliferation and synthesis of matrix proteins, proteinases, and cytokines are observed. The metabolic potential of these cells is also indicated by their capacity to proliferate in culture and synthesize matrix proteins after enzymatic release from the cartilage of even elderly individuals.

TABLE 13–1 • CARTILAGE-MATRIX COMPONENTS SYNTHESIZED BY CHONDROCYTES*

Collagens
Type II
Type IX
Type XI
Type VI
Types XII, XIV
Type X (hypertrophic chondrocyte)
Proteoglycans
Aggrecan
Versican
Link protein
Biglycan (DS-PGI)
Decorin (DS-PGII)
Epiphycan (DS-PGIII)
Fibromodulin
Lumican
Proline/arginine-rich and leucine-rich repeat protein (PRELP)
Chondroadherin
Perlecan
Lubricin (SZP)
Other Noncollagenous Proteins (structural)
Cartilage oligomeric matrix protein (COMP), or thrombospondin-5
Thrombospondin-1 and -3
Cartilage matrix protein (matrilin-1); matrilin-3
Fibronectin
Tenascin-c
Cartilage intermediate layer protein (CILP)
Fibrillin
Elastin
Other Noncollagenous Proteins (regulatory)
Glycoprotein (gp)-39, YKL-40
Matrix Gla protein (MGP)
Chondromodulin-I (SCGP) and -II
Cartilage-derived retinoic acid-sensitive protein (CD-RAP)
Growth factors
Membrane-Associated Proteins
Integrins (α1β1, α2β1, α3β1, α5β1, α6β1, α10β1, αvβ3, αvβ5)
Anchorin CII (annexin V)
Cell determinant 44 (CD44)
Syndecan-3

*The collagens, proteoglycans, and other noncollagenous proteins in the cartilage matrix are synthesized by chondrocytes at different stages during development and growth of cartilage, and the mature articular chondrocyte may have a limited capacity to maintain and repair some of the matrix components, particularly proteoglycans. Proteins that are associated with chondrocyte cell membranes are also listed because they permit specific interactions with extracellular matrix proteins. The specific structure-function relationships are discussed in Chapter 1 and described in Table 1-1.

Abbreviations: DS-PG, dermatan sulfate proteoglycan; SCGP, small cartilage-derived glycoprotein; SZP, superficial zone protein; YKL-40, 40KD chitinase 3-like glycoprotein.

Attempts to map the abnormal occurrence and distribution of matrix proteins in OA cartilage and other cartilage pathologies have provided insights into pathogenesis of joint disease. Thus, phenotypic alterations have been reported, such as the appearance of the chondroprogenitor collagen type IIA, the splice variant of the normal cartilage-specific type IIB collagen (COL2B1), as well as a reactivation of COL2A1 and aggrecan expression in the middle zones of OA cartilage.[29,30] A recapitulation of the fetal skeletal development also occurs in the deep and calcified zones where the hypertrophic chondrocyte-specific type X collagen is expressed and in the upper middle zone where type III collagen expression is detected.[31] The increase in pericellular type VI collagen microfibrils also indicates that the chondrocyte is able to respond to changes in its microenvironment.[32] The early response of the chondrocytes in the OA lesion is to increase the synthesis of type II collagen and aggrecan.[33] However, the capacity of the adult articular chondrocyte to regenerate the normal cartilage matrix architecture is limited, and the damage becomes irreversible unless the degradative process is interrupted.

Culture Models for Studying Chondrocyte Metabolism

Primary cultures of articular chondrocytes isolated from various animal and human sources have served as useful models for studying the mechanisms controlling responses to growth factors and cytokines.[34-36] In monolayer, chondrocytes maintain a rounded, polygonal morphology in primary culture (Fig. 13–2), but there is a progressive loss of cartilage phenotype with passage of time. High-density monolayer cultures maintain the cartilage-specific phenotype until they are subcultured, although gene expression of type II collagen is generally more labile than that of aggrecan. This loss of phenotype is termed *dedifferentiation,* during which chondrocytes lose the rounded, polygonal morphology and express some, but not all, characteristics of the fibroblast phenotype, such as type I collagen. It is possible to expand the cultures through a limited number of subcultures and "redifferentiate" the cells in fluid or gel suspension cultures, in which the chondrocytes regain morphology and the cessation of proliferation is associated with increased expression of cartilage-specific matrix proteins.[37] Alternatively, explant cultures of articular cartilage in which the chondrocytes remain encased within their own ECM have been used as in vitro models to study cartilage biochemistry and metabolism, as described in the following section.

ARTICULAR CHONDROCYTES

Cartilage Explant (Organ) Cultures

Based on the pioneering work of Fell,[38] who showed that it was possible to maintain pieces of cartilage in culture, the explant culture system was used to characterize chondrocyte function in cartilage from various species, including humans, at different ages. The early work in bovine cartilage established the mechanisms of biosynthesis of cartilage proteoglycans under the influence of different serum concentrations and determined the turnover rate whereby the chondrocyte could maintain the balance between anabolic and catabolic pathways.[39] Methods developed for measuring the proteoglycan content in cartilage and the incorporation of ^{35}S-sulfate into newly synthesized proteoglycans are used widely as the standard assays for assessing cartilage metabolism.[40-42] Cartilage organ cultures also maintain constant levels of type II collagen during several weeks of culture, as well as the characteristic morphology and banding pattern of

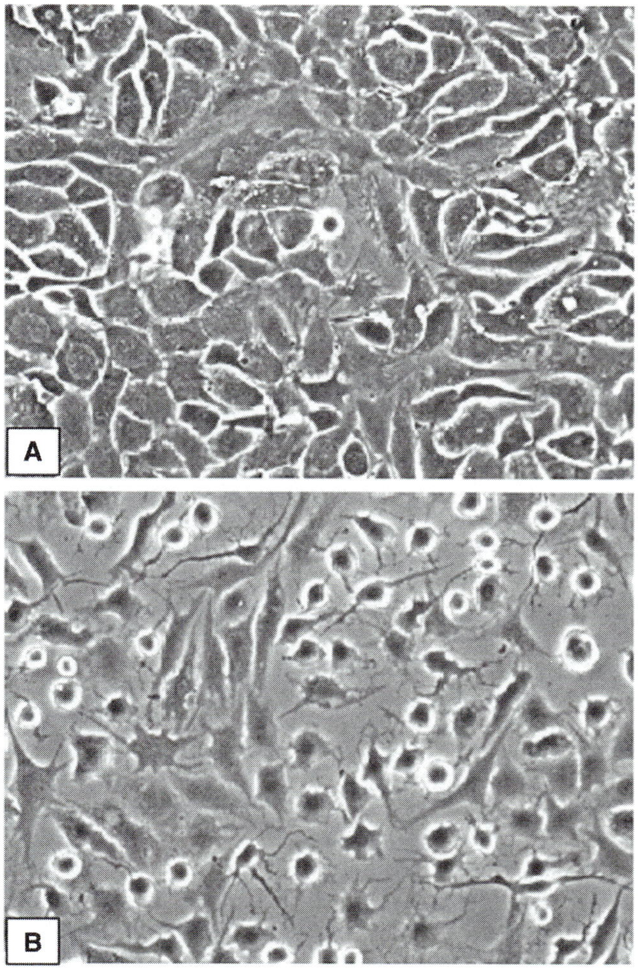

FIGURE 13–2 · Morphology of Human Articular Chondrocytes Grown in Monolayer Culture on Plastic. Chondrocytes were isolated from articular cartilage and cultured in growth medium containing 10 percent fetal calf serum until confluent. The cultures were changed to serum-free defined medium, interleukin-1β (IL-1β) was added the next day, and incubation continued for 24 hours. *A*, Untreated chondrocytes display the characteristic cobblestone morphology. *B*, IL-1β–treated cultures respond with a dramatic morphologic change.

collagen fibers. Thus, they have been useful for studying the responses to damage by proteinases,[43] lipopolysaccharides,[44] interleukin-1,[41,45,46] retinoic acid,[47] and anabolic responses to growth factors.[48-50]

Monolayer Cultures

Primary monolayer cultures of chondrocytes isolated from young animals that maintain the cartilage-specific phenotype at least throughout primary culture are easily obtained and have been used widely to assess differentiated chondrocyte functions. Early attempts to culture chondrocytes from various animal and human sources were frustrated by the tendency of these cells to acquire a fibroblast-like morphology[51,52] associated with the appearance of type I collagen synthesis.[53,54] Freshly isolated human articular or costal chondrocytes express cartilage-specific type II collagen and continue to do so for several days to weeks in primary monolayer culture.[55,56] Other markers expressed in primary chondrocyte cultures include chondromodulin and protein S-100.[13,57,58] During prolonged culture and serial subculture, monolayer cultures begin to express type I and type III collagens. This dedifferentiation is associated with a decrease in the expression of one or more chondrocyte markers, particularly type II collagen,[55,59,60] and can be accelerated by plating the cells at low densities or by treatment with cytokines such as interleukin-1 (IL-1)[56,61] or retinoic acid. The use of chondrocytes of adult-human origin in studies related to the pathogenesis of joint diseases has been problematic, because the source of the cartilage cannot be controlled, sufficient numbers of cells are not readily obtained from random operative procedures, and the phenotypic stability of adult-human chondrocytes is lost more quickly upon expansion in serial monolayer cultures than in cells of juvenile-human[55] or embryonic- or postnatal-animal origin.[62,63] Because the stability of the phenotype of isolated chondrocytes is critically dependent on cell shape and cell density,[53,64] high-density micromass cultures is useful if sufficient numbers of chondrocytes can be obtained,[65,66] particularly for studying proteoglycan biosynthesis.[67] Collagen-containing matrix preparations, in which chondrocytes can be grown as monolayers, may also support phenotype, probably because of presence of growth and differentiation factors such as TGF-β that copurify with the matrix proteins.[68] Serum-free defined media of varying compositions, but usually including insulin, have also been used, frequently in combination with monolayer and other culture systems mentioned in the following section.[69]

Three-Dimensional Culture Systems

Early studies showed that phenotype could be maintained if the isolated chondrocytes are placed in suspension cultures in spinner flasks[51,70-73] or in dishes coated with nonadherent substrates.[74-76] Freshly isolated or subcultured chondrocytes can also be embedded in solid support matrices such as collagen gels[77] or sponges,[78,79] agarose,[5,6,10,59,80] or alginate.[81-86] In these three-dimensional (3D) matrices, chondrocytes have the normal spherical shape, synthesize and secret abundant cell-associated ECM components, and maintain phenotypic stability for several months. Because articular chondrocytes are unable to proliferate in fluid- or gel-suspension culture, expansion in monolayer culture followed by transfer to alginate or other suspension culture has been used as a strategy to obtain sufficient numbers of differentiated chondrocytes for study.[87] However, after prolonged culture in monolayer, dedifferentiated chondrocytes may lose irreversibly their chondrogenic potential.[88] The high-density pellet culture system, originally developed to study growth plate hypertrophy,[89] has also been used as a 3D model, because it permits articular chondrocytes to deposit a well-organized ECM containing type II collagen and aggrecan.[90-92] Isolated chondrons containing one or more chondrocytes within a capsule of pericellular matrix have also been used for in vitro studies of chondrocyte metabolism within a 3D environment.[93]

PREHYPERTROPHIC AND HYPERTROPHIC CHONDROCYTES: MODELS OF THE GROWTH PLATE AND TERMINAL DIFFERENTIATION

Tissues or cells from embryonic or young animals at specific developmental stages or with different developmental fates have been used widely to recapitulate in vitro the transitional stages of chondrogenesis, chondrocyte hypertrophy, and endochondral ossification.[62,63,94-98] A common feature of these models is the requirement for deposition of a collagenous matrix by sufficient numbers of cells following cessation of proliferation of chondrogenic cells in high-density monolayer cultures or their entrapment within a gel or suspension culture. Epiphyseal chondrocytes isolated from the long bones of postnatal immature rats and rabbits and cultured at high density progress through a differentiation pathway that mimics the transition from a type II collagen-producing, proliferating chondrocyte phenotype to the terminally differentiated type X collagen–producing hypertrophic phenotype associated with growth plate formation and endochondral ossification. Alkaline phosphatase, osteocalcin, and osteopontin have also been used as markers of terminal differentiation.[99] The pellet-culture system has been used widely to study terminal differentiation and hypertrophy, because it mimics the distribution of cells within the growth plate and is sufficiently organized to permit calcification in situ.[89,100-103] Arrest of cell proliferation and activation of type X collagen expression occurs when the serum concentration is reduced from 10 percent to 2 percent or lower. Insulin-like growth factor-I (IGF-I) or insulin added in serum-free medium or as a constituent of serum appears to be a universal basal requirement in these culture systems.[69,104-106] Ascorbic acid[107-109] and retinoic acid[110,111] have been used to promote terminal differentiation in vitro. The chondrocytes do not enter the later hypertrophic stage observed in vivo, which is characterized by type X collagen synthesis, cessation of type II collagen synthesis, and matrix mineralization, unless a steroid hormone, such as thyroxine, vitamin D_3 metabolite, or dexamethasone, is added to the medium.[105,106,112,113] Ectopic matrix mineralization may require a phosphate donor such as β-glycerophosphate (BGP).[103] However, in the presence of thyroxine, retinoic acid, or 1,25$(OH)_2$, vitamin D3 may inhibit chondrocyte hypertrophy.[114] In contrast, certain bone morphogenetic proteins (BMPs) (see following) alone or in the presence of ascorbic acid can induce hypertrophy in the absence of other additives, if the appropriate progenitor-cell population is used.[115]

IMMORTALIZED CHONDROCYTE CELL LINES

Several different approaches have been used in the attempt to develop cell lines that maintain the chondrocyte phenotype. Immortalization of avian, rabbit, mouse, and rat chondrocytes with viral oncogenes has generated cell lines with high proliferative capacities and at least some differentiated chondrocyte properties.[116-120] Chondrocyte cell lines have also arisen spontaneously from fetal rat calvaria[98,121] or have been derived from transgenic mice harboring the temperature-sensitive mutant of simian virus 40 (SV40) large T antigen (TAg).[122,123] Human chondrosarcoma cell lines express some aspects of the chondrocyte phenotype but are tumorigenic.[124,125]

Stable expression of SV40-TAg using plasmid or retroviral vectors has been a popular method for immortalizing human chondrocytes. However, clonal expansion usually results in type II collagen–negative cell lines that express types I and III collagens in monolayer culture,[126,127] whereas the loss of phenotype may be reversible if established monolayer cultures are maintained as nonclonal populations and selected by passaging through suspension cultures.[128,129] Human articular chondrocyte cell lines have also been established using the human papilloma virus type 16 (HPV-16) early function genes E6 and E7[130] and telomerase.[131] A general observation is that phenotypic stability of immortalized chondrocytes is lost during serial subculture in monolayer but can be restored by transfer to 3D culture in alginate[129] or hyaluronan[130] or to suspension culture in poly-(2-hydroxyethyl methacrylate) (polyHEMA)-coated dishes.[131]

Interactions of Chondrocytes with the Extracellular Matrix

INTEGRINS

Chondrocytes in vivo respond to structural changes in the ECM. The ECM provides not only a framework for the chondrocytes suspended within it, but its constituents also interact with cell-surface receptors and provide signals that regulate a number of chondrocyte functions. The most prominent of the ECM receptors are the integrins, which bind specifically with different ECM ligands and thereby induce the formation of intracellular signaling complexes that regulate cell proliferation, differentiation, survival, and matrix remodeling. Integrins may also serve as mechanoreceptors and mediate responses to normal and abnormal loading of cartilage. Chondrocytes express a number of different integrins that interact with cartilage ECM ligands, although they are not specific to this cell type. They include α1β1 that interacts with type I, type II, or type VI collagen,; α3β1 that interacts with type II collagen; α5β1 that interacts with fibronectin; and α10β1, another collagen-binding integrin.[132-136] The α5β1 integrin is the prominent integrin in human, adult articular cartilage.[132] Depending on the method of analysis, adult chondrocytes also express α1β1 and αvβ5 integrins accompanied by weaker expression of α3β1 and αvβ3.[134] Normal adult articular chondrocytes express little or no α2β1, whereas the expression of α2β1 and α6β1 integrins is associated with a proliferative phenotype, as in fetal chondrocytes, and in chondrosarcoma and immortalized chondrocyte cell lines.[137-139]

Because α1β1, α2β1, and α10β1 can all serve as receptors for cartilage-specific type II collagen,[133,135,136,139,140] there is great interest in determining whether they mediate differential responses of chondrocytes to changes in the ECM due to normal loading or pathologic changes.[141-144] The α1β1 has a broader ligand specificity than the other collagen-binding integrins and also mediates chondrocyte adhesion to the pericellular type VI collagen and to the cartilage matrix protein, matrilin-1.[142,145] The α2β1 integrin also binds to chondroadherin.[146] A general increase in integrin expression has been noted in OA chondrocytes in situ compared to those in normal adult articular cartilage.[135] The αv-containing integrins bind to vitronectin and osteopontin and may serve as alternative fibronectin (FN) receptors.[147] Because α5β1 acts as the primary fibronectin receptor, its modulation by FN fragments, which stimulate cartilage degradation via upregulation of metalloproteinases (MMPs) such as MMP-3 and MMP-13, may play a role in the pathogenesis of joint disease.[148-150]

Cellular binding to immobilized ECM proteins or integrin receptor aggregation with antibodies can promote a number of intracellular signaling events. As in other cell types, integrin signaling is mediated by interaction with nonreceptor protein tyrosine kinases such as pp125 focal-adhesion kinase and pyk2, which interact with the integrin cytoplasmic tail and induce a conformational change in the receptor subunits. Formation of these integrin-associated signaling complexes is associated with changes in organization of the cytoskeleton. Other signaling kinases, such as Src, Ras/Raf, Sos, and Mek family members may be associated with integrin signaling complexes and mediate downstream signaling cascades in a cell type– and ligand-specific manner.

Cooperation between integrins and growth-factor signaling appears to be a fundamental mechanism in the regulation of cellular functions. Integrin aggregation and receptor occupancy has been shown to enhance phosphorylation of growth factor receptors and mitogen-activated protein (MAP) kinase activation in many cell types. The anchorage-dependent mitogenic response to growth factors is thought to be due to synergy between integrin and growth-factor signaling. For example, the induction of chondrocyte proliferation by fibroblast growth factor (FGF) requires FN binding to α5β1 integrin.[151] The β1 integrin subunit also interacts with the IGF-I receptor upon treatment of chondrocytes with IGF-I.[152] Further-more, FN increases FGF-and IGF-I–stimulated proteoglycan synthesis in chondrocytes, and nitric oxide, which disrupts focal-adhesion signaling complexes, inhibits this process.[153] Type II collagen also increases TGF-β–induced type II collagen and aggrecan synthesis by a mechanism that is mediated by βl-integrin.[154,155]

Chondrocyte adhesion to FN or binding to FN fragments increases the production of cytokines such as IL-1, tumor necrosis factor (TNF), IL-6 and granulocyte-macrophage colony-stimulating factor (GM-CSF).[156,157] Synergies between FN/α5β1 and IL-1 action or production have been demonstrated in chondrocytes.[158,159] Normal chondrocytes use α5β1 as a mechanoreceptor and, subsequent to activation of the integrin-signaling cascade by mechanic stimulation, there is secretion of IL-4, which acts in an autocrine manner via the janus activating kinase (JAK)/signal transducer and activator of transcription (STAT) pathway to increase aggrecan mRNA and decrease MMP-3 mRNA levels.[143] However, OA chondrocytes appear to respond to α5β1 ligation by production of IL-1β and other proinflammatory mediators, whereas αvβ3 integrin ligation attenuates these responses.[159] Recent work indicates that FN fragments or blocking antibodies to α2β1 and α5β1 integrins can directly stimulate signaling via extracellular signal-regulated kinase (Erk) 1 or -2, c-Jun N-terminal kinase (JNK), and p38 MAP kinase (MAPK) in chondrocytes and increase MMP-13 production independent of autocrine production of IL-1β.[150] Collagen binding to α1β1 and α2β1 integrins also results in activation of distinct signaling pathways and may lead to opposite cellular responses.[160] Thus, the specificity of the response may depend on the relative expression of α-integrin subunits on the chondrocyte cell surface.

ANNEXINS

The annexins are a large family of proteins with diverse functions in nearly all eukaryotic cells that include calcium-, phospholipid-, and matrix-binding proteins. Three types, annexins II, V, and VI, have been detected in or on chondrocytes or associated with matrix vesicles.[161-164] Annexin V, or anchorin CII, was first detected in chick cartilage and described as a type II collagen–binding protein that anchors the chondrocytes to the ECM.[161,162] The expression of functionally deficient annexin V on the cell surface of chondrosarcoma cells may account for the inability of these cells to bind to the ECM.[165] In growth plate chondrocytes, annexins are required for calcium ion uptake and subsequent mineralization.[166] Annexin V expression is increased in OA cartilage, where it may have a role in apoptosis.[167] Annexin V antibodies block chondrocyte attachment to immobilized type II collagen more effectively than integrin antibodies,[168] but not to a cut cartilage surface, where the N-terminal collagen binding site may not be exposed.[169]

CELL DETERMINANT 44

Another cell surface receptor expressed in chondrocytes is cell determinant 44 (CD44), the hyaluronan-binding protein.[170,171] Through specific interactions with hyaluronan, CD44 has a role in assembly, organization, and maintenance of the chondrocyte pericellular matrix.[172-175] In chondrocyte cultures, the assembly of a newly synthesized pericellular matrix can be prevented or reversed by incubation with hyaluronan hexasaccharides or with a CD44 monoclonal antibody.[174,175] Although blocking CD44 has no effect on attachment of chondrocytes to a cut-cartilage surface,[169] recent evidence indicates that CD44 mediates the induction of MMP-1, -2, -9, and -13 by the heparin-binding FN fragment in articular cartilage.[176] Because FN fragments, as well as IL-l, enhance CD44 expression in chondrocytes,[177] cell-matrix interactions mediated by such cell surface receptors represent alternative mechanisms for cartilage damage in joint disease.

Angiogenic and Antiangiogenic Factors

Adult articular cartilage is among the few avascular tissues in mammalian organisms, and this property makes it resistant to vascular angiogenesis and invasion by inflammatory and neoplastic cells[178,179] Angiogenic inhibitors have been purified from normal cartilage.[180,181] However, in conditions where there is extensive remodeling of ECM, as in arthritis and during development, the cartilage becomes susceptible to invasion by vascular mesenchymal cells. In OA, angiogenic factors may contribute to chondrocyte activation and mineralization,[182] and in rheumatoid arthritis (RA), the ingrowth of blood vessels and synovial pannus into cartilage contributes to the degradation of the cartilage matrix.[183] Troponin I, MMP inhibitors, and chondromodulin-I have been proposed as cartilage-derived angiogenic inhibitors.[184,185] A recent study demonstrates that endostatin, a 20-kD proteolytic fragment of type XVIII collagen that is a potent angiogenesis inhibitor,[186] is expressed in human cartilage and fibrocartilage.[187] Vascular endothelial cell growth factor (VEGF), which is an essential mediator of angiogenesis during endochondral ossification[188,189] (see Chapter 1), is expressed in OA cartilage[190,191] and induced by IL-1, TNF-α, and hypoxia.[192] Thus, in OA in which abnormal biomechanics and joint effusions cause severe hypoxia, chondrocytes may produce VEGF, thereby inducing angiogenesis at the chondro-osseous junction and contributing to cartilage destruction.

TABLE 13–2 • ANABOLIC FACTORS INVOLVED IN CHONDROCYTE DIFFERENTIATION

Condensation and limb bud formation	FGF-2, 4, 8, 10 Wnt-3A, Wnt-7A Sonic hedgehog TGF-β
Chondrogenesis	BMP-2, 4, 7 IGF-I FGFs Wnt-14 GDF-5 (CDMP-1, BMP-14)
Chondrocyte hypertrophy	FGFs BMP-6 PTHrP TGF-β Indian hedgehog Noggin Chordin VEGF
Phenotypic stability of articular chondrocyte	BMP-2, -7, -13 IGF-I

Abbreviations: BMP, bone morphogenetic protein; CDMP, cartilage-derived morphogenetic protein; FGF, fibroblast growth factor; GDF, growth and differentiation factor; IGF, insulin-like growth factor; PTHrP, parathyroid hormone related protein; TGF-β, transforming growth factor-β; VEGF, vascular endothelial growth factor; Wnt, wingless type.

The Roles of Growth and Differentiation, or Anabolic, Factors in Normal Cartilage Metabolism

Growth and differentiation factors, such as IGF-I and members of the TGF-β or BMP family have been implicated as important regulators of cartilage-specific gene expression during development, growth and differentiation[34,193,194] (see Chapter 1). Because they oppose cartilage destruction by stimulating chondrocyte differentiation or proliferation and increasing the synthesis of matrix proteins and proteinase inhibitors,[195] they are also considered major anabolic factors for cartilage that can participate in matrix repair responses (Table 13–2). Different combinations of basic FGF (bFGF), TGF-β, and insulin or IGF-I have been used to promote chondrogenic differentiation and maintain type II collagen and proteoglycan synthesis by chondrocytes in vitro.[50,196,197]

INSULIN-LIKE GROWTH FACTOR

IGF-I, also known as somatomedin C, was first discovered as a serum factor controlling sulfate incorporation by articular cartilage in vitro[198] and was later found to have the capacity to specifically stimulate or maintain chondrocyte phenotype in vitro by promoting the synthesis of type II collagen and aggrecan.[48,50,199-204] IGF-I is more appropriately categorized as a differentiation factor, as its limited mitogenic activity appears to be dependent on the presence of other growth factors such as bFGF.[205] IGF-I may also serve as a survival factor for chondrocytes.[206] Both IGF-I and insulin can activate either the cell surface IGF-I tyrosine kinase receptor or the type I insulin receptor at concentrations proportional to their binding affinities. Further regulation of IGF-I activity is provided by specific IGF-binding proteins (IGFBPs) that do not recognize insulin. Chondrocytes at different stages of differentiation express IGF-I and IGF receptors, as well as different arrays of IGFBPs,[207-212] thus providing a unique system by which IGF-I can exert different regulatory effects on these cells. For example, IGFBP-2 appears to be a positive regulator in chondrocytes, because its induction by TGF-β or estrogen is associated with increased proteoglycan synthesis.[212,213] Binding of IGFBP-3 to IGF-I is thought to negatively regulate the anabolic functions of IGF-I,[206] although IGFBP-3 may directly inhibit chondrocyte proliferation in an IGF-independent manner.[214]

In OA cartilage, the normal anabolic function of IGF-I may be disrupted, because chondrocytes from animals with experimental arthritis and from patients with OA are hyporesponsive to IGF-I, despite normal or increased IGF-I receptor levels. This has been attributed to increased levels of IGFBPs that may interfere with IGF-I actions.[215-220] Disturbances in the balance of IGF-I to IGFBP-3, in particular, that have been reported in OA and RA joints[211,221-223] may contribute to defective chondrocyte responses to IGF-I.[206,224] Although IGF-I can oppose the effects of inflammatory cytokines that promote cartilage degradation and inhibit proteoglycan synthesis,[225] these cytokines also increase the production of IGFBP-3 by chondrocytes.[226] Overproduction of nitric oxide may also contribute to IGF-I resistance by chondrocytes.[227,228] The age-associated decline in the capacity of chondrocytes to synthesize proteoglycans in response to IGF-1 has also been attributed to increased IGFBP-3.[224,229]

FIBROBLAST GROWTH FACTOR

The FGF superfamily at present encompasses more than 20 distinct, but related, gene products that signal through four related receptor tyrosine kinases that are expressed on most types of cells in tissue culture.[230,231] Until recently, cartilage biologists have focused on bFGF, or FGF-2, which has distinct effects on type II collagen and proteoglycan synthesis by chondrocytes depending on the stage of differentiation and the culture conditions.[232,233] Identified originally as cartilage-derived growth factor,[234] bFGF is the most potent mitogen for chondrocytes[235] and may interact with IGF-I and TGF-β, which are not mitogenic, to promote or maintain specific chondrocyte functions, depending on the stage of differentiation of the cell population.[196,197,205,233,236] By itself, bFGF may have opposite effects compared to IGF-I, including inhibiting the expression and synthesis of cartilage-specific matrix proteins by mature chondrocytes.[237] For example, bFGF stimulates, whereas IGF-1 inhibits, expression of matrix Gla protein,[238] which is a marker for the chondrogenic lineage during development.[239-241] In proliferating, type II collagen–producing epiphyseal chondrocytes, bFGF stabilizes the phenotype and inhibits terminal differentiation to hypertrophic chondrocytes.[232] Thus, it is clear that FGFs and FGF receptors have important roles in chondrocyte differentiation and cartilage formation during development (see Chapter 1).

TABLE 13–3 • THE BONE MORPHOGENETIC PROTEIN SUPERFAMILY

Bone Morphogenic Protein	Other Names	Potential Function
BMP-2	BMP-2A	Cartilage and bone morphogenesis
BMP-3	Osteogenin, GDF-10	Bone formation
BMP-4	BMP-2B	Cartilage and bone morphogenesis
BMP-5		Bone morphogenesis
BMP-6	Vegetal-related-1 (Vgr-1)	Cartilage hypertrophy
BMP-7	Osteogenic protein-1 (OP-1)	Cartilage and bone morphogenesis
BMP-8	Osteogenic protein-2 (OP-2)	Bone morphogenesis
BMP-9	GDF-2	Cartilage morphogenesis
BMP-10		Unknown
BMP-11	GDF-11	Unknown
BMP-12	GDF-7, CDMP-3	Cartilage morphogenesis
BMP-13	GDF-6, CDMP-2	Cartilage morphogenesis
BMP-14	GDF-5, CDMP-1	Cartilage morphogenesis

Abbreviations: CDMP, cartilage-derived morphogenetic protein; GDF, growth and differentiation factor.

THE TRANSFORMING GROWTH FACTOR-β/BONE MORPHOGENETIC PROTEIN SUPERFAMILY

Activities of the TGF-β/BMP superfamily in the skeleton were first discovered as constituents of demineralized bone that induced new bone formation when implanted into extraskeletal sites in rodents.[242] These bioactive morphogens were subsequently extracted, purified, and cloned[243-250] and found to regulate the early commitment of mesenchymal cells to the chondrogenic and osteogenic lineages during cartilage development and endochondral bone formation[193] (Table 13–3). In addition to BMPs, the TGF-β superfamily includes activins, inhibins, müllerian duct inhibitory substance, nodal, glial-derived neurotrophic factor, and growth-differentiation factors (GDFs),[251-253] including the cartilage-derived morphogenetic proteins (CDMPs).[254] In addition to regulating cartilage condensation and chondrocyte differentiation, members of this superfamily also play key roles in site specification and cavitation of synovial joints[255,256] (see Chapter 1) and may also participate in the development of other organ systems.[257]

Many of these factors, including BMP-2, -6, -7, and -9, TGF-β, and CDMP-1, are able to induce chondrogenic differentiation of mesenchymal progenitor cells in vitro.[258-269] They also may have direct effects on mature articular chondrocytes in vivo and in vitro.[270-275]

Transforming Growth Factor-β

TGF-β was named based on its discovery as a factor that could transform cells to grow in soft agar. However, it is not a potent inducer of chondrocyte proliferation; rather, it may promote differentiation of chondroprogenitors at different stages (see Chapter 1). Both inhibition and stimulation of the synthesis of aggrecan and type II collagen by TGF-β have been observed in vitro.[50,272,276-280] However, TGF-β, by itself, cannot rescue the type II collagen phenotype once the cells have undergone dedifferentiation during serial passaging.[281]

Although early studies identified TGF-β as an inhibitor of protease release and inducer of tissue inhibitors of MMP (TIMP) expression, more recent work has shown it to be a potent inducer of MMP-13 expression.[282] The levels of TGF-β measured in synovial fluids of OA and RA patients[283] may reflect anabolic processes in cartilage and other joint tissues. This assumption is also supported by the detection of TGF-β mRNA in the articular cartilage in a murine model of spontaneous OA.[284] These and other studies in animals have implicated a dual role for TGF-β in OA. Single injections of TGF-β in the murine knee joint increase cartilage proteoglycan synthesis and IL-1 receptor antagonist (IL-1Ra) production, thereby protecting against IL-1–induced cartilage damage.[285,286] However, repeated injections of TGF-β produce long-term OA changes associated with severe proteoglycan depletion in the deep cartilage layers and increased osteophyte formation.[286]

Bone Morphogenetic Proteins

The BMPs, which include at least 13 individual molecules, may be divided into four distinct subfamilies based on the similarity of primary amino acid sequences: (1) BMP-2 and -2B (BMP-4), which are 92-percent identical in the 7-cysteine region; (2) BMP-3 (osteogenin) and BMP-3B (GDF-10); (3) BMP-5, -6, -7 (osteogenic protein-1, or OP-1), -8 (OP-2), -9 (GDF-2), -10, and -11 (GDF-11); and (4) BMP-12 (GDF-7 or CDMP-3), -13 (GDF-6 or CDMP-2), -14 (GDF-5, or CDMP-1), and -15.[193,251] BMP-1 is not a member of this family but is an astacin-related MMP that cleaves the BMP inhibitor chordin and acts as a procollagen C-proteinase.[287-289]

Several BMPs, including BMP-2, -4, -6, -7, and -9, have been shown to be capable of maintaining or enhancing expression of cartilage-specific matrix proteins in articular chondrocytes in vitro.[91,261,270,272,273,275,290-292] BMP-7 is expressed in mature articular cartilage[293] and is possibly the strongest anabolic stimulus for adult chondrocytes in vitro, because it increases aggrecan and type II collagen synthesis more strongly than IGF-I.[291] BMP-2 is also expressed in both normal and OA articular cartilage,[294] and it is a molecular marker, along with type II collagen and FGF receptor 3 (FGFR3), of the capacity of adult articular chondrocyte cultures to form stable cartilage in vivo.[295] BMP-2, BMP-7, and BMP-9 are able to oppose many of the detrimental effects of IL-1 on chondrocyte metabolism in vitro[296-299] and in vivo.[300] BMP-7 can prevent retinoic acid–induced dedifferentiation of articular chondrocytes.[292] However, BMPs have pleiotropic effects in vivo, acting in a concentration-dependent manner. While initiating chondrogenesis in the limb bud, they generally set the stage for bone morphogenesis (see Chapter 1). Furthermore, several BMPs are also true morphogens for other tissues, such as kidney, eye, heart, and skin.[193]

Because all BMPs first induce chondrogenesis during endochondral ossification, they may be termed *cartilage morphogenetic proteins*. However, whether they stimulate chondrocyte differentiation, rather than osteogenesis, depends on the cell type and culture conditions.[301] For example, C3H10T1/2 cells, which are multipotential progenitor cells, show dose-dependent differentiation into fat, cartilage, or bone cells in response to BMP-2 or -4.[260,302] BMP-2 strongly induces chondrogenesis in micromass cultures of the C3H10T1/2 cells.[303] The chondrogenic cell line, ATDC5, can be induced by BMP-2, -4, -7, or -14 (GDF-5) to undergo sequential chondrogenesis, which may continue through the stages of hypertrophy and matrix mineralization.[260,264,304,305] Cell lines that are already committed as osteoprogenitors, such as ROS17/2.8,[306] ROB-C26,[307,308] MC3T3-E1,[309] and C2C12[310,311] cells, cannot be induced to express the chondrogenic phenotype with BMP treatment.

Cartilage-Derived Morphogenetic Proteins

The isolation and cloning of the first BMP family members from bone prompted a search for cartilage morphogenetic proteins produced by articular cartilage. Three novel CDMPs, CDMP-1, -2, and -3, have been identified and cloned[254] and are classified as GDF-5, -6, and -7. CDMP-2 is found in articular cartilage, skeletal muscle, and placenta. CDMP-2 is also localized in the hypertrophic chondrocytes of the epiphyseal growth plate. CDMP-1 is a potent stimulator of chondrogenesis in vivo.[255,312] CDMP-1 and CDMP-2 maintain the synthesis of type II collagen and aggrecan in mature articular chondrocytes,[274,304,313] although they are less-effective initiators of chondrogenesis than other BMPs in early progenitor cell populations in vitro.[268,314,315]

Receptors, Signaling Molecules, and Antagonists That Mediate Chondrocyte Responses to Transforming Growth Factor-β/Bone Morphogenetic Protein Family Members

TGF-β/BMP family members, including CDMPs, transduce signals from the membrane to the nucleus via two types of membrane-bound serine-threonine kinase receptors, type I and type II, both of which are required for signal transduction[316-319] (Fig. 13–3). Seven types of type I receptors, termed *activin receptor-like kinases* (ALK), have been identified in mammals and have similar structures. TGF-β interacts with the type II receptor (TβRII), which, in turn, recruits a TGF-β type I receptor (principally TβRI) to form a heterotrimeric receptor complex. The constitutively active TβRII kinase phosphorylates TβRI at serine and threonine residues. Three type I receptors, BMP type IA (BMPR-IA or ALK-3), BMPR-IB (ALK-6), and ALK-2 mediate BMP signaling.[320] Although type I BMP receptors are able to bind ligand in the absence of type II BMP receptors, cooperativity has been demonstrated in binding assays. Upon ligand binding, analogous to TβRI and TβRII, BMP type I receptors are phosphorylated by the BMP type II receptors, which include activin (Act) RII, ActRIIB, and T-ALK. Thus, spatial and temporal differences in the distribution of these receptors in different tissues can govern the response patterns to different members of the TGF-β/BMP family.

The specificity of subsequent signals is mainly determined by the type I receptors. The phosphorylated BMP or TGF-β type I receptor in turn phosphorylates signal-transducing acceptor proteins, SMADs, which are related to the *Drosophila* mothers against decapentaplegic (MAD) and nematode SMA signaling molecules.[193,321] Smads 1 and 5 are activated by BMPs and Smads 2 and 3 are activated by TGF-β/activin.[321,322] Smad 4, which is distantly related to the ligand-specific SMADs, acts as a common partner for the BMP- or TGF-β–induced SMADs and forms heteromeric complexes that translocate to the nucleus and induce transcriptional activity.[323] Smads 6 and 7 act as inhibitors of phosphorylation of Smads 1 and 5. Cytoskeletal compartmentation of SMAD signaling complexes may regulate the differentiation of chondroprogenitor cells into chondrocytes.[298]

Noggin, chordin, and other BMP-binding proteins provide an additional mechanism for determining biologic responses to BMPs. Originally discovered in *Xenopus*, they act as antagonists by determining the bioavailability of BMPs for binding to BMP receptors.[324,325] The roles of noggin and chordin appear to be critical for determining boundaries during joint morphogenesis. They display different spatial and temporal patterns of expression, binding affinities, and susceptibility to proteinases that

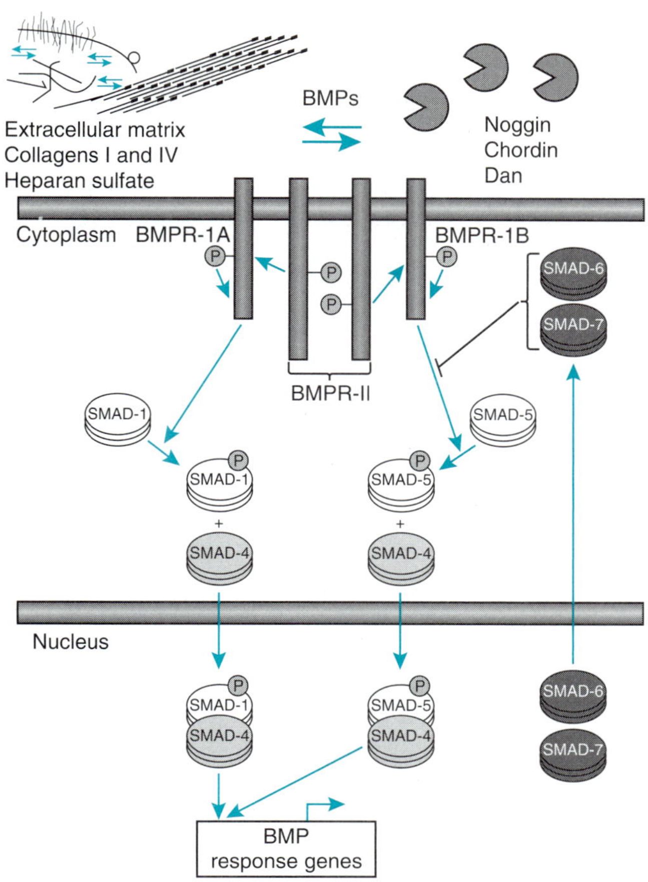

FIGURE 13–3 · **Bone Morphogenetic Protein (BMP) Receptors and Signaling Cascade.** BMPs are dimeric ligands with a single interchain, disulfide bond. BMPs interact with type I and II BMP receptors (BMP-RI and BMP-RII). BMP-RII phosphorylates BMP-RI and activates the serine/threonine kinase receptor. The BMP-RI protein serine/threonine kinase phosphorylates cytoplasmic signaling substrates Smad 1 or Smad 5. This phosphorylation is modulated and inhibited by inhibitory Smads 6 and 7. Phosphorylated Smads 1 and 5 interact with a common co-Smad 4 and are translocated into the nucleus to initiate the transcription of BMP-response genes. A Smad interacting protein (SIP) modulates binding of the Smad 1/4 complex to DNA. The bioavailability of BMP for interaction with cognate receptors is critically dependent on BMP binding proteins and antagonists, such as noggin and chordin, and also extracellular matrix components such as collagens I and IV and heparan sulfate. (Reprinted with permission from Reddi AH: Role of morphogenetic proteins in skeletal tissue engineering and regeneration. Nature Biotech 16:247-252, 1998.)

release BMP.[326-328] BMPs bind to chordin and noggin via cysteine-rich domains that are similar to domains in the N-terminal–propeptides of fibrillar procollagens I, II, II, and V that also bind BMPs and are susceptible to cleavage by MMPs.[329,330] BMP may be released from chordin by cleavage with MMPs or BMP-1/tolloid, whereas noggin binds BMP with high affinity and cannot be cleaved to release BMP. Thus, there are several mechanisms by which bioavailability of BMPs may be controlled during chondrogenesis. Whether the interactions between BMPs and BMP antagonists have roles in mature cartilage or in cartilage regeneration are the subject of current investigations.[195]

The Role of the Chondrocyte in Cartilage Pathology

The chondrocyte, the unique cell type in mature cartilage, maintains a stable equilibrium between the synthesis and the degradation of matrix components. During aging and joint diseases, such as RA and OA, this equilibrium is disrupted and the rate of loss of collagens and proteoglycans from the matrix exceeds the rate of deposition of newly synthesized molecules. Cartilage destruction in RA occurs primarily in areas contiguous with the proliferating synovial pannus due to the release and activation of proteinases from the synovial cells and, to some extent, at the cartilage surface exposed to matrix-degrading enzymes from polymorphonuclear leukocytes in the synovial fluids. In addition to the direct action of proteinases, the RA synovial tissues contribute indirectly to cartilage loss by releasing cytokines and other mediators that act on the chondrocytes to produce dysregulation of chondrocyte function.[331] The role of cytokines in cartilage destruction in RA is well established based on studies in animal models.[332] There is some evidence that the chondrocytes themselves may participate not only by responding to but also by producing various proinflammatory, inhibitory, and anabolic cytokines. The cartilage destruction in OA is believed to be chondrocyte-mediated in response to biomechanic insult, which may occur directly or indirectly through generation of cytokines that stimulate the production of cartilage matrix–degrading proteinases. The impact of cytokines on chondrocyte function, particularly with respect to their various roles in cartilage destruction, has been reviewed extensively[35,36,333-337] (Fig. 13–4).

CARTILAGE MATRIX–DEGRADING PROTEINASES

A large body of research has established that cartilage degradation is mediated by matrix MMPs, aggrecanases, and other proteinases produced by the chondrocytes themselves in OA or by the synovial cells along the cartilage-pannus junction in RA. MMPs are localized in regions of cartilage degradation[338-341] and detected in synovial fluids and cartilage from OA and RA patients[342-344] and in animal models of arthritis.[345] In early studies, chondrocytes were among the first identified sources of TIMP-1,[346,347] and they are now known to synthesize additional TIMPs.[348,349] Chondrocytes, therefore, are assumed to be a major source of the TIMPs, as well as MMPs, detected in synovial fluids from OA and RA patients, where they reflect an adaptive response to the local imbalance due to increased production of active MMPs by chondrocytes and other joint tissues.[350,351]

The MMPs of the collagenase and stromelysin families have been given greatest attention because they are produced by chondrocytes and can specifically degrade native collagens and proteoglycans in cartilage matrix[352] (Table 13–4). The collagenases implicated in collagen degradation include collagenases 1-, -2, and -3 (MMP-1, -8, -13) and membrane type I MMP (MT1)-MMP, or MMP-14).[353-356] The expression of MMP-13 in OA and RA cartilage and its ability to more effectively degrade type II

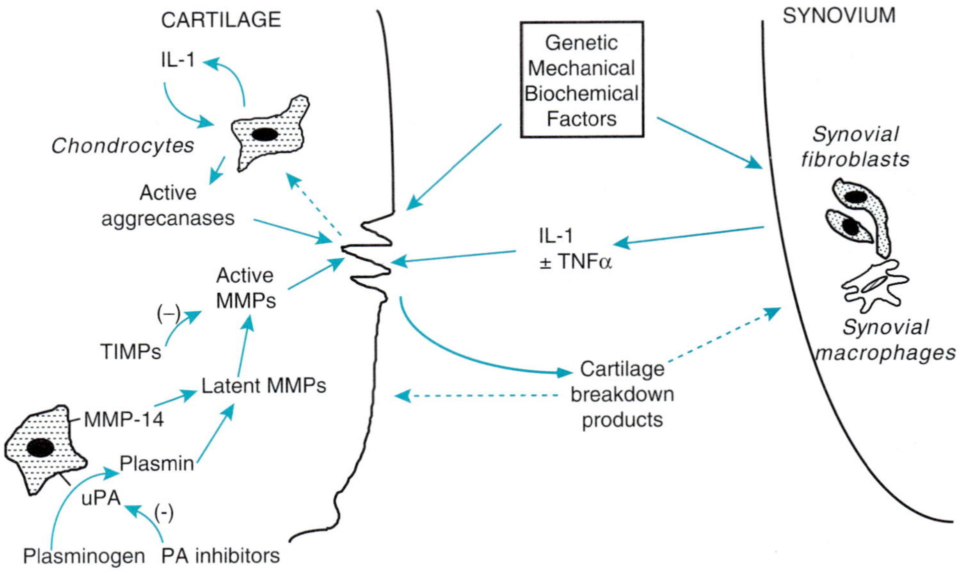

FIGURE 13–4 • **The Role of Chondrocyte-Derived Proteinases in Cartilage Destruction in Osteoarthritis.** Although studies in vitro and in vivo have shown that the chondrocyte can respond directly to mechanic loading, to catabolic cytokines such as interleukin-1 (IL-1) and tumor necrosis factor-α (TNF-α), and to cartilage breakdown products, the initiating signals and their relative importance have not been defined clearly. (Reprinted with permission from Goldring MB: Osteoarthritis and cartilage: the role of cytokines. Curr Rheumatol Rep 2:459-465, 2000.)

TABLE 13–4 • **CHONDROCYTE PROTEINASES THAT MEDIATE DEGRADATION OF CARTILAGE MATRIX**

Proteinase Class	Cartilage Matrix Substrates	Activity
Matrix Metalloproteinases		
Collagenases-1, -2, -3 (MMP-1, -8, -13)	Collagen II	Fibrillar domain, 3/4 from N-terminus N-telopeptide (MMP-13)
	Aggrecan core protein	Asn^{341}–Phe^{342} IGD
Stromelysins-1 (MMP-3)	Aggrecan core protein	Asn^{341}–Phe^{342} IGD
	Collagens IX, XI	Telopeptide region
	Link protein, FN proMMPs, proTNF	
Gelatinases (MMP-2, -9)	Collagens II, XI Proteoglycans, link protein	Telopeptide or denatured collagen chains
MT-MMP-1, -2, -3, -4 (MMP-14, -15, -16, -17)	Collagen II FN, aggrecan, proMMP-2, -13 ProTNF	Telopeptide
Matrilysin (MMP-7)	Link protein	
Enamelysin (MMP-20)	COMP, link protein	
Aggrecanases		
(ADAM-TS1, -4, -5)	Aggrecan core protein IGD	Glu^{373}–Ala^{374}, Glu^{1545}–Gly^{1546}, Glu^{1714}–Gly^{1715}, Glu^{1819}–Ala^{1820}, Glu^{1919}–Leu^{1920}
Serine		
Plasminogen activators (tPA, uPA)	Aggrecan, FN, proMMPs	Activation of plasminogen gives rise to plasmin
Cathepsin G	Aggrecan, collagen II, proMMPs	
Cysteine		
Cathepsins B, L, S	Collagens IX, XI Link protein; aggrecan	Telopeptides (optimal pH 4.0–6.5)
Aspartate		
Cathepsin D	Phagocytosed ECM components	In lysosomes (optimal pH 3.0–6.0)

Abbreviations: ADAM-TS1, a distintegrin and metalloproteinase with thrombospondin-1 domains; COMP, cartilage oligomeric matrix protein; ECM, extracellular matrix; FN, fibronectin; IGD, interglobular domain; MMP, matrix metalloproteinase; MT-MMP, membrane-type MMP; proMMP, proenzyme form of MMP; TNF, tumor necrosis factor.

collagen suggest a major role for this enzyme in cartilage degradation.[354,357] MMP-3 (stromelysin-1), MMP-8, MMP-14, MMP-19, and MMP-20 also have the capacity to degrade the aggrecan core protein.[358-363]

Cleavage at the Asn341-Phe342 bond of aggrecan has been attributed to the actions of MMPs.[46,358,364] There is, however, evidence that degradation at the "aggrecanase" cleavage site at Glu373-Phe342 is the primary event in chondrocyte-mediated catabolism of aggrecan.[46,365,366] Candidate aggrecanases are the reprolysin-related proteinases of the a disintegrin and metalloproteinase (ADAM) family. ADAM mRNAs were first reported in human articular chondrocytes by McKie and colleagues.[367] ADAM-like aggrecanase activities were identified on chondrocyte membranes,[368] where they were proposed to be involved in proteolytic processing of cell-surface integrins, membrane fusion, and cell–cell and cell-matrix interactions.[369] Later, aggrecanase-1 and -2 were cloned and characterized as ADAM with thrombospondin-1 domains (ADAMTS)-4 and -5.[370-372] Subsequently, ADAMTS-1, which was characterized originally as an inflammation-associated protein,[373] was also found to be expressed by chondrocytes in cartilage as an aggrecanase.[374,375] TIMP-3, but not TIMP-1, -2, or -4, is a potent inhibitor of ADAMTS-4 and -5 in vitro.[376,377]

Other proteinases that may have roles in the degradation of various matrix components or participate in the proteinase-activation cascade include the gelatinases, MMP-2 and -9, the cathepsins, and plasminogen activator. The cysteine proteinases, cathepsins B and L and the aspartic proteinase, cathepsin D, are lysosomal enzymes thought to play a secondary role in cartilage degradation via intracellular digestion of products released by other proteinases.[378-381] Cathepsin B may also have a role in extracellular degradation of collagen telopeptides, collagens IX and XI, and aggrecan.[382,383] Chondrocytes synthesize and secrete MMPs in latent forms, which are activated outside the cells via activation cascades.[384-386] An important cascade in cartilage is initiated by plasmin, the product of plasminogen activator activity, which may be produced by the chondrocyte; plasmin, in turn, activates latent stromelysin (MMP-3), an activator of latent collagenases. The MT1-MMP (MMP-14) may also serve as an activator of other MMPs produced by chondrocytes.[339,387]

Identification of the precise roles of these proteinases and their endogenous inhibitors in chondrocyte-mediated cartilage degradation has provided the opportunity to develop targeted therapies that interfere with the activities of aggrecanases[388] or MMPs[389-392] without disrupting physiologic homeostasis.

THE BALANCE OF CYTOKINES IN CARTILAGE DESTRUCTION

Of the cytokines that affect cartilage metabolism, most were identified originally according to the cells of origin, the biologic effects on target cells, or both. Molecular cloning of genes encoding cytokines and information available through the Human Genome Project has permitted more rigorous classification of the individual cytokines into families on the basis of gene and protein structure. A systematic examination of the full spectrum of the biologic activities of individual cytokines and their family members has revealed several general principles regarding their functional properties and activities, which are also applicable to chondrocytes. First, the activities of individual cytokines are pleiotropic. For example, cytokines that were originally identified as immunomodulators, such as IL-1 and TNF-α, are now known to induce the synthesis of catabolic and inflammatory proteins, but they also regulate matrix protein synthesis and cell proliferation in chondrocytes. Second, cytokines do not act alone, but rather in synergy or partnership with or in opposition to other cytokines via cytokine networks to regulate cell and tissue responses. For example, IL-1 alone or together with TNF-α stimulates the synthesis of almost all of the proteinases described previously. The actions of destructive cytokines in cartilage may be counteracted by modulatory cytokines or anabolic factors also produced by the chondrocytes themselves or by other cells in damaged or inflamed joint tissues. Third, there is considerable redundancy and overlap in the biologic activities of individual cytokines. For example, IL-1, TNF-α, IL-17,and IL-18 have been characterized as catabolic cytokines with respect to their capacities to stimulate chondrocytes to synthesize cartilage matrix-degrading proteinases (Table 13–5). Other naturally occurring cytokines may have modulatory or inhibitory effects on chondrocyte responses to the catabolic cytokines. Investigations in vitro and in vivo have begun to sort out the complexities of the cytokine networks and to determine how the balance in normal homeostasis can be restored once it is disrupted (Fig. 13–5). Examination of type II collagen-induced arthritis (CIA) and other types of induced arthritis in transgenic animals with overexpressed or deleted genes encoding cytokines, their receptors, or activators has provided further insights into the role of these factors in cartilage destruction.[393-396]

Interleukin-1 and Tumor Necrosis Factor-α

Extensive studies in vitro and in vivo have established that IL-1 and TNF-α are the major monocyte-macrophage products responsible for inducing chondrocytes to synthesize catabolic and inflammatory proteins. The first description of IL-1 as a regulator of chondrocyte function stems largely from the early work of Fell and coworkers who identified a soluble factor, termed *catabolin*, in supernatants of normal, noninflamed porcine synovial fragment cultures that stimulated chondrocytes to breakdown the surrounding cartilage matrix.[397,398] Similar activities in culture supernatants from mononuclear cells and synovium[399,400] were later attributed to IL-1.[401-403] Subsequently, the catabolin isoforms were identified as IL-1α and IL-1β.[404] Since those early studies, the capacity of IL-1 to stimulate the production of most, if not all, of the proteinases involved in cartilage destruction has been established in many studies in vitro and in vivo. Chondrocytes can produce IL-1 at concentrations that induce the

TABLE 13–5 • CYTOKINES THAT REGULATE CARTILAGE DESTRUCTION

Catabolic	Interleukin-1 (IL-1) Tumor necrosis factor-α (TNF-α) Interleukin-17 Interleukin-18
Modulatory	Interleukin-6 Leukemia inhibitory factor (LIF) Oncostatin M Interleukin-11
Inhibitory	Interleukin-4 Interleukin-10 Interleukin-13 Interleukin-1 receptor antagonist (IL-1Ra)

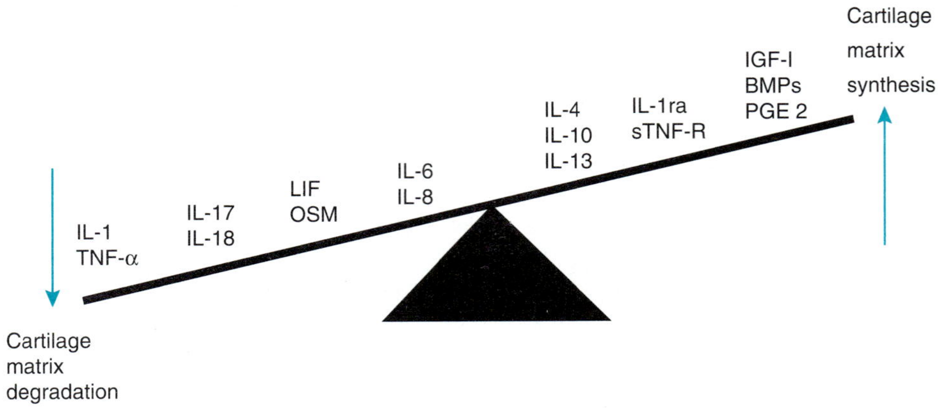

FIGURE 13–5 · The Cytokine Balance in Cartilage Metabolism. The soluble mediators toward the left of the balance promote the loss of cartilage matrix. The mediators on the right side prevent the synthesis or actions of the catabolic cytokines and thereby prevent the loss of cartilage matrix. The anabolic factors, including insulin-like growth factor I (IGF-I) and bone morphogenic proteins (BMPs), as well as prostaglandin E_2 (PGE_2) maintain or promote cartilage matrix synthesis. (Adapted with permission from Goldring MB: Osteoarthritis and cartilage: the role of cytokines. Curr Rheumatol Rep 2:459-465, 2000.)

expression of MMPs and other proinflammatory and catabolic genes.[405-407] IL-1β and TNF-α colocalize with MMPs in superficial regions of OA cartilage.[340] However, the initial inducers of cartilage catabolism in OA have not been identified. Potential stimuli include mechanic stress[408] and degradation products of ECM components, including FN fragments, which stimulate the production of matrix-degrading proteinases in chondrocytes by both IL-1–dependent and –independent mechanisms.[149,156]

Originally known as cachectin, TNF-α has effects in vitro similar to those of IL-1 on chondrocyte functions, such as stimulation of the production of matrix-degrading proteinases.[409-413] Although IL-1 is 100-to 1000-fold more potent on a molar basis than TNF-α, strong synergies can be demonstrated both in vitro and in vivo.[336,414] Thus, intra-articular injection of recombinant IL-1 alone in the joints of rats, mice, and rabbits stimulates destruction of the articular cartilage,[415,416] in some cases without antecedent inflammation.[417] However, injection of recombinant preparations of both TNF-α and IL-1, or of purified preparations containing both cytokines, elicits more severe cartilage damage than injection of either cytokine alone.[418,419] Nevertheless, studies in animal models of RA using cytokine-specific neutralizing antibodies, soluble receptors, or receptor antagonists indicate that TNF-α is sufficient to drive inflammation at the onset of arthritis, whereas IL-1 has a pivotal role in sustaining both inflammation and cartilage erosion.[336]

Both IL-1 and TNF-α can also inhibit the synthesis of proteoglycans and type II collagen by chondrocytes,[56,409,420-422] thereby promoting chondrocyte dedifferentiation and preventing cartilage repair. IL-1 and TNF-α also induce chondrocytes to synthesize prostaglandin E_2 (PGE_2) due to increased cyclooxygenase (COX)-2 activity, nitric oxide (NO) via inducible nitric oxide synthetase (iNOS), soluble phospholipase A2 (sPLA2), and other cytokines such as IL-6, leukemia inhibitory factor (LIF), IL-17, and IL-18, and the chemokine IL-8. Interestingly, the IL-1–induced COX-2 response is dependent on the differentiated phenotype of the chondrocytes,[423] and PGE_2 opposes the effects of IL-1 on cartilage matrix synthesis by inhibiting type I and stimulating type II collagen gene expression.[56,61,422,424]

Recent studies indicate that ligands that activate the peroxisome proliferator-activated receptor-γ (PPAR-γ), such as the prostaglandin D_2 metabolite, 15d-PGJ_2, and certain nonsteroidal anti-inflammatory drugs (NSAIDs) are capable of opposing many of the actions of IL-1 on chondrocytes, including stimulation of iNOS, MMP-1, and MMP-13 and inhibition of proteoglycan synthesis.[425-428]

Following the first reports that IL-1 and TNF-α induce NO in chondrocytes,[429,430] the role of NO as a mediator of other IL-1–induced responses, including the inhibition of aggrecan synthesis,[431] enhancement of MMP activity,[432] and reduction in IL-1 receptor antagonist (IL-1Ra) synthesis,[433] has been suggested.[434] NO may also increase chondrocyte susceptibility to injury by other oxidants such as H_2O_2 and contribute to the resistance to the anabolic effects of IGF-I.[227,228,435,436] NO has also been implicated as an important mediator in chondrocyte apoptosis, and an association between NO production and apoptosis in OA cartilage has been proposed.[437,438] Recent evidence indicates that PGE_2 directly mediates the induction of apoptosis by NO,[439] or that PGE_2 sensitizes chondrocytes to NO-induced apoptosis.[440] Inhibition of chondrocyte apoptosis using iNOS or caspase inhibitors has been proposed as a therapeutic strategy for OA.[441,442] However, there is evidence that NO may inhibit cytokine production or activity in chondrocytes.[443] Furthermore, IL-1 appears to protect chondrocytes from CD95-induced apoptosis by a mechanism that is independent of IL-1–induced NO.[444] Thus, the balance of mediators determining normal homeostasis is complex, and modulation of their activities may produce positive or negative effects on chondrocyte function.

IL-6 Family of Cytokines

Of the cytokines induced by IL-1 and TNF-α, IL-6 appears to play a dual role by increasing IL-1Ra, soluble TNF receptor (sTNFR), and TIMP, while also enhancing immune cell function and inflammation. Although IL-1 induces IL-6 synthesis and release, and antisense IL-6 blocks the IL-1–induced inhibition of proteoglycan synthesis in chondrocytes,[445] direct effects of IL-6 on chondrocyte responses are difficult to observe.[446] Recent studies have shown that the soluble IL-6 receptor α (sIL-6Rα) is required for full responses to IL-6 in chondrocytes in vitro[447,448] and permits synergistic stimulation of collagenase activity by IL-1 and IL-6.[449]

Other members of the IL-6 family, which all act via receptors associated with the gp130 domain, may also serve modulatory roles (Table 13–5). IL-11 shares several actions of IL-6, including stimulation of TIMP production without affecting MMP production by chondrocytes.[449,450] LIF may participate in a positive feedback loop in that it increases the production of IL-6 by chondrocytes, and treatment with IL-1, IL-6, or TNF-α stimulates its production.[451,452] Oncostatin M (OSM) is another product of macrophages and activated T cells that is a member of the IL-6 family of cytokines. OSM is a potent stimulator of chondrocyte production of MMPs and aggrecanases and can synergize with IL-1.[453] Adenoviral overexpression of OSM in mouse knee joints increases cartilage damage due to synovial inflammation and hyperplasia.[454] Furthermore, a study using neutralizing OSM antibodies to demonstrate amelioration of cartilage damage in CIA and pristane-induced arthritis indicates that endogenously produced OSM may have a role distinct from that of IL-1 and TNF-α.[455] OSM stimulates MMP expression in chondrocytes via the JAK/STAT pathway, rather than by the stress-activated, p38, and JNK pathways that mediate the effects of IL-1 and TNF-α.[456]

Interleukin-17 and Interleukin-18

Two recently discovered cytokines, IL-17 and IL-18, are potent inducers of catabolic responses in chondrocytes.[457] IL-18 is produced by macrophages, induces IL-1 and TNF-α, and promotes arthritis and T cell differentiation. IL-17 is produced by activated T helper type 1 (Th1), or CD4+, lymphocytes in RA synovial fluid and tissue. The IL-17 receptor is unique in that it is not related to any known cytokine receptor family, whereas the IL-18 receptor shares homology with IL-1RI and has a Toll-like receptor family signaling domain. Both IL-17 and IL-18 increase the expression of IL-1β by human chondrocytes, as well as stimulating many of the same responses such as the production of IL-6, iNOS, COX-2, and MMPs.[458-463] Both in vitro and in vivo, IL-17 increases degradation and suppresses the synthesis of cartilage proteoglycans independent of IL-1,[464,465] and aggrecanases rather than MMPs are responsible for the IL-17–induced cartilage destruction.[466] Adenoviral overexpression of IL-17 induces cartilage proteoglycan loss in the joint with minor cartilage erosion in the absence of CIA and enhancement of the cartilage erosions induced by CIA.[464] Although IL-17 blockade significantly suppresses CIA- and antigen-induced arthritis (AIA)-induced joint destruction, the enhancement of this effect by concomitant TNF blockade demonstrates the requirement for synergy with other cytokines.[464,467] In animal models, IL-18 deficiency and or blockade with IL-18–neutralizing antibody or IL-18–binding protein reduces cartilage destruction, as well as inflammation.[468]

Inhibitory Cytokines

IL-4, IL-10, and IL-13, as well as the naturally occurring IL-1Ra, are classified as inhibitory cytokines, because they decrease the production and activities of the catabolic and proinflammatory cytokines in chondrocytes in vitro and suppress cartilage destruction in vivo[35,334,336,457,469] (Table 13–5). IL-4 and IL-10 inhibit cartilage-degrading proteinases and reverse some effects of the catabolic cytokines in vitro,[470-475] and together they produce a synergistic suppression of cartilage destruction in vivo.[476-478] IL-1Ra is capable of blocking the actions of IL-1 if added at sufficiently high concentrations in vitro and is among the first agents to be developed for anticytokine therapy.[479,480] IL-1Ra can be produced by the same cells that secrete IL-1 and exists as at least three isoforms, including an intracellular form.[481] IL-4, IL-10, and IL-13 have all been shown to increase IL-1Ra production and decrease the production and actions of proinflammatory cytokines.[482,483] Thus, the inhibitory cytokines may have both direct effects on cartilage metabolism and indirect effects by mediating the production and actions of catabolic cytokines.

Chemokines

The role of chemokines in RA tissues is well established; their induction by proinflammatory cytokines, including IL-1, TNF-α, IL-17, IL-18, and OSM, is associated with recruitment of leukocytes to sites of inflammation and modulation of synovial fibroblast responses and actions. Recent work indicates that chemokines are capable of modulating chondrocyte functions associated with cartilage degradation. Chondrocytes, when activated by IL-1 and TNF-α, express several chemokines present at high levels in arthritic joints and also have receptors that enable responses to some of these chemokines (Table 13–6). The first report of expression of functional CC and CXC chemokine receptors (CCR and CXCR), including CCR1, CCR2, CCR3, CCR5, CXCR1, and CXCR2, on chondrocytes was by Borzi and coworkers,[484] who showed that interaction of these receptors with their corresponding ligands, monocyte chemoattractant protein (MCP)-1, regulated on activation normal T-cell expressed and secreted (RANTES), and gro-related oncogene (GRO)α, results in upregulation of MMP-3. Yuan and colleagues[485] showed that both normal and OA chondrocytes express the C-C chemokines, MCP-1, macrophage inhibitory factor (MIF)-1α, MIP-1β, and RANTES, the levels of which are increased by IL-1β or TNF-α, and that RANTES increases expression of its own receptor, CCR5. They also showed that MCP-1 and RANTES increase MMP-3 expression, inhibit proteoglycan synthesis, and enhance proteoglycan release from the chondrocytes.[485] The RANTES receptors CCR3 and CCR5, but not CCR1, are expressed in normal cartilage, whereas all three receptors are expressed in OA cartilage or after stimulation of normal chondrocytes by IL-1β.[486] Furthermore, RANTES induces the expression of iNOS, IL-6, and MMP-1.[486] More-recent work has demonstrated the expression of an additional chemokine receptor, CXCR4, by chondrocytes but not synovial fibroblasts, and that its ligand, stromal cell–derived factor 1 (SDF-1), increases the synthesis of MMP-3 but not MMP-1.[487]

SIGNALING PATHWAYS AND TRANSCRIPTION FACTORS INVOLVED IN CARTILAGE METABOLISM

Although the receptors for IL-1 and TNF-α and associated adaptor molecules are distinct, they share the capacity to activate some of the same signaling pathways

TABLE 13–6 • CHEMOKINES AND RECEPTORS IN CHONDROCYTES

Functional Name	Systematic Name	Chemokine Receptor
Groα	CXCL1	CXCR1, CXCR2
IL-8	CXCL8	CXCR1, CXCR2
MCP-1	CCL2	CCR2
MIP-1α	CCL3	CCR1, CCR5
MIP-1β	CCL4	CCR5
RANTES	CCL5	CCR1, CCR3, CCR5
SDF-1	CXCL12	CXCR4

Abbreviations: Groα, growth-related oncogene α; IL-8; interleukin-8; MCP-1, monocyte chemoattractant protein-1; MIP-1, macrophage inhibitory protein-1; RANTES, regulated upon activation, normal T-cell expressed and secreted; SDF-1, stromal-derived growth factor-1. Chemokines are classified according to the positions of the first two cysteines (C) of the 4 conserved N-terminal cysteines: CC chemokine ligand (CCL), first 2 cysteines are adjacent; CXC chemokine ligand (CXCL), first 2 cysteines are separated by amino acid X other than cysteine. CXCR, CXC chemokine receptor; CCR, CC chemokine receptor.

(Fig. 13–6). These pathways include the stress-activated protein kinase (SAPKs), also termed C-jun N-terminal kinase (JNK) and p38 mitogen-activated protein kinase (MAPK)[488]; IκB kinases[489,490]; and phosphatidylinositol-3′-kinase (PI-3K) pathways,[491-493] and there is cross-talk among these pathways.[494,495] Specific adaptor molecules involved in the pathways induced by TNF-α receptors, which are members of the TNF receptor superfamily, are different from those used by IL-1 signaling pathways.[496] The TNF receptor pathway uses TNF receptor associated factor (TRAF2), TRAF6, and the receptor interacting protein (RIP) kinase, whereas the IL-1 receptor pathway uses TRAF6, IL-1 receptor-associated kinase (IRAK), and evolutionarily conserved signaling intermediate in Toll pathways (ECSIT) as adaptor molecules.[491,497,498] Signaling through TNF-RI associated with TNF receptor-associated death domain receptor (TRADD) activates apoptosis, whereas TNF-RII signaling through TRAF2 activates JNK and nuclear factor kappa B (NFκB).[499]

The SAPKs are a subfamily of the extracellular signal-regulated kinase (ERK) family of serine/threonine kinases, but unlike the MAPKs, Erk-1 and Erk-2, they are weakly activated by growth factors. In chondrocytes, the p38 MAPK cascade is involved in the signaling pathways that mediate induction of the expression of several different genes by IL-1 and TNF-α,[423,500-504] as well as by IL-17.[458,505] In a culture model of cartilage breakdown, short-term IL-1–induced degradation of glycosaminoglycans (GAGs) and inhibition of proteoglycan synthesis is unaffected by the p38 MAPK inhibitor, SB203580, in 24-hour incubations, although collagen breakdown is prevented after 2 weeks.[506] However, a more selective p38 MAPK inhibitor has been shown to be somewhat protective against cartilage destruction in the rat AIA model.[507] Inhibition of p38 MAPK also reverses partially the IL-1–mediated suppression of type II collagen gene expression in chondrocytes.[129] Changes in cell surface integrin profiles and regulation of matrix-binding

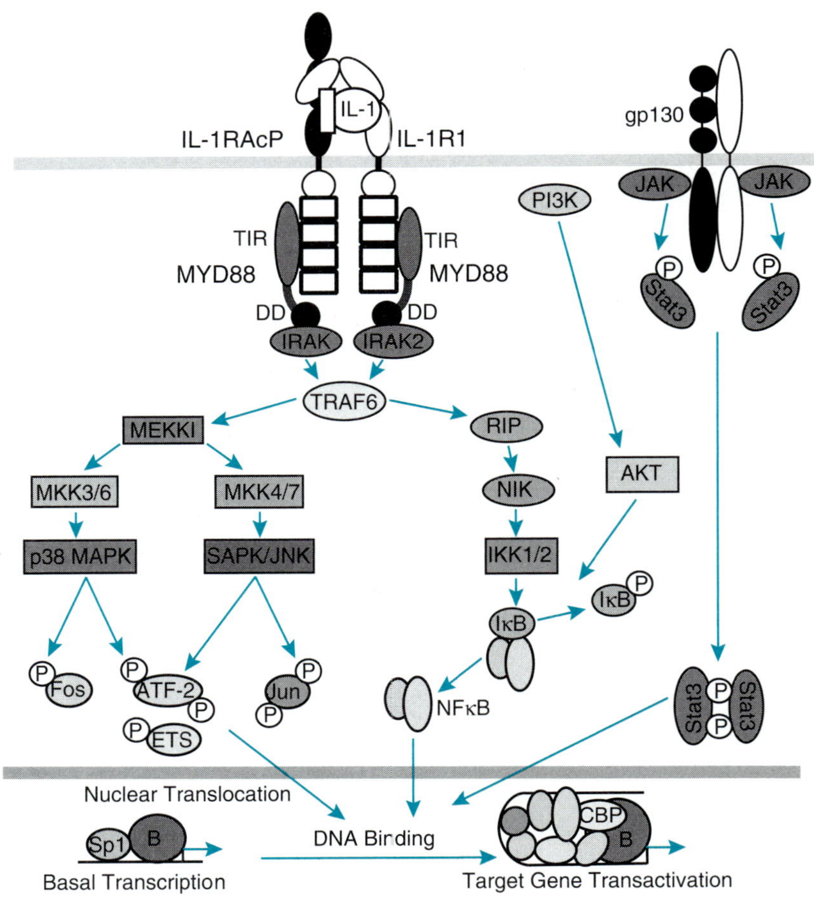

FIGURE 13–6 • **Intracellular Signaling Pathways Activated by Interleukin-1 (IL-1) in Chondrocytes.** Binding of IL-1 to the type I IL-1 receptor (IL-1R1) leads to the recruitment of the IL-1R accessory protein (IL-1RAcP). The cytoplasmic Toll/IL-1 receptor (TIR) domains of the receptor then recruit the MyD88 via its TIR, and the MyD88 death domain (DD) recruits, in turn, the IL-1 receptor-associated kinases (IRAK and IRAK2) to the receptor complex before being rapidly phosphorylated and degraded. The IRAKs mediate TNF receptor associated factor (TRAF)6 oligomerization, initiating various protein kinase cascades, the major ones of which involve (1) the stress-activated protein kinases, p38 mitogen-activated protein kinase (MAPK), and c-Jun N-terminal kinase (JNK), which lead to activation of activator protein-1 (AP-1) (c-Fos/c-Jun), activating transcription factor-1 (ATF-2), and E Twenty Six (ETS) factors, among other transcription factors; and (2) inhibitor of kappa B (IκB) kinases (IKK)-1 and -2, which lead to activation of nuclear factor kappa B (NFκB). Tumor necrosis factor-α (TNF-α) also stimulates these pathways, but via TRAF2 and -5. Other signaling pathways may also influence the target gene responses, such as the growth factor– or chemokine-induced phosphatylinositol 3-kinase (PI3K) via the serine/threonine kinase, Akt/protein kinase B, and the gp130 cytokine-induced janus activating kinase (JAK)/signal transducer and activator of transcription (STAT) pathway. The responses of the target genes depend on the presence of DNA sequences within the respective promoters that bind to the various transcription factors.

proteins may also influence chondrocyte-matrix interactions that regulate alternate signaling pathways.[508]

In articular chondrocytes, promoter or enhancer regions of chondrocyte-specific genes, such as type II collagen and aggrecan, interact with positive or negative transcription factors that determine developmental stage- and tissue-specific expression during chondrogenesis (Table 13–7). Binding motifs for the ubiquitous transcription factor Sp1 were among the first identified in type II collagen genes,[509-511] and recent work has shown that Sp3 represses Sp1-mediated transactivation of the promoter activity.[512] E-box sites, which are consensus binding sites for basic helix-loop-helix (HLH) proteins, are present in both promoter and enhancer regions, and a conserved E-box site (CAGGTG) in the promoter also interacts with the zinc finger homeodomain protein, E2-box binding factor (δEF1), which represses constitutive activity of the rat collagen type II promoter.[513] The zinc finger protein, cKrox, activates collagen type II transcription in differentiated chondrocytes but inhibits constitutive activity in subcultured cells.[514] The high-mobility group (HMG) protein Sox9 plays a key role in cartilage formation and maintenance by permitting transcription of cartilage-specific genes such as type II and type IX collagens, aggrecan, and cartilage-derived retinoic acid sensitive protein (CD-RAP).[515-518] Sox9 activates collagen type II transcription by binding to the first intron enhancer through itsHMG DNA-binding domain and acts cooperatively with L-Sox5 and Sox6 to regulate chondrogenesis in vivo.[519,520] The anabolic effects of IGF-I, BMP-2, and bFGF appear to be mediated, at least in part, by Sox9.[519,521-524] The homeobox protein, distal-less (Dlx)-2, which is stimulated by BMP-2, also acts via the intronic enhancer to increase collagen type II expression.[525]

Downstream activation of transcription factors of the NFκB, CCAAT enhancer binding protein (C/EBP), STAT, ETS, and Jun/Fos families have been shown to be important for expression of IL-1– and TNF-α–inducible genes, including MMPs, COX-2, and iNOS.[504,526-530] IL-1–induced transcription factors may also suppress expression of COL2A1 and other chondrocyte-specific genes[531,532] (Table 13–7). Studies showing that gene deletions or overexpression of IL-1 or TNF-α does not lead to abnormal skeletal development suggest that these cytokines are not involved in the formation of articular cartilage. However, the cartilage remodeling initiated in response to trauma or inflammation may involve inactivation of some the chondrogenic transcription factors. The regulation by cytokine-induced transcription factors may involve direct or indirect interactions with other regulatory factors that promote chondrogenic phenotype, such as members of the SRY-related HMG-box protein (SOX)[533,534] and HLH families[513,535-537] and those that suppress chondrocyte differentiation, such as c-Fos,[538,539] the nuclear factor of activated T cells p(c2) (NFATp[c2]),[540] the retinoic acid receptor,[541] the zinc finger transcription factors, zinc finger protein 60 (Zfp60)[542] and αA-crystalline binding protein 1 (CRYBP1),[543] and activator protein-2 (AP-2).[544,545] Different ETS factors may have positive or negative effects on cartilage-specific gene transcription.[546] It has been proposed that inhibition of Sox9 expression by IL-1 determines the regulation of COL2A1 gene transcription by these cytokines,[523,534,547] although downregulation of Sox9 and COL2A1 expression does not always correlate.[532,539,548] Recent evidence indicates that Sox9 overexpression in chondrocytes may either increase or decrease COL2A1 transcription, depending on its concentration and the differentiation state of the cells.[549]

The observation that Cbfa1/Runx2, δEF-1, C/EBP, and AP-2 are highly expressed in hypertrophic cartilage[550] suggests that downregulation of chondrocyte-specific genes is necessary before mineralization can occur. For example, Cbfa1/Runx2, the so-called osteoblastic-specific gene, stimulates chondrocyte terminal differentiation[551,552] and increases the expression of type X collagen and MMP-13 in hypertrophic chondrocytes.[553-555] Also, Cbfa1/Runx2 is required for IL-1 induction of MMP-13 gene transcription in articular chondrocytes,[527] and it partners with SMADs to regulate the type X collagen gene in response to BMPs.[556] Cross-talk occurs between Smad2 and the Erk1/2 and p38 MAPK pathways during TGF-β–induced aggrecan gene expression in the chondroprogenitor ATDC5 cell line.[557] The T-box transcription factor, *Brachyury*, another factor that is upregulated by BMP-2 during FGFR3-induced differentiation of the C3H10T1/2 cell line to chondrocytes.[558] Together, these and other findings suggest the complexity of the signaling pathways and downstream transcription factors involved in regulation of the gene expression in chondrocytes.

TABLE 13–7 • TRANSCRIPTION FACTORS INVOLVED IN THE REGULATION OF CHONDROCYTE RESPONSES

Cytokine-Induced	Differentiation-Modulated
NFκB	HMG (Sox9, L-Sox5, Sox6)
AP-1 family (c-Fos/c-Jun)	Runx2 (Cbfa1)
C/EBPβ, C/EBPδ	bHLH (scleraxis, twist, δEF1)
ETS (Ets-1, PEA-3, ESE-1)	Homeobox (Hox-C8, Msx2, Dlx-2)
Egr-1	Retinoic acid receptors
(RAR/RXR)	
STATs	SMADs
	Zinc finger proteins (cKrox, AP2, Sp1/3, CRYBP1)
	ETS (Erg, C-1-1)
	NFATp(c2)

Abbreviations: AP-1, activator protein-1; AP-2, activator protein-2; ATF-2, activating transcription factor-1; BHLH, basic helix-loop-helix; Cbfa1, core binding factor a1; C/EBP, CCAAT-enhancer binding protein; CRYBP1, αA-crystalline binding protein 1; δEF-1, E2-box binding factor; Dlx, distal-less; Egr-1, early growth response gene; ETS, E Twenty Six; ESE-1, epithelial-specific ETS factor; HMG, high mobility group protein; mammalian homologues of *Drosophila* mothers against decapentaplegic (Mad) gene; NFAT, nuclear factor of activated T cells; NF-κB, nuclear factor kappa B; PEA, polyoma enhancer A binding protein; Runx, runt domain binding protein; SMADs, signal transducers and activators of transcription; SOX, SRY-related HMG-box protein; STATs, signal transducers and activators of transcription.

The Role of the Chondrocyte in Cartilage Repair

THE AGING CHONDROCYTE

Chondrocyte function, including mitotic and synthetic activity, deteriorates with age.[559] Changes in matrix synthesis lead to small and irregular proteoglycan aggregates due to decreased size of aggrecan molecules and less functional link proteins.[560] There is also a stiffening of the collagen network due to nonenzyme-mediated pentosidine cross-linking.[561] Degradative changes are generally due to the actions of proteinases and are, at least partially, the cumulative consequences of adverse conditions, such as mechanic insults or inflammation, to which the chondrocyte is exposed throughout life. Deficiencies in cartilage matrix proteins may also disrupt chondrocyte-matrix interactions that are important to cell survival.[562] Chondrocytes also show an age-related decline in the anabolic response to IGF-I,[224] possibly due to increased synthesis of IGFBP-3, which is itself antiproliferative.[214] Indeed, chondrocytes from elderly donors depend strongly upon IGF-I and IGF-II for survival.[206] The decline in chondrocyte number may also be attributed to increased cell death with age. Although programmed cell death, or apoptosis, increases with age in adult rats and mice, this may be due to skeletal growth that occurs throughout life in these animals.[563] However, in human adult cartilage, apoptotic cell removal does not appear to be a widespread phenomenon.[564] Recent work suggests that aging chondrocytes, similar to other cells, undergo progressive replicative senescence, detected as β-galactosidase activity and decreased telomere length.[565] Epidemiologic studies showing a strong association between age and OA suggest that the decline in the capacity of aging chondrocytes to maintain and restore articular cartilage contributes to development and progression of this joint disease.[566]

THERAPEUTIC STRATEGIES THAT TARGET CHONDROCYTES

Growth and differentiation factors are obvious tools for enhancing cartilage repair.[567] For example, injection of BMP-2 into murine knee joints stimulates cartilage proteoglycan synthesis without counteracting the deleterious effects of IL-1 on proteoglycan synthesis and content.[300] Similarly, IGF-I is an effective inducer of cartilage repair in a canine OA model if administered with the catabolic inhibitor pentosan polysulfate.[568] Although injection of free TGF-β or adenovirus-mediated delivery of TGF-β into joint cavities may have deleterious effects,[286,569] introduction of liposome-encapsulated TGF-β in a fibrin matrix directly into partial-thickness defects produces healing in adult articular cartilage.[570]

Autologous chondrocyte transplantation has been used somewhat successfully to repair small cartilage lesions in young adults with sports injuries.[571] However, surgical intervention required to remove cartilage may produce further damage, and expansion of the isolated chondrocytes causes dedifferentiation. Thus, ex vivo gene transfer has been proposed as a strategy for enhancing this procedure. Approaches for delivery of BMPs and other factors in synthetic or natural-carrier scaffolds have been developed.[572-574] BMP-2 implanted in a collagen carrier promotes the repair of full-thickness defects of articular cartilage in an animal model.[575] The transfer of genes encoding anabolic factors to chondrocytes prior to transplantation has been proposed as an additional strategy for promoting cartilage-specific matrix synthesis.[576] Indeed, the induction of the synthesis of IGF-I, TGF-β, BMP-2, and BMP-7 by gene transfer increases the synthesis of cartilage proteoglycans and collagens in cultured chondrocytes.[281,574,577-579]

IL-1 and TNF-α have been targeted for gene therapy in RA. Initial clinical trials tested the delivery ex vivo of IL-1Ra using retroviral vectors.[580,581] However, the ex vivo delivery via synoviocytes targets type B synoviocytes, whereas ex vivo delivery via chondrocytes results in transient gene expression. In vivo gene delivery is a more promising strategy for inhibiting cartilage destruction.[582] Promising results have been obtained via intra-articular delivery of adenoviral vectors expressing soluble receptors of IL-1, TNF-α, IL-4, and IL-10, alone and in combination.[477,583-587] Gene transfer of combinations of anabolic factors and inhibitory cytokines combined with cartilage engineering approaches may make it possible to repair the extensive defects in RA or late-OA patients and also prevent further damage.[573,582] The use of bone marrow–derived chondroprogenitor cells as gene-delivery vehicles to the site of cartilage damage is a promising strategy for the future.[588]

Summary and Conclusion

As the single cellular component in adult articular cartilage, chondrocytes are responsible for maintaining the ECM components in a low-turnover state. The composition and organization of matrix macromolecules, which are unique to this tissue, are determined during chondrocyte differentiation in embryonic and postnatal development of cartilage. Adult chondrocytes exist in a hypoxic environment within articular cartilage, are relatively inactive metabolically (due in part to an absence of blood vessels and nerves), and display a rounded morphology that reflects their quiescent state. Chondrocyte culture models have been developed with the aim of maintaining differentiated phenotypes, characterized by the major collagen and proteoglycan constituents, type II collagen and aggrecan. Chondrocytes interact with specific ECM components via integrins, annexins, and CD44 on the cell surface. Studies in vitro and in vivo have shown that adult articular chondrocytes are capable of responding to biologic and mechanical stimuli that are either anabolic or catabolic. Anabolic factors include members of the TGF-β/BMP family and IGF-I. Catabolic factors include proinflammatory cytokines, such as IL-1, TNF-α, IL-17, and IL-18, which stimulate the synthesis of matrix-degrading proteinases, such as MMPs and aggrecanases, and inhibit cartilage matrix–protein synthesis. Members of the IL-6 family of cytokines, including IL-6 itself, OSM, and LIF, and chemokines, including IL-8, synergize with the catabolic cytokines or modulate the chondrocyte responses. Inhibitory cytokines, including IL-4, IL-10, IL-13, and IL-1Ra attenuate the actions of the catabolic cytokines. Many of the signaling pathways and transcription factors that mediate the responses of chondrocytes to these cytokines have been elucidated, but how they orchestrate the specific chondrocyte functions is complex and not fully understood. Although chondrocytes in situ are able to respond to both catabolic and anabolic factors, they are not capable of mediating effective repair of extensive cartilage lesions. Thus, further understanding of how the adult articular chondrocyte functions within its unique environment will aid in the development of rational strategies for protecting cartilage from damage resulting from joint disease.

REFERENCES

1. Stockwell RA, Meachim G: The chondrocytes. *In* Freeman MAR (ed): Adult Articular Cartilage. Tunbridge Wells, England, Pitman Medical, 1979, pp 69-144.
2. Rothwell AG, Bentley G: Chondrocyte multiplication in osteoarthritic articular cartilage. J Bone Joint Surg Br 55:588-594, 1973.
3. Hunziker EB, Michel M, Studer D: Ultrastructure of adult human articular cartilage matrix after cryotechnical processing. Microsc Res Tech 37:271-284, 1997.
4. Poole AR, Kojima T, Yasuda T, et al: Composition and structure of articular cartilage: A template for tissue repair. Clin Orthop (391 suppl):S26-S33, 2001.
5. Aydelotte MB, Kuettner KE: Differences between sub-populations of cultured bovine articular chondrocytes. I. Morphology and cartilage matrix production. Conn Tiss Res 18:205-222, 1988.
6. Aydelotte MB, Greenhill RR, Kuettner KE: Differences between sub-populations of cultured bovine articular chondrocytes. II. Proteoglycan metabolism. Conn Tiss Res 18:223-234, 1988.
7. Maroudas A, Venn M: Chemical composition and swelling of normal and osteoarthrotic femoral head cartilage. II. Swelling. Ann Rheum Dis 36:399-406, 1977.
8. Bush PG, Hall AC: The volume and morphology of chondrocytes within non-degenerate and degenerate human articular cartilage. Osteoarthritis Cartilage 11:242-251, 2003.
9. Poole CA, Jensen CG, Snyder JA, et al: Confocal analysis of primary cilia structure and colocalization with the Golgi apparatus in chondrocytes and aortic smooth muscle cells. Cell Biol Int 21:483-494, 1997.
10. Benya PD, Shaffer JD: Dedifferentiated chondrocytes reexpress the differentiated collagen phenotype when cultured in agarose gels. Cell 30:215-224, 1982.
11. Horton W, Hassell JR: Independence of cell shape and loss of cartilage matrix production during retinoic acid treatment of cultured chondrocytes. Dev Biol 115:392-397, 1986.
12. Mallein-Gerin F, Ruggiero F, Garrone R: Proteoglycan core protein and type II collagen gene expressions are not correlated with cell shape changes during low density chondrocyte cultures. Differentiation 43:204-211, 1990.
13. Schnabel M, Marlovits S, Eckhoff G, et al: Dedifferentiation-associated changes in morphology and gene expression in primary human articular chondrocytes in cell culture. Osteoarthritis Cartilage 10:62-70, 2002.
14. Hall BK, Miyake T: All for one and one for all: condensations and the initiation of skeletal development. Bioessays 22:138-147, 2000.
15. DeLise AM, Fischer L, Tuan RS: Cellular interactions and signaling in cartilage development. Osteoarthritis Cartilage 8:309-334, 2000.
16. Grimshaw MJ, Mason RM: Modulation of bovine articular chondrocyte gene expression in vitro by oxygen tension. Osteoarthritis Cartilage 9:357-364, 2001.
17. Rajpurohit R, Koch CJ, Tao Z, et al: Adaptation of chondrocytes to low oxygen tension: relationship between hypoxia and cellular metabolism. J Cell Physiol 168:424-432, 1996.
18. Jubb RW: Effect of hyperoxia on articular tissues in organ culture. Ann Rheum Dis 38:279-286, 1979.
19. Wilkins RJ, Browning JA, Ellory JC: Surviving in a matrix: membrane transport in articular chondrocytes. J Membr Biol 177:95-108, 2000.
20. Lee RB, Wilkins RJ, Razaq S, Urban JP: The effect of mechanical stress on cartilage energy metabolism. Biorheology 39:133-143, 2002.
21. Stockwell RA: Metabolism of cartilage. *In* Hall BK (ed): Cartilage: Structure, Function and Biochemistry. New York, Academic Press, 1983, pp 253-280.
22. Kim JJ, Conrad HE: Kinetics of mucopolysaccharide and glycoprotein synthesis by chick embryo chondrocytes. Effect of D-glucose concentration in the culture medium. J Biol Chem 251:6210-6217, 1976.
23. Mason RM, Sweeney C: The relationship between proteoglycan synthesis in Swarm chondrocytes and pathways of cellular energy and UDP-sugar metabolism. Carbohydr Res 255:255-270, 1994.
24. Shikhman AR, Brinson DC, Valbracht J, Lotz MK: Cytokine regulation of facilitated glucose transport in human articular chondrocytes. J Immunol 167:7001-7008, 2001.
25. Mobasheri A, Neama G, Bell S, et al: Human articular chondrocytes express three facilitative glucose transporter isoforms: GLUT1, GLUT3 and GLUT9. Cell Biol Int 26:297-300, 2002.
26. Maroudas A, Palla G, Gilav E: Racemization of aspartic acid in human articular cartilage. Connect Tissue Res 28:161-169, 1992.
27. Verzijl N, DeGroot J, Thorpe SR, et al: Effect of collagen turnover on the accumulation of advanced glycation end products. J Biol Chem 275:39027-39031, 2000.
28. Maroudas A, Bayliss MT, Uchitel-Kaushansky N, et al: Aggrecan turnover in human articular cartilage: use of aspartic acid racemization as a marker of molecular age. Arch Biochem Biophys 350:61-71, 1998.
29. Aigner T, Zhu Y, Chansky HH, et al: Reexpression of type IIA procollagen by adult articular chondrocytes in osteoarthritic cartilage. Arthritis Rheum 42:1443-1450, 1999.
30. Sandell LJ, Aigner T: Articular cartilage and changes in arthritis. An introduction: cell biology of osteoarthritis. Arthritis Res 3: 107-113, 2001.
31. Aigner T, Dudhia J: Phenotypic modulation of chondrocytes as a potential therapeutic target in osteoarthritis: a hypothesis. Ann Rheum Dis 56:287-291, 1997.
32. Soder S, Hambach L, Lissner R, et al: Ultrastructural localization of type VI collagen in normal adult and osteoarthritic human articular cartilage. Osteoarthritis Cartilage 10:464-470, 2002.
33. Aigner T, Gluckert K, von der Mark K: Activation of fibrillar collagen synthesis and phenotypic modulation of chondrocytes in early human osteoarthritic cartilage lesions. Osteoarthritis Cartilage 5:183-189, 1997.
34. Goldring MB: Degradation of articular cartilage in culture: Regulatory factors. *In* Woessner JF Jr., Howell DS (eds): Joint Cartilage Degradation: Basic and Clinical Aspects. New York, Marcel Dekker, 1993, pp 281-345.
35. Goldring MB: The role of the chondrocyte in osteoarthritis. Arthritis Rheum 43:1916-1926, 2000.
36. Goldring MB: Osteoarthritis and cartilage: the role of cytokines. Curr Rheumatol Rep 2:459-465, 2000.
37. Hauselmann HJ, Hedbom E: In vitro models of cartilage metabolism. *In* Seibel MJ, Robins SP, Bilezekian JP (eds): Dynamics of Bone and Cartilage Metabolism. New York, Academic Press, 1999, pp 325-338.
38. Poole AR: Honor Bridgett Fell, Ph.D., D.Sc. F.R.S., D.B.E., 1900-1986. The scientist and her contributions. In Vitro Cell Dev Biol 25:450-453, 1989.
39. Hascall VC, Handley CJ, McQuillan DJ, et al: The effect of serum on biosynthesis of proteoglycans by bovine articular cartilage in culture. Arch Biochem Biophys 224:206-223, 1983.
40. Morales TI: Articular organ cultures. *In* Woessner JF Jr., Howell DS (eds): Joint Cartilage Degradation: Basic and Clinical Aspects. New York, Marcel Dekker, 1993, pp 261-280.
41. Campbell MA, Handley CJ, Hascall VC, et al: Turnover of proteoglycans in cultures of bovine articular cartilage. Arch Biochem Biophys 234:275-289, 1984.
42. Hascall VC, Morales TI, Hascall GK, et al: Biosynthesis and turnover of proteoglycans in organ culture of bovine articular cartilage. J Rheumatol 11(Suppl):45-52, 1983.
43. Bartholomew JS, Lowther DA, Handley CJ: Changes in proteoglycan biosynthesis following leukocyte elastase treatment of bovine articular cartilage in culture. Arthritis Rheum 27:905-912, 1984.
44. Morales TI, Wahl LM, Hascall VC: The effect of bacterial lipopolysaccharides on the biosynthesis and release of proteoglycans from calf articular cartilage cultures. J Biol Chem 259: 6720-6729, 1984.

45. Tyler JA: Chondrocyte-mediated depletion of articular cartilage proteoglycans in vitro. Biochem J 225:493-507, 1985.
46. Sandy JD, Neame PJ, Boynton RE, Flannery CR: Catabolism of aggrecan in cartilage explants. Identification of a major cleavage site within the interglobular domain. J Biol Chem 266:8683-8685, 1991.
47. Handley CJ, Winter GM, Ilic MZ, et al: Distribution of newly synthesized aggrecan in explant cultures of bovine cartilage treated with retinoic acid. Matrix Biol 21:579-592, 2002.
48. Luyten FP, Hascall VC, Nissley SP, et al: Insulin-like growth factors maintain steady-state metabolism of proteoglycans in bovine articular cartilage explants. Arch Biochem Biophys 267:416-425, 1988.
49. Barone-Varelas J, Schnitzer TJ, Meng Q, et al: Age-related differences in the metabolism of proteoglycans in bovine articular cartilage explants maintained in the presence of insulin-like growth factor I. Connect Tissue Res 26:101-120, 1991.
50. Morales TI: Transforming growth factor-β and insulin-like growth factor-1 restore proteoglycan metabolism of bovine articular cartilage after depletion by retinoic acid. Arch Biochem Biophys 315:190-198, 1994.
51. Holtzer J, Abbott J, Lash J, Holtzer A: The loss of phenotypic traits by differentiated cells in vitro. I. Dedifferentiation of cartilage cells. Proc Natl Acad Sci U S A 46:1533-1542, 1960.
52. Sokoloff L, Malemud CJ, Srivastava VM, Morgan WD: In vitro culture of articular chondrocytes. Fed Proc 32:1499-1502, 1973.
53. von der Mark K, Gauss V, von der Mark H, Muller P: Relationship between cell shape and type of collagen synthesised as chondrocytes lose their cartilage phenotype in culture. Nature 267: 531-532, 1977.
54. Benya PD, Padilla SR, Nimni ME: Independent regulation of collagen types by chondrocytes during the loss of differentiated function in culture. Cell 15:1313-1321, 1978.
55. Goldring MB, Sandell LJ, Stephenson ML, Krane SM: Immune interferon suppresses levels of procollagen mRNA and type II collagen synthesis in cultured human articular and costal chondrocytes. J Biol Chem 261:9049-9056, 1986.
56. Goldring MB, Birkhead J, Sandell LJ, et al: Interleukin 1 suppresses expression of cartilage-specific types II and IX collagens and increases types I and III collagens in human chondrocytes. J Clin Invest 82:2026-2037, 1988.
57. Hiraki Y, Mitsui K, Endo N, et al: Molecular cloning of human chondromodulin-I, a cartilage-derived growth modulating factor, and its expression in Chinese hamster ovary cells. Eur J Biochem 260:869-878, 1999.
58. Tetlow LC, Woolley DE: Expression of vitamin D receptors and matrix metalloproteinases in osteoarthritic cartilage and human articular chondrocytes in vitro. Osteoarthritis Cartilage 9:423-431, 2001.
59. Aulthouse AL, Beck M, Friffey E, et al: Expression of the human chondrocyte phenotype in vitro. In Vitro Cell Devel Biol 25: 659-668, 1989.
60. Kolettas E, Buluwela L, Bayliss MT, Muir HI: Expression of cartilage-specific molecules is retained on long-term culture of human articular chondrocytes. J Cell Sci 108(Pt 5):1991-1999, 1995.
61. Goldring MB, Krane SM: Modulation by recombinant interleukin 1 of synthesis of types I and III collagens and associated procollagen mRNA levels in cultured human cells. J Biol Chem 262:16724-16729, 1987.
62. Gerstenfeld LC, Kelly CM, Von Deck M, Lian JB: Comparative morphological and biochemical analysis of hypertrophic, non-hypertrophic and $1,25(OH)_2D_3$ treated non-hypertrophic chondrocytes. Conn Tiss Res 24:29-39, 1990.
63. Adams SL, Pallante KM, Niu Z, et al: Rapid induction of type X collagen gene expression in cultured chick vertebral chondrocytes. Exp Cell Res 193:190-197, 1991.
64. Watt FM: Effect of seeding density on stability of the differentiated phenotype of pig articular chondrocytes in culture. J Cell Sci 89(Pt 3):373-378, 1988.
65. Kuettner KE, Pauli BU, Gall G, et al: Synthesis of cartilage matrix by mammalian chondrocytes in vitro. I. Isolation, culture characteristics, and morphology. J Cell Biol 93:743-750, 1982.
66. Bassleer C, Gysen P, Foidart JM, Bassleer R, Franchimont P: Human chondrocytes in tridimensional culture. In Vitro Cell Devel Biol 22:113-119, 1986.
67. Thonar EJ, Buckwalter JA, Kuettner KE: Maturation-related differences in the structure and composition of proteoglycans synthesized by chondrocytes from bovine articular cartilage. J Biol Chem 261:2467-2474, 1986.
68. Vukicevic S, Kleinman HK, Luyten FP, et al: Identification of multiple active growth factors in basement membrane Matrigel suggests caution in interpretation of cellular activity related to extracellular matrix components. Exp Cell Res 202:1-8, 1992.
69. Adolphe M, Froger B, Ronot X, et al: Cell multiplication and type II collagen production by rabbit articular chondrocytes cultivated in a defined medium. Exp Cell Res 155:527-536, 1984.
70. Ham RG, Sattler GL: Clonal growth of differentiated rabbit cartilage cells. J Cell Physiol 72:109-114, 1968.
71. Green WT Jr: Behavior of articular chondrocytes in cell culture. Clin Orthopaed Rel Res 75:248-260, 1971.
72. Deshmukh K, Kline WH: Characterization of collagen and its precursors synthesized by rabbit-articular-cartilage cells in various culture systems. Eur J Biochem 69:117-123, 1976.
73. Norby DP, Malemud CJ, Sokoloff L: Differences in the collagen types synthesized by lapine articular chondrocytes in spinner and monolayer culture. Arthritis Rheum 20:709-716, 1977.
74. Glowacki J, Trepman E, Folkman J: Cell shape and phenotypic expression in chondrocytes. Proc Soc Exp Biol Med 172:93-98, 1983.
75. Castagnola P, Moro G, Descalzi-Cancedda F, Cancedda R: Type X collagen synthesis during in vitro development of chick embryo tibial chondrocytes. J Cell Biol 102:2310-2317, 1986.
76. Reginato AM, Iozzo RV, Jimenez SA: Formation of nodular structures resembling mature articular cartilage in long-term primary cultures of human fetal epiphyseal chondrocytes on hydrogel substrate. Arthritis Rheum 37:1338-1349, 1994.
77. Gibson GJ, Schor SL, Grant ME: Effects of matrix macromolecules on chondrocyte gene expression: Synthesis of a low molecular weight collagen species by cells cultured within collagen gels. J Cell Biol 93:767-774, 1982.
78. Mizuno S, Allemann F, Glowacki J: Effects of medium perfusion on matrix production by bovine chondrocytes in three-dimensional collagen sponges. J Biomed Mater Res 56:368-375, 2001.
79. Wu QQ, Chen Q: Mechanoregulation of chondrocyte proliferation, maturation, and hypertrophy: Ion-channel dependent transduction of matrix deformation signals. Exp Cell Res 256:383-391, 2000.
80. Buschmann MD, Gluzband YA, Grodzinsky AJ, et al: Chondrocytes in agarose culture synthesize a mechanically functional extracellular matrix. J Orthop Res 10:745-758, 1992.
81. Guo J, Jourdian GW, MacCallum DK: Culture and growth characteristics of chondrocytes encapsulated in alginate beads. Conn Tiss Res 19:277-297, 1989.
82. Hauselmann HJ, Aydelotte MB, Schumacher BL, et al: Synthesis and turnover of proteoglycans by human and bovine adult articular chondrocytes cultured in alginate beads. Matrix 12:116-129, 1992.
83. Hauselmann HJ, Fernandes RJ, Mok SS, et al: Phenotypic stability of bovine articular chondrocytes after long-term culture in alginate beads. J Cell Sci 107(Pt 1):17-27, 1994.
84. Liu H, Lee YW, Dean MF: Re-expression of differentiated proteoglycan phenotype by dedifferentiated human chondrocytes during culture in alginate beads. Biochim Biophys Acta 1425: 505-515, 1998.
85. Bonaventure J, Kadhom N, Cohen-Solal L, et al: Reexpression of cartilage-specific genes by dedifferentiated human articular chondrocytes cultured in alginate beads. Exp Cell Res 212: 97-104, 1994.
86. Lemare F, Steimberg N, Le Griel C, et al: Dedifferentiated chondrocytes cultured in alginate beads: Restoration of the differentiated phenotype and of the metabolic responses to interleukin-1beta. J Cell Physiol 176:303-313, 1998.
87. Srivastava VM, MaleMud CJ, Sokoloff L: Chondroid expression by lapine articular chondrocytes in spinner culture following monolayer growth. Connect Tissue Res 2:127-136, 1974.
88. Schulze-Tanzil G, de Souza P, Villegas Castrejon H, et al: Redifferentiation of dedifferentiated human chondrocytes in high-density cultures. Cell Tissue Res 308:371-379, 2002.
89. Kato Y, Iwamoto M, Koike T, et al: Terminal differentiation and calcification in rabbit chondrocyte cultures grown in centrifuge

tubes: regulation by transforming growth factor beta and serum factors. Proc Natl Acad Sci U S A 85:9552-9556, 1988.

90. Xu C, Oyajobi BO, Frazer A, et al: Effects of growth factors and interleukin-1 alpha on proteoglycan and type II collagen turnover in bovine nasal and articular chondrocyte pellet cultures. Endocrinology 137:3557-3565, 1996.
91. Stewart MC, Saunders KM, Burton-Wurster N, Macleod JN: Phenotypic stability of articular chondrocytes in vitro: The effects of culture models, bone morphogenetic protein 2, and serum supplementation. J Bone Miner Res 15:166-174, 2000.
92. Croucher LJ, Crawford A, Hatton PV,et al: Extracellular ATP and UTP stimulate cartilage proteoglycan and collagen accumulation in bovine articular chondrocyte pellet cultures. Biochim Biophys Acta 1502:297-306, 2000.
93. Lee GM, Poole CA, Kelley SS, et al: Isolated chondrons: A viable alternative for studies of chondrocyte metabolism in vitro. Osteoarthritis Cartilage 5:261-274, 1997.
94. Gibson GJ, Beaumont BW, Flint MH: Synthesis of a low molecular weight collagen by chondrocytes from the presumptive calcification region of the embryonic chick sterna: The influence of culture with collagen gels. J Cell Biol 99:208-216, 1984.
95. Solursh M, Jensen KL, Reiter RS, et al: Environmental regulation of type X collagen production by cultures of limb mesenchyme, mesectoderm, and sternal chondrocytes. Dev Biol 117:90-101, 1986.
96. Franzen A, Heinegard D, Solursh M: Evidence for sequential appearance of cartilage matrix proteins in developing mouse limbs and in cultures of mouse mesenchymal cells. Differentiation 36:199-210, 1987.
97. Boyan BD, Schwartz Z, Swain LD, et al: Differential expression of phenotype by resting zone and growth region costochondral chondrocytes in vitro. Bone 9:185-194, 1988.
98. Grigoriadis AE, Heersche JN, Aubin JE: Differentiation of muscle, fat, cartilage, and bone from progenitor cells present in a bone-derived clonal cell population: Effect of dexamethasone. J Cell Biol 106:2139-2151, 1988.
99. Lian JB, McKee MD, Todd AM, Gerstenfeld LC: Induction of bone-related proteins, osteocalcin and osteopontin, and their matrix ultrastructural localization with development of chondrocyte hypertrophy in vitro. J Cell Biochem 52:206-219, 1993.
100. Kato Y, Nakashima K, Iwamoto M, et al: Effects of interleukin-1 on syntheses of alkaline phosphatase, type X collagen, and 1,25-dihydroxyvitamin D3 receptor, and matrix calcification in rabbit chondrocyte cultures. J Clin Invest 92:2323-2330, 1993.
101. Ballock RT, Heydemann A, Wakefield LM, et al: TGF-beta 1 prevents hypertrophy of epiphyseal chondrocytes: Regulation of gene expression for cartilage matrix proteins and metalloproteases. Dev Biol 158:414-429, 1993.
102. Jikko A, Aoba T, Murakami H, et al: Characterization of the mineralization process in cultures of rabbit growth plate chondrocytes. Dev Biol 156:372-380, 1993.
103. Alini M, Carey D, Hirata S, et al: Cellular and matrix changes before and at the time of calcification in the growth plate studied in vitro: Arrest of type X collagen synthesis and net loss of collagen when calcification is initiated. J Bone Miner Res 9:1077-1087, 1994.
104. Glaser JH, Conrad HE: Properties of chick embryo chondrocytes grown in serum-free medium. J Biol Chem 259:6766-6772, 1984.
105. Ballock RT, Reddi AH: Thyroxine is the serum factor that regulates morphogenesis of columnar cartilage from isolated chondrocytes in chemically defined medium. J Cell Biol 126:1311-1318, 1994.
106. Bohme K, Conscience-Egli M, Tschan T, et al: Induction of proliferation or hypertrophy of chondrocytes in serum-free culture: The role of insulin-like growth factor-I, insulin, or thyroxine. J Cell Biol 116:1035-1042, 1992.
107. Habuchi H, Conrad HE, Glaser JH: Coordinate regulation of collagen and alkaline phosphatase levels in chick embryo chondrocytes. J Biol Chem 260:13029-13034, 1985.
108. Tacchetti C, Quarto R, Nitsch L,et al: In vitro morphogenesis of chick embryo hypertrophic cartilage. J Cell Biol 105:999-1006, 1987.
109. Leboy PS, Vaias L, Uschmann B, et al: Ascorbic acid induces alkaline phosphatase, type X collagen, and calcium deposition in cultured chick chondrocytes. J Biol Chem 264:17281-17286, 1989.
110. Pacifici M, Golden EB, Iwamoto M, Adams SL: Retinoic acid treatment induces type X collagen gene expression in cultured chick chondrocytes. Exp Cell Res 195:38-46, 1991.
111. Iwamoto M, Shapiro IM, Yagami K, et al: Retinoic acid induces rapid mineralization and expression of mineralization-related genes in chondrocytes. Exp Cell Res 207:413-420, 1993.
112. Quarto R, Campanile G, Cancedda R, Dozin B: Thyroid hormone, insulin, and glucocorticoids are sufficient to support chondrocyte differentiation to hypertrophy: a serum-free analysis. J Cell Biol 119:989-995, 1992.
113. Alini M, Kofsky Y, Wu W, et al: In serum-free culture thyroid hormones can induce full expression of chondrocyte hypertrophy leading to matrix calcification. J Bone Miner Res 11: 105-113, 1996.
114. Ballock RT, Zhou X, Mink LM, et al: Both retinoic acid and 1,25(OH)2 vitamin D3 inhibit thyroid hormone-induced terminal differentiaton of growth plate chondrocytes. J Orthop Res 19:43-49, 2001.
115. Leboy PS, Sullivan TA, Nooreyazdan M, Venezian RA: Rapid chondrocyte maturation by serum-free culture with BMP-2 and ascorbic acid. J Cell Biochem 66:394-403, 1997.
116. Alema S, Tato F, Boettiger D: Myc and src oncogenes have complementary effects on cell proliferation and expression of specific extracellular matrix components in definitive chondroblasts. Mol Cell Biol 5:538-544, 1985.
117. Gionti E, Pontarelli G, Cancedda R: Avian myelocytomatosis virus immortalizes differentiated quail chondrocytes. Proc Natl Acad Sci U S A 82:2756-2760, 1985.
118. Horton WE Jr, Cleveland J, Rapp U, et al: An established rat cell line expressing chondrocyte properties. Exp Cell Res 178: 457-468, 1988.
119. Thenet S, Benya PD, Demignot S, et al: SV40-immortalization of rabbit articular chondrocytes: Alteration of differentiated functions. J Cell Physiol 150:158-167, 1992.
120. Mallein-Gerin F, Olsen BR: Expression of simian virus 40 large T (tumor) oncogene in chondrocytes induces cell proliferation without loss of the differentiated phenotype. Proc Natl Acad Sci U S A 90:3289-3293, 1993.
121. Bernier SM, Goltzman D: Regulation of expression of the chondrogenic phenotype in a skeletal cell line (CFK2) in vitro. J Bone Miner Res 8:475-484, 1993.
122. Lefebvre V, Garofalo S, deCrombrugghe B: Type X collagen gene expression in mouse chondrocytes immortalized by a temperature-sensitive simian virus 40 large tumor antigen. J Cell Biol 128:239-245, 1995.
123. Mataga N, Tamura M, Yanai N, et al: Establishment of a novel chondrocyte-like cell line derived from transgenic mice harboring the temperature-sensitive simian virus 40 large T-antigen. J Bone Min Res 11:1646-1654, 1996.
124. Block JA, Inerot SE, Gitelis S, Kimura JH: Synthesis of chondrocytic keratan sulphate-containing proteoglycans by human chondrosarcoma cells in long-term cell culture. J Bone Joint Surg Am 73:647-658, 1991.
125. Takigawa M, Pan HO, Kinoshita A, et al: Establishment from a human chondrosarcoma of a new immortal cell line with high tumorigenicity in vivo, which is able to form proteoglycan-rich cartilage-like nodules and to respond to insulin in vitro. Int J Cancer 48:717-725, 1991.
126. Benoit B, Thenet-Gauci S, Hoffschir F, et al: SV40 large T antigen immortalization of human articular chondrocytes. In Vitro Cell Dev Biol 31:174-177, 1995.
127. Steimberg N, Viengchareun S, Biehlmann F, et al: SV40 large T antigen expression driven by col2a1 regulatory sequences immortalizes articular chondrocytes but does not allow stabilization of type II collagen expression. Exp Cell Res 249:248-259, 1999.
128. Goldring MB, Birkhead JR, Suen L-F, et al: Interleukin-1β-modulated gene expression in immortalized human chondrocytes. J Clin Invest 94:2307-2316, 1994.
129. Robbins JR, Thomas B, Tan L, et al: Immortalized human adult articular chondrocytes maintain cartilage-specific phenotype and responses to interleukin-1β. Arthritis Rheum 43:2189-2201, 2000.

130. Grigolo B, Roseti L, Neri S, et al: Human articular chondrocytes immortalized by HPV-16 E6 and E7 genes: Maintenance of differentiated phenotype under defined culture conditions. Osteoarthritis Cartilage 10:879-889, 2002.
131. Piera-Velazquez S, Jimenez SA, Stokes D: Increased life span of human osteoarthritic chondrocytes by exogenous expression of telomerase. Arthritis Rheum 46:683-693, 2002.
132. Salter DM, Hughes DE, Simpson R, Gardner DL: Integrin expression by human articular chondrocytes. Br J Rheumatol 31:231-234, 1992.
133. Durr J, Goodman S, Potocnik A, et al: Localization of beta 1-integrins in human cartilage and their role in chondrocyte adhesion to collagen and fibronectin. Exp Cell Res 207:235-244, 1993.
134. Woods VL Jr., Schreck PJ, Gesink DS, et al: Integrin expression by human articular chondrocytes. Arthritis Rheum 37:537-544, 1994.
135. Loeser RF, Carlson CS, McGee MP: Expression of beta 1 integrins by cultured articular chondrocytes and in osteoarthritic cartilage. Exp Cell Res 217:248-257, 1995.
136. Camper L, Hellman U, Lundgren-Akerlund E: Isolation, cloning, and sequence analysis of the integrin subunit alpha10, a beta1-associated collagen binding integrin expressed on chondrocytes. J Biol Chem 273:20383-20389, 1998.
137. Holmvall K, Camper L, Johansson S, et al: Chondrocyte and chondrosarcoma cell integrins with affinity for collagen type II and their response to mechanical stress. Exp Cell Res 221:496-503, 1995.
138. Salter DM, Godolphin JL, Gourlay MS: Chondrocyte heterogeneity: immunohistologically defined variation of integrin expression at different sites in human fetal knees. J Histochem Cytochem 43:447-457, 1995.
139. Loeser RF, Sadiev S, Tan L, Goldring MB: Integrin expression by primary and immortalized human chondrocytes: Evidence of a differential role for alpha1beta1 and alpha2beta1 integrins in mediating chondrocyte adhesion to types II and VI collagen. Osteoarthritis Cartilage 8:96-105, 2000.
140. Enomoto M, Leboy PS, Menko AS, Boettiger D: Beta 1 integrins mediate chondrocyte interaction with type I collagen, type II collagen, and fibronectin. Exp Cell Res 205:276-285, 1993.
141. Homandberg GA: Potential regulation of cartilage metabolism in osteoarthritis by fibronectin fragments. Front Biosci 4:D713-730, 1999.
142. Loeser RF: Chondrocyte integrin expression and function. Biorheology 37:109-116, 2000.
143. Salter DM, Millward-Sadler SJ, Nuki G, Wright MO: Integrin-interleukin-4 mechanotransduction pathways in human chondrocytes. Clin Orthop 391:S49-S60, 2001.
144. Mobasheri A, Carter SD, Martin-Vasallo P, Shakibaei M: Integrins and stretch activated ion channels; putative components of functional cell surface mechanoreceptors in articular chondrocytes. Cell Biol Int 26:1-18, 2002.
145. Makihira S, Yan W, Ohno S, et al: Enhancement of cell adhesion and spreading by a cartilage-specific noncollagenous protein, cartilage matrix protein (CMP/Matrilin-1), via integrin alpha1beta1. J Biol Chem 274:11417-11423, 1999.
146. Camper L, Heinegard D, Lundgren-Akerlund E: Integrin alpha2beta1 is a receptor for the cartilage matrix protein chondroadherin. J Cell Biol 138:1159-1167, 1997.
147. Loeser RF: Integrin-mediated attachment of articular chondrocytes to extracellular matrix proteins. Arthritis Rheum 36: 1103-1110, 1993.
148. Homandberg GA, Costa V, Wen C: Fibronectin fragments active in chondrocytic chondrolysis can be chemically cross-linked to the alpha5 integrin receptor subunit. Osteoarthritis Cartilage 10:938-949, 2002.
149. Yasuda T, Poole AR: A fibronectin fragment induces type II collagen degradation by collagenase through an interleukin-1-mediated pathway. Arthritis Rheum 46:138-148, 2002.
150. Forsyth CB, Pulai J, Loeser RF: Fibronectin fragments and blocking antibodies to alpha2beta1 and alpha5beta1 integrins stimulate mitogen-activated protein kinase signaling and increase collagenase 3 (matrix metalloproteinase 13) production by human articular chondrocytes. Arthritis Rheum 46:2368-2376, 2002.
151. Enomoto-Iwamoto M, Iwamoto M, Nakashima K, et al: Involvement of alpha5beta1 integrin in matrix interactions and proliferation of chondrocytes. J Bone Miner Res 12:1124-1132, 1997.
152. Shakibaei M, John T, De Souza P, et al: Signal transduction by beta1 integrin receptors in human chondrocytes in vitro: Collaboration with the insulin-like growth factor-I receptor. Biochem J 342(Pt 3):615-623, 1999.
153. Clancy RM, Rediske J, Tang X, et al: Outside-in signaling in the chondrocyte. Nitric oxide disrupts fibronectin-induced assembly of a subplasmalemmal actin/rho A/focal adhesion kinase signaling complex. J Clin Invest 100:1789-1796, 1997.
154. Scully SP, Lee JW, Ghert PMA, Qi W: The role of the extracellular matrix in articular chondrocyte regulation. Clin Orthop 391:S72-S89, 2001.
155. Qi WN, Scully SP: Type II collagen modulates the composition of extracellular matrix synthesized by articular chondrocytes. J Orthop Res 21:282-289, 2003.
156. Homandberg GA, Hui F: Association of proteoglycan degradation with catabolic cytokine and stromelysin release from cartilage cultured with fibronectin fragments. Arch Biochem Biophys 334:325-331, 1996.
157. Yonezawa I, Kato K, Yagita H, et al: VLA-5-mediated interaction with fibronectin induces cytokine production by human chondrocytes. Biochem Biophys Res Commun 219:261-265, 1996.
158. Arner EC, Tortorella MD: Signal transduction through chondrocyte integrin receptors induces matrix metalloproteinase synthesis and synergizes with interleukin-1. Arthritis Rheum 38:1304-1314, 1995.
159. Attur MG, Dave MN, Clancy RM, et al: Functional genomic analysis in arthritis-affected cartilage: yin-yang regulation of inflammatory mediators by alpha 5 beta 1 and alpha V beta 3 integrins. J Immunol 164:2684-2691, 2000.
160. Heino J: The collagen receptor integrins have distinct ligand recognition and signaling functions. Matrix Biol 19:319-323, 2000.
161. Mollenhauer J, von der Mark K: Isolation and characterization of a collagen-binding glycoprotein from chondrocyte membranes. Embo J 2:45-50, 1983.
162. Mollenhauer J, Bee JA, Lizarbe MA, von der Mark K: Role of anchorin CII, a 31,000-mol-wt membrane protein, in the interaction of chondrocytes with type II collagen. J Cell Biol 98:1572-1579, 1984.
163. Pfaffle M, Ruggiero F, Hofmann H, et al: Biosynthesis, secretion and extracellular localization of anchorin CII, a collagen-binding protein of the calpactin family. Embo J 7:2335-2342, 1988.
164. Genge BR, Cao X, Wu LN, et al: Establishment of the primary structure of the major lipid-dependent Ca2+ binding proteins of chicken growth plate cartilage matrix vesicles: Identity with anchorin CII (annexin V) and annexin II. J Bone Miner Res 7:807-819, 1992.
165. King KB, Chubinskaya S, Reid DL, et al: Absence of cell-surface annexin V is accompanied by defective collagen matrix binding in the Swarm rat chondrosarcoma. J Cell Biochem 65:131-144, 1997.
166. Kirsch T, Harrison G, Golub EE, Nah HD: The roles of annexins and types II and X collagen in matrix vesicle-mediated mineralization of growth plate cartilage. J Biol Chem 275:35577-35583, 2000.
167. Mollenhauer J, Mok MT, King KB, et al: Expression of anchorin CII (cartilage annexin V) in human young, normal adult, and osteoarthritic cartilage. J Histochem Cytochem 47:209-220, 1999.
168. Reid DL, Aydelotte MB, Mollenhauer J: Cell attachment, collagen binding, and receptor analysis on bovine articular chondrocytes. J Orthop Res 18:364-373, 2000.
169. Kurtis MS, Tu BP, Gaya OA, et al: Mechanisms of chondrocyte adhesion to cartilage: Role of beta1-integrins, CD44, and annexin V. J Orthop Res 19:1122-1130, 2001.
170. Hua Q, Knudson CB, Knudson W: Internalization of hyaluronan by chondrocytes occurs via receptor-mediated endocytosis. J Cell Sci 106:365-375, 1993.
171. Salter DM, Godolphin JL, Gourlay MS, et al: Analysis of human articular chondrocyte CD44 isoform expression and function in health and disease. J Pathol 179:396-402, 1996.

172. Aguiar DJ, Knudson W, Knudson CB: Internalization of the hyaluronan receptor CD44 by chondrocytes. Exp Cell Res 252:292-302, 1999.
173. Chow G, Nietfeld JJ, Knudson CB, Knudson W: Antisense inhibition of chondrocyte CD44 expression leading to cartilage chondrolysis. Arthritis Rheum 41:1411-1419, 1998.
174. Knudson CB: Hyaluronan receptor-directed assembly of chondrocyte pericellular matrix. J Cell Biol 120:825-834, 1993.
175. Knudson W, Aguiar DJ, Hua Q, Knudson CB: CD44-anchored hyaluronan-rich pericellular matrices: An ultrastructural and biochemical analysis. Exp Cell Res 228:216-228, 1996.
176. Yasuda T, Poole AR, Shimizu M, et al: Involvement of CD44 in induction of matrix metalloproteinases by a COOH-terminal heparin-binding fragment of fibronectin in human articular cartilage in culture. Arthritis Rheum 48:1271-1280, 2003.
177. Chow G, Knudson CB, Homandberg G, Knudson W: Increased expression of CD44 in bovine articular chondrocytes by catabolic cellular mediators. J Biol Chem 270:27734-27741, 1995.
178. Eisenstein R, Kuettner KE, Neapolitan C, et al: The resistance of certain tissues to invasion. III. Cartilage extracts inhibit the growth of fibroblasts and endothelial cells in culture. Am J Pathol 81:337-347, 1975.
179. Brem H, Folkman J: Inhibition of tumor angiogenesis mediated by cartilage. J Exp Med 141:427-439, 1975.
180. Moses MA, Sudhalter J, Langer R: Identification of an inhibitor of neovascularization from cartilage. Science 248:1408-1410, 1990.
181. Moses MA, Sudhalter J, Langer R: Isolation and characterization of an inhibitor of neovascularization from scapular chondrocytes. J Cell Biol 119:475-482, 1992.
182. Brown RA, Weiss JB: Neovascularisation and its role in the osteoarthritic process. Ann Rheum Dis 47:881-885, 1988.
183. Colville-Nash PR, Scott DL: Angiogenesis and rheumatoid arthritis: pathogenic and therapeutic implications. Ann Rheum Dis 51:919-925, 1992.
184. Moses MA, Wiederschain D, Wu I, et al: Troponin I is present in human cartilage and inhibits angiogenesis. Proc Natl Acad Sci U S A 96:2645-2650, 1999.
185. Shukunami C, Hiraki Y: Role of cartilage-derived anti-angiogenic factor, chondromodulin-I, during endochondral bone formation. Osteoarthritis Cartilage 9(Suppl A):S91-S101, 2001.
186. O'Reilly MS, Boehm T, Shing Y, et al: Endostatin: An endogenous inhibitor of angiogenesis and tumor growth. Cell 88:277-285, 1997.
187. Pufe T, Petersen W, Goldring MB, et al: Endostatin–an inhibitor of angiogenesis–is expressed in human cartilage and fibrocartilage. Matrix Biol (in press).
188. Carlevaro MF, Cermelli S, Cancedda R, et al: Vascular endothelial growth factor (VEGF) in cartilage neovascularization and chondrocyte differentiation: Auto-paracrine role during endochondral bone formation. J Cell Sci 113(Pt 1):59-69, 2000.
189. Schipani E, Ryan HE, Didrickson S, et al: Hypoxia in cartilage: HIF-1alpha is essential for chondrocyte growth arrest and survival. Genes Dev 15:2865-2876, 2001.
190. Pufe T, Petersen W, Tillmann B, Mentlein R: The splice variants VEGF121 and VEGF189 of the angiogenic peptide vascular endothelial growth factor are expressed in osteoarthritic cartilage. Arthritis Rheum 44:1082-1088, 2001.
191. Pfander D, Kortje D, Zimmermann R, et al: Vascular endothelial growth factor in articular cartilage of healthy and osteoarthritic human knee joints. Ann Rheum Dis 60:1070-1073, 2001.
192. Berse B, Hunt JA, Diegel RJ, et al: Hypoxia augments cytokine (transforming growth factor-beta (TGF-beta) and IL-1)-induced vascular endothelial growth factor secretion by human synovial fibroblasts. Clin Exp Immunol 115:176-182, 1999.
193. Reddi AH: Role of morphogenetic proteins in skeletal tissue engineering and regeneration. Nature Biotech 16:247-252, 1998.
194. van den Berg WB: The role of cytokines and growth factors in cartilage destruction in osteoarthritis and rheumatoid arthritis. Zeitschrift fur Rheumatologie 58:136-141, 1999.
195. Reddi AH: Interplay between bone morphogenetic proteins and cognate binding proteins in bone and cartilage development: noggin, chordin and DAN. Arthritis Res 3:1-5, 2001.
196. Nataf V, Tsagris L, Dumontier MF, et al: Modulation of sulfated proteoglycan synthesis and collagen gene expression by chondrocytes grown in the presence of bFGF alone or combined with IGF1. Reprod Nutr Dev 30:331-342, 1990.
197. O'Keefe RJ, Crabb ID, Puzas JE, Rosier RN: Effects of transforming growth factor-β1 and fibroblast growth factor on DNA synthesis in growth plate chondrocytes are enhanced by insulin-like growth factor-I. J Orthopaed Res 12:299-310, 1994.
198. Daughaday WH, Hall K, Raben MS, et al: Somatomedin: proposed designation for sulphation factor. Nature 235:107, 1972.
199. McQuillan DJ, Handley CJ, Campbell MA, et al: Stimulation of proteoglycan biosynthesis by serum and insulin-like growth factor-I in cultured bovine articular cartilage. Biochem J 240:423-430, 1986.
200. Fosang AJ, Tyler JA, Hardingham TE: Effect of interleukin-1 and insulin like growth factor-1 on the release of proteoglycan components and hyaluronan from pig articular cartilage in explant culture. Matrix 11:17-24, 1991.
201. Trippel SB: Growth factor actions on articular cartilage. J Rheumatol 43(Suppl):129-132, 1995.
202. Trippel SB, Corvol MT, Dumontier MF, et al: Effect of somatomedin-C/insulin-like growth factor I and growth hormone on cultured growth plate and articular chondrocytes. Pediatr Res 25:76-82, 1989.
203. Nixon AJ, Lillich JT, Burton-Wurster N, et al: Differentiated cellular function in fetal chondrocytes cultured with insulin-like growth factor-I and transforming growth factor-beta. J Orthop Res 16:531-541, 1998.
204. Fortier LA, Lust G, Mohammed HO, Nixon AJ: Coordinate upregulation of cartilage matrix synthesis in fibrin cultures supplemented with exogenous insulin-like growth factor-I. J Orthop Res 17:467-474, 1999.
205. Trippel SB, Whelan MC, Klagsburn M, Doctrow SR: Interaction of basic fibroblast growth factor with bovine growth plate chondrocytes. J Orthop Res 10:638-646, 1992.
206. Loeser RF, Shanker G: Autocrine stimulation by insulin-like growth factor 1 and insulin-like growth factor 2 mediates chondrocyte survival in vitro. Arthritis Rheum 43:1552-1559, 2000.
207. Bhaumick B: Insulin-like growth factor (IGF) binding proteins and insulin-like growth factor secretion by cultured chondrocyte cells: identification, characterization and ontogeny during cell differentiation. Regul Pept 48:113-122, 1993.
208. Morales TI: The role and content of endogenous insulin-like growth factor-binding proteins in bovine articular cartilage. Arch Biochem Biophys 343:164-172, 1997.
209. Sunic D, McNeil JD, Rayner TE, et al: Regulation of insulin-like growth factor-binding protein-5 by insulin-like growth factor I and interleukin-1alpha in ovine articular chondrocytes. Endocrinology 139:2356-2362, 1998.
210. Bhakta NR, Garcia AM, Frank EH, et al: The insulin-like growth factors (IGFs) I and II bind to articular cartilage via the IGF-binding proteins. J Biol Chem 275:5860-5866, 2000.
211. Morales TI: The insulin-like growth factor binding proteins in uncultured human cartilage: Increases in insulin-like growth factor binding protein 3 during osteoarthritis. Arthritis Rheum 46:2358-2367, 2002.
212. Morales TI, Hunziker EB: Localization of insulin-like growth factor binding protein-2 in chondrocytes of bovine articular cartilage. J Orthop Res 21:290-295, 2003.
213. Fernihough JK, Richmond RS, Carlson CS, et al: Estrogen replacement therapy modulation of the insulin-like growth factor system in monkey knee joints. Arthritis Rheum 42:2103-2111, 1999.
214. Spagnoli A, Hwa V, Horton WA, et al: Antiproliferative effects of insulin-like growth factor-binding protein-3 in mesenchymal chondrogenic cell line RCJ3.1C5.18. relationship to differentiation stage. J Biol Chem 276:5533-5540, 2001.
215. Middleton JF, Tyler JA: Upregulation of insulin-like growth factor I gene expression in the lesions of osteoarthritic human articular cartilage. Ann Rheum Dis 51:440-447, 1992.
216. Dore S, Pelletier JP, DiBattista JA, et al: Human osteoarthritic chondrocytes possess an increased number of insulin-like growth factor 1 binding sites but are unresponsive to its stimulation. Possible role of IGF-1-binding proteins. Arthritis Rheum 37:253-263, 1994.

217. Olney RC, Tsuchiya K, Wilson DM, et al: Chondrocytes from osteoarthritic cartilage have increased expression of insulin-like growth factor I (IGF-I) and IGF-binding protein-3 (IGFBP-3) and -5, but not IGF-II or IGFBP-4. J Clin Endocrinol Metab 81:1096-1103, 1996.
218. Chevalier X, Tyler JA: Production of binding proteins and role of the insulin-like growth factor I binding protein 3 in human articular cartilage explants. Br J Rheumatol 35:515-522, 1996.
219. Tardif G, Reboul P, Pelletier JP, et al: Normal expression of type 1 insulin-like growth factor receptor by human osteoarthritic chondrocytes with increased expression and synthesis of insulin-like growth factor binding proteins. Arthritis Rheum 39:968-978, 1996.
220. Fernihough JK, Billingham ME, Cwyfan-Hughes S, Holly JM: Local disruption of the insulin-like growth factor system in the arthritic joint. Arthritis Rheum 39:1556-1565, 1996.
221. Whellams EJ, Maile LA, Fernihough JK, et al: Alterations in insulin-like growth factor binding protein-3 proteolysis and complex formation in the arthritic joint. J Endocrinol 165:545-556, 2000.
222. Neidel J: Changes in systemic levels of insulin-like growth factors and their binding proteins in patients with rheumatoid arthritis. Clin Exp Rheumatol 19:81-84, 2001.
223. Matsumoto T, Tsurumoto T: Inappropriate serum levels of IGF-I and IGFBP-3 in patients with rheumatoid arthritis. Rheumatology (Oxford) 41:352-353, 2002.
224. Loeser RF, Shanker G, Carlson CS, et al: Reduction in the chondrocyte response to insulin-like growth factor 1 in aging and osteoarthritis: studies in a non-human primate model of naturally occurring disease. Arthritis Rheum 43:2110-2120, 2000.
225. Tyler JA: Insulin-like growth factor 1 can decrease degradation and promote synthesis of proteoglycan in cartilage exposed to cytokines. Biochem J 260:543-548, 1989.
226. Olney RC, Wilson DM, Mohtai M, et al: Interleukin-1 and tumor necrosis factor-alpha increase insulin-like growth factor-binding protein-3 (IGFBP-3) production and IGFBP-3 protease activity in human articular chondrocytes. J Endocrinol 146:279-286, 1995.
227. van de Loo FA, Arntz OJ, van Enckevort FH, et al: Reduced cartilage proteoglycan loss during zymosan-induced gonarthritis in NOS2-deficient mice and in anti-interleukin-1-treated wild-type mice with unabated joint inflammation. Arthritis Rheum 41:634-646, 1998.
228. Loeser RF, Carlson CS, Del Carlo M, Cole A: Detection of nitrotyrosine in aging and osteoarthritic cartilage: Correlation of oxidative damage with the presence of interleukin-1beta and with chondrocyte resistance to insulin-like growth factor 1. Arthritis Rheum 46:2349-2357, 2002.
229. Martin JA, Ellerbroek SM, Buckwalter JA: Age-related decline in chondrocyte response to insulin-like growth factor-I: The role of growth factor binding proteins. J Orthop Res 15:491-498, 1997.
230. Mason IJ: The ins and outs of fibroblast growth factors. Cell 78:547-552, 1994.
231. Nishimura T, Nakatake Y, Konishi M, Itoh N: Identification of a novel FGF, FGF-21, preferentially expressed in the liver. Biochim Biophys Acta 1492:203-206, 2000.
232. Kato Y, Iwamoto M: Fibroblast growth factor is an inhibitor of chondrocyte terminal differentiation. J Biol Chem 265:5903-5909, 1990.
233. Sah RL, Chen AC, Grodzinsky AJ, Trippel SB: Differential effects of bFGF and IGF-I on matrix metabolism in calf and adult bovine cartilage explants. Arch Biochem Biophys 308:137-147, 1994.
234. Davidson JM, Klagsbrun M, Hill KE, et al: Accelerated wound repair, cell proliferation and collagen accumulation are produced by a cartilage-derived growth factor. J Cell Biol 100:1219-1227, 1985.
235. Kato Y, Gospodarowicz D: Growth requirements of low-density rabbit costal chondrocyte cultures maintained in serum-free medium. J Cell Physiol 120:354-363, 1984.
236. Sah RL, Trippel SB, Grodzinsky AJ: Differential effects of serum, insulin-like growth factor-I, and fibroblast growth factor-2 on the maintenance of cartilage physical properties during long-term culture. J Orthop Res 14:44-52, 1996.
237. Jingushi S, Scully SP, Joyce ME, et al: Transforming growth factor-beta 1 and fibroblast growth factors in rat growth plate. J Orthop Res 13:761-768, 1995.
238. Stheneur C, Dumontier MF, Guedes C, et al: Basic fibroblast growth factor as a selective inducer of matrix Gla protein gene expression in proliferative chondrocytes. Biochem J 369:63-70, 2003.
239. Luo G, D'Souza R, Hogue D, Karsenty G: The matrix Gla protein gene is a marker of the chondrogenesis cell lineage during mouse development. J Bone Miner Res 10:325-334, 1995.
240. Yagami K, Suh JY, Enomoto-Iwamoto M, et al: Matrix GLA protein is a developmental regulator of chondrocyte mineralization and, when constitutively expressed, blocks endochondral and intramembranous ossification in the limb. J Cell Biol 147: 1097-1108, 1999.
241. Newman B, Gigout LI, Sudre L, et al: Coordinated expression of matrix Gla protein is required during endochondral ossification for chondrocyte survival. J Cell Biol 154:659-666, 2001.
242. Urist MR: Bone: formation by osteoinduction. Science 150:893, 1965.
243. Urist MR, Huo YK, Brownell AG, et al: Purification of bovine bone morphogenetic protein by hydroxyapatite chromatography. Proc Natl Acad Sci U S A 81:371, 1984.
244. Sampath TK, Reddi AH: Dissociative extraction and reconstitution of extracellular matrix components involved in local bone differentiation. Proc Natl Acad Sci U S A 78:7599-7603, 1981.
245. Wozney JM, Rosen V, Celeste AJ, et al: Novel regulators of bone formation: molecular clones and activities. Science 242:1528-1534, 1988.
246. Wang EA, Rosen V, Cordes P, et al: Purification and characterization of other distinct bone-inducing factors. Proc Natl Acad Sci U S A 85:9484-9488, 1988.
247. Rosen V, Wozney JM, Wang EA, et al: Purification and molecular cloning of a novel group of BMPs and localization of BMP mRNA in developing bone. Connect Tissue Res 20:313-319, 1989.
248. Reddi AH: Bone morphogenetic proteins: An unconventional approach to isolation of first mammalian morphogens. Cytokine Growth Factor Rev 8:11-20, 1997.
249. Rosen DM, Stempien SA, Thompson AY, Seyedin SM: Transforming growth factor-beta modulates the expression of osteoblast and chondroblast phenotypes *in vitro*. J Cell Physiol 134:337-346, 1988.
250. Celeste AJ, Iannazzi JA, Taylor RC, et al: Identification of transforming growth factor beta family members present in bone-inductive protein purified from bovine bone. Proc Natl Acad Sci U S A 87:9843-9847, 1990.
251. Kingsley DM: The TGF-β superfamily: New members, new receptors, and new genetic tests of function in different organisms. Genes Devel 8:133-146, 1994.
252. Erlebacher A, Filvaroff EH, Gitelman SE, Derynck R: Toward a molecular understanding of skeletal development. Cell 80: 371-378, 1995.
253. Rosen V, Thies RS: The BMP proteins in bone formation and repair. Trends Genet 8:97-102, 1992.
254. Chang SC, Hoang B, Thomas JT, et al: Cartilage-derived morphogenetic proteins. New members of the transforming growth factor-beta superfamily predominantly expressed in long bones during human embryonic development. J Biol Chem 269:28227-28234, 1994.
255. Hall BK, Miyake T: Divide, accumulate, differentiate: Cell condensation in skeletal development revisited. Int J Dev Biol 39:881-893, 1995.
256. Edwards CJ, Francis-West PH: Bone morphogenetic proteins in the development and healing of synovial joints. Semin Arthritis Rheum 31:33-42, 2001.
257. Hogan BL: Bone morphogenetic proteins: Multifunctional regulators of vertebrate development. Genes Dev 10:1580-1594, 1996.
258. Carrington JL, Chen P, Yanagishita M, Reddi AH: Osteogenin (bone morphogenetic protein-3) stimulates cartilage formation by chick limb bud cells in vitro. Developmental Biology (Orlando) 146:406-415, 1991.
259. Chen P, Carrington JL, Hammonds RG, Reddi AH: Stimulation of chondrogenesis in limb bud mesoderm cells by recombinant human bone morphogenetic protein 2B (BMP-2B) and modu-

lation by transforming growth factor beta 1 and beta 2. Experimental Cell Research 195:509-515, 1991.
260. Asahina I, Sampath TK, Nishimura I, Hauschka PV: Human osteogenic protein-1 induces both chondroblastic and osteoblastic differentiation of osteoprogenitor cells derived from newborn rat calvaria. J Cell Biol 123:921-933, 1993.
261. Rosen V, Nove J, Song JJ, et al: Responsiveness of clonal limb bud cell lines to bone morphogenetic protein 2 reveals a sequential relationship between cartilage and bone cell phenotypes. J Bone Miner Res 9:1759-1768, 1994.
262. Johnstone B, Hering TM, Caplan AI, et al: In vitro chondrogenesis of bone marrow-derived mesenchymal progenitor cells. Exp Cell Res 238:265-272, 1998.
263. Klein-Nulend J, Semeins CM, Mulder JW, et al: Stimulation of cartilage differentiation by osteogenic protein-1 in cultures of human perichondrium. Tissue Eng 4:305-313, 1998.
264. Shukunami C, Ohta Y, Sakuda M, Hiraki Y: Sequential progression of the differentiation program by bone morphogenetic protein-2 in chondrogenic cell line ATDC5. Exp Cell Res 241:1-11, 1998.
265. Pittenger MF, Mackay AM, Beck SC, et al: Multilineage potential of adult human mesenchymal stem cells. Science 284:143-147, 1999.
266. Kramer J, Hegert C, Guan K, et al: Embryonic stem cell-derived chondrogenic differentiation in vitro: Activation by BMP-2 and BMP-4. Mech Dev 92:193-205, 2000.
267. Majumdar MK, Banks V, Peluso DP, Morris EA: Isolation, characterization, and chondrogenic potential of human bone marrow-derived multipotential stromal cells. J Cell Physiol 185:98-106, 2000.
268. Gruber R, Mayer C, Bobacz K, et al: Effects of cartilage-derived morphogenetic proteins and osteogenic protein-1 on osteochondrogenic differentiation of periosteum-derived cells. Endocrinology 142:2087-2094, 2001.
269. Sekiya I, Colter DC, Prockop DJ: BMP-6 enhances chondrogenesis in a subpopulation of human marrow stromal cells. Biochem Biophys Res Commun 284:411-418, 2001.
270. Luyten FP, Yu YM, Yanagishita M, et al: Natural bovine osteogenin and recombinant human bone morphogenetic protein-2B are equipotent in the maintenance of proteoglycans in bovine articular cartilage explant cultures. J Biol Chem 267:3691-3695, 1992.
271. Chen P, Vukicevic S, Sampath TK, Luyten FP: Bovine articular chondrocytes do not undergo hypertrophy when cultured in the presence of serum and osteogenic protein-1. Biochem Biophys Res Commun 197:1253-1259, 1993.
272. Luyten FP, Chen P, Paralkar V, Reddi AH: Recombinant bone morphogenetic protein-4, transforming growth factor-beta 1, and activin A enhance the cartilage phenotype of articular chondrocytes in vitro. Exper Cell Res 210:224-229, 1994.
273. Lietman SA, Yanagishita M, Sampath TK, Reddi AH: Stimulation of proteoglycan synthesis in explants of porcine articular cartilage by recombinant osteogenic protein-1 (bone morphogenetic protein-7). J Bone Joint Surg Am 79:1132-1137, 1997.
274. Erlacher L, Ng CK, Ullrich R, et al: Presence of cartilage-derived morphogenetic proteins in articular cartilage and enhancement of matrix replacement in vitro. Arthritis Rheum 41:263-273, 1998.
275. Valcourt U, Ronziere MC, Winkler P, et al: Different effects of bone morphogenetic proteins 2, 4, 12, and 13 on the expression of cartilage and bone markers in the MC615 chondrocyte cell line. Exp Cell Res 251:264-274, 1999.
276. Morales TI, Roberts AB: Transforming growth factor-β regulates the metabolism of proteoglycans in bovine cartilage organ cultures. J Biol Chem 263:12828-12831, 1988.
277. Rosier RN, OKeefe RJ, Crabb ID, Puzas JE: Transforming growth factor beta: an autocrine regulator of chondrocytes. Connect Tissue Res 20:295-301, 1989.
278. Horton WEJ, Higginbotham JD, Chandrasekhar S: Transforming growth factor-beta and fibroblast growth factor act synergistically to inhibit collagen II synthesis through a mechanism involving regulatory DNA sequences. J Cell Physiol 141:8-15, 1989.
279. Hardingham TE, Bayliss MT, Rayan V, Noble DP: Effects of growth factors and cytokines on proteoglycan turnover in articular cartilage. Br J Rheumatol 31(Suppl 1):1-6, 1992.
280. Frazer A, Bunning RA, Thavarajah M, et al: Studies on type II collagen and aggrecan production in human articular chondrocytes in vitro and effects of transforming growth factor-beta and interleukin-1beta. Osteoarthritis Cartilage 2:235-245, 1994.
281. Shuler FD, Georgescu HI, Niyibizi C, et al: Increased matrix synthesis following adenoviral transfer of a transforming growth factor beta1 gene into articular chondrocytes. J Orthop Res 18:585-592, 2000.
282. Moldovan F, Pelletier JP, Hambor J, et al: Collagenase-3 (matrix metalloprotease 13) is preferentially localized in the deep layer of human arthritic cartilage in situ: in vitro mimicking effect by transforming growth factor β. Arthritis Rheum 40:1653-1661, 1997.
283. Schlaak JF, Pfers I, Meyer Zum Buschenfelde KH, Marker-Hermann E: Different cytokine profiles in the synovial fluid of patients with osteoarthritis, rheumatoid arthritis and seronegative spondylarthropathies. Clin Exp Rheumatol 14:155-162, 1996.
284. Chambers MG, Bayliss MT, Mason RM: Chondrocyte cytokine and growth factor expression in murine osteoarthritis. Osteoarthritis Cartilage 5:301-308, 1997.
285. Bakker AC, van de Loo FA, van Beuningen HM, et al: Overexpression of active TGF-beta-1 in the murine knee joint: evidence for synovial-layer-dependent chondro-osteophyte formation. Osteoarthritis Cartilage 9:128-136, 2001.
286. van Beuningen HM, Glansbeek HL, van der Kraan PM, van den Berg WB: Osteoarthritis-like changes in the murine knee joint resulting from intra-articular transforming growth factor-β injections. Osteoarthritis Cartilage 8:25-33, 2000.
287. Kessler E, Takahara K, Biniaminov L, et al: Bone morphogenetic protein-1: The type I procollagen C-proteinase. Science 271:360-362, 1996.
288. Li SW, Sieron AL, Fertala A, et al: The C-proteinase that processes procollagens to fibrillar collagens is identical to the protein previously identified as bone morphogenic protein-1. Proc Natl Acad Sci U S A 93:5127-5130, 1996.
289. Goodman SA, Albano R, Wardle FC, et al: BMP1-related metalloproteinases promote the development of ventral mesoderm in early Xenopus embryos. Dev Biol 195:144-157, 1998.
290. Sailor LZ, Hewick RM, Morris EA: Recombinant human bone morphogenetic protein-2 maintains the articular chondrocyte phenotype in long-term culture. J Orthop Res 14:937-945, 1996.
291. Flechtenmacher J, Huch K, Thonar EJ, et al: Recombinant human osteogenic protein 1 is a potent stimulator of the synthesis of cartilage proteoglycans and collagens by human articular chondrocytes. Arthritis Rheum 39:1896-1904, 1996.
292. Nishihara A, Fujii M, Sampath TK, et al: Bone morphogenetic protein signaling in articular chondrocyte differentiation. Biochem Biophys Res Commun 301:617-622, 2003.
293. Chubinskaya S, Merrihew C, Cs-Szabo G, et al: Human articular chondrocytes express osteogenic protein-1. J Histochem Cytochem 48:239-250, 2000.
294. Nakase T, Miyaji T Tomita T, et al: Localization of bone morphogenetic protein-2 in human osteoarthritic cartilage and osteophyte. Osteoarthritis Cartilage 11:278-284, 2003.
295. Dell'Accio F, De Bari C, Luyten FP: Molecular markers predictive of the capacity of expanded human articular chondrocytes to form stable cartilage in vivo. Arthritis Rheum 44:1608-1619, 2001.
296. Huch K, Wilbrink B, Flechtenmacher J, et al: Effects of recombinant human osteogenic protein 1 on the production of proteoglycan, prostaglandin E2, and interleukin-1 receptor antagonist by human articular chondrocytes cultured in the presence of interleukin-1beta. Arthritis Rheum 40:2157-2161, 1997.
297. Majumdar MK, Wang E, Morris EA: BMP-2 and BMP-9 promotes chondrogenic differentiation of human multipotential mesenchymal cells and overcomes the inhibitory effect of IL-1. J Cell Physiol 189:275-284, 2001.
298. Vinall RL, Lo SH, Reddi AH: Regulation of articular chondrocyte phenotype by bone morphogenetic protein 7, interleukin 1, and cellular context is dependent on the cytoskeleton. Exp Cell Res 272:32-44, 2002.
299. Takegami K, Thonar EJ, An HS, et al: Osteogenic protein-1 enhances matrix replenishment by intervertebral disc cells previously exposed to interleukin-1. Spine 27:1318-1325, 2002.

300. Glansbeek HL, van Beuningen HM, Vitters EL, et al: Bone morphogenetic protein 2 stimulates articular cartilage proteoglycan synthesis in vivo but does not counteract interleukin-1α effects on proteoglycan synthesis and content. Arthritis Rheum 40:1020-1028, 1997.
301. Dieudonne SC, Semeins CM, Goei SW, et al: Opposite effects of osteogenic protein and transforming growth factor beta on chondrogenesis in cultured long bone rudiments. J Bone Miner Res 9:771-780, 1994.
302. Wang EA, Israel DI, Kelly S, Luxenberg DP: Bone morphogenetic protein-2 causes commitment and differentiation in C3H10T1/2 and 3T3 cells. Growth Factors 9:57-71, 1993.
303. Izzo MW, Pucci B, Tuan RS, Hall DJ: Gene expression profiling following BMP-2 induction of mesenchymal chondrogenesis in vitro. Osteoarthritis Cartilage 10:23-33, 2002.
304. Erlacher L, McCartney J, Piek E, et al: Cartilage-derived morphogenetic proteins and osteogenic protein-1 differentially regulate osteogenesis. J Bone Miner Res 13:383-392, 1998.
305. Shukunami C, Akiyama H, Nakamura T, Hiraki Y: Requirement of autocrine signaling by bone morphogenetic protein-4 for chondrogenic differentiation of ATDC5 cells. FEBS Lett 469: 83-87, 2000.
306. Macias D, Ganan Y, Sampath TK, et al: Role of BMP-2 and OP-1 (BMP-7) in programmed cell death and skeletogenesis during chick limb development. Development 124:1109-1117, 1997.
307. Yamaguchi A, Katagiri T, Ikeda T, et al: Recombinant human bone morphogenetic protein-2 stimulates osteoblastic maturation and inhibits myogenic differentiation in vitro. J Cell Biol 113:681-687, 1991.
308. Gitelman SE, Kirk M, Ye JQ, et al: Vgr-1/BMP-6 induces osteoblastic differentiation of pluripotential mesenchymal cells. Cell Growth Differ 6:827-836, 1995.
309. Takuwa Y, Ohse C, Wang EA, et al: Bone morphogenetic protein-2 stimulates alkaline phosphatase activity and collagen synthesis in cultured osteoblastic cells, MC3T3-E1. Biochem Biophys Res Commun 174:96-101, 1991.
310. Nishimura R, Kato Y, Chen D, et al: Smad5 and DPC4 are key molecules in mediating BMP-2-induced osteoblastic differentiation of the pluripotent mesenchymal precursor cell line C2C12. J Biol Chem 273:1872-1879, 1998.
311. Yamamoto N, Akiyama S, Katagiri T, et al: Smad1 and smad5 act downstream of intracellular signalings of BMP-2 that inhibits myogenic differentiation and induces osteoblast differentiation in C2C12 myoblasts. Biochem Biophys Res Commun 238:574-580, 1997.
312. Hotten GC, Matsumoto T, Kimura M, et al: Recombinant human growth/differentiation factor 5 stimulates mesenchyme aggregation and chondrogenesis responsible for the skeletal development of limbs. Growth Factors 13:65-74, 1996.
313. Bobacz K, Gruber R, Soleiman A, et al: Cartilage-derived morphogenetic protein-1 and -2 are endogenously expressed in healthy and osteoarthritic human articular chondrocytes and stimulate matrix synthesis. Osteoarthritis Cartilage 10:394-401, 2002.
314. Gruber R, Mayer C, Schulz W, et al: Stimulatory effects of cartilage-derived morphogenetic proteins 1 and 2 on osteogenic differentiation of bone marrow stromal cells. Cytokine 12:1630-1638, 2000.
315. De Bari C, Dell'Accio F, Luyten FP: Human periosteum-derived cells maintain phenotypic stability and chondrogenic potential throughout expansion regardless of donor age. Arthritis Rheum 44:85-95, 2001.
316. Massagué J, Hata A, Fang L: TGF-β signalling through the Smad pathway. Trends Cell Biol 7:187-192, 1997.
317. Kawabata M, Imamura T, Miyazono K: Signal transduction by bone morphogenetic proteins. Cytokine Growth Factor Rev 9:49-61, 1998.
318. Massague J: TGF-beta signal transduction. Annu Rev Biochem 67:753-791, 1998.
319. Balemans W, Van Hul W: Extracellular regulation of BMP signaling in vertebrates: A cocktail of modulators. Dev Biol 250: 231-250, 2002.
320. Rosen V, Thies RS, Lyons K: Signaling pathways in skeletal formation: a role for BMP receptors. Ann N Y Acad Sci 785:59-69, 1996.
321. Sakou T: Bone morphogenetic proteins: From basic studies to clinical approaches. Bone 22:591-603, 1998.
322. Heldin CH, Miyazono K, ten Dijke P: TGF-beta signalling from cell membrane to nucleus through SMAD proteins. Nature 390:465-471, 1997.
323. Wrana JL: Regulation of Smad activity. Cell 100:189-192, 2000.
324. Smith WC, Harland RM: Expression cloning of noggin, a new dorsalizing factor localized to the Spemann organizer in Xenopus embryos. Cell 70:829-840, 1992.
325. Piccolo S, Sasai Y, Lu B, De Robertis EM: Dorsoventral patterning in Xenopus: inhibition of ventral signals by direct binding of chordin to BMP-4. Cell 86:589-598, 1996.
326. Zimmerman LB, De Jesus-Escobar JM, Harland RM: The Spemann organizer signal noggin binds and inactivates bone morphogenetic protein 4. Cell 86:599-606, 1996.
327. Brunet LJ, McMahon JA, McMahon AP, Harland RM: Noggin, cartilage morphogenesis, and joint formation in the mammalian skeleton. Science 280:1455-1457, 1998.
328. Larrain J, Oelgeschlager M, Ketpura NI, et al: Proteolytic cleavage of Chordin as a switch for the dual activities of Twisted gastrulation in BMP signaling. Development 128:4439-4447, 2001.
329. Zhu Y, McAlinden A, Sandell LJ: Type IIA procollagen in development of the human intervertebral disc: regulated expression of the NH(2)-propeptide by enzymic processing reveals a unique developmental pathway. Dev Dyn 220:350-362, 2001.
330. Fukui N, Purple CR, Sandell LJ: Cell biology of osteoarthritis: the chondrocyte's response to injury. Curr Rheumatol Rep 3:496-505, 2001.
331. Dayer JM: The pivotal role of interleukin-1 in the clinical manifestations of rheumatoid arthritis. Rheumatology (Oxford) 42(Suppl 2):ii3-ii10, 2003.
332. van den Berg WB: Lessons for joint destruction from animal models. Curr Opin Rheumatol 9:221-228, 1997.
333. Goldring MB: The role of cytokines as inflammatory mediators in osteoarthritis: lessons from animal models. Connect Tissue Res 40:1-11, 1999.
334. Goldring MB: Anticytokine therapy for osteoarthritis. Expert Opin Biol Ther 1:817-829, 2001.
335. Fukui N, Purple DR, Sandell LJ: Cell biology of osteoarthritis: The chondrocyte's response to injury. Curr Rheum Rep 3: 496-505, 2001.
336. van den Berg WB: Uncoupling of inflammatory and destructive mechanisms in arthritis. Semin Arthritis Rheum 30:7-16, 2001.
337. Goldring MB, Goldring SR: Role of cytokines and chemokines in cartilage and bone destruction in arthritis. Curr Opin Orthopaed 13:351-362, 2002.
338. Stahle-Backdahl M, Sandstedt B, Bruce K, et al: Collagenase-3 (MMP-13) is expressed during human fetal ossification and re-expressed in postnatal bone remodeling and in rheumatoid arthritis. Lab Invest 76:717-728, 1997.
339. Konttinen YT, Salo T, Hanemaaijer R, et al: Collagenase-3 (MMP-13) and its activators in rheumatoid arthritis: Localization in the pannus-hard tissue junction and inhibition by alendronate. Matrix Biol 18:401-412, 1999.
340. Tetlow LC, Adlam DJ, Woolley DE: Matrix metalloproteinase and proinflammatory cytokine production by chondrocytes of human osteoarthritic cartilage. Arthritis Rheum 44:585-594, 2001.
341. Wu W, Billinghurst RC, Pidoux I, et al: Sites of collagenase cleavage and denaturation of type II collagen in aging and osteoarthritic articular cartilage and their relationship to the distribution of matrix metalloproteinase 1 and matrix metalloproteinase 13. Arthritis Rheum 46:2087-2094, 2002.
342. Cunnane G, Fitzgerald O, Beeton C, et al: Early joint erosions and serum levels of matrix metalloproteinase 1, matrix metalloproteinase 3, and tissue inhibitor of metalloproteinases 1 in rheumatoid arthritis. Arthritis Rheum 44:2263-2274, 2001.
343. Ishiguro N, Ito T, Ito H, et al: Relationship of matrix metalloproteinases and their inhibitors to cartilage proteoglycan and collagen turnover: analyses of synovial fluid from patients with osteoarthritis. Arthritis Rheum 42:129-136, 1999.
344. Yoshihara Y, Nakamura H, Obata K, et al: Matrix metalloproteinases and tissue inhibitors of metalloproteinases in synovial

fluids from patients with rheumatoid arthritis or osteoarthritis. Ann Rheum Dis 59:455-461, 2000.
345. Flannelly J, Chambers MG, Dudhia J, et al: Metalloproteinase and tissue inhibitor of metalloproteinase expression in the murine STR/ort model of osteoarthritis. Osteoarthritis Cartilage 10: 722-733, 2002.
346. Murphy G, Cartwright EC, Sellers A, Reynolds JJ: The detection and characterisation of collagenase inhibitors from rabbit tissues in culture. Biochim Biophys Acta 483:493-498, 1977.
347. Murphy G, McGuire MB, Russell RG, Reynolds JJ: Characterization of collagenase, other metallo-proteinases and an inhibitor (TIMP) produced by human synovium and cartilage in culture. Clin Sci (Lond) 61:711-716, 1981.
348. Apte SS, Hayashi K, Seldin MF, et al: Gene encoding a novel murine tissue inhibitor of metalloproteinases (TIMP), TIMP-3, is expressed in developing mouse epithelia, cartilage, and muscle, and is located on mouse chromosome 10. Dev Dyn 200:177-197, 1994.
349. Ellis AJ, Curry VA, Powell EK, Cawston TE: The prevention of collagen breakdown in bovine nasal cartilage by TIMP, TIMP-2 and a low molecular weight synthetic inhibitor. Biochem Biophys Res Commun 201:94-101, 1994.
350. Dean DD, Martel-Pelletier J, Pelletier JP, et al: Evidence for metalloproteinase and metalloproteinase inhibitor imbalance in human osteoarthritic cartilage. J Clin Invest 84:678-685, 1989.
351. Martel-Pelletier J, McCollum R, Fujimoto N, et al: Excess of metalloproteases over tissue inhibitor of metalloprotease may contribute to cartilage degradation in osteoarthritis and rheumatoid arthritis. Lab Invest 70:807-815, 1994.
352. Clark IM, Murphy G: Matrix proteinases. *In* Seibel MJ, Robins SP, Bilezekian JP (eds): Dynamics of Bone and Cartilage Metabolism. New York, Academic Press, 1999, pp 137-150.
353. Billinghurst RC, Dahlberg L, Ionescu M, et al: Enhanced cleavage of type II collagen by collagenases in osteoarthritic articular cartilage. J Clin Invest 99:1534-1545, 1997.
354. Mitchell PG, Magna HA, Reeves LM, et al: Cloning, expression, and type II collagenolytic activity of matrix metalloproteinase-13 from human osteoarthritic cartilage. J Clin Invest 97:761-768, 1996.
355. Shlopov BV, Lie WR, Mainardi CL, et al: Osteoarthritic lesions: involvement of three different collagenases. Arthritis Rheum 40:2065-2074, 1997.
356. Imai K, Ohta S, Matsumoto T, et al: Expression of membrane-type 1 matrix metalloproteinase and activation of progelatinase A in human osteoarthritic cartilage. Am J Pathol 151:245-256, 1997.
357. Knauper V, Lopez-Otin C, Smith B, et al: Biochemical characterization of human collagenase-3. J Biol Chem 271:1544-1550, 1996.
358. Flannery CR, Lark MW, Sandy JD: Identification of a stromelysin cleavage site within the interglobular domain of human aggrecan. Evidence for proteolysis at this site in vivo in human articular cartilage. J Biol Chem 267:1008-1014, 1992.
359. Lark MW, Bayne EK, Flanagan J, et al: Aggrecan degradation in human cartilage. Evidence for both matrix metalloproteinase and aggrecanase activity in normal, osteoarthritic, and rheumatoid joints. J Clin Invest 100:93-106, 1997.
360. Fosang AJ, Last K, Neame PJ, et al: Neutrophil collagenase (MMP-8) cleaves at the aggrecanase site E373-A374 in the interglobular domain of cartilage aggrecan. Biochem J 304:347-351, 1994.
361. Buttner FH, Hughes CE, Margerie D, et al: Membrane type 1 matrix metalloproteinase (MT1-MMP) cleaves the recombinant aggrecan substrate rAgg1mut at the 'aggrecanase' and the MMP sites. Characterization of MT1-MMP catabolic activities on the interglobular domain of aggrecan. Biochem J 333:159-165, 1998.
362. Stracke JO, Fosang AJ, Last K, et al: Matrix metalloproteinases 19 and 20 cleave aggrecan and cartilage oligomeric matrix protein (COMP). FEBS Lett 478:52-56, 2000.
363. Little CB, Hughes CE, Curtis CL, et al: Matrix metalloproteinases are involved in C-terminal and interglobular domain processing of cartilage aggrecan in late stage cartilage degradation. Matrix Biol 21:271-288, 2002.
364. Fosang AJ, Last K, Knauper V, et al: Fibroblast and neutrophil collagenases cleave at two sites in the cartilage aggrecan interglobular domain. Biochem J 295(Pt 1):273-276, 1993.
365. Hughes CE, Caterson B, Fosang AJ, et al: Monoclonal antibodies that specifically recognize neoepitope sequences generated by 'aggrecanase' and matrix metalloproteinase cleavage of aggrecan: application to catabolism in situ and in vitro. Biochem J 305:799-804, 1995.
366. Lark MW, Gordy JT, Weidner JR, et al: Cell-mediated catabolism of aggrecan. Evidence that cleavage at the "aggrecanase" site (Glu373-Ala374) is a primary event in proteolysis of the interglobular domain. J Biol Chem 270:2550-2556, 1995.
367. McKie N, Edwards T, Dallas DJ, et al: Expression of members of a novel membrane linked metalloproteinase family (ADAM) in human articular chondrocytes. Biochem Biophys Res Commun 230:335-339, 1997.
368. Billington CJ, Clark IM, Cawston TE: An aggrecan-degrading activity associated with chondrocyte membranes. Biochem J 336:207-212, 1998.
369. Wolfsberg TG, Primakoff P, Myles DG, White JM: ADAM, a novel family of membrane proteins containing a disintegrin and metalloprotease domain: Multipotential functions in cell-cell and cell-matrix interactions. J Cell Biol 131:275-278, 1995.
370. Tortorella MD, Burn TC, Pratta MA, et al: Purification and cloning of aggrecanase-1: a member of the ADAMTS family of proteins. Science 284:1664-1666, 1999.
371. Abbaszade I, Liu RQ, Yang F, et al: Cloning and characterization of ADAMTS11, an aggrecanase from the ADAMTS family. J Biol Chem 274:23443-23450, 1999.
372. Hurskainen TL, Hirohata S, Seldin MF, Apte SS: ADAM-TS5, ADAM-TS6, and ADAM-TS7, novel members of a new family of zinc metalloproteases. General features and genomic distribution of the ADAM-TS family. J Biol Chem 274:25555-25563, 1999.
373. Kuno K, Terashima Y, Matsushima K: ADAMTS-1 is an active metalloproteinase associated with the extracellular matrix. J Biol Chem 274:18821-18826, 1999.
374. Flannery CR, Little CB, Hughes CE, Caterson B: Expression of ADAMTS homologues in articular cartilage. Biochem Biophys Res Commun 260:318-322, 1999.
375. Kuno K, Okada Y, Kawashima H, et al: ADAMTS-1 cleaves a cartilage proteoglycan, aggrecan. FEBS Lett 478:241-245, 2000.
376. Kashiwagi M, Tortorella M, Nagase H, Brew K: TIMP-3 is a potent inhibitor of aggrecanase 1 (ADAM-TS4) and aggrecanase 2 (ADAM-TS5). J Biol Chem 276:12501-12504, 2001.
377. Hashimoto G, Aoki T, Nakamura H, Tanzawa K, Okada Y: Inhibition of ADAMTS4 (aggrecanase-1) by tissue inhibitors of metalloproteinases (TIMP-1, 2, 3 and 4). FEBS Lett 494:192-195, 2001.
378. Hembry RM, Knight CG, Dingle JT, Barrett AJ: Evidence that extracellular cathepsin D is not responsible for the resorption of cartilage matrix in culture. Biochim Biophys Acta 714:307-312, 1982.
379. Maciewicz RA, Wotton SF, Etherington DJ, Duance VC: Susceptibility of the cartilage collagens types II, IX and XI to degradation by the cysteine proteinases, cathepsins B and L. FEBS Lett 269:189-193, 1990.
380. Buttle DJ, Handley CJ, Ilic MZ, et al: Inhibition of cartilage proteoglycan release by a specific inactivator of cathepsin B and an inhibitor of matrix metalloproteinases. Evidence for two converging pathways of chondrocyte-mediated proteoglycan degradation. Arthritis Rheum 36:1709-1717, 1993.
381. Baici A, Lang A, Horler D, et al: Cathepsin B in osteoarthritis: cytochemical and histochemical analysis of human femoral head cartilage. Ann Rheum Dis 54:289-297, 1995.
382. Lang A, Horler D, Baici A: The relative importance of cysteine peptidases in osteoarthritis. J Rheumatol 27:1970-1979, 2000.
383. Mort JS, Magny MC, Lee ER: Cathepsin B: an alternative protease for the generation of an aggrecan 'metalloproteinase' cleavage neoepitope. Biochem J 335(Pt 3):491-494, 1998.
384. Gavrilovic J, Hembry RM, Reynolds JJ, Murphy G: Tissue inhibitor of metalloproteinases (TIMP) regulates extracellular type I collagen degradation by chondrocytes and endothelial cells. J Cell Sci 87(Pt 2):357-362, 1987.
385. Springman EB, Angleton EL, Birkedal-Hansen H, Van Wart HE: Multiple modes of activation of latent human fibroblast

collagenase: evidence for the role of a Cys73 active-site zinc complex in latency and a "cysteine switch" mechanism for activation. Proc Natl Acad Sci U S A 87:364-368, 1990.
386. Murphy G, Knauper V: Relating matrix metalloproteinase structure to function: Why the "hemopexin" domain? [Review]. Matrix Biology 15:511-518, 1997.
387. Murphy G, Knauper V, Cowell S, et al: Evaluation of some newer matrix metalloproteinases. Ann N Y Acad Sci 878:25-39, 1999.
388. Arner EC: Aggrecanase-mediated cartilage degradation. Curr Opin Pharmacol 2:322-329, 2002.
389. Bottomley KM, Borkakoti N, Bradshaw D, et al: Inhibition of bovine nasal cartilage degradation by selective matrix metalloproteinase inhibitors. Biochem J 323(Pt 2):483-488, 1997.
390. Dahlberg L, Billinghurst RC, Manner P, et al: Selective enhancement of collagenase-mediated cleavage of resident type II collagen in cultured osteoarthritic cartilage and arrest with a synthetic inhibitor that spares collagenase 1 (matrix metalloproteinase 1). Arthritis Rheum 43:673-682, 2000.
391. Mix KS, Mengshol J, Benbow U, et al: A synthetic triterpenoid selectively inhibits the induction of matrix metalloproteinases 1 and 13 by inflammatory cytokines. Arthritis Rheum 44:1096-1104, 2001.
392. Baker AH, Edwards DR, Murphy G: Metalloproteinase inhibitors: biological actions and therapeutic opportunities. J Cell Sci 115: 3719-3727, 2002.
393. Horai R, Saijo S, Tanioka J, et al: Development of chronic inflammatory arthropathy resembling rheumatoid arthritis in interleukin 1 receptor antagonist-deficient mice. J Exp Med 191:313-320, 2000.
394. Campbell IK, O'Donnell K, Lawlor KD, Wicks IP: Severe inflammatory arthritis and lymphadenopathy in the absence of TNF. J Clin Invest 107:1519-1527, 2001.
395. Matsuno H, Yudoh K, Katayama R, et al: The role of TNF-alpha in the pathogenesis of inflammation and joint destruction in rheumatoid arthritis (RA): a study using a human RA/SCID mouse chimera. Rheumatology (Oxford) 41:329-337, 2002.
396. Bendele AM, Chlipala ES, Scherrer J, et al: Combination benefit of treatment with the cytokine inhibitors interleukin-1 receptor antagonist and PEGylated soluble tumor necrosis factor receptor type I in animal models of rheumatoid arthritis. Arthritis Rheum 43:2648-2659, 2000.
397. Fell HB, Jubb RW: The effect of synovial tissue on the breakdown of articular cartilage in organ culture. Arthritis Rheum 20:1359-1371, 1977.
398. Dingle JT, Saklatvala J, Hembry R, et al: A cartilage catabolic factor from synovium. Biochem J 184:177-180, 1979.
399. Dayer J-M, Russell RGG, Krane SM: Collagenase production by rheumatoid synovial cells: stimulation by a human lymphocyte factor. Science 195:181-183, 1977.
400. Meats JE, McGuire MB, Russell RGG: Human synovium releases a factor which stimulates chondrocyte production of PGE and plasminogen activator. Nature 286:891-892, 1980.
401. Dayer JM, Zavadil-Grob C, Ucla C, Mach B: Induction of human interleukin 1 mRNA measured by collagenase-and prostaglandin E2-stimulating activity in rheumatoid synovial cells. Eur J Immunol 14:898-901, 1984.
402. McGuire-Goldring MB, Meats JE, Wood DD, et al: In vitro activation of human chondrocytes and synoviocytes by a human interleukin-1-like factor. Arthritis Rheum 27:654-662, 1984.
403. Stephenson ML, Goldring MB, Birkhead JR, et al: Stimulation of procollagenase synthesis parallels increases in cellular procollagenase mRNA in human articular chondrocytes exposed to recombinant interleukin 1 beta or phorbol ester. Biochem Biophys Res Commun 144:583-590, 1987.
404. Saklatvala J, Pilsworth LM, Sarsfield SJ, et al: Pig catabolin is a form of interleukin 1. Cartilage and bone resorb, fibroblasts make prostaglandin and collagenase, and thymocyte proliferation is augmented in response to one protein. Biochem J 224:461-466, 1984.
405. Middleton J, Manthey A, Tyler J: Insulin-like growth factor (IGF) receptor, IGF-I, interleukin-1 beta (IL-1 beta), and IL-6 mRNA expression in osteoarthritic and normal human cartilage. J Histochem Cytochem 44:133-141, 1996.
406. Moos V, Fickert S, Muller B, et al: Immunohistological analysis of cytokine expression in human osteoarthritic and healthy cartilage. J Rheumatol 26:870-879, 1999.
407. Attur MG, Dave M, Cipolletta C, et al: Reversal of autocrine and paracrine effects of interleukin 1 (IL-1) in human arthritis by type II IL-1 decoy receptor. Potential for pharmacological intervention. J Biol Chem 275:40307-40315, 2000.
408. Millward-Sadler SJ, Wright MO, Lee H, et al: Integrin-regulated secretion of interleukin 4: A novel pathway of mechanotransduction in human articular chondrocytes. J Cell Biol 145:183-189, 1999.
409. Saklatvala J: Tumour necrosis factor α stimulates resorption and inhibits synthesis of proteoglycan in cartilage. Nature 322:547-549, 1986.
410. Bunning RA, Russell RGG: The effect of tumor necrosis factor α and γ-interferon on the resorption of human articular cartilage and on the production of prostaglandin E and of caseinase activity by human articular chondrocytes. Arthritis Rheum 32:780-784, 1989.
411. Lefebvre V, Peeters-Joris C, Vaes G: Modulation by interleukin 1 and tumor necrosis factor α of production of collagenase, tissue inhibitor of metalloproteinases and collagen types in differentiated and dedifferentiated articular chondrocytes. Biochim Biophys Acta 1052:366-378, 1990.
412. Campbell IK, Piccoli DS, Roberts MJ, et al: Effects of tumor necrosis factor α and β on resorption of human articular cartilage and production of plasminogen activator by human articular chondrocytes. Arthritis Rheum 33:542-552, 1990.
413. Meyer FA, Yaron I, Yaron M: Synergistic, additive, and antagonistic effects of interleukin-1 beta, tumor necrosis factor alpha, and gamma-interferon on prostaglandin E, hyaluronic acid, and collagenase production by cultured synovial fibroblasts. Arthritis Rheum 33:1518-1525, 1990.
414. van den Berg WB: Anti-cytokine therapy in chronic destructive arthritis. Arthritis Res 3:18-26, 2001.
415. Pettipher ER, Higgs GA, Henderson B: Interleukin 1 induces leukocyte infiltration and cartilage proteoglycan degradation in the synovial joint. Proc Natl Acad Sci U S A 83:8749-8753, 1986.
416. O'Byrne E, Blancuzzi V, Wilson DE, et al: Elevated substance P and accelerated cartilage degradation in rabbit knees injected with interleukin-1 and tumor necrosis factor. Arthritis Rheum 33:1023-1028, 1990.
417. van Beuningen HM, Arntz OJ, van den Berg WB: In vivo effects of interleukin-1 on articular cartilage. Arthritis Rheum 34:606-615, 1991.
418. Henderson B, Pettipher ER: Arthritogenic actions of recombinant IL-1 and tumor necrosis factor alpha in the rabbit: Evidence for synergic interactions between cytokines *in vivo*. Clin Exp Immunol 75:306-310, 1989.
419. Page-Thomas DP, King B, Dingle JT: In vivo studies of cartilage regeneration after damage induced by catabolin/interleukin-1. Ann Rheum Dis 50:75-80, 1991.
420. Goldring MB, Birkhead J, Sandell LJ, Krane SM: Synergistic regulation of collagen gene expression in human chondrocytes by tumor necrosis factor-α and interleukin-1β. Ann N Y Acad Sci 580:536-539, 1990.
421. Reginato AM, Sanz-Rodriguez C, Diaz A, et al: Transcriptional modulation of cartilage-specific collagen gene expression by interferon gamma and tumour necrosis factor alpha in cultured human chondrocytes. Biochem J 294:761-769, 1993.
422. Goldring MB, Fukuo K, Birkhead JR, et al: Transcriptional suppression by interleukin-1 and interferon-γ of type II collagen gene expression in human chondrocytes. J Cell Biochem 54:85-99, 1994.
423. Thomas B, Thirion S, Humbert L, et al: Differentiation regulates interleukin-1β-induced cyclo-oxygenase-2 in human articular chondrocytes: Role of p38 mitogen-activated kinase. Biochem J 362:367-373, 2002.
424. Riquet RB, Lai W-FT, Birkhead JR, et al: Suppression of type I collagen gene expression by prostaglandins in fibroblasts is mediated at the transcriptional level. Molec Med 6:705-719, 2000.
425. Bordji K, Grillasca JP, Gouze JN, et al: Evidence for the presence of peroxisome proliferator-activated receptor (PPAR) alpha and gamma and retinoid Z receptor in cartilage. PPARgamma activation modulates the effects of interleukin-1beta on rat chondrocytes. J Biol Chem 275:12243-12250, 2000.
426. Fahmi H, Di Battista JA, Pelletier JP, et al: Peroxisome proliferator–activated receptor gamma activators inhibit interleukin-

1beta-induced nitric oxide and matrix metalloproteinase 13 production in human chondrocytes. Arthritis Rheum 44:595-607, 2001.
427. Fahmi H, Pelletier JP, Di Battista JA, et al: Peroxisome proliferator-activated receptor gamma activators inhibit MMP-1 production in human synovial fibroblasts likely by reducing the binding of the activator protein 1. Osteoarthritis Cartilage 10:100-108, 2002.
428. Kalajdzic T, Faour WH, He QW, et al: Nimesulide, a preferential cyclooxygenase 2 inhibitor, suppresses peroxisome proliferator-activated receptor induction of cyclooxygenase 2 gene expression in human synovial fibroblasts: Evidence for receptor antagonism. Arthritis Rheum 46:494-506, 2002.
429. Stadler J, Stefanovic-Racic M, Billiar TR, et al: Articular chondrocytes synthesize nitric oxide in response to cytokines and lipopolysaccharide. J Immunol 147:3915-3920, 1991.
430. Palmer RM, Hickery MS, Charles IG, et al: Induction of nitric oxide synthase in human chondrocytes. Biochem Biophys Res Commun 193:398-405, 1993.
431. Taskiran D, Stefanovic-Racic M, Georgescu H, Evans C: Nitric oxide mediates suppression of cartilage proteoglycan synthesis by interleukin-1. Biochem Biophys Res Commun 200:142-148, 1994.
432. Sasaki K, Hattori T, Fujisawa T, et al: Nitric oxide mediates interleukin-1-induced gene expression of matrix metalloproteinases and basic fibroblast growth factor in cultured rabbit articular chondrocytes. J Biochem (Tokyo) 123:431-439, 1998.
433. Maneiro E, Lopez-Armada MJ, Fernandez-Sueiro JL, et al: Aceclofenac increases the synthesis of interleukin 1 receptor antagonist and decreases the production of nitric oxide in human articular chondrocytes. J Rheumatol 28:2692-2699, 2001.
434. Abramson SB, Attur M, Amin AR, Clancy R: Nitric oxide and inflammatory mediators in the perpetuation of osteoarthritis. Curr Rheumatol Rep 3:535-541, 2001.
435. Clancy RM, Abramson SB, Kohne C, Rediske J: Nitric oxide attenuates cellular hexose monophosphate shunt response to oxidants in articular chondrocytes and acts to promote oxidant injury. J Cell Physiol 172:183-191, 1997.
436. Studer RK, Levicoff E, Georgescu H, et al: Nitric oxide inhibits chondrocyte response to IGF-I: inhibition of IGF-IRbeta tyrosine phosphorylation. Am J Physiol Cell Physiol 279:C961-969, 2000.
437. Blanco FJ, Ochs RL, Schwarz H, Lotz M: Chondrocyte apoptosis induced by nitric oxide. Am J Pathol 146:75-85, 1995.
438. Hashimoto S, Takahashi K, Amiel D, et al: Chondrocyte apoptosis and nitric oxide production during experimentally induced osteoarthritis. Arthritis Rheum 41:1266-1274, 1998.
439. Miwa M, Saura R, Hirata S, et al: Induction of apoptosis in bovine articular chondrocyte by prostaglandin E(2) through cAMP-dependent pathway. Osteoarthritis Cartilage 8:17-24, 2000.
440. Notoya K, Jovanovic DV, Reboul P, et al: The induction of cell death in human osteoarthritis chondrocytes by nitric oxide is related to the production of prostaglandin E2 via the induction of cyclooxygenase-2. J Immunol 165:3402-3410, 2000.
441. Pelletier JP, Jovanovic DV, Lascau-Coman V, et al: Selective inhibition of inducible nitric oxide synthase reduces progression of experimental osteoarthritis in vivo: possible link with the reduction in chondrocyte apoptosis and caspase 3 level. Arthritis Rheum 43:1290-1299, 2000.
442. Lee D, Long SA, Adams JL, et al: Potent and selective nonpeptide inhibitors of caspases 3 and 7 inhibit apoptosis and maintain cell functionality. J Biol Chem 275:16007-16014., 2000.
443. Henrotin YE, Zheng SX, Deby GP, et al: Nitric oxide downregulates interleukin 1beta (IL-1beta) stimulated IL-6, IL-8, and prostaglandin E2 production by human chondrocytes. J Rheumatol 25:1595-1601, 1998.
444. Kuhn K, Hashimoto S, Lotz M: IL-1 beta protects human chondrocytes from CD95-induced apoptosis. J Immunol 164:2233-2239, 2000.
445. Nietfeld JJ, Duits AJ, Tilanus MG, et al: Antisense oligonucleotides, a novel tool for the control of cytokine effects on human cartilage. Focus on interleukins 1 and 6 and proteoglycan synthesis. Arthritis Rheum 37:1357-1362, 1994.
446. Seckinger P, Yaron I, Meyer FA, et al: Modulation of the effects of interleukin-1 on glycosaminoglycan synthesis by the urine-derived interleukin-1 inhibitor, but not by interleukin-6. Arthritis Rheum 33:1807-1814, 1990.
447. Silacci P, Dayer JM, Desgeorges A, et al: Interleukin (IL)-6 and its soluble receptor induce TIMP-1 expression in synoviocytes and chondrocytes, and block IL-1-induced collagenolytic activity. J Biol Chem 273:13625-13629, 1998.
448. Guerne PA, Desgeorges A, Jaspar JM, et al: Effects of IL-6 and its soluble receptor on proteoglycan synthesis and NO release by human articular chondrocytes: comparison with IL-1. Modulation by dexamethasone. Matrix Biol 18:253-260, 1999.
449. Rowan AD, Koshy PJ, Shingleton WD, et al: Synergistic effects of glycoprotein 130 binding cytokines in combination with interleukin-1 on cartilage collagen breakdown. Arthritis Rheum 44:1620-1632, 2001.
450. Maier R, Ganu V, Lotz M: Interleukin-11, an inducible cytokine in human articular chondrocytes and synoviocytes, stimulates the production of the tissue inhibitor of metalloproteinases. J Biol Chem 268:21527-21532, 1993.
451. Villiger PM, Geng Y, Lotz M: Induction of cytokine expression by leukemia inhibitory factor. J Clin Invest 91:1575-1581, 1993.
452. Henrotin YE, De Groote DD, Labasse AH, et al: Effects of exogenous IL-1β, TNFα, IL-6, IL-8 and LIF on cytokine production by human articular chondrocytes. Osteoarthritis Cartilage 4:163-173, 1996.
453. Koshy PJ, Lundy CJ, Rowan AD, et al: The modulation of matrix metalloproteinase and ADAM gene expression in human chondrocytes by interleukin-1 and oncostatin M: a time-course study using real-time quantitative reverse transcription-polymerase chain reaction. Arthritis Rheum 46:961-967, 2002.
454. Langdon C, Kerr C, Hassen M, et al: Murine oncostatin M stimulates mouse synovial fibroblasts in vitro and induces inflammation and destruction in mouse joints in vivo. Am J Pathol 157: 1187-1196, 2000.
455. Plater-Zyberk C, Buckton J, Thompson S, et al: Amelioration of arthritis in two murine models using antibodies to oncostatin M. Arthritis Rheum 44:2697-2702, 2001.
456. Li WQ, Dehnade F, Zafarullah M: Oncostatin M-induced matrix metalloproteinase and tissue inhibitor of metalloproteinase-3 genes expression in chondrocytes requires Janus kinase/STAT signaling pathway. J Immunol 166:3491-3498, 2001.
457. van den Berg WB: Lessons from animal models of arthritis. Curr Rheumatol Rep 4:232-239, 2002.
458. Shalom-Barak T, Quach J, Lotz M: Interleukin-17-induced gene expression in articular chondrocytes is associated with activation of mitogen-activated protein kinases and NF-κB. J Biol Chem 273:27467-27473, 1998.
459. Olee T, Hashimoto S, Quach J, Lotz M: IL-18 is produced by articular chondrocytes and induces proinflammatory and catabolic responses. J Immunol 162:1096-1100, 1999.
460. Martel-Pelletier J, Mineau F, Jovanovic D, et al: Mitogen-activated protein kinase and nuclear factor kappaB together regulate interleukin-17-induced nitric oxide production in human osteoarthritic chondrocytes: Possible role of transactivating factor mitogen-activated protein kinase-activated proten kinase (MAPKAPK). Arthritis Rheum 42:2399-2409, 1999.
461. Boileau C, Martel-Pelletier J, Moldovan F, et al: The in situ up-regulation of chondrocyte interleukin-1-converting enzyme and interleukin-18 levels in experimental osteoarthritis is mediated by nitric oxide. Arthritis Rheum 46:2637-2647, 2002.
462. Benderdour M, Tardif G, Pelletier JP, et al: Interleukin 17 (IL-17) induces collagenase-3 production in human osteoarthritic chondrocytes via AP-1 dependent activation: Differential activation of AP-1 members by IL-17 and IL-1beta. J Rheumatol 29:1262-1272, 2002.
463. Pacquelet S, Presle N, Boileau C, et al: Interleukin 17, a nitric oxide-producing cytokine with a peroxynitrite-independent inhibitory effect on proteoglycan synthesis. J Rheumatol 29:2602-2610, 2002.
464. Lubberts E, Joosten LA, Oppers B, et al: IL-1-independent role of IL-17 in synovial inflammation and joint destruction during collagen-induced arthritis. J Immunol 167:1004-1013, 2001.
465. Dudler J, Renggli-Zulliger N, Busso N, et al: Effect of interleukin 17 on proteoglycan degradation in murine knee joints. Ann Rheum Dis 59:529-532, 2000.
466. Cai L, Yin JP, Starovasnik MA, et al: Pathways by which interleukin 17 induces articular cartilage breakdown in vitro and in vivo. Cytokine 16:10-21, 2001.

467. Chabaud M, Lubberts E, Joosten L, et al: IL-17 derived from juxta-articular bone and synovium contributes to joint degradation in rheumatoid arthritis. Arthritis Res 3:168-177, 2001.
468. Plater-Zyberk C, Joosten LA, Helsen MM, et al: Therapeutic effect of neutralizing endogenous IL-18 activity in the collagen-induced model of arthritis. J Clin Invest 108:1825-1832, 2001.
469. Fernandes JC, Martel-Pelletier J, Pelletier JP: The role of cytokines in osteoarthritis pathophysiology. Biorheology 39:237-246, 2002.
470. Shingu M, Miyauchi S, Nagai Y, et al: The role of IL-4 and IL-6 in IL-1-dependent cartilage matrix degradation. Br J Rheumatol 34:101-106, 1995.
471. Cawston TE, Ellis AJ, Bigg H, et al: Interleukin-4 blocks the release of collagen fragments from bovine nasal cartilage treated with cytokines. Biochim Biophys Acta 1314:226-232, 1996.
472. Salter DM, Nuki G, Wright MO: IL-4 inhibition of cartilage breakdown in bovine articular explants. J Rheumatol 23:1314-1315, 1996.
473. Iannone F, De Bari C, Dell'Accio F, et al: Interleukin-10 and interleukin-10 receptor in human osteoarthritic and healthy chondrocytes. Clin Exp Rheumatol 19:139-145, 2001.
474. Wang Y, Lou S: Direct protective effect of interleukin-10 on articular chondrocytes in vitro. Chin Med J (Engl) 114:723-725, 2001.
475. Guicheux J, Palmer G, Relic B, et al: Primary human articular chondrocytes, dedifferentiated chondrocytes, and synoviocytes exhibit differential responsiveness to interleukin-4: Correlation with the expression pattern of the common receptor gamma chain. J Cell Physiol 192:93-101, 2002.
476. Lubberts E, Joosten LAB, van de Loo FAJ, et al: Reduction of interleukin-17-induced inhibition of chondrocyte proteoglycan synthesis in intact murine articular cartilage by interleukin-4. Arthritis Rheum 43:1300-1306, 2000.
477. Lubberts E, Joosten LA, Van Den Bersselaar L, et al: Intra-articular IL-10 gene transfer regulates the expression of collagen-induced arthritis (CIA) in the knee and ipsilateral paw. Clin Exp Immunol 120:375-383., 2000.
478. van Roon JAG, Lafeber FPJG, Bijlsma JWJ: Synergistic activity of interleukin-4 and interleukin-10 in suppression of inflammation and joint destruction in rheumatoid arthritis. Arthritis Rheum 44:3-12, 2001.
479. Evans CH, Ghivizzani SC, Herndon JH, et al: Clinical trials in the gene therapy of arthritis. Clin Orthop 379:S300-S307, 2000.
480. Bresnihan B: The safety and efficacy of interleukin-1 receptor antagonist in the treatment of rheumatoid arthritis. Semin Arthritis Rheum 30(Suppl 2):17-20, 2001.
481. Arend WP, Gabay C: Physiologic role of interleukin-1 receptor antagonist. Arthritis Res 2:245-248, 2000.
482. Chabaud M, Page G, Miossec P: Enhancing effect of IL-1, IL-17, and TNF-alpha on macrophage inflammatory protein-3alpha production in rheumatoid arthritis: Regulation by soluble receptors and Th2 cytokines. J Immunol 167:6015-6020, 2001.
483. Woods JM, Katschke KJ Jr., Tokuhira M,et al: Reduction of inflammatory cytokines and prostaglandin E2 by IL-13 gene therapy in rheumatoid arthritis synovium. J Immunol 165:2755-2763, 2000.
484. Borzi RM, Mazzetti I, Cattini L, et al: Human chondrocytes express functional chemokine receptors and release matrix-degrading enzymes in response to C-X-C and C-C chemokines. Arthritis Rheum 43:1734-1741, 2000.
485. Yuan GH, Masuko-Hongo K, Sakata M, et al: The role of C-C chemokines and their receptors in osteoarthritis. Arthritis Rheum 44:1056-1070, 2001.
486. Alaaeddine N, Olee T, Hashimoto S,et al: Production of the chemokine RANTES by articular chondrocytes and role in cartilage degradation. Arthritis Rheum 44:1633-1643, 2001.
487. Kanbe K, Takagishi K, Chen Q: Stimulation of matrix metalloprotease 3 release from human chondrocytes by the interaction of stromal cell-derived factor 1 and CXC chemokine receptor 4. Arthritis Rheum 46:130-137, 2002.
488. Saklatvala J, Dean J, Finch A: Protein kinase cascades in intracellular signalling by interleukin-I and tumour necrosis factor. Biochem Soc Symp 64:63-77, 1999.
489. Ding GJF, Fischer PA, Boltz RC, et al: Characterization and quantitation of NF-κB nuclear translocation induced by interleukin-1 and tumor necrosis factor-α. J Biol Chem 273:28897-28905, 1998.
490. Mercurio F, Manning AM: NF-kappaB as a primary regulator of the stress response [Review]. Oncogene 18:6163-6171, 1999.
491. Auron PE: The interleukin 1 receptor: Ligand interactions and signal transduction. Cytokine Growth Factor Rev 9:221-237, 1998.
492. Reddy SA, Huang JH, Liao WS: Phosphatidylinositol 3-kinase in interleukin 1 signaling. Physical interaction with the interleukin 1 receptor and requirement in NFκB and AP-1 activation. J Biol Chem 272:29167-29173, 1997.
493. Reddy SA, Huang JH, Liao WS: Phosphatidylinositol 3-kinase as a mediator of TNF-induced NF-κB activation. J Immunol 164:1355-1363, 2000.
494. Malinin NL, Boldin MP, Kovalenko AV, Wallach D: MAP3K-related kinase involved in NF-kappaB induction by TNF, CD95 and IL-1. Nature 385:540-544, 1997.
495. Ozes ON, Mayo LD, Gustin JA,et al: NF-κB activation by tumour necrosis factor requires the Akt serine-threonine kinase. Nature 401:82-85, 1999.
496. Arch RH, Gedrich RW, Thompson CB: Tumor necrosis factor receptor-associated factors (TRAFS)–a family of adapter proteins that regulates life and death. Genes Develop 12:2821-2830, 1998.
497. Wesche H, Cao X, Li X, et al: IRAK-M is a novel member of the Pelle/interleukin-1 receptor-associated kinase (IRAK) family. J Biol Chem 274:19403-19410, 1999.
498. Kopp E, Medzhitov R, Carothers J, et al: ECSIT is an evolutionarily conserved intermediate in the Toll/IL-1 signal transduction pathway. Genes Devel 13:2059-2071, 1999.
499. Baud V, Liu ZG, Bennett B, et al: Signaling by proinflammatory cytokines: oligomerization of TRAF2 and TRAF6 is sufficient for JNK and IKK activation and target gene induction via an amino-terminal effector domain. Genes Develop 13:1297-1308, 1999.
500. Geng Y, Maier R, Lotz M: Tyrosine kinases are involved with the expression of inducible nitric oxide synthase in human articular chondrocytes. J Cell Physiol 163:545-554, 1995.
501. Scherle PA, Pratta MA, Feeser WS, et al: The effects of IL-1 on mitogen-activated protein kinases in rabbit articular chondrocytes. Biochem Biophys Res Commun 230:573-577, 1997.
502. Badger AM, Cook MN, Lark MW, et al: SB203580 inhibits, p38 mitogen-activated protein kinase, nitric oxide production, and inducible nitric oxide synthase in bovine cartilage-derived chondrocytes. J Immunol 161:467-473, 1998.
503. Mengshol JA, Vincenti MP, Coon CI, et al: Interleukin-1 induction of collagenase 3 (matrix metalloproteinase 13) gene expression in chondrocytes requires p38, c-Jun N-terminal kinase, and nuclear factor κB. Arthritis Rheum 43:801-811, 2000.
504. Liacini A, Sylvester J, Li WQ, Zafarullah M: Inhibition of interleukin-1-stimulated MAP kinases, activating protein-1 (AP-1) and nuclear factor kappa B (NF-kappa B) transcription factors down-regulates matrix metalloproteinase gene expression in articular chondrocytes. Matrix Biol 21:251-262, 2002.
505. Martel-Pelletier J, Mineau F, Jovanovic D, et al: Mitogen-activated protein kinase and nuclear factor κB together regulate interleukin-17-induced nitric oxide production in human osteoarthritic chondrocytes: Possible role of transactivating factor mitogen-activated protein kinase-activated proten kinase (MAPKAPK). Arthritis Rheum 42:2399-2409, 1999.
506. Ridley SH, Sarsfield SJ, Lee JC, et al: Actions of IL-1 are selectively controlled by p38 mitogen-activated protein kinase: regulation of prostaglandin H synthase-2, metalloproteinases, and IL-6 at different levels. J Immunol 158:3165-3173, 1997.
507. Badger AM, Griswold DE, Kapadia R, et al: Disease-modifying activity of SB 242235, a selective inhibitor of p38 mitogen-activated protein kinase, in rat adjuvant-induced arthritis. Arthritis Rheum 43:175-183, 2000.
508. Parkar AA, Kahmann JD, Howat SL, et al: TSG-6 interacts with hyaluronan and aggrecan in a pH-dependent manner via a common functional element: Implications for its regulation in inflamed cartilage. FEBS Letters 428:171-176, 1998.
509. Ryan MC, Sieraski M, Sandell LJ: The human type II procollagen gene: Identification of an additional protein-coding domain

and location of potential regulatory sequences in the promoter and first intron. Genomics 8:41-48, 1990.
510. Dharmavaram RM, Liu G, Mowers SD, Jimenez SA: Detection and characterization of Sp1 binding activity in human chondrocytes and its alterations during chondrocyte dedifferentiation. J Biol Chem 272:26918-26925, 1997.
511. Savagner P, Krebsbach PH, Hatano O, et al: Collagen II promoter and enhancer interact synergistically through Sp1 and istinct nuclear factors. DNA Cell Biol 14:501-519, 1995.
512. Ghayor C, Chadjichristos C, Herrouin J-F, et al: Sp3 represses the Sp1-mediated transactivation of the human COL2A1 gene in primary and de-differentiated chondrocytes. J Biol Chem 276:36881-36895, 2001.
513. Murray D, Precht P, Balakir R, Horton WE Jr: The transcription factor deltaEF1 is inversely expressed with type II collagen mRNA and can repress Col2a1 promoter activity in transfected chondrocytes. J Biol Chem 275:3610-3618, 2000.
514. Ghayor C, Herrouin J-F, Chadjichristos C, et al: Regulation of human COL2A1 gene expression in chondrocytes. Identification of C-Krox-responsive elements and modulation by phenotype alteration. J Biol Chem 275:27421-27438, 2000.
515. Stokes DG, Liu G, Dharmavaram R, et al: Regulation of type-II collagen gene expression during human chondrocyte dedifferentiation and recovery of chondrocyte-specific phenotype in culture involves Sry-type high-mobility-group box (SOX) transcription factors. Biochem J 360:461-470, 2001.
516. Zhang P, Jimenez SA, Stokes DG: Regulation of human COL9A1 gene expression. Activation of the proximal promoter region by SOX9. J Biol Chem 278:117-123, 2003.
517. Sakano S, Zhu Y, Sandell LJ: Cartilage-derived retinoic acid-sensitive protein and type II collagen expression during fracture healing are potential targets for Sox9 regulation. J Bone Miner Res 14:1891-1901, 1999.
518. Bridgewater LC, Walker MD, Miller GC, et al: Adjacent DNA sequences modulate Sox9 transcriptional activation at paired Sox sites in three chondrocyte-specific enhancer elements. Nucleic Acids Res 31:1541-1553, 2003.
519. Lefebvre V, Li P, de Crombrugghe B: A new long form of Sox5 (L-Sox5), Sox6 and Sox9 are coexpressed in chondrogenesis and cooperatively activate the type II collagen gene. EMBO J 17:5718-5733, 1998.
520. Leung KK, Ng LJ, Ho KK, et al: Different cis-regulatory DNA elements mediate developmental stage- and tissue-specific expression of the human COL2A1 gene in transgenic mice. J Cell Biol 141:1291-1300, 1998.
521. Zehentner BK, Dony C, Burtscher H: The transcription factor Sox9 is involved in BMP-2 signaling. J Bone Miner Res 14:1734-1741, 1999.
522. Murakami S, Kan M, McKeehan WL, de Crombrugghe B: Up-regulation of the chondrogenic Sox9 gene by fibroblast growth factors is mediated by the mitogen-activated protein kinase pathway. Proc Natl Acad Sci U S A 97:1113-1118, 2000.
523. Kolettas E, Muir HI, Barrett JC, Hardingham TE: Chondrocyte phenotype and cell survival are regulated by culture conditions and by specific cytokines through the expression of Sox-9 transcription factor. Rheumatology (Oxford) 40:1146-1156, 2001.
524. Uusitalo H, Hiltunen A, Ahonen M, et al: Accelerated up-regulation of L-Sox5, Sox6, and Sox9 by BMP-2 gene transfer during murine fracture healing. J Bone Miner Res 16:1837-1845, 2001.
525. Xu SC, Harris MA, Rubenstein JLR, et al: Bone morphogenetic protein-2 (BMP-2) signaling to the *Col2a1* gene in chondroblasts requires the homeobox gene *Dlx-2*. DNA Cell Biol 20:359-365, 2001.
526. Thomas B, Berenbaum F, Humbert L, et al: Critical role of C/EBPδ and C/EBPβ factors in the stimulation of cyclooxygenase-2 gene transcription by interleukin-1β in articular chondrocytes. Eur J Biochem 267:1-13, 2000.
527. Mengshol JA, Vincenti MP, Brinckerhoff CE: IL-1 induces collagenase-3 (MMP-13) promoter activity in stably transfected chondrocytic cells: Requirement for Runx-2 and activation by p38 MAPK and JNK pathways. Nucleic Acids Res 29:4361-4372, 2001.
528. Catterall JB, Carrere S, Koshy PJ, et al: Synergistic induction of matrix metalloproteinase 1 by interleukin-1alpha and oncostatin M in human chondrocytes involves signal transducer and activator of transcription and activator protein 1 transcription factors via a novel mechanism. Arthritis Rheum 44:2296-2310, 2001.
529. Legendre F, Dudhia J, Pujol JP, Bogdanowicz P: JAK/STAT but not ERK1/ERK2 pathway mediates interleukin (IL)-6/soluble IL-6R down-regulation of Type II collagen, aggrecan core, and link protein transcription in articular chondrocytes. Association with a down-regulation of SOX9 expression. J Biol Chem 278:2903-2912, 2003.
530. Grall F, Gu X, Tan L, et al: Responses to the pro-inflammatory cytokines interleukin-1 and tumor necrosis factor-α in cells derived from rheumatoid synovium and other joint tissues involve NF-κB-mediated induction of the Ets transcription factor ESE-1. Arthritis Rheum 2003.
531. Okazaki K, Li J, Yu H, et al: CCAAT/Enhancer-binding proteins β and δ mediate the repression of gene transcription of cartilage-derived retinoic acid-sensitive protein Induced by interleukin-1β. J Biol Chem 277:31526-31533, 2002.
532. Tan L, Peng H, Osaki M, et al: Egr-1 mediates transcriptional repression of COL2A1 promoter activity by interleukin-1beta. J Biol Chem 278:17688-17700, 2003.
533. Lefebvre V, Behringer RR, de Crombrugghe B: L-Sox5, Sox6 and Sox9 control essential steps of the chondrocyte differentiation pathway. Osteoarthritis Cartilage 9(Suppl A):S69-S75, 2001.
534. Murakami S, Lefebvre V, de Crombrugghe B: Potent inhibition of the master chondrogenic factor Sox9 gene by interleukin-1 and tumor necrosis factor-α. J Biol Chem 275:3687-3692, 2000.
535. Cerjesi P, Brown D, Ligon KL, et al: Scleraxis: A basic helix-loop-helix protein that prefigures skeletal formation during mouse embyrogenesis. Development 121:1099-1110, 1995.
536. Asp J, Thornemo M, Inerot S, Lindahl A: The helix-loop-helix transcription factors Id1 and Id3 have a functional role in control of cell division in human normal and neoplastic chondrocytes. FEBS Lett 438:85-90, 1998.
537. Shen M, Yoshida E, Yan W, et al: Basic helix-loop-helix protein DEC1 promotes chondrocyte differentiation at the early and terminal stages. J Biol Chem 277:50112-50120, 2002.
538. Tsuji M, Funahashi S, Takigawa M, et al: Expression of c-fos gene inhibits proteoglycan synthesis in transfected chondrocyte. FEBS Lett 381:222-226, 1996.
539. Thomas DP, Sunters A, Gentry A, Grigoriadis AE: Inhibition of chondrocyte differentiation in vitro by constitutive and inducible overexpression of the c-fos proto-oncogene. J Cell Sci 113(Pt 3):439-450, 2000.
540. Ranger AM, Gerstenfeld LC, Wang JW, et al: The nuclear factor of activated T cells (NFAT) transcription factor (NFATc2) is a repressor of chondrogenesis. J Exp Med 191:9-21, 2000.
541. De Luca F, Uyeda JA, Mericq V, et al: Retinoic acid is a potent regulator of growth plate chondrogenesis. Endocrinology 141:346-353, 2000.
542. Ganss B, Kobayashi H: The zinc finger transcription factor Zfp60 is a negative regulator of cartilage differentiation. J Bone Miner Res 17:2151-2160, 2002.
543. Tanaka K, Matsumoto Y, Nakatani F, et al: A zinc finger transcription factor, alphaA-crystallin binding protein 1, is a negative regulator of the chondrocyte-specific enhancer of the alpha1(II) collagen gene. Mol Cell Biol 20:4428-4435, 2000.
544. Xie WF, Kondo S, Sandell LJ: Regulation of the mouse cartilage-derived retinoic acid-sensitive protein gene by the transcription factor AP-2. J Biol Chem 273:5026-5032, 1998.
545. Tuli R, Seghatoleslami MR, Tuli S, et al: p38 MAP kinase regulation of AP-2 binding in TGF-beta1-stimulated chondrogenesis of human trabecular bone-derived cells. Ann N Y Acad Sci 961:172-177, 2002.
546. Iwamoto M, Higuchi Y, Koyama E, et al: Transcription factor ERG variants and functional diversification of chondrocytes during limb long bone development. J Cell Biol 150:27-40, 2000.
547. Schaefer JF, Millham ML, de Crombrugghe B, Buckbinder L: FGF signaling antagonizes cytokine-mediated repression of Sox9 in SW1353 chondrosarcoma cells. Osteoarthritis Cartilage 11:233-241, 2003.
548. Kulyk WM, Franklin JL, Hoffman LM: Sox9 expression during chondrogenesis in micromass cultures of embryonic limb mesenchyme. Exp Cell Res 255:327-332, 2000.

549. Kypriotou M, Fossard-Demoor M, Chadjichristos C, et al: SOX9 exerts a bifunctional effect on type II collagen gene (COL2A1) expression in chondrocytes depending on the differentiation state. DNA Cell Biol 22:119-129, 2003.
550. Davies SR, Sakano S, Zhu Y, Sandell LJ: Distribution of the transcription factors Sox9, AP-2, and [delta]EF1 in adult murine articular and meniscal cartilage and growth plate. J Histochem Cytochem 50:1059-1065, 2002.
551. Stricker S, Fundele R, Vortkamp A, Mundlos S: Role of Runx genes in chondrocyte differentiation. Dev Biol 245:95-108, 2002.
552. Lengner CJ, Drissi H, Choi JY, et al: Activation of the bone-related Runx2/Cbfa1 promoter in mesenchymal condensations and developing chondrocytes of the axial skeleton. Mech Dev 114:167-170, 2002.
553. Enomoto H, Enomoto-Iwamoto M, Iwamoto M, et al: Cbfa1 is a positive regulatory factor in chondrocyte maturation. J Biol Chem 275:8695-8702, 2000.
554. Jimenez MJ, Balbin M, Alvarez J, et al: A regulatory cascade involving retinoic acid, Cbfa1, and matrix metalloproteinases is coupled to the development of a process of perichondrial invasion and osteogenic differentiation during bone formation. J Cell Biol 155:1333-1344, 2001.
555. Wu CW, Tchetina EV, Mwale F, et al: Proteolysis involving matrix metalloproteinase 13 (collagenase-3) is required for chondrocyte differentiation that is associated with matrix mineralization. J Bone Miner Res 17:639-651, 2002.
556. Leboy P, Grasso-Knight G, D'Angelo M, et al: Smad-Runx interactions during chondrocyte maturation. J Bone Joint Surg Am 83(Suppl 1):S15-S22, 2001.
557. Watanabe H, de Caestecker MP, Yamada Y: Transcriptional cross-talk between Smad, ERK1/2, and p38 mitogen-activated protein kinase pathways regulates transforming growth factor-beta-induced aggrecan gene expression in chondrogenic ATDC5 cells. J Biol Chem 276:14466-14473, 2001.
558. Hoffmann A, Czichos S, Kaps C, et al: The T-box transcription factor Brachyury mediates cartilage development in mesenchymal stem cell line C3H10T1/2. J Cell Sci 115:769-781, 2002.
559. Meachim G: Age changes in articular cartilage. Clin Orthop 64:33-44, 1969.
560. Roughley PJ: Age-associated changes in cartilage matrix: implications for tissue repair. Clin Orthop 391:S153-S160, 2001.
561. Bank RA, Bayliss MT, Lafeber FP, et al: Ageing and zonal variation in post-translational modification of collagen in normal human articular cartilage. The age-related increase in non-enzymatic glycation affects biomechanical properties of cartilage. Biochem J 330(Pt 1):345-351, 1998.
562. Yang C, Li SW, Helminen HJ, et al: Apoptosis of chondrocytes in transgenic mice lacking collagen II. Exp Cell Res 235:370-373, 1997.
563. Adams CS, Horton WE Jr.: Chondrocyte apoptosis increases with age in the articular cartilage of adult animals. Anat Rec 250:418-425, 1998.
564. Aigner T, Hemmel M, Neureiter D, et al: Apoptotic cell death is not a widespread phenomenon in normal aging and osteoarthritis human articular knee cartilage: a study of proliferation, programmed cell death (apoptosis), and viability of chondrocytes in normal and osteoarthritic human knee cartilage. Arthritis Rheum 44:1304-1312, 2001.
565. Martin JA, Buckwalter JA: Telomere erosion and senescence in human articular cartilage chondrocytes. J Gerontol A Biol Sci Med Sci 56:B172-B179, 2001.
566. Martin JA, Buckwalter JA: The role of chondrocyte senescence in the pathogenesis of osteoarthritis and in limiting cartilage repair. J Bone Joint Surg Am 85(Suppl 2):106-110, 2003.
567. van den Berg WB, van der Kraan PM, Scharstuhl A, van Beuningen HM: Growth factors and cartilage repair. Clin Orthop 391:S244-S250, 2001.
568. Rogachefsky RA, Dean DD, Howell DS, Altman RD: Treatment of canine osteoarthritis with insulin-like growth factor-1 (IGF-1) and sodium pentosan polysulfate. Osteoarthritis Cartilage 1:105-114, 1993.
569. Mi Z, Ghivizzani SC, Lechman ER, et al: Adverse effects of adenovirus-mediated gene transfer of human transforming growth factor beta 1 into rabbit knees. Arthritis Res 5:R132-R139, 2003.
570. Hunziker EB: Growth-factor-induced healing of partial-thickness defects in adult articular cartilage. Osteoarthritis Cartilage 9:22-32, 2001.
571. Brittberg M, Lindahl A, Nilsson A, et al: Treatment of deep cartilage defects in the knee with autologous chondrocyte transplantation. N Engl J Med 331:889-895, 1994.
572. Hunziker EB, Driesang IM, Morris EA: Chondrogenesis in cartilage repair is induced by members of the transforming growth factor-beta superfamily. Clin Orthop S171-S181, 2001.
573. Li RH, Wozney JM: Delivering on the promise of bone morphogenetic proteins. Trends Biotechnol 19:255-265, 2001.
574. Gooch KJ, Blunk T, Courter DL, et al: Bone morphogenetic proteins-2, -12, and -13 modulate in vitro development of engineered cartilage. Tissue Eng 8:591-601, 2002.
575. Sellers RS, Peluso D, Morris EA: The effect of recombinant human bone morphogenetic protein-2 (rhBMP-2) on the healing of full-thickness defects of articular cartilage. J Bone Joint Surg 79A:1452-1463, 1997.
576. Kang R, Marui T, Ghivizzani SC, et al: Ex vivo gene transfer to chondrocytes in full-thickness articular cartilage defects: a feasibility study. Osteoarthritis Cartilage 5:139-143, 1997.
577. Mi Z, Ghivizzani SC, Lechman ER, et al: Adenovirus-mediated gene transfer of insulin-like growth factor 1 stimulates proteoglycan synthesis in rabbit joints. Arthritis Rheum 43:2563-2570, 2000.
578. Smith P, Shuler FD, Georgescu HI, et al: Genetic enhancement of matrix synthesis by articular chondrocytes: Comparison of different growth factor genes in the presence and absence of interleukin-1. Arthritis Rheum 43:1156-1164, 2000.
579. Kaps C, Bramlage C, Smolian H, et al: Bone morphogenetic proteins promote cartilage differentiation and protect engineered artificial cartilage from fibroblast invasion and destruction. Arthritis Rheum 46:149-162, 2002.
580. Evans CH, Robbins PD, Ghivizzani SC, et al: Clinical trial to assess the safety, feasibility, and efficacy of transferring a potentially anti-arthritic cytokine gene to human joints with rheumatoid arthritis. Human Gene Therapy 7:1261-1280, 1996.
581. Evans CH, Robbins PD, Ghivizzani SC, et al: Results from the first human clinical trial of gene therapy for arthritis. Arthritis Rheum 44(Suppl):S170, 1999.
582. Gouze E, Ghivizzani SC, Robbins PD, Evans CH: Gene therapy for rheumatoid arthritis. Curr Rheumatol Rep 3:79-85, 2001.
583. Ghivizzani SC, Lechman ER, Kang R, et al: Direct adenovirus-mediated gene transfer of interleukin 1 and tumor necrosis factor alpha soluble receptors to rabbit knees with experimental arthritis has local and distal anti-arthritic effects. Proc Natl Acad Sci U S A 95:4613-4618, 1998.
584. Whalen JD, Lechman EL, Carlos CA, et al: Adenoviral transfer of the viral IL-10 gene periarticularly to mouse paws suppresses development of collagen-induced arthritis in both injected and uninjected paws. J Immunol 162:3625-3632, 1999.
585. Lechman ER, Jaffurs D, Ghivizzani SC, et al: Direct adenoviral gene transfer of viral IL-10 to rabbit knees with experimental arthritis ameliorates disease in both injected and contralateral control knees. J Immunol 163:2202-2208, 1999.
586. Lubberts E, Joosten LA, van Den Bersselaar L, et al: Adenoviral vector-mediated overexpression of IL-4 in the knee joint of mice with collagen-induced arthritis prevents cartilage destruction. J Immunol 163:4546-4556, 1999.
587. Kim SH, Evans CH, Kim S, et al: Gene therapy for established murine collagen-induced arthritis by local and systemic adenovirus-mediated delivery of interleukin-4. Arthritis Res 2:293-302, 2000.
588. Yoo JU, Mandell I, Angele P, Johnstone B: Chondrogenitor cells and gene therapy. Clin Orthop 379:S164-S170, 2000.

14 Neutrophils and Eosinophils

NATHALIE BURG • MICHAEL H. PILLINGER • STEVEN B. ABRAMSON

Polymorphonuclear leukocytes constitute a family of hematopoietically derived cells that share the feature of a multilobed nucleus. These leukocytes also share the property of possessing highly developed populations of intracytoplasmic granules, which are divisible into subsets and distinct between cell types. The presence of these granules permits the further designation of polymorphonuclear leukocytes as granulocytes. Based on the histocytochemical staining properties of their respective granules, three classes of polymorphonuclear, leukocytes have been identified: neutrophils, eosinophils, and basophils. Whereas neutrophil, also known as polymorphonuclear neutrophil (PMN), granules stain with neutral dyes, the granules of eosinophils, are most effectively stained with acidic dyes, such as eosin, and basophils stain with basic dyes. In a standard polychromatic Wright stain of a peripheral blood smear, the cytoplasm of neutrophils, eosinophils, and basophils will appear blue-pink, pink, and blue, respectively. These classes of polymorphonuclear leukocytes differ not only with respect to appearance, but also to biochemistry and function. Polymorphonuclear leukocytes comprise an important part of the organism's system of innate immunity: their responses to foreign organisms, antigens, or both are preprogrammed and do not depend on prior exposure to the particle. This chapter will review the salient features of neutrophils and eosinophils.

The Neutrophil

Neutrophils are the body's first line of defense against foreign invaders and constitute the major cell type involved in acute, as well as some forms of chronic, inflammatory disease. The importance of neutrophils in bacterial defense is demonstrated by patients who have hereditary defects in neutrophil function and are prone to repeated and often life-threatening infections. Neutrophils are the most prevalent leukocyte in the blood stream, typically constituting more than 50 percent of all blood-stream leukocytes. During bacterial infection the percentage of neutrophils may increase to 80 percent or more. In contrast, tissue concentrations of resting (inactive) neutrophils appear to be quite low. Thus, neutrophils may be thought of as surveillance cells—sweeping through the blood stream, scanning for infections or other inflammatory events. However, the capacity of neutrophils to destroy foreign organisms is matched, in some circumstances, by a capacity for host-tissue destruction.

NEUTROPHIL MYELOPOIESIS AND CLEARANCE

The neutrophil majority in the blood stream is also present in the bone marrow, where up to 60 percent of hematopoietic capacity may be dedicated to neutrophil production. As many as 10^{11} neutrophils per day may be released into the blood stream. Neutrophil development in the bone marrow takes about 14 days, originating with the hematopoietic stem cell. Stem cells fated to become neutrophils first differentiate into myeloblasts, which retain the capacity to develop into eosinophils and basophils, as well as neutrophils. Subsequent differentiation leads to the neutrophilic promyelocyte, a dedicated precursor of the neutrophil, and then proceeds through the stages of the neutrophilic myelocytes, metamyelocyte, band cell, and mature neutrophil. It is at the metamyelocyte stage that neutrophil mitosis ceases, while neutrophil development and organization of granules continues. Neutrophils are terminally differentiated; they neither divide nor mature after their release from the marrow.

Given the origin of neutrophils in a pluripotent stem cell and the precise phases of their development, the mechanisms regulating neutrophil differentiation are of considerable interest. Although incompletely understood, studies have emphasized the role of a particular complement of cytokines that appear to direct the early cells toward neutrophil development. Principal among those described to date are granulocyte colony-stimulating factor (G-CSF) and granulocyte-macrophage colony-stimulating factor (GM-CSF).[1]

Neutrophils released from the marrow have a blood-stream half-life of approximately 6 hours, with a tissue half-life only marginally longer. The high output and short half-life of neutrophils implies that neutrophil clearance mechanisms must exist. Neutrophils, when exposed to appropriate stimuli, such as tumor necrosis factor-α (TNF-α) and Fas (CD95) ligand, undergo apoptosis, or programmed cell death.[2,3] Senescent or apoptotic blood-stream neutrophils are cleared largely by liver and spleen macrophages (reticuloendothelial system). Whether tissue neutrophils are cleared primarily via local macrophages remains a matter of speculation.

NEUTROPHIL MORPHOLOGY AND CONTENT

Neutrophil nuclei tend to have a greater number of lobes than those of other polymorphs, typically three to five. The multilobed nature of this nucleus reflects a condensation of chromatin, which suggests that neutrophils might be incapable of transcription. However, it is now appreciated that neutrophils retain the capacity for consitutive and stimulated protein synthesis, albeit at a limited rate.

Neutrophil granules identifiable by classic histochemical staining constitute two classes. Neutrophil primary granules form first and, by virtue of their staining tendencies, are also referred to as azurophilic granules. These granules are oval or round and vary in size. They are similar, and functionally equivalent, to the lysosomes of other cells. In contrast, neutrophil secondary granules constitute a population unique to neutrophils, a fact reflected in the alternative nomenclature of *specific granules* often used to describe these structures. Characteristic of azurophilic granules is the presence of myeloperoxidase, an enzyme that catalyzes the formation of hypochlorous acid from chloride in the presence of superoxide anion (O_2^-).[4] Indeed, the presence of large amounts of this enzyme in azurophilic granules lends collections of neutrophils (pus) their typical greenish-yellow color. Consistent with their role as lysosomes, azurophilic granules also contain a variety of proteases and other enzymes, including elastase, lysozyme, acid phosphatase, and cathepsins, as well as enzymes directed at nucleic acids and sugars. One particularly important family of proteinases found in neutrophils are the matrix metalloproteinases (MMPs), including neutrophil collagenase-2 (MMP-8), gelatinase-B (MMP-9), and stromelysin (MMP-3). In contrast to azurophilic granules, specific granules possess an extensive array of membrane-associated proteins including cytochromes, signaling molecules, and receptors. Specific granules thus constitute a reservoir of proteins destined for topologically external surfaces of both phagocytic vacuoles themselves and the plasma membrane.[4]

Further study has confirmed the existence of two additional classes of vesicles.[5] Gelatinase granules are almost identical in size to specific granules and share some proteins in common with them. As their name implies, however, gelatinase granules are noteworthy for their high concentrations of gelatinase, a latent enzyme with the capacity for tissue destruction.[6] Secretory vesicles are smaller and lighter than the other classes and do not appear to contain proteolytic enzymes.[4] Rather, they are noteworthy for an extensive series of membrane-associated proteins, including receptors otherwise identified with the plasma membrane.[7] These and other data suggest that the secretory vesicle is a reservoir of neutrophil plasma membrane proteins.

Both azurophilic and specific granules also contain antimicrobial proteins and peptides that are the cornerstone of innate immunity. Detailed description of the neutrophil's armamentarium against foreign invaders is beyond the scope of this review, but a few whose mechanisms of action have more recently been elucidated deserve mention. Elastase, mentioned previously, aids in the killing of gram-negative bacteria via degradation of bacterial outer membrane protein A (OMP A), as shown by Belaaouaj and colleagues.[8] Elastase-deficient mice are more susceptible to infection with gram-negative (but not gram-positive) organisms than are wild-type mice. The defensins, normally located in azurophilic granules, are found in mg/ml concentrations in the phagocytic vacuole (see following) and permeabilize target cell membranes. Bactericidal permeability-inducing protein (BPI), also located in azurophilic granules, acts in concert with the defensins; it potently neutralizes endotoxin and is cytotoxic to gram-negative bacteria.[9] BPI also enhances the activity of secretory phospholipase A_2 ($sPLA_2$), which has activity against both gram-negative and -positive bacteria. Lactoferrin (found in specific granules) deprives microorganisms of iron and has both antiviral and antibacterial effects.

Neutrophil proteases play important roles beyond their antimicrobial effects: They may also amplify or dampen the innate, as well as adaptive, immune response. For example, lactoferrin released during phagocytosis may inhibit proliferation of mixed lymphocyte cultures by decreasing release of interleukin (IL)-2, as well as TNF-α and IL-1.[9a] Proteinase 3 (PR3) has been found to augment release of active TNF-α and IL-1 in monocyte/neutrophil cocultures by releasing the membrane-bound forms of these cytokines.[10] Gelatinase B has been shown to convert latent IL-1 into its active form,[11] and to potentiate IL-8 activity by truncating this chemoattractant and increasing its release, thereby amplifying neutrophilic influx.[12] In an interesting and eloquent series of studies, Fadok and coworkers have recently proposed that neutrophil elastase may play a proinflammatory role by virtue of its ability to cleave and disrupt phosphatidyl serine receptors on macrophages. Apoptotic cells undergo membrane alterations that lead to expression of phosphatidyl serine on their outer membrane surface, and interaction of phosphatidyl serine with its receptor leads to macrophage responses that downregulate inflammation through the generation of TGF-β.[13] By disrupting these interactions, the presence of neutrophil elastase may permit inflammation to continue.[14]

NEUTROPHIL ACTIVATION AND FUNCTION

For blood-stream neutrophils to destroy foreign targets in the periphery, they must sense the presence of such targets at a distance. They must then adhere to and pass through the endothelium of postcapillary venules (diapedesis) and migrate to the source of the signal (chemotaxis). Finally, neutrophils must encounter a target, engulf it, and destroy it. Collectively, these processes are referred to as *neutrophil activation*. Because of the potential for tissue destruction, neutrophil activation must be carefully regulated. The internal responses through which a cell translates an encounter with a stimulus into particular phenotypic response have been termed *signal transduction*. In neutrophils, as in other cells, the study of signal transduction has made extraordinary advances in the last decade.[15,16]

Stimuli and Receptors

Classic chemoattractants include both lipid mediators, such as leukotriene B_4 (LTB_4) and platelet activating factor, and proteins/peptides, such as formylated peptides, the complement split product C5a, and IL-8. Chemoattractants in vivo are formed at sites of inflammation; they are either produced at the site by inflammatory cells (LTB_4, IL-8) or liberated from already-synthesized proteins, as in the case of C5a. The ability of formylated peptides such as formyl-methionyl-leucyl-phenylalanine (FMLP) to stimulate neutrophils probably represents a particularly ancient arm of the innate immune response because prokaryotic, but not eukaryotic, cells synthesize proteins whose first amino acid is a formylated methionine. Chemoattractants also have the capacity to stimulate most other aspects of neutrophil activation. However, their individual potencies for particular responses may differ, suggesting that they may serve overlapping, but distinct, functions in neutrophil activation.[17]

Blood-stream activation of neutrophils depends on the presence of specific surface receptors. Chemoattractant receptors belong to a class known as seven-transmembrane-domain receptors, or "serpentine seven" receptors, which are composed of a single protein chain whose seven hydrophobic domains span the plasma membrane. Binding of a particular chemoattractant occurs in a pocket on the cytoplasmic face, close to or below the level of the plasma membrane.

Receptors for soluble ligands other than chemoattractants have also been identified on neutrophils, including receptors for growth factors, colony-stimulating factors, and cytokines. These receptors fall into several families distinct from the serpentine sevens. For instance, growth-factor receptors are members of the protein tyrosine kinase receptor (PTKR) family, in which ligand interaction with two identical or related receptors brings them into proximity, causing their phosphorylation and activation. Some nonchemoattractant ligands do not directly activate neutrophils but may modulate their function. For example, pretreatment of neutrophils with either insulin or GM-CSF results in amplification of subsequent neutrophil responses to chemoattractants, a process referred to as *priming*.

Guanosine Triphosphate–binding Proteins

Ligation of seven-transmembrane-domain receptors results in the interaction of cytoplasmic elements of the receptor with a class of effectors known as heterotrimeric guanosine triphosphate (GTP)-binding proteins (G proteins). G proteins are composed of α, β, and γ subunits, and individual G protein types are distinguished by their particular combination of subunits. In neutrophils, the predominant G proteins are of the G_i family.[15] G protein g subunits are modified by the addition of prenyl (polyisoprene) and carboxyterminal methyl groups, which serve to anchor them to the plasma membrane. All G proteins share the capacity, localized to their α subunits, to bind GTP and subsequently hydrolyze it to guanine diphosphate (GDP). G proteins are active when GTP bound, but they are inactive in the GDP-bound form. Engagement of the appropriate seven-transmembrane-domain receptor results in the binding of GTP on a subunit. As a consequence of GTP binding, heterotrimeric G proteins dissociate into α and β/γ components, each with specific effector functions.[18]

A monomeric class of low molecular weight (20 to 25 kD) GTP-binding proteins (LMW-GBPs) has also been described. Because the first, prototypical LMW-GBP to be described was the protooncogene *ras*, these are also referred to as *ras*-related proteins. LMW-GBPs combine, in one molecule, the prenyl and methyl modifications of the G protein γ subunit with the GTP-binding capacity of the α. At least four families of LMW-GBPs have been described: the ras family, whose members play roles in cell growth and division; the rho family, functioning in cytoskeletal rearrangements; and the rab and arf families, critical for vesicular and endomembrane trafficking. All four classes of LMW-GBPs appear to be represented in neutrophils.[19]

Second Messengers

Second messengers are small, diffusible molecules generated in response to stimuli that transmit signals from membrane receptors to downstream effector proteins. In the classic model of neutrophil activation, engagement of receptors results in the activation of phospholipase C (PLC), which cleaves phosphoinositol trisphosphate (PIP_3) into diacyl glycerol (DAG) and inositol trisphosphate (IP_3). DAG and IP_3 then mediate the influx of cytosolic calcium and the activation of protein kinase C. Other phospholipases present in the neutrophil include PLA_2, which cleaves phosphatidylcholine, ethanolamine, or both and is responsible for the generation of arachidonic acid, and phospholipase D, which cleaves phosphatidylcholine into phosphatidic acid and choline.[17] Whereas the second messengers described previously have all been implicated in neutrophil activation, other lipid mediators may have negative regulatory effects. For instance, sphingosine and ceramide each inhibit neutrophil phagocytosis.[20]

In addition to lipids, other organic and inorganic messenger molecules have been characterized. Intracellular concentrations of cyclic adenosine monophosphate (cAMP), a classic second messenger, rise rapidly in neutrophils exposed to both stimuli and inhibitors. cAMP in these settings is likely to provide a negative regulatory (off) signal because direct exposure to cAMP inhibits neutrophil responses, probably through the activation of protein kinase A.[21,22] In contrast, rising levels of cyclic guanosine 3′, 5′ monophosphate (cGMP) have a modest enhancing effect on some neutrophil responses. Nitric oxide (NO), an important molecule in the regulation of host defense, is also produced in neutrophils, albeit at low levels.[23] Endogenously produced NO in neutrophils is likely to play an important role in signal transduction, as several studies have documented the capacity of exogenously added NO to exert a variety of effects, including inhibition of the NADPH oxidase, actin polymerization, and chemotaxis (see following). Moreover, excessive NO production has been implicated in a number of rheumatic diseases.[24]

Kinases and Kinase Cascades

The last decade has seen explosive growth in our understanding of how kinases—proteins capable of enzymatically adding phosphate groups to target molecules—contribute to signaling in myeloid and nonmyeloid cells. Nonetheless, portion of the molecules involved. Protein kinase C (PKC), the best characterized kinase (actually a family of kinases) in neutrophil activation, is activated in response to chemoattractants. The ability of phorbol myristate acetate—a synthetic activator of PKC—to stimulate neutrophil responses including adhesion and $O_2^{-\cdot}$ generation supports a role for PKC in neutrophil activation.[25] In addition, inhibitors of PKC block stimulation of neutrophil functions.

The mitogen-activated protein kinases (MAPKs) are a family of serine threonine kinases including p38, jun kinase (JNK), and the prototypic MAPK, extracellular signal-regulated kinase (ERK). ERK activation has been best studied in mitotic cells, where it plays a role in cell growth and division. Strikingly, it has recently been appreciated that in neutrophils, chemoattractants and other stimuli are able to activate p38, JNK and ERK on time courses consistent with neutrophil activation.[26,27] A role for ERK activation in signaling for neutrophil O_2^- has been proposed but remains controversial; a role in neutrophil adhesion and phagocytosis appears to be better established.[22,28]

Phosphatidylinositol 3-kinase (PI3k) is a set of related enzymes found in abundance in neutrophils and that primarily catalyze the phosphorylation, not of proteins, but of the 3-position of phosphatidylinositol phospholipids. The main active product of PI3ks appears to be phosphatidylinositol trisphosphate (PIP_3). Chemoattr-actants rapidly activate PI3k in neutrophils, where it appears to play a role in diverse neutrophil functions, including O_2^- generation, adhesion, and degranulation.[29] PI3k may also regulate neutrophil survival and apoptosis.[30]

Neutrophil Adhesion

One of the earliest, critical aspects of the inflammatory response is the ability of blood-stream neutrophils to adhere to vascular endothelium to prepare for movement into the tissues (Fig. 14–1). Stimulated neutrophils also possess the ability to adhere to each other, a process termed *homotypic aggregation*, which may in vivo bring blood-stream neutrophils into proximity with neutrophils already adherent to the vessel or concentrate them at a site of inflammation. Extensive work has provided significant insight into the mechanisms involved in neutrophil adhesion. Several families of interacting adhesion molecules have been shown to exist on both neutrophils and endothelial cells. These include the selectins, the integrins, and the intercellular adhesion molecules (ICAMs), as well as sialylated glycoproteins.

The selectins consist of three related molecules (L-selectin on leukocytes, E-selectin on endothelial cells, and P-selectin on activated platelets and endothelial cells) sharing a common structure of two or more complement regulatory (CR) domains, an epidermal growth-factor–like domain, and a lectin domain. Each binds to a sialylated glycoprotein on the surface of its interacting cell. Thus, E-selectin binds to the sialyl Lewis^x antigen on neutrophils, P-selectin binds P-selectin glycoprotein-1 (PSGL-1) on neutrophils, and L-selectin binds both PSGL-1 on neutrophils and glycosylation-dependent cell adhesion molecule-1 (GlyCAM-1) on the endothelium. Selectin expression is largely constitu-

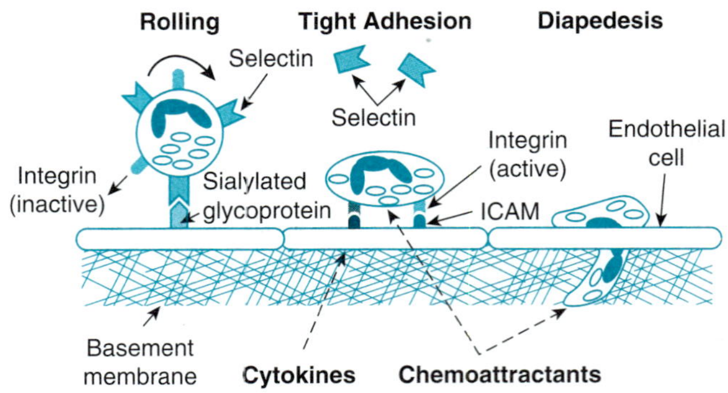

FIGURE 14–1 · A model of neutrophil adhesion and diapedesis. *Left,* Rolling. An unstimulated neutrophil adheres with low affinity to the unstimulated endothelium of a postcapillary venule, a process mediated by the interaction of selectins (on both neutrophil and endothelium) with sialylated glycoproteins and resulting in the rolling of neutrophils along the vessel wall. *Center,* Tight adhesion. Exposure of the neutrophil to chemoattractants results in activation of integrins (CD11a/CD18, CD11b/CD18); exposure of endothelium to cytokines results in the expression of ICAMs. These molecules then interact, resulting in tight adhesion. Concurrently, selectins may be shed from the cell surfaces. *Right,* Diapedesis. A neutrophil undergoes diapedesis, passing across the endothelium and making its way through the basement membrane. Thus, blood stream neutrophils have the capacity to adhere to and move out of the vasculature in response to tissue signals for inflammation.

tive, but selectin/sialylated-glycoprotein interactions are transient. The result of these interactions is that a pool of blood-stream neutrophils is, at any one time, loosely marginated to the vascular surface and moving along it slowly in a rolling, tumbleweed-like motion. Exposure of neutrophils and endothelium to appropriate stimuli leads to shedding of selectins and neutrophil release (stress demargination), with apparent increases in the peripheral neutrophil count.

The integrins are a large family of heterodimeric molecules generated by various combinations of α- and β-chains. Like the selectins, they require divalent cations (Ca^{2+} or Mg^{2+}) to engage their ligands. Neutrophils express three β_2-type integrins, each constructed from a distinct subcomponent (CD11a, CD11b, or CD11c) and a common, β_2-chain (CD18). Integrins use the ICAMs as their counterligands. CD11b/CD18 (also called Mac-1 or CR3) binds to fibrinogen, factor X, heparin, and the complement component iC3b, in addition to ICAM, and is most strongly implicated in both neutrophil-endothelial and neutrophil-neutrophil interactions. In contrast to the selectins, neutrophil CD11b/CD18 is constitutively expressed but inactive; stimulation of neutrophils by chemoattractants and other agents results in changes in the activation state of CD11b/CD18 and increases its affinity for ICAMs and other ligands. On the other hand, stimulation of endothelium with cytokines such as IL-1 results in increased expression of ICAM-1 and ICAM-2, providing a coordinate mechanism for the regulation of adhesion. In contrast to selectin-mediated adhesion, integrin-ICAM interactions are high affinity and persistent. Thus, stimulation of rolling neutrophils results in their tight adhesion to vessel walls and constitutes the first committed step in the movement of neutrophils into the tissues. Additionally, engagement of integrins by their counterligands sends signals into the cell ("outside-in" signaling), regulating selective cell responses such as cytoskeletal reorganization, oxidant production, and degranulation. Outside-in signaling through CD11b/CD18 also coordinates with signaling through FcγRIII (see following) to mediate phagocytosis of particles opsonized by immunoglobulin G (IgG) and the complement component iC3b. Cross-talk between neutrophils and endothelial cells has also been shown to be a CD11b/CD18-dependent event: Cross-linking of CD18 on neutrophils leads to increased permeability of endothelial cells, probably through the release of neutrophil proteases.[31]

Although the function of CD11a/CD18 on neutrophils has been more controversial, some studies suggest that this molecule may be both necessary and sufficient in mediating neutrophil emigration.[32,33] Others indicate that both CD11b/Cd18 and CD11a/CD18 are important in neutrophil adhesion, with CD11a/CD18 playing an earlier, but more transient, role.[34] In addition, CD11b/CD18 may be critical for bacterial killing. The function of CD11c/CD18 remains obscure, although it may contribute to neutrophil activation via outside-in signaling.

Diapedesis and Chemotaxis

The mechanism by which neutrophils pass through the endothelial barrier is not entirely clear. One report supports a model in which neutrophils pass directly through pores generated within the endothelial cells themselves, rather than around them by disruption of cell-cell junctions.[35] Other studies have clearly shown that diapedesis occurs via homotypic interactions bet-ween adhesion molecules found on both neutrophils and endothelial cells, known as platelet-endothelial cell adhesion molecules (PECAMs). These molecules are concentrated at endothelial cell junctions, and antibodies that block PECAMs inhibit transmigration in vitro by limiting neutrophils to the apical surface of the endothelium. Transmigrating neutrophils undergo upregulation of $\alpha_6\beta_1$, an integrin that mediates binding to laminin (a key component of the perivascular basement membrane). Antibodies to $\alpha_6\beta_1$ generally block neutrophil transmigration, but they fail to do so in a PECAM knockout mouse, implicating $\alpha_6\beta_1$/ PECAM as critical to the passage of neutrophils out of the vasculature.[36]

CD47, otherwise known as integrin-associated protein (IAP), has also been implicated in neutrophil transmigration across both endothelium and epithelium.[37] CD99, a protein highly expressed at endothelial junctions, has been directly implicated in monocyte passage through the endothelium, once homotypic PECAM interations have occurred. A role for CD99 in neutrophil transmigration has yet to be defined.[38] Once beyond the endothelium, most neutrophils pause for a time before essaying the basement membrane (basal lamina). In vitro studies by Weiss and colleagues suggest that neutrophils pass through the basement membrane by disrupting its patency, without elucidation of known proteases or oxygen radicals. The disruptions are then rapidly repaired by an unknown mechanism, probably involving the endothelium[39] (Fig. 14–2).

Chemotaxis in the direction of a gradient is achieved by the extension of membrane ruffles (lamellipodia), followed by anchorage of the ruffles to the substrate and withdrawal of the trailing edge of the cell in the direction of movement. These changes are accomplished primarily through rearrangement of the actin cytoskeleton. Actin is a 41-kD protein that exists as a soluble, globular monomeric form (g-actin) and as an insoluble linear polymer (f-actin). F-actin may be assembled (extended) at one end (barbed end) and disassembled at the other, under the control of regulatory molecules. During chemotaxis, f-actin formation and extension are concentrated at the leading edge of the neutrophil, permitting extension of the cell membrane. Chemoattractant receptors also concentrate at the leading edge, defining the cell's directional response to the gradient (headlight phenomenon). As the neutrophil moves along, receptors that were formerly at the leading edge are swept to the tail and internalized.[40]

Phagocytosis and Degranulation

Neutrophil phagocytosis of an encountered bacterium or other particle requires direct contact. Neutrophils are generally poor at phagocytosing unmodified targets, particularly encapsulated bacteria. Optimal phagocytosis depends on opsonization (from the Greek, meaning to prepare for the table), the modification of a target via its adornment with immunoglobulin, complement components, or both. Neutrophils express two families of receptors for the crystallizable (Fc) portion of complexed or aggregated IgG: low-affinity FcγRIIa and high-affinity FcγRIIIb. During some infections, or after in vitro stimulation with interferon or G-CSF, neutrophils also express the high-affinity receptor FcγRI, which binds monomeric IgG.

FcγRIIa binds subclasses of IgG with varying efficiency depending on a polymorphism at amino acid position 131. Confusingly, the "low responder" allotype (so named because of its weak interaction with *mouse* IgG_1) binds human IgG_2 efficiently, and the "high responder" allotype (which binds *mouse* IgG_1 efficiently) does not. FcγRIIIb polymorphisms of neutrophil antigens (NA)1 and NA2 also determine binding to IgG subclasses. Individuals homozygous for the NA2 allele have a lower capacity to mediate phagocytosis than those homozygous for the NA1. These differences have important implications for rheumatic diseases, in which immune complexes play an important role (see following).

Phagocytosis is an active process that involves both extension of the neutrophil membrane (filopodia and ruffle formation) and invagination of the neutrophil at the locus of the target. Engagement of FcγR and complement receptors results in the activation of diverse signaling pathways. Elegant studies by Caron and Hall indicate that FcγR and complement receptors play distinct roles in phagocytosis.[40a] Whereas engagement of CR3 (CD11b/CD18) results in actin stress-fiber formation and invagination, engagement of FcγRII results primarily in extension of membranes out from and around the target (filopodia and lamellipodia formation). Signaling by these receptors depends on the activation of distinct members of the Rho family of LMW-GBPs. However,

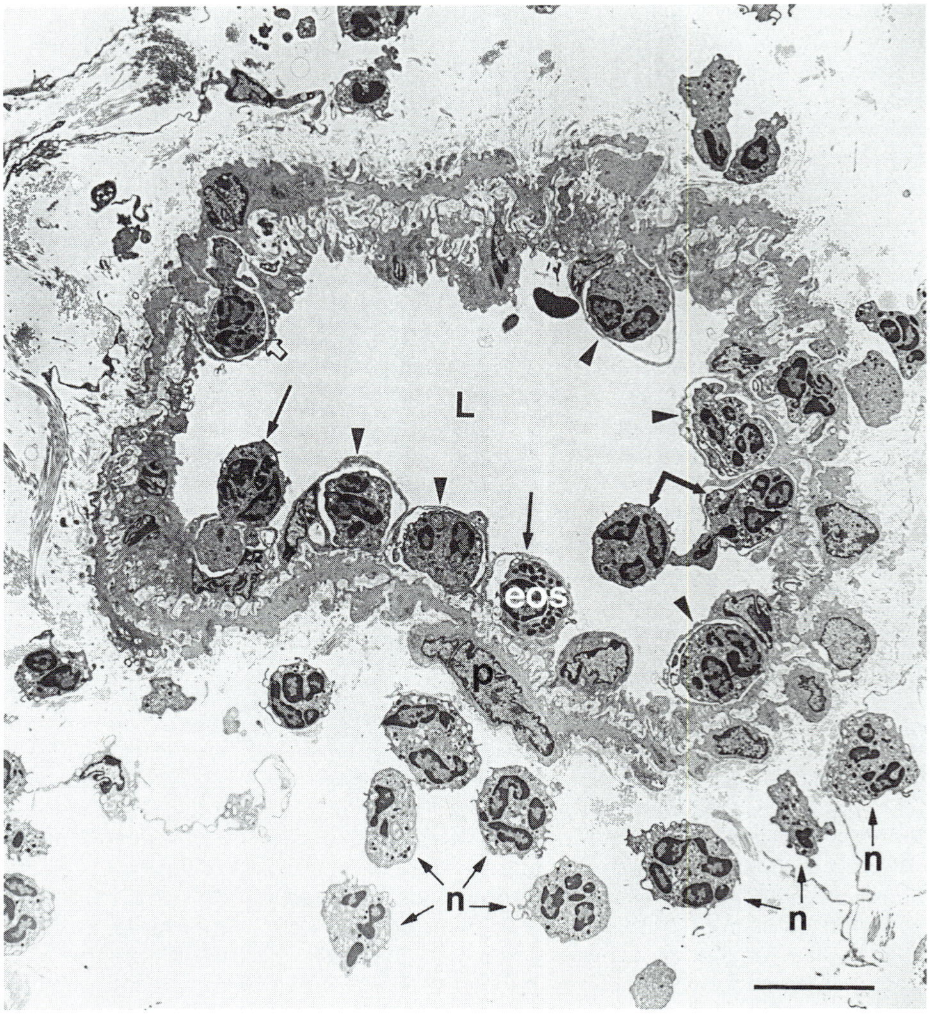

FIGURE 14-2 • This micrograph shows the adhesion and diapedesis of neutrophils in a venule after exposure of the tissue to a formylated peptide. Neutrophils can be seen in various stages of extravasation. The neutrophil indicated by the *long arrow* has adhered to an underlying endothelial cell and begun to project a cytoplasmic extension into the body of that cell. The *joined arrows* indicate a neutrophil that has partly passed through the endothelium but is simultaneously adherent to a second neutrophil still within the vascular lumen, L. (i.e., homotypic aggregation of two neutrophils). *Arrowheads* indicate multiple neutrophils that have crossed through the endothelium but have not ye! penetrated the basement membrane. The *open arrow* indicates a neutrophil that has passed through the endothelium and is extending a process into the basement membrane. Still other neutrophils (labeled n with arrows) have moved completely through the basement membrane and have reached the surrounding connective tissues. Finally, a single eosinophil (labeled eos) has also passed through the endothelium but has not yet crossed the basement membrane. P, pericyte. (From Feng D, Nagy JA, Pyne K, et al: Neutrophils emigrate from venules by a transendothelial cell pathway in response to FMLP. J Exp Med 187:903–915, 1998.)

these observations remain to be specifically confirmed for neutrophils.

Upon activation, neutrophils *degranulate*, a term actually reflecting two distinct processes. Vesicles can either fuse with the plasma membrane, thus spilling their contents into the extracellular space, or they can fuse with the phagocytic vacuole to form a phagolysosome. The former type of degranulation is regulated differently from the latter and favors mobilization of lighter granules in response to stimuli. Secretory granules are mobilized first, followed by gelatinase, specific, and azurophilic granules; (secretory vesicles > gelatinase granules > specific granules > azurophilic granules). In the latter type of degranulation (phagolysosome formation), fusion of azurophilic granules with the phagocytic vacuole results in the delivery of proteolytic enzymes, myeloperoxidase, and antibacterial proteins to the site of the ingested bacterium. Fusion of specific granules with the phagocytic vacuole permits the delivery of collagenase, as well as the appropriate localization of cytochrome-b_{558}, a requisite for the NADPH oxidase (see following). Containment of potentially toxic substrates within the phagolysosome keeps host-tissue damage and neutrophil autodestruction in check.[41] However, as will be discussed later in the chapter, in several of the rheumatic diseases, neutrophilic activation plays an important role in abetting inflammation and host-tissue damage.

The NADPH Oxidase System

In addition to the collection of proteases and other antibacterial proteins contained in their granules, neutrophils also have the capacity to kill bacteria through the generation of toxic oxygen metabolites. This process, frequently referred to as the respiratory burst, is extremely potent and requires tight regulation to prevent neutrophil autodestruction. Studies in broken cell preparations, and in cell-free systems consisting of recombinant proteins, have established the so-called "minimal system" required for O_2^- generation: the NADPH oxidase.[42,43] The central component of the NADPH oxidase is cytochrome, b_{558}, which is localized to the membranes of specific granules and consists of two subunits: a 22-kDa component (gp22^{phox}, for *ph*agocyte *ox*idase) and a 91-kD component (gp91^{phox}). However, this cytochrome lacks independent activity. Three cytosolic proteins are also required: a 47-kD and a 67-kD component (p47^{phox} and p67^{phox}), and a low molecular weight GTP-binding protein, p21^{rac}. Upon neutrophil stimulation, the p47^{phox} and p67^{phox} components translocate to the membrane to form an active complex with the cytochrome.[44] Although p21^{rac} also translocates in response to stimuli, the significance of its translocation is more controversial.[45] A fifth protein, p40^{phox}, has also recently been reported to be associated with p47/p67 in the cytosol. It remains unclear

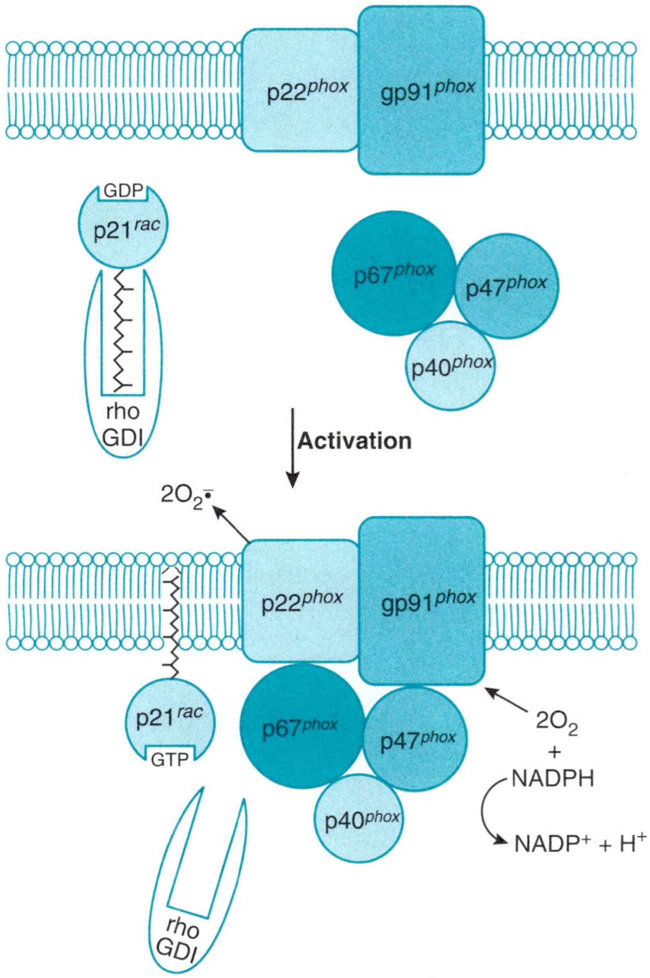

FIGURE 14-3 · Assembly of the neutrophil NADPH oxidase system. *Top*, Basic components of the NADPH oxidase as they are distributed in a resting state. The cytochrome-b_{558}, composed of the two subunits gp91^{phox} and p22^{phox}, are membrane associated, whereas p47^{phox}, p67^{phox}, and the recently identified p40^{phox} exist as a complex in the cytoplasm. p21^{rac} in an inactive, GDP-bound form also resides in the cytoplasm, in association with a chaperon (Rho-GDI) that sheaths its hydrophobic tail to permit solubility. *Bottom*, Activation of the neutrophil leads to translocation of the cytosolic components of the oxidase to the neutrophil membrane, where they form an active complex with the cytochrome, resulting in the generation of O_2. Thus, the potentially damaging oxidase system is carefully regulated through the segregation and assembly of its component parts.

whether p40^{phox} positively or negatively regulates the respiratory burst[46] (Fig. 14–3).

Once assembled and activated, the NADPH oxidase transfers electrons from NADPH to generate O_2^-:

$$2O_2 + NADPH \xrightarrow{\text{NADPH Oxidase}} O_2^- + NADP^+ + H^+$$

A subsequent, spontaneous dismutase reaction rapidly produces hydrogen peroxide:

$$O_2^- + 2\,H^+ \rightarrow H_2O_2 + O_2$$

Although both $O_2^{-\cdot}$ and H_2O_2 can kill organisms in vitro, they are short-lived and probably do not account for most of the bacteria-killing capacity of the system under normal circumstances. (Indeed, many bacteria have catalase, an enzyme that degrades H_2O_2.) Rather, the production of H_2O_2 within the same space into which the myeloperoxidase (MPO) has been released permits the generation of large quantities of hypochlorous acid (HOCl, which is chlorine bleach), a powerful oxidant with potent killing capacity. HOCl may further interact with proteins to form chloramines, which are less potent but longer-lived oxidants.[41]

Neutrophil oxidant production plays a key role in the body's defense. However, the current view that oxidant production, via the production of HOCl by MPO, is the neutrophil's most powerful tool against microbes has recently been challenged. Mice lacking either NADPH oxidase or elastase and cathepsin G are equally susceptible to infection, implying that both arms of defense, oxidant production and protease-mediated microbial destruction, are equally critical. Superoxide production in phagocytic vacuoles causes the pH to rise (secondary to the consumption of protons necessary to make H_2O_2), which in turn causes an influx of K^+. The resulting increase in ionicity liberates cationic proteases from the anionic proteoglycan matrix, freeing them to kill bacteria. Thus, in this new model, oxidants are not directly destructive to microbes but are necessary to facilitate proteolytic damage.[47] In support of this model is the fact that MPO deficiency is common (1 in 2000), and surprisingly benign.

NEUTROPHIL PRODUCTION OF PROINFLAMMATORY MEDIATORS

Arachidonic Acid Metabolites

The capacity of stimulated neutrophils to liberate arachidonic acid from membranes has implications for the propagation of acute inflammation. Although arachidonic acid itself has chemoattractant and neutrophil-stimulatory properties,[28,48,49] its metabolites are more critical to regulation of inflammation. Best recognized among these are the leukotrienes (LTs). Neutrophils have the capacity to produce LTB_4,[48] a highly potent lipid mediator for the chemoattraction of other neutrophils. Intermediates of leukotriene production such as 5-hydroxyeicosatetraenoic acid are also produced by neutrophils and may have stimulatory properties.[28,50] Interestingly, an alternative class of lipoxygenase products, the lipoxins, has also been identified. Synthesis of lipoxins requires coordinate activity of neutrophil 5-lipoxygenase and a related enzyme (either 12- or 15-lipoxygenase) in another cell type, either platelets or endothelial cells. In contrast to leukotrienes, lipoxins inhibit neutrophil function and may be anti-inflammatory.[51,52] The capacity of aspirin to stimulate lipoxin generation suggests a previously unappreciated mechanism for its anti-inflammatory action.[53]

The cyclooxygenase (COX), or endoperoxide synthase, pathway is the other major pathway of arachidonic-acid metabolism. Arachidonic acid metabolized by COX is converted into prostaglandin H (PGH),[54] which undergoes further, cell-type–specific conversion to a variety of other prostaglandins. The prostaglandins of most relevance to inflammation are those of the E series, particularly PGE_2. PGEs have numerous proinflammatory effects, including increased vasodilatation, vascular permeability, and pain. Interestingly, the direct effects of PGEs on neutrophils appear to be inhibitory, probably through elevations of intracellular cAMP.[55,56] Although resting neutrophils exhibit little cyclooxygenase activity, persistent neutrophil activation results in upregulation of COX-2,[57] suggesting that neutrophils may contribute PGE_2 to both the proinflammatory brew and the down-regulation of their own activity.

Cytokine Production

Although the relative amount of cytokine production by neutrophils is small, the large numbers of neutrophils present in infected or inflammatory sites suggest that overall neutrophil cytokine production may play a role in recruiting additional neutrophils to the target area. Among the cytokines produced by neutrophils are IL-1, IL-8, IL-12, TNF-α, TNF-β, macrophage inhibitory protein-1 (MIP-1α), oncostatin M, monocyte chemoattractant protein-1 (MCP-1), and transforming growth factor-β (TGF-β).[58,59] TGF-β is a powerful neutrophil chemoattractant,[60] and its recruitment of neutrophils into an inflammatory space may lead to additional neutrophil cytokine production, including further production of TGF-β.[61] However, TGF-β also has potent anti-inflammatory effects,[13] suggesting that neutrophils may also participate in the resolution of inflammation. Moreover, activated neutrophils also produce an antagonist to IL-1, the IL-1 receptor antagonist (IL-1Ra).[62,63]

HERITABLE DISORDERS OF NEUTROPHIL FUNCTION

A wide variety of acquired conditions result in neutrophil dysfunction, depletion, or both, including malignancies (myeloid leukemias), metabolic abnormalities (diabetes), and drugs (corticosteroids, chemotherapy). In addition, a number of rare, congenital disorders of neutrophils have been identified. In general, patients with impaired neutrophil function are prone to infection by bacteria (predominantly *Staphylococcus aureus*, *Pseudomonas* species, *Burkholderia*) and fungi (*Aspergillus*, *Candida*),[64,65] but not viruses and parasites. The major sites of infection include skin, mucus membranes, and lungs, but any site may be affected, and spreading abcesses are common. Most of these diseases are potentially life-threatening in the absence of available effective therapy (Table 14–1).

Diseases of Diminished Neutrophil Number

Severe congenital neutropenia (Kostmann's syndrome) is an autosomal recessive disorder resulting in marrow maturation arrest of myelopoiesis and leading to neutrophil counts persistently below 0.5×10^9 cells/L. Patients are prone, from early infancy, to severe bacterial infections, including omphalitis, pneumonia, otitis, gingivitis, and perirectal infections. Because acute inflammation is lacking, infections tend to spread extensively before coming to anyone's attention. Mortality has been high. Therapy formerly consisted of antibiotics, but it has recently been appreciated that long-term therapy with recombinant human granulocyte colony stimulating factor (RhG-CSF) may help maintain normal or near-normal neutrophil counts.[66] A milder form of neutropenia (benign congenital neutropenia) with somewhat higher neutrophil counts and fewer infections has also been observed. Another variant is cyclic neutropenia, which causes transient, recurrent neutropenia on a 21-day cycle.[67] Recent studies suggest that a defect in neutrophil elastase affects neutrophil survival in the marrow and is responsible for cyclic neutropenia.[68]

Leukocyte Adhesion Deficiencies

Leukocyte adhesion deficiency type 1 (LAD1) results from an autosomal recessive defect in production of the CD18 chain of β_2 integrins. In consequence, neutrophil β_2 integrins fail to form,[69] and blood-stream neutrophils are unable to adhere firmly to vascular endothelium and transmigrate to sites of infection. Phagocytosis is also impaired. The clinical picture is similar to that of the neutropenias, with recurrent life-threatening infections. Complete LAD1 manifests in infancy.[64,65] Leukocyte adhesion deficiency 2 (LAD2) results from an autosomal recessive defect in the glycosylation of sialyl Lewis^x, the neutrophil counterligand for endothelial selectins. Patients with LAD2 have neutrophils that are unable to roll along the endothelium and have symptoms similar to LAD1, but they may also have mental retardation, short stature, distinctive facies, and the Bombay (hh) blood type.[64,70]

Neutrophil Granule Defects

The best-known defect in neutrophil granule formation is Chediak-Higashi syndrome. Chediak-Higashi is an autosomal recessive disorder in which granule subtypes—in neutrophils, but also in lymphocytes, melanocytes, Schwann cells, and others—undergo disordered fusion, resulting in giant, dysfunctional granules.[64] The cause appears to relate to a defect in the gene for lysosomal transport protein (Lyst).[71] Chediak-Higashi patients present with partial occulocutaneous albinism, neutropenia, frequent infection, mild bleeding diathesis, and neurologic abnormalities.[65] Approximately 85 percent of patients who survive childhood will enter a so-called accelerated phase, a lymphoma-like infiltration of lymphocytes and histiocytes throughout the body, which is generally fatal. Other diseases of neutrophil granules have somewhat less ominous prognoses.

Oxidase Deficiencies: Chronic Granulomatous Disease

Chronic granulomatous disease (CGD) resembles other diseases of neutrophil dysfunction in that it results in severe, recurrent infections of the skin and mucus membranes. Osteomyelitis and intra-abdominal abcesses are common. In contrast to the other defects, infection in patients with CGD generally results in a delayed, but quantitatively normal, neutrophil response. However, because of an incapacity to kill organisms, the accumu-

TABLE 14–1 • HERITABLE DISORDERS OF NEUTROPHIL FUNCTION

Disorder	Defect	Inheritance	Presentation	Therapy	Typical Prognosis
Neutropenia					
Severe congenital neutropenia (Kostmann's syndrome)	Maturation arrest (<0.5 × 10^9 PMN/L)	AR	Bacterial infections (omphalitis, abscesses, gingivitis, UTIs)	RhG-CSF	Improved with treatment
Chronic benign neutropenia	(0.2-2 × 10^9 PMN/L)	?	Mild infections	None	Good
Cyclic neutropenia	Stem cell defect (nadir every 21 d)	?	Infection during nadirs	RhG-CSF	Improved with treatment
Adhesion Deficiency					
Leukocyte adhesion deficiency type 1	Absent or abnormal CD18; defects of PMN/eosinophil adhesion	AR	Leukocytosis; recurrent infections (skin, mucous, membranes, gastrointestinal tract)	Marrow transplant	Fair-poor
Leukocyte adhesion deficiency type 2	Absent sialyl-Lewis^x	AR	Neutrophilia; infection; retardation, short stature		Poor
Granule Disorders					
Chédiak-Higashi syndrome	Defective lysosomal transport	AR	Albinism, infection	Marrow transplant	Poor
Specific granule deficiency	Abnormal/reduced specific and azurophilic granules	AR?	Infection of skin, mucous membranes, lungs	Antibiotics	Fair-good
Myeloperoxidase deficiency	Myeloperoxidase absent	?	None	None	Excellent
Oxidase Defects					
Chronic granulomatous disease (multiple types)	gp91^{phox} absent p22^{phox} absent p47^{phox} absent p67^{phox} absent	X-linked (50%) AR (5%) AR (35%) AR (5%)	Early childhood infections, especially skin and mucous membranes, abscesses	Interferon-γ	Improved with treatment

Abbreviations: AR, Autosomal recessive; PMN, polymorphonuclear neutrophil; RhG-CSF, recombinant human granulocyte colony-stimulating factor; UTIs, urinary tract infections.

lation of neutrophils at a site of infection generally results in granuloma formation rather than rapid clearance of the target. Cutaneous infections tend to demonstrate persistent drainage and scarring. On the other hand, the presence of even partially responsive neutrophils results in a lower frequency of sepsis in these patients, relative to those with absolute neutropenia. CGD is typically a disease of early childhood, although some milder cases may be recognized later in life.[64,65]

CGD is actually a group of diseases. In each, a genetic defect in a different component of the NADPH oxidase results in failure of neutrophils (as well as other phagocytes) to generate O_2^-. Previously, treatment for CGD consisted of aggressive antibiotic prophylaxis and therapy. Recently, the addition of chronic therapy with recombinant human interferon-γ has significantly improved the outcome for patients with this disease.[72]

THE NEUTROPHIL IN RHEUMATIC DISEASE

Neutrophil-mediated Tissue Destruction

Despite sophisticated regulatory mechanisms, tissue destruction by neutrophils is common. Several mechanisms may permit the release of neutrophil proteases and oxygen radicals into the extracellular milieu. First, necrosis or destruction of neutrophils may liberate cellular contents indiscriminately. Second, studies have revealed that degranulation and O_2^- generation may begin before complete closure of the phagocytic vacuole, releasing products either into the external environment or against a target surface. Thus, neutrophils may destroy host tissues they have been misdirected to attack. Although both serum and joint fluid contain antiproteases and antioxidants, the "protected space" between a neutrophil and a surface (such as cartilage) may exclude these factors. Moreover, release of HOCl, myeloperoxidase, and proteinases into the extracellular milieu may inactivate the protective compounds and act as an "antiproteinase shield."[41]

Neutrophil Fc Receptor Polymorphisms and Rheumatic Diseases

Given that polymorphisms of the FcγRs determine phagocytic capacity of IgG isotypes, it is not surprising that they determine susceptibity to diseases in which autoantibodies play a key role. Phagocytes from individuals with the

FcγRIIa polymorphism (H131) allele are able to bind and phagocytose IgG_2; phagocytes from individuals with a different polymorphism (R131) cannot. In white European and African American populations, respectively, patients with lupus nephritis have a higher frequency of the FcγRIIa-R131 allele than control groups; their relative inability to clear immune complexes may make them more susceptible to renal disease.[73,74] Not surprisingly, the significance of different Fc-receptor polymorphisms may vary between rheumatologic diseases: Tse and collegues found no association between FcγRIIa polymorphisms and likelihood of developing antineutrophil cytoplasmic antibodies (ANCA)-associated vasculitides, but they found an overrepresentation of homozygosity for the FcγRIIIb NA1 allele among patients with anti-MPO antibodies.[75,76] Surprisingly few studies have been published on Fc polymorphisms and susceptibity or severity of rheumatoid arthritis. A recent study found no association between FcγRIIa type and rheumatoid-arthritis susceptibility but a correlation between patients with extra-articular disease and the homozygous R131 genotype.[77]

Gout

Gout may be the quintessential neutrophilic rheumatic disease. Although the initiation of the acute gouty attack appears to involve the phagocytosis of urate crystals by synovial macrophages and the generation of cytokines, such as IL-1 and IL-8, the hallmark of acute gout is the presence of enormous numbers of neutrophils, sometimes more than $100,000/mm^3$ in the affected joint space. Urate crystals in the joint are capable of nonspecifically binding immunoglobulin, as well as fixing complement by the classic and alternative pathways. C5a liberated from the complement fixation process attracts neutrophils to the joint space, where they phagocytose opsonized crystals via receptor-dependent mechanisms, resulting in further activation of the neutrophil and production of LTB_4, IL-8, and other mediators. Thus, activation of neutrophils results in the ingress of additional neutrophils. Neutrophils in the gouty joint may damage joint structures through discharge of contents directly into the joint fluid during crystal phagocytosis or directly against cartilage during attempted phagocytosis of urate crystals embedded in or adherent to cartilage. In addition, interaction of phagocytosed urate crystals with lysosomal membranes results in the dissolution of the latter, spilling lysosomal proteases into the cytoplasm and, eventually, into the extracellular space.[78]

Rheumatoid Arthritis

Although the focus in rheumatoid arthritis over the past decade has been on the role of T cells, synovial fibroblasts, and mononuclear cells, the first inflammatory cell type to be appreciated in rheumatoid arthritis was the neutrophil. Rheumatoid arthritis in the joint may be conceptualized as a two-compartment inflammatory disease: In the synovium, lymphocytes, fibroblasts, and macrophages predominate, but neutrophils usually predominate in the joint space. Although the numbers of neutrophils in the rheumatoid joint are usually less than are found in gout, as many as 10 billion cells per day can cycle through a 30-ml effusion. The classic model suggests that rheumatoid factor-based immune complexes, produced in the pannus and present in the joint space in high concentrations, can fix complement and draw neutrophils into the joint space in high numbers.

Once in the articular cavity, in vitro studies have documented the ability of neutrophils to bind to cartilage surfaces embedded with immune complexes and damage them via incomplete phagocytosis. However, no adequate in situ demonstration of direct neutrophil attack on cartilage has yet been offered. Moreover, the fact that seronegative arthritides, such as psoriatic arthritis, lack rheumatoid factor but nonetheless share with rheumatoid arthritis the presence of both pannus and a large neutrophilic infiltrate in the joint space suggests that immune-complex formation may be important, but not absolutely required, for neutrophil influx. The ability of rheumatoid synovial monocytic leukocytes to secrete both IL-1 and IL-8, as well as other cytokines, indicates that pannus itself may play an important role in the attraction of neutrophils out of the blood stream and into the joint. It should also be noted that, although few in number, neutrophils within the pannus have been documented to concentrate at the pannus-cartilage border, suggesting a possible role in pannus-driven marginal erosion.[18]

In addition to promoting joint destruction, neutrophils in the rheumatoid joint may also contribute to the propagation of pannus and rheumatoid inflammation. As noted previously, neutrophils produce proinflammatory cytokines; several such cytokines, including oncostatin M, are expressed in rheumatoid but not nonrheumatoid neutrophils. Injection of lysates of neutrophil granules into joints in animal models produces a synovitis indistinguishable histologically from rheumatoid synovitis, an effect that can be reproduced by injection with purified active or inactive myeloperoxidase.[79,80] Neutrophil proteins may also regulate synovial proliferation through effects on other resident or immigrant cell populations. Neutrophil proteinase 3 may enhance the proinflammatory effects of monocytes by cleaving and releasing active IL-1 and TNF-α from the surface of the latter. Neutrophil defensins enhance phagocytosis by macrophages and stimulate the activation and degranulation of mast cells, an interesting observation in light of a recent report that mice deficient in mast cells are resistant to the initiation of inflammatory arthritis in one model.[81] Neutrophil proteases also enhance the adherence of rheumatoid synovial fibroblasts to articular cartilage,[82] and neutrophils may regulate synovial vascularization through the production of vascular endothelial growth factor, leading to endothelial proliferation.[83] Finally, several recent studies have raised the intriguing possibility that, under certain condition of stimulation, neutrophils may actually express class II major histocompatibility complex (MHC) and serve as antigen-presenting cells.[84] The importance of neutrophils to the rheumatoid process may be underscored by a rheumatoid arthritis animal model in which mice deficient in neutrophils were completely resistant to the arthritis.[85]

Vasculitis

Neutrophils may be identified, to a greater or lesser degree, in the lesions of virtually all kinds of vasculitis. The mechanisms of neutrophil accumulation may vary, however, with different mechanisms predominating in different conditions. The early observation that infusions of allospecies serum produced acute inflammation in skin and joints (serum sickness), together with the appreciation that subcutaneous rechallenge with previously administered antigen leads to intense local inflammation (Arthus reaction), led to the development of a model in which immune-complex deposition in the blood vessels results in complement activation and an influx of neutrophils to the affected site. As immune-complex formation is a hallmark of a number of primary rheumatic vasculitides (essential mixed cryoglobulinemia, hypersensitivity vasculitis, Henoch-Schönlein purpura, and others), it is likely that immune-complex deposition is critical to the genesis of these diseases. In several of these vasculitides, neutrophil disruption and fragmentation—*clasis*—is a prominent pathologic finding, leading to their designation under the rubric leukocytoclastic vasculitis. In some rheumatic diseases in which vasculitis is a secondary phenomenon, such as rheumatoid arthritis and systemic lupus erythematosus, the role of immune-complex deposition is also implicit. Patients with lupus may experience transient accumulations of neutrophils (leukoaggregation) in small vessels of the lungs and other tissues, in consequence of complement activation within these vessels or in the soluble phase.[86]

Induction of adhesion molecules on endothelial cells or neutrophils themselves is an alternative mechanism through which neutrophil accumulation in vessels may be propagated. The Schwartzmann phenomenon, in which reinjection of cellular material leads to vascular inflammation via a cytokine-dependent, immune complex-independent mechanism, is a model for this avenue to vasculitis. Adhesion-molecule upregulation may be particularly relevant to vasculitides in which immune-complex formation is not a hallmark, such as giant cell (temporal) arteritis. Indeed, a detailed analysis of the inflammatory cells involved in giant cell arteritis showed the presence of T cells, producing IL-1β and IL-6, which may act on vascular endothelium.[87] It is likely that many rheumatic diseases employ both immune-complex-dependent and –independent mechanisms in the pathogenesis of neutrophil ingress into vascular structures. For instance, in addition to the role of immune complexes, increased expression of adhesion molecules occurs in patients with lupus.[88]

Several vasculitides are noteworthy for the presence, in the serum of affected patients, of antibodies directed at cytoplasmic components of neutrophils, or ANCA.[89] ANCA-positive vasculitides are discussed in detail elsewhere in this textbook.

Neutrophilic Dermatoses

Sweet's syndrome, named after the physician who first described it in 1964, is characterized by fever, neutrophilia, and painful erythematous papules, nodules, and plaques. It can be subdivided into five groups: idiopathic, parainflammatory (associated with inflammatory bowel disease or infection), paraneoplastic (most commonly in the setting of leukemia), pregnancy related, and drug associated (usually after treatment with G-CSF). Sweet's syndrome is primarily a diagnosis of exclusion. It frequently appears after an upper respiratory-tract infection and has a propensity to involve the face, neck, and upper extremities. When found on the legs, lesions can be confused with erythema nodosum. Histopathology is characterized by dense neutrophilic infiltrate in the superficial dermis and edema of the dermal papillae and papillary dermis. Leukocytoclasia may suggest leukocytoclastic vascultitis, though vascular damage is absent. It is typically accompanied by peripheral neutrophilia. Treatment with systemic corticosteroids usually induces a dramatic resolution of the lesions and the systemic symptoms. Although the etiology of the disease is unclear, many believe Sweet's syndrome may represent a form of hypersensitivity reaction to microbial or tumor antigens. Notably, antibiotics do not influence the course of the disease in most patients.

Pyoderma gangrenosum is characterized by painful ulcerating cutaneous lesions over the lower extremities, usually in patients with an underlying inflammatory illness. Inflammatory bowel disease, rheumatoid arthritis, and seronegative arthritis are the most common associations, though an association with malignancy has also been reported. Fifteen percent of patients have a benign monoclonal gammopathy, usually IgA. Like Sweet's syndrome, pyoderma gangrenosum is a diagnosis of exclusion, is characterized on biopsy by neutrophilic infiltrate, and usually remits with systemic corticosteroids, though topical and intralesional injections of corticosteroids may also be beneficial. Other rare neutrophilic dermatoses include rheumatoid neutrophilic dermatitis, described as symmetric erythematous nodules on extensor surfaces of joints; the bowel-associated dermatosis-arthritis syndrome, occurring after bowel-bypass surgery for obesity; and neutrophilic eccrine hidradenitis, linked to acute myelogenous leukemia.

EFFECTS OF ANTIRHEUMATIC DRUGS ON NEUTROPHIL FUNCTIONS

Although recent research in anti-inflammatory and immunosuppressive therapy has tended to emphasize interventions at the T cell or cytokine level, many antirheumatic therapies currently in use have been documented to act, at least in part, at the level of the neutrophil. The most frequently used class of antirheumatic agents are the nonsteroidal anti-inflammatory drugs (NSAIDs). By virtue of their ability to inhibit COX activity and prostaglandin production, moderate doses of NSAIDS have diverse effects on inflammation, including the inhibition of vascular permeability and the modulation of pain. At higher, clinically anti-inflammatory concentrations, NSAIDs inhibit chemoattractant-stimulated neutrophil CD11b/CD18-dependent adhesion, as well as degranulation and NADPH oxidase activity.[18,90,91] However, it is unlikely that these effects are due solely to COX inhibition because 1) as noted earlier, neutrophils exhibit little COX activity under normal circumstances; and 2) concentrations of NSAIDs required to inhibit neutrophil function exceed those required to inhibit COX. Moreover, high-dose NSAIDs appear to have other, pleiotropic effects on neutrophil signaling. Recently, both aspirin and the poor COX-inhibitor sodium salicylate were shown to block ERK activation in a manner consistent with inhibition of adhesion. Whether similar effects will be observed with the selective COX2 inhibitors currently coming into use remains to be determined.

Like NSAIDs, glucocorticoids also exert potent effects on neutrophils, including inhibition of neutrophil phagocytic activity and adhesive function. The ability of steroids to raise peripheral blood neutrophil counts acutely—an effect known as demargination—may be directly attributable to the release of neutrophils adherent to vessel walls. In addition, glucocorticoids inhibit phospholipase A_2, and therefore leukotriene and prostaglandin, production. Glucocorticoids may also regulate the expression of COX2 and stimulate the release of lipocortins, which are compounds with anti-inflammatory effects on neutrophils. Although the ability of glucocorticoids to interact with cytosolic receptors and regulate transcription is unlikely to be directly relevant to neutrophil function, these longer term effects may have indirect relevance in that steroids possess the capacity to reduce production of IL-1 and other cytokines at inflammatory sites.

Other anti-inflammatory/immunomodulatory agents also have well-established effects on neutrophils. Methotrexate, widely used in rheumatoid arthritis, has no direct neutrophil effect but is able to produce indirect effects, possibly by virtue of its ability to stimulate the release of adenosine from surrounding cells. Methotrexate-induced adenosine release can inhibit phagocytosis and O_2^-. production and adhesion, and treatment of patients with methotrexate inhibits the capacity of neutrophils to generate LTB_4.

Colchicine, a standard agent in the treatment of gout, inhibits microtubule formation and has pleiotropic effects on neutrophils, including the inhibition of adhesion via decrements in selectin expression.[92] Interestingly, colchicine also stimulates the expression of pyrin in neutrophils. Because pyrin is the protein whose abnormalities are implicated in familial Mediterranean fever, and because it is presumed to have anti-iflammatory effects on neutrophils, this observation suggests that colchicine might have a unique mechanism of action in cases of neutrophilic disease.[93]

Sulfasalazine also inhibits neutrophil responsiveness to chemoattractants and suppresses chemotaxis, degranulation, O_2^- production, and LTB_4 production. Like sulfasalazine, gold salts may scavenge toxic metabolites. Gold salts also decrease neutrophil collagenase activity and lower E-selectin expression on endothelium.[18]

The current era of biologic therapies has been ushered in through the introduction of agents designed to block the effects of IL-1 or TNF-α. As noted previously, both IL-1 and TNF-α directly affect neutrophil function, including priming for stimulus-induced responses such as O_2^- production, cartilage destruction, and the production of cytokines such as IL-8 and LTB_4.[94] Nonetheless, one study showed no difference in stimulated neutrophil function tested ex vivo in patients treated with the anti-TNF agent etanercept for 6 months versus controls.[95] Thus, treatment with cytokine blockade may reduce the stimulation, proliferation, or both of neutrophils in vivo, rather than intrinsically altering the neutrophils themselves. Consistent with this suggestion, patients receiving the anti-TNF antibody infliximab show decreases in peripheral blood neutrophil, but not other leukocyte populations.[96]

Eosinophils

The eosinophil line shares many features with the other families of polymorphonuclear granulocytes. In contrast to the neutrophil, however, the eosinophil is primarily a tissue-localized cell. Eosinophils are produced in fewer numbers than neutrophils, and their half-life in the blood is shorter (3 to 8 hours), owing to higher rates of diapedesis. Thus, normal blood-stream levels of eosinophils tend to be low—typically less than 5 percent of blood leukocytes. Once in the tissues, eosinophils are more long-lived than their neutrophil cousins, with life estimates ranging from 2 to 14 days. Tissue eosinophils are found in greatest concentrations in gastrointestinal mucosa, suggesting that they participate in barrier, rather than blood stream, surveilance.[97-100]

EOSINOPHIL DEVELOPMENT AND MORPHOLOGY

Like neutrophils, eosinophils follow a classic pattern of granulocyte differentiation, passing through blast, promyelocyte, myelocyte, metamyelocyte, and band stages before reaching maturity.[99] Along the way, eosinophils successively acquire morphologically distinct classes of granules. The factors required for eosinophil differentiation include GM-CSF and IL-3, which are also required for neutrophil differentiation and therefore cannot account for eosinophil commitment. More recently, an essential role for IL-5 in eosinophil development has been described, supported by the observation that intravenous administration of IL-5 rapidly results in peripheral eosinophilia. However, IL-5 may not be completely eosinophil specific; studies in animal models suggest that it is also trophic for B cells. Like IL-5, IL-2 (used in the treatment of some malignancies) can also stimulate eosinophilia. However, the IL-2 effect appears to be mediated via production of IL-5.

When viewed under hematoxylin and eosin staining, the eosinophil appears slightly larger than the neutrophil (12 to 17 μm). Its nucleus is typically bilobed. Most striking is the presence of large, pink-staining granules. In addition, lipid bodies may occasionally be seen—nonvesicular accumulations of arachidonic acid and other lipids, presumably liberated from plasma membrane. These are not unique, however, and may occasionally be detected in neutrophils as well.

Like neutrophils, eosinophils contain at least four distinguishable classes of granules. Primary granules form first and are analagous to the primary (azurophilic) granules of neutrophils. Because eosinophil primary granules have not been isolated, their repertoire of proteins is not well elucidated. In contrast to neutrophils, however, eosinophils lack myeloperoxidase. Eosinophil primary granules are most numerous in eosinophiliic promyelocytes and persist in lesser numbers in mature forms. In mature eosinophils, a lysophospholipase, which is present in large quantities (7 to 10 percent of total eosinophil protein), has been tentatively localized to specific granules, and when it is released extracellularly it precipitates into bipyramidal structures known as Charcot-Leyden crystals.[101] The deposit of these crystals in tissues is frequently taken as evidence of present or past eosinophilia.

The large granules visible in mature eosinophils are specific granules, which form in approximately the myelocyte stage. When viewed under scanning electron microscopy, specific granules demonstrate a unique appearance consisting of a dense crystalline core surrounded by an intermediate-density matrix. Because of their greater size and number, eosinophil specific granules have yielded to both isolation and immunocytochemic examination, and their contents are at least partially evaluated. Among the contents localized to the specific granules are lysosomal enzymes (acid and neutral hydrolases, collagenase, cathepsin, and gelatinase) and lectins, as well as components of the oxidase system.

A distinctive characteristic of eosinophils is the presence of four highly basic proteins that lend the granule its tinctorial properties. Most prevalent is major basic protein (MBP), an 11,000-kD protein with an isoelectric point (pI) greater than or equal to 10. MBP accounts for more than 50 percent of the total granule protein and is the major, or possibly sole, component of the crystalline core. Trace amounts of MBP (less than 0.1 percent of that found in eosinophils) may also be observed in basophils. Eosinophil cationic protein (ECP), actually a heterogeneous group of several related proteins (with molecular weights of 18 to 21 kD), is also present in large amounts, but less than that of MBP (less than or equal to 10 percent on weight-to-weight basis). ECP and the remaining eosinophil cationic proteins are localized to the granule matrix. Eosinophil-derived neurotoxin (EDN)kD, the third of the basic granular proteins, has a molecular weight of 18 kD, is slightly less basic (pI 8.9) than the aforementioned proteins, and is present in still smaller quantities. In contrast to MBP and ECP, which have likely roles in host defense, EDN is mainly recognized for its function as a neurotoxin for myelinated neurons, the evolutionary advantage of which remains unclear. The Gordon phenomenon, in which injection of eosinophil-laden tissue into an animal produces profound neurologic deficits, is likely due to EDN. Finally, eosinophil specific granules contain large quantities of eosinophil peroxidase, an enzyme distinctly different from neutrophil myeloperoxidase but probably subsuming the same function of generating hypohalides for cell killing and the activation of latent proteinases.[102]

A third population of smaller eosinophilic granules has been identified by virtue of its acid phosphatase arylsulfatase B content, and a fourth distinct population of small granules has been identified by morphology alone.

EOSINOPHIL ACTIVATION AND DISTRIBUTION

Like neutrophils, eosinophils undergo activation in response to stimuli and are capable of adhesion, chemotaxis, and phagocytosis, as well as degranulation and O_2^- generation. Eosinophils respond to many of the same chemoattractant stimuli as neutrophils, although perhaps with different sensitivities. In addition, eosinophils respond to a number of stimuli that do not affect neutrophils, including IL-3, IL-5, RANTES, and MIP-1α. Whether the distribution of these factors is sufficient to explain the tissue distribution of eosinophils relative to other granulocytes is uncertain; however, both eosinophils and mast cells secrete IL-3 and IL-5, suggesting their capacity to attract additional eosinophils to sites of atopy. Eosinophils express adhesion molecules identified on neutrophils—CD11a/CD18, CD11b/CD18, and L-selectin—but also others not shared by neutrophils, such as the $\alpha_4\beta_1$ integrin very late antigen (VLA)-4. Indeed, although IL-4 has no direct effect on eosinophils, local production of this cytokine leads to eosinophil influx, probably though the endothelial upregulation of the VLA-4 ccounterligand, vascular cell adhesion molecule-1 (VCAM-1). Finally, eosinophils also differ from neutrophils in their repertoire of immunoglobulin receptors. Although eosinophils do possess IgG receptors, they are relatively sparse. Instead, the predominant Ig receptors on the eosinophil surface are high-affinity for IgA and IgE, consistent with the eosinophil's roles in barrier defense and atopy.[103]

NORMAL EOSINOPHIL FUNCTION

Although a number of studies have demonstrated the capacity of eosinophils to phagocytose bacteria, others have indicated that these cells are poor at such phagocytosis, and it is likely that antibacterial defense is not a primary eosinophil function. MBP does have the capacity to stimulate neutrophils, but the relevance of this observation is not clear. Rather, eosinophils appear to be particularly adept at host defense against multicellular, helminthic parasites. Host eosinophilia in response to parasitic, but not bacterial, infection supports such an interpretation. Although eosinophils can phagocytose small parasitic forms, more typically they attach, in a polarized manner, to the surface of larger parasites and discharge their granular contents into the protected space between the parasite and the eosinophil. O_2^- generation and proteinase release might play a role in this attack, but the specific granule-associated, basic proteins are the major weapon in the eosinophil's antiparasitic armamentarium. In vitro studies have demonstrated the capacities of these proteins—particularly ECP and MBP—to kill protozoa. Whereas ECP is about tenfold more potent, the higher concentration of MBP present in the granules has led to the consensus that it is the dominant parasite toxin. Parasitic killing by each of the proteins appears to depend on its capacity to disrupt the plasma membrane; in the case of ECP, membrane disruption occurs through the formation of pores or channels.[97,98] Interestingly, eosinophils have been reported to present antigen to T cells; whether antigen presentation plays any role in the antiparasitic effect has not been established.[104] Finally, it should be noted that, despite a large literature to the contrary, several recent studies have questioned the central role of eosinophils in parasitic defense. In particular, ablation of eosinophilia through IL-5 depletion had no effect on the course of parasite infections in mice. Possibly this reflects the presence of redundant antiparasitic defenses.[100]

THE EOSINOPHIL IN DISEASE

Although the presence of blood and pulmonary eosinophilia in asthma has been appreciated for a century,[97] the role of eosinophils in the pathogenesis of this disease remains a subject of intense study. Asthmatic eosinophilia is presumably stimulated by high levels of IL-5 and other cytokine production, and the ability of eosinophils to bind IgE almost certainly contributes to their specificity for the disease. Moreover, eosinophils possess multiple mechanisms through which they can, at least potentially, enhance the asthmatic response. Like neutrophils, stimulated eosinophils synthesize LTA_4, leukotriene A_4 from arachidonic acid. In contrast to neutrophils, however, eosinophil metabolism of LTA_4 leads to the production, not of LTB_4, but of LTC_4 and LTD_4, both potent bronchoconstrictors.[105] Eosinophils themselves are exquisitely sensitive to the effects of these cysteinyl leukotrienes, which have been shown to stimulate eosinophil adhesion, migration, and degranulation, as well as the proliferation of eosinophil progenitor cells.[106-108] The recently developed leukotriene receptor antagonists (lukasts) are effective in the treatment of asthma and have been shown to have direct effects on eosinophils in vivo and in vitro, including reduction of eosinophil transmigration and reduction of pulmonary and peripheral eosinophilia.[109-111] Indeed, lukasts appear to have beneficial effects on other diseases characterized by eosinophilia, including cystic fibrosis, eosinophilic gastroenteritis, and atrophic dermatitis.[112-114]

Platelet-activating factor is also produced by stimulated eosinophils and has bronchoconstricting activities. Release of specific granule proteins per se have multiple proasthmatic effects, including epithelial damage due to membrane perturbations similar to those seen in parasites and activation of mast cells with subsequent histamine and leukotriene production.[97] Interestingly, MBP may also act specifically as an antagonist of muscarinic M2 receptors, resulting in enhanced vagal tone and increased bronchospasm.[115]

Although hypereosinophilia can occasionally be observed in virtually all rheumatic diseases, it is a characteristic of just a few. In Churg-Strauss vasculitis, hypereosinophilia is the classic laboratory abnormality accompanying a constellation of pulmonary and renal vasculitis and asthma. In some cases peripheral eosinophil counts in Churg-Strauss have been reported to exceed 50 percent of total leukocytes. The cluster of asthma and eosinophilia accompanying Churg-Strauss vasculitis suggests that this syndrome may represent an atopic response to a foreign antigen. However, IgE response is variable, and asthma may precede the rest of the disease by years. Moreover, the presence of antimyeloperoxidase antibodies (pANCA)—an IgG class antibody—is common, suggesting a broader autoimmune response.

Eosinophilia-myalgia syndrome (EMS) was first observed in the 1989 in New Mexico and was defined by the Centers for Disease Control (CDC) for surveillance purposes as peripheral eosinophilia and muscle pains, unexplained by other illnesses. Rash and skin edema are common findings. Follow-up of cases over time revealed the frequent appearance of fibrosing fasciitis, which, in more severe disease, results in skin retraction, particularly over the veins where it gives rise to a traintrack appearance. Intensive epidemiologic investigation pinpointed the likely cause of the epidemic to the consumption of L-tryptophan supplements produced by a single manufacturer, probably owing to trace contaminants. Discontinuation of the sales of the supplement has led to resolution of the epidemic—although sporadic, tryptophan-independent cases continue to be reported.[116]

Eosinophilic fasiitis, a condition first described in 1975, resembles EMS in that it involves fasciitis and eosinophilia, but it differs in that myalgias are not a prominent feature and organ involvement is unusual. Clinically, the skin of patients with eosinophilic fasciitis bears some resemblance to that of systemic sclerosis, but the distribution is typically on the distal extremities, with sparing of the hands and feet. An epidemic similar to eosinophilia-myalgia syndrome was seen in Spain in 1981, relating to the consumption of adulterated grapeseed oil (toxic oil syndrome). Although in these syndromes it is unclear whether the eosinophils act as mediators of fasciitis or merely as reporters of exposure to an atopic antigen, the capacity of eosinophils to produce TGF-β suggests a potential role for these cells in the generation of fibrous tissue. However, the presence of eosinophils in the affected tissues is variable, with most of the infiltrates comprised of other leukocytes.[117] A single study has demonstrated indirect evidence for the presence of increased numbers of eosinophils (Charcot-Leyden crystal deposition) in progressive systemic sclerosis; the relevance of this observation remains to be determined.

The idiopathic hypereosinophilic syndrome has been defined as: 1) persistent eosinophils,1500/mm^3 or more for 6 or more months (or until death); 2) absence of parasites, allergy, or other cause of eosinophilia; and 3) signs and symptoms of organ involvement relating directly to eosinophils or eosinophil accumulation. Morbidity is largely from eosinophil tissue infiltration, and granuloma formation may occur.[118] Löffler's syndrome is a self-limiting eosinophilic pneumonitis with peripheral eosinophilia, presumably a hypersensitivity reaction. Allergic bronchopulmonary aspergillosis also represents a hypersensitivity reaction and may be indistinguishable from Löffler's.[119] A novel eosinophilic syndrome was recently described, consisting of nodules, eosinophilia, rheumatism, dermatitis, and swelling (NERDS); as only a few cases have been reported to date, the clinical identity of this illness awaits validation.[120]

Addison's disease is a disorder of adrenal failure, resulting in underproduction of steroid hormones. Addison's disease is frequently accompanied by peripheral eosinophilia. In contrast to increases in peripheral neutrophil counts, the ability of glucocorticoids to reverse the eosinophilia of Addison's disease implicates that class of agents as a key regulator in the downregulation of eosinophil numbers. Indeed, glucocoticoids rapidly reduce eosinophil numbers in most hypereosinophilic as well as nonhypereosinophilic patients, a fact enshrined in the clinic maxim that detectable levels of eosinophils in a patient on chronic glucocorticoid therapy may be evidence of noncompliance with medication. Whether glucocorticoids have their effect on eosinophil production, release, or survival remains to be determined. Regardless of the mechanism of their effect, the use of glucocoticoids to reduce eosinophil count is an important strategy in reducing morbidity from hypereosinophilic diseases.

ACKNOWLEDGMENTS

The authors would like to express their gratititude to Dr. Gerald Weissmann and Dr. Harold Ballard for generously sharing their images for figures. The authors also thank Ms. Madeline Rios for her excellent judgment and tireless editorial support. Finally, the authors express their gratititude to the Arthritis Foundation, New York Chapter, for their ongoing support of our research and academic activities.

REFERENCES

1. Bainton DF: Phagocytic cells: developmental biology of neutrophils and eosinophils. *In* Gallin JI, Goldstein IM, Snyderman R (eds): Inflammation: Basic Principles and Clinical Correlates. New York: Raven Press, 1988, pp 265-280.
2. Barbara MJ, Dunkley SA, Lopez AF, et al: Regulation of neutrophil apoptosis by tumor necrosis factor-alpha:requirement for TNFR55 and TNFR75 for the induction of apoptosis in vitro. Blood 90(7):2772-2783, 1997.
3. Tortorella C, Piazzolla G, Spaccavento F, et al: Spontaneous and Fas-induced apoptotic cell death in aged neutrophils. J Clin Immunol 18(5):321-329, 1998.
4. Borregaard N, Lollike K, Kjeldsen L, et al: Human neutrophil granules and secretory vesicles [review]. Eur J Hem 51:187-198, 1993.
5. Borregaard N, Miller LJ, Springer TA: Chemoattractant-regulated mobilization of a novel intracellular compartment in human neutrophils. Science 237:1204-1206, 1987.
6. Dewald B, Bretz U, Baggiolini M: Release of gelatinase from a novel secretory compartment of human neutrophils. J Clin Invest 70:518-525, 1982.
7. Calafat J, Kuijpers TW, Janssen H, et al: Evidence for small intracellular vesicles in human blood phagocytes containing cytochrome b558 and the adhesion molecule cd11b/cd18. Blood 81:3122-3129, 1993.
8. Belaaouaj A, Kim KS, Shapiro SD: Degradation of outer membrane protein A in *Escherichia coli* killing by neutrophil elastase. Science 289:1185-1188, 2000.
9. Elsbach P: The bactericidal/permeability-increasing protein (BPI) in antibacterial host defense. J Leukoc Biol 64:14-18, 1998.
9a. Crouch SP, Slater KJ, Fletcher J: Regulation of cytokine release from mononuclear cells by the iron-binding protein lactoferrin. Blood 80:235-240, 1992.
10. Coeshott C, Ohnemus C, Pilyavskaya A, et al: Converting enzyme-independent release of tumor necrosis factor alpha and IL-1beta from a stimulated human monocytic cell line in the presence of activated neutrophils or purified proteinase 3. Proc Natl Acad Sci U S A 96(11):6261-6266, 1999.
11. Schonbeck U, Mach F, Libby P: Generation of biologically active IL-1 beta by matrix metalloproteinases: a novel caspase-1-independent pathway of IL-1 beta processing. J Immunol 161(7):3340-3346, 1998.
12. Van den Steen PE, Proost P, Wuyts A, et al: Neutrophil gelatinase B potentiates interleukin-8 tenfold by aminoterminal processing, whereas it degrades CTAP-III, PF-4 and GRO-alpha and leaves RANTES and MCP-2 intact. Blood 96(8):2673-2681, 2000.
13. Huynh ML, Fadok VA, Henson PM: Phosphatidyl serine-dependent ingestion of apoptotic cells promotes TGF-beta1 secretion and the resolution of inflammation. J Clin Invest 109(1):41-50, 2002.
14. Vandivier RW, Fadok VA, Hoffmann PR, et al: Elastase-mediated phosphatidylserine receptor cleavage impairs apoptotic cell clearance in cystic fibrosis and bronchiectasis. J Clin Invest 109(5):661-670, 2002.
15. Bokoch GM: Chemoattractant signaling and leukocyte activation. Blood 86:1649-1660, 1995.
16. McLeish KR, Knall C, Ward RA, et al: Activation of mitogen-activated protein kinase cascades during priming of human neutrophils by TNF-alpha and GM-CSF. J Leukoc Biol 64(4): 537-545, 2003.
17. McPhail LC, Harvath L: Signal transduction in neutrophil oxidative metabolism and chemotaxis. *In* Abramson JS,Wheeler JG (eds): The Neutrophil. Oxford: IRL Press at Oxford University Press, 1993, pp 63-107.
18. Pillinger MH, Abramson SB: The neutrophil in rheumatoid arthritis. Rheum Dis Clin North Am 21:691-714, 1995.
19. Bokoch GM, Knaus UG: The role of small GTP-binding proteins in leukocyte function. Curr Opin Immunol 6:98-105, 1994.
20. Raeder EMB, Mansfield PJ, Hiskovska-Galcheva V, et al: Sphingosine blocks human polymorphonuclear leukocyte phagocytosis through inhibition of mitogen-activated protein kinase activation. Blood 93(2):686-693, 1999.
21. Smolen JE, Stoehr SJ, Kuczynski B: Cyclic AMP inhibits secretion from electroporated human neutrophils. J Leukoc Biol 49: 172-179, 1991.
22. Pillinger MH, Feoktistov AS, Capodici C, et al: Mitogen-activated protein kinase in neutrophils and enucleate neutrophil cytoplasts: evidence for regulation of cell-cell adhesion. J Biol Chem 271(20):12049-12056, 1996.
23. Amin AR, Attur M, Vyas P, et al: Expression of nitric oxide synthase in human peripheral blood mononuclear cells and neutrophils. J Inflamm 47(4):190-205, 1995.
24. Clancy RM, Abramson SB: Nitric oxide: a novel mediator of inflammation. Proc Soc Exp Biol Med 210(2):93-101, 1995.
25. Nauseef WM, Volpp BD, McCormick S, et al: Assembly of the neutrophil respiratory burst oxidase: protein kinase C promotes cytoskeletal and membrane association of cytosolic oxidase components. J Biol Chem 266:5911-5917, 1991.
26. Nick JA, Avdi NJ, Young SK, et al: Selective activation and functional significance of p38alpha mitogen-activated protein kinase in lipopolysaccharide-stimulated neutrophils. J Clin Invest 103(6): 851-858, 1999.
27. Avdi NJ, Nick JA, Whitlock BB, et al: Tumor necrosis factor-alpha activation of the c-Jun N-terminal kinase pathway in human neutrophils. Integrin involvement in a pathway leading from cytoplasmic tyrosine kinases to apoptosis. J Biol Chem 276(3): 2189-2199, 2001.
28. Capodici C, Pillinger MH, Han G, et al: Integrin-dependent homotypic adhesion of neutrophils: arachidonic acid activates Raf-1/Mek/Erk via a 5-lipoxygenase-dependent pathway. J Clin Invest 102(1):165-175, 1998.
29. Capodici C, Hanft SJ, Feoktistov M, et al: Phosphatidylinositol 3-kinase mediates chemoattractant-stimulated, CD11b/CD18-dependent cell-cell adhesion of human neutrophils: and Erk-independent pathway. J Immunol 160:1901-1909, 1998.
30. Kilpatrick LE, Lee JY, Haines KM, et al: A role for PKC-delta and PI 3-kinase in TNF-alpha-mediated antiapoptotic signaling in the human neutrophil. Am J Physiol Cell Physiol 283(1):C48-C57, 2002.

31. Gautam N, Herwald H, Hedqvist P, et al: Signaling via beta(2) integrins triggers neutrophil-dependent alteration in endothelial barrier function. J Exp Med 191(11):1829-1839, 2000.
32. Lu H, Smith CW, Perrard J, et al: LFA-1 is sufficient in mediating neutrophil emigration in Mac-1-deficient mice. J Clin Invest 99(6):1340-1350: 1997.
33. Andrew DP, Spellberg JP, Takimoto H, et al: Transendothelial migration and trafficking of leukocytes in LFA-1-deficient mice. Eur J Immunol 28(6):1959-1969, 1998.
34. Neelamegham S, Taylor AD, Burns AR, et al: Hydrodynamic shear shows distinct roles for LFA-1 and Mac-1 in neutrophil adhesion to intercellular adhesion molecule-1. Blood 92(5):1626-1638, 1998.
35. Feng D, Nagy JA, Pyne K, et al: Neutrophils emigrate from venules by a transendothelial cell pathway in response to FMLP. J Exp Med 187(6):903-915, 1998.
36. Dangerfield J, Larbi KY, Huang MT, et al: PECAM-1 (CD31) homophilic interaction up-regulates alpha6beta1 on transmigrated neutrophils in vivo and plays a functional role in the ability of alpha6 integrins to mediate leukocyte migration through the perivascular basement membrane. J Exp Med 196(9):1201-1211, 2002.
37. Liu Y, Merlin D, Burst SL, et al: The role of CD47 in neutrophil transmigration: Increased rate of migration correlates with increased cell surface expression of CD47. J Biol Chem 276(43):40156-40166, 2001.
38. Schenkel AR, Mamdouh Z, Chen X, et al: CD99 plays a major role in the migration of monocytes through endothelial junctions. Nat Immunol 3(2):143-150, 2002.
39. Huber AR,Weiss SJ. Disruption of the subendothelial basement membrane during neutrophil diapedesis in an in vitro construct of a blood vessel wall. J Clin Invest 83:1122-1136, 1989.
40. Hallett MB: Controlling the molecular motor of neutrophil chemotaxis. Bio Essays 19(7):615-621, 1997.
40a. Caron E, Hall A: Identification of two distinct Mechanisms of phagocytosis controlled by different Rho GTPases. Science 282: 1717-1721, 1998.
41. Weiss SJ: Tissue destruction by neutrophils. N Engl J Med 320(6):365-376, 1989.
42. DeLeo FR, Quinn MT. Assembly of the phagocyte NADPH oxidase: molecular interaction of oxidase proteins. J Leukoc Biol 60(6):677-691, 1996.
43. Nauseef WM. Cytosolic oxidase factors in the NADPH-dependent oxidase of human neutrophils. Eur J Hem 51(5):301-308, 1993.
44. Clark RA, Volpp BD, Leidal KG, et al: Two cytosolic components of the human neutrophil respiratory burst oxidase translocate to the plasma membrane during cell activation. J Clin Invest 85:714-721, 1990.
45. Philips MR, Feoktistov A, Pillinger MH, et al: Translocation of p21rac2 from cytosol to plasma membrane is neither necessary nor sufficient for neutrophil nadph oxidase activity. J Biol Chem 270:11514-11521, 1995.
46. Sathyamoorthy M, deMendez I, Adams AG, et al: p40(phox) down-regulates NADPH oxidase activity through interactions with its SH3 domain. J Biol Chem 272(14):9141-9146, 1997.
47. Reeves EP, Lu H, Jacobs HL, et al: Killing activity of neutrophils is mediated through activation of proteases by K+ flux. Nature 416:291-297, 2002.
48. Samuelsson B, Dahlen SE, Lindgren JA, et al: Leukotrienes and lipoxins: structures, biosynthesis, and biological effects. Science 237:1171-1176, 1987.
49. Abramson SB, Leszczynska-Piziak J,Weissmann G. Arachidonic acid as a second messenger: interactions with a GTP-binding protein of human neutrophils. J Immunol 147:231-236, 1991.
50. O'Flaherty JT,Rossi AG. 5-Hydroxyicosatetraenoate stimulates neutrophils by a sterospecific, G protein-linked mechanism. J Biol Chem 268(20):14708-14714, 1993.
51. Lee TH, Horton CE, Kyan-Aung U, et al: Lipoxin A_4 and lipoxin B_4 inhibit chemotactic responses of human neutrophils stimulated by leukotriene B_4 and N-formyl-methionyl-L-leucyl-L-phenylalanine. Clin Sci 77:195-203, 1989.
52. Papayianni A, Serhan CN, Brady HR. Lipoxin A_4 and B_4 inhibit leukotriene-stimulated interactions of human neutrophils and endothelial cells. J Immunol 156:2264-2272, 1996.
53. Claria J,Serhan CN: Aspirin triggers previously undescribed bioactive eicosanoids by human endothelial cell-leukocyte interactions. Proc Natl Acad Sci U S A 92:9475-9479, 1995.
54. Hamberg M, Svensson J, Samuelsson B. Prostaglandin endoperoxides: A new concept concerning the mode of action and release of prostaglandins. Proc Natl Acad Sci U S A 79:3711, 1974.
55. Kitsis EA, Weissmann G, Abramson SB. The prostaglandin paradox: additive inhibition of neutrophil function by aspirin-like drugs and the prostaglandin E_1 analog misoprostol. J Rheum 18(10):1461-1465, 1991.
56. Pillinger MH, Philips MR, Feoktistov A, et al: Crosstalk in signal transduction via EP receptors: prostaglandin E_1 inhibits chemoattractant-induced mitogen-activated protein kinase activity in human neutrophils. *In* Samuelsson B (ed): Advances in Prostaglandin, Thromboxane, and Leukotriene Research. Vol. 23. New York: Raven Press, 1995, pp 311-316.
57. Maloney CG, Kutchera WA, Albertine KH, et al: Inflammatory agonists induce cyclooxygenase type 2 expression by human neutrophils. J Immunol 160:1402-1410, 1998.
58. Lord PCW, Wilmoth LMG, Mizel SB, et al: Expression of interleukin-1a and ß genes by human blood polymorphonuclear leukocytes. J Clin Invest 87:1312-1321, 1991.
59. Cassatella MA, Bazzoni F, Ceska M, et al: IL-8 production by human polymorphonuclear leukocytes: the chemoattractant formyl-methionyl-leucyl-phenylalanine induces the gene expression and release of IL-8 through a pertussis toxin-sensitive pathway. J Immunol 148:3216-3220, 1992.
60. Reibman J, Meixler S, Lee TC, et al: Transforming growth factor β1, a potent chemoattractant for neutrophils, bypasses classic signal transduction pathways. Proc Natl Acad Sci U S A 88:6805-6809, 1991.
61. Fava RA, Olsen NJ, Postlethwaite AE, et al: Transforming growth factor 1 (TGF-β1) induced neutrophil recruitment to synovial tissues: implications for TGF-β-driven synovial inflammation and hyperplasia. J Exp Med 173:1121-1132, 1991.
62. McColl SR, Paquin R, Menard C, et al: Human neutrophils produce high levels of the interleukin 1 receptor antagonist in response to granulocyte/macrophage colony-stimulating factor and tumor necrosis factor alpha. J Exp Med 176(1):593-598, 1992.
63. Malyak M, Swaney RE, Arend WP: Levels of synovial fluid interleukin-1 receptor antagonist in rheumatoid arthritis and other arthropathies: Potential contribution from synovial fluid neutrophils. Arthritis Rheum 36(6):781-789, 1993.
64. Holland SM,Gallin JI: Evaluation of the patient with recurrent bacterial infections. Annu Rev Med 49:185-199, 1998.
65. Mills EL, Noya FJD: Congenital neutrophil deficiencies. *In* Abramson JS,Wheeler JG (eds): The Neutrophil. Oxford: IRL Press and Oxford University Press, 1993, pp 183-227.
66. Welte K,Dale D: Pathophysiology and treatment of severe chronic neutropenia. Ann Hematol 72:158-165, 1996.
67. Hammon WP, Price TH, Souza LM, et al: Treatment of cyclic neutropenia with granulocyte colony-stimulating factor. N Eng J Med 320:1306-1311, 1989.
68. Aprikyan AAG, Dale DC: Mutations in the neutrophil elastase gene in cyclic and congenital neutropenia. Curr Opin Immun 13:535-538, 2001.
69. Anderson DC, Springer TA: Leukocyte adhesion deficiency: an inherited defect in the Mac-1, LFA-1 and p150/95 glycoproteins. Annu Rev Med 38:175-194, 1987.
70. Etzioni A, Frydman M, Pollack S, et al. Brief report: recurrent severe infections caused by a novel leukocyte adhesion deficiency. N Engl J Med 327:1789-1792, 1992.
71. Barbosa MD, Nguyen QA, Tchernev VT, et al. Identification of the homologous beige and Chediak-Higashi syndrome genes. Nature 382(6588):262-265, 1996.
72. Gallin JI, Farber JM, Holland SM, et al: Interferon-g in the management of infectious diseases. Ann Intern Med 123:216-224, 1995.
73. Duits AJ, Bootsma H, Derksen RH, et al: Skewed distribution of IgG Fc receptor IIa (CD32) polymorphism is associated with renal disease in systemic lupus erythematosus patients. Arthritis Rheum 38(12):1832-1836, 1995.
74. Salmon JE, Millard S, Schachter LA, et al: Fc gamma RIIA alleles are heritable risk factors for lupus nephritis in African Americans. J Clin Invest 97(5):1348-1354, 1996.
75. Tse WY, Abadeh S, McTiernan A, et al: No association between neutrophil Fc gamma RIIa allelic polymorphism and anti-neutrophil cytoplasmic antibody (ANCA)-positive systemic vasculitis. Clin Exp Immun 117(1):198-205, 1999.

(ANCA)-positive vasculitis. Clin Exp Immun 119(3):574-577, 2000.
77. Pawlik A, Ostanek L, Brzosko I, et al: FC gamma RIIa polymorphism in patients with rheumatoid arthritis. Clin Exp Rheum 20(6):841-844, 2002.
78. Mandel NS: The structural basis of crystal-induced membranolysis. Arthritis Rheum 19(3):439-445, 1976.
79. Lefkowitz DL, Gelderman MP, Fuhrmann SR, et al: Neutrophilic myeloperoxidase-macrophage interactions perpetuate chronic inflammation associated with experimental arthritis. Clin Immunol 91(2):145-155, 1999.
80. Weissmann G, Spilberg I,Krakauer K: Arthritis induced in rabbits by lysates of granulocyte lysosomes. Arthritis Rheum 12(2):103-116, 1969.
81. Befus AD, Gilchrist M, Hu J, et al: Neutrophil defensins induce histamine secretion from mast cells: mechanisms of action. J Immunol 163(2):947-953, 1999.
82. McCurdy L, Chatham WW, Blackburn WD Jr: Rheumatoid synovial fibroblast adhesion to human articular cartilage: Enhancement by neutrophil proteases. Arthritis Rheum 38:1694-1700, 1995.
83. Kasama T, Kobayashi K, Yajima N, et al: Expression of vascular endothelial growth factor by synovial fluid neutrophils in rheumatoid arthritis (RA). Clin Exp Immun 121:533-538, 2000.
84. Cross A, Bucknall RS, Edwards SW, et al: Expression of MHC class II molecules by synovial fluid neutrophils. Arthritis Rheum 44(9):S303, 2001.
85. Wipke BT, Allen PM: Essential role of neutrophils in the initiation and progression of a murine model of rheumatoid arthritis. J Immunol 167:1601-1608, 2001.
86. Abramson SB, Dobro J, Eberle MA, et al: Acute reversible hypoxemia in systemic lupus erythematosus. Ann Intern Med 114(11):941-947, 1991.
87. Brack A, Geisler A, Martinez-Taboada VM, et al: Giant cell vasculitis is a T cell-dependent disease. Mol Med 3(8):530-543, 1997.
88. Belmont HM, Buyon J, Giorno R, et al: Upregulation of endothelial cell adhesion molecules characterizes disease activity in systemic lupus erythematosus: the Schwartzman phenomenon revisited. Arthritis Rheum 37(3):376-383, 1994.
89. van der Woude FJ, Rasmussen N, Lobatto S, et al: Autoantibodies against neutrophils and monocytes: tool for diagnosis and marker of disease activity in Wegener's granulomatosis. Lancet 1(8426): 425-429, 1985.
90. Cronstein BN, Van De Stouwe M, Druska L, et al: Nonsteroidal antiinflammatory agents inhibit stimulated neutrophil adhesion to endothelium: adensosine dependent and independent mechanisms. Inflammation 18(3):323-335, 1994.
91. Neal TM, Vissers MC, Winterbourn CC: Inhibition by nonsteroidal antiinflammatory drugs of superoxide production and granule enzyme release by polymorphonuclear leukocytes stimulated with immune comoplexes or formyl-methionyl-leucyl-phenylalanine. Biochem Pharmacol 36(15):2511-2517, 1987.
92. Cronstein BN, Molad Y, Reibman J, et al: Colchicine alters the quantitative and qualitative display of selectins on endothelial cells and neutrophils. J Clin Invest 96(2):994-1002, 1995.
93. Centola M, Wood G, Frucht DM, et al: The gene for famililal Mediterranean fever, MEFV, is expressed in early leukocyte development and is regulated in response to inflammatory mediators. Blood 95(10):3223-3231, 2000.
94. Lo SK, Janakidevi K, Lai L, et al: Hydrogen peoxide-induced increase in endothelial adhesiveness is dependent on ICAM-1 activation. Am J Physiol 264:L406-L412, 1993.
95. Ambruso DR, Bolscher BG, Stokman PM, et al: Assembly and activation of the NADPH:O_2 oxidoreductase in human neutrophils after stimulation with phorbol myristate acetate. J Biol Chem 265:924-930, 1990 [erratum in J Biol Chem 265(31):19370-1, 1990].
96. Heyworth PG, Knaus UG, Settleman J, et al: Regulation of NADPH oxidase activity by Rac GTPase activating protein(s). Mol Biol Cell 4:1217-1223, 1993.
97. Gleich GJ, Adolphson CR,Leiferman KM: The biology of the eosinophilic leukocyte. Annu Rev Med 44:85-101, 1993.
98. Gleich GJ, Adolphson CR, Leiferman KM: Eosinophils. *In* Gallin JI, Goldstein IM, Snyderman R (eds): Inflammation: Basic Principles and Clinical Correlates, ed 2. New York: Raven Press, 1992, pp 663-700.
99. Bainton DF: Developmental biology of neutrophils and eosinophils. *In* Gallin JI, Goldstein IM, Snyderman R (eds): Inflammation: Basic Principles and Clinical Correlates, ed 2. New York: Raven Press, 1992, pp 303-324.
100. Weller PF: Eosinophils: structure and functions. Curr Opin Immun 6:85-90, 1994.
101. Weller PF, Bach DS, Austen KF: Biochemical characterization of human eosinophil Charcot-Leyden crystal protein (lysophospholipase). J Biol Chem 259:15100-15105, 1984.
102. Abu-Ghazaleh RI, Dunnette SL, Loegering DA, et al: Eosinophil granule proteins in peripheral blood granulocytes. J Leukoc Biol 52:611-618, 1992.
103. Nourshargh S: Mechanisms of neutrophil and eosinophil accumulation in vivo. Am Rev Resp Dis 148:S60-S64, 1993.
104. Weller PF, Rand TH, Barrett T, et al: Accessory cell function of human eosinophils: HLA-DR dependent, MHC-restricted antigen presentation and interleukin-1a formation. J Immunol 150:2554-2562, 1993.
105. Weller PF: Lipid, peptide and cytokine mediators elaborated by eosinophils. *In* Smith JH, Cook RM (eds): The Handbook of Immunopharmacology. London: Academic Press, 1993, pp 25-42.
106. Nagata M, Saito K, Tsuchiya K, et al: Leukotriene D4 upregulates eosinophil adhesion via the cysteinyl leukotriene 1 receptor. J Allergy Clin Immunol 109(4):676-680, 2002.
107. Ohshima N, Nagase H, Koshino T, et al: A functional study on CysLT(1) receptors in human eosinophils. Int Arch Allergy Immunol 129(1):67-75, 2002.
108. Braccioni F, Dorman SC, O'Byrne P, et al: The effect of cysteinyl leukotrienes on growth of eosinophil progenitors from peripheral blood and bone marrow of atopic subjects. J Allergy Clin Immunol 110:96-101, 2002.
109. Virchow JC Jr, Faehndrich S, Nassenstein C, et al: Effect of a specific cysteinyl leukotriene-receptor 1-anatgonist (montelukast) on the transmigration of eosinophils across human umbilical vein endothelial cells. Clin Exp Allergy 31(6):836-844, 2001.
110. Finsnes F, Lyberg T, Christensen G, et al: Leukotriene antagonism reduces the generation of endothelin-1 and interferon-gamma and inhibits eosinophilic airway inflammation. Respir Med 96(11):901-906, 2002.
111. Minoguchi K, Kohno Y, Minoguchi H, et al: Reduction of eosinophilic inflammation in the airways of patients with asthma using montelukast Chest 121(3):732-738, 2002.
112. Daikh BE, Ryan CK, Schwartz RH: Montelukast reduces peripheral blood eosinophilia but not tissue eosinophilia or symptoms in a patient with eosinophilic gastroenteritis and esophageal stricture. Ann All Asthma Immunol 90(1):23-27, 2003.
113. Capella GL, Grigerio E, Altomare G: A randomized trial of leukotriene receptor antagonist montelukast in moderate-to-severe atopic dermatitis of adults. Eur J Dermatol 11(3):209-213, 2001.
114. Schmitt-Grohe S, Eickmeier O, Schubert R, et al: Anti-inflammatory effects of montelukast in mild cystic fibrosis. Ann All Asthma Immunol 89(6):599-605, 2002.
115. Jacoby DB, Gleich GJ, Fryer AD: Human eosinophil major basic protein is an endogenous allosteric antagonist at the inhibitory muscarinic M2 receptor. J Clin Invest 91:1314-1318, 1993.
116. Varga J, Uitto J, Jimenez SA: The cause and pathogenesis of the eosinophilia-myalgia syndrome. Ann Intern Med 116:140-147, 1992.
117. Clauw DJ, Crofford LJ: Eosinophilic rheumatic disorders. Rheum Dis Clin North Am 21(1):231-243, 1995.
118. Fauci AS, Harley JB, Roberts WC, et al: The idiopathic hypereosinophilic syndrome: clinical, pathophysiologic, and therapeutic considerations. Ann Intern Med 97:78-92, 1982.
119. Enright T, Chua S, Lim DT: Pulmonary eosinophilic syndromes. Ann Allergy 62:277-283, 1989.
120. Butterfield JH, Leiferman KM, Gleich GJ: Nodules, eosinophilia, rheumatism, dermatitis and swelling (NERDS): a novel eosinophilic disorder. Clin Exp Allergy 23:571-580, 1993.

15 Platelets and Rheumatic Diseases

FEDERICO DÍAZ-GONZÁLEZ · MARK H. GINSBERG

Platelets are small circulating cytoplasmic fragments that play a critical role in hemostasis. They are produced in the bone marrow by megakaryocytes. Single platelets circulate freely in the blood stream; following vascular injury, platelets adhere to the subendothelium, triggering responses that contribute to the formation of the hemostatic plug, including aggregation, secretion of platelet agonists, and production of procoagulant activity. Platelets also secrete soluble factors that contribute to wound repair by altering vascular tone and permeability, promoting cell growth, and stimulating scavenger cells such as monocytes. During the inflammatory response, many of the same activities that lead to hemostasis contribute to inflammation. Thus, platelets release chemotactic factors that promote leukocyte adhesion, which facilitates their extravasation into inflammatory foci. Further-more, platelets secrete a variety of factors that can alter vascular tone and permeability. Lastly, platelets are a major source of transforming growth factor β, a potent stimulus of fibrosis. Taken together, these activities make platelets contributors to the inflammatory response and, hence, to the pathogenesis of systemic rheumatic diseases.[1] This chapter is focused on platelet functions, particularly as they pertain to the inflammatory response and rheumatic diseases.

General Characteristics of Platelets

Platelets are the smallest blood cells and are cytoplasmic fragments derived from their bone marrow precursor, the megakaryocyte. Resting platelets have a smooth, disk shape and are 3.6 (± 0.7) μm in diameter. Upon activation, platelets undergo a shape change, becoming a compact sphere with numerous long dendritic extensions, which markedly increases their surface area. In humans, normal platelet counts range from 150,000 to 450,000 per μl. The main function of platelets is to maintain vascular integrity, playing a critical role in hemostasis.

The plasma membrane of platelets is a typical lipid bilayer, having an extensive series of complex invaginations termed the *canalicular system*. The role of this surface-connected tubular system seems to be to facilitate the quick release of secreted substances to the extracellular environment. The platelet membrane bears a number of glycoprotein (GP) receptors.[2] Platelet surface phospholipids play an important role in coagulation[3] and are a source of arachidonic acid, a precursor of important vasoactive substances such as thromboxane A2, a potent vasoconstrictor and platelet-aggregating agent, and leukotrienes, which can amplify the inflammatory response. Platelet surface GPs are receptors that mediate both the adhesion to subendothelial tissue and the subsequent aggregation to form the hemostatic plug.[4-6] The largest GP is termed I and the smallest IX. Letters a and b distinguish between two separate electrophoretic bands that were initially considered one (e.g., GP I became GP Ia and Ib). The platelet GPIb-IX-V is an important receptor that binds to the von Willebrand factor (vWf) exposed in the subendothelial matrix, causing the attachment of platelets.[7] Deficiency of components of the GPIb-IX-V complex or of vWf leads to the congenital bleeding disorders Bernard-Soulier disease[6] and von Willebrand disease,[8] respectively. ADAMTS-13 is a plasma protease that cleaves vWf into smaller multimers, thus reducing its hemostatic potency.[9] Deficiency of A Disintegrin-like And Metalloprotease with Thrombo Spoudin type 1 motif (ADAMTS-13) or antibodies against it lead to intravascular platelet aggregation, and thus the syndrome of thrombotic thrombocytopenic purpura.[10] Other interactions that contribute to the initial platelet adhesion are mediated by collagen receptors GPIa-IIa (integrin α2β1) and GPVI, which bind to collagen in the subendothelial matrix.[11] The most abundant surface receptor, GPIIb-IIIa (integrin αIIbβ3), is activated by adhesion to collagen or vWf, or by soluble agonists such as thrombin. Following activation, GPIIb-IIIa binds fibrinogen, leading to platelet aggregation.[4] Deficiency of this GP results in Glanzmann thrombasthenia, a disorder characterized by petechial bleeding and the absence of platelet aggregation and clot retraction.[12]

The cytoplasm of platelets is rich in actin and myosin, which provide platelets with the ability to change shape and to retract clots. Platelet cytoplasm contains mitochondria, lysosomes, glycogen stores, and three types of granules that contain a vast number of biologically active molecules (Table 15–1). These granules are classified—according to their ultrastructure, density, and contents—as alpha (α)-granules, lysosomes, and dense granules. Although most of the contents of these granules are made in megakaryocytes, some are taken up from the plasma by both megakaryocytes and platelets.

α-Granules contain numerous proteins and growth factors, such as platelet-derived growth factor (PDGF), transforming growth factor-β (TGF-β), platelet factor-4, and vWf, which are synthesized in the megakaryocyte.[13] However, other proteins, such as fibrinogen, enter the alpha-granules from the plasma via GPIIb-IIIa receptor-mediated endocytosis.[14,15] P-selectin (CD62P), an adhesion

TABLE 15–1 • PLATELET GRANULE COMPOUNDS AND GRANULE MEMBRANE COMPONENTS WITH ROLE IN THE HEMOSTATIC/INFLAMMATORY RESPONSE

Platelet Granules	Actions	Contents
Dense granule	Proaggregating factors	Serotonin, histamine, ADP, ATP, Ca^{2+}, Mg^{2+}
Alpha-granule	Adhesive glycoproteins	P-selectin, CD31, GPIIb-IIIa, fibronectin, vitronectin, thrombospondin
	Growth factors	TGF-β
		PDGF
	Platelet aggregation and chemotaxis	β-thromboglobulin, PF4
	Hemostasis factors	Fibrinogen, vWf
Lysosome	Tissue destruction	Hydrolasas, collagenase, catepsins D,E

Abbreviations: ADP, Adenosine diphosphate; ATP, adenosine triphosphate; PDGF, platelet-derived growth factor; PF4 platelet factor-4; TGF-β, transforming growth factor-β vWf, von Willebrand factor.
Modified from Rendu F, Brohard-Bohn B: The platelet release reaction: granules' constituents, secretion and functions. Platelets 12:261, 2001.

molecule, is also localized in the membrane of α-granules[16,17] and redistributes to the cell surface during platelet activation. Platelet P-selectin has been implicated in stabilizing platelet aggregates.[18] The best documented high-affinity counter-receptor for P-selectin is P-selectin glycoprotein ligand-1 (PSGL-1), a transmembrane sialomucin found on leukocytes and lymphoid cells,[19] through whose interaction platelets participate in the inflammatory response.[20]

Dense granules contain serotonin, adenosine diphosphate (ADP), adenosine triphosphate (ATP), and calcium. The dense-granule membrane bodies are made in megakaryocytes, but they do not acquire their content of serotonin and calcium until the platelets are released into the circulation.[21] Another series of intracellular membrane vesicles serves as a reserve to increase membrane surface area upon platelet activation.

As stated previously, platelets are small cytoplasmic fragments derived from megakaryocytes. Although megakaryocytes are rare in the bone marrow (approximately 0.1 percent of all nucleated cells), megakaryocytes are easily recognized by their giant size (50- to 100-μm diameter) and large, multilobed nucleus. Megakaryo-cytes have two unique characteristics: They undergo a process known as endomitosis in which the nucleus accumulates many times the normal number of chromosomes, and they have specialized structures in the cytoplasm that permit fragments to be shed, as platelets, into the blood stream.[22]

In humans, as in other species, there is an inverse relationship between the platelet count and the mean platelet volume.[23] This suggests that platelet production by bone-marrow megakaryocytes is regulated to maintain a constant total platelet mass. The tendency toward a stable platelet mass explains the wide variation in the platelet count in healthy donors (150,000/μl to 450,000/μl).[24] Megakaryocytes normally replace about 10 percent of the platelet mass daily.[25] In response to the increased need for platelets, megakaryocytes alter their number, size, and ploidy.[26,27] Changes in free-thrombopoietin levels, the main physiologic regulator of platelet production, are responsible for these morphologic and functional adaptations in megakaryocytes.

Thrombopoietin is an 80- to 90-kD glycoprotein produced mainly by the liver[28] and released at a constant rate into the circulation. Thrombopoietin acts through its receptor, the thrombopoietin receptor, also known as c-Mpl, which is present in platelets, megakaryocytes, and, to a lesser extent, in most other hematopoietic precursor cells. Thrombopoietin prevents apoptosis of megakaryocytes, while increasing their number, size, and ploidy,[26,27] but it does not appear to increase the rate of shedding of platelets into circulation.[29] On circulating platelets, thrombopoietin exerts a moderate functional effect, reducing the threshold for activation by other agonists such as ADP. However, binding to the platelet thrombopoietin receptor is the major route of catabolism of circulating thrombopoietin. When the platelet production rate decreases, the platelet mass and the quantity of thrombopoietin receptor also decrease, thrombopoietin concentrations rise, and megakaryocyte growth is stimulated. In conditions of high platelet mass (e.g., hypertransfusion of platelets), the number of thrombopoietin receptors increases, thrombopoietin concentrations fall, and megakaryocyte growth decreases. In addition to thrombopoietin, other soluble factors, such as interleukin (IL)-3 and IL-11, seem to promote megakaryocyte maturation, and these cytokines may play a relevant role in thrombocytosis conditions.[30,31]

The life span of platelets in circulation is between 7 and 10 days. Under normal conditions, the spleen stores about one third of circulating platelets. Circumstances that increase the spleen volume, such as hepatic cirrhosis and portal hypertension, cause a reduction in the circulating platelet count by a sequestration within the splenic sinusoids.[32] However, hypersplenism does not reduce platelet life span; rather, it reduces the circulating platelets available for effective hemostasis. After senescence, platelets are removed from circulation by the reticuloendothelial system. In addition, a small fraction of circulating platelets is consumed in forming hemostatic plugs to maintain vascular integrity.

Function of Platelets

In response to vascular injury, platelets adhere to the subendothelium, secreting a variety of potent agonists and aggregating to form a hemostatic plug.

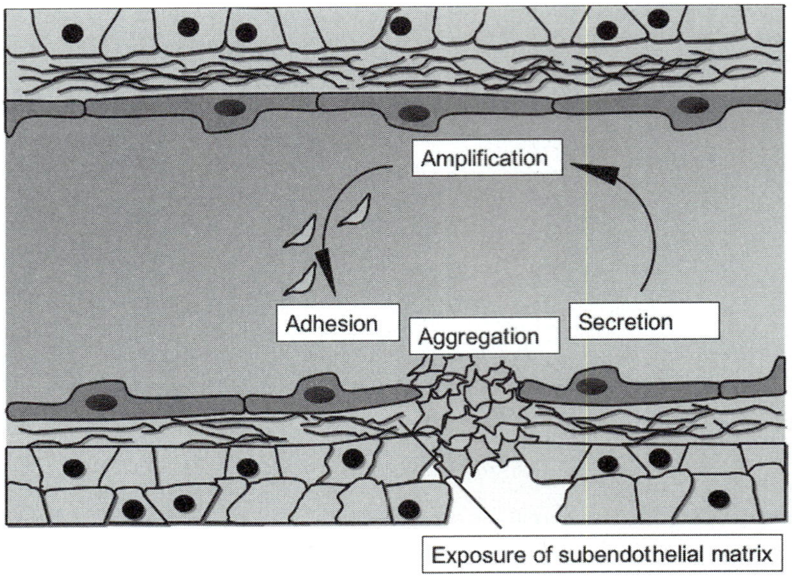

FIGURE 15–1 · **Platelet Plug Formation.** Platelet activation can be initiated by several mechanic (vessel-wall injury, disruption of atherosclerotic plaques) or chemic (adenosine diphosphate [ADP], epinephrine, thromboxane A2, thrombin) stimuli. In response to vessel-wall injury, platelets attach to subendothelial matrix (adhesion), which is followed by fibrinogen-mediated platelet–platelet interaction (aggregation). Simultaneously, platelets release their intracellular granule contents (secretion), which lead to the recruitment of additional circulating platelets (amplification).

During the inflammatory response, these physiologic responses of platelets can promote and exacerbate inflammation. In this sense, platelets are authentic inflammatory cells.

HEMOSTASIS

When a blood vessel is injured, a complex process, which involves both biochemical reactions and cell–cell and cell-matrix interactions, known as hemostasis, takes place. The initial hemostatic response is mediated by platelets that form the platelet plug (Fig. 15–1).

Under physiologic conditions, the undamaged endothelium prevents the adherence of platelets by several mechanisms. These include a cell-associated ecto-ADPase (CD39) and the production of both nitric oxide and prostacyclin.[33] When blood vessel integrity is disrupted, the first reaction is vasoconstriction, which reduces blood loss. Simultaneously, subendothelial matrix elements are exposed, and platelets are rapidly transformed into sticky cellular elements capable of adhering to the underlying surface. Platelet adhesion is initially mediated by the interaction of GPIb-IX-V receptor complex to vWf in the subendothelial matrix.[7] This interaction transduces signals through the GPIb-IX-V complex that activates platelet integrins.[34,35] The activation of GPIa-IIa and GPIIb-IIIa integrins allows binding to collagen and vWf, respectively, mediating the stable adhesion of platelets to subendothelial surface. In addition to vWf, the active form of GPIIb-IIIa binds fibrinogen.[36] The association of soluble fibrinogen with GPIIb-IIIa creates bridges between platelets that result in platelet aggregation and thrombus growth. In concert with aggregation, platelets release their intracellular granules, amplifying the hemostatic response[37,38] (see Table 15–1). The final outcome is the formation of a platelet plug and the triggering of the coagulation cascade, which leads to thrombin activation and fibrin clot formation (Fig. 15–2).

One response of platelets to activation by stimuli such as shear stress or collagen is the shedding of microparticles, fragments 0.1 to 0.2 μm in diameter, that carry some antigens present in intact platelets. These platelet-derived microparticles may play a role in normal hemostasis.[39] Increases in circulating microparticles have been associated with several rheumatic diseases.[40-42] However, the relevance of platelet-derived microparticles in the physiopathology of those disorders remains to be fully clarified.

GPIIb-IIIa

GPIIb-IIIa is a member of a family of cell-adhesion receptors called *integrins*. It is also referred to as integrin αIIbβ3. Although integrins are expressed on virtually all nucleated cells, GPIIb-IIIa is restricted to megakaryocytes

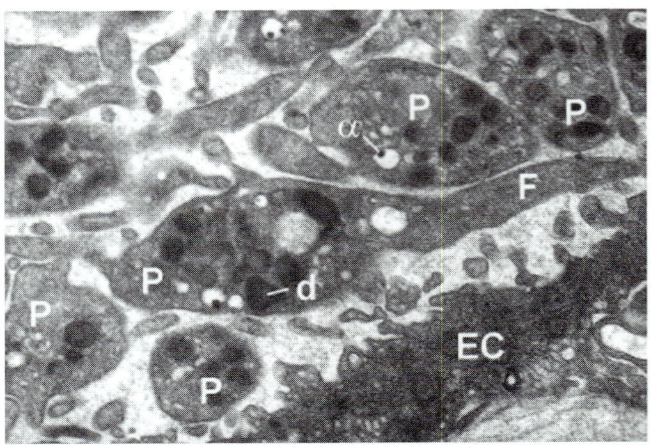

FIGURE 15–2 · **Anatomy of a Platelet Plug.** Electron microscopy of a group of platelets (P) attached to an endothelial cell (EC) in the initial platelet plug formation. Several dense (d) and α-granules (a) are visible. The central platelet shows a long dendritic extensions, or filopodia (F).

and platelets. It is the most abundant receptor on the platelet surface, averaging 80,000 complexes per platelet. GPIIb-IIIa recognizes at least five different adhesive ligands[43]: fibronectin, fibrinogen, vWf, thrombospondin, and vitronectin. Integrins can modify their adhesion through dynamic modulation of receptor affinity.[43] On resting platelets, GPIIb-IIIa does not bind soluble fibrinogen. However, following platelet stimulation (e.g., by thrombin, collagen, or ADP), GPIIb-IIIa undergoes a conformational change and is converted from a low to a high-affinity fibrinogen receptor, a process known as "inside-out" signaling. In this situation, fibrinogen bridges the activated platelets, and platelet aggregation takes place. Simultaneously, the cytosolic portion of the activated GPIIb-IIIa binds to platelet cytoskeleton proteins and mediates platelet spreading and clot retraction in what is referred to as "outside-in" integrin signaling. Thus, GPIIb-IIIa integrates receptor–ligand interactions on the external face of the membrane with cytosolic events in a bidirectional fashion.[4] This is the final common pathway for platelet aggregation, irrespective of the mode of platelet stimulation. The importance of GPIIb-IIIa integrin is illustrated by Glanzmann thrombasthenia, a bleeding disorder caused by mutations in the gene for either the αIIb or β3 subunit,[12] and by the clinical utility of GPIIb-IIIa antagonists as antithrombotic agents in the treatment of thrombotic diseases.

ROLE OF PLATELETS IN THE INFLAMMATORY RESPONSE

The accumulation of leukocytes in tissue is an essential event for the inflammatory response. The current paradigm of leukocyte extravasation requires a multistep cascade of sequential leukocyte–endothelial cell interactions, in which members of three different families of adhesion receptors participate: selectins, integrins, and the immunoglobulin superfamily.[44] Platelets contribute in many ways to leukocyte accumulation (Table 15–2).

In flowing blood, leukocytes roll on adherent activated platelets, mainly through the interaction of platelet P-selectin with its major leukocyte ligand, PSGL-1.[45-47] This initial rolling of leukocytes on platelet P-selectin is followed by their firm adhesion and subsequent migration, processes that are dependent on the leukocyte integrin Mac-1 (αMβ2, CD11b/CD18).[47,48] Furthermore, Mac-1 adheres firmly to platelets through direct binding to GPIbα.[49] These interactions provide molecular mechanisms for leukocyte recruitment to hemostatic plugs where platelets have been previously deposited in response to vascular injury.[50,51] Parallel lines of investigation have demonstrated that resting platelets are able to roll on activated endothelial cells,[52] apparently through an interaction between PSGL-1 expressed in platelets and the endothelial P-selectin.[53] The physiologic function of platelet rolling on stimulated endothelial cells remains to be clarified. However, if this contact results in activation of platelets, then those platelets may release proinflammatory mediators such as cytokines, chemokines,[54,55] and eicosanoid precursors,[56-58] or growth factors that stimulate tissue healing.

In addition to the adhesion molecules, activated platelets express on their surface two major proinflammatory mediators: the platelet-activating factor (PAF) and CD40 ligand (CD154). PAF is a potent platelet aggregating phospholipid produced by macrophages, mast cells, platelets, endothelial cells, neutrophils, and monocytes. Upon platelet activation, PAF is rapidly synthesized and translocated to the plasma membrane of endothelial cells where, by a juxtacrine mechanism, it recognizes its receptor in neutrophils, resulting in β2 integrin-mediated adhesion of leukocytes to endothelial surface.[59] In the same way, PAF can signal neutrophils when it is displayed on the surface of adherent activated platelets acting in cooperation with P-selectin to tether neutrophis.[59] The biologic action of PAF is physiologically inactivated by a plasma and cellular acetylhydrolase.[60] A role of PAF in the pathogenesis of chronic inflammatory arthritis has been proposed[61,62]; however, a well-controlled clinical trial failed to show any beneficial effect of a PAF antagonist in patients with active rheumatoid arthritis (RA).[63]

CD40 is a transmembrane protein member of the tumor necrosis factor (TNF) receptor family. CD40 is present on many cells, including B cells, monocytes, macrophages, dendritic cells, and vascular endothelial cells.[64] Platelets are the major peripheral blood source of CD154, the ligand of CD40, and they express it on their surface within seconds of exposure to an agonist.[65]

TABLE 15–2 • PLATELET COMPONENTS IMPLICATED IN THE INFLAMMATORY RESPONSE

	Platelet Component	Actions
Surface molecules	P-selectin (CD62-P), PECAM (CD31), GPIbα	Adhesive targets for leukocytes
	PAF	Neutrophil activation
	CD154 (CD40 ligand)	Agonist for endothelial cells
Soluble factors	Serotonin, histamine	Regulators of vascular permeability
	β-Thromboglobulin, PF4	Chemotaxis
	Acid hydrolases	Tissue digestion
	PDGF, TGF-β	Cellular mitogens, chemoattractant
End products of platelet procoagulant activity	Thrombin, fibrin	Promote leukocyte accumulation

Abbreviations: GPI, Glycosylphosphatidylinositol; PAF, platelet-activating factor; PDGF, platelet-derived growth factor; PECAM, platelet-endothelial cell adhesion molecule; PF4, platelet factor-4; TGF-β, transforming growth factor-β.

The interaction of CD154 on activated platelets with CD40 on endothelial cells causes a proinflammatory reaction of the endothelium, characterized by the expression of inflammatory adhesion molecules such as E-selectin, vascular cell adhesion molecule (VCAM)-1, and intercellular adhesion molecule (ICAM)-1, and the secretion of the chemokines IL-8 and monocyte chemoattractant protein (MCP)-1.[65] Thus, CD154 expressed on activated platelets can provide a potent stimulus to the inflammatory response. Recent clinical data suggest that the blockade of CD154 may induce a prothrombotic state in patients with lupus[66] through a mechanism that needs to be clarified.

When platelets adhere, they release a number of growth factors, such as PDGF, TGF-β, and other factors that are chemotactic for monocytes, macrophages, and fibroblasts. These may play an important role in the chronic inflammatory response by mediating a fibroproliferative response. PDGF is a homo- or heterodimer molecule of A and B chains[67] produced by platelets, monocytes or macrophages, endothelial cells, and vascular smooth muscle cells (under some conditions). This molecule plays an essential role in tissue repair and wound healing.[68] PDGF is a potent mitogen and chemoattractant for smooth muscle cells, connective tissue cells, and macrophages,[69-72] which contributes to the formation of lesions of atherosclerosis,[72,73] a disorder strongly related to the inflammatory response.[74] TGF-β has three isoforms (TGF-β1, -β2, and -β3) secreted by virtually all cell types as latent complexes that need to be processed to exhibit biologic activity.[75] Several effects have been associated with TGF-β: 1) It is chemotatic for various cell types, including leukocytes; 2) it inhibits proliferation of most cells; 3) it induces the synthesis and deposition of extracellular matrix; and 4) it stimulates the formation of granulation tissue.[76] The net result is that TGF-β is mainly an inhibitor of the inflammatory response.[77,78] In this regard, the systemic administration of TGF-β1 antagonizes the development of polyarthritis in susceptible rats.[79] Thus, carefully regulated expression of active TGF-β is essential for resolution of inflammation and repair. Overproduction of this cytokine can be associated with fibrosis.[80-82]

Platelets and Rheumatic Diseases

ALTERATIONS IN PLATELET NUMBERS IN RHEUMATIC DISEASES

Increases in platelet counts have three major causes: 1) reactive or secondary thrombocytosis, 2) familial thrombocytosis, and 3) clonal thrombocytosis, including essential thrombocythemia and related myeloproliferative disorders. The platelet count is frequently elevated in patients with active RA and juvenile RA due to reactive thrombocytosis. The level of thrombocytosis correlates with both clinic and laboratory parameters of disease activity. Relapses of RA are often accompanied by increases in platelet count, whereas remissions are associated with their reduction to normal limits.[83] This indicates that the thrombocytosis observed in patients with rheumatic disease is reactive or secondary to the chronic inflammatory process. Although the mechanism involved in this thrombocytosis is uncertain, increased intravascular coagulation with a compensatory increase in platelet production has been suggested as a possible cause.[84] More recently, several studies have suggested that inflammatory cytokines with a minor role in the physiologic production of platelets, such as IL-6, IL-1, or TNF-α,[85-87] may be active mediators in the regulation of thrombopoiesis during the reactive thrombocytosis that occurs in the inflammatory process.

Reduced platelet count, or thrombocytopenia, is not uncommon in rheumatic diseases. The mechanisms involved in thrombocytopenic states are reduction in platelet production, sequestration, and rapid platelet destruction. Several drugs used in rheumatic diseases are able to suppress the bone marrow. Among the drugs that can produce thrombocytopenia as a result of a megakaryocytic hypoplasia are gold, cyclophosphamide, methotrexate, penicillamine, and azathioprine. The effect these compounds have on suppressing megakaryocyte replication depends on the time and dose of exposure; thus, reduced elimination of these drugs places patients at increased risk for this complication.[88]

The normal spleen contains about 30 percent of the platelet mass, and splenomegaly can result in a low circulating count without reduction in the platelet life span.[89] Several rheumatic diseases may lead to this type of thrombocytopenia. The most characteristic is Felty's syndrome, an uncommon but severe subset of seropositive RA complicated by granulocytopenia and splenomegaly. In this disorder, thrombocytopenia is usually not life threatening.

Another related disease is immune-mediated platelet destruction,[90] a disorder termed idiopathic thrombocytopenic purpura (ITP). Autoantibodies cause ITP, and platelet surface proteins, including GPIIb/IIIa, Ib/IX, Ia/IIa, IV, and V, can be antigenic targets of such autoantibodies.[91,92] Circulating platelets coated with immunoglobulin G (IgG) autoantibodies suffer an accelerated clearance through fragment crystallizable gamma (Fcγ) receptors expressed by macrophages in the spleen and liver. In some cases of ITP, platelet production appears to be reduced, either by intramedullary destruction of antibody-coated platelets or by the inhibition of megakaryocytopoiesis.[93] The level of thrombopoietin is not increased,[94] suggesting a normal megakaryocyte mass. ITP is present in 15 to 25 percent of patients with systemic lupus erythematosus[95] and in about 25 percent of patients with antiphospholipid syndrome.[96] The outcome in these cases is rarely severe. In contrast, the thrombopenia that occurs during episodes of systemic vasculitis has a more complex pathogenesis, a worse clinical course, and a poorer outcome.[97,98] Immune thrombocytopenia is rare in RA, except when related to therapy. Among the drugs that can produce thrombocytopenia in RA, intramuscular gold salts are the most clearly associated with drug-induced immune thrombocytopenia. About 1 to 3 percent of patients receiving intramuscular gold salts for the treatment of RA develop a thrombocytopenia, which may be life threatening. Although bone-marrow suppression can occur in patients undergoing gold treatment, thrombocytopenia is usually due to immune destruction of platelets associated with an active marrow.[99,100]

ROLE OF PLATELETS IN THE PATHOGENESIS OF RHEUMATIC DISEASES

The role platelets play in the amplification of the inflammatory response provides a basis for their involvement in rheumatic diseases. However, most of the available evidence implicating platelets in the pathogenesis of rheumatic disorders is indirect and circumstantial.

Platelets have been implicated in the pathogenesis of RA,[1] based mainly on the observation that labeled platelets only localize to joints with clinically active inflammation.[101] A direct correlation has been described between platelet-derived microparticle levels and disease activity in RA patients, which suggests that platelet microparticle generation[42] contributes to the pathogenesis of RA. Patients with essential thrombocythemia have an increased prevalence of antiphospholipid antibodies, which may be associated with a higher risk of thrombosis.[102] Several studies have focused on the presence of activated platelets in patients with systemic lupus erythematosus,[103,104] antiphospholipid syndrome,[104] and systemic sclerosis.[105]

INHIBITION OF PLATELET FUNCTION BY PHARMACOLOGIC AGENTS

Nonsteroidal anti-inflammatory drugs (NSAIDs) are a foundation of therapy in many rheumatic diseases. These agents inhibit prostaglandin synthesis[106] through the blockade of cyclooxygenase (COX). These agents can interfere with platelet aggregation and secretion[107,108] through the inactivation of platelet COX. This enzyme is a rate-limiting step in the transformation of arachidonic acid into thromboxane A2, a potent platelet-aggregating agent. In addition, some NSAIDs are able to reduce platelet aggregation by interfering with the activation of GPIIb-IIIa through a COX-independent mechanism.[109] Thus, the NSAIDs inhibit platelet function and can lead to bleeding complications in patients with rheumatic diseases.

The recent development of potent new antithrombotic agents may also provide new weapons in the treatment of rheumatic diseases. Among these are ticlopidine and its analogue, clopidogrel, two inhibitors of the P2Y12 ADP receptor. These agents have greater efficacy than aspirin for prevention of recurrent stoke[110] and may find a place in the antirheumatic armamentarium. Agents that interfere directly with the adhesive function of integrin GPIIb-IIIa[111] also have come into therapeutic use. This new group of agents includes monoclonal antibodies, peptides, and other small molecules that have been approved for intravenous coronary angioplasty and stent procedures. Orally active GPIIb-IIIa blockers have been developed for chronic therapy, including secondary and even primary prevention of thrombotic diseases. However, available data from the clinic trials of these oral agents have failed to show clinic benefits, but they have shown unexplained increased mortality.[112]

ACKNOWLEGMENTS

This is publication 15953-CB From The Scripps Research Institute and was supported by grants AR27214, HL48728, and FIS 01/1024 from Instituto de Salud Carlos III of Spain.
Authors are indebted with Dr. Juan C. Quevedo for the artwork and to Dr. Lucio Díaz-Flores for the platelet electron micrograph.

REFERENCES

1. Ginsberg MH: Role of platelets in inflammation and rheumatic disease. Adv Inflamm Res 2:53, 1986.
2. Isenberg WH, Bainton DF: Megakaryocyte and platelet structure. *In* Hoffman R, Benz EJ, Shattil SJ, et al (eds): Hematology: Basic Principles and Practice. New York, Churchill Livingstone, 1994, p 1516.
3. Shattil SJ, Bennett JS: Platelets and their membranes in hemostasis: physiology and pathophysiology. Ann Intern Med 94:108, 1981.
4. Shattil SJ, Kashiwagi H, Pampori N: Integrin signaling: the platelet paradigm. Blood 91:2645, 1998.
5. Santoro SA, Zutter MM: The alpha 2 beta 1 integrin: a collagen receptor on platelets and other cells. Thromb Haemost 74:813, 1995.
6. Lopez JA, Andrews RK, Afshar-Kharghan V, Berndt MC: Bernard-Soulier syndrome. Blood 91:4397, 1998.
7. Clemetson KJ: Platelet GPIb-V-IX complex. Thromb Haemost 78:266, 1997.
8. Schneppenheim R, Budde U, Ruggeri ZM: A molecular approach to the classification of von Willebrand disease. Best Pract Res Clin Haematol 14:281, 2001.
9. Chung DW, Fujikawa K: Processing of von Willebrand factor by ADAMTS-13. Biochemistry 41:11065, 2002.
10. Ashida A, Nakamura H, Yoden A, et al: Successful treatment of a young infant who developed high-titer inhibitors against VWF-cleaving protease (ADAMTS-13): important discrimination from Upshaw-Schulman syndrome. Am J Hematol 71:318, 2002.
11. Sixma JJ, van Zanten GH, Huizinga EG, et al: Platelet adhesion to collagen: an update. Thromb Haemost 78:434, 1997.
12. Tomiyama Y: Glanzmann thrombasthenia: integrin alpha IIb beta 3 deficiency. Int J Hematol 72:448, 2000.
13. Greenberg SM, Kuter DJ, Rosenberg RD: In vitro stimulation of megakaryocyte maturation by megakaryocyte stimulatory factor. J Biol Chem 262:3269, 1987.
14. Handagama PJ, Amrani DL, Shuman MA: Endocytosis of fibrinogen into hamster megakaryocyte alpha granules is dependent on a dimeric gamma A configuration. Blood 85:1790, 1995.
15. Harrison P, Wilbourn B, Debili N, et al: Uptake of plasma fibrinogen into the alpha granules of human megakaryocytes and platelets. J Clin Invest 84:1320, 1989.
16. Stenberg PE, McEver RP, Shuman MA, et al: A platelet alpha-granule membrane protein (GMP-140) is expressed on the plasma membrane after activation. J Cell Biol 101:880, 1985.
17. Berman CL, Yeo EL, Wencel-Drake JD, et al: A platelet alpha granule membrane protein that is associated with the plasma membrane after activation: characterization and subcellular localization of platelet activation-dependent granule-external membrane protein. J Clin Invest 78:130, 1986.
18. Smyth SS, Reis ED, Zhang W, et al: Beta(3)-integrin-deficient mice but not P-selectin-deficient mice develop intimal hyperplasia after vascular injury: correlation with leukocyte recruitment to adherent platelets 1 hour after injury. Circulation 103:2501, 2001.

19. Norman KE, Moore KL, McEver RP, Ley K: Leukocyte rolling in vivo is mediated by P-selectin glycoprotein ligand-1. Blood 86:4417, 1995.
20. McEver RP: Adhesive interactions of leukocytes, platelets, and the vessel wall during hemostasis and inflammation. Thromb Haemost 86:746, 2001.
21. Schick PK, Weinstein M: A marker for megakaryocytes: serotonin accumulation in guinea pig megakaryocytes. J Lab Clin Med 98:607, 1981.
22. Cramer EM: Megakaryocyte structure and function. Curr Opin Hematol 6:354, 1999.
23. Bessman JD, Williams LJ, Gilmer PR Jr: Mean platelet volume: the inverse relation of platelet size and count in normal subjects, and an artifact of other particles. Am J Clin Pathol 76:289, 1981.
24. Giles C: The platelet count and mean platelet volume. Br J Haematol 48:31, 1981.
25. Gurney AL, Carver-Moore K, de Sauvage FJ, Moore MW: Thrombocytopenia in c-mpl-deficient mice. Science 265:1445, 1994.
26. Penington DG, Olsen TE: Megakaryocytes in states of altered platelet production: cell numbers, size and DNA content. Br J Haematol 18:447, 1970.
27. Kuter DJ, Rosenberg RD: Regulation of megakaryocyte ploidy in vivo in the rat. Blood 75:74, 1990.
28. Nomura S, Ogami K, Kawamura K, et al: Cellular localization of thrombopoietin mRNA in the liver by in situ hybridization. Exp Hematol 25:565, 1997.
29. Choi ES, Hokom MM, Chen JL, et al: The role of megakaryocyte growth and development factor in terminal stages of thrombopoiesis. Br J Haematol 95:227, 1996.
30. Kobayashi S, Teramura M, Hoshino S, et al: Circulating megakaryocyte progenitors in myeloproliferative disorders are hypersensitive to interleukin-3. Br J Haematol 83:539, 1993.
31. Cairo MS, Plunkett JM, Nguyen A, et al: Effect of interleukin-11 with and without granulocyte colony-stimulating factor on in vivo neonatal rat hematopoiesis: induction of neonatal thrombocytosis by interleukin-11 and synergistic enhancement of neutrophilia by interleukin-11 + granulocyte colony-stimulating factor. Pediatr Res 34:56, 1993.
32. Aster RH: Pooling of platelets in the spleen: role in the pathogenesis of "hypersplenic" thrombocytopenia. J Clin Invest 45:645, 1966.
33. Marcus AJ, Safier LB, Broekman MJ, et al: Thrombosis and inflammation as multicellular processes: significance of cell-cell interactions. Thromb Haemost 74:213, 1995.
34. Zaffran Y, Meyer SC, Negrescu E, et al: Signaling across the platelet adhesion receptor glycoprotein Ib-IX induces alpha IIbbeta 3 activation both in platelets and a transfected Chinese hamster ovary cell system. J Biol Chem 275:16779, 2000.
35. Yap CL, Hughan SC, Cranmer SL, et al: Synergistic adhesive interactions and signaling mechanisms operating between platelet glycoprotein Ib/IX and integrin alpha IIbbeta 3: studies in human platelets ans transfected Chinese hamster ovary cells. J Biol Chem 275:41377, 2000.
36. Savage B, Saldivar E, Ruggeri ZM: Initiation of platelet adhesion by arrest onto fibrinogen or translocation on von Willebrand factor. Cell 84:289, 1996.
37. Kroll MH, Schafer AI: Biochemical mechanisms of platelet activation. Blood 74:1181, 1989.
38. Harrison P, Savidge GF, Cramer EM: The origin and physiological relevance of alpha-granule adhesive proteins. Br J Haematol 74:125, 1990.
39. Sims PJ, Wiedmer T, Esmon CT, et al: Assembly of the platelet prothrombinase complex is linked to vesiculation of the platelet plasma membrane. Studies in Scott syndrome: an isolated defect in platelet procoagulant activity. J Biol Chem 264:17049, 1989.
40. Nomura S, Suzuki M, Katsura K, et al: Platelet-derived microparticles may influence the development of atherosclerosis in diabetes mellitus. Atherosclerosis 116:235, 1995.
41. Jy W, Horstman LL, Arce M, Ahn YS: Clinical significance of platelet microparticles in autoimmune thrombocytopenias. J Lab Clin Med 119:334, 1992.
42. Knijff-Dutmer EA, Koerts J, Nieuwland R, et al: Elevated levels of platelet microparticles are associated with disease activity in rheumatoid arthritis. Arthritis Rheum 46:1498, 2002.
43. Ginsberg MH, Díaz-González F: Cell adhesion molecules and endothelial cells in arthritis. *In* Koopman WJ (ed): Arthritis and Allied Conditions: A Textbook of Rheumatology, 13th ed. Baltimore, Williams & Wilkins, 1997, p 479.
44. Springer TA: Traffic signals for lymphocyte recirculation and leukocyte emigration: the multistep paradigm. Cell 76:301, 1994.
45. Buttrum SM, Hatton R, Nash GB: Selectin-mediated rolling of neutrophils on immobilized platelets. Blood 82:1165, 1993.
46. Yeo EL, Sheppard JA, Feuerstein IA: Role of P-selectin and leukocyte activation in polymorphonuclear cell adhesion to surface adherent activated platelets under physiologic shear conditions (an injury vessel wall model). Blood 83:2498, 1994.
47. Diacovo TG, Roth SJ, Buccola JM, et al: Neutrophil rolling, arrest, and transmigration across activated, surface-adherent platelets via sequential action of P-selectin and the beta 2-integrin CD11b/CD18. Blood 88:146, 1996.
48. Evangelista V, Manarini S, Rotondo S, et al: Platelet/polymorphonuclear leukocyte interaction in dynamic conditions: evidence of adhesion cascade and cross talk between P-selectin and the beta 2 integrin CD11b/CD18. Blood 88:4183, 1996.
49. Simon DI, Chen Z, Xu H, et al: Platelet glycoprotein ibalpha is a counterreceptor for the leukocyte integrin Mac-1 (CD11b/CD18). J Exp Med 192:193, 2000.
50. Rinder CS, Bonan JL, Rinder HM, et al: Cardiopulmonary bypass induces leukocyte-platelet adhesion. Blood 79:1201, 1992.
51. Rogers C, Edelman ER, Simon DI: A mAb to the beta2-leukocyte integrin Mac-1 (CD11b/CD18) reduces intimal thickening after angioplasty or stent implantation in rabbits. Proc Natl Acad Sci U S A 95:10134, 1998.
52. Frenette PS, Johnson RC, Hynes RO, Wagner DD: Platelets roll on stimulated endothelium in vivo: an interaction mediated by endothelial P-selectin. Proc Natl Acad Sci U S A 92:7450, 1995.
53. Frenette PS, Denis CV, Weiss L, et al: P-Selectin glycoprotein ligand 1 (PSGL-1) is expressed on platelets and can mediate platelet-endothelial interactions in vivo. J Exp Med 191:1413, 2000.
54. Schenk BI, Petersen F, Flad HD, Brandt E: Platelet-derived chemokines CXC chemokine ligand (CXCL)7, connective tissue-activating peptide III, and CXCL4 differentially affect and cross-regulate neutrophil adhesion and transendothelial migration. J Immunol 169:2602, 2002.
55. Schober A, Manka D, von Hundelshausen P, et al: Deposition of platelet RANTES triggering monocyte recruitment requires P-selectin and is involved in neointima formation after arterial injury. Circulation 106:1523, 2002.
56. Marcus AJ, Hajjar DP: Vascular transcellular signaling. J Lipid Res 34:2017, 1993.
57. Serhan CN, Haeggstrom JZ, Leslie CC: Lipid mediator networks in cell signaling: update and impact of cytokines. Faseb J 10:1147, 1996.
58. Marcus AJ, Broekman MJ, Safier LB, et al: Formation of leukotrienes and other hydroxy acids during platelet-neutrophil interactions in vitro. Biochem Biophys Res Commun 109:130, 1982.
59. Zimmerman GA, McIntyre TM, Prescott SM: Adhesion and signaling in vascular cell-cell interactions. J Clin Invest 98:1699, 1996.
60. Prescott SM: Inflammatory actions of platelet-activating factor: control by PAF acetylhydrolase. J Investig Allergol Clin Immunol 7:416, 1997.
61. Gutierrez S, Palacios I, Egido J, et al: IL-1 beta and IL-6 stimulate the production of platelet-activating factor (PAF) by cultured rabbit synovial cells. Clin Exp Immunol 99:364, 1995.
62. Palacios I, Miguelez R, Sanchez-Pernaute O, et al: A platelet activating factor receptor antagonist prevents the development of chronic arthritis in mice. J Rheumatol 26:1080, 1999.
63. Hilliquin P, Chermat-Izard V, Menkes CJ: A double blind, placebo controlled study of a platelet activating factor antagonist in patients with rheumatoid arthritis. J Rheumatol 25:1502, 1998.
64. Karmann K, Hughes CC, Schechner J, et al: CD40 on human endothelial cells: inducibility by cytokines and functional regulation of adhesion molecule expression. Proc Natl Acad Sci U S A 92:4342, 1995.
65. Henn V, Slupsky JR, Grafe M, et al: CD40 ligand on activated platelets triggers an inflammatory reaction of endothelial cells. Nature 391:591, 1998.

66. Boumpas DT, Furie R, Manzi S, et al: A short course of BG9588 (anti-CD40 ligand antibody) improves serologic activity and decreases hematuria in patients with proliferative lupus glomerulonephritis. Arthritis Rheum 48:719, 2003.
67. Hart CE, Bailey M, Curtis DA, et al: Purification of PDGF-AB and PDGF-BB from human platelet extracts and identification of all three PDGF dimers in human platelets. Biochemistry 29:166, 1990.
68. Pierce GF, Mustoe TA, Altrock BW, et al: Role of platelet-derived growth factor in wound healing. J Cell Biochem 45:319, 1991.
69. Ross R, Raines EW, Bowen-Pope DF: The biology of platelet-derived growth factor. Cell 46:155, 1986.
70. Grotendorst GR, Chang T, Seppa HE, et al: Platelet-derived growth factor is a chemoattractant for vascular smooth muscle cells. J Cell Physiol 113:261, 1982.
71. Deuel TF, Senior RM, Huang JS, Griffin GL: Chemotaxis of monocytes and neutrophils to platelet-derived growth factor. J Clin Invest 69:1046,1982.
72. Ross R, Masuda J, Raines EW, et al: Localization of PDGF-B protein in macrophages in all phases of atherogenesis. Science 248:1009, 1990.
73. Wilcox JN, Smith KM, Williams LT, et al: Platelet-derived growth factor mRNA detection in human atherosclerotic plaques by in situ hybridization. J Clin Invest 82:1134, 1988.
74. Ridker PM, Rifai N, Rose L, et al: Comparison of C-reactive protein and low-density lipoprotein cholesterol levels in the prediction of first cardiovascular events. N Engl J Med 347:1557, 2002.
75. Lawrence DA: Transforming growth factor-beta: a general review. Eur Cytokine Netw 7:363, 1996.
76. Wahl SM: Transforming growth factor-b (TGF-b) in the resolution and repair of inflammation. *In* Gallin JI, Snyderman R (eds): Inflammation: Basic Principles and Clinical Correlates, 3rd ed. Philadelphia, Lippincott Williams & Wilkins, 1999, p 883.
77. McCartney-Francis NL, Mizel DE, Redman RS, et al: Autoimmune Sjogren's-like lesions in salivary glands of TGF-beta1-deficient mice are inhibited by adhesion-blocking peptides. J Immunol 157:1306, 1996.
78. Christ M, McCartney-Francis NL, Kulkarni AB, et al: Immune dysregulation in TGF-beta 1-deficient mice. J Immunol 153:1936, 1994.
79. Brandes ME, Allen JB, Ogawa Y, Wahl SM: Transforming growth factor beta 1 suppresses acute and chronic arthritis in experimental animals. J Clin Invest 87:1108, 1991.
80. Bernasconi P, Torchiana E, Confalonieri P, et al: Expression of transforming growth factor-beta 1 in dystrophic patient muscles correlates with fibrosis: pathogenetic role of a fibrogenic cytokine. J Clin Invest 96:1137, 1995.
81. Border WA, Noble NA, Yamamoto T, et al: Natural inhibitor of transforming growth factor-beta protects against scarring in experimental kidney disease. Nature 360:361, 1992.
82. Varga J: Scleroderma and Smads: dysfunctional Smad family dynamics culminating in fibrosis. Arthritis Rheum 46:1703, 2002.
83. Hutchinson RM, Davis P, Jayson MI: Thrombocytosis in rheumatoid arthritis. Ann Rheum Dis 35:138, 1976.
84. Ehrenfeld M, Penchas S, Eliakim M: Thrombocytosis in rheumatoid arthritis. Recurrent arterial thromboembolism and death. Ann Rheum Dis 36:579, 1977.
85. Wang JC, Chen C, Novetsky AD, et al: Blood thrombopoietin levels in clonal thrombocytosis and reactive thrombocytosis. Am J Med 104:451, 1998.
86. Dan K, Gomi S, Inokuchi K, et al: Effects of interleukin-1 and tumor necrosis factor on megakaryocytopoiesis: mechanism of reactive thrombocytosis. Acta Haematol 93:67, 1995.
87. Hsu HC, Tsai WH, Jiang ML, et al: Circulating levels of thrombopoietic and inflammatory cytokines in patients with clonal and reactive thrombocytosis. J Lab Clin Med 134:392, 1999.
88. Calvo-Romero JM: Severe pancytopenia associated with low-dose methotrexate therapy for rheumatoid arthritis. Ann Pharmacother 35:1575, 2001.
89. Warkentin TE, Trimble MS, Kelton JG: Thrombocytopenia due to platelet destruction and hypersplenism. *In* Hoffman R, Benz EJ, Shattil SF, et al (eds): Hematology: Basic Principles and Practice. New York, Churchill Livingstone, 1995, p 1889.
90. Cines DB, Blanchette VS: Immune thrombocytopenic purpura. N Engl J Med 346:995, 2002.
91. McMillan R: Autoantibodies and autoantigens in chronic immune thrombocytopenic purpura. Semin Hematol 37:239, 2000.
92. He R, Reid DM, Jones CE, Shulman NR: Spectrum of Ig classes, specificities, and titers of serum antiglycoproteins in chronic idiopathic thrombocytopenic purpura. Blood 83:1024, 1994.
93. Gernsheimer T, Stratton J, Ballem PJ, Slichter SJ: Mechanisms of response to treatment in autoimmune thrombocytopenic purpura. N Engl J Med 320:974, 1989.
94. Emmons RV, Reid DM, Cohen RL, et al: Human thrombopoietin levels are high when thrombocytopenia is due to megakaryocyte deficiency and low when due to increased platelet destruction. Blood 87:4068, 1996.
95. Gladman DD, Urowitz MB, Tozman EC, Glynn MF: Haemostatic abnormalities in systemic lupus erythematosus. Q J Med 52:424, 1983.
96. Cuadrado MJ, Hughes GR: Hughes (antiphospholipid) syndrome: clinical features. Rheum Dis Clin North Am 27:507, 2001.
97. Pistiner M, Wallace DJ, Nessim S, et al: Lupus erythematosus in the 1980s: a survey of 570 patients. Semin Arthritis Rheum 21:55, 1991.
98. Reveille JD, Bartolucci A, Alarcon GS: Prognosis in systemic lupus erythematosus: negative impact of increasing age at onset, black race, and thrombocytopenia, as well as causes of death. Arthritis Rheum 33:37, 1990.
99. Adachi JD, Bensen WG, Kassam Y, et al: Gold induced thrombocytopenia: 12 cases and a review of the literature. Semin Arthritis Rheum 16:287, 1987.
100. von dem Borne AE, Pegels JG, van der Stadt RJ, et al: Thrombocytopenia associated with gold therapy: a drug-induced autoimmune disease? Br J Haematol 63:509, 1986.
101. Farr M, Scott DL, Constable TJ, et al: Thrombocytosis of active rheumatoid disease. Ann Rheum Dis 42:545, 1983.
102. Harrison CN, Donohoe S, Carr P, et al: Patients with essential thrombocythaemia have an increased prevalence of antiphospholipid antibodies which may be associated with thrombosis. Thromb Haemost 87:802, 2002.
103. Nagahama M, Nomura S, Ozaki Y, et al: Platelet activation markers and soluble adhesion molecules in patients with systemic lupus erythematosus. Autoimmunity 33:85, 2001.
104. Joseph JE, Harrison P, Mackie IJ, et al: Increased circulating platelet-leucocyte complexes and platelet activation in patients with antiphospholipid syndrome, systemic lupus erythematosus and rheumatoid arthritis. Br J Haematol 115:451, 2001.
105. Silveri F, De Angelis R, Poggi A, et al: Relative roles of endothelial cell damage and platelet activation in primary Raynaud's phenomenon (RP) and RP secondary to systemic sclerosis. Scand J Rheumatol 30:290, 2001.
106. Vane JR: Inhibition of prostaglandin synthesis as a mechanism of nonsteroidal antiinflammatory drugs. Nature 231:232, 1971.
107. O'Brien JR: Effect of anti-inflammatory agents on platelets. Lancet 1:894, 1968.
108. McQueen EG, Facoory B, Faed JM: Non-steroidal anti-inflammatory drugs and platelet function. N Z Med J 99:358, 1986.
109. Dominguez-Jimenez C, Diaz-Gonzalez F, Gonzalez-Alvaro I, et al: Prevention of alphaII(b)beta3 activation by non-steroidal anti-inflammatory drugs. FEBS Lett 446:318, 1999.
110. Sharis PJ, Cannon CP, Loscalzo J: The antiplatelet effects of ticlopidine and clopidogrel. Ann Intern Med 129:394, 1998.
111. Topol EJ, Byzova TV, Plow EF: Platelet GPIIb-IIIa blockers. Lancet 353:227, 1999.
112. Newby LK, Califf RM, White hd, et al: The failure of orally administered glycoprotein IIb/IIIa inhibitors to prevent recurrent cardiac events. Am J Med 112:647, 2002.

S E C T I O N

III

Effector Mechanisms in Autoimmunity and Inflammation

16

Autoimmunity

BRIAN L. KOTZIN

Overview of Autoimmune Disease Pathogenesis

The human immune system has evolved to defend us from infection with potentially harmful microorganisms. One major component of this response depends on the specific recognition of foreign antigens by T and B lymphocytes. T cells (see Chapter 9) are distinguished by the presence of the T cell receptor for antigen (TCR) and recognize antigens presented by major histocompatibility complex (MHC) molecules on antigen-presenting cells. B cells (see Chapter 10) are identified by the expression of surface immunoglobulin (Ig), which functions as the specific B cell receptor (BCR) for antigen. The TCR and BCR repertoires are extremely diverse, and an individual's immune cells can collectively respond to an almost unlimited number of foreign antigens. Remarkably, these lymphocytes do not normally respond to the individual's own tissues. This selective unresponsiveness to self antigens, called *self-tolerance*, has long been recognized as a fundamental feature of the normal immune system. When self-tolerance fails, the resulting autoimmune reaction can be the basis for certain diseases, including certain systemic rheumatic diseases.

REQUIREMENTS FOR SELF-RECOGNITION AND TISSUE DAMAGE

Autoimmune diseases are a heterogeneous group of disorders in which recognition of self antigens by lymphocytes is centrally involved in pathologic organ damage. Not all immune-mediated destruction of self organs is autoimmune in nature. For example, the liver damage that occurs in hepatitis B infection is related primarily to immune responses directed at the virus and not at self liver antigens. In contrast, some autoimmune diseases, such as rheumatic heart disease, may initially be triggered by the immune response to an infectious organism, but the pathologic response is autoimmune in nature. In other situations, it is not clear whether the disease process is autoimmune. In chronic Lyme arthritis, for example, disease progression may be antibiotic resistant, and *Borrelia burgdorferi* antigens may be undetectable, but the T cells isolated from joints continue to show reactivity to this bacteria's outer surface protein-A antigens.[1] A subset of these T cells can cross-react with a normal lymphocyte protein, lymphocyte function–associated protein-1.[2] Whether chronic Lyme arthritis depends on T cells directed to undetectable but present bacterial antigens or depends on autoimmune responses has yet to be determined. Rheumatoid arthritis (RA), systemic sclerosis, Sjögren's syndrome, and polymyositis are marked by the production of various autoantibodies. However, antigens recognized by T cells at the sites of pathology have yet to be clearly defined as self or foreign.

CLASSIFYING AUTOIMMUNE DISEASES: ORGAN-SPECIFIC VERSUS SYSTEMIC AND ANTIBODY VERSUS T CELL MEDIATED

Autoimmune diseases can be divided into two broad categories: organ specific and systemic. Examples of relatively common organ-specific autoimmune diseases include thyroiditis, in which damage to thyroid cells may lead to hypothyroidism; type I diabetes, in which the insulin-secreting beta cells in pancreatic islets are destroyed; and multiple sclerosis, in which central nervous system myelin is damaged. There is an organ-specific autoimmune disease for almost every organ in the body (Table 16–1). Autoimmune diseases are also divided by whether pathology is mediated primarily through autoantibodies or autoreactive T cells (see Table 16–1). For example, in myasthenia gravis, autoantibodies to the muscle acetylcholine receptor are primarily responsible for receptor degradation and dysfunction leading to muscle weakness. In Graves' dis-

TABLE 16–1 • EXAMPLES OF ORGAN-SPECIFIC AUTOIMMUNE DISEASES

Organ	Disease(s)	Self Antigen (example)	Major Autoimmune Mechanism
Adrenal cells	Addison's disease	Cytochrome P450 antigens	Autoantibodies
Brain/spinal cord	Multiple sclerosis	Myelin proteins (myelin basic protein)	T cells
Eye	Uveitis	Uveal antigens	T cells
Gastrointestinal tract			
Stomach	Pernicious anemia	Gastric parietal cell antigens (H^+/ATPase, intrinsic factor)	Autoantibodies/T cells
Small bowel	Celiac sprue (gluten enteropathy)	Transglutaminase	Autoantibodies/T cells
Large bowel	Ulcerative colitis or Crohn's disease	Unknown	T cells
Heart	Myocarditis	Myocardial cell proteins (myosin)	Autoantibodies/T cells
	Rheumatic heart disease	Myocardial antigens	Autoantibodies
Hematopoietic system			
Platelets	Idiopathic thrombocytopenic purpura	Platelet antigens (GP IIb/IIIa)	Autoantibodies
Red blood cells	Autoimmune hemolytic anemia	Red blood cell membrane proteins	Autoantibodies
Neutrophils	Autoimmune neutropenia	Neutrophil membrane proteins	Autoantibodies
Kidney/lung	Goodpasture's disease	Basement membrane antigens (type IV collagen α3 chain)	Autoantibodies
Liver			
Bile duct cells	Primary biliary cirrhosis	Intrahepatic bile duct/ mitochondrial antigens/ 2-oxoacid dehydrogenase complexes (pyruvate dehydrogenase complex proteins)	Autoantibodies/T cells
Hepatocytes	Autoimmune hepatitis	Hepatocyte antigens (cytochrome P450IID6)	T cells/autoantibodies
Muscle	Myasthenia gravis	Acetylcholine receptors	Autoantibodies
Pancreatic islets	Type 1 diabetes	Beta-cell antigens (glutamic acid decarboxylase, insulin)	T cells (autoantibodies present)
Skin	Pemphigus/other bullous diseases	Desmogleins	Autoantibodies
Testis/ovaries	Orchitis/oophoritis	Unknown/multiple	Autoantibodies
Thyroid	Hashimoto's thyroiditis	Thyroid cell antigens (e.g., thyroglobulin)	T cells/autoantibodies
	Grave's disease	Thyroid-stimulating hormone receptor	Autoantibodies

Abbreviations: ATPase, adenosine triphosphatase; GP glycoprotein.

ease, autoantibodies bind to the thyroid-stimulating hormone receptor and cause hyperthyroidism. In contrast, T cells appear to be primarily responsible for the myelin damage and neurologic deficits in multiple sclerosis. The presence of autoantibodies does not necessarily imply a role in pathogenesis, because autoantibodies can just be a marker of the underlying T helper cell response. Such a scenario may occur in type 1 diabetes, in which IgG autoantibodies to insulin and other pancreatic islet cell antigens are generated, but islet cell destruction is mediated by $CD4^+$ and $CD8^+$ T cells.[3]

The best examples of systemic autoimmune diseases are certain rheumatic diseases such as systemic lupus erythematosus (SLE), RA, systemic sclerosis, Sjögren's syndrome, and polymyositis or dermatomyositis. SLE is considered to be the prototypic systemic autoimmune disease, and IgG autoantibodies directed to different autoantigens are primarily responsible for the multitude of possible clinical manifestations (see Chapter 74). Although $CD4^+$ T cells may not directly cause tissue damage in SLE, they clearly provide help for pathogenic autoantibodies. RA is commonly characterized as an organ- or joint-selective disease process, but it is systemic in that autoantibodies to organ-nonselective autoantigens, such as rheumatoid factor and citrulline-containing proteins, are usually present. Severe arthritis in RA is also frequently accompanied by extra-articular manifestations. The prevailing model of RA pathogenesis has been that synovial CD4+ T cells specific for self antigens are central to driving the disease process in the joint (see Chapter 65). Recent studies have also focused attention on B cells and on pathogenic autoantibodies, including those directed to systemic (widely expressed) antigens.[4]

MODEL FOR THE PATHOGENESIS OF AUTOIMMUNE DISEASE

The development of autoimmune disease in humans appears to be a multistep process. Figure 16–1 presents a conceptual framework for the pathogenesis of autoimmune disease. Considerable evidence from genetic epidemiology, association, and linkage studies indicates that the development of most autoimmune diseases has a strong genetic basis[5] (see Chapter 17). Studies in patients and animal models have emphasized that these diseases are complex genetic traits, usually with contributions from MHC genes and multiple non-MHC genes. Evidence also suggests that certain environmental influences may interact with this genetic predisposition to result in disease, although for most autoimmune diseases, environmental triggers remain undefined. Key to the pathogenesis of most autoimmune diseases seems to be the emergence of functional autoreactive CD4$^+$ T cells (see Fig. 16–1). In SLE and other autoantibody-mediated diseases, the development of disease also involves the emergence and activation of autoreactive B cells. Pathogenic autoantibody production in these diseases is CD4$^+$ T cell dependent. In other autoimmune diseases such as multiple sclerosis, autoreactive CD4$^+$ T cells and recruited macrophages appear to mediate end-organ damage directly or indirectly with CD8$^+$ T cells to cause pathology. The contribution of susceptibility genes may occur at several levels, from the breakdown of tolerance to the immune-mediated end-organ damage.[5]

AUTOIMMUNE DISEASE VERSUS AUTOIMMUNE CELLS

Self-reactive T cells and B cells are components of the normal immune system. A subset of these cells are potentially pathogenic, and they must be eliminated or maintained in an inactivated state to prevent a pathologic response to self tissues. Other self-reactive cells may actually function as part of the normal immune response. In experimental animal models, there is evidence that CD4$^+$ (particularly CD4$^+$CD25$^+$), CD8$^+$, and $\gamma\delta$ T cells may be involved in the downregulation of certain immune responses, and their absence may be associated with pathologic autoimmune responses. Although the specificity of most regulatory T cell populations has not been defined, some regulatory CD4$^+$CD25$^+$ cells have been shown to be self antigen–specific, and some regulatory CD8$^+$ T cells have been demonstrated to recognize peptides derived from the TCR.[6-9] Such protective autoreactive T cells should not be confused with those that drive autoimmune disease.

Even stronger arguments can be made for the presence of nonpathogenic, autoreactive B cells in the normal immune system, because they can be more easily marked by the antibodies that they secrete. A relatively large fraction of serum Igs in healthy animals and humans bind to self antigens, and a major subset of these autoantibodies has been labeled natural autoantibodies[10,11] (see Chapter 10). Most of these antibodies are IgM, bind to self antigens with relatively low affinity, frequently cross-react with multiple antigens, and are independent of T cell help for production. Natural autoantibodies appear to be an important component of the normal immune system, and B cells with these self specificities are positively selected during development.[11] Their cross-reactivity to bacterial glycoproteins or glycolipids may be part of the early immune response to pathogens. Natural autoantibodies also function to help in the clearance of senescent cells or cell constituents after cell death or in the removal of immune complexes.[12] Studies in humans and mice also suggest that a major portion of these autoantibodies are secreted by the B-1 B cell lineage, including CD5$^+$ B cells[10,11] (see Chapter 10). The genetic origin and characteristics of pathogenic autoantibodies, as in SLE, are mostly different from those of natural autoantibodies. B cells producing natural autoantibodies should be recognized as another component of the normal immune system and distinguished from potentially pathologic B cells.

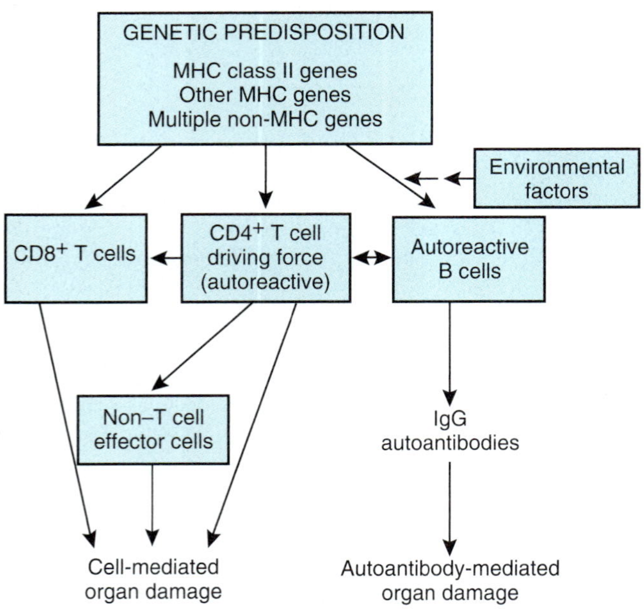

FIGURE 16–1 · **Steps Involved in the Pathogenesis of Autoimmune Disease.** Though not shown here, the contribution of susceptibility genes may occur at several levels, from the breakdown of tolerance to immune-mediated end-organ damage.

Experimental Animal Models

Studies using animal models have contributed greatly to our understanding of the immunopathogenesis of autoimmune disease. Models of disease can be divided into three broad categories based on how or why disease developed: spontaneously occurring and dependent on the combination of genes in an inbred strain; induced by immunization, cell transfer, thymectomy, viral infection, or chemical exposure; and developing after genetic manipulation, usually by transgenic expression or knockout of single genes. In addition to these models of disease, genetically manipulated TCR and BCR transgenic mice have also been invaluable in studies of self-reactive T cells and B cells.

ANIMAL MODELS WITH SPONTANEOUS DISEASE

The animal models most similar to human autoimmune disease include strains that develop a very high incidence of disease spontaneously. Examples include the nonobese diabetic (NOD) mouse,[13] which develops a disease similar to type I diabetes, and several models of lupus-like disease.[14-17] The best characterized lupus-prone strains are New Zealand hybrid mice, in which crosses or inbred recombinant strains of New Zealand black (NZB) and New Zealand white (NZW) mice develop lupus-like disease; the MRL strain; and the BXSB strain. MRL-*lpr/lpr* (also referred to as MRL-Fas^{lpr}) mice, which are homozygous for the *lymphoproliferation (lpr)* mutation in the gene encoding Fas, demonstrate an accelerated form of disease compared with non-*lpr* littermates.[18] *Lpr* and related mutations affecting apoptosis are discussed in Chapter 26. All of these murine lupus models develop a progressive immune complex–mediated glomerulonephritis associated with high levels of IgG autoantibodies to nuclear antigens, including double-stranded DNA (dsDNA). Extrarenal disease manifestations variably occur in these models and include lymphoproliferation with splenomegaly and lymphadenopathy, hemolytic anemia, autoimmune thrombocytopenia, vasculitis, and thrombosis. A subset of MRL-*lpr/lpr* mice also develop arthritis associated with rheumatoid-factor production. All of these lupus-prone strains exhibit premature thymic atrophy, the significance of which is unknown. Several different autoimmune strains (NOD, NZB, MRL-*lpr/lpr*) also demonstrate salivary and lacrimal gland pathology that is characteristic of Sjögren's syndrome.

The spontaneous animal models of human autoimmune disease have provided systems to dissect genetic contributions to disease.[15,16,19,20] The ability to study many related offspring with similar disease manifestations after directed breeding of autoimmune and nonautoimmune strains is a great advantage compared to genetic studies of the human disease. Studies of these animal models, in contrast to patients, also offer the opportunity to control environmental exposures. Expression of disease in experimental crosses can be made to be solely a reflection of the genes inherited, their penetrance, and how the products of these genes interact. Spontaneous animal models also permit the characterization of immunologic changes before, during, and after disease development. Early immunologic abnormalities that are central to disease development can be distinguished from later defects that are secondary to disease.

ANIMAL MODELS IN WHICH DISEASE IS INDUCED BY IMMUNOLOGIC MANIPULATION

A second category of the experimental models depends on induction of disease in susceptible strains, such as after immunization with a self antigen. Although most of these immunization models use organ-specific antigens (e.g., myelin basic protein, acetylcholine receptor, thyroglobulin, retinal antigens, type II collagen), some models have used ubiquitous nuclear antigens to induce lupus-like autoantibodies and disease.[21-23] One of the best characterized organ-specific models is experimental autoimmune encephalomyelitis (EAE), in which central nervous system demyelination and paralysis are induced in animals after immunization with myelin proteins (e.g., myelin basic protein) or peptides derived from these antigens.[24,25] EAE is studied as a model of multiple sclerosis. Effective immunization frequently requires that antigen be administered in the presence of adjuvant, usually complete Freund's adjuvant, which is a mixture of mineral oil and mycobacterial protein. EAE has provided important insight into the mechanisms by which myelin-specific T cells, recruited macrophages, and their various cytokines mediate myelin destruction. Studies of multiple sclerosis patients have also indicated that the antigens used to induce EAE are likely targeted in the human disease.[25] Whether they represent initiating immune responses or late autoimmune reactions in response to released myelin antigens is unclear.

One well-studied model possibly relevant to inflammatory arthritis in humans is collagen-induced arthritis in which mice or rats are usually immunized with type II collagen isolated from bovine, chicken, or human cartilage.[26,27] In susceptible mouse strains, cross-reactivity of immune responses to murine type II collagen, involving autoreactive T cells and autoantibodies, results in the development of a peripheral arthritis. This model has provided insight into the effector mechanisms that lead to inflammation in patients with arthritis.[28] Other cartilage proteins can also be used to induce arthritis in susceptible mice.[29] Despite reminiscent synovial pathology, it is not clear whether these rodent models of induced arthritis are recapitulating the specific immune responses in RA. None result in rheumatoid-factor production. A modification in studies of collagen-induced arthritis involved the use of mice expressing transgenes encoding RA-relevant human MHC class II molecules, including HLA-DRB1* 0401 and *0101.[27] Whether these transgenic mice will provide more insight into T cell recognition in RA depends on whether collagen epitopes are truly recognized by synovial CD4$^+$ T cells in RA, which remains an unresolved issue.[30]

A variety of other induced models of disease have been developed. Several involve the transfer of CD4$^+$ T cell populations in rodents. For example, induction of chronic graft-versus-host disease in rodents has been used to study lupus-like autoantibody production and immune complex glomerulonephritis.[31] Another example of induced autoimmunity is the development of multiorgan autoimmunity (i.e., gastritis, oophoritis/orchitis, and thyroiditis) when thymectomy is performed within the first few days of life. Studies have indicated that thymectomy removes a population of CD4$^+$ CD25$^+$ regulatory T cells that normally prevents the development of autoimmunity.[6,7] Overall, the relevance of the induced animal models to spontaneous human autoimmune disease remains to be demonstrated. Still, the induced models of disease have provided important lessons regarding the immune mechanisms that lead to autoimmune pathologic damage. One recurring principle is that potentially pathogenic autoreactive T and B cells are components of the normal peripheral lymphocyte repertoires. Preventing autoreactive cells normally present in peripheral lymphoid organs from responding to self tissues must therefore be key to the maintenance of self-tolerance.

ANIMAL MODELS WITH AUTOIMMUNE DISEASE AFTER GENETIC MANIPULATION

A third category of experimental disease model involves genetically engineering a single gene deficiency (gene knockout) or single gene overexpression (by transgene). It is remarkable how many gene perturbations have resulted in the development of an autoimmune syndrome. For example, lupus-like disease has resulted from genetic deficiencies that cause defects in lymphocyte apoptosis, unregulated B cell or T cell activation, defects in the ability to clear apoptotic cells or cellular debris, and altered cytokine production.[5] Knockouts of interleukin 2 (IL-2), IL-2 receptor (IL-2R), IL-10, various T cell subsets, and certain TCR gene complexes have been shown to cause inflammatory colitis.[5,32] In some cases, the background of the strain in which the knockout is placed can greatly alter the form of immunopathology. For example, IL-2 gene knockouts can lead to inflammatory colitis or autoimmune hemolytic anemia, depending on the genetic background to which the mutation is bred.[32] Knockout of the gene that encodes the type IIB low affinity receptor for IgG (FcγRIIB) results in a severe lupus-like syndrome when bred on one type of non-autoimmune (C57BL/6) background but almost no pathology on a different non-autoimmune (BALB/c) background.[33] This genetic deficiency results in unregulated B cell activation, and the reason for the different expression on the two different genetic backgrounds is currently unclear. The single gene models do not recapitulate the complex genetics of human autoimmune disease, but are useful to point to particular genes and mechanistic pathways for study in human disease. For example, knockout mice have provided at least a partial basis for genetic studies in humans that have identified SLE patients with deficient DNAse I genes [34,35] and with variant alleles of the gene encoding programmed death-1 (PD-1), which negatively regulates T cells and B cells after activation.[36,37]

Genetic manipulations have produced surprising systems to study the development of autoimmune disease, including arthritis. For example, a model generating wide interest (referred to as the K/B × N model)[38,39] involves mice with transgenes encoding a TCR that recognizes a foreign antigen (bovine ribonuclease) in the context of the mouse MHC class II allele, I-A^{k}. As in other TCR transgenics, nearly all of the T cells in these mice express one type of TCR. Remarkably, when these TCR transgenic mice are bred with mice expressing a different MHC class II molecule (I-A^{g7} from the NOD strain), the progeny develop a severe and destructive arthritis with histologic features reminiscent of RA.[38] These investigators subsequently showed that in the context of I-A^{g7}, the transgenic TCR recognizes a peptide derived from a self glycolytic enzyme (glucose-6-phosphate isomerase [GPI]), and this unexpected cross-reactivity allows for a T cell–dependent IgG antibody response to this ubiquitous cytoplasmic antigen.[39] The arthritis in these mice is mediated by autoantibodies, and transfer of a small amount of anti-GPI autoantibody causes severe arthritis in recipients. Recent studies have shown that the arthritogenic antibodies form immune complexes that mediate damage through activation of the alternative pathway of complement on the articular surface.[40] Damage also requires mast cells and other cells with type III low affinity receptors for IgG (FcγRIII), neutrophils, and the production of inflammatory cytokines such as IL-1 and tumor necrosis factor-α (TNF-α).[41] Recent studies have also provided insight into how an immune response to a widely expressed autoantigen drives a disease limited to progressive destructive arthritis.[40] Although GPI may not be an autoantigen relevant to RA, this model may have important implications for pathogenic mechanisms in the human disease.

Genetically manipulated mice have also been useful for study of mechanisms of tolerance, the initiation of autoimmune responses, and molecules required for the development of autoimmune disease.[42] The insights have been tremendous and could not have been accomplished in human studies. Experimental systems have frequently used mice expressing transgenes that encode a TCR or BCR specific for one autoantigen or for an exogenous antigen introduced genetically so as to become an autoantigen. In these mice, large numbers of T or B cells with the same autoreactive receptor can be easily identified and tracked, greatly facilitating their characterization. Transgenes encoding autoreactive TCR and BCR transgenes have also been bred onto autoimmune backgrounds to help elucidate the mechanisms by which self-tolerance may fail in autoimmune disease. Results from these systems have provided important insight into the multiple checkpoints involved in T cell and B cell tolerance.

Genetic Basis of Autoimmune Disease

Considerable evidence indicates that all of the common autoimmune diseases (e.g., SLE, RA, type I diabetes, multiple sclerosis) have a strong genetic predisposition.[5,15-16,19-20,43-45] Much of this evidence has come from genetic epidemiology studies that determine disease prevalence within families in which there is an affected individual compared to the prevalence in the general population and from analyses of disease prevalence in identical versus nonidentical twins (see Chapter 17). Autoimmune diseases are complex genetic traits, which, by definition, are not inherited in a simple Mendelian way. Multiple genes determine susceptibility to autoimmune disease, and no particular gene is necessary or sufficient for disease expression. The low penetrance of each contributing gene (i.e., the small increase in probability of disease expression given a particular disease allele) is the main reason why autoimmune diseases are so complex genetically. Overt autoimmune disease frequently does not occur even in the presence of a full complement of susceptibility alleles, as in the identical twin of an affected individual. Genetic complexity in autoimmunity is also determined by genetic heterogeneity, in which the same phenotype (e.g., anti-dsDNA autoantibody production or lupus nephritis) is the result of a different set of genes. Gene alleles that increase the risk of autoimmune disease also can be frequent in the general population, making their identification as a disease allele difficult.

Most genetic studies of human patients have focused on the association of particular alleles with disease. MHC genes and other immunologically relevant genes have been the main targets for intensive scrutiny (see Chapter 17). Association studies are, however, potentially subject to inherent biases such that spurious associations are revealed because of the lack of appropriate controls. The interpretation of associations may be further complicated by the presence of linkage disequilibrium with the actual causal gene. Trying to identify the gene that underlies the association of type I diabetes, RA, and SLE with particular MHC haplotypes exemplifies this difficulty (discussed later).[43,46] Association studies also require an a priori hypothesis that a particular candidate gene is involved in the disease process and, therefore, are not suitable to investigate the many unknown non-MHC genetic contributions to disease.

A significant advance in recent years has been the development of techniques to map the position of disease susceptibility loci in genome-wide screens without regard to candidate genes.[5,15,19-20,43] The availability of easy to use maps of markers that cover the entire mouse and human genomes has revolutionized the study of non-MHC genes that predispose to autoimmunity. These markers can be used in linkage analyses to map the chromosomal positions of genetic loci linked with disease and therefore identify regions of the genome that contain disease-susceptibility genes. Genetic mapping studies have been reported in many of the common autoimmune diseases, including type I diabetes, multiple sclerosis, SLE, and RA, as well as murine models of these diseases[5,15-16,19-20,38,43-45,47] (see Chapter17).

In studies of patients with autoimmune diseases, some investigators have observed that different autoimmune diseases appear to be increased in frequency in the same families.[5] This is exemplified by the patient with SLE or with myositis who has family members with other systemic rheumatic diseases or organ-specific autoimmune diseases. It is also true that autoimmune type I diabetes, autoimmune thyroiditis, Addison's disease, autoimmune polyendocrine syndromes, vitiligo, and celiac disease are increased in frequency in some families. These observations have raised a question about whether there are autoimmunity genes that may contribute to separate autoimmune diseases in different individuals. Polymorphism in the autoimmune regulator (*AIRE*) gene leads to autoimmune polyendocrine syndrome-1 (APS-1), in which patients can demonstrate autoimmune disease affecting different endocrine organs.[48] Furthermore, studies suggest that an allelic variation of the gene encoding cytotoxic T lymphocyte-associated antigen-4 (CTLA-4) contributes to type I diabetes, Graves' disease, and autoimmune thyroiditis.[49] The idea that one gene variation can lead to different autoimmune diseases has also been supported by studies in animal models.[5,50]

ASSOCIATION OF MAJOR HISTOCOMPATIBILITY COMPLEX GENES WITH AUTOIMMUNE DISEASE

Molecules encoded by genes within the MHC have a powerful influence on immune responses, and the association between particular MHC haplotypes and different autoimmune diseases has been repeatedly confirmed (see Chapter 17). In humans, the human leukocyte antigen (HLA) region spans approximately 3.6 megabases and encompasses more than 200 genes. Tight linkage of genes in this region has made it difficult to identify the specific HLA genes (and alleles) that explain the association of a particular haplotype (usually identified by its HLA-DR and DQ genes) with autoimmune disease. Within a given ethnic group, certain HLA-DR alleles are frequently inherited with a similar set of DQ alleles. A disease associated with one DR type could be related to the DRB1 gene encoding the DR β-chain or to other MHC genes inherited with it. In whites, for example, type I diabetes and RA have been associated with DR4, but the molecular basis for these associations is different in each disease.

Although type I diabetes is clearly polygenic in inheritance, it has been estimated that class II MHC molecules (e.g., HLA-DR and DQ contribute to more than 50 percent of this heritability.[3] About 95 percent of diabetic patients possess either HLA-DR3 or DR4 compared with 45 to 55 percent of the normal population. The increased risk of disease related to each DR type is approximately fivefold. Individuals who carry both DR3 and DR4 have the greatest risk (relative risk greater than 20), whereas individuals who carry DR2 are protected from developing disease. Studies investigating disease associations showed that only those DR4 individuals with an associated DQB1*0302 allele (HLA-DQ8) are predisposed to develop disease. Additional studies, including those in different ethnic populations, have supported the conclusion that positive and negative associations of DR types with disease are primarily explained by the DQ allele, especially DQB1 allele, inherited in linkage disequilibrium with DR.

The major genetic contribution to RA involves particular DRB1 alleles[43,51] (see chapters 17 and 65). DRB1*0401 and *0404 predominate in white patients, but other DR4 subtypes (*0405, *0408), as well as DRB1*0101, *1402, and *1001, also have been implicated in disease susceptibility. In contrast to type I diabetes, linked DQ alleles do not explain these associations with disease. Instead, the disease-associated DR alleles all share a sequence motif at positions 67 to 74 (L-L-E-Q-R/K-R-A-A) in the third hypervariable region of the DRB1 gene. This shared segment has been called the shared epitope.[43] The increased risk for disease development has been estimated to be fivefold to sixfold for DRB1*0404 and *0401, with absolute risks of 1 in 20 and 1 in 35, respectively. For individuals carrying both alleles (i.e., *0401/*0404), the increased risk for developing RA has been estimated to be about 30-fold, with an absolute risk of 1 in 7.[51] Individuals with two *04 alleles also appear to have an increased risk of more severe destructive joint disease and extra-articular involvement. The association of particular DR alleles with RA is frequently cited as the most compelling evidence for the important role of CD4+ T cells in this disease.

Until recently, a clear association between particular MHC haplotypes and development of SLE in general had been difficult to establish. For example, modest associations of HLA-DR3 (DRB1*0301) and DR2 (DRB1*1501) have been demonstrated in white individuals with SLE. The increased risk from haplotypes with these HLA-DR alleles has been recently confirmed in transmission disequilibrium studies in families with SLE.[46] Although it has been suggested that the association of particular haplotypes with SLE relates to genes away from DR and DQ genes, such as the genes encoding complement component C4A and tumor neciosis factor-α (TNF-α), studies using a dense map of markers across the HLA region strongly suggested that it is the class II genes (e.g., DR and DQ) that underlie the increased risk of disease from a particular HLA haplotypes.[46] A strong association of SLE with particular class II alleles has also been demonstrated when patients are grouped according to the specific types of autoantibodies produced. Autoantibodies to Ro/SS-A (plus La/SS-B), U1RNP, Sm, phospholipids (i.e., anticardiolipin antibodies or the lupus anticoagulant), and dsDNA have been associated with particular DQ alleles. These data suggest that the contribution of class II MHC molecules in SLE is predominantly at the level of specific autoantibody production, consistent with an effect on CD4+ T cell help.

ASSOCIATION OF NON–MAJOR HISTOCOMPATIBILITY COMPLEX GENES WITH AUTOIMMUNE DISEASE

Multiple non-MHC genes have been studied for associations with autoimmune diseases. For example, studies of SLE have addressed genes encoding complement genes, Fc receptor alleles, mannose-binding protein, various cytokines such as IL-10 and TNF-α, and gene segments of the TCR and Ig gene complexes. A review of these studies and their implications is not possible in this chapter (see Chapter 74).

Alleles determining deficiencies of classic pathway complement components have demonstrated strong associations with SLE[52] (see Chapter 22). For example, most individuals with genetically determined complete deficiencies of complement C1q or C1r/C1s develop a syndrome resembling SLE. C2 and C4, encoded within MHC, also have alleles that result in deficiencies, and complete deficiencies of these molecules markedly increase the risk of disease. The association of these deficiency states and SLE is likely to be an etiologic one, but the mechanism for the influence of genetic complement deficiencies in SLE is unknown. Studies have suggested that complement deficiencies may lead to lupus through defects in the clearance of apoptotic cells and cellular debris (as in DNase I–deficient humans and mice[34,35]) or alternatively through defects in the clearance of immune complexes.[52] These genetic contributions may allow enhanced deposition or formation of immune complexes in the kidney or possibly affect the inflammatory response or end-organ response to complexes.

Associations have also been demonstrated between SLE and alleles of the genes encoding cell surface low-affinity receptors for IgG (i.e., Fcγ receptors).[53,54] For example, investigators have demonstrated an association between SLE and alleles of the gene encoding FcγRIIA (CD32), expressed on monocytes or macrophages and neutrophils.[53] Alleles of this gene differ substantially in the ability to bind human IgG2, and studies found a decrease in the prevalence of the high-affinity binding allele in SLE, particularly in patients with lupus nephritis. Thus, possibly similar to complement deficiencies, the genetic contribution of this Fcγ receptor deficiency may reflect a relatively late event in the pathophysiologic scheme of SLE-related immune complex damage, such as in lupus nephritis. Consistent with this hypothesis, other studies have noted the underrepresentation of a high-binding FcγRIIIA allele (expressed on natural killer [NK] cells and monocytes) in patients with SLE, especially with lupus nephritis.[54] The Fcγ receptor molecules and related pathways appear to be extremely important in immune complex–mediated glomerulonephritis and the generation of lupus-like disease. In studies of the (NZB × NZW)F_1 mouse model, knockout of FcγRIII function had no apparent effect on the deposition of immune complexes in glomeruli but markedly reduced the development of severe lupus nephritis.[55] In contrast, knockout of the gene encoding FcγRIIB, which negatively regulates B cell activation, causes lupus-like disease in normal mice.[33]

LINKAGE ANALYSES AND THE IDENTIFICATION OF OTHER GENES IN AUTOIMMUNE DISEASE

The chromosomal positions of various susceptibility loci have been mapped in backcross or intercross analyses of NOD mice, murine models of lupus, and induced models of autoimmune disease (e.g., collagen-induced arthritis and EAE).[5,15-16,19-20,26] Linkage analyses of families with affected siblings have also been reported in human type I diabetes, autoimmune polyendocrine syndromes, autoimmune thyroid diseases, multiple sclerosis, SLE, and RA.[5,15-16,19-20,43-49] Although the susceptibility genes underlying most of these mapped loci have not been identified, recent studies suggest that interesting variants of molecules involved in immune function will underlie the contribution of certain loci and that the elucidation of these alleles will provide new insight into normal immune functioning and the development of autoimmune disease. For example, a chromosome 2q33 locus mapped in human families with type 1 diabetes and autoimmune thyroid disease has led to the identification of a variant allele of the gene encoding CTLA-4 and points to an important role for alternative splice forms of this gene.[49,50] Furthermore, studies of a susceptibility locus in NOD mice, mapped to the analogous region in the mouse genome (proximal chromosome-1), has led to a newly discovered form of the CTLA-4 molecule.[49] Studies of the *AIRE* gene, which is responsible for autoimmune disease of different endocrine organs, suggest that defects in this gene may lead to autoimmunity by affecting central tolerance of organ-specific antigens.[48,56,57] In type 1 diabetes, other identified susceptibility genes based on linkage analyses include the insulin gene in the human disease and probably the gene encoding IL-2 in the NOD mouse model.[5]

Gene identification following linkage studies in human SLE and mouse models of lupus have also begun to provide new insight into the immunopathogenesis of disease. For example, one study of human families has suggested that a locus on chromosome 2 is related to a polymorphism in the gene encoding PD-1 (*PDCD1* gene), which provides a downregulatory signal after T cell activation.[37] In mouse lupus, the interferon-inducible gene *Ifi202* has been proposed as the major candidate gene for a NZB lupus-susceptibility locus on mouse distal chromosome 1.[58] Studies suggest that increased expression of this transcription factor leads to lupus through inhibition of B lymphocyte apoptosis (see below). Identification of an interferon-inducible gene in lupus susceptibility may also relate to recent studies in both human SLE and mouse models of lupus that have emphasized the potential role of type 1 interferons (IFN-α/β) in the pathogenesis of this disease.[59,60]

An important step forward in understanding genetic contributions in lupus also relates to the identification of *lpr* and *gld* in murine studies as mutations in Fas and Fas ligand, respectively. These genes are involved in programmed cell death (i.e., apoptosis), and the traits resulting from these mutations have been described extensively (see Chapter 26). Homozygosity for these mutations results in the acceleration of lupus-like autoimmunity and in a massive accumulation of $CD4^-$ $CD8^-$ (double negative) T cells.[18] Although the mechanism by which mutations in Fas lead to accelerated autoimmunity is unknown, the strongest hypothesis is that self-reactive T and B cells arise when they fail to undergo apoptosis normally. Studies have shown that T cells and B cells must carry the *lpr* mutation for maximal autoantibody production to occur. Fas may not be so important in central (intrathymic) tolerance during T cell development. Instead, studies support the contention that peripheral T cell tolerance mechanisms are primarily affected by the *lpr* mutation. Studies also suggest that central B cell tolerance may be relatively independent of Fas, and surface expression of Fas on B cells may be most important in preventing inappropriate CD4 T cell–dependent expansion of autoreactive B cells in the periphery.[61] *Fas* mutations have been identified in a few children with lymphoproliferative syndromes and evidence of autoimmunity[62] (see Chapter 26). However, there is no counterpart to the *lpr* or *gld* phenotype in human SLE, and studies have found defects of these genes in SLE patients. There is a belief that other genes involved only in very rare apoptosis or related cell-signaling pathways may be involved in the genetic susceptibility and pathogenesis of the human disease.

Overall, there is great optimism that many more of the non-MHC genes that contribute to autoimmunity will be defined in the next few years. Because the genes that predispose to autoimmunity are almost certainly related to primary events in pathogenesis, their identification will provide additional insight into the development of autoimmunity and the cause of autoimmune disease.

Environmental Triggers and Influences

It seems likely that environmental triggers or influences interact with susceptibility genes to result in autoimmune disease (see Fig. 16–1). However, the effect of environment in autoimmune disease has been extremely difficult to define. In some diseases, this may reflect the fact that such a trigger does not exist or that it is ubiquitous in different populations. Relevant to rheumatic diseases, one example of the latter may be infection with Epstein-Barr virus (EBV), which is highly prevalent in most adult populations worldwide.

Geographic clustering not explained by genetic variation is strongly suggestive of an environmental effect. Clustering has been documented in multiple sclerosis and type I diabetes but not in SLE or RA.[3,5,25,63] Case reports and epidemiologic studies suggest that infection with particular viruses, such as congenital rubella or enteroviruses, is associated with an increased risk of developing type I diabetes in susceptible individuals.

Studies of animal models have also emphasized that stochastic events are important in the development of autoimmunity and expression of autoimmune disease. The fact that approximately 75 percent of monozygotic twins are discordant for SLE has been used as evidence to support the existence of an environmental trigger in this disease. However, lupus-prone strains of mice can also be created such that 25 percent reproducibly develop disease or produce particular autoantibodies, and careful examination of positive mice has excluded environmental effects as the major factor in variable expression.[5,15] In these mice, the probability of disease appears to be almost totally genetically determined, and unknown stochastic (random) events appear to determine which mouse will develop disease. The mechanism for this stochastic expression of disease remains unknown.

The most important environmental agents to consider in the triggering of autoimmune diseases are infectious microorganisms.[5] Infections of target tissues could result in the release or expression of normally sequestered antigens or in the ability to present self antigens that are normally prevented from being exposed to the immune system.[64] Closely tied to this effect may be the release of inflammatory cytokines at the infected site and surrounding lymphoid tissues, which mobilizes and activates inflammatory cells to allow effective presentation of foreign and also self antigens. The release of IL-12, IFN-γ, and IFN-α/β, for example, may promote the development of a pathologic T helper type 1 (Th1)-type response with resulting tissue damage (see below). Infections may also induce an immune response to the pathogen that cross-reacts with some host antigen.[5] Examples of this molecular mimicry leading to human autoimmune disease are described later. It is also possible that an immune response to an infectious pathogen may affect the immune system in a general manner, tipping the balance toward pathogenic autoimmunity. This may involve the release of various inflammatory cytokines systemically, a shift from Th2 to Th1 T cell responses (see Chapter 9), or interference with normal regulatory pathways.

The possible viral cause of RA and SLE has been vigorously pursued. Data showing the presence of an etiologic virus in the joints of patients have been elusive. One agent that continues to generate interest in RA and SLE is EBV.[65,66] Studies have shown that RA patients generate increased and qualitatively different antibody responses, as well as different T cell responses to the virus and its effects. Studies have also shown that a subset of clonally expanded CD8+ T cells in the joints of patients are directed to EBV proteins. One study showed that children with SLE have a higher prevalence of EBV infection than control groups.[67] Which condition is predisposing to the other has yet to be clarified.

Environmental influences on the expression of disease manifestations are also seen in autoimmune diseases. In SLE, for example, exacerbation of rash or systemic symptoms after sun exposure and exacerbations of disease after viral or bacterial infections have been readily observed in patients. It is possible that the latter associations are related to the exacerbating influence of interferons on disease activity in SLE.[59,60] Changes in disease activity have also been noted after administration of exogenous hormones. Epidemiologic data and studies of animal models support the contention that estrogens can increase the risk of developing SLE or exacerbate disease. The mechanism for how disease is affected in these situations is unknown.

Long-term treatment of patients with certain drugs (e.g., procainamide, hydralazine) can induce the production of antinuclear antibodies and a lupus-like disease. Understanding how this occurs, perhaps through studies of animals given these drugs, may provide insights into the development of autoimmunity in SLE. However, drug-induced lupus is not the same as induction of SLE in individuals predisposed to develop SLE. It appears to be a different disease in a different subset of the population who have different genetic predispositions.

Cellular Mechanisms of Autoimmune Disease

T CELL DEPENDENCE OF DISEASE

A large body of evidence suggests that $CD4^+$ T cells are required for the full expression of most autoimmune diseases. For example, essentially all spontaneous murine models of lupus, models of type I diabetes, and models of induced autoimmune disease have shown the importance of $CD4^+$ T cells.[68] Treatment of these animals with monoclonal antibodies to the CD4 surface molecule results in the deletion or blocking of these cells and prevents disease. Similar studies in human patients have been difficult to accomplish, but the same conclusion seems likely based on associations of disease with MHC class II genes, the presence of infiltrating $CD4^+$ T cells at the sites of pathology in various organ-specific autoimmune diseases, and the pattern of IgG autoantibody production in autoantibody-mediated diseases. Pathogenic autoantibodies in SLE, for example, reflect isotype switching and somatic mutation.[68] These B cell differentiation events require the presence of $CD4^+$ T cell help (see Chapter 10). Table 16–2 presents the most frequently cited evidence to support a primary role of $CD4^+$ T cells in RA. The importance of $CD4^+$ T cells in the initiation and perpetuation of RA has been a controversial issue, mostly related to studies showing that T cell–derived cytokines are scarce in synovium compared to those derived from macrophage or fibroblast cells, and related to the failure to define the antigens to which the synovial T cells are responding.[69] Although therapies directed against T cells and T cell products have shown some efficacy in RA, the effects have been weak compared to therapies directed against TNF-α. (see chapters 61 and 67).

ORIGIN OF AUTOREACTIVE T CELLS IN AUTOIMMUNE DISEASE

The TCR repertoire of early immature T cells appears to depend solely on the random rearrangement of TCR genes. Subsequently, two major processes in the thymus modify this repertoire (see Chapter 9). One process positively selects cells that have some TCR affinity for self-MHC/peptides and allows mature cells to eventually recognize foreign antigens in the context of self-MHC (i.e., self-MHC restriction). Cells that are not positively selected undergo programmed cell death within the thymus. The other intrathymic process deletes T cells that have a high level of self-reactivity (i.e., negative selection). In the most prevalent model, cells that are positively selected by an interaction with class II MHC molecules mature into the $CD4^+$ pop-

TABLE 16–2 • EVIDENCE FOR A CENTRAL ROLE FOR CD4+ T CELLS IN THE PATHOGENESIS OF RHEUMATOID ARTHRITIS

1. Association of disease susceptibility, disease severity, or both with particular class II major histocompatibility complex (MHC) alleles (i.e., HLA-DRB1 shared epitope)
2. Infiltration of synovial tissue with T cells, including activated $CD4^+$ T cells
3. Studies of T cell receptor (TCR) repertoire showing TCR $V\beta^+$ subset expansions, oligoclonal expansions, and accumulation of related T cell clones
4. Association of disease with TCR gene–complex alleles
5. Role of T cells in the production of cytokines by non–T cells
6. Improvement of disease with therapies directed against T cells or T cell products
7. Role of T cells in experimental models of inflammatory arthritis

ulation, whereas cells that are positively selected on class I MHC molecules become the CD8+ population. Mature thymocytes subsequently migrate to peripheral lymphoid tissues, where they maintain these surface characteristics.

There is little evidence to support the contention that defects in central (intrathymic) tolerance lead to systemic autoimmune disease such as SLE.[68] Studies using lupus mice have repeatedly shown that high-affinity responses to self antigens are tolerized normally in the thymus. In contrast, accumulating data suggest that defects in central tolerance may underlie disease in some individuals with organ-specific autoimmunity, such as patients with autoimmune endocrine diseases.[56,57] In addition, studies in the NOD mouse model of type 1 diabetes suggest that a component of the non-MHC genetic contribution may be at the level of central tolerance.[70]

Clonal deletion in the thymus may be the major process for eliminating T cells reactive to self antigens with high affinity, as long as the antigen is present or expressed in the thymus during T cell development. Studies have indicated that a number of antigens previously thought to be organ specific and organ sequestered are indeed expressed and presented in the thymus presumably for the purpose of self tolerance.[56,57] Still, a number of organ-sequestered antigens are never presented adequately in the thymus, and intrathymic tolerance is inadequate for antigens modified in the peripheral organs. T cells specific for such autoantigens can reach the peripheral lymph nodes and spleen, and peripheral self-tolerance mechanisms must prevent activation of these autoreactive T cells. Any self antigen needs to be processed and presented with MHC molecules to allow for negative selection in the thymus. Dominant determinants of an antigen are presented efficiently. In contrast, other determinants are not presented adequately, and cells capable of recognizing these peptides can escape central tolerance and be part of the normal peripheral T cell repertoire. This would include determinants that are created only in the periphery by proteolysis during inflammation and also by post-translational modifications of peptides, such as glycosylation or citrullination.[71,72] Studies have shown that T cells with self-reactive TCRs are present in the peripheral lymphoid organs and circulation of healthy individuals, but they are not sufficient for the development of autoimmune disease. As discussed previously, several well-studied animal models are generated by immunization of animals with peripheral organ antigens, such as type II collagen in collagen-induced arthritis and myelin proteins in EAE. In addition, immunization of normal mice with nuclear antigens has resulted in lupus-like autoantibody production.[21-23,73-75]

A number of mechanisms appear to help prevent peripheral self-reactive T cells from mediating autoimmune responses[42] (Table 16–3). Perhaps most important is the maintenance of autoreactive T cells in an ignorant state. This self-tolerance process appears to prevent the T cell from recognizing its autoantigen or to prevent the self antigen from being effectively presented to a self-reactive T cell. For example, resting T cells with self-reactive potential may not be able to

TABLE 16–3 • PROPOSED MECHANISMS OF PERIPHERAL TOLERANCE AND ACTIVATION OF AUTOREACTIVE T CELLS

Tolerance	Activation
Immune ignorance	Release of sequestered antigens Breakdown in immune privilege Aberrant expression of MHC class II Increased expression of autoantigen/MHC class II Molecular mimicry Epitope spreading
Deletion	Defects in apoptosis
Anergy (functional inactivation)	Release of inflammatory mediators (e.g., after infection) Inadequate tolerance promoting costimulation
Lack of costimulation	Increased expression or function of costimulatory molecules
Regulatory T cells	Decreased cell number or function
Regulatory cytokine pattern (Immune deviation)	Release of inflammatory mediators (e.g., after infection) Altered Th1/Th2 pattern in cytokine production
Downregulation of TCR or coreceptors	

Abbreviations: MHC, major histocompatibility complex; TCR, T cell receptor.

traffic to certain tissues or find their target antigens presented by the type of antigen-presenting cells necessary for T cell activation. Infiltrating T cells may also be silenced or induced to die at a site of immune privilege, such as the eye. Bypassing these protective mechanisms can lead to autoimmune disease. Examples may include the release of organ-sequestered antigens, aberrant expression of class II antigens, and autoreactive T cell activation triggered by an infectious agent. In the latter case, autoreactive T cells may then be able to traffic to tissues and be activated inappropriately by self antigens presented by macrophages or B cells.

A number of mechanisms participate in the peripheral tolerance process (see Table 16–3). To effectively present antigenic peptides, antigen-presenting cells must be capable of performing at least two functions: processing and displaying peptides together with MHC molecules on their cell surface for interaction with the TCR (signal 1) and providing the other accessory signals (costimulation) necessary for T cell activation (signal 2)[76-78] (see Chapter 9). Autoreactive T cells that recognize self antigen without effective antigen-presenting cells and costimulation may be functionally deactivated (or anergized) and prevented from any subsequent stimulation by that self antigen. These cells continue to be present in the peripheral T cell repertoire, but their prior contact with self antigen prevents any subsequent response. There is also evidence that the encounter of self-reactive T cells with antigen but without effective costimulation sometimes leads to death of the autoreactive T cell rather than to anergy. Recent studies have also shown that a different set of costimulatory signals are required for the induction of self-tolerance.[50,76-78] The absence of these tolerogenic signals would, therefore, leave the T cell available to generate autoimmunity. Another mechanism to prevent the activation of self-reactive T cells involves suppressor or regulatory T cells that control T cells with self-reactive potential. Considerable evidence indicates that one of these subsets can be recognized by the CD4+ CD25+ surface phenotype.[6-8] In some systems, regulatory CD4+ T cells appear to release cytokines, such as transforming growth factor-β (TGF-β) or IL-10, that suppress a possible autoreactive and damaging T cell response.[6-8,79] Studies of transgenic TCR mice have suggested that downregulation of TCR or coreceptor (CD4 or CD8) expression may be another mechanism to help prevent autoimmune responses.

ROLE OF MAJOR HISTOCOMPATIBILITY COMPLEX CLASS II MOLECULES

CD4+ T cells recognize peptides complexed to class II MHC molecules on antigen-presenting cells, and T cell stimulation in autoimmune disease could be enhanced by increased or altered expression of class II or self antigen in target organs or in lymphoid tissues. Various autoimmune diseases are also associated with particular MHC class II alleles. The most straightforward explanation for this association is that the disease-associated (versus nonassociated) MHC molecules can bind and present particular self peptides to autoreactive T cells. In the analysis of DRB1 molecules associated with RA, the crystal structures have confirmed that the shared epitope encodes a segment of the DR β-chain α-helix bordering the antigen-binding site and that variation in this region might profoundly influence peptide binding and T cell recognition of the MHC/peptide complex[5,51] (see Chapter 9). A model of disease pathogenesis entailing the selective binding and presentation of possible arthritogenic peptides has been used as a conceptual framework for understanding the shared epitope association with RA.[51,69] However, because the antigens (peptides) recognized by synovial CD4+ T cells in RA are unknown, the relevance of differences in peptide-binding motifs to disease pathogenesis remains theoretical.

It has also been proposed that disease-associated class II molecules may contribute to the pathogenesis of disease through an effect on T cell development[5] (see Chapter 9). Certain class II alleles might predispose to autoimmunity by increasing positive selection or decreasing negative selection of autoreactive T cells in the thymus. They might also act by inhibiting selection in the thymus of the regulatory CD4+ T cells that are thought to prevent autoantigen-specific responses. Finally, class II alleles might inhibit autoimmunity by deleting potentially autoreactive cells. Sometimes a single individual MHC might act in several of these ways.[5]

The evidence strongly suggests that MHC class II effects in autoimmune disease are antigen-specific in nature.[5] As discussed in an earlier section, the class II alleles predisposing to autoimmunity vary from one human disease to another, suggesting that class II alleles act in autoimmunity via specific antigens rather than comprehensively. Some investigators have proposed that I-A^{g7}, because of its poor peptide-binding properties, enhances autoimmunity in NOD mice in a global fashion. However, a defect in central tolerance in NOD mice has been shown to be independent of I-A^{g7},[70] and pancreatic islet cell autoimmunity in this strain switches to thyroiditis when a different class II molecule without these properties is exchanged for I-A^{g7}.[50] The most straightforward explanation for the effects of I-A^{g7} is that it predisposes to islet-specific autoimmunity and not system-wide reactivity.

ROLE OF SELF ANTIGEN

Considerable evidence indicates that pathogenic T cells and B cells in autoimmune disease are specific for certain self antigens and are driven by those antigens in the disease process.[5] In the NOD mouse model of type I diabetes, the induction of T cell tolerance at birth or early in life to particular islet antigens, such as glutamic acid decarboxylase (GAD) or insulin, prevents the development of disease. For example, the intrathymic injection or expression of GAD prevented the emergence of GAD-reactive T cells and responses, development of other anti-islet responses, and development of disease.[80] In addition, the suppression of GAD expression in islet cells or elimination of autoantigenic insulin by gene manipulation prevented anti-islet cell responses and the development of disease in NOD mice. In studies of other organ-specific diseases, the presence of the specific, targeted self antigens has been shown to be required for development and perpetuation of disease.[81]

Studies have also shown that pathogenic IgG autoantibody production in SLE is selective for only certain self antigens and is driven by self antigen at the B cell level.[5,68] In SLE and lupus mice, studies have repeatedly shown that a subset of anti-DNA–producing B cells are driven by a process that mimics a normal T cell–dependent response to foreign antigen, involving common mechanisms of somatic mutation, affinity maturation, and IgM to IgG class switching (see Chapter 10). That self antigen is involved in ANA production in lupus is further supported by studies showing that multiple epitopes on the same autoantigen particle (e.g., chromatin, Sm/U1RNP) are targeted by the autoantibody response. The specificities of the autoreactive T cells in SLE have been much more difficult to characterize, and the nature of T cell help in SLE may differ from conventional responses. In the anti-DNA response, it seems unlikely that T cells directed to DNA determinants are operative, and studies in murine lupus have suggested that T cells directed to other components of chromatin may be important. Thus, a DNA-specific B cell could bind and internalize nucleosomes, with subsequent class II MHC presentation of histone or other chromosomal peptides to T cells. Apoptotic cells are strong candidates as sources of the autoantigens that drive autoantibody responses in SLE. Studies suggest that defects in the physiologic mechanisms involved in the clearance of dying cells and cellular debris may promote disease susceptibility in SLE.[5,34,35,52]

The abnormal release of sequestered antigen with subsequent presentation to autoreactive T cells in surrounding lymphoid tissues may be one mechanism that overcomes immunologic ignorance. This may be the mechanism for autoimmunity in sympathetic ophthalmia, in which a penetrating injury to one eye results in the release of uveal antigens, T cell activation, and an immune-mediated attack on the other eye. It has also been proposed that virus-induced inflammatory responses resulting in release of self antigen may trigger autoreactive T cells.[5] One example may be the autoimmune myocarditis induced in animals or even humans after coxsackievirus B3 infection. The release of sequestered antigens may also be important in the expansion of autoimmune responses to additional determinants after the initial damage has occurred.

MOLECULAR MIMICRY AND ACTIVATION OF AUTOREACTIVE CELLS BY EXOGENOUS ANTIGENS

One proposed mechanism for how infection can initiate an autoimmune disease is that determinants of an infectious agent mimic a host antigen and trigger self-reactive T cell clones to attack host tissues. This is referred to as *molecular mimicry*.[5,82] In animal studies, certain viral peptides that cross-react with self peptides can be used to immunize animals, stimulate autoreactive T cells, and cause disease. Mice genetically engineered to express a viral protein as a self antigen can be shown to develop autoimmune responses and tissue damage after infection with the relevant virus.[42] More direct evidence has been presented for the role of molecular mimicry in animal and human autoimmune diseases. Herpes stromal keratitis is a disorder induced by herpes simplex virus type 1 and characterized by autoreactive T cell destruction of corneal tissue. In an animal model of this disorder, an epitope of the viral coat protein was shown to be recognized by autoreactive T cells and required for infection-induced disease.[83] Molecular mimicry was also implicated in a murine model of *Chlamydia*-induced heart damage, mediated by cross-reaction to heart muscle–specific α-myosin.[84] Relevant to rheumatic disease, molecular mimicry has been implicated as a mechanism for the perpetuation of arthritis in patients with chronic Lyme arthritis.[1,2] Molecular mimicry has also been used to explain how coxsackievirus might induce autoimmunity to GAD in type I diabetes, how EBV might stimulate an autoimmune response to the nuclear antigen Sm, and how the DR4 shared epitope might be associated with disease development in RA.[5,69,75,82] Although many cross-reactions have been suggested to cause autoimmune disease, many studies have also failed to confirm the cross-reactions reported.[5]

EPITOPE SPREADING

Molecular mimicry would be unlikely to trigger an autoimmune response unless an initial response to one self determinant (one peptide) could expand to involve additional determinants on the same molecule and additional self proteins.[85] This process of epitope spreading has been well studied in induced animal models such as EAE.[85,86] Initial immunization to one myelin basic protein peptide can be shown to spread to other determinants on the same protein and to spread to other myelin proteins such as proteolipid protein. In models relevant to SLE, immunization of normal animals to a cryptic epitope on a nuclear complex demonstrates spreading to other determinants on the same molecule and to other molecules in the same complex (e.g., anti-Sm to anti-U1RNP, anti-Ro/SS-A to anti-La/SS-B) and may lead to lupus-like disease.[21-23,73-75,87] Epitope spreading explains how a response to one epitope can mature into a full-blown autoimmune response. Studies have also emphasized an important role for B cells in epitope spreading, probably related to the effectiveness of antigen-specific B cells to present additional determinants after binding and internalizing antigenic complexes.[87-89]

ROLE OF B CELLS

B cell repertoire formation in the fetal liver and adult bone marrow is random, and B cells with self-reactivity are generated. Negative selection of some autoreactive B cells, involving both deletion and anergy, is a normal part of B cell development (see Chapter 10). A separate mechanism has been described in which immature B cells with specificity for self antigens can modify their receptors through a process called receptor editing.[88] Unlike T cells, mature B cells also have the ability to modify their BCRs in the peripheral lymphoid tissues through a process of somatic mutation (see Chapter 10). This allows a secondary immune response to generate antibodies with higher affinity for the stimulating antigen but offers additional opportunity for the generation of self-reactive B cells. Multiple checkpoints are involved in the prevention of activation of autoreactive B cells in the peripheral lymphoid tissues.[61]

Autoreactive B cells are part of the normal peripheral B cell repertoire, and defects in central B cell tolerance do not appear to be necessary to allow for pathogenic autoantibody production.[68] For example, the escape of autoreactive T cells secondary to intrathymic deficiency of *Aire* is sufficient for the subsequent development of autoantibodies to multiple organs.[56] The transfer of alloreactive $CD4^+$ T cells and generation of chronic graft-versus-host disease causes pathogenic lupus-like autoantibody production in normal recipient animals.[31] The ability of normal animals to generate spreading antinuclear autoantibody responses after immunization with one peptide further supports this conclusion.[21-23,73-75,87] Similar to regulation of autoreactive T cells, studies suggest that regulation of B cells in the peripheral lymphoid tissues may be important for the prevention of B cell autoimmunity.

B cells, however, appear to be more important in the development of autoimmune disease than just as a source of autoantibodies.[89] Studies in murine lupus have indicated that $CD4^+$ T cell activation probably depends on the presence of B cells. This may also be one of the mechanisms why B cells are important for continued disease activity in RA. The process of epitope spreading also appears to be dependent on the B cells.[87] After resting T cells are activated, which frequently requires specialized antigen-presenting cells such as dendritic cells, antigen-specific B cells may be the most efficient presenters of determinants from that antigen. Studies in murine lupus have also suggested that, even though autoantibody production is specific for certain self antigens, polyclonal B cell activation may predispose to disease development.

IMPORTANCE OF COSTIMULATION

Autoreactive T cells, such as T cells specific for foreign antigens, must receive several signals to be activated.[76-78] One signal is antigen specific and provided by engagement of the TCR (signal 1). Additional signals are provided by costimulatory molecules and their interactions (signal 2). Frequently, antigen-presenting cells, such as resting B cells, do not express significant levels of costimulatory molecules, and interaction with T cells does not lead to T cell activation. To be immunogenic, the antigen may need to be presented by antigen-presenting cells activated in an inflammatory context, and this may be one mechanism that links infection with autoimmunity. In addition, costimulatory signals appear to be involved in the active generation of self tolerance and defects in these interactions could also lead to autoimmunity.[50,76-78]

In the response to foreign and self determinants, two of the most important costimulatory interactions involve CD28 and CD40 ligand on the T cell, which bind to B7 (B7-1 [CD80] and B7-2 [CD86]) and CD40, respectively, on antigen-presenting cells and B cells.[76-78] The interaction of CD40 ligand with CD40 is bidirectional, providing signals important for T cell and B cell activation. Engagement of the TCR on a naïve autoreactive T cell in the absence of costimulation can result in different outcomes. In some situations, the cell continues to remain ignorant of its self antigen. At other times, recognition can induce apoptosis of the responding T cells or anergy, in which case the T cells are unable to respond to a subsequent encounter with the same antigen. Activation of memory T cells appear to depend less on the CD28-B7 costimulation, although antagonists that interrupt these cellular interactions can have profound effects even late in the course of an established autoimmune response.[90] For example, blocking the CD28-B7 or the CD40 ligand–CD40 interaction separately, and especially together, suppresses disease activity in murine lupus[90] and other models of autoimmune disease and is being developed to treat human autoimmune diseases. Additional costimulatory pathways relevant to autoimmunity include the CTLA-4 interaction with B7 and the PD-1 interaction with its ligand.[76-78] Alterations in the gene encoding CTLA-4 have been associated with autoimmune endocrine diseases,[49] and deficiencies of PD-1 have been implicated in lupus-like disease in animals[36] and as a possible gene contribution to SLE.[37] Both of these pathways result in negative-regulatory signals being delivered to the T cell.[76-78]

HELPER T CELL SUBSETS AND CYTOKINE DEPENDENCE OF AUTOIMMUNE DISEASE

Although more sharply defined in mice than humans, it is clear that T cells, after activation, may evolve into two major subsets of helper T cells, distinguished by the cytokines that they produce[79] (see Chapter 9). Th1 cells mainly synthesize IL-2 and IFN-γ, as well as other inflammatory cytokines such as lymphotoxin and TNF. Th2 cells are primarily distinguished by their secretion of IL-4, IL-5, IL-10, and IL-13. Th1 cells primarily enhance cell-mediated inflammatory immune responses such as delayed-type hypersensitivity reactions, which frequently involve activation of macrophages and effector T cells. The ability to mediate an effective immune response against certain intracellular pathogens appears to strongly depend on the generation of a Th1 response. In contrast, Th2 cells mainly provide help for B cells by promoting class switching and enhancing the production of certain IgG isotypes and production of IgE, including in allergic diseases.

Studies using animals have shown that Th1 cells have much greater potential to mediate organ damage in various organ-specific autoimmune diseases such as EAE (multiple sclerosis), NOD mice (type I diabetes), and other induced diseases.[25,79,91-95] Studies of patients with RA have also supported the contention that Th1 cells are primarily involved in pathogenesis, a conclusion consistent with the important role of TNF-α in this disease.[28,96] Crohn's disease is another process in which Th1-type cytokines appear to be paramount. In SLE, Th2-type responses may be more important in disease development compared to the other more organ-specific diseases. However, in spontaneous murine models, the IgG isotypes most important for pathogenicity suggest the additional influence of Th1-type cytokines and the importance of IFN-γ. IFN-γ appears to be required for the full expression of disease in murine models of lupus,[97] and this cytokine is known to exacerbate disease in SLE patients. The precise mechanism of this influence is unknown.

The cytokines present when the T cell is first activated greatly influence whether the response will be polarized toward Th1 or Th2 differentiation.[79] IL-12 and IFN-γ have been shown to be most important in directing the development of Th1 cells that then go on to produce IFN-γ. Infection may lead to the production of IL-12 by macrophages or dendritic cells and cause NK cells to release IFN-γ, which may be a mechanism by which infection leads to autoimmune disease. In a similar but opposite manner, the presence of IL-4 early in the immune response directs the development of Th2 cells from naïve precursors. If IL-4 levels exceed a threshold, Th2 development ensues, which leads to additional IL-4 production. Evidence also suggests that differences in the type of dendritic cell presenting to a naïve T cell may control Th1 and Th2 development, and different costimulatory pathways are operative as well.

The cytokines produced by Th1 and Th2 subsets cross-regulate each other's development and function. For example, IFN-γ produced by Th1 cells inhibits the development of Th2 cells, as well as certain humoral responses. In a similar but opposite manner, IL-4 and IL-10 produced by Th2 cells inhibit Th1 development and activation, as well as macrophage activation by Th1 cytokines. These considerations are the basis for how a shift from Th1 to Th2 pattern of cytokine production, especially early in the immune response, can alter a damaging Th1 autoimmune response. The shift in cytokine pattern, which may involve regulatory T cells, is referred to as immune deviation.

REGULATORY T CELLS

In experimental animal models, there is evidence that $CD4^+$, $CD8^+$, and $\gamma\delta$ T cells (see Chapter 9) may be involved in the downregulation of certain immune responses, and their absence may be associated with pathologic autoimmune responses. Examples of this phenomenon include the development of organ-specific autoimmunity after thymectomy in early life, which prevents the emergence of $CD4^+CD25^+$ regulatory cells, and the worsening of organ-specific autoimmunity with deliberate elimination of this subset.[6-8] Worsening of autoimmune disease in animal models has also been reported after the elimination of $CD8^+$ or $\gamma\delta$ T cells. In most situations, the specificity of the regulatory cell has not been defined. NK T cells, restricted by CD1, have also been noted to suppress organ-specific autoimmunity after activation with α-galactosylceramide, and deficiency of this subset may also contribute to organ-specific autoimmunity in some models.[98,99] Regulatory $CD4^+$ T cell subsets frequently inhibit cell-mediated immune responses and inflammatory pathologies based on the cytokines they produce. Some subsets release IL-10, downregulating the development and further activation of Th1-type cells involved in the autoimmune process. Regulatory $CD4^+$ and $CD8^+$ cells that release TGF-β have also been described. TGF-β is capable of suppressing both Th1 and Th2 T cell responses.[79] Tissue production of TGF-β with local immunosuppression may also be one of several mechanisms that lead to immune privilege and the prevention of autoimmune responses in a particular organ. Mice made deficient in TGF-β by gene knockout techniques show evidence of progressive inflammation and autoimmunity involving multiple organs, and T cells (regulatory) with receptor for TGF-β appear to be required to prevent systemic autoimmunity.

Conclusions

The development of autoimmune disease is a complex process. Although our knowledge regarding different aspects of the immunopathogenesis of disease, especially related to studies of animal models, seems so much greater than just a few years ago, major black boxes persist. WD Perhaps most poorly understood are the mechanisms involved in the initial breakdown of self-tolerance. The cellular immunologic abnormalities involved in the initiation and perpetuation of disease also need much greater definition. The identification and understanding of susceptibility genes and etiologic triggers should provide insights into these questions. Understanding these processes will also provide new directions for prophylaxis and treatment of disease.

Much better understood are the later events in autoimmune disease pathogenesis, such as how autoantibodies or cellular immune-mediated damage leads to disease manifestations. Other chapters in this textbook address these aspects of disease in much greater detail, but many critical details remain unknown. What is the role of $CD4^+$ T cells or autoantibody in established RA, and what leads to exacerbations of disease in SLE or multiple sclerosis? Considering the remarkable increase in information regarding the normal immune system, immunity, and the genetic basis of complex traits, it seems likely that our understanding of autoimmunity will greatly increase in the near future.

REFERENCES

1. Kamradt T, Lengl-Janssen B, Strauss AF, et al: Dominant recognition of a Borrelia burgdorferi outer surface protein A peptide by T helper cells in patients with treatment-resistant Lyme arthritis. Infect Immun 64:1284, 1996.
2. Gross DM, Forsthuber T, Tary-Lehmann M, et al: Identification of LFA-1 as a candidate autoantigen in treatment-resistant Lyme arthritis (See comments). Science 281:703, 1998.
3. Notkins AL, Lernmark A: Autoimmune type 1 diabetes: resolved and unresolved issues. J Clin Invest 108:1247, 2001.
4. Matsumoto I, Maccioni M, Lee DM, et al: How antibodies to a ubiquitous cytoplasmic enzyme may provoke joint-specific autoimmune disease. Nat Immunol 3:360, 2002.
5. Marrack P, Kappler J, Kotzin BL: Autoimmune disease: Why and where it occurs. Nature Medicine 7:899, 2001.
6. Sakaguchi S, Sakaguchi N, Shimizu J, et al: Immunologic tolerance maintained by CD25+ CD4+ regulatory T cells: Their common role in controlling autoimmunity, tumor immunity, and transplantation tolerance. Immunol Rev 182:18, 2001.
7. Shevach EM, McHugh RS, Piccirillo CA, Thornton AM: Control of T-cell activation by CD4+ CD25+ suppressor cells. Immunol Rev 182:58, 2001.
8. Maloy KJ, Powrie F: Regulatory T cells in the control of immune pathology. Nature Immunol 2:816, 2001.
9. Jiang H, Braunstein NS, Yu B, et al: CD8+ T cells control the TH phenotype of MBP-reactive CD4+ T cells in EAE mice. Proc Natl Acad Sci U S A 98: 6301, 2001.
10. Coutinho A, KazatchkineMD, Avrameas S: Natural autoantibodies. Curr Opin Immunol 7:812, 1995.
11. Hayakawa K, Asano M, Shinton SA, et al: Positive selection of anti-Thy-1 autoreactive B-1 Cells and natural serum autoantibody production independent from bone marrow development. J Exp Med 197: 87, 2003.
12. Boes M, Schmidt T, Linkermann K, et al: Accelerated development of IgG autoantibodies and autoimmune disease in the absence of secreted IgM. Proc Natl Acad Sci U S A 97:1184, 2000.
13. Wicker LS, Todd JA, Peterson LB: Genetic control of autoimmune diabetes in the NOD mouse. Annu Rev Immunol 13:179, 1995.
14. Theofilopoulos AN, Dixon FJ: Murine models of systemic lupus erythematosus. Adv Immunol 37:269, 1985.
15. Vyse TJ, Kotzin BL: Genetic susceptibility to systemic lupus erythematosus. Annu Rev Immunol 16:261, 1998.
16. Theofilopoulos AN: The basis of autoimmunity: Part II. Genetic predisposition. Immunol Today 16:150, 1995.
17. Hahn BH: Animal models of systemic lupus erythematosus. *In* Wallace DJ, Hahn BH (eds): Dubois' Lupus Erythematosus, 5th ed. Baltimore, Williams & Wilkins, 1997, p 339.
18. Cohen PL, Eisenberg RA: Lpr and gld: Single gene models of systemic autoimmunity and lymphoproliferative disease. Annu Rev Immunol 9:243, 1991.

19. Theofilopoulos AN, Kono DH: The genes of systemic autoimmunity. Proc Assoc Am Physicians 111:228, 1999.
20. Wakeland EK, Liu K, Graham RR, Behrens TW: Delineating the genetic basis of systemic lupus erythematosus. Immunity 15:397, 2001.
21. Topfer F, Gordon T, McCluskey J: Intra-and intermolecular spreading of autoimmunity involving the nuclear self-antigens La (SS-B) and Ro (SS-A). Proc Natl Acad Sci U S A 92:875, 1995.
22. James JA, Harley JB: B-cell epitope spreading in autoimmunity. Immunol Rev 164:185, 1998.
23. Mamula MJ: Epitope spreading: The role of self peptides and autoantigen processing by B lymphocytes. Immunol Rev 164:231, 1998.
24. Wekerle H, Kojima K, Lannes-Vieira J, et al: Animal models. Ann Neurol 36:S47, 1994.
25. Steinman L: Multiple sclerosis: A coordinated immunological attack against myelin in the central nervous system. Cell 85:299, 1996.
26. Remmers EF, Longman RE, Du Y, et al: A genome scan localizes five non-MHC loci controlling collagen-induced arthritis in rats. Nat Genet 14:82, 1996.
27. Rosloniec EF, Brand DD, Myers LK, et al: Induction of autoimmune arthritis in HLA-DR4 (DRB1*0401) transgenic mice by immunization with human and bovine type II collagen. J Immunol 160:2573, 1998.
28. Feldmann M, Brennan FM, Maini RN: Rheumatoid arthritis. Cell 85:307, 1996.
29. Zhang Y, Guerassimov A, Leroux JY, et al: Arthritis induced by proteoglycan aggrecan G1 domain in BALB/c mice: Evidence for T cell involvement and the immunosuppressive influence of keratan sulfate on recognition of T and B cell epitopes. J Clin Invest 101:1678, 1998.
30. Kotzin BL, Falta MT, Crawford F, et al: Use of soluble peptide-DR4 tetramers to detect synovial T cells specific for cartilage antigens in patients with rheumatoid arthritis. Proc Natl Acad Sci U S A 97:291, 2000.
31. Via CS, Shearer GM: T-cell interactions in autoimmunity: Insights from a murine model of graft-versus-host disease. Immunol Today 9:207, 1988.
32. Horak I, Lohler J, Ma A, et al: Interleukin-2 deficient mice: A new model to study autoimmunity and self-tolerance. Immunol Rev 148:35, 1995.
33. Bolland S, Ravetch JV: Spontaneous autoimmune disease in FcγRIIB-deficient mice results from strain-specific epistasis. Immunity 13:277, 2000.
34. Napirei M, Karsunky H, Zevnik B, et al: Features of systemic lupus erythematosus in Dnase I-deficient mice. Nature Genet 25:177, 2000.
35. Yasutomo K, Horiuchi T, Kagami S, et al: Mutations of *DNASE1* in people with systemic lupus erythematosus. Nature Genet 28:313, 2001.
36. Nishimura H, Nose M, Hiai H, et al: Development of lupus-like autoimmune diseases by disruption of the PD-1 gene encoding an ITIM motif-carrying immunoreceptor. Immunity 11:141, 1999.
37. Prokunina L, Castillejo-Lopez C, Oberg F, et al: A regulatory polymorphism in *PDCD1* is associated with susceptibility to systemic lupus erythematosus in humans. Nature Genet 32:666, 2002.
38. Kouskoff V, Korganow AS, Duchatelle V, et al: Organ-specific disease provoked by systemic autoimmunity. Cell 87:811, 1996.
39. Matsumoto I, Staub A, Benoist C, Mathis D: Arthritis provoked by linked T and B cell recognition of a glycolytic enzyme. Science 286:1732, 1999.
40. Matsumoto I, Maccioni M, Lee DM, et al: How antibodies to a ubiquitous cytoplasmic enzyme may provoke joint-specific autoimmune disease. Nature Immunol 3:360, 2002.
41. Lee DM, Friend DS, Gurish MF, et al: Mast cells: A cellular link between autoantibodies and inflammatory arthritis. Science 297:1689, 2002.
42. Basten A: Basis and mechanisms of self-tolerance. *In* Rose NR, Mackay IR (eds): The Autoimmune Diseases, 3rd ed. San Diego, Academic Press, 1998, p 9.
43. Gregersen PK: Teasing apart the complex genetics of human autoimmunity: Lessons from rheumatoid arthritis. Clin Immunol 107:1, 2003.
44. Onengut-Gumuscu S, Concannon P: Mapping genes for autoimmunity in humans: type 1 diabetes as a model. Immunol Rev 190:182, 2002.
45. Oksenberg JR, Barcellos LF, Hauser SL: Genetic aspects of multiple sclerosis. Semin Neurol 19:281, 1999.
46. Graham RR, Ortmann WA, Langefeld CD, et al: Visualizing human leukocyte antigen class II risk haplotypes in human systemic lupus erythematosus. Am J Hum Genet 71:543, 2002.
47. Kelly JA, Moser KL, Harley JB: The genetics of systemic lupus erythematosus: putting the pieces together. Genes Immun 1:S71, 2002.
48. Peterson P, Nagamine K, Scott H, et al: APECED: A monogenic autoimmune disease providing new clues to self-tolerance. Immunol Today 19:384, 1998.
49. Ueda H, Howson JMM, Esposito L, et al: Association of the T-cell regulatory gene *CTLA4* with susceptibility to autoimmune disease. Nature 423:506, 2003.
50. Lesage S, Goodnow CC: Organ-specific autoimmune disease: a deficiency of tolerogenic stimulation. J Exp Med 194:F31, 2001.
51. Nepom GT: Major histocompatibility complex–directed susceptibility to rheumatoid arthritis. Adv Immunol 68:315, 1998.
52. Walport MJ: Complement. New Engl J Med 344:1058, 2001.
53. Salmon JE, Millard S, Schachter LA, et al: Fc gamma RIIA alleles are heritable risk factors for lupus nephritis in African Americans. J Clin Invest 97:1348, 1996.
54. Edberg JC, Langefeld CD, Wu J, et al: Genetic linkage and association of Fcgamma receptor IIA (CD16A) on chromosome 1q23 with human systemic lupus erythematosus. Arthritis Rheum 46:2132, 2002.
55. Clynes R, Dumitru C, Ravetch JV: Uncoupling of immune complex formation and kidney damage in autoimmune glomerulonephritis. Science 279:1052, 1998.
56. Anderson MS, Venanzi ES, Klein L, et al: Projection of an immunological self shadow within the thymus by the Aire protein. Science 298: 1395, 2002.
57. Liston A, Lesage S, Wilson J, et al: Aire regulates negative selection of organ-specific T cells. Nature Immunol 4:350, 2003.
58. Rozzo SJ, Allard JD, Choubey D, et al: Evidence for an interferon-inducible gene, Ifi202, in the susceptibility to systemic lupus. Immunity 15:435, 2001.
59. Ronnblom L, Alm GV: An etiopathogenic role for the type 1 IFN system in SLE. Trends Immunol 22:427, 2001.
60. Blanco P, Palucka AK, Gill M, et al: Induction of dendritic cell differentiation by IFN-α in systemic lupus erythematosus. Science 294:150, 2001.
61. Rathmell JC, Goodnow CC: The in vivo balance between B cell clonal expansion and elimination is regulated by CD95 both on B cells and in their micro-environment. Immunol Cell Biol 76:387, 1998.
62. Straus SE, Sneller M, Lenardo MJ, et al: An inherited disorder of lymphocyte apoptosis: The autoimmune lymphoproliferative syndrome. Ann Intern Med 130:591, 1999.
63. Wynn DR, Rodriguez M, O'Fallon WM, et al: Update on the epidemiology of multiple sclerosis. Mayo Clin Proc 64:808, 1989.
64. Matzinger P: The danger model: A renewed sense of self. Science 296:301, 2002.
65. Saal JG, Krimmel M, Steidle M, et al: Synovial Epstein-Barr virus infection increases the risk of rheumatoid arthritis in individuals with the shared HLA-DR4 epitope. Arthritis Rheum 42:1485, 1999.
66. Vaughan JH: Viruses and autoimmune disease (editorial). J Rheumatol 23:1831, 1996.
67. James JA, Kaufman KM, Farris AD, et al: An increased prevalence of Epstein-Barr virus infection in young patients suggests a possible etiology for systemic lupus erythematosus. J Clin Invest 100:3019, 1997.
68. Kotzin BL: Systemic lupus erythematosus. Cell 85:303, 1996.
69. Bennett SR, Falta MT, Bill J, Kotzin BL: Antigen-specific T cells in rheumatoid arthritis. Curr Rheum Rep, 5:255, 2003.
70. Kishimoto H, Sprent J: A defect in central tolerance in NOD mice. Nature Immunol 2:1025, 2001.
71. Casciola-Rosen L, Andrade F, Ulanet D,et al: Cleavage by granzyme B is strongly predictive of autoantigen status: implications for initiation of autoimmunity. J Exp Med 190:815, 1999.
72. Backlund J, Carlsen S, Hoger T, et al: Predominant selection of T cells specific for the glycosylated collagen type II epitope (263-270)

in humanized transgenic mice and in rheumatoid arthritis. Proc Natl Acad Sci U S A 99:9960, 2002.
73. Bockenstedt LK, Gee RJ, Mamula MJ: Self-peptides in the initiation of lupus autoimmunity. J Immunol 154:3516, 1995.
74. Craft J, Fatenejad S: Self antigens and epitope spreading in systemic autoimmunity. Arthritis Rheum 40:1374, 1997.
75. James JA, Gross T, Scofield RH, et al: Immunoglobulin epitope spreading and autoimmune disease after peptide immunization: Sm B/B′-derived PPPGMRPP and PPPGIRGP induce spliceosome autoimmunity. J Exp Med 181:453, 1995.
76. Salomon B, Bluestone JA: Complexities of CD28/B7: CTLA-4 costimulatory pathways in autoimmunity and transplantation. Annu Rev Immunol 19:225, 2001.
77. Chitnis T, Khoury SJ: Role of costimulatory pathways in the pathogenesis of multiple sclerosis and experimental autoimmune encephalomeulitis. J Allergy Clin Immunol, 112:837, 2003.
78. Goodnow CC: Pathways for self-tolerance and the treatment of autoimmune diseases. Lancet 357:2115, 2001.
79. O'Garra A: Cytokines induce the development of functionally heterogeneous T helper cell subsets. Immunity 8:275, 1998.
80. Kaufman DL, Clare-Salzler M, Tian J, et al: Spontaneous loss of T cell tolerance to glutamic acid decarboxylase in murine insulin-dependent diabetes (See comments). Nature 366:69, 1993.
81. Bach JF, Koutouzov S, van Endert PM: Are there unique autoantigens triggering autoimmune diseases? Immunol Rev 164:139, 1998.
82. Albert LJ, Inman RD: Molecular mimicry and autoimmunity N Engl J Med 341:2068, 1999.
83. Zhao ZS, Granucci F, Yeh L, et al: Molecular mimicry by herpes simplex virus-type 1: Autoimmune disease after viral infection (See comments). Science 279:1344, 1998.
84. Bachmaier K, Neu N, de la Maza LM, et al: Chlamydia infections and heart disease linked through antigenic mimicry (See comments). Science 283:1335, 1999.
85. Lehmann PV, Sercarz EE, Forsthuber T, et al: Determinant spreading and the dynamics of the autoimmune T-cell repertoire (See comments). Immunol Today 14:203, 1993.
86. Vanderlugt CL, Begolka WS, Neville KL, et al: The functional significance of epitope spreading and its regulation by co-stimulatory molecules. Immunol Rev 164:63, 1998.
87. Mamula MJ, Fatenejad S, Craft J: B cells process and present lupus autoantigens that initiate autoimmune T cell responses. J Immunol 152:1453, 1994.
88. Nussenzweig MC: Immune receptor editing: Revise and select. Cell 95:875, 1998.
89. Chan OT, Madaio MP, Shlomchik MJ: The central and multiple roles of B cells in lupus pathogenesis. Immunol Rev 169:107, 1999.
90. Daikh DI, Finck BK, Linsley PS, et al: Long-term inhibition of murine lupus by brief simultaneous blockade of the B7/CD28 and CD40/gp39 costimulation pathways. J Immunol 159:3104, 1997.
91. Bradley LM, Asensio VC, Schioetz LK, et al: Islet-specific Th1, but not Th2, cells secrete multiple chemokines and promote rapid induction of autoimmune diabetes. J Immunol 162:2511, 1999.
92. Katz JD, Benoist C, Mathis D: T helper cell subsets in insulin-dependent diabetes. Science 268:1185, 1995.
93. O'Garra A, Steinman L, Gijbels K: CD4+ T-cell subsets in autoimmunity. Curr Opin Immunol 9:872, 1997.
94. Liblau RS, Singer SM, McDevitt HO: Th1 and Th2 CD4+ T cells in the pathogenesis of organ-specific autoimmune diseases (See comments). Immunol Today 16:34, 1995.
95. King C, Sarvetnick N: Organ-specific autoimmunity. Curr Opin Immunol 9:863, 1997.
96. Miossec P: Interleukin 17 in rheumatoid arthritis: If T cells were to contribute to inflammation and destruction through synergy. Arthritis Rheum 48:594, 2003.
97 Lawson BR, Prud'homme GJ, Chang Y, et al: Treatment of murine lupus with cDNA encoding IFN-γR/Fc. J Clin Invest 106:207, 2000.
98. Beaudoin L, Laloux V, Novak J, et al: NKT cells inhibit the onset of diabetes by impairing the development of pathogenic T cells specific for pancreatic β cells. Immunity 17:725, 2002.
99. Sharif S, Arreaza GA, Zucker P, et al: Activation of natural killer T cells by α-galactosylceramide treatment prevents the onset and recurrence of autoimmune type 1 diabetes. Nature Med 7:1057, 2001.

17 Genetics of Rheumatic Diseases

PETER K. GREGERSEN

Genetic analysis is being widely applied to the problem of human disease, including rheumatic disease, reflecting the unprecedented advances in technology and a more sophisticated approach to interpreting the role of genetic variation in the origin of disease. The completion of the Human Genome Project[1,2] has accelerated this process, and rheumatologists need to understand the basic principles and concepts that underlie the genetic approach to rheumatic disease. Comprehension of these principles should permit practitioners and researchers to interpret the wealth of new genetic findings that are likely to emerge over the next few years.

Until recently, most research on genetic susceptibility to rheumatic diseases involved gene families that control the immune response. The major histocompatibility complex (MHC), which encodes the human leukocyte antigens (HLAs), is by far the most studied of these gene families. There are a large number of HLA genes within the MHC, and they exhibit an enormous degree of structural variability (i.e., polymorphism). Many of these polymorphisms influence immune-response patterns and are associated with susceptibility to a wide spectrum of autoimmune diseases, although the exact mechanisms underlying these associations remain obscure. The genetics of the human MHC are, therefore, covered in some detail in this chapter.

The Multifactorial Nature of Rheumatic Diseases

In the case of simple dominant or recessive mendelian inheritance, the correlation between the inheritance of the relevant disease genes and the presence of the disease phenotype in the affected individual is usually straightforward. For example, homozygosity for the sickle hemoglobin allele usually is associated with the clinical syndrome of sickle cell anemia. In contrast, inheritance of genes that predispose to autoimmunity do not give rise to the clinical syndrome of autoimmunity in most cases. This is most directly demonstrated by the data on disease concordance rates in monozygotic (MZ) twins with autoimmune diseases.

When one MZ twin is affected with an autoimmune disease, the probability that the other twin of the pair will develop the same illness is approximately 1 in 4 (25 percent), although the exact concordance rates vary somewhat for different rheumatic diseases. The concordance rate for clinic lupus in identical twins has been reported at 24 percent.[3] Similar concordance rates have been observed in other autoimmune diseases, such as multiple sclerosis and type I (juvenile) diabetes.[4,5] Early studies of twin concordance for rheumatoid arthritis (RA) also suggested that approximately 30 percent of MZ twin pairs were concordant for RA.[6] However, large studies of twins in the Finnish and British populations have reported concordance rates in the range of 12 to 15 percent.[7,8] In most cases, only one member of an MZ twin pair is affected with these rheumatic diseases, despite the identical genetic inheritance. Other factors must come into play in causing the development of autoimmunity. These factors can be attributed to two other general sources of variation among individuals: differences in exposure to disease-related environmental factors[9] and differences arising out of developmental processes, many of which have a stochastic component.[10,11]

Disease is a phenomenon that occurs in populations, as well as individuals, and the historic and evolutionary factors that have shaped populations should be taken into account when trying to understand the ultimate causes of disease. The clinical expression of disease is an outcome of a complex interactive process that occurs over time in both individuals and populations. When searching for genetic factors that may predispose to autoimmune diseases, it must be kept in mind that these effects are obscured by the multifactorial nature of disease etiology.

Genetic Susceptibility

The genetic influences on rheumatic diseases are usually described in terms of conferring susceptibility to, or risk for, the disease. The degree of risk conferred by a given genetic polymorphism can be calculated as the estimated relative risk, which is described in a later section. This pattern of conferring genetic susceptibility for disease is typical of the associations between HLA genes and rheumatic disease and is revealed by a higher frequency of such genes in populations of patients, compared to normal subjects. Nevertheless, the relatively low concordance rate in MZ twins suggests that even those genes directly involved in causing autoimmunity will be found in a substantial number of normal individuals who will never develop the disease.

At first consideration, the relatively weak relationship between inheritance and autoimmunity may appear to have limited utility. However, the analysis of HLA associations with autoimmune disease has revealed the power of detailed genetic studies to suggest new hypotheses about the causes of autoimmunity. Even if particular genetic factors play a role in only a small subset of patients, or only in certain environmental settings, they may nevertheless provide important insights into disease pathogenesis and provide for diagnostic and therapeutic specificity. This is a major rationale for continuing to search for additional genetic factors underlying autoimmunity.

The Major Histocompatibility Complex

The chromosomal region containing the MHC was originally identified because of the ability of genes in this region to regulate transplant rejection[12] and to control the immune responses of mice and guinea pigs to simple antigens,[13] a series of observations that led to the 1980 Nobel prize. The human MHC encodes the HLAs. The HLA molecules and their counterparts in rodents were subsequently shown to be directly responsible for immune response differences between individuals and for determining the likelihood of graft rejection.[12-15] A large number of studies indicate that genetic variants of HLA molecules are associated with a wide variety of disorders, many of which appear to have an autoimmune origin.[16]

The entire MHC region on chromosome 6 has been sequenced, revealing the presence of many new genes in this region.[17] This information has prompted a reevaluation of the significance of the HLA associations with disease. Although the "classic" MHC molecules are undoubtedly of major importance in regulating immune responsiveness, other genes within the MHC are also relevant to immune function and are likely to be important for disease susceptibility.

HUMAN LEUKOCYTE ANTIGEN MOLECULES AND ANTIGEN-SPECIFIC T CELL RECOGNITION

The primary function of HLA molecules is the presentation of antigenic peptides to T cells. In the case of α/β T cells, most antigen recognition events involve the formation of a trimolecular complex consisting of the HLA molecule, its bound peptide, and the α/β T cell receptor (see Chapters 7 and 9). When this recognition occurs in the appropriate context, it may result in signal transduction and activation of the T cell. The requirement for MHC molecules to present antigenic peptides to T cells is frequently referred to as MHC-restricted T cell recognition. In each individual, T cells are generally restricted to recognize antigens presented by the person's own HLA molecules. The allelic differences between different HLA molecules may result in differences in the types of antigenic peptides to which an individual responds or in the types of T cells that are used in an immune response.

HUMAN LEUKOCYTE ANTIGEN CLASS I AND CLASS II MOLECULES

The original serologic and biochemic studies of HLA molecules revealed the presence of two major isotypes: HLA class I and HLA class II. The basic structural features of these classic HLA molecules are summarized in Figure 17–1. HLA class I molecules consist of a 45-kD α-chain encoded within the MHC that is noncovalently associated with the 12-kD β_2-microglobulin chain (encoded on chromosome 15). HLA class II molecules consist of noncovalently associated α– (32 kD) and β– (28 kD) chains, both of which are encoded within the MHC. HLA class I and class II molecules are cell-surface glycoproteins, anchored to the membrane by hydrophobic transmembrane segments.

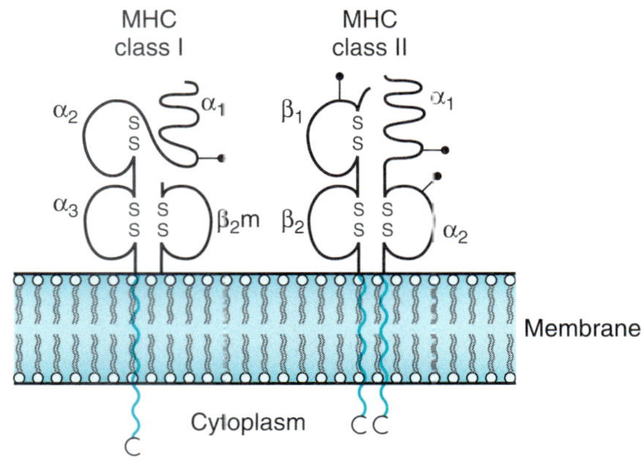

FIGURE 17–1 · Comparison of the Structural Features of Major Histocompatibility Complex (MHC) Class I and Class II Molecules. MHC class I molecules are anchored in the membrane by a single transmembrane segment contained in the 45kD α-chain. The MHC class I α-chain is noncovalently associated with β2 microglobulin. There are four external domains, three of which contain intramolecular disulfide bonds, as indicated. In contrast, MHC class II molecules consist of noncovalently associated α– (32kD) and β– (28kD) chains, both of which are anchored within the membrane by a transmembrane segment. The overall domain organization of the two molecules is highly similar, however. Glycosylation sites on both molecules are indicated (•).

A major breakthrough in the understanding of HLA molecules came in 1987, when Bjorkman and colleagues reported the crystal structure of the HLA class I molecule, HLA-A2.[18,19] This work was followed by the solution of other MHC class I and class II structures relevant to rheumatic diseases.[20,21] A side view of the class I molecule taken from Bjorkman's original paper is shown in Figure 17–2*A*. The base of the molecule (directly adjacent to the cell membrane) is formed by β_2-microglobulin and the immunoglobulin-like α_3 domain. The α_1 and α_2 domains form a distinct cleft or groove at the top of the molecule. The function of this cleft is to bind antigenic peptides for presentation to T cells. A top view of this cleft is shown in Figure 17–2*B*. The "floor" of the peptide-binding cleft consists of β-sheets, whereas the "walls" of the cleft are bounded by extended regions of α-helical structure. The size of the HLA class I cleft is approximately 10 to 20 angstroms and generally can accommodate antigenic peptides that are nine amino acids long.[22,23]

HLA class II molecules have a structure that is highly similar to that of class I molecules, with a prominent peptide-binding cleft at the membrane distal portion, sitting on top of a base formed by the α_2 and β_2

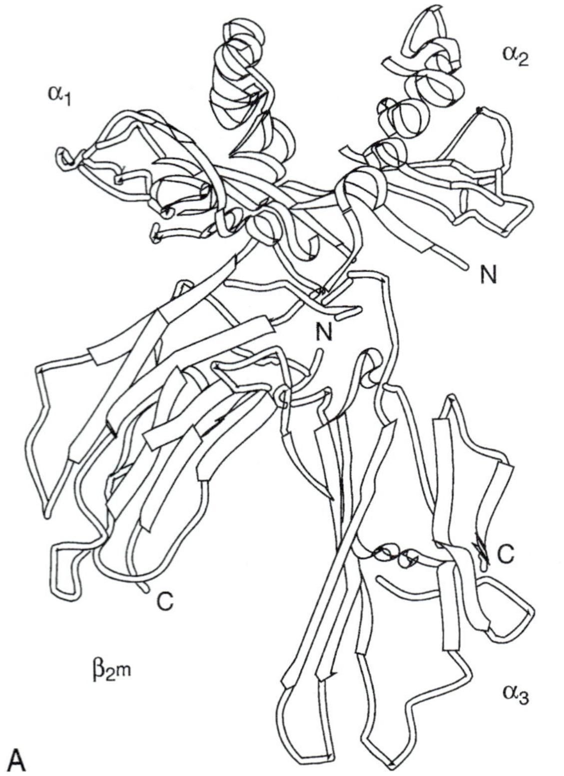

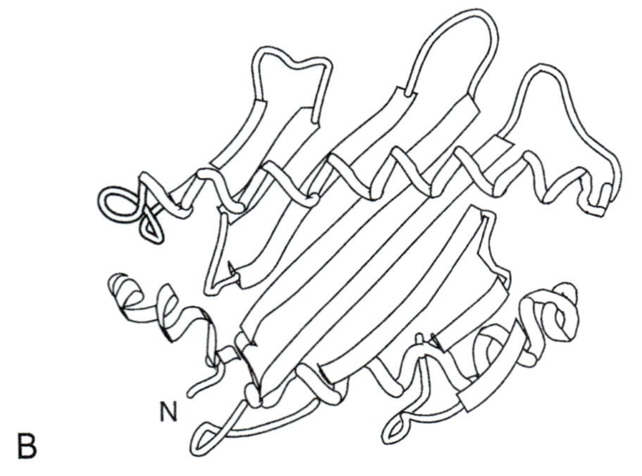

FIGURE 17–2 · Three-Dimensional Stucture of an HLA Class I Molecule, Based on the X-ray Crystallographic Analysis of Bjorkman.[19] *A*, Side view. A peptide binding cleft is formed by the α1 and α2 domains at the top of the molecule. The α3 and β2 microglobulin domains are similar in structure to immunoglobulin domains; essentially, they act as a platform on which the peptide-binding cleft rests, as well as providing contact sites for the CD8 molecule during CD8+ T cell recognition. *B*, Top view of the empty peptide-binding cleft. This "T cell view" of the major histocompatibility complex (MHC) molecule would normally include a peptide bound within the cleft.

immunoglobulin-like domains. The overall size and shape of the cleft in the two classes of HLA molecules are almost superimposable. However, subtle differences exist, particularly at the ends of the cleft, and this allows for some differences in the sizes of antigenic peptides that are presented by HLA class II molecules, compared to class I. Direct analysis of peptides bound to HLA class II molecules has shown that their size commonly varies from 12 to 19 amino acids.[23] Thus, relatively longer peptides lie in the cleft of class II molecules, possibly extending beyond the ends of the cleft, whereas class I molecules contain much shorter peptides that are buried within the cleft at either end.

Finally, x-ray crystallographic analyses of the entire trimolecular complex have revealed that it consists of an HLA molecule, its bound peptide, and the T cell receptor. Figure 17–3 shows an example of this structure for a HLA-DRB1*0401 allele presenting influenza hemagglutinin peptide to its cognate α/βT cell receptor.[24] These structures are now freely available at *http://www.rcsb.org/pdb*, as well as *http://www.imtech.res. in/raghava/mhcbn/tsmhc.html*. These Web sites enable users to view and understand these structures by rotating them in three dimensions using downloadable software.

Human Leukocyte Antigen Class I and Class II Isotypes: Functional Correlates

HLA class II molecules have a restricted tissue distribution, generally limited to antigen-presenting cells of the immune system such as B cells, macrophages, dendritic cells, and some subsets of T cells. This reflects the fact that HLA class II molecules are primarily involved in presenting foreign antigens to CD4-positive (CD4+) T cells during the initiation and propagation of the immune response. However, the expression of HLA class II molecules can also be induced on a variety of other cell types by inflammatory cytokines such as interferon-γ, enabling these cells to engage in antigen presentation to $CD4^+$ T cells. In contrast, HLA class I molecules are widely distributed on all somatic cells, with the exception of red blood cells. This distribution reflects their predominant role in presenting antigen to $CD8^+$ effector or cytotoxic T cells.

Another major functional difference between class I and class II molecules is related to the source of peptide antigens found in the antigen-binding cleft. In general, class I molecules present peptide antigens derived from proteins that are actively synthesized within the endoplasmic reticulum, whereas HLA class II molecules present antigens that are taken up from outside the cell by endocytosis. These differences are reflected in the antigen-processing machinery and the different trafficking patterns of class I and class II molecules inside the cell. This complex process is discussed in some detail in Chapter 7.

GENETIC ORGANIZATION OF THE HUMAN MAJOR HISTOCOMPATIBILITY COMPLEX

The human MHC extends over approximately 4 million base pairs on the short arm of chromosome 6 (6p21.3). The HLA class I and class II gene clusters are found in distinct locations, as indicated on the highly abridged genetic map shown in Figure 17–4. Only those genes that are traditionally associated with immune function are shown in Figure 17–4. More than 200 genes have been identified in the MHC, one of the most gene-rich regions in the human genome.[17] Detailed genetic maps with the complete DNA sequence of the MHC and a

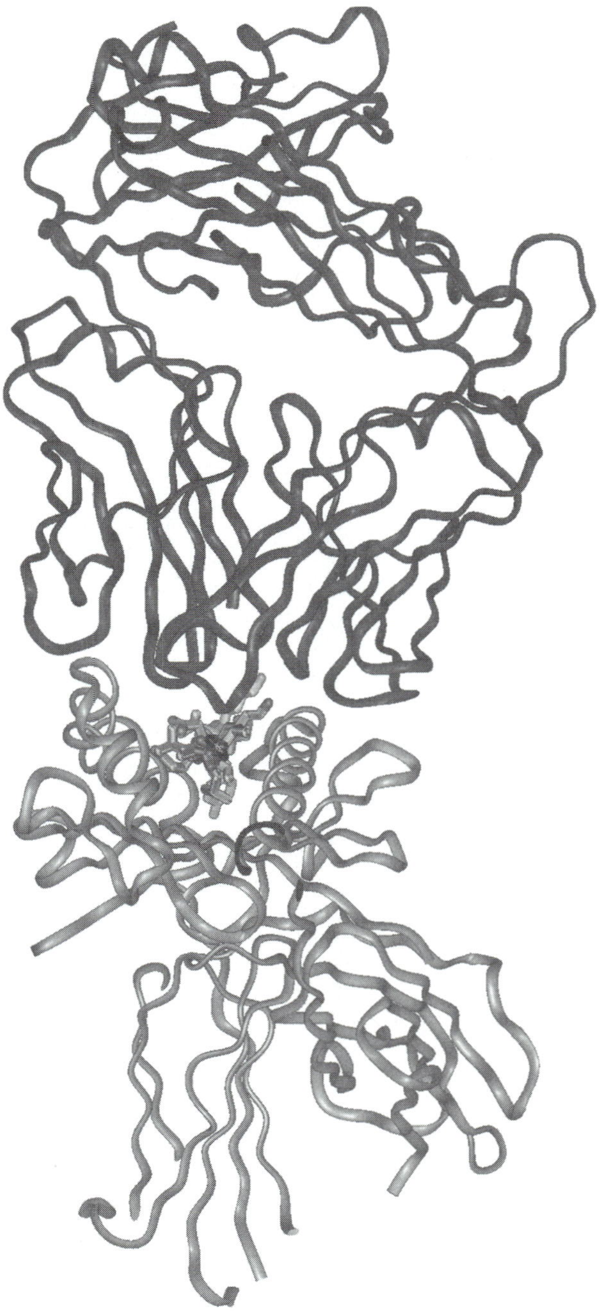

FIGURE 17–3 · Ribbon diagram derived from the three-dimensional crystal structure of the trimolecular complex of a human α/β-T cell receptor (*top, green*), influenza hemaglutinin (Ha) antigen peptide, and the MHC class II molecule, DRB1*0401.[24] Note that the peptide is contained with the peptide binding cleft of the HLA-DR molecule. The polymorphisms associated with the "shared epitope" are located on α-helical rim (DRB1 chain) of the peptide-binding cleft where they may interact with either the bound peptide antigen or the T cell receptor. (See color plate 4.)

complete list of genes in the region can be found online at *http://www.sanger.ac.uk/HGP/Chr6/MHC.shtml.*

The HLA class I α-chain genes are found on the telomeric side of the MHC, including the classic class I genes, HLA-A, HLA-B, and HLA-C; these three genes are also referred to as the class Ia genes. Several other class I genes have been defined. These include the HLA-G, HLA-E, and HLA-F loci, also known as class Ib genes. Initially, these class Ib genes were thought to be nonfunctional because they exhibit limited polymorphism. However, some of these genes do have significant immune functions. For example, HLA-G and HLA-E can act as ligands for natural killer (NK) cell inhibitory receptors.[25] In a surprising twist, HLA-E molecules bind and present peptides that are derived from the leader peptide of the class Ia genes and HLA-G.[26]

The HLA class II genes are situated centromeric to the class I region and have a somewhat more complicated organization. The three major subregions of the class II cluster are designated DR, DQ, and DP. Each of these subregions contains a variable number of α- and β-chain genes. Particularly in the case of the DR subregion, this variability has led to confusion regarding the nomenclature of these genes. However, an international standard for this nomenclature has been formalized.[27]

The DR subregion contains a single α-chain gene, designated DRA, which does not exhibit significant allelic variation. In contrast, the genes encoding the DRβ chains (DRB) are highly polymorphic and vary in number among different individuals in the population. This is shown in the box at the lower right of Figure 17–4, in which several examples of common DR haplotypes are displayed. (A *haplotype* refers to a group of alleles at closely linked loci that are commonly inherited together.) Many of these DRB genes are nonfunctional pseudogenes (indicated by the symbol ψ), although all haplotypes contain at least one functional DRB1 gene, and many haplotypes contain a second functional DRB gene (DRB3, DRB4, or DRB5).

The DQ subregion contains one pair of functional α- and β-chain genes, designated DQA1 and DQB1. These two genes encode all the known HLA-DQ molecules. Protein products of the DQA2 and DQB2 loci have not been reported. A similar situation exists in the DP subregion, in which only the DPA1 and DPB1 genes give rise to known protein products, the HLA-DP molecules.

In addition to the HLA class II molecules, several other genes distributed within the class II region are involved in peptide-antigen processing. The transport associated with antigen processing (TAP)1 and TAP2 genes have been of particular interest, because they exhibit a modest degree of polymorphism and are involved in delivering peptides for loading onto HLA class I molecules.[28] Other proteins encoded in this region are involved in peptide loading onto class II molecules, such as the DM molecule (encoded by the DMA and DMB genes) and the DO/DN heterodimer (encoded by DOB and DNA).

The "central" MHC is located in between the MHC class I and class II regions. It contains several genes involved in immune function, including those for tumor necrosis factor (TNF) -α and TNF-β, as well as the complement components C4A, C4B, C2, and factor B. This region also contains a number of other genes with potential relevance to immune function and disease susceptibility.[29]

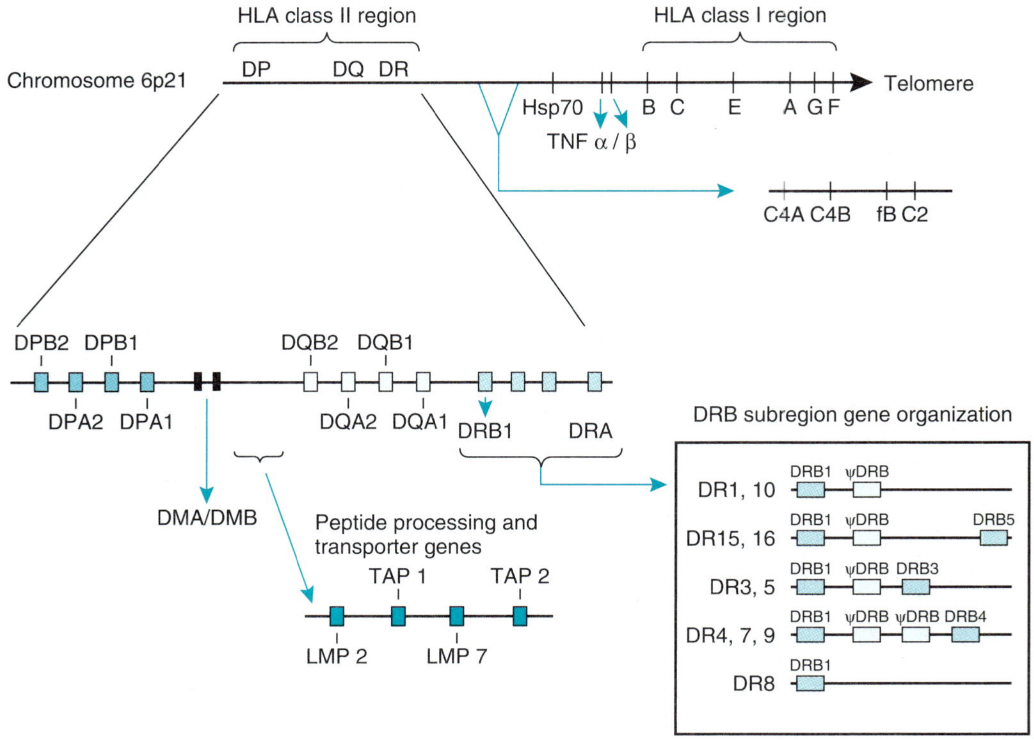

FIGURE 17–4 · Map of the Human Major Histocompatibility Complex (MHC). The HLA class I and class II molecules are encoded in distinct regions of the MHC. The HLA class II region contains three subregions, DR, DQ, and DP. Each of these contains a variable number of α- and β-chain genes. HLA class II loci with known functional protein products are labeled in **bold**. In the case of DR, different numbers of DRB genes are present in different haplotypes. A summary of the most common is shown in the box. The DQ and DP subregions each contain one pair of functional α- and β-chain genes. A number of genes involved in antigen processing and presentation by class I molecules are situated between the DP and DQ subregions. The HLA class I region contains the three "classic" class I genes—HLA-A, -B, and -C—as well as other related class I molecules (see text). The central MHC also contains a number of genes related to immune function, including the complement components (C4A, C4B, C2, and factor B), tumor necrosis factors (TNF) -α and -β and several heat-shock proteins such as HSP70.

POLYMORPHIC NATURE OF HUMAN LEUKOCYTE ANTIGEN MOLECULES

One of the most dramatic aspects of the HLA system is the extreme degree of polymorphism at most of these loci. The formal definition of polymorphism (Table 17–1) usually requires that the most common allele at the locus not exceed a frequency of 98 percent. In contrast, at many HLA loci, it is uncommon for a single HLA allele to exceed a frequency of 50 percent in the population. The number of different alleles present in the population is much larger than in any other known polymorphic locus encoding functional genes. For example, at the HLA-A locus, more than 100 different alleles have been reported; at HLA-B, the number of reported alleles is well over 200. A similar degree of allelic diversity is seen at the DRB1 locus and, to a lesser degree, at DQA and DQB.

The naming of these various HLA alleles has been a major source of confusion in the literature. The difficulty with the nomenclature stems in part from the different methods that have been used to define HLA polymorphisms. Originally, HLA class I alleles were detected through the use of alloantisera (see Table 17–1); the prefix "allo-" refers to genetic differences that exist between individuals of the same species. Alloantisera directed toward HLA molecules are commonly found in the context of pregnancy, in which the mother mounts an immune response against the "foreign" HLA molecules carried by the fetus (derived from the father). Anti-HLA responses are also seen after blood transfusion because the HLA molecules on the donor cells are highly immunogenic. In the case of HLA class II alleles, differences were originally detected using mixed lymphocyte responses. When T cells from a responder are mixed with lymphocytes from another individual, differences in HLA class II alleles cause the responder's T cells to proliferate. Data on mixed lymphocyte culture (MLC) typing dominated the early HLA literature, and it was the method first used to detect the HLA class II associations with RA.[30] Subsequently, serologic methods were also employed to detect class II polymorphisms.

TABLE 17–1 • GLOSSARY OF TERMS

Allele	Alternative form, or variant, of a gene at a particular locus.
Alloantisera	Antisera that detect antigenic differences between individuals in the population. The term is most often used to refer to sera that detect antigenic (i.e., structural) differences among human leukocyte antigen (HLA) molecules carried by different individuals.
Haplotype	A group of alleles at adjacent or closely linked loci on the same chromosome that are usually inherited together as a unit.
Heterozygote	An individual who inherits two different alleles at a given locus on two homologous chromosomes.
Heterozygosity	A measure, at a particular locus, of the frequency with which heterozygotes occur in the population.
Linkage	The tendency toward the coinheritance within a family of two genes that lie near each other on the genome. Complete linkage occurs when parents who are heterozygous at each locus are unable to produce recombinant gametes.
Linkage disequilibrium (LD)	The preferential association in a population of two or more alleles or mutations that occurs together more frequently than predicted by chance. Linkage disequilibrium is detected statistically, and except in unusual circumstances, it implies that the, associated alleles lie near to each other on the genome.
Polymorphism	The degree of allelic variation at a locus within a population. Specific criteria differ, but a locus is said to be polymorphic if the most frequent allele does not occur in more than 98% of the population. Occasionally, the term polymorphism can be used in the same way as allele to refer to a particular genetic variant.
Penetrance	The conditional probability of disease (or phenotype) given the presence of a risk genotype.

The current names of the HLA class I and class II alleles are attached to the specific DNA sequence and locus for each allele and are definitive.[27] However, many older publications have used the serologically derived names for alleles. It is therefore important to have some concept of how these naming conventions are related. The modern, definitive (sequence-based) allele names are derived from the older serologic names because the serologic techniques frequently detected whole groups of related alleles. Two examples of this are shown in Table 17–2. The designation HLA-B27 was developed for people carrying an HLA-B allele recognized by the B27-specific alloantisera. However, sequencing of the HLA-B alleles carried by these individuals revealed the existence of at least 17 different alleles, five of which are listed in Table 17–2. A similar situation exists for HLA class II allele families, such as HLA-DR4, also shown in Table 17–2. In this case, the DR4 allospecificity was already known to detect a number of different alleles that could be further discriminated on the basis of MLC typing.[31] These have been defined and named by their sequence, as shown in Table 17–2. A full list of all HLA alleles at the major loci can be found on the Internet at *http://www.ebi.ac.uk/imgt/hla/*.

Despite the precision of the molecular definition of HLA alleles, the old serologic names are often used in oral discussion because they are less cumbersome. For example, the DRB1*03011 allele is common in white populations (up to 10 percent in some populations) and is often referred to as simply DR3, after its original serologic designation. There are at least 16 distinct alleles detected by such DR3 alloantisera, and therefore the term DR3 is imprecise. However, when used in the context of a discussion about white populations, DR3 is assumed to refer to the predominant DRB1*03011 allele.

LINKAGE DISEQUILIBRIUM OF HUMAN LEUKOCYTE ANTIGEN ALLELES

In addition to their highly polymorphic nature, a characteristic feature of HLA genes is the tendency for cer-

TABLE 17–2 • COMPARISON BETWEEN MODERN, SEQUENCE-BASED NOMENCLATURE AND OLDER NAMING CONVENTIONS FOR CLASS I AND CLASS II ALLELES BELONGING TO THE HLA-B27 AND HLA-DR4 SEROLOGIC GROUPS

HLA-B locus: HLA-B27 alleles*		HLA-DRB1 locus: HLA-DR4 alleles*		
Definitive Nomenclature Based on DNA Sequence	*Serologic Designation (Defined by Alloantisera)*	*Definitive Nomenclature Based on DNA Sequence*	*Serologic Designation (Defined by Alloantisera)*	*Cellular Typing (Based on MLC)*
B*2701	B27	DRB1*0401	DR4	Dw4
B*2702	B27	DRB1*0402	DR4	Dw10
B*2703	B27	DRB1*0403	DR4	Dw13
B*2704	B27	DRB1*0404	DR4	Dw14
B*2705	B27	DRB1*0405	DR4	Dw15

*This list of alleles is incomplete. The B27 allele family contains at least 17 members, and the HLA-DR4 allele family contains at least 35 members. See *http://www.ebi.ac.uk/imgt/hla/* for a complete list of all HLA alleles.

Abbreviations: HLA, Human leukocyte antigen; MLC, mixed lyphocyte culture.

tain HLA alleles to be found together on the same haplotype. This phenomenon is referred to as *linkage disequilibrium* (LD), and it is central to understanding the significance of HLA associations with disease. LD exists when the frequency of two alleles occurring together on the same haplotype exceeds that predicted by chance. For example, a common haplotype that exhibits LD in the white population carries a certain combination of alleles, A*0101-B*0801-DRB1*03011, commonly referred to as the A1-B8-DR3 haplotype. This haplotype is present in about 9 percent of the Danish population, a typical white Northern European group. To understand why this reflects the presence of LD, consider the fact that the A1 allele is present in 17 percent of Danes, and the B8 allele is present in 12.7 percent of Danes. They could statistically be expected to be found together 12.7 percent × 17 percent = 2.1 percent of the time, much less than what is observed (9 percent). A simple way to express the extent of LD is the Δ value:

$$\Delta = 0.09 \text{ (observed value)} - 0.021 \text{ (expected value)} = 0.069$$

There are three likely explanations for LD. First, the population may have originated from a mixture of two populations, one of which had a very high frequency of a particular haplotype (in this case, A1-B8-DR3). If this happened recently, there would not have been time (i.e., a sufficient number of generations) to randomize alleles at closely linked loci by recombination at meiosis. Inasmuch as human history is marked by large population migrations,[32] it is probable that population admixture explains many examples of LD.

A second explanation, related to the first, rests on the observation that certain regions of the genome tend to exhibit relatively low levels of meiotic recombination. Thus, genetic variants within these regions tend to stay together on the same haplotype over many generations, even if haplotypes were introduced into a population in the distant past. The importance of this concept for understanding LD is still under active debate in the genetics community and is discussed further in a later section.

A third explanation for LD posits that the alleles in LD may be maintained together because of a selective advantage. For example, A1 and B8 (and other genes closely linked to them) could confer an advantage for immune defense when they are present together in the same individual. Although plausible, this hypothesis is difficult to prove for any particular haplotype, and there is no direct evidence for it.

Human Leukocyte Antigen Associations with Rheumatic Disease

POPULATION-ASSOCIATION STUDIES AND THE CALCULATION OF THE ODDS RATIO

The scientifically ideal way to establish whether a gene (allele) confers risk for a disease is by performing a prospective cohort study. In this kind of study, a group of individuals carrying (exposed to) the allele is compared with a matched control group that does not carry the allele. These two groups are followed over time (preferably over a lifetime) to see if disease develops more frequently in the exposed group. The results can be displayed in a contingency table (Table 17–3). By examining the upper half of Table 17–3, it is apparent that the fraction of exposed individuals who get the disease is a ÷ (ab), whereas the fraction of unexposed individuals who develop the disease is c ÷ (c + d). The ratio of these two fractions is known as the relative risk (RR).

$$RR = [a \div (a + b)] \div [c \div (c \times d)] = (ac \times ad) \div (ac \times bc)$$

If the disease is rare in the population, ac is very small, and the RR is approximated by (a × d) ÷ (b × c), also referred to as the cross product.

In reality, such prospective cohort studies are often impractical; therefore, a retrospective case-control design is used. In this type of study, subjects are initially identified according to whether they have the disease, and individuals without the disease are the controls. The data can be tabulated as in the lower half of Table 17–3. In this case, the cross product, or (a × d) ÷ (b × c), is known as the odds ratio (OR). In practice, this quantity is often reported as the estimated relative risk, because the cross product is close to the RR when the disease is rare. An odds ratio of 1 indicates that the genetic factor confers no risk for the disease. An odds ratio less than 1 suggests that the genetic factor under study is negatively associated with the disease. Odds ratios of less than 1 are occasionally reported as the negative inverse value; an odds ratio of 0.5 may also be reported −2.0. With the exception of HLA-B27–associated diseases, most HLA associations with rheumatic diseases have odds ratios of less than 10. Several examples of typical HLA associations with rheumatic and autoimmune disorders are shown in Table 17–4.

HUMAN LEUKOCYTE ANTIGEN CLASS I ASSOCIATIONS

One of the strongest and earliest-reported[33] HLA associations with the rheumatic diseases is the association of HLA-B27 with ankylosing spondylitis (AS). In white pop-

TABLE 17–3A • CONTINGENCY TABLE FOR COHORT STUDY*

	Disease	No Disease
Exposed	a	b
Not Exposed	c	d

TABLE 17–3B • CONTINGENCY TABLE FOR CASE-CONTROL STUDY*

	Exposed	Not Exposed
Disease	a	b
No Disease	c	d

*a, b, c, d = number of individuals observed in each category

TABLE 17–4 • SOME COMMON HLA ASSOCIATIONS WITH RHEUMATIC AND AUTOIMMUNE DISEASES

Disease	HLA Allele (Serologically Defined)	Approximate Allele Frequency in Caucasian Patients (%)	Approximate Allele Frequency in Caucasian Controls (%)	Approximate Relative Risk
Ankylosing spondylitis	B27	90%	8%	90
Reiter's syndrome	B27	70%	8%	40
Spondylitis in inflammatory bowel disease	B27	50%	8%	10
Rheumatoid arthritis	DR4	70%	30%	6
Systemic lupus	DR3	45%	20%	3
Multiple sclerosis	DR2	60%	20%	4
Juvenile diabetes (Type 1)	DR4	75%	30%	6

Abbreviation: HLA, Human leukocyte antigen.

ulations, more than 90 percent of patients with AS carry HLA-B27, in contrast to approximately 8 percent of normal individuals, giving estimated RR values of 50 to 100 or higher. The consistency of this finding across most ethnic groups lends support to the contention that the HLA-B27 alleles are directly involved in the pathogenesis of AS.[34] HLA-B27 is also associated with reactive arthritis, including Reiter's syndrome, and with the arthritis seen in the context of inflammatory bowel disease. As shown in Table 17–4, the strength of these associations is lower in terms of estimated RR compared to AS.

The serologic specificity of HLA-B27 actually encompasses many distinct HLA class I alleles. These alleles differ from one another at a number of amino acid positions, most of which involve amino acid substitutions in and around the peptide-binding pocket. This fact leads naturally to the question of whether there are differences among these B27 alleles in terms of disease association. Most data indicate that this is not the case, although there may be exceptions in some populations.[34] These exceptions may provide clues to the role of the HLA-B27 molecule in pathogenesis. Overall, however, it appears that most of the structural differences among the B27 alleles do not affect disease risk.

Some hypotheses can be derived by combining the sequence information on the various B27 alleles with structural information about the HLA-B27 molecule and the peptides bound to it.[20,35] The structure of the B*2705 allele (the most common allele in white populations) has been solved by x-ray crystallography and reveals the presence of a characteristic "pocket" in the floor of the peptide-binding cleft. This has been referred to as the "45 pocket" because amino acid position 45 is situated at the base of this pocket, and, in the case of the B27 alleles, it contains a negatively charged glutamic acid.[35] The peptides that bind to B27 alleles are all 9 amino acids long and invariably contain a positively charged arginine at the second position from the N-terminus.[35] This arginine appears to be situated within the 45 pocket when a peptide is bound to the HLA-B27 molecule. This sequence motif is distinct from peptides bound to other HLA class I alleles, such as HLA-A2, which lacks a glutamic acid in the 45 pocket. A number of other sequence motifs of B27-associated peptides have also been described.

These data suggest that the reason for the HLA-B27 association with AS may be related to the specific peptides bound and presented to CD8 T cells by these molecules. However, because a negatively charged 45 pocket is not uniquely present in B27 alleles but is also found in class I molecules not associated with spondyloarthropathies, this feature cannot be a complete explanation for the B27 associations with AS.

Human Leukocyte Antigen Class Antigen Class II Associations with Autoimmune Diseases

A large number of HLA class II associations with autoimmune diseases have been described.[14] Generally, the disease associations with HLA class II alleles are weaker and more complex than those seen with HLA-B27. RA has received particularly intense scrutiny, but the precise mechanisms underlying the HLA associations with this disease are still unknown. In the case of systemic lupus erythematosus (SLE) and related illnesses, many of the HLA class II alleles are associated with the presence of specific autoantibodies or clinical phenotypes. These differences suggest that different mechanisms may be involved in the HLA associations with these diseases.

RHEUMATOID ARTHRITIS: HLA-DRB1 ASSOCIATIONS AND THE "SHARED EPITOPE"

The first associations of RA with HLAs were reported in the 1970s by Stastny.[30] This was done using cellular[36] and antibody reagents[37] that are no longer routinely used for HLA typing; however, as discussed previously, the nomenclature for HLA alleles still derives from these early typing methods. The DRB1*0401 allele (corresponding to the "Dw4" type in Stastny's original report[36]) was the first HLA polymorphism to be associated with RA. Numerous studies have generally confirmed that this allele is the most strongly associated with RA, at least in Caucasian populations.[38-40] However, several other HLA-DRB1 alleles have also been associated with RA, although the strength of these associations varies.[39,41,42] In some ethnic groups, RA is not associated with HLA-DR4 alleles, but rather with HLA-

DR1[43] or HLA-DR10.[44] It is now widely accepted that the following alleles are the major contributors to RA risk at the DRB1 locus: DRB1*0401, -0404, -0405, -0101, and -1001. In addition, minor variants of these alleles, as well as others (DRB1*1402),[45] may also contribute to susceptibility. All of these risk alleles share a common sequence, as shown in Table 17–5. This predicted amino acid sequence,[70] Q–K or R–R–A–A[74] has been termed the "shared epitope" (SE).[46] (In the case of the DRB1*1001 risk allele, one amino acid varies from this consensus by a conservative change, with an R at position 70.) This structural feature is located on the α-helical portion of the DR β-chain, in a position where it may influence both peptide binding and T cell receptor interactions with the DRB1 molecule.

A number of different hypotheses have been advanced to explain the SE association with RA.[47,48] Two of these follow directly from knowledge of the role of HLA molecules in antigen presentation and immune regulation. Thus, it has been suggested that a particular peptide antigen, or set of related antigens, may be involved in the initiation or propagation of RA, and that SE-positive DRB1 alleles possess a unique, or enhanced, ability to bind or present these peptides to the immune system.[47] It has been difficult to address this hypothesis directly because the identity of these putative disease-causing peptide antigens is unknown. A second hypothesis posits that these risk alleles regulate the formation of the peripheral T cell repertoire by acting to select for particular T cell receptors (TCR) during thymic selection.[48] There is elegant experimental evidence in humans to support a role for DR4 alleles in shaping the peripheral T cell repertoire.[49] However, it is unclear whether this effect on the TCR repertoire is responsible for disease risk. In general, attempts to define the T cell repertoire involved in RA pathogenesis have yielded highly complex results that are difficult to interpret.

Several alternative hypotheses have also been proposed to explain the SE association with RA. Roudier and colleagues[50] noted the similarity of the SE sequence to viral antigens, leading to further proposals of molecular mimicry as a mechanism for the disease association with the SE.[51] Murine and human studies have provided evidence that peptides derived from MHC molecules can act as nominal antigen and can play a role in thymic selection and tolerance induction.[52,53] There is also evidence that the SE may influence patterns of intracellular trafficking of HLA-DR molecules.[54] However, these intriguing observations have not yet been supported by definitive experimentation that shows how the SE is actually involved in RA susceptibility.

More recently, the SE hypothesis itself has come under renewed scrutiny, with some investigators proposing a direct role for HLA-DQ polymorphisms,[55,56] in part based on studies in transgenic mice.[57] As can be seen in Figure 17-4, the HLA DQ α- and β-chains are encoded just centromeric to DRB1, and alleles at this locus are in strong LD with DRB1 alleles. The strong LD between the DR and DQ loci makes it difficult to tease apart the effects of DR versus DQ based solely on population genetic studies; the arguments for a DQ effect generally depend on showing the enrichment of relatively rare genotypes in the RA patient group compared with controls. Overall, a primary role for DQ alleles is not strongly supported by large HLA-association studies that have examined this issue.[58]

Regardless of whether HLA-DQ alleles are involved in RA susceptibility, it is quite clear that the SE hypothesis is not a complete explanation for the HLA associations with RA. This has been shown by formal analysis,[59] but it also is evident based on the fact that not all SE+ alleles carry the same degree of genetic risk, and the strength of the association varies in different populations. In general, DRB1*0101 alleles carry lower levels of RR for RA than the DRB1*0401 and 0404 alleles,[40] and yet DRB1*0101 is the major risk allele in some ethnic groups.[60,61] In contrast, the SE itself does not appear to associate with RA in African American and some Hispanic populations.[62,63] Furthermore, certain combinations of DRB1 alleles carry especially high risk, as originally observed by Nepom and colleagues.[64] Thus, the combination of DRB1*0401 with *0404 carries an RR of more than 30 in white populations.[40] This compares with RR values in the range of 4 or 5 for either allele alone. Some of these relationships are summarized in Table 17–6. It is unclear whether these interactive effects are mediated by the HLA-DR molecules themselves or reflect the action of other genes on these haplotypes.

TABLE 17–5 • AMINO ACID SUBSTITUTIONS COMPRISING THE SHARED EPITOPE AT POSITIONS 70-74 OF DRB1 ALLELES ASSOCIATED WITH RHEUMATOID ARTHRITIS

	Amino Acid Position				
DRB1 Alleles	70	71	72	73	74
0101	Gln	Arg	Arg	Ala	Ala
0401	-	Lys	-	-	-
0404	-	-	-	-	-
0405	-	-	-	-	-
0408	-	-	-	-	-
1402	-	-	-	-	-
1001	Arg	-	-	-	-

TABLE 17–6 • GENOTYPE RELATIVE RISKS OF DRB1 GENOTYPES FOR RHEUMATOID ARTHRITIS

DRB1 Genotype	Relative Risk	P value
0101/DRX	2.3	10^{-3}
0401/DRX	4.7	10^{-12}
0404/DRX	5.0	10^{-9}
0101/0401	6.4	10^{-4}
0401/0404	31.3	10^{-33}

Data from Hall FC, Weeks DE, Camilleri JP, et al: Influence of the HLA-DRB1 locus on susceptibility and severity in rheumatoid arthritis. QJM 89:821-829, 1996.

HLA-DQ ASSOCIATIONS WITH AUTOIMMUNE DISEASES

Many of the first HLA class II associations with autoimmune disorders were detected using alloantisera for HLA-DR alleles, as indicated in Table 17–4. However, as knowledge increased about the genetic organization of the class II region, it became apparent that for some diseases, the genetic associations are stronger with HLA-DQ alleles. For example, although juvenile diabetes does exhibit HLA associations with both HLA-DR4 and HLA-DR3, it is likely that a group of associated HLA-DQ alleles actually are responsible for these observations.[65] As discussed in the following paragraphs, the HLA associations with particular autoantibodies in systemic lupus also probably reflect the effects of HLA-DQ alleles.

The DQ subregion presents special challenges for the newcomer to HLA because the old serologic nomenclature does not usually have a simple correlation with a group of alleles at a single locus. Because most of the HLA correlations with autoantibodies in lupus involve the DQ loci, it is important to understand this at the outset. The problem arises because the α- and β-chains are both polymorphic in DQ molecules. The serologic specificity of DQ2 may detect one of three closely related DQB1 alleles: DQB1*0201, DQB1*0202, or DQB1*0203. This is similar to the DR serologic specificity detecting a group of related DRB1 alleles (see Table 17–2). However, in the case of DQ, the DQ2 serologic specificity also detects these alleles on several different haplotypes that may encode quite different DQ α-chains. (This is different from HLA-DR molecules, in which the DR α-chain structure is constant and does not vary between haplotypes.) In white populations, the DQB1*0201 allele is commonly found on DR3 haplotypes (associated with DQA1*0501) and DR7 haplotypes (associated with DQA1*0201), but both these haplotypes would type serologically as DQ2 (Fig. 17–5). Especially when reading the older literature and discussing DQ polymorphisms, it is important to distinguish serologically defined polymorphisms, which may vary within the group of alleles on the α- and β-chains, from polymorphisms defined by sequence at a specific locus (DQA1 or DQB1).

The HLA associations with the Ro (SS-A) and La (SS-B) autoantibody systems have been thoroughly studied. The anti-Ro response is present in 25 to 50 percent of patients with lupus[66] and even more frequently in the setting of primary Sjogren's syndrome.[67] Although early serologic studies indicated an association with HLA-DR3 and DR2, a detailed molecular analysis of these HLA haplotypes has provided evidence that HLA-DQ alleles in LD with DR2 and DR3 are responsible for controlling this autoantibody response; heterozygous individuals who inherit a DR2-DQ1 haplotype and a DR3-DQ2 haplotype tend to have very high anti-Ro antibody titers in the setting of lupus or Sjogren's syndrome.[68] The strongest associations involve a DQA1*0501DQB1*0201 haplotype (frequently found in linkage disequilibrium with DR3) and a DQA1*06-DQB1*06 haplotype (frequently found in linkage disequilibrium with DR2).

Reveille and colleagues[69] attempted to further refine these associations by looking at DQ alleles in Ro antibody–positive patients who do not inherit one of these two associated haplotypes. These data led to the hypothesis that particular amino acid substitutions in the DQ α-chain (glutamine at position 34) and DQ β-chain (leucine at position 26) may be involved in risk for developing a Ro-antibody response. Proof of this hypothesis is unlikely to come solely from additional genetic studies, but also from experiments that directly test the influence of these DQ polymorphisms on the immune response to specific autoantigens.[70,71] HLA-DQ associations have also been reported for other autoantibody systems, such as antiphospholipid antibodies[72] and anti-Sm responses.[73] The overall pattern of HLA-DQ associations with these antibody responses is similar to those seen for anti-Ro responses, although the alleles involved are quite different.

POPULATION-ASSOCIATION STUDIES: WHAT DO THEY MEAN?

Almost all the studies on HLA and disease involve population associations that are detected by means of retrospective case-control studies. It is essential to understand the strengths and weaknesses of this approach to genetic analysis to judge the significance

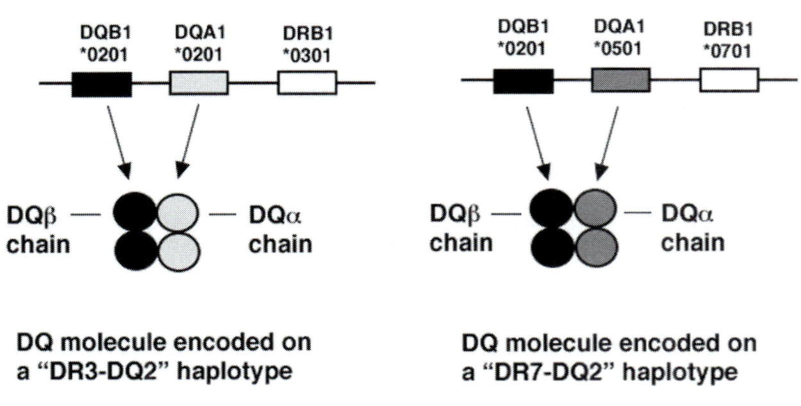

FIGURE 17–5 · Combinatorial Diversity of HLA-DQ Molecules. The serologically defined DQ2 molecule may contain the same DQ β-chain paired with different DQ α-chain alleles. This is different from HLA-DR molecules, in which the DR α-chain does not vary among different MHC haplotypes.

these HLA associations. In general, there are three possible reasons for detecting an association between a particular allele and a disease.

First, the allele under investigation may be directly involved in the pathogenesis of the disease. This assumption actually underlies most of the foregoing discussion on HLA and rheumatic disease. The studies described reflect the search for ever-more-precise definitions of particular amino acid substitutions or structural characteristics of disease-associated alleles. This effort derives from the belief that HLA alleles directly predispose to disease by virtue of their ability to control the immune response.[15] As discussed previously, this may involve a number of mechanisms, including preferential peptide binding and the influence of MHC on thymic selection of the peripheral T cell repertoire.

The second possible reason for observing an HLA association is that a gene in LD with HLA may be the disease gene. LD over long distances is a particularly prominent feature of the HLA region. There are a number of genes with immunologic function within the MHC complex that may themselves be directly involved in predisposing to autoimmunity. As shown in Figure 17–4, genes involved in antigen processing (TAP1 and TAP 2), complement activation (C4, C2, factor B), and cytokines such as TNF are all encoded in this region and could be responsible for disease risk. As discussed in a later section, it is likely that for many autoimmune diseases, MHC genes other than, or in addition to, the classical HLA alleles are involved in disease susceptibility.

A third reason to consider with any HLA association is the possibility that the result is an artifact of population stratification of patients and controls. The potential for population stratification can be a significant problem for population-association studies. The concern is that the control group may not be genetically matched to the disease group at loci unrelated to disease. This can result from a failure to study a control group ethnically matched to the disease group. To take an extreme example, when studying the frequency blue eyes in Scandinavian patients with RA, it would be inappropriate to use a random sample of New Yorkers as the control population, because blue eyes are much less common in that population. This mismatch would lead to the incorrect conclusion that blue eye color is associated with RA. Because of this problem, retrospective use of published control frequencies for HLA alleles is not acceptable methodology, and all good HLA-association studies go to great efforts to match patients and controls with regard to ethnicity. Nevertheless, it is difficult to be certain that the two populations are not stratified in some subtle way, particularly in the U.S. population, in which ethnic admixture is common. One solution to this difficulty is to rely on repeated studies in a new set of patients and controls and to look at HLA associations in a variety of ethnic groups. However, several approaches have been developed that get around the problem of population stratification. These are described in the next section.

ALTERNATIVES TO THE CASE-CONTROL METHOD FOR DETECTING DISEASE ASSOCIATION

To avoid the confounding effects of population stratification in case-control studies, family-based controls can also be used for association studies. Consider the family shown in Figure 17–6. The affected child carries DR4 and DR3, each of which is inherited from one parent. The laws of mendelian inheritance specify that one DR haplotype from each parent is not inherited by any given offspring—in this example, DR2 in the father and DR5 in the mother. These two noninherited haplotypes can be thought of as forming a genotype for a "control" individual. In this manner, issues of population stratification are eliminated because patients and controls are sampled from the identical (parental) gene pool. This approach to disease association was originally proposed by Falk and Rubinstein[74] and was called the "haplotype relative risk" method. Its validity depends on a number of assumptions, including that the genetic marker under study does not influence mating preference or the production of gametes.

A popular extension of this approach is called the transmission disequilibrium test (TDT).[75] Using the family in Figure 17–6, for a given heterozygous parent (such as the father carrying DR2 and DR4), there is a probability of 0.5 that any given allele, such as DR4, will be transmitted to the child. If the DR4 allele has no bearing on disease risk, the probability of transmission (T) to an affected child is equal to the probability of nontransmission (NT). This can be stated simply as $P(T|D) = P(NT|D)$, in which D indicates the presence of disease in the offspring. However, if the allele being examined is associated with disease risk, then $P(T|D) > P(NT|D)$. If large numbers of heterozygous parents with affected offspring are examined, TDT can establish an association between disease and the test allele, compared to the (noninherited) control alleles.

The TDT has been used to confirm HLA associations and to investigate the role of other MHC-linked genes, such as TNF, in rheumatic diseases.[76] The advantages of this approach for avoiding the problem of population stratification are appealing. However, it does require the availability of parents, and case-control studies still have a major role to play in genetic analysis.[77]

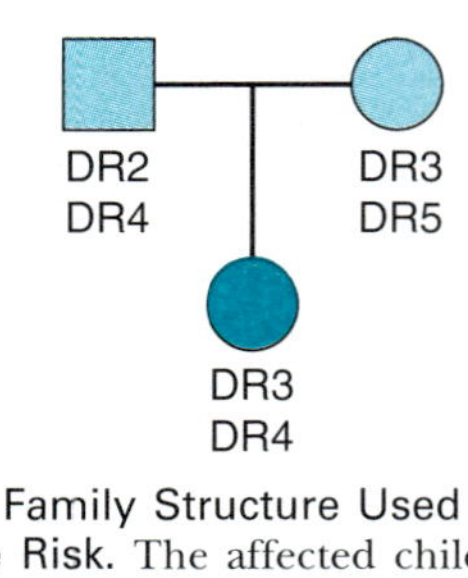

FIGURE 17–6 · Family Structure Used for Determination of Haplotype Relative Risk. The affected child carries the DR3 and DR4 alleles. A fictitious "control" individual can be contructed from the noninherited DR2 and DR5 alleles and used for a relative risk (RR) calculation. Such families can also be used for transmission disequilibrium testing (TDT), as discussed in the text.

COMPLEXITY OF HLA ASSOCIATIONS WITH RHEUMATIC DISEASES

The foregoing discussion has emphasized the assumption that for a given disease or autoimmune phenotype, a set of alleles at a single HLA locus is likely to explain the association. However, for at least some autoimmune diseases it appears likely that multiple genes within the MHC may contribute independently to disease risk. In the case of RA, a number of studies have indicated that a separate locus in the central MHC may associate with the disease, independent of the HLA-DRB1 locus.[76,78-80] In addition, there is evidence that genes in the class I region may influence the risk conferred by certain HLA-DRB1*0404 haplotypes[79] or may interact with other non-MHC genes.[81] Similar analyses in lupus,[82] juvenile arthritis,[83] and multiple sclerosis[84] all point to the possibility that multiple genes within the MHC can contribute to disease susceptibility. This issue will likely be a focus of future research efforts on the HLA region in rheumatic diseases.

Other Approaches to Analysis of Genetically Complex Disease

Although the MHC is important for susceptibility to rheumatic diseases, non–MHC-linked genes also must be involved. How do we know this? In the absence of knowledge about specific genes, the evidence for a genetic contribution to a complex phenotype such as autoimmunity depends almost entirely on epidemiologic data. These data involve the comparison of disease prevalence in groups of individuals with different degrees of genetic relatedness. The most common types of groups used for such studies are genetically identical individuals (MZ twins), individuals who share approximately 50 percent of their genes in common (DZ twins and siblings), and unrelated individuals in the population whose overall degree of genetic similarity (at polymorphic loci) is relatively low, with about 0.1 percent difference over the entire genome. (A 0.1 percent difference among unrelated subjects implies approximately 3 million base pair differences over the entire genome of 3.2 billion base pairs, assuming only single nucleotide polymorphisms.)

The use of such family and background population prevalence data to calculate risk ratios has become a popular means of estimating the size of the genetic component in complex diseases.[85] This method uses prevalence rates to calculate the relative risk of disease between two comparison populations, most often siblings of affected individuals compared to the general population. This leads to a value called λ_s, or relative risk to siblings, which is calculated as follows:

λ_s = disease prevalence in siblings of affected individuals ÷ disease prevalence in general population

Obtaining a reliable value of λ_s depends on having accurate estimates of disease prevalence in the two comparison groups. This is not a trivial matter. In the case of RA, the estimation of population prevalence is fraught with potential sources of error. A firm diagnosis of RA is difficult to make in large surveys, with errors in both directions possible. Underestimation may occur because of the lack of reporting of disease that is no longer active. Overestimation may result from inadequate distinction between RA and other forms of polyarthritis. Similar problems may occur in estimates of population prevalence of lupus, in which mild disease may be overlooked, or variability in phenotypic expression may confound the issue. Accurate detection and assessment of disease phenotype are also involved in the determination of sibling affection rates.

Despite these difficulties, a range of values for λ_s has been established for many of the common autoimmune disorders.[86] Representative examples are shown in Table 17–7. With the exception of AS, most autoimmune disorders appear to have a λ_s in the range of 10 to 20. Table 17–7 also shows the estimates for λ_{MZ}. Analogous to the calculation for λ_s, λ_{MZ} is calculated by the following:

λ_{MZ} = disease prevalence in identical (MZ) twins of affected individuals ÷ disease prevalence in general population

The value λ_{MZ} can be interpreted as an estimate of the maximal genetic risk for the disease. This assumes that all the increased risk to an MZ twin of an affected individual results from the fact that the two share the same genetic polymorphisms. This is clearly not the case, because at least some environmental sharing probably contributes to the risk. However, it is notable that the estimated value for λ_{MZ} is quite high for many autoimmune disorders, and this emphasizes the fact that MZ-twin concordance rates must be interpreted in light of the background population prevalence of the disease. A relatively low MZ-twin concordance rate does not necessarily imply a low genetic component to the disorder. For most diseases, only a fraction of the total genetic risk can be ascribed to MHC-linked genes. Other genes must be involved.

SEARCHING FOR NON–HUMAN LEUKOCYTE ANTIGEN GENES

Population-association studies have been the primary means of detecting the involvement of HLA or other genetic loci in the rheumatic diseases. Two other methods of genetic analysis offer powerful alternatives to

TABLE 17–7 • FAMILIAL CLUSTERING OF SELECTED AUTOIMMUNE DISEASES, AS MEASURED BY THE RELATIVE RISK TO SIBLINGS (λ_s) AND TWINS(λ_{MZ})

Disease	λ_s	λ_{MZ}
Type 1 diabetes	15	60
Rheumatoid arthritis	3-10	20-60
Multiple sclerosis	20	250
Systemic lupus erythematosus	20	250
Ankylosing spondylitis	54	500

From Vyse TJ, Todd JA: Genetic analysis of autoimmune disease. Cell 85: 311-318, 1996.

this approach: classic linkage analysis of multiplex families and the analysis of allele sharing between affected individuals (usually siblings) within a family. Allele-sharing methods are being used extensively to search for susceptibility genes outside the MHC. It is important for the rheumatologist to have some understanding of the concepts underlying these methods, including their advantages and limitations.

The basic purpose of linkage analysis is to determine whether a particular genetic marker and a disease (or phenotype) tend to be inherited together in families. The power of this approach depends on the occurrence of recombination during the first meiotic division. This first meiotic division leads to the production of gametes containing different combinations of the disease gene and any given marker locus. The frequency of these combinations depends on the relative locations of the disease gene and the genetic marker being examined.

Figure 17–7 illustrates the possible outcome of meiosis for two genes situated at different distances from each other on the same chromosome. One of the genes may carry a disease allele, D, or the corresponding wild-type (normal) allele, d, at the disease gene locus, designated *D*. A second marker gene can also carry one of two alleles, M and m, at locus *M*. In Figure 17–7*A*, the two loci are very widely separated from one another at different ends of the chromosome. In this case the four possible meiotic products also occur with equal frequency because the likelihood of a crossover (recombination) event occurring between the two loci is very high, effectively producing random combinations of marker and disease alleles in the meiotic products. (At least one recombination event occurs in every chromosome at every meiosis. On average, approximately 66 recombination events at each meiosis are spread over the 23 chromosomes. This number is slightly higher for females than males.)

The situation in Figure 17–7*B* is slightly different. In this case, the *D* and *M* loci are very close together on the same arm of the chromosome. The likelihood that recombination will occur between them is very low, but not zero. The same four meiotic products can occur, but at different frequencies. Two of the meiotic products are recombinants, and in this case they constitute 10 percent of the total. This quantity is called the recombination fraction, θ. When 10 percent of the meiotic products are recombinants, $\theta = 0.1$. If the marker gene is extremely close to or is identical with the disease gene, $\theta = 0$; no recombinants would be observed in the meiotic products.

These principles can be applied to the two families with an autosomal dominant disease shown in Figure 17–8. In family A, two of the four children with the disease inherit the marker allele, M, from their affected father (through the grandmother), whereas the unaffected children do not inherit the M allele. In this family, marker M segregates with the disease. Can we conclude that marker M is linked to the disease locus? We do not know at the outset whether the *M* locus is near to the disease locus or not. It could be that *D* and *M* are very far apart ($\theta = 0.5$). If this is the case, what is

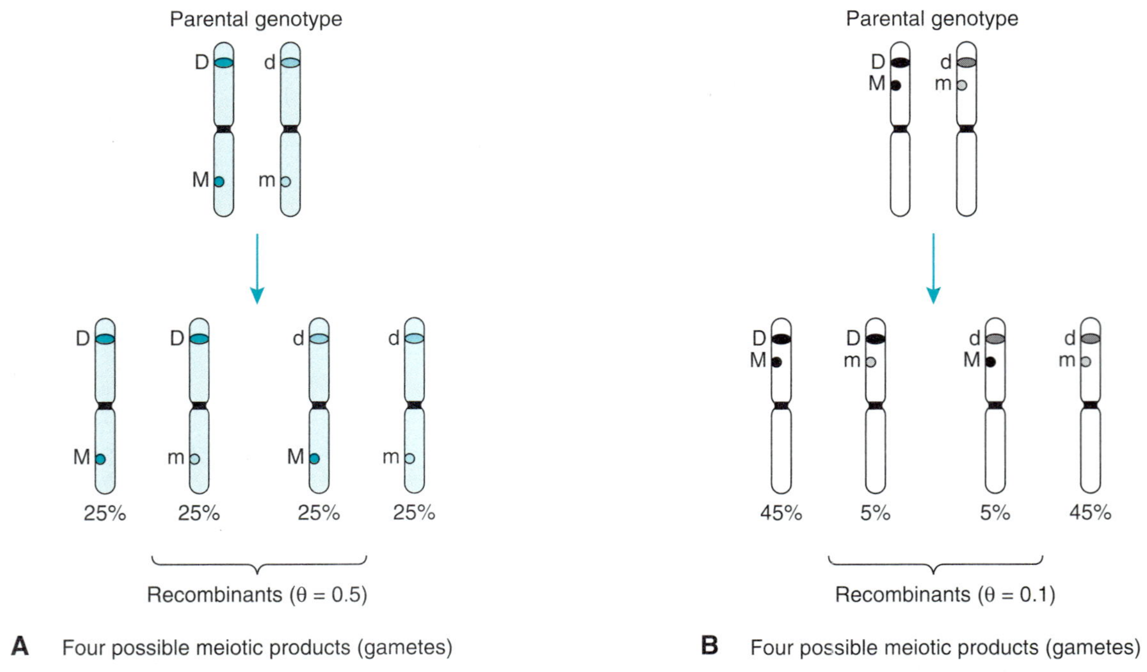

FIGURE 17–7 · Segregation of Alleles at the *M* and *D* Loci Depends on Their Relative Locations. *A*, the *M* and *D* loci are located very far apart on the same chromosome; thus, recombination during the first meiotic division will result in an equal distribution of the four meiotic products. *B*, the *M* and *D* loci are located very close to one another in the same chromosomal region, making recombination between them an uncommon event during meiosis. The frequency of recombination, in this case 10 percent, is expressed as the recombination fraction, $\theta = 0.1$.

the probability that the cosegregation of disease with marker M happened by chance in family A? In Figure 17–7*A*, half of the father's meiotic products that carry the disease allele (D) are expected to also carry M, if *D* and *M* are unlinked ($\theta = 0.5$). The probability that D will always segregate with M (and d with m) in four of four offspring is $(1/2)^4 = 1/16$, even if the *M* and *D* loci are on different chromosomes. We cannot conclude anything with certainty on the basis of family A alone. However, if 10 offspring were available for analysis, as shown in family B, with the same pattern of complete cosegregation between the disease and the marker allele M, chance alone would be unlikely to explain it. In this case the probability would be $(1/2)^{10} = 1/1024$, and linkage between M and the disease would be very likely, although not certain.

In practice, the calculation of a likelihood ratio is used to derive conclusions from such family data. In the case of family B (see Fig. 17–8), the best fit for the data is that the disease locus and marker M are very close to or identical to one another ($\theta = 0$). If this is the case, the probability of observing the outcome shown in family B is 1. If the disease gene and the marker allele M are nowhere near each other ($\theta = 0.5$), the likelihood of observing the pattern of segregation in family B is 1/1024. The ratio of these two probabilities is called the likelihood ratio, $Z(\theta)$

$$Z(\theta) = L(\theta) \div L(1/2) = \text{likelihood of the data if } \theta = 0 \div \text{likelihood of the data if } \theta = 0.5$$

$$= 1/(1/1024) = 1024$$

The $\log_{10}$ of this ratio is referred to as the LOD score. In this case, the LOD score is slightly greater than 3. For the purpose of linkage analysis, an LOD score of 3 is considered a statistically significant result and is used as a cutoff. Family B provides enough information to conclude that the marker locus is very near to the disease locus.

When performing linkage studies, a candidate genetic marker is often near but not immediately adjacent to the disease gene ($0 < \theta < 0.5$). Suppose, for example, that one of the 10 offspring in family B was affected in the absence of the marker allele M. Assuming that the *M* and *D* loci are linked, this would imply that recombination between the marker locus and the disease locus occurs in 10 percent of the cases. In this case, the maximal LOD score would be calculated on the basis of using the probability of the data if $\theta = 0.1$ in the numerator of the likelihood ratio, $Z(\theta)$. In practice, the calculations for a large amount of family data are done with various values of θ to determine which θ gives the best fit for the data and therefore the highest LOD score. A detailed discussion of how these calculations are done is beyond the scope of this chapter but can be found in a classic textbook on this topic.[87]

Several major discoveries in rheumatic diseases have resulted from the use of classic linkage analysis. In 1992, familial Mediterranean fever was mapped to chromosome 16,[88] and this led to the identification of the gene for this disease in 1997.[89] In addition, an entirely new class of familial periodic fever syndromes has been localized to mutations in the TNF-receptor 1 gene on chromosome 12.[90,91] Thus, for highly penetrant mendelian disorders, linkage analysis is a powerful means of identifying the underlying molecular basis of disease.

ALLELE-SHARING METHODS

One of the drawbacks to classic linkage analysis is that, to be most useful, it should be applied to disorders with a high penetrance and a known genetic model (e.g., dominant or recessive). Classic linkage analysis is of limited utility for investigating the more common rheumatic diseases, in which the penetrance is low and the genetic models are highly uncertain. An alternative

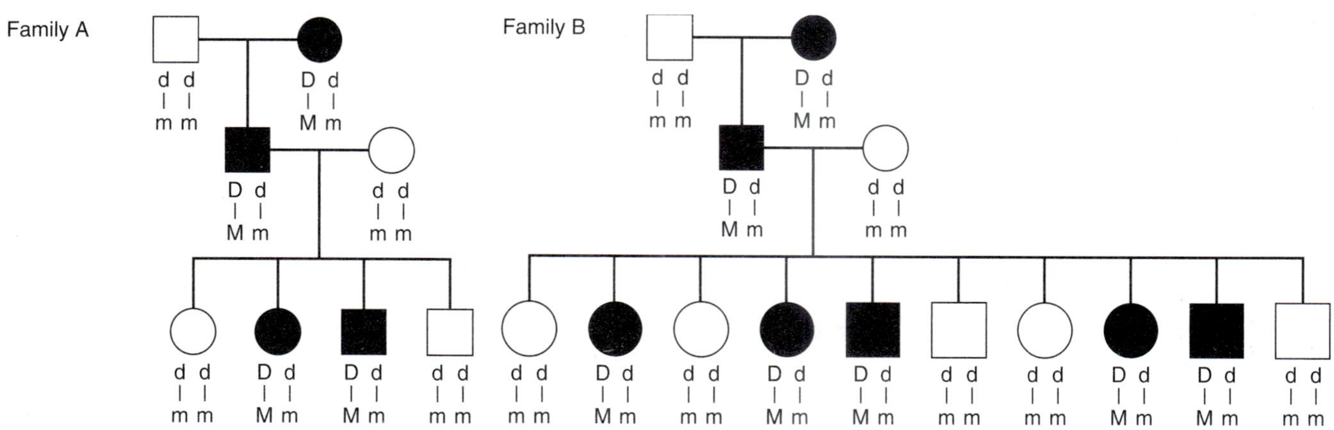

FIGURE 17–8 · Two families are shown in which a marker allele (M) and the disease allele (D) are inherited through the father on a haplotype derived from the the paternal grandmother. In both families, the disease always segregates with M allele in the children. In family A, the likelihood of this happening by chance is 1⁄16, if the *M* and *D* loci are unlinked ($\theta = 0.5$). However, when more meioses are available for inspection (i.e., siblings of known phenotype), as in family B, the likelihood of this pattern of segregation occuring by chance (in the absence of linkage) is much lower, with a probability calculated at 1/1024 (see text).

approach based on linkage, broadly called allele sharing, is preferred for the study of autoimmune diseases that have a complex genetic basis.[92]

The most common approach to allele sharing is the affected sibling pair (ASP) method. This method is based on a simple question: When two siblingss are both affected with a disease, do they share alleles at particular genetic markers more frequently than would be expected by chance? The basic approach is illustrated in Figure 17–9. In this family two siblings are affected, and the first-born sibling (sib 1) has inherited alleles 1 and 3 at a marker locus, X. By the laws of mendelian inheritance, sibling 2 has a 25 percent chance of inheriting these same two alleles and has a 25 percent chance of inheriting neither of these alleles (i.e., sib 2 inherits 2, 4 and shares nothing with sib 1 at locus X). By similar reasoning, there is a 50 percent chance that these two siblings will share one allele in common. This 25:50:25 distribution of sharing zero, one, or two haplotypes is expected if there is no linkage between the disease and the marker locus. However, if a gene that lies very near the marker locus is involved in disease risk, a significant deviation toward increased sharing among affected siblings will be observed. The closer the marker is to the disease locus (θ close to 0), the greater the deviation will be from a 25:50:25 distribution. By examining large numbers of affected sibling pairs in this manner, the investigator can develop statistical evidence that this is the case using a standard χ^2 analysis, with the null hypothesis being that there is no increased sharing at the marker locus.

ASP analysis has a number of distinct advantages and disadvantages. In contrast to linkage analysis, only affected individuals are used, and the problem of falsely assigning a family member as "unaffected" is eliminated. This is a major issue for diseases such as RA, because the disease may not express itself until later in life. ASP analysis can be done without committing to a specific model of inheritance (i.e., recessive or dominant). The ASP methods suffer from having relatively low power to detect genes that confer only modest risk. This means that quite large numbers (hundreds or thousands) of families may need to be studied to obtain statistically significant results.

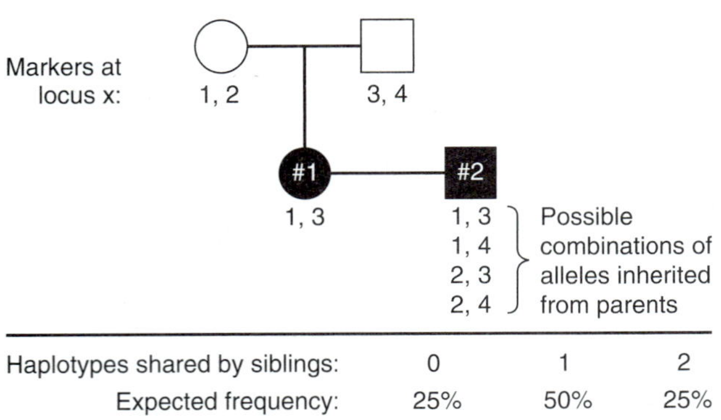

FIGURE 17–9 · **A Nuclear Family with Two Affected Children (affected sibling pair).** The possible distribution of alleles at an autosomal locus, X, is shown for sibling 2, along with the predicted frequency of shared haplotypes among the siblings. Such families can be used to detect linkage using affected sibling pair analysis (see text).

ASP methods have become increasing popular and are being applied to the study of a variety of autoimmune and rheumatic diseases, including lupus,[93-95] RA,[96-99] and AS.[100] This approach has also been used successfully in Crohn's disease and has led to the identification of a gene on chromsome 16, NOD2, that is involved in susceptibility to inflammatory bowel disease.[101,102] Thus, it is not unreasonable to expect that successful gene identification will be forthcoming in some of the major rheumatic disorders.

THE NATURE OF GENETIC MARKERS

A discussion of genetics would not be complete without some details about genetic markers. Markers can be chosen for study for a number of reasons. They may constitute polymorphisms that are known to have functional significance, such as the amino acid substitutions found in HLA molecules. Alternatively, the marker itself may have no biologic relevance but is used because of its location near a candidate gene of interest. When scanning the entire genome for linkage using ASP analysis, the need is for markers that are spread at intervals throughout the genome and are sufficiently informative (polymorphic) to allow sharing among sibling pairs to be assessed. In general, 300 to 400 markers are required for a genome scan.

Microsatellite Markers and the Calculation of Heterozygosity

The most common type of marker used for linkage studies is called a microsatellite.[103] Microsatellites are short sequences that contain variable numbers of tandem repeats (VNTRs), generally consisting of dinucleotide, trinucleotide, or tetranucleotide repeats. These repeated elements are flanked by unique sequences that define the location of the microsatellite. This allows the investigator to design polymerase chain reaction (PCR) primers that specifically amplify a particular microsatellite at a particular location in the genome, as shown in Figure 17–10*A*. Many thousands of these microsatellite markers have been defined and are widely used for genetic-mapping purposes.

In addition to their uniquely defined locations, the utility of microsatellite markers depends on their variability (length polymorphism), which allows the researcher to follow the segregation of particular chromosomal regions in families. The degree to which a marker is informative by virtue of this variability is reflected in a parameter-designated heterozygosity (H). Heterozygosity can be assessed in two ways. An empiric estimate can be derived by directly measuring the frequency of heterozygous individuals in the population. However, for many markers and populations, this information is not available. Alternatively, heterozygosity can be estimated by calculation from the estimated frequency of each allele at the marker locus:

$$H = 1 - \Sigma p_i^2$$

in which p_i is the frequency of the ith allele at the marker locus. For example, if there are three alleles at

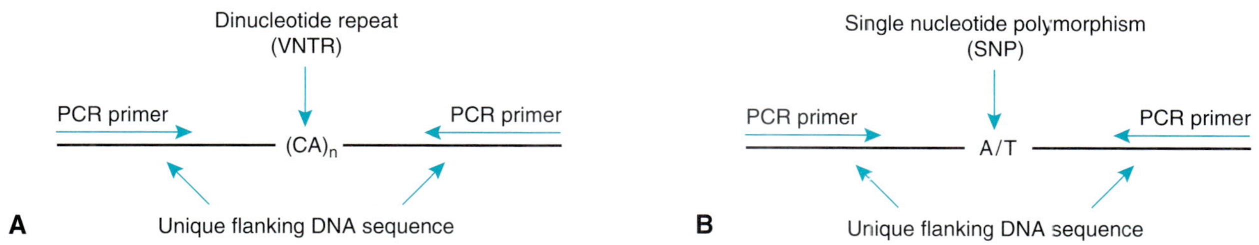

FIGURE 17–10 · Comparison of Microsatellite and SNP Markers. *A*, Microsatellite markers consist of variable numbers of tandem repeats (VNTRs), also known as short tandem repeats (STRs), in this case a dinucleotide repeat of $(CA)_n$. The flanking DNA sequence is unique to a specific location in the genome, and these sequences can be used for polymerase chain reaction (PCR) to rapidly analyze the number of repeats in a given individual. *B*, Single nucleotide polymorphisms (SNPs) consist of single base-pair changes at a particular base-pair positions. In this case, either A or T can be present. Similar to the situation for VNTRs, the SNP polymorphism is flanked by unique sequences that can be PCR amplified.

the locus with a frequency of 0.1, 0.4, and 0.5, the heterozygosity would be 1 – (0.01 + 0.16 + 0.25) = 0.68. That is, 68 percent of the population will be heterozygous, and 42 percent will be homozygous for one of these three alleles. The probability of being homozygous for a particular allele is the square of the frequency of that allele in all of the chromosomes present in the population under study. The level of heterozygosity primarily depends on two factors: the number of different alleles and their pattern of distribution. The higher the number of alleles and the more evenly distributed they are, the higher the level of heterozygosity. For a locus with five alleles, equally frequent, $H = 1 - 5 (0.2^2) = 0.8$. Many microsatellite loci have H values of 0.8 or higher, and these highly informative markers are preferred for genetic-mapping studies.

Single Nucleotide Polymorphisms and Haplotype Blocks

In recent years, the genetics community has focused an enormous amount of attention on the utility of markers called single nucleotide polymorphisms (SNPs, pronounced "snips"). Like microsatellites, these DNA markers occur at unique positions in the genome, but consist of only a single base pair change, generally A/T or G/C variations (see Figure 17–10*B*). Because any given SNP has only two alleles, the maximum heterozygosity (H) value is only 0.5. However, unlike microsatellites, there are millions of SNPs in the genome, approximately one every 1000 base pairs. SNPs may occur within coding regions and lead to amino acid changes, or they may have functional effects by changing promoter function. Most SNPs lie outside genes and probably have no functional signficance. Nevertheless, they can be useful for mapping disease, particularly using association methods.

SNPs have been most commonly used in the context of candidate gene-association studies. However, it is becoming apparent that combinations of SNPs can be used to define common haplotype "blocks" that exist by virtue of strong LD between alleles at adjacent SNP markers.[104,105] Current data suggest that a large portion of the sequence variation in the human genome actually consists of a patchwork of several hundred thousand such blocks of common haplotypes, with each block ranging from several thousand base pairs to more than 100,000 base pairs in length.[104,105] For each haplotype block, there may be only a few major combinations of SNPs. This holds out the possibility of simplifying the problem of mapping disease genes by association, at least for common genetic variants. However, there is considerable controversy on this point, and it remains to be seen whether current efforts to define a "haplotype map" of the genome will actually be useful for gene mapping.[106,107]

The Future of Genetics in the Rheumatic Diseases

This chapter has discussed some of the fundamental genetic concepts and techniques applied to the study of rheumatic diseases in the last decade. Although the underlying concepts will not change, it is likely that mapping strategies, statistical methods, and approaches to gene identification will undergo a rapid evolution in the coming years. The appearance of new technologies such as DNA "chips"[108] is already opening up new possibilities for efficient massive screening for genetic variation in human populations. Particularly for the genetically complex rheumatic disorders, one of the major challenges will be to define and integrate the multiple genetic and environmental factors into an overall understanding of disease pathogenesis. This will likely lead to a new appreciation for the underlying heterogeneity of many rheumatic diseases and provide opportunities for new and more specific approaches to diagnosis and treatment.

REFERENCES

1. Lander ES, Linton LM, Birren B, et al: Initial sequencing and analysis of the human genome. Nature 409:860-921, 2001.
2. Venter JC, Adams MD, Myers EW, et al: The sequence of the human genome. Science 291:1304-1351, 2001.
3. Deapen D, Escalante A, Weinrib L, et al: A revised estimate of twin concordance in systemic lupus erythematosus. Arthritis Rheum 35:311-318, 1992.
4. Olmos P, A'Hern R, Heaton DA, et al: The significance of the concordance rate for type 1 (insulin-dependent) diabetes in identical twins. Diabetologia 31:747-750, 1988.

5. Ebers GC, Bulman DE, Sadovnick AD, et al: A population-based study of multiple sclerosis in twins. N Engl J Med 315:1638-1642, 1986.
6. Lawrence JS: Heberden Oration, 1969. Rheumatoid arthritis—nature or nurture? Ann Rheum Dis 29:357-379, 1970.
7. Silman AJ, MacGregor AJ, Thomson W, et al: Twin concordance rates for rheumatoid arthritis: results from a nationwide study. Br J Rheumatol 32:903-907, 1993.
8. Aho K, Koskenvuo M, Tuominen J, Kaprio J: Occurrence of rheumatoid arthritis in a nationwide series of twins. J Rheumatol 13:899-902, 1986.
9. Jarvinen P, Aho K: Twin studies in rheumatic diseases. Semin Arthritis Rheum 24:19-28, 1994.
10. Gregersen PK: Discordance for autoimmunity in monozygotic twins. Are "identical" twins really identical? Arthritis Rheum 36:1185-1192, 1993.
11. Gregersen PK: Genetics of rheumatoid arthritis: Confronting complexity. Arthritis Res 1:37-44, 1999.
12. Snell G, Dausset J, Nathanson S: Histocompatibility. New York, Academic Press, 1976.
13. Benacerraf B: Role of MHC gene products in immune regulation. Science 212:1229-1238, 1981.
14. Schwartz RH: T-lymphocyte recognition of antigen in association with gene products of the major histocompatibility complex. Annu Rev Immunol 3:237-261, 1985.
15. McDevitt HO, Benacerraf B: Genetic control of specific immune responses. Adv Immunol 11:31-74, 1969.
16. Tiwari J, Terasaki P: HLA and Disease Associations. Berlin, Springer-Verlag, 1985.
17. Complete sequence and gene map of a human major histocompatibility complex. The MHC sequencing consortium. Nature 401:921-923, 1999.
18. Bjorkman PJ, Saper MA, Samraoui B, et al: The foreign antigen binding site and T cell recognition regions of class I histocompatibility antigens. Nature 329:512-518, 1987.
19. Bjorkman PJ, Saper MA, Samraoui B, et al: Structure of the human class I histocompatibility antigen, HLA-A2. Nature 329:506-512, 1987.
20. Madden DR, Gorga JC, Strominger JL, Wiley DC: The three-dimensional structure of HLA-B27 at 2.1 A resolution suggests a general mechanism for tight peptide binding to MHC. Cell 70:1035-1048, 1992.
21. Dessen A, Lawrence CM, Cupo S, et al: X-ray crystal structure of HLA-DR4 (DRA*0101, DRB1*0401) complexed with a peptide from human collagen II. Immunity 7:473-481, 1997.
22. Rammensee HG, Falk K, Rotzschke O: Peptides naturally presented by MHC class I molecules. Annu Rev Immunol 11:213-244, 1993.
23. Engelhard VH: Structure of peptides associated with class I and class II MHC molecules. Annu Rev Immunol 12:181-207, 1994.
24. Hennecke J, Wiley DC: Structure of a complex of the human alpha/beta T cell receptor (TCR) HA1.7, influenza hemagglutinin peptide, and major histocompatibility complex class II molecule, HLA-DR4 (DRA*0101 and DRB1*0401): Insight into TCR cross-restriction and alloreactivity. J Exp Med 195:571-581, 2002.
25. O'Callaghan CA, Bell JI: Structure and function of the human MHC class Ib molecules HLA-E, HLA-F and HLA-G. Immunol Rev 163:129-138, 1998.
26. Llano M, Lee N, Navarro F, et al: HLA-E-bound peptides influence recognition by inhibitory and triggering CD94/NKG2 receptors: Preferential response to an HLA-G-derived nonamer. Eur J Immunol 28:2854-2863, 1998.
27. Marsh SG, Albert ED, Bodmer WF, et al: Nomenclature for factors of the HLA system, 2002. Hum Immunol 63:1213-1268, 2002.
28. van Endert PM: Genes regulating MHC class I processing of antigen. Curr Opin Immunol 11:82-88, 1999.
29. Price P, Witt C, Allcock R, et al: The genetic basis for the association of the 8.1 ancestral haplotype (A1, B8, DR3) with multiple immunopathological diseases. Immunol Rev 167:257-274, 1999.
30. Stastny P: Mixed lymphocyte cultures in rheumatoid arthritis. J Clin Invest 57:1148-1157, 1976.
31. Reinsmoen NL, Bach FH: Five HLA-D clusters associated with HLA-DR4. Hum Immunol 4:249-258, 1982.
32. Cavalli-Sforza LL, Cavalli-Sforza F: The Great Human Diasporas. Reading, Mass, Addison-Wesley, 1995.
33. Brewerton DA, Hart FD, Nicholls A, et al: Ankylosing spondylitis and HL-A 27. Lancet 1:904-907, 1973.
34. Reveille JD, Ball EJ, Khan MA: HLA-B27 and genetic predisposing factors in spondyloarthropathies. Curr Opin Rheumatol 13:265-272, 2001.
35. Madden DR, Gorga JC, Strominger JL, Wiley DC: The structure of HLA-B27 reveals nonamer self-peptides bound in an extended conformation. Nature 353:321-325, 1991.
36. Stastny P: HLA-D and Ia antigens in rheumatoid arthritis and systemic lupus erythematosus. Arthritis Rheum 21:S139-S143, 1978.
37. Stastny P: Association of the B-cell alloantigen DRw4 with rheumatoid arthritis. N Engl J Med 298:869-871, 1978.
38. Weyand CM, Hicok KC, Conn DL, Goronzy JJ: The influence of HLA-DRB1 genes on disease severity in rheumatoid arthritis. Ann Intern Med 117:801-806, 1992.
39. Nepom GT: Major histocompatibility complex-directed susceptibility to rheumatoid arthritis. Adv Immunol 68:315-332, 1998.
40. Hall FC, Weeks DE, Camilleri JP, et al: Influence of the HLA-DRB1 locus on susceptibility and severity in rheumatoid arthritis. QJM 89:821-829, 1996.
41. Ollier W, Winchester R: The germline and somatic genetic basis for rheumatoid arthritis. Curr Dir Autoimmun 1:166-193, 1999.
42. Gregersen PK: T-cell receptor-major histocompatibility complex genetic interactions in rheumatoid arthritis. Rheum Dis Clin North Am 18:793-807, 1992.
43. Nichol FE, Woodrow JC: HLA DR antigens in Indian patients with rheumatoid arthritis. Lancet 1:220-221, 1981.
44. Sanchez B, Moreno I, Magarino R, et al: HLA-DRw10 confers the highest susceptibility to rheumatoid arthritis in a Spanish population. Tissue Antigens 36:174-176, 1990.
45. Willkens RF, Nepom GT, Marks CR, et al: Association of HLA-Dw16 with rheumatoid arthritis in Yakima Indians. Further evidence for the "shared epitope" hypothesis. Arthritis Rheum 34:43-47, 1991.
46. Gregersen PK, Silver J, Winchester RJ: The shared epitope hypothesis. An approach to understanding the molecular genetics of susceptibility to rheumatoid arthritis. Arthritis Rheum 30:1205-1213, 1987.
47. Buckner JH, Nepom GT: Genetics of rheumatoid arthritis: is there a scientific explanation for the human leukocyte antigen association? Curr Opin Rheumatol 14:254-259, 2002.
48. Roudier J: Association of MHC and rheumatoid arthritis. Association of RA with HLA-DR4: The role of repertoire selection. Arthritis Res 2:217-220, 2000.
49. Walser-Kuntz DR, Weyand CM, Weaver AJ, et al: Mechanisms underlying the formation of the T cell receptor repertoire in rheumatoid arthritis. Immunity 2:597-605, 1995.
50. Roudier J, Petersen J, Rhodes GH, et al: Susceptibility to rheumatoid arthritis maps to a T-cell epitope shared by the HLA-Dw4 DR beta-1 chain and the Epstein-Barr virus glycoprotein gp110. Proc Natl Acad Sci U S A 86:5104-5108, 1989.
51. Albani S, Keystone EC, Nelson JL, et al: Positive selection in autoimmunity: Abnormal immune responses to a bacterial dnaJ antigenic determinant in patients with early rheumatoid arthritis. Nat Med 1:448-452, 1995.
52. Roudier J, Sette A, Lamont A, et al: Tolerance to a self peptide from the third hypervariable region of the Es beta chain. Implications for molecular mimicry models of autoimmune disease. Eur J Immunol 21:2063-2067, 1991.
53. Salvat S, Auger I, Rochelle L, et als: Tolerance to a self-peptide from the third hypervariable region of HLA DRB1*0401 in rheumatoid arthritis patients and normal subjects. J Immunol 153:5321-5329, 1994.
54. Auger I, Toussirot E, Roudier J: HLA-DRB1 motifs and heat shock proteins in rheumatoid arthritis. Int Rev Immunol 17:263-271, 1998.
55. Zanelli E, Huizinga TW, Guerne PA, et al: An extended HLA-DQ-DR haplotype rather than DRB1 alone contributes to RA predisposition. Immunogenetics 48:394-401, 1998.
56. Zanelli E, Gonzalez-Gay MA, David CS: Could HLA-DRB1 be the protective locus in rheumatoid arthritis? Immunol Today 16:274-278, 1995.
57. Taneja V, Griffiths MM, Luthra H, David CS: Modulation of HLA-DQ-restricted collagen-induced arthritis by HLA-DRB1 polymorphism. Int Immunol 10:1449-1457, 1998.

58. Milicic A, Lee D, Brown MA, et al: HLA-DR/DQ haplotype in rheumatoid arthritis: novel allelic associations in UK Caucasians. J Rheumatol 29:1821-1826, 2002.
59. Dizier MH, Eliaou JF, Babron MC, et al: Investigation of the HLA component involved in rheumatoid arthritis (RA) by using the marker association-segregation chi-square (MASC) method: Rejection of the unifying-shared-epitope hypothesis. Am J Hum Genet 53:715-721, 1993.
60. Gao X, Gazit E, Livneh A, Stastny P: Rheumatoid arthritis in Israeli Jews: Shared sequences in the third hypervariable region of DRB1 alleles are associated with susceptibility. J Rheumatol 18:801-803, 1991.
61. Gao XJ, Brautbar C, Gazit E, et al: A variant of HLA-DR4 determines susceptibility to rheumatoid arthritis in a subset of Israeli Jews. Arthritis Rheum 34:547-551, 1991.
62. Teller K, Budhai L, Zhang M, et al: HLA-DRB1 and DQB typing of Hispanic American patients with rheumatoid arthritis: The "shared epitope" hypothesis may not apply. J Rheumatol 23:1363-1368, 1996.
63. McDaniel DO, Alarcon GS, Pratt PW, Reveille JD: Most African-American patients with rheumatoid arthritis do not have the rheumatoid antigenic determinant (epitope). Ann Intern Med 123:181-187, 1995.
64. Nepom BS, Nepom GT, Mickelson E, et al: Specific HLA-DR4-associated histocompatibility molecules characterize patients with seropositive juvenile rheumatoid arthritis. J Clin Invest 74:287-291, 1984.
65. Todd JA, Bell JI, McDevitt HO: HLA-DQ beta gene contributes to susceptibility and resistance to insulin-dependent diabetes mellitus. Nature 329:599-604, 1987.
66. Hamilton RG, Harley JB, Bias WB, et al: Two Ro (SS-A) autoantibody responses in systemic lupus erythematosus. Correlation of HLA-DR/DQ specificities with quantitative expression of Ro (SS-A) autoantibody. Arthritis Rheum 31:496-505, 1988.
67. Harley JB, Alexander EL, Bias WB, et al: Anti-Ro (SS-A) and anti-La (SS-B) in patients with Sjogren's syndrome. Arthritis Rheum 29:196-206, 1986.
68. Harley JB, Reichlin M, Arnett FC, et al: Gene interaction at HLA-DQ enhances autoantibody production in primary Sjögren's syndrome. Science 232:1145-1147, 1986.
69. Reveille JD, Macleod MJ, Whittington K, Arnett FC: Specific amino acid residues in the second hypervariable region of HLA-DQA1 and DQB1 chain genes promote the Ro (SS-A)/La (SS-B) autoantibody responses. J Immunol 146:3871-3876, 1991.
70. Mamula MJ, Fatenejad S, Craft J: B cells process and present lupus autoantigens that initiate autoimmune T cell responses. J Immunol 152:1453-1461, 1994.
71. Talken BL, Schafermeyer KR, Bailey CW, et al: T cell epitope mapping of the Smith antigen reveals that highly conserved Smith antigen motifs are the dominant target of T cell immunity in systemic lupus erythematosus. J Immunol 167:562-568, 2001.
72. Arnett FC, Thiagarajan P, Ahn C, Reveille JD: Associations of anti-beta2-glycoprotein I autoantibodies with HLA class II alleles in three ethnic groups. Arthritis Rheum 42:268-274, 1999.
73. Olsen ML, Arnett FC, Reveille JD: Contrasting molecular patterns of MHC class II alleles associated with the anti-Sm and anti-RNP precipitin autoantibodies in systemic lupus erythematosus. Arthritis Rheum 36:94-104, 1993.
74. Falk CT, Rubinstein P: Haplotype relative risks: an easy reliable way to construct a proper control sample for risk calculations. Ann Hum Genet 51:227-233, 1987.
75. Spielman RS, McGinnis RE, Ewens WJ: Transmission test for linkage disequilibrium: the insulin gene region and insulin-dependent diabetes mellitus (IDDM). Am J Hum Genet 52:506-516, 1993.
76. Mulcahy B, Waldron-Lynch F, McDermott MF, et al: Genetic variability in the tumor necrosis factor-lymphotoxin region influences susceptibility to rheumatoid arthritis. Am J Hum Genet 59:676-683, 1996.
77. Morton NE, Collins A: Tests and estimates of allelic association in complex inheritance. Proc Natl Acad Sci U S A 95:11389-11393, 1998.
78. Ota M, Katsuyama Y, Kimura A, et al: A second susceptibility gene for developing rheumatoid arthritis in the human MHC is localized within a 70-kb interval telomeric of the TNF genes in the HLA class III region. Genomics 71:263-270, 2001.
79. Jawaheer D, Li W, Graham RR, et al: Dissecting the genetic complexity of the association between human leukocyte antigens and rheumatoid arthritis. Am J Hum Genet 71:585-594, 2002.
80. Okamoto K, Makino S, Yoshikawa Y, et al: Identification of IkappaBL as the second major histocompatibility complex-linked susceptibility locus for rheumatoid arthritis. Am J Hum Genet 72:303-312, 2003.
81. Yen JH, Moore BE, Nakajima T, et al: Major histocompatibility complex class I-recognizing receptors are disease risk genes in rheumatoid arthritis. J Exp Med 193:1159-1167, 2001.
82. Graham RR, Ortmann WA, Langefeld CD, et al: Visualizing human leukocyte antigen class II risk haplotypes in human systemic lupus erythematosus. Am J Hum Genet 71:543-553, 2002.
83. Zeggini E, Donn RP, Ollier WE, Thomson W: Evidence for linkage of HLA loci in juvenile idiopathic oligoarthritis: Independent effects of HLA-A and HLA-DRB1. Arthritis Rheum 46:2716-2720, 2002.
84. Rubio JP, Bahlo M, Butzkueven H, et al: Genetic dissection of the human leukocyte antigen region by use of haplotypes of Tasmanians with multiple sclerosis. Am J Hum Genet 70:1125-1137, 2002.
85. Risch N: Linkage strategies for genetically complex traits. II. The power of affected relative pairs. Am J Hum Genet 46:229-241, 1990.
86. Vyse TJ, Todd JA: Genetic analysis of autoimmune disease. Cell 85:311-318, 1996.
87. Ott J: Analysis of Human Genetic Linkage. Baltimore, Johns Hopkins University Press, 1999.
88. Pras E, Aksentijevich I, Gruberg L, et al: Mapping of a gene causing familial Mediterranean fever to the short arm of chromosome 16. N Engl J Med 326:1509-1513, 1992.
89. Ancient missense mutations in a new member of the RoRet gene family are likely to cause familial Mediterranean fever. The International FMF Consortium. Cell 90:797-807, 1997.
90. McDermott MF, Aksentijevich I, Galon J, et al: Germline mutations in the extracellular domains of the 55 kDa TNF receptor, TNFR1, define a family of dominantly inherited autoinflammatory syndromes. Cell 97:133-144, 1999.
91. Hull KM, Drewe E, Aksentijevich I, et al: The TNF receptor-associated periodic syndrome (TRAPS): Emerging concepts of an autoinflammatory disorder. Medicine (Baltimore) 81:349-368, 2002.
92. Lander ES, Schork NJ: Genetic dissection of complex traits. Science 265:2037-2048, 1994.
93. Gaffney PM, Kearns GM, Shark KB, et al: A genome-wide search for susceptibility genes in human systemic lupus erythematosus sib-pair families. Proc Natl Acad Sci U S A 95:14875-14879, 1998.
94. Rao S, Olson JM, Moser KL, et al: Linkage analysis of human systemic lupus erythematosus-related traits: A principal component approach. Arthritis Rheum 44:2807-2818, 2001.
95. Kelly JA, Moser KL, Harley JB: The genetics of systemic lupus erythematosus: Putting the pieces together. Genes Immun 3(Suppl 1):S71-S85, 2002.
96. Cornelis F, Faure S, Martinez M, et al: New susceptibility locus for rheumatoid arthritis suggested by a genome-wide linkage study. Proc Natl Acad Sci U S A 95:10746-10750, 1998.
97. MacKay K, Eyre S, Myerscough A, et al: Whole-genome linkage analysis of rheumatoid arthritis susceptibility loci in 252 affected sibling pairs in the United Kingdom. Arthritis Rheum 46:632-639, 2002.
98. Jawaheer D, Seldin MF, Amos CI, et al: A genomewide screen in multiplex rheumatoid arthritis families suggests genetic overlap with other autoimmune diseases. Am J Hum Genet 68:927-936, 2001.
99. Jawaheer D, Seldin MF, Amos CI, et al: Screening the genome for rheumatoid arthritis susceptibility genes: A replication study and combined analysis of 512 multicase families. Arthritis Rheum, 48:906-916, 2003.
100. Brown MA, Pile KD, Kennedy LG, et al: A genome-wide screen for susceptibility loci in ankylosing spondylitis. Arthritis Rheum 41:588-595, 1998.
101. Hugot JP, Chamaillard M, Zouali H, et al: Association of NOD2 leucine-rich repeat variants with susceptibility to Crohn's disease. Nature 411:599-603, 2001.

102. Ogura Y, Bonen DK, Inohara N, et al: A frameshift mutation in NOD2 associated with susceptibility to Crohn's disease. Nature 411:603-606, 2001.
103. Todd JA: La carte des microsatellites est arrivee! [The map of microsatellites has arrived!]. Hum Mol Genet 1:663-666, 1992.
104. Rioux JD, Daly MJ, Silverberg MS, et al: Genetic variation in the 5q31 cytokine gene cluster confers susceptibility to Crohn disease. Nat Genet 29:223-228, 2001.
105. Jeffreys AJ, Kauppi L, Neumann R: Intensely punctate meiotic recombination in the class II region of the major histocompatibility complex. Nat Genet 29:217-222, 2001.
106. Wang N, Akey JM, Zhang K, et al: Distribution of recombination crossovers and the origin of haplotype blocks: the interplay of population history, recombination, and mutation. Am J Hum Genet 71:1227-1234, 2002.
107. Pritchard JK, Cox NJ: The allelic architecture of human disease genes: Common disease-common variant . . . or not? Hum Mol Genet 11:2417-2423, 2002.
108. Warrington JA, Shah NA, Chen X, et al: New developments in high-throughput resequencing and variation detection using high density microarrays. Hum Mutat 19:402-409, 2002.

18 Signal Transduction in Rheumatic Diseases

EDWARD M. SCHWARZ

The biologic processes of activation, suppression, replication, differentiation, and apoptosis occur in response to extracellular signals. The biochemic events by which cells internalize these signals to orchestrate the appropriate response is referred to as *signal transduction*. Over the last decade, extensive research has elucidated many of the critical signal transduction pathways operant in rheumatic diseases.[1] Remarkably, this information has been translated into therapeutic interventions, both small molecules, such as cyclooxygenase 2 (COX2) selective inhibitors, and biologics, such as tumor necrosis factor (TNF) antagonists, which have completely transformed rheumatology and our ability to effectively treat arthritis. This chapter will review the fundamental basis of signal transduction using the TNF, interleukin (IL), interferon (IFN), T cell receptor (TCR), and steroid and tumor growth factor–beta (TGF-β) signaling pathways as examples (Table 18–1).

The goal of signal transduction is the alteration of gene expression to allow the cell to respond to the environmental signals. There are five fundamental components to every signal transduction pathway, which cells use to modulate both immediate and long-term changes in gene expression. They are: (1) the ligand, (2) the receptor, (3) the cytoplasmic transduction molecule(s), (4) the transcription factor(s), and (5) the negative regulator(s). These proteins can be enzymes (i.e., kinases, phosphatases, ubiquitin ligases), or they can function solely by physical association to activate a transcription factor such that it will bind to its specific DNA recognition sequence in the promoter of the target gene and facilitate transcription by RNA polymerase II. In inflammatory responses, these target genes include the cytokines, adhesion molecules, oxygenases, and proteases that precipitate tissue destruction. Thus, another critical target gene is the negative regulator, which functions to autoregulate the pathway to inhibit constitutive activation and a chronic response. Because a growing paradigm to explain chronic diseases like rheumatoid arthritis (RA) posits that the central etiologic mechanism is the inability to downregulate proinflammatory signal transduction pathways, this chapter places special emphasis on these negative regulators.

The Tumor Necrosis Factor Signal Transduction Pathway

Although the clinic success of anti-TNF therapy has attracted a lot of attention since its inception in 1995, this pathway has long been recognized for its importance in inflammatory and immune responses.[2] The importance of this pathway for innate immunity is also highlighted by its extraordinary conservation during evolution (Fig. 18–1), as homologues for all five components of the pathway have been identified from drosophilla to humans. It is also noteworthy to mention the resolution of our knowledge of TNF signaling, in that the three-dimensional structure and the in vivo function of most of the molecules in this pathway have been defined by radiographic crystallography and targeted gene disruption (knockout) in mice, respectively.

TNF was originally discovered based on its anticancer activity in the nineteenth century.[3] It is now known that there is a large family of TNF ligands, which are characterized by homologous C-terminal domains. TNF receptors are type I membrane proteins characterized by cysteine-rich extracellular domains. Three salient features distinguish TNF-receptor signaling from all other pathways. First, ligand binding mediates activation by oligomerization of three identical receptors to form a homotrimer. Second, TNF receptors lack catalytic activity. TNF signal transduction occurs via the recruitment of adaptor proteins, called TNF receptor–associated factors (TRAFs), that bind to sites in the TNF receptors created by homotrimerization.[4] TRAF binding allows for the recruitment and activation of mitogen-activated protein kinases (MAPKs), which triggers nuclear factor kappa B (NFκB) and activator protein-1 (AP-1)–mediated transcription.[5] Finally, TNF signaling is the only receptor-mediated pathway known to directly trigger programmed cell death, known as apoptosis. This feature of TNF signaling is arguably the most dominant and has been demonstrated to be central in disease pathogenesis in many different organ systems (Table 18–2).

Death Receptor Signaling Through Caspases

Although all TNF receptors can influence apoptosis, only a subset, known as the death receptors (DR), can activate this process directly.[6] This property is engendered by a unique amino-acid motif in the cytoplasmic tail called the death domain (DD). TNF receptors containing a DD trigger apoptosis by recruiting adapter proteins (TNF Receptor Associated Death Domain [TRADD] and Fas Associated Death Domain [FADD]) that associate with the receptor via mutual DD binding. Instead of recruiting MAPKs like the TRAFs, DD-adapter proteins recruit cysteine proteases called caspases. The

TABLE 18–1 • SIGNAL TRANSDUCTION PATHWAYS CRITICAL TO RHEUMATIC DISEASE

Signaling Pathway	Cytoplasmic Transduction Molecules	Transcription Factors	Negative Regulators
TNF	TRAFs, MAPKs	NFκB, AP-1	IκB, Fra-1, Fra-2
DR	TRADD, FADD, caspase	None	IAPs
IL + IFN	JAKs, STATs	STATs	SOCS, PIAS
TCR	PKC, calmodulin, calcineurin,	NF-AT, AP-1	JNK
SR	SR	SR	SR
TGF-β + BMP	Common Smads	Receptor-specific Smads	Inhibitory Smads, Smurfs

Abbreviations: AP-1, activator protein-1; BMP, bone morphogenetic protein;DR, death receptor: FADD, Fas-associated death domain; Fra-1, Fos-related antigen 1; Fra-2, Fos-related antigen 2; IAP, inhibitors of apoptosis; IFN, interferon; IκB, inhibitor of NFκB; IL, interleukin; JAKs, Janus kinases; JNK, Jun kinase; MAPKs, mitogen-activated protein kinases;NF-AT, nuclear factor of activated T cells; NFκB, nuclear factor kappa B; PIAS, protein inhibitors of activated STATs; PKC, protein kinase C; SOCS, suppressors of cytokine signaling; SR, steroid receptor; STAT, signal transducer and activator of transcription; TGF-β, tumor growth factor-β; TCR, T cell receptor; TNF, tumor necrosis factor; ; TRADD, TNF-receptor associated death domain; TRAFs, TNF-receptor associated factors.

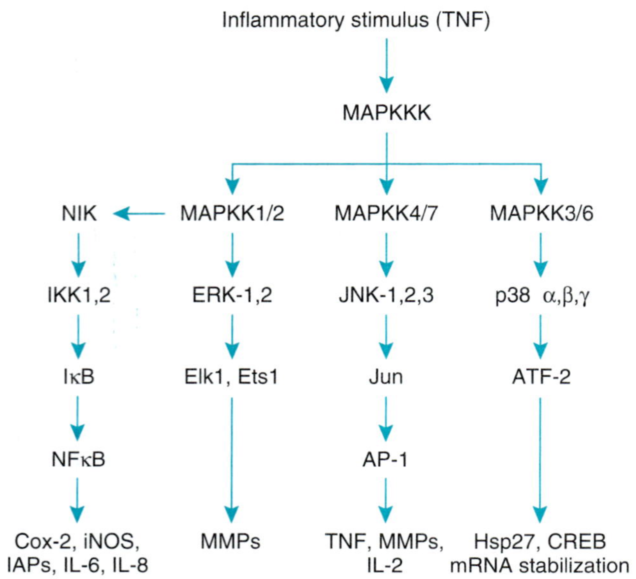

FIGURE 18–1 • Schematic representation of the tumor necrosis factor (TNF)/nuclear factor kappa B (NFκB) signal transduction pathway. TNF signaling commences when the ligand (*1*) binds to its receptor (*2*) on the plasma membrane of the cell (*A*). This ligation results in trimerization of the TNF receptor in a conformation that generates high-affinity binding sites for the TNF receptor-associated factors (TRAFs), which then recruit the intracellular signaling molecules (*3*) receptor interacting protein (RIP) and a yet-to-be identified kinase that phosphorylates the IKKs. This activation triggers the phosphorylation of inhibitor of NFκB (IκB), targeting it for proteasomal degradation, which allows the NFκB transcription factor (*4*) to translocate to the nucleus, where it binds to its DNA element to mediate transcription of various proinflammatory target genes (*B*). In addition to the proinflammatory genes, NFκB also mediates the transcription of it negative regulator IκB (*5*). Following IκB resynthesis, the protein binds to NFκB in the nucleus and translocates it to the cytoplasm, resetting the cell for another round of signal transduction (*C*).

binding of caspase-8 or -10 results in autoproteolytic processing and the release of the active enzyme, which mediates a cleavage cascade of family members, culminating in the processing of caspase-3. Once caspase-3 is processed, apoptosis is irreversible, as this enzyme directly activates the DNases, lipases, and proteases that destroy the cell. Prior to caspase-3 cleavage, apoptosis can be prevented by the synthesis of inhibitor of apoptosis proteins (IAPs) via NFκB-dependent signaling.

TABLE 18–2 • TNF RECEPTORS ASSOCIATED WITH ORGAN SPECIFIC DISEASES

TNF Receptor	Organ System	Disease Process
TNFRI	CD8+ T-cells	Autoimmunity[30]
FAS	CD4+ T-cells	Autoimmunity[30]
CD30	Thymocytes	Autoimmunity[31]
CD40	B-cells	X-linked hyper-IgM syndrome[32]
RANK	Osteoclasts	Osteopetrosis[33]
NGFR	Neurons	Neuropathy[34]
NOD2	Gut mucosa	Crohn's disease[35,36]

MAPK Signal Transduction

Protein phosphorylation is the most common mechanism used by cells to respond to extracellular signals. The MAPK family is responsible for transducing the majority of inflammatory signals that ultimately lead to NFκB-, AP-1–, and signal transducer and activator of transcription (STAT)-mediated transcription.[1] The phosphorylation cascade consists of a three- or four-tiered signaling module in which the MAPK is activated by a MAP kinase kinase (MAPKK), which in turn is activated by a MAP kinase kinase kinase, (MAPKKK). The MAPKKK is itself activated by a small G protein, such as Ras, directly, or by an intermediate kinase, as a direct consequence of membrane receptor activation.

One area of active investigation is the effort to understand how identical MAPK signals in the same cell, derived from different receptors can have opposing biologic outcomes.[7] One example is the response of neuroendocrine cells to epidermal growth factor (EGF) and nerve growth factor (NGF).[7] Although both of these signals require Raf (the MAPKKK), MEK (the MAPKK), and extracellular signal-regulated kinase (ERK) (the MAPK), EGF signals for proliferation, while NGF signals for differentiation. There are two theories to explain this phenomenon. The first is the concept of "cross-talk," which posits that different signaling pathways, such as MAPK and cyclic adenosine monophosphate (cAMP), that are simultaneously active can interact with each other at some point to produce an effect that is different from either one alone. The other mechanism is the duration of the signal. MAPK activity is negatively regulated by protein phosphatases that dephosphorylate the kinases. Thus, the time interval from when the MAPKs become phosphorylated to the time they are dephosphorylated may control the strength of the signal and the ultimate biologic response.

NFκB Signal Transduction

NFκB is a transcription factor that was first described as a B cell–specific protein that bound to a short DNA sequence motif located in the immunoglobulin κ light-chain enhancer.[8] Subsequently, it was discovered that NFκB is expressed in virtually all cell types and is involved in the transcription of a wide array of genes.[9] NFκB is comprised of a family of proteins (termed Rel) that share a Rel homology domain. This region mediates dimerization and DNA binding of the transcription factor. The most ubiquitious form of NFκB is a heterodimer of RelA (p65) and NFκB1 (p50), but almost all combinations of homo- and heterodimers are known to exist. It is believed that through these different combinations, target-gene specificity is derived. Among these are genes known to play a critical role in rheumatic diseases, including cytokines, such as TNF, IL-1β, IL-6; adhesion molecules, such as intercellular adhesion molecules-1 (ICAM-1), vascular cell adhesion molecule-1 (VCAM-1), and E-selectin; oxygenases, such as inducible nitric oxide synthase (iNOS) and COX2; and matrix metalloproteinases (MMPs). Furthermore, the efficacy of aspirin, gold compounds, sulfasalazine, and corticosteroids in the treatment of RA has been attributed to their inhibitory effects on NFκB.

The fundamental regulation of NFκB occurs via post-translational modifications by phosphorylation and proteolysis. In resting cells, NFκB is sequestered in the cytoplasm by proteins termed inhibitor of NFκB (IκB). This protein family is characterized by common, ankyrin-like repeat domains, which function by binding to NFκB in a manner that masks the nuclear localization (NLS). Following the appropriate signal (i.e., TNF), activation of the transcription factor occurs through the signal-induced proteolytic degradation of IκB in the cytoplasm, which liberates NFκB to translocate to the nucleus. The critical MAPKKK like proteins in this pathway are the IκB kinases (IKK1,2), which directly phosphorylate IκB to trigger ubiquitination and degradation by the proteosome.[10] Although the true MAPKK that phophorylates the IKKs in response to TNF has yet to be determined, several upstream kinases have been identified, including receptor interacting protein (RIP), NFκB inducing kinase (NIK), and MEKK-1. Phosphorylation of NFκB is also important in the regulation of this pathway. The transcriptional activity of NFκB is stimulated upon phosphorylation of its p65 subunit by protein kinase A (PKA).[11] This phosphorylation is required for efficient association with the transcriptional coactivator CBP/p300 and high transcriptional activity.

NFκB signaling is negatively autoregulated by the induction of three different NFκB target genes, IκB, IAP, and A20. One of the first genes transcribed by NFκB following nuclear translocation is IκBα.[12] This resynthesized IκB enters the nucleus, binds to NFκB, and relocates it to the cytoplasm, thus extinguishing NFκB activity.[13] As described previously, NFκB-mediated transcription of IAP genes is required to protect cells from TNF-induced apoptosis via caspase inhibition.[14] Similarly, NFκB-mediated transcription of A20 is also required to downregulate TNF responses, including apoptosis.[15] Although the mechanism of A20 activity is unclear, there is evidence that it plays a role in the inactivation of the IKK complex. In vivo loss of these negative feedback pathways has severe consequences, as seen in the embryonic lethal phenotype of the RelA[16] and IKK-2 knockout mice[17] and the severe runting and postnatal wasting observed in the RIP[18] and A20[15] knockout mice. It has also been shown that the chronic inflammation found in RA synovium is associated with constitutive NFκB activity.[19]

AP-1 Signal Transduction

Although AP-1 is a distinct signaling pathway from NFκB, it is activated by many of the same signals and mediates a similar gene expression profile. Thus, AP-1 is also a central regulator of the inflammatory responses that control rheumatic diseases. The AP-1 transcription factor is also composed of family of proteins that are subdivided into two groups: Jun (c-Jun, Jun B, Jun D) and Fos (c-Fos, Fos B, Fra-1, Fra-2).[20] Structurally, AP-1 proteins have two characteristic domains, a basic domain for transactivation, and a leucine-zipper domain for dimerization and DNA binding, which is referred to as bZIP. These motifs are also shared by activating transcription factor-2 (ATF-2), which can heterodimerize with Jun. Although AP-1 complexes can bind to DNA as Jun homodimers, Jun-Jun heterodimers, and Jun-Fos heterodimers, the prototypic AP-1 is a c-Jun/c-Fos heterodimer. Three distinct MAPK pathways, the ERKs, Jun N-terminal kinases (JNK), and the p38 kinases, activate AP-1. The ERKs are activated by mitogens and growth factors via a Ras-dependent pathway, and the JNK and p38 kinases are activated in response to the proinflammatory cytokines and cellular stress (e.g., reactive oxygen metabolites, ultraviolet light, heat, and osmotic shock). Based on these stimuli, the JNKs and p38 kinases have been termed stress-activated protein kinases (SAPKs).

The MAPKs activate the AP-1 pathway by two distinct mechanisms. First, they directly phosphorylate c-Jun and ATF-2, which markedly increases their transcriptional activity by allowing for efficient association with CBP/p300 and the RNA polymerase II complex. They also signal for c-Fos de novo synthesis. This c-Fos binds with phosphorylated c-Jun to generate the AP-1 transcription factor that is responsible for the induction of the inflammatory response genes. Negative regulation of the AP-1 pathway is tripartite, which involves dephosphorylation of the MAPKs, proteolysis of c-Fos, and de novo synthesis of Fos-related antigens (Fra-1 and 2). After their synthesis, Fra-1 and -2 bind to Jun to make a DNA-binding AP-1 complex, but because they lack the potent transactivation domain of c-Fos, they act as transcriptional inhibitors.

Nuclear Factor of Activated T cell Signal Transduction

The discovery of the nuclear factor of activated T cell (NF-AT) signaling pathway was the culmination of an intense investigation to understand the molecular mechanism of cyclosporine/FK506 activity and the independent Ca^{++} and protein kinase C (PKC)-derived signals from the T cell receptor.[21] These studies revealed that PKC activation leads to c-Fos expression and inducible AP-1 activity. Ca^{++} mobilization activates the calmodulin-dependent phosphatase calcineurin, which functions to dephosphorylate NF-AT in the cytoplasm of resting cells. This cyclosporine/FK506-sensitive step allows the active transcription factor to translocate to the nucleus, where it binds to its cognate DNA-binding site, which is usually adjacent to an AP-1 binding site. As a complex, NF-AT and AP-1 cooperate to mediate transcription of a large set of target genes that are critical for antigen and fragment crystallizable (Fc) receptor-mediated response. This activation is autoregulated by the proteolysis of c-Fos, as described previously, and the nuclear activity of JNK, which phosphorylates NF-AT, relocating it back to the cytoplasm.[22]

Subsequent studies have found that NF-AT is a family of transcription factors that are encoded by at least four genes (NF-AT 1-4). Although there are immune cell–specific isoforms, NF-AT is also ubiquitously expressed to activate a wide array of genes. Interestingly, NF-AT has been shown to be a repressor of cartilage cell growth and differentiation and may be a critical regulator of the changes seen in osteoarthritis.[23]

Stat Signal Transduction

Interferons and interleukins are the critical cytokines produced to orchestrate a protective immune response against virulent pathogens and tumors. As these factors bind to different kinds of receptors, they heavily rely on the signal transducer and activator of transcription (STAT) pathways to mediate their responses.[24] The STATs are a highly conserved family of proteins for which seven mammalian homologues are known, and the family contains three functional domains. The C-terminus contains the transactivation domain, and the DNA-binding domain is in the center of the molecule. The unique STAT feature is its Src-homology 2 (SH2) domain, which is a protein motif that specifically binds to phosphorylated tyrosine residues. The STAT SH2 domain functions by binding to the activated receptor after ligation to the cytokine. This activation occurs through phosphorylation by a novel family of cytoplasmic tyrosine kinases, termed Janus kinases (JAKs). JAKs bind specifically to intracellular domains of cytokine receptor signaling chains and catalyze ligand-induced phosphorylation of themselves and the receptor, generating STAT binding sites. Then, STAT phosphorylation on activating tyrosine residues leads to the formation of STAT homo- and heterodimers, which rapidly translocate to the nucleus to mediate transcription of the target genes.

Negative regulation of the STAT pathway is mediated by common mechanisms such as receptor internalization and dephosphorylation. It is also downregulated specifically by de novo synthesis of the pathway inhibitors: suppressors of cytokine signaling (SOCS) and protein inhibitors of activated STATs (PIAS). The SOCS family consists of eight proteins: SOCS1 through SOCS7 and CIS, each of which contains a central SH2 domain and a C-terminal SOCS box.[25] SOCS are STAT target genes that function in a negative feedback loop by occupying the STAT binding site on the cytokine receptor and preventing further activation. SOCS proteins also function to direct a response to a particular cytokine when the cell is in the presence of other cytokines. For example, T helper type 1 (Th1) responses are mediated in part by IFN-γ induction of SOCS-1 through the STAT-1 pathway, which binds to the IL-4 receptor inhibiting signaling through STAT-6 and preventing Th2 responses.[26] The PIASs function by associating with phosphorylated STAT dimers and preventing DNA binding.[24]

Steroid Receptor Signal Transduction

The steroid receptor family of transcription factors, which includes the sex hormone receptors (i.e., estrogen and androgen) and the glucocorticoid receptors (the targets of steroidal drug therapy), mediates a very simple signal transduction that is completely void of intermediate molecules. Because steroids are hydrophobic and can readily diffuse through membranes, receptor ligation can occur in the nucleus, triggering immediate DNA binding and transactivation. In the case of inflammatory diseases, the inhibitory functions of steroid receptors are perhaps more important than their transcriptional activity. This inhibition occurs through two mechanisms. First, after ligand binding, steroid receptors can inhibit other transcription factors (i.e., NFκB) through direct interaction.[27] They also inhibit transcription through a process known as "squelching," whereby the steroid receptors occupy a large proportion of the available coactivators, CBP/p300 and RNA polII complexes, thereby creating a shortage for other transcription factors.

Steroid receptor signaling is downregulated primarily by proteolysis of the receptors and de novo synthesis of steroid receptors with limited transactivation potential. As an example, the effects of estrogens are manifested almost entirely by estrogen receptor-alpha (ERα). One ERα target gene is ERβ, which acts as an efficient dominant inhibitor of ERα transcriptional activity in cells in which both receptors are expressed.[28] Thus, this pathway is also tightly controlled in an autoregulatory loop.

Signal Transduction by the TGF-β Superfamily

Following the establishment of a concrete understanding of proinflammatory/catabolic signal transduction, which occurred in the 1990s, a new thrust of research has been focused toward understanding the signal transduction events that mediate tissue regeneration and repair. Based on the cytokines and signal transduction pathways involved, it has become clear that regeneration and repair processes are essentially a recapitulation of embryonic development at the tissue level. With respect to mesenchymal cells and the repair of skeletal tissue, the transforming growth factor–β (TGF-β)/bone morphogenetic protein (BMP) superfamily has been defined as central to this process. Two of its members (BMP-2 and BMP-7) are already in clinical use to facilitate fracture healing and spinal fusion.

The first member of the superfamily, TGF-β1, was discovered in the early 1980s.[29] Currently there are more than 30 known vertebrate members, and many of these have invertebrate homologues. TGF-β signaling plays a critical role in development and homeostasis. TGF-β and BMP ligands signal by binding to a transmembrane heterodimer composed of a type I and a type II receptor. Both receptor subunits are serine-threonine kinase receptors. Following ligand binding, the type II receptor phosphorylates the type I receptor. This activates its kinase domain and leads to the phosphorylation of bound transcription factors known as receptor-associated Smads (Smads 2 and 3 for TGF-β, Smads 1, 5, and 8 for BMP). This signal allows the receptor-associated Smads to dissociate and bind the common Smad (Smad 4), which then triggers the heteromeric complex to translocate to the nucleus where it binds to its cognate DNA sequence. Like NF-AT, Smad-mediated transcription is virtually always mediated by cooperation with other transcription factors (i.e., AP-1, ATF-2). This can be accomplished by direct activation of the MAPKKK TGF-β receptor–associated kinase (TAK), which leads to the activation of IKK, JNK, and p38.

Two of the target genes activated by TFG-β and BMP signaling are the "inhibitory Smads," Smad-6 and Smad-7. These proteins contain the receptor-binding domain but lack the phosphorylation domain of the receptor-associated Smads. Thus, they act like dominant-negatives by binding the receptor irrespective of its activation state, and they prevent the phosphorylation of the receptor-associated Smads. The Smads are also negatively regulated by the induction of the E3-ubiquitin ligases Jab1, Roc1, and Smad Ubitquitin Regulatory Factors (Smurfs), which mediate their proteolysis.

Another elegant component of this pathway is the mechanism by which opposing signals in the cell are avoided by direct competition for Smad 4. Thus, in mesenchymal stem cells, the TGF-β signal for proliferation prevents a subsequent BMP signal for differentiation by consuming the cytoplasmic Smad 4 in TGF-β receptor–specific Smad complexes, and vice versa.

Conclusions

The elucidation of the signal transduction pathways involved in inflammation and immunity has provided a biochemic basis for the etiology of rheumatic diseases. From this information we now understand how overactivation or defective inhibition of selective receptors, kinases, and transcription factors can convert a normal phlogisitc or immune response into a chronic disease state. Furthermore, targets for intervention have been identified and the promise of rational drug design has come to fruition. As the gaps in our knowledge of signal transduction continue to be filled, and new advances in drug development are made, it is likely that our ability to treat patients will also markedly improve. From this approach we may also see the development of the first therapeutics designed for tissue repair and regeneration.

REFERENCES

1. Firestein GS, Manning AM: Signal transduction and transcription factors in rheumatic disease. Arthritis Rheum 42:609, 1999.
2. Smith CA, Farrah T, Goodwin RG: The TNF receptor superfamily of cellular and viral proteins: activation, costimulation, and death. Cell 76:959, 1994.
3. Locksley RM, Killeen N, Lenardo MJ: The TNF and TNF receptor superfamilies: integrating mammalian biology. Cell 104:487, 2001.
4. Arch RH, Gedrich RW, Thompson CB: Tumor necrosis factor receptor-associated factors (TRAFs): a family of adapter proteins that regulates life and death. Genes Dev 12:2821, 1998.
5. Chen G, Goeddel DV: TNF-R1 signaling: a beautiful pathway. Science 296:1634, 2002.
6. Wajant H: The Fas signaling pathway: more than a paradigm. Science 296:1635, 2002.
7. Vaudry D, Stork PJ, Lazarovici P, Eiden LE: Signaling pathways for PC12 cell differentiation: making the right connections. Science 296:1648, 2002.
8. Sen R, Baltimore D: Multiple nuclear factors interact with the immunoglobulin enhancer sequences. Cell 46:705, 1986.
9. Verma IM, Stevenson JK, Schwarz EM, et al: Rel/NF-kappa B/I kappa B family: intimate tales of association and dissociation. Genes Dev 9:2723, 1995.
10. Verma IM, Stevenson J: IkappaB kinase: beginning, not the end. Proc Natl Acad Sci U S A 94:11758, 1997.
11. Zhong H, Voll RE, Ghosh S: Phosphorylation of NF-kappa B p65 by PKA stimulates transcriptional activity by promoting a novel bivalent interaction with the coactivator CBP/p300. Mol Cell 1:661, 1998.
12. Chiao PJ, Miyamoto S, Verma IM: Autoregulation of I kappa B alpha activity. Proc Nat Acad Sci U S A 91:28, 1994.
13. Arenzana-Seisdedos F, Turpin P, Rodriguez M, et al: Nuclear localization of I kappa B alpha promotes active transport of NF-kappa B from the nucleus to the cytoplasm. Cell Sci 110:369, 1997.
14. Wang CY, Mayo MW, Korneluk RG, et al: NF-kappaB antiapoptosis: induction of TRAF1 and TRAF2 and c-IAP1 and c-IAP2 to suppress caspase-8 activation. Science 281:1680, 1998.
15. Lee EG, Boone DL, Chai S, et al: Failure to regulate TNF-induced NF-kappaB and cell death responses in A20-deficient mice. Science 289:2350, 2000.
16. Beg AA, Sha WC, Bronson RT, et al: Embryonic lethality and liver degeneration in mice lacking the RelA component of NF-kappa B. Nature 376:167, 1995.
17. Li QD, Van Antwerp F, Mercurio KF, et al: Severe liver degeneration in mice lacking the IkappaB kinase 2 gene. Science 284:321, 1999.

18. Kelliher MA, Grimm S, Ishida Y, et al: The death domain kinase RIP mediates the TNF-induced NF-kappaB signal. Immunity 8:297, 1998.
19. Marok R, Winyard PG, Coumbe A, et al: Activation of the transcription factor nuclear factor-kappaB in human inflamed synovial tissue. Arthritis Rheum 39:583, 1996.
20. Ransone LJ, Verma IM: Nuclear proto-oncogenes fos and jun. Annu Rev Cell Biol 6:539, 1990.
21. Rao A, Luo C, Hogan PG: Transcription factors of the NFAT family: regulation and function. Annu Rev Immunol 15:707, 1997.
22. Chow CW, Rincon M, Cavanagh J, et al: Nuclear accumulation of NFAT4 opposed by the JNK signal transduction pathway. Science 278:1638, 1997.
23. Ranger AM, Gerstenfeld LC, Wang J, et al: The nuclear factor of activated T cells (NFAT) transcription factor NFATp (NFATc2) is a repressor of chondrogenesis. J Exp Med 191:9, 2000.
24. Aaronson DS, Horvath CM: A road map for those who know JAK-STAT. Science 296:1653, 2002.
25. Krebs DL, Hilton DJ: SOCS: physiological suppressors of cytokine signaling. J Cell Sci 113:2813, 2000.
26. Dickensheets HL, Venkataraman C, Schindler U, Donnelly RP: Interferons inhibit activation of STAT6 by interleukin 4 in human monocytes by inducing SOCS-1 gene expression. Proc Natl Acad Sci U S A 96:10800, 1999.
27. Doucas V, Shi Y, Miyamoto S, et al: Cytoplasmic catalytic subunit of protein kinase A mediates cross-repression by NF-kappa B and the glucocorticoid receptor. Proc Natl Acad Sci U S A 97:11893, 2000.
28. McDonnell DP, Norris JD: Connections and regulation of the human estrogen receptor. Science 296:1642, 2002.
29. Attisano L, Wrana JL: Signal transduction by the TGF-beta superfamily. Science 296:1646, 2002.
30. Zheng L, Fisher G, Miller RE, et al: Induction of apoptosis in mature T cells by tumour necrosis factor. Nature 377:348, 1995.
31. Amakawa R, Hakem A, Kundig TM, et al: Impaired negative selection of T cells in Hodgkin's disease antigen CD30-deficient mice. Cell 84:551, 1996.
32. Allen RC, Armitage RJ, Conley ME, et al: CD40 ligand gene defects responsible for X-linked hyper-IgM syndrome [see comments]. Science 259:990, 1993.
33. Dougall WC, Glaccum M, Charrier K, et al: RANK is essential for osteoclast and lymph node development. Genes Dev 13:2412, 1999.
34. Lee KF, Davies AM, Jaenisch R: p75-Deficient embryonic dorsal root sensory and neonatal sympathetic neurons display a decreased sensitivity to NGF. Development 120:1027, 1994.
35. Hugot JP, Chamaillard M, Zouali H, et al: Association of NOD2 leucine-rich repeat variants with susceptibility to Crohn's disease. Nature 411:599, 2001.
36. Ogura Y, Bonen DK, Inohara N, et al: A frameshift mutation in NOD2 associated with susceptibility to Crohn's disease. Nature 411:603, 2001.

19 Rheumatoid Factor

HELEN TIGHE • DENNIS A. CARSON

Rheumatoid factors (RFs) are autoantibodies directed against antigenic determinants on the fragment crystallizable (Fc) fragment of immunoglobulin G (IgG) molecules (Fig. 19–1). Although RFs have generally been associated with rheumatoid arthritis (RA), they also can be present in normal individuals (particularly following antigenic challenge) and are elevated in a proportion of patients with a variety of other diseases, including other rheumatic diseases, viral infections, acute and chronic inflammatory diseases, and lymphoproliferative diseases such as chronic lymphocytic leukemia, Wäldenström's macroglobulinemia, and mixed cryoglobulinemia.[1-7] Many of these conditions also are associated with hypergammaglobulinemia, indicative of polyclonal B lymphocyte activation, or circulating immune complexes. The RFs associated with RA are generally specific for human IgG and are of higher affinity. They include not only IgM RFs but also IgG, IgA, and IgE RF variants. In contrast, RFs associated with other diseases are frequently of lower affinity, are generally of the IgM isotype, and are polyspecific (Table 19–1).

Incidence of Rheumatoid Factor

Table 19–2 is a partial list of diseases in which an increased incidence of RF has been reported. The exact incidence of RF in a population depends on the assay system and the titer chosen to separate positive and negative reactors. The titer of RF in a population, whether measured by the sensitized sheep-cell agglutination test or by latex fixation, usually behaves as a continuous variable, but differs among various ethnic groups.[2,3,8] With increasing age, both the percentage of individuals with a particular titer and the mean titer of a population as a whole increase.[9] Some studies have shown that the prevalence of RFs and other autoantibodies in the general population tends to decline beyond the age of 70 to 80.[8] This decrease may be related to an increased mortality among autoantibody-positive individuals.

In most, but not all, nonrheumatic conditions, titers of RF are lower than in RA. Thus, the specificity of the RF reaction for RA increases with serum titer.[3] At a dilution of serum at which 95 percent of the normal population will be RF negative, 70 percent of patients with RA (as diagnosed by other criteria) will assay RF positive by latex agglutination. This number increases to 90 percent when the more sensitive enzyme-linked immunosorbent assay (ELISA) is used.[10] The remaining patients are considered seronegative, that is, having RF titers falling within the normal range. Some of the latter sera, particularly from patients with juvenile rheumatoid arthritis, may contain hidden IgM RFs,[8,11,12] which are IgM RFs whose detection is masked by nonspecifically aggregated IgG in improperly treated sera or specific immune complexes. A few have IgG RFs in the absence of IgM. Some seronegative patients, on repeated testing, convert to seropositive. Although high titers of RF are generally associated with RA, elevation of more than one RF isotype, particularly in the joint, is considered highly specific for RA and is rarely found in other rheumatic diseases.[19] IgG RFs are abundant in the sera, and particularly the synovial fluids, of many patients with severe RA.[13-15] Furthermore, the presence of IgA RFs in RA patients is associated with rapidly progressive, more severe disease and bone erosion, and both IgG and IgA RF are associated with systemic manifestations such as vasculitis.[9,16-19] The presence of IgE RF, as measured by ELISA, also correlates with extra-articular manifestations in RA patients.[9,10,20] In general, the specificity of RF for the diagnosis of RA is increased by demonstration of a positive RF test on two or more consecutive occasions, by high titer, by reactivity with both human and rabbit IgG, and by association with the IgM, IgG, and IgA isotypes. Serial measurements of IgM RF modestly correlate with disease activity, but they are far less useful than erythrocyte sedimentation rate (ESR) or measurement of C-reactive protein in this respect.[21]

A variable percentage of adult RA patients, who in the authors' experience represent not more than 10 percent of the total, remain seronegative by the usual criteria. These patients generally display milder synovitis than the seropositive patients and seldom develop extra-articular rheumatoid disease, which may implicate a contributory role for RF in pathogenesis.[12] Furthermore, asymptomatic individuals with persistently raised RFs have greatly increased risk of developing RA, suggesting that disregulation of RF production is a predisposing factor in the development of RA.[22] However, although elevated expression of RF may have significant effects on immune regulation through the production of immune complexes and complement activation, its absence in patients with seronegative RA argues against it being a causative factor in joint disease. This is also supported by the finding of elevated RF titers in other diseases, for example, congenital human immunodeficiency virus (HIV) infection in which the infected children do not manifest clinical rheumatic disease in spite of the presence of circulating IgA RF in 50 percent of cases.[6]

TABLE 19–1 • COMPARISON OF RHEUMATOID FACTORS OF THE IMMUNOGLOBULIN M AND IMMUNOGLOBULIN G CLASSES

Property	IgM Rheumatoid Factor	IgG Rheumatoid Factor
Effective valence for IgG	5	2
Intrinsic affinity for antigen (liters/mole)	10^4–10^6	10^4–10^6
Agglutination of IgG-coated latex particles	Strong	Weak
Enhanced binding to aggregated IgG	Marked	Moderate
Usual sedimentation constants in ultracentrifuge	19S–22S	10S–18S
Self-association	No	Yes
Binding to IgG after treatment with reducing agents	Decreased	Unchanged
Binding to IgG after treatment with pepsin	Decreased	Unchanged or increased

TABLE 19–2 • DISEASES COMMONLY ASSOCIATED WITH RHEUMATOID FACTOR

Rheumatic diseases	Rheumatoid arthritis, systemic lupus erythematosus, scleroderma, mixed connective tissue disease, Sjögren's syndrome
Viral infections	Acquired immune deficiency syndrome (AIDS), mononucleosis, hepatitis, influenza, and many others; after vaccination (may yield falsely elevated titers of antiviral antibodies)
Parasitic infections	Trypanosomiasis, kala-azar, malaria, schistosomiasis, filariasis, etc.
Chronic bacterial infections	Tuberculosis, leprosy, yaws, syphilis, brucellosis, subacute bacterial endocarditis, salmonellosis
Neoplasms	Lymphoproliferative diseases
Other hyperglobulinemic states	Hypergammaglobulinemic purpura, cryoglobulinemia, chronic liver disease, sarcoid, other chronic pulmonary diseases

Immunochemical Properties of Rheumatoid Factor

ANTIGEN SPECIFICITY

A number of studies have analyzed the fine antigen specificity of RFs derived from patients with RA and compared them to those from normal immunized volunteers and to monoclonal IgM RFs from patients with Waldenstrom's macroglobulinemia. Specificity for the IgG1/2/4 subclasses (termed the Ga specificity) was associated with RFs derived from all sources. By comparison, the RFs from RA patients were relatively enriched for reactivity with IgG3.[7,23] Furthermore, RFs derived from rheumatoid synovia exhibit higher binding activity with IgG3 than serum RFs, which mainly react with IgG1/2/4 subclasses.[17] Consequently the IgG3 binding specificity of RFs appears to be relatively disease associated. The antigenic determinant recognized by IgM RFs appears primarily localized to the Fc portion of the IgG molecule in both the CH_2 and CH_3 domains[23-25] (see Fig 19–1). Analysis of the crystal structure of a complex of a human RA synovial RF with the Fc portion of IgG confirms contacts with the CH_2/CH_3 cleft. This study also shows that the ratio of Fab to Fc fragments within the crystal is 2:1, implying that monomeric IgG can cross-link two RF molecules.[26,27]

A number of years ago it was discovered that RA patients have significantly fewer galactose residues on their IgG Fc compared to age-matched healthy controls[28] as a result of reduced B cell galactosyltransferase activity.[29] A lack of terminal galactose residues early in disease is associated with a worse prognosis.[30] However, in different cases, glycosylation differences in IgGs have no effect on binding of IgM RFs, can enhance binding of RFs (particularly those of high affinity), or reduce the solubility of the immune complex.[31-33] RA patients differ most significantly from controls with respect to the galactosylation of IgG2 antibodies, less with IgG1 and IgG4 antibodies, and not at all in IgG3.[34] The defect in the IgG1/2/4 subclasses is intriguing, as the Ga antigenic specificity for RF is also associated with

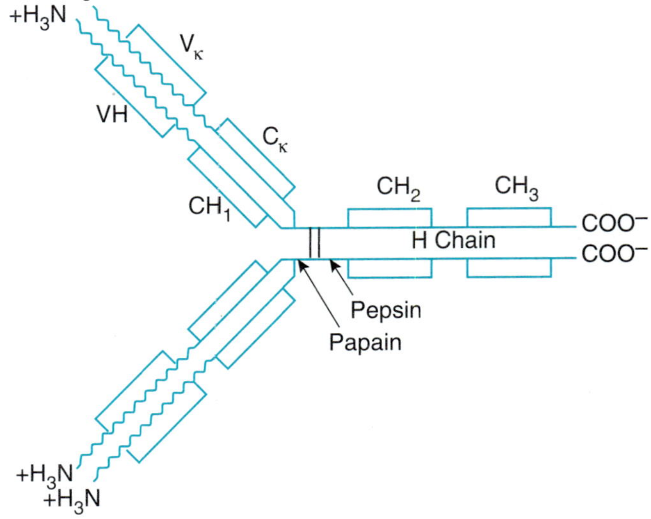

FIGURE 19–1 • Structure of an Immunoglobulin G (IgG) molecule of the G1 subclass containing κ light chains. The antigens reacting with rheumatoid factor (RF) are in the fragment crystallizable (Fc) region.

the same subclasses.[35] Because some RFs secreted by synovial cells react preferentially with IgG3,[7,36] it is possible that galactose-deficient IgG3 is produced by RA patients but is preferentially cleared from the circulation in complexes with RF. IgG RFs from synovial fluid show elevated binding to degalactosylated Fc fragments.[37] In contrast, serum IgG RFs and certain monoclonal IgG RFs have been reported to require intact carbohydrate for binding.[37,38]

KINETICS OF INTERACTION OF RHEUMATOID FACTOR WITH IGG

The affinity of RF for IgG depends on the source of the RF. Monoclonal IgM RFs isolated from patients with mixed cryoglobulinemia or lymphoproliferative disease, or from normal immunized donors, tend to have low affinities in the range of kD = 10^{-4} to 10^{-5} M.[39-41] In contrast, patients with RA produce a high proportion of IgM RFs that react more avidly with human IgG (kD = 10^{-7} M)[39,42,43] However, even lower-affinity RFs can produce stable complexes with IgG under appropriate conditions. For multivalent IgM RF, this occurs when the IgG antigen is aggregated. Although each individual antigen-antibody bond in such an IgM-IgG aggregate probably is individually of insufficient energy to yield a long-lived complex, the sum total of multiple interactions produces a stable structure.[44]

IgG RFs have unique kinetic properties that distinguish them from all other antibodies: The antigenic determinants they target reside on the antibody molecule itself. Hence, IgG RFs can self-associate and form immune complexes in the absence of exogenous antigen.[45-47] The ability of IgG RF to form high-molecular-weight complexes probably depends on the concentration and affinity of the autoantibody and the ratio of IgG RF to normal IgG. IgM RF may, in addition, enhance the formation of IgG RF–containing complexes by cross-linking the reversibly aggregated IgG.

Stimuli for Rheumatoid Factor Synthesis

At least three types of environmental stimuli potentially can trigger active RF synthesis in normal adults. They are 1) immunization with antigen-antibody complexes during anamnestic immune responses,[48-50] 2) polyclonal B cell activation,[51,52] and 3) chronic viral infection.[53-55]

Adoptive transfer experiments have elucidated the cellular requirements for the induction of RF synthesis during murine secondary immune responses.[48,56] Optimal RF production requires the presence of T cells sensitized to the specific antigen being administered, as well as antibodies against the antigen. The RF precursor B cells can come from nonimmunized or T cell–deficient mice. Importantly, the RF elicited during secondary immune responses is directed against the IgG isotype that is dominant in the antigen-antibody complex. These results are explainable by the ability of RF-expressing B cells to present immune-complexed antigen to antigen-specific helper T lymphocytes. During secondary immune responses, antigen-antibody complexes are taken up and processed by RF-precursor B lymphocytes, as well as by antigen-specific B cells.[57,58] Subsequently, peptides derived from the antigens appear on the cell surface in association with class II histocompatibility molecules. Unlike antibodies, the antigen receptors of T lymphocytes (i.e., T cell receptors [TCR]) recognize small linear peptides associated with cell surface major histocompatibility complex (MHC) molecules. When RF-expressing B cells present antigenic peptides derived from immune complexes, the antigen-specific T lymphocytes can trigger RF production. This phenomenon is a form of linked recognition, insofar as the helper T cell and the RF-expressing B cell recognize different antigens. The frequency of RF precursor cells in mouse spleen is remarkably high and may approach the frequency of cells producing specific antibody.[49]

The production of RFs is induced during the course of many acute and chronic inflammatory diseases.[59,60] IgM RFs predominate in most of these conditions, but IgG RFs are occasionally produced. As in the experimental models, sustained RF production usually depends on the continual presence of the immunologic stimuli. A well-studied example is subacute bacterial endocarditis, in which elimination of bacteria by antibiotics leads to a subsequent decline in RF titers.[59,60] With few exceptions, the nonrheumatic diseases and the animal models associated with RF induction are characterized by elevated levels of non–RF-containing immune complexes and/or a diffuse elevation of serum immunoglobulins, indicating polyclonal B lymphocyte activation.

Experimental induction of graft versus host disease has been shown to stimulate production of a variety of autoantibodies, including RFs from host B cells.[61,62] In this model, donor T cells reactive with host MHC class II molecules provide T cell help for a population of self-reactive B cells. Studies of transgenic mice expressing low affinity, polyreactive autoantibodies have similarly shown that such B cells are hyperresponsive to allogeneic T cell help, resulting in the secretion of autoantibodies in the absence of exogenously added antigen.[63]

The potential importance of polyclonal B lymphocyte activation in inducing RF production in humans has been emphasized.[51,52] Polyclonal B lymphocyte activators are mitogens that stimulate lymphocytes to secrete immunoglobulins in the absence of specific antigenic stimulation. They are widespread and include bacterial proteins and lipopolysaccharides, mycoplasma components, and certain viruses such as the Epstein-Barr virus (EBV). Lymphocytes from many normal adult humans will release low-affinity IgM RFs after mitogenic stimulation by EBV.[51] These RFs commonly express the major cross-reactive idiotypes found on Wäldenstrom's macroglobulins with anti-IgG autoantibody activity, and they may also derive from the minor subset of B lymphocytes that express the CD5 antigen.[64]

RFs potentially could be induced by cross-reactive epitopes on foreign antigens, although this has never been proven experimentally. Herpes simplex virus and cytomegalovirus encode Fc receptors on infected cells.

Consequently the production of RF may be part of an anti-idiotypic response against antibody to the viral Fcγ receptor.[53] Increasing evidence supports a role for Hepatitis C virus (HCV) infection in both type II mixed cryoglobulinemia (MC) and certain subsets of B cell non-Hodgkin's lymphoma (NHL).[54,65-67] MC is a systemic vasculitis characterized by the presence in serum of monoclonal cryoprecipitable Ig with RF activity. MC frequently evolves into NHL.[67a] Heavy-chain variable/diversity/joining (VDJ) usage and heavy- and light-chain pairing in both MC and certain NHLs show notable similarities to those used by RFs, as well as anti-HCV E2 antibodies.[65,66,68] This, together with the demonstration that HCV binds to CD81, a molecule that can interact with B cell–signaling molecules CD19 and CD21, may be an important clue to the B cell abnormalities associated with this infection.[55]

Genetic Basis

The question of which particular inherited immunoglobulin variable (V)-region genes encode autoantibodies in disease states and in healthy individuals, and whether these are in germline configuration or are somatically mutated, has concerned investigators for a number of years. A relative paucity of somatic point mutations has been assumed to reflect nonspecific polyclonal B cell activation, whereas multiple mutations usually indicate selection by antigen.

Until recently, our knowledge of the structure and specificities of RFs was largely based on monoclonal IgM RFs isolated from patients with MC or the other lymphoproliferative diseases described previously.[6,69-75] Nearly 10 percent of monoclonal IgM from unrelated individuals with MC or Waldenström's macroglobulinemia have anti-IgG autoantibody activity.[76] These RFs are generally encoded by a restricted set of V-region genes in germline or near to germline configuration, and as such, they have restricted idiotypic specificities with a relatively high percentage expressing either the 17.109 or 6B6.6 idiotypes that are markers for the human subgroup genes, Vκ325 or Vκ328, respectively.[40,76-78] The light-chain genes are preferentially associated with members of the V_H1 and V_H4 heavy-chain gene families respectively.[76,78a] Such natural antibodies have low affinity for human IgG (kD = 10^{-4} to 10^{-5} M),[39,40] tend to be produced by the $CD5^+$ B lymphocyte subpopulation, and are generally polyspecific, reacting with a wide variety of both self and exogenous antigens.[39,40,79-81]

B cells capable of producing IgM RFs are present in the periphery of normal individuals. These RFs can be germline encoded and tend to be polyspecific, cross-reacting with a variety of other antigens.[79,82] Production of RF occurs following secondary immunization or infection and requires the presence of both immune-complexed antigen and T cells specific for the antigen present in the immune complex.[48,49,56,83] However, in contrast to RA patients, RF production in normal individuals is transient and regulated. These physiologic RFs are encoded predominantly by Vκ3 light chains and either V_H1, V_H3, or V_H4 V-region genes, similar to IgM RFs derived from MC patients.[84] The IgM RF-secreting lines derived from patients following secondary immunization have undergone extensive somatic mutation, but with no evidence of affinity maturation and with an apparent selection against amino acid–replacement mutations in the antibody-combining site.[41,85] These data imply that, under normal circumstances, there are efficient peripheral mechanisms that prevent the expression of higher-affinity, potentially pathologic RFs.

Many studies have analyzed RFs derived from either the peripheral blood or synovium of patients with RA. Low affinity, polyspecific RFs (kD = 10^{-4} to 5×10^{-5} M) can be derived from RA patients.[39,42] However, in contrast to normal individuals, the patients produce a high proportion of IgM RFs that react avidly with human IgG (kD = 10^{-7} M).[39,42,43] Monoreactive IgM RFs can form large immune aggregates and activate complement more efficiently than the lower-affinity polyspecific RFs.[86] Such complement activation undoubtedly contributes to joint inflammation, and there is evidence for selective enrichment of these high-affinity clones in the synovium.[87] IgM RF-secreting lines use many different heavy- and light-chain variable region genes and gene combinations.[42,43,78,88-94] A commonly expressed type of RF uses a Vκ325-encoded light chain paired with a V_H1-family heavy chain with a specific somatically created CDR3.[95] These autoantibodies occur in healthy individuals, in cryoglobulins, and in RA patients, but usually with a higher frequency of somatic replacement mutations in RA RFs.[41] However, in RA, there is a general trend away from the $V_H1/4$ and Vκ3 genes common in natural antibodies in favor of predominant use of V_H3 genes and a wide variety of light chains including V-lambda subgroups.[41,43,89,92,93,96-99] When V_H3 genes are utilized by low-affinity RFs from normal individuals, they appear to be encoded by different V_H3 family members compared to RA-associated RFs.[41] The relevance of many reported RF B cell lines has been questioned, as they were derived from peripheral blood and may not be representative of the disease, but V_H3-encoded RFs have been suggested to predominate in rheumatoid synovium and be most contributory to pathogenesis.[41]

Together, these data indicate that the RFs in RA have undergone antigen-induced expansion and affinity maturation, together with recruitment of new clones of B cells. Studies of IgG RFs derived from RA patients support this conclusion. Some IgG RFs use the same V genes as IgM RFs but exhibit a much greater degree of somatic mutation than IgM RFs, indicating a further affinity maturation of the autoantibody response.[100,101] Sequencing of synovial RFs indicate that class switching and subsequent somatic mutation occur within the synovium, supporting the view that synovial tissue becomes a type of secondary lymphoid tissue containing germinal center–like lymphoid aggregates.[102]

Structural analysis of the Fab fragment of an RA synovium-derived IgM RF complexed with human IgG suggests that an antigen-driven response to IgG Fc was involved in production of this pathologic RF, as one of the important contact residues in IgG binding is somatically mutated.[26] Moreover, the antibody residues involved in recognition of self IgG are all located at the edge of the conventional antigen-combining surface, which leaves much of the latter available to potentially bind to another ligand. These findings have lead to the proposal that this autoantibody may have arisen in response to an entirely different antigen and that binding to self IgG was an unfortunate cross-reactivity.[26]

Physiologic Role of Rheumatoid Factors

The majority of the RF B lymphocytes in normal lymphoid tissues are in the mantle zone regions.[103] In experimental animals, antigen-antibody complexes that reach lymphoid tissues via the afferent lymphatic vessels often localize to the mantle and marginal zones.[104] Studies of transgenic mice expressing low-affinity RFs have shown that such RF B cells remain ignorant of the presence of monomeric IgG under normal circumstances.[105] They may, however, serve as excellent antigen-presenting cells for immune-complexed antigen, resulting in expansion of antigen-reactive T cells.[57,58] It is likely that early in a secondary immune response, when very small amounts of antigen are available, most of the antigen arrives in the draining lymph nodes in the form of an immune complex. Low levels of immune-complexed antigen may not bind efficiently to conventional antigen-presenting cells. Moreover, the interaction of IgG with Fc receptors on B cells may inhibit antigen presentation.[106] Under these circumstances, IgM RF-expressing B cells may act as highly efficient antigen-presenting cells for immune-complexed antigen, able to enhance an antigen-specific T cell expansion early in a secondary immune response. One would expect that this would in turn lead to expansion, somatic mutation, and affinity maturation of the RF B cell Ig receptor such that it may now be able to bind soluble, as well as immune-complexed, IgG. Indeed, such an increase in RF precursor B cells normally accompanies a secondary immune response.[83] However, RFs derived from healthy immunized volunteers are of low affinity and have few replacement mutations in the antibody-combining site, indicating an efficient process for prevention of long-term expression and expansion of high-affinity RFs.[41,85]

Studies of transgenic mice expressing high-affinity disease-associated RFs have shown that encounter with soluble IgG leads to deletion of the RF B cells.[107-109] Deletion occurs by apoptosis via a Fas/Fas ligand independent pathway as a result of the lack of appropriate survival signals provided by T cell help.[108,110] The ability of IgG to bind to FcγRII on the B cell surface also appears to play a role in the deletion process.[111] Thus, as specific antigen is cleared and T cell help becomes limiting, encounter of somatically mutated high-affinity RF B cells with soluble IgG should lead to apoptosis of clones of B cells with binding affinities above a certain threshold. This would leave only those RF B cell clones whose somatic mutations have not resulted in substantially increased affinities, accounting for the type of RFs detected in healthy immunized donors.[41,85]

The common appearance of IgM RFs during acute infections also suggests that the secreted, as well as surface-bound, autoantibodies have an important physiologic function. The RFs produced by polyclonal B lymphocyte activation can potentially amplify the early response of the humoral immune system to bacterial or parasitic exposure. IgM RFs have the ability to cross-link low-affinity IgG antibodies aligned on a surface of a viral or bacterial particle. The net result is the formation of a relatively stable, multivalent, and multispecific complex.

When bound to aggregated IgG, RFs of the IgM class activate complement remarkably efficiently.[112] If the IgG is bound to a bacterium or parasite, the end result probably is either the lysis of the invading organism or its clearance from the circulation via the abundant complement receptors of the reticuloendothelial system. For this reason, IgM RF synthesis may represent an essential component of an effective polyclonal antibody response.

Under certain conditions, complexes of IgG and antigen potently inhibit immune responses.[113] The immune complexes can bind to the FcγRII class of membrane receptors for the Fc fragment of IgG, which are expressed by most B lymphocytes. This interaction inhibits B lymphocyte activation by antigen and thereby impedes antibody production. IgM RFs may prevent immune complexes from binding to Fc receptors and so substantially amplify IgG antibody responses.[114]

The physiologic functions of IgM-RF are summarized in Table 19–3.

Role of Rheumatoid Factor in Rheumatoid Arthritis

In patients with RA, Sjögren's syndrome, and MC, RFs persist in the circulation in the absence of any known exogenous antigenic stimulus. Understanding the regulation of RF production may therefore yield clues concerning the immune pathogenesis of these diseases.

As discussed previously, the RFs produced in lymphoproliferative and autoimmune diseases are structurally dissimilar (Table 19–4). In lymphoproliferative disease, such as chronic lymphocytic leukemia, Wäldenström's macroglobulinemia, and MC, as well as in some cases of Sjögren's syndrome, the RFs are monoclonal or oligoclonal and display cross-reactive idiotypic antigens.[73,75,115,116] The restricted nature of these RFs is uncommon for antigen-driven immune responses, which typically undergo time-dependent diversification. The accumulation of somatic mutations, immunoglobulin class switching, and the recruitment of new antibody-secreting clones all contribute to antibody heterogeneity.

TABLE 19–3 • PHYSIOLOGIC FUNCTIONS OF IgM RHEUMATOID FACTOR

1. Cell-associated rheumatoid factor
   a. Antigen processing and presentation
2. Secreted rheumatoid factor
   a. Stabilization of low-affinity IgG antigen complexes
   b. Immune-complex clearance
   c. Enhancement of opsonization

TABLE 19–4 • COMPARISON OF RHEUMATOID FACTORS IN LYMPHOPROLIFERATIVE AND AUTOIMMUNE DISEASES

Lymphoproliferative:	1. Restricted variable-region gene usage, cross-reactive idiotypes 2. Limited or no somatic mutations 3. Low affinity 4. Mainly Immunoglobulin M (IgM)
Autoimmune:	1. Many genes, private idiotypes 2. Multiple somatic mutations 3. Higher affinity 4. All Ig classes

These processes are controlled by helper T cells. In contrast, RF synthesis in lymphoproliferative diseases may result from unrestrained proliferation of immature B lymphocyte clones. In this regard, clinical studies have shown that a significant fraction of patients with MC eventually develop overt lymphoma.[116] Neoplastic transformation of B lymphocytes is an established complication of Sjögren's syndrome.[117] A possible role for HCV in the pathogenesis of some cases of Sjögren's syndrome[54, 117a] and in the development of non-Hodgkin's lymphoma, has become a topic of active investigation.[66-68]

The RFs in the sera of patients with RA are heterogeneous.[78,93,115] The autoantibodies contain light and heavy chains distributed among all the variable-region subgroups and among the IgM, IgG, and IgA classes. Sequence analyses indicate that these RFs are the products of multiple B cell clones, whose immunoglobulin genes contain many somatic mutations[41-43,78,87-91,93,96,100] RA-associated RFs can be derived from the immunoglobulin genes encoding the low-affinity RFs, as well as other Ig genes. It is possible that the normal process of somatic mutation in additional immunoglobulin genes may generate antibodies, which cross-react with human IgG. The simplest interpretation of these results, however, is that the production of RFs in RA is part of an antigen-specific response and is driven by helper T lymphocytes reactive with a foreign antigen trapped in an immune complex. However, immune complexes containing exogenous antigens have never been detected in RA. In addition, although some patients have been demonstrated to have T cell reactivity to IgG, this is not generally the case.[118] Studies of transgenic mice expressing high-affinity RFs have shown that encounter with soluble IgG results in deletion of the autoreactive B cell in the absence of T cell help.[107-110] However, in the presence of allospecific T cell help, high-affinity RF B cells differentiate and secrete RF in response to soluble IgG and do not require immune-complexed antigen.[108] The presence of two binding sites for RF on the Fc portion of IgG is presumably sufficient to cross-link surface RF.[27] Consequently, it is interesting that RA patients were reported several years ago to have T cells responsive to autologous macrophages and other antigen-presenting cells.[119-121] Potentially this weak T cell responsiveness may be sufficient to promote RF B cell survival within the environment of the rheumatoid joint, where adhesion molecules are abundant and sludging of cells delays migration. Furthermore, in the confined environment of the rheumatoid joint, the relative proportion of complexed to soluble IgG is increased. In this unique situation, T cell help may be amply supplied by a localized weak graft versus host reaction. Alternatively, CD40L (CD154) or anti-CD40 antibodies have been shown to substitute for T cell help in induction of RF synthesis in transgenic mice. T cell cytokines are not required. CD40L is expressed nonspecifically by T cells within the synovium, as well as by activated platelets and endothelium.[122-124] Hence, the inflamed rheumatoid synovium contains all the prerequisites for sustained RF synthesis, and it is not surprising that RF synthesis primarily occurs within the joints. The recent finding that RF B cells can be activated to proliferate by dual engagement of both surface Ig and Toll-like receptors by IgG-chromatin immune complexes provides an alternative pathway for RF B cell expansion.[125,126] Toll-like receptor 9 (TLR9) primarily recognizes unmethylated CpG mofifs common in pathogen DNA.[127] However, such motifs can also occur in certain regions of mammalian DNA. Consequently, the need for T cell help is bypassed and substituted for by stimulation of TLR9 and simultaneous activation of surface RF by IgG-DNA complexes. These data may also provide an alternative explanation for the production of RF during acute bacterial infections.[59,60]

High levels of serum RF are associated with a worse prognosis in RA.[12] High titers of RF, particularly IgG RF, are a risk factor for the development of vasculitis,[16,18] and elevated IgA RFs may correlate with bone erosions, vasculitis, and a more severe disease course.[9,10,17,19] Although it is unlikely that prolonged production of high-affinity RFs are responsible for the joint involvement in RA, they probably exacerbate joint inflammation and promote immune disregulation. During established disease, the synovium may convert to lymphoid granulation tissue. B lymphocytes with RF specificity, particularly IgG RF, are abundant in the rheumatoid synovium[128] where they can lead to complement activation and contribute to the inflammatory process.[129] The synovial fluids of RA patients, unlike their sera, frequently have markedly depressed complement levels and contain high-molecular-weight IgG aggregates as detected in the analytic ultracentrifuge or by cryoprecipitation.[14] Partial isolation and characterization of the immune complexes from rheumatoid synovial fluids and tissues have yielded IgG RFs, sometimes complexed with IgM RFs, in the absence of other known antigens.[14,130,131] Consequently, the synovium becomes a major source of the RFs, which appear in copious amounts in the circulation of RA patients, although lymphoid tissues such as bone marrow also produce the autoantibody.[132] A number of provocative reports have indicated alternative mechanisms by which some RFs may affect immune regulation. For example, both monoclonal and polyclonal RFs can cross-react weakly with human β_2-microglobulin, a member of the immunoglobulin supergene family, at residues 57-63,[133,134] and with some human leukocyte antigen (HLA) molecules.[133] β_2-Microglobulin shares considerable sequence homology and three-dimensional structure with immunoglobulin domains.

Consequently, RF B cells may be involved in the pathogenesis of RA through their role in the afferent arm of immune synovitism functioning as antigen-presenting cells,[57,58] and also in the efferent arm of the response. As efficient antigen-presenting cells, RF B lymphocytes may further increase the chance of T cell autosensitization to self-components that are released from necrotic joint tissues, such as collagen, proteoglycans, and heat shock proteins. In this way, the abnormal conglomeration of activated RF B cells at synovial sites would create a vicious cycle that promotes T cell–dependent joint inflammation through a variety of mechanisms. Secreted RF can play a role in the efferent arm of immune synovitis by complement fixation and through cytokine induction (tumor necrosis factor-α [TNF-α]) via IgG RF complexes binding to Fc receptors (FcγRIIIa) on macrophages.[135] Whether the primary involvement of RF in the course of disease is as RF B cell antigen-presenting cells or secreted RF antibody, B cell depletion would be expected to have a positive effect on the disease process. Preliminary data from clinical trials in both RA and systemic lupus erythematosis (SLE) using anti-CD20 antibodies to deplete B cells support this assumption.[136-139] In addition, they provide a rationale to pursue in the future more precise targeting strategies. Clinical trials targeting the CD40-CD40L interaction failed due to the presence of side effects, but other potential targets for future studies include BAFF-R, TACI and BCMA.

REFERENCES

1. Kunkel HG, Simon HJ, Fudenberg H: Observations concerning positive serologic reactions for rheumatoid factor in certain patients with sarcoidosis and other hyperglobulinemic states. Arthritis Rheum 1:289, 1958.
2. Mikkelsen WM, et al: Estimates of the prevalence of rheumatic diseases in the population of Tecumseh, Michigan, 1959-60. J Chronic Dis 20(6):351-369, 1967.
3. Lawrance JS: Rheumatism in Populations. London, William Heinemann, 1977.
4. Procaccia S, et al: IgM, IgG and IgA rheumatoid factors and circulating immune complexes in patients with AIDS and AIDS-related complex with serological abnormalities. Clin Exp Immunol 67(2):236-244, 1987.
5. Jarvis JN, et al: Rheumatoid factor expression and complement activation in children congenitally infected with human immunodeficiency virus. Clin Immunol Immunopathol 67(1):50-54, 1993.
6. Chen PP, Carson DA: New insights on the physiological and pathological rheumatoid factors in humans. *In* Coutinho A, Kazatchkinc M (eds): Autoimmunity: Physiology and Disease. New York, Wiley-Liss, 1994, pp 247-266.
7. Bonagura VR, et al: Mapping IgG epitopes bound by rheumatoid factors from immunized controls identifies disease-specific rheumatoid factors produced by patients with rheumatoid arthritis. J Immunol 160(5):2496-2505, 1998.
8. Hooper B, et al: Autoimmunity in a rural community. Clin Exp Immunol 12(1):79-87, 1972.
9. Pai S, Pai L, Birkenfeldt R: Correlation of serum IgA rheumatoid factor levels with disease severity in rheumatoid arthritis. Scand J Rheumatol 27(4):252-256, 1998.
10. Jonsson T, et al: Combined elevation of IgM and IgA rheumatoid factor has high diagnostic specificity for rheumatoid arthritis. Rheumatol Int 18(3):119-122, 1998.
11. Nykanen M, et al: Improved immunoturbidimetric method for rheumatoid factor testing. J Clin Pathol 46(11):1065-1066, 1993.
12. Masi AT, et al: Prospective study of the early course of rheumatoid arthritis in young adults: comparison of patients with and without rheumatoid factor positivity at entry and identification of variables correlating with outcome. Semin Arthritis Rheum 4(4):299-326, 1976.
13. Winchester RJ, Kunkel HG, Agnello V: Occurrence of -globulin complexes in serum and joint fluid of rheumatoid arthritis patients: use of monoclonal rheumatoid factors as reagents for their demonstration. J Exp Med 134(3 Suppl):286S, 1971.
14. Winchester RJ, Agnello V, Kunkel HG: Gamma globulin complexes in synovial fluids of patients with rheumatoid arthritis. Partial characterization and relationship to lowered complement levels. Clin Exp Immunol 6(5):689-706, 1970.
15. Hannestad K: Presence of aggregated gamma-G-globulin in certain rheumatoid synovial effusions. Clin Exp Immunol 2(4):511-529, 1967.
16. Scott DG, et al: IgG rheumatoid factor, complement and immune complexes in rheumatoid synovitis and vasculitis: Comparative and serial studies during cytotoxic therapy. Clin Exp Immunol 43(1):54-63, 1981.
17. Houssien DA, et al: Rheumatoid factor isotypes, disease activity and the outcome of rheumatoid arthritis: Comparative effects of different antigens. Scand J Rheumatol 27(1):46-53, 1998.
18. Westedt ML, et al: Rheumatoid factors in rheumatoid arthritis and vasculitis. Rheumatol Int 5(5):209-214, 1985.
19. Arnason JA, et al: Relation between bone erosions and rheumatoid factor isotypes. Ann Rheum Dis 46(5):380-384, 1987.
20. Gioud-Paquet M, et al: IgM rheumatoid factor (RF), IgA RF, IgE RF, and IgG RF detected by ELISA in rheumatoid arthritis. Ann Rheum Dis 46(1):65-71, 1987.
21. Wolfe F: A comparison of IgM rheumatoid factor by nephelometry and latex methods: clinical and laboratory significance. Arthritis Care Res 11(2):89-93, 1998.
22. Halldorsdottir HD, et al: A prospective study on the incidence of rheumatoid arthritis among people with persistent increase of rheumatoid factor. Ann Rheum Dis 59(2):149-151, 2000.
23. Artandi SE, et al: Molecular analysis of IgM rheumatoid factor binding to chimeric IgG. J Immunol 146(2):603-610, 1991.
24. Natvig JB, Gaarder PI, Turner MW: IgG antigens of the C gamma 2 and C gamma 3 homology regions interacting with rheumatoid factors. Clin Exp Immunol 12(2):177-184, 1972.
25. Williams RC Jr, Malone CC: Rheumatoid-factor-reactive sites on CH2 established by analysis of overlapping peptides of primary sequence. Scand J Immunol 40(4):443-456, 1994.
26. Corper AL, et al: Structure of human IgM rheumatoid factor Fab bound to its autoantigen IgG Fc reveals a novel topology of antibody-antigen interaction. Nat Struct Biol 4(5):374-381, 1997.
27. Sohi MK, et al: Crystallization of a complex between the Fab fragment of a human immunoglobulin M (IgM) rheumatoid factor (RF-AN) and the Fc fragment of human IgG4. Immunology 88(4):636-641, 1996.
28. Parekh RB, et al: Association of rheumatoid arthritis and primary osteoarthritis with changes in the glycosylation pattern of total serum IgG. Nature 316(6027):452-457, 1985.
29. Axford JS, et al: Reduced B-cell galactosyltransferase activity in rheumatoid arthritis. Lancet 2(8574):1486-1488, 1987.
30. van Zeben D, et al: Early agalactosylation of IgG is associated with a more progressive disease course in patients with rheumatoid arthritis: results of a follow-up study. Br J Rheumatol 33(1):36-43, 1994.
31. Tsuchiya N, et al: Effects of galactose depletion from oligosaccharide chains on immunological activities of human IgG. J Rheumatol 16(3):285-290, 1989.
32. Newkirk MM, Lemmo A, Rauch J: Importance of the IgG isotype, not the state of glycosylation, in determining human rheumatoid factor binding. Arthritis Rheum 33(6):800-809, 1990.
33. Soltys AJ, et al: The binding of synovial tissue-derived human monoclonal immunoglobulin M rheumatoid factor to immunoglobulin G preparations of differing galactose content. Scand J Immunol 40(2):135-143, 1994.
34. Tsuchiya N, et al: Distribution of glycosylation abnormality among serum IgG subclasses from patients with rheumatoid arthritis. Clin Immunol Immunopathol 70(1):47-50, 1994.
35. Jefferis R, Mageed RA: The epitope specificity and idiotypy of monoclonal rheumatoid factors. Scand J Rheumatol 75(Suppl): 89-92, 1988.
36. Robbins DL, et al: Estimation of the relative avidity of 19S IgM rheumatoid factor secreted by rheumatoid synovial cells for human IgG subclasses. Arthritis Rheum 29(6):722-729, 1986.

37. Chou CT: Binding of rheumatoid and lupus synovial fluids and sera-derived human IgG rheumatoid factor to degalactosylated IgG. Arch Med Res 33(6):541-544, 2002.
38. Newkirk MM, Rauch J: Binding of human monoclonal IgG rheumatoid factors to Fc is influenced by carbohydrate. J Rheumatol 20(5):776-780, 1993.
39. Burastero SE, et al: Monoreactive high affinity and polyreactive low affinity rheumatoid factors are produced by CD5+ B cells from patients with rheumatoid arthritis. J Exp Med 168(6):1979-1992, 1988.
40. Chen PP, et al: Idiotypic and molecular characterization of human rheumatoid factors. Chem Immunol 48:63-81, 1990.
41. Borretzen M, et al: Differences in mutational patterns between rheumatoid factors in health and disease are related to variable heavy chain family and germ-line gene usage. Eur J Immunol 27(3):735-741, 1997.
42. Harindranath N, et al: Complete sequence of the genes encoding the VH and VL regions of low- and high-affinity monoclonal IgM and IgA1 rheumatoid factors produced by CD5+ B cells from a rheumatoid arthritis patient. Int Immunol 3(9):865-875, 1991.
43. Mantovani L, Wilder RL, Casali P: Human rheumatoid B-1a (CD5+ B) cells make somatically hypermutated high affinity IgM rheumatoid factors. J Immunol 151(1):473-488, 1993.
44. Eisenberg R: The specificity and polyvalency of binding of a monoclonal rheumatoid factor. Immunochemistry 13(4):355-359, 1976.
45. Pope RM, Teller DC, Mannik M: The molecular basis of self-association of antibodies to IgG (rheumatoid factors) in rheumatoid arthritis. Proc Natl Acad Sci U S A 71(2):517-521, 1974.
46. Nardella FA, Teller DC, Mannik M: Studies on the antigenic determinants in the self-association of IgG rheumatoid factor. J Exp Med 154(1):112-125, 1981.
47. Lu EW, et al: Generation and characterization of two monoclonal self-associating IgG rheumatoid factors from a rheumatoid synovium. Arthritis Rheum 35(1):101-105, 1992.
48. Nemazee DA Sato VL: Induction of rheumatoid antibodies in the mouse. Regulated production of autoantibody in the secondary humoral response. J Exp Med 158(2):529-545, 1983.
49. Van Snick J, Coulie P: Rheumatoid factors and secondary immune responses in the mouse. I. Frequent occurrence of hybridomas secreting IgM anti-IgG1 autoantibodies after immunization with protein antigens. Eur J Immunol 13(11):890-894, 1983.
50. Welch MJ, et al: Increased frequency of rheumatoid factor precursor B lymphocytes after immunization of normal adults with tetanus toxoid. Clin Exp Immunol 51(2):299-304, 1983.
51. Slaughter L, et al: In vitro effects of Epstein-Barr virus on peripheral blood mononuclear cells from patients with rheumatoid arthritis and normal subjects. J Exp Med 148(5):1429-1434, 1978.
52. Izui S, Eisenberg RA, Dixon FJ: IgM rheumatoid factors in mice injected with bacterial lipopolysaccharides. J Immunol 122(5):2096-2102, 1979.
53. Tsuchiya N, Williams RC Jr, Hutt-Fletcher LM: Rheumatoid factors may bear the internal image of the Fc gamma-binding protein of herpes simplex virus type 1. J Immunol 144(12): 4742-4748, 1990.
54. Ramos-Casals M, et al: Cryoglobulinemia in primary Sjögren's syndrome: Prevalence and clinical characteristics in a series of 115 patients. Semin Arthritis Rheum 28(3):200-205, 1998.
55. Pileri P, et al: Binding of hepatitis C virus to CD81. Science 282(5390):938-941, 1998.
56. Coulie PG, Van Snick J: Rheumatoid factor (RF) production during anamnestic immune responses in the mouse. III. Activation of RF precursor cells is induced by their interaction with immune complexes and carrier-specific helper T cells. J Exp Med 161(1):88-97, 1985.
57. Roosnek E, Lanzavecchia, A: Efficient and selective presentation of antigen-antibody complexes by rheumatoid factor B cells. J Exp Med 173(2):487-489, 1991.
58. Tighe H, et al: Function of B cells expressing a human immunoglobulin M rheumatoid factor autoantibody in transgenic mice. J Exp Med 177(1):109-118, 1993.
59. Williams RC Jr, Kunkel HG: Rheumatoid factor, complement and conglutinin aberrations in patients with subactute bacterial endocarditis. J Clin Invest 41:666, 1962.
60. Carson DA, et al: IgG rheumatoid factor in subacute bacterial endocarditis: relationship to IgM rheumatoid factor and circulating immune complexes. Clin Exp Immunol 31(1):100-103, 1978.
61. Gelpi C, et al: Different strains of donor parental lymphoid cells induce different models of chronic graft-versus-host disease in murine (Balb/c × A/J)F1 hybrid hosts. Clin Immunol Immunopathol 56(3):298-310, 1990.
62. Morris SC, et al: Allotype-specific immunoregulation of autoantibody production by host B cells in chronic graft-versus host disease. J Immunol 144(3):916-922, 1990.
63. Widhopf G, Tighe H. unpublished data.
64. Casali P, Notkins AL: CD5+ B lymphocytes, polyreactive antibodies and the human B-cell repertoire. Immunol Today 10(11): 364-368, 1989.
65. Sasso EH: The rheumatoid factor response in the etiology of mixed cryoglobulins associated with hepatitis C virus infection. Ann Med Interne (Paris) 151(1):30-40, 2000.
66. Gasparotto D, De Re V, Boiocchi M: Hepatitis C virus, B-cell proliferation and lymphomas. Leuk Lymphoma 43(4):747-751, 2002.
67. Zignego AL, et al: Hepatitis C virus infection in mixed cryoglobulinemia and B-cell non-Hodgkin's lymphoma: evidence for a pathogenetic role. Arch Virol 142(3):545-555, 1997.
67a. La Civita L, Zignego AL, Monti M, et al: Mixed cryoglobulinemia as a possible preneoplastic disorder. Arthritis Rheum 38(12): 1859-1860, 1995.
68. De Re V, et al: Sequence analysis of the immunoglobulin antigen receptor of hepatitis C virus-associated non-Hodgkin lymphomas suggests that the malignant cells are derived from the rheumatoid factor-producing cells that occur mainly in type II cryoglobulinemia. Blood 96(10):3578-3584, 2000.
69. Kunkel HG, et al: Cross-idiotypic specificity among monoclonal IgM proteins with anti-globulin activity. J Exp Med 137(2):331-342, 1973.
70. Capra JD, Kehoe JM: Structure of antibodies with shared idiotypy: the complete sequence of the heavy chain variable regions of two immunoglobulin M anti-gamma globulins. Proc Natl Acad Sci U S A 71(10):4032-4036, 1974.
71. Carson DA, Fong S: A common idiotope on human rheumatoid factors identified by a hybridoma antibody. Mol Immunol 20(10):1081-1087, 1983.
72. Chen PP, et al: Characterization of human rheumatoid factors with seven antiidiotypes induced by synthetic hypervariable region peptides. J Exp Med 162(2):487-500, 1985.
73. Carson DA, et al: Idiotypic and genetic studies of human rheumatoid factors. Arthritis Rheum 30(12):1321-1325, 1987.
74. Liu MF, et al: Characterization of four homologous L chain variable region genes that are related to 6B6.6 idiotype positive human rheumatoid factor L chains. J Immunol 142(2):688-694, 1989.
75. Kipps TJ, et al: Molecular characterization of a major autoantibody-associated cross-reactive idiotype in Sjogren's syndrome. J Immunol 142(12):4261-4268, 1989.
76. Silverman GJ, et al: Idiotypic and subgroup analysis of human monoclonal rheumatoid factors. Implications for structural and genetic basis of autoantibodies in humans. J Clin Invest 82(2):469-475, 1988.
77. Chen PP, et al: Cross-reacting idiotypes on cryoprecipitating rheumatoid factor. Springer Semin Immunopathol 10(1):35-55, 1988.
78. Schrohenloher RE, et al: Monoclonal antibody 6B6.6 defines a cross-reactive kappa light chain idiotope on human monoclonal and polyclonal rheumatoid factors. Arthritis Rheum 33(2): 187-198, 1990.
78a. Silverman GJ, Schrohenloher RE, Accavitti MA, et al: Structural characterization of the second major cross-reactive idiotype group of human rheumatoid factors. Association with the VH4 gene family. Arthritis Rheum 33(9):1347-1360, 1990.
79. Nakamura M, et al: Human monoclonal rheumatoid factor-like antibodies from CD5 (Leu-1)+ B cells are polyreactive. J Immunol 140(12):4180-4186, 1988.
80. Hardy RR: Variable gene usage, physiology and development of Ly-1+ (CD5+) B cells. Curr Opin Immunol 4(2):181-185, 1992.
81. Riboldi P, et al: Natural antibodies. *In* Bona CA, et al (eds): The Molecular Pathology of Autoimmune Diseases. Philadelphia, Gordon and Breach Science Publishers, 1993, p 45.
82. Casali P, et al: Human lymphocytes making rheumatoid factor and antibody to ssDNA belong to Leu-1+ B-cell subset. Science 236(4797):77-81, 1987.

83. Nemazee DA: Immune complexes can trigger specific, T cell-dependent, autoanti-IgG antibody production in mice. J Exp Med 161(1):242-256, 1985.
84. Thompson KM, et al: Variable region gene usage of human monoclonal rheumatoid factors derived from healthy donors following immunization. Eur J Immunol 24(8):1771-1778, 1994.
85. Borretzen M, et al: Control of autoantibody affinity by selection against amino acid replacements in the complementarity-determining regions. Proc Natl Acad Sci U S A 91(26):12917-12921, 1994.
86. Sato Y, et al: Complement activating properties of monoreactive and polyreactive IgM rheumatoid factors. Ann Rheum Dis 52(11):795-800, 1993.
87. Hakoda M, et al: Selective infiltration of B cells committed to the production of monoreactive rheumatoid factor in synovial tissue of patients with rheumatoid arthritis. Clin Immunol Immunopathol 69(1):16-22, 1993.
88. Randen I, et al: Clonally related IgM rheumatoid factors undergo affinity maturation in the rheumatoid synovial tissue. J Immunol 148(10):3296-3301, 1992.
89. Pascual V, et al: Nucleotide sequence analysis of rheumatoid factors and polyreactive antibodies derived from patients with rheumatoid arthritis reveals diverse use of VH and VL gene segments and extensive variability in CDR-3. Scand J Immunol 36(2):349-362, 1992.
90. Lee SK, et al: The immunoglobulin kappa light chain repertoire expressed in the synovium of a patient with rheumatoid arthritis. Arthritis Rheum 35(8):905-913, 1992.
91. Soto-Gil RW, et al: A systematic approach to defining the germline gene counterparts of a mutated autoantibody from a patient with rheumatoid arthritis. Arthritis Rheum 35(3):356-363, 1992.
92. Sasso EH: Immunoglobulin V genes in rheumatoid arthritis. Rheum Dis Clin North Am 18(4):809-836, 1992.
93. Youngblood K, et al: Rheumatoid factors from the peripheral blood of two patients with rheumatoid arthritis are genetically heterogeneous and somatically mutated. J Clin Invest 93(2):852-861, 1994.
94. Newkirk MM, et al: Restricted immunoglobulin variable region gene usage by hybridoma rheumatoid factors from patients with systemic lupus erythematosus and rheumatoid arthritis. Mol Immunol 30(3):255-263, 1993.
95. Borretzen M, et al: Structural restriction in the heavy chain CDR3 of human rheumatoid factors. J Immunol 155(7): 3630-3637, 1995.
96. Victor KD, et al: Rheumatoid factors isolated from patients with autoimmune disorders are derived from germline genes distinct from those encoding the Wa, Po, and Bla cross-reactive idiotypes. J Clin Invest 87(5):1603-1613, 1991.
97. Robbins DL, et al: Serologic and molecular characterization of a human monoclonal rheumatoid factor derived from rheumatoid synovial cells. Arthritis Rheum 33(8):1188-1195, 1990.
98. Ermel RW, et al: Molecular analysis of rheumatoid factors derived from rheumatoid synovium suggests an antigen-driven response in inflamed joints. Arthritis Rheum 36(3):380-388, 1993.
99. Ermel RW, et al: Preferential utilization of a novel V lambda 3 gene in monoclonal rheumatoid factors derived from the synovial cells of rheumatoid arthritis patients. Arthritis Rheum 37(6): 860-868, 1994.
100. Randen I, et al: Synovial IgG rheumatoid factors show evidence of an antigen-driven immune response and a shift in the V gene repertoire compared to IgM rheumatoid factors. Eur J Immunol 23(6):1220-1225, 1993.
101. Deftos M, et al: Defining the genetic origins of three rheumatoid synovium-derived IgG rheumatoid factors. J Clin Invest 93(6):2545-2553, 1994.
102. Williams DG, Moyes SP, Mageed RA: Rheumatoid factor isotype switch and somatic mutation variants within rheumatoid arthritis synovium. Immunology 98(1):123-136, 1999.
103. Axelrod O, et al: Idiotypic cross-reactivity of immunoglobulins expressed in Waldenström's macroglobulinemia, chronic lymphocytic leukemia, and mantle zone lymphocytes of secondary B-cell follicles. Blood 77(7):1484-1490, 1991.
104. Kumararatne DS, Bazin H, MacLennan IC: Marginal zones: The major B cell compartment of rat spleens. Eur J Immunol 11(11):858-864, 1981.
105. Hannum LG, et al: A disease-related rheumatoid factor autoantibody is not tolerized in a normal mouse: Implications for the origins of autoantibodies in autoimmune disease. J Exp Med 184(4):1269-1278, 1996.
106. Phillips NE, Parker DC: Fc-dependent inhibition of mouse B cell activation by whole anti-mu antibodies. J Immunol 130(2): 602-606, 1983.
107. Tighe H, et al: Human immunoglobulin (IgG) induced deletion of IgM rheumatoid factor B cells in transgenic mice. J Exp Med 181(2):599-606, 1995.
108. Tighe H, et al: Peripheral deletion of rheumatoid factor B cells after abortive activation by IgG. Proc Natl Acad Sci U S A 94(2):646-651, 1997.
109. Wang H, Shlomchik MJ: High affinity rheumatoid factor transgenic B cells are eliminated in normal mice. J Immunol 159(3):1125-1134, 1997.
110. Warnatz K, et al: Rheumatoid factor B cell tolerance via autonomous Fas/FasL-independent apoptosis. Cell Immunol 191(1):69-73, 1999.
111. Warnatz K and Tighe H, unpublished data.
112. Sabharwal UK, et al: Activation of the classical pathway of complement by rheumatoid factors. Assessment by radioimmunoassay for C4. Arthritis Rheum 25(2):161-167, 1982.
113. Rigley KP, Harnett MM, Klaus GG: Co-cross-linking of surface immunoglobulin Fc gamma receptors on B lymphocytes uncouples the antigen receptors from their associated G protein. Eur J Immunol 19(3):481-485, 1989.
114. Panoskaltis A, St Clair NR: Rheumatoid factor blocks regulator Fc signals. Cellular Immunol 123:177, 1989.
115. Fong S, et al: Expression of three cross-reactive idiotypes on rheumatoid factor autoantibodies from patients with autoimmune diseases and seropositive adults. J Immunol 137(1):122-128, 1986.
116. Brouet JC, et al: Biologic and clinical significance of cryoglobulins. A report of 86 cases. Am J Med 57(5):775-788, 1974.
117. Talal N, Bunim J: The development of malignant lymphoma in Sjögren's syndrome. Am J Med 36:529, 1964.
117a. Ramos-Casals M, Garcia-Carrasco M, Cervera R, et al: Hepatitis C virus infection mimicking primary Sjögren syndrome. A clinical and immunologic description of 35 cases. Medicine (Baltimore) 80(1):1-8, 2001.
118. Lang AK, et al: Ability of T cells from patients with rheumatoid arthritis to respond to immunoglobulin G. Immunology 98(1):116-122, 1999.
119. Duke O, Gordon Y, Panayi GS: Synovial fluid mononuclear cells exhibit a spontaneous HLA-DR driven proliferative response. Clin Exp Immunol 70(1):10-17, 1987.
120. Hazelton RA, et al: Analysis of the responding and stimulating cells in the AMLR of patients with rheumatoid arthritis using limiting dilution. Clin Exp Immunol 74(1):94-99, 1988.
121. Duke-Cohan JS, et al: The reaction against autologous lymphoblasts as an indicator of lymphocyte hyperreactivity in rheumatoid arthritis. Clin Immunol Immunopathol 54(2):298-308, 1990.
122. MacDonald KP, et al: Functional CD40 ligand is expressed by T cells in rheumatoid arthritis. J Clin Invest 100(9):2404-2414, 1997.
123. Mach F, et al: Functional CD40 ligand is expressed on human vascular endothelial cells, smooth muscle cells, and macrophages: implications for CD40-CD40 ligand signaling in atherosclerosis. Proc Natl Acad Sci U S A 94(5):1931-1936, 1997.
124. Berner B, et al: Increased expression of CD40 ligand (CD154) on CD4+ T cells as a marker of disease activity in rheumatoid arthritis. Ann Rheum Dis 59(3):190-195, 2000.
125. Rifkin IR, et al: Immune complexes present in the sera of autoimmune mice activate rheumatoid factor B cells. J Immunol 165(3):1626-1633, 2000.
126. Leadbetter EA, et al: Chromatin-IgG complexes activate B cells by dual engagement of IgM and Toll-like receptors. Nature 416(6881):603-607, 2002.
127. Bernasconi NL, Onai N, Lanzavecchia A: A role for Toll-like receptors in acquired immunity: Upregulation of TLR9 by BCR triggering in naive B cells and constitutive expression in memory B cells. Blood 30:30, 2003.

128. Youinou PY, et al: Specificity of plasma cells in the rheumatoid synovium. I. Immunoglobulin class of antiglobulin-producing cells. Scand J Immunol 20(4):307-315, 1984.
129. Brown PB, Nardella FA, Mannik M: Human complement activation by self-associated IgG rheumatoid factors. Arthritis Rheum 25(9):1101-1107, 1982.
130. Winchester RJ: Characterization of IgG complexes in patients with rheumatoid arthritis. Ann N Y Acad Sci 256:73-81, 1975.
131. Mannik M, Nardella FA: IgG rheumatoid factors and self-association of these antibodies. Clin Rheum Dis 11(3):551-572, 1985.
132. Panush RS, et al: IgM rheumatoid factor elaboration by blood, bone marrow, and synovial mononuclear cells in patients with rheumatoid arthritis. Clin Immunol Immunopathol34(3):387-391, 1985.
133. Williams RC Jr, Malone CC: Human IgM rheumatoid factors react with class I HLA molecules. Arthritis Rheum 36:S265, 1993.
134. van Eyndhoven WG, Malone CC, Williams RC Jr: Changes in rheumatoid factor and monoclonal IgG antibody specificity after site-specific mutations in antigenic region of beta 2-microglobulin. Clin Immunol Immunopathol 72(3):362-372, 1994.
135. Edwards JC, Cambridge G: Rheumatoid arthritis: The predictable effect of small immune complexes in which antibody is also antigen. Br J Rheumatol 37(2):126-130, 1998.
136. Edwards JC, Cambridge G: Sustained improvement in rheumatoid arthritis following a protocol designed to deplete B lymphocytes. Rheumatology (Oxford) 40(2):205-211, 2001.
137. De Vita S, et al: Efficacy of selective B cell blockade in the treatment of rheumatoid arthritis: Evidence for a pathogenetic role of B cells. Arthritis Rheum 46(8):2029-2033, 2002.
138. Leandro MJ, Edwards JC, Cambridge G: Clinical outcome in 22 patients with rheumatoid arthritis treated with B lymphocyte depletion. Ann Rheum Dis 61(10):883-888, 2002.
139. Leandro MJ, et al: An open study of B lymphocyte depletion in systemic lupus erythematosus. Arthritis Rheum 46(10):2673-2677, 2002.

20 Antinuclear Antibodies

STANFORD L. PENG • JOE CRAFT

In the strictest sense, antinuclear antibodies (ANAs) are autoantibodies directed against nuclear specificities, such as deoxyribonucleic acid (DNA) or small nuclear ribonucleoproteins (snRNPs); but since the advent of the now widely used fluorescent antinuclear antibody test (FANA), which detects autoantigens throughout the entire cell, the spectrum of ANAs has vastly expanded to include a diverse spectrum of both nuclear and cytoplasmic specificities.[1] The ANA diseases (Table 20–1) consist of several syndromes whose patients are characterized by an unusually high prevalence of antinuclear antibody activity: systemic lupus erythematosus (SLE), systemic sclerosis (SSc), and mixed connective tissue disease (MCTD). The prevalence of ANAs in polymyositis, dermatomyositis, and Sjögren's syndrome (SS) have been reported to be somewhat lower than in the other ANA diseases,[2,3] but they are grouped together here because they share similar target-antigen structures and, therefore, presumably share similar etiologies. For decades, ANAs have remained important diagnostic and prognostic tools for these connective tissue diseases and have become almost routine assays in the evaluation of patients with suspected rheumatic diseases. Nevertheless, these autoantibodies appear in a variety of infectious, inflammatory, and neoplastic diseases, as well as in normal individuals. Therefore, this chapter describes the more-common ANA specificities, outlining their history, methods of detection, clinical disease associations, and the molecular biology of their target autoantigens, in an effort to delineate clearly the clinical efficacy of testing for these specificities.

History

Over the past six decades, ANAs have cultivated an ever-growing collaboration between clinical immunology and molecular biology. In 1948, the concentrated bone marrow specimens of SLE patients were found to contain lupus erythematosus ("LE") cells, the first formal description of an ANA-related phenomenon.[4,5] The "LE cell" was subsequently used as an adjunct tool in the diagnosis of SLE and drug-induced lupus, as well as SS and rheumatoid arthritis (RA).[6] LE cells were soon discovered to be due to a plasma factor,[7,8] autoantibody against deoxyribonucleoprotein,[9] which opsonized, induced apoptosis, or both in free-cell nuclei, which were then antibody-sensitized and subsequently phagocytosed by polymorphonuclear neutrophils.[10] In 1957, the new technique of indirect immunofluorescence allowed the development of the FANA, which offered a more sensitive assay for autoimmunity in SLE as well as other diseases and, thus, brought a new method of choice for the screening of autoimmune disease.[11] The introduction of immunodiffusion permitted a finer distinction of autoantibody specificities to soluble components of whole cells[12] and subsequently led to the identification of new ANA specificities, including Smith, (Sm),[13] nuclear ribonucleoprotein (nRNP),[14] and Ro/Sjögrens syndrome SS-A and La/SS-B.[15] Later studies brought further biologic significance to these findings by demonstrating that these autoantigens play prominent roles in cellular homeostasis: snRNPs, for example, targets of the anti-Sm and anti-nRNP antibodies, play essential roles in the splicing of premessenger ribonucleic acid.[16] These discoveries subsequently led to the elucidation of many autoantigens (Table 20–2), many of which have yet to be fully characterized. As a result of such clinical-biochemical concordances, ANAs have not only served as helpful diagnostic markers in autoimmune diseases but have also greatly aided molecular biologic studies on intracellular metabolism.

Methods OF Detection

IMMUNOFLUORESCENCE

The indirect immunofluorescence ANA test (FANA) provides a rapid, yet highly sensitive screening method for ANA detection. Test sera at varying dilutions (typically serially increasing by twofold) are incubated with substrate cells, and bound antibodies are detected by fluorescein-conjugated anti–human immunoglobulin G (IgG), followed by visualization via a fluorescence microscope. Results typically are reported by two parameters: pattern and titer, with any pattern of reactivity at a titer of 1:40 or greater being considered positive.[2] The former includes one or more morphologic descriptors that reflect the localization of the respective autoantigen(s): Homogeneous and rim nuclear patterns, for example, often reflect anti-DNA autoantibodies, whereas speckled patterns often reflect ribonucleoprotein autoantibodies (see Table 20–2, Fig. 20–1 and 20–2). Other easily discernable patterns include nucleolar, nuclear membrane, cytoplasmic, mitotic spindle apparatus, and centromere. Notably, these patterns may vary with serum dilution. Sera containing antibodies to DNA and snRNPs, for example, may produce the homogeneous pattern of anti-DNA antibodies at lower dilutions but produce the speckled pattern of anti-snRNP antibodies at higher dilutions.

TABLE 20–1 • THE ANTINUCLEAR ANTIBODY (ANA) DISEASES AND RELATED CONDITIONS

Condition	Patients with ANAs (%)
Diseases for which ANA Testing is helpful for Diagnosis	
SLE	99-100
Systemic sclerosis	97
Polymyositis/Dermatomyositis	40-80
Sjögren's syndrome	48-96
Diseases in which ANA is Required for the Diagnosis	
Drug-induced lupus	100
MCTD	100
Autoimmune hepatitis	100
Diseases in which ANA may be useful for Prognosis	
Juvenile rheumatoid arthritis	20-50
Antiphospholipid antibody syndrome	40-50
Raynaud's phenomenon	20-60
Some Diseases in which ANA is Typically not useful	
Rheumatic disease	
Discoid lupus erythematosus	5-25
Fibromyalgia	15-25
Rheumatoid arthritis	30-50
Relatives of patients with autoimmune diseases	5-25
Multiple sclerosis	25
Idiopathic thrombocytopenic purpura	10-30
Thyroid disease	30-50
Patients with silicone breast implants	15-25
Infectious diseases	varies widely
Malignancies	varies widely
Normal Persons	
≥ 1:40	20-30
≥ 1:80	10-12
≥ 1:160	5
≥ 1:320	3

Abbreviations: SLE, Systemic Lupus Erythematosus; MCTO, mixed connective tissue disease.

Adapted from Kavanaugh A, Tomar R, Reveille J, et al: Guidelines for clinical use of the antinuclear antibody test and tests for specific autoantibodies to nuclear antigens. American College of Pathologists. Arch Pathol Lab Med 124:71, 2000.

On the other hand, the clinical utility of these patterns has been largely supplanted by tests for specific antinuclear antibody specificities, such as autoantigen-specific enzyme-linked immunosorbent assays (see following).

Most laboratories report titer as the last dilution at which an ANA pattern is detectable.[2] This technique has been considered somewhat imprecise and variable due to its subjectivity,[17] so several laboratories have attempted to standardize the protocol via computer-based fluorescent image quantitation.[18,19] Alternatively, some laboratories have suggested the use of a 0, 1+, 2+, 3+, 4+ subjective optical scale,[20] whereas others, such as the World Health Organization (WHO) and the Center for Disease Control (CDC) and Prevention, have advocated the use of standardized sera to define ANA activity in terms of international units (IU/mL).[21,22] Nonetheless, interlaboratory standardization of FANA results has not been widely instituted.

Not surprisingly, although the FANA remains a widely used diagnostic test, its results must always be interpreted in light of the particular method used by individual clinical laboratories.[2] Indeed, the substrate used for assessment may vary from frozen sections of rodent liver or kidney to cultured proliferating cell lines, most commonly the human epithelial tumor line HEp-2. Although tissue sections possess the advantage of eliminating interference from blood-group antibodies, heterophile antibodies, or passenger viruses, cultured cell lines remain a common substrate due to their higher concentration of nuclear and cytoplasmic antigens and standardization of use.[3,23] Different ANA test substrates are usually comparable in their ability to detect common ANAs, but differ substantially in the quantitation of antibody titer,[20] such that HEp-2 substrates often yield higher sensitivities in the detection of ANA-associated diseases at the cost of lower specificities.[3] Additional sources of variability include the subjective nature of the test, the quality of reagents (e.g., fluorescein-conjugated anti–human IgG) used, and the microscope used for visualization. As such, the several organizations, including the College of American Pathologists and the National Committee for Clinical Laboratory Standards, recommend several laboratory practices:[2,24] 1) performance of the test on serum, which may be stored at 4°C for up to 72 hours or at – 20°C or below indefinitely; 2) use of acetone-fixed HEp-2 cells as substrate, because ethanol and methanol fixation may remove the Ro/SS-A antigen, and mouse or rat tissues contain little Ro/SS-A and do not reveal antibodies to several organelles, such as centromere; 3) use of IgG-specific anti-Ig FITC conjugates with a FITC-to-protein ratio of approximately 3.0, antibody-to-protein ratio of ≥ 0.1, specific antibody content of 30 to 60μg/mL, and working dilution determined by titration of reference sera with known patterns and endpoint titers; and 4) use of reference sera, as by the WHO or CDC.

Finally, normal individuals, usually older and female persons, or relatives of persons with connective-tissue diseases, produce positive FANAs at a frequency of up to 30 percent[25] (see Table 20–1). These patients often possess titers of less than 1:320 with homogeneous staining patterns, though several patients possess higher titers yet remain clinically asymptomatic for years.[26] Conversely, rare SLE patients may demonstrate negative FANAs, for example, if they possess isolated anti-Ro antibodies, the test uses rat or mouse tissues, or both, because they contain very low concentrations of Ro antigen.[27,28] Additional false negatives occur for sera with isolated anti–single-stranded DNA or cytoplasmic specificities.[27,29] Such phenomena warrant further caution in the interpretation of FANA titer and pattern and suggest that the FANA, although an effective screening test, requires clinical correlation.

IMMUNODIFFUSION

The double-immunodiffusion Ouchterlony technique provides a crude method for the detection, confirmation, or both of autoimmune serum specificity via the comparison of precipitin activity with prototype antisera. It consists of the placement of control and test sera in agarose wells adjacent to disrupted rabbit- or calf-tissue extract, which contains extractable nuclear antigens (ENA), but retains very little DNA and DNA-associated proteins, due to the insolubility of chromatin. Over the next 24 to 48 hours, the antibodies and antigens diffuse outward from the wells, forming precipitin lines as the autoantibodies bind their epitopes and form an insoluble lattice. Sera that share specificity with the prototype sera produce precipitin lines that fuse with that of the prototype; heterologous specificities spur across one another or form lines of nonfusion (Fig. 20–3). This method remains insensitive in comparison to other assays, requiring large quantities (0.1 mg) of IgG and IgM to form visible precipitin lines. In addition, immunodiffusion fails to detect antibodies directed against rare or unstable antigens, such as the nucleolar Th and U3 RNPs, as well as insoluble antigens, such as DNA and histones. At the same time, immunodiffusion can detect autoantibodies to all soluble ENAs, such as snRNPs, Ro, and La; chromatin components that dissociate from DNA in saline buffer, such as topoisomerase I, proliferating cell nuclear

TABLE 20–2 • DIAGNOSTIC CHARACTERISTICS OF THE ANTINUCLEAR ANTIBODIES (ANAS)

Specificity	ANA Pattern(s)	Other Tests	Primary Rheumatic Disease Associations
Nuclear			
Chromatin-Associated Antigens			
ds-DNA	Rim, homogeneous	RIA, ELISA, CIF, Farr	SLE
ss-, ds-DNA	Rim, homogeneous	RIA, ELISA, CIF	SLE
ss-DNA	Undetectable	ELISA	SLE, DIL, RA
Histones		IB, RIA, ELISA	
H1, H2A, H2B, H3, H4	Homogeneous, rim		SLE, DIL, RA, PBC, Scl
H3	Large speckles		SLE, UCTD
Kinetochore (centromere)	Speckles*	IF, ELISA	Scl, SLE, SS
CENP-A			
CENP-B			
CENP-C			
CENP-D			
Ku	Diffuse-speckled nuclear/nucleolar*	ID, IPP, IB	SLE, PM/Scl overlap
PCNA/Ga/LE-4	Nuclear/nucleolar speckles*	ELISA, ID, IB, IPP	SLE
Spliceosomal components	Speckled	ID, ELISA, IB, IPP	
Sm			SLE
U1 snRNP			SLE, MCTD
U2 snRNP			SLE, MCTD, overlap
U4/U6 snRNP			SS, Scl
U5 snRNP			SLE, MCTD
U7 snRNP			SLE
U11 snRNP			Scl
SR		ELISA, IB, IPP	SLE
Other Ribonucleoproteins			
Ro/SS-A	Speckled or negative**	ID, ELISA, IB, IPP	SS, SCLE, NLE, SLE, PBC, Scl
La/SS-B/Ha	Speckled	ID, ELISA, IB, IPP	SS, SCLE, NLE, SLE
Mi-2	Homogeneous	ID, IPP	DM
p80-coilin	Speckled		SS
MA-I	Speckled*		SS, Scl
Nucleolar			
RNA polymerases (RNAP)	Punctate	IPP, IB	
RNAP I	Nucleolar		Scl
RNAP II	Nuclear/nucleolar***		Scl, SLE, overlap
RNAP III	Nuclear/nucleolar***		Scl
Ribosomal RNP	Nucleolar, cytoplasmic	ID, IB, IPP, ELISA	SLE
Topoisomerase I (Scl-70)	Diffuse, grainy nuclear/nucleolar	ID, IB, ELISA	Scl
Topoisomerase II	?	ELISA	Scl
U3 snoRNP (fibrillarin)	Clumpy	IB, IPP	Scl
Th snoRNP (RNase MRP)	Diffuse with sparse nuclear	IPP	Scl
NOR 90 (hUBF)	10-20 discrete spots, nuclear*	IB, IPP	Scl
PM-Scl (PM-1)	Homogeneous nuclear/nucleolar	ID, IPP, IB	PM, DM, Scl, overlap
Nucleobindin-2 (Wa)	?	ELISA	Scl, SLE, PM/DM
Cytoplasmic			
tRNA Synthetases			
$tRNA^{His}$ (Jo-1)	Diffuse	ID, IPP, IB, ELISA, AAI	PM, DM
$tRNA^{Thr}$ (PL-7)	Diffuse	ID, IPP, IB, ELISA, AAI	PM, DM

Continued

TABLE 20–2 • DIAGNOSTIC CHARACTERISTICS OF THE ANTINUCLEAR ANTIBODIES (ANAS)—cont'd

Specificity	ANA Pattern(s)	Other Tests	Primary Rheumatic Disease Associations
tRNA^{Ala} (PL-12)	Diffuse	ID, IPP, IB, ELISA, AAI	PM, DM
tRNA^{Gly} (EJ)	Diffuse	ID, IPP, IB, ELISA, AAI	PM, DM
tRNA^{Ile} (OJ)	Diffuse	ID, IPP, IB, ELISA, AAI	PM, DM
tRNA^{Asn} (KS)	Diffuse	ID, IPP, IB, ELISA, AAI	UCTD, ?
Fodrin	Diffuse subplasmalemmal	ELISA	SS
Signal recognition particle (SRP)	?	IPP, IB	PM
KJ	?	ID, IB	myositis
Elongation factor 1α (Fer)	?	IPP	myositis
tRNA^{Ser} (Mas)	?	IPP	myositis

*Cell cycle–dependent

**In cell studies, Ro RNP associates with cytoplasmic fractions (O'Brien CA, Wolin SL: A possible role for the 60-kD Ro autoantigen in a discard pathway for defective 5S rRNA precursors. Genes Dev 8: 2891, 1994).

***May also stain nucleoli because of an association with antibodies to RNA polymerase I

Adapted from Fritzler MJ: Immunofluorescent antinulear antibody test. *In* Rose, NR, de Macario EC, Fakey JL, el al (eds): Manual of Clinical Laboratory Immunology. Washington, DC, American Society for Microbiology, 1992, p 724.

Abbreviations: AAI, aminoacylation inhibition; CIE, counterimmunoelectrophoresis; CIF, *Crithidia luciliae* immunofluorescence; DIL, drug-induced lupus erythematosus; DM, dermatomyositis; ELISA, enzyme-linked immunosorbent assay; Farr, Farr radioimmunoassay; IB, immunoblot; ID, immunodiffusion; IPP, immunoprecipitation; MCTD, mixed connective tissue disease; NLE, neonatal lupus erythematosus; overlap, overlap syndromes; PBC, primary biliary cirrhosis; PM, polymyositis; RA, rheumatoid arthritis; RIA, radioimmunoassay; Scl, systemic sclerosis; SCLE, subacute cutaneous lupus erythematosus; SLE, systemic lupus erythematosus; SS, Sjögren's syndrome; RNA, transfer RNA; UCTD, undifferentiated connective tissue disease.

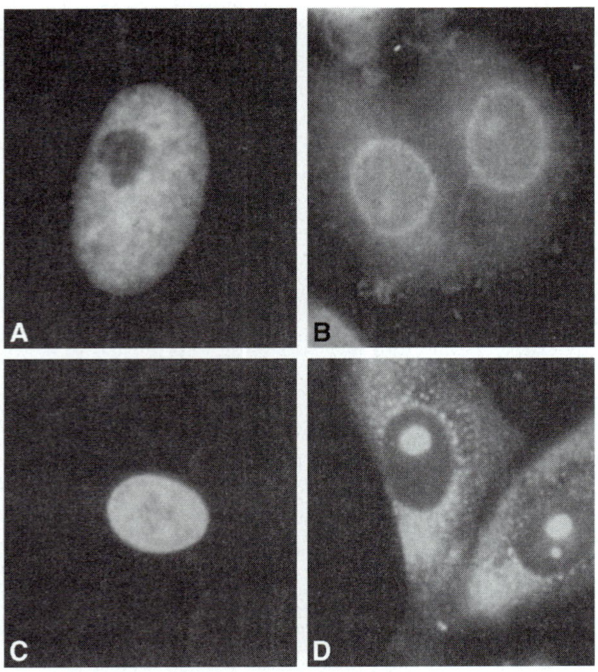

FIGURE 20–1 • The Fluorescent Antinuclear Antibody Test: Specificities of Systemic Lupus Erythematosus. *A*, Speckled nuclear pattern of anti-Sm antibodies. *B*, Nuclear rim pattern of anti-DNA antibodies. *C*, Homogeneous nuclear pattern of anti-DNA antibodies. *D*, Discrete cytoplasmic and nucleolar pattern of antiribosome antibodies.

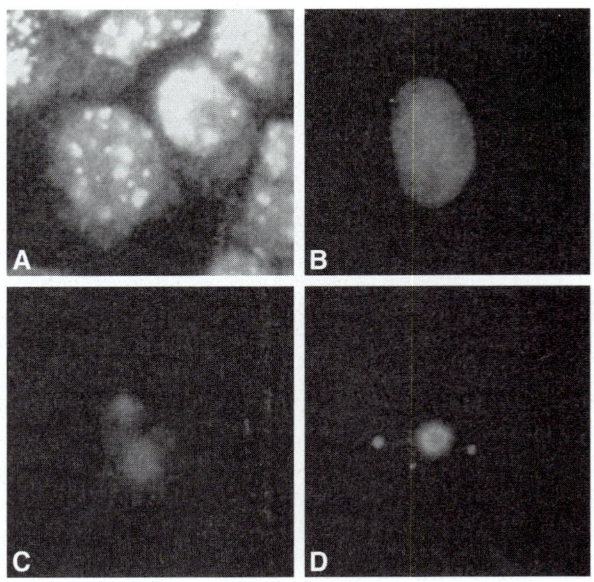

FIGURE 20–2 • The Fluorescent Antinuclear Antibody Test: Specificities of Systemic Sclerosis. *A*, Discrete speckled nuclear pattern of antikinetochore (centromere) antibodies. *B*, Grainy nuclear and nucleolar pattern of anti–topoisomerase I (Scl-70) antibodies. *C*, Diffuse nucleolar and sparse nucleoplasmic pattern of anti-Th (RNase MRP, 7-2) antibodies. *D*, Punctate nucleolar staining of anti–RNA polymerase antibodies. (*A*, Reprinted from the Clinical Slide Collection on the Rheumatic Diseases, copyright 1991; used by permission of the American College of Rheumatology.)

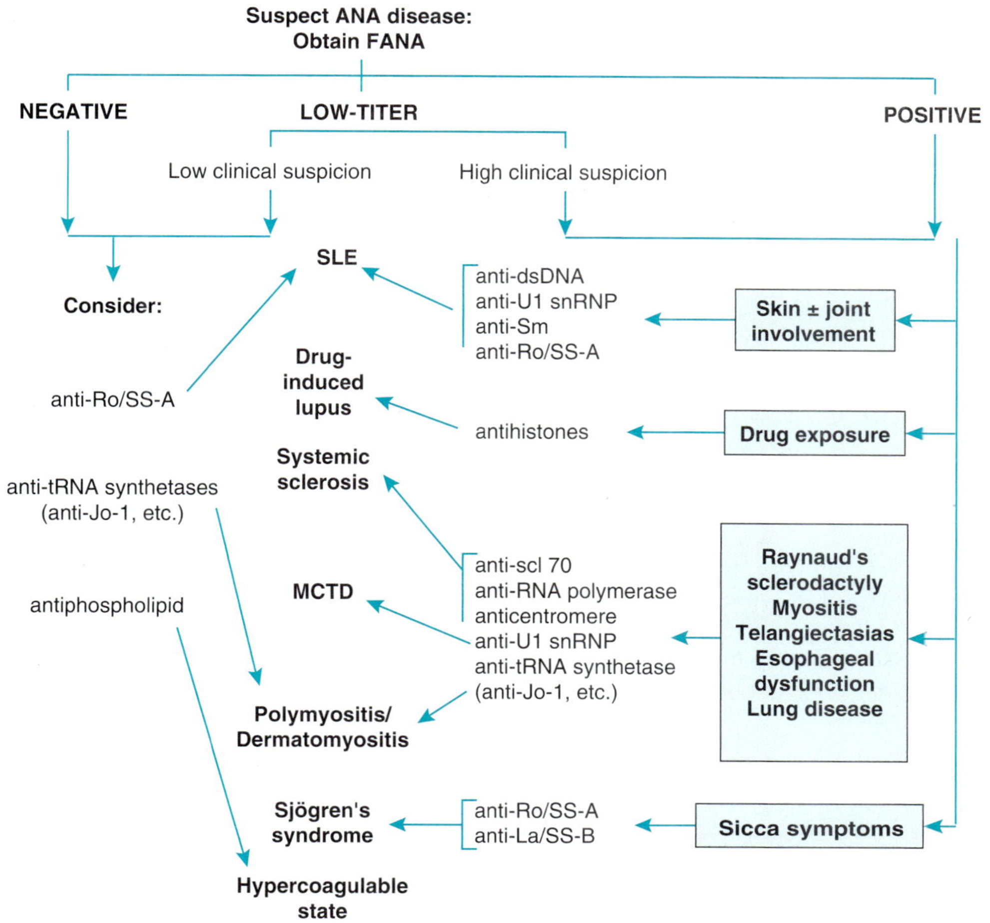

FIGURE 20–3 • Algorithm for the use of antinuclear antibodies (ANAs) in the diagnosis of connective tissue disorders. See text for details. (Modified from Craft J, Hardin JA: Antinuclearantibodies. In Kelly WN, Harris ED, Ruddy S, Sledge CB [eds]:Textbook of Rheumatology, 4th ed. Philadelphia, WB Saunders, 1993, p 164.)

antigen, and Ku; and soluble nucleolar components, such as Polymyositis Scleroderma, (Pm-Scl) (Table 20–3). Thus, although immunodiffusion provides a simple, straightforward method for the detection of specific autoantibodies, its repertoire, lengthy time requirements, and low sensitivity compared to newer assays limit its widespread use. Nevertheless, because it does not require special instrumentation or highly purified antigen, immunodiffusion gained wide acceptance in past clinical studies, from which many clinical antibody correlations have been drawn.

COUNTERIMMUNOELECTROPHORESIS

The counterimmunoelectrophoresis (CIE) technique modifies the immunodiffusion technique to generate somewhat greater sensitivity.[30] Acidic antigens, such as DNA or RNA, are electrophoresed from a cathode (–) well, whereas antibodies are electrophoresed from an anode (+) well. A precipitin line forms as specific autoantibodies encounter antigen, similar to immunodiffusion. CIE requires less antibody (0.01 to 0.05 mg), but cannot measure basic proteins or antibodies that move cathodally by endosmosis, such as IgM or IgA. Because this technique also provides limited sensitivity with a limited repertoire of autoantibody detection, it has largely become supplanted by other methods of ANA detection.

ENZYME-LINKED IMMUNOSORBENT ASSAY

The enzyme-linked immunosorbent assay (ELISA) provides a highly sensitive and rapid technique for the detection of ANAs and determination of antibody specificity. Test sera are incubated in wells precoated with purified target antigen; bound antibodies are detected

TABLE 20–3 • DETECTION OF MAJOR AUTOANTIGENS BY IMMUNODIFFUSION

Detectable	Undetectable
snRNPs	Double-stranded DNA
Ro	Single-stranded DNA
La	Histones
Ku	Deoxyribonucleoprotein
PCNA	Centromere/kinetochore
ribosomes	RNA polymerases
topoisomerase I	Th snoRNP (RNase MRP, 7-2 RNA)
PM/Scl	U3 snoRNP (fibrillarin)
tRNA synthetases	NOR 90 (hUBF)
Ki/SL	Signal recognition particle
Mi-2	MA-I
Ma	p80-coilin

Abbreviations: hUBF, Human upstream binding factor, NOR, nucleolar organizer region; PCNA, proliferating cell nuclear antigen; snoRNP, small nucleolar ribonucleoprotein; snRNPs, small nuclear ribonucleoproteins; t RNA, transfer RNA.

via an enzyme-conjugated anti–human immunoglobulin antibody, followed by color visualization with the appropriate enzyme substrate. Although these assays require highly purified antigen, many clinical laboratories have begun to utilize ELISAs for the routine determination of ANA specificity after positive FANA results. Indeed, their popularity has further resulted from the commercial availability of ELISA kits for the detection of specific autoantibodies, as well as the cloning and bacterial overexpression of recombinant autoantigens, such as Sm, U1 snRNP, Ro, La, tRNA synthetases, and topoisomerase I, making easier the development of various specificity-determining ELISAs. Unfortunately, ELISAs tend to produce some false-positive results, and confirmation sometimes requires further testing. Still, ELISAs continue to play a prominent role in the identification of ANAs.

IMMUNOPRECIPITATION

Radioimmunoprecipitation assays provide sensitive, specific means by which to determine autoantibody specificity. In these techniques, radiolabeled cell extracts are incubated with test sera, and the resulting autoantibody-autoantigen complexes are precipitated by an insoluble carrier, such as protein A–conjugated sepharose. Subsequent resolution by electrophoresis and visualization by autoradiography allows for the detection of radiolabeled proteins or nucleic acids bound by the autoimmune serum[31]. This technique, through the use of radiolabeled extracts, increases the sensitivity of detection for antibodies against minor cellular components, such as the Ro autoantigen, as well as for more abundant antigens, such as the U1 snRNP. In addition, with the use of whole cell extracts, simultaneous specificities are tested at once. Still, immunoprecipitations require the use of radioactivity and present a more laborious procedure than ELISA or immunodiffusion. Its use has thus remained predominantly in research settings, but it may occasionally offer important information in determining or confirming serum specificities not defined by other assays.

IMMUNOBLOT

Western blotting techniques provide particularly efficacious information concerning antibody specificity. These assays use autoimmune serum as probes against membranes containing electrophoretically resolved purified or crude antigens. Bound antibodies are detected via an enzyme-linked anti–human immunoglobulin antibody and substrate-dependent color development. Such resolution of various autoantigens allows determination of all relevant polypeptides targeted by a given serum. Unfortunately, immunoblot techniques remain somewhat less sensitive than ELISA and more laborious. In addition, some autoantigens possess conformational epitopes disrupted by gel electrophoresis, as in the case of the Ro autoantigen.[32] Thus, like immunoprecipitation assays, immunoblotting techniques remain predominantly confined to research settings, but sometimes are used to determine or confirm the specificity of difficult sera.

ENZYME INHIBITION ASSAYS

Enzymatic inhibition assays are quite specific for the characterization of individual ANAs. Unlike the majority of other autoantibody tests, such assays require that the tested autoantibody inhibit native protein function, versus simply recognizing denatured autoantigen, such as on an ELISA plate or on a Western blot. For example, anti-topoisomerase I (Scl-70) activity in systemic sclerosis can dramatically inhibit DNA relaxation in vitro, probably providing a more specific clinical predictor than results based on ELISA or immunoblot.[33,34] Similarly, antisynthetase antibodies in myositis can inhibit tRNA synthetase activity,[35] and anti-snRNP antibodies in lupus can inhibit in vitro splicing.[36] However, like immunoblot and immunoprecipitation techniques, enzyme inhibition assays require somewhat specialized training, so are often confined to research laboratories with specific biochemical interests in the autoantigens.

ANTI-DNA ANTIBODY TESTS

Anti-DNA antibodies warrant special diagnostic consideration due to their wide range of autoantigenic epitopes and their concomitant assay difficulties.[37] Antibodies that recognize denatured, single-stranded (ss) DNA bind the free purine and pyrimidine base sequences, and appear in several different diseases, including SLE, drug-induced lupus, chronic active hepatitis, infectious mononucleosis, and RA. On the other hand, SLE-specific anti-DNA antibodies recognize native, double-stranded (ds) DNA, binding the deoxyribose phosphate backbone, or the rarer, conformation-dependent left-handed helical Z-form. With these differences in epitope and disease associations, anti-DNA assays most importantly must clearly distinguish between ss-DNA and ds-DNA substrates. Two methods to ensure the use of native ds-DNA include digestion with S1 nuclease, which removes overhanging ss-DNA ends, or chromatography on a hydroxyapatite column, which separates large single-stranded segments from ds-DNA. Unfortunately, native DNA may spontaneously denature, especially when bound to plastic ELISA plates; this may account for the results of several reports that revealed a relative lack of specificity of anti–ds-DNA antibodies for SLE. Reliable assays, therefore, must ensure the integrity of the ds-DNA substrate.

Two assays offer greater assurance for anti–ds-DNA testing. The Farr radioimmunoassay, which resembles immunoprecipitation assays, involves the binding of autoantibodies to radiolabeled ds-DNA in solution. Precipitation of the antibody-DNA complexes by ammonium sulfate allows a quantification of the percentage of incorporated (antibody-bound) radioactive ds-DNA. Normal sera typically bind a small fraction of added DNA (usually less than 20%), whereas SLE sera often bind nearly 100 percent of added DNA. The specificity of this assay, however, still depends on the quality of ds-DNA and the removal of contaminating ss-DNA; but because the assay requires autoantibodies to bind antigen in solution, the Farr assay is generally considered the gold standard for anti–ds-DNA analysis.

One alternative to the Farr assay, the *Crithidia luciliae* test, provides an inherently reliable ds-DNA substrate. In this assay, the hemoflagellate *C. luciliae* serves as a substrate for indirect immunofluorescence. Its kinetoplast, a modified giant mitochondrion, contains a concentrated focus of stable, circularized ds-DNA, without contaminating RNA or nuclear proteins, providing a sensitive and specific fluorescence substrate by which to establish anti–ds-DNA activity. For these reasons, many laboratories have adopted the *Crithidia* immunofluorescence test for routine use. Radioimmunoassays and *Crithidia luciliae* immunofluorescence tests thus provide effective, complementary mechanisms to distinguish anti–ss-DNA from anti–ds-DNA activities.

PRACTICAL ASPECTS OF ANTINUCLEAR ANTIBODY TESTING

In most clinical laboratories, serum specimens are first tested by indirect immunofluorescent microscopy on human epithelial-2 (Hep-2) cells, with a positive result often prompting "cascade" testing by the laboratory, ordering physician, or both of ELISAs or other assays for specific autoantibody specificities, such as anti–ds-DNA, anti-Ro, anti-La, anti-RNP, and anti-Sm.[2,3] In contrast, negative tests generally do not warrant additional testing.[38] However, because the clinical and research studies upon which most autoantibody-disease associations have been developed often use more refined detection methods, such as immunoprecipitation or immunoblot, and different laboratories often vary somewhat in technique and test reproducibility, the relevance of many antibody-test results in specific clinical settings continues to require careful, individualized interpretation by the referring physician.

Diseases associated with Antinuclear Antibodies

SYSTEMIC LUPUS ERYTHEMATOSUS

Antinuclear antibodies are a hallmark of SLE: The FANA is likely to test positive in more than 99 percent of patients using current methods.[39] Past studies have reported frequencies as low as 90 percent, probably due to differences in substrate and technique.[27] The majority of autoantigens reside in the nucleus, but SLE often evokes autoantibodies against a seemingly endless range of antigens in many cellular locations. Nonetheless, these autoantigens may be broadly categorized into chromatin-associated versus ribonucleoprotein antigens (Table 20–4). Significant individual specificities are discussed in the following sections.

Chromatin-Associated Antigens

Though antibodies against DNA remain one of the most widely recognized specificities in SLE, recent studies suggest that its more physiologic forms, nucleosomes, chromatin, or both, provide more relevant information regarding the pathogenesis and antibody response.[37] SLE sera may target several DNA-associated molecules, including histones, and, indeed, higher prevalences of antibodies that recognize nucleosomes and subnucleosomes, which contain both DNA and histone proteins, are found among SLE patients than those that recognize DNA alone.[40] In fact, antichromatin antibodies, reactive against native chromatin, appear at the highest described frequency for autoantibodies in SLE (88%), providing further support for a role of native structures in the genesis of the autoantibody response. Still, the majority of clinical literature regarding antichromatin autoantibodies remains linked to classic anti-DNA antibodies, antihistone antibodies, or both, so these are detailed here.

Anti-DNA

Anti-DNA antibodies include anti–ss-DNA antibodies, which target the purine and pyrimidine bases of denatured DNA; anti–ds-DNA antibodies, which target the ribose phosphate backbone of native DNA; and anti–Z-DNA antibodies, which target the left-handed helical Z form of DNA. Interestingly, these antibodies may preferentially target the matrix attachment regions[41] or telomeres[42] of chromosomes, or the other anti-DNA antibodies themselves (anti-idiotype).[43] Detection of anti–ds-DNA antibodies usually involves FANA, in which these antibodies produce nuclear staining in a homogeneous or rim pattern, followed by confirmation via ELISA,

TABLE 20–4 • ANTINUCLEAR ANTIBODIES (ANAs) IN SYSTEMIC LUPUS ERYTHEMATOSUS (SLE)

Antibody Specificity	Prevalence (%)
Chromatin-Associated Antigens	
ds-DNA	73
Histone	50-70
Chromatin	88
Ku	20-40
PCNA	3-6
RNA polymerase II	9-14
Kinetochore	6
Ribonucleoproteins	
snRNPs	
Sm core	20-30
U1 snRNP	30-40
U2 snRNP	15
U5 snRNP	?
U7 snRNP	?
Ro/SS-A	40
La/SS-B	10-15
Ribosomes	
P0, P1, P2 protein	10-20
28S rRNA	?
S10 protein	?
L5 protein	?
L12 protein	?
Proteasome	58

Abbreviations: dsDNA, Double-stranded DNA; PCNA, proliferating cell nuclear antigen, snRNP, small nuclear ribonucleoprotein.

C. luciliae immunofluorescence, Farr radioimmunoassay, or some combination of these tests. Anti–ss-DNA antibodies, on the other hand, do not elicit positive FANA and, therefore, require separate testing for detection, such as ELISA.[27,29]

Although a variety of diseases produce anti–ss-DNA activity, only SLE sera possess high-titer anti–ds-DNA activity, anti–Z-DNA activity, or both. Anti–ds-DNA antibodies appear in approximately 73 percent of SLE patients, whereas low titers appear much less often in patients with SS, RA, other disorders, or in normal individuals. In SLE, anti-DNA antibodies strongly correlate with nephritis and disease activity, in contrast to all other currently studied antinuclear autoantibody specificities; they appear to contribute to disease pathology through high avidity to DNA, immune-complex formation, complement fixation, renal antigen cross-reactivity, direct cellular toxicity upon intracellular penetration, or some combination of these.[37] Interestingly, some anti-DNA antibodies may cross-react with nonrenal antigens, such as the neuronal N-methyl-D-aspartate (NMDA) receptor or ribosomal P antigens, potentially mediating pathologic effects, as in the central nervous system.[44,45] At the same time, several reports describe lupus nephritis in the absence of anti-DNA antibodies, and others describe persistence of high-titer anti-DNA antibodies in the absence of renal injury, suggesting that other antibody specificities may contribute to end-organ disease. Indeed, some studies suggest that the observed anti-DNA activities of these antibodies are experimental artifacts and that these antibodies instead recognize antigens distinct from DNA.[46] Furthermore, other investigations have found that these antibodies cross-react with other antigens, such as snRNPs or foreign proteins, suggesting that the immunologically relevant antigen for anti-DNA antibodies may not, in fact, be DNA.[47] Thus, although most clinicians and researchers agree that antibodies reactive with DNA often correlate strongly with lupus nephritis, they do not concur on their precise ontogeny or phylogeny.[37]

Antihistone (Nucleosome)

Antihistone antibodies target the protein components of nucleosomes, the DNA-protein complexes that form the substructure of transcriptionally inactive chromatin. Each nucleosome consists of approximately 200 bp of chromatin DNA, wrapped around a central core of the histone proteins H2A, H2B, H3, and H4, in association with the linker histone H1.[48] These antibodies may be detected by FANA, ELISA, or immunoblot; non-H3 antihistone antibodies produce a homogenous or rim nuclear pattern by FANA, whereas anti-H3 histone antibodies produce large speckles.[23] In the 50 to 70 percent of SLE patients with antihistone antibodies, they predominantly target the H1 and H2B protein, followed by H2A, H3, and H4, usually in association with anti–ds-DNA. These antibodies appear consistently in drug-induced lupus, where they associate with anti–ss-DNA antibodies and appear at lower frequency in other diseases such as RA or juvenile arthritis, primary biliary cirrhosis,[49] inflammatory myositis,[50] autoimmune hepatitis,[51] scleroderma,[52-54] Epstein-Barr virus infection,[55] Chagas' disease,[56] schizophrenia,[57] sensory neuropathy,[58] monoclonal gammopathies,[59] and cancer.[60] Some consider autoantibodies against histones as sensitive markers for drug-induced lupus and autoantibodies against native chromatin structures as specific for SLE; however, due to the wide clinical spectrum in which antihistone antibodies appear, studies have not consistently upheld any significant clinical correlations for antihistone antibodies, such as with disease activity,[61] in contrast to anti-DNA antibodies.

Anti-Ku

Antibodies to the Ku antigen target a chromatin-associated heterodimer that includes the catalytic subunit of the 470-kD DNA-dependent protein kinase implicated in DNA repair and V(D)J recombination. Ku controls these processes through the recognition and protection of ds-DNA termini, telomeres, nicks, hairpins, and gaps, perhaps recruiting, activating, or both other repair proteins, including the kinase-dependent regulation of transcription factors and the RNA polymerases I and II.[62] It includes two subunits, p70 and p80, each targeted in various diseases. In FANA, anti-Ku antibodies demonstrate cell-cycle-dependent diffuse nuclear staining, nucleolar staining, or both, reflective of its biologic activity.[63] Originally described in scleroderma-polymyositis overlap syndrome,[64] anti-Ku has been found in a highly variable percentage (0 to 40%) of SLE sera (perhaps in association with anti-RNA polymerase II antibodies[65]),[66] more than 20 percent of sera from patients with primary pulmonary hypertension,[67] and more than 50 percent of Graves' disease sera,[49] as well as other connective tissue diseases including RA.[68] The significance of these antibodies remains largely uninvestigated, although one study suggests an association with Raynaud's phenomenon, arthralgia, skin thickening, and esophageal reflux,[68] whereas another suggests that anti-p70 antibodies correlate with features of scleroderma-polymyositis overlap, and anti-p80 antibodies correlate with features of scleroderma or SLE.[69]

Anti–Proliferating Cell Nuclear Antigen

Proliferating cell nuclear antigen (PCNA) is a 36-kD ring-like sliding clamp protein that participates in a DNA scaffold to facilitate the attachment of DNA nucleases, polymerases, ligases, and other proteins involved in replication, recombination, and repair, thereby regulating not only DNA replication, but also cell-cycle progression, DNA repair, and cellular apoptosis.[70] Anti-PCNA autoantibodies appear in approximately 3 to 6 percent of SLE patients.[71] These autoantibodies had been considered specific for the disease until recent investigations demonstrated their presence in other conditions, such as viral hepatitis.[72] These antibodies may be detected by FANA, which reveals variable speckled nucleoplasmic and nucleolar patterns depending on the cell-cycle state of the stained cell, reflecting its bulk expression during late G1 and early S phase of the cell cycle just before DNA synthesis.[73] The clinical significance of these antibodies continues to remain unclear at this time.

Anti-RNA Polymerase

Anti-RNA polymerase (RNAP) antibodies target the eukaryotic RNA polymerases, which consist of three classes of synthetic enzymes containing two distinct high-molecular-weight polypeptides, as well as at least six smaller subunits. RNA polymerase I synthesizes ribosomal RNA precursors in the nucleolus; RNA polymerase II transcribes some small nuclear RNA genes as well as all protein-encoding genes; and RNA polymerase III synthesizes some small nuclear RNAs as well as the 5S rRNA and tRNAs. By FANA, these antibodies produce punctate nucleolar staining in resting cells, and dots in areas of condensed chromosomes in metaphase cells.[74] Although anti-RNA polymerase I antibodies originally were described in SLE, MCTD and RA, subsequent work suggests that these antibodies are more specific for scleroderma.[75] Anti-RNAP II antibodies, however, appear in 9 to 14 percent of SLE and overlap syndromes, where they tend to be accompanied by anti-Ku or antiribonucleoprotein antibodies.[65] Because of the paucity of information regarding these antibodies, their significance in SLE remains purely observational.

Ribonucleoproteins

Anti–small nuclear ribonucleoproteins

In SLE, autoantibodies against snRNPs generally target the RNAs or proteins of the spliceosome, a complex of RNP particles involved in the splicing of premessenger RNA. These particles include the U1, U2, U4/U6, U5, U7, U11, and U12 snRNPs, each of which consists of its respective uridine-rich (thus U) small nuclear RNA (snRNA) and a set of polypeptides, including a common core of "Sm" polypeptides (B/B', D1, D2, D3, E, F, and G) as well as particle-specific polypeptides.[76] All anti-snRNP antibodies produce a distinct speckled nuclear pattern in FANA, reflective of the focal distribution of spliceosomal snRNPs in the nucleoplasm;[77] individual particle or protein epitopes may be determined by immunoprecipitation or immunoblot.[76] Anti-Sm antibodies target proteins of the Sm core, the B/B' and one of the D polypeptides, as well as the like-Sm protein LSm4;[78] they are considered specific antibodies in the diagnosis of SLE, although they appear in only 20 to 30 percent of patients. Their presence has been associated with milder renal disease, central nervous system disease, or both, organic brain syndrome, disease flares, or paradoxically more active disease, but additional studies have not upheld these findings, reporting no correlations with disease manifestations.[76]

Other specific anti-snRNP antibodies target polypeptides or RNAs particular to respective U snRNPs. Anti–U1 snRNP (anti-nRNP [nuclear RNP] or anti-U1 RNP, historically), for example, targets the 70 K, A, or C polypeptides specific to the U1 snRNP. These antibodies occur in 30 to 40 percent of SLE patients and are associated with disease activity, myositis, esophageal hypomotility, Raynaud's phenomenon, lack of nephritis, arthralgias or arthritis, sclerodactyly, and interstitial changes on chest radiographs.[79] Other anti-snRNP antibodies, targeting U2-, U5-, or U7 snRNP–specific proteins, have been described in SLE, but with low frequency and often in overlap syndromes.[76] Likewise, some studies have suggested non-rheumatologic disease associations for the anti-snRNP antibodies, such as with monoclonal gammopathies[80] or psychiatric diseases,[81] but these findings remain unconfirmed. In addition, several investigators have described substantial cross-reactivity of some anti-snRNP antibodies with other specificities, such as anti-DNA or anti-ribosomal P.[47,82] Thus, although anti-Sm has generally remained a specific marker for SLE, and anti–U1 snRNP maintains strong associations with SLE, many studies continue to report disease associations with other anti-snRNP specificities, whose significances await determination.

Anti-Ro/SS-A and La/SS-B

These two antibody specificities target distinct ribonucleoprotein particles. Ro is composed of a 60-kD and 52-kD protein component as well as small RNAs known as the hY1, hY3, hY4, and hY5 RNAs. Extensive molecular biologic work continues to define the biologic role of the Ro ribonucleoproteins: The 60-kD protein contains a zinc-finger motif, and the 52-kD protein resembles the *rfp* protein, a homologue of the transforming protein *ret*, and *rpt-1*, a murine transcription factor.[83] The 60-kD protein may partake in a discard pathway for 5S rRNA precursors,[84] in a nucleocytoplasmic shuttling pathway for RNA polymerase III transcripts, or both[85] La, a 43- to 52-kD RNP, partakes in the transcriptional regulation of RNA polymerase III as well as some messenger RNAs.[86] Along with other nucleoproteins, such as cellular nuclear acid binding protein (CNBP), these two particles likely exist in a macromolecular complex, where the 60-kD autoantigen provides a stabilizing or docking function for La as it recognizes ribosomal RNA sequences.[87] Anti-Ro antibodies have posed difficulty in detection in the past, sometimes testing negative by FANA due to the low concentration of Ro in substrate cells.[2,3,27,28]

Although most commonly associated with SS, approximately 40 percent of SLE patients possess anti-Ro activity, and 10 to 15 percent possess anti-La. In SLE, anti-La correlates with late-onset SLE, secondary SS, the neonatal lupus syndrome, and protection from anti-Ro–associated nephritis.[88,89] Anti-Ro is associated with photosensitive skin rash and cutaneous lupus erythematosus,[90] pulmonary disease, lymphopenia,[91] the neonatal lupus syndrome, and cardiac fibroelastosis;[92,93] less-discussed associations include chilblain lupus erythematosus,[94] the presence of rheumatoid factors, nephritis, thrombocytopenia, anti-La, and complement (particularly C4) deficiencies.[95,96] The presence of anti–52-kD without anti–60-kD antibodies has been correlated with Sjögren's syndrome, whereas the presence of both anti–52-kD and 60-kD antibodies, or anti–60-kD antibodies alone, has been correlated with SLE, RA, or other connective tissue diseases; however, these have not remained consistent findings.[97-101] Further significant clinical associations of anti-Ro antibodies also include the neonatal lupus syndrome, as well as SS-SLE overlap, subacute cutaneous lupus erythematosus, multiple sclerosis, and primary biliary cirrhosis;[102,103] less-described disease associations include human immunodeficiency virus (HIV) infection,[104] glaucoma,[105] multiple myeloma, RA, polymyositis, and scleroderma.[95]

Antiribosome

Antiribosome antibodies in SLE target protein or RNA components of the eukaryotic 80S ribosome, the ribonucleoprotein complex involved in the translation of mRNA into protein. The mammalian ribosome includes two subunits of 40S and 60S, comprised of 28S, 18S, 5.8S, and 5S ribosomal (r) RNAs, in addition to at least 80 different proteins.[106] Antiribosomal P protein (anti-P) antibodies target the P0, P1, and P2 alanine-rich ribosomal proteins (38-, 19-, and 17-kD, respectively), which are part of the large 60S subunit. Antibodies against these antigens produce FANA staining in both the cytoplasm, where protein translation occurs, and the nucleolus, where ribosome biogenesis occurs. They occur in 10 to 20 percent of SLE patients and have proven to be highly specific for SLE among connective-tissue disease patients, even though these specificities also have been found among seemingly normal individuals.[107] Although analyses of SLE populations have failed to reveal definite clinical associations with anti-P antibodies, most investigators consider these specificities significantly associated with neuropsychiatric lupus, including psychosis.[108-111] Correlation with active disease, liver disease, and renal disease, as well as anti-Sm, anti-DNA, and anticardiolipin antibodies has also been suggested,[112] although some of these apparent associations may result from cross-reacting antibodies whose significance remains unclear.[45,82,113] Other, less prevalent antiribosomal antibodies target rRNA, such as the 28S rRNA, or other ribosomal proteins, such as the S10, L5, and L12 subunit proteins.[112] The clinical significance of these latter antibodies remains unclear, although recent studies suggest that all antiribosomal antibodies appear in association with each other and, therefore, may represent a cluster of disease autoantibodies.[114]

Anti-SR

The SR proteins comprise a family of arginine/serine-rich pre-mRNA splicing factors that partake in spliceosome assembly and alternative splice-site selection.[115] One study has reported a 50 to 52–percent prevalence of autoantibodies against SR family members in SLE,[116] in which they have been speculated to regulate the alternative splicing of apoptotic effector molecules.[117] However, because these specificities have not been extensively studied in SLE or other ANA diseases, their clinical associations and disease specificities remain incompletely determined.

Anti-RNA

Autoantibodies that bind deproteinized RNA have been described for anti-U snRNAs and antiribosomal RNAs,[118] as well as to transfer RNAs[119] in both SLE and myositis. Because their prevalence and disease associations have not been well characterized, their significance remains largely unknown. One study, however, suggests that these antibodies associate with SLE and overlap syndromes.[120]

Other Autoantibodies

A wide number of other autoantibody specificities have been described in SLE, but because comprehensive studies have not been performed, their clinical significance remains undetermined. These include specificities such as Ki-67, a cell proliferation–associated, alternatively spliced protein of 395-kD and 320-kD whose autoantibodies are associated with lupus with sicca,[121,122] the nuclear matrix,[123] kinetochore,[124] 90-kD or 70-kD heat-shock proteins,[125-127] neutrophil cytoplasmic antigens perinuclear-anti neutrophil cytoplasmic antigen (p-ANCA), cytoplasmic-anti neutrophil cytoplasmic antigen (c-ANCA)),[128,129] carbonic anhydrase,[130] proteasome,[131,132] cyclophilin,[133] hn-RNP A1,[134] fimbrin,[135] microfilaments,[136] nuclear lamina,[137] transcription factor TFIIF,[138] the tumor suppressor p53,[139] non-Ku DNA double-strand break repair proteins such as XRCC4 and DNA ligase IV,[140] topoisomerase I,[141] and Su.[142]

SCLERODERMA OR SYSTEMIC SCLEROSIS

Antinuclear antibodies against nucleolar antigens characterize the autoantibody response in systemic sclerosis. Positive FANAs, sometimes speckled in appearance, appear in as high as 97 percent of sera,[143] although percentages vary depending on the substrate used for detection. Unlike SLE sera, however, systemic sclerosis sera usually contain monospecific autoantibody specificities, targeting such structures as the kinetochore, topoisomerase I, or RNA polymerases[144,145] (Table 20–5).

Antikinetochore (Centromere)

Antikinetochore antibodies target integral components of the mitotic spindle apparatus, which promotes chromosome separation during mitosis. Although these specificities were initially named anticentromere antibodies (ACA),[146] refined ultrastructural studies have defined the centromere as the primary constriction of mitotic chromosomes containing the genetic locus for partitioning,

TABLE 20–5 • ANTINUCLEAR ANTIBODIES (ANAs) IN SYSTEMIC SCLEROSIS

Antibody Specificity	Prevalence (%)
Kinetochore (centromere)	22-36
Topoisomerase I	22-40
Topoisomerase II	22
Wa (NEFA/Nucleobindin-2)	33
RNA polymerases	4-23
U3 snoRNP (fibrillarin)	6-8
Th snoRNP (RNase MRP, 7-2 RNA)	4-11
PM-Scl	3
NOR 90 (hUBF)	?

Abbreviations: hUBF, Human upstream binding factor, NOR, nucleolar Organizer region; snoRNP, small nucleolar ribonucleoprotein and defined the kinetochore, whose components are targeted by these antibodies, as the specialized trilaminar structure to which the spindle microtubules attach.[147] These autoantibodies target at least four constitutive centromere (kinetochore) antigens (CENPs): CENP-B (the predominant kinetochore autoantigen recognized by all ACA sera), CENP-A, CENP-C, and CENP-D, which provide essential roles in the packaging of centromere DNA through various protein-protein and protein-nucleic acid interactions.[75,144,147] These antibodies produce weak, fluorescent, speckled patterns with titers less than 1:32 when metabolically inactive cells, such as rodent tissues, are used as substrate; laboratories that use such FANA substrates as a screening test may report such sera as negative.[75,144] Therefore, screening for ACA typically involves immunofluorescence of mitotically active cells, such as HEp-2 cells, or ELISA.

ACAs occur in 22 to 36 percent of systemic sclerosis patients. Their presence correlates with Raynaud's phenomenon; CREST (calcinosis, Raynaud's phenomenon, esophageal dysmotility, sclerodactyly, and telangiectasias), with which as many as 98 percent of patients have ACA;[148] and limited skin involvement, as well as the development of mat-like telangiectasias; the signs of systemic sclerosis, including pulmonary or vascular disease;[149] and ACAs may be associated with an increased risk of malignancy.[150] Indeed, several studies have reported significant prevalences of ACA in diffuse scleroderma (22 to 36%) and scleroderma with proximal skin involvement (26%),[151] as well as Hashimoto's thyroiditis with Raynaud's syndrome,[152] primary biliary cirrhosis associated with systemic sclerosis,[153] SS,[154] and RA.[151] Most investigators consider ACAs specific for systemic sclerosis and CREST, as well as primary and secondary Raynaud's phenomenon, although not all agree.[75,151,154]

Antitopoisomerase I

Antitopoisomerase (Scl-70) autoantibodies predominantly target the catalytic carboxy-terminal region of DNA topoisomerase I, a 100-kD helicase that relieves superhelical strain during the transcription or replication of DNA.[155] Although studies to reveal its true molecular weight have caused much dispute in the past, most workers now agree that the initial 70-kD protein recognized by these sera represents a proteolytic product of the intact helicase.[1] This specificity produces a diffusely grainy nucleoplasmic and nucleolar staining pattern in FANAs; typical follow-up testing includes immunodiffusion, immunoblot, or ELISA.[156] Antitopoisomerase I antibodies appear in 22 to 40 percent of scleroderma patients and generally predict diffuse cutaneous disease and proximal skin involvement,[75,144,157] longer disease duration, association with cancer, or both,[151] pulmonary fibrosis, digital pitting scars, and cardiac involvement.[158] In conjunction with antikinetochore antibodies, antitopoisomerase antibodies constitute major diagnostic tools in the subclassification of diffuse versus limited scleroderma; however, approximately 40 percent of all systemic sclerosis patients may lack either antibody,[151] and a minority (less than 1%) of SSc patients may possess both antibodies.[159] Finally, like ACAs, antitopoisomerase antibodies may occasionally be found in other connective-tissue diseases.

Anti-RNA Polymerases

Anti-RNA polymerase (RNAP) antibodies target the eukaryotic RNA polymerases (see section on SLE: anti-RNA polymerase). These antibodies appear in 4 to 23 percent of scleroderma patients and are associated with diffuse cutaneous involvement.[160] Although anti-RNAP II antibodies appear in other diseases, such as SLE or overlap syndrome, and may be associated with other autoantibody specificities against Ku or ribonucleoproteins, anti-RNAP I and III antibodies remain specific for scleroderma,[65,160] in which they may be useful for the diagnosis of renal crisis.[161]

Antifibrillarin

Antifibrillarin antibodies predominantly target the N^G, N^G-dimethylarginine-rich 34-kD protein of the U3 small nucleolar ribonucleoprotein (snoRNP), which participates in the processing of preribosomal RNA.[162] This protein has been termed *fibrillarin* for its association with the nucleolar fibrillar component. FANA reveals clumpy nucleolar staining in resting cells and significant condensed chromosome staining in metaphase cells. Antifibrillarin antibodies appear in 6 to 8 percent of scleroderma patients. Although their clinical significance remains unclear, they appear generally to associate with diffuse disease, including internal organ involvement.[163,164]

Antitopoisomerase II

DNA topoisomerase II, both an enzyme and a structural component of the nuclear matrix, regulates the topologic states of DNA, as well as DNA replication.[165] Antitopoisomerase II antibodies are seen in approximately 22 percent of SSc patients, where they associate with pulmonary hypertension, as opposed to pulmonary fibrosis.[166]

Anti-Wa

Anti-Wa antibodies bind nucleobindin-2, a calcium-binding protein implicated in apoptosis, calcium homeostasis, and Golgi apparatus function. Preliminary reports indicate that these specificities occur in 33 percent of SSc patients and to a lesser extent in SLE, polymyositis/dermatomyositis (PM/DM), and RA, associated with hypocomplementemia and hypergammaglobulinemia.[167]

Anti-Th Small Nucleolar Ribonucleoprotein

Anti-Th antibodies bind the Th snoRNP, now known to be identical to the mitochondrial RNA processing (MRP) RNase MRP, which contains the 7-2 RNA.[168] This RNP resides predominantly in the nucleus and is implicated in the processing of precursor tRNAs, as well in ribosome biogenesis and mitochondrial DNA replication.[144] This specificity, appearing in 4 to 16 percent of scleroderma patients, may predict limited cutaneous disease, puffy fingers, small-bowel involvement, hypothyroidism, and reduced arthritis or arthralgias, or perhaps disease similar to anticentromere antibody–positive systemic sclerosis.[169-171]

Anti–Nucleolar Organizer Regions 90

Anti–nucleolar organizer regions (NOR) 90 antibodies were originally named for their immunoblotting of a 90-kD protein doublet and immunofluorescent staining of NORs, which comprise the secondary constriction sites on chromosomes 13, 14, 15, 21, and 22. These sites consist of multiple rRNA gene clusters around which nucleoli reform after mitosis.[172] More recently, the molecular target of these antibodies has been demonstrated as the RNA polymerase human upstream binding transcription factor (hUBF), which exists as spliced variants of 97-kD and 94-kD.[173,174] These sera produce 10 to 20 discrete, tiny spots per nucleolus by FANA, changing to nucleoplasmic staining in a cell cycle–dependent fashion. Although generally associated with scleroderma, anti-hUBF antibodies have been demonstrated in patients with SLE, SS, RA, and cancer.[175] Their overall clinical significance and prevalence remain particularly unknown, because they may potentially be confused with antibodies against another poorlyvcharacterized fibrillar NOR protein, ASE-1 (antisense to ERCC-1).[176]

Anti Polymyositis-Scleroderma, (Pm-Scl)

Anti–PM-Scl antibodies, typically identified by immunodiffusion or ELISA, target the exosome, a complex of 11 to 16 nucleolar proteins, of which the 100-kD, 70- to 75-kD, and 37-kD proteins predominate, that possesses 3′ to 5′ exoribonuclease activity and participates in ribosomal RNA processing and degradation.[177] Three percent of scleroderma patients possess this antibody, which produces homogenous nucleolar staining by FANA. Its presence associates with myositis-scleroderma overlap without SLE features: Fifty percent of anti–PM-Scl antibody–positive patients have the overlap, and 25 percent of the overlap patients have the antibody.[178,179] Also, anti–PM-Scl appears associated with arthritis and skin lesions of dermatomyositis, calcinosis, mechanic's hands, and eczema;[178,180] compared to other antinucleolar antibody–positive patients, anti–PM-Scl patients have a higher incidence of muscle, tendon, and renal disease.[181]

Other Autoantibodies

Other antibodies sometimes found in scleroderma include antihistone,[52,182] antinucleolar B23,[183] anticarbonic anhydrase,[130] anti–high mobility group antigens,[184] antilaminin,[185] anti-hsp90,[126] anti-Ku,[144] anti-Ro,[186] anticentriole,[187] anti–Ki-67,[122] antineutrophil cytoplasmic antibodies (ANCA),[188] anti-tRNA,[189] antimicrofilament,[136] anti–nuclear lamina,[137] antitrimethylguanosine,[190] anti–U1 snRNP,[191-193] anti–U4/U6 snRNP (anti-MaS),[194] anti–U11 snRNP,[195] anti-Su,[142] and anti-NuMA[196] antibodies. The RNAP II transcription activator Sp1 has been recently described as an autoantigen. Its presence seems to correlate with Raynaud's phenomenon and other signs of undifferentiated connective-tissue diseases.[197]

INFLAMMATORY MUSCLE DISEASES

Inflammatory muscle diseases comprise a diverse group of illnesses often characterized by autoantibody responses against cytoplasmic antigens. Although between 40 and 80 percent of PM/DM patients have positive ANA,[198] as many as 90 percent of patients with all types of inflammatory muscle diseases have autoantibodies to cellular antigens.[199] Autoantibodies in myositis are generally categorized into myositis-specific autoantibodies (MSAs), which are found almost exclusively in inflammatory myositis, and those associated with overlap syndromes that include myositis. MSAs include the antisynthetase antibodies, antisignal recognition particle, and anti–Mi-2; overlap antibodies include anti-snRNP and anti–PM-Scl[200,201] (Table 20–6).

Anti-tRNA Synthetase

The antisynthetase MSAs comprise a group of highly antigen-specific, disease-associated reactivities that produce cytoplasmic FANA. At least five different antisynthetase activities target different aminoacyl-tRNA synthetases, which are cytoplasmic enzymes that catalyze the binding of amino acids to their respective tRNAs. These include anti–Jo-1, –PL-7, –PL-12, -EJ, and -OJ, which target the synthetases for histidine, threonine, alanine, glycine, and isoleucine, respectively, and produce characteristic tRNA immunoprecipitation patterns.[202] Anti-OJ represents the only specificity targeting

TABLE 20–6 • ANTINUCLEAR ANTIBODIES (ANAS) IN INFLAMMATORY MUSCLE DISEASES

Antibody Specificity	Prevalence (%)
Myositis-Specific Antibodies:	
Anti-tRNA Synthetases	
Histidyl (Jo-1)	20-30
Threonyl (PL-7)	1-5
Alanyl (PL-12)	1-5
Glycyl (EJ)	1-5
Isoleucyl (OJ)	1-5
Mi-2	8 (15-20% of DM)
Signal recognition particle	4
KJ	<1
Other Associated Antibodies:	
Proteasome	62
Histone	17
snRNPs:	
U1 snRNP	12
U2 snRNP	3
Ro	10
PM-Scl	8
Elongation factor 1α (Fer)	1
tRNA$^{[Ser]Sec}$ (Mas)	1-2
Described Only in Overlap Syndromes:	
Ku	?
U3 snoRNP	?

Abbreviations: DM: dermatomyositis; snoRNP, small nucleolar ribonucleoprotein, snRNP, small nuclear ribonucleoprotein; tRNA, transfer RNA.

a class I tRNA synthetase (isoleucyl); the other antisynthetase antibodies target class II tRNA synthetases.[203] Some of these antibodies target the tRNA anticodon loop, which explains their ability to specifically inhibit synthetase enzymatic activity; but other epitopes may be conformational. These antibodies may, therefore, be identified by FANA, ELISA, immunoprecipitation, immunoblot, and also by inhibition of in vitro aminoacylation reactions.[200]

Although the individual prevalences of these antibodies vary, their clinical associations remain similar. Anti–Jo-1, the most common, appears in 20 to 30 percent of PM/DM populations, whereas the non–Jo-1 autoantibodies vary in prevalences of up to 5 percent, depending on geographic location.[198,200] PM appears more commonly with anti–Jo-1, and DM is more common with the other synthetases, but these specificities together correlate with the "antisynthetase syndrome," which includes interstitial lung disease, arthritis, Raynaud's phenomenon, mechanic's hands, hyperkeratotic lines, sclerodactyly, facial telangiectasia, calcinosis, and sicca. One study has associated anti–threonyl-tRNA synthetase antibodies with fetal loss, severe relapsing myositis, and pregnancy,[204] and a recently discovered, rare, antisynthetase activity, anti-KS, has been described against the asparaginyl-tRNA synthetase in a few patients with interstitial lung disease and inflammatory arthritis or undifferentiated connective-tissue disease.[205] Despite these common associations, different antisynthetase antibodies have not been found to coexist within a patient. Indeed, the antisynthetases present a unique immunologic phenomena: Their autoantigens are each associated with the same syndrome and perform similar cellular functions, yet these specificities never cross-react or appear simultaneously in a single patient.

Anti–Signal Recognition Particle

Anti–signal recognition particle (SRP) MSAs target the SRP, which is the cytoplasmic ribonucleoprotein involved in the translocation of nascent proteins across the endoplasmic reticulum.[206] They occur in 4 percent of myositis patients, in the absence of other MSAs, and associate with acute onset, severe disease, resistance to therapy, cardiac involvement, and higher mortality, but a lower frequency of interstitial lung disease and arthritis.[198]

Anti–Mi-2

Anti–Mi-2 MSAs target a 240-kD nuclear component of a complex responsible for the control of cellular proliferation via chromatin remodeling.[207] Mi-2 may play a critical role in this complex, because it functionally associates with members of the Ikaros gene family, which are zinc finger proteins essential for lymphoid lineage determination and proliferation,[208] as well as transforming proteins such as human papillomavirus E7.[209] Additional proteins of 150-, 72-, 65-, 63-, 50-, and 34-kD, which were initially described as part of the autoantigen, may represent members of this multisubunit complex.[210] FANA reveals homogeneous nuclear fluorescence. The antibody occurs in 15 to 20 percent of DM patients, but more than 95 percent of patients with anti–Mi-2 have DM rather than PM. In addition, anti–Mi-2 has been associated with the "shawl" and "V" signs of dermatomyositis.[198,211] Thus, anti–Mi-2 appears generally associated with greater dermatologic involvement.

Anti-Mas

Anti-Mas has been found to target a UGA suppressor serine tRNA that carries selenocysteine ($tRNA^{[Ser]Sec}$), which is distinct from seryl-tRNA synthetase. Among connective tissue diseases, it is considered an MSA despite associations with autoimmune hepatitis.[212] Still, because it appears in only 1 to 2 percent of myositis patients, its prognostic utility remains undetermined.[198,213]

Anti-snRNP

Generally present in overlap syndromes, anti-snRNP antibodies in inflammatory muscle diseases predominantly consist of anti–U1 snRNP–specific antibodies, although a few anti-Sm and anti–U2 snRNP–specific antibodies have been described (see SLE: anti-snRNP). Anti–U1 snRNP antibodies generally associate with features of MCTD (i.e., PM/DM, scleroderma, and SLE), SLE-myositis overlap, myositis-scleroderma overlap, undifferentiated features (Raynaud's phenomenon, puffy fingers, arthritis) later progressing to myositis, and possibly response to corticosteroids.[214] Anti–U2 snRNP antibodies associate with myositis and sclerodactyly, sometimes with SLE and usually without interstitial lung disease.[76] These antibodies may coexist with MSAs.[198]

Anti–PM-Scl

Anti–PM-Scl antibodies target the exosome (see systemic sclerosis: anti-PM-Scl) and are found in approximately 8 percent of PM patients. As stated previously, its presence associates with myositis-scleroderma overlap without SLE features. Fifty percent of anti–PM-Scl antibody–positive patients have the overlap, and 25 percent of the overlap patients have the antibody.[178] Anti–PM-Scl also appears to be associated with arthritis, DM skin lesions, calcinosis, mechanic's hands, and eczema.[178,180] Unlike anti-snRNP antibodies in myositis overlap syndromes, PM-Scl and MSA autoantibodies have been found to be mutually exclusive.[178,180]

Other Overlap Antibodies

Other antibodies associated with myositis in overlap syndromes include several specificities found in other diseases. Anti-Ku antibodies, found more commonly in SLE and scleroderma, have been described in Japanese but not American patients with myositis-scleroderma overlap.[215] Anti–U3 RNP (fibrillarin) antibodies are associated with an increased incidence of inflammatory myositis among scleroderma patients, especially of the diffuse type.[216] Anti-Ro and anti-La antibodies, typically associated with SLE and SS, may appear occasionally, but their association with myositis remains unclear.[198]

Miscellaneous Antibodies

Other autoantibodies rarely or occasionally found in inflammatory muscle diseases include anti-KJ, which blocks in vitro translation;[217] anti-Fer, which targets translation elongation factor 1α;[218] antihistone;[50] antibody to a 56-kD Syrian Hamster nucleoprotein, which remains uncharacterized in terms of both molecular biology and clinical significance; anticarbonic anhydrase;[130] anti-Ro;[101,219] anti–U3 snRNP (Myo 22/25);[220] anti-hsp60, anti-hsp73, and anti-hsp90, whose antigens include three heat-shock proteins involved in the cellular stress response;[127,221,222] anti–transcription factor;[138] antiproteasome,[131,132] and antilaminin and antimicrofilament, which target nuclear and cytoplasmic cytoskeletal proteins.[136,185]

SJÖGREN'S SYNDROME

Antinuclear antibodies comprise a common finding among patients with SS. Reported incidences of positive FANAs range widely, reflecting differences in study populations and disease criteria, and depend heavily on the inclusion or exclusion of secondary, connective-tissue disease–related disease, which increases the likelihood and amplitude of a positive test.[3] Thus, although as low as 40-percent ANA positivity has been reported, many studies report frequencies of 90 to 96 percent,[223] with a diverse range of autoantibodies including both ubiquitous and tissue-specific reactivities such as antithyroid, gastric parietal cell, and muscarinic receptor. In this chapter we focus on the nuclear autoimmune targets, of which the Ro (SS-A) and La (SS-B) autoantigens remain the most thoroughly investigated (Table 20–7).

Anti-Ro and Anti-La

These two antibodies target two nuclear RNPs involved in RNA metabolism (see SLE: anti-Ro/SS-A and anti-La/SS-B). Anti-Ro antibodies appear in approximately 40 to 95 percent of SS patients and are associated with extraglandular manifestations such as neurologic involvement,[224] vasculitis,[225] glandular dysfunction,[226,227] anemia, lymphopenia, thrombocytopenia, anti-La, rheumatoid factor, and hypergammaglobulinemia.[223] Interestingly, they may result from genetically linked alternative processing of the Ro mRNA.[228] Anti-La antibodies appear in as many as 87 percent of SS patients and are associated with extraglandular manifestations such as neurologic involvement and vasculitis,[225] glandular dysfunction,[227] purpura, leukopenia, lymphopenia, hypergammaglobulinemia, and rheumatoid factor.[223]

TABLE 20–7 • ANTINUCLEAR ANTIBODIES (ANAs) IN SJÖGREN'S SYNDROME (SS)

Antibody Specificity	Prevalence (%)
Ro/SS-A	40-95
La/SS-B	87
Fodrin	64-100
Proteasome	39
MA-I	8
pp75 (Ro-associated protein)	6
Kinetochore	4
p80-coilin	4

Abbreviations: SS-A; SS-B, Sjögrens Syndrome-A -B.

Antifodrin

Fodrin (nonerythroid spectrin), a cytoskeletal heterodimer composed of α and β subunits structurally and functionally similar to erythroid spectrin, contributes to cellular mechanic support, shape, and membrane reorganization, including exocytosis.[229] In secretory cells, cellular stimulation results in its reorganization from a uniform subplasmalemmal localization into discrete patches,[230] and cytotoxic lymphocyte granule-induced apoptosis induces its fragmentation.[231] In SS, antibodies against α-fodrin have been detected in 64 to 67 percent of patients,[232-234] and in up to 100 percent of patients in small pediatric series,[235,236] but they are relatively uncommon in other connective tissue diseases such as SLE. Preliminary analyses suggest that they associate with pernio, hyperglobulinemia, rheumatoid factor positivity, and anti–SS-B (La) antibody, but not with annular erythema, photosensitivity, vasculitis, or renal disorder. Antibodies against β-fodrin have been described in as many as 70 percent of patients, but clinical associations have not been reported.[237]

Anti–MA-I

Anti–MA-I antibodies target a 200-kD protein localized to the mitotic apparatus in dividing cells. During interphase, it produces fine, speckled nucleoplasmic staining with nucleolar sparing, which changes to bright staining of centrosome rims and proximal spindles during metaphase. It appears in 8 percent of SS patients, but its clinical significance remains unknown. This specificity may be similar or identical to anti-NuMA, which targets a 240-kD coiled-coil protein localized at the mitotic apparatus, but such conclusions await further biochemical characterization.[83,238]

Anti–p80-Coilin

Anti–p80-coilin antibodies target an 80-kD nuclear protein associated with coiled bodies, which are noncapsular nuclear bodies of 0.3 to 1 micron that partake in snRNP biogenesis.[239,240] They appear in 4 percent of SS patients and rarely in scleroderma or other skin diseases,[241,242] but their clinical significance remains unclear.

Miscellaneous Antibodies

Other ANAs described in SS patients include antikinetochore, typically associated with scleroderma but found infrequently in SS;[154,243] perinuclear antineutrophil cytoplasmic antibodies (p-ANCA), classically associated with polyarteritis nodosa but found in 11 to 40 percent of SS patients;[244-246] antimitochondrial antibodies and anti–pyruvate dehydrogenase antibodies, typically associated with primary biliary cirrhosis but found in 6.6 and 27 percent of SS patients, respectively;[247] anti–U4/U6 snRNP, described in a single SS patient;[248] antimicrofilament;[136] anti–carbonic anhydrase;[130] anti–nuclear lamina;[137] anti–transcription factor TFIIF;[138] anti–Golgi apparatus,[249] antiproteasome,[132,250] and antibody against the Ro-associated pp75 protein.[251]

MIXED CONNECTIVE TISSUE DISEASE AND OVERLAP SYNDROMES

Although overlap syndromes of connective tissue disease have remained matters of nosological debate for decades, virtually all investigators agree that the presence of antinuclear antibodies are universal in these conditions.[252,253] Indeed, since the initial formal description of MCTD in 1972, the presence of anti–U1 snRNP antibodies has been consistently required for classification, diagnosis, or both, and associated ANA titers typically exceed 1:1000 and often exceed 1:10,000.[252,253]

However, several investigations have noted that a significant proportion of such patients develop manifestations that allow the diagnosis of a defined connective tissue disease, such as SLE, RA, SSc, or PM/DM,[254,255] and, therefore, the accuracy of specific clinical associations of specific ANAs in these settings is significantly hindered by issues of disease classification. As a result, for MCTD and overlap syndromes, clinicians most generally base the importance of individual autoantibody specifcities upon their primary disease association (e.g., anti–topoisomerase I as predictive of eventual diffuse scleroderma-like skin disease or pulmonary fibrosis, or anti-dsDNA as predictive of eventual lupus-like glomerulonephritis, despite the lack of definitive, well-codified evidence).

MISCELLANEOUS DISEASES

In contrast to the traditional ANA diseases, the presence of a positive ANA in Raynaud's phenomenon, juvenile rheumatoid arthritis (JRA), and antiphospholipid antibody syndrome (APS) is unhelpful for diagnosis, but may offer prognostic information (see Table 20–1). In Raynaud's phenomenon, a positive result increases the likelihood, from 19 percent to 30 percent, of the development of a systemic rheumatic disease, including SLE, RA, and SSc. In contrast, a negative result decreases the likelihood to approximately 7 percent, which is often helpful for patient reassurance.[256,257] In JRA, ANA positivity may predict the development of uveitis;[258-260] and in APS, it may predict the development or presence of underlying SLE.[261]

ANAs have also been found in several other conditions both related and unrelated to rheumatologic illnesses. These include such rheumatic conditions as Henoch-Schonlein purpura,[262] JRA,[263] relapsing polychondritis,[264] and sarcoidosis;[265] other autoimmune diseases such as multiple sclerosis,[266] myasthenia gravis,[267] inflammatory bowel disease,[268] autoimmune hepatitis,[269] interstitial cystitis,[270] and thyroid disease;[271] infectious diseases such as viral hepatitis[272,273] or leprosy;[274] psychiatric conditions such as schizophrenia,[275] Tourette's syndrome,[276] or dementia;[277] dermatologic conditions such as polymorphous light eruption,[278] lichen planus,[279] and atopic dermatitis;[280] and many miscellaneous conditions including liver disease,[281] severe coronary atherosclerosis,[282] epilepsy,[283] chronic neutropenia,[284] silicone-gel implants,[285] mercury intoxication,[286] eosinophilia-myalgia syndrome,[287] and pregnancy.[288] Even with the vast numbers of such diverse reports of antinuclear antibodies in unexpected situations, these studies lack comprehensive analyses regarding the significance of these antibodies in these diseases. The role of such ANAs in the clinical evaluation of such patients therefore remains largely unexplored.

Clinical Evaluation of Antinuclear Antibodies

Figure 20–3 describes an algorithm for the rheumatologic evaluation of a patient for ANAs. In general, the FANA serves as a screening test, with subsequent specific autoantigen testing depending on the clinical situation. A negative FANA, or a low-titer FANA, in the setting of a low clinical suspicion of rheumatic disease usually indicates the absence of ANAs and argues against the diagnosis of one of the ANA diseases (see Table 20–1). Still, if the clinical picture strongly suggests connective tissue disease, further investigation may involve specific assays for antigens that commonly test negative in FANA, such as Ro, Jo-1, or phospholipids. On the other hand, because some specific ANAs possess diagnostic significance, positive FANA results usually warrant follow-up with specialized assays. Thus, if SLE is suspected, further work may assay for anti-DNA, anti-Sm, anti–U1 snRNP, and anti-Ro antibodies. Similarly, if MCTD, SS, scleroderma, or polymyositis are suspected, the serum may be tested, respectively, for anti–U1 snRNP; anti-Ro or anti-La; anti–topoisomerase I, anticentromere, or antinucleoli; or anti–tRNA synthetases. Positive results in these more-specialized assays do not alone signify specific diseases, but rather add weight to diagnoses that should throughout the evaluation rely heavily on other clinical information.[289]

Conclusion

The ANAs continue to encompass an ever-widening range of nuclear, nucleolar, and cytoplasmic autoantigen specificities. Within the ANA diseases, including SLE, SSc, PM/DM, SS, and MCTD, each autoantibody possesses its own unique rheumatologic associations, but the specificity of these associations has diminished as the sensitivity of clinical studies has increased in the detection of these specificities. Consequently, tests for ANAs can greatly aid in the clinical evaluation of patients in the context of their particular disease associations, but these studies retain only an adjunct role in rheumatologic diagnosis. Hopefully future studies will more clearly elucidate the clinical and biochemical nuances that have caused these tests to be widely accepted yet inadequately understood. Until then, clinical acumen continues to direct the utility of the test for ANAs.

REFERENCES

1. Peng SL, Hardin JA, Craft J: Antinuclear antibodies. *In* Kelly WN, Harris ED, Ruddy S, Sledge CB, (eds): Textbook of Rheumatology. Philadelphia, PA, W. B. Saunders, 1997, p 250.
2. Kavanaugh A, Tomar R, Reveille J, et al: Guidelines for clinical use of the antinuclear antibody test and tests for specific autoantibodies to nuclear antigens. American College of Pathologists. Arch Pathol Lab Med 124:71, 2000.
3. Solomon DH, Kavanaugh AJ, Schur PH, American College of Rheumatology Ad Hoc Committee on Immunologic Testing: Evidence-based guidelines for the use of immunologic tests: antinuclear antibody testing. Arthritis Rheum 47:434, 2002.
4. Hargraves MM, Richmond H, Morton R: Presentation of two bone marrow elements: the "tart" cell and "L.E. cell." Proc Staff Meet Mayo Clin 23:25, 1948.
5. Tan EM: The L.E. cell and its legacy. Clin Exp Rheum 16:652, 1998.
6. Beck J: Antinuclear antibodies: methods of detection and significance. Mayo Clin Proc 44:600, 1960.
7. Hargraves MM: Production in vitro of the LE cell phenomenon: use of normal bone marrow elements and blood plasma from patients with acute disseminated lupus erythematosus. Proc Staff Meet Mayo Clin 24:234, 1949.
8. Haserick JR, Bortz DW: Normal bone marrow inclusion phenomena induced by lupus erythematosus plasma. J Invest Dermatol 13:47, 1949.
9. Holman HR, Kunkel HG: Affinity between the lupus erythematosus serum factor and cell nuclei and nucleoprotein. Science 126:162, 1957.
10. Schmidt-Acevedo S, Perez-Romano B, Ruiz-Arguelles A: 'LE cells' result from phagocytosis of apoptotic bodies induced by antinuclear antibodies. J Autoimmun 15:15, 2000.
11. Friou GJ: Clinical application of lupus serum nucleoprotein reaction using fluorescent antibody technique. J Clin Invest 36:890, 1957.
12. Deicher HRG, Holman HR, Kunkel HG: The precipitin reaction between DNA and a serum factor in systemic lupus erythematosus. J Exp Med 109:97, 1959.
13. Tan EM, Kunkel HG: Characteristics of a soluble nuclear antigen precipitating with sera of patients with systemic lupus erythematosus. J Immunol 96:464, 1966.
14. Mattioli M, Reichlin M: Characterization of a soluble nuclear ribonucleoprotein antigen reactive with SLE sera. J Immunol 107:1281, 1971.
15. Clark G, Reichlin M, Tomasi TB Jr.: Characterization of a soluble cytoplasmic antigen reactive with sera from patients with systemic lupus erythmatosus. J Immunol 102:117, 1969.
16. Lerner MR, Steitz JA: Antibodies to small nuclear RNAs complexed with proteins are produced by patients with systemic lupus erythematosus. Proc Natl Acad Sci U S A 76:5495, 1979.
17. Hollingsworth PN, Bonifacio E, Dawkins RL: Use of a standard curve improves precision and concordance of antinuclear antibody measurement. J Clin Lab Immunol 22:197, 1987.
18. Nakabayashi T, Kumagai T, Yamauchi K, et al: Evaluation of the automatic fluorescent image analyzer, Image Titer, for quantitative analysis of antinuclear antibodies. Am J Clin Pathol 115:424, 2001.
19. Flessland KA, Landicho HR, Borden KK, Prince HE: Performance characteristics of the PolyTiter Immunofluorescent Titration system for determination of antinuclear antibody endpoint dilution. Clin Diagn Lab Immunol 9:329, 2002.
20. Molden DP, Nakamura RM, Tan EM: Standardization of the immunofluorescence test for autoantibody to nuclear antigens (ANA): use of reference sera of defined antibody specificity. Am J Clin Pathol 82:57, 1984.
21. Johnson GD, Holborow EJ: Standardisation of tests for antinuclear antibody. Ann Rheum Dis 39:529, 1980.
22. James K, Carpenter AB, Cook L, et al: Development of the antinuclear and anticytoplasmic antibody consensus panel by the Association of Medical Laboratory Immunologists. Clin Diagn Lab Immunol 7:436, 2000.
23. Fritzler MJ: Immunofluorescent antinuclear antibody test. *In* Rose NR, de Macario EC, Fahey JL, et al (eds): Manual of Clinical Laboratory Immunology. Washington, DC, American Society for Microbiology, 1992, p 724.
24. Nakamura RM: Quality Assurance for the Indirect Immunofluorescence Test for Autoantibodies to Nuclear Antigen (IF-ANA): Approved Guideline. National Committee for Clinical Laboratory Standards, Wayne, PA, 1996.
25. Tan EM, Feltkamp TE, Smolen JS, et al: Range of antinuclear antibodies in "healthy" individuals. Arthritis Rheum 40:1601, 1997.
26. Vaile JH, Dyke L, Kherani R, et al: Is high titre ANA specific for connective tissue disease? Clin Exp Rheum 18:433, 2000.
27. Maddison PJ, Provost TT, Reichlin M: Serological findings in patients with "ANA-negative" systemic lupus erythematosus. Medicine 60:87, 1981.
28. Bylund DJ, Nakamura RM: Importance of detection of SS-A/Ro autoantibody in screening immunofluorescence tests for autoantibodies to nuclear antigens. J Clin Lab Anal 5:212, 1991.
29. Wasicek CA, Maddison PJ, Reichlin M: Occurrence of antibodies to single-stranded DNA in ANA negative patients. Clin Exp Immunol 37:190, 1979.
30. Tilton RC: Counterimmunoelectrophoresis in biology and medicine. CRC Crit Rev Clin Lab Sci 9:347, 1978.
31. Craft J, Hardin JA: Immunoprecipitation assays for the detection of soluble nuclear and cytoplasmic nucleoproteins. *In* Rose NR, de Macario EC, Fahey JL, et al (eds): Manual of Clinical Laboratory Immunology. Washington, DC, American Society for Microbiology, 1992, p 47.
32. Boire G, Lopez-Longo FJ, Lapointe S, Menard HA: Sera from patients with autoimmune disease recognize conformational determinants on the 60-kd Ro/SS-A protein. Arthritis Rheum 34:722, 1991.
33. Maul GG, French BT, van Venrooij WJ, Jimenez SA: Topoisomerase I identified by scleroderma 70 antisera: enrichment of topoisomerase I at the centromere in mouse mitotic cells before anaphase. Proc Natl Acad Sci U S A 83:5145, 1986.
34. Samuels DS, Tojo T, Homma M, Shimizu N: Inhibition of topoisomerase I by antibodies in sera from scleroderma patients. FEBS Lett 209:231, 1986.
35. Yang DC, Dang CV, Arnett FC: Rat liver histidyl-tRNA synthetase. Purification and inhibition by the myositis-specific anti-Jo-1 autoantibody. Biochem Biophys Res Commun 120:15, 1984.
36. Padgett RA, Mount SM, Steitz JA, Sharp PA: Splicing of messenger RNA precursors is inhibited by antisera to small nuclear ribonucleoprotein. Cell 35:101, 1983.
37. Hahn BH: Antibodies to DNA. New Engl J Med 338:1359, 1998.
38. Thomson KF, Murphy A, Goodfield MJ, Misbah SA: Is it useful to test for antibodies to extractable nuclear antigens in the presence of a negative antinuclear antibody on Hep-2 cells? J Clin Pathol 54:413, 2001.
39. Tan EM, Cohen AS, Fries JF, et al: The 1982 revised criteria for the classification of systemic lupus erythematosus. Arthritis Rheum 25:1271, 1982.
40. Burlingame RW, Boey ML, Starkebaum G, Rubin RL: The central role of chromatin in autoimmune responses to histones and DNA in systemic lupus erythematosus. J Clin Invest 94:184, 1994.
41. Tohge H, Tsutsui K, Sano K, Isik S: High incidence of antinuclear antibodies that recognize the matrix attachment region. Biochem Biophys Res Commun 285:64, 2001.
42. Wallace DJ, Salonen EM, Avaniss-Aghajani E, et al: Anti-telomere antibodies in systemic lupus erythematosus: a new ELISA test for anti-DNA with potential pathogenetic implications. Lupus 9:328, 2000.
43. Eivazova ER, McDonnell JM, Sutton BJ, Staines NA: Cross-reactivity of antiidiotypic antibodies with DNA in systemic lupus erythematosus. Arthritis Rheum 43:429, 2000.
44. DeGiorgio LA, Konstantinov KN, Lee SC, et al: A subset of lupus anti-DNA antibodies cross-reacts with the NR2 glutamate receptor in systemic lupus erythematosus. Nature Med 7:1189, 2001.
45. Takeda I, Rayno K, Movafagh FB, et al: Dual binding capabilities of anti-double-stranded DNA antibodies and anti-ribosomal phosphoprotein (P) antibodies. Lupus 10:857, 2001.
46. Zack DJ, Yamamoto K, Wong AL, et al: DNA mimics a self-protein that may be a target for some anti-DNA antibodies in systemic lupus erythematosus. J Immunol 154:1987, 1995.
47. Reichlin M, Martin A, Taylor-Albert E, et al: Lupus autoantibodies to native DNA cross-react with the A and D SnRNP polypeptides. J Clin Invest 93:443, 1994.

48. Ramakrishnan V: Histone structure and the organization of the nucleosome. Ann Rev Biophys Biomolec Struct 26:83, 1997.
49. Reeves WH, Satoh M, Wang J, et al: Antibodies to DNA, DNA-binding proteins, and histones. Rheum Dis Clin North Am 20:1, 1994.
50. Kubo M, Ihn H, Yazawa N, et al: Prevalence and antigen specificity of anti-histone antibodies in patients with polymyositis/dermatomyositis. J Invest Dermatol 112:711, 1999.
51. Chen M, Shirai M, Czaja AJ, et al: Characterization of anti-histone antibodies in patients with type 1 autoimmune hepatitis. J Gastroenterol Hepatol 13:483, 1998.
52. Martin L, Pauls JD, Ryan JP, Fritzler MJ: Identification of a subset of patients with scleroderma with severe pulmonary and vascular disease by the presence of autoantibodies to centromere and histone. Ann Rheum Dis 52:780, 1993.
53. Sato S, Fujimoto M, Ihn H, et al: Antigen specificity of antihistone antibodies in localized scleroderma. Arch Derm 130:1273, 1994.
54. Sato S, Ihn H, Kikuchi K, Takehara K: Antihistone antibodies in systemic sclerosis. Association with pulmonary fibrosis. Arthritis Rheum 37:391, 1994.
55. Garzelli C, Incaprera M, Bazzichi A, et al: Epstein-Barr virus-transformed human B lymphocytes produce natural antibodies to histones. Immunol Lett 39:277, 1994.
56. Bonfa E, Viana VS, Barreto AC, et al: Autoantibodies in Chagas' disease. An antibody cross-reactive with human and Trypanosoma cruzi ribosomal proteins. J Immunol 150:3917, 1993.
57. Chengappa KN, Carpenter AB, Yang ZW, et al: Elevated IgG anti-histone antibodies in a subgroup of medicated schizophrenic patients. Schiz Res 7:49, 1992.
58. Monestier M, Fasy TM, Bohm L, Lieberman FS: Anti-histone antibodies in subacute sensory neuropathy. J Neuro-Onc 11:71, 1991.
59. Shoenfeld Y, el-Roeiy A, Ben-Yehuda O, Pick AI: Detection of anti-histone activity in sera of patients with monoclonal gammopathies. Clin Immunol Immunopathol 42:250, 1987.
60. Kamei M, Kato M, Mochizuki K, et al: Serodiagnosis of cancers by ELISA of anti-histone H2B antibody. Biotherapy 4:17, 1992.
61. Viard JP, Choquette D, Chabre H, et al: Anti-histone reactivity in systemic lupus erythematosus sera: a disease activity index linked to the presence of DNA: anti-DNA immune complexes. Autoimmunity 12:61, 1992.
62. Tuteja R, Tuteja N: Ku autoantigen: a multifunctional DNA-binding protein. Crit Rev Biochem Mol Biol 35:1, 2000.
63. Reeves WH: Antibodies to the p70/p80 (Ku) antigens in systemic lupus erythematosus. Rheum Dis Clin North Am 18:391, 1992.
64. Mimori T, Akizuki M, Yamagata H, et al: Characterization of a high molecular weight acidic nuclear protein recognized by autoantibodies in sera from patients with polymyositis-scleroderma overlap. J Clin Invest 68:611, 1981.
65. Satoh M, Ajmani AK, Ogasawara T, et al: Autoantibodies to RNA polymerase II are common in systemic lupus erythematosus and overlap syndrome. Specific recognition of the phosphorylated (IIO) form by a subset of human sera. J Clin Invest 94:1981, 1994.
66. Wang J, Satoh M, Kabir F, et al: Increased prevalence of autoantibodies to ku antigen in African American versus white patients with systemic lupus erythematosus. Arthritis Rheum 44:2367, 2001.
67. Isern RA, Yaneva M, Weiner E, et al: Autoantibodies in patients with primary pulmonary hypertension: association with anti-Ku. Am J Med 93:307, 1992.
68. Cooley HM, Melny BJ, Gleeson R, et al: Clinical and serological associations of anti-Ku antibody. J Rheum 26:563, 1999.
69. Suwa A: Studies on the antigenic epitopes reactive with autoantibody in patients with PSS-PM overlap syndrome. Keio Igaku 67:865, 1990.
70. Paunesku T, Mittal S, Protic M, et al: Proliferating cell nuclear antigen (PCNA): ringmaster of the genome. Int J Radiat Biol 77:1007, 2001.
71. Takeuchi K, Kaneda K, Kawakami I, et al: Autoantibodies recognizing proteins copurified with PCNA in patients with connective tissue diseases. Mol Biol Rep 23:243, 1996.
72. Tzang BS, Chen TY, Hsu TC, et al: Presentation of autoantibody to proliferating cell nuclear antigen in patients with chronic hepatitis B and C virus infection. Ann Rheum Dis 58:630, 1999.
73. Kurki P, Vanderlaan M, Dolbeare F, et al: Expression of proliferating cell nuclear antigen (PCNA)/cyclin during the cell cycle. Exp Cell Res 166:209, 1986.
74. Reimer G, Rose KM, Scheer U, Tan EM: Autoantibody to RNA polymerase I in scleroderma sera. J Clin Invest 79:65, 1987.
75. Rothfield NF: Autoantibodies in scleroderma. Rheum Dis Clin North Am 18:483, 1992.
76. Peng SL, Craft J: Spliceosomal snRNPs autoantibodies. *In* Peter JB, Shoenfeld Y (eds): Autoantibodies. Amsterdam, Elsevier, 1996, p 774.
77. Matera AG, Ward DC: Nucleoplasmic organization of small nuclear ribonucleoproteins in cultured human cells. J Cell Biol 121:715, 1993.
78. Eystathioy T, Peebles CL, Hamel JC, et al: Autoantibody to hLSm4 and the heptameric LSm complex in anti-Sm sera. Arthritis Rheum 46:726, 2002.
79. Margaux J, Hayem G, Palazzo E, et al: Clinical usefulness of antibodies to U1snRNP proteins in mixed connective tissue disease and systemic lupus erythematosus. Rev Rhum Engl Ed 65:378, 1998.
80. Abu-Shakrah M, Krupp M, Argov S, et al: The detection of anti-Sm-RNP activity in sera of patients with monoclonal gammopathies. Clin Exp Immunol 75:349, 1989.
81. de Vries E, Schipperijn AJ, Breedveld FC: Antinuclear antibodies in psychiatric patients. Acta Psych Scand 89:289, 1994.
82. Hasegawa H, Uchiumi T, Sato T, et al: Anti-Sm autoantibodies cross-react with ribosomal protein S10: a common structural unit shared by the small nuclear RNP proteins and the ribosomal protein. Arthritis Rheum 41:1040, 1998.
83. Chan EK, Andrade LE: Antinuclear antibodies in Sjogren's syndrome. Rheum Dis Clin North Am 18:551, 1992.
84. O'Brien CA, Wolin SL: A possible role for the 60-kD Ro autoantigen in a discard pathway for defective 5S rRNA precursors. Genes Dev 8:2891, 1994.
85. Campos-Almaraz M, Barbosa-Cisneros O, Herrera-Esparza R: Ro60 ribonucleoprotein inhibits transcription by T3 RNA polymerase in vitro. Rev Rhum 66:310, 1999.
86. Maraia RJ, Intine RV: Recognition of nascent RNA by the human La antigen: conserved and divergent features of structure and function. Molec Cell Biol 21:367, 2001.
87. Pellizzoni L, Lotti F, Rutjes SA, Pierandrei-Amaldi P: Involvement of the Xenopus laevis Ro60 autoantigen in the alternative interaction of La and CNBP proteins with the 5'UTR of L4 ribosomal protein mRNA. J Molec Biol 281:593, 1998.
88. St. Clair EW: Anti-La antibodies. Rheum Dis Clin North Am 18:359, 1992.
89. Wasicek CA, Reichlin M: Clinical and serological differences between systemic lupus erythematosus patients with antibodies to Ro versus patients with antibodies to Ro and La. J Clin Invest 69:835, 1982.
90. Weston WL, Morelli JG, Lee LA: The clinical spectrum of anti-Ro-positive cutaneous neonatal lupus erythematosus. J Amer Acad Derm 40:675, 1999.
91. Sibilia J: Ro(SS-A) and anti-Ro(SS-A): an update. Rev Rhum Engl Ed 65:45, 1998.
92. Brucato A, Buyon JP, Horsfall AC, et al: Fourth international workshop on neonatal lupus syndromes and the Ro/SSA-La/SSB System. Clin Exp Rheum 17:130, 1999.
93. Nield LE, Silverman ED, Smallhorn JF, et al: Endocardial fibroelastosis associated with maternal anti-Ro and anti-La antibodies in the absence of atrioventricular block. J Am Coll Cardiol 40:796, 2002.
94. Franceschini F, Calzavara-Pinton P, Valsecchi L, et al: Chilblain lupus erythematosus is associated with antibodies to SSA/Ro. Adv Exp Med Biol 455:167, 1999.
95. Harley JB, Scofield RH, Reichlin M: Anti-Ro in Sjogren's syndrome and systemic lupus erythematosus. Rheum Dis Clin North Am 18:337, 1992.
96. Scofield RH, Frank MB, Neas BR, et al: Cooperative association of T cell beta receptor and HLA-DQ alleles in the production of anti-Ro in systemic lupus erythematosus. Clin Immunol Immunopathol 72:335, 1994.
97. Lopez-Longo FJ, Rodriguez-Mahou M, Escalona M, et al: Heterogeneity of the anti-Ro(SSA) response in rheumatic diseases. J Rheum 21:1450, 1994.

98. Cho CS, Park SH, Min JK, et al: Clinical significances of antibodies to Ro/SS-A autoantigens and its subtypes in primary Sjogren's syndrome. Korean J Int Med 12:176, 1997.
99. Fujimoto M, Shimozuma M, Yazawa N, et al: Prevalence and clinical relevance of 52-kDa and 60-kDa Ro/SS-A autoantibodies in Japanese patients with systemic sclerosis. Ann Rheum Dis 56:667, 1997.
100. Cavazzana I, Franceschini F, Belfiore N, et al: Undifferentiated connective tissue disease with antibodies to Ro/SSa: clinical features and follow-up of 148 patients. Clin Exp Rheum 19:403, 2001.
101. Kubo M, Ihn H, Asano Y, et al: Prevalence of 52-kd and 60-kd Ro/SS-A autoantibodies in Japanese patients with polymyositis/dermatomyositis. J Amer Acad Derm 47:148, 2002.
102. McCauliffe DP: Cutaneous diseases in adults associated with anti-Ro/SS-A autoantibody production. Lupus 6:158, 1997.
103. de Andres C, Guillem A, Rodriguez-Mahou M, Lopez Longo FJ: Frequency and significance of anti-Ro (SS-A) antibodies in multiple sclerosis patients. Acta Neurol Scand 104:83, 2001.
104. Hansen A, Feist E, Hiepe F, et al: Diffuse infiltrative lymphocytosis syndrome in a patient with anti-52-kd Ro/SSA and human immunodeficiency virus type 1. Arthritis Rheum 42:578, 1999.
105. Wax MB, Tezel G, Saito I, et al: Anti-Ro/SS-A positivity and heat shock protein antibodies in patients with normal-pressure glaucoma. Am J Opthal 125:145, 1998.
106. Doudna JA, Rath VL: Structure and function of the eukaryotic ribosome: the next frontier. Cell 109:153, 2002.
107. Pan ZJ, Anderson CJ, Stafford HA: Anti-idiotypic antibodies prevent the serologic detection of antiribosomal P autoantibodies in healthy adults. J Clin Invest 102:215, 1998.
108. Golombek SJ, Graus F, Elkon KB: Autoantibodies in the cerebrospinal fluid of patients with systemic lupus erythematosus. Arthritis Rheum 29:1090, 1986.
109. Bonfa E, Golombek SJ, Kaufman LD, et al: Association between lupus psychosis and anti-ribosomal P protein antibodies. New Engl J Med 317:265, 1987.
110. Schneebaum AB, Singleton JD, West SG, et al: Association of psychiatric manifestations with antibodies to ribosomal P proteins in systemic lupus erythematosus. Am J Med 90:54, 1991.
111. Ghirardello A, Doria A, Zampieri S, et al: Anti-ribosomal P protein antibodies detected by immunoblotting in patients with connective tissue diseases: their specificity for SLE and association with IgG anticardiolipin antibodies. Ann Rheum Dis 59:975, 2000.
112. Elkon KB, Bonfa E, Brot N: Antiribosomal antibodies in systemic lupus erythematosus. Rheum Dis Clin No Am 18:377, 1992.
113. Caponi L, Bombardieri S, Migliorini P: Anti-ribosomal antibodies bind the Sm proteins D and B/B'. Clin Exp Immunol 112:139, 1998.
114. Sato T, Uchiumi T, Arakawa M, Kominami R: Serological association of lupus autoantibodies to a limited functional domain of 28S ribosomal RNA and to the ribosomal proteins bound to the domain. Clin Exp Immunol 98:35, 1994.
115. Valcarcel J, Green MR: The SR protein family: pleiotropic functions in pre-mRNA splicing. Trends Biochem Sci 21:296, 1996.
116. Neugebauer KM, Merrill JT, Wener MH, et al: SR proteins are autoantigens in patients with systemic lupus erythematosus. Importance of phosphoepitopes. Arthritis Rheum 43:1768, 2000.
117. Utz PJ, Hottelet M, van Venrooij WJ, Anderson P: Association of phosphorylated serine/arginine (SR) splicing factors with the U1-small ribonucleoprotein (snRNP) autoantigen complex accompanies apoptotic cell death. J Exp Med 187:547, 1998.
118. Craft J, Hardin JA: Antinuclear antibodies. *In* Kelly WN, Harris ED, Ruddy S, Sledge CB (eds): Textbook of Rheumatology. Philadelphia, PA, W. B. Saunders, 1993, p 164.
119. Ohosone Y, Ishida M, Takahashi Y, et al: Spectrum and clinical significance of autoantibodies against transfer RNA. Arthritis Rheum 41:1625, 1998.
120. van Venrooij WJ, Hoet R, Castrop J, et al: Anti-(U1) small nuclear RNA antibodies in anti-small nuclear ribonucleoprotein sera from patients with connective tissue diseases. J Clin Invest 86:2154, 1990.
121. Yamanaka K, Takasaki Y, Nishida Y, et al: Detection and quantification of anti-Ki antibodies by enzyme-linked immunosorbent assay using recombinant Ki antigen. Arthritis Rheum 35:667, 1992.
122. Muro Y, Kano T, Sugiura K, Hagiwara M: Low frequency of autoantibodies against Ki-67 antigen in Japanese patients with systemic autoimmune diseases. J Autoimmun 10:499, 1997.
123. Fritzler MJ, Salazar M: Diversity and origin of rheumatologic autoantibodies. Clin Microbiol Rev 4:256, 1991.
124. Nakano M, Ohuchi Y, Hasegawa H, et al: Clinical significance of anticentromere antibodies in patients with systemic lupus erythematosus. J Rheum 27:1403, 2000.
125. Kindas-Mugge I, Steiner G, Smolen JS: Similar frequency of autoantibodies against 70-kD class heat-shock proteins in healthy subjects and systemic lupus erythematosus patients. Clin Exp Immunol 92:46, 1993.
126. Conroy SE, Faulds GB, Williams W, et al: Detection of autoantibodies to the 90 kDa heat shock protein in systemic lupus erythematosus and other autoimmune diseases. Br J Rheum 33:923, 1994.
127. Minota S, Koyasu S, Yahara I, Winfield J: Autoantibodies to the heat-shock protein hsp90 in systemic lupus erythematosus. J Clin Invest 81:106, 1988.
128. Pauzner R, Urowitz M, Gladman D, Gough J: Antineutrophil cytoplasmic antibodies in systemic lupus erythematosus. J Rheum 21:1670, 1994.
129. Schnabel A, Csernok E, Isenberg DA, et al: Antineutrophil cytoplasmic antibodies in systemic lupus erythematosus. Prevalence, specificities, and clinical significance. Arthritis Rheum 38:633, 1995.
130. Itoh Y, Reichlin M: Antibodies to carbonic anhydrase in systemic lupus erythematosus and other rheumatic diseases. Arthritis Rheum 35:73, 1992.
131. Feist E, Dorner T, Kuckelkorn U, et al: Proteasome a-type subunit C9 is a primary target of autoantibodies in sera of patients with myositis and systemic lupus erythematosus. J Exp Med 184:1313, 1996.
132. Feist E, Dorner T, Kuckelkorn U, et al: Diagnostic importance of anti-proteasome antibodies. Int Arch Allergy Immunol 123:92, 2000.
133. Kratz A, Harding MW, Craft J, et al: Autoantibodies against cyclophilin in systemic lupus erythematosus and Lyme disease. Clin Exp Immunol 90:422, 1992.
134. Montecucco C, Caporali R, Cobianchi F, et al: Antibodies to hn-RNP protein A1 in systemic lupus erythematosus: clinical association with Raynaud's phenomenon and esophageal dysmotility. Clin Exp Rheum 10:223, 1992.
135. De Mendonca Neto EC, Kumar A, Shadick NA, et al: Antibodies to T- and L-isoforms of the cytoskeletal protein, fimbrin, in patients with systemic lupus erythematosus. J Clin Invest 90:1037, 1992.
136. Girard D, Senecal JL: Anti-microfilament IgG antibodies in normal adults and in patients with autoimmune diseases: immunofluorescence and immunoblotting analysis of 201 subjects reveals polyreactivity with microfilament-associated proteins. Clin Immunol Immunopathol 74:193, 1995.
137. Konstantinov K, Foisner R, Byrd D, et al: Integral membrane proteins associated with the nuclear lamina are novel autoimmune antigens of the nuclear envelope. Clin Immunol Immunopathol 74:89, 1995.
138. Cai Y, Kitajima S, Etoh F, et al: Autoantibody reactive with the human general transcription factor TFIIF in sera from patients with autoimmune disorders. Clin Exp Immunol 109:488, 1997.
139. Herkel J, Mimran A, Erez N, et al: Autoimmunity to the p53 protein is a feature of systemic lupus erythematosus (SLE) related to anti-DNA antibodies. J Autoimmun 17:63, 2001.
140. Takeda Y, Dynan WS: Autoantibodies against DNA double-strand break repair proteins. Front Biosci 6:D1412, 2001.
141. Gussin HA, Ignat GP, Varga J, Teodorescu M: Anti-topoisomerase I (anti-Scl-70) antibodies in patients with systemic lupus erythematosus. Arthritis Rheum 44:376, 2001.
142. Satoh M, Langdon JJ, Chou CH, et al: Characterization of the Su antigen, a macromolecular complex of 100/102 and 200-kDa proteins recognized by autoantibodies in systemic rheumatic diseases. Clin Immunol Immunopathol 73:132, 1994.
143. Bernstein RM, Steigerwald JC, Tan EM: Association of antinuclear and antinucleolar antibodies in progressive systemic sclerosis. Clin Exp Immunol 48:43, 1982.
144. Lee B, Craft JE: Molecular structure and function of autoantigens in systemic sclerosis. Int Rev Immunol 12:129, 1995.

145. Bunn CC, Denton CP, Shi-Wen X, et al: Anti-RNA polymerases and other autoantibody specificities in systemic sclerosis. Br J Rheum 37:15, 1998.
146. Moroi Y, Peebles C, Fritzler MJ, et al: Autoantibody to centromere (kinetochore) in scleroderma sera. Proc Natl Acad Sci U S A 77:1627, 1980.
147. Dobie KW, Hari KL, Maggert KA, Karpen GH: Centromere proteins and chromosome inheritance: a complex affair. Curr Opin Gene Dev 9:206, 1999.
148. Fritzler MJ, Kinsella TD: The CREST syndrome: a distinct serologic entity with anticentromere antibodies. Am J Med 69:520, 1980.
149. Weiner ES, Hildebrandt S, Senecal JL, et al: Prognostic significance of anticentromere antibodies and anti-topoisomerase I antibodies in Raynaud's disease. A prospective study. Arthritis Rheum 34:68, 1991.
150. Higuchi M, Horiuchi T, Ishibashi N, et al: Anticentromere antibody as a risk factor for cancer in patients with systemic sclerosis. Clin Rheumatol 19:123, 2000.
151. Spencer-Green G, Alter D, Welch HG: Test performance in systemic sclerosis: anti-centromere and anti-Scl-70 antibodies. Am J Med 103:242, 1997.
152. Weiner ES, Earnshaw WC, Senecal JL, et al: Clinical associations of anticentromere antibodies and antibodies to topoisomerase I. A study of 355 patients. Arthritis Rheum 31:378, 1988.
153. Akimoto S, Ishikawa O, Takagi H, Miyachi Y: Immunological features of patients with primary biliary cirrhosis (PBC) overlapping systemic sclerosis: a comparison with patients with PBC alone. J Gastroenterol Hepatol 13:897, 1998.
154. Tubach F, Hayem G, Elias A, et al: Anticentromere antibodies in rheumatologic practice are not consistently associated with scleroderma. Rev Rhum Engl Ed 64:362, 1997.
155. Pommier Y: Diversity of DNA topoisomerases I and inhibitors. Biochimie 80:255, 1998.
156. Hildebrandt S, Weiner ES, Senecal JL, et al: Autoantibodies to topoisomerase I (Scl-70): analysis by gel diffusion, immunoblot, and enzyme-linked immunosorbent assay. Clin Immunol Immunopathol 57:399, 1990.
157. Steen VD, Powell DL, Medsger TA, Jr.: Clinical correlations and prognosis based on serum autoantibodies in patients with systemic sclerosis. Arthritis Rheum 31:196, 1988.
158. Murata I, Takenaka K, Shinohara S, et al: Diversity of myocardial involvement in systemic sclerosis: an 8-year study of 95 Japanese patients. Am Heart J 135:960, 1998.
159. Dick T, Mierau R, Bartz-Bazzanella P, et al: Coexistence of antitopoisomerase I and anticentromere antibodies in patients with systemic sclerosis. Ann Rheum Dis 61:121, 2002.
160. Kuwana M, Kaburaki J, Mimori T, et al: Autoantibody reactive with three classes of RNA polymerases in sera from patients with systemic sclerosis. J Clin Invest 91:1399, 1993.
161. Phan TG, Cass A, Gillin A, et al: Anti-RNA polymerase III antibodies in the diagnosis of scleroderma renal crisis sine scleroderma. J Rheum 26:2489, 1999.
162. Dragon F, Gallagher JE, Compagnone-Post PA, et al: A large nucleolar U3 ribonucleoprotein required for 18S ribosomal RNA biogenesis. Nature 417:967, 2002.
163. Tormey VJ, Bunn CC, Denton CP, Black CM: Anti-fibrillarin antibodies in systemic sclerosis. Rheumatology (Oxford) 40:1157, 2001.
164. Yimane K, Ihn H, Kubo M, et al: Anti-U3 snRNP antibodies in localised scleroderma. Ann Rheum Dis 60:1157, 2001.
165. Larsen AK, Skladanowski A, Bojanowski K: The roles of DNA topoisomerase II during the cell cycle. Prog Cell Cycle Res 2:229, 1996.
166. Grigolo B, Mazzetti I, Meliconi R, et al: Anti-topoisomerase II alpha autoantibodies in systemic sclerosis-association with pulmonary hypertension and HLA-B35. Clin Exp Immunol 121:539, 2000.
167. Yamauchi Y, Nojima T, Shirai Y, et al: Molecular Cloning of the Wa Autoantigen and Clinical Features of Anti-Wa Autoantibodies [Abstract]. Arthritis Rheum 46:S130, 2002.
168. Lindahl L, Zengel JM: RNase MRP and rRNA processing. Mol Biol Rep 22:69, 1995.
169. Okano Y, Medsger TA Jr.: Autoantibody to Th ribonucleoprotein (nucleolar 7-2 RNA protein particle) in patients with systemic sclerosis. Arthritis Rheum 33:1822, 1990.
170. Falkner D, Wilson J, Medsger TA Jr., Morel PA: HLA and clinical associations in systemic sclerosis patients with anti-Th/To antibodies. Arthritis Rheum 41:74, 1998.
171. Yamane K, Ihn H, Kubo M, et al: Antibodies to Th/To ribonucleoprotein in patients with localized scleroderma. Rheumatology (Oxford) 40:683, 2001.
172. Ochs RL, Lischwe MA, Shen E, et al: Nucleologenesis: composition and fate of prenucleolar bodies. Chromosoma 92:330, 1985.
173. Chan EK, Imai H, Hamel JC, Tan EM: Human autoantibody to RNA polymerase I transcription factor hUBF. Molecular identity of nucleolus organizer region autoantigen NOR-90 and ribosomal RNA transcription upstream binding factor. J Exp Med 174:1239, 1991.
174. Imai H, Fritzler MJ, Neri R, et al: Immunocytochemical characterization of human NOR-90 (upstream binding factor) and associated antigens reactive with autoimmune sera. Two MR forms of NOR-90/hUBF autoantigens. Mol Biol Rep 19:115, 1994.
175. Fujii T, Mimori T, Akizuki M: Detection of autoantibodies to nucleolar transcription factor NOR 90/hUBF in sera of patients with rheumatic diseases, by recombinant autoantigen-based assays. Arthritis Rheum 39:1313, 1996.
176. Whitehead CM, Fritzler MJ, Rattner JB: The relationship of ASE-1 and NOR-90 in autoimmune sera. J Rheum 25:2126, 1998.
177. Brouwer R, Pruijn GJ, van Venrooij WJ: The human exosome: an autoantigenic complex of exoribonucleases in myositis and scleroderma. Arthritis Res 3:102, 2001.
178. Oddis CV, Okano Y, Rudert WA, et al: Serum autoantibody to the nucleolar antigen PM-Scl. Clinical and immunogenetic associations. Arthritis Rheum 35:1211, 1992.
179. Hausmanowa-Petrusewicz I, Kowalska-Oledzka E, Miller FW, et al: Clinical, serologic, and immunogenetic features in Polish patients with idiopathic inflammatory myopathies. Arthritis Rheum 40:1257, 1997.
180. Marguerie C, Bunn CC, Copier J, et al: The clinical and immunogenetic features of patients with autoantibodies to the nucleolar antigen PM-Scl. Medicine 71:327, 1992.
181. Reimer G, Steen VD, Penning CA, et al: Correlates between autoantibodies to nucleolar antigens and clinical features in patients with systemic sclerosis (scleroderma). Arthritis Rheum 31:525, 1988.
182. Satoh M, Akizuki M, Kuwana M, et al: Genetic and immunological differences between Japanese patients with diffuse scleroderma and limited scleroderma. J Rheum 21:111, 1994.
183. Li XZ, McNeilage LJ, Whittingham S: Autoantibodies to the major nucleolar phosphoprotein B23 define a novel subset of patients with anticardiolipin antibodies. Arthritis Rheum 32:1165, 1989.
184. Ayer LM, Senecal JL, Martin L, et al: Antibodies to high mobility group proteins in systemic sclerosis. J Rheum 21:2071, 1994.
185. Cohen DE, Kaufman LD, Varma AA, et al: Anti-laminin autoantibodies in collagen vascular diseases: the use of adequate controls in studies of autoimmune responses to laminin. Ann Rheum Dis 53:191, 1994.
186. Parodi A, Puiatti P, Rebora A: Serological profiles as prognostic clues for progressive systemic scleroderma: the Italian experience. Dermatologica 183:15, 1991.
187. Sato S, Fujimoto M, Ihn H, Takehara K: Antibodies to centromere and centriole in scleroderma spectrum disorders. Dermatology 189:23, 1994.
188. Endo H, Hosono T, Kondo H: Antineutrophil cytoplasmic autoantibodies in 6 patients with renal failure and systemic sclerosis. J Rheum 21:864, 1994.
189. Miyachi K, Takano S, Mimori T, et al: A novel autoantibody reactive with a 48 kDa tRNA associated protein in patients with scleroderma. J Rheum 18:373, 1991.
190. Okano Y, Medsger TA, Jr.: Novel human autoantibodies reactive with 5'-terminal trimethylguanosine cap structures of U small nuclear RNA. J Immunol 149:1093, 1992.
191. Hietarinta M, Lassila O, Hietaharju A: Association of anti-U1RNP- and anti-Scl-70-antibodies with neurological manifestations in systemic sclerosis (scleroderma). Scand J Rheum 23:64, 1994.
192. Ihn H, Yamane K, Yazawa N, et al: Distribution and antigen specificity of anti-U1RNP antibodies in patients with systemic sclerosis. Clin Exp Immunol 117:383, 1999.

193. Yamane K, Ihn H, Kubo M, et al: Anti-U1RNP antibodies in patients with localized scieroderma. Arch Dermatol Res 293:455, 2001.
194. Okano Y, Medsger TA Jr.: Newly identified U4/U6 snRNP-binding proteins by serum autoantibodies from a patient with systemic sclerosis. J Immunol 146:535, 1991.
195. Gilliam AC, Steitz JA: Rare scleroderma autoantibodies to the U11 small nuclear ribonucleoprotein and to the trimethylguanosine cap of U small nuclear RNAs. Proc Natl Acad Sci U S A 90:6781, 1993.
196. Herrera-Esparza R, Avalos-Diaz E, Barbosa-Cisneros O: Anti-NuMA antibodies: an uncommon specificity in scleroderma sera. Rev Rhum Engl Ed 66:315, 1999.
197. Spain TA, Sun R, Gradzka M, et al: The transcriptional activator Sp1, a novel autoantigen. Arthritis Rheum 40:1085, 1997.
198. Love LA, Leff RL, Fraser DD, et al: A new approach to the classification of idiopathic inflammatory myopathy: myositis-specific autoantibodies define useful homogeneous patient groups. Medicine 70:360, 1991.
199. Reichlin M, Arnett FC Jr.: Multiplicity of antibodies in myositis sera. Arthritis Rheum 27:1150, 1984.
200. Targoff IN: Immune manifestations of inflammatory muscle disease. Rheum Dis Clin North Am 20:857, 1994.
201. Vazquez-Abad D, Rothfield NF: Sensitivity and specificity of anti-Jo-1 antibodies in autoimmune diseases with myositis. Arthritis Rheum 39:292, 1996.
202. Targoff IN: Autoantibodies to aminoacyl-transfer RNA synthetases for isoleucine and glycine. Two additional synthetases are antigenic in myositis. J Immunol 144:1737, 1990.
203. Plotz PH, Rider LG, Targoff IN, et al: NIH conference. Myositis: immunologic contributions to understanding cause, pathogenesis, and therapy. Ann Int Med 122:715, 1995.
204. Satoh M, Ajmani AK, Hirakata M, et al: Onset of polymyositis with autoantibodies to threonyl-tRNA synthetase during pregnancy. J Rheum 21:1564, 1994.
205. Hirakata M, Suwa A, Nagai S, et al: Anti-KS: identification of autoantibodies to asparaginyl-transfer RNA synthetase associated with interstitial lung disease. J Immunol 162:2315, 1999.
206. Bui N, Strub K: New insights into signal recognition and elongation arrest activities of the signal recognition particle. Biol Chem 380:135, 1999.
207. Zhang Y, LeRoy G, Seelig HP, et al: The dermatomyositis-specific autoantigen Mi2 is a component of a complex containing histone deacetylase and nucleosome remodeling activities. Cell 95:279, 1998.
208. Kim J, Sif S, Jones B, et al: Ikaros DNA-binding proteins direct formation of chromatin remodeling complexes in lymphocytes. Immunity 10:345, 1999.
209. Brehm A, Nielsen SJ, Miska EA, et al: The E7 oncoprotein associates with Mi2 and histone deacetylase activity to promote cell growth. EMBO J 18:2449, 1999.
210. Nilasena DS, Trieu EP, Targoff IN: Analysis of the Mi-2 autoantigen of dermatomyositis. Arthritis Rheum 38:123, 1995.
211. Targoff IN, Nilasena DS, Trieu EP, al. e: Clinical features and immunologic testing of patients with anti-Mi-2 antibodies [abstract]. Arthritis Rheum 33:S72, 1990.
212. Gelpi C, Sontheimer EJ, Rodriguez-Sanchez JL: Autoantibodies against a serine tRNA-protein complex implicated in cotranslational selenocysteine insertion. Proc Natl Acad Sci U S A 89:9739, 1992.
213. Brouwer R, Hengstman GJ, Vree Egberts W, et al: Autoantibody profiles in the sera of European patients with myositis. Ann Rheum Dis 60:116, 2001.
214. Lundberg I, Nennesmo I, Hedfors E: A clinical, serological, and histopathological study of myositis patients with and without anti-RNP antibodies. Sem Arth Rheum 22:127, 1992.
215. Hirakata M, Mimori T, Akizuki M, et al: Autoantibodies to small nuclear and cytoplasmic ribonucleoproteins in Japanese patients with inflammatory muscle disease. Arthritis Rheum 35:449, 1992.
216. Okano Y, Steen VD, Medsger TA, Jr.: Autoantibody to U3 nucleolar ribonucleoprotein (fibrillarin) in patients with systemic sclerosis. Arthritis Rheum 35:95, 1992.
217. Targoff IN, Arnett FC, Berman L, et al: Anti-KJ: a new antibody associated with the syndrome of polymyositis and interstitial lung disease. J Clin Invest 84:162, 1989.
218. Targoff IN, Hanas J: The polymyositis-associated Fer antigen is elongation factor 1a [Abstract]. Arthritis Rheum 32:S81, 1989.
219. Frank MB, McCubbin V, Trieu E, et al: The association of anti-Ro52 autoantibodies with myositis and scleroderma autoantibodies. J Autoimmun 12:137, 1999.
220. Kubo M, Ihn H, Kuwana M, et al: Prevalence in myositis of antibodies recognizing anti-U3 RNA probably in a novel complex with 22/25 kD protein and not fibrillarin. Clin Exp Immunol 126:339, 2001.
221. Jarjour WN, Jeffries BD, Davis JSt, et al: Autoantibodies to human stress proteins. A survey of various rheumatic and other inflammatory diseases. Arthritis Rheum 34:1133, 1991.
222. Appelboom T, Kahn MF, Mairesse N: Anti-73 kDa heat shock protein (hsp 73) in mixed connective tisue disease (MCTD) (abstract). Arthritis Rheum 36:S252, 1993.
223. Harley JB, Alexander EL, Bias WB, et al: Anti-Ro (SS-A) and anti-La (SS-B) in patients with Sjogren's syndrome. Arthritis Rheum 29:196, 1986.
224. Alexander EL, Ranzenbach MR, Kumar AJ, et al: Anti-Ro(SS-A) autoantibodies in central nervous system disease associated with Sjogren's syndrome (CNS-SS): clinical, neuroimaging, and angiographic correlates. Neurology 44:899, 1994.
225. Molina R, Provost TT, Alexander EL: Two types of inflammatory vascular disease in Sjogren's syndrome. Differential association with seroreactivity to rheumatoid factor and antibodies to Ro (SS-A) and with hypocomplementemia. Arthritis Rheum 28:1251, 1985.
226. Tsuzaka K, Fujii T, Akizuki M, et al: Clinical significance of antibodies to native or denatured 60-kd or 52-kd Ro/SS-A proteins in Sjogren's syndrome. Arthritis Rheum 37:88, 1994.
227. Tsuzaka K, Ogasawara T, Tojo T, et al: Relationship between autoantibodies and clinical parameters in Sjogren's syndrome. Scand J Rheum 22:1, 1993.
228. Nakken B, Jonsson R, Bolstad AI: Polymorphisms of the Ro52 gene associated with anti-Ro 52-kd autoantibodies in patients with primary Sjogren's syndrome. Arthritis Rheum 44:638, 2001.
229. Nakano M, Nogami S, Sato S, et al: Interaction of syntaxin with a-fodrin, a major component of the submembranous cytoskeleton. Biochem Biophys Res Commun 288:468, 2001.
230. Perrin D, Aunis D: Reorganization of a-fodrin induced by stimulation in secretory cells. Nature 315:589, 1985.
231. Nagaraju K, Cox A, Casciola-Rosen L, Rosen A: Novel fragments of the Sjogren's syndrome autoantigens a-fodrin and type 3 muscarinic acetylcholine receptor generated during cytotoxic lymphocyte granule-induced cell death. Arthritis Rheum 44:2376, 2001.
232. Haneji N, Nakamura T, Takio K, et al: Identification of a-fodrin as a candidate autoantigen in primary Sjogren's syndrome. Science 276:604, 1997.
233. Watanabe T, Tsuchida T, Kanda N, et al: Anti-a-fodrin antibodies in Sjogren syndrome and lupus erythematosus. Arch Derm 135:535, 1999.
234. Witte T, Matthias T, Arnett FC, et al: IgA and IgG autoantibodies against a-fodrin as markers for Sjogren's syndrome. Systemic lupus erythematosus. J Rheum 27:2617, 2000.
235. Kobayashi I, Kawamura N, Okano M, et al: Anti-a-fodrin autoantibody is an early diagnostic marker for childhood primary Sjogren's syndrome. J Rheum 28:363, 2001.
236. Maeno N, Takei S, Imanaka H, et al: Anti-a-fodrin antibodies in Sjogren's syndrome in children. J Rheum 28:860, 2001.
237. Kuwana M, Okano T, Ogawa Y, et al: Autoantibodies to the amino-terminal fragment of b-fodrin expressed in glandular epithelial cells in patients with Sjogren's syndrome. J Immunol 167:5449, 2001.
238. Yang CH, Lambie EJ, Snyder M: NuMA: an unusually long coiled-coil related protein in the mammalian nucleus. J Cell Biol 116:1303, 1992.
239. Hebert MD, Szymczyk PW, Shpargel KB, Matera AG: Coilin forms the bridge between Cajal bodies and SMN, the spinal muscular atrophy protein. Genes Dev 15:2720, 2001.
240. Tucker KE, Berciano MT, Jacobs EY, et al: Residual Cajal bodies in coilin knockout mice fail to recruit Sm snRNPs and SMN, the spinal muscular atrophy gene product. J Cell Biol 154:293, 2001.
241. Fujimoto M, Kikuchi K, Tamaki T, et al: Distribution of anti-p80-coilin autoantibody in collagen diseases and various skin diseases. Br J Derm 137:916, 1997.

242. Onouchi H, Muro Y, Tomita Y: Clinical features and IgG subclass distribution of anti-p80 coilin antibodies. J Autoimmun 13:225, 1999.
243. Katano K, Kawano M, Koni I, et al: Clinical and laboratory features of anticentromere antibody positive primary Sjogren's syndrome. J Rheum 28:2238, 2001.
244. Fukase S, Ohta N, Inamura K, et al: Diagnostic specificity of antineutrophil cytoplasmic antibodies (ANCA) in otorhinolaryngological diseases. Acta Otolaryngol (Stockholm) 511(Suppl):204, 1994.
245. Font J, Ramos-Casals M, Cervera R, et al: Antineutrophil cytoplasmic antibodies in primary Sjogren's syndrome: prevalence and clinical significance. Br J Rheum 37:1287, 1998.
246. Nishiya K, Chikazawa H, Hashimoto K, Miyawaki S: Antineutrophil cytoplasmic antibody in patients with primary Sjogren's syndrome. Clin Rheumatol 18:268, 1999.
247. Skopouli FN, Barbatis C, Moutsopoulos HM: Liver involvement in primary Sjogren's syndrome. Br J Rheum 33:745, 1994.
248. Fujii T, Mimori T, Hama N, et al: Characterization of autoantibodies that recognize U4/U6 small ribonucleoprotein particles in serum from a patient with primary Sjogren's syndrome. J Biol Chem 267:16412, 1992.
249. Kooy J, Toh BH, Pettitt JM, et al: Human autoantibodies as reagents to conserved Golgi components. Characterization of a peripheral, 230-kDa compartment-specific Golgi protein. J Biol Chem 267:20255, 1992.
250. Feist E, Kuckelkorn U, Dorner T, et al: Autoantibodies in primary Sjogren's syndrome are directed against proteasomal subunits of the a and b type. Arthritis Rheum 42:697, 1999.
251. Wang D, Buyon JP, Zhu W, Chan EK: Defining a novel 75-kDa phosphoprotein associated with SS-A/Ro and identification of distinct human autoantibodies. J Clin Invest 104:1265, 1999.
252. Maddison PJ: Mixed connective tissue disease: overlap syndromes. Baillieres Best Pract Res Clin Rheumatol 14:111, 2000.
253. Smolen JS, Steiner G: Mixed connective tissue disease: to be or not to be? Arthritis Rheum 41:768, 1998.
254. Nimelstein SH, Brody S, McShane D, Holman HR: Mixed connective tissue disease: a subsequent evaluation of the original 25 patients. Medicine 59:239, 1980.
255. van den Hoogen FH, Spronk PE, Boerbooms AM, et al: Long-term follow-up of 46 patients with anti-(U1)snRNP antibodies. Br J Rheum 33:1117, 1994.
256. Kallenberg CG, Wouda AA, Hoet MH, van Venrooij WJ: Development of connective tissue disease in patients presenting with Raynaud's phenomenon: a six year follow up with emphasis on the predictive value of antinuclear antibodies as detected by immunoblotting. Ann Rheum Dis 47:634, 1988.
257. Spencer-Green G: Outcomes in primary Raynaud phenomenon: a meta-analysis of the frequency, rates, and predictors of transition to secondary diseases. Arch Intern Med 158:595, 1998.
258. Moore TL, Osborn TG, Weiss TD, et al: Autoantibodies in juvenile arthritis. Sem Arth Rheum 13:329, 1984.
259. Rosenberg AM, Romanchuk KG: Antinuclear antibodies in arthritic and nonarthritic children with uveitis. J Rheum 17:60, 1990.
260. Manzotti F, Orsoni JG, Zavota L, et al: Autoimmune uveitis in children: clinical correlation between antinuclear antibody positivity and ocular recurrences. Rheumatol Int 21:127, 2002.
261. Petri M: Diagnosis of antiphospholipid antibodies. Rheum Dis Clin North Am 20:443, 1994.
262. Garber ME, Mohr BW, Calabrese LH: Henoch-Schonlein purpura associated with anti-Ro (SSA) and antiphospholipid antibody syndrome. J Rheum 20:1964, 1993.
263. Lawrence JM, Moore TL, Osborn TG, et al: Autoantibody studies in juvenile rheumatoid arthritis. Sem Arth Rheum 22:265, 1993.
264. Piette JC, El-Rassi R, Amoura Z: Antinuclear antibodies in relapsing polychondritis. Ann Rheum Dis 58:656, 1999.
265. Weinberg I, Vasiliev L, Gotsman I: Anti-dsDNA antibodies in sarcoidosis. Sem Arth Rheum 29:328, 2000.
266. Barned S, Goodman AD, Mattson DH: Frequency of anti-nuclear antibodies in multiple sclerosis. Neurology 45:384, 1995.
267. Lindsey JW, Albers GW, Steinman L: Recurrent transverse myelitis, myasthenia gravis, and autoantibodies. Ann Neurol 32:407, 1992.
268. Folwaczny C, Noehl N, Endres SP, et al: Antinuclear autoantibodies in patients with inflammatory bowel disease. High prevalence in first-degree relatives. Dig Dis Sci 42:1593, 1997.
269. Mackay IR: Antinuclear (chromatin) autoantibodies in autoimmune hepatitis. J Gastroenterol Hepatol 16:245, 2001.
270. Ochs RL, Stein TW, Jr., Peebles CL, et al: Autoantibodies in interstitial cystitis. J Urol 151:587, 1994.
271. Morita S, Arima T, Matsuda M: Prevalence of nonthyroid specific autoantibodies in autoimmune thyroid diseases. J Clin Endo Metab 80:1203, 1995.
272. Gutierrez A, Chinchilla V, Espasa A, Perez-Mateo M: Transient detection of antinuclear and anti-smooth muscle antibodies in hepatitis A virus infection. Am J Gastroenterol 90:171, 1995.
273. Peng YC, Hsieh SC, Yang DY, et al: Expression and clinical significance of antinuclear antibody in hepatitis C virus infection. J Clin Gastroenterol 33:402, 2001.
274. Garcia-De La Torre I: Autoimmune phenomena in leprosy, particularly antinuclear antibodies and rheumatoid factor. J Rheum 20:900, 1993.
275. Sirota P, Firer MA, Schild K, et al: Autoantibodies to DNA in multicase families with schizophrenia. Biol Psych 33:450, 1993.
276. Morshed SA, Parveen S, Leckman JF, et al: Antibodies against neural, nuclear, cytoskeletal, and streptococcal epitopes in children and adults with Tourette's syndrome, Sydenham's chorea, and autoimmune disorders. Biol Psych 50:566, 2001.
277. Mecocci P, Ekman R, Parnetti L, Senin U: Antihistone and anti-dsDNA autoantibodies in Alzheimer's disease and vascular dementia. Biol Psych 34:380, 1993.
278. Kiss M, Husz S, Dobozy A: The occurrence of antinuclear, anti-SSA/Ro and anti-SSB/La antibodies in patients with polymorphous light eruption. Acta Derm Venereol 71:341, 1991.
279. Carrizosa AM, Elorza FL, Camacho FM: Antinuclear antibodies in patients with lichen planus. Exp Derm 6:54, 1997.
280. Taniguchi Y, Yamakami A, Sakamoto T, et al: Positive antinuclear antibody in atopic dermatitis. Acta Derm Venereol 176:62, 1992.
281. Imai H, Nakano Y, Kiyosawa K, Tan EM: Increasing titers and changing specificities of antinuclear antibodies in patients with chronic liver disease who develop hepatocellular carcinoma. Cancer 71:26, 1993.
282. Grainger DJ, Bethell HW: High titres of serum antinuclear antibodies, mostly directed against nucleolar antigens, are associated with the presence of coronary atherosclerosis. Ann Rheum Dis 61:110, 2002.
283. Peltola JT, Haapala A, Isojarvi JI, et al: Antiphospholipid and antinuclear antibodies in patients with epilepsy or new-onset seizure disorders. Am J Med 109:712, 2000.
284. Papadaki HA, Psyllaki M, Eliopoulos DG, et al: Increased frequency and specific reactivity of serum antinuclear antibodies in patients with nonimmune chronic idiopathic neutropenia of adults. Acta Haematol 105:13, 2001.
285. Bridges AJ: Autoantibodies in patients with silicone implants. Sem Arth Rheum 24:54, 1994.
286. Schrallhammer-Benkler K, Ring J, Przybilla B, et al: Acute mercury intoxication with lichenoid drug eruption followed by mercury contact allergy and development of antinuclear antibodies. Acta Derm Venereol 72:294, 1992.
287. Varga J, Maul GG, Jimenez SA: Autoantibodies to nuclear lamin C in the eosinophilia-myalgia syndrome associated with L-tryptophan ingestion. Arthritis Rheum 35:106, 1992.
288. Kiuttu J, Hartikainen-Sorri AL, Makitalo R: Occurrence of antinuclear antibodies in an unselected pregnancy population. Gyn Obst Invest 33:21, 1992.
289. Illei GG, Klippel JH: Why is the ANA result positive? Bull Rheum Dis 48:1, 1999.

21 Immune Complexes

URS E. NYDEGGER

The close encounter between antigen and antibody has been studied for many decades, but scientists have not yet reached completion in their knowledge—and perhaps never will. On one hand, novel antigens will appear, some known ones will change, and not all the currently known, clinically important ones will remain the same. On the other hand, the polyclonal antibody synthesis destined to interact with antigen is subject to interindividual and antigen-dependent diversity. In addition to immunoglobulins, both the T cell receptor and the major histocompatibility complex (MHC) are further examples of specific antigen-binding molecular types that bind peptides only, whereas antibodies often bind three-dimensional structures that been instructed by the immunizing antigens, including proteins, lipids, and polysaccarides. All antibody molecules share the same basic structural characteristics but display remarkable variability in the regions that bind antigens, due to continually better-understood pathways in immunoglobulin-specific modification reactions, such as somatic hypermutation, class-switch recombination, and gene conversion.[1,2]

The classic model of serum sickness, which was extensively studied in the last century in laboratory animals, set the stage for elucidation of human immune complex diseases, which emerged as a broad spectrum of disparate clinical entities. We now know that low levels of transient circulating immune complexes represent a healthy reaction of the organism against invasive antigens, and that higher concentrations of chronically circulating immune complexes lead to overflow of removal capacity and ensuing tissue deposition. Such types of immune complex diseases, due to local formation of such complexes, require adequate therapy. Engagements of humoral and cellular receptors and of complement determine the severity of immune complex diseases, and knowledge of their functional capacity allows for adapting of therapeutic strategy.

Physicochemical Properties

The binding of any antigen to antibodies occurs on the basis of electrostatic forces that cause exclusion of cations from the interface site. On the antigen, this site is the epitope, and on the antibody it is the cleft at the N-terminus of the variable portions of the light and heavy chains. Intermolecular attractions of electrical nature (van der Waals forces) hold the two together, and the absence of covalent bonding makes the antigen-antibody handshake a dynamic process equilibrium, which follows the binding constant:

$$K = \frac{[AbAg]}{[Ab]\ [Ag]}$$

where Ab represents free antibody sites, Ag the free antigen, and AbAg the antibody-antigen complex. Temperature, concentrations of Ab and Ag, and pH conditions influence the overall affinity. An association constant can be measured using two chambers on either side of a semipermeable membrane with a tracer-labeled antigen in known concentration on one side and the antibody with known concentration on the other, allowing them to interact with defined conditions. Such a simple approach is not suitable for the study of the reaction between antibody and multivalent antigen. One monoclonal antibody molecule, immunoglobulin G (IgG), has two identical combining sites and can combine with two separate homologous hapten molecules (Fig. 21–1). Recent procedures include flow-enzyme systems with immobilizing biotinylated antigens on streptavidin-coated sensor chips.[3] The quantity of the complex on the surface of the flow cell is monitored by measurement intensity of chemiluminiscence. Such an approach is attractive, bearing the potential to more precisely estimate the interaction of specific cell-surface antibody with antigen on carrier cells. Other approaches focus on the multivalency of the binding reactions using immunoaffinity electrophoresis, which allows the study of valence.[4] The size of the complexes goes from a 150-kD starting point to macromolecular complexes arranged in a three-dimensional lattice that are almost visible with the naked eye. The three-dimensional structure of such a lattice depends on the antigen, the isotype of the antibody, the antigen/antibody ratio, and the clonality of the immune response, and it might be represented by a fractal-type repeating pattern, as was recently proposed in the context of chaos theory.[5] Quite often, the valence of the antigen is so great that several thousand epitopes are united on a single-cell carrier, bacterium, or virus. Such complexes then acquire the dimension of visible agglutinates/multicellular congregations in vivo or in vitro during analytic testing. In the hemagglutination system, this phenomenon is referred to as prozone and postzone phenomenona. Equally important, the complex's size is determined by the ratio of antigen to antibody (Fig. 21–2). For every antigen/antibody system, this ratio also determines complement-activating capacity and the removal properties of circulating immune complexes. In any event, the in vitro addition of antibody to a fixed amount of antigen, or vice versa, will lead to formation of a lattice structure. Very small antigens, such as glycosaminoglycans or oligosaccharides,

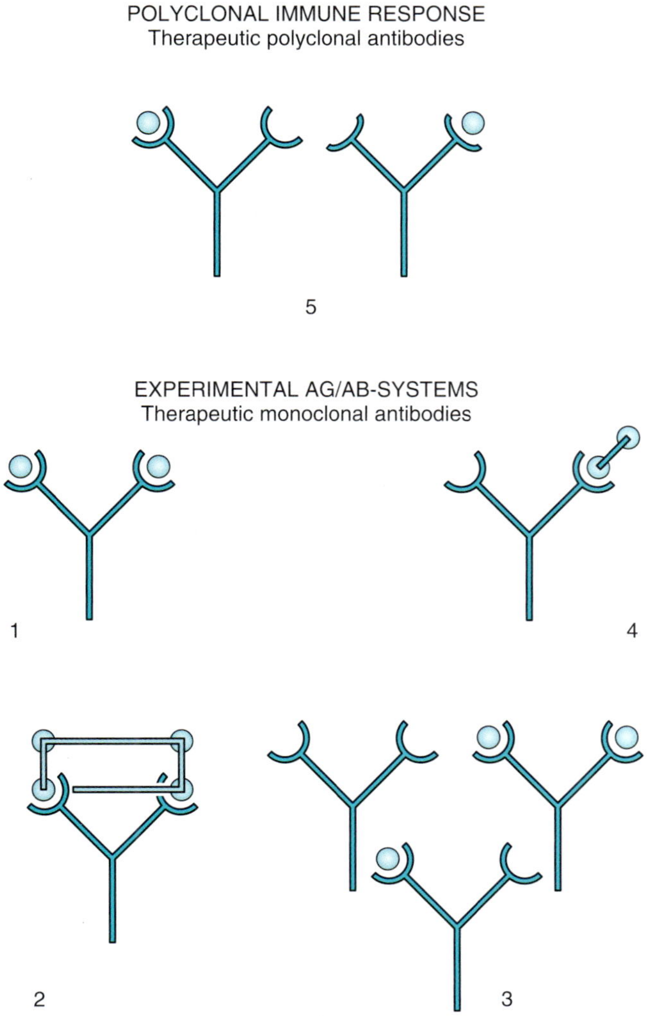

FIGURE 21–1 · **The Antigen-Antibody Interaction on a Molecular Level.** Interaction of monoclonal (**1-4**) and polyclonal (**5**) antibodies with haptens or epitopes. *1*, Both Fab portions of a monoclonal antibody bind a small, soluble antigen with an Ag_2Ab relationship. *2*, The same antibody type binds to homopolymeric antigen (an antigen carrier that bears multiple identical epitopes). *3*, Cooperativity of two binding sites of divalent mAb are shown with the examples of unoccupied (*Ab*), singly occupied (*AgAb*), and doubly occupied ($Ag_2 Ab$) form. Assumption of fast dissociation rates K_{off} is made, in part from,[4] with extensions. Ab, antibody; Ag, antigen.

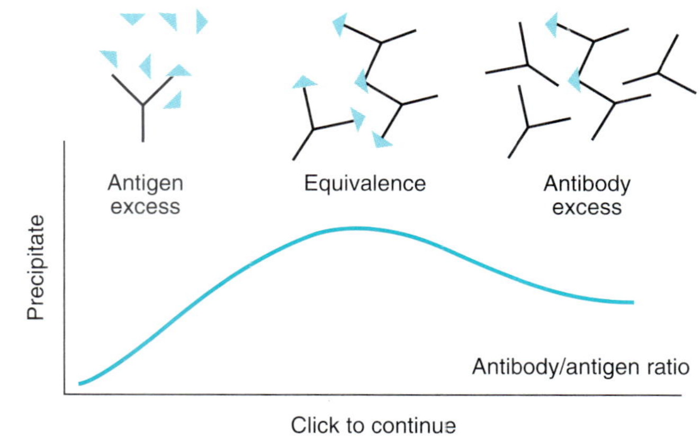

FIGURE 21–2 · **Importance of Antigen/Antibody Ratio in Immune Complexes.** Addition of incremental amounts of antibody to equal amounts of antigen shifts antigen/antibody ratio to from antigen to antibody excess, passing through equivalence. During in vitro experiments, after 1 hour at 37°C and overnight at 2° to 6°C, such samples may precipitate with trichloroacetic acid, and quantitative estimation of proteins in the precipitate follows the pattern of the bell-shaped curve. (From the Macromedia Flash presentation at *www.immune-complex.unibe.ch* and *www.immunecomplex.cu.)*

might do nothing other than neutralize the antibodies without being able to induce lattice formation; whether neutralized antibodies will form a lattice is to be determined for every system.

The presence of complement near circulating or locally formed immune complexes contributes to the physicochemical properties. Sufficient complement at the outset of antigen/antibody interaction prevents formation of sizeable lattice or, once formed, complexes added to fresh serum with complement might bring insoluble complexes into solution again.[6,7] The temperature dependency of physicochemical properties of circulating immune complexes is best understood in the example of cryoglobulins, which are complexes that precipitate at cooler temperatures in serum and plasma stored between 2° and 6°C. The physicochemical property that underlies this phenomenon is still poorly understood. A similar situation occurs with cryofibrinogen as well, but part of the question may be answered as the carbohydrate composition of the involved proteins is better known; thus, glycosylation of antibody molecules is now acknowledged as decisively influencing their physicochemical makeup. Rheumatoid factors display atypical glycosylation, a property that decisively determines some functional properties of antibody molecules.[8,9]

ANTIBODY ACTIVITY OF IGG SUBCLASSES IN IMMUNE COMPLEXES

The IgG subclass distribution in specific antibody responses has been found to vary with the structure of the antigen (nature of the carrier, number and composition of the epitopes, physicochemical properties), its dose and route of entry, and with the genetic constitution of the host. In contrast to T cell–independent (thymus-independent) antigens, T cell–dependent antigens do require interaction with helper T lymphocytes to stimulate B lymphocytes to antibody production. Stimulation of antibody responses toward certain antigens may result in a selective increase in IgG antibodies of certain subclasses. IgG_1 and IgG_3 are the prevailing isotypes against bacterial and viral protein antigens, such as tetanus toxoid or outer-membrane components (e.g., T cell–dependent antigen); antibodies of the IgG_2 subclass often provide only a marginal contribution. In contrast, IgG antibodies against polysaccharide antigens, generally T cell–independent, show a much more pronounced subclass distribution. Immunization with several encapsulated bacteria (*Neisseria meningitidis, Haemophilus influenzae*, and *Streptococcus pneumoniae*) leads to an almost exclusive IgG_2 antipolysaccharide response. An exception is seen in children under the age of 2 or 3 years, as their antipolysaccharide antibodies have been found to be of the IgG_1 subclass. Patients with hemophilia who are regularly treated with clotting factor VIII develop antibodies against the administered proteins, which are mostly of the IgG_4 subclass. In general, antiviral IgG antibodies are highly restricted to IgG_1 and IgG_3, with IgG_3 appearing first during the course of infection. Whereas the antigen-binding capacity of the four subclasses is roughly the same, their complement-activation capacities differ, such that the poorly complement-activating IgG_3 will form larger immune-complex lattices because complement will poorly solubilize them.

Physiologic Necessity

INTERACTION OF IMMUNE COMPLEXES WITH THE CELL-RECEPTOR NETWORK

The binding of specific proteins to their cognate receptors in cell plasma membranes has broad biologic significance. With immune complexes, receptor-mediated functions are manifold; they include 1) their transport from one site to another, 2) endocytosis followed by digestion, and 3) induction of specific effector functions of the receptor carrier cell. The performance of the receptor network that is able to interact with immune complexes plays a decisive role in their handling by the cellular immune system. Decoration of the lattice with complement components C4b or, more importantly, with C3b,[10] provides for an interface with complement-receptor expressing cells (Table 21–1). These receptors thus serve to link humoral immune responses with cellular effector mechanisms.

The receptor network recognizes cross-linked fragment crystallizable (Fc) portions or complement on the complexes (Fig. 21–3), and the cognate components remain attached to the receptor-bearing cell where the complex can experience several fates: It may share the destiny of the receptor-bearing cell; when bound to red blood cells carrying CR1, immune complexes are carried throughout the body and remain trapped in the reticuloendothelial system (RES) of liver, spleen, or both (see later discussion). Complement-decorated complexes or cell surfaces decorated with complement deposited on the cell-bound complexes, as in cold agglutinin disease,[11] will predominantly remain in the RES of the liver, whereas IgG-composed complexes, decorated with complement or not, are largely cleared by the spleen.

Soluble Fcγ receptors, equivalents of IgG-binding factors, can be identified in serum-free supernatants of T cells, and they may play a role in the regulation of immune complex–mediated activation of phagocytes and platelets. This becomes evident when an intradermal injection of sFcγRII mixed with rabbit antiovalbu-

TABLE 21–1 • THE IMMUNE COMPLEX EFFECTOR-CELL RECEPTOR SYSTEM

Ligand Specificity	Cluster of Differentiation Nomenlature	Effector-Cell Carrier	Characteristic of Cluster of Differentiation Molecule	Functional Consequence of Ligand Binding	Role in Immune-Complex Handling
I. Fc Receptors					
FcγRIIIa, gp50-65	16	NK, G, Mac	Low-affinity receptor for complexed IgG	Mediate neutrophil cytolysis	Trigger phagocytosis and ADCC
FcγRII, gp40	32	M, G, B, Eo	6 isoforms originating from splicing of three genes on ch1	Low affinity for IgG, bind immune complexes only (ITAM and ITIM)	Enhancement or inhibition
FcγRI, gp75	64	M, G act	6 potential sites for *N*-linked glycosylation	Occupied by IgG under physiologic conditions	Phagocytic signaling
FcαR, gp 55-70	89	G, M, DC, smooth muscle cells		Occupied by IgA under physiologic conditions	Important in the mucosal immune response
II. Complement Receptors					
C3b/C4b complement receptor (CR) 1	35	G, M, B, some T/NK		C3b-decorating immune-complex lattices bind loosely and briefly (approximately 2 min)	Transport of immune complexes, mainly on red blood cells
CR3: iC3b receptor	11b/18	M, G, NK, T sub	β2-Integrin member		
CR4	11c/18	M, G, NK, B sub, T sub	β2-Integrin member		
Decay-accelerating factor (DAF)	75	Broad	Prevents complement activation on the cell surface	Locally downregulates complement activation	Increases mobility in the membrane facilitating apical targeting

Abbreviations: Act, Activated; ADCC, antibody dependent cellular cytotoxicity; B, B cells; Eo, eosinophilic G; G, granulocytes; ITAM, immunoreceptor tyrosine-based activation motif; ITIM, immunoreceptor typosine-based inhibition motif; M, monocytes; Mac, macrophage; NK, natural killer.

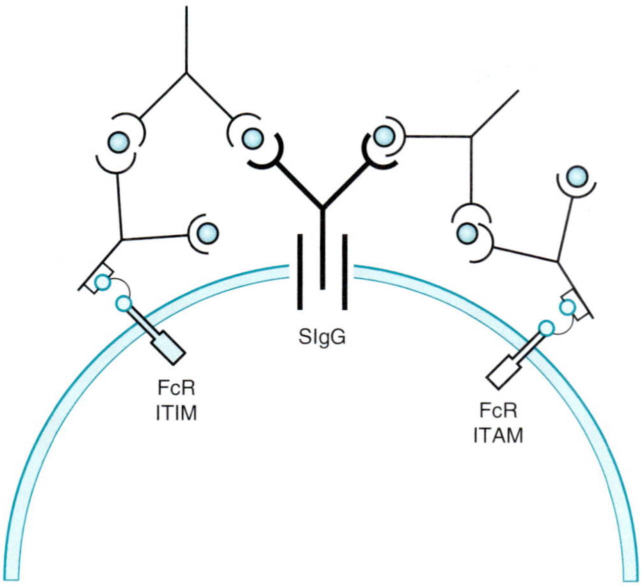

FIGURE 21–3 · B Cell Receptor Coligation by Immune Complexes. When immune complexes assemble on Fc receptor-bearing cells (FcR) that simultaneously express surface IgG, a portion of the antigen is bound by IgG (SIgG, bold). Ligation of IgG Fc portions cross-linked within immune complexes to inhibitory FcγRBII (immunoreceptor tyrosine-based inhibitory motif [ITIM]) receptor is followed by reduction of Ca^{++} influx and cell proliferation. When ligation occurs to an immunoreceptor tyrosine-based activation motif (ITAM)-type FcR, the contrary occurs. On many cell clones both receptor types are expressed and the effect of either type prevailing is the subject of current research.

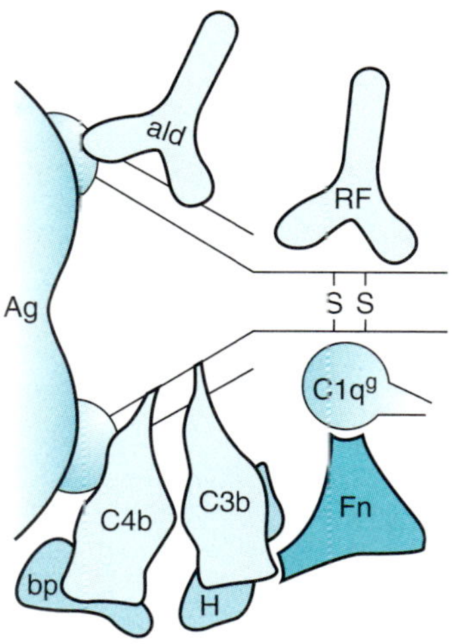

FIGURE 21–4 · Decoration of Immune Complexes with Humoral Bystanders. Once antigen (Ag) and antibody combine, a number of humoral bystanders assemble on the structure and might override physicochemical properties based on mere antigen/antibody ratio, temperature, molarity, and pH. Covalent ligation of C4b and C3b to the Fab portion of the heavy chains, assembly of C1q (one of the six heads of the macromolecule shown here), rheumatoid factor, and anti-idiotypic IgG are important modifiers of immune-complex properties. Fibronectin and histidine-rich glycoprotein (not shown) are further contenders.

min (OVA) antibodies—after an intravenous injection of OVA—inhibits vascular leakage in rats.[12]

The receptors relating to immune complexes listed in Table 21–1, are widely distributed. The immune-complex lattice expresses different possible ligands (Fig. 21–4) for numerous receptors on different cell types that bind to each other when proximity, concentration, pH, molarity, and affinity constants are optimal. One can determine the affinity constant of these receptors in vitro via Scatchard plots,[13] which relate the proportion of free to bound soluble immune-complex ligands. Similar to antigen-antibody interactions, the ligand-receptor interaction is noncovalent, and ligand might also dissociate from its receptor. A striking example of such reversible binding is C3b with immune complexes, which associates, then dissociates, from CR1 or red blood cells.

Immune Complex Transport

Migration of immune complexes from one site to another reflects their antigen-removing capacity from entry sites with consecutive systemic spreading. Both antigen and antibodies express their organ tropism (e.g., viruses that prefer the liver, such as hepatitis B virus, the heart and bone marrow, such as parvovirus P19, or the joints); these organs become damaged by excessive immune complexes not appropriately cleared. Antibodies contained in immune complexes follow a tropism determined by the receptor system, which can include the RES and lymphoid systems, but also circulating blood cells, such as lymphocytes, neutrophils,[14] mononuclear cells, and red blood cells. Immune-complex binding to mononuclear cells can lead to cell activation, such as super oxide production, activation of the pentose-shunt,[15] interleukin (IL)-6 release,[16] and thrombocytopenia due to platelets bearing FcR. In addition to occasionally causing immune hemolytic anemia, circulating immune complexes use red blood cells as carriers under physiologic conditions. They are endowed with transport receptors CR1 and CR3 and are ready to bind immune complexes anywhere on their passage[17] and discharge them in the RES.[18] Using time-lapse cameras, it was observed recently that the immune complexes are on the red blood cell surface for a short time (approximately 2 min) and then take 1 to 4 hours to be internalized by the Fc receptor–bearing macrophages.[19]

Endocytosis/Phagocytosis

The primary goal of immune complex formation lies in two-step (binding and ingestion) endocytosis (soluble antigens) or phagocytosis (particulate antigens) of the antigen-antibody complex. The Fc receptor apparatus on phagocytes, consisting of at least FcγRI (CD64), FcγRIIA (CD32), and FcγRIIIB (CD16), catches cross-linked Fc fragments. The attached antigens complexed to the Fab portion thus are pulled toward the cell surface where coated pits and clathrin-stabilized cell-surface organelles provide optimal ingestion of the whole complex by professional phagocytes, such as polymorphonuclear neutrophilic leukocytes, monocytes, and macrophages.[20]

The complement receptors CR3 and CD4 found on phagocytes have a low capacity to bind C3b-opsonized particles, but the binding capacity of polymorphonuclear leukocytes is rapidly upregulated during activation.

However, in rheumatic diseases, this receptor apparatus may be functionally deficient.

Induction of Effector Functions

The receptor apparatus engaged upon formation of immune complexes has been identified with the endocytosis/phagocytosis phenomenon described previously. Its involvement in the overall immune response as an additional major function has only emerged in recent years.[20,20b]

A complex interplay unfolds to augment the efficacy of our immune defense. It is a homeostatic system that should be perceived as analogous to the acid-base equilibrium or the cytokine network. Elucidation of single steps using specific knockout mice has led to revision of the significance of many receptor types. Two general classes of IgG Fc Rs are now recognized: the activation receptors displaying a cytoplasmic immunoreceptor tyrosine-based activation motif (ITAM) amino acid sequence and the inhibitory receptor with its immunoreceptor tyrosine-based inhibition motif (ITIM) sequence (see Fig. 21–3). The two classes function in concert and are often coexpressed, with coengagement of both signaling pathways being the rule.[21] Many of the ITIMs belong to the immunoglobulins superfamily (IgSF), which includes surface molecules such as CD5, CD22, and FcγIIR/CD32. The ITAM-based receptors, such as FcγRI, RIIA and IIIA, bind IgG with high affinity (R I: 10^{-9}) or with low affinity (RIIA and RIIIA: 10^{-6}, that is, free ligand concentration is higher in binding studies using scratchard plots); the ITIM-based RIIB interacts with low affinity at physiologic antibody concentrations, reflecting the low-grade constant, hence physiologic, engagement. The physiologic role of monomeric and low-grade particular form of immune-complexed IgG, even as small as dimers, cannot be underestimated because immune complexes help to present antigen to helper T cells, such as by follicular dendritic cells in germinal centers, but not in primary follicles expressing high levels of IgG Fc RIIB.[22] Logical consequence, underlined by experiments with Fc RIIB-deficient inbred DBA mouse strains, is loss of peripheral tolerance with emergence of autoantibodies, a finding validated for the rheumatologist with bovine type II collagen-induced arthritis in Fc RγIIB-deficient mice.[23] The dermatologic equivalent of such models is the Arthus reaction: Intradermally injected antibody triggers inflammation in antigen-primed animals. Locally formed immune complexes are the hallmark of the Arthus reaction, and complement activation attracts neutrophils that immediately induce inflammation. One question researchers could not answer for a long time is why fibrinogen is, in addition to Ig and complement, part of the abnormal deposits in early immune complex–mediated inflammatory sites. Now, release of tissue factor by immune complex–stimulated macrophages is a plausible explanation of this phenomenon.[24] Activation products of blood clotting (e.g., thrombin and fibrinopeptides) have various proinflammatory activities and are suggested to modulate inflammation. The macrophage expression of tissue factor has been shown to cause clotting at the site of the delayed-type hypersensitivity reaction, a cellular immune response. Tissue factor antigen was expressed on polymorphonulear neutrophilic leukocytes of Arthus infiltrates.[25]

An actual dermatologic Arthus model is autoimmune vitiligo, in which a membrane protein of melanocytes is targeted, resulting in autoimmune hypopigmentation, dependent on FcγR.[26] That such receptors also display importance in local immune-complex reactions, such as Arthus, becomes clear when IgG immune complexes trigger cutaneous reactions even in the absence of complement. Finally, FcγRIIb modulates the magnitude of the response with enhanced Arthus reactions observed in FcγRII-deficient mouse strains, with the effector cell being the mast cell.[21] Commercial intravenous immunoglobulin (IVIG) preparations, in such experimental systems, come to attenuate such reactions because they appease the low-affinity Fc receptor system.

What, then, is the reason complement components deposit in immune complex–induced inflammatory tissues, including joints? Complement is the most important humoral effector of immune complexes interacting simultaneously with the formation of (antigen-) complexed IgG. Whereas the 1980s were rich in discoveries of immune complex-complement interactions,[27] newer work has sought other proteins that interact with complexes, such as histidine-rich glycoproteins,[28] now known to also inhibit insoluble immune-complex formation. Not merely a reactive system engaged upon antigen-antibody encounter, complement may indeed actively counteract immune-complex deposition through engagement of downregulators of complement activation. A typical example would be the factor H–related proteins; during in vitro and in vivo models of complement activation on glomerular epithelial cells, factor H became upregulated three- to sixfold to ameliorate glomerular immune-complex diseases.[29] This is where the complement-receptor network must be considered more loosely. Early work has identified these receptors through their protective role for cells against complement activation. Ruddy's,[29a] Fearon's, and Nicholson Weller's[29b] work was pivotal and lead to the discovery of membrane proteins, specific for complement ligands, which were able to prevent assembly of or destroy membrane attack complexes. Although the interaction of FcγRs and complement remains to be fully elucidated (and for some remains controversial[30,31]), focus now centers on C5a and its receptor, C5aR. Pharmacologic inbition of C5aR has beneficial effects in tissue damage, ischemia/reperfusion injury, and sepsis,[32–34] which suggests that C5a-C5aR interaction is essential for the majority of complement-mediated inflammatory reactions. C5a anaphylatoxin has several tissue effects, such as vasodilatation, increased vascular permeability, and edema formation.

The interplay between FcγF and C5aR was recently studied.[35] This work quite clearly points to the functional interplay of C5a/C5aR with activating FcγRIII and inhibitory FcγRII receptor pair in vivo. In fact, C5a/C5aR induce FcγRIII and suppress FcγRII. Absence of FcγR regulation in C5aR mutant mice indicates that C5a-C5aR interation may exert a causative role in immune complex–induced changes of FcγR expression.

Cytokines and Immune Complexes

Cytokines mediate interactions between the immune and inflammatory systems and represent a homeostatic system, with concentrations in biologic fluids interpreted by taking into account the levels of other synergistic cytokines, their respective inhibitors, and of each cytokine receptor.[36] Cellular phenotypes associated with FcγR activation receptors include degranulation, phagocytosis, antibody-dependent cellular cytotoxicity (ADCC), transcription of cytokine genes, and release of inflammatory mediators. FcγRII displays its inhibitory activity in part by preventing calcium signaling, which leads to downregulation of cytokine release. Therefore, immune-complex interaction influences cytokine profile.[37] This author has recently reviewed the impact of immune complexes on the cytokine network[38] (Fig. 21–5). Briefly, immune complexes increase production of IL-4 and IL-10, and they suppress IFNγ. In rheumatoid disease, cytokines play a crucial role in the local inflammatory process[36,39] (see also Chapters 25 and 61). New work during the last few years has centered on the question: What is first, immune-complex stimulation of FcγR or cytokine release?[40,40a] Because plasma concentrations of macrophage-colony stimulating factor and IL-10 are significantly higher in rheumatoid arthritis patients, it comes as a little surprise that expression of FcγRIIB is markedly elevated in synovial fluid mononuclear cells compared with their circulating blood counterparts. We are still at a loss for appreciating the significance of normal serum concentrations and circadian variations of some cytokines,[41] as well as the short-term elevations under particular circumstances following invasive procedures on the vessels and heart.[42]

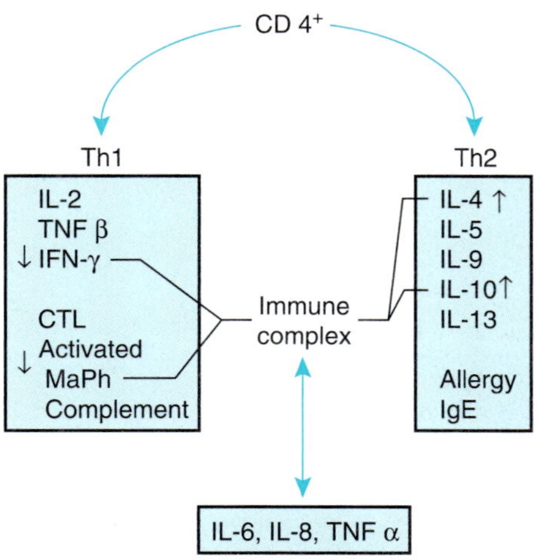

FIGURE 21–5 · Immune Complexes and Cytokines. Intervetion of immune complexes with opposing sets of cytokines. Immune complex–induced increased production of interleukin (IL)-4 and IL-10 suppresses interferon (IFN)-γ production by helper T cells and natural killer (NK) cells. Upregulation of IFN-γ production by 2A treatment of immune-complex diseases might attenuate their unfavorable effect of IFN-γ suppression.[56] Immune complex–induced IL-10 suppresses the production of several proinflammatory, macrophage-derived cytokines, including tumor necrosis factor α (TNFα), IL-1α, IL-1β, IL-6, IL-8, granulocyte macrophage, and granulocyte colony-stimulating factors. IL-10 also inhibits expression of major histocompatibility complex (MHC) class II antigen on monocytes and upregulates inducible nitric oxide synthease in macrophages. Exogenously admiminstered IL-10 has been shown to protect rats from lung injury after intrapulmonary deposition of IgG immune complexes. CTL, cytotoxic T lymphocytes.

Clinical Practice with Immune Complexes

A list of disases associated with circulating and tissue-bound immune complexes is given in Table 21–2. The term *immune-complex diseases* is not confined to soluble, circulating immune complexes; rather, blood cell–bound and tissue-bound complexes comprise a significant portion of this list. The possible destiny of immune complexes is shown by an algorithm in Figure 21–6.

In the 1970s and 1980s, recognition of such widespread involvement of immune complexes in disease was achieved through a variety of methods for their detection, both in the form of soluble immune complexes in bodily fluids and deposited in biopsy tissues.

SOLUBLE IMMUNE COMPLEXES: METHODS FOR DETECTION

Emerging from the detection of complexed antibodies in tissues, and with the developing knowledge of cellular (Raji cells) and humoral (C1q) receptor systems for immune complexes, researchers began to develop radioimmunoassays, now replaced by ELISA systems, to detect soluble immune complexes. Using such technology, it was recognized that insufficient removal or overproduction of soluble complexes induces tissue damage by triggering inflammatory processes lead by complement, especially in rheumatic diseases.[43,44] Today, detection of soluble immune complexes is part of diagnostic workup in a sizeable number of diseases, and this procedure is questioned only by a few.[45] Because of the large array of possible antigens contained in such complexes, the variable antigen-antibody ratios, and their variable decoration with different serum proteins, standardization of detection techniques[46] remains difficult, and validation is achieved as much by reproducibility as by specific assays.[47]

A decisive step toward clinical importance of soluble immune complex diagnostic procedures in human disease came with the breakthrough work of Agnello and colleagues,[48] who showed that hepatitis C virus formed part of circulating cryoglobulins, the cold, precipitable form of some soluble immune complexes.[49] Furthermore, presence of cryoglobulins was a significant risk factor at disease onset for the development of thromboembolic events in patients with systemic lupus erythematosus.[50] Low-density lipoprotein (LDL)–anti-LDL complexes were significantly higher in diabetic patients than in healthy volunteers.[51] Equally important,

TABLE 21–2 • DISEASES ASSOCIATED WITH SOLUBLE IMMUNE COMPLEXES

Disease	Levels of Chronically Circulating Complexes	Predominance of Antigen Specificity	Predominance of Organ Deposition/Damage
Idiopathic inflammatory Diseases			
Systemic lupus erythematosus	Low	DNA	Skin
Rheumatoid arthritis	Low	IgG	Joints
Ankylosing spondylitis (seropositive form)			
Wegener's granulomatosis			
Infectious Diseases			
Bacterial	Intermediate	Streptococcal, staphylococcal, pneumococcal, *Mycoplasma pneumoniae, M. leprae*	Pneumonia, vasculitis, subacute endocarditis
Viral	High	Hepatitis B, hepatitis C, AIDS, dengue fever, infectious mononucleosis, cytomegalovirus of the newborn	Hepatitis, pneumonia
Parasitic	Low	Toxoplasma, schistosoma, trypanosoma	Intestines, heart
Renal Diseases			
Acute glomerulonephritis	High	Multivariate	Glomeruli
IgA nephropathy	High	Intestinal antigens	Glomeruli
Renal transplantation	Low	HLA	Glomeruli
Hematologic Diseases			
Immune hemolytic anemia	High	Red blood cell auto- cr alloantigens	Red blood cell surface
Immune thrombocytopenia	High	Platelet auto- or alloantigens	Platelet surfaces
Iatrogenic Disesaes			
Gold nephropathy	Intermediate	Aureum	Glomeruli, synovium
Acute serum sickness	High	Antilymphocyte immunoglobulin	Pneumonia

Abbreviations: AIDS, Acquired immunodeficiency syndrome; DNA, deoxyribonucleic acid; HLA, human leukocyte antigen; IgG, immunoglobulin G.

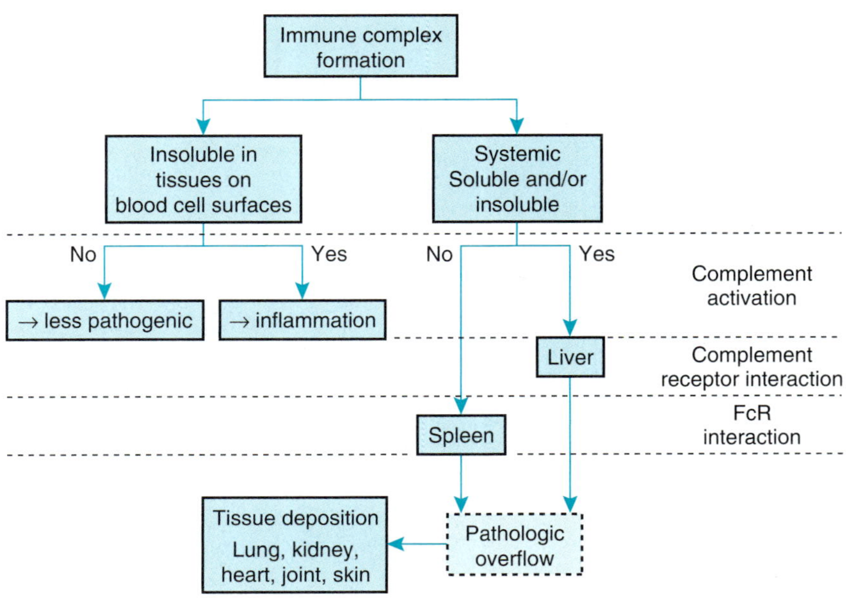

FIGURE 21–6 • Algorithm of Immune-Complex Fate. As antigen and antibody assemble, their fate is highly varied. Immune-complex pathology after excessive production or insufficient removal is manifold. The algorithm illustrates the different possibilities with one common denominator: systemic inflammatory disease.

the acute stroke was significantly associated with chlamydial lipopolysaccharide and anticytomegalovirus antibodies in immune complexes. These are typical examples of other recent observations that underline the still-ongoing quest to define the antigen contained in the circulating immune complexes.[52]

Collectively, these findings underscore the potential value of clinical measurement of immune complexes. Further simplifications and improvements of detection techniques are under way.[53,54] The autoimmune hemolytic anemia syndrome can be diagnosed more clearly by antiglobulin testing profiles, which detect red blood cell–bound immune complexes in which the antigen is an epitope of the normal red blood cell surface or erythrocyte-associated drugs.[55]

Therapeutic Approach for Diseases Associated with Circulating Immune Complexes

ANTIGEN SPECIFIC

Identification of the pathogenetic antigen contained in soluble immune complexes is the ultimate goal; no therapeutic regimen will be better than eradication of a putative infectious antigen or downregulation of a putative autoantigen. For rheumatic diseases the former option is more promising because autoantigens in these diseases are either ubiquitous (DNA) or structural components (collagen). Thus, more selective approaches use monoclonal antibodies directed at cytokines or their receptors. For example, 2A (anti-CD137, the cognate antigen being a member of the tumor necrosis factor [TNF] receptor superfamily) was used to activate T cells to restore the balance of cytokines in a murine model of lupus. In this study, suppression of IFNγ induced by immune complexes (see Fig. 21–5) became counterbalanced in that A2 treatment rapidly augmented IFNγ production.[56,57] This may be beneficial as it leads to depletion of autoreactive B cells via early stage T cell activation. Sudden and robust IFNγ production resulting from CD137 stimulation could contribute to activated autoreactive lymphocyte apoptosis, while avoiding global immunosuppression.[58] Removal of free auto- or alloantibody in anticipation of the undesired immune-complex formation with the antigen is an option in immunohematologic diseases and transplantation medicine.[59]

In chronic infectious diseases with circulating immune complexes containing the infectious antigen, disappearance of the antigen upon antimicrobial treatment is a more direct approach to eliminate immune complexes. However, with severe systemic manifestations at stake, such as vasculitis, pneumonia, carditis, arthritis, and glomerulonephritis, the patient cannot wait for completion of immune-complex removal and must benefit from standard anti-inflammatory protocols. Certainly, new approaches must be addressed, such as using 3-hydroxy-3-methylglutaryl coenzyme A (HMG-CoA) reductase inhibitors (statins) as immunomodulators[60] or deliberately anti-inflammatory agents.[61]

ANTIGEN NONSPECIFIC

Antigen-nonspecific treatment of diseases associated with circulating immune complexes may be divided in immunosuppressive treatment, using steroids and antimetabolites. Attempts are under way to transfect cells with human Fcγ receptor constructs so that the desired cell line becomes macrophage-like. Should the encouraging results with mouse experiments result in improvement of immune-complex removal capacity, its application to human immune-complex disease will be a matter of time.[62] Modulation of FcR system to downregulate autoantibody production may also be achieved with IVIG therapy (*www.ivig.com*).[63] Conversely, immune-complex formation might be a desired phenomenon in situations where the antibody needs to be neutralized. An example is injecting trisaccharide GAS 914 or soluble blood type A substance contained in human plasma for plasma exchange therapy[64] to accelerate antigen-specific elimination of the αGal antibodies or anti-A antibodies.[65] Removal of immune complexes by plasma exchange therapy, as well as absorption by protein A or C1q-coated plasma absorbers[66] might be worthwhile, but it has not seen the expected large-scale application, perhaps because of poor cost-benefit ratio[67] and because of side effects.[68] However, the rationale for introducing this treatment option for immune-complex diseases is strong. Attempts to treat immune-complex damage to organs directly has been attempted. Once immune complexes have formed or deposited in tissues, it is conceivable to withdraw them at the inflammatory site by reducing their concentration, or that of autoantibodies in the circulating blood, by plasmaphoresis. A typical example of such an approach is the removal of antiganglioside M1 autoantibodies by plasma exchange therapy in cases of Guillain-Barré syndrome.[69,70]

ACKNOWLEDGMENTS

The author's research laboratory is sponsored by the University Clinic for Cardiovascular Surgery (Prof. T. Carrel) and currently under the guidance of Marie-Noelle. The Octapharma company, CH-Lachen Giraud-Fluck, PhD. is kindly acknowledged for financial support. The art work by Christian Langenegger (figures), FotoGrafikZentrum, Inselspital, and by Beatrice Boog (Flash presentation), Abteilung für Unterrichtsmedien, University of Bern, is kindly acknowledged.

REFERENCES

1. Papavasiliou FN, Schatz DG: Somatic hypermutation of immunoglobulin genes: Merging mechanisms for genetic diversity. Cell 109:S35-S44, 2002.
2. Di Noia J, Neuberger MS: Altering the pathway of immunoglobulin hypermutation by inhibiting uracil-DNA glycosylase. Nature 419:43-48, 2002.
3. Osipov AP, Zaitseva NV, Egorov AM: Chemiluminescent immunoenzyme biosensor with a thin-layer flow-through cell. Application for study of a real-time bimolecular antigen-antibody interaction. Biosens Bioelectron 11:881-887, 1996.

4. Tseng WL, Chang HT, Hsu SM, et al: Immunoaffinity capillary electrophoresis: Determination of binding constant and stoichiometry for antibody-antigen interaction. Electrophoresis 23:836-846, 2002.
5. Taylor RP: Order in Pollock's chaos. Sci Am 287:116-121, 2002.
6. Spycher MO, Spath PJ, Hafsig A, Nydegger UE: Immunoglobulin-mediated shifting of immune complexes to increased complement-dependent solubility and immunoadherence. Mol Immunol 21:497-505, 1984.
7. Schifferli JA, Peters DK: Complement-mediated inhibition of immune precipitation. II. Analysis by sucrose density gradient ultracentrifugation. Clin Exp Immunol 47:563-569, 1982.
8. Kuroki A, Kuroda Y, Kikuchi S, et al: Level of galactosylation determines cryoglobulin activity of murine IgG3 monoclonal rheumatoid factor. Blood 99:2922-2928, 2002.
9. Saphire EO, Stanfield RL, Crispin MD, et al: Contrasting IgG structures reveal extreme asymmetry and flexibility. J Mol Biol 319:9-18, 2002.
10. Traustadottir KH, Sigfusson A, Steinsson K, Erlendsson K: C4A deficiency and elevated level of immune complexes: The mechanism behind increased susceptibility to systemic lupus erythematosus. J Rheumatol 29:2359-2366, 2002.
11. Nydegger UE, Kazatchkine MD, Miescher PA: Immunopathologic and clinical features of hemolytic anemia due to cold agglutinins. Semin Hematol 28:66-77, 1991.
12. Ierino FL, Powell MS, McKenzie IF, Hogarth PM: Recombinant soluble human Fc gamma RII: Production, characterization, and inhibition of the Arthus reaction. J Exp Med 178:1617-1628, 1993.
13. Bobrovnik SA: Ligand-receptor interaction. Klotz-Hunston problem for two classes of binding sites and its solution. J Biochem Biophys Methods 52:135-143, 2002.
14. Scott-Zaki P, Purkall D, Ruddy S: Neutrophil chemotaxis and superoxide production are induced by cross-linking FcgammaRII receptors. Cell Immunol 201:89-93, 2000.
15. Nydegger UE, Anner RM, Gerebtzoff A, et al: Polymorphonuclear leukocytes stimulation by immune complexes. Assessment by nitroblue tetrazolium dye reduction. Eur J Immunol 3:465-470, 1973.
16. Ling ZD, Webb BT, Yeoh E, Matheson DS: Regulation of Fc-induced IL-6 from human peripheral blood mononuclear cells. Cytokine 5:379-385, 1993.
17. Pascual M, Schifferli JA: Another function of erythrocytes: Transport of circulating immune complexes. Infusionsther Transfusionsmed 22:310-315, 1995.
18. Henderson AL, Lindorfer MA, Kennedy AD, et al: Concerted clearance of immune complexes bound to the human erythrocyte complement receptor: Development of a heterologous mouse model. J Immunol Methods 270:183-197, 2002.
19. Craig ML, Bankovich AJ, Taylor RP: Visualization of the transfer reaction: Tracking immune complexes from erythrocyte complement receptor 1 to macrophages. Clin Immunol 105:36-47, 2002.
20. Fossati G, Moots RJ, Bucknall RC, Edwards SW: Differential role of neutrophil Fcgamma receptor IIIB (CD16) in phagocytosis, bacterial killing, and responses to immune complexes. Arthritis Rheum 46:1351-1361, 2002.
20a. Underhill DM, Ozinsky A: Phagocytosis of microbes: Complexity in action. Annu Rev Immunol 20:825-852, 2002.
20b. Tan Sardjono C, Mottram PL, Hogarth PM: The role of FcgammaRIIa as an inflammatory mediator in rheumatoid arthritis and systemic lupus erythematosus. Immunol Cell Biol 81: 374-381, 2003.
21. Ravetch JV, Bolland S: IgG Fc receptors. Annu Rev Immunol 19:275-290, 2001.
22. Qin D, Wu J, Vora KA, et al: Fc gamma receptor IIB on follicular dendritic cells regulates the B cell recall response. J Immunol 164:6268-6275, 2000.
23. Yuasa T, Kubo S, Yoshino T, et al: Deletion of fcgamma receptor IIB renders H-2(b) mice susceptible to collagen-induced arthritis. J Exp Med 189:187-194, 1999.
24. Bokarewa MI, Morrissey JH, Tarkowski A: Tissue factor as a proinflammatory agent. Arthritis Res 4:190-195, 2002.
25. Imamura T, Kaneda H, Nakamura S: New functions of neutrophils in the arthus reaction: Expression of tissue factor, the clotting initiator, and fibrinolysis by elastase. Lab Invest 82:1287-1295, 2002.
26. Trcka J, Moroi Y, Clynes RA, et al: Redundant and alternative roles for activating Fc receptors and complement in an antibody-dependent model of autoimmune vitiligo. Immunity 16:861-868, 2002.
27. Davis KA, Walport MJ: Processing and clearance of immune comlpexes by compement and the role of complement in immune complex diseases. *In* Volanakis JE, Frank MM (eds): The Human Complement System in Health and Disease. New York, Marcel Dekker, 1998, pp 423-454.
28. Gorgani NN, Parish CR, Easterbrook Smith SB, Altin JG: Histidine-rich glycoprotein binds to human IgG and C1q and inhibits the formation of insoluble immune complexes. Biochemistry 36:6653-6662, 1997.
29. Ren G, Doshi M, Hack BK, et al: Isolation and characterization of a novel rat factor H-related protein that is up-regulated in glomeruli under complement attack. J Biol Chem 277:48351-48358, 2002.
29a. Ruddy S, Austen KF: C3b inactivator of man. II. Fragments produced by C3b inactivator cleavage of cell-bound or fluid phase C3b. J Immunol 107:742-750, 1971.
29b. Nicholson-Weller A, Burge J, Fearon DT, et al: Isolation of a human erythrocyte membrane glycoprotein with decay-accelerating activity for C3 convertases of the complement system. J Immunol 129:184-189, 1982.
30. Ravetch JV, Clynes RA: Divergent roles for Fc receptors and complement in vivo. Annu Rev Immunol 16:421-432, 1998.
31. Kohl J, Gessner JE: On the role of complement and Fc gamma-receptors in the Arthus reaction. Mol Immunol 36:893-903, 1999.
32. Nydegger UE, Carrel T, Laumonier T, Mohacsi P: New concepts in organ preservation. Transpl Immunol 9:215-225, 2002.
33. Heller T, Hennecke M, Baumann U, et al: Selection of a C5a receptor antagonist from phage libraries attenuating the inflammatory response in immune complex disease and ischemia/reperfusion injury. J Immunol 163:985-994, 1999.
34. Riedemann NC, Guo RF, Neff TA, et al: Increased C5a receptor expression in sepsis. J Clin Invest 110:101-108, 2002.
35. Shushakova N, Skokowa J, Schulman J, et al: C5a anaphylatoxin is a major regulator of activating versus inhibitory FcgammaRs in immune complex-induced lung disease. J Clin Invest 110:1823-1830, 2002.
36. Burger D, Dayer JM: Cytokines, acute-phase proteins, and hormones: IL-1 and TNF-alpha production in contact-mediated activation of monocytes by T lymphocytes. Ann N Y Acad Sci 966:464-473, 2002.
37. Ronnelid J, Tejde A, Mathsson L, et al: Immune complexes from SLE sera induce IL10 production from normal peripheral blood mononuclear cells by an FcgammaRII dependent mechanism: implications for a possible vicious cycle maintaining B cell hyperactivity in SLE. Ann Rheum Dis 62:37-42, 2003.
38. Nydegger UE. Immune complexes. *In* Delves PJ, Roitt IM (eds): Encyclopedia of Immunology. Vol. 3. San Diego, Academic Press, 1998, pp 1220-1225.
39. Kawanaka N, Yamamura M, Aita T, et al: CD14+,CD16+ blood monocytes and joint inflammation in rheumatoid arthritis. Arthritis Rheum 46:2578-2586, 2002.
40. Nordstrom E, Abedi-Valugerdi M, Moller E: Immune complex-induced chronic and intense IL-4 independent IgG1-rheumatoid factor production in NZB mice. Scand J Immunol 53:32-39, 2001.
40a. Dinaerello CA: Setting the cytokine trap for autoimmunity. Nature Medicine 9:20-22, 2003.
41. Berdat PA, Wehrle TJ, Kueng healthy A, et al: Age-specific analysis of normal cytokine levels in infants. Clin Chem Lab Med 41:1335-1339, 2003.
42. Schulze PC, Kluge E, Schuler G, Lauer B: Periprocedural kinetics in serum levels of cytokines and adhesion molecules in elective PTCA and stent implantation: impact on restenosis. Arterioscler Thromb Vasc Biol 22:2105-2107, 2002.
43. Nydegger UE, Zubler RH, Gabay R, et al: Circulating complement breakdown products in patients with rheumatoid arthritis. Correlation between plasma C3d, circulating immune complexes, and clinical activity. J Clin Invest 59:862-868, 1977.
44. Agarwal V, Misra R, Aggarwal A: Immune complexes contain immunoglobulin A rheumatoid factor in serum and synovial fluid of patients with polyarticular juvenile rheumatoid arthritis. Rheumatology (Oxford) 41:466-467, 2002.

45. Lock RJ, Unsworth DJ. Measurement of immune complexes is not useful in routine clinical practice. Ann Clin Biochem 37:253-256, 2000.
46. Nydegger UE, Svehag SE. Improved standardization in the quantitative estimation of soluble immune complexes making use of an international reference preparation. Results of a collaborative multicentre study. Clin Exp Immunol 58:502-509, 1984.
47. Rose N, DeMacario EC, Folds JD, et al (eds): Manual of Clinical Laboratory Immunology. London, Blackwell, 1997, p 1300.
48. Agnello V: The etiology and pathophysiology of mixed cryoglobulinemia secondary to hepatitis C virus infection. Springer Semin Immunopathol 19:111-129, 1997.
49. Corvetta A, Spaeth PJ, Ghirelli PA, et al: Complement activation and impaired capacity to solubilize immune complexes or to prevent their formation in essential mixed cryoglobulinemia. Diagn Immunol 1:315-323, 1983.
50. Manger K, Manger B, Repp R, et al: Definition of risk factors for death, end stage renal disease, and thromboembolic events in a monocentric cohort of 338 patients with systemic lupus erythematosus. Ann Rheum Dis 61:1065-1070, 2002.
51. Tarnacka B, Gromadzka G, Czlonkowska A: Increased circulating immune complexes in acute stroke: the triggering role of Chlamydia pneumoniae and cytomegalovirus. Stroke 33:936-940, 2002.
52. Turk Z, Sesto M, Skodlar J, et al: Soluble LDL-immune complexes in type 2 diabetes and vascular disease. Horm Metab Res 34:196-201, 2002.
53. Soares NM, Santiago MB, Pontes deCarvalho LC: An improved anti-C3/IgG ELISA for quantification of soluble immune complexes. J Immunol Methods 249:199-205, 2001.
54. Yoshinoya S, Mizoguchi Y, Aotsuka S, et al: Circulating immune complex levels measured by new ELISA kits utilizing monoclonal anti-C1q and anti-C3d antibodies correlate with clinical activities of SLE but not with those of RA. J Clin Lab Immunol 38:161-173, 1992.
55. Arndt PA, Garratty G, Hill J, et al: Two cases of immune haemolytic anaemia, associated with anti-piperacillin, detected by the 'immune complex' method. Vox Sang 83:273-278, 2002.
56. Sun Y, Chen HM, Subudhi SK, et al: Costimulatory molecule-targeted antibody therapy of a spontaneous autoimmune disease. Nat Med 8:1405-1413, 2002.
57. Kammer GM. Immunotherapy tackles lupus. Nat Med 8:1356-1358, 2002.
58. Gescuk BD, Davis JC Jr: Novel therapeutic agents for systemic lupus erythematosus. Curr Opin Rheumatol 14:515-521, 2002.
59. Sawada T, Fuchinoue S, Teraoka S: Successful A1-to-O ABO-incompatible kidney transplantation after a preconditioning regimen consisting of anti-CD20 monoclonal antibody infusions, splenectomy, and double-filtration plasmapheresis. Transplantation 74:1207-1210, 2002.
60. Mach F: Statins as immunomodulators. Transpl Immunol 9:197-200, 2002.
61. Meroni PL, Luzzana C, Ventura D: Anti-inflammatory and immunomodulating properties of statins. An additional tool for the therapeutic approach of systemic autoimmune diseases? Clin Rev Allergy Immunol 23:263-277, 2002.
62. Jones BA, Moo-Kyung K, Schreiber AD: Enhanced clearance of immune complexes following adenoviral mediated gene transfer of Fcgamma receptors [abstract]. Blood 100 5555, 2002.
63. Nydegger UE, Mohacsi P: Immunoglobulins in clinical medicine. *In* Simon TL, Dzik WH, Snyder EL, et al (eds): Rossi's Principles of Transfusion Medicine. Philadelphia, Lippincott Williams & Wilkins, 2002, pp 316-332.
64. Nydegger UE, Julmy F, Achermann F, Carrel T: Soluble ABO-blood group A-substance (SAS) in fresh frozen plasma (FFP) [abstract]. Vox Sang 83(suppl 2):667, 2002.
65. Katopodis AG, Warner RG, Duthaler RO, et al: Removal of anti-Galalpha1,3Gal xenoantibodies with an injectable polymer. J Clin Invest 110:1869-1877, 2002.
66. Kunkel S, Holtz M, Grossjohann B, et al: Selective removal of circulating immune complexes from patient plasma. Artif Organs 26:124-132, 2002.
67. Berner B, Scheel AK, Schettler V, et al: Rapid improvement of SLE-specific cutaneous lesions by C1q immunoadsorption. Ann Rheum Dis 60:898-899, 2001.
68. Deodhar A, Allen E, Daoud K, Wahba I: Vasculitis secondary to staphylococcal protein A immunoadsorption (Prosorba column) treatment in rheumatoid arthritis. Semin Arthritis Rheum 32:3-9, 2002.
69. Raphael JC, Chevret S, Hughes RAC: Plasma exchange for Guillain-Barré syndrome. Cochrane Database Systemic Review 2001:Update Software (2):CD001798.
70. Uetz-von Allmen E, Sturzenegger M, Rieben R, et al: Antiganglioside GM1 antibodies and their complement activating capacity in central and peripheral nervous system disorders and in controls. Eur Neurol 39:103-110, 1998.

22 Complement System

JOHN P. ATKINSON

In this chapter, the "workings" of the complement system will be reviewed with a focus on how the system functions in rheumatic diseases. In that regard, the involvement of complement has long been recognized in two of the most common inflammatory diseases treated by rheumatologists, systemic lupus erythematosus (SLE) and rheumatoid arthritis (RA). Further, what has been learned about complement's role in these two diseases also applies to closely related syndromes that mimic and are in the differential diagnosis of vasculitis or polyarthritis. Therefore, the goal of this chapter is to provide an understanding of the system so the rheumatologist may appreciate its biologic relevance and clinical role in the rheumatic diseases. This information will also assist in the interpretation of laboratory tests for complement proteins and in the determination of the significance of complement fragments in pathologic specimens.

Discovery and Other Historical Aspects

Today *complement* is used as a collective term to designate a group of plasma and membrane proteins that play a key role in innate and adaptive immunity. The complement system is ancient, as it predates chordates[1] such as the lamprey and hagfish. Complement was discovered in the late nineteenth century as experimental pathologists were trying to understand the biologic basis of vaccination and blood specialists the cause of transfusion reactions.[2] In these studies, it became apparent that the cell-free portion of blood contained a lytic substance for bacteria and for the transfused red blood cells (RBCs). The factor was heat labile (i.e., destroyed by heating at 56° C for 30 minutes or by leaving it out overnight) and was innate or nonspecific (i.e., all individuals had it and it lysed many types of bacteria and cells). This substance was contrasted to antibody (Ab), which was heat stable and specific because only immunized animals contained this substance. Through mixing experiments, two factors were found to be required for lysis: a specific recognition piece antibody, (Ab) and a nonspecific lytic piece (complement). In retrospect, this was the discovery of the classical complement pathway and led to its initial characterization as a heat-labile bactericidal factor that "complemented" the acquired factor raised by immunization. Similarly, in the blood of patients who recovered from transfusion reactions a heat-stable substance was found that recognized transfused blood cells. However, it did not lyse the transfused cells directly but required another substance, which was present in fresh serum.

From this discussion, it is also apparent why lysis became tightly associated with the complement system and why the study of Ab and complement dominated the field of immunology for the next half century. Of interest, the first autoimmune disease to be recognized was a hemolytic anemia (paroxysmal cold hemoglobinuria) in which the same pair of factors, Ab and complement, were shown to mediate RBC lysis.[3] This "double-edged sword" aspect of the complement system has been demonstrated repeatedly. For example, compared to normal mice, C5-deficient mice are 100-fold more sensitive to death from a pneumococcal infection but 100-fold less sensitive to tissue destruction by autoantibodies. Also, congenital deficiencies of C1, C4, and C2 strongly predispose to SLE, yet immune complex (IC) deposition and complement activation contribute to tissue damage in SLE.

Function

A major function of the complement system is to modify membranes and soluble antigens to which its activation fragments become tightly (covalently) bound (Fig. 22–1). As part of this proteolytic activation process, smaller fragments are liberated in the local milieu to activate cells with the overall goal of preparing the host for an inflammatory and immune response (see next paragraph). Activated fragments of complement proteins deposit in large amounts on a target such as microbes and IC. For example, several million C3b molecules attach to one bacterial surface in less than 2 minutes. The goal of these deposited complement proteins is to *opsonize* the target. They also further activate the cascade on the surface of the cellular target. C3b (and its degradation fragments) and C4b are ligands for complement receptors on peripheral blood cells, tissue macrophages, and antigen-presenting cells such as follicular-dendritic cells. This coupling process, known as *immune adherence*, is a phenomenon at which complement ligands and their receptors are particularly adept. On phagocytic cells, this leads to ingestion of the infectious particle, IC, or tissue debris. Additionally, the membranes of some microorganisms (e.g., gram negative) and most host cells can be disrupted by the terminal complement components (C5b-C9) resulting in lysis. In many cases, however, microbes feature thick capsules that make them resistant to lysis (e.g., as gram-positive organisms). In human diseases featuring autoantibodies, cells and tissues are similarly opsonized and membrane integrity is compromised. A recent extension of this opsonic function relates to a

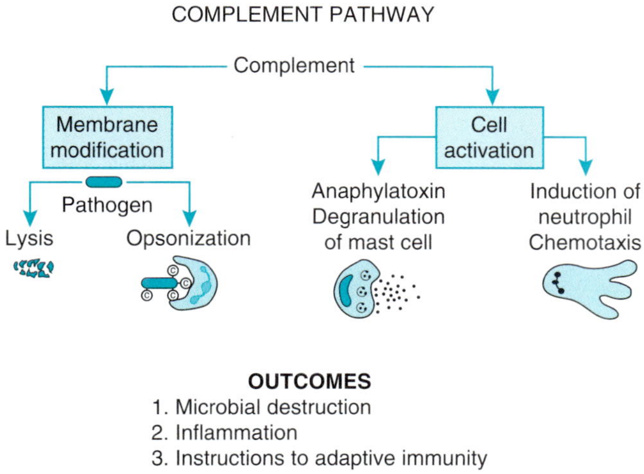

FIGURE 22–1 · Function of the Complement System. The most important function of complement is to alter the membrane of a pathogen by coating its surface with clusters of complement-activation fragments (the phenomenon of opsonization). These, in turn, facilitate interactions with complement receptors and, in some cases, such as with certain gram-negative bacteria and viruses, lead to lysis. The second critical function of complement is to activate cells to promote inflammatory and immune responses. The complement fragments C3a and C5a (termed *anaphylatoxins*) stimulate many cell types, such as mast cells, which release their contents, and phagocytic cells, which migrate to an inflammatory site (chemotaxis). Through opsonization and cell activation, complement serves as nature's adjuvant to prepare, facilitate, and instruct the host for an adaptive immune response. (Adapted with permission from Liszewski, M.K., and Atkinson, J.P.: Fundamental Immunology, 3rd ed. 1993, pp 917-939.)

role for complement in clearance of cellular debris following necrosis or apoptosis. In particular, one hypothesis to explain autoantibody formation in SLE is a failure to properly clear apoptotic cells by the complement system.[4]

A second functional activity of complement is cellular activation that prepares the local environment for defense against infection (see Fig. 22–1). In the proteolytic steps of the early part of complement-activation process, mediators are released that activate nearby cells. These low molecular weight fragments (C4a, C3a, C5a) are termed *anaphylatoxins* because, if released in excessive amounts, they induce a reaction resembling anaphylaxis. C3a and C5a, the two most powerful mediators, bind to their respective receptors at sites of complement activation (also known as a complement-fixing site). This causes phenomena at the site of activation such as histamine release by mast cells and chemotaxis of phagocytic cells. With improved reagents and newer technology, receptors for C3a and C5a have now been shown to be much more widely expressed than initially thought; for example, they are expressed by most epithelial cells, immunocomplement cells, hepatocytes, endothelial cells, neurons, and other cell types. Thus, some manifestations of central nervous system (CNS) lupus may be caused by C3a and C5a engaging their receptors on endothelial and neuronal cells.

Nomenclature

There are three activation cascades: the classic pathway (CP), the alternative pathway (AP), and the lectin pathway (LP) (Fig. 22–2). These converge to activate C3 and the common membrane attack complex (MAC).

The nine proteins of the CP are designated by the uppercase letter "C" followed by a number (Table 22–1). These numbered components generally act in numeric order, except C4, which acts before C2 and C3. Components of the AP are designated by capital letters (e.g., factor B). Regulatory proteins are designated by a descriptive title (e.g., C4 binding protein) or, in the case of the AP, a letter (e.g., factor H). Single components or multimer complexes that have enzymatic activity are often designated by a bar (e.g., $C\overline{1s}$). The loss of hemolytic activity by a component is usually designated by a lower case suffix (e.g., C3bi). Fragments generated during complement activation are designated by a lowercase letter suffix (e.g., C3a, C3b), except for the fragments of C2 which are just the opposite. In these fragments, the "a" fragment is smaller and is liberated into the surrounding milieu, whereas the larger "b" fragment becomes cell bound and continues the cascade.

Receptors were named in order of their discovery, but they also are commonly noted relative to their ligand specificity and cell determinant (CD) number. For example, complement receptor type one is noted in the literature as CR1, C3b/C4b, or immune adherence receptor, and as CD35.

Activation Cascades

Because many rheumatic diseases feature autoantibodies and IC, an understanding of the general principles of the activation cascades is particularly essential to characterizing complement's role in diseases such as SLE[2,5-8] (Figs. 22–2 to 22–4).

CLASSICAL PATHWAY

The classical pathway, (CP) is activated primarily by immune complexes, (IC) and a few other substances including CRP.[9] Once C1 is bound to an activator, via the Fc portion of immunoglobulin G (IgG) or IgM

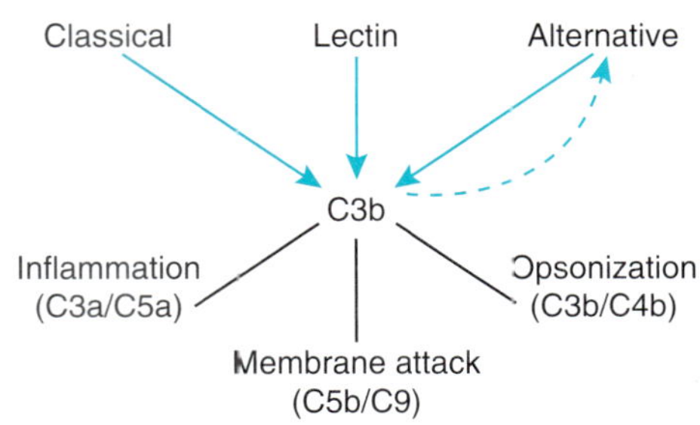

FIGURE 22–2 · The Three Pathways of Complement Activation. Deposition of clusters of C3b on a target is the primary goal. As shown by the broken line, the alternative pathway (AP) also serves as a feedback loop to amplify C3b deposition (regardless of which cascade deposited the C3b).

TABLE 22–1 • PLASMA COMPONENTS OF THE COMPLEMENT CASCADES

Component	Serum Concentration (μg/ml)	Function
Classical Pathway (CP)		
C1	50	Binds IC to trigger CP
C1q		Binds Fc portion of IgG/IgM
C1r		Protease: cleaves C1s
C1s		Protease: cleaves C4 and C2
C4	200-500	Opsonin* (C4b), C4a release
C2	20	Protease: cleaves C3 and C5
Lectin Pathway (LP)		
MBL	150 (wide range)	Binds sugars to trigger LP
MASP-1	5	Protease
MASP-2	5	Protease: cleaves C4 and C2
Alternative Pathway (AP)		
Factor B	150-250	Protease: cleaves C3 and C5
Factor D	1-2	Protease: cleaves factor B
Properdin (P)	25	Stabilizes AP convertases
Central Protein		
C3	550-1200	Opsonin* (C3b), C3a release
Terminal Pathway (TP)		
C5	70	MAC component (C5b), C5a release
C6	60	MAC component
C7	60	MAC component
C8	60	MAC component (pore formation)
C9	60	MAC component (pore formation)

*C4b and C3b also form part of the C3 and C5 convertases.

Abbreviations: IC, immune complexes; Ig, immunoglobulin; MAC, membrane attack complex; MASP, MBL-associated serine protease; MBL, mannan-binding lectin.

interacting with C1q subunit (see Fig. 22–4), the C1r enzymatic subcomponent autoactivates by proteolysis and then cleaves C1s to form C1 within the C1 complex. C4 is a substrate for C1s̄ and is cleaved by C1s̄ to C4b, releasing the C4a fragment (Fig. 22–5). The C4b fragment, having had its thioester bond disrupted, now has the transient (a few microseconds) ability to covalently bind to a hydroxyl or amino group on a nearby target. C2 is also a substrate for C1s̄, and C2 is cleaved by C1s̄ to yield C2a and C2b. C2a interacts with 10 to 20 percent of the target-bound C4b to form the CP C3 convertase, C4bC2a (Fig. 22–6). The enzymatic or catalytic domain of this complex is C2a, which cleaves C3 to form C3a and activated C3b (Fig. 22–7). Activated C3b attaches to the target by binding covalently to a hydroxyl group (analogous interaction of C4b with a hydroxyl group). Newly formed C3b also has two other fates. First, it is rapidly inactivated if it does promptly bind to the target. Second, it binds covalently to a specific region of C4b thereby forming the CP C5 convertase, C4bC2aC3b (see Fig. 22–6).

The rapidity and magnitude of the CP activation process is remarkable (as it should be on a microbial target). In a few cases, the reactants in a model system have been quantitated. In one such study in which complement was activated by IgG binding to a membrane antigen of nucleated cells, approximately 2.5 million C4b molecules and about 500,000 C2a molecules subsequently attached to C4b molecules.[10] Within 5 minutes, 21 million (10 × amplification over the number of attached C4b molecules) C3b molecules were deposited. Further, only about 10 to 20 percent of the C4b and C3b molecules generated bound to the target. The rest were by hydrolysis in the fluid phase and then degraded by fluid-phase inhibitors. Concomitantly, C4a, C3a, and C5a anaphylatoxins were generated, equal to the number of C4b, C3b, and C5b fragments. Approximately one million MACs

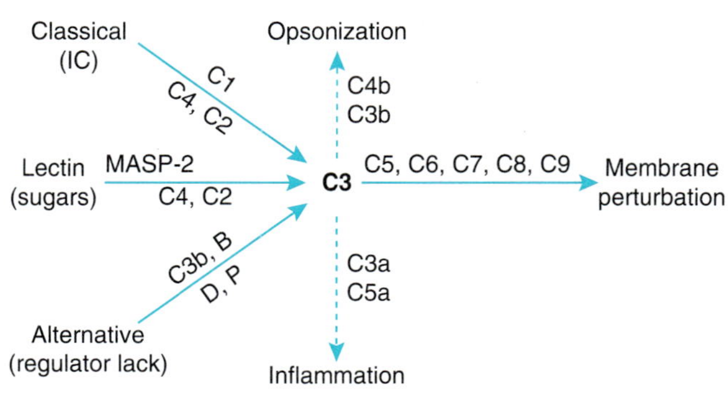

FIGURE 22–3 • The Initiation Step and Reaction Cascade of the Three Complement Pathways. Note that C4 and C2 serve in both the classic and lectin pathways. They are cleaved identically by MASP-2 or C1. The convertases for C3 and C5 are shown in Figure 22–6.

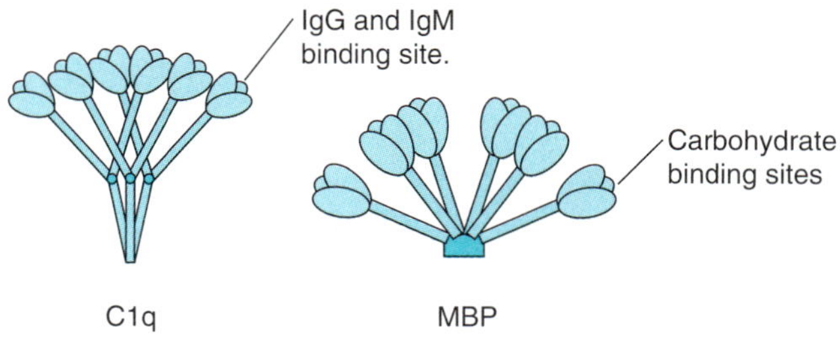

FIGURE 22–4 • Similarity of C1q and MBP (MBL) Structure. Ficolins, surfactins, and other members of the collectin family of proteins share this general structure. Many activate the lectin pathway (LP) upon interaction with their ligands. (Modified from: Frank, Atkinson J.P.: Sampter's Immunologic Diseases, 6th ed. Lippincott, Williams, & Wilkins, Baltimore, MD 2001, p 285.)

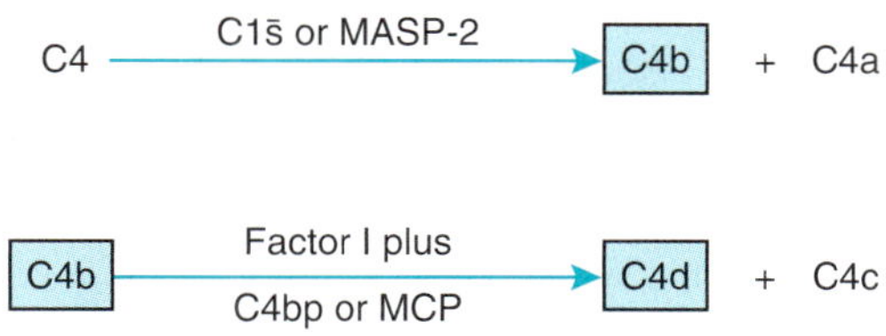

FIGURE 22–5 • C4 Activation and Degradation. The boxed activation fragment is the one that remains covalently attached to the target. The other fragments are released into the surrounding milieu. C4a is a anaphylatoxin. (Modified from: Liszewski, M.K. Atkinson, J.P.: The Complement System. Primer on the Rheumatic Diseases 12th ed., page 66, 2001).

Convertase	Classical/lectin	Alternative
C3	C4bC2a	C3bBbP
C5	C3b/C4bC2a	C3b/C3bBbP

FIGURE 22–6 • Proteins of the C3 and C5 Convertases. C4b or C3b anchors the enzyme to the target. The catalytic domains are the serine proteases C2a and Bb. The C3 convertase becomes a C5 convertase when a C3b attaches to a preferred acceptor site on C4b or C3b. Properdin (P) stabilizes the alternative pathway (AP) convertases.

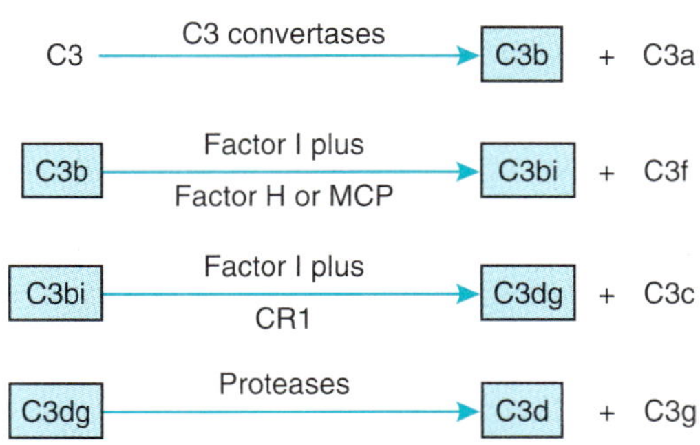

FIGURE 22–7 • C3 Activation and Degradation. The boxed activation fragment is the one that remains covalently attached to the target. The other fragments are released into the surrounding milieu. C3a is a potent anaphylatoxin. C3f may be a marrow mobilizing factor for neutrophils. C3c and C3g have no known function.

were formed. Fragment attachment to and the amplification on soluble antigens is a less-efficient process.

A single IgM can activate the CP. On the other hand, two IgGs in close proximity (side by side) are required before C1 is fixed. On an RBC this means that several thousand IgGs must bind before activation can occur. Consequently, antigenic density and display can play a role in whether or not complement is activated. For example, in warm Ab (IgG)-mediated autoimmune hemolytic anemia, complement is usually not fixed (despite the autoantibody being of an appropriate IgG subclass) because the density of the antigen is too low.

LECTIN PATHWAY

Lectins are carbohydrate-binding proteins[11,12] (see Fig. 22–4). They initially were described as proteins capable of agglutinating RBCs. They are important players in innate immunity and in rheumatic diseases. In particular, mannan-binding lectin (MBL) is a hepatocyte-synthesized serum protein that preferentially binds to repeating mannoses and certain other oligosaccharides of pathogens. MBL resembles C1q (belongs to the same family of proteins known as *collectins*) in that it is an oligomer with a terminal collagenous domain on one end and a globular domain on the other. The main difference is that the carboxyl-terminus of MBL possesses a carbohydrate-recognition domain, whereas C1q has an immunoglobulin-binding domain. Like C1q binding to the Fc portion of IgG, MBL engagement with a sugar leads to activation of serine proteases similar to C1r and C1s, called mannan-associated serine proteases (MASPs). MASP-2 cleaves C4 and C2. MBL was discovered during an investigation of the cause of bacterial infections in young children. Accumulating evidence suggests that MBL deficiency is also a predisposing factor for SLE and RA and is associated with more severe disease.[13]

The LP shares many features with the CP.[11,12] The few differences are at the initial steps in which MBL binds to an activating surface, such as yeast cell walls with the appropriate repeating oligosaccharides. Two serine esterases are associated with MBL, MASP-1, and MASP-2. Each element of the MBL-MASP complex is structurally and functionally homologous to the corresponding elements in the CP. C1q and MBL have globular ends through which they attach to their respective substrates. The MASP-2 in the complex cleaves C4 to form C4a and C4b and cleaves C2 to form C2a and C2b; this is analogous to C1 cleaving C4 and C2. The C4b2a complex formed is the same C3 convertase as that generated in the CP (see Fig. 22–6). The LP is a key player in innate immunity where MBL and related lectins, such as surfactants and ficollins, bind to their cognate residues on microbes to trigger C activation. At one time MASPs and possibly C1 directly activated C3, but, through the evolution of C4 and C2, further amplification of the C3 activating process was engineered through these intermediates.[12,14]

ALTERNATIVE PATHWAY

The AP was the second complement activation pathway discovered (hence the name), but it is phylogenetically the most ancient.[1,12] In contrast to CP and LP, the AP does not require Ab or a lectin to be triggered. It likely plays a larger role in rheumatic diseases than previously appreciated because of its so-called feedback or amplification loop. Thus, if C3b is deposited on a target by CP or LP, the AP can enhance C3b deposition manyfold. The alternative pathway is also continuously active at a low level under normal circumstances (similar to an idling car). The process accounts for most of the 1 to 2 percent per hour turnover of C3. Inhibitors such as factor H and factor I and host cell surface regulators keep the system in check. In the absence of these regulators, the system fires to exhaustion, as in inherited deficiencies of the fluid-phase regulators. The AP routinely "kicks into gear" in the setting of substances that lack regulators. If C3b deposits on an activating (i.e., one that lacks regulators) surface such as that of most microbes, the system's feedback loop allows for several million C3b molecules to be deposited on a surface in less than 5 minutes. In this pathway, factor B, structurally and functionally homologous to C2, binds to the deposited C3b and is then cleaved by the constitutively active factor D to Bb and Ba. C3bBb is the alternative pathway C3 convertase (see Fig. 22–6). It is stabilized by properdin (P). The catalytic serine protease Bb component of C3bBbP then cleaves C3 to C3a and C3b (a feedback loop has been set up). Some of the newly generated C3b molecules bind covalently to C3b already deposited on the target to form a C5 convertase ([(C3b)$_2$Bb]). The C5 convertase is also stabilized by P. In vivo, neither the C3 or C5 AP convertases are efficient without P because they spontaneously decay before amplification occurs.

MEMBRANE ATTACK COMPLEX

The terminal pathway begins with the cleavage of C5 by either the CP, LP, or AP C5 convertase. The C5a generated is a potent cell activator and chemotactic factor. The C5b binds C6 which, in turn, binds C7 to yield fluid phase C5b67. This lipophilic complex can now interact with cell membranes. Following membrane insertion, it next recruits C8. The C5b678 forms an initial pore in the plasma membrane and then recruits multiple (five to 10) C9 molecules to yield C5b6789n. This complex is an efficient membrane channel–former and is responsible for cell lysis. Many organisms and cell types, however, are not easily lysed. However, the MAC has multiple nonlytic effects on cells as well. The majority of these seem to be activation of signaling pathways such as those observed for neurons and kidney cells.[5,7] Some of the organ dysfunction observed in SLE, especially if transient or correctable with treatment, may be secondary to these nonlytic effects of the MAC.

Regulators

PHYSIOLOGIC REGULATION

Unregulated, the complement system would fire to exhaustion, a point illustrated by inborn errors of plasma regulatory proteins.[15-17] The complement system evolved to allow unimpeded activation on a microbe but also to limit the process in time and space. The reaction must be finite in time to avoid excessive consumption of components in any one reaction and finite in space to minimize damage to surrounding host tissue. Thus, a typical complement reaction on a microbial target occurs within a few minutes and during this time, self tissue is protected by plasma and membrane regulators. These inhibitors function at the critical steps of initiation, convertase assembly and stability, and membrane attack. The convertase enzyme complexes also intrinsically have short half-lives.

FLUID PHASE AND MEMBRANE INHIBITORS

These inhibitors, (Table 22–21) distributed both in plasma and on cells, regulate primarily at 1) initiating events (see Fig. 22–3); 2) the C3 and C5 convertases (see Fig. 22–6); and 3) the MAC. The major activity of the plasma inhibitors is to prevent fluid-phase activation (no target) and the membrane inhibitors' activation on self tissue (wrong target). Furthermore, they prevent excessive activation on one target, and, in some cases, the fluid-phase inhibitors bind to damaged cells and tissues where they then function as a membrane regulator.[6,7,18]

In the early phase of the CP, C1 inhibitor prevents excessive fluid-phase C1 activation.[19] C1-inhibitor is a serine protease inhibitor SERPIN and binds to C1r and C1s the inactivation process. The C1 complex is thereby disrupted, leaving C1q bound to Ab in the immune complex. C1q may then interact with C1q receptors to facilitate disposal of the IC. The C3 and C5 convertases are regulated by a family of proteins that include the membrane proteins decay-accelerating factor (CD55) and membrane cofactor protein (CD46), and the serum inhibitors C4-binding protein and factor H.[15-17] These proteins function in two ways: They dissemble the convertases (decay-accelerating activity) and serve as cofactors for the proteolytic inactivation of C4b and C3b cofactor activity (Fig. 22–8). The latter process is mediated by the plasma serine protease factor I. The MAC also is regulated by distinct serum and cell-anchored proteins. CD59 is a glycolipid-anchored membrane protein that binds C8 and C9 to prevent MAC insertion, whereas the plasma protein vitronectin (S-protein) binds to and thereby inactivates fluid-phase MAC.

As a result of this regulatory activity, complement attack is focused on foreign surfaces (which usually lack complement regulators) and is held in check on host cells and in body fluids. Interestingly, a number of microorganisms have "captured" complement regulators (e.g., pox viruses) or have evolved proteins (Herpes simplex viruses) that inhibit complement activation (virulence factors).[20] However, the activation of the CP by antibody is extremely rapid and efficient such that the inhibitors, in general, have modest effects on limiting damage by complement-fixing antibodies. The inhibitors are efficient at preventing fluid phase activation and amplification by the feedback loop on host tissue.

TABLE 22–2 • COMPLEMENT REGULATORY PROTEINS

	Tissue Distribution	Function	Disease Association
Initiation			
C1 inhibitor	Plasma	Inactivates C1r, C1s, and MASPs; a SERPIN	Hereditary angioedema
Convertases			
Factor I	Plasma	Cleaves C3b and C4b; requires a cofactor protein	Infections (secondary C3 deficiency)
Membrane cofactor protein	Most cells	Cofactor for cleavage of C4b and C3b	Hemolytic uremic syndrome*
Decay-accelerating factor	Most cells	Destabilizes C3 and C5 convertases	NA†
C4-binding protein	Plasma	Cofactor for cleavage of C4b; decays CP C3 and C5 convertases	NA†
Factor H	Plasma	Cofactor for cleavage of C3b; destabilizes AP C3 and C5 convertases	Hemolytic uremic syndrome*; glomerulonephritis
Complement receptor type one (CR1)	Blood cells	Receptor for C3b and C4b; cofactor activity for C3b and C4b and decays C3 and C5 convertases	NA‡
Membrane Attack			
S protein	Plasma	Blocks fluid-phase MAC	Unknown
CD59	Most cells	Blocks MAC on host cells	Paroxysmal nocturnal hemoglobinuria
Other			
Anaphylatoxin inactivator	Plasma	Inactivates C3a, C4a, and C5a	Hives

*Most patients are heterozygous for function-altering mutations.[18]
†Insufficient number of cases described of complete deficiency to establish an association.
‡A complete deficiency has not been reported.

Abbreviations: AP, alternative pathway; CP, classical pathway; MAC, membrane attack complex; MASPs, MBL-associated serine proteases; SERPIN, serine protease inhibitor.

Complement Receptors

The complement system exerts many of its effects through receptors. (Tables 22–3 and 22–4) During the activation process, target-bound and locally released fragments serve as ligands. For example, the vasomodulatory and chemotactic effects of C3a and C5a are due to interaction with their respective receptors. The opsonic fragments C4b and C3b mediate clearance of ICs and bacteria through complement receptors. Degradation of C3b by regulators leads to formation of iC3b and then C3dg, which, in turn, interact with additional complement receptors CR3/CR4 and CR2, respectively.

Complement receptor one (CR1) plays an important role in IC clearance. CR1 on erythrocytes binds C3b/C4b-coated ICs for processing and transport to the liver and spleen.[21] In these organs, the ICs are transferred from the erythrocyte to tissue macrophages, allowing the erythrocyte to return to the circulation for another round of clearance. CR1 on granulocytes and monocytes promotes IC adherence and phagocytosis, whereas CR1 on B lymphocytes, tissue macrophages, and follicular-dendritic cells facilitates trapping and processing of IC in lymphoid organs. CR2 is expressed by B lymphocytes and follicular-dendritic cells where it

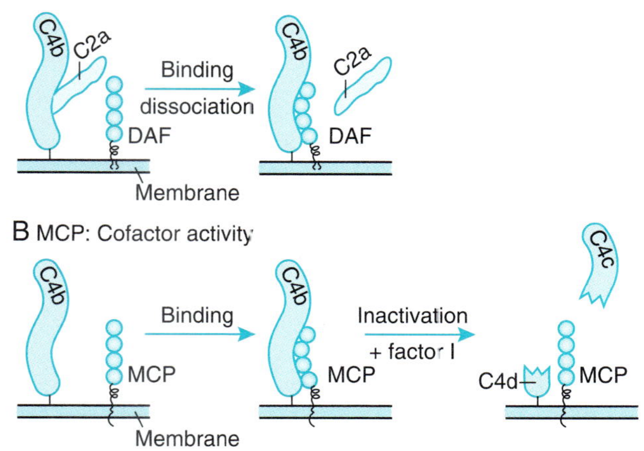

FIGURE 22–8 • Regulation of Convertases. The classic pathway (CP) C3 convertase is shown. Decay-accelerating factor (DAF) irreversibly displaces the protease, C2a, from C4b. To prevent C4b from interacting with a newly formed C2a, C4b is cleaved by membrane cofactor protein (MCP) in concert with the serine protease factor I. The residual bound C4d has no known biologic activity. CP C5 convertase is similarly inactivated. Moreover, the alternative pathway (AP) C3 and C5 convertases are also disassembled in an identical fashion by DAF and MCP, except that C3b is cleaved to C3bi rather than to C3dg. (From: Liszewski et al. Advances in Immunology Control of the Complement System 61: 201-283, 1996, with permission).

TABLE 22–3 • COMPLEMENT RECEPTORS FOR C3 AND C4

Name*	Primary Ligand	Location	Function
Complement receptor type 1 (CR1)	C3b/C4b	Peripheral blood cells (except for platelets), FDC, B cells, podocytes	Immune adherence, phagocytosis, antigen localization, regulation
CR2	C3dg/C3d	B lymphocytes, FDC	Coreceptor for Bcell–signaling, antigen localization
CR3/CR4	C3bi	Myeloid lineage	Phagocytosis, adherence

*The CD numbers are CR1, CD35; CR2, CD21; CR3, CD11b/CD18; CR4, CD11c/CD18.
Abbreviations: FDC, follicular-dendritic cells.

TABLE 22–4 • COMPLEMENT RECEPTORS FOR ANAPHYLATOXINS

Receptor	Ligand	Distribution	Function
C3aR	C3a	Myeloid lineage including mast cells, smooth-muscle cells, epithelial cells, endothelial cells, neuronal cells	Cell activation including granule exocytosis, upregulation of adhesins, chemotaxis, cytoskeletal effects
C5aR	C5a	Similar to C3aR	Similar to C3a but with more chemotactic effects

facilitates antigen trapping and is a coreceptor for activation of the B cell antigen receptor.[22]

Complement in the Innate and Adaptive Immune Response

INNATE IMMUNITY

The complement system is activated by three mechanisms independent of an adaptive immune response, namely, natural Abs, lectins, and the AP itself (Fig. 22–9). Complement activation is, therefore, one of the earliest reactions at sites of infection. This complement response opsonizes organisms for adherence, phagocytosis, and antigen processing while released fragments trigger immunocompetent cells and set up an inflammatory milieu (Table 22–5).

TABLE 22–5 • COMPLEMENT SYSTEM IN IMMUNITY

1. Serves as first line of defense as part of an innate immunity
2. Mediates an inflammatory response
3. Modifies membranes of microbes
4. Has an instructive role to adaptive immunity
5. Participates in antigen identification, processing, transportation, and retention
6. Involved in cellular activation and induction of costimulatory molecules, cytokines, and other mediators of an immune response; lowers threshold for B lymphocyte signaling
7. Serves as effector arm of humoral immunity
8. Handles clearance of necrotic debris and apoptotic cells

ADAPTIVE IMMUNITY

As pointed out at the beginning of this chapter, complement was discovered through its role as an effector arm of humoral immunity. IgM and IgG activate the CP and in so doing opsonize and lyse targets. This important effector activity is one aspect of complement function in adaptive immunity. More recently, an important role for complement in the afferent side has been "rediscovered."[2,22] Accumulating evidence indicates that complement is an "instructor" of adaptive immunity.[2,22] Nearly 30 years ago, the injection of cobra venom factor to destroy normal plasma-complement activity was demonstrated to attenuate immune response of a mouse. A weak primary response and no class switching to IgG were the results. Moreover, these mice did not generate memory B cells. Similarly, in multiple subsequent studies, C4- or C2-deficient guinea pigs and humans did not respond efficiently to intravenous administration of a phage antigen. Although they did produce IgM Ab, they did *not* class switch from IgM to IgG Ab or demonstrate immunologic memory. In other studies, blocking CR2 reduced the Ab response to T cell–dependent Ags and inhibited isotype switching. Further, animals with a targeted gene deletion of complement receptor CR1/CR2 also had a decreased response to Ag and a failure to isotype switch. Taken together, these data imply a role for the CP and complement receptors in mounting an adaptive immune response. Finally, coating of antigen with C3d increased its immunogenicity up to 10,000-fold.[23,24] Consequently, vaccines containing complement-coated antigens are likely to be more immunogenic. This linkage of innate to adaptive immunity occurs through complement coating of an antigen.

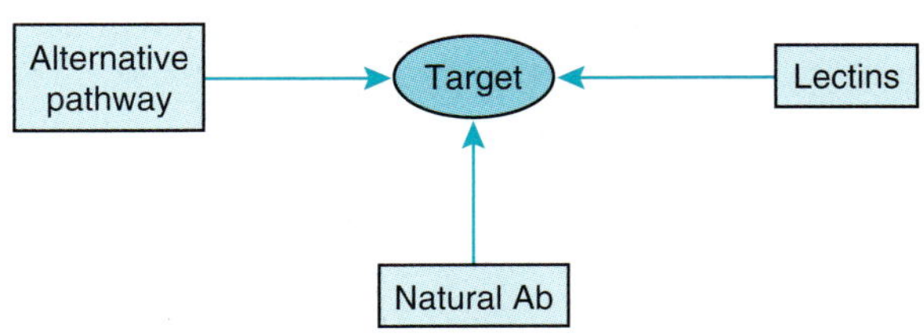

FIGURE 22–9 • Three potential means of complement activation on a target novel to the immune system.

CLEARANCE OF DEAD, DAMAGED, AND APOPTOTIC CELLS

The complement, (C) system likely plays an important role in facilitating the removal of injured cells and their cellular debris.[4-7] Natural antibodies, lectins, and the AP recognize altered surface characteristics of damaged cells and, through opsonization, promote their proper removal. Such a system probably evolved to remove injured tissue, especially traumatized skin and apoptotic cells. If this system fails, as might happen in C1q or C4 deficiency, the individual may be predisposed to developing autoantibodies (the so-called "garbage or waste disposal hypothesis" for explaining autoimmunity in SLE).[6,7] Ischemia-reperfusion injury may also be a related situation.[25] In this situation, complement activation has clearly been shown to mediate damage of viable (but at-risk) tissue surrounding a myocardial infarction.

Immune Complex Clearance

The C system is important for the processing and clearance of IC.[5,6,8,21] As IC form, activation of the CP leads to C3b deposition that, in turn, prevents the IC from precipitating in a vessel wall or tissue site (this is called maintenance of IC solubility). The deposition of C3b on the Ab and antigen may reduce the ability of Ab to cross-link and, therefore, precipitate the IC. Even preformed immune complexes can be solubilized by exposure to fresh serum. The soluble immune complexes, bearing clusters of C3b, next become bound to peripheral blood cells, especially erythrocytes. This phenomenon is called immune adherence. Erythrocytes, (E) possess more than 80 percent of the CR1 in blood and serve as a taxi or shuttle, taking the IC to the liver and spleen, where they are dissociated from the RBC. Most IC are destroyed in the liver or the spleen. This transfer of IC from the E to tissue macrophages may be mediated by simple affinity differences (multiple types of receptors with higher affinity for C3 fragments) and also by a proteolytic cleavage event that occurs near the stalk of CR1. The E returns to the circulation, possibly minus a few of its receptors, but ready for another round of immune adherence and immune clearance. This processing system for IC evolved to prevent IC from depositing in undesirable locations such as the kidney glomerulus. Based on the previous discussion, this mechanism would fail due to: 1) a CP component deficiency up to and including C3; 2) C receptor deficiency; 3) synthesis of a non–CP fixing Ab such as IgG_4 or IgA; 4) severe hepatic dysfunction; or 5) following splenectomy.[26] This concept of IC clearance is part of most infectious diseases in which an Ab response is made and is especially relevant to syndromes featuring IC such as in SLE, cryoglobulinemia, serum sickness, and certain other vasculitic syndromes.

Complement Measurement

Complement is assessed by antigenic and functional assays (Tables 22–6 and 22–7). In clinical practice, the most commonly used, functional measurement is the total hemolytic complement assay (THC or CH_{50}). The assay is based on the ability of the patient's serum sample to lyse sheep erythrocytes optimally sensitized with rabbit antibody. All nine components of the CP (i.e., C1 through C9) are required for a normal THC. A result of "200 units" means that at a dilution of 1:200, the test serum lysed 50 percent of the antibody-coated (sensitized) sheep erythrocytes. THC is a useful screening tool for detecting a homozygous deficiency of single component (C1 through C8) because a total deficiency of a component will produce a score of less than 10, or undetectable, THC. Deficiency of C9 will give a low but detectable THC. This assay should probably be performed at the time of initial evaluation of appropriate patients. It provides a screen for a total deficiency as well as an assessment of whether complement activation is occurring.

More commonly used tests are antigenic assays for C4 and C3. They are widely available, relatively inexpensive, and more simply and accurately measured by nephelometric-based immunoassays. They are useful in the initial diagnosis of lupus and related syndromes and for following the course of patients undergoing treatment whose values were low when their disease process was active. Upon treatment, the return of the values to normal correlates with clinical improvement and bodes a better outcome. Table 22–6 provides examples of serum-complement test results and their interpretation in rheumatic diseases.

Becoming more widely utilized and available are tests for the detection of activation fragments (such as C3a and C5a), neoantigens, and activation fragments (C4d, C3d, Bb). Their clinical utility relates to the fact that they are dynamic parameters and, thus, reflect ongoing turnover of the system. Also, the tests are not affected by partial inherited deficiencies or alterations in synthetic rates. However, they are more costly, not widely available, and unnecessary in most clinical situations.

Complement Deficiency

Inherited deficiencies of complement components predispose to bacterial infections (as expected) or autoimmunity (this was unexpected), especially SLE[14,27] (Tables 22–8, 22–9 and 22–10). Most are inherited as autosomal codominant (recessive) traits, except for the C1 inhibitor, which is autosomal dominant, and P and factor D, which are sex-linked. A thorough and well-reasoned analysis of this subject can be found in Pickering and colleagues' 2000 article in *Advances in Immunology*,[14] which also includes tables listing every published case of early complement component deficiency in humans. Several other reviews have been recently published.[27-30]

CLASSIC PATHWAY

The prevalence of lupus in homozygous C1q, C4, or C2 deficiency is approximately 90, 75, and 10 to 30 percent, respectively.[14,27-30] The female-to-male ratio is approximately 1 to 1 in C1q or C4 deficiency but approximates

TABLE 22–6 • ASSAYS FOR COMPLEMENT ACTIVATION IN HUMAN DISEASE

Method	Use	Comments
CH_{50} or THC	Screen for a component deficiency or activation of classical pathway	Functional assay—requires appropriate sample handling
AP_{50}	Screen for component deficiency or activation of alternative pathway	Functional assay—requires appropriate sample handling
Antigenic (ELISA, immunodiffusion, nephelometry)	Standard method for C3, C4, factor B, C1-inhibitor, and MBL determinations	Widely available, easy to perform, reliable, inexpensive
Antigenic or hemolytic assay of individual components	Further define a suspected deficiency	Samples usually sent to laboratories specializing in complement assays
Activation fragments C3a, C5a, Bb, C1r/C1s, C5b-9 (neoantigen)	May be positive with normal complement levels	Expensive, sample collection important, commercial labs often do these assays; more sensitive than static levels
C1-inhibitor function	Clinical picture consistent with HAE but C1-inhibitor levels by antigenic assay are normal or elevated	15% of HAE kindreds have normal or elevated levels of a nonfunctional protein
Immunofluorescence	Demonstration of complement activation fragments in tissue	C1q, C4, and C3 are most commonly studied in kidney and skin biopsies
Antiglobulin testing (non-gamma Coombs)	Demonstration of C3 fragments on erythrocytes	Usual fragment detected is C3d

Abbreviations: AP_{50}, alternative pathway equivalent of THC or CH_{50}; CH_{50} or THC, total hemolytic assay for classic pathway; ELISA, enzyme-linked immunosorbent assay; HAE, hereditary angioedema; MBL, mannan-binding lectin.

TABLE 22–7 • INTERPRETATION OF THE RESULTS OF COMPLEMENT DETERMINATIONS

THC (units/ml)	C4 (mg/dl)	C3 (mg/dl)	Interpretation
150-250	16-40	100-180	Normal range
250	40	200	Acute-phase response
100	10	80	Classical pathway activation
100	30	50	Alternative pathway activation
<10 or 0	30	140	Inherited deficiency or in vitro activation*
50	<8	100	Partial C4 deficiency or fluid-phase activation†

*In vitro activation is more common than an inherited deficiency state. The lack of activity (<10 THC) in the setting of normal C4 and C3 antigenic levels suggests: 1) an improperly handled sample; 2) cold activation (such as by cryoglobulins) following collection of the sample; or 3) homozygous component deficiency (most commonly C2 with a lupus presentation or, if a *Neisseria* infection, of an alternative pathway [AP] or membrane attack complex [MAC] component).

†Because THC is detectable, this cannot be a complete deficiency of C4. A partial C4 deficiency, such as of C4A, could give this result. Some types of immune complexes, especially cryoglobulins, and a deficiency of the C1-inhibitor (hereditary angioedema) also give this pattern. In these cases, measurement of C2 is often helpful; a low value suggests activation, whereas a normal value suggests an inherited, partial C4 deficiency. Also, C4A and C4B alleles can be assessed by commercial laboratories.

Modified from: Liszewski, M.K., Atkinson, J.P.: The complement, system. Primer on the Rheumatic Diseases 12th ed., page 66, 2001.

Abbreviations: THC, total hemolytic complement or CH_{50}.

7 to 1 in C2 deficiency. Concordance rates for SLE among dizygotic twins is 2 percent and 24 percent for monozygotic twins, whereas concordance of SLE among siblings with C1q, C4, or C2 deficiency is 90, 80, and 58 percent, respectively. Those complement deficient with SLE usually begin having symptoms before age 20 and often have prominent cutaneous (90%) and renal (50%) manifestations. Antinuclear antibody (ANA) tests are positive in about 75 percent of patients. Most patients are DNA negative, whereas antibodies to ENA are detected in approximately 70 percent. The disease process tends to be more severe in C1q and C4 than C2 deficiency. About 1 percent of lupus patients have a complete complement component deficiency, most commonly C2 deficiency.

About one third of SLE patients develop a deficiency of C1q secondary to anti-C1q Ab. These Abs probably develop after the onset of SLE and, therefore, are a secondary phenomenon.[14] These patients tend to have renal disease and low complements (C4, C2, C3).

The C4 genes are duplicated (all four must be deleted or defective to give a total C4 deficiency) giving rise to C4A (acidic) and C4B (basic) types.[31] C4A deficiency occurs in up to 15 percent of Caucasian SLE patients (vs. 1 to 3% of controls). C4A preferentially binds amino groups and because of this reacts more efficiently with some types of IC than C4b. This may explain why homozygous C4A deficiency has been shown to be an independent risk factor for SLE. The association generally

TABLE 22–8 • CLINICAL MANIFESTATIONS OF COMPLEMENT-COMPONENT DEFICIENCY

Deficient Component	Clinical Syndrome
Classical Pathway	
C1q	SLE, infections
C1r/C1s	SLE, infections
C4	SLE, infections
C2	SLE, infections
Lectin Pathway	
Mannan Binding Lectin, (MBL)	Infections
Central Component	
C3	Severe infections, GN, SLE
Membrane Attack Component	
C5, C6, C7, C8, or C9	*Neisseria* infections
Alternative Pathway	
Properdin, factor D	*Neisseria* infections

*With the early component deficiency of the classical pathway, C1, C4, and C2, the infections tend to be with commonly encountered pyogenic organisms. With a late component (C5-9) and an alternative pathway component deficiency, *Neisseria* infections predominate, especially with the meningococcus.

Abbreviations: GN, glomerulonephritis; SLE, systemic lupus erythematosus.

occurs across multiple ethnic backgrounds, as well as in the absence of the European ancestral "autoimmune" haplotype (HLA-A1, C7, B8, C4AQ*0, C4B1, DR3, DQ2). The clinical course is similar to idiopathic lupus, but there may be less renal disease.[32-34] In fact, one group has argued for caution in the use of immunosuppressive therapy because of the generally favorable course of renal disease in most patients.[32] C4A measurements are available through commercial laboratories.

The most common homozygous complement component deficiency state is that of C2 (1:10-20,000 individuals). Heterozygotes are present in 1 to 2 percent of the Caucasian population. SLE occurs in 10 to 30 percent of homozygous C2-null individuals. Notable differences in associations of SLE with C2 deficiency relate to less renal and cerebral but more cutaneous (prominent photosensitivity) involvement, earlier age of onset, and a higher frequency of anti-Ro antibodies. Heterozygosity for C2 deficiency does not appear to be at an increased risk for SLE.

ALTERNATIVE PATHWAY

C3 deficiency is associated with recurrent pyogenic infections and, less commonly, glomerulonephritis. For the latter, ANAs are usually not detected, and other systemic features of SLE are lacking. P, Factor B (one case), and factor D deficiency are strongly associated with meningococcal infections but not autoimmunity.[35]

LECTIN PATHWAY

Polymorphisms producing low serum-MBL levels demonstrate an association with SLE across several ethnic backgrounds. In one series, the incidence of SLE was increased twofold in MBL deficiency.[36] Impressively, infectious complications, particularly severe pneumonias in association with immunosuppressive therapy, were much more frequent in the MBL-deficient patients. The combination of an MBL and a C4 gene deficiency may be a particularly predisposing combination to SLE. In RA, MBL deficiency may be a modest risk factor for getting the disease.[13,37] Of perhaps greater interest, MBL deficiency was associated with earlier age of onset, more severe erosive disease, and increased frequency of infectious complications during treatment.

ACQUIRED COMPLEMENT-DEFICIENCY STATES

Acquired complement deficiency usually results from accelerated consumption. CP activation is observed in more than 50 percent of lupus patients. Generally, the more active the disease process, the more likely complement levels will be low as consumption outstrips the liver's synthetic capacity. Low complement values (C4, C3, or THC) are a poor prognostic factor and correlate with antibodies to native DNA, nephritis, and, overall, more severe disease. Complement deposition in tissue, especially in the glomerulus as detected by immunofluorescence, assists in the diagnosis and classification of lupus nephritis. Antibodies to C1q occur in 15 to 30 percent of SLE patients, but their contribution to disease pathogenesis is not well understood.

"C3 nephritic factor" is an autoantibody against the AP C3 convertase. The autoantibody stabilizes the convertase

TABLE 22–9 • AUTOIMMUNE DISORDERS IN COMPLETE COMPLEMENT-COMPONENT DEFICIENCIES

Component	Cases (n)	Dominant Phenotype (%)	Autoimmune Phenotype (%)	Other Phenotypes
C1q	35	94 SLE	94 SLE	Infection
C1r/s	11	55 SLE	55 SLE 9 GN	Infection
C4	24	75 SLE	75 SLE 8 HSP 4 Scl 4 SS 4 GN	Infection
C2	110	32 SLE	32 SLE	Infection
C3	21	75 Severe infections	23 GN 14 SLE 14 vasculitis	Arthritis

Modified from: Sullivan K.E.: Complement deficiency and autoimmunity Current Opinion In Pediatrics 10:600, 1998.

Abbreviations: GN, glomerulonephritis; SLE, systemic lupus erythematosus.

TABLE 22–10 • WHAT IS THE DEFECT IN A CLASSICAL PATHWAY COMPLEMENT COMPONENT DEFICIENCY THAT LEADS TO AUTOIMMUNITY? THE TWO LEADING HYPOTHESIS ARE LISTED HERE. THEY ARE NOT MUTUALLY EXCLUSIVE

Defective Immune Complex Handling
Of foreign antigens
Of self antigens (apoptotic and necrotic debris)
Defective Immune Response
Reduced humoral immune responsiveness
Failure to regulate autoreactive B cells

to the point that excessive C3 cleavage and a secondary deficiency of C3 results. Patients with C3 nephritic factor are predominantly children who may present with glomerulonephritis, partial lipodystrophy, or frequent infections with encapsulated bacteria.

Models of Inflammatory Disease Featuring Complement Activation

In general, these in vivo models have explored C activation 1) in mediating tissue damage in diseases featuring complement as an immune effector (autoantibodies); 2) in producing inflammation; or 3) enhancing the afferent limb of the immune response.

DEFICIENT ANIMALS

Before knockout mice were available, guinea pigs deficient in C4 or C2 or with very low levels of C3, rats and rabbits deficient in C6, dogs deficient in C3, and pigs deficient in factor H had been characterized.[2] Further, in the 1960s, many strains of inbred mice were shown to be deficient in C5. Experiments with these species clearly indicated the double-edged sword aspects of the C system. In general, the deficient animals were more sensitive to challenges with bacteria but more resistant to antibody-mediated tissue damage. These animals were also widely used to determine the role of complement in inflammatory or immune models (i.e, the Arthus reaction, serum sickness, and Forssman shock). These will be briefly discussed in the following paragraphs because they demonstrate the range of reactions caused in part by complement activation.

In the Arthus model, antibodies to a foreign antigen are raised, and then the antigen is reinjected into the immune host. If the antigen is injected in a joint, IC form in the joint space, complement is activated, Fcγ receptors engaged, and an inflammatory reaction ensues. It is a transient and nondestructive process unless antigen is repeatedly injected.

Emphasis has recently been placed on separating the effects of IgG antibody working through Fcγ receptors on phagocytes and B cells from those induced by complement.[2,38-41] For example, it had generally been believed that the Arthus reaction was mediated by local C activation. The immigration of neutrophils in this process was thought to be caused primarily by the local formation of C5a. This concept was challenged when it became possible to generate mice by homologous recombination with C3 deficiency on one hand and FcγRI and FcγRIII deficiency on the other. In the mouse, FcγRIII was required for Arthus reaction in the skin but not C. However, complement was of critical importance in IC-mediated peritonitis in mice and in IC-mediated lung disease in rats. Interestingly, C is also of major importance in the IC-mediated skin disease of guinea pigs and rats. Thus, the species, the experimental conditions, and genetic backgrounds are of critical importance.

In the usual serum-sickness model in the rabbit employing the BSA-anti-BSA, synovitis develops, which is mediated by the deposition of IC in association with complement activation in joints. In the preantibiotic era, a serum-sickness reaction was observed in children receiving horse serum containing antibodies to treat infectious diseases. The human or rabbit clinical illness lasted 1 to 2 weeks, resolving as the host went into Ab excess and cleared the foreign protein. Of course, if more antigen was injected, an accelerated serum-sickness reaction developed. These conditions are likely to be met in SLE and mixed cryoglobulinemia secondary to chronic hepatitis B or hepatitis C infection.

Another model of complement-dependent pathologic damage is that of Forssman shock.[2] Forssman antigen is a widely distributed lipopolysaccharide. Species, such as the rabbit, that are Forssman negative develop an immune response to sheep RBCs, as sheep are a Forssman-positive species. The rabbit responds to the injection of sheep E with high titer anti-Forssman antibody. Upon intravenous injection of this rabbit Ab into guinea pigs, a Forssman-positive species, the Ab travels from the vein into the lung where it causes massive damage that is CP dependent with alveolar capillary fluid leakage and hemorrhage. Phagocytes are not important in this cataclysmic reaction, in which death occurs within a few minutes, but the lytic activities of C appear to be essential. This model and the Arthus reaction have been used, for example, to test the effect of anticomplement reagents in preventing tissue damage.

GENE-TARGETED DEFICIENCIES

Over the past decade, C1q, factor B, factor D, factor B/C2, C3, C4, CR1/CR2, C5aR, MCP, and DAF have all been deleted by targeted insertional mutagenesis.[5-7,27,42,43] C1q, C4, C2, C3, and CR1/CR2 mice demonstrated substantial defects in T cell–dependent immune responses and have the expected defects in IC clearance. Thus, for most strains with a defect in the CP or AP, defective clearance of bacteria and viruses could be shown. The C1q- and C4-deficient mice (depending on their genetic background) have enhanced humoral immunity and glomerulonephritis (lupus-like picture) with problems in clearance of apoptotic bodies. The C5aR-deficient mice have a decrease in inflammatory cell infiltrates. Most of these knockout mice have only been developed since the mid 1990s. Over the next decade, they will be used to clarify C's role in host defense against infection, in the immune response, and in autoimmunity.

Complement Activation in Polyarthritis

HUMAN RHEUMATOID ARTHRITIS

A major observation in RA and juvenile rheumatoid arthritis (JRA) is that complement is activated locally (i.e., in synovial fluid and joint tissue).[13,44,45] Thus, if the functional activity of joint fluid C4, C2, or C3 is determined, it is low versus that obtained for a parallel antigenic level. These types of data have established that complement components in RA joint fluid are antigenically intact but functionally inactive. In other words, the components have been engaged in an immune reaction. Further, essentially every known complement activation fragment is elevated in RA joint fluid. The activation profile is primarily that of the CP (low C4 and C2), but there is substantial evidence for an AP contribution. The clinical correlations established with these measures of complement activation in RA are erosive, seropositive disease. B cells, rheumatoid factors, and complement were postulated to play a critical role in mediating synovial inflammation in these early days (1950 to 1980) of investigations into immune basis of RA.[18] However, from then until the turn of the 20th century, T cell–mediated immunity was considered to be the predominant system responsible for the synovial-based reaction in RA. A more prominent role for B cells, autoantibodies, and complement has arisen again with recognition of the critical role in animal models of RA (see following).

COLLAGEN-INDUCED ARTHRITIS

Complement activation products are prominent in the joint fluid and synovial tissue of rats and mice in this model of collagen injection.[45-47] The disease is mild or absent in C5-deficient mice, mice treated with a mAb to C5, and mice treated with the potent complement inhibitor, soluble CR1. The C5 mAb treatment also ameliorated established disease. These results implicate C5a or C5b-C9 (MAC) or some combination of the two as being responsible for the synovitis. One might have suspected a major contribution to disease pathogenesis from C3-activation products.

K/BXN MOUSE MODEL

This spontaneous mouse model was generated by crossing the T cell receptor (TCR) transgenic mouse line (known as KRNxC56B1/6) with the nonobese diabetic (NOD) mouse strain.[48,49] Autoantibodies that arise in the K/BxN mouse recognize the ubiquitously expressed intracellular enzyme glucose-6-phosphate isomerase (GPI). The important points are as follows:

1. A destructive small joint arthritis develops in these mice.
2. The autoantibodies are pathogenic.
3. The disease can be transferred to other strains by antibody.
4. Complement is required for the arthritis to develop.

Surprisingly, the CP is not necessary, as mice deficient in C1q or C4 were susceptible. Mice deficient in C3 or AP component factor B did not develop arthritis. Moreover, C5-deficient mice or mice treated with a mAb to C5 did not develop arthritis (in the transfer model). C5a receptor–deficient mice were studied, and they were protected from developing arthritis. In this new model then, AP activation produces C5a, which interacts with its receptor to mediate the "complement effect" required for disease development.

Another lesson from this model is the role of the complement regulatory proteins in "allowing" the disease to develop. Thus, the pathogenic Ab also binds to the kidney glomerulus, but there was no excessive C3b deposition or development of glomerulonephritis. A likely explanation for this lack of renal disease is that it requires both antigen accessibility and a permissive environment for complement activation. Cartilage may be relatively devoid of complement-regulatory proteins, so the AP can be engaged. The CP is not activated in this model because the Ab is predominantly of the IgG1 subclass, which, in the mouse, is poorly complement fixing. Nevertheless, Abs bound to an antigen can protect the cascade from regulation by inhibitors and thereby trigger the AP.[50] Therefore, although it remains unclear as to clear why the autoantibody arises, this model has provided provocative insights into how an autoantibody-mediated inflammatory arthritis that mimics RA could occur, and it establishes a role for the complement system.

Therapeutic Implications

Study of the complement system has undergone a renaissance over the past decade. Much of this revival relates to: 1) identification of complement regulatory and receptor proteins; 2) development of inhibitors for experimental and clinical use; 3) association of deficiency states with autoimmunity (especially the C1q, C4, or C2 lupus association); 4) greater appreciation of the importance of complement as part of the innate immune system in instructing the adaptive immunity; and 5) availability of gene-targeted mice to more precisely define the role of complement in the normal immune response and in mouse models of autoimmunity. The development of complement inhibitors for clinical use is a long-sought goal. Currently, two such compounds, a humanized monoclonal antibody to C5 and a solubilized version of complement receptor one, (sCR1) are in clinical trials[51-54] (Table 22–11). They effectively attenuate tissue destruction and inflammatory responses in animal models in which considerable evidence has already accumulated relative to complement's participation (e.g., Arthus reaction, serum sickness, SLE, and many others). Complement inhibition, however, also reduced infarct size in experimental models of myocardial infarction and tissue damage in many other types of ischemia-reperfusion injury.

TABLE 22–11 • COMPLEMENT ACTIVATION INHIBITORS UNDERGOING CLINICAL TRIALS

Product	Description	Actions	Company
TP10	Soluble recombinant CR1 (sCR1)	Degrades C3b/C4b (CA) and decays C3/C5 convertases (DAA)	Avant Immunotherapeutics (Needham, Mass.)
H5G1.1; h5G1.1-scFv	Humanized, high-affinity anti-C5 mAb; single-chain version	Blocks cleavage of C5 by C5 convertases	Alexion Pharmaceuticals (New Haven, Conn.)

Abbreviations: CA, cofactor activity; DAA, decay-accelerating activity; mAb, monoclonal antibody.

Further, a role for complement in clearing apoptotic cells is also likely. These remarkable results suggest that the complement system removes damaged tissue. Unfortunately, these two recombinantly produced inhibitors are not commercially available but are in phase II and phase III trials. A complement inhibitor for clinical use is much anticipated.

REFERENCES

1. Zarkadis IK, Mastellos D, Lambris JD: Phylogenetic aspects of the complement system. Dev Comp Immunol 25:745-762, 2001.
2. Frank MM, Atkinson JP: Complement system. *In* Austen KF, Frank MM, Atkinson JP, Cantor H (eds): Samter's Immunologic Diseases, 6th ed, vol. 1. Baltimore, Lippincott, Williams and Wilkins, 2001, pp 281-299.
3. Silverstein AM: A History of Immunology. San Diego, Calif., Academic Press, 1989.
4. Nauta AJ, MDaha M, R., van Kooten C, et al: Recognition and clearance of apoptitic cells: a role for complement and pentraxins. Trend Immunol 24:148-154, 2003.
5. Volanakis JE: Overview of the complement system. *In* Volanakis JE, Frank MM (eds): The Human Complement System in Health and Disease, 10th ed. New York, Marcel Dekker, 1998, pp 9-32.
6. Walport MJ: Complement: First of two parts. N Engl J Med 344:1058-1066, 2001.
7. Walport MJ: Complement: Second of two parts. N Engl J Med 344:1140-1144, 2001.
8. Morgan BP: Complement: Clinical Aspects and Relevance to Disease. London, Harcourt Brace Jovanovich, 1990.
9. DuClos TW: Function of C-reactive protein. Ann Med 32:274-278, 2000.
10. Ollert MW, Kadlec JV, David K, et al: Antibody-mediated complement activation on nucleated cells: A quantitative analysis of the individual reaction steps. J Immunol 153:2213-2221, 1994.
11. Turner MW: Mannose-binding lectin: The pluripotent molecule of the innate immune system. Immunol Today 17:532-540, 1996.
12. Fujita T: Evolution of the lectin-complement pathway and its role in innate immunity. Nat Rev. Immunol 2:346-353, 2002.
13. Atkinson JP: Complement and other aspects of innate immunity. *In* St. Clair EW (ed): RA: Textbook of Rheumatoid Arthritis, in press.
14. Pickering MC, Botto M, Taylor PR, et al: Systemic lupus erythematosus, complement deficiency, and apoptosis. Adv Immunol 76:227-324, 2000.
15. Liszewski MK, Farries TC, Lublin DM, et al: Control of the complement system. Adv Immunol 61:201-283, 1996.
16. Morgan BP, Harris CL: Complement Regulatory Proteins. San Diego, Calif., Harcourt Brace, 1999.
17. Parker CM: Membrane Defenses Against Attack by Complement and Perforins. Berlin, Springer-Verlag, 1992.
18. Zipfel PF, Skerka C, Caprioli J, et al: Complement factor H and hemolytic uremic syndrome. Int Immunopharmacol 1:461-468, 2001.
19. Davis AE III: C1 inhibitor gene and hereditary angioedema. *In* Volanakis JE, Frank MM (eds): The Human Complement System in Health and Disease. New York, Marcel Dekker, 1998, pp 455-480.
20. Kotwal GJ: Poxviral mimicry of complement and chemokine system components: what's the end game? Immunol Today 21:242-248, 2000.
21. Hebert LA: The clearance of immune complexes from the circulation of man and other primates. Am J Kidney Dis 17:353-361, 1991.
22. Nielsen CH, Leslie RG: Complement's participation in acquired immunity. J Leukocyte Biol 72:249-261, 2002.
23. Fearon DT, Locksley RM: The instructive role of innate immunity in the acquired immune response. Science 272:50-54, 1996.
24. Dempsey PW, Allison ME, Akkaraju S, et al: C3d of complement as a molecular adjuvant: bridging innate and acquired immunity. Science 271:348-350, 1996.
25. Moore FD Jr.: Therapeutic regulation of the complement system in acute injury states. Adv Immunol 56:267-299, 1994.
26. Atkinson JP, Schifferli JA: Complement system and systemic lupus erythematosus. *In* Kammer GM and Tsokos, G.C. (eds): Lupus: Molecular and Cellular Pathogenesis. Totowa, NJ, Humana Press, 1999, pp 529-540.
27. Barilla-LaBarca ML, Atkinson JP: Rheumatic syndromes associated with complement deficiency. Curr Opin Rheum 15:55-60, 2003.
28. Welch TR: The complement system in renal diseases. Nephron 88:199-204, 2001.
29. Sullivan KE: Complement deficiency and autoimmunity. Curr Opin Pediatrics 10:600-606, 1998.
30. O'Neil KM: Complement deficiency. Clin Rev Allergy Immunol 19:83-108, 2000.
31. Atkinson JP, Schneider PM: Genetic susceptibility and class III complement genes. *In* Lahita RG (ed): Systemic Lupus Erythematosus, 3rd ed. San Diego, Calif., Academic Press, 1999, pp 91-104.
32. Welch TR, Frenzke M: Glomerulonephritis associated with deficiencies and polymorphisms of complement components encoded in the class III region of the MHC. Front Biosci 6:D898-903, 2001.
33. Welch TR, Brickman C, Bishof N, et al: The phenotype of SLE associated with complete deficiency of complement isotype C4A. J Clin Immunol 18:48-51, 1998.
34. Petri M, Watson R, Winkelstein JA, et al: Clinical expression of systemic lupus erythematosus in patients with C4A deficiency. Medicine 72:236-244, 1993.
35. Figueroa JE, Densen P: Infectious diseases associated with complement deficiencies. Clin Microbiol Rev 4:359-395, 1991.
36. Garred P, Madsen HO, Halberg P, et al: Mannose-binding lectin polymorphisms and susceptibility to infection in systemic lupus erythematosus. Arthritis Rheum 42:2145-2152, 1999.
37. Garred P, Madsen HO, Halberg P, et al: The association of variant mannose-binding lectin genotypes with radiographic outcome in rheumatoid arthritis. Arthritis Rheum 43:515-521, 2000.
38. Takai T: Roles of Fc receptors in autoimmunity. Nat Rev Immunology 2:580-592, 2002.
39. Ravetch JV, Bolland S: IgG Fc receptors. Ann Rev Immunol 19:275-290, 2001.
40. Baumann U, Chouchakova N, Gewecke B, et al: Distinct tissue site-specific requirements of mast cells and complement components C3/C5a receptor in IgG immune complex-induced injury of skin and lung. J Immunol 167:1022-1027, 2001.
41. Shushakova N, Skokowa J, Schulman J, et al: C5a anaphylatoxin is a major regulator of activating versus inhibitory Fc gamma

receptors in immune complex-induced lung disease. J Clin Invest 110:1823-1830, 2002.
42. Holers VM: Phenotypes of complement knockouts. Immunopharmacology 49:125-131, 2000.
43. Einav S, Pozdnyakova OO, Ma M, et al: Complement C4 is protective for lupus disease independent of C3. J Immunol 168:1036-1041, 2002.
44. Neumann E, Barnum SR, Tarner IH, et al: Local production of complement proteins in rheumatoid arthritis synovium. Arthritis Rheum 46:934-945, 2002.
45. Linton SM, Morgan BP: Complement activation and inhibition in experimental models of arthritis. Molecular Immunol 36:905-914, 1999.
46. Wang Y, Kristan J, Hao L, et al: A role for complement in antibody-mediated inflammation: C5-deficient DBA/1 mice are resistant to collagen-induced arthritis. J Immunol 164:4340-4347, 2000.
47. Wang Y, Rollins SA, Madri JA, et al: Anti-C5 monoclonal antibody therapy prevents collagen-induced arthritis and ameliorates established disease. Proc Nat Acad Sci U S A 92:8955-8959, 1995.
48. Ji H, Ohmura K, Mahmood U, et al: Arthritis critically dependent on innate immune system players. Immunity 16:157-168, 2002.
49. Matsumoto I, Maccioni M, Lee DM, et al: How antibodies to a ubiquitous cytoplasmic enzyme may provoke joint-specific autoimmune disease. Nat Immunol 3:360-365, 2002.
50. Fearon DT, Austen KF: Current concepts of immunology: The alternative pathway of complement - a system for host defense to microbial infection. N Engl J Med 303:259-263, 1980.
51. Liszewski MK, Atkinson JP: Complement inhibition. *In* Smolen J, Lipsky P (eds): Biological Therapy in Rheumatology. London, Martin Dunitz, 2002, pp 453-461.
52. Klickstein LB, Moore FD Jr., Atkinson JP: Therapeutic inhibition of complement activation with emphasis on drugs in clinical trials. *In* Austen KF, Burakoff SJ, Strom TB, Rosen FS (eds): Therapeutic Immunology. Malden, Mass., Blackwell Science, 2000, pp 287-301.
53. Kirshfink M: Targeting complement in therapy. Immunol Rev 180:177-189, 2001.
54. Bhole D, Stahl GL: Therapeutic potential of targeting the complement cascade in critical care medicine. Crit Care Med 31:S97-104, 2003.

23 Prostaglandins, Leukotrienes, and Related Compounds

ROBERT B. ZURIER

The addition of oxygen to arachidonic acid and other polyunsaturated fatty acids not bound to membrane phospholipids in nearly all human cell types results in formation of several classes of bioactive products called eicosanoids. These include prostaglandins, prostacyclin, thromboxanes, leukotrienes, and lipoxins. All of these compounds are critical to the regulation of immunity and inflammation, among other physiologic and pathologic processes. Although eicosanoids are derived from C20 polyunsaturated fatty acids (eicosa = 20), only a small percentage of these polyenoic acids form the eicosanoids: dihomogamma linolenic acid (DGLA), which is 8,11,14-eicosatrienoic acid); arachidonic acid (AA), which is 5,8,11,14-eicosatetraenoic acid; and eicosapentaenoic acid (EPA), which is 5,8,11,14,17 eicosapentaenoic acid (Fig. 23–1).

Two groups of fatty acids are essential to the body: the omega-6 series derived from linoleic acid (18:2 n-6) and the omega-3 series derived from alpha linolenic acid (18:3 n-3). The n refers to the number of carbon atoms from the methyl (omega) end of the fatty acid chain to the first double bond (i.e., omega-3 and omega-6 designations). Using this notation, 18 refers to the number of carbon atoms in the fatty acid. The degree of unsaturation (the number of double carbon-carbon bonds) follows the number of carbon atoms. Fatty acids are metabolized by an alternating sequence of desaturation (i.e., removal of two hydrogens) and elongation (i.e., addition of two carbons). Membrane phospholipids are the main storage site for polyunsaturated fatty acids and are particularly rich in eicosanoid precursors, which are located at the sn-2 position (Fig. 23–2). Because mammalian cells cannot interconvert n-3 and n-6 fatty acids, the composition of membrane phospholipids is determined by exogenous sources of fatty acids.

Biosynthesis of Eicosanoids

PHOSPHOLIPASES

Phospholipase A_2 (PLA_2) in lysosomes or bound to cell membranes catalyses the breaking of the sn-2 bond, facilitating release of arachidonic acid or other polyunsaturated fatty acids (see Fig. 23–2). The enzyme is crucial to eicosanoid-synthesis regulation, because it is in the nonesterified state that the polyunsaturated precursors enter into the cascades leading to eicosanoid formation. Only a scant amount of oxidation at carbon 15 of arachidonic acid occurs catalytically when the fatty acid is still covalently bound as part of a phospholipid.[1] Lysophospholipids "left over" after the action of PLA_2 are direct precursors of platelet-activating factor (PAF), a potent mediator of inflammation, which is generated by acylation in the open sn-2 position of the lysophospholipid.

Four distinct types of PLA_2 activities hydrolyze fatty acids esterified at the sn-2 position: secretory PLA_2 ($sPLA_2$), with small disulfide cross-linked proteins that require mM Ca^{2+} for optimal activity; cytoplasmic PLA_2 ($cPLA_2$), with larger proteins requiring μM Ca^{2+}, which are arachidonic-acid selective and can deacylate diacylphospholipids completely, thereby preventing accumulation of potentially toxic lysophospholipids; Ca^{2+}-independent PLA_2 ($iPLA_2$) that exhibits specificity for plasmalogen substrates; and PAF acetylhydrolase (PAF-AH or PAF-PLA_2), with a series of isozymes specific for short chains.[2]

Under basal conditions, arachidonic acid is liberated by $iPLA_2$, then reincorporated into cell membranes (reacylated), and, therefore, is not available for appreciable eicosanoid biosynthesis. Thus, the acylase enzymes competitively inhibit the cyclooxygenase (COX) isoenzymes. Following receptor activation and cell stimulation, intracellular Ca^{2+} levels rise, the Ca^{2+} dependent of $cPLA_2$ liberates arachidonate at a rate that exceeds the rate of reacylation, leading to arachidonate metabolism by COX isoenzymes. Initial formation of PGE_2, for example, appears to be due to preferential coupling between $cPLA_2$, COX-1, and cytosolic PGH-PGE isomerase. More intense inflammation leads to participation of inducibles, a secreted $sPLA_2$ and amplification of PGE_2 biosynthesis by inducible COX-2. It is, of course, an oversimplification to regard availability of arachidonic acid as the sole rate-limiting step in cellular eicosanoid biosynthesis. The coordinated action of phospholipases and the restricted expression and altered activation of COX isoenzymes are also important.[3]

Phospholipase C (PLC) hydrolyzes the polar head group (e.g., inositol, choline) from phospholipids to yield diacyl glycerol (DAG) and the polar head group. Direct protein isolation and molecular-cloning studies have revealed multiple PLC isozymes in mammalian tissues. Phosphatidylinositol (PI)-PLC occurs in cytosolic (cPLC) and secreted (sPLC) forms and can be divided into three major classes (PLC-β, PLC-γ, PLC-δ) based on substrate specificity. PLC with specificity for PI and phosphorylated PI is a key component of PI-mediated signaling pathways. DAG is an activator of protein kinase C (PKC), and rapid production of this lipid by PI-PLC hydrolysis of the phosphorylated PI pool is a primary step in signaling. Further arachidonic acid is made available

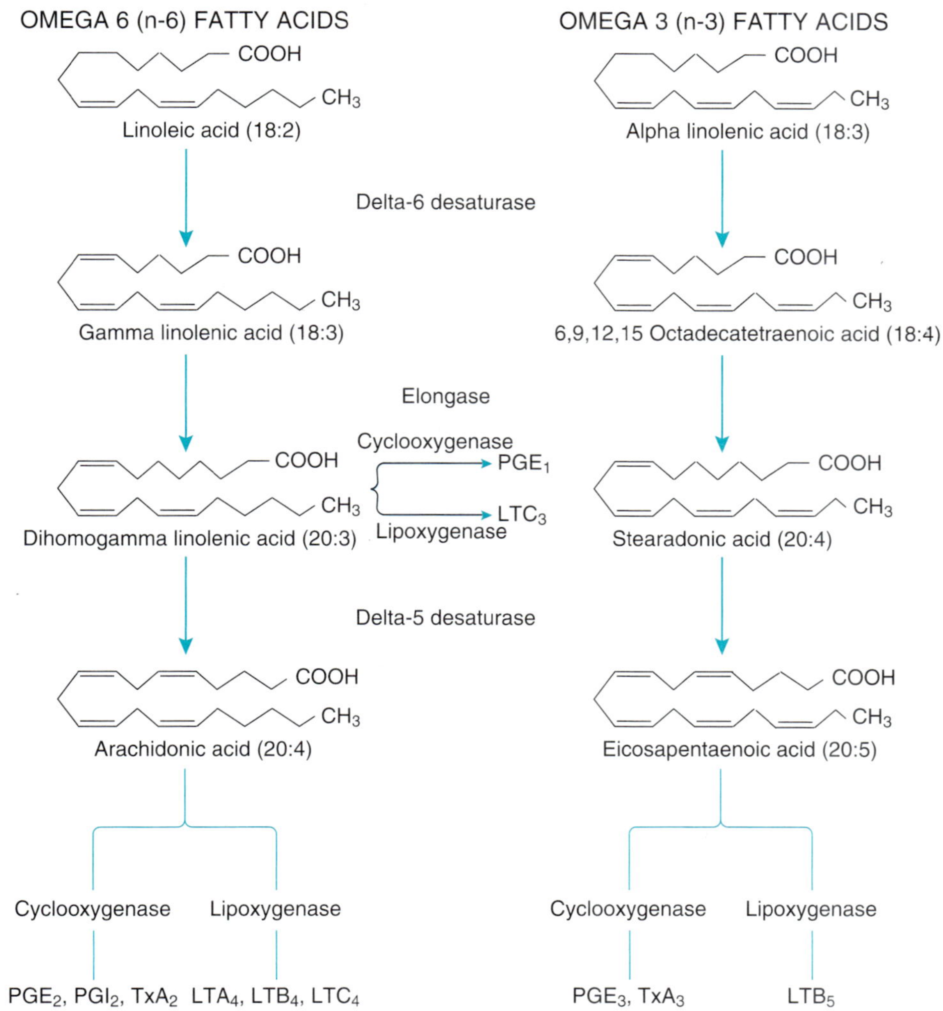

FIGURE 23–1 · Metabolic pathways of essential fatty acids. The pathways are ones of progressive desaturation alternating with elongation. Eicosanoid precursors include dihomogamma linolenic acid, arachidonic acid, and eicosapentaenoic acid.

by the sequential actions of diglyceride lipase and monoglyceride lipase.[4] PLC with activity on phosphatidylcholine has also been identified. Peripheral blood monocytes from patients with rheumatoid arthritis (RA) exhibit greater PLA_2 and PLC activity than cells from healthy volunteers. The greatest increases in enzyme activity were seen in cells from patients with the most severe, persistent, proliferative disease and not necessarily in cells from patients with the most active disease at the time the cells were studied.[5]

Hydrolysis of phospholipids by phospholipase D (PLD) produces phosphatidic acid (PA) and the respective polar head groups. The capacity of cells to interconvert PA and DAG through the action of specific cellular phosphatases and kinases (Fig. 23–3) suggests that arachidonic-acid release from DAG and a variety of intracellular-signaling and protein-trafficking events may be regulated by PLD activity. PLD may be activated after or independent of PLC activation.

The tetraenoic precursor (arachidonic acid) is the most abundant of the three precursor fatty acids in cells of people who eat usual diets in western culture. Metabolites of arachidonic acid constitute the "2" series (dienoic) prostaglandins (two double bonds in the molecule), and the metabolic pathway has acquired the familiar name *arachidonic acid cascade*. Figure 23–4 illustrates the COX and 5-lipoxygenase pathways of the cascade.

CYCLOOXYGENASE PATHWAY

The first step in the biosynthesis of the "prostanoids" (e.g., prostaglandins, thromboxanes, prostacyclin) is catalyzed by prostaglandin endoperoxide synthase isozyme (PGHS)-1 (COX-1) and PGHS-2 (COX-2). To form the characteristic five-carbon ring structure (thromboxanes contain a six-member ring), the precursor fatty acids must have double bonds at carbons 8, 11, and 14 (numbering from the carboxyl group). When a molecule of oxygen is inserted across carbons 9 and 11, ring closure takes place enzymatically across C8 and C12, creating the unstable prostaglandin endoperoxides PGG and PGH and forming the cyclopentane ring. PGH serves as the common precursor for prostaglandins, prostacyclin, and thromboxanes (see Fig. 23–4). In addition to the activity of phospholipases, regulation of prostaglandin synthesis also occurs at the level of PGHS gene expression. PGHS levels are increased by interleukin-1 (IL-1), platelet-derived growth factor (PDGF), and epidermal growth factor (EGF), agents that increase prostaglandin synthesis.

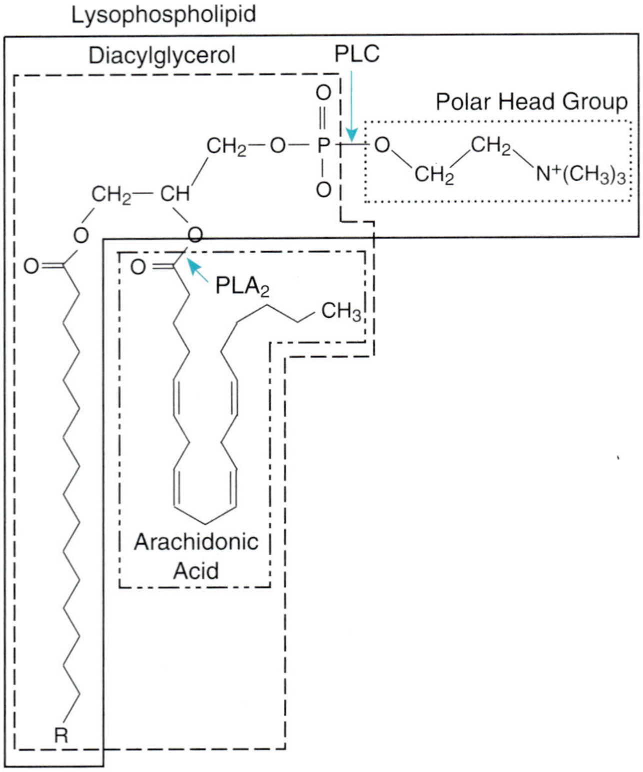

FIGURE 23–2 • Arachidonic acid release from phospholipid. Shown here is phosphatidylcholine, the major membrane storage site for polyunsaturated fatty acids. PLA_2, phospholipase A_2; PLC, phospholipase C.

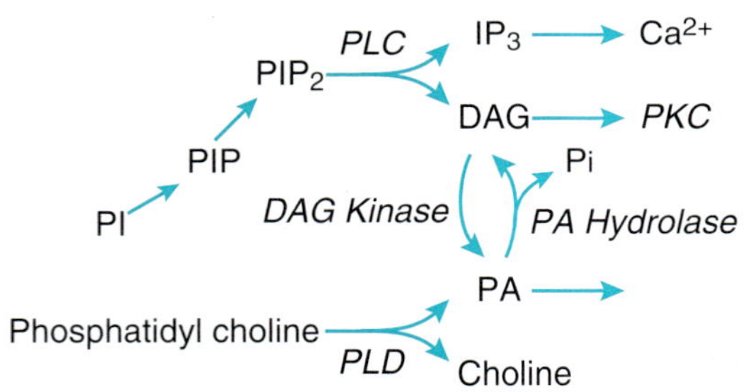

FIGURE 23–3 • Reactions catalyzed by phospholipases C and D, illustrating interconversion of diacylglycerol (DAG) and phosphatidic acid (PA).

Cell membranes constitute the source of substrate arachidonic acid and the site of action of eicosanoid-forming enzymes. However, prostaglandin synthesis can also form at lipid bodies, which are non–membrane-bound, lipid-rich cytoplasmic inclusions that develop in cells associated with inflammation. Lipid bodies isolated from human monocytes express PGHS activity, are reservoirs of arachidonyl phospholipids, and can function as domains of prostaglandin synthesis during an inflammatory reaction.[6]

PGHS, the well-known target of nonsteroidal anti-inflammatory drugs (NSAIDs) exists in two isoforms that are similar in terms of amino acid identities (about 60%), catalytic properties, and substrate specificity, but they differ in their genomic regulation.[7]

Regulation Of Cyclooxygenase-1 Expression

COX-1 is preferentially expressed constitutively at high levels in selected cells, including endothelium, monocytes, platelets, renal collecting tubules, and seminal vesicles. Because the expression level of the enzyme does not vary greatly, it has been difficult to study its transcriptional regulation. The gene has a TATA-less promoter that contains multiple start sites for transcription.[8] It is also known that Sp1/*Cis* regulatory elements in the promoter band the Sp1 transcription factor to induce COX-1 gene expression.[9] The localization of COX-1 in nearly all tissues under basal conditions suggests that its major function is to provide eicosanoids for physiologic regulation. This is seen clearly in platelets that do not have nuclei and cannot produce an inducible enzyme on activation. Rather, thromboxanes are produced constitutively so that platelet aggregation can be completed.

Regulation Of Cyclooxygenase-2 Expression

The regulated formation of eicosanoids implies that cells have an appreciable ability to amplify the rate and amount of eicosanoid synthesis. Several processes contribute to that regulation, including silencing of $sPLA_2$ expression by COX-2 and autoinactivation ("suicide inactivation") of COX-2 and other oxygenases and synthases. In addition, the COX-2 transcript contains at least 12 copies of the AUUUA RNA motif, which makes it unstable and subject to rapid degradation.[10] Factors that regulate COX-2 expression are specific for the physiologic processes involved. For example, expression of COX-2 in the macula densa in the kidney depends on lumenal salt concentrations. Transcriptional activation of the COX-2 gene by mediators of inflammation such as IL-1β and tumor necrosis factor-α (TNF-α) is likely regulated by the transcription factors nuclear factor kappa B (NFκB) and C/EBP.[11] Perhaps the most critical of the several demonstrated regulatory sequences in the 5′flanking regions of the COX-2 gene is the ATF/CRE, a site that is activated by the transcriptional activator protein-1 (AP-1) and the cyclic adenosine monophosphate (cAMP) regulatory binding protein (CREB).[12]

COX-1 and COX-2 effect a balance in several physiologic and pathologic situations. Of particular interest are their actions in kidney and stomach. During times of low blood volume, the kidney releases angiotensin and other factors to maintain blood pressure by systemic vasoconstriction. Angiotensin also provokes prostaglandin synthesis in the kidney. COX-1, expressed in vessels, glomeruli, and collecting ducts, produces vasodilating prostaglandins, which maintain renal plasma flow and glomerular filtration during conditions of systemic vasoconstriction. In the antrum of the stomach, COX-1 leads to production of prostaglandins, which increase gastric blood flow and mucus secretion. Inhibition of COX-1 by NSAIDs prevents these protective mechanisms and results in renal ischemia and damage and gastric ulcers (mainly antral) in susceptible individuals. These observations have led to development of NSAIDs that selectively inhibit COX-2 and spare COX-1. Arachidonic acid gains access to the active site of the COX via a hydrophobic

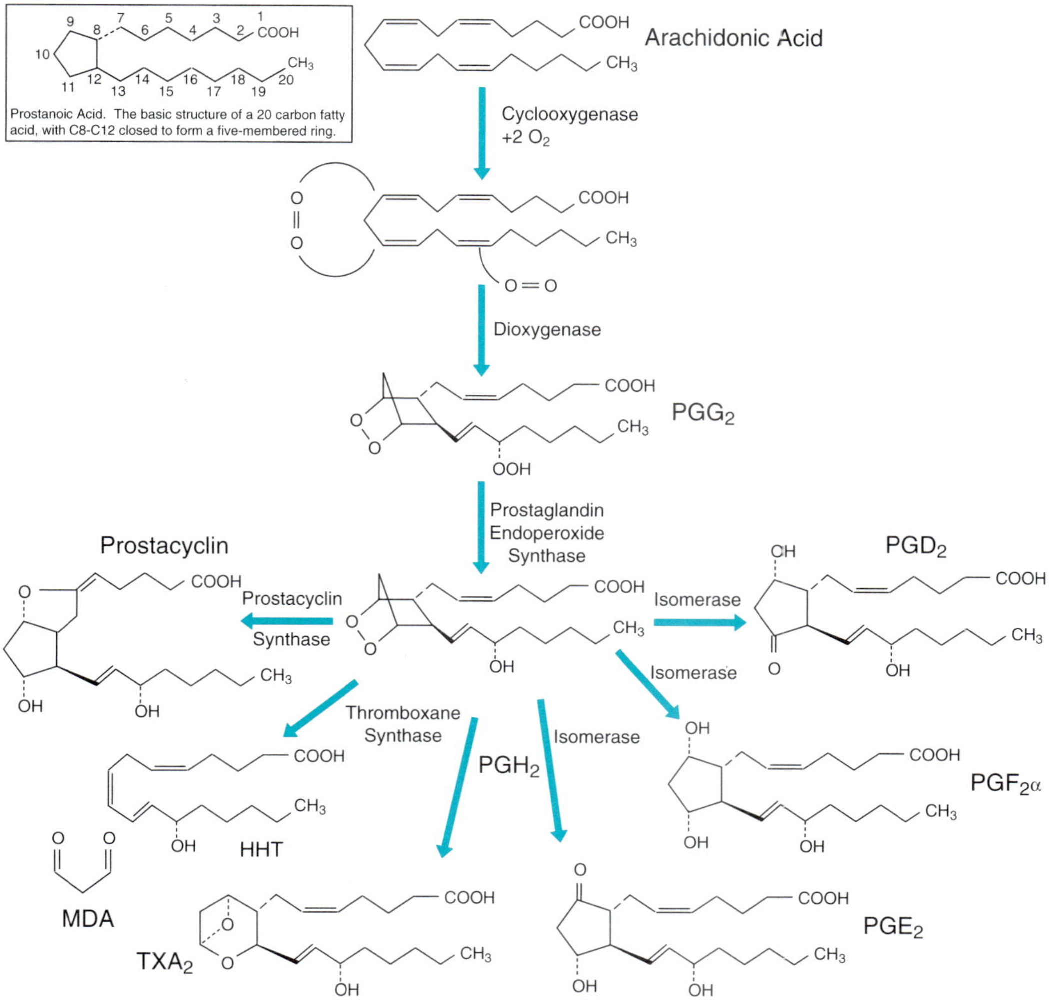

FIGURE 23–4 • Cyclooxygenase (COX) pathway of arachidonic acid metabolism.

channel, and access is blocked by insertion of an acetyl residue on Ser 530 in COX-1 and Ser 516 in COX-2. The irreversibility of the interaction and the unique expression of COX-1 in the anucleate platelet is the reason for the clinical efficacy of low-dose aspirin. Nonacetylated NSAIDs compete with arachidonate for the active site and can also interfere with the sustained effects of aspirin.[13] Although the structures of COX isozymes are similar, COX-2 is characterized by a side-pocket extension to the hydrophobic channel, which is where the selective COX-2 inhibitors localize.[7]

The major adverse effects of NSAIDs, gastroduodenal injury and impaired renal function, are caused by inhibition of COX-1, whereas the analgesic and anti-inflammatory activities of NSAIDs rest in part on their ability to inhibit COX-2. However, COX-2 appears also to have a regulating role in renal, brain, gastrointestinal, ovarian, and bone function.[14] COX-2 is also expressed in endothelial cells, and inhibition of COX-2 suppresses prostacyclin synthesis by endothelial cells.[12] It is not yet known whether long-term use of COX-2 inhibitors can accelerate vasculitis or atherosclerosis. COX-2 acts in both the initiation and resolution of inflammation. COX-2 expression increases transiently early in the course of carageenan-induced pleurisy in rats. Later in the response, COX-2 is expressed at even higher levels, leading to synthesis of the anti-inflammatory prostaglandins PGD_2 and 15-deoxy-Δ^{12-14}-PGJ2.[16] Early expression of COX-2 is associated with production of inflammatory prostaglandins, whereas the later peak may result in production of prostaglandins that suppress inflammation. Inflammation occurs in COX-2 knockout mice.[17] As Lewis Thomas informed us,[18] "inflammation will take place at any cost." Widespread use of the selective COX-2 inhibitors will undoubtedly help define the function of each COX isoform in health and disease.

Cyclooxygenase-3

Acetaminophen, like NSAIDs, suppresses pain and fever. It is not an anti-inflammatory agent, and its mechanism of action—despite its extensive use—has not been apparent. The finding that acetaminophen inhibits COX activity more in dog-brain homogenates than in spleen homogenates gave rise to the concept that variants of the COX enzyme exist that are differentially sensitive to acetaminophen. It turns out that a distinct COX isoenzyme, COX-3, is made from the COX-2 gene and is expressed in canine brain.[19] In humans, COX-3 mRNA is expressed as an approximately 5.2-kb transcript most abundant in cerebral cortex and heart. COX-3 possesses gylcosylation-dependent COX activity that is selectively inhibited by analgesic or antipyretic drugs such as acetaminophen and phenacetin. Further, experimental evidence suggests that additional acetaminophen-inhibitable COX forms exist that are likely also derived from COX-2.

Products of the Cyclooxygenase Pathway

PROSTAGLANDINS

The basic structure of all prostaglandins is a "prostanoic acid" skeleton, a 20-carbon fatty acid with a five-membered ring at C8 through C12 (see Fig. 23–4, inset). The term *prostaglandins* is employed widely but should be used to describe only those oxygenation products that contain the five-membered carbon ring. A family of acidic lipids found first in human seminal fluid, they were misnamed because it was thought they were produced in the prostate gland, rather than in the seminal vesicles.[20-22] The alphabetic prostaglandin nomenclature (e.g., PGE, PGF, PGD) is related to the chemical architecture of the cyclopentane ring. For example, PGE and PGF differ only in the presence of a ketone or hydroxyl function at C9 (see Fig. 23–4). These compounds are made by a variety of cells (e.g., PGE_2 and PGD_2 by isomerases, $PGF_{2\alpha}$ by a reductase). In the nomenclature, a subscript numeral after the letters indicates the degree of unsaturation in the alkyl and carboxylic acid side chains. The numeral 1 indicates the presence of a double bond at C13–C14 (PGE_1), 2 marks the presence of an additional double bond at C5–C6 (PGE_2), and 3 denotes a third double bond at C17–C18 (PGE_3).

Prostaglandins are produced on demand and appear to exert their effects on the cell of origin or nearby structures. Abundant experimental evidence supports the view that prostaglandins participate in development of the inflammatory response. Administration to rats of a monoclonal antibody to PGE_2 prevents carrageenan-induced pain and inflammation.[23] Prostaglandins are probably better at potentiating the effects of other mediators of inflammation than they are at inducing inflammation directly.[24] PGE compounds and intermediate hydroperoxides of arachidonic acid increase pain sensitivity to bradykinin and histamine. The effects of PGE are cumulative, depending on concentration and time. Even very small amounts of prostaglandins, if allowed to persist at the site of injury, may in time cause pain.

PGE_2 stimulates bone resorption,[25] and its 13,14-dihydro derivative is nearly as potent, which is of interest because derivatives of the biologically active prostaglandins are usually assumed not to be of functional significance. Addition of serum to the culture medium stimulates bone resorption, a process that is complement dependent and prostaglandin mediated. The mechanism may help explain bone erosion in joints of patients with RA, in which complement is activated and PGE_2 concentrations are high. However, the observation[26] that PGE_1 can stimulate bone formation suggests that prostaglandins physiologically participate in coordination of bone formation and resorption. Many effects of IL-1 and TNF-α on cells are associated with stimulation of prostaglandin production and inflammation. Cartilage explants from osteoarthritis (OA) patients express COX-2 (but not COX-1) and release 50 times more PGE_2 in culture than cartilage from healthy subjects and 18 times more PGE_2 than normal cartilage stimulated with cytokines plus lipopolysaccharide.[27] Explants from OA patients release IL-1β, whereas normal cartilage does not express mRNA for pro—IL-1β nor release IL-1β spontaneously. It appears that in OA—and probably in RA—upregulation of cartilage IL-1β and subsequent production of PGE_2 leads to cartilage degradation.

Mast cells, often overlooked as important in inflammatory responses, are seen in large numbers in synovium from patients early in the course of RA. PGD_2, the major prostaglandin formed by mast cells, can also mediate histamine release from mast cells exposed to anti-IgE antibody.

PGJ_2, formed from the dehydration of PGD_2, appears to function as a brake on the inflammatory response. It reduces macrophage activation, reduces nitric oxide (NO) production from stimulated cells, and induces apoptosis in tumor cell lines.[28] PGJ_2 is metabolized to Δ^{12}-PGJ_2 and ultimately to $\Delta^{12,14}$-PGJ_2, which are also biologically active.

PROSTACYCLIN

Prostacyclin, discovered in 1976,[29] has been purified, and the cDNA for prostacyclin synthase has been cloned.[30] In addition to a cyclopentane ring, a second ring is formed by an oxygen bridge between carbons 6 and 9. It is generated from PGH_2 by a distinct prostacyclin synthase, a 56-kD member of the cytochrome P-450 superfamily of enzymes found predominantly in endothelial and vascular smooth-muscle cells.[31] Production of prostacyclin can be stimulated by thrombin or generated by transfer of PGH_2 from platelets (the endoperoxide steal), contact with activated leukocytes, or stretching of the arterial wall. It is a powerful vasodilator and inhibits platelet aggregation through activation of adenylate cyclase, which leads to an increase in intracellular cAMP. It is metabolized rapidly (half-life in plasma is less than one circulation time) to the more stable, less biologically active 6-keto-prostaglandin $F_{1\alpha}$. The enzymatic products of its conversion—2,3-dinor-6 keto-$PGF_{1\alpha}$ and 6,15-di-keto-2,3-dinor $PGF_{1\alpha}$—are also chemically stable and have very little biologic activity. They are the major metabolites of prostacyclin excreted in urine, in which they can be assayed as indicators of prostacyclin generation.[32]

Prostacyclin generated in the vessel wall has antiplatelet and vasodilator actions, whereas thromboxane A_2 (TXA_2) generated by platelets from the same precursors induces platelet aggregation and vasoconstriction.[33] These two eicosanoids represent biologically opposite poles of a mechanism for regulating the interaction between platelets and the vessel wall and, therefore, of formation of hemostatic plugs and intra-arterial thrombi. Given the central role of platelets in inflammatory reactions, an appropriate prostacyclin-thromboxane balance is important to regulation of inflammation. The balance may be altered in patients with the antiphospholipid antibody syndrome and in patients treated with cyclosporine.

Endotoxin-mediated lung injury depends on neutrophil and platelet activation and on activation of the clotting system and fibrin deposition. Prevention of lung-tissue injury by prostacyclin infusion is associated with increased numbers of circulating platelets and a decrease in fibrin-degradation products. Intravascular infusion of prostacyclin also reduces some of the clinical changes associated with pulmonary embolism. The instability of prostacyclin makes it cumbersome to administer therapeutically. Nonetheless, it has been used with limited success to treat peripheral vascular disease, including Raynaud's phenomenon.[34] In addition to its vasodilator effects, prostacyclin suppresses endothelial cell proliferation. Thus, prostacyclin analogs administered subcutaneously may prove useful for treatment of pulmonary hypertension.[35]

THROMBOXANES

The endoperoxide PGH_2 can be converted into thromboxanes after the action of the enzyme thromboxane synthase, a microsomal 60-kD member of the cytochrome P-450 family, which is quite active in the platelet. The gene that encodes the enzyme has been cloned. Thromboxanes contain a six-member oxane ring instead of the cyclopentane ring of the prostaglandins. Thromboxane synthase converts PGH_2 into equal amounts of TXA_2 and 12L-hydroxy-5,8,10-heptadecatrienoic acid (HHT). TXA_2 stimulates platelet activation, contributes to intravascular aggregation of platelets, and contracts arteriolar and bronchiolar smooth muscles. It is hydrolyzed rapidly ($t_{(1/2)}$ = 30 seconds) to the inactive, stable, measurable product TXB_2; its actions are limited to the microenvironment of its release.[31]

The extraordinary rapidity with which platelets adhere to damaged tissue, aggregate, and release potent biologically active materials suggests that the platelet is well suited to be a cellular trigger for the inflammatory process. Efforts directed at suppression of thromboxane synthesis and platelet aggregation may result in limitation of inflammatory responses. Inhibition of platelet aggregation may be important to the anti-inflammatory effects of aspirin and other NSAIDs. Long-term administration of low doses of aspirin (40 mg/day)—the lowest dose predicted to cause total inhibition of thromboxane formation in serum, according to mathematic modeling—has inhibitory effects on platelet function ex vivo that are indistinguishable from those caused by giving 325 mg/day of aspirin.[36] Even low-dose aspirin, however, has some depressive effect on prostacyclin synthesis. This means recovery of vascular prostacyclin production may be more difficult to attain in elderly patients.[37]

Selective inhibition of thromboxane synthase represents an approach that may be effected without depressing prostacyclin formation. The endoperoxide steal appears to function in vivo after administration of a thromboxane synthase inhibitor. Antagonists of the receptors shared by endoperoxide and TXA_2 have been developed, and these agents inhibit platelet aggregation in patients recalcitrant to thromboxane synthase inhibition. More specific inhibition of thromboxane action may become possible now that two thromboxane receptors have been cloned and characterized.[38]

LIPOXYGENASE PATHWAYS

In contrast to the COX pathway, in which stable products have three atoms of oxygen covalently attached to arachidonic acid from 2 moles of molecular oxygen, lipoxygenases insert a single oxygen atom into the molecular structure of arachidonic acid. Separate lipoxygenases exist in certain cells and have strict structural requirements for their substrates. Three major mammalian lipoxygenases exist that insert their oxygen atoms into the 5, 12, or 15 position of arachidonic acid, with formation of a new double bond and hydroperoxy group. The hydroperoxy fatty acids (HPETE) can be reduced by peroxidases in the cell to yield the corresponding hydroxy fatty acids (HETE). For example, the exclusive lipoxygenase product of the human platelet is 12(*S*)-hydroperoxyeicosatetraenoic acid (12HPETE), which on reduction of the hydroperoxy group yields 12-hydroxyeicosatetraenoic acid (12HETE). In contrast, the human neutrophil makes predominantly 5HPETE, but when high concentrations of arachidonic acid are added, 15-lipoxygenase can be demonstrated. Lipoxygenases that act on arachidonic acid are found in the cytosol fraction of cells. The human 5-lipoxygenase gene has been isolated and characterized[39] and produces a 78-kD enzyme. In myeloid cells, the 5-lipoxygenase pathway leads to formation of the biologically active leukotrienes (Fig. 23–5) that were originally found in leukocytes and that contain three conjugated double bonds (trienes). Cell activation leads to translocation of 5-lipoxygenase from cytosol to the nuclear membrane, where it encounters the 18-kD 5-lipoxygenase–activating protein (FLAP). Arachidonic acid is also translocated to FLAP for presentation to 5-lipoxygenase.[40]

The unstable HPETE is the initial metabolite of each lipoxygenase pathway. HPETE is reduced to the more stable HETE or is converted by 5-lipoxygenase to leukotriene A_4 (LTA_4). LTA_4 can then be converted to LTB_4 (in neutrophils and macrophages) or conjugated with reduced glutathione to form LTC_4 (in eosinophils, mast cells, endothelial cells, and macrophages). Unlike lipoxygenase, which is mainly distributed in myeloid cells, LTA_4 hydrolase (5,12-dihydroxyeicosatetraenoic acid), a zinc-requiring enzyme that converts LTA_4 to LTB_4, is widely distributed. From the cDNA sequence, it was suggested that mRNA for LTA_4 may have a short half-life, which could account for the interesting properties of extremely rapid production and shutdown of LTB_4 and other eicosanoid biosynthesis.

LTA_4 can be exported from the cell of origin and converted in other cells by LTA_4 hydrolase to LTB_4. This variation on the endoperoxide steal—perhaps better called *transcellular metabolism*—also applies to conversion of LTA_4 to LTC_4 by LTC_4 synthase, a glutathione-*S*-transferase.[41] Although human endothelial cells do not produce terminal products of the 5-lipoxygenase system, they

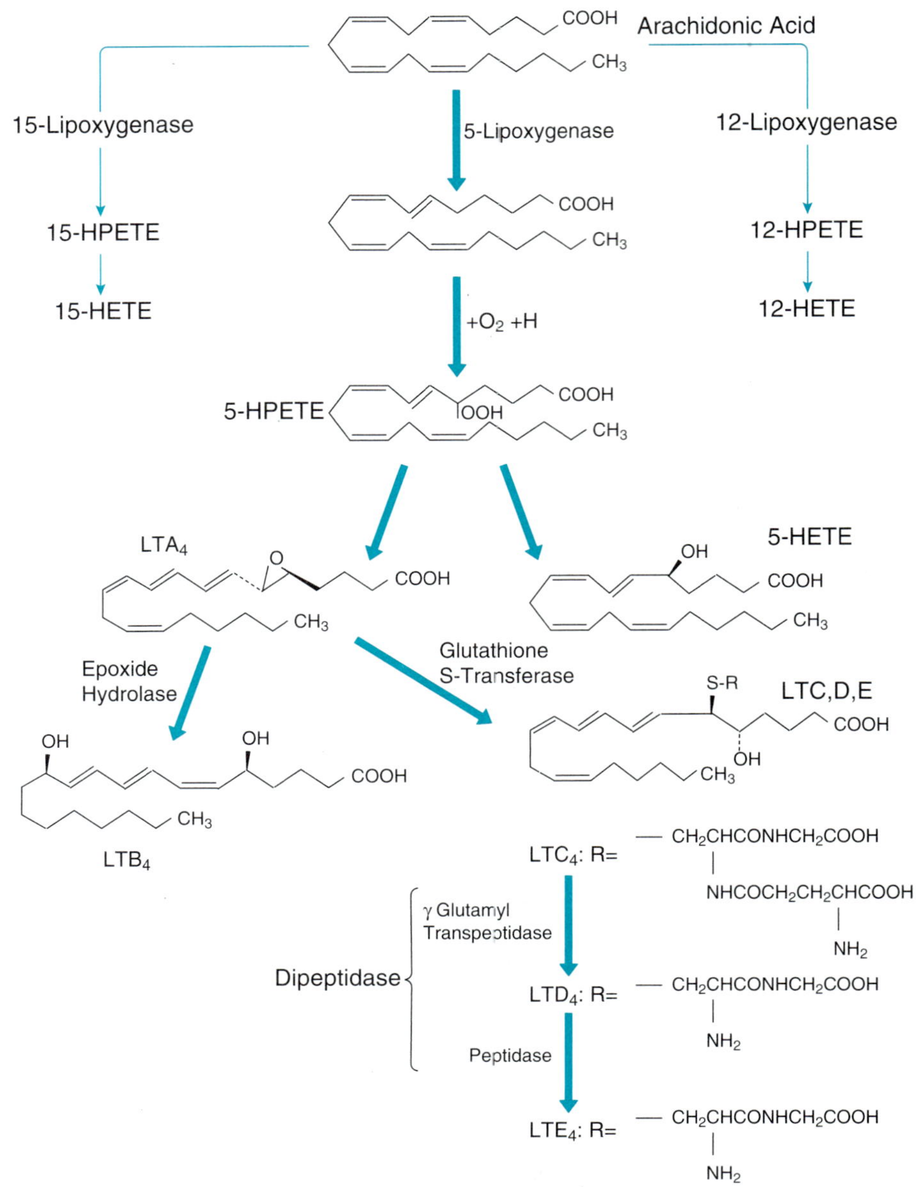

FIGURE 23–5 • 5-lipoxygenase pathway of arachidonic acid metabolism.

do generate LTC_4 from LTA_4 provided by neutrophils. LTC_4 and its products, LTD_4 and LTE_4, make up the biologic mixture previously known as slow-reacting substance of anaphylaxis. LTD_4 and LTE_4 arise from LTC_4 after sequential removal of γ-glutamic acid and glycine from LTC_4. The enzyme γ-glutamyl transpeptidase is present in many cells as part of a complex enzymatic system involved in glutathione biosynthesis and amino acid transport. In many systems, the major sulfidopeptide leukotriene has been reported to be LTD_4 rather than the precursor LTC_4. Removal of glycine from LTD_4 results in LTE_4 with concomitant loss of a significant amount of biologic activity. The principal route of inactivation of LTB_4 is by omega oxidation.

PRODUCTS OF THE LIPOXYGENASE PATHWAYS

The biologic effects of compounds produced in the lipoxygenase pathway indicate their importance in inflammatory diseases. They have displaced the products of the COX pathway as candidates for the major mediators of inflammation formed by the oxygenation of arachidonic acid and are implicated as key mediators in several diseases, including inflammatory bowel disease, psoriasis, bronchial asthma, and RA.

5HETE and 5HPETE stimulate the generation of superoxide in human neutrophils. These compounds also augment intracellular calcium levels, facilitating protein kinase C–dependent activation of a superoxide generating system of neutrophils.[42] LTB_4 increases adherence of leukocytes to endothelial cells, a response that is augmented by exposure of the endothelial cells to TNF-α. LTB_4 does not appear to have a direct vascular contractile action, because it is inactive in the hamster cheek pouch preparation and several other microvasculature systems. In rabbit skin, administration of LTB_4 with a vasodilator prostaglandin induces plasma exudation, which suggests that LTB_4 may facilitate enhanced vascular permeability. Increased venule permeability does occur in response to

LTC_4, LTD_4, and LTE_4. LTB_4 is a potent chemotactic factor for neutrophils and is weakly chemotactic for eosinophils. LTB_4, and to a lesser extent 5HETE, enhance migration of T lymphocytes in vitro. Synovial cells produce 5HETE but do not appear to produce significant amounts of LTB_4. However, macrophages that invade the synovium in RA patients generate substantial quantities of 5- and 15-lipoxygenation products, including LTB_4. In addition to the local signs of inflammation induced by products of the lipoxygenase pathway, these compounds may contribute to the pain, tenderness, and aching so common in RA patients. LTB_4 also appears to serve an immunoregulatory function. For example, it stimulates differentiation of competent CD8 T lymphocytes from precursors lacking the CD8 marker. LTB_4 also stimulates interferon-γ (IFN-γ) and IL-2 production by T cells and biosynthesis of IL-1 by monocytes.[43]

Synovial-cell and endothelial-cell proliferation are central to propagation of the rheumatoid joint lesion. LTB_4 and the cysteinyl leukotrienes act as growth or differentiation factors for a number of cell types in vitro. For example, LTC4 and $LTD4_4$ promote proliferation of human glomerular epithelial cells in vitro. These compounds also increase proliferation of fibroblasts when prostaglandin synthesis is inhibited,[44] findings that emphasize the importance of interactions between the COX and lipoxygenase pathways and that suggest limitations to NSAID therapy for RA patients.

Strategies for inhibiting production or antagonizing the actions of leukotrienes include development of selective leukotriene receptor antagonists and inhibition of the production of leukotriene by blocking the action of 5-lipoxygenase. Inhibition of enzymes distal in the leukotriene cascade, such as LTA_4 hydrolase,[45] is also a promising strategy for development of anti-inflammatory drugs. A compound that inhibits binding of 5-lipoxygenase to FLAP exhibits anti-inflammatory effects in animal models.

Lipoxygenase activities do not lead solely to production of mediators of inflammation. DGLA is converted by 15-lipoxygenase into 15-hydroxyeicosatrienoic acid (15HETrE), which is incorporated into DAG and exerts anti-inflammatory effects in part by interfering with PKC-β activity. A lipoxygenase product of linoleic acid, 13-hydroxyoctadecadienoic acid (13-HODE), also suppresses inflammation and cell proliferation by means of a similar mechanism.[46] EPA is converted by lipoxygenase into 15-hydroxyeicosapentaenoic acid (15HEPE), which also exhibits anti-inflammatory properties.[47]

LIPOXINS

Another large family of arachidonic acid metabolites arises from the sequential action of 5- and 15-lipoxygenases. Addition of 15HPETE and 15HETE to human leukocytes results in formation of a pair of oxygenated products containing a unique conjugated tetraene. One compound (lipoxin A_4) was identified as 5,6,15L-trihydroxy-7,9,11,13-eicosatetraenoic acid, and the other proved to be its positional isomer (lipoxin B_4), 5D-14,15-trihydroxy-6,8,10,12-eicosatetraenoic acid (Fig. 23–6). Because both of these compounds can arise through an interaction between lipoxygenase pathways, the trivial name lipoxins (i.e., lipoxygenase interaction products) was introduced. Platelet 12-lipoxygenase can transform neutrophil LTA_4 to lipoxins. The complete stereochemistry and multiple routes of biosynthesis for the biologically active lipoxin A_4 (LXA_4) and lipoxin B_4 (LXB_4) have been determined.[48]

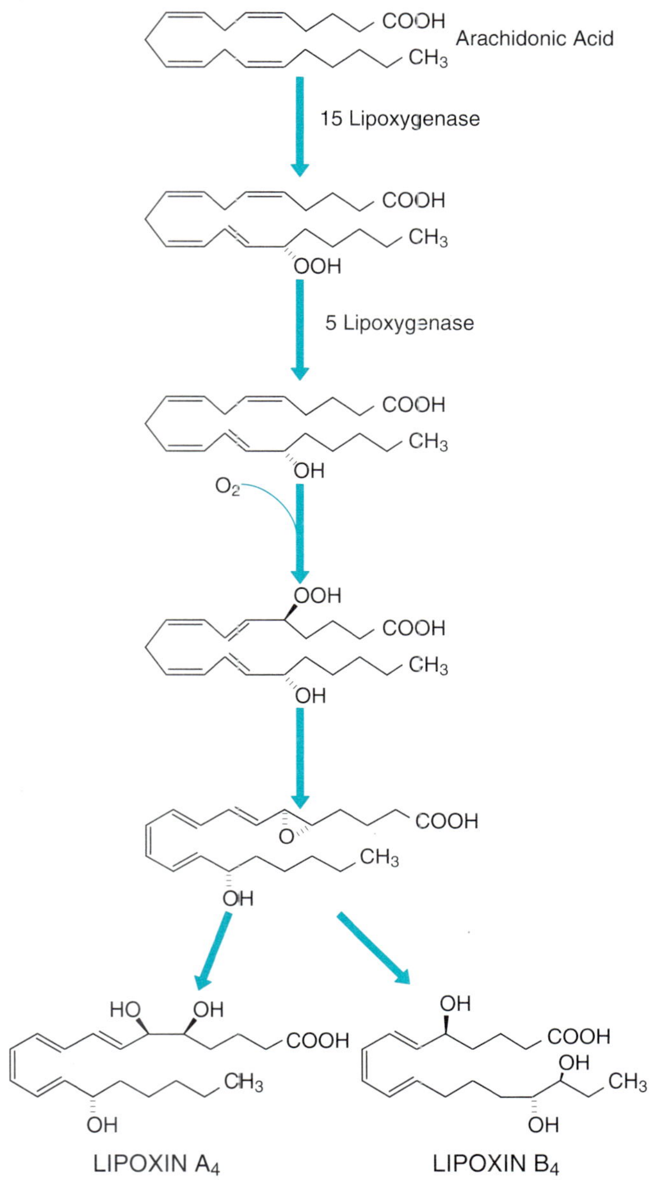

FIGURE 23–6 · Lipoxin biosynthesis. The lipoxins result from the sequential action of 15-lipoxygenase and 5-lipoxygenase on arachidonic acid.

That macrophages of rainbow trout generate lipoxins rather than leukotrienes or prostaglandins as their major products of arachidonic acid metabolism indicates that lipoxins have a long evolutionary history. Leukotrienes and lipoxins can be generated in parallel in fish. In humans, the process has diverged to a two-cell system. Biosynthesis of eicosanoids by transcellular and cell-cell interactions is recognized as an important way to generate and amplify lipid-derived mediators. Lipoxins can be generated within the vascular lumen during platelet-leucocyte interactions and at mucosal surfaces via leucocyte-epithelial cell interactions. Thus, in humans, lipoxins are formed in vivo during multicellular responses such as inflammation, atherosclerosis, and in asthma. These tetraene-containing products serve as stop signals in that they prevent leucocyte-mediated tissue injury. A major problem in joints of patients with RA is that inflammation usually does not resolve. Lipoxins and aspirin-induced 15-epi lipoxins are endogenous components of events governing resolution of inflammation. Aspirin acetylation of COX-2 in endothelial cells suppresses prostaglandin synthesis, but leads to generation of 15R-HETE from arachidonic acid, which is transformed to 15-epi-lipoxin by leukocytes in a transcellular biosynthetic route involving vascular endothelial cells or epithelial cells. These 15-epi-lipoxins exhibit anti-inflammatory and antiproliferative actions in vitro and in vivo. Stable analogs of LXA_4 and of aspirin-triggered lipoxin also suppress inflammation in animal models.[49] These observations may lead to development of new anti-inflammatory drugs.

Lipoxins block human polymorphonuclear leukocyte chemotaxis but stimulate monocyte chemotaxis and adherence. However, monocytes do not release mediators of inflammation in response to lipoxins, and lipoxins are converted rapidly by monocytes to inactive compounds. This selective effect on chemotaxis suggests that lipoxins can play a role in wound healing. LXA_4 antagonizes LTD_4-induced vasoconstriction in vivo and blocks binding of LTD_4 to its receptors on mesangial cells. LXA_4 suppresses LTB_4-induced plasma leakage and leucocyte migration and blocks LTB_4-induced neutrophil inositol triphosphate generation and calcium mobilization but not superoxide anion generation. Conversely, LXA_4 activates PKC and is more potent in this regard than DAG and arachidonic acid. LXA_4 appears to be specific for the γ subspecies of PKC. These results indicate that lipoxins may regulate the actions of vasoconstrictor leukotrienes and suggest that LXA_4 may be an important modulator of intracellular signal transduction.

ISOEICOSANOIDS

Isoeicosanoids, isomers of enzymatically derived eicosanoids, are free radical–catalyzed products of arachidonic acid. They include members of the F, D, and E isoprostanes, isothromboxanes, and isoleukotrienes. Analysis of the isoprostanes indicates that they reflect lipid peroxidation in vivo. Theoretically, up to 64 F-type isoprostanes (iPFs) may be formed, although few have been characterized. As more isoprostanes are identified, the nomenclature probably will continue to change. One iPF, $iPF_{2\alpha}$ III (formerly 8-iso$PGF_{2\alpha}$) has been studied in detail because of its biologic activity in vitro. Isoprostane $F_{2\alpha}$-III (Fig. 23–7) is a potent vasoconstrictor and may function as a mitogen, with actions that are blocked by thromboxane receptor antagonists. Although isoprostanes may act as ligands at thromboxane or prostaglandin receptors (8,12-iso-$iPF_{2\alpha}$ III activates the $PGF_{2\alpha}$ receptor), they may also activate specific isoprostane receptors. However, no such receptors have been cloned.

Isoprostanes

What all iPs have in common, and what distinguishes them from the prostaglandins is the fact that the top (α) and the bottom (ω) side chains are always syn—that is, crowded together on the same face of the cyclopentane ring. The minimum requirement for generation of an isoprostane is a polyunsaturated fatty acid with three contiguous methylene-interrupted double bonds, a requirement met by dozens of naturally occurring polyunsaturated fatty acids. Those formed from docosahexaenoic acid (DHA), for example, might be important markers for brain disorders. Unlike conventional, enzymatically derived prostaglandins that are formed intracellularly and released immediately, isoprostanes are formed in the cell membrane, cleaved by phospholipases, circulate in plasma, and are excreted in urine.[50] They are increased in several diseases, including adult respiratory distress syndrome in which polymorphonuclear leukocytes generate reactive oxygen species that damage pulmonary epithelium. The immune cells in inflamed tissues are exposed to reactive oxygen intermediates produced by neutrophils and other phagocytic cells. Oxidants are also generated as mediators in intracellular signaling pathways by cytokines such as IL-1β and TNF-α.

It is likely that isoprostanes will prove to be important in inflammatory conditions such as vasculitis and RA. Because isoprostanes are released preformed, their production is not blocked by NSAIDs, which suppress

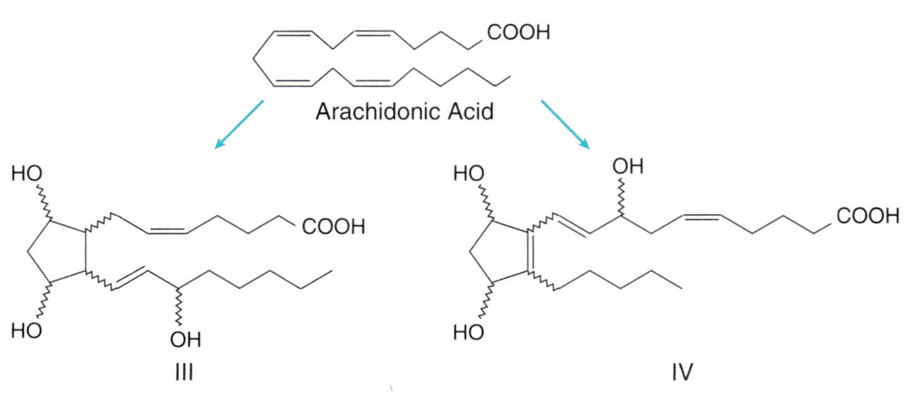

FIGURE 23–7 · Isoprostane $F_{2\alpha}$ structures. *Jagged lines* indicate that the stereochemistry is uncertain.

metabolism of free arachidonic acid. It is possible that inflammation unresponsive to NSAIDs may yield to inhibition of isoprostanes.

Oxidant stress has been implicated in vascular reperfusion after a period of ischemia. Examples include the myocardial dysfunction seen after coronary artery bypass surgery. Urinary excretion of $iPF_{2\alpha}$ III and $iPF_{2\alpha}$ VI are increased substantially coincident with reperfusion in patients treated with thrombolytic agents or coronary angioplasty for acute myocardial infarction. Recurrent vasospasm and vasodilation (Raynaud's phenomenon) probably lead to reperfusion injury in patients with systemic sclerosis. Urinary isoprostanes may prove to be useful markers of lipid peroxidation and tissue injury in a variety of inflammatory diseases.[48]

ANANDAMIDES

The molecule called *anandamide* (from the Sanskrit word for bliss) is the ethanolamide derivative of arachidonic acid (arachidonoyl ethanolamide) and may, therefore, be considered a novel member of the eicosanoid family (Fig. 23–8). Of much interest is the identification of the molecule as a putative endogenous ligand for the two known G protein–coupled transmembrane cannabinoid (CB) receptors. Anandamide binds weakly to the CB1 receptor in the brain but has a higher affinity for the CB2 receptor on peripheral cells. Anandamides can modulate muscarinic acetylcholine receptor binding properties unrelated to actions on CB receptors.[51] Discovery of naturally occurring and synthetic analogs and metabolites of anandamide suggest that a family of such biologically active substances exists. The polyunsaturated amides dihomogammalinolenoyl (20:3 n-6) and adrenoyl (22:4 n-6) ethanolamides have been found in mammalian brain.[52] It is likely that n-3 fatty acid ethanolamides also exist in mammalian tissues.

Two pathways have been proposed for the production of fatty acid ethanolamides: direct condensation of ethanolamide with free fatty acid in an adenosine triphosphate (ATP)- and CoA-independent process and the formation of *N*-acylphosphatidyl ethanolamine precursors, with release of ethanol amide by receptor-coupled PLD activity in stimulated cells. Anandamide is not stored in cells; rather, it is believed to be synthesized rapidly in response to stimuli in the manner of prostaglandins and leukotrienes.

Stimulated macrophages produce anandamide, and anandamides reduce activation of macrophages and reduce production of TNF-α by stimulated human monocytes.[53] They act outside the brain through the CB2 receptor on cells involved in inflammation and immune responses. That anandamide can enhance its own synthesis in macrophages suggests the presence of a rapid response to counter excessive inflammatory or immune responses. Anandamide is converted by COX-2 (but not by COX-1) into PGE_2 ethanolamide directly, without going through free arachidonic acid.[54] This novel prostaglandin ("prostamide") is pharmacologically active, but its physiologic relevance has not been established.[55] Because anandamide is a substrate for COX-2, inhibitors of COX-2 may reduce anandamide metabolism with a subsequent increase in concentration of the anti-inflammatory anandamide.

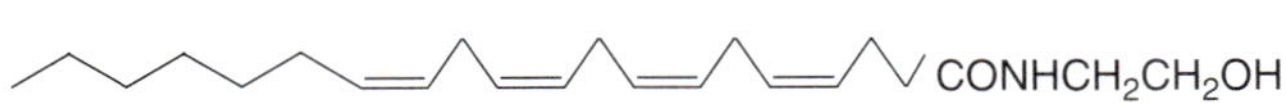

FIGURE 23–8 · The chemical structure of anandamide (arachidonoyl ethanolamide).

Eicosanoid Receptors

For many years, it was thought that the lipophilic eicosanoids—in contrast to the peptide molecules for which receptors were routinely characterized—simply "diffused" into cell membranes or were carried in by a binding protein. The isolation and cloning of eicosanoid receptors changed that thinking.[54]

PROSTAGLANDIN RECEPTORS

G Protein–Coupled Prostaglandin Receptors

The eight receptors for the COX products are designated P receptors, depending on the prostanoid that has most affinity for them.[56] These receptors are: the PGD receptor (DP); four subtypes of the PGE receptor (EP1-EP4); the PGF receptor (FP); the PGI receptor (IP); and the thromboxane receptor (TP). All are G protein–coupled rhodopsin-type receptors with seven transmembrane domains, and each is encoded by different genes. The IP, DP, EP2, and EP4 receptors mediate increases in cellular cAMP, whereas TP, FP, and EP1 receptors induce calcium mobilization. Thus, EP2, EP4, and IP regulate macrophage cytokine production in a similar manner. As might be expected, signaling through these receptors is actually more complicated. For example, although PGI_2 analogs are ligands for IP and increase cAMP, high concentrations of PGI_2 analogs activate phospholipase C and induce calcium mobilization.[57] It does seem clear that modification of immune cell and surrounding cell functions by prostanoids during immune or inflammatory responses is influenced by the different repertoire of prostaglandin receptors expressed on these cells. Knowledge of the roles of the P receptors in physiologic and pathologic processes has been advanced by experiments with mice deficient in the receptors (knockout mice).[58] For example, as noted previously, PGE can suppress or induce bone formation. EP2 and EP4 knockout mice exhibit impaired osteoclastogenesis and inflammation-induced bone resorption. The receptor mediating PGE-induced bone formation is not known. In animal models, both acute inflammation and pain are completely absent in IP-deficient mice. The profile of prostaglandin formation changes as the inflammatory response evolves to a more chronic state, so other receptors are probably involved. Thus, it is unlikely that blockade of one receptor will block completely an inflammatory response. More encouraging is the fact that prostaglandins participate in allodynia, a pain response to a usually nonpainful stimulus. Knowing the contribution of P receptors to allodynia might lead to better treatment of neuropathic pain and the myofascial pain syndromes such as fibromyalgia.

The availability of cloned P receptors should facilitate development of more effective receptor-active compounds. The PGI_2 analog iloprost is somewhat useful for treatment of peripheral vascular disease and pulmonary hypertension. However, although iloprost binds to IP with high affinity, it also binds EPI and EP3. It may be that targeting activation, blockade, or both of a single P receptor or a specific set of P receptors will provide advantages over compounds that work "upstream," such as the COX-2 inhibitors or traditional NSAIDs. The implications for therapy derived from this new knowledge are clear and exciting, but prostanoid analogs with very selective binding properties will have to be developed. Some progress has been made, and it appears that deletion of P receptors, with the exception of EP4, is not associated with serious problems of fetal development or physiologic function in animals.

LEUKOTRIENE RECEPTORS

Less is known about the surface receptors for leukotrienes. However, two receptors for LTB_4 (BLT_1 and BLT_2) have been cloned and characterized.[56] Both are coupled to G protein and contain seven transmembrane domains. BLT_1 is activated only by LTB_4 whereas BLT_2 is activated by HETEs as well.[59] High-affinity LTB_4 receptors transduce chemotaxis and adhesion responses, whereas the low-affinity receptors are responsible for secretion of granule contents and superoxide generation. The receptor for cysteinyl leukotrienes includes two subtypes—Lys LT_1 and Cys LT_2—that have been identified pharmacologically, although their molecular structures are unknown. Most actions of the cysteinyl leukotrienes are mediated by Cys LT_1. More than a dozen chemically distinct, specific, and selective antagonist drugs that block the binding of leukotriene to Cys LT_1 have been identified. Clinical use of these compounds has mainly been in the treatment of asthma. A 5-lipoxygenase–specific inhibitor reduced whole blood LTB_4 production but did not suppress synovitis in a 4-week trial of RA patients.[60]

LIPOXIN RECEPTORS

Lipoxins can act at their own specific receptors for LXA_4 and LXB_4, and LXA_4 can interact with a subtype of LTD_4 receptors. Lipoxins can also act at intracellular targets within their cell of origin or after uptake by another cell. The cDNA for the seven transmembrane spanning G protein–coupled LXA_4 receptor has been cloned and characterized. Its signaling involves a novel polyisoprenyl-phosphate pathway that regulates phospholipase D.[61] Lipoxin actions are cell-type specific. The monocyte and neutrophil LXA_4 receptors are identical at the cDNA level, but they evoke different responses, and the LXA_4 receptor on endothelial cells appears to be a structurally distinct form.

Nuclear Receptors

Peroxisome proliferator-activated receptors (PPARs) are members of the nuclear receptor family of transcription factors, a large and diverse group of proteins that mediate ligand-dependent transcriptional activation and repression. PPARs were first cloned as nuclear receptors that mediate the effects on gene transcription of synthetic compounds called peroxisome proliferators. Interest in PPARs increased dramatically when they were shown to be activated by medically relevant compounds including NSAIDs, and PGD_2 and its metabolite 15-deoxy-Δ12, 14 PGJ_2 (15d PGJ_2).[62] Most information available on a potential role of PPARs in inflammation relates to PPARγ. Upregulation of PPARγ reduces expression of several mediators of inflammation, raising the possibility that PPARγ ligands may be therapeutic for diseases characterized by inflammation. However, 15dPGJ_2 can also exhibit anti-inflammatory activity in a PPARγ-independent manner.[63] It also is not clear whether eicosanoids other than PGD_2 and PGJ_2 are bona fide PPARγ ligands. PPARα is expressed mainly in tissues that have a high fatty-acid catabolism, including liver and the immune system. LTB_4 is an activator and natural ligand of PPARα.[64] Activation of PPARα results in induction of genes involved in fatty acid oxidation pathways that degrade fatty acids and derivatives including LTB_4. Thus, a feedback mechanism is established that controls inflammation. Experiments with PPAR knockout (−/−) mice indicate that PPARα suppresses LTB_4-induced inflammation.

Platelet-Activating Factor

Platelet-activating factor (PAF), 1-0-alkyl-2-acetyl-sn-glycero-3-phosphocholine, is a potent mediator of inflammation that causes neutrophil activation, increased vascular permeability, vasodilation, and bronchoconstriction in addition to platelet activation. PAF is formed by a smaller number of cell types than the eicosanoids—mainly leukocytes, platelets, and endothelial cells. However, because of the extensive distribution of these cells, the actions of PAF can manifest in virtually every organ system. In contrast to the two long-chain acyl groups present in phosphatidyl choline, PAF contains a long-chain alkyl group joined to the glycerol backbone in an ether linkage at position 1 and an acetyl group at position 2 (Fig. 23–9). PAF actually represents a family of phospholipids because the alkyl group at position 1 can vary in length from 12 to 18 carbons.

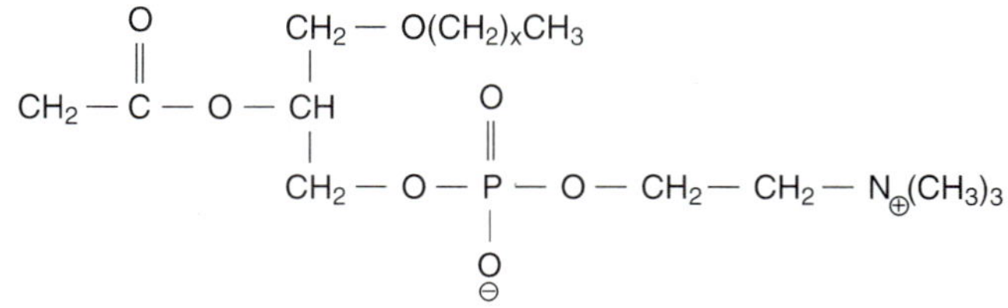

FIGURE 23–9 • The chemical structure of platelet-activating factor (PAF).

PAF, like the eicosanoids, is not stored in cells, but is synthesized on stimulation of cells, at which time the composition of the alkyl group may change. Despite the potent inflammatory effects of PAF, its inhibition in animal models does not lead to marked suppression of inflammatory responses. Plasma PAF acetylhydrolase, an enzyme that hydrolyzes PAF, may be a particularly important terminator of PAF-induced tissue injury and may find a place among strategies designed to suppress inflammation.[65] Given the involvement of PAF in immediate-hypersensitivity reactions and inflammation, further search for PAF antagonists is warranted.

Eicosanoids as Regulators of Inflammation and Immune Responses

The role of prostaglandins in the inflammatory process is not as well defined as once supposed, because the stable prostaglandins PGE and PGI_2 have anti-inflammatory and inflammatory effects.[66] PGJ and lipoxins appear to act as brakes to protect against runaway inflammatory responses. Even LTB_4 appears capable of modulating inflammation and immune responses.[43] The observation that PGE_1 inhibits platelet aggregation led to the notion that COX products of arachidonic acid metabolism might have anti-inflammatory activity. As it becomes more clear that NSAIDs have anti-inflammatory effects other than interference with COX production and subsequent prostaglandin inhibition, the potential protective effects of prostaglandins are being considered.

PGE_1 has remained a bit of an orphan among the eicosanoids, mainly because of a long-held notion that not enough of it is made by human cells to be of use and that its biologic effects are no different from those of PGE_2 and PGI_2. Contrary to popular belief, PGE_1 is found in physiologically important amounts in humans. Lost in the vast literature on the "arachidonic acid cascade" are the early observations of Bygdeman and Samuelson[67] who found (using bioassay) the concentration of PGE_1 in human seminal plasma (16 μg/ml) to be higher than PGE_2 (13 μg/ml), PGE_3 (3 μg/ml), $PGF_{1\alpha}$ (2 μg/ml), and $PGF_{2\alpha}$ (12 μg/ml). Karim found PGE_1 to be the sole PGE in the human thymus.[68] Prostaglandin immunoassays usually do not distinguish between PGE_1 and PGE_2. To identify PGE_1, it must first be separated from PGE_2 by thin-layer or high-performance liquid chromatography. When such methods have been used, PGE_1 has been identified consistently in platelets, leukocytes, macrophages, vas deferens, oviducts, uterus, heart, and skin.[69]

Evidence from in vitro and in vivo experiments indicates that prostaglandins, notably PGE compounds, can suppress diverse effector systems of inflammation. PGE can enhance and diminish cellular and humoral immune responses, observations that reinforce a view of these compounds as regulators of cell function. These actions of eicosanoids depend on the stimulus to inflammation, the predominant eicosanoid produced at a particular time in the host response, and the profile of eicosanoid-receptor expression.[70,71]

Modulation of Eicosanoid Synthesis by Administration of Precursor Fatty Acids

The relationship between essential fatty acids and prostaglandins was discovered simultaneously and independently by van Dorp and coworkers[72] and Bergstrom and associates.[73] Both groups reported that arachidonic acid was converted to PGE_2, and, shortly thereafter, they showed that PGE_1 is formed from DGLA.[74] Attempts to modulate eicosanoid production have been directed at providing fatty acids other than arachidonic acid as substrates for oxygenation enzymes in an effort to generate a unique eicosanoid profile with different biologic effects. The fatty acids themselves, by virtue of their incorporation into signal-transduction elements, also have effects that are independent of eicosanoid effects on cells involved in inflammation and immune responses.[75]

Experiments directed at suppression of thromboxane synthesis, enhancement of prostacyclin production, and inhibition of platelet aggregation have been done in an effort to limit inflammatory responses. EPA is not found in appreciable amounts in cells from people who eat a western diet. Fish-oil lipids, rich in EPA (20:5 n-3), inhibit formation of COX products (e.g., TXA_2, PGE_2) derived from arachidonic acid, and the newly formed TXA_3 has much less ability than TXA_2 to constrict vessels and aggregate platelets. Production of prostaglandin I_2 (prostacyclin) by endothelial cells is not reduced appreciably by increased EPA content, and the physiologic activity of newly synthesized PGI_3 is added to that of PGI_2. Administration of fish oil to humans leads to reduced production of LTB_4 by means of 5-lipoxygenase in stimulated neutrophils and monocytes and induces EPA-derived LTB_5, which is far less biologically active than LTB_4. Fish oil also reduces production of IL-1β, TNF-α, and PAF by activated blood monocytes. Fish oil supplements in the treatment of RA for 6 to 12 months result in significant reductions in number of tender joints and time of morning stiffness compared to the same measures done at baseline. Fish oil treatment allowed patients to reduce or stop NSAID treatment.[76] Human endothelial cells treated with aspirin in vitro convert EPA to anti-inflammatory lipoxins; these novel compounds are also found in inflammatory exudates from animals administered aspirin and fish oil.[49]

The other "alternative" eicosanoid precursor fatty acid, DGLA (20:3 n-6), can also be increased by administration of certain plant-seed oils, notably those extracted from the seeds of *Oenothera biennis* (evening primrose) and *Boragio officianalis* (borage), which contain relatively large amounts of gamma-linolenic acid (GLA). GLA is converted to DGLA, the immediate precursor of PGE_1, and is an eicosanoid with known anti-inflammatory and immunoregulating properties. Administration of GLA to volunteers and RA patients results in increased production of PGE_1 and reduced production of the inflammatory eicosanoids PGE_2, LTB_4, and LTC_4 by stimulated peripheral blood monocytes. In addition to competing with arachidonic acid for oxidative enzymes, DGLA cannot be converted to inflammatory leukotrienes. Rather, it is converted by means of 15-lipoxygenase to a 15-hydroxy-DGLA, which has the capacity to inhibit 5- and 12-lipoxygenase activities. DGLA should, therefore, have anti-inflammatory actions because of its capacity to reduce synthesis of oxygenation products of arachidonic acid through the COX and lipoxygenase pathways.[77]

In addition to their roles as precursors of eicosanoids, essential fatty acids are important for the maintenance of cell membrane structure and function. DGLA can modulate immune responses in an eicosanoid-independent manner. For example, DGLA suppresses IL-2 production by human peripheral blood monocytes in vitro, suppresses proliferation of IL-2–dependent human peripheral blood and synovial tissue T lymphocytes, and reduces expression of activation markers on T lymphocytes directly in a manner that is independent of its conversion to eicosanoids. Oral administration of oils enriched in GLA, but not administration of oils enriched in linoleic acid (the parent n-6 fatty acid) or α-linolenic acid (the parent n-3 fatty acid) reduce proliferation of human lymphocytes activated through the T cell–receptor complex.[78]

Addition to peripheral blood mononuclear cells in vitro or administration of GLA in vivo reduces secretion of IL-1β and TNF-α from lipopolysaccharide-stimulated human cells. GLA also reduces autoinduction of IL-1β in human monocytes, thereby preserving the protective effects of IL-1β while suppressing excessive production of the cytokine.[79,80] IL-1β and TNF-α are important polypeptide mediators of inflammation and joint-tissue injury in patients with RA, and both cytokines have become targets of therapy for patients with RA. GLA suppresses acute and chronic inflammation, including arthritis, in several animal models, and randomized, double-blind, placebo-controlled trials of GLA in patients with RA and active synovitis indicate that GLA treatment results in statistically significant and clinically relevant reduction in signs and symptoms of disease activity compared to baseline and placebo.[81]

EPA suppresses conversion of DGLA to arachidonic acid, and a combination of EPA- and GLA-enriched oils exhibits synergy in its capacity to reduce synovitis in animal models. GLA and EPA treatment of RA patients reduces the need for NSAIDs and corticosteroids,[76,81,82] and both protect the gastric mucosa from NSAID-induced injury. A combination of GLA and EPA may be useful therapy for RA patients. Continued study of the eicosanoids and their precursor fatty acids should delineate the mechanisms by which these lipids influence the function of cells that participate in immune responses and inflammatory reactions.

REFERENCES

1. Brash AR: Specific lipoxygenase attack on arachidonic acid and linoleate esterified in phosphatidylcholine: Precedent for an alternative mechanism in activation of eicosanoid biosynthesis. Adv Prostaglandin Thromboxane Leukot Res 15:197, 1985.
2. Roberts MF: Phospholipases: Structural and functional motifs for working at an interface. FASEB J 10:1159, 1996.
3. Fitzpatrick FA, Soberman R: Regulated formation of eicosanoids. J Clin Invest 107:1347, 2001.
4. Bell RI, Kennerly DA, Dianford N: Diglyceride lipase: A pathway for arachidonate release from human platelets. Proc Natl Acad Sci U S A 76:3238, 1979.
5. Bomalaski JS, Clark MA, Zurier RB: Enhanced phospholipase activity in peripheral blood monocytes from patients with rheumatoid arthritis. Arthritis Rheum 29:312, 1986.
6. Bozza PT, YU W, Penrose JF, et al: Eosinophil lipid bodies: Specific, inducible intracellular sites for enhanced eicosanoid formation. J Exp Med 186:909, 1997.
7. Smith WL, DeWitt DL, Garavito RM: Cyclooxygenases: Structural, cellular, and molecular biology. Annu Rev Biochem 69:145, 2000.
8. Reed DW, Bradshaw WS, Xie W, Simmons DL: In vivo and in vitro expression of a non-mammalian cyclooxygenase-1. Prostaglandins 52:269, 1996.
9. Kulmacz RJ, Pendleton RB, Lands WE: Interaction between peroxidose and cyclooxygenase activities in prostaglandin-endoperoxide synth. Interpretation of reaction kinetics, J Biol Chem 269: 5527-36, 1994.
10 Shaw G. Kamen R.: A conserved AU sequence from the 3 untranslated region of GM-CSF mRNA mediates selective mRNA degradation. Cell 29:659, 1986.
11. Nakao S, Ogata Y, Shimizu-Sasaki E, et al: Activation of NFkappaB is necessary for IL-1beta-induced cyclooxygenase-2 (COX-2) expression in human gingival fibroblasts. Mol Cell Biochem 209:113-118, 2000.
12. Debey S, Meyer-Kirchrath J, Schror K: Regulation of cyclooxygenase-2 expression in iloprost in human vascular smooth muscle cells. Role of transcription factors CREB and ICER. Biochem Pharmacol 65:979-988, 2003.
14. Dubois RN, Abramson SB, Crofford L, et al: Cyclooxygenase in biology and disease. FASEB J 12:1063, 1998.
15. McAdam BF, Catella-Lawson F, Mardini IA, et al: Systemic biosynthesis of prostacyclin by cyclooxygenase (COX)-2: The human pharmacology of a selective inhibitor of COX-2. Proc Natl Acad Sci U S A 96:272, 1999.
16. Gilroy DW, Colville-Nash PR, Willis D, et al: Inducible cyclooxygenase may have antiinflammatory properties. Nature Med 5:968-701, 1999.
17. Dinchuk JE, Car BD, Focht RJ, et al: Renal abnormalities and an altered inflammatory response in mice lacking cyclooxygenase II. Nature 378:406, 1995.
18. Thomas L: The Lives of a Cell. New York, Penguin, 1995.
19. Chandreskharan NV, Dai H, Roos KL, et al: COX-3, a cyclooxygenase-1 variant inhibited by acetaminophen and other analgesic/antipyretic drugs: cloning, structure, and expression. Proc Natl Acad Sci U S A 99:13371, 2002.
20. Kurzrock R, Lieb CC: Biochemical studies of human semen. II. The action of semen on the human uterus. Proc Soc Exp Biol Med 28:268, 1930.
21. von Euler US: On the specific vasodilating and plain muscle stimulating substances from accessory genital glands in man and certain animals (prostaglandin and vesiglandin). J Physiol (Lond) 88:213, 1936.
22. Bergstrom S, Ryhage R, Samuelsson B: The structure of prostaglandins E_1, F_1, and F_2. Acta Chem Scand 16:501, 1962.
23. Portanova JP, Zhang Y, Anderson GD, et al: Selective neutralization of prostaglandin E_2 blocks inflammation, hyperalgesia, and interleukin-6 production in vivo. J Exp Med 184:883, 1996.
24. Ferreira SH: Prostaglandins, aspirin-like drugs and analgesia. Nat New Biol 240:200, 1972.
25. Raisz LG: Recent advances in bone cell biology: Interactions of vitamin D with other local and systemic factors. Bone Miner 9:191, 1990.
26. Marks SC, Miller SC: Prostaglandins and the skeleton: The legacy and challenges of two decades of research. Endocr J 1:337, 1993.
27. Amin AR, Attur M, Patel RN, et al: Superinduction of cyclooxygenase-2 activity in human osteoarthritis-affected cartilage: Influence of nitric oxide. J Clin Invest 99:1231, 1997.
28. Jiang C, Ting AT, Seed B: PPAR-gamma agonists inhibit production of monocyte inflammatory cytokines. Nature 391:82, 1998.
29. Moncada S, Gryglewski R, Bunting S, Vane JR: An enzyme isolated from arteries transforms prostaglandin endoperoxides to an unstable substance that inhibits platelet aggregation. Nature 263:633, 1976.

30. Miyata A, Hara S, Yokoyama C, et al: Molecular cloning and expression of human prostacyclin synthase. Biochem Biophys Res Commun 200:1728, 1994.
31. Baenziger NL, Becherer PR, Majerus PJ: Characterization of prostacyclin synthesis in cultured human smooth muscle cells, venous endothelial cells and skin fibroblasts. Cell 16:967, 1979.
32. Vane JR, Anggard EE, Botting RM: Regulatory function of the vascular endothelium. N Engl J Med 323:27, 1990.
33. Hamberg M, Svensson J, Samuelsson B: Thromboxanes: A new group of biologically active compounds derived from prostaglandin endoperoxides. Proc Natl Acad Sci U S A 72:2994, 1975.
34. Wigley FM, Wise RA, Seibold JR, et al: Intravenous iloprost infusion in patients with Raynaud phenomenon secondary to systemic sclerosis: A multicenter, placebo-controlled, double-blind study. Ann Intern Med 120:199, 1994.
35. Horn EM, Barst RJ: Trepostinil therapy for pulmonary artery hypertension. Expert Opin Investig Drugs 11:1615, 2002.
36. Remuzzi G, Fitzgerald GA, Patrono C: Thromboxane synthesis and action within the kidney. Kidney Int 41:1483, 1992.
37. Oates JA, Fitzgerald G, Branch RA, et al: Clinical implications of prostaglandin and thromboxane A_2 formation. N Engl J Med 219:761, 1988.
38. Kinsella BT: Thromboane A_2 signalling in humans: a 'Tail' of two receptors. Biochem Soc Trans 29641, 2001.
39. Funk CD, Hoshiko S, Matsumoto T, et al: Characterization of the human 5-lipoxygenase gene. Proc Natl Acad Sci U S A 86:2587, 1989.
40. Brock TG, McNish RW, Peters-Golden M: Rapid import of cytosolic 5-lipoxygenase into the nucleus of neutrophils after in vivo recruitment and in vitro adherence. J Biol Chem 272:8276, 1997.
41. Lewis RA, Austen KF, Soberman RJ: Leukotrienes and other products of the 5-lipoxygenase pathway: Biochemistry and relation to pathobiology in human disease. N Engl J Med 323:645, 1990.
42. Heyworth PG, Karnovsky ML, Badwey JA: Protein phosphorylation associated with synergistic stimulation of neutrophils. J Biol Chem 2674:14935, 1989.
43. Haeggstrom JZ, Wetterholm A: Enzymes and receptors in the leukotriene cascade. Cell Mol Life Sci 59:742-753, 2002.
44. Baud L, Perez J, Denis M, Ardaillous R: Modulation of fibroblast proliferation by sulfidopeptide leukotrienes: Effect of indomethacin. J Immunol 138:1190, 1987.
45. Haeggstrom JZ, Kull F, Rudberg, PC, et al: Leukotriene A4 hydrolase. Prostaglandins Other Lipid Mediat 68-69:495-510, 2002.
46. Mani I, Iversen L, Ziboh VA: Upregulation of nuclear PKC and MAP-kinase during hyperproliferation of guinea pig epidermis: modulation by 13-(s) hydroxyoctadecadienoic acid (13-HODE). Cell Signal 10:143, 1998.
47. Ziboh VA: The role of n-3 fatty acids in psoriasis. *In* Kremer JM (ed): Medicinal Fatty Acids in Inflammation. Basel, Birkha_user-Verlag, 1998, p 45.
48. Serhan CN, Oliw E: Unorthodox routes to prostanoid formation: new twists in cyclooxygenase-initiated pathways. J Clin Invest 107:1481, 2001.
49. Serhan CN, Cish CB, Brannon J, et al: Anti-microinflammatory lipid signals generated from dietary N-3 fatty acids via cyclooxygease-2 and transcellular processing: a novel mechanism for NSAID and N-3 PUFA therapeutic actions. J Physiol Pharmacol 51:643, 2000.
50. Pratico D, Barry OP, Lawson JA, et al: IPF_2: An index of lipid peroxidation in humans. Proc Natl Acad Sci U S A 95:3449, 1998.
51. Christopoulos A,Wilson K: Interaction of ananamide with the M(1) and M(4) muscarinic acetylcholine receptors. Brain Res 915:70, 2001.
52. DiMarzo V, DePetrocellis L, Sepe N, Buono A: Biosynthesis of anandamide and related acylethanolamides in mouse J774 macrophages and N_{18} neuroblastoma cells. Biochem J 316:977, 1996.
53. Burstein S: The cannabinoid acids: Nonpsychoactive derivatives with therapeutic potential. Pharmacol Ther 82:87, 1999.
54. Burstein SH, Rossetti RG, Yagen B, Zurier RB: Oxidative metabolism of anandamide. Prostaglandins Other Lipid Mediat 61:29, 2000.
55. Ross RA, Craib SJ, Stevenson LA, et al: Pharmacological characterization of the anandamide cyclooxygenase metabolite: Prostaglandin E_2 ethanolamide. J Pharmacol Exp. Therap 301:900, 2002.
56. Ushikubi F, Hirata M, Naurmiya S: Molecular biology of prostanoid receptors: An overview. J Lipid Mediat Cell Signal 12:343, 1995.
57. Smith EM, Austin SC, Reilly MP, Fitzgerald GA: Internalization and sequestration of the human prostacyclin receptor. J Biol Chem 275:32037, 2000.
58. Narumiya S, Fitzgerald GA: Genetic and pharmacological analysis of prostanoid receptor function. J Clin Invest 108:25, 2001.
59. Yokomizo T, Kato K, Hagiya H, et al: Hydroxyeicosanoids bind to and activate the low affinity leukotrine B4 receptor. J Biol Chem 276:12454, 2001.
60. Weinblatt ME, Kremer JM, Coblyn JS, et al: Zileuton, a 5-lipoxygenase inhibitor in rheumatoid arthritis. J Rheumatol 19:1537, 1992.
61. Levy BD, Serhan CN: Polyisoprenyl phosphates: natural anti-inflammatory lipid signals. Cell Mol Life Sci 59:729-741, 2002.
62. Ricote M, Li AC, Willson TM, et al: The peroxisome-proliferator-activated receptor-gamma is a negative regulator of macrophage activation. Nature 391:79, 1998.
63. Tsubouchi Y, Kawahito Y, Kohno M, et al: Biochem Biophys Res Comm 283:750, 2001.
64. Devchand PR, Keller H, Peters JM, et al: The PPARα-leukotriene B_4 pathway to inflammation control. Nature 384:39, 1996.
65. Zimmerman GA, McIntyre TM, Prescott SM, et al: The platelet activating factor signaling system and its regulators in syndromes of inflammation and thrombosis. Crit Care Med 30(Suppl 5):S294, 2002.
66. Zurier RB: Prostaglandins, fatty acids, and arthritis. *In* Cunningham-Rundles S (ed): Nutrient Modulation of the Immune Response. New York, Marcel Dekker, 1993, p 201.
67. Bygdeman M, Samuelsson B: Quantitative determination of prostaglandins in human semen. Clin Chim Acta 10:566, 1964.
68. Karim SMM, Soindler M, Williams ED: Distribution of prostaglandins in human tissues. Br J Pharmacol Chemother 31:340, 1967.
69. Horrobin DF: The roles of essential fatty acids in the development of diabetic neuropathy and other complications of diabetes mellitus. Prostaglandins Leukot Essent Fatty Acids 31:181, 1988.
70. Tilley SL, Coffman TM, Koller BH: Mixed messages: modulation of inflammation and immune responses b prostaglandins and thromboxanes. J Clin Invest 108:15, 2001.
71. Brash AR: Arachidonic acid as a bioactive molecule. J Clin Invest 107:7700-7705, 2001.
72. van Dorp DA, Beer Thuis RK, Nugteren DH: The biosynthesis of prostaglandins. Biochem Biophys Acta 90:204, 1964.
73. Bergstrom S, Daniellson H, Samuelsson B: The enzymatic formation of prostaglandin E_2 from arachidonic acid. Biochem Biophys Acta 90:207, 1964.
74. Bergstrom S, Daniellson H, Klenberg D, Samuelsson B: The enzymatic conversion of essential fatty acids into prostaglandins. J Biol Chem 239:4006, 1964.
75. Vassilopoulos D, Zurier RB, Rossetti RG, Tsokos GC: Gammalinolenic acid and dihomogammalinolenic acid suppress the CD3 mediated signal transduction pathway in human T cells. Clin Immunol Immunopathol 83:237, 1997.
76. Kremer JM: Effects of modulation of inflammatory and immune parameters in patients with rheumatic and inflammatory disease receiving dietary supplementation of n-3 and n-6 fatty acids. Lipids 31:S253, 1996.
77. DeLuca P, Rothman D, Zurier RB: Marine and botanical lipids as immunomodulatory and therapeutic agents in the treatment of rheumatoid arthritis. Rheum Dis Clin North Am 21:759, 1995.
78. Rossetti RG, Seiler CM, DeLuca P, Zurier RB: Oral administration of unsaturated fatty acids: Effects on human peripheral blood T lymphocyte proliferation. J Leukoc Biol 62:438, 1997.
79. Furse RK, Rossetti RG, Zurier RB: Gammalinolenic acid, an unsaturated fatty acid with antiinflammatory properties, blocks amplification of IL-1β production by human monocytes. J Immunol 167:490, 2001.
80. Furse RK, Rossetti, RG, Seiler CM, Zurier RB: Oral administration of gammalinolenic acid, an unsaturated fatty acid with anti-inflammatory properties, modulates interleukin-1β production by human monocytes. J Clin Immunol 22:83, 2002.
81. Zurier RB, Rossetti RG, Jacobson EW, et al: Gammalinolenic acid treatment of rheumatoid arthritis: A randomized, placebo-controlled trial. Arthritis Rheum 39:1808, 1996.
82. Belch JJF, Madhok AR, O'Dowd A, Sturrock RD: Effects of altering dietary essential fatty acids on requirements for nonsteroidal anti-inflammatory drugs in patients with rheumatoid arthritis: A double blind placebo controlled study. Ann Rheum Dis 47:96, 1988.

24 Endothelial Cell Biology, Angiogenesis, and Recruitment of Cells

ZOLTAN SZEKANECZ • ALISA E. KOCH

A number of factors, including inflammatory cells, soluble mediators, cell adhesion molecules (CAMs), and proteolytic enzymes are involved in the pathogenesis of inflammatory synovitis, such as in rheumatoid arthritis (RA). In RA, inflammatory leukocytes invade the synovium by transmigrating through the vascular endothelium (Figs. 24–1 and 24–2). The formation of blood vessels, termed *angiogenesis*, is a key event underlying RA that perpetuates the recruitment of leukocytes into the inflamed synovium[1-6] (Fig. 24–3). Several CAMs interacting with soluble inflammatory mediators, such as cytokines and chemokines, are involved in leukocyte extravasation, as well as angiogenesis.[1-6]

Endothelial cells (ECs) line the lumina of arteries, veins, and capillaries, thus separating—and also connecting—the blood and the extravascular tissues. In inflammatory reactions, such as RA synovitis, ECs are not only passive bystanders, but they interact with cells and soluble mediators found in the surrounding tissues. ECs are active responders to external stimuli, and they also produce a number of mediators and express CAMs, thereby influencing the action of leukocytes and the outcome of the inflammatory response.[7,8]

Angiogenesis is a crucial event in a number of physiologic processes, such as reproduction, development, and tissue repair. Among disease states, enhanced neovascularization is present in, among others, RA and other inflammatory diseases, as well as malignancies. The angiogenic process, its mediators and inhibitors, cellular and molecular interactions underlying neovascularization, and the role of angiogenesis and the possibilities of angiostatic targeting in RA have been recently reviewed.[1,2,9-13] The increased number of blood vessels produced during angiogenesis further perpetuates the extravasation of leukocytes, and thus synovitis, in RA.[1,11,12] Several growth factors, cytokines, chemokines, CAMs, extracellular matrix (ECM) components, and other factors involved in neovascularization have been detected in significant amounts in the RA synovium[1-4,11-13] (see Fig. 24–3).

In this chapter, we review the role of blood vessels in the pathogenesis of RA. The role of endothelium in two major processes, leukocyte extravasation and angiogenesis, also will be discussed. The regulation of leukocyte recruitment and neovascularization will be reviewed as well. Some data on the clinical relevance of these important processes will also be presented here.

Endothelial Morphology and Function in Inflammatory Synovitis

The endothelium may undergo numerous morphologic changes during inflammation. Extensive vasodilatation and increased vascular permeability (vascular leakage) occurs in rheumatoid synovitis. Vascular leakage can result from EC contraction and retraction, as well as leukocyte- or anti-EC antibody (AECA)-mediated vascular injury.[8] Most vasodilatory mediators originate from the plasma or blood cells. However, ECs also release vasodilators, including prostacyclin (PGI_2), nitric oxide (NO), and platelet-activating factor (PAF).[14]

A number of key mechanisms may play a role in increased vascular permeability. The most important morphologic basis for vascular leakage is the formation and widening of intercellular gaps between ECs induced by, among other mediators, histamine, serotonin, C3a, C5a, bradykinin, leukotrienes, and PAF.[8,15] This type of leakage, also termed *histamine-mediated injury*, occurs mostly in smaller venules.[8] EC retraction, associated with cytoskeletal reorganization, occurs in vitro upon exposure to cytokines, including tumor necrosis factor-α (TNF-α), interleukin-1 (IL-1), or interferon-γ (IFN-γ).[16] EC retraction is a good example of EC stimulation, but EC contraction is a manifestation of EC activation.[8,15]

Leukocytes interacting with the vascular wall may themselves cause EC injury, leading to increased vascular permeability. The key mediators in this process are reactive oxygen intermediates and some matrix metalloproteinases (MMPs).[17] Resting leukocytes extravasate without causing vascular leakage, but activated white blood cells trigger increased vascular permeability.[18,19] The production of AECAs has been described in several inflammatory rheumatic diseases, including RA.[20,21] AECA may be a marker of vascular damage.

Capillary regeneration after vascular injury and angiogenesis is also associated with leakage. Increased permeability of newly formed vessels is due to open intercellular junctions and the incomplete basement membranes of ECs.[1,2,13,22]

Cellular Adhesion Molecules

Adhesion of peripheral blood inflammatory leukocytes to endothelium is a key event in inflammation, leading to the process of leukocyte transendothelial emigration

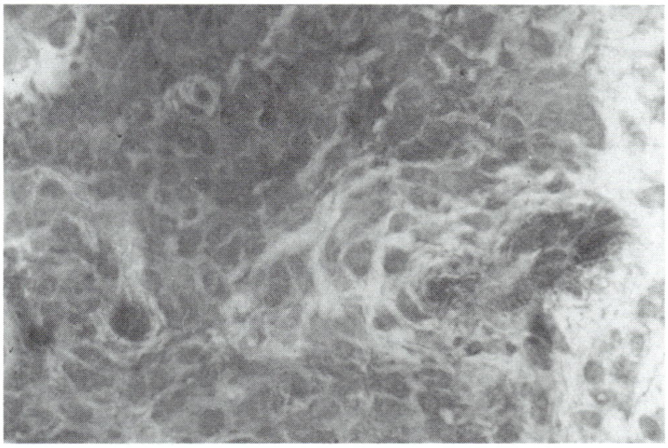

FIGURE 24–1 · Indirect immunoperoxidase staining of frozen rheumatoid synovial tissue showing endothelial intercellular adhesion molecule-1 (ICAM-1) expression as indicated by the dark color. (× 696). (See color plate 5.)

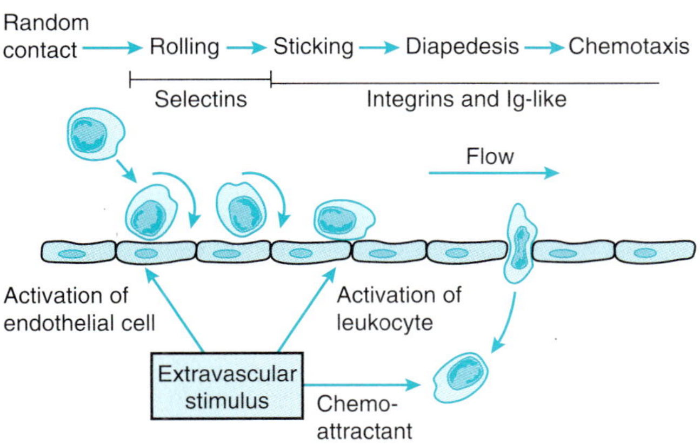

FIGURE 24–2 · The steps of leukocyte extravasation into the synovium.

into inflammatory sites[4,23-26] (see Figs. 24–1 and 24–2; Table 24–1). For example, in rheumatoid synovitis, the cascade of events begins with the adhesion of neutrophils, lymphocytes, and monocytes to the specialized, fenestrated synovial EC.[4] High endothelial venule (HEV)-like microvessels, similar to HEV in the primary lymphoid organs involved in "lymphocyte homing," are present in the synovial tissue[4] (see Fig. 24–1). Thus, leukocyte recruitment to inflammatory sites may be considered a type of "pathologic homing." Leukocyte adhesion to EC is followed by the transmigration of inflammatory cells through the vessel wall into the synovium[4,26] (see Fig. 24–2 and Table 24–1; Table 24–2).

EC adhesion to leukocytes and to the ECM, as well as numerous steps of angiogenesis, are mediated by CAMs. CAMs have been classified into a number of superfamilies. However, CAMs that are most relevant for the adhesive events and angiogenesis underlying inflammation belong to three familes: the integrins, selectins, and immunoglobulin supergene family[23-26] (see Table 24–1). Integrins are mainly involved in EC adhesion to ECM macromolecules, and immunoglobulin supergene family members and selectins play a role in EC adhesion to other cells.[23-26]

Selectins contain an extracellular N-terminal domain related to lectins, an epidermal growth factor–like domain, and moieties related to complement regulatory proteins.[23-26] This CAM family includes E-, P-, and L-selectin. E- and P-selectin are present on endothelia.[23-26]

E-selectin is usually not expressed on resting cultured ECs. However, IL-1 and TNF-α stimulate EC E-selectin expression within a few hours.[27] Maximal endothelial E-selectin expression is seen after 4 to 6 hours of cytokine treatment, followed by downregulated expression.[27] In addition, cytokine-activated EC shed E-selectin, thus releasing soluble E-selectin from the EC surface. Soluble E-selectin is a good marker for cytokine-induced EC

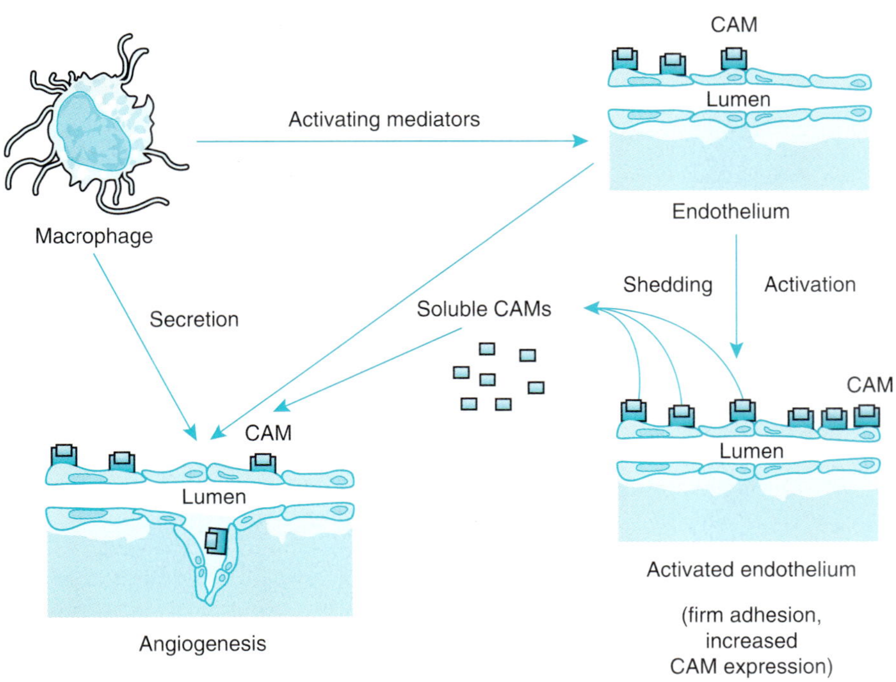

FIGURE 24–3 · The involvement of soluble mediators, as well as soluble and surface-bound adhesion molecules, in angiogenesis.

TABLE 24–1 • SOME IMPORTANT ENDOTHELIAL ADHESION MOLECULES IN SYNOVIAL INFLAMMATION

Adhesion Molecule Superfamily	Endothelial Adhesion Molecule	Ligand(s)
Integrins	β_1 integrins (most)	ECM components (laminin, fibronectin, collagen, vitronectin, etc.)
	$\alpha_4\beta_1$ integrin	VCAM-1, fibronectin
	$\alpha_V\beta_3$ integrin	ECM components (fibronectin, fibrinogen, thrombospondin)
Immunoglobulins	ICAM-1	β_2 integrins: LFA-1, Mac-1
	VCAM-1	$\alpha_4\beta_1$ and $\alpha_4\beta_7$
	LFA-3	CD2
	PECAM-1 (CD31)	Homophilic, $\alpha_V\beta_3$
Selectins	E-selectin	ESL-1, PSGL-1, CLA
	P-selectin	PSGL-1
Cadherins	VE-cadherin	Homophilic
Others	CD44	Hyaluronic acid
	Endoglin	TGF-β
	VAP-1	?

Abbreviations: CLA, cutaneous leukocyte antigen; ECM, extracellular matrix; ESL-1, E-selectin ligand-1; LFA, lymphocyte function–associated antigen; Mac, macrophage; PECAM-1, platelet-endothelial cell adhesion molecule-1; PSGL-1, P-selectin glycoprotein ligand-1; TGF-β, transforming growth factor-β; VAP-1, vascular adhesion protein-1; VCAM-1, vascular cell adhesion molecule-1; VE, vascular endothelial.

TABLE 24–2 • DISTINCT STEPS DURING LEUKOCYTE EMIGRATION

Step	Factors on Endothelium	Factors on Leukocytes
Rolling	P-selectin	PSGL-1
	E-selectin	ESL-1
	L-selectin ligand ?	Sialyl Lewis-X
		CLA
		L-selectin
Activation	Chemokines (IL-8, MCP-1, etc)	Cytokine and chemokine receptors
	PAF	
	PECAM-1	PECAM-1
	E-selectin	PSGL-1, ESL-1
Firm adhesion	ICAM-1	β_1, β_2, and β_7 integrins
	VCAM-1	
Diapedesis	ICAM-1	β_1, β_2, and β_7 integrins
	VCAM-1	PECAM-1
	PECAM-1	

Abbreviations: CLA, cutaneous leukocyte antigen; ESL-1, E-selectin ligand-1; ICAM-1, intercellular adhesion molecule-1; IL, interleukin; PAF, platelet-activating factor; PECAM-1, platelet-endothelial cell adhesion molecule-1; PSGL-1, P-selectin glycoprotein ligand-1; VCAM-1, vascular cell adhesion molecule-1.

activation.[4,28] Ligands for E-selectin, such as E-selectin ligand-1 (ESL-1), P-selectin glycoprotein ligand-1 (PSGL-1), and cutaneous leukocyte antigen (CLA), contain sialylated glycan motifs, such as sialyl Lewis-X (sLe^x).[29,30] E-selectin has been associated with RA synovitis, as well as dermal and pulmonary inflammation[4,19,28,31]; abundant expression of E-selectin in RA synovial tissues and increased production of soluble E-selectin in RA synovial fluids were described.[28,31] In addition, soluble E-selectin mediates monocyte chemotaxis.[32] Antibodies to E-selectin reduce neutrophil influx in animal models of airway and skin inflammation.[19,26,33]

P-selectin is constitutively present on the membrane of EC Weibel-Palade bodies.[4,34] P-selectin is involved in leukocyte-EC adhesion in vitro.[35] PSGL-1 is a known ligand for P-selectin.[30] Proinflammatory cytokines upregulate P-selectin expression on EC within seconds. Thus, P-selectin is involved in the very early phases of adhesion.[36] In contrast to E-selectin, the induction of P-selectin on ECs is an example of endothelial stimulation rather than activation.[30,36] P-selectin has also been implicated in synovial inflammation and is expressed on RA synovial ECs.[37] In addition, soluble P-selectin concentrations are increased in RA versus osteoarthritic synovial fluids.[38] Anti-PSGL-1 antibody blocked the migration of T cells into inflammatory sites.[30]

L-selectin is absent from ECs, but present on most leukocytes. L-selectin serves as a lymphocyte homing receptor, and it mediates the physiologic recirculation of naïve lymphocytes through specialized HEV-expressing L-selectin ligands, including CD34, MadCAM-1, and GlyCAM-1.[23-26] In addition, L-selectin is also involved in leukocyte-EC interactions underlying arthritis.[4,26] However, L-selectin expression on leukocytes is downregulated upon cytokine activation[39]; therefore, the exact role of L-selectin in inflammation is not yet fully clear.

Integrins are αβ heterodimers, and each of the common β subunits is associated with one or more α chains.[23-26] β_1 and β_3 integrins are expressed on EC. These integrins ($\alpha_{1\text{-}9}\beta_1$, $\alpha_V\beta_3$) mediate cell adhesion to ECM components including types I and IV collagen, laminin, fibronectin, fibrinogen, tenascin, vitronectin, and thrombospondin. Integrins containing the β_1 subunit are also termed *very late antigens* (VLA). The $\alpha_1\beta_1$ (VLA-1) and $\alpha_2\beta_1$ (VLA-2) integrins mediate EC adhesion to collagen and laminin.[23-26,40] However, the main EC laminin receptor is $\alpha_6\beta_1$ (VLA-6). There are two important receptors for fibronectin: $\alpha_4\beta_1$ (VLA-4) and $\alpha_5\beta_1$ (VLA-5).[23-26,40] All these integrins, as well as $\alpha_3\beta_1$ (VLA-3), a receptor for laminin, collagen, and fibronectin, are also expressed on EC.[40] β_3 integrins mediate EC adhesion to ECM components, including fibronectin, vitronectin, thrombospondin, von Willebrand factor, and fibrinogen. The α_V integrin subunit can be associated with several β-chains (β_1, β_3, β_5, β_6, β_8) and thus is involved in EC adhesion to the various ECM molecules, depending on the β subunit.[23-26,40] In addition, most β_1 integrins, as well as $\alpha_V\beta_3$ are involved in EC migration and angiogenesis (see later discussion) and are required for the survival and maturation of new blood vessels.[40,41] Integrin-mediated adhesion has been implicated in leukocyte-EC interactions during inflammation. For example, there is an abundant expression of EC integrins in RA and other types of arthritis.[4,37]

Regarding members of the *immunoglobulin superfamily* of CAMs, VCAM-1, a ligand for the integrins $\alpha_4\beta_1$ and $\alpha_4\beta_7$, is expressed on resting EC, and its expression is markedly upregulated by proinflammatory cytokines.[4,42] Abundant VCAM-1 expression has been associated with synovitis and various other types of inflammation.[4,31,43] ICAM-1 is a ligand for β_2 integrins, including lymphocyte function–associated antigen-1 (LFA-1), Mac-1, and p150,95.[23-26] The expression of ICAM-1 on EC can be induced by IL-1, TNF-α, and IFN-γ,[44] and the maximal expression of ICAM-1 on ECs is observed later than (more than 24 hours after) that of E-selectin.[7] ICAM-1 is expressed on EC in inflammatory sites, including RA synovium in situ.[4,31]

Vascular addressins are CAMs expressed by HEVs in lymphoid organs, as well as by HEV-like structures in the arthritic synovium. These addressins are recognized by leukocyte integrins and selectins and are involved in physiologic homing, as well as in the transendothelial migration of inflammatory leukocytes. Addressins recognized by L-selectin, such as CD34, MadCAM-1, and GlyCAM-1, were discussed previously. In addition, a family of junctional CAMs (JAMs) expressed on HEVs and recognized by leukocyte integrins has recently been described.[45-47] JAM-1, JAM-2, and JAM-3 are ligands for the β_2 integrin LFA-1, the $\alpha_4\beta_1$ integrin (VLA-4), and the β_2 integrin Mac-1, respectively.[45-47] All these JAMs may be involved in leukocyte migration during inflammation.[45-47]

Other CAMs mediating leukocyte-EC adhesion during synovitis include LFA-3, CD2, platelet-endothelial cell adhesion molecule-1 (PECAM-1, also known as CD31), CD44, vascular adhesion protein-1 (VAP-1), endoglin, VE-cadherin, certain glycoconjugates, CD99, and possibly ICAM-3.[4,23-26,48-57] LFA-3, an EC CAM, and its counterreceptor on T cells, CD2, are members of the immunoglobulin superfamily. The CD2/LFA-3 adhesion pathway is involved in various inflammatory responses, including arthritis.[4,51] PECAM-1, another member of the immunoglobulin superfamily, mediates homotypic adhesion by binding to PECAM-1, as well as heterotypic adhesion by recognizing the $\alpha_V\beta_3$ integrin.[23-26] PECAM-1 is found in large quantities in the RA synovium.[4,37] CD44 is a receptor for hyaluronate[23-26] and is present on activated ECs in inflammatory synovitis.[37,52] VAP-1 was originally isolated from synovial ECs. The expression of VAP-1 is increased in inflammation.[48] Endoglin is a receptor for transforming growth factor (TGF)-β_1 and TGF-β_3 and is involved in EC adhesion. Endoglin is expressed by most ECs in the RA synovium.[50] VE-cadherin, a major constituent of EC junctions, mediates homophilic binding between ECs and is involved in EC migration and polarization.[53] Certain glycoconjugates may also be involved in cell adhesion. For example, MUC18 (CD146) has been detected in RA synovial fluids.[55] CD99 is a heavily glycosylated protein expressed on most leukocytes and is involved in leukocyte migration through EC junctions.[56] ICAM-3 is a leukocyte CAM, which is a known ligand for LFA-1. It is usually absent from resting ECs; however, it has been detected on some RA synovial ECs.[49,57] Thus, a number of CAMs may play a role in the adhesive interactions of EC (see Figs. 24–1 and 24–2 and Tables 24–1 and 24–2).

The Process of Leukocyte Recruitment

The process of leukocyte adhesion to and migration through endothelia occurs in at least four distinct steps[26,58] (see Fig. 24–2 and Table 24–2).

1. An early, weak adhesion, termed *rolling*, occurs within the first 1 to 2 hours. This step is mediated mostly by selectins and their ligands.
2. Leukocyte activation and triggering occurs next due to the interactions between chemokine receptors on leukocytes and proteoglycans on EC. PECAM-1 and PAF are also involved in this step.
3. Activation-dependent, firm adhesion occurs within 4 to 6 hours, mediated mostly by $\alpha_4\beta_1$ (VLA-4) integrin/VCAM-1 and LFA-1/ICAM-1 interactions; this is also accompanied by the secretion of various chemokines.
4. Transendothelial migration, or diapedesis, involving integrins occurs when secreted chemokines bind to EC heparan sulphate. Chemokines preferentially attract endothelium-bound leukocytes. The $\alpha_4\beta_1$ (VLA-4) and $\alpha_5\beta_1$ (VLA-5) integrins recognize EC fibronectin, and $\alpha_6\beta_1$ (VLA-6) binds to laminin.

The possible role of JAMs in integrin-mediated transendothelial migration was discussed previously. These adhesive interactions enable leukocyte ingress into the synovium.[4,26,45-47,58]

Angiogenesis: Its Mediators and Inhibitors

Angiogenesis, the formation of new blood vessels, is pathologically enhanced in a number of inflammatory diseases, such as RA and psoriasis, as well as in malignancies. The neovascularization process and the outcome of such angiogenic diseases are dependent on the balance or imbalance between angiogenic mediators and inhibitors. A number of cytokines, growth factors, chemokines, and certain CAMs, as well as other mediators, can modulate capillary formation. The suppression of neovascularization by blocking the action of angiogenic mediators, or by the administration of angiostatic compounds, may be useful for suppressing various inflammatory processes, such as arthritis[1,2,11-13,59-61] (see Fig. 24–3; Table 24–3).

New vessels are generated following a program of several distinct steps. First, ECs are activated by different angiogenic stimuli. In response, ECs secrete proteases, which degrade the underlying basement membrane and ECM. The emigration of loose ECs results in the formation of primary capillary sprouts. Sprouting ECs then further proliferate, migrate, and synthesize new basement membrane. This process is followed by lumen formation within the sprouts. Two sprouts may link to form capillary loops. Finally, the emigration of ECs from these sprouts results in the development of second and further generations of capillary sprouts.[1,2,12,13,59]

Preferential EC precursors may exist within the population of blood stem cells. Some CD34$^+$ cells carrying receptors for vascular endothelial growth factor (VEGF) may, under some circumstances, develop into ECs.[62-64] These cells may be important in the induction and perpetuation of angiogenesis, as well as EC differentiation.[62-64] In addition, they may also be used for the induction of neovascularization in future therapeutic trials in certain vascular disorders.[65-67] VEGF and basic fibroblast growth factor (bFGF) have been introduced into clinical trials to induce angiogenesis by stimulating EC morphogenesis from stem cells in ischemic heart disease,[65] as well as obliterative arteriosclerosis.[66,67]

TABLE 24–3 • SOME ANGIOGENIC MEDIATORS AND ANGIOGENESIS INHIBITORS IN RHEUMATOID ARTHRITIS

	Mediators	Inhibitors
1. Growth factors	BFGF, aFGF VEGF HGF PDGF, PD-ECGF EGF IGF-1 TGF-β*	TGF-β*
2. Cytokines	TNF-β IL-1* IL-6* IL-13 IL-15 IL-18	IL-1* IL-4 IL-6* IFN-α,-γ
3. Chemokines	IL-8 ENA-78 Gro CTAP-III MCP-1 Fractalkine SDF-1	PF4 IP-10 MIG
4. Matrix molecules	Type I collagen Fibronectin, laminin heparin, heparan sulphate	RGD sequence Thrombospondin
5. Proteolytic	Matrix metalloproteinases Plasminogen activators	Metalloproteinase inhibitors Plasminogen activator inhibitors
6. Adhesion molecules	β1, β3 integrins Soluble E-selectin Soluble VCAM-1 Endoglin CD31 (PECAM-1) MUC18	RGD sequence
7. Others	Angiogenin PAF Substance P SLe^y/H Prolactin Prostaglandin E2	Some antirheumatic drugs Some antibiotics SPARC Angiostatin Endostatin

*Mediators with both pro- and antiangiogenic effects.

See text for abbreviations.

A number of in vitro and in vivo models are available to study angiogenesis. In vitro systems include EC cultures grown on ECM substrata, such as the laminin-containing Matrigel, tissue culture systems, or EC chemotaxis assays.[1,2,11-13] In vivo capillary formation has been investigated using the rat, murine, rabbit, and guinea pig corneal micropocket, the chick embryo chorioallantoic membrane, the hamster cheek pouch, the mesenteric, the aortic ring, implanted matrix assays, sponge models, and other systems.[1,2,11-13] These models are suitable to investigate the role of angiogenesis in the pathogenesis of certain diseases, as well asto design strategies for therapies based on angiogenesis suppression.[1,2]

Angiogenic factors may act directly on EC proliferation and migration (see Fig. 24–3). ECs express receptors for these mediators.[1,2,5,13] In contrast, indirect angiogenic mediators act by stimulating macrophages or other cells to release angiogenic growth factors.[1,2,11,59] Soluble forms of certain EC CAMs described previously, such as E-selectin or VCAM-1, can also induce angiogenesis.[41,68,69] Only those angiogenic and angiostatic factors that may be involved in inflammatory synovitis, particularly in RA, will be discussed in this chapter (see Table 24–3).

Angiogenic mediators involved in the progression of RA are released by ECs and macrophages, cells present in high quantities in the RA synovium[1,2,10-13] (see Fig. 24–3 and Table 24–3). Among growth factors, VEGF, bFGF, acidic fibroblast growth factor (aFGF), and hepatocyte growth factor (HGF)/scatter factor are bound to heparin or heparan sulfate in the ECM. During angiogenesis, these mediators are released from the ECM by EC-derived heparanase and plasmin.[1,2,11-13] VEGF, at least in part, stimulates angiogenesis via the cyclooxygenase-2 (COX-2) pathway.[70] The role of VEGF receptor 2–expressing CD34$^+$, EC precursor cells in vascular morphogenesis was discussed previously. Hypoxia-inducible factor 1α (HIF-1α) is an important regulator of hypoxia-induced VEGF production. This molecule has been implicated in the pathogenesis of various vascular disorders, and it may be involved in synovitis-associated angiogenesis.[67,71]

Other growth factors that mediate neovascularization, such as platelet-derived growth factor (PDGF), platelet-derived endothelial cell growth factor (PD-ECGF), epidermal growth factor (EGF), insulin-like growth factor I (IGF-I), and TGF-ß, do not bind to heparin. However, these growth factors may also promote capillary formation.[1,2,11-13,72]

Among proinflammatory cytokines, which also play a role in RA, TNF-α, IL-1, IL-8, IL-13, IL-15, IL-18, and maybe IL-6 are involved in angiogenesis.[1,2,11-13,73,74]

Chemotactic cytokines, termed *chemokines*, may also stimulate neovascularization.[1,2,5] Among C-X-C (Cys-X-Cys) chemokines, IL-8 (CXCL8), epithelial neutrophil-activating protein-78 (ENA-78; CXCL5), groα (CXCL1), and connective tissue–activating protein-III (CTAP-III; CXCL6) promote angiogenesis.[1,2,5,75,76] IL-8, ENA-78, groα, and CTAP-III all contain the ELR (glutamyl-leucyl-arginyl) amino acid sequence, the motif responsible for their angiogenic activity.[75,76] The only ELR lacking, but angiogenic C-X-C chemokine is stromal cell–derived factor-1 (SDF-1).[2] In the RA synovium, chemokine-expressing cells are localized in the proximity of factor VIII-related antigen–expressing endothelial cells. In a rat cornea assay, RA synovial tissue homogenates produced significantly more ENA-78 and IL-8, exhibited increased chemotactic activity toward ECs, and showed increased angiogenic capacity than did homogenates prepared from normal synovial tissues.[77] There is relatively little information available on the possible role of C-C (Cys-Cys) chemokines in RA-associated angiogenesis. Nevertheless, monocyte chemoattractant protein-1 (MCP-1) induces EC chemotaxis in vitro, as well as angiogenesis in animal systems in vivo. MCP-1–induced neovascularization has been associated with abundant EC expression of the CCR2 chemokine receptor.[78] Fractalkine is the only characterized C-X3-C chemokine and is expressed on cytokine-activated ECs.[79,80] Fractalkine enhances neovascularization both in vitro and in vivo.[79,80]

Regarding the possible role of chemokine receptors in angiogenesis, a number of these receptors may be detected on ECs, thus playing a role in chemokine-derived angiogenesis. There is a growing body of evidence that CXCR2 may be the most important EC receptor for C-X-C chemokines containing the ELR amino acid sequence.[76,81]

In addition to growth factors, cytokines, and chemokines, ECM components, including type I collagen, fibronectin, heparin, laminin, and tenascin; proteolytic enzymes, such as matrix metalloproteinases (MMP) and plasminogen activators; some CAMs, including soluble E-selectin and soluble VCAM-1; some ECβ_1, β_3 and β_5 integrins; PECAM (CD31); and endoglin (CD105) have been implicated in angiogenesis. As described previously, these CAMs play an important role in the cell adhesion and migration underlying synovial inflammation.[1,2,10-13] Among glycoconjugates also present in the arthritic synovium, Le^y/H promoted neovascularization using both in vitro and in vivo models.[54] MUC18 (CD146) has also been implicated in synovial angiogenesis.[55] The role of most MMPs has been widely studied in the pathogenesis of inflammatory synovitis. A novel family of MMPs, termed ADAMTS proteinases, includes aggrecanase-1 and -2. These aggrecanases are expressed in the RA synovium, mostly at sites of neovascularization.[82]

The COX/prostaglandin system is also involved in angiogenesis. Prostaglandin E2 is angiogenic.[1,2,13] COX-2 has been implicated in VEGF-dependent neovascularization.[70]

Other angiogenic molecules also produced by synovial cells, including angiogenin, platelet-activating factor (PAF), and substance P have been suggested to play a role in RA-associated angiogenesis.[1,2,11-13] Recently, prolactin and prolactin-like polypeptides were detected in RA synovial tissues. Prolactin was found to play an important role in T cell activation, cell communication, and synovial angiogenesis.[83]

Angiogenesis inhibitors in RA include some cytokines and growth factors, some of which may also stimulate neovascularization under different circumstances, such as TGF-ß, IL-1α, IL-1ß, IL-4, IL-6, IL-12, IFN-α, IFN-γ and leukemia inhibitory factor (LIF).[1,2,11-13,60] C-X-C chemokines lacking the ELR motif, such as platelet factor-4 (PF4; CXCL4), monokine induced by interferon-γ (MIG; CXCL9) and interferon-γ–inducible protein (IP-10; CXCL10) also inhibit neovascularization.[5,75,76] Regarding chemokine receptors, as angiostatic chemokines such as IP-10, MIG, and the recently described SLC all bind to CXCR3, this receptor may play a role in chemokine-mediated angiogenesis inhibition.[2,5,84]

In addition to these angiostatic factors, a number of antirheumatic drugs used in the treatment of arthritides inhibit angiogenesis. These drugs include corticosteroids, chloroquin, sulfasalazine, cyclosporine A, gold salts, cyclophosphamide, azathioprine, methotrexate, thalidomide, and anti-TNF biologics. Neovascularization may also be blocked by protease inhibitors, including tissue inhibitors of metalloproteinases (TIMPs) and plasminogen activator inhibitors (PAI); thrombospondin-1; derivatives of antibiotics, including fumagillin and minocyclin; some cartilage-derived inhibitors; cytoskeleton-dissembling agents, including Taxol; secreted protein acidic and rich in cysteine (SPARC)/osteonectin; and several other compounds.[1,2,11-13,60,85-87] Tumor-derived angiostatic agents, such as endostatin and angiostatin gene transfer, inhibit murine arthritis and arthritis-associated angiogenesis.[88,89] Troponin I is present in the joint and inhibits neovascularization.[90]

The Regulation of Leukocyte-Endothelial Adhesion and Angiogenesis

A number of soluble and cell surface–bound factors may be involved in leukocyte adhesion to and migration through endothelium (see Fig. 24–3 and Table 24–3). As described previously, proinflammatory cytokines, including IL-1, TNF-α, and in some cases IFN-γ may upregulate EC CAM expression and stimulate leukocyte-EC adhesion.[4,42,44,58] ECs themselves also release a number of inflammatory mediators. Some of these endogenous mediators may also be involved in EC adhesion. For example, PAF and chemokines have been implicated in P-selectin–dependent rolling and integrin-dependent firm adhesion, respectively.[58,91] Certain CAMs can also cross-talk with each other, resulting in strengthened intercellular adhesion. For example, E- and P-selectin stimulate the adhesive activity of β_2 integrins on neutrophils.[91,92] EC selectins not only mediate adhesion, but they are also signaling receptors.[93] The cross-talk between selectins and integrins is crucial for the transition from rolling to firm adhesion. Finally, intercellular contact itself may result in increased cytokine release and CAM expression.[4,94] These mechanisms may be important in the perpetuation of leukocyte extravasation.

The angiogenic process and the outcome of angiogenesis, and thus the extent of leukocyte ingress into the synovium, depends on the balance between angiogenic and angiostatic mediators, which are mostly produced by synovial macrophages, ECs, and fibroblasts[1,2,11-13] (see Fig. 24–3 and Table 24–3). Several intermolecular interactions and feedback loops exist in the RA synovial tissue, as well as in other inflamed tissues, which regulate capillary formation. Possibly the most important mechanisms in the regulation of angiogenesis are as follows[1,13,59,60]:

1. balance between antagonistic angiogenic and angiostatic couples
2. concentration-dependent regulation of neovascularization by bifunctional mediators
3. direct or indirect interactions between soluble and cell-bound angiogenic factors
4. stimulation of angiostatic factor production by angiogenic mediators
5. downregulation of the production of angiogenic mediators by angiostatic agents
6. angiogenesis stimulation or inhibition by administered drugs or other compounds

In conclusion, a regulatory network of leukocytes and ECs, as well as soluble inflammatory mediators, CAMs, and other factors, exists in the inflamed synovium. Antiadhesive and antiangiogenic agents can interfere with pathologically enhanced inflammatory cell recruitment, indicating potentially new strategies in antirheumatic therapy.

Inhibition of Cell Adhesion and Angiogenesis: Future Perspectives in Antirheumatic Therapy

Clinical trials using antiadhesion therapy have provided an important perspective on the role of cell adhesion and CAMs in the pathogenesis of RA. In one trial, an anti–human ICAM-1 antibody (enlimomab) was used to treat refractory RA. Many patients reported improvement in their status. A transient increase in the number of circulating T cells after the administration of the antibody suggested that leukocyte extravasation into the RA synovium was inhibited.[4,95] Anti–ICAM-1 antibodies may activate blood neutrophils, evidenced by increased β_2 integrin and decreased L-selectin expression on these cells, which may at least in part account for the side effects observed during antibody treatment.[96] In addition, anti–ICAM-1 and anti-β_2 integrin antibodies prevent the development of arthritis in rats and rabbits, respectively. RGD (arginyl-glycyl-aspartate) peptide, a motif recognized by several integrins, has suppressed arthritis in rats.[1,4] There have been several attempts in animal models of arthritis, as well as in human RA, to target CAMs involved in the pathogenesis of synovitis.[4]

Angiogenesis research may also have important therapeutic relevance in rheumatology. In general, two central mechanisms may be targeted when developing antiangiogenic therapy. First, switch from the resting to the angiogenic EC phenotype could be inhibited by blocking the secretion, transport, and ECM binding of angiogenic factors. Alternatively, vascular EC response to these mediators could be suppressed.[97] As discussed previously, a number of antirheumatic drugs currently used in RA inhibit angiogenesis or the production of macrophage-derived angiogenic mediators.[1,2,12,60] The inhibition of several soluble cytokines, growth factors, and chemokines can suppress the pathologic angiogenesis underlying RA. At this moment TNF-α seems to be a primary target for biologic therapy, although IL-1, IL-8, and other angiogenic mediators have recently been targeted in clinical trials.[98] For example, trials with infliximab showed that blocking TNF-α reduced the synovial expression of VEGF and numerous CAMs.[99] A humanized anti-VEGF antibody successfully suppressed neovascularization.[99] Collagen-induced arthritis in rats was suppressed by a fumagillin-derivative antibiotic angiogenesis inhibitor, as well as by the microtubule stabilizer taxol.[1,2,60] MMP inhibitors have been tried in several models of angiogenesis.[100] Theoretically, most angiogenesis inhibitors described previously may undergo trials in animal or human arthritis.

Summary

In this chapter we discussed the putative role of vascular endothelium, including leukocyte recruitment and angiogenesis, in the pathogenesis of rheumatic diseases, particularly RA. ECs play a central role in leukocyte extravasation. A number of CAMs regulate the sequence of distinct steps. These CAMs interact with soluble inflammatory mediators, such as cytokines and chemokines. The presence of various CAM pairs and the existence of distinct steps of rolling, activation, adhesion, and migration account for the diversity and specificity of leukocyte-endothelial interactions. ECs are active participants in angiogenesis. A number of soluble and cell-bound factors may stimulate or inhibit angiogenesis. The outcome of inflammatory and other angiogenic diseases, such as various forms of arthritis, depends on the imbalance between angiogenic and angiostatic mediators. There have been several attempts to therapeutically interfere with the cellular and molecular mechanisms described in this chapter. Specific targeting of pathologic endothelial function, leukocyte recruitment, angiogenesis, or all three may be useful for the future management of numerous inflammatory rheumatic conditions.

REFERENCES

1. Szekanecz Z, Szegedi G, Koch AE: Angiogenesis in rheumatoid arthritis: Pathogenic and clinical significance. J Invest Med 46:27, 1998.
2. Szekanecz Z, Koch AE: Chemokines and angiogenesis. Curr Opin Rheumatol 13:202, 2001.

3. Szekanecz Z, Koch AE: Cytokines. *In* Ruddy S, Harris ED Jr, Sledge CB, et al (eds): Textbook of Rheumatology, 6th ed. Philadelphia, WB Saunders, 2001, p 275.
4. Szekanecz Z, Szegedi G, Koch AE: Cellular adhesion molecules in rheumatoid arthritis. Regulation by cytokines and possible clinical importance. J Invest Med 44:124, 1996.
5. Szekanecz Z, Kunkel SL, Strieter RM, et al: Chemokines in rheumatoid arthritis. Springer Semin Immunopathol 20:115, 1998.
6. Dayer JM, Arend WP: Cytokines and growth factors. *In* Ruddy S, Harris ED Jr, Sledge CB, et al (eds): Textbook of Rheumatology, 5th ed. Philadelphia, WB Saunders, 1997, p 267.
7. Pober JS, Cotran RS: Cytokines and endothelial cell biology. Physiology Rev 70:427, 1990.
8. Cotran RS: Endothelial cells. *In* Kelley WN, Harris ED Jr, Ruddy S, Sledge C (eds): Textbook of Rheumatology, 4th ed. Philadelphia, WB Saunders, 1993, p 327.
9. Brenchley PE: Angiogenesis in inflammatory joint disease: a target for therapeutic intervention [Editorial]. Clin Exp Immunol 121:426, 2000.
10. Walsh DA: Angiogenesis and arthritis. Rheumatology 38:103, 1999.
11. Koch AE: Angiogenesis: implications for rheumatoid arthritis. Arthritis Rheum 41:951, 1998.
12. Colville-Nash PR, Scott DL: Angiogenesis in rheumatoid arthritis: pathogenic and therapeutic implications. Ann Rheum Dis 51:919, 1992.
13. Szekanecz Z, Halloran MM, Haskell CJ, et al: Mediators of angiogenesis: the role of cellular adhesion molecules. Trends Glycosci Glycotechnol (TIGG) 11:73, 1999.
14. Brenner BM, Troy JL, Ballermann BJ: Endothelium-dependent vascular responses. Mediators and mechanisms. J Clin Invest 84:1373, 1989.
15. Joris I, Majno G, Corey EJ, et al: The mechanism of vascular leakage induced by leukotriene E4. Endothelial contraction. Am J Pathol 126:19, 1987.
16. Brett J, Gerlach H, Nawroth P, et al: Tumor necrosis factor/cachectin increases permeability of endothelial cell monolayers by a mechanism involving regulatory G proteins. J Exp Med 169:1977, 1989.
17. Varani J, Ginsburg I, Schuger L, et al: Endothelial cell killing by neutrophils. Synergistic interaction of oxygen products and proteases. Am J Pathol 135:435, 1989.
18. Hurley JV: Acute Inflammation. Baltimore, Williams & Wilkins, 1972.
19. Mulligan MS, Varani J, Dame MK, et al: Role of endothelial-leukocyte adhesion molecule 1 (ELAM-1) in neutrophil-mediated lung injury in rats. J Clin Invest 88:1396, 1991.
20. Antibodies to endothelial cells [Editorial]. Lancet 337:649, 1991.
21. Westphal JR, Boerbooms AMTh, Schalkwijk CJM, et al: Anti-endothelial cell antibodies in sera of patients with autoimmune diseases: Comparison between ELISA and FACS analysis. Clin Exp Immunol 96:444, 1994.
22. Schoefl G: Studies on inflammation. III. Growing capillaries. Virchows Arch A337:97, 1963.
23. Albelda SM, Buck CA: Integrins and other cell adhesion molecules. FASEB J 4:2868, 1990.
24. Springer TA: Adhesion receptors of the immune system. Nature 346:425, 1990.
25. Szekanecz Z, Szegedi G: Cell surface adhesion molecules: structure, function, clinical importance. Orv Hetil 133:135, 1992.
26. Carlos TM, Harlan JM: Leukocyte-endothelial adhesion molecules. Blood 84:2068, 1994.
27. Bevilacqua MP, Pober JS, Mendrick DL, et al: Identification of an inducible endothelial-leukocyte adhesion molecule. Proc Natl Acad Sci U S A 84:9238, 1987.
28. Koch AE, Turkiewicz W, Harlow LA, et al: Soluble E-selectin in arthritis. Clin Immunol Immunopathol 69:29, 1993.
29. Walz G, Aruffo A, Kolanus W, et al: Recognition by ELAM-1 of the sialyl-Lex determinant on myeloid and tumor cells. Science 250:1132, 1990.
30. Borges E, Tietz W, Steegmaier M, et al: P-selectin glycoprotein ligand-1 (PSGL-1) on T helper 1 but not on T helper 2 cells binds to P-selectin and supports migration into inflamed skin. J Exp Med 185:573, 1997.
31. Koch AE, Burrows JC, Haines GK, et al: Immunolocalization of leukocyte and endothelial adhesion molecules in human rheumatoid and osteoarthritic synovial tissue. Lab Invest 64:313, 1991.
32. Kumar P, Hosaka S, Koch AE: Soluble E-selectin induces monocyte chemotaxis through Src family of tyrosine kinases. J Biol Chem 276:21039, 2001.
33. Kavanaugh A: Adhesion molecules as therapeutic targets in the treatment of allergic and immunologically mediated diseases. Clin Immunol Immunopathol 80:S15, 1996.
34. McEver RP, Beckstead JH, Moore KL, et al: GMP-140, a platelet alpha-granule membrane protein, is also synthesized by vascular endothelial cells and is localized in Weibel-Palade bodies. J Clin Invest 84:92, 1989.
35. Geng JG, Bevilacqua MP, Moore KL, et al: Rapid neutrophil adhesion to activated endothelium mediated by GMP-140. Nature 343:757, 1990.
36. Lawrence MB, Springer TA: Leukocytes roll on a selectin at physiologic flow rates: Distinction from and prerequisite for adhesion through integrins. Cell 65:859, 1991.
37. Johnson B, Haines GK, Harlow LA, et al: Adhesion molecule expression in human synovial tissues. Arthritis Rheum 36:137, 1993.
38. Hosaka S, Shah MR, Pope RM, et al: Soluble forms of P-selectin and intercellular adhesion molecule-3 in synovial fluids. Clin Immunol Immunopathol 78:276, 1996.
39. Ichikawa Y, Shimizu H, Yoshida M, et al: Accessory molecules expressed on the peripheral blood or synovial fluid T lymphocytes from patients with Sjogren's syndrome or rheumatoid arthritis. Clin Exp Rheumatol 10:447, 1992.
40. Bischoff J: Approaches to studying cell adhesion molecules in angiogenesis. Trends Cell Biol 5:69, 1995.
41. Brooks PC, Clark RA, Cheresh DA: Requirement of vascular integrin alpha v beta 3 for angiogenesis. Science 264:569, 1994.
42. Thornhill MH, Haskard DO: IL-4 regulates endothelial cell activation by IL-1, tumor necrosis factor, or IFN-gamma. J Immunol 145:865, 1990.
43. Wilkinson LS, Edwards JC, Poston RN, et al: Expression of vascular cell adhesion molecule-1 in normal and inflamed synovium. Lab Invest 68:82, 1993.
44. Pober JS, Gimbrone MA Jr, Lapierre LA, et al: Overlapping patterns of activation of human endothelial cells by interleukin 1, tumor necrosis factor, and immune interferon. J Immunol 137:1893, 1986.
45. Ostermann G, Weber KS, Zernecke A, et al: JAM-1 is a ligand of the beta-2 integrin LFA-1 involved in transendothelial migration of leukocytes. Nat Immunol 3:151, 2002.
46. Cunningham SA, Rodriguez JM, Arrate MP, et al: JAM2 interacts with $\alpha_4\beta_1$. Facilitation by JAM3. J Biol Chem 277:27589, 2002.
47. Santoso S, Sachs UJ, Kroll H, et al: The junctional adhesion molecule 3 (JAM-3) on human platelets is a counterreceptor for the leukocyte integrin Mac-1. J Exp Med 196:679, 2002.
48. Salmi M, Kalimo K, Jalkanen S: Induction and function of vascular adhesion protein-1 at sites of inflammation. J Exp Med 178:2255, 1993.
49. Szekanecz Z, Haines GK, Lin TR, et al: Differential distribution of ICAM-1, ICAM-2 and ICAM-3, and the MS-1 antigen in normal and diseased human synovia. Arthritis Rheum 37:221, 1994.
50. Szekanecz Z, Haines GK, Harlow LA, et al: Increased synovial expression of transforming growth factor (TGF)-ß receptor endoglin and TGF-ß1 in rheumatoid arthritis: Possible interactions in the pathogenesis of the disease. Clin Immunol Immunopathol 76:187, 1995.
51. Haynes BF, Hale LP, Denning SM, et al: The role of leukocyte adhesion molecules in cellular interactions: Implications for the pathogenesis of inflammatory synovitis. Springer Semin Immunopathol 11:163, 1989.
52. Haynes BF, Hale LP, Patton KL, et al: Measurement of an adhesion molecule as an indicator of inflammatory disease activity. Up-regulation of the receptor for hyaluronate (CD44) in rheumatoid arthritis. Arthritis Rheum 34:1434, 1991.
53. Dejana E: Endothelial adherens junctions: Implications in the control of vascular permeability and angiogenesis. J Clin Invest 98:1949, 1996.

54. Halloran MM, Carley WW, Polverini PJ, et al: Ley/H: An endothelial-selective, cytokine-inducible, angiogenic mediator. J Immunol 164:4868, 2000.
55. Neidhart M, Wehrli R, Bruhlmann P, et al: Synovial fluid CD146 (MUC18), a marker for synovial membrane angiogenesis in rheumatoid arthritis. Arthritis Rheum 42:622, 1999.
56. Schenkel AR, Mamdouh Z, Chen X, et al: CD99 plays a major role in the migration of monocytes through endothelial junctions. Nat Immunol 3:143, 2002.
57. Szekanecz Z, Koch AE: Intercellular adhesion molecule (ICAM)-3 expression on endothelial cells. Am J Pathol 151:313, 1997.
58. Butcher EC: Leukocyte-endothelial cell recognition: Three (or more) steps to specificity and diversity. Cell 67:1033, 1991.
59. Folkman J, Klagsbrun M: Angiogenic factors. Science 235:442, 1987.
60. Auerbach W, Auerbach R: Angiogenesis inhibition: A review. Pharmacotherapy 63:265, 1994.
61. Schweigerer L: Antiangiogenesis as a novel therapeutic concept in pediatric oncology. J Mol Med 73:497, 1995.
62. Peichev M, Naiyer AJ, Pereira D, et al: Expression of VEGFR-2 and AC133 by circulating human CD34(+) cells identifies a population of functional endothelial precursors. Blood 95:952, 2000.
63. Gehling UM, Ergun S, Schumacher U, et al: In vitro differentiation of endothelial cells from AC133-positive progenitor cells. Blood 95:3106, 2000.
64. Eichmann A, Corbel C, Nataf V, et al: Ligand-dependent development of the endothelial and hemopoetic lineages from embryonic mesodermal cells expressing vascular endothelial growth factor receptor 2. Proc Natl Acad Sci U S A 94:5141, 1997.
65. Freedman SB, Isner JM: Therapeutic angiogenesis for ischemic cardiovascular disease. J Mol Cell Cardiol 33:379, 2001.
66. Shyu KG, Manor O, Magner M, et al: Direct intramuscular injection of plasmid DNA encoding angiopoietin-1 but not angiopoietin-2 augments revascularization in the rabbit ischemic hindlimb. Circulation 98:2081, 1998.
67. Isner JM, Baumgartner I, Rauh G, et al: Treatment of thromboangiitis obliterans (Buerger's disease) by intramuscular gene transfer of vascular endothelial growth factor: Preliminary clinical results. J Vasc Surg 28:964, 1998.
68. Szekanecz Z, Koch AE: Adhesion molecules: potent inducers of endothelial cell chemotaxis. *In* Zilla PP, Greisler HP (eds): Tissue Engineering of Prosthetic Vascular Grafts. Austin, Tex, RG Landes, 1999, p 271.
69. Koch AE, Halloran MM, Haskell CJ, et al: Angiogenesis mediated by soluble forms of E-selectin and vascular cell adhesion molecule-1. Nature 376:517, 1995.
70. Hernandez GL, Volpert OV, Iniguez MA, et al: Selective inhibition of vascular endothelial growth factor-mediated angiogenesis by cyclosporin A: Roles of the nuclear factor of activated T cells and cyclooxygenase 2. J Exp Med 193:607, 2001.
71. Hollander AP, Corke KP, Freemont AJ, et al: Expression of hypoxia-inducible factor 1 alpha by macrophages in the rheumatoid synovium: Implications for targeting of therapeutic genes to the inflamed joint. Arthritis Rheum 44:1540, 2000.
72. Koch AE, Harlow LA, Haines GK, et al: Vascular endothelial growth factor. A cytokine modulating endothelial function in rheumatoid arthritis. J Immunol 152:4149, 1994.
73. Angiolillo AL, Kanegane H, Sgadari C, et al: Interleukin-15 promotes angiogenesis in vivo. Biochem Biophys Res Commun 233:231, 1997.
74. Park CC, Morel JC, Amin MA, et al: Evidence of IL-18 as a novel angiogenic mediator. J Immunol 167:1644, 2001.
75. Strieter RM, Polverini PJ, Kunkel SL, et al: The functional role of the ELR motif in CXC chemokine-mediated angiogenesis. J Biol Chem 270:27348, 1995.
76. Strieter RM, Kunkel SL, Shanafelt AM, et al: The role of C-X-C chemokines in regulation of angiogenesis. *In* Koch AE, Strieter RM (eds): Chemokines in Disease. Austin, Tex, RG Landes, 1996, p 196.
77. Koch AE, Volin MV, Woods JM, et al: Regulation of angiogenesis by the C-X-C chemokines interleukin-8 and epithelial neutrophil activating peptide-78 in the rheumatoid joint. Arthritis Rheum 44:31, 2001.
78. Salcedo R, Ponce ML, Young HA, et al: Human endothelial cells express CCR2 and respond to MCP-1: Direct role of MCP-1 in angiogenesis and tumor progression. Blood 96:34, 2000.
79. Ruth JH, Volin MV, Haines GK III, et al: Fractalkine, a novel chemokine in rheumatoid arthritis and rat adjuvant-induced arthritis. Arthritis Rheum 44:1568, 2001.
80. Volin MV, Woods JM, Amin MA, et al: Fractalkine: A novel angiogenic chemokine in rheumatoid arthritis. Am J Pathol 159:1521, 2001.
81. Walz A, Kunkel SL, Strieter RM: C-X-C chemokines—an overview. *In* Koch AE, Strieter RM (eds): Chemokines in Disease. Austin,Tex., RG Landes, 1996, p 1.
82. Vankemmelbeke MN, Holen I, Wilson AG, et al: Expression and activity of ADAMTS-5 in synovium. Eur J Biochem 268:1259, 2001.
83. Neidhart M, Gay RE, Gay S: Prolactin and prolactin-like polypeptides in rheumatoid arthritis. Biomed Pharmacother 53:218, 1999.
84. Vicari AP, Ait-Yahia S, Chemin K, et al: Antitumor effects of the mouse chemokine 6Ckine/SLC through angiostatic and immunological mechanisms. J Immunol 165:1992, 2000.
85. Calabrese L, Fleischer AB: Thalidomide: Current and potential clinical applications. Am J Med 108:487, 2000.
86. Fishman SJ, Feins NR, D'Amoto RJ, et al: Thalidomide for Crohn's disease. Gastroenterology 119:596, 2000.
87. Oliver SJ, Cheng TP, Banquerigo ML, et al: The effect of thalidomide and two analogs on collagen induced arthritis. J Rheumatol 25:964, 1998.
88. Yin G, Liu W, An P, et al: Endostatin gene transfer inhibits joint angiogenesis and pannus formation in inflammatory arthritis. Mol Ther 5:547, 2002.
89. Kim JM, Ho SH, Park EJ, et al: Angiostatin gene transfer as an effective treatment strategy in murine collagen-induced arthritis. Arthritis Rheum 46:793, 2002.
90. Moses MA, Wiederschain D, Wu I, et al: Troponin I is present in human cartilage and inhibits angiogenesis. Proc Natl Acad Sci U S A 96:2645, 1989.
91. Lorant DE, Patel KD, McIntyre TM, et al: Coexpression of GMP-140 and PAF by endothelium stimulated by histamine or thrombin: A juxtacrine system for adhesion and activation of neutrophils. J Cell Biol 115:223, 1991.
92. Lo SK, Lee S, Ramos RA, et al: Endothelial-leukocyte adhesion molecule 1 stimulates the adhesive activity of leukocyte integrin CR3 (CD11b/CD18, Mac-1) on human neutrophils. J Exp Med 173:1493, 1991.
93. Lorenzon P, Vecile E, Nardon E, et al: Endothelial cell E- and P-selectin and vascular cell adhesion molecule-1 function as signaling receptors. J Cell Biol 142:1381, 1998.
94. Bombara MP, Webb DL, Conrad P, et al: Cell contact between T cells and synovial fibroblasts causes induction of adhesion molecules and cytokines. J Leukoc Biol 54:399, 1993.
95. Kavanaugh AF, Davis LS, Nichols LA, et al: Treatment of refractory rheumatoid arthritis with a monoclonal antibody to intercellular adhesion molecule-1. Arthritis Rheum 37:992, 1994.
96. Vuorte J, Lindsberg PJ, Kaste M, et al: Anti-ICAM-1 monoclonal antibody R6.5 (Enlimomab) promotes activation of neutrophils in whole blood. J Immunol 162:2353, 1999.
97. Folkman J: Angiogenesis: Retrospect and outlook. EXS 59:4, 1991.
98. Strand CV, Keystone E: Biologic agents for the treatment of rheumatoid arthritis. *In* Ruddy S, Harris ED Jr, Sledge CB, et al (eds): Kelley's Textbook of Rheumatology, 6th ed. Philadelphia, WB Saunders, 2001, p 899.
99. Lin YS, Nguyen C, Mendoza JL, et al: Preclinical pharmacokinetics, interspecies scaling, and tissue distribution of a humanized monoclonal antibody against vascular endothelial growth factor. J Pharmacol Exp Ther 288:371, 1999.
100. Skotnicki JS, Zask A, Nelson FC, et al: Design and synthetic considerations of matrix metalloproteinase inhibitors. Ann NY Acad Sci 878:61, 1999.

25 Cytokines

IAIN B. MCINNES

Immune function depends on the biological activities of numerous small glycoprotein messengers, termed *cytokines.* Originally discovered and defined on the basis of their functional activities, cytokines are now designated primarily by structure. Typically, cytokines exhibit broad functional activities that mediate not only effector and regulatory immune function, but also wider effects across a range of tissues and biologic systems. As such, cytokines play a role not only in host defense, but also in a variety of normal physiologic and metabolic processes. The human genome project has facilitated discovery of large numbers of cytokines, posing considerable challenges in resolving their respective and synergistic functions in complex tissues in health and disease. Such understanding is, however, essential with the advent of cytokine-targeting therapies in the clinic. This chapter will review general features of cytokine biology and the cellular and molecular networks within which cytokines operate, and it will focus on the effector functions of cytokines that are important in chronic inflammation and in rheumatic diseases.

Classification of Cytokines

In the absence of a unified classification system, cytokines are variously identified by numeric order of discovery (currently interleukin [IL]-1 through -29), by a given functional activity (e.g., tumor necrosis factor [TNF], granulocyte colony stimulating factor [G-CSF]), by kinetic or functional role in inflammatory responses (early or late, innate or adaptive, proinflammatory or anti-inflammatory [Fig. 25–1]), by primary cell of origin (*monokine* = monocyte derivation, *lymphokine* = lymphocyte derivation), and—recently—by structural homologies shared with related molecules. Superfamilies of cytokines share sequence similarity and also exhibit homology and some promiscuity in their reciprocal receptor systems. Cytokine superfamilies also contain important regulatory cell membrane receptor-ligand pairs, reflecting evolutionary pressures that use common structural motifs in diverse immune functions in higher mammals. For example, the TNF/TNF receptor superfamily[1] contains immune regulatory cytokines, including TNFα, lymphotoxins, and cellular ligands such as CD40L, which mediates B cell and T cell activation, and FasL (CD95), which promotes apoptosis. Similarly, the IL-1/IL-1 receptor superfamily[2] contains cytokines including IL-1β, IL-1α, IL-receptor antagonist, and IL-18, which mediate physiologic and host-defense function, but this family also includes the Toll-like receptors, a series of mammalian pattern-recognition molecules with a crucial role in recognition of microbial species early in innate responses.

Assessing Cytokine Function In Vitro and In Vivo

Although originally identified by bioactivity and quantified by bioassay, most cytokines are now identified via homologous receptor binding or sequence homology in gene databases. Function is thereafter assessed by identification of the cellular source of cytokine, determination of native stimuli, characterization of receptor distribution, and determination of function in target cells. Experimental in vivo models utilize the addition of neutralizing cytokine-specific antibodies or soluble receptors (often as fragment crystallizable [Fc] fusion or pegylated proteins to enhance half-life and modulate functional interaction with leukocytes) to modulate cytokine function. Genetically modified knockout mice (cytokine or receptor rendered deficient by embryonic stem (ES) cell technology) or transgenic mice (tissue/cell lineage-specific overexpression) have proven particularly useful. Conditional gene-targeting approaches (e.g., using the *cre* system) facilitate circumvention of embryonic lethal deficiencies or allow kinetic evaluation of the relative contribution of a cytokine throughout a response. Cytokine function is assessed in vitro in primary or transformed cell lines stimulated in the presence or absence of recombinant cytokine or specific anticytokine antibody or soluble receptor.

This general approach has proven critical in rheumatic disease research. Studies in which cytokine addition and neutralization takes place in synovial tissue explants or disaggregated cell populations, chondrocyte explants, bone culture models, skin, and renal tissue explants and lines have all proven informative. Moreover, ex vivo methodologies now include intracellular fluorescence activated cell sorter (FACS) methods, confocal and laser scanning microscopy, and quantitative histologic evaluation using automated image analysis. Such modalities, particularly when employed in human therapeutic cytokine neutralization studies in which inflammatory tissues are obtained through therapy, are considerably advancing the understanding of basic and pathogenetic cytokine function. Analysis of synovial biopsies obtained during infliximab, IL-1Ra, IL-10, and interferon β (IFNβ) administration in rheumatoid arthritis (RA) provide the strongest evidence for the success of this approach.[3,4]

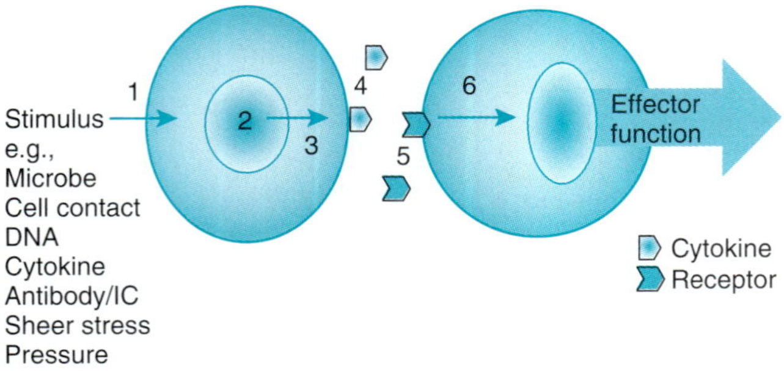

FIGURE 25–1 • An Overview of Cytokine Regulatory Function. Numerous and diverse stimuli (*1*) promote cytokine expression arising either from novel gene expression (*2*) or from activation of preformed cytokine (*3*). Cytokine proteins are thereafter expressed in the cytosol, on the cell membrane, or in soluble form in the extracellular environment (*4*). Cytokines, in turn, bind to reciprocal receptors that reside either on the membrane of a target cell or in the soluble phase (*5*). Membrane receptors, upon cytokine ligation, signal to the recipient cell nucleus (*6*) and drive novel gene expression to promote effector function. Each phase of cytokine function offers rich therapeutic potential.
Abbreviations: IC, immune complexes.

Cytokine receptors

Cytokine receptors exist in structurally related superfamilies and comprise high-affinity molecular signaling complexes that facilitate cytokine-mediated communication. Such complexes often include heterodimeric or heterotrimeric structures that use unique, cytokine-specific recognition receptors together with common receptor chains shared across a cytokine superfamily. Examples include the use of the common γ-chain receptor by IL-2, IL-4, IL-9, IL-15, IL-21, and glycoprotein 130 (gp130) by members of the IL-6 family.[5,6] Alternatively, distinct receptors may utilize shared signaling domains. Thus, homologous death domains are found in many TNF-receptor (TNF-R) family members. Similarly, the IL-1 signaling domain is common to not only IL-1R, but also to other IL-1R superfamily members, including IL-18R, ST2, and the Toll-like receptors (TLRs).[2] Signaling pathways dependent upon these are discussed in detail elsewhere.

Cytokine receptors can operate via several mechanisms. Membrane receptors, with intracellular signaling domains intact, can transmit signals to the target cell nucleus following soluble cytokine binding and thereby promote effector function. Membrane receptors may bind cell membrane cytokines facilitating cross-talk between adjacent cells. Membrane-bound and soluble cytokines may promote distinct receptor function. For example, TNFα binds TNF-RI and TNF-RII with similar affinity, but it has a slower rate of dissociation from TNF-RI. Soluble TNFα may rapidly dissociate from TNF-RII to bind TNF-RI, promoting preferential signaling by the latter (ligand passing).[1] In contrast, during cell–cell contact, stable TNFα/TNF-RI and TNFα/TNF-RII complexes form, allowing for differential signaling contribution by TNF-RI and TNF-RII. Cytokine receptor/cytokine complexes may also operate in *trans*, whereby component parts of the ligand-receptor complex are derived from adjacent cells. Thus, IL-15/IL-15Rα complexed on one cell may bind IL-15Rβ/γ on another.[7] Receptors also exist in soluble form, derived either from alternative mRNA processing to generate receptor-lacking transmembrane or intracellular domains, or by enzymatic cleavage of receptor from the cell surface (e.g., sTNF-R, sIL-1R1). Soluble receptors may act to antagonize cytokine function, thereby regulating responses. Soluble receptors may also preform complexes with cytokine to promote subsequent ligand-receptor assembly on the target cell membrane, and thereby enhance function. Finally, soluble receptors can deliver cytokine to the cell membrane via ligand passing.

Regulation of Cytokine Expression

Cytokines are synthesized in the golgi and may traffic through the endoplasmic reticulum to be released as soluble mediators, or they may remain membrane bound, or they may be processed into cytosolic forms that can traffic intracellularly. Cytokines, therefore, mediate autocrine function either through release or membrane expression and immediate receptor ligation on the source cell, or intracellularly within the source cell. Alternatively, cytokines operate in a paracrine manner, allowing cellular communication beyond that facilitated by local cell–cell contact. However, the distance and kinetics for effective function may be limited[8] by numerous factors, including physicochemical considerations of the peptide structure itself, extracellular matrix binding (e.g., to heparan sulphate), enzymatic degradation (e.g., serine protease degradation of IL-18), or the presence of soluble receptors (e.g., TNFα/soluble TNF-RI and TNF-RII, IL-2/soluble IL-2Rα) or novel cytokine-binding proteins (e.g., IL-18/IL-18 binding protein) in the inflammatory milieu.

Numerous factors promote cytokine expression in vivo (Fig. 25–2), including cell–cell contact, immune complexes/autoantibodies, local complement activation, microbial species and their soluble products, reactive oxygen and nitrogen intermediates, trauma, sheer stress, ischemia, radiation, ultraviolet light, extracellular matrix components, DNA (mammalian or microbial), heat-shock proteins, and cytokines themselves in autocrine loops. Commonly used in vitro stimuli include many of these, as well as chemical entities, including phorbol esters, calcium ionophores, lectins (e.g., phytohaemaglutinin), and receptor-specific antibodies such as anti-CD3 and anti-CD28 for T cell activation or anti-immunoglobulin and anti-CD40 for B cells.

Cytokine regulation within the cell can be usefully considered at several levels. Transcriptional regulation depends on the recruitment of discrete transcription factors (TFs) to the cytokine promoter region. TF binding allows for numerous signal pathways to regulate cytokine expression across a range of stimuli. Several transcription factors (e.g., nuclear factor kappa B [NF-κB], activator protein-1 [AP-1], nuclear factor of activated T cell [NF-AT]) have critical importance in cytokine production. Inhibition of NF-kB activity using either chemical inhibitors or adenoviral delivery of regulatory peptides

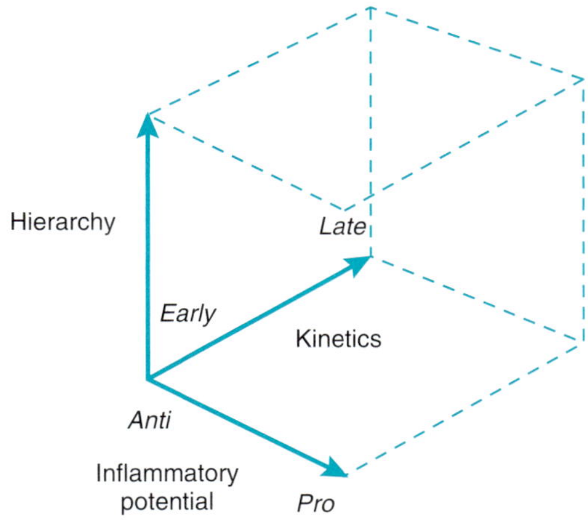

FIGURE 25–2 · Placing Cytokines in Functional Context. Cytokines often exhibit pleiotropic functions that vary throughout an immune response and according to the nature of a stimulus. Cytokines could be envisaged at one point in three-dimensional space, representing their hierarchic capacity to contribute to an inflammatory lesion over time. For example, a given cytokine might have early proinflammatory function but late, net anti-inflammatory function within an evolving immune response. Similarly, at an early stage a cytokine might function atop a hierarchy but later function primarily as an effector downstream moiety. Moreover, cytokines may have roles in both innate and acquired responses that are discrete. A cytokine might have distinct functions in different tissues and in response to different stimuli. This has important implications for predicting the effect of cytokine targeting in vivo.

leads to amelioration of inflammatory synovitis in vivo and in vitro.[9] Sequence polymorphism within cytokine promoters offers potential for differential cytokine expression between individuals that could confer selective advantage against infection, but could also increase susceptibility to, or progression of, autoimmunity. This is best exemplified in the TNFα and IL-1 promoters.[10,11] Thus, single nucleotide polymorphisms (SNP) in the TNFα promoter region (e.g., –308) are associated with altered TNFα release upon leukocyte stimulation in vitro. Similarly, homozygotes for the A2 allele at +3954 in the IL-1β gene produce more IL-1β with lipopolysaccharide (LPS) stimulation. Polymorphisms also exist in the IL-1Ra gene, rendering the functional significance of individual SNPs on IL-1 protein release difficult to interpret. In general, the net effect of haplotypes may be more important at the functional level, particularly when their relevance to disease entities is considered.

Post-transcriptional regulation isimportant in determining longevity of cytokine expression. This may operate by promoting translational initiation, mRNA stability, and polyadenylation. AU-rich elements (ARE) within the 5′ or 3′ untranslated regions (UTR) of cytokine mRNA are crucial for stability. For example 3′ UTR ARE downregulate TNF expression such that transgenic knockin mice that lack TNFα ARE develop spontaneous inflammatory arthritis and bowel disease.[12] Regulatory proteins bind ARE to mediate such effects. For example, HuR and AUF1 exert opposing effects, respectively stabilizing or destabilizing ARE-containing transcripts.[13] TIA-1 and TIAR have been identified as RNA recognition motif family members[14] that function as translational silencers. Macrophages from TIA-1–deficient macrophages produce excess TNFα, whereas TIA-1–deficient lymphocytes exhibit normal TNFα release, suggesting distinctions in mRNA regulation in discrete cell types.[15] Alternatively, cytokines may generate stable mRNA a priori to facilitate subsequent rapid response in tissues. IL-15 mRNA 5′ UTR contains 12 AUG triplets that significantly reduce the efficiency of IL-15 translation. Deletion of this sequence permits IL-15 secretion. IL-15 mRNA can thereby produce a 48-aa signal peptide that allows IL-15 release and a shorter 21-aa signal peptide that targets intracellular distribution. IL-15 forms thus generated exhibit discrete functions.[16]

Post-translational regulation also regulates cytokine expression via several mechanisms. Patterns of glycosylation are important for cytokine function and may regulate intracellular trafficking.[16] Modified leader sequences may alter intracellular trafficking of cytokines. Some cytokines are translated without functional leader sequences. Their secretion depends on nonconventional secretory pathways that are thus far poorly understood. IL-1β, for example, employs a purine receptor–dependent pathway (P_2X_7) for cellular release.[17] Enzymatic activation of cytokines is common, whereby nonfunctional promolecules are cleaved to generate functional subunits. Examples include the cleavage by caspase 1 of pro-IL-1β to generate active IL-1β and, similarly, of pro-IL-18 to generate an active 18-kD species.[18] Alternative processing pathways for cytokines include the serine proteases, proteinase 3 and elastase, and adamolysin family members. Enzyme cleavage pathways operate within and outside cells, providing for extracellular cytokine activation. Similarly, cell membrane enzymes serve to cleave membrane-expressed cytokine. Thus, members of the adamolysin family regulate TNFα release; for example, TNFα-conversing enzyme (TACE) cleaves and mediates the release of both TNFα and its receptors.[19] In summary, extensive molecular machinery exists to tightly regulate not only the production and stability of cytokine mRNA, but also its translation and cellular expression and distribution. At each level, opportunities exist for intervention and therapeutic cytokine modulation.

Effector Function of Cytokines

Cytokines possess pleiotropic and potent effector function in both acute and chronic inflammatory responses. The identity, receptor specificity, and key effects of cytokines understood to have particular importance in pathogenesis of human autoimmunity and chronic inflammation are summarized in Tables 25–1 through 25–7.

CYTOKINES IN ACUTE INFLAMMATION

Cytokines operate at every stage in the critical early events that promote acute inflammation. Thus, cells that comprise the innate immune response, including neutrophils, natural killer (NK) cells, macrophages, mast

TABLE 25–1 • IL-1 SUPERFAMILY CYTOKINES WITH ROLES IN RHEUMATIC DISEASE

Cytokine	Size*	Receptor(s)	Major Cell Sources	Key Functions
IL-1β	35 kD (pro) 17 kD (active)	IL-1RI IL-1RAcP IL-1RII (decoy)	Monocytes, B cells, fibroblasts, chondrocytes, keratinocytes	Fibroblast cytokine, chemokine, MMP, iNOS, PG release ↑ Monocyte cytokine, ROI, PG ↑ Osteoclast activation Chondrocyte GAG synthesis ↓, iNOS, MMP and aggrecanase ↑ Endothelial adhesion-molecule expression
IL-1α	35 kD (pro)† 17 kD (active)	IL-1RI IL-1RAcP IL-1RII (decoy)	Monocytes, B cells, PMN, epithelial cells, keratinocytes	Similar to IL-1β Autocrine growth factor (e.g., keratinocytes)
IL-1Ra	22 kD	IL-1RI IL-1RAcP IL-1RII	Monocytes	Antagonize effects of IL-1β and IL-1α
IL-18	23 kD (pro) 18 kD (active)	IL-18R IL-18Rβα	Monocytes, PMNs dendritic cells, platelets, endothelial cells	T cell effector polarization (Th1 with IL-12 /Th2 with IL-4) Chondrocyte GAG synthesis ↓, iNOS expression NK activation, cytokine release, cytotoxicity Monocyte cytokine release, adhesion molecule expression PMN activation, cytokine release, migration Endothelial cells—proangiogenic

*Pro forms cleaved to active moieties by proteases including caspase-1, calpain, elastase, cathepsin G.
†Pro-IL-1α retains bioactivity prior to cleavage.

Abbreviations: GAG, Glycosaminoglycan; iNOS, inducibile nitric oxide synthase; MMP, matrix metalloproteinase; NK, natural killer; PG, peptidoglycan; PMN, polymorphonuclear; ROI, reactive oxygen intermediates.

TABLE 25–2 • TNF SUPERFAMILY CYTOKINES* WITH POTENTIAL ROLE IN RHEUMATIC DISEASE

Cytokine	Size	Receptor(s)	Major Cell Sources	Selected Functions
TNFα	26 kD (pro)	TNF-RI (p55) TNF-RII (p75)	Monocytes, T/B/NK cells, PMNs, eosinophils, mast cells, fibroblasts, keratinocytes, glial cells, osteoblasts, smooth muscle	Monocyte activation, cytokine, and PG ↑ PMN priming, apoptosis, oxidative burst ↑ Endothelial cell adhesion molecule, cytokine release ↑ Fibroblast proliferation and collagen synthesis ↓, MMP and cytokine ↑ T cell apoptosis, clonal (auto)regulation, TCR dysfunction Adipocyte FFA release ↑ Endocrine effects – ACTH, prolactin ↑; TSH, FSH, GH ↓
LTα	22-26 kD	TNF-RI TNF-RII	T cells, monocytes, fibroblasts, astrocytes, myeloma, endothelial cells, epithelial cells	Peripheral lymphoid development Otherwise similar bioactivities to TNFα
RANK ligand	35 kD	RANK	Stromal cells, osteoblasts, T cells	Stimulates bone resorption via osteoclast maturation and activation Modulation of T cell–dendritic cell interaction
OPG	55 kD	RANKL	Stromal cells, osteoblasts	Soluble decoy receptor for RANKL
BLyS†	18-32 kD	TACI BCMA BLyS-R	Monocytes, T cells, DCs	B cell proliferation, Ig secretion, isotype switching, survival T cell costimulation
APRIL	—	TACI BCMA	Monocytes, T cells, tumor cells	B cell proliferation Tumor proliferation

*Additional members of importance include TRAIL, TWEAK, CD70, FasL, and CD40L.
†Also called BAFF.

Abbreviations: APRIL, A proliferation inducing ligand; BAFF, B cell activating factor belonging to the TNF family; BCMA, B cell maturation protein; BlyS, B lymphocyte stimulator protein; DC, dendritic cell; FFA, free fatty acid; GAG, glycosaminoglycan; LT, lymphotoxin; MMP, matrix metalloproteinase; NK, natural killer; OPG, osteoprotogerin; PG, peptidoglycan; PMN, polymorphonuclear cell; RANK, receptor activator of NFκB ligand; TACI, transmembrane activator and calcium modulator and cyclophilin ligand; TNF, tumor necrosis factor; TRAIL, TNF related apoptosis inducing ligand; TWEAK, TNF-like weak inducer of apoptosis.

TABLE 25–3A • CYTOKINES ASSOCIATED PREDOMINANTLY WITH EFFECTOR FUNCTION FOR T CELLS[*]

Cytokine	Size	Receptor(s)	Major Cell Sources	Key Functions
Type II Interferon				
IFNγ	20-25 kD	IFNγR	Th/c1 cells, NK cells γδT cells, B cells macrophage / dendritic cells	Macrophage activation, dendritic cell APC function ↑ Endothelial adhesion molecule ↑ MHC class II expression ↑ T cell growth ↓, opposes Th2 responses Bone resorption ↓, fibroblast collagen synthesis
4a-helix Family				
IL-2	15 kD	IL-2Rα IL-2/15Rβ γ-chain	Th/c cells, NK cells	T cell division, maturation, cytokine release, cytotoxicity NK cell cytokine release, cytotoxicity; monocyte activation Lymphocyte apoptosis ↓
IL-4	20 kD	IL-4Rα/ γ-chain IL-4Rα/ IL-13R1	Th/c cells (Th2), NK cells	Th2 differentiation, maturation, apoptosis ↓ B cell maturation, isotype switch (IgE) Eosinophil migration, apoptosis ↓ Endothelial activation, adhesion-molecule expression
IL-5	25 kD monomer 50 kD homodimer	IL-5Rα IL-5Rβ	Th/c2 cells, NK cells mast cells, epithelial cells	B cell differentiation, Ig production (IgA) Eosinophil differentiation and activation Tc maturation
IL-17 Family[†]				
IL-17	20-30 kD	IL-17R	T cells (Th1)	Fibroblast cytokine release, MMP release ↑ Osteoclastogenesis; hemopoiesis Chondrocyte GAG synthesis ↓ Leukocyte cytokine production ↑

[*]Additional T cell derived cytokines of potential interest include IL-13 from Th2 and NK2 cells.
[†]IL-17 family also contains IL-17B, IL-17C, IL-17E, and IL-17F, the distinct functions of which are currently unclear.
Abbreviations: APC, Antigen-presenting cell; CAG, glycosaminoglycan; FB, fibroblast; IFN, interferon; MHC, major histocompatibility complex; MMP, matrix metalloproteinase; NK, natural killer; PMN, polymorphonuclear cell; Th/c, T helper/cytotoxic.

TABLE 25–3B • CYTOKINES DESCRIBED INITIALLY WITH PRIMARY ROLE IN REGULATION OF T CELLS[‡]

Cytokine	Size	Receptor(s)	Major Cell Sources	Key Functions
IL-12	IL-12p40 IL-12p35	IL-12Ra IL-12Rβ1 IL-12Rβ2	Macrophages, dendritic cells	Th1 cell proliferation, maturation T cell cytotoxicity B cell activation
IL-15	15 kD	IL-15Rα IL-2/15Rβ γ-chain	Monocytes, FB, mast cells B cells, PMN, dendritic cells	T cell chemokinesis, activation, memory maintenance NK cell maturation, activation, cytotoxicity Macrophage activation, suppression (dose dependent) PMN activation, adhesion molecule, oxidative burst Fibroblast activation B cell differentiation and isotype switching
IL-21	15 kD	IL-21R γ-chain	Activated T cells, others?	B cell activation

[‡]Cytokines included in this table are now understood to exhibit considerable functional heterogeneity as shown. Novel T cell regulatory cytokines have recently been described, including IL-23 and IL-27, the functions of which are currently under investigation.
Abbreviations: APC, Antigen-presenting cell; CAG, glycosaminoglycan; FB, fibroblast; IFN, interferon; MHC, major histocompatibility complex; MMP, matrix metalloproteinase; NK, natural killer; PMN, polymorphonuclear cell; Th/c, T helper/cytotoxic.

cells, and eosinophils, all produce and respond to cytokines generated within seconds of tissue insult. Cytokines prime leukocytes for response to microbial and chemical stimuli, upregulate adhesion-molecule expression on migrating leukocytes and endothelial cells, and amplify the release of reactive oxygen intermediates, nitric oxide (NO), vasoactive amines, and neuropeptides, and the activation of kinins and arachidonic acid derivatives, prostaglandins, and leukotrienes, which in turn regulate cytokine release. Similarly, cytokines regulate the expression of complement processing and membrane defense molecules, scavenger receptors, and TLRs. Moreover, cytokines, particularly IL-1, TNFα, and IL-6, are critical in driving the acute phase response. Tables 25–1 through 25–7 provide descriptions of the function of cytokines expressed within the acute inflammatory response.

CYTOKINES IN CHRONIC INFLAMMATION

Cytokines critically modulate the cellular interactions that characterize chronic inflammation. Studies using real-time image analytic techniques, such as two-photon microscopy and confocal scanning, suggest continuous

TABLE 25–4 • IL-10 SUPERFAMILY CYTOKINES*

Cytokine	Receptor(s)	Cellular Sources	Key Functions
IL-10	IL-10R1 IL-10R2	Monocytes, T cells, B cells, dendritic cells, epithelial cells, keratinocytes	Macrophage cytokine release, iNOS, ROI ↓, soluble receptor ↑ T cell cytokine release, MHC expression ↓, anergy induction Treg cell maturation, effector function? Dendritic cell activation, cytokine release ↓ Fibroblast MMP, collagen release ↓, no effect on TIMP B cell isotype switching enhanced
IL-19	IL-20R1/IL-20R2	Monocytes, others?	Monocyte cytokine and ROI release, monocyte apoptosis
IL-20	IL-22R/IL-20R2 IL-20R1/IL-20R2	Keratinocytes, others?	Autocrine keratinocyte growth regulation
IL-22	IL-22R/IL-10R2	Th1 cells, NK cells	Acute-phase response ↑
IL-24	IL-22R/IL-20R2 IL-20R1/IL-20R2	Monocytes, T cells	Tumor apoptosis, Th1 cytokine release by PBMC

*Additional members include IL-26, IL-28, and IL-28A. Many functions of IL-10 superfamily are as yet poorly understood, but they likely reside beyond the immune system.

Abbreviations: iNOS, Inducible nitric oxide synthase; MMP, matrix metalloproteinase; NK, natural killer cell; PBMC, peripheral blood mononuclear cells; ROI, reactive oxygen intermediates; TIMP, tissue inhibitor of MMP.

TABLE 25–5 • IL-6 SUPERFAMILY CYTOKINES*

Cytokine	Size	Receptor(s)	Major Cell Sources	Key Functions
IL-6	21-28 kD	IL-6R† gp130	Monocytes, fibroblasts, B cells T cells	B cell proliferation, Ig production Hemopoiesis, thrombopoiesis T cell proliferation, differentiation, cytotoxicity Hepatic acute phase response Hypothalamic/pituitary/adrenal axis Variable effects on cytokine release by monocytes
Oncostatin M	28 kD	OMR gp130	Monocytes, activated T cells	Megakaryocyte differentiation Fibroblast TIMP and cytokine release, Acute phase reactants ↑, Fibroblast protease inhibitors ↑ Monocyte TNF release ↓, IL-1 effector function ↓ Hypothalamic-pituitary axis ↑, corticosteroid release Modulatory effect on osteoblast? Proinflammatory effects in some models?
Leukemia inhibitory factor (LIF)	58 kD	LIFR gp130	Fibroblasts, monocytes lymphocytes, mesangial cells smooth muscle, epithelial cells mast cells	Acute-phase reactants ↑ Hemopoiesis, thrombopoiesis Role in neural development, neural effector function, implantation Bone metabolism, extracellular matrix regulation Eukocyte adhesion-molecule expression Eosinophil priming Mixed pro v anti-inflammatory effects in models

*Additional members of potential importance include IL-11, cardiotrophin-1, ciliary neurotrophic factor. Note overlapping effects within family.
†Membrane or soluble form can dimerise gp130 to promote signaling that in turn promotes signal transduction

Abbreviations: LIFR, Leukemia inhibitory factor receptor; OMR, oncostatin M receptor.

cellular motility during inflammation. Inflammatory lesions might properly be considered fluid states in which individual cells under cytokine control transiently contribute to organized functional subunits—such as the ectopic germinal center, synovial lining layer, or renal interstitial nephritis—yet remain competent to migrate thereafter under the influence of chemotactic gradients on the extracellular matrix. Cytokines may also promote cell death (apoptosis) either by withdrawal (e.g., IL-2, IL-15) or by binding cytokine receptors containing death domains (e.g., TNF-R1). Therefore, cytokines contribute at every stage of inflammatory lesion development in a dynamic equilibrium, rather than in a static, linear manner. Chronic inflammation in rheumatic disease usually contains cytokine activities reminiscent of both innate and acquired immune responses. For convenience, cytokines can therefore be considered by their effect on cell subsets and cellular interactions (Fig. 25–2 describes a notional positioning for cytokine activity in a developing and chronic lesion). Investigation of cytokine-regulated pathways in several rheumatic diseases has identified several common pathways.

T Cell Effector Function in Chronic Inflammation

T cells are dependent on cytokine function at every developmental stage from bone marrow stem cell maturation, through thymic education, to functional determination

TABLE 25–6 • GROWTH FACTORS RELEVANT TO RHEUMATIC DISEASES

Cytokine	Receptor(s)	Cellular Sources	Key Functions
TGFβ* Isoforms 1-3†	Type I TGFβR Type 0II TGFβR Others	Broad—including fibroblasts, monocytes, T cells, platelets	Wound repair, matrix maintenance, and fibrosis Initial activation then suppression of inflammatory responses T cell and NK cell proliferation and effector function ↓ Early phase leukocyte chemoattractant, gelatinase, and integrin expression ↑ Early macrophage activation then suppression, reduced iNOS expression
BMP family (BMP2-15)	BMPRI BMPRII	Varied (e.g., epithelial and mesenchymal embryonic tissues) Bone-derived cell lineages	Regulate critical chemotaxis, mitosis, and differentiation processes during chondrogenesis and osteogenesis, tissue morphogenesis (e.g., heart, skin, eye)
PDGF	PDGFRα PDGFRβ	Platelets, macrophages, endothelial cells, fibroblasts, glial cells, astrocytes, myoblasts, smooth muscle cells	Local paracrine or autocrine growth factor for variety of lineages Wound healing
FGF family	FGFR (various) Basic FGF Acidic FGF	Widespread	Growth and differentiation of mesenchymal, epithelial, and neuroectodermal cells

*Members of TGFβ superfamily include bone morphogenetic proteins (BMP), growth and differentiation factor, inhibinA, inhibinB, mullerian inhibitory substance, glial-derived neurotrophic factor, and macrophage inhibitory cytokine.
†Bound to latency-associated peptide (LAP) to form small latency complex and to latent TGFβ binding protein (LTBP) to form large latent complex; activated by proteolytic and nonproteolytic pathways.

Abbreviations: BMP, Bone morphogenic protein; FGF, fibroblast growth factor; iNOS, inducible nitric oxide synthase; PDGF, platelet derived growth factor; TFG, transforming growth factor.

TABLE 25–7 • MISCELLANEOUS CYTOKINES WITH POTENTIAL ROLES IN RHEUMATIC DISEASES

Cytokine	Size	Receptor(s)	Cellular Sources	Key Functions
MIF	12 kD	Unclear	Macrophages, activated T cells, fibroblasts (synoviocytes)	Macrophage cytokine release, phagocytosis, NO release ↑ T cell activation, DTH Fibroblast proliferation, COX expression, PLA2 expression Intrinsic oxidoreductase activity ("cytozyme")
HMGB1	30 kD	RAGE, dsDNA others?	Widespread expression Necrotic cells Macrophages Pituicytes	DNA-binding transcription factor Necrosis-induced inflammation Macrophage activation—delayed proinflammatory cytokine Smooth muscle chemotaxis Disrupts epithelial barrier function Bacteriocidal (direct)
GM-CSF	14-35 kD	GM-CSFRα GM-CSFRβ	T cells, macrophages, endothelial cells, fibroblasts	Granulocyte and monocyte maturation, hemopoietic effects Leukocyte PG release, DC maturation Pulmonary surfactant turnover
G-CSF	19kD	G-CSFR	Monocytes, PMN, endothelial cells, fibroblasts, various tumor cells, stromal cells	Granulocyte maturation, promotes PMN function
M-CSF	28-44 kD	M-CSFR	Monocytes, fibroblasts endothelial cells	Monocyte activation, maturation
Type I interferons IFNα/β family	IFNαβR		Widespread	Antiviral response Broad immune modulatory effects (promotes MHC expression) Macrophage activation, lymphocyte activation and survival Antiproliferative, cytoskeletal alteration, differentiation ↑

Abbreviations: COX, Cyclooxygenase; DC, dendritic cell; DTH, delayed type hypersensitivity; G-CSF, granulocyte colony stimulating factor; GM-CSF, granulocyte macrophage colony stimulating factor; HMGB, high mobility group box chromosomal protein; IFN, interferon; M-CSF, macrophage colony stimulating factor; MIF, macrophage migration inhibitory factor; NO, nitric oxide; PG, prostaglandin; PLA, phospholipase A; PMN, polymorphonuclear cell; RAGE, receptor for advanced glycation endproducts.

and maturation following primary or secondary antigen exposure. The latter is of prime importance because reeducation of phenotypic T cell responses may be achieved through alteration of the ambient cytokine milieu. T cell receptor (TCR)-peptide–major histocompatibility complex(MHC) interactions during T cell–dendritic cell (DC) interaction rely on costimulatory molecule and local cytokine expression to determine functional outcome (see Table 25–3). Thus, IL-12 or IL-23, in the presence of IL-18, promotes type 1 phenotypic development, characterized ultimately by IFNγ– and IL-17–producing T1 effector cells.[20] IFNγ drives macrophage priming and activation and adhesion-molecule expression and thereby promotes granuloma formation and microbial killing. However, IFNγ has a complex role in tissue destruction, with contradictory data obtained in inflammation models in IFNγ– and IFNγR-deficient mice. IFNγ may ultimately retard tissue destruction, perhaps by suppressing osteoclast activation.[21] IL-17, in contrast, provides a direct and rapid route to tissue damage via such means as osteoclast activation or FLS activation.[22] On the other hand, IL-4 dominance during T cell–dendritic cell (DC) interactions in the presence of IL-18 leads to type 2 responses, which promote humoral immunity driven by T2 cells synthesizing primarily IL-4, IL-5, IL-10, and IL-13. Resulting pathogenesis may more likely be B cell mediated. Cytokines that predispose to regulatory T cell development are unclear, although high levels of IL-10 or transforming growth factor (TGF)β have been suggested in this context.[23] In summary, effector T cells can operate via secretion of cytokines to patterns determined by their prior activatory conditions.

Cognate Cellular Interactions

In many inflammatory lesions there is relative paucity of inducer T cell–derived cytokines (especially IFNγ), despite abundant proinflammatory cytokine expression. Cell–cell membrane interactions between leukocyte subsets and between tissue cells and leukocytes have emerged as a dominant mechanism sustaining chronic inflammation. Cytokines contribute to these interactions at several levels (Fig. 25–3), including directly as membrane-expressed ligands, indirectly via activating cells, and synergistically by enhancing their subsequent cognate activities. The importance of cytokine–cell contact interactions is best studied in synovial tissues, but applies to many inflammatory lesions. Many data now

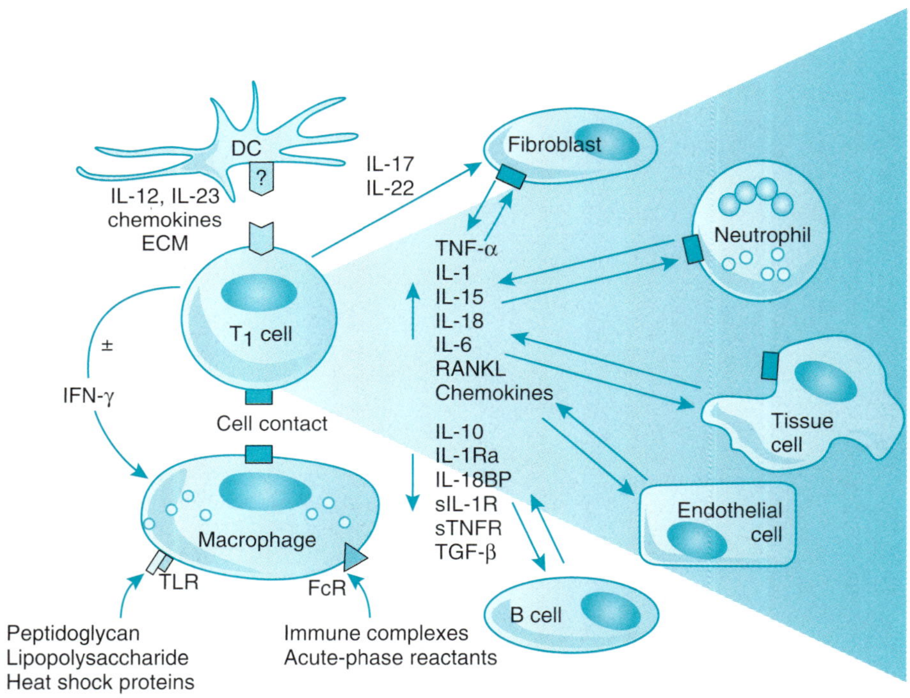

FIGURE 25–3 · Cytokines Regulate Complex Cellular Networks in Chronic Inflammation. Cytokines regulate interactions between T_1 cells and antigen-presenting cells (dendritic cells) and thereafter they promote cell–cell contact and soluble interactions between T cells, macrophages, neutrophils, endothelial cells, fibroblasts, B cells, and target tissue cells (e.g., mesangial cells, renal tubular epithelial cells, keratinocytes). Note that tissue cells may make substantial contributions to organ dysfunction through inflammatory mediator release. Critical to these pathways are the synergistic combinations of cytokines that operate as "cassettes" (synergistic teams) or together with cell-cell contact–dependent interactions. The latter are mediated via membrane cytokine expression or through cell surface receptors, including integrin and immunoglobulin superfamily adhesion molecules and members of the interleukin (IL)-1R and tumor necrosis factor-receptor (TNF-R) superfamilies. Chronicity is maintained on the basis of overproduction of proinflammatory moieties *(red arrow)* relative to the presence of anti-inflammatory mediators *(green arrow)*. Soluble cytokines also regulate activation of additional effector leukocytes (see Tables 25–1 through 25–7), including mast cells and eosinophils, which are not shown here because they may not be characteristic of the T helper type 1 (Th1) response shown. They may, however, be relevent in inflammatory arthritis.

show that cognate interactions between T cells and adjacent macrophages constitute a major pathway driving cytokine release and that cytokines, in turn, sustain this pathway (see Fig. 25–3).

Dayer first observed monocyte activation via cell contact with mitogen-stimulated T cells.[24] Freshly isolated synovial T cells activate macrophages by this mechanism, confirming that contact-induced cellular activation is a fundamental property of inflammatory T cells.[25] Antigen-independent, cytokine-mediated bystander activation confers this capacity on human CD4$^+$ memory T cells.[26] Studies using synovial T cells from RA and psoriatic arthritis (PsA) tissues reveal that exposure of memory T cells to synergistic combinations of cytokines are most potent in this respect, particularly IL-15, TNFα, and IL-6.[27,28] Cytokine activities also operate directly on macrophages to synergize with T cell contact. IFNγ and IL-18, for example, are most potent in this respect, acting via increased adhesion-molecule expression.

Activated memory CD4$^+$ T cells promote cytokine release from macrophages via diverse membrane ligands, including LFA-1/ICAM-1, CD69, and CD40/CD154.[27,29] Following contact with T cells, macrophages release increased concentrations of TNFα and IL-1, but not IL-10, and they exhibit reduced levels of IL-1Ra. Importantly, T helper type 1 (Th1) cells promote relatively greater proinflammatory cytokine release than do Th2 cells following coculture. This suggests that their functional phenotype extends beyond cytokine secretion to include a differential membrane-receptor array.[30] This is borne out further in the relative phenotypic distinctions between Th1 (CD40L, CCR5, IL-18Ra) and Th2 (ST2, CXCR3) cells. Signaling pathways engaged in monocytes following such T cell–membrane interactions are distinct from those activated by conventional cytokine-inducing agents. Thus, distinct utilization of phosphatidylinositol 3-kinase, NF-κB, and p38 mitogen-activated protein kinase (MAPK) pathways is observed.[31] Similarly, discrete macro-phage signals follow contact with cytokine-activated T cells (which resemble synovial T cells) as compared with TCR-activated T cells.[32] Such distinctions offer therapeutic potential in targeting cytokine-activated T cell– driven pathways, leaving antigen-driven responses relatively intact. Finally, the activation state of memory T cells necessary for the previously discussed interactions to proceed remains controversial. Purified resting T cell subsets activate synovial fibroblasts to release IL-6, IL-8, matrix metalloproteinase 3 (MMP3), and prostanoids, in synergy with IL-17.[33]

It is likely that T cells may be activated by interactions with diverse moieties, including extracellular matrix components—and potentially autoantigens. Nevertheless, it is now clear that cytokines can promote chronicity by activating T cells to promote inflammation irrespective of local (auto)antigen recognition and that this has enormous therapeutic potential (see Fig. 25–3).

Agonist/Antagonist Cytokine Activities in Chronic Inflammation

Complex regulatory interactions exist to suppress ongoing inflammatory responses. This is often achieved via parallel secretion of antagonistic cytokines and soluble receptors to regulate cytokine effector pathways. Thus, T1 responses are suppressed in part by cytokines of T2 type (e.g., IL-4 or IL-10), and in consequence, exaggerated Th1 responses arise in models in which the Th2 response is deficient.[20] Similar regulatory loops operate for other leukocytes, exemplified by the yin-yang effects of TNFα and IL-10 on macrophage cytokine release and effector function.[34]

Inhibitory cytokine activities are usually defined with respect to a proinflammatory cytokine, and in other contexts they may have quite distinct function, rendering prediction of their net contribution to an inflammatory response difficult. Thus, IL-10 opposes many of the proinflammatory effects of TNFα and IL-1β, (e.g., reduces adhesion-molecule expression, MHC expression, and MMP release), but it potently activates B cell activation and immunoglobulin secretion.[34] Similarly, TNFα, which is normally considered a proinflammatory moiety, may have an important role in regulating T cell function because T cells removed from sites of chronic inflammation exhibit suppressed capacity to signal via their TCR that recovers upon TNFα neutralization.[35] Such regulation is further complicated by the precise ratio of cytokine to soluble receptor, such as TNF to sTNFR or IL-10 to sIL-10R within the local environment. Commensurate with this, administration of anti-inflammatory cytokines such as IL-4, IL-10, and IL-11 has, in general, proven disappointing in the context of clinical inflammatory diseases. An important caveat to this is the potential requirement of combinations of cytokines to optimally suppress inflammation (e.g., combinations including IL-4, IL-10, and IL-11). Further functional antagonism is exemplified in the antagonistic activities of IL-1β and IL-1Ra, of IL-18, and of IL-18 binding protein in regulating macro-phage activation.

Recently, the role of cytokines in regulating cognate interactions between leukocytes has also emerged. Thus, although anti-inflammatory pathways are poorly induced following cell contact, cytokine-activated T cells can induce IL-10 release by monocytes.[32] For example, RA synovial membrane IL-10 release, which is partially T cell dependent, will feedback to regulate TNFα release. Cytokine production from adjacent cell lineages within an inflammatory lesion may also be suppressive. IFNβ reduces mitogen-activated T cell–induced macrophage release of TNFα and IL-1, whereas IL-1Ra release is enhanced.[36] This provides a mechanism whereby type I interferons could modify proinflammatory cytokine production. Regulation extends beyond conventional cytokine activities. Prostaglandins and lipoprotein moieties, particularly high density lipoprotein (HDL), can suppress cytokine-mediated T cell–macrophage interactions.[37]

Conventional DMARDs

Conventional disease modifying antirheumatic drug (DMARDs) can also act via modulation of cytokine production. Methotrexate modulates release of various cytokines in vitro, in part mediated via adenosine-cyclic adenosine monophosphate (cAMP) pathway.[38] A77 11726, the active metabolite of the dihydroorotate dehydrogenase inhibitor leflunomide, reduces TNFα, IL-1β,

IL-6, and MMP-1, but it does not reduce IL-1Ra release by monocytes after mitogen-activated T cell contact.[39,40] Leflunomide may mediate these activities through modulation of inhibitor of NF-κB (IκB)α phosphorylation and degradation and AP-1 and c-Jun N-terminal protein kinase activation.[41] Finally, sulfasalazine is an inhibitor of proinflammatory cytokine-induced NF-κB.

Cellular Interactions Across Diverse Tissues

Cytokines promote cognate cellular interactions across a range of tissues. In contrast to T cell–macrophage and T cell–DC interactions, in which adhesion molecule and costimulatory pathways are often implicated, cell–cell membrane communication apart from leukocyte-leukocyte interactions are often mediated through membrane cytokine expression (see Fig. 25–3). Thus, T cell–contact mediated activation of fibroblasts operates via membrane TNFα and IFNγ to enhance fibroblast cytokine release and MMP—but not tissue inhibitors of metalloproteinase (TIMP)—expression, thereby favoring tissue destruction.[29] The source and activation status of the fibroblast is vital; fibroblast-like synoviocytes, but not cutaneous fibroblasts, are potently activated by this route. Other studies have shown T cell–contact mediated activation of neutrophils, keratinocytes, mesangial cells (via a combination of membrane cytokine and CD40L expression), platelets, and renal tubule epithelial cells. Furthermore, cytokine-activated macrophages (via IFNγ and sCD40L) may interact via cell contact with mesangial cells to activate adhesion molecule and chemokine release by the latter. Thus, cell–cell contact between cells of the immune system and beyond likely represents a ubiquitous mechanism whereby perpetuation of chronic inflammation is potently influenced by local production of cytokines.

B Cells and Cytokine Release in Chronic Inflammation

Cytokines are critical to B cell maturation, proliferation, activation, isotype switching, and survival (see Chapter 10). Cytokine-mediated B cell activation is therefore of importance in immune complex generation, B cell antigen presentation, B cell–T cell interactions, and germinal center formation. B cells have, in turn, been considered important inducers of macrophage-derived cytokine release. This process may operate primarily via immune complex formation[42] or through regulation of T cell activation (with B cell help). Thus, complex regulatory feedback loops involving cytokine expression and B cells are likely of importance in a range of rheumatic diseases in which B cells are of paramount pathophysiologic importance.

Innate Cell Lineages in Chronic Inflammation

Cytokines potently activate innate response cells that contribute to the chronic inflammatory lesion of a variety of rheumatic diseases. Tables 25–1 through 25–7 document relevant examples in which neutrophils, NK cells, eosinophils, and mast cells may be recruited and activated by the presence of appropriate cytokine combinations.

Growth Factors in Chronic Inflammation

Many data document the importance of growth factor families in chronic inflammation. WD TGFβ superfamily members, including TGFβ isoforms and bone morphogenic protein (BMP) family members, deserve particular reference. TGFβ is critically involved in processes of cell proliferation, differentiation, inflammation, and wound healing.[43] BMPs, in addition to regulating inflammatory responses, are of primary importance in determining cartilage and bone tissue development and remodeling.[44] As such, they are of increasing interest in the pathogenesis of several rheumatic diseases.

Cytokine Effects Beyond Immune Regulation

A striking feature of the cytokine field concerns the broad functional pleiotropy exemplified in the effects of cytokines in normal physiologic and adaptive processes. Cytokine activities are found in muscle, adipose tissue, the central nervous system, the liver, and beyond, mediating both normal regulation of metabolic pathways and also modulation imposed by altered tissue conditions. Examples are found in the release of adipokines that regulate adipose metabolic pathways, but also in the release of conventional cytokines by fat pads in inflammatory synovitis.

Summary

Cytokines represent a diverse family of glycoproteins active across a broad range of tissues. Their pleiotropic functions and propensity for synergistic interactions and functional redundancy render them intriguing therapeutic targets. Thus far, single cytokine targeting has proven useful in several rheumatic disease states. Further elucidation of the biology and functional interactions within this expanding family of bioactive moieties will likely prove informative, both in resolving pathogenesis and in generating novel therapeutic options.

REFERENCES

1. Locksley RM, Killeen N, Lenardo MJ: The TNF and TNF receptor superfamilies: Integrating mammalian biology. Cell 104:487, 2001.
2. Bowie A, O'Neill LA: The interleukin-1 receptor/Toll-like receptor superfamily: Signal generators for pro-inflammatory interleukins and microbial products. J Leukoc Biol 67:508, 2000.
3. Tak PP, Bresnihan B: The pathogenesis and prevention of joint damage in rheumatoid arthritis: Advances from synovial biopsy and tissue analysis. Arthritis Rheum 43:2619, 2000.
4. Ulfgren AK, Andersson U, Engstrom M, et al: Systemic anti-tumor necrosis factor alpha therapy in rheumatoid arthritis down-regulates synovial tumor necrosis factor alpha synthesis. Arthritis Rheum 43:2391, 2000.
5. Gadina M, Hilton D, Johnston JA, et al: Signaling by type I and II cytokine receptors: Ten years after. Curr Opin Immunol 13:363, 2001.
6. Bravo J, Heath JK: Receptor recognition by gp130 cytokines. Embo J 19:2399, 2000.

7. Dubois S, Mariner J, Waldmann TA, et al: IL-15Ralpha recycles and presents IL-15 In trans to neighboring cells. Immunity 17:537, 2002.
8. Francis K, Palsson BO: Effective intercellular communication distances are determined by the relative time constants for cyto/chemokine secretion and diffusion. Proc Natl Acad Sci U S A 94:12258, 1997.
9. Feldmann M, Andreakos E, Smith C, et al: Is NF-kappaB a useful therapeutic target in rheumatoid arthritis? Ann Rheum Dis 61(Suppl 2):13, 2002.
10. Hajeer AH, Hutchinson IV: TNF-alpha gene polymorphism: clinical and biological implications. Microsc Res Tech 50:216, 2000.
11. Hurme M, Lahdenpohja N, Santtila S: Gene polymorphisms of interleukins 1 and 10 in infectious and autoimmune diseases. Ann Med 30:469, 1998.
12. Kontoyiannis D, Pasparakis M, Pizarro TT, et al: Impaired on/off regulation of TNF biosynthesis in mice lacking TNF AU-rich elements: implications for joint and gut-associated immunopathologies. Immunity 10:387, 1999.
13. Anderson P: Post-transcriptional regulation of tumour necrosis factor alpha production. Ann Rheum Dis 59:3, 2000.
14. Gueydan C, Droogmans L, Chalon P, et al: Identification of TIAR as a protein binding to the translational regulatory AU-rich element of tumor necrosis factor alpha mRNA. J Biol Chem 274: 2322, 1999.
15. Saito K, Chen S, Piecyk M, et al: TIA-1 regulates the production of tumor necrosis factor in macrophages, but not in lymphocytes. Arthritis Rheum 44:2879, 2001.
16. Waldmann TA, Tagaya Y: The multifaceted regulation of interleukin-15 expression and the role of this cytokine in NK cell differentiation and host response to intracellular pathogens. Annu Rev Immunol 17:19, 1999.
17. Ferrari D, Chiozzi P, Falzoni S, et al: Extracellular ATP triggers IL-1 beta release by activating the purinergic P2Z receptor of human macrophages. J Immunol 159:1451, 1997.
18. Fantuzzi G, Dinarello CA: Interleukin-18 and interleukin-1 beta: Two cytokine substrates for ICE (caspase-1). J Clin Immunol 19:1, 1999.
19. Wallach D, Varfolomeev EE, Malinin NL, et al: Tumor necrosis factor receptor and Fas signaling mechanisms. Annu Rev Immunol 17:331, 1999.
20. Liew FY: T(H)1 and T(H)2 cells: A historical perspective. Nat Rev Immunol 2:55, 2002.
21. Takayanagi H, Kim S, Taniguchi T: Signaling crosstalk between RANKL and interferons in osteoclast differentiation. Arthritis Res 4(Suppl 3):S227, 2002.
22. Aggarwal S, Gurney AL: IL-17: prototype member of an emerging cytokine family. J Leukoc Biol 71:1, 2002.
23. Shevach EM: Regulatory T cells in autoimmmunity. Annu Rev Immunol 18:423, 2000.
24. Vey E, Zhang JH, Dayer JM: IFN-gamma and 1,25(OH)2D3 induce on THP-1 cells distinct patterns of cell surface antigen expression, cytokine production, and responsiveness to contact with activated T cells. J Immunol 149:2040, 1992.
25. McInnes IB, Leung BP, Sturrock RD, et al: Interleukin-15 mediates T cell-dependent regulation of tumor necrosis factor-alpha production in rheumatoid arthritis. Nat Med 3:189, 1997.
26. Unutmaz D, Pileri P, Abrignani S: Antigen-independent activation of naive and memmory resting T cells by a cytokine combination. J Exp Med 180:1159, 1994.
27. McInnes IB, Leung BP, Liew FY: Cell-cell interactions in synovitis. Interactions between T lymphocytes and synovial cells. Arthritis Res 2:374, 2000.
28. Sebbag M, Parry SL, Brennan FM, et al: Cytokine stimulation of T lymphocytes regulates their capacity to induce monocyte production of tumor necrosis factor-alpha, but not interleukin-10: Possible relevance to pathophysiology of rheumatoid arthritis. Eur J Immunol 27:624, 1997.
29. Dayer JM, Burger D: Cytokines and direct cell contact in synovitis: Relevance to therapeutic intervention. Arthritis Res 1:17, 1999.
30. Ribbens C, Dayer JM, Chizzolini C: CD40-CD40 ligand (CD154) engagement is required but may not be sufficient for human T helper 1 cell induction of interleukin-2- or interleukin-15-driven, contact-dependent, interleukin-1beta production by monocytes. Immunology 99:279, 2000.
31. Hayes AL, Smith C, Foxwell BM, et al: CD45-induced tumor necrosis factor alpha production in monocytes is phosphatidylinositol 3-kinase-dependent and nuclear factor-kappaB-independent. J Biol Chem 274:33455, 1999.
32. Foey A, Green P, Foxwell B, et al: Cytokine-stimulated T cells induce macrophage IL-10 production dependent on phosphatidylinositol 3-kinase and p70S6K: implications for rheumatoid arthritis. Arthritis Res 4:64, 2002.
33. Yamamura Y, Gupta R, Morita Y, et al: Effector function of resting T cells: Activation of synovial fibroblasts. J Immunol 166:2270, 2001.
34. Fickenscher H, Hor S, Kupers H, et al: The interleukin-10 family of cytokines. Trends Immunol 23:89, 2002.
35. Cope AP: Studies of T-cell activation in chronic inflammation. Arthritis Res 4(Suppl 3):S197, 2002.
36. Jungo F, Dayer JM, Modoux C, et al: IFN-beta inhibits the ability of T lymphocytes to induce TNF-alpha and IL-1beta production in monocytes upon direct cell-cell contact. Cytokine 14:272, 2001.
37. Hyka N, Dayer JM, Modoux C, et al: Apolipoprotein A-I inhibits the production of interleukin-1beta and tumor necrosis factor-alpha by blocking contact-mediated activation of monocytes by T lymphocytes. Blood 97:2381, 2001.
38. Chan ES, Cronstein BN: Molecular action of methotrexate in inflammatory diseases. Arthritis Res 4:266, 2002.
39. Breedveld FC, Dayer JM: Leflunomide: mode of action in the treatment of rheumatoid arthritis. Ann Rheum Dis 59:841, 2000.
40. Burger D, Begue-Pastor N, Benavent S, et al: The active metabolite of leflunomide, A77 1726, inhibits the production of prostaglandin E(2), matrix metalloproteinase 1 and interleukin 6 in human fibroblast-like synoviocytes. Rheumatology (Oxford) 42:89, 2003.
41. Manna SK, Mukhopadhyay A, Aggarwal BB: Leflunomide suppresses TNF-induced cellular responses: Effects on NF-kappa B, activator protein-1, c-Jun N-terminal protein kinase, and apoptosis. J Immunol 165:5962, 2000.
42. Chantry D, Winearls CG, Maini RN, et al: Mechanism of immune complex-mediated damage: induction of interleukin 1 by immune complexes and synergy with interferon-gamma and tumor necrosis factor-alpha. Eur J Immunol 19:189, 1989.
43. Chen W, Wahl SM: TGF-beta: receptors, signaling pathways and autoimmunity. Curr Dir Autoimmun 5:62, 2002.
44. Wozney JM: Overview of bone morphogenetic proteins. Spine 27:S2, 2002.

26 Apoptosis

KEITH B. ELKON

History and Concepts

APOPTOSIS

Illustrations of cells undergoing apoptosis were made almost as soon as stains were used to examine the appearance of cells in different tissues. Drawings of ovarian follicles undergoing cell death made more than 100 years ago demonstrate cell shrinkage and nuclear condensation. Subsequent descriptions of "pyknosis," chromatin margination, and other terms used to convey the appearance of subcellular particles during cell death included many features now recognized as apoptosis. The history of this subject is reviewed elsewhere.[1]

The modern understanding of apoptosis began with the electron microscopic descriptions of morphologic changes characterized by shrinkage of hepatocytes (i.e., shrinkage necrosis) after ischemic or toxic injury to the liver. The name *apoptosis* was coined by Kerr, Wyllie, and Currie in 1972 to describe the form of death that was "consistent with an active, inherently controlled phenomenon" characterized by cell shrinkage, nuclear condensation, and cell blebbing[2] (Fig. 26–1). This term also conveyed the concept of cell death that was similar to leaves falling from a tree (*apo* means "from" and *ptosis* "a fall" in Greek), implying a regulated "mechanism of cell deletion, which is complementary to mitosis."[2]

Further developments in apoptosis paralleled advances in molecular biology, genetics, and biochemistry. The detection of a nucleosomal ladder[3] was of considerable importance, because it defined a biochemical event (i.e., nucleosomal cleavage) and provided a simple electrophoretic test for detection of apoptotic cell death that remains a standard in the field (see "Methods of Detection" section later in this chapter). Another landmark was the discovery, in the 1980s, that the death of cells during the development of the nematode *Caenorhabditis elegans* was under strict genetic control. Remarkably, the death of these cells could be perturbed by mutation of a small number of genes called cell death abnormal (*ced*) genes.[4] Horvitz and colleagues determined that two *ced* genes, *ced3* and *ced4,* encoded death effectors, whereas *ced9* was an antiapoptotic gene. Most of the remaining *ced* genes were responsible for engulfment and removal of the "corpses." This simple model, in which CED-3 is the main death protease activated by CED-4 and inhibited by CED-9, has served as a paradigm for defining apoptotic pathways in mammalian cells (see Fig. 26–2). In 2002, Robert Horwitz was awarded the Nobel Prize for "discoveries concerning the genetic regulation of ...programmed cell death" (http://www.nobel.se/medicine/laureates/2002/index.html).

Mammalian cells are more complex and, as will be discussed in detail, have multiple defined pathways that follow the basic *C. elegans* model. The molecules within these pathways, the downstream effectors of apoptosis, the caspases (cysteine aspartate proteases), and the proteins implicated in the clearance of apoptotic cells will also be discussed in detail. Regulation of cell death is of seminal importance in a number of diseases, including cancers, autoimmune diseases, and degenerative disorders.[5,6] The relevance of apoptosis to rheumatic disorders is summarized at the end of the chapter.

PROGRAMMED CELL DEATH

Whereas "apoptosis" originally referred to the appearance of dying cells in certain contexts, as explained previously, the concepts of atrophy, cellular or tissue involution or regression, and degeneration have also been appreciated for hundreds of years. However, the two phenomena were not associated until relatively recently. Perhaps the most precise descriptions of cells that died in an orderly and apparently programmed fashion have been documented in developmental biology. Examples include the involution of cells between digits, metamorphosis of insect larvae, and the death of specific cells during the development of *C. elegans.*

NECROSIS

Necrosis is distinguished from apoptosis predominantly by morphologic appearances.[7] Necrotic cells are swollen, and electron microscopy reveals disorderly fragmentation of chromatin and severe damage to the mitochondria (see Fig. 26–1). The cellular membrane loses integrity and becomes permeable to vital dyes such as trypan blue as well as propidium iodide (see Fig.26–5). The distinction between apoptosis and necrosis remains important from a number of perspectives. In contrast to the genetic and biochemical programs that regulate apoptosis, necrotic cells usually result from death "by accident"—from thermal or drug injury, infection, or infarction of an organ. Because of the uncontrolled release of lysosomal and granular contents, necrotic cells induce a proinflammatory immune response, whereas apoptotic cells normally elicit an anti-inflammatory response.

The same inducers (e.g., ischemia, hydrogen peroxide) may produce apoptosis or necrosis, depending on the severity of the injury and the rapidity of cell death. The cell's fate is determined in part by cellular energy

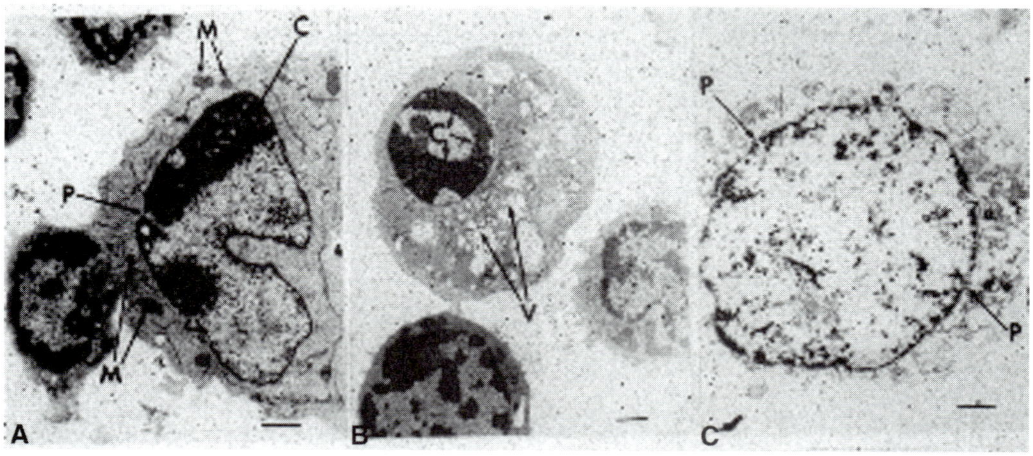

FIGURE 26–1 · Electron Microscopic Morphology of Apoptosis. *A*, A cytotoxic T cell (*lower left*) conjugated to its target, P815 (a murine mast cell), before the initiation of cell death. *B*, Induction of apoptotic changes in P815. Note the reduction in target cell size, nuclear condensation, and vacuoles with the relative preservation of organelles. *C*, Osmotic lysis and necrosis in P815 induced by antibody and complement. Note the increased size of the nucleus and apparently random fragmentation of the chromatin. Organelles are severely disrupted. C, dense chromatin; M, mitochondria; P, nuclear pore; V, vacuoles. (Adapted from Russell JH, Masakowski V, Rucinsky T, et al: Mechanisms of immune lysis III. Characterization of the nature and kinetics of the cytotoxic T lymphocyte induced nuclear lesion in the target. J Immunol 128:2087, 1982 with permission.)

reserves such as adenosine triphosphate (ATP).[8] Some inducers may initially cause apoptosis followed by necrosis (postapoptotic necrosis). This is likely to occur when removal of the apoptotic cells is delayed.

Biochemistry of Apoptosis

A schematic diagram of the cell death program is shown in Figure 26–3. A brief outline of each major functional component within the program, from the signals for death to removal of the apoptotic cells, is discussed here, but space limitations preclude a detailed analysis of the layers of regulation at each step of the pathway. For example, postranslational protein modifications such as phosphorylation, nitrosylation, and oxidation provide additional complexities that are under intense study, and a series of reviews in the November 24 and 27, 2003 Issues of Oncogene offer a more detailed review of structure and function relationships and the broad role of these pathways in biologic systems.

The specialized proteins involved in apoptosis and its regulation contain a number of modules or domains predominantly involved in promoting protein-protein interactions (Table 26–1). These domains may be found in receptors, adaptors, effectors, or inhibitors. Furthermore, as will be discussed, these domains occur in proteins involved in apoptosis, as well as inflammation. It has been suggested that death domain (DD), death effector domain (DED), caspase recruitment domain (CARD), and Pyrin domains all evolved from the prototypic DD

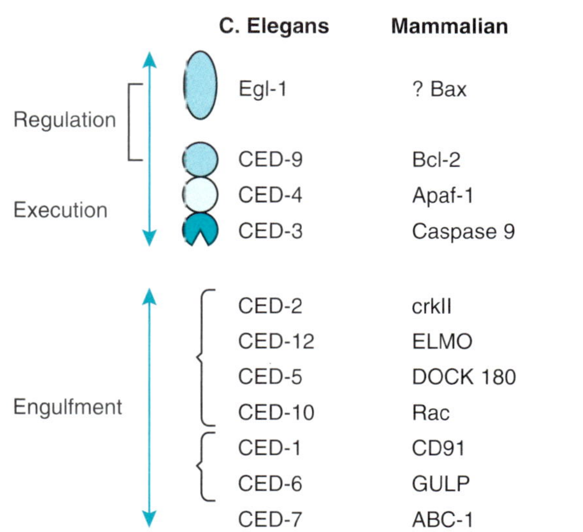

FIGURE 26–2 · *Caenorhabditis elegans* paradigm of apoptosis. Genes involved in the regulation, execution, and clearance of apoptotic cells during the development of *C. elegans* and their mammalian homologues are shown. In this figure, only the most closely related homologues are indicated, but, as described in the text and shown in Figs. 27–3 and 27–4, the complexity in mammalian cells is much greater. Note that at least half of the CED proteins are involved in engulfment and removal of apoptotic corpses. There are two distinct but partially overlapping pathways of engulfment in *C. elegans*: CED-2, –12, –5 and –10, which most likely regulate cytoskeletal changes, and CED-1 and –6, which may be involved in recognition (CED-1) and upstream signal transduction (CED-6). CED-7 is homologous to the mammalian ATP-binding cassette transporter-1 (ABC-1), but it is unclear at present what is transported during apoptosis and which other protein it interacts with. The grey symbols represent inhibitory proteins.

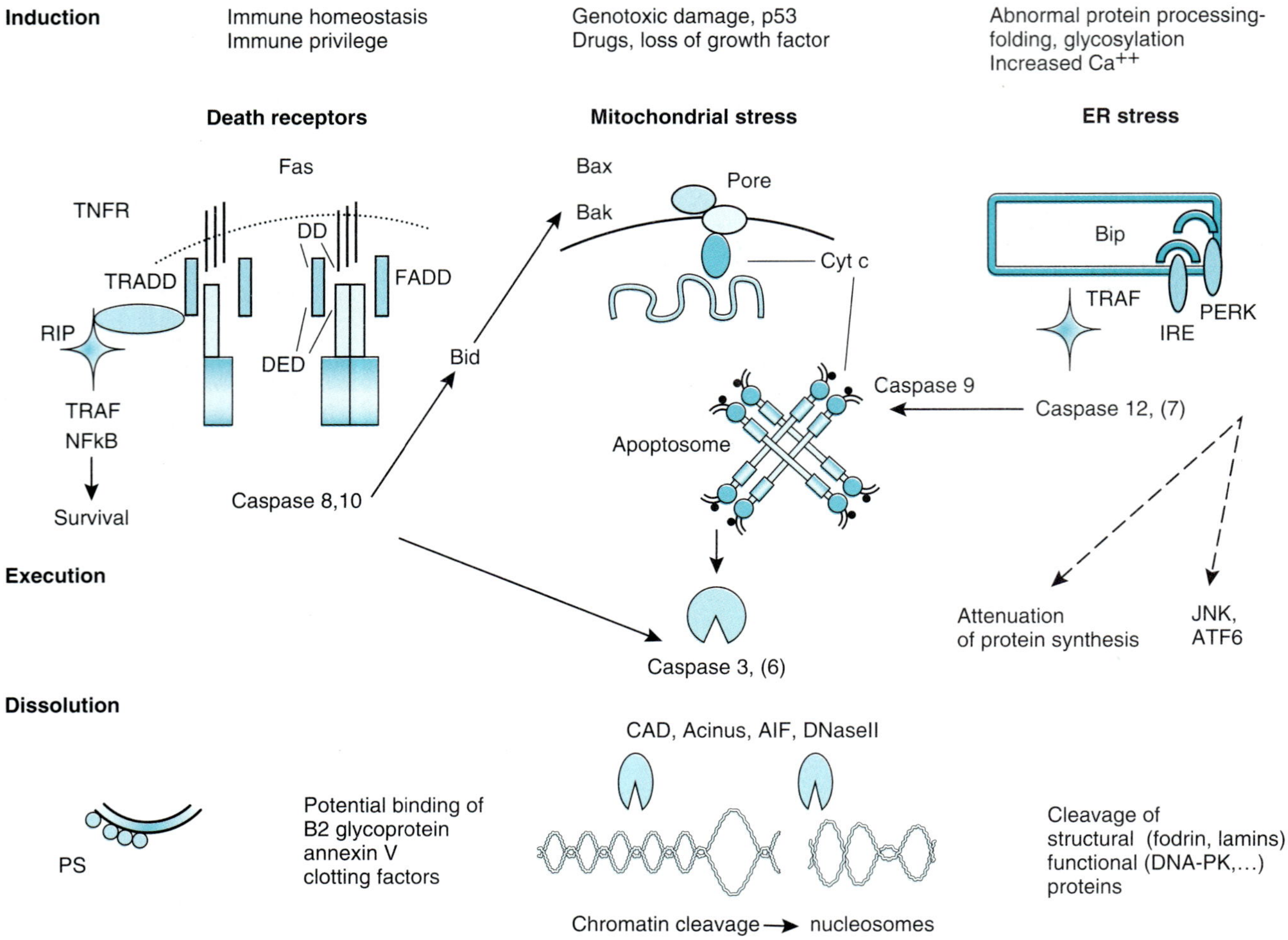

FIGURE 26–3 · Mammalian apoptotic pathways. Cell death can be initiated by multiple pathways, including an extrinsic ligand-induced pathway *(left panel)*, an intrinsic pathway mediated by the mitochondria (*middle panel*), and an intrinsic pathway mediated through the endoplasmic reticulum (ER) (*right panel*). Examples of stimuli that can induce each of these pathways are shown and discussed in further detail in the text. Note that these pathways differ in the upstream caspases activated but converge to cleave the effector caspases, such as caspase 3, during execution of apoptosis. Tumor necrosis factor receptor (TNF-R) and other "death receptors" can also signal cell survival by activation of nuclear factor kappa B (NFκB). During ER stress, unfolded proteins release the ER chaperone protein, Bip, from binding to the stress sensor proteins, IRE, PERK, and ATF6. PERK attenuates protein synthesis, whereas ATF6 and JNK are transcription factors that upregulate the expression of proapoptotic proteins such as CHOP (GADD 153) and caspases.

The alterations that occur during dissolution of the cell are too numerous to mention, but a few are highlighted in view of their potential relevance to autoimmunity (see text). Exposure of phosphatidylserine (PS) on the cell surface *(left lower panel)* provides a simple means for detection of apoptotic cells through binding annexin V and may be relevant to the generation of antiphospholipid autoantibodies and coagulation disorders in vivo. Cleavage products of chromatin *(lower middle panel)* as well as proteins, such as lamins and DNA-PK, may be antigenic. AIF, apoptosis inducing factor; CAD, caspase activated DNAse; Cyt C, cytochrome c; DD, death domain; DED, death effector domain.

fold, corresponding to an antiparallel six helix bundle.[9] In general, like domains bind so as to facilitate homotypic interactions leading to oligomerization of the same protein or binding to different proteins in a signaling pathway. These changes usually lead to conformational alterations, which lead to further protein recruitment. Other domains such as nucleotide binding site, (NBS) specify nucleotide binding.

Death Ligands, Receptors, and Signals

Death of a cell may result from intracellular stress activating an intrinsic death program or may be forced on the cell by the interaction of a death ligand with a death receptor (see Fig. 26–3). Death receptors (DRs) belong to the tumor necrosis factor receptor (TNF-R) superfamily of proteins, which has approximately 25 members.[10,11] This family of receptors is responsible for diverse biologic responses such as inflammation, proliferation, antiviral activity, and cell death. Receptors in the TNF family include at least six receptors capable of transmitting apoptosis (see following), as well as receptors such as CD40, CD30, BlyS/BAFF/TALL, and TACI[10] that trigger survival, proliferation, or both, in part through activation of nuclear factor kappa B (NFκB). Although most receptors of the TNF-R family exert their effects primarily within the immune system, some members

TABLE 26–1 • MODULAR COMPONENTS OF PROTEINS INVOLVED IN APOPTOSIS AND INFLAMMATION

Module	Component of	Function
DD	Death receptors, adaptors, kinases	P-P I
DED	Adaptors, caspases,	P-P I
CARD	Caspases, adaptors, Nod	P-P I
BH (1-4)	Bcl-2 family	P-P I
Pyrin	Pyrin family	P-P I
LRR	Pyrin family, NODs	P-P I
NBS / NOD	Pyrin family, NODs	Nucleotide binding, oligomerization

Abbreviations: BH, Bcl-2 homology; CARD, caspase recruitment domain; DD, death domain; DED, death effector domain; LRR, leucine-rich repeats; NBS, nucleotide binding site; NOD, nucleotide oligomerization domain; P-P I, protein-protein interaction. See [145, 150] for further discussion.

(e.g., p75 nerve growth factor receptor [NGF-R], TNF-RI, and TNF-RII) appear to serve important functions in the nervous system and other organs. Some TNF-R–like proteins, such as PV-T2, PV-A53R, and CAR1, are encoded by viruses and may contribute to their virulence.[10]

DEATH RECEPTORS

The DRs identified, including Fas, TNF-RI, DR-3 (TRAMP/wsl/APO-3), DR-4 (TRAIL-R1), DR-5 (TRAIL-R2), and DR-6, share homology in their intracellular domains throughout a 70-amino acid region called the *death domain*(DD).[12] Three decoy receptors have been identified, two (DcR1 and DcR2) that bind and inhibit their ligand, TRAIL, and one (DcR3) that binds Fas ligand. These decoy receptors presumably modulate cytotoxic function of the ligands, but the biologic contexts remain to be fully defined. Alternative splice forms and shedding of the receptors and ligands also downmodulate their function.

TNF-R family members are characterized by two to six cysteine-rich domains (CRDs) in their extracellular regions.[10] The cocrystal structure of TNF-RI and lymphotoxin-α indicates that the CRDs project from the cell surface in a linear array, making distinct contacts with ligands at subunit interfaces. The first CRD may also be responsible for preassembly of the receptor as trimers that undergo further conformational alterations upon ligand engagement.

The three-dimensional structure of the DD has been solved by nuclear magnetic resonance spectroscopy and consists of six amphipathic α-helices that create a unique fold.[13] Functionally, the DD appears to be a novel protein-protein association motif that facilitates homotypic interactions. For example, the DD of Fas and TNF-RI self-associate, thereby recruiting adaptor proteins that also contain DD and that directly or indirectly mediate receptor signal transduction (see Fig. 26–3).

DEATH RECEPTOR SIGNAL TRANSDUCTION

This section will focus predominantly on signaling from Fas and TNF-R, as these are the best-characterized members of the death receptor subfamily, and it is likely that other death receptors signal through similar pathways. As illustrated in Figure 26–3, Fas and TNF-R1 share a common death pathway. Binding of Fas ligand to Fas causes conformational changes in the receptor cluster, leading to recruitment of intracellular adaptor molecules. Initially, aggregation of Fas induces uptake of the adaptor protein, FADD, to the DD of Fas. FADD has two structural domains: a C-terminal DD, which mediates Fas binding, and an N-terminal death effector domain (DED). The FADD DED allows recruitment of procaspase 8[14,15] and procaspase 10[16] through DED-DED interactions. Procaspases 8 and 10 have a bipartite structure consisting of a DED and an enzymatic caspase domain, the latter linking Fas aggregation with the execution phase of apoptosis. The apposition of procaspases 8 and 10 to the activated Fas complex leads to autocatalytic cleavage and conversion of the proenzymes to activated proteases, which are released and able to initiate a proteolytic cascade, leading to programmed cell death. In some cell lines, caspase 8 cleavage also results in cleavage of the proapoptotic molecule Bid, which activates the mitochondrial amplification cascade (type II pathway)[17] (see Fig. 26–3).

Although the six DD-containing receptors initiate cell death in certain contexts, all may signal cell survival or proliferation in different cell types, in different contexts, or both. The ability to signal an opposite cell fate depends on the recruitment of proteins such as the tumor necrosis factor receptor–associated factors (TRAFs) that activate NFκB, thereby promoting cell survival (see following).

DEATH LIGANDS

FasL (CD178) is a 40-kD type II transmembrane protein that shares 15 to 35 percent of its amino acid identity with the TNF superfamily of ligands. FasL is expressed constitutively in the anterior chamber of the eye and in the testis, but it is induced when CD8, T helper type 1 (Th1) CD4 T cells, and some natural killer (NK) cell populations become activated.[18] In lymphocytes, expression of ligand is tightly regulated, and activity on the cell surface short lived because metalloproteases cleave the extracellular portion of the ligand into soluble, functional molecules. The zinc metalloprotease, TNF-α-converting enzyme (TACE) is a membrane-anchored member of the disintegrin family of proteases that cleaves active TNF-α from the cell surface.[19,20]

FUNCTION IN IMMUNE REGULATION

Although the role of Fas and FasL interactions in the thymus remains controversial,[21] this pathway is involved in the maintenance of immune privilege in the eye and the testis, in the pathogenesis of graft-versus-host disease, and in immune evasion by tumors.[18] The major physiologic function of Fas and FasL in the immune system is the preservation of peripheral tolerance. This is achieved by the phenomenon of activation-induced cell death (AICD), whereby CD8 T cells, Th1 CD4 T cells, and possibly NK cells induce apoptosis of activated T cells, B cells, and macrophages. The deletion of activated immune cells removes the source of proinflammatory molecules, prevents the continued presentation of self peptides by primed (with high levels of costimulatory molecules) antigen-presenting cells, and eliminates B cells that have mutated to self-specificity in the germinal centers.[22] These topics are discussed in greater detail elsewhere in this textbook, and the consequences of Fas deficiency are described later in this chapter.

It should be noted that, whereas TRAIL signals apoptosis through DR4 and DR5 predominantly in tumor cells, recent evidence suggests that TRAIL plays a role in negative selection of thymocytes.[23] Similarly, DR3 (the receptor for the ligand ,TWEAK) has also been implicated in negative selection.[24] Finally, DR6 plays a role in immunologic homeostasis as evidenced by enhanced T and B cell proliferation in DR6-deficient mice.[25]

Intrinsic Cell Death Pathways: Initiation and Execution of Apoptosis

Cells need constant sources of nutrition and depend on a variety of signals for active survival. Loss of signals from neighboring cells[26] or withdrawal of growth factors or cytokines results in initiation of a cell death program. Damage or stress to intracellular organelles may be induced from outside or from within the cell.

GENOTOXIC INJURY

Mutations occur frequently in mammalian DNA and are usually promptly repaired. However, if repair fails or DNA is severely damaged by radiation or drugs, the transcription factor p53 ("guardian of the genome") is upregulated and phosphorylated by DNA damage sensors such as ATM. Activated p53 induces a cell cycle arrest through induction of the cyclin-dependent kinase inhibitor, p21. If the DNA damage is repaired, cell cycle arrest is abrogated, whereas if the injury cannot be repaired, the cell undergoes apoptosis. The critical importance of p53 as a tumor suppressor is illustrated by the high frequency of p53 mutations in cancers.[27] p53 induces apoptosis, in part by transcription of death effectors, such as Bax, that cause mitochondrial stress.

MITOCHONDRIAL STRESS

Mitochondria are cytoplasmic organelles that contain their own 16-kb genome encased by inner and outer membranes with a number of proteins, including cytochrome-*c*, situated between these membranes (see Fig. 26–3). Mitochondria help to maintain redox potential and are the energy powerhouse of the cell through the generation of ATP by oxidative phosphorylation. These biochemical pathways create an electrochemical gradient ($\Delta\psi$) that is positive and acidic on the outside and alkaline on the inner side of the mitochondrial membrane. Spanning the inner membrane is the adenine nuclear translocator (ANT) that transports the ATP. On the outer mitochondrial membrane (OMM) is the voltage-dependent anion channel (VDAC) that is permeable to solutes of approximately 5,000 kD.[28]

Genotoxic injury, reduced supply of nutritional or growth factors, and exposure to certain chemicals such as staurosporine, cause mitochondrial stress. These initiating factors lead to selective mitochondrial membrane permeabilization (MMP) with the resulting dissipation of the proton gradient responsible for the $\Delta\psi$, as well as permeabilization of the outer membrane. Once initiated, cytochrome-*c* is released from the intermitochondrial space into the cytosol (see Fig. 26–3). In the cytosol, cytochrome *c* and the cofactors Apaf-1 and ATP or dATP assemble with caspase 9 to form a molecular aggregate called the apoptosome that promotes the cleavage of procaspase 9 into its active form.[29] Caspase 9 acts on effector caspases such as caspase 3, resulting in the caspase cascade that leads to the cleavage and inactivation of a wide variety of substrates within the cell (see Fig. 26–3). A caspase-independent apoptosis-inducing factor (AIF) is also be released from the mitochondria and induces nuclear changes and cell death by less well-defined pathways.[30]

ENDOPLASMIC RETICULUM STRESS

The main functions of the endoplasmic reticulum (ER) are to regulate intracellular calcium flux and to promote proper folding of nascent proteins. In the contiguous conduit, the Golgi apparatus, post-translation modifications such as glycosylation and isoprenylation are executed. As in the nucleus, elaborate mechanisms are in place to ensure that errors do not occur, but if they do and cannot be repaired, a cell death program is initiated. The ER/ Golgi initiates apoptosis if calcium flux is excessive, if unfolded proteins persist, or if post-translational protein modification is abnormal[31] (see Fig. 26–3). Release of the cleaved IRE protein leads to degradation of 28S RNA and termination of protein synthesis. In contrast to the DR or mitochondrial pathways, apoptosis is executed through caspase 12.[32]

ANTIAPOPTOTIC PROTEINS

Cellular homeostasis within each body system is carefully regulated. Excessive cell growth or premature cell death translate into diseases, as will be discussed in the last part of this chapter. The death and survival pathways are finely balanced and each cell death program is may be attenuated, often at multiple levels. Prior to discussion about how the death program is executed, the way in which cell death is regulated by inhibitors of apoptosis will be discussed.

Inhibition of Death Receptors

In most resting cell types that express Fas on their cell surface (e.g., lymphocytes), the receptor is nonfunctional. Resistance to death is explained by low levels of expression of the receptor, as well as by active inhibition by a protein called FLIP. FLIP resembles the structure of caspase 8 and competes with it for binding to FADD, thus diverting a Fas signal away from caspase activation and death. When lymphocytes become activated, FLIP is usually degraded, allowing Fas signal transduction to occur unimpeded. Similarly, a protein called silencer of death domain (SODD), attenuates TNF-R1 signal transduction.

The B Cell Lymphoma-2 (Bcl-2) Family of Cell Death Regulators

The B cell lymphoma (Bcl) family, includes more than 15 members.[33] Bcl-2 is the prototype antiapoptotic protein first discovered to be overexpressed in certain B cell lymphomas. Of particular significance, Bcl-2 overexpression did not enhance cell proliferation (most cells were in the G_0/G_1 phase of the cell cycle) but rendered the cells more resistant to death. Bcl-2 homologues, such as Bcl-XL (other homologues include mammalian proteins Bcl-w, Mcl-1, A1, and virus-encoded proteins, BHRF1, LMW5-HL, ORF16, KS-Bcl-2, and E1B-19K), have at least one of the characteristic Bcl-2 homology (BH) domain motifs, and most possess a hydrophobic C-terminal membrane anchor, accounting for their attachment to mitochondrial and nuclear membranes. The proapoptotic members of this family such as Bax (others include Bak, Bok, Bik, Blk, Hrk, BNIP3, Bim, Bad, and Bid) also contain BH domains. How do Bcls regulate apoptosis? One level of regulation is conferred by binding interactions (homodimerization or heterodimerization) between members[34] and their BH1, BH2, and BH3 domains. Although the outcomes vary for each specific pair, homodimerization of Bcl-2 or Bax potentiates their antiapoptotic or proapoptotic function, respectively, whereas heterodimers may potentiate or abrogate function of one member of the pair. Bcls such as Bcl-2 and Bcl-XL may also bind to Apaf-1 and prevent it from activating caspase 9, analogous to the regulation of CED-4 by CED-9 in *C. elegans* (see Fig. 26–1).

Bcl regulation of cell death is closely connected to mitochondrial function. The physical association of Bcl-2 family proteins with the outer mitochondrial membrane, as well as the close structural similarity between the BH1 and BH2 domains and bacterial pore-forming proteins such as colicin,[35] allows them to regulate ion fluxes or the transfer of small molecules from the membrane. In vitro models suggest that Bax and Bak promote opening of the VDAC, allowing the release of cytochrome-*c* into the cytosol, whereas Bcl-2 binds directly to VDAC and closes it.[28]

Intracellular Inhibitors of Apoptosis

Intracellular inhibitors of apoptosis (IAPs) are a separate family of antiapoptotic proteins that have been highly conserved through evolution. The neuronal apoptosis inhibitory protein (NAIP) was discovered through the association of NAIP mutations in patients with the severe form of spinal muscular atrophy. Four additional members of the family (i.e., c-IAP-1, c-IAP-2, X-IAP, and survivin) that share a baculovirus IAP repeat domain have subsequently been identified. Although IAPs were shown to bind to TRAFs and, therefore, were thought to function upstream in the apoptotic pathway, subsequent studies suggested that IAPs inhibited effector caspases.[36] IAPs block apoptosis induced by a variety of stimuli, including Fas, TNF-α, ultraviolet irradiation, and serum withdrawal, and survivin is overexpressed in certain cancers and in the rheumatoid arthritis synovium.[37] In some cells, the antiapoptotic effect of IAPs is eliminated by the release of a protein called Smac/Diablo from the mitochondria.

Caspases

Caspases are cysteine-containing proteases that have an unusual substrate specificity for peptidyl sequences with a P1 aspartate residue.[38,39] These proteases are 30 to 55 kD and comprise an amino-terminal prodomain, with a large subunit domain and a small subunit domain (see Figure 26–2). The active-site cysteine residue is contained within the conserved pentapeptide, QACxG, on the large subunit of the enzyme, whereas most of the substrate specificity is determined by the small subunit. The upstream caspases 8, 9, 10, 2, and 4 have large prodomains that interact with regulatory proteins such as FADD for caspases 8 and 10 and Apaf-1 for caspase 9 (see Fig. 26–3). Presumably, clustering of these complexes allows autocatalytic cleavage of the large and small subdomains to form the active tetramer. However, more recent findings show that the upstream caspases 8 and 9 can become activated even in their full-length form, through dimerization with themselves or related proteins. Effector caspases such as 3, 6, and 7 have small prodomains and are thought to be cleaved into their active forms by the upstream caspases.

Members of the caspase family can be divided into three functional subgroups based on their substrate specificities.[40] Group I members (caspases 1, 4, and 5) are potently inhibited by the serpin CrmA; group II members (caspases 2, 3, and 7) are specific for DExD; and group III members (caspases 6, 8, 9, and 10) are specific for I/V/LExD, a sequence that is also contained at the junctions of the caspase subunits themselves. Significantly, granzyme B produced by cytotoxic T cells has a substrate specificity similar to that of group III caspases and is capable of inducing apoptosis through this pathway. Identification of the substrate specificity of caspases has led to a number of practical applications, including the ability to quantify activity using fluorogenic tetrapeptide substrates and blockade of proteolytic activity with noncleavable cell-permeable tetrapeptide analogues.

The effector caspases are necessary for the execution of apoptosis. They cleave specific substrates such as the structural proteins fodrin, gelsolin, and lamins, key intracellular enzymes involved in DNA repair (e.g., poly adenosine diphosphate [ADP] ribose polymerase, DNA-PK) (see Fig. 26–3). These changes facilitate inactivation of synthetic functions of the cell, dissolution of the nuclear membrane, and packaging of cellular proteins into apoptotic blebs on the cell surface. Caspases also cleave regulatory proteins such as Bcl family members and the inhibitor of caspase-activated DNase (ICAD). Cleavage of ICAD leads to the release of active CAD, which enters the nucleus and cleaves nucleosomes at the linker region, yielding the characteristic "DNA ladder"[41,42] (see Fig. 26–3 and Fig. 26–5G).

Not all caspases are involved in the execution of apoptosis. Human caspases 1, 4, 5, and mouse caspase 11 and

12 are most likely involved in inflammation. Caspase 1 was originally defined as the enzyme that cleaves interleukin-1 (IL-1)–converting enzyme (ICE) into its active form. Recently, it has been shown that caspase 1 and caspase 5 interact and form a multiprotein complex that has been called the inflammasome (analogous to the apoptosome).[43] Caspase 1 and 5 bind to the adaptor proteins, ASC (PYCARD) and NALP1 (DECAP), respectively, by their CARD domains. ASC and NALP1 are mutidomain proteins that contain many of the protein-interaction domains listed in Table 26–1. The protein, pyrin, that is mutated in familial Mediterranean fever (FMF), binds to ASC. Mutation of pyrin, therefore, most likely leads to inflammation through uncontrolled activation of caspase 1 and IL-1β.[44]

Caspases are tightly regulated by their own prodomains and by Bcl and IAP family members. In addition, viral proteins such as the serpin CrmA, produced by cowpox, and p35, produced by baculovirus, are potent inhibitors of caspases.

Removal of Apoptotic Cells

Of the 14 *C. elegans* death genes (*ced1* through *ced14*), at least half encode proteins that are required for engulfment of apoptotic cells[45] (see Fig. 26–2). CED 7 is present in the membranes of both the apoptotic cell and phagocyte, whereas the remaining proteins function in the phagocyte to execute two partially overlapping pathways of engulfment. CED 1 is a receptor that recognizes changes in the apoptotic cell and signals through CED 6 to activate the phagocyte. CED2, 5, 10, and 12 most likely form a functional complex that promotes the cytoskeletal changes required to engulf the apoptotic prey.[46]

Within the immune system alone, more than 10^8 apoptotic cells are removed from the body each day. These apoptotic cells are generated in vast numbers in the central lymphoid organs such as the thymus and bone marrow by out-of-frame rearrangements of antigen receptors, negative selection, or simple "neglect." A significant load of apoptotic cells is produced in the peripheral immune system because of the relatively short life span of lymphocytes and myeloid cells and secondary selection of high-affinity B cells in germinal centers. The specialized sites of selection (i.e., thymus, bone marrow, and lymphoid follicles) have remarkably efficient phagocytes that rapidly remove the dying cells.

An early event during apoptosis is the appearance of phosphatidylserine (PS) on the cell surface membrane (see Fig. 26–3). This membrane asymmetry (PS is usually located on the inner surface of the membrane) is caused by the reduced function of a translocase and possibly by activation of a lipid scramblase.[47] PS is an important ligand for phagocytosis of apoptotic cells,[48] and the receptor has been identified as a 70-kD member of the cupin family of metalloenzymes.[49] Similarly, sugars such as N-acetyl-glucosamine and N-acetyl-galactosamine may be selectively exposed on the apoptotic membrane, triggering ingestion of the cell.[50]

Despite the detection of only limited chemical alterations on the apoptotic cell membrane, blockade of a

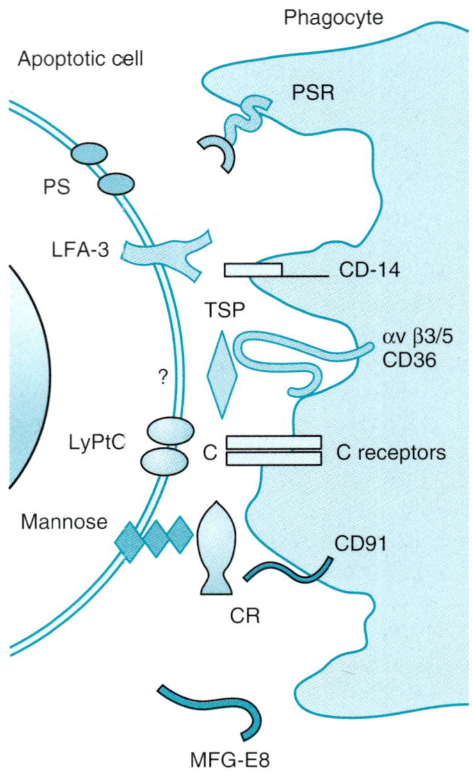

FIGURE 26–4 • Receptors and ligands implicated in recognition or phagocytosis of apoptotic cells. For receptors shown at in the bottom half of the diagram, serum opsonins are required for optimal phagocytosis. C, complement; CR, calreticulin; LyPtC, lysophosphatidylcholine; PS, phosphatidylserine; TSP, thrombospondin.

large and diverse number of receptors on phagocytes can impair the uptake of apoptotic cells (Fig. 26–4). This diversity may in part be explained by the different cells and conditions used for phagocytic assays, but it undoubtedly also reflects the overlapping and partially redundant function of each individual receptor. All the receptors identified have other functions, perhaps reflecting an evolution from receptors designed to remove apoptotic cells during development to pattern-recognition receptors useful for host defense.[51] Many of the receptors are integrins comprising the vitronectin receptor, $\alpha_v\beta_3$,[52] $\alpha_v\beta5$,[53] complement receptors 3 (CD11b/CD18) and 4 (CD11c/CD18),[54] and class A and B scavenger receptors.[55-57] Nonintegrin receptors include the ATP-binding cassette transporter (ABC1)[58] and CD14.[59] In some cases, phagocytosis of apoptotic cells requires serum factors such as thrombospondin to bridge the $\alpha_v\beta_3$ and CD36 receptors,[60] as well as serum complement,[54] which is amplified on apoptotic cell membranes by natural immunoglobulin M (IgM) antibodies,[61] mannose-binding protein, and acute phase proteins such as C-reactive protein (CRP). Other proteins, such as calreticulin, MFG-E8, and Gas6, have been implicated in promoting the phagocytosis of apoptotic cells in certain contexts. Finally, engagement of the closely related Tyro 3–family receptor tyrosine kinases, MER, TYRO, and Axl, by their ligands, such as Gas6, protein S, appear to be required to prevent production of IL-12 or TNF-α from macrophages that have ingested apoptotic cells.[62]

The precise mechanisms by which apoptotic cells are taken up, processed, and eliminated are not well characterized. Of considerable interest is their effect on the phagocyte. In vitro[63,64] and some in vivo[65] studies suggest that uptake of apoptotic cells induces the expression of immunosuppressive cytokines such as transforming growth factor–β1 (TGF-β1), prostaglandin E_2, and possibly IL-10, by macrophages. These cytokines tend to dampen an immune response to self antigens. In contrast, if cells become necrotic, ingestion by phogocytes induces TNF-α and other proinflammatory cytokines.[63,66] Because some peptides derived from apoptotic cells can be presented to lymphocytes by dendritic cells and possibly by macrophages through cross-priming,[53,67] a question of critical importance to studies of autoimmunity is whether self peptides are presented after phagocytosis of apoptotic cells and under what conditions they induce tolerance or immunity.

Detection of Apoptosis

Numerous methods have been devised to detect cells undergoing apoptosis. These methods depend on the biochemical changes in the cell described previously and are depicted in Fig. 26–5.

CELL MEMBRANE ALTERATIONS

Annexin V binds to negatively charged phospholipids in a calcium-dependent manner and therefore can readily detect the flip of phosphatidylserine to the outer surface of the cell membrane (see Fig. 26–5A). When annexin V is conjugated to FITC, biotin or other markers, it provides a convenient tag for detecting apoptotic cells by flow cytometry.[68] Flow cytometry detection with Annexin V is simple, sensitive, and detects cells at an early stage of apoptosis. Annexin V will also bind to necrotic cell membranes before complete rupture of the cell. Entry of trypan blue, as seen by light microscopy, or propidium iodide, as quantified by flow cytometry, into the cell indicates profound damage to the cell membrane, which is indicative of necrosis.

LOSS OF MITOCHONDRIAL MEMBRANE POTENTIAL

As discussed previously, multiple stimuli lead to apoptosis through the intrinsic mitochondrial pathway, resulting in a loss of membrane potential. Several dyes, including rhodamine 123, TMRM (see Fig 26–5B), and DiOC6, bind relatively selectively to mitochondria, and thus provide a fairly sensitive measure of membrane potential.

CASPASE ACTIVATION

As discussed previously, caspases are normally present in an inactive state, but once activated, they recognize specific tetrapetide sequences. Therefore, caspase activity can be quantified directly in intact cells by flow-cytometry analysis with cell-permeable fluorochrome tetrapeptide conjugates, or in cell extracts by enzyme-linked immunosorbent assay (ELISA) that detect release of colorimetric dyes conjugated to the tetrapeptides. Caspase activation can also be quantified indirectly, by western blot analysis of cleavage of specific caspase substrates. Cleavage of the nuclear protein, poly-(ADP-ribose) polymerase (PARP), is frequently used to evaluate activation of caspase 3 (see Fig. 26–5C).

CHROMATIN CONDENSATION AND DNA FRAGMENTATION

Condensation of chromatin can be seen by light microscopy following nuclear staining (see Fig. 26–5D). This can be a sensitive screening method, depending on the experience of the viewer, but confirmation with a more specific assay is usually required for verification. Chromatin condensation is more easily seen by staining with vital dyes such as Hoechst No. 33342 bisBENZIMIDE (2′-(4-Ethoxyphenyl)-5-(4-methyl-1-piperazinyl)-2,5′-bi-1H-benzimidazole) or DAPI (4′,6-diamidino-2-phenylindole) and inspection under fluorescence microscopy (see Fig. 26–5E). For precise quantification of nuclear condensation, DNA staining with propidium iodide and flow-cytometry analysis of condensed (subdiploid) DNA is widely used[69] (see Fig. 26–5F).

As mentioned previously, DNA is cleaved by multiple DNAses, leading to the cleavage of nucleosomes at the linker region, and yielding the characteristic "DNA ladder" (see Fig. 26–5G). DNA fragmentation results in free 3′-OH groups, which can be detected within the nuclei in tissue sections using biotinylated dNTPs (TUNEL assay)[70] (see Fig. 26–5H). Whereas formation of the ladder is specific to apoptosis, generation of free ends of DNA is not, and it may also be detected in DNA damaged by necrosis.

Apoptosis in Relation to Rheumatic Disorders

The regulation of apoptosis is highly relevant to the pathogenesis and treatment of rheumatic disorders. Pertinent examples are discussed in the following sections and are reviewed elsewhere.[71]

APOPTOTIC CELLS IN TOLERANCE AND AUTOIMMUNITY

Autoantibodies were discovered in the 1940s and 1950s and their molecular and functional identities have been characterized in the 1980s and 1990s. Why the immune system targets a select subset of self antigens in each disease has never been satisfactorily explained. One hypothesis to explain antigen selection is that alterations occurring during cell death render the byproducts of dying cells, such as negatively charged phospholipids and nucleosomes (see Fig. 26–3), more antigenic. A number of clinical and experimental observations lend support to this hypothesis.

Nucleosomes are detected in the circulation of systemic lupus erythematosus (SLE) patients with active disease.[72] Autoantibodies to nucleosomes precede those to DNA and histones,[73,74] and nucleosomes are more

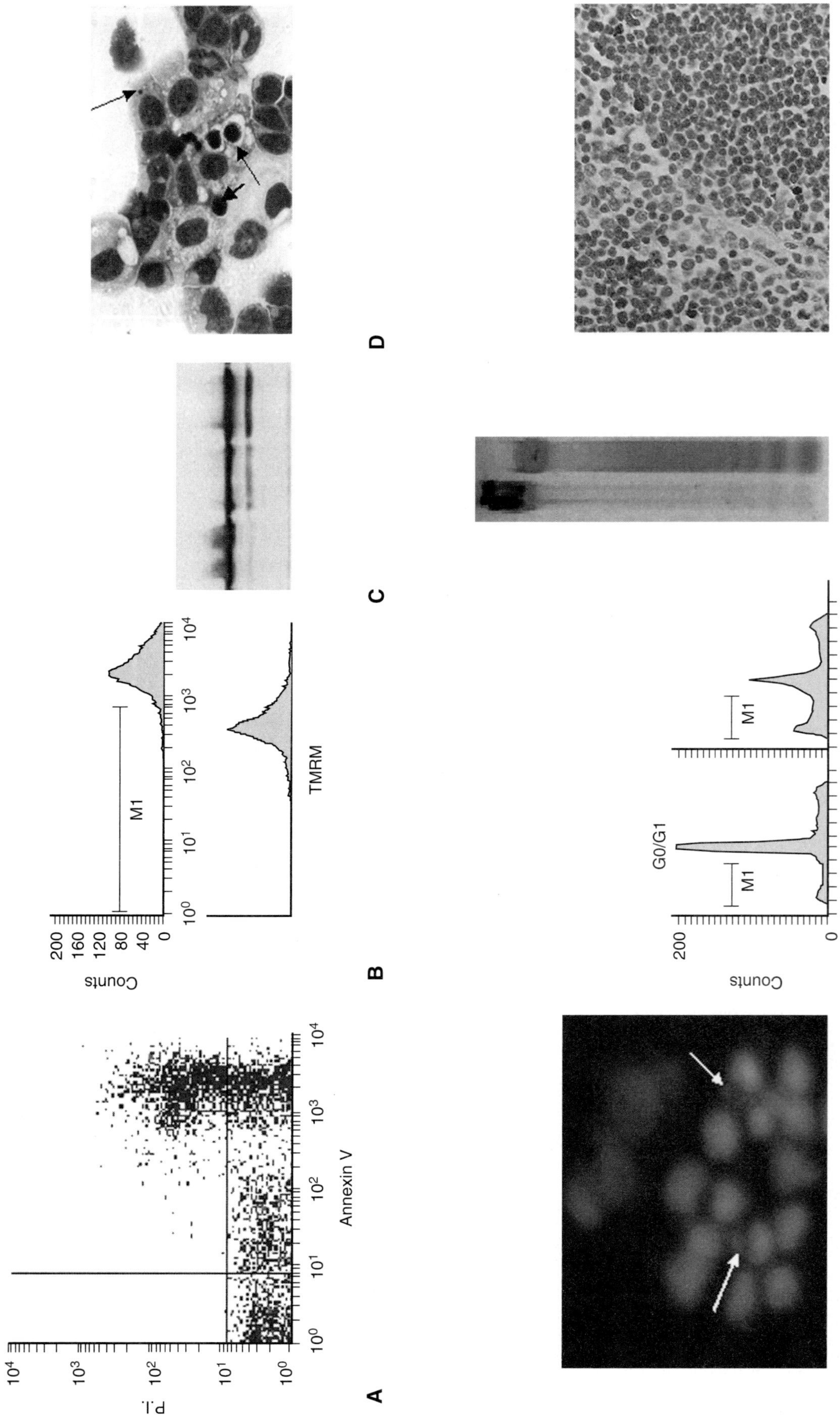
A
B
C
D
E
F
G
H
P.I.
Annexin V
Counts
M1
TMRM
G0/G1

FIGURE 26–5 · Methods for detection of apoptotic cells. A variety of methods are available for the identification and quantification of dying cells, a sampling is shown here. A through C depend on changes to the cell surface membrane, mitochondria, and caspase activation, whereas D through H detect changes in the nucleus.

A, Apoptotic thymocytes were incubated with FITC-conjugated annexin V in the presence of the dye propidium iodide (PI) that permeates cells with severely damaged cell membranes. Note that cells in the bottom left quadrant (not stained for annexin or PI) are live; cells in the lower right quadrant are early apoptotic; and cells in the upper right quadrant are late apoptotic (stain with annexin and admit PI). For cells in suspension, such as lymphocytes, annexin V binding to phosphatidylserine (PS) is the most commonly used method to detect early apoptotic cells.

B, Human embryonic kidney cells were incubated in medium alone (*upper panel*) or medium containing valinomycin, an ionophore that increases ionic permeability of the inner mitochondrial membrane (*lower panel*). The cells were then incubated with tetramethylrhodamine methyl ester (TMRM), a cell-permeable dye that binds to the outer mitochondrial membrane proportional to its membrane potential ($\Delta\psi$), and analyzed by flow cytometry. Note that the fluorescence intensity for the apoptotic cells is lower due to loss of mitochondrial membrane potential (MMP). Other probes used in similar assays for mitochondrial potential are rhodamine 123 and the carbocyanine dye, DiOC6.

C, Cells were induced to undergo apoptosis by anti-Fas antibodies. Cell extracts taken at 0, 4, and 6 hours postinduction were analyzed for poly-ADP ribose polymerase (PARP) cleavage by western blot analysis. Note that the 4- and 6-hour samples show partial cleavage of PARP (*arrow*).

D, Mouse peritoneal macrophages were incubated with apoptotic thymocytes, cytocentrifuged onto glass slides, and stained with Diffquik (Dade Behring, AG). The arrows indicate ingested apoptototic cells with condensed nuclei.

E, Jurkat T cells were induced to undergo apoptosis, stained with the dye bisBENZIMIDE (Hoechst No.33342. Sigma, St. Louis) and viewed by immunofluorescence microscopy. The arrows indicate condensed nuclei.

F, Normal (*left panel*) or apoptotic (*right panel*) cells were permeabilized, incubated with RNase, and their DNA stained with P.I. according to the method of Nicoletti and colleagues.[69] The cells were analyzed by flow cytometry, and staining in the subdiploid peak (smaller than the G0/G1 peak and labeled M1 in the histogram) reflects the extent of apoptosis.

G, Normal and apoptotic cells were lysed and the nuclei removed by centrifugation. Cytosolic extracts were then applied to agarose gels and components resolved by electrophoresis. Ethidium bromide staining of the extract made from live cells reveals high-molecular-weight DNA that remains close to the application well (*left lane*), whereas the extract from apoptotic cells demonstrates loss of high-molecular-weight DNA and the appearance of the typical ladder of nucleosomes.

H, Six-micron sections were made from a normal mouse thymus. The cells were permeabilized and incubated with biotinylated deoxyuridine triphosphate (d-UTP) in the presence of terminal deoxynucleotidyl transferase (TdT). Nicked DNA incorporated the labeled deoxynucleotide and was detected by staining with peroxidase-labeled streptavidin and substrate (*dark color*).

strongly antigenic for T cells[75] and B cells than DNA or histones alone. Nucleosomes, but not isolated DNA or histones, deposit in the glomeruli, suggesting that the in situ fixation of nucleosomes, rather than DNA/anti-DNA immune complexes, causes lupus nephritis.[76,77] Many of the SLE antigens redistribute to apoptotic blebs when cells such as keratinocytes undergo programmed cell death.[78] Some of these antigens undergo modification, including cleavage and phosphorylation.[79-81] A particularly relevant antigen in this context is PS, which translocates to the cell surface during apoptosis and is recognized by certain anticardiolipin antibodies.[82] An increase in the rate of apoptosis of SLE peripheral blood mononuclear cells has been observed in vitro,[83,84] suggesting that accelerated apoptosis occurs in vivo. This may explain lymphopenia in SLE patients.[85]

Because apoptosis occurs on a vast scale in the central lymphoid organs and should tolerize the host, under what conditions would apoptotic cells immunize? Several possibilities should be considered. One or more death receptors or biochemical pathways of apoptosis could be dysfunctional, leading to aberrant response to or processing of the apoptotic material, subsequently leading to immune-cell activation. If apoptosis occurs in the presence of an adjuvant (virus, bacteria, or chemicals) tolerance may be lost, at least transiently. Abnormalities leading to the accelerated apoptosis of cells in the periphery or reduced uptake of dying cells will allow cells to undergo postapoptotic necrosis which, in turn, will provoke a proinflammatory cytokine response from phagocytes,[63] as explained previously. Experiments in mice and in human cells in culture indicate that phagocytosis of apoptotic cells is impaired in the absence of early complement components,[54,86] and it is well known that deficiencies of early complement components predispose to human SLE.[87] Knockout of members of the Tyro 3–receptor tyrosine kinases is associated with defective clearance of apoptotic cells and the expression of a lupus-like disease.[62,88] It is also likely that the lupus-like diseases that occur in mice deficient in DNase 1 or the acute-phase protein serum amyloid P protein (SAP) result from reduced clearance of apoptotic cell debris.[89,90]

MUTATIONS IN DEATH RECEPTORS

Mice with mutations of Fas or Fas ligand (FasL) develop a syndrome characterized by lymphoproliferation (*lpr*) and generalized lymphadenopathy (*gld*) together with systemic autoimmunity.[91] As might be expected from the key role described for Fas in AICD, lymphadenopathy and splenomegaly are the consequence of failure of activated lymphocytes to die, resulting in an absolute increase in the numbers of T and B lymphocytes, as well as by the accumulation of an unusual subset of T cells that do not express CD4 or CD8 coreceptors (i.e., double-negative T cells). These double-negative cells are derived from previously activated T cells that have failed to undergo apoptosis but have downregulated expression of their coreceptor. The nature and extent of systemic autoimmunity varies according to the strain into which the Fas or FasL mutation has been bred.[91]

A syndrome of massive lymphadenopathy with systemic autoimmunity in children was reported by Canale and Smith in 1967. Subsequently, these and other *lpr* patients were found to have mutations in Fas.[92-94] The syndrome (called Canale-Smith syndrome [CSS] or autoimmune lymphoproliferative syndrome [ALPS]) is characterized by lymphadenopathy or splenomegaly, autoimmune cytopenias (most commonly affecting platelets and red cells), and an increase (of more than 5 percent) in circulating double-negative T cells. These patients had defective lymphocyte apoptosis in response to anti-Fas antibodies or FasL when tested in vitro, and most had heterozygous mutations in Fas affecting the DD. These mutations impair Fas-mediated apoptosis through a dominant negative effect.[95,96]

Although isolated cases of SLE patients with Fas[97] or FasL[98] mutations have been described, Fas and FasL are not mutated in the majority of SLE patients.[99] Nevertheless, the ALPS/Canale-Smith syndrome is informative because it suggests that defective apoptosis of cells of the immune system can cause systemic autoimmune diseases such as SLE, idiopathic thrombocytopenic purpura, autoimmune hemolytic anemia, and Guillain-Barré syndrome. It illustrates (as do the mouse models) that even when a single gene has a powerful effect on predisposition to systemic autoimmunity, the clinical expression of disease depends on the precise nature of the mutation[95,96] and the interaction of modifiers.

There are several other examples of genetic alterations in death or survival genes that lead to lupus-like diseases in mice. [100] Of particular interest is the overexpression of the ligand for the BlyS/BAFF/TALL/zTNF receptor that promotes the survival of B lymphocytes,[101] because increased expression of this ligand has been reported in SLE as well as in Sjogren's syndrome.[102] Finally, mutations in the p55/TNF-R1/CD120a receptor in humans results in a periodic autoinflammatory syndrome called tumor necrosis factor receptor associated periodic syndrome (TRAPS). Mutations predominantly occur in the first two CRDs of the receptor, resulting in reduced shedding of the extracellular domain of the receptor and reduced neutralization of circulating TNF-α.[44]

PROLONGED EXPOSURE TO GROWTH FACTORS

Histologically, rheumatoid arthritis (RA) is characterized by an accumulation of inflammatory cells in the synovium, leading to pannus formation and destruction of cartilage and bone. Although Fas and FasL can be detected in RA synovium, and evidence of apoptosis has been detected in RA synoviocytes,[103,104] the extent of synoviocyte apoptosis is not adequate to counteract ongoing proliferation. This imbalance is explained by a number of factors. First, FasL is expressed at relatively low levels on synovial T cells,[105] and soluble Fas or FasL competitors may impede Fas-induced apoptosis. Cytokines, such as TNF-α, IL-1β, and TGF-β1, that are overexpressed in the joints of patients with RA, favor synoviocyte proliferation and inhibit susceptibility to apoptosis.[106-108] These and other signals reduce apoptosis of synoviocytes through activation of NFκB and increased expression of antiapoptotic proteins.[109-111] Growth of the pannus is compounded by inflammatory changes such as oxidation that result in upregulation and mutations of the growth suppressor protein p53[112] (Fig. 26–6).

The observations regarding apoptosis regulators in RA are significant because they provide an opportunity for therapeutic manipulation. Local administration of anti-Fas monoclonal antibodies to human T cell lymphotropic virus-1 *tax* transgenic mice or Fas ligand to collagen arthritis (mouse models of RA) led to an improvement in arthritis.[113,114] Several strategies to modulate NFκB attenuate the growth of synovial cells. Interestingly, administration of TRAIL also attenuated experimental arthritis, although this was not thought to be due to apoptosis.[115]

Evidence is accumulating that fibroblasts in scleroderma may also be more resistant to apoptosis and that TGF-β may promote this phenotype.[116]

TISSUE INJURY IN ORGAN-SPECIFIC AUTOIMMUNITY

In contrast to systemic autoimmune diseases characterized by B lymphocyte stimulation that leads to antibody and immune complex–mediated tissue injury, many organ-specific autoimmune diseases are caused by a cell-mediated attack, leading to the death of specific cell types within the organ. Cell targets are β cells of the islets of Langerhans of the pancreas in insulin-dependent diabetes mellitus, oligodendrocytes in the brain in multiple sclerosis, the salivary and lacrimal glands in Sjögren's syndrome, and myocytes in polymyositis.[117] Programmed pathways of apoptosis can be implicated in disease pathogenesis, as illustrated by the resistance

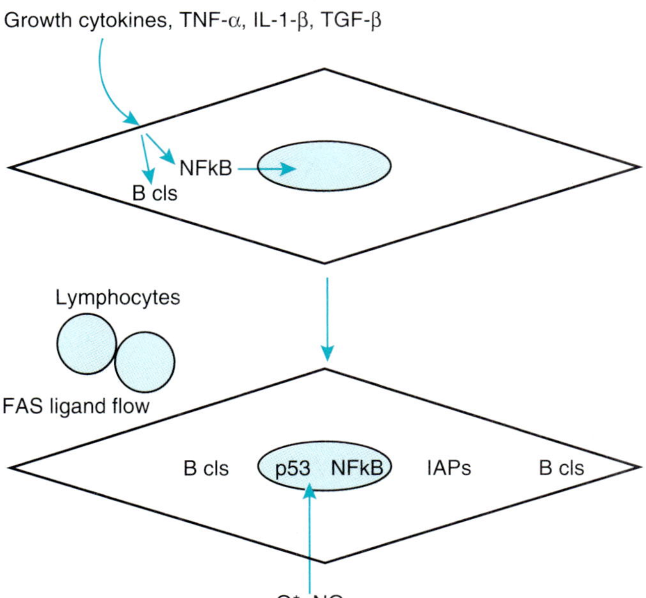

FIGURE 26–6 · Antiapoptotic Phenotype of Rheumatoid Synovial Fibroblasts. Cytokines and growth factors lead to activation of nuclear factor kappa B(NFκB) and overexpression of antiapoptotic proteins such B cell lymphoma-2 (Bcl-2). Inflammatory stimuli, release of nitric oxide (NO), and reactive oxygen intermediates (O*) upregulate and induce mutations of p53. Infiltrating lymphocytes have a Fas ligand "low" phenotype.

of Fas-deficient (*lpr*) mice to diseases such as diabetes and experimental encephalomyelitis. In many of these diseases, cell death at the site of injury can also be directly demonstrated by DNA fragmentation (TUNEL staining) in situ. Apoptosis is usually considered noninflammatory but, as discussed previously, the context of cell death influences the immune response. For example, cytotoxic T lymphocytes (CTL), which induce cell death predominantly by perforin-mediated cell lysis (necrosis), or macrophage defects, which lead to delayed clearance of dying cells, will promote the release of proinflammatory cytokines such as TNF-α.

In most organ-specific autoimmune diseases, especially those for which adoptive transfers have been performed in animal models, $CD4^+$ T cells have been shown to be critically involved in disease pathogenesis. The disease-promoting CD4 T cells are restricted by major histocompatibility complex (MHC) class II molecules and are therefore unlikely to exert a direct cytotoxic action on the class I–bearing target cell. CD4 cells may arm other effectors through the production of cytokines (γ-interferon); they may induce tissue injury through a "bystander pathway" involving macrophages or induce receptors for cell death on the target cell "assisted suicide pathway." In Hashimoto's thyroiditis in humans,[118] as well as a mouse model of Sjogren's syndrome in nonobese diabetic (NOD) *scid* mice[119] (i.e., diabetes-prone mice lacking mature T and B lymphocytes), glandular cells constitutively express FasL, and it is the regulated expression of Fas that allows for pathologic cell death and expression of disease. In Sjögren's syndrome in humans, there is controversy about whether Fas or FasL is constitutively expressed in normal salivary glands, but the coexpression of both molecules in patients with Sjögren's syndrome presumably causes cell death of acinar and ductal cells.[120]

Inflammatory myopathies, such as polymyositis (PM) and dermatomyositis (DM), are autoimmune diseases that result in destruction of skeletal muscle fibers. Although Fas is upregulated on the myocytes in these diseases, expression is also increased in nonautoimmune muscle disorders such as metabolic myopathies, denervating disorders, and muscular dystrophies, but not in normal human muscle tissue.[121] Detection of FasL on mononuclear cells invading the muscles in PM and DM patients with apoptosis of muscle cells implicates Fas/FasL in tissue injury in myositis.[122] Increased expression of the T cell cytotoxic mediator perforin in some PM and DM patients[123] indicates that granzyme-mediated myocyte injury is also involved. Intriguingly, the tRNA synthetase antigens or their cleavage products may perpetuate inflammation by exerting chemotactic recruitment of immune cells through chemokine receptors.[124]

ACCELERATED APOPTOSIS IN DEGENERATIVE RHEUMATIC DISORDERS

Apoptosis of chondrocytes occurs during normal development of joints, and accelerated cell death may also be important in diseases such as osteoarthritis (OA). The main mechanism underlying primary or secondary osteoarthritis is degradation of cartilage. Degradation is mediated by enzymatic and nitric oxide (NO)-induced breakdown of the extracellular matrix and insufficient new matrix synthesis. Normal and OA-derived chondrocytes in the superficial and middle cartilage zones, the major areas involved in early cartilage degeneration, express Fas and are sensitive to Fas-mediated death.[125] Chondrocytes obtained from patients with OA have enhanced spontaneous apoptosis in these zones, compared to normal controls.[126,127] Although NO is also capable of inducing apoptosis in chondrocytes, it does not seem to act through the Fas pathway.[125] In an experimental model of OA, transgenic mice lacking type II collagen, the main constituent of the extracellular matrix in cartilage, had high levels of apoptosis in their chondrocytes.[128] Together, these findings suggest that apoptosis of chondrocytes plays a role in OA and that inhibitors of NO synthesis may be of value in treating this disease. The therapeutic use of intra-articular Fas agonists in RA may be deleterious to chondrocytes.

Osteoporosis is a common disorder resulting from increased bone resorption, decreased bone synthesis, or a combination of the two. Several reports support the concept that estrogen exerts its beneficial effect in preventing osteoporosis by the induction of apoptosis in the bone-resorbing osteoclasts,[129,130] and glucocorticoid-induced osteoporosis may also be explained by an increased rate of apoptosis of osteoblasts and osteocytes.[131] In the presence of M-CSF, osteoclasts differentiate from a myeloid precursor common to macrophages and dendritic cells. In addition to the numerous factors influencing bone turnover,[132] a soluble member of the TNF-R family, osteoprotegerin (OPG) or osteoclastogenesis-inhibitory factor (OCIF), inhibits osteoclast activity after binding to its cognate ligand OPGL (OPG ligand/TRANCE/RANKL).[133,134] OPG/RANK ligand is expressed on osteoblasts and on activated T cells. Engagement of the membrane form of the receptor induces activation of NFκB, thereby enhancing the formation, survival, and resorptive activity of osteoclasts.

DRUGS THAT AFFECT APOPTOTIC PATHWAYS

Until very recently, therapy for inflammatory rheumatic disorders had been largely empiric. The types of drugs used include anti-inflammatory agents, such as corticosteroids and nonsteroidals (NSAIDs); immunomodulatory drugs, such as cyclosporine; and cytotoxic drugs, such as cyclophosphamide and azathioprine. Because most of these drugs impinge on critical biochemical events within the cell, it is not surprising that they have effects on pathways of apoptosis.

Anti-inflammatory Drugs

Glucocorticoids at high doses induce the death of lymphoid cells. Involvement of caspases[135] suggests that apoptotic programs are activated. Corticosteroids modulate expression of a large number of molecules that affect apoptotic programs—cytokines, cell cycle control proteins, c-myc, Bcl-2—and inhibit NFκB activation, but the precise pathways relevant to clinical efficacy remain to be defined. Patients on long-term steroid therapy are also susceptible to osteoporosis and osteonecrosis, which may be explained by bone loss caused by apoptosis of osteoblasts and osteocytes.[131]

NSAIDs' major mechanism of action is inhibition of cyclooxygenases (COXs), which reduce the production of proinflammatory cytokines and prostaglandins (see Chapter 56). NSAIDs also are effective in the chemoprevention of colorectal tumors in genetically susceptible individuals. Their antineoplastic properties may be explained by an increase of the prostaglandin precursor arachidonic acid and by conversion of sphingomyelin to ceramide, a proapoptotic lipid.[136,137]

Immunomodulatory Drugs

Cyclosporine and a closely related macrolide antibiotic, FK506, have potent immunosuppressive properties and are used to prevent allograft rejection. Both drugs modulate T and B cell immune responses by interfering with NFAT-mediated IL-2 gene transcription, NO synthase activation, cell degranulation, and apoptosis.[138] The reduced cytotoxic T lymphocyte activity is explained in part by impaired FasL induction, secondary to the effect on NFAT,[139,140] but effects on mitochondrial function have also been demonstrated. Certain cell types, such as renal proximal tubules and synoviocytes or endothelial cells in RA, may be more susceptible to the proapoptotic effects of cyclosporine.[141]

Cytotoxic Drugs

Many cytotoxic or immunosuppressive drugs that induce the suicide of lymphocytes, mostly through the p53 pathway (see Fig.26–3), exert some anti-inflammatory effect. Although methotrexate has effects on adenosine receptors, even low-dose methotrexate induces apoptosis of activated lymphocytes in vitro and in RA patients, probably in a Fas-independent manner.[142] Cyclophosphamide is an alkylating agent commonly used to treat many human cancers and severe autoimmune disease. Its efficacy has partly been attributed to apoptosis of tumor cells and perhaps of mesangial cells in glomerulonephritis.[143] Induction of apoptosis may also account for certain adverse effects, such as oligospermia or azoospermia and pancreatic β cell destruction.

Biphosphonates are the most potent antiresorptive drugs available and are widely used to treat various metabolic bone diseases, such as Paget's disease, bone tumors, ectopic calcification, and osteoporosis. Although individual members of this family differ somewhat in their effects, their general mechanisms of action include direct and indirect effects on osteoclast recruitment, function, and survival[144] (see also Chapter 90).

Tumor Necrosis Factor-α Blockade

The remarkable success of anti–TNF-α therapy for the treatment of RA, other arthritides, and Crohn's disease is generally attributed to blockade of TNF-α stimulation of the proinflammatory NFκB pathway (see Fig 26–3).[145] However, in Crohn's disease, it has also been suggested that anti–TNF-α monoclonal antibodies ameliorate disease through binding to cell associated TNF-α and induction of apoptosis of macrophages.[146,147]

Potential for Therapeutic Intervention

Understanding the biochemical pathways that regulate apoptosis offers new opportunities for therapeutic intervention (Fig. 26–7). In some situations, such as Sjögren's syndrome or polymyositis, it may be beneficial to induce apoptosis of the cytotoxic effector cell or of the target cell itself (e.g., the rheumatoid pannus) (see Fig. 26–7A, 1). If a death receptor is selectively expressed on the cell to be killed, a death ligand could be administered.

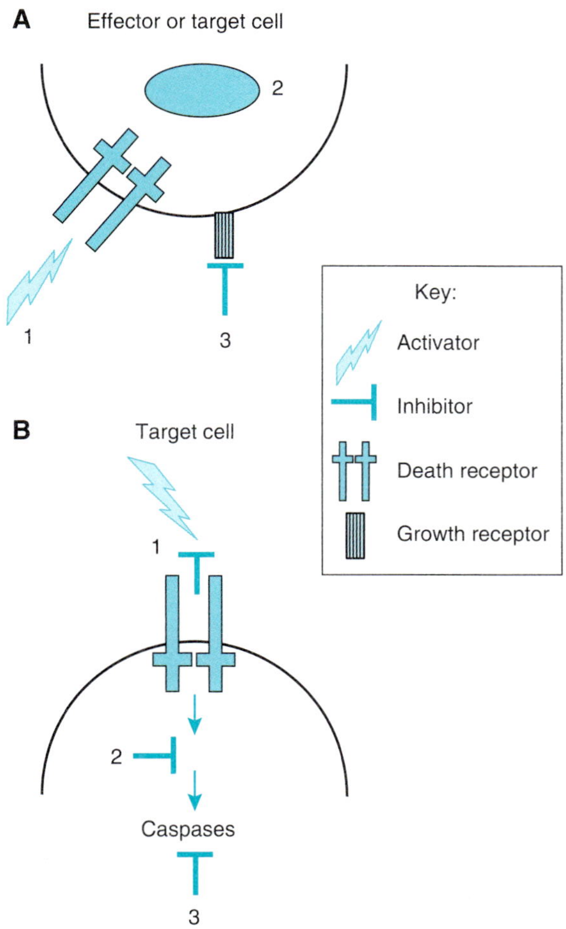

FIGURE 26–7 · Avenues for Therapeutic Manipulation of Apoptosis. *A*, To eliminate effector cells that cause disease, such as cytotoxic lymphocytes, or to kill unwanted target cells (e.g., activated fibroblasts in rheumatoid arthritis [RA] or osteoclasts in osteoarthritis [OA]), apoptosis can be directly induced by an appropriate death ligand or agonist antibody (*1*). Alternatively, the intrinsic death pathway can be initiated from within the cell (*2*) by gene-therapy approaches (e.g., expressing a proapoptotic protein such as Bax or blocking NFκB) or by using drugs that induce apoptosis, frequently through the p53 pathway. Finally, cells can be eliminated by blocking essential growth receptors or ligands with antibodies or soluble receptor fusion proteins (*3*) An example is blockade of tumor necrosis factor (TNF)-α in RA. *B*, To protect or rescue cells from apoptosis, death receptors or ligands can be blocked with soluble fusion proteins (*1*), antiapoptotic genes (such as B cell lymphoma-2 [Bcl-2]) can be introduced into the cell (*2*), or, farther downstream, cell-permeable caspase inhibitors (*3*) can block the execution phase of apoptosis.

Examples of such a strategy are the use of Fas agonists in experimental arthritis and TRAIL to selectively kill cancer cells in vivo.[148] Proapoptotic pathways could also be initiated from within the cell by gene-therapy approaches (see Fig. 26–7A, 2). Examples include blockade of NFκB or overexpression of Bax. Similarly, as discussed previously, if a cytokine or growth promoter such as TNF-α in RA or OPG/RANK ligand in osteoporosis contributes to disease, it can be blocked by a monoclonal antibody or soluble receptor fusion protein (see Fig.26–7A, 3).

In diseases in which apoptotic cell death leads to loss of organ function, the death ligand could be blocked by a monoclonal antibody or soluble receptor fusion protein (see Fig. 26–7B, 1). Even when the death pathway has not been fully determined, attempts can be made to interfere with upstream components of apoptosis well before the "point of no return." Antiapoptotic genes with limited (e.g., the protein FLIP blocks the Fas pathway) or broad (e.g., Bcl-2 family) specificity can be introduced into the cell (see Fig. 26–7B, 2). Further downstream, cell-permeable caspase inhibitors (see Fig. 26–7B, 3) can block the execution phase of apoptosis in vivo, as has been illustrated experimentally.[149] All these approaches are feasible, but they are limited by their potential adverse effects. Therapy must be relatively specific for the target cell, because widespread prevention of cell death for sustained periods is likely to predispose to neoplasia.

Conclusions

Death and survival of cells are highly regulated and, the dissection of the biochemical pathways activated by different modes of intracellular stress have made an enormous contribution to our understanding of the pathophysiology of human disease. Inherited mutations of apoptosis-regulatory molecules may cause systemic autoimmunity, dysregulation, or misdirection of other cell death and survival molecules, contributing to a whole range of musculoskeletal disorders. Many of the drugs used to treat musculoskeletal disorders exert potent effects on apoptotic programs. All these findings suggest that further understanding of the regulation of apoptosis will have widespread implications for the pathogenesis and therapeutic manipulation of rheumatic disorders.

ACKNOWLEDGEMENTS

Help and discussion from current and past laboratory members is gratefully acknowledged.

REFERENCES

1. Majno G, Joris I: Apoptosis, oncosis, and necrosis: An overview of cell death. Am J Pathol 146:3, 1995.
2. Kerr J, Wyllie A, Currie A: Apoptosis: A basic biological phenomenon with wide-ranging implications in tissue kinetics. Brit J Cancer 26:239, 1972.
3. Wyllie AH, Morris RG, Smith AL, et al: Chromatin cleavage in apoptosis: Association with condensed chromatin morphology

and dependence on macromolecular synthesis. J Pathol 142:67, 1984.
4. Ellis H, Horvitz H: Genetic control of programmed cell death in the nematode C. elegans. Cell 44:817, 1986.
5. Thompson CB: Apoptosis in the pathogenesis and treatment of disease. Science 267:1456, 1995.
6. Vaishnaw AK, McNally JD, Elkon KB: Apoptosis in the rheumatic diseases. Arthritis Rheum 40:1917, 1997.
7. Duvall E, Wyllie AH: Death and the cell. Immunol Today 7:115, 1986.
8. Leist M, Single B, Castoldi AF, et al: Intracellular adenosine triphosphate (ATP) concentration: a switch in the decision between apoptosis and necrosis. J Exp Med 185:1481, 1997.
9. Aravind L, Dixit VM, Koonin EV: The domains of death: evolution of the apoptosis machinery. Trends Biochem Sci 24:47, 1999.
10. Smith C, Farrah T, Goodwin R: The TNF receptor superfamily of cellular and viral proteins: activation, costimulation, and death. Cell 76:959, 1994.
11. Locksley RM, Killeen N, Lenardo MJ: The TNF and TNF receptor superfamilies: integrating mammalian biology. Cell 104:487, 2001.
12. Ashkenazi A, Dixit VM: Apoptosis control by death and decoy receptors. Curr Opin Cell Biol 11:255, 1999.
13. Huang B, Eberstadt M, Olejniczak E, et al: NMR structure and mutagenesis of the Fas (APO-1/CD95) death domain. Nature 384:638, 1996.
14. Muzio M, Chinnaiyan A, Kischkel F, et al: FLICE, a novel FADD-homologous ICE/CED-3-like protease, is recruited to the CD95 (Fas/APO-1) death-inducing signaling complex. Cell 85:817, 1996.
15. Boldin M, Goncharov T, Goltsev Y, et al: Involvement of MACH, a novel MORT1/FADD-interacting protease, in Fas/APO-1- and TNF receptor-induced cell death. Cell 85:803, 1996.
16. Vincenz C, Dixit V: Fas-associated death domain protein interleukin-1b-converting enzyme 2 (FLICE2), an ICE/Ced-3 homologue, is proximally involved in CD95- and p55-mediated death signaling. J Biol Chem 272:6578, 1997.
17. Scaffidi C, Fulda S, Srinivasan A, et al: Two CD95 (APO-1/Fas) signaling pathways. EMBO J 17:1675, 1998.
18. Nagata S: Apoptosis by death factor. Cell 88:355, 1997.
19. Black R, Rauch C, Kozlosky C, et al: A metalloproteinase disintegrin that releases tumor necrosis factor-a from cells. Nature 385:729, 1997.
20. Moss M, Jin S-LC, Milla M, et al: Cloning of a disintegrin metalloproteinase that processes precursor tumor necrosis factor-a. Nature 385:733, 1997.
21. Kishimoto H, Sprent J: Negative selection in the thymus includes semimature T cells. J Exp Med 185:263, 1997.
22. Elkon KB, Marshak-Rothstein A: B cells in systemic autoimmune disease: recent insights from Fas-deficient mice and men. Curr Opin Immunol 8:852, 1996.
23. Lamhamedi-Cherradi SE, Zheng SJ, Maguschak KA, et al: Defective thymocyte apoptosis and accelerated autoimmune diseases in TRAIL(-/-) mice. Nat Immunol 4:255, 2003.
24. Wang EC, Thern A, Denzel A, et al: DR3 regulates negative selection during thymocyte development. Mol Cell Biol 21:3451, 2001.
25. Schmidt CS, Liu J, Zhang T, et al: Enhanced B cell expansion, survival, and humoral responses by targeting death receptor 6. J Exp Med 197:51, 2003.
26. Raff M: Social controls on cell survival and cell death. Nature 356:397, 1992.
27. Levine AJ: P53, the cellular gatekeeper for growth and division. Cell 88:323, 1997.
28. Kroemer G, Reed JC: Mitochondrial control of cell death. Nat Med 6:513, 2000.
29. Zou H, Henzel W, Liu Z, et al: Apaf-1, a human protein homologous to C. elegans CED-4, participates in cytochrome c-dependent activation of caspase 3. Cell 90:405, 1997.
30. Susin SA, Lorenzo HK, Zamzami N, et al: Molecular characterization of mitochondrial apoptosis-inducing factor. Nature 397:441, 1999.
31. Kaufman RJ: Orchestrating the unfolded protein response in health and disease. J Clin Invest 110:1389, 2002.
32. Nakagawa T, Zhu H, Morishima N, et al: Caspase-12 mediates endoplasmic-reticulum-specific apoptosis and cytotoxicity by amyloid-beta. Nature 403:98, 2000.
33. Adams JM, Cory S: The Bcl-s protein family: arbiters of cell survival. Science 281:1322, 1998.
34. Oltvai ZN, Korsmeyer SJ: Checkpoints of dueling dimers foil death wishes. Cell 79:189, 1994.
35. Muchmore SW, Sattler M, Liang H, et al: X-ray and NMR structure of human Bcl-xL, an inhibitor of programmed cell death. Nature 381:335, 1996.
36. Roy N, Deveraux QL, Takahashi R, et al: The c-IAP-1 and c-IAP-2 proteins are direct inhibitors of specific caspases. EMBO J 16:6914, 1997.
37. Deveraux QL, Reed JC: IAP family proteins—suppressors of apoptosis. Genes Dev 13:239, 1999.
38. Thornberry NA, Lazebnik Y: Caspases: Enemies within. Science 281:1312, 1998.
39. Los M, Wesselborg S, Schulze-Osthoff K: The role of caspases in development, immunity, and apoptotic signal transduction: lessons from knockout mice. Immunity 10:629, 1999.
40. Garcia-Calvo M, Peterson EP, Leiting B, et al: Inhibition of human caspases by peptide-based and macrophage inhibitors. J Biol Chem 273:32608, 1998.
41. Enari M, Sakahira H, Yokoyama H, et al: A caspase-activated DNase that degrades DNA during apoptosis, and its inhibitor ICAD. Nature 391:43, 1998.
42. Sakahira H, Enari M, Nagata S: Cleavage of CAD inhibitor in CAD activation and DNA degradation during apoptosis. Nature 391:96, 1998.
43. Martinon F, Burns K, Tschopp J: The inflammasome: a molecular platform triggering activation of inflammatory caspases and processing of proIL-beta. Mol Cell 10:417, 2002.
44. Hull KM, Shoham N, Chae JJ, et al: The expanding spectrum of systemic autoinflammatory disorders and their rheumatic manifestations. Curr Opin Rheumatol 15:61, 2003.
45. Ellis RE, Jacobson DM, Horvitz R: Genes required for the engulfment of cell corpses during programmed cell death in Caenorhabditis elegans. Genetics 129:79, 1991.
46. Hengartner MO: Apoptosis: corralling the corpses. Cell 104:325, 2001.
47. Verhoven B, Schlegel RA, Williamson P: Mechanisms of phosphatidylserine exposure, a phagocyte recognition signal, on apoptotic T lymphocytes. J Exp Med 182:1597, 1995.
48. Fadok VA, Savill JS, Haslett C, et al: Different populations of macrophages use either the vitronectin receptor or the phosphatidylserine receptor to recognize and remove apoptotic cells. J Immunol 149:4029, 1992.
49. Fadok VA, Bratton DL, Rose DM, et al: A receptor for phosphatidylserine-specific clearance of apoptotic cells [see comments]. Nature 405:85, 2000.
50. Duvall E, Wyllie AH, Morris RG: Macrophage recognition of cells undergoing programmed cell death. Immunology 56:351, 1985.
51. Franc NC, Dimarcq J-L, Lagueux M, et al: Croquemort, a novel drosophila hemocyte/macrophage receptor that recognizes apoptotic cells. Immunity 4:431, 1996.
52. Savill J, Dransfield Hogg N, Haslett C: Vitronectin receptor-mediated phagocytosis of cells undergoing apoptosis. Nature 343:170, 1990.
53. Albert ML, Pearce SFA, Francisco LM, et al: Immature dendritic cells phagocytose apoptotic cells via alpha-v-beta-5 and CD36, and cross-present antigens to cytotoxic T lymphocytes. J Exp Med 188:1359, 1998.
54. Mevorach D, Mascarenhas J, Gershov DA, et al: Complement-dependent clearance of apoptotic cells by human macrophages. J Exp Med, 188:2313, 1998.
55. Platt N, Suzuki H, Kurihara Y, et al: Role for the class A macrophage scavenger receptor in the phagocytosis of apoptotic thymocytes in vitro. Proc Natl Acad Sci U S A 93:12456, 1996.
56. Sambrano GR, Steinberg D: Recognition of oxidatively damaged and apoptotic cells by an oxidized low density lipoprotein receptor on mouse peritoneal macrophages: Role of membrane phosphatidylserine. Proc Natl Acad Sci U S A 92:1396, 1995.
57. Fukasawa M, Adachi H, Hirota K, et al: SRB1, a class B scavenger receptor, recognizes both negatively charged liposomes and apoptotic cells. Exper Cell Res 222:246, 1996.
58. Luciani M-F, Chimini G: The ATP binding cassette transporter, ABC1, is required for the engulfment of corpses generated by apoptotic cell death. EMBO J 15:226, 1996.
59. Devitt A, Moffatt OD, Raykundalia C, et al: Human CD14 mediates recognition and phagocytosis of apoptotic cells. Nature 392:505, 1998.

60. Ren Y, Silverstein RL, Allen J, et al: CD36 gene transfer confers capacity for phagocytosis of cells undergoing apoptosis. J Exp Med 181:1857, 1995.
61. Kim G, Jun JB, Elkon KB: Necessary role of phosphatidylinositol 3-kinase in transforming growth factor beta-mediated activation of Akt in normal and rheumatoid arthritis synovial fibroblasts. Arthritis Rheum 46:1504, 2002.
62. Lu Q, Lemke G: Homeostatic regulation of the immune system by receptor tyrosine kinases of the Tyro 3 family. Science 293:306, 2001.
63. Fadok VA, Bratton DL, Konowal A, et al: Macrophages that have ingested apoptotic cells in vitro inhibit proinflammatory cytokine production through autocrine/paracrine mechanisms involving TGF-beta, PGE2, and PAF. J Clin Invest 101:890, 1998.
64. Voll RE, Herrmann M, Roth EA, et al: Immunosuppresive effects of apoptotic cells. Nature 390:350, 1997.
65. Huynh ML, Fadok VA, Henson PM: Phosphatidylserine-dependent ingestion of apoptotic cells promotes TGF-beta1 secretion and the resolution of inflammation. J Clin Invest 109:41, 2002.
66. Gallucci S, Lolkema M, Matzinger P: Natural adjuvants: endogenous activators of dendritic cells. Nat Med 5:1249, 1999.
67. Bellone M, Iezzi G, Rovere P, et al: Processing of engulfed apoptotic bodies yields T cell epitopes. J Immunol 159:5391, 1997.
68. Vermes I, Haanen C, Steffens-Nakken H, et al: A novel assay for apoptosis: Flow cytometric detection of phosphatidylserine expression on early apoptotic cells using fluorescein-labeled Annexin V. J Immunol Methods 184:39, 1995.
69. Nicoletti I, Migliorati G, Pagliacci MC, et al: A rapid and simple method for measuring thymocytes apoptosis by propidium iodide staining and flow cytometry. J Immunol Meth 139:1173, 1991.
70. Gavrieli Y, Sherman Y, Ben-Sasson SA: Identification of programmed cell death in situ via specific labeling of nuclear DNA fragmentation. J Cell Biol 119:493, 1992.
71. Grodzicky T, Elkon KB: Apoptosis in rheumatic diseases. Am J Med 108:73, 2000.
72. Rumore PM, Steinman CR: Endogenous circulating DNA in systemic lupus erythematosus, occurrence as multimeric complexes bound to histone. J Clin Invest 86:69, 1990.
73. Burlingame RW, Rubin RL, Balderas RS, et al: Genesis and evolution of anti-chromatin autoantibodies in murine lupus implicates T-dependent immunization and self antigen. J Clin Invest 91:1687, 1993.
74. Amoura Z, Chabre H, Koutouzov S, et al: Nucleosome restricted antibodies are detected before anti-ds DNA and/ or anti-histone antibodies in serum of MRL-Mp lpr/lpr and +/+ mice, adn are present in kidney eluates of lupus mice with proteinuria. Arthritis Rheum 37:1684, 1994.
75. Mohan C, Adams S, Stanik V, et al: Nucleosome: A major immunogen for pathogenic autoantibody-inducing T cells of lupus. J Exp Med 177:1367, 1993.
76. Termaat RM, Assmann KJ, Dijkman HB, et al: Anti-DNA antibodies can bind to the glomerulus via two distinct mechanisms. Kidney Int 42:1363, 1992.
77. Kramers C, Hylkema MN, van Bruggen MCJ, et al: Anti-nucleosome antibodies complexed to nucleosomal antigens show anti-DNA reactivity and bind to rat glomerular basement membrane in vivo. J Clin Invest 94:568, 1994.
78. Casciola-Rosen LA, Anhalt G, Rosen A: Autoantigens targeted in systemic lupus erythematosus are clustered in two populations of surface structures on apoptotic keratinocytes. J Exp Med 179:1317, 1994.
79. Casciola-Rosen LA, Anhalt GJ, Rosen A: DNA-dependent protein kinase is one of a subset of autoantigens specifically cleaved early during apoptosis. J Exp Med 182:1625, 1995.
80. Casiano CA, Martin SJ, Green DR, et al: Selective cleavage of nuclear autoantigens during CD95 (Fas/APO-1)-mediated T cell apoptosis. J Exp Med 184:765, 1996.
81. Utz PJ, Hottelet M, Schur PH, et al: Proteins phosphorylated during stress-induced apoptosis are common targets for autoantibody production in patients with systemic lupus erythematosus. J Exp Med 185:843, 1997.
82. Price BE, Rauch J, Shia MA, et al: O'Laughlin T, Koh JS, Levine JS. Antiphospholipid autoantibodies bind to apoptotic, but not viable, thymocytes in a beta2-glycoprotein I-dependent manner. J Immunol 157:2201, 1996.
83. Emlen W, Niebur J-A, Kadera R: Accelerated in vitro apoptosis of lymphocytes from patients with systemic lupus erythematosus. J Immunol 152:3685, 1994.
84. Perniok A, Wedekind F, Herrmann M, et al: High levels of circulating early apoptotic peripheral blood mononuclear cells in systemic lupus erythematosus. Lupus 7:113, 1998.
85. Georgescu L, Vakkalanka RK, Elkon KB, et al: Interleukin-10 promotes activation-induced cell death of SLE lymphocytes mediated by Fas ligand. J Clin Invest 100:2622, 1997.
86. Botto M, Dell'Agnola C, Bygrave AE, et al: Homozygous C1q deficiency causes glomerulonephritis associated with multiple apoptotic bodies. Nature Gen 19:56, 1998.
87. Morgan BP, Walport MJ: Complement deficiency and disease. Immunol Today 12:301, 1991.
88. Scott RS, McMahon EJ, Pop SM, et al: Phagocytosis and clearance of apoptotic cells is mediated by MER. Nature 411:207, 2001.
89. Bickerstaff MCM, Botto M, Hutchinson WL, et al: Serum amyloid P component controls chromatin degradation and prevents antinuclear autoimmunity. Nature Medicine 5:694, 1999.
90. Napirei M, Karsunky H, Zevnik B, et al: Features of systemic lupus erythematosus in Dnase1-deficient mice [see comments]. Nat Genet 25:177, 2000.
91. Cohen PL, Eisenberg RA: lpr and gld: single gene models of systemic autoimmunity and lymphoproliferative disease. Annu Rev Immunol 9:243, 1991.
92. Fisher GH, Rosenberg FJ, Straus SE, et al: Dominant interfering Fas gene mutations impair apoptosis in a human lymphoproliferative syndrome. Cell 81:935, 1995.
93. Rieux-Laucat F, Le Deist F, Hivroz C, et al: Mutations in Fas associated with human lymphoproliferative syndrome and autoimmunity. Science 268:1347, 1995.
94. Drappa J, Vaishnaw AK, Sullivan KE, et al: The Canale Smith syndrome: an inherited autoimmune disorder associated with defective lymphocyte apoptosis and mutations in the Fas gene. N Engl J Med 335:1643, 1996.
95. Vaishnaw AK, Orlinick JR, Chu JL, et al: Molecular basis for the apoptotic defects in patients with CD95 (Fas/Apo-1) mutations. J Clin Invest 103:355, 1999.
96. Martin DA, Zheng L, Siegel RM, et al: Defective CD95/APO-1/Fas signal complex formation in the human autoimmune lymphoproliferative syndrome, type Ia [In Process Citation]. Proc Natl Acad Sci U S A 96:4552, 1999.
97. Vaishnaw AK, Toubi E, Ohsako S, et al: Both quantitative and qualitative apoptotic defects are associated with the clinical spectrum of disease, including systemic lupus erythematosus in humans with Fas (APO-1/CD95) mutations. Arthritis Rheum 42:1833, 1999.
98. Wu J, Wilson J, He J, et al: Fas ligand mutation in a patient with systemic lupus erythematosus and lymphoproliferative disease. J Clin Invest 98:1107, 1996.
99. Mysler E, Bini P, Drappa J, et al: The APO-1/Fas protein in human systemic lupus erythematosus. J Clin Invest 93:1029, 1994.
100. Kim S, Gershov D, Ma X, et al: Opsonization of apoptotic cells and its effects on macrophage and T cell immune responses. Ann NY Acad Sci 987:1 2003.
101. Khare SD, Sarosi I, Xia XZ, et al: Severe B cell hyperplasia and autoimmune disease in TALL-1 transgenic mice. Proc Natl Acad Sci U S A 97:3370, 2000.
102. Groom J, Kalled SL, Cutler AH, et al: Association of BAFF/BLyS overexpression and altered B cell differentiation with Sjogren's syndrome. J Clin Invest 109:59, 2002.
103. Nakajima T, Aono H, Hasunuma T, et al: Apoptosis and functional Fas antigen in rheumatoid arthritis synoviocytes. Arthritis Rheum 38:485, 1995.
104. Firestein GS, Yeo M, Zvaifler NJ: Apoptosis in rheumatoid arthritis synovium. J Clin Invest 96:1631, 1995.
105. Cantwell MJ, Hua T, Zvaifler NJ, et al: Deficient Fas ligand expression by synovial lymphocytes from patients with rheumatoid arthritis. Arthritis Rheum 40:1644, 1997.
106. Kawakami A, Eguchi K, Matsuoka N, et al: Thyroid-stimulating hormone inhibits Fas antigen-mediated apoptosis of human thyrocytes in vitro. Endocrinology 137:3163, 1996.
107. Tsuboi M, Eguchi K, Kawakami A, et al: Fas antigen expression on synovial cells was downregulated by interleukin 1. Biochem Biophys Res Comm 218:280, 1996.

108. Salmon M, Scheel-Toellner D, Huissoon AP, et al: Inhibition of T cell apoptosis in the rheumatoid synovium. J Clin Invest 99:439, 1997.
109. Fujisawa K, Aono H, Hasunuma T, et al: Activation of transcription factor NF-kB in human synovial cells in response to tumor necrosis factor. Arthritis Rheum 39:197, 1996.
110. Marok R, Winyard PG, Coumbe A, et al: Activation of the transcription factor nuclear factor k-B in human inflamed synovial tissue. Arthritis Rheum 39:583, 1996.
111. Sugiyama M, Tsukazaki T, Yonekura A, et al: Localization of apoptosis and expression of apoptosis-related proteins in the synovium of patients with rheumatoid arthritis. Ann Rheum Dis 55:442, 1996.
112. Tak PP, Smeets TJ, Boyle DL, et al: P53 overexpression in synovial tissue from patients with early and longstanding rheumatoid arthritis compared with patients with reactive arthritis and osteoarthritis. Arthritis Rheum 42:948, 1999.
113. Fujisawa K, Asahara H, Okamoto K, et al: Therapeutic effect of the anti-Fas antibody on arthritis in HTLV-1 tax transgenic mice. J Clin Invest 98:271, 1996.
114. Zhang H, Yang Y, Horton JL, et al: Amelioration of collagen-induced arthritis by CD95 (Apo-1/Fas)-ligand gene transfer. J Clin Invest 100:1951, 1997.
115. Song K, Chen Y, Goke R, et al: Tumor necrosis factor-related apoptosis-inducing ligand (TRAIL) is an inhibitor of autoimmune inflammation and cell cycle progression. J Exp Med 191:1095, 2000.
116. Jelaska A, Korn JH: Role of apoptosis and transforming growth factor beta1 in fibroblast selection and activation in systemic sclerosis. Arthritis Rheum 43:2230, 2000.
117. Ohsako S, Elkon KB: Apoptosis in the effector phase of autoimmune diabetes, multiple sclerosis and thyroiditis. Cell Death Differe 6:13, 1999.
118. Giordano C, Stassi G, de Maria R, et al: Potential involvement of Fas and its ligand in the pathogenesis of Hashimoto's thyroiditis. Science 275:960, 1997.
119. Robinson CP, Yamachika S, Alford CE, et al: Elevated levels of cystein protease activity in saliva and salivary glands of the nonobese diabetic (NOD) mouse model for Sjogren syndrome. Proc Natl Acad Sci U S A 94:5767, 1997.
120. Kong L, Ogawa N, Masago R, et al: Bcl-2 family in salivary gland from Sjogren's syndrome: Bax may be involved in the destruction of SS salivary glandular epithelium. Arthritis Rheum 39:S289, 1996.
121. Behrens L, Bender A, Johnson MA, et al: Cytotoxic mechanisms in inflammatory myopathies. Co-expression of Fas and protective Bcl-2 in muscle fibres and inflammatory cells. Brain 120:929, 1997.
122. Sugiura T, Murakawa Y, Nagai A, et al: Fas and Fas ligand interaction induces apoptosis in inflammatory myopathies: CD4+ T cells injury in polymyositis. Arthritis Rheum 42:291, 1999.
123. Goebels N, Michaelis D, Engelhardt M, et al: Differential expression of perforin in muscle-infiltrating T cells in myositis and dermatomyositis. J Clin Invest 97:2905, 1996.
124. Howard OM, Dong HF, Yang D, et al: Histidyl-tRNA synthetase and asparaginyl-tRNA synthetase, autoantigens in myositis, activate chemokine receptors on T lymphocytes and immature dendritic cells. J Exp Med 196:781, 2002.
125. Hashimoto S, Setareh M, Ochs RL, et al: Fas/Fas ligand expression and induction of apoptosis in chondrocytes. Arthritis Rheum 40:1749, 1997.
126. Hashimoto S, Ochs RL, Komiya S, et al: Linkage of chondrocyte apoptosis and cartilage degradation in human osteoarthritis. Arthritis Rheum 41:1632, 1998.
127. Blanco FJ, Guitian R, Vazquez ME, et al: Osteoarthritis chondrocytes die by apoptosis. A possible pathway for osteoarthritis pathology. Arthritis Rheum 41:284, 1998.
128. Yang C, Li SW, Helminen HJ, et al: Apoptosis of chondrocytes in transgenic mice lacking collagen II. Exp Cell Res 235:370, 1997.
129. Kameda T, Mano H, Yuasa T, et al: Estrogen inhibits bone resorption by directly inducing apoptosis of the bone-resorbing osteoclasts. J Exp Med 186:489, 1997.
130. Okahashi N, Koide M, Jimi E, et al: Caspases (interleukin-1beta-converting enzyme family proteases) are involved in the regulation of the survival of osteoclasts. Bone 23:33, 1998.
131. Weinstein RS, Jilka RL, Parfitt AM, et al: Inhibition of osteoblastogenesis and promotion of apoptosis of osteoblasts and osteocytes by glucocorticoids. Potential mechanisms of their deleterious effects on bone. J Clin Invest 102:274, 1998.
132. Jilka RL, Weinstein RS, Bellido T, et al: Osteoblast programmed cell death (apoptosis): modulation by growth factors and cytokines. J Bone Miner Res 13:793, 1998.
133. Yasuda H, Shima N, Nakagawa N, et al: Osteoclast differentiation factor is a ligand for osteoprotegerin/ osteoclastogenesis-inhibitory factor and is identical to TRANCE/RANKL. Proc Natl Acad Sci U S A 95:3597, 1998.
134. Kong YY, Yoshida H, Sarosi I, et al: OPGL is a key regulator of osteoclastogenesis, lymphocyte development and lymph-node organogenesis. Nature 397:315, 1999.
135. McColl KS, He H, Zhong H, et al: Apoptosis induction by the glucocorticoid hormone dexamethasone and the calcium-ATPase inhibitor thapsigargin involves Bc1-2 regulated caspase activation. Mol Cell Endocrinol 139:229, 1998.
136. Chan TA, Morin PJ, Vogelstein B, et al: Mechanisms underlying nonsteroidal antiinflammatory drug-mediated apoptosis. Proc Natl Acad Sci U S A 95:681, 1998.
137. Schwenger P, Bellosta P, Vietor I, et al: Sodium salicylate induces apoptosis via p38 mitogen-activated protein kinase but inhibits tumor necrosis factor-induced c-Jun N-terminal kinase/stress-activated protein kinase activation. Proc Natl Acad Sci U S A 94:2869, 1997.
138. Thomson AW, Bonham CA, Zeevi A: Mode of action of tacrolimus (FK506): molecular and cellular mechanisms. Ther Drug Monit 17:584, 1995.
139. Anel A, Buferne M, Boyer C, et al: T cell receptor-induced Fas ligand expression in cytotoxic T lymphocyte clones is blocked by protein tyrosine kinase inhibitors and cyclosporin A. Eur J Immunol 24:2469, 1994.
140. Migita K, Eguchi K, Kawabe Y, et al: FK506 augments activation-induced programmed cell death of T lymphocytes in vivo. J Clin Invest 96:727, 1995.
141. Cutolo M, Barone A, Accardo S, et al: Effect of cyclosporin on apoptosis in human cultured monocytic THP-1 cells and synovial macrophages. Clin Exp Rheumatol 16:417, 1998.
142. Genestier L, Paillot R, Fournel S, et al: Immunosuppressive properties of methotrexate: apoptosis and clonal deletion of activated peripheral T cells. J Clin Invest 102:322, 1998.
143. Cha DR, Feld SM, Nast C, et al: Apoptosis in mesangial cells induced by ionizing radiation and cytotoxic drugs. Kidney Int 50:1565, 1996.
144. Hughes DE, Wright KR, Uy HL, et al: Bisphosphonates promote apoptosis in murine osteoclasts in vitro and in vivo. J Bone Miner Res 10:1478, 1995.
145. Tak PP, Taylor PC, Breedveld FC, et al: Decrease in cellularity and expression of adhesion molecules by anti-tumor necrosis factor à monoclonal antibody treatments in patients with rheumatoid arthritis. Arthritis Rheum 39:1077, 1996.
146. Lugering A, Schmidt M, Lugering N, et al: Infliximab induces apoptosis in monocytes from patients with chronic active Crohn's disease by using a caspase-dependent pathway. Gastroenterology 121:1145, 2001.
147. ten Hove T, van Montfrans C, Peppelenbosch MP, et al: Infliximab treatment induces apoptosis of lamina propria T lymphocytes in Crohn's disease. Gut 50:206, 2002.
148. Walczak H, Miller RE, Ariail K, et al: Tumoricidal activity of tumor necrosis factor-related apoptosis-inducing ligand in vivo. Nat Med 5:157, 1999.
149. Rodriguez I, Matsuura K, Ody C, et al: Systemic injection of a tripeptide inhibits the intracellular activation of CPP32-like proteases in vivo and fully protects mice against Fas-mediated fulminant liver destruction and death. J Exp Med 184:2067, 1996.
150. Gumucio DL, Diaz A, Schaner P, et al: Fire and ICE: the role of pyrin domain-containing proteins in inflammation and apoptosis. Clin Exp Rheumatol 20:S45, 2002.
151. Russell JH, Masakowski V, Rucinsky T, et al: Mechanisms of immune lysis III. Characterization of the nature and kinetics of the cytotoxic T lymphocyte induced nuclear lesion in the target. J Immunol 128:2087, 1982.
152. Karin M, Lin A: NF-kappaB at the crossroads of life and death. Nat Immunol 3:221, 2002.
153. Datta SR, Brunet A, Greenberg ME: Cellular survival: a play in three Akts. Genes Dev 13:2905, 1999.

SECTION

IV

Broad Issues in the Approach to Rheumatic Diseases

27 Epidemiology of the Rheumatic Diseases

HILAL MARADIT KREMERS • SHERINE E. GABRIEL

The Role of Epidemiology in Improving Our Understanding of the Rheumatic Diseases

Epidemiology is the study of the distribution and determinants of disease in human populations.[1] This definition is based on two fundamental assumptions: First, human disease does not occur at random; and second, human disease has causal and preventive factors that can be identified through systematic investigation of different populations, or subgroups of individuals within a population, in different places or at different times. Thus, epidemiologic studies include simple descriptions of the manner in which disease appears in a population (i.e., levels of disease frequency [incidence and prevalence], mortality, trends over time, geographic distributions, and clinical characteristics) and analyses that attempt to quantify the role of putative risk factors for disease occurrence. Incidence studies include all new cases of a specified condition arising in a defined population, and prevalence studies include all cases with the condition who are present in a population at a particular point in time (Fig. 27–1). In this chapter, we will review data on the descriptive epidemiology (incidence, prevalence, and survival) and risk factors associated with the major rheumatic diseases.

The Epidemiology of Rheumatoid Arthritis

The most reliable estimates of incidence, prevalence, and mortality in rheumatoid arthritis (RA) are those derived from population-based studies. Several of these have been conducted in a variety of geographically and ethnically diverse populations (Table 27–1).

One hundred four newly diagnosed cases of RA, which fulfilled the 1987 American College of Rheumatology (ACR) criteria for RA at the time of presentation between 1990 and 1991, were identified using the Norfolk Arthritis Register.[2] The annual incidence rate per 100,000 population was 35.9 for females and 14.3 for males (see Table 27–1). RA was rare in men under 45 years of age. The incidence of RA in men rose steeply with age, whereas in women, the incidence rose up to age 45 and plateaued until 75 years, after which it declined.[2]

Numerous studies describing the epidemiology of RA have been undertaken in Finland. Estimates of the incidence and prevalence have been derived from several surveys based on computerized data registers covering the entire Finnish population.[3-7] The incidence of clinically significant RA in these surveys was approximately 29 to 35.5 per 100,000 adult population over the study years (1975, 1980, 1985, 1990, and 1995) (see Table 27–1). Trends in RA incidence between 1975 and 1995 were also examined.[4,7] The authors noted an 8.8-year increase in the mean age at onset (from 50.2 to 59.0 years) between 1975 and 1995 and a simultaneous decline in the age-specific incidence rates in the younger individuals.[4] The same investigators studied the incidence of rheumatoid factor (RF)-positive RA and RF-negative polyarthritis.[6] In that study, they demonstrated a decline of approximately 40 percent in the number of RF-negative RA cases in 1990 compared to the earlier years. This declining trend was statistically significant ($p = 0.008$), and the decline in incidence was noted to affect, nearly exclusively, RF-negative disease.

The overall age- and sex-adjusted annual incidence of RA among Rochester, Minnesota, residents 18 years of age or older (1955 through 1994) was 44.6 per 100,000 (95 percent, confidence interval [CI]: 41.0 to 48.2).[8,9] The incidence was approximately double in women compared to that in men, and incidence increased steadily with age until age 85, after which it decreased. Incidence peaked earlier in women than in men. Although the incidence rate fell progressively over the four decades of study, from 61.2 per 100,000 in 1955 through 1964, to 32.7 per 100,000 in 1985 through 1994, there were indications of cyclic trends over time (Fig. 27–2). Birth-cohort analysis showed diminishing incidence rates

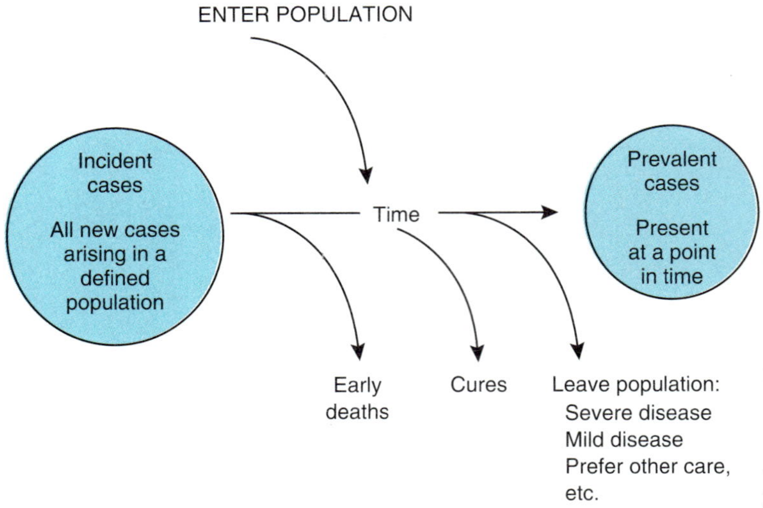

FIGURE 27–1 • The difference in cases for incidence and prevalence studies. (Adapted from Fletcher RH, Fletcher SW, Wagner EH (eds): Clinical Epidemiology–The Essentials, Vol 2. Baltimore, Williams & Wilkins, 1988, p 87; with permission.)

TABLE 27–1 • INCIDENCE OF RHEUMATOID ARTHRITIS

Author	County/Region	Years of Study	Age Range	Sample Size	Annual Incidence Rate per 100,000
Dugowson et al, 1991[12]	Seattle, Wash., USA	1987-1989	18-64	81*	23.9 – F (95% CI: 18.5, 29.3)
Chan et al, 1993[311]	Massachusetts, USA	1987-1990	18-70+	81	42 – O (95% CI: 23, 60) 60 – F (95% CI: 46, 75) 22 – M (95% CI: 13, 32)
Symmons et al, 1994[2]	Manchester, UK	1990-1991	15-85+	104*	35.9 – F (95% CI: 26.9, 43.1) 14.3 – M (95% CI: 8.2, 18.7)
Jacobsson et al, 1994[10]	Pima Indian Reservation AZ, USA	1965-1990	25-65+	78	1966-73 – 890 (95% CI: 590, 1190) 1974-82 – 620 (95% CI: 380, 860) 1983-90 – 380 (95% CI: 170, 590)
Aho et al, 1998[3]; Kaipiainen-Seppanen and Aho, 2000[4]; Kaipiainen et al, 1996[6,7]	Finland	5 (1-yr periods) 1975, 1980, 1985, 1990, 1995	16-85+	1321* 366*	1975: 29.0 1980: 35.5 1985: 35.0 1990: 29.5 1995: 33.7 – O (95% CI: 30.4, 37.4) 43.2 – F (95% CI: 37.9, 49.0) 23.5 – M (95% CI: 19.6, 28.1)
Drosos et al, 1997[11]	Northwest	1987-1995 Greece (Ioannina)	16-75+	428*	24 – O (95% CI: 15, 33) 36 – F (95% CI: 21, 51) 12 – M (95% CI: 4, 20)
Uhlig et al, 1998[312]	Oslo, Norway	1988-1993	20-79	550*	25.7 – O (95% CI: 23.6, 28.0)) 36.7 – F (95% CI: 33.4, 40.6) 13.8 – M (95% CI: 11.6, 16.2)
Shichikawa et al, 1999[313]	Wakayama, Japan	1965-1996		16	1965-75 – 39 (95% CI: 12, 66) 1975-85 – 24 (95% CI: 3, 46) 1985-96 – 8 (95% CI: 0, 17)
Riise et al, 2000[24]	Troms County, Norway	1987-1996	20+	316*	28.7 – O (95% CI: 25.6, 32.0) 34.9 – F (95% CI: 30.2, 40.1) 22.2 – M (95% CI: 18.4, 26.6)
Gabriel et al, 1999[8]; Doran et al, 2002[9]	Olmsted County, Minn., USA		18-85+	609*	44.6 – O (95% CI: 41.0, 48.2) 57.8 – F (95% CI: 52.4, 63.2) 30.4 – M (95% CI: 25.6, 35.1)

*American College of Rheumatology (ACR) 1987 criteria.
Abbreviations: CI, Confidence interval; F, female; M, male; O, overall.

through successive cohorts following a peak in the 1880 through 1890 cohorts.[9]

Seventy-eight cases of RA were identified among a population-based cohort of 2894 Pima Indians in Arizona during the period from 1965 through 1990.[10] The total age- and sex-adjusted incidence rate per 100,000 population was 890 (95 percent, CI: 590 to 1190) in 1966 through 1973, 620 (95 percent, CI: 380 to 860) in 1974 through 1982, and 380 (95 percent, CI: 170 to 590) in 1983 through 1990. The age-adjusted incidence declined by 55 percent in men (p trend = 0.225) and by 57 percent in women (p trend = 0.017) after controlling for all contraceptive use, estrogen use, and pregnancy experience. Drosos and colleages,[11] in Ioannina,

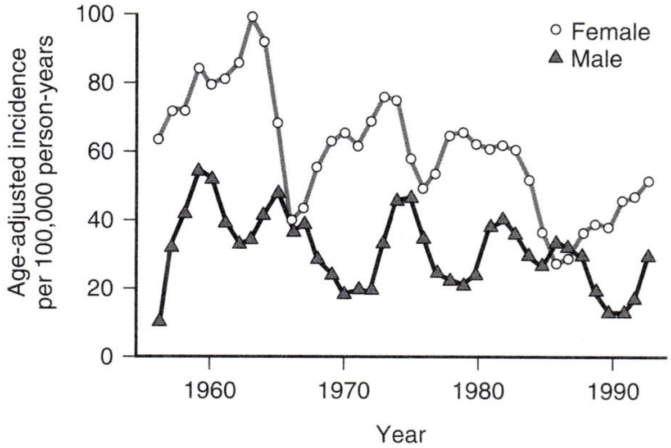

FIGURE 27–2 · **Annual Incidence of Rheumatoid Arthritis (RA) in Rochester, Minnesota.** Annual incidence rate per 100,000 population by gender, 1955 to 1995. Each rate was calculated as a 3-year centered moving average. (From Doran MF, Pond GR, Crowson CS, et al: Trends in incidence and mortality in rheumatoid arthritis in Rochester, Minnesota, over a forty-year period. Arthritis Rheum 46(3):625-631, 2002 with permission.)

Greece, identified 428 cases of RA with annual incidence rates fluctuating between 12 and 36 per 100,000.

A review of the incidence rates from the 10 major population-based epidemiologic studies (see Table 27–1) reveals substantial variation in incidence rates across the different studies and across time periods within the studies. These data emphasize the dynamic nature of the epidemiology of RA. A substantial decline in RA incidence over time with a shift toward a more elderly age of onset was a consistent finding across various studies.[6,7,9,10,12-14]

Several studies in the literature provide estimates of the number of people with current disease (prevalence) in a defined population. Although these studies suffer from a number of methodologic limitations,[15] the remarkable finding across these studies is the uniformity of RA prevalence rates in developed populations, approximately 0.5 to 1 percent of the adult population.[3,8,10,11,16-25]

The first mortality study of RA was published by Cobb.[26] The reported mortality rates among the RA patients and non-RA controls were 24.4 and 18.9 deaths per 1000 patients per year, respectively. Subsequent studies have consistently demonstrated an increased mortality in patients with RA when compared to expected rates in the general population[9,10,26-57] (Table 27–2). The standardized mortality ratios (SMR) in these studies varied from 1.28 to 2.98. Two studies have specifically examined trends in mortality over time using a population-based design. Unfortunately, both concluded that the excess mortality associated with RA has remained unchanged over the past two to three decades.[29,32] Although some referral-based studies have reported an apparent improvement in survival, a recent critical review indicates that these observations are likely due to referral selection bias.[58]

TABLE 27–2 · **SUMMARY OF RESULTS OF RHEUMATOID ARTHRITIS (RA) MORTALITY STUDIES**

Author, Publication Year	No. of RA Cases	Standardized Mortality Ratio
Cobb et al, 1953[26]	583	1.29
van Dam et al, 1961[41]	231	1.66
Duthie et al, 1964[42]	307	1.66
Uddin et al, 1970[55]	475	1.29
Isomaki et al, 1975[34]	1000	1.77
Monson and Hall, 1976[30]*	1035	1.86
Linos et al, 1980[45]*	521	1.16
Lewis et al, 1980[44]	311	1.40
Allebeck et al, 1981[37]*	293	1.32
Allebeck, 1982[38]	1165	2.48
Prior et al, 1984[39]	489	2.98
Pincus et al, 1984[36]	75	1.31
Vandenbroucke et al, 1984[35]	209	1.14
Mutru et al, 1985[57]	1000	1.64
Mitchell et al, 1986[46]	805	1.51
Reilly et al, 1990[43]	100	1.40
Jacobsson et al, 1993[40]*	2979	1.28
Wolfe et al, 1994[27]	3501	2.26
Myllykangas-Luosujarvi et al, 1995[33]*	1666	1.37
Callahan et al, 1996[56]	1384	1.54
Wallberg-Jonsson et al, 1997[47]	606	1.57
Symmons et al, 1998[49]	448	2.7
Lindquist and Eberhardt, 1999[314]	183	0.87
Sokka et al, 1999[48]	135	1.28
Gabriel et al, 1999[32]	425	1.38
Kvalvik et al, 2000[50]	149	1.49
Cheheta et al, 2001[51]	309	1.65
Krause et al, 2000[52]	271	2.6
Martinez et al, 2001[53]	182	1.85
Riise et al, 2001[54]	187	2.0
Doran et al, 2002[9]*	609	1.27

*Population-based studies.

A number of investigators have examined the underlying causes for the observed excess mortality in RA.[29,39,44,46,47,57,59,60] These reports suggest increased risk from cardiovascular, infectious, hematologic, gastrointestinal, and respiratory diseases among RA patients compared to controls. Various disease severity and disease activity markers in RA (e.g., extra-articular manifestations, erythrocyte sedimenation rate [ESR], RF-positive status, higher joint count, functional status) have also been shown to be associated with increased mortality.[61-66]

RISK FACTORS FOR RHEUMATOID ARTHRITIS

Several factors have been suggested as important contributors to the development or progression of RA. Of these, perhaps the most important are formal education, smoking, coffee consumption, use of oral contraceptives, infectious agents, and genetics.

The risk of self-reported arthritis, as well as several other chronic diseases, has been found to be inversely related to the level of formal education.[67] Low levels of formal education have also been associated with increased mortality,[68] as well as poor clinical status,[68-70] in patients with RA. No relationship was found between the onset of RA and indicators of socioeconomic deprivation using employment categories as indicators for social class.[71] Thus, although some evidence points to low formal education as a risk factor for RA, there is no apparent association with socioeconomic deprivation. Moreover, the mechanism for this possible excess risk is unknown.

Several studies have assessed the relationship between smoking and the development and severity of RA.[72-77] Uhlig and colleagues[73] identified a significant association for the development of RA among male cigarette smokers compared to nonsmokers (odds ratio [OR] 2.38, 95 percent, CI: 1.45 to 3.92), especially for seropositive (RF+) males (OR 4.77, 95 percent, CI: 2.09 to 10.9). Evidence for an independent effect of cigarette smoking was further strengthened in a study of twins with an odds ratio of 12.0 (95 percent, CI: 1.78 to 515) in monozygotic pairs.[75] Karlson and coworkers[77] studied the association of cigarette smoking with risk of RA among 377,481 female health professionals in the Women's Health Cohort Study. After adjusting for potential confounders, duration (but not intensity) of smoking was associated with a significantly increased risk of RA ($p < 0.01$). Wolfe and colleagues[74] reported that the RF concentration was linearly related to the number of years the person had smoked. Smoking was related to rheumatoid nodule formation and radiographic abnormalities, but it had no effect on disease process variables such as ESR, pain, joint count, global severity, or functional ability. These findings add to the growing body of evidence suggesting that smoking is an independent risk factor in the development of RA.[75,76] The increased risk of RA associated with smoking is speculated to be mediated through antiestrogenic effects of smoking.

Two studies examined the association between coffee consumption and the development of RA.[78,79] In a cross-sectional survey of almost 7000 people, the number of cups of coffee consumed daily was directly proportional to the prevalence of RF positivity.[78] The same authors also prospectively followed-up nearly 20,000 people for the development of RA and reported that subjects consuming four or more cups of coffee per day were more than twice as likely to develop seropositive RA, compared to those drinking less (relative risk [RR] 2.2, 95 percent, CI: 1.13 to 4.27).[78] Mikuls and colleagues[79] examined the types of coffee consumed and found that decaffeinated coffee intake is positively associated with RA onset (RR 3.1, 95 percent, CI: 1.75 to 5.48), whereas tea consumption is protective (RR 0.24, 95 percent, CI: 0.06 to 0.98).

The possibility that oral contraceptives (OC) offer a protective effect against the development of RA has been proposed by numerous investigators. Brennan and coworkers[80] reviewed the 17 studies investigating this association and noted that 11 showed a protective effect and six did not. These authors also provided their own results, based on 115 incident cases of inflammatory polyarthritis, which showed that current oral contraceptive use does protect against the development of RA (OR 0.22, 95 percent, CI: 0.06 to 0.85). Doran and colleagues[81] observed an inverse association between ever use of oral contraceptives and the risk of RA, even after adjusting for potential confounders (OR 0.54, 95 percent, CI: 0.32, 0.89). Exposure to OC in earlier calendar years, when higher doses of estrogen and progestins were used in the formulations, is associated with a further lowering of risk, such that women who received OC prior to 1970 have only one quarter the risk of unexposed women. There was no evidence of an association of estrogen replacement therapy with RA risk (OR 1.11, 95 percent, CI: 0.69, 1.78).[81] Overall, the bulk of the evidence points to a protective role for estrogens in the etiology of RA. Additional research is needed to elucidate the mechanism underlying this association.

A feature of disease occurrence that might point to an environmental component is evidence of secular trends or disease clusters in time or space. Data from the population-based incidence studies in Olmsted County, Minn., demonstrate secular trends in the incidence of RA[8,9] (Fig. 27–3). Silman and coworkers[82] conducted time trend and spatial clustering analyses on 687 incident cases of inflammatory joint disease and demonstrated no evidence of a consistent seasonal variation in the onset of disease. Modest evidence for spatial clustering was demonstrated with nonrandom distribution observed in one geographic area. Unfortunately, the small sample size precluded any definitive conclusions. Further investigation into local factors that might explain this finding is underway.[82,83] The observation of high incidence rates of RA among certain North American Indian populations[10] and the unusually low incidence of RA in the population of northwest Greece[11] lend support to the hypothesis of a host environment interaction. Human parvovirus infection has also been linked to the occurrence of inflammatory polyarthritis, but its role in the development of RA is less clear. Data from the Norfolk Arthritis Register, which has the benefit of ascertaining cases close in time to disease onset, showed that only 2.7 percent of patients with polyarthri-

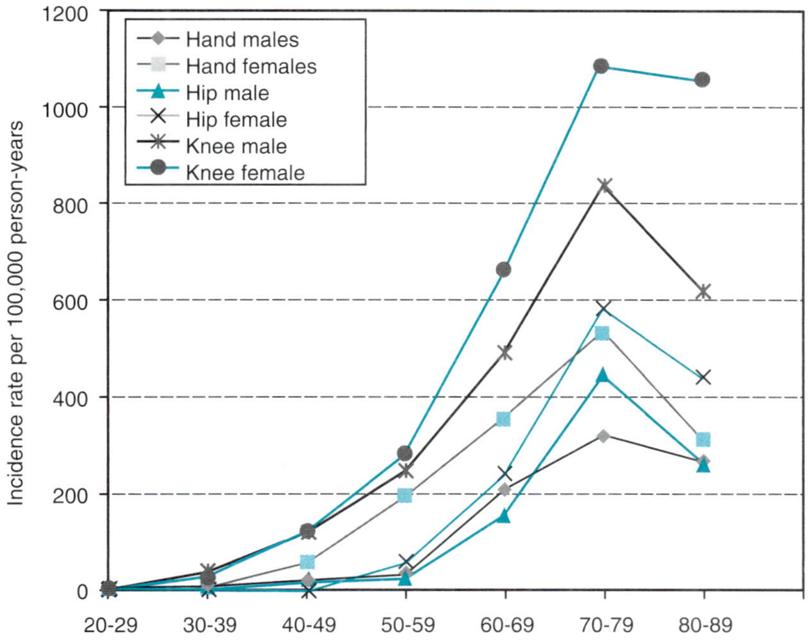

FIGURE 27–3 · Incidence of osteoarthritis of the hand, hip, and knee, in members of the Fallon Community Health Plan, 1991-1992, by age and sex. (Adapted from Oliveria SA, Felson DT, Reed JI, et al: Incidence of symptomatic hand, hip, and knee osteoarthritis among patients in a health maintenance organization. Arthritis Rheum 38(8):1134-1141, 1995 with permission.)

tis had evidence of recent human parvovirus B19 infection, suggesting that such infection could not explain more than a very small proportion of RA cases.[84]

The familiality of RA has long been recognized,[85,86] suggesting that genetic risk factors are important in the etiology of this disease. Several investigators have demonstrated important associations between specific human leukocyte antigen (HLA) alleles (i.e., HLA-DR4 and HLA-DR1) and susceptibility to RA.[87-95] The magnitude of the genetic contribution of RA has been estimated using twin studies and first-degree relatives of affected individuals. The concordance rates in monozygotic twins is around 15 percent,[96-98] which is four to five times greater than the rates observed among dizygotic twins and siblings of RA probands.[99,100] The heritability of RA is estimated at 65 percent (95percent, CI: 50 to 77),[101] suggesting that genetic factors account for a substantial portion of the disease risk.

The Epidemiology of Juvenile Rheumatoid Arthritis

A number of studies have examined the epidemiology of chronic arthritis in childhood.[102-105] Oen and Cheang[102] conducted a comprehensive review of descriptive epidemiology studies of chronic arthritis in childhood and analyzed factors that may explain differences in the reported incidence and prevalence rates. As this review illustrates, the large majority of available studies are clinic-based and thus are susceptible to numerous biases. The few population-based estimates available indicate that the prevalence of juvenile rheumatoid arthritis (JRA) is approximately 1 to 2 per 1000 children, and the incidence is 11 to 14 new cases per 100,000 children. This analysis revealed that reports of the descriptive epidemiology of chronic arthritis in childhood differ in methods of case ascertainment, data collection, source population, geographic location, and ethnic background of the study population. These analyses further demonstrated that the use of different diagnostic criteria had no effect on the reported incidence or prevalence rates. The strongest predictors of disease frequency were source population (with the highest rates being reported in population studies and the lowest in clinic-based cohorts) and geographic origin of the report. The former is consistent with more complete case ascertainment in population-based studies compared to clinic-based studies; although the latter suggests possible environmental or genetic influences in the etiology of juvenile chronic arthritis. A review in 1999 concurred that the variations in incidence over time indicate environmental influences, whereas ethnic and familial aggregations suggest the role of genetic factors.[103] The genetic component of juvenile arthritis is complex, likely involving the effects of multiple genes. The best evidence pertains to certain HLA loci (HLA-A, -DR/DQ, and -DP), but there are marked differences according to disease subtypes.[106,107] Environmental influences are also suggested by five studies that demonstrated secular trends in the yearly incidence of JRA and two in which a seasonal variation in systemic JRA was documented.[105,108-113]

Various studies examined long-term outcomes of JRA.[114-121] Adults with a history of JRA have been shown to have a lower life expectancy compared to members of the general population of the same age and sex. Throughout 25 years of follow-up of a cohort of 57 adults with a history of RA, the mortality rate among JRA cases was 0.27 deaths per 100 years of patient follow-up, compared to an expected mortality rate of 0.068 deaths per 100 years of follow-up in the general population. All deaths were associated with autoimmune disorders.[122] In another study, a clinic-based cohort of 215 juvenile idiopathic arthritis patients were followed-up for a median of 16.5 years.[123] The majority of the patients had a favorable outcome and no deaths were observed. Half of the patients had low levels of disease activity and few physical signs of disease (e.g., tender, swollen joints; restrictions in joint motion; local growth disturbances). Ocular involvement was the most common extra-articular manifestation and affected 14 percent of the patients.

The Epidemiology of Psoriatic Arthritis

Three studies have provided population-based data on the incidence of psoriatic arthritis.[124-126] Kaipiainen-Seppanen[4] examined all subjects who were entitled, under the nationwide Finnish sickness insurance scheme, to receive specially reimbursed medication for psoriatic arthritis in 1990[124] and 1995. A total of 65 incident cases of psoriatic arthritis were identified in the 1990 study, resulting in an annual incidence of 6 per 100,000 of the adult population 16 years of age or older. The mean age at diagnosis was 46.8 years, with the peak incidence occurring in the 45- to 54-year-old age-group. There was a slight male-to-female predominance (1.3:1). Incidence in the 1995 study was of the same order of magnitude at 6.8 per 100,000 (95 percent, CI: 5.4 to 8.6).[4] Another study reported the incidence in southern Sweden to be similar to Finland.[125]

A study by Shbeeb and colleagues[126] from Olmsted County, Minnesota, used the population-based data resources of the Rochester Epidemiology Project to identify all cases of inflammatory arthritis associated with a definite diagnosis of psoriasis. Sixty-six cases of psoriatic arthritis were first diagnosed between 1982 and 1991. The average age- and sex-adjusted incidence rate per 100,000 was 6.59 (95 percent, CI: 4.99 to 8.19), a rate remarkably similar to that reported in the Finnish study. The average age at diagnosis was 40.7 years. At diagnosis, 91 percent of cases had oligoarthritis. Over the 477.8 person-years of follow-up, only 25 patients developed extra-articular manifestations, and survival was not significantly different from the general population. The prevalence rate on January 1, 1992, was 1 per 1000 (95 percent, CI: 0.81 to 1.21). The American study reported a higher prevalence rate and lower disease severity than other similar studies.[4,124,125,127,128] These differences may be explained by differences in the case definition and ascertainment methods. Although the Finnish cohort was population based, the study's ascertainment methods relied on receipt of medication for psoriatic arthritis. Thus, mild cases not requiring medication may not have been identified in the Finnish cohort. Gladman and coworkers[129-132] have published extensively on the clinical characteristics, outcomes, and mortality experience of large groups of patients with psoriatic arthritis seen in a single tertiary referral center. The results of these studies differ from those of the population-based analyses in that they demonstrate significantly increased mortality and morbidity among patients with psoriatic arthritis compared to the general population. However, because all patients in these studies are referred to a single outpatient, tertiary referral center, these findings could represent selection referral bias. Clearly, additional population-based data are needed to resolve these discrepancies.[128]

The Epidemiology of Osteoarthritis

Osteoarthritis (OA) is the most common form of arthritis, affecting every population and ethnic group investigated thus far. It accounts for more dependency in walking, stair climbing, and other lower-extremity tasks than any other disease, particularly in the elderly.[133] The economic impact of OA, both in terms of direct medical costs and lost wages, is substantial.[134-136] Indeed, the cost of OA in the United States has been estimated at $15.5 billion dollars (in 1994 dollars).[137] Moreover, given that preventive interventions and therapeutic options for OA are limited, we can expect the morbidity and economic impact of OA to increase with the aging of the developed world.

HIP OSTEOARTHRITIS

Although hip OA is less common than knee OA, symptoms can be more frequent and are often more severe.[138] The age- and sex-standardized incidence rate for hip OA is approximately 88 per 100,000 person-years (95 percent, CI: 75 to 101).[139] Hip OA rarely occurs before the age of 50, after which the incidence rises rapidly and declines again slightly at approximately age 80[139] (see Fig. 27–3).

Several population-based prevalence surveys have provided estimates of the prevalence of radiographic hip OA. Kellgren[140] and Lawrence and colleagues[141] reported a prevalence of 16 percent for men and 6 percent for women, both between the ages of 65 and 74 years among a population in England. They also noted an increase in prevalence with age. A survey of a farming community in Switzerland also reported higher prevalence rates in men.[142] However, other studies of Caucasian populations in Jerusalem and Sweden have reported equivalent rates in older men and women and lower rates in general, compared to those found in England (between 4 to 7 percent).[143,144] The prevalence of hip OA of severity grade 2 or greater in those aged 55 to 74 was estimated at 3.1 percent.[145] The prevalence of mild and severe radiologic OA was investigated in a random sample of 6585 inhabitants of a Dutch village.[146] These data indicated that prevalence of mild hip OA in men over age 55 was approximately 5 to 11 percent, and the prevalence of severe OA in the same age-group of men varied from approximately 1 to 3.5 percent. Likewise, in women 55 years and older, the prevalence of mild hip OA varied from 2 to 26 percent with marked increases in prevalence with increasing age; and the prevalence of severe OA ranged from approximately 0.5 to 10 percent. Marked increases in prevalence were noted in older compared to younger subjects and in women compared to men.[146] Prevalence can clearly vary based on the population studied, as the prevalence is very high in Iceland—estimated to be at least fivefold higher than the prevalence found in southern Scandinavia.[147] In contrast, the prevalence in a population-based group of Chinese subjects aged 60 years or older was 80 to 90 percent lower than the US Caucasian population.[148]

KNEE OSTEOARTHRITIS

Although knee OA is more common than other forms, it rarely occurs before the age of 50 (see Fig. 27–3). The age- and sex-standardized incidence rate for knee OA is approximately 240 per 100,000 person-years (95 percent, CI: 218 to 262).[139] It has been estimated that 3.1 percent of adult women develop knee joint-space narrowing each year.[149] The prevalence of knee OA is approximately 30 percent among those aged 75 and older. It is higher in men than in women up to age 45, after which the reverse is true.[139,150,151] Autopsy studies report much higher estimates of knee OA prevalence compared to studies using radiographs (i.e., 60 to 100 percent vs. 4 to 29 percent).[141,145,152,153] All studies that provide age-specific prevalence rates demonstrate a marked increase in prevalence with age.

HAND OSTEOARTHRITIS

The age- and sex-standardized incidence rate for hand OA is approximately 100 per 100,000 person-years (95 percent, CI: 86 to 115).[139] Among women, the incidence rates ranged from a low of 0 per 100,000 person-years among those aged 20 to 39 to a high of 529 per 100,000 person-years among those aged 70 to 79. For men, the incidence rates ranged from 0 per 100,000 person-years among those aged 20 to 29 to 319 per 100,000 person years among those 70 to 79 years of age. The incidence rates for OA of the thumb and fingers are similar to the distribution of rates of OA in the hand, overall.

A large-scale, comprehensive incidence study of symptomatic hand, hip, and knee OA demonstrated that the incidence of hand OA increased with age and that women had higher rates than men, especially after the age of 50.[139] The study authors noted that the incidence of knee OA was twice that of hand or hip OA and that the annual incidence of clinical knee OA was more than 1 percent per year in women aged 70 to 79. The female-to-male sex ratio for hand, hip, and knee OA was approximately 2:1, and the epidemiologic profiles of hip and knee OA were similar (i.e., the incidence rates of both increased up to age 79 and were more common in women after approximately age 50). Together, these results suggest that there may be more similarity in hand, hip, and knee OA epidemiology than has been previously thought and that future epidemiologic investigations should consider these disorders together, rather than separately.

RISK FACTORS FOR OSTEOARTHRITIS

A number of risk factors have been associated with the incidence and prevalence of OA. Aging is the strongest risk factor for the development of OA.[149] The increase in incidence and prevalence of OA with age is likely related to several biologic changes that occur with aging, including decreased responsiveness of chondrocytes to growth factors that stimulate repair; an increase in ligamentous laxity, making older joints relatively unstable and thus, more susceptible to injury; and a failure of major shock absorbers or protectors of the joint with age, such as gradual decrease in strength and slowing of peripheral neurologic responses.[154,155] In addition, as the joint ages, the rim of noncalcified cartilage becomes thinner, increasing cartilage vulnerability.

The role of race as a risk factor for OA has been difficult to elucidate because of conflicting study results. Some studies have suggested a low prevalence of hip OA among black populations in Jamaica, South Africa, Nigeria, and Liberia compared to the European population; but a community-based study of hip OA in North Carolina did not confirm racial differences in prevalence.[156-158] According to the National Health and Nutritution Examination Survey and a cross-sectional study in Michigan, the prevalence of knee OA was higher in black females compared to white females, whereas there were no real ethnic differences in the prevalence of hip and hand OA.[156,159,160] Several reports indicate that the prevalence of hip OA may be very low in Asians and in Blackfeet and Pima Native Americans.[148,158,161-164] However, a recent study reported very high prevalence of knee OA in elderly (60 years or older) Chinese women in Beijing, China, whereas the prevalence in men was comparable to white men.[165]

Several studies have demonstrated that persons whose parents had OA (especially polyarticular OA or if the onset was in middle age or earlier) are at a higher risk of developing OA themselves.[166-168] It has also been suggested that the heritability of OA may be higher in women than in men.[169] There is growing evidence of the genetic component of OA,[170-172] especially for hip OA.[168,173,174]

Before the age of 50 years, men have a higher incidence and prevalence of OA than women, but after age 50, women have a higher incidence and prevalence. This sex difference in prevalence increases with age.[133,146] Both incidence and prevalence appear to plateau or decline at around age 80 (see Fig. 27–3). The sex- and age-related incidence and prevalence patterns of OA are consistent with the hypothesis that postmenopausal hormone deficiency increases the risk of OA. In fact, a number of epidemiologic studies suggest that estrogen replacement therapy is associated with a reduction in the risk of knee and hip OA,[149,175-181] whereas evidence is conflicting in other studies.[182-184]

Osteoporosis and OA are inversely associated.[185,186] Bone density in patients with OA is greater than in age-matched controls, even at sites distanced from the joint affected by OA.[187,188] The association of OA with high bone density appears to be independent of body weight.[189] In addition, women with OA have greater bone-mineral density and less bone turnover over time than women without OA,[189-191] and high bone-mineral density might actually slow down disease progression in established OA by reducing joint-space loss.[192]

Damage from reactive oxygen radicals have been implicated in the pathogenesis of OA.[193] It has been suggested that antioxidants from diet or other sources may prevent or delay the occurrence of OA. Vitamins C and E are among the most potent dietary antioxidants.

Among subjects in the Framingham, Massachusettes, OA study, persons in the lowest tertile of vitamin C intake, as assessed by a food frequency questionnaire, had a threefold greater risk of progression of knee OA, joint-space loss, and onset of knee pain, compared to those with a higher intake.[194] Vitamin D status may also affect OA occurrence and progression, because vitamin D is active in bone remodeling. High levels of vitamin D have been shown to protect against incident hip OA.[195] The development of joint-space narrowing was increased for those in the lowest tertile of serum 25-hydroxyvitamin D intake compared to the highest tertile (OR 3.34, 95 percent, CI: 1.13 to 9.86). In the Framingham OA study, no effect of vitamin D on incident OA was demonstrated. However, among individuals with radiographic OA at baseline, those in the lowest tertile of serum 25 hydroxyvitamin D intake had a much higher rate of radiographic progression (OR for radiographic progression 2.9, 95 percent, CI: 1.01 to 8.25) compared to those in the highest tertile of serum 25-hydroxyvitamin D intake.[196]

Knee OA can be experimentally induced in animals by major joint trauma. In humans, major injury is also a common risk factor for OA.[197-199] In the Framingham study, men with a history of major knee injury had five to six times the risk of knee OA of those without such a history; for women, the risk is increased more than threefold.[197] In particular, cruciate ligament damage and meniscal tears have been strongly associated with knee OA.

Repetitive joint use also appears to be a risk factor for OA in the hand,[200] knee,[201-205] and hip.[206-210] Jobs that require kneeling and squatting appear to be associated with a higher-than-expected prevalence of knee OA.[201,204] Men with jobs that require carrying and kneeling or squatting have more than twice the risk of later knee OA development than do men whose jobs did not require these physical activities.[202,203] Repetitive use may also play a role in causing hip OA. Several studies have consistently shown a high rate of hip OA among farmers[206,207] and of knee and hip OA among miners and floorlayers.[204,208] Athletes are at high risk of later development of OA, especially in the weight-bearing joints.[211,212] In fact, individuals with a high lifetime level of general physical activity have been shown to have a high risk of hip OA.[213] Low to moderate physical activity has low, if any, risk of OA.[214]

Overweight persons more often develop knee OA than persons who are not overweight.[149,155] This finding has been shown repeatedly and has been confirmed in longitudinal studies.[198,215-217] Moreover, obesity increases the risk for OA progression, and weight loss is associated with a reduction in the risk of developing symptomatic knee OA.[215,218-220] The relationship of increased body weight with hip and hand OA is not as strong as it is with knee OA.[221,222] In fact, some studies show no association between obesity and hip OA.[140,223-225]

Three uncommon developmental abnormalities—congenital dislocation, Legg-Calvé-Perthes disease, and slipped femoral capital epiphysis—invariably lead to hip OA in later life.[226] More research is needed to determine whether milder developmental abnormalities also increase the risk of hip OA.

Both the quantity and quality of evidence describing the epidemiology and risk factors of OA is growing rapidly. Together, these data will serve as the foundation for new interventions aimed at preventing the onset and progression of this disabling condition.

The Epidemiology of Systemic Lupus Erythematosus

A population-based study examined the incidence and mortality of systemic lupus erythematosus (SLE) in a geographically defined population over a 42-year period.[227] These results indicated that, over the past four decades, the incidence of SLE has nearly tripled and that the survival rate for individuals with this condition (although still poorer than expected for the general population) has significantly improved. The average incidence rate (age- and sex-adjusted to the 1970 US white population) was 5.56 per 100,000 (95 percent CI: 3.93 to 7.19) in the 1980 through 1992 period, compared to an incidence of 1.51 (95 percent, CI: 0.85 to 2.17) in the 1950 through 1979 period. These results compare favorably with previously reported SLE incidence rates of between 1.5 and 7.6 per 100,000.[228,229] In general, studies reporting higher incidence rates used more comprehensive case-retrieval methods. The reported prevalence of SLE has also varied significantly. One study reported an age- and sex-adjusted prevalence, as of January 1, 1992, at approximately 122 per 100,000 (95 percent, CI: 97 to 147).[227] This prevalence is higher than other reported prevalence rates in the continental United States, which have ranged between 14.6 and 50.8 per 100,000.[230,231] However, two studies of self-reported diagnoses of SLE indicated that the actual prevalence of SLE in the United States may be much higher than previously reported.[232,233] One of these studies validated the self-reported diagnoses of SLE by reviewing available medical records.[232] The prevalence rate in that study was 124 cases per 100,000.

There is good evidence that the survival of SLE patients has improved significantly over the past four decades.[227,234-237] Explanations for the improved survival rate included earlier diagnosis of SLE, recognition of mild disease, increased use of antinuclear antibody testing, and better approaches to therapy. Walsh and DeChello[238] demonstrated considerable geographic variation of SLE mortality within the United States. Although it is difficult to distinguish whether the observed variation reflects clustering of risk factors for SLE or regional differences in diagnosis and treatment, there is a clear pattern of elevated mortality in clusters with high poverty rates and greater concentrations of ethnic Hispanics compared to those with lower mortality. Moreover, although improvements in survival have also been demonstrated in some Asian and African countries, these are not as significant as those in the United States.[239-241]

Numerous risk factors have been purported to be involved in the etiology of SLE[242-247] (Fig. 27–4). Because the risk of developing SLE is substantially higher in women than men, differences in hormonal profiles have been suggested as a possible explanation for these differing risks. Unfortunately, the evidence concerning estrogen exposure in relation to the risk of developing SLE is mixed.[243]

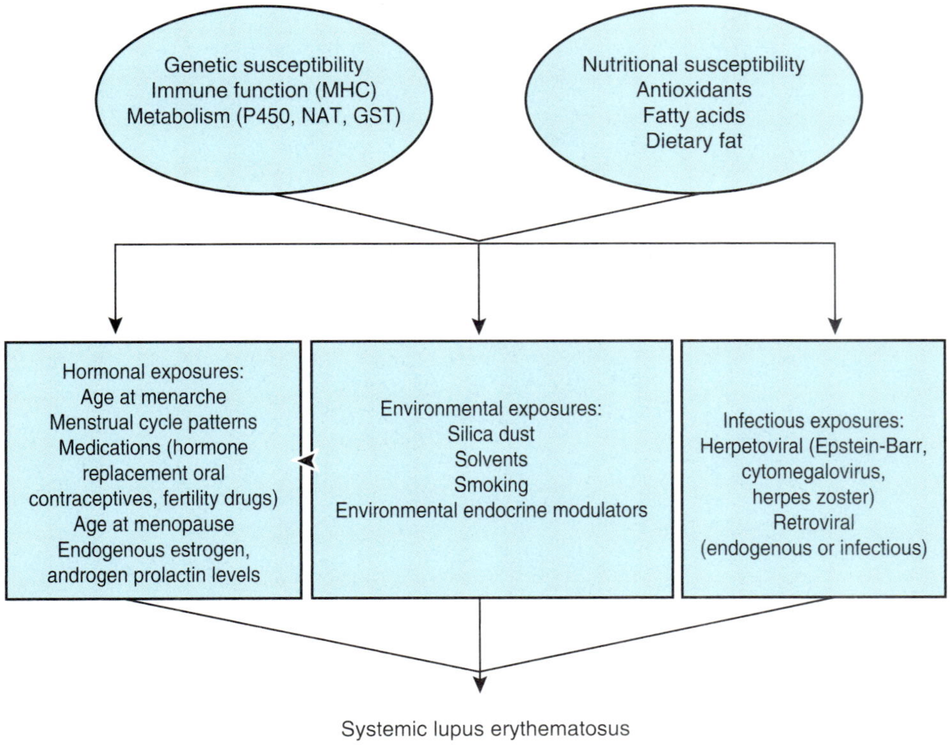

FIGURE 27–4 · Possible interactions between some of the genetic, dietary, hormonal, environmental, and infectious risk factors that are potentially involved in the etiology of systemic lupus erythematosus (SLE). These factors are not firmly established etiologic agents. MHC, major histocompatibility complex; NAT *N*-acetyltransferase; GST, glutathione *S*-transferase. (Adapted from Cooper GS, Dooley MA, Treadwell EL,et al: Hormonal, environmental, and infectious risk factors for developing systemic lupus erythematosus. Arthritis Rheum 41(10):1714-1724, 1998 with permission.)

There are also well-documented racial differences in the risk of developing SLE.[229,248-252] This disease develops at a younger age in blacks, and a higher prevalence of antibodies to Sm and to ribonucleoprotein (RNP) antigens is seen in African American patients compared to white patients in the United States and compared to Latin Americans in Colombia. Discoid lupus is more common in blacks, and white patients more frequently manifest symptoms of photosensitivity and sicca.[253,254] Chinese patients are less likely to have serositis or a hematologic disorder at diagnosis and are more likely to develop proteinuria or central nervous system or other major organ involvement over the course of the disease compared to Caucasian patients.[255] These differences may reflect differences in socioeconomic status, environmental exposures, or genetic susceptabilities. Environmental and infectious exposures currently under study include silica dust, solvents, hair dyes, smoking, environmental endocrine modulators, herpes viruses (including Epstein Barr, cytomegalovirus, and herpes zoster), and retroviruses (both endogenous and exogenous).[245,256-261] Ultimately, the etiology of SLE may unfold as a complex interplay between numerous genetic, hormonal, and environmental risk factors.[262-264]

The Epidemiology of Giant-Cell Arteritis and Polymyalgia Rheumatica

Polymyalgia rheumatica (PMR) and giant cell arteritis (GCA) are closely related conditions.[265] Numerous studies have been conducted that describe the epidemiology of PMR and GCA in a variety of population groups (Table 27–3). As shown in Table 27–3, GCA appears to be most frequent in the Scandinavian countries, with an incidence rate of approximately 27 per 100,000,[266] and in the northern United States, with an incidence rate of approximately 19 per 100,000,[267] compared to southern Europe and the southern United States, where the reported incidence rates have been approximately 7 per 100,000.[268] Such remarkable differences in incidence rates according to geographic variation and latitude are suggestive of a common environmental exposure. However, these differences do not rule out common genetic predisposition.

The average annual age- and sex-adjusted incidence of PMR per 100,000 population 50 years of age or older has been estimated at 58.7 (95 percent, CI: 52.8 to 64.7) with a significantly higher incidence in females (69.8; 95 percent, CI: 61.2 to 78.4) than in males (44.8; 95 percent, CI: 37.0 to 52.6).[269] The prevalence of PMR among persons older than 50 years of age on January 1, 1992, has been estimated at 6 per 1000.[270] The incidence rate in Olmsted County, Minnesota, (58.7 per 100,000) is similar to that reported in a Danish County (68.3 per 100,000)[271] but is somewhat higher than that reported in Goteborg, Sweden (28.6 per 100,000),[272] in Reggio Emilia, Italy (12.7 per 100,000),[268] and in Lugo, Spain (18.7 per 100,000).[273]

Secular trends in incidence rates can provide important etiologic clues. Two studies have examined secular trends in the incidence of GCA and PMR. Nordborg and Bengtsson,[274] from Sweden, examined trends in the incidence of GCA between 1977 and 1986 and showed a near doubling of the incidence rate over this time period, particularly in women. Data from Olmsted County have also shown important secular trends in the incidence of

TABLE 27–3 • GEOGRAPHIC VARIATION IN THE INCIDENCE OF GIANT-CELL ARTERITIS

Author	Region	Years of Study	Annual Incidence*
Huston et al, 1978[276]	Olmsted County, Minn., USA	1950-1974	11.7
Machado et al, 1988[275]	Olmsted County, Minn., USA	1950-1985	17.0
Salvarani et al, 1995[267]	Olmsted County, Minn., USA	1950-1991	17.8
Nordborg and Bengtsson, 1990[274]	Göteborg, Sweden	1977-1986	18.3
Petursdottir et al, 1999[315]	Göteborg, Sweden	1976-1995	22.2
Boesen and Sorensen, 1987[271]	Ribe County, Denmark	1982	23.3
Elling et al, 1996[279]	13 counties, Denmark	1982-1994	20.4
Franzen et al, 1992[316]	Western Nyland, Finland	1987-1988	33.7
Noltorp and Svensson, 1991[317]	Helsingborg, Sweden	1986-1987	33.6
Baldursson et al, 1994[266]	Reykjavik, Iceland	1984-1990	27.0
Friedman et al, 1982[318]	Israel	1960-1978	10.2
Sonnenblick et al, 1994[319]	Jerusalem, Israel	1980-1991	0.5
Smith et al, 1983[320]	Tennessee, USA	1971-1980	1.58
Salvarani et al, 1991[268]	Reggio Emilia, Italy	1980-1988	6.9
Gonzales-Gay et al, 1992[321]	Lugo, Spain	1986-1990	8.3
Gonzales-Gay et al, 1997[322]	Lugo, Spain	1991-1995	10.5
Gran and Myklebust, 1997[323]	Aust Agder, Norway	1987-1994	29
Haugeberg et al, 2000[324]	Vest Agder, Norway	1992-1996	32.8

*Per 100,000 population, > 50 years of age.

GCA.[267] The annual incidence rates increased significantly from 1970 to 2000 and appeared to have clustered in five peak periods, which occurred about every 7 years. A significant calendar-time effect was identified that predicted an increase in incidence of 2.6 percent (CI, 0.9 percent to 4.3 percent) every 5 years.[267] Similarly, Machado and colleagues[275] demonstrated an increase in incidence rates between 1950 and 1985. Notably, these secular trends were quite different in women, in whom the rate increased steadily over the time period compared to males, in whom the rate increased steadily from 1950 to 1974 and then began to decline in the late 1970s and early 1980s. The same finding of different secular trends according to gender were also observed in a Swedish study.[274] Such secular trends may be the result of increased recognition of GCA. In fact, there have been reports demonstrating that the observed frequency of classic disease manifestations in patients with a subsequent diagnosis of GCA is actually declining. This suggests that awareness of the less typical manifestations has improved, resulting in the diagnosis of previously unrecognized cases. However, if improved diagnosis were the only factor accounting for the increase in incidence rate, comparable changes in both sexes would have been expected. This was not so.

Increased use of a diagnostic test could also result in a rise in reported incidence rate of a disease. Huston and coworkers[276] examined the use of temporal artery biopsy between 1965 and 1985 in an effort to examine the effect of a possible detection bias on the divergent sex-specific GCA incidence rates. For women, the biopsy rate increased from 31.9 per 100,000 in 1965 through 1969 to 76.0 per 100,000 in 1980 through 1985. The biopsy rate in men was approximately one half the biopsy rate in women throughout this time period. The proportion of patients 50 years of age or older who had a positive biopsy result did not change significantly over time in women (41 percent) or men (26 percent). This finding suggests that the increased use of temporal artery biopsies does not fully account for the observed rise in GCA incidence over time.

Epidemiologic data can also provide evidence for or against the role of environmental factors in disease pathogenesis. O'Brien and Regan,[277] in the late 1970s, proposed that actinic irradiation could cause GCA by causing transcutaneous damage to the elastin of the internal elastic lamina of the temporal artery. The degeneration of the internal elastic lamina of elderly people was found to be morphologically virtually indistinguishable from the degeneration found in clinically damaged dermal elastic fibers. Thus, these investigators argued that normal aging may predispose to an autoimmune reaction against arterial constituents leading to GCA. In this case, the epidemiologic data is directly contrary to this hypothesis, because the incidence of GCA is markedly lower in warmer climates compared to colder climates.

Of the conditions that occur with a higher frequency in colder climates, respiratory infections are perhaps the most common. The clinical characteristics of PMR and GCA share many characteristics with those of an infectious disease. In addition, there have been a number of anecdotal reports that show an increased frequency of seemingly trivial infections prior to the onset of GCA. Together these data raised the hypothesis of an infectious etiology for GCA. Epidemiologic data from two different sources support this hypothesis.[278,279] Elling and colleagues[279] analyzed data on 10,818 patients from 13 counties and 2651 temporal artery biopsy from two counties in Denmark, which were collected over a 14-year period between 1982 and 1994. These investigators reported an incidence rate of 20.4 for GCA and 41.3 for PMR per 100,000 population. Secular trends in incidence were demonstrated with pronounced quarterly and annual variations in rate. The same study also showed close concurrence of the peaks in incidence of GCA with epidemics of parvovirus B19, *Chlamydia pneumoniae*, and *Mycoplasma pneumoniae*, but not with influenza A or B, hepatitis A or B, or rubella. In a 42-year study of the epidemiology of GCA, the authors reported a regular cyclic pattern in incidence over time, with peaks occurring every 6 to 7 years. This data indicated a statistically significant association between histologic evidence of GCA and the presence of parvovirus B19 DNA in temporal artery biopsy tissue.[280] In spite of these consistent observations, such epidemiologic associations do not necessarily imply causation. Another study failed to identify any seasonal patterns or association with infections.[279] For example, parvovirus B19 may be an innocent bystander that is latent in inflammatory cells, resulting in an increased frequency of B19 in GCA patients compared to biopsy-negative controls. It is also possible that even if parvovirus infection is occurring in patients with GCA, it is a coinfection in these elderly individuals with inflammatory disease, rather than the cause of the underlying disease. These results do illustrate, however, that epidemiologic data can provide unique insights in disease pathogenesis.

The Epidemiology of Gout

There have been very few studies on the epidemiology of gout. In 1967, a study using the Framingham data reported the prevalence of gout at 1.5 percent (2.8 percent in men and 0.4 percent in women).[281] In England, Currie[282] reported the prevalence of gout in 1975 at 0.26 percent, and a multicenter study reported the prevalence in 1995 at 0.95 percent.[283] Various studies revealed that both gout and hyperuricemia have been increasing in the United States, Finland, New Zealand, and Taiwan.[284-288] The most recent study of the incidence of gout was a longitudinal cohort study of 1337 eligible medical students who received a standardized medical examination and questionnaire during medical school.[289] Sixty cases (47 primary and 13 secondary) were identified among the 1216 men in the study. None occurred among the 121 women in the study. The cumulative incidence of all gout was 8.6 percent among men (95 percent, CI: 5.9 to 11.3). Body mass index at age 35 ($p = 0.01$), excessive weight gain (more than 1.88 kg/m^2) between cohort entry and age 35 years ($p = 0.007$), and the development of hypertension ($p = 0.004$) were significant risk factors for the development of gout in univariate analyses. Multivariate Cox proportional hazards models confirmed the association of body mass index at age 35 years (RR 1.12; $p = .02$), excessive weight gain (RR = 2.07; $p = 0.02$), and hypertension (RR = 3.26; $p = 0.002$) as risk factors for all gout. Epidemiologic studies in various non-Western countries also confirm that factors influencing the development of gouty arthritis are similar to those observed in Western countries.[290] Although more research needs to be done, it is clear that the prevention of obesity, particularly in young adulthood, and hypertension may decrease the incidence of and morbidity of gout.

The Epidemiology of Fibromyalgia

Although there have been many studies discussing various clinical aspects of fibromyalgia, there have been few population-based analyses describing the epidemiology of this condition. Since the seminal paper by Smythe and Moldofsky in 1977,[291] interest in fibromyalgia and chronic widespread pain syndromes has grown considerably. In 1992, the annual meeting of the Standing Committee on Epidemiology of the European League against Rheumatism (EULAR) was organized as a workshop to discuss to the concept, definition, and occurrence of fibromyalgia from an epidemiologic perspective.[292] The prevalence of fibromyalgia was reviewed, and wide variation in the reported prevalence of this condition was demonstrated. It varied from a prevalence of 0.7 percent from a study in Denmark to a prevalence of 10.5 percent in a study in Norway. Since that review, additional studies have reported the prevalence at between 1.2 and 4.9 percent, with a peak prevalence in middle-aged women.[151,293-295] Wolfe and coworkers[295] reported a prevalence of 2.0 percent (95 percent, CI: 1.4 to 2.7) overall, 3.4 percent (95 percent, CI: 2.3 to 4.6) for women, and 0.5 percent (95 percent, CI: 0 to 1.0) for men. Another study, based on a screening questionnaire sent to 2498 females aged 20 to 49 living in south Norway, reported an incidence of fibromyalgia in females of 583 per 100,000.[296] All these studies suffer from important methodologic limitations, and thus, the results are not directly comparable. For example, not only is the approach to diagnosis of this condition different across investigators and across sites, but many of these studies use different approaches for case identification.[292,297] Another concern is that many studies on fibromyalgia were derived from clinical populations, and thus, suffer from referral bias. A third concern is the lack of reliability of the measurements employed in these studies. An international group of fibromyalgia investigators all reported significant difficulties in conducting epidemiologic studies of fibromyalgia and concluded that fibromyalgia may be too heterogeneous and may, in fact, represent more than one disease state.[292]

Croft and colleagues[298] have taken a slightly different approach to this condition by studying chronic widespread pain, rather than fibromyalgia, per se. In a cross-sectional postal survey of 2034 adults in the north of England, they reported a point prevalence of 11.2 percent. Both chronic widespread pain and fibromyalgia have been shown to be strongly associated with somatic complaints, as well as measures of depression and anxiety. In addition, fibromyalgia is frequently associated with other musculoskeletal and rheumatic conditions, such as RA and SLE.[299]

The Epidemiology of Sjögren's Syndrome

There have been very few studies performed describing the epidemiology of Sjogren's syndrome and keratoconjunctivitis sicca. Moreover, interpretation of existing studies is complicated by differences in the definition and application of diagnostic criteria. In a population based study from Olmsted County, Minnesota, the average annual age- and sex-adjusted incidence of physician-diagnosed Sjögren's syndrome per 100,000 population was estimated at 3.9 (95 percent, CI: 2.8 to 4.9) with a significantly higher incidence in females (6.9; 95 percent, CI: 5.0 to 8.8) than in males (0.5; 95 percent, CI: 0.0 to 1.2).[300] The prevalence of dry eyes or dry mouth and of primary Sjögren's syndrome among 52- to 72-year-old residents of Malmo, Sweden, according to the Copenhagen criteria, were established in 705 randomly selected subjects who answered a simple questionnaire.[301] The calculated prevalence for the population of keratoconjunctivitis sicca was 14.9 percent (95 percent, CI: 7.3 to 22.2) and of xerostomia was 5.5 percent (3.0 to 7.9), and the prevalence of autoimmune sialoadenitis and primary Sjögren's syndrome was 2.7 percent (1.0 to 4.5). In a Danish study, the frequency of keratoconjunctivitis sicca in persons aged 30 to 60 years was estimated at 11 percent, according to the Copenhagen criteria, and the frequency of Sjögren's syndrome in the same age-group was estimated to be between 0.2 and 0.8 percent.[302] In another study from China, the prevalence was 0.77 percent using Copenhagen criteria and 0.33 percent by the San Diego criteria.[303] Two studies from Greece and Slovenia reported a prevalence of 0.6 percent using the criteria adopted by the Epidemiology Committee of the European Community.[304,305] Sjögren's syndrome has also been reported to be associated with other rheumatic and autoimmune conditions, including fibromyalgia, autoimmune thyroid disease, multiple sclerosis, and spondyloarthropathy, as well as several malignancies, especially non-Hodgkin's lymphoma.

The Epidemiology of Ankylosing Spondylitis

Two large population-based studies provide estimates of the incidence and prevalence of ankylosing spondylitis.[306,307] Using the population-based data resources of the Rochester Epidemiology Project, Carbone and colleagues[306] determined the incidence and prevalence of ankylosing spondylitis first diagnosed between 1935 and 1989 among residents of Rochester, Minnesota. The overall age- and sex-adjusted incidence was 7.3 per 100,000 person-years (95 percent, CI: 6.1 to 8.4). This incidence rate tended to decline between 1935 and 1989; however, there was little change in the age at symptom onset or at diagnosis over the 55-year study period. Overall survival was not decreased up to 28 years following diagnosis. Using the population-based data resources of the Finland sickness insurance registry, Kaipiainen-Seppanen and coworkers[4,307] estimated the annual incidence of ankylosing spondylitis requiring antirheumatic medication at 6.9 per 100,000 adults (95 percent, CI: 6.0 to 7.8) with no change over time. They reported a prevalence of 0.15 percent (95 percent, CI: 0.08 to 0.27). Together, these results indicate a constancy in the epidemiologic characteristics of ankylosing spondylitis.

The incidence of spondyloarthropathies mirrors the prevalence of HLA-B27 seropositivity. HLA-B27 is present throughout Eurasia, but it is virtually absent among the genetically unmixed native populations of South America, Australia, and in certain regions of equatorial and southern Africa.[308] It has a very high prevalence among the native peoples of the circumpolar arctic and the subarctic regions of Eurasia and North America and in some regions of Melanesia. The prevalence of spondyloarthropathies are known to be very high in certain North American Indian populations.[309,310]

REFERENCES

1. Fletcher RH, Fletcher SW, Wagner EH: Clinical epidemiology: The essentials, 3rd ed. Baltimore, Williams & Wilkins, 1996.
2. Symmons DPM, Barrett EM, Bankhead CR, et al: The incidence of rheumatoid arthritis in the United Kingdom: Results from the Norfolk Arthritis Register. Br J Rheumatol 33:735-739, 1994.
3. Aho K, Kaipiainen-Seppanen O, Heliovaara M, Klaukka T: Epidemiology of rheumatoid arthritis in Finland. Semin Arthritis Rheum 27:325-334, 1998.
4. Kaipiainen-Seppanen O, Aho K: Incidence of chronic inflammatory joint diseases in Finland in 1995. J Rheumatol 27(1):94-100, 2000.
5. Kaipiainen-Seppanen O, Aho K, Nikkarinen M: Regional differences in the incidence of rheumatoid arthritis in Finland in 1995. Ann Rheum Dis 60(2):128-132, 2001.
6. Kaipiainen-Seppanen O, Aho K, Isomaki H, Laakso M: Incidence of rheumatoid arthritis in Finland during 1980-1990. Ann Rheum Dis 55:608-611, 1996.
7. Kaipiainen-Seppanen O, Aho K, Laakso M: Shift in the incidence of rheumatoid arthritis toward elderly patients in Finland during 1975-1990. Clin Exp Rheumatol 14:537-542, 1996.
8. Gabriel SE, Crowson CS, O'Fallon WM: The epidemiology of rheumatoid arthritis in Rochester, Minnesota, 1955-1985. Arthritis Rheum 42(3):415-420, 1999.
9. Doran MF, Pond GR, Crowson CS, et al: Trends in incidence and mortality in rheumatoid arthritis in Rochester, Minnesota, over a forty-year period. Arthritis Rheum 46(3):625-631, 2002.
10. Jacobsson LTH, Hanson RL, Knowler WC, et al. Decreasing incidence and prevalence of rheumatoid arthritis in Pima Indians over a twenty-five-year period. Arthritis Rheum 37:1158-1165, 1994.
11. Drosos AA, Alamanos I, Voulgari PV, et al: Epidemiology of adult rheumatoid arthritis in northwest Greece 1987-1995. J Rheumatol 24:2129-2133, 1997.
12. Dugowson CE, Koepsell TD, Voigt LF, et al: Rheumatoid arthritis in women. Incidence rates in Group Health Cooperative, Seattle, Washington, 1987-1989. Arthritis Rheum 34:1502-1507, 1991.
13. Hochberg MC: Changes in the incidence and prevalence of rheumatoid arthritis in England and Wales, 1970-1982. Semin Arthritis Rheum 19(5):294-302, 1990.
14. Imanaka T, Shichikawa K, Inoue K, et al: Increase in age at onset of rheumatoid arthritis in Japan over a 30 year period. Ann Rheum Dis 56(5):313-316, 1997.
15. MacGregor AJ, Silman AJ: A reappraisal of the measurement of disease occurrence in rheumatoid arthritis. J Rheumatol19:1163-1165, 1992.
16. Boyer GS, Benevolenskaya LI, Templin DW, et al: Prevalence of rheumatoid arthritis in circumpolar native populations. J Rheumatol 25(1):23-29, 1998.
17. Cimmino MA: Prevalence of rheumatoid arthritis in Italy: The Chiavari study. Ann Rheum Dis 57(5):315-318, 1998.
18. Stojanovic R, Vlajinac H, Palic-Obradovic D, et al: Prevalence of rheumatoid arthritis in Belgrade, Yugoslavia. Br J Rheumatol 37(7):729-732, 1998.
19. Kvien TK, Glennas A, Knudsrod OG, et al: The prevalence and severity of rheumatoid arthritis in Oslo. Results from a county register and a population survey. Scand J Rheumatol 26(6): 412-418, 1997.
20. Power D, Codd M, Ivers L, et al: Prevalence of rheumatoid arthritis in Dublin, Ireland: A population based survey. Ir J Med Sci 168(3):197-200, 1999.
21. Saraux A, Guedes C, Allain J, et al: Prevalence of rheumatoid arthritis and spondyloarthropathy in Brittany, France. Societe de Rhumatologie de l'Ouest. J Rheumatol 26(12):2622-2627, 1999.
22. Simonsson M, Bergman S, Jacobsson LT, et al: The prevalence of rheumatoid arthritis in Sweden. Scand J Rheumatol 28(6): 340-343, 1999.

23. Carmona L, Villaverde V, Hernandez-Garcia C, et al: The prevalence of rheumatoid arthritis in the general population of Spain. Rheumatology 41(1):88-95, 2002.
24. Riise T, Jacobsen BK, Gran JT: Incidence and prevalence of rheumatoid arthritis in the county of Troms, northern Norway. J Rheumatol 27(6):1386-1389, 2000.
25. Symmons D, Turner G, Webb R, et al: The prevalence of rheumatoid arthritis in the United Kingdom: New estimates for a new century. Rheumatology (Oxford) 41:793-800, 2002.
26. Cobb S, Anderson F, Bauer W: Length of life and cause of death in rheumatoid arthritis. New Engl J Med 249(14):553-556, 1953.
27. Wolfe F, Mitchell DM, Sibley JT, et al: The mortality of rheumatoid arthritis. Arthritis Rheum 37(4):481-494, 1994.
28. Pincus T, Brooks RH, Callahan LF: Prediction of long-term mortality in patients with rheumatoid arthritis according to simple questionnaire and joint count measures. Ann Intern Med 120:26-34, 1994.
29. Coste J, Jougla E: Mortality from rheumatoid arthritis in France, 1970-1990. Int J Epidemiol 23:545-552, 1994.
30. Monson RR, Hall AP: Mortality among arthritics. J Chron Dis 29:459-467, 1976.
31. Myllykangas-Luosujarvi RA, Aho K, Isomaki HA: Mortality in rheumatoid arthritis. Semin Arthritis Rheum 25(3):193-202, 1995.
32. Gabriel SE, Crowson CS, O'Fallon WM: Mortality in rheumatoid arthritis: Have we made an impact in 4 decades? J Rheumatol 26(12):2529-2533, 1999.
33. Myllykangas-Luosujarvi R, Aho K, Kautiainen H, Isomaki H: Shortening of life span and causes of excess mortality in a population-based series of subjects with rheumatoid arthritis. Clin Exp Rheumatol 13(2):149-153, 1995.
34. Isomaki HA, Mutru O, Koota K: Death rate and causes of death in patients with rheumatoid arthritis. Scand J Rheumatol 4(4):205-208, 1975.
35. Vandenbroucke JP, Hazevoet HM, Cats A: Survival and cause of death in rheumatoid arthritis: A 25-year prospective followup. J Rheumatol 11(2):158-161, 1984.
36. Pincus T, Callahan LF, Sale WG, et al: Severe functional declines, work disability, and increased mortality in seventy-five rheumatoid arthritis patients studied over nine years. Arthritis Rheum 27(8):864-872, 1984.
37. Allebeck P, Ahlbom A, Allander E: Increased mortality among persons with rheumatoid arthritis, but where RA does not appear on death certificate. Eleven-year follow-up of an epidemiological study. Scand J Rheumatol 10(4):301-306, 1981.
38. Allebeck P: Increased mortality in rheumatoid arthritis. Scand J Rheumatol 11(2):81-86, 1982.
39. Prior P, Symmons DPM, Scott DL, et al: Cause of death in rheumatoid arthritis. Br J Rheumatol 23(2):92-99, 1984.
40. Jacobsson LTH, Knowler WC, Pillemer S, et al: Rheumatoid arthritis and mortality: A longitudinal study in Pima Indians. Arthritis Rheum 36(8):1045-1053, 1993.
41. van Dam G, Lezwign A, Bos JG: Death rate in patients with rheumatoid arthritis. Minerva Med 1:161-164, 1961.
42. Duthie JJR, Brown PE, Truelove LH, et al: Course and prognosis in rheumatoid arthritis. A further report. Ann Rheum Dis 23: 193-204, 1964.
43. Reilly PA, Cosh JA, Maddison PJ, et al: Mortality and survival in rheumatoid arthritis: A 25 year prospective study of 100 patients. Ann Rheum Dis 49(6):363-369, 1990.
44. Lewis P, Hazleman BL, Hanka R, Roberts S: Cause of death in patients with rheumatoid arthritis with particular reference to azathioprine. Ann Rheum Dis 39(5):457-461, 1980.
45. Linos A, Worthington JW, O'Fallon WM, Kurland LT: The epidemiology of rheumatoid arthritis in Rochester, Minnesota: A study of incidence, prevalence, and mortality. Am J Epidemiol 111(1):87-98, 1980.
46. Mitchell DM, Spitz PW, Young DY, et al: Survival, prognosis, and causes of death in rheumatoid arthritis. Arthritis Rheum 29(6):706-714, 1986.
47. Wallberg-Jonsson S, Ohman ML, Dahlqvist SR: Cardiovascular morbidity and mortality in patients with seropositive rheumatoid arthritis in Northern Sweden. J Rheumatol 24:445-451, 1997.
48. Sokka T, Mottonen T, Hannonen P: Mortality in early "sawtooth" treated rheumatoid arthritis patients during the first 8-14 years. Scan J Rheumatol 28(5):282-287, 1999.
49. Symmons DP, Jones MA, Scott DL, Prior P: Longterm mortality outcome in patients with rheumatoid arthritis: Early presenters continue to do well. J Rheumatol 25(6):1072-1077, 1998.
50. Kvalvik AG, Jones MA, Symmons DP: Mortality in a cohort of Norwegian patients with rheumatoid arthritis followed from 1977 to 1992. Scand J Rheumatol 29(1):29-37, 2000.
51. Chehata JC, Hassell AB, Clarke SA, et al: Mortality in rheumatoid arthritis: Relationship to single and composite measures of disease activity. Rheumatology 40(4):447-452, 2001.
52. Krause D, Schleusser B, Herborn G, Rau R: Response to methotrexate treatment is associated with reduced mortality in patients with severe rheumatoid arthritis. Arthritis Rheum 43(1):14-21, 2000.
53. Martinez MS, Garcia-Monforte A, Rivera J: Survival study of rheumatoid arthritis patients in Madrid (Spain). A 9-year prospective follow-up. Scand J Rheumatol 30(4):195-198, 2001.
54. Riise T, Jacobsen BK, Gran JT, et al: Total mortality is increased in rheumatoid arthritis. A 17-year prospective study. Clin Rheumatol 20(2):123-127, 2001.
55. Uddin J, Kraus AS, Kelly HG: Survivorship and death in rheumatoid arthritis. Arthritis Rheum 13(2):125-130, 1970.
56. Callahan LF, Cordray DS, Wells G, Pincus T: Formal education and five-year mortality in rheumatoid arthritis: Mediation by helplessness scale score. Arthritis Care Research 9(6):463-472, 1996.
57. Mutru O, Laakso M, Isomaki H, Koota K: Ten year mortality and causes of death in patients with rheumatoid arthritis. Br Med J (Clin Res Educ) 290(6484):1797-1799, 1985.
58. Ward MM: Recent improvements in survival in patients with rheumatoid arthritis: Better outcomes or different study designs? Arthritis Rheum 44(6):1467-1469, 2001.
59. Goodson NJ, Wiles NJ, Lunt M, et al: Mortality in early inflammatory polyarthritis: Cardiovascular mortality is increased in seropositive patients. Arthritis Rheum 46(8):2010-2019, 2002.
60. Gabriel SE, Crowson CS, O'Fallon WM: Comorbidity in arthritis. J Rheumatol 26(11):2475-2479, 1999.
61. Soderlin MK, Nieminen P, Hakala M: Functional status predicts mortality in a community based rheumatoid arthritis population. J Rheumatol 25(10):1895-1899, 1998.
62. Wallberg-Jonsson S, Johansson H, Ohman ML, Rantapaa-Dahlqvist S: Extent of inflammation predicts cardiovascular disease and overall mortality in seropositive rheumatoid arthritis. A retrospective cohort study from disease onset. J Rheumatol 26(12):2562-2571, 1999.
63. Leigh JP, Fries JF: Mortality predictors among 263 patients with rheumatoid arthritis. J Rheumatol 18(9):1307-1312, 1991.
64. Turesson C, O'Fallon WM, Crowson CS, et al: Occurrence of extraarticular disease manifestations is associated with excess mortality in a community based cohort of patients with rheumatoid arthritis. J Rheumatol 29(1):62-67, 2002.
65. Erhardt CC, Mumford PA, Venables PJ, Maini RN: Factors predicting a poor life prognosis in rheumatoid arthritis: An eight year prospective study. Ann Rheum Dis 48(1):7-13, 1989.
66. Gabriel SE, Crowson CS, Maradit Kremers H, et al: Survival in rheumatoid arthritis: A population-based analysis of trends over 40 years. Arthritis Rheum, in press.
67. Pincus T, Callahan LF, Burkhauser RV: Most chronic diseases are reported more frequently by individuals with fewer than 12 years of formal education in the age 18-64 United States population. J Chron Dis 40:865-874, 1987.
68. Pincus T, Callahan LF: Formal education as a marker for increased mortality and morbidity in rheumatoid arthritis. J Chron Dis 38(12):973-984, 1985.
69. Callahan LF, Pincus T: Formal education level as a significant marker of clinical status in rheumatoid arthritis. Arthritis Rheum 31(11):1346-1357, 1988.
70. Pincus T, Callahan LF: Taking mortality in rheumatoid arthritis seriously - predictive markers, socioeconomic status and comorbidity. J Rheumatol 13(5):841-845, 1986.
71. Bankhead C, Silman A, Barrett B, et al: Incidence of rheumatoid arthritis is not related to indicators of socioeconomic deprivation. J Rheumatol 23:2039-2042, 1996.
72. Harrison BJ: Influence of cigarette smoking on disease outcome in rheumatoid arthritis. Curr Opin Rheumatol 14(2):93-97, 2002.

73. Uhlig T, Hagen KB, Kvien TK: Current tobacco smoking, formal education, and the risk of rheumatoid arthritis. J Rheumatol 26:47-54, 1999.
74. Wolfe F: The effect of smoking on clinical, laboratory, and radiographic status in rheumatoid arthritis. J Rheumatol 27(3):630-637, 2000.
75. Silman AJ, Newman J, MacGregor AJ: Cigarette smoking increases the risk of rheumatoid arthritis. Results from a nationwide study of disease-discordant twins. Arthritis Rheum 39:732-735, 1996.
76. Heliovaara M, Aho K, Aromaa A, et al: Smoking and risk of rheumatoid arthritis. J Rheumatol 20:1830-1835, 1993.
77. Karlson EW, Lee IM, Cook NR, et al: A retrospective cohort study of cigarette smoking and risk of rheumatoid arthritis in female health professionals. Arthritis Rheum 42(5):910-917, 1999.
78. Heliovaara M, Aho K, Knekt P, et al: Coffee consumption, rheumatoid factor, and the risk of rheumatoid arthritis. Ann Rheum Dis 59(8):631-635, 2000.
79. Mikuls TR, Cerhan JR, Criswell LA, et al: Coffee, tea, and caffeine consumption and risk of rheumatoid arthritis: results from the Iowa Women's Health Study. Arthritis Rheum 46(1):83-91, 2002.
80. Brennan P, Bankhead C, Silman A, Symmons D: Oral contraceptives and rheumatoid arthritis: results from a primary care-based incident case-control study. Semin Arthritis Rheum 26:817-823, 1997.
81. Doran M: The Effect of Oral Contraceptives and Estrogen Replacement Therapy on the Risk of Rheumatoid Arthritis: A Population-Based Study J Rheumatol 31(2), 2004. In press.
82. Silman A, Bankhead C, Rowlingson B, et al: Do new cases of rheumatoid arthritis cluster in time or in space? Int J Epidemiol 26(3):628-634, 1997.
83. Silman A, Harrison B, Barrett E, Symmons D: The existence of geographical clusters of cases of inflammatory polyarthritis in a primary care based register. Ann Rheum Dis 59(2):152-154, 2000.
84. Harrison B, Silman A, Barrett E, Symmons D: Low frequency of recent parvovirus infection in a population-based cohort of patients with early inflammatory polyarthritis. Ann Rheum Dis 57(6):375-377, 1998.
85. Hochberg MC: Adult and juvenile rheumatoid arthritis: current epidemiologic concepts. Epidemiol Rev 3:27-44, 1981.
86. Deighton CM, Walker DJ: The familial nature of rheumatoid arthritis. Ann Rheum Dis 50(1):62-65, 1991.
87. Stastny P: Association of the B-cell alloantigen DRw4 with rheumatoid arthritis. N Engl J Med 298(16):869-871, 1978.
88. Gregerson P, Silver J, Winchester R: The shared epitope hypothesis: an approach to understanding the molecular genetics of susceptibility to rheumatoid arthritis. Arthritis Rheum 30:1205-1213, 1987.
89. Nepom GT, Hansen JA, Nepom BS: The molecular basis for HLA class II associations with rheumatoid arthritis. J Clin Immunol 7(1):1-7, 1987.
90. Willkens RF, Nepom GT, Marks CR, et al: Association of HLA-Dw16 with rheumatoid arthritis in Yakima Indians. Further evidence for the "shared epitope" hypothesis. Arthritis Rheum 34(1):43-47, 1991.
91. del Rincon I, Escalante A: HLA-DRB1 alleles associated with susceptibility or resistance to rheumatoid arthritis, articular deformities, and disability in Mexican Americans. Arthritis Rheum 42(7):1329-1338, 1999.
92. Pascual M, Nieto A, Lopez-Nevot MA, et al: Rheumatoid arthritis in southern Spain: Toward elucidation of a unifying role of the HLA class II region in disease predisposition. Arthritis Rheum 44(2):307-314, 2001.
93. Tuokko J, Nejentsev S, Luukkainen R, et al: HLA haplotype analysis in Finnish patients with rheumatoid arthritis. Arthritis Rheum 44(2):315-322, 2001.
94. Gonzalez-Gay MA, Garcia-Porrua C, Hajeer AH: Influence of human leukocyte antigen-DRB1 on the susceptibility and severity of rheumatoid arthritis. Semin Arthritis Rheum 31(6):355-360, 2002.
95. Ioannidis JP, Tarassi K, Papadopoulos IA, et al: Shared epitopes and rheumatoid arthritis: Disease associations in Greece and meta-analysis of Mediterranean European populations. Semin Arthritis Rheum 31(6):361-370, 2002.
96. Aho K, Koskenvuo M, Tuominen J, Kaprio J: Occurrence of rheumatoid arthritis in a nationwide series of twins. J Rheumatol 13:899-902, 1986.
97. Silman AJ, MacGregor AJ, Thomson W, et al: Twin concordance rates for rheumatoid arthritis: Results from a nationwide study. Br J Rheumatol 32(10):903-907, 1993.
98. Jarvinen P, Aho K: Twin studies in rheumatic diseases. Semin Arthritis Rheum 24(1):19-28, 1994.
99. Wolfe F, Kleinheksel SM, Khan MA: Familial vs sporadic rheumatoid arthritis: A comparison of the demographic and clinical characteristics of 956 patients. J Rheumatol 15(3):400-404, 1988.
100. Hasstedt SJ, Clegg DO, Ingles L, Ward RH: HLA-linked rheumatoid arthritis. Am J Hum Genet 55(4):738-746, 1994.
101. MacGregor AJ, Snieder H, Rigby AS, et al: Characterizing the quantitative genetic contribution to rheumatoid arthritis using data from twins. Arthritis Rheum 43(1):30-37, 2000.
102. Oen KG, Cheang M: Epidemiology of chronic arthritis in childhood. Semin Arthritis Rheum 26(3):575-591, 1996.
103. Andersson Gare B: Juvenile arthritis–who gets it, where and when? A review of current data on incidence and prevalence. Clin Exp Rheumatol 17(3):367-374, 1999.
104. von Koskull S, Truckenbrodt H, Holle R, Hormann A: Incidence and prevalence of juvenile arthritis in an urban population of southern Germany: A prospective study. Ann Rheum Dis 60(10):940-945, 2001.
105. Kaipiainen-Seppanen O, Savolainen A: Changes in the incidence of juvenile rheumatoid arthritis in Finland. Rheumatology 40(8):928-932, 2001.
106. Prahalad S, Ryan MH, Shear ES, et al: Juvenile rheumatoid arthritis: linkage to HLA demonstrated by allele sharing in affected sibpairs. Arthritis Rheum43(10):2335-2338, 2000.
107. Forre O, Smerdel A: Genetic epidemiology of juvenile idiopathic arthritis. Scand J Rheumatol 31(3):123-128, 2002.
108. Oen K, Fast M, Postl B: Epidemiology of juvenile rheumatoid arthritis in Manitoba, Canada, 1975-92: cycles in incidence. J Rheumatol 22(4):745-750, 1995.
109. Gare BA, Fasth A: Epidemiology of juvenile chronic arthritis in southwestern Sweden: A 5-year prospective study. Pediatrics 90:950-958, 1992.
110. Aredarczyk Z: Rheumatoid arthritis in children up to 15 years of age in Poland. Pediatr Pol LII:73-78, 1977.
111. Lindsley CB: Seasonal variation in systemic onset juvenile rheumatoid arthritis. Arthritis Rheum 30:838-839, 1987.
112. Feldman B: Is there a seasonal onset to systemic juvenile rheumatoid arthritis? Arthritis Rheum 36:S60, 1993.
113. Peterson LS, Mason T, Nelson AM, et al: Juvenile rheumatoid arthritis in Rochester, Minnesota 1960-1993. Arthritis Rheum 39(8):1385-1390, 1996.
114. Koivuniemi R, Leirisalo-Repo M: Juvenile chronic arthritis in adult life: a study of long-term outcome in patients with juvenile chronic arthritis or adult rheumatoid arthritis. Clin Rheumatol 18(3):220-226, 1999.
115. David J, Cooper C, Hickey L, et al: The functional and psychological outcomes of juvenile chronic arthritis in young adulthood. Br J Rheumatol 33(9):876-881, 1994.
116. Gare BA, Fasth A: The natural history of juvenile chronic arthritis: a population based cohort study. II. Outcome. J Rheumatol 22(2):308-319, 1995.
117. Peterson LS, Mason T, Nelson AM, et al: Psychosocial outcomes and health status of adults who have had juvenile rheumatoid arthritis: a controlled, population-based study. Arthritis Rheum 40(12):2235-2240, 1997.
118. Ruperto N, Levinson J, Ravelli A, et al: Long-term health outcomes and quality of life in American and Italian inception cohorts of patients with juvenile rheumatoid arthritis. I. Outcome status. J Rheumatol 24:945-951, 1997.
119. Zak M, Pedersen FK: Juvenile chronic arthritis into adulthood: a long-term follow-up study. Rheumatology 39(2):198-204, 2000.
120. Arguedas O, Fasth A, Andersson-Gare B: A prospective population based study on outcome of juvenile chronic arthritis in Costa Rica. J Rheumatol 29(1):174-183, 2002.
121. Flato B, Smerdel A, Johnston V, et al: The influence of patient characteristics, disease variables, and HLA alleles on the development of radiographically evident sacroiliitis in juvenile idiopathic arthritis. Arthritis Rheum 46(4):986-994, 2002.

122. French AR, Mason T, Nelson AM, et al: Increased mortality in adults with a history of juvenile rheumatoid arthritis: A population-based study. Arthritis Rheum 44(3):523-527, 2001.
123. Minden K, Niewerth M, Listing J, et al: Long-term outcome in patients with juvenile idiopathic arthritis. Arthritis Rheum 46(9):2392-2401, 2002.
124. Kaipiainen-Seppanen O. Incidence of psoriatic arthritis in Finland. Br J Rheumatol 35:1289-1291, 1996.
125. Soderlin MK, Borjesson O, Kautiainen H, et al: Annual incidence of inflammatory joint diseases in a population based study in southern Sweden. Ann Rheum Dis 61(10):911-915, 2002.
126. Shbeeb M, Uramoto KM, Gibson LE, et al: The epidemiology of psoriatic arthritis in Olmsted County, Minnesota, USA, 1982-1991. J Rheumatol 27(5):1247-1250, 2000.
127. Gladman DD: Natural history of psoriatic arthritis. Baillière's Clin Rheumatol 8(2):379-393, 1994.
128. Taylor WJ: Epidemiology of psoriatic arthritis. Curr Opin Rheumatol 14(2):98-103, 2002.
129. Gladman DD, Farewell VT, Wong K, Husted J: Mortality studies in psoriatic arthritis: results from a single outpatient center. II. Prognostic indicators for death. Arthritis Rheum 41(6):1103-1110, 1998.
130. Wong K, Gladman DD, Husted J, et al: Mortality studies in psoriatic arthritis: results from a single outpatient clinic. I. Causes and risk of death. Arthritis Rheum 40(10):1868-1872, 1997.
131. Gladman DD, Hing EN, Schentag CT, Cook RJ: Remission in psoriatic arthritis. J Rheumatol 28(5):1045-1048, 2001.
132. Husted JA, Gladman DD, Farewell VT, Cook RJ: Health-related quality of life of patients with psoriatic arthritis: A comparison with patients with rheumatoid arthritis. Arthritis Rheum 45(2):151-158, 2001.
133. Felson DT, Zhang Y: An update on the epidemiology of knee and hip osteoarthritis with a view to prevention. Arthritis Rheum 41(8):1343-1355, 1998.
134. Gabriel SE, Crowson CS, O'Fallon WM: Costs of osteoarthritis: estimates from a geographically-defined population. J Rheumatol 22(suppl 43):23-25, 1995.
135. Gabriel SE, Crowson CS, Campion ME, O'Fallon WM: Direct medical costs unique to people with arthritis. J Rheumatol 24:719-725, 1997.
136. Gabriel SE, Crowson CS, Campion ME, O'Fallon WM: Indirect and nonmedical costs among people with rheumatoid arthritis and osteoarthritis compared with nonarthritic controls. J Rheumatol 24:43-48, 1997.
137. Yelin E: The economics of osteoarthritis. *In* Brandt K, Doherty M, Lohmander LS (eds): Osteoarthritis. New York, Oxford University Press, 1998, pp 23-30.
138. Felson DT: Epidemiology of hip and knee osteoarthritis. Epidemiol Rev 10:1-28, 1988.
139. Oliveria SA, Felson DT, Reed JI, et al: Incidence of symptomatic hand, hip, and knee osteoarthritis among patients in a health maintenance organization. Arthritis Rheum 38(8):1134-1141, 1995.
140. Kellgren J: Osteoarthritis in patients and populations. Br Med J 7:1-6, 1961.
141. Lawrence JS, Bremner JM, Bier F: Osteo-arthrosis. Prevalence in the population and relationship between symptoms and x-ray changes. Ann Rheum Dis 25(1):1-24, 1966.
142. Zinn WM: Reflections on degenerative hip disease. Ann Phys Med 10(5):209-217, 1970.
143. Pogrund H, Rutenberg M, Makin M, et al: Osteoarthritis of the hip joint and osteoporosis: a radiological study in a random population sample in Jerusalem. Clin Orthop 164:130-135, 1982.
144. Danielsson L, Lindberg H, Nilsson B: Prevalence of coxarthrosis. Clin Orthop 191:110-115, 1984.
145. Maurer K: Basic Data on Arthritis, Knee, Hip, and Sacroiliac Joints in Adults Ages 25–74 Years: United States, 1971–1975. National Center for Health Statistics. Vital Health Stat Series No. 11(213). 1979.
146. van Saase JL, van Romunde LK, Cats A, et al: Epidemiology of osteoarthritis: Zoetermeer survey. Comparison of radiological osteoarthritis in a Dutch population with that in 10 other populations. Ann Rheum Dis 48(4):271-280, 1989.
147. Ingvarsson T, Hagglund G, Lohmander LS: Prevalence of hip osteoarthritis in Iceland. Ann Rheum Dis 58(4):201-207, 1999.
148. Nevitt MC, Xu L, Zhang Y, et al: Very low prevalence of hip osteoarthritis among Chinese elderly in Beijing, China, compared with whites in the United States: The Beijing osteoarthritis study. Arthritis Rheum 46(7):1773-1779, 2002.
149. Hart DJ, Doyle DV, Spector TD: Incidence and risk factors for radiographic knee osteoarthritis in middle-aged women. Arthritis Rheum 42(1):17-24, 1999.
150. Felson DT, Naimark A, Anderson J, et al: The prevalence of knee osteoarthritis in the elderly. The Framingham Osteoarthritis Study. Arthritis Rheum 30(8):914-918, 1987.
151. Carmona L, Ballina J, Gabriel R, et al: The burden of musculoskeletal diseases in the general population of Spain: results from a national survey. Ann Rheum Dis 60(11):1040-1045, 2001.
152. Heine J: Uber die arthritis deformans. Arch Pathol Anat 260:521, 1926.
153. Stankovic A, Mitrovic D: Prevalence of the degenerative lesions in articular cartilage of the human knee joint: Relationship with age. *In* Peyron JG (ed): Epidemiologie de L'arthrose. Paris, Geigy, 1980, pp 94-98.
154. Sharma L, Pai YC, Holtkamp K, Rymer WZ: Is knee joint proprioception worse in the arthritic knee versus the unaffected knee in unilateral knee osteoarthritis? Arthritis Rheum 40(8):1518-1525, 1997.
155. Felson DT, Lawrence RC, Dieppe PA, et al: Osteoarthritis: new insights. Part I: The disease and its risk factors. Ann Intern Med 133(8):635-646, 2000.
156. Anderson JJ, Felson DT: Factors associated with osteoarthritis of the knee in the first national Health and Nutrition Examination Survey (HANES I). Evidence for an association with overweight, race, and physical demands of work. Am J Epidemiol 128(1):179-189, 1988.
157. Jordan JM, Linder GF, Renner JB, Fryer JG: The impact of arthritis in rural populations. Arthritis Care Res 8(4):242-250, 1995.
158. Lawrence JS, Sebo M: The geography of osteoarthritis. *In* Nuki G (ed): The Aetiopathogenesis of Osteoarthrosis. Baltimore, University Park Press, 1980, pp 155-183.
159. Sowers M, Lachance L, Hochberg M, Jamadar D: Radiographically defined osteoarthritis of the hand and knee in young and middle-aged African American and Caucasian women. Osteoarthritis Cartilage 8(2):69-77, 2000.
160. Tepper S, Hochberg MC: Factors associated with hip osteoarthritis: data from the First National Health and Nutrition Examination Survey (NHANES-I). Am J Epidemiol 137(10):1081-1088, 1993.
161. Hoaglund FT, Yau AC, Wong WL: Osteoarthritis of the hip and other joints in southern Chinese in Hong Kong. J Bone Joint Surg Am 55(3):545-557, 1973.
162. Hoaglund FT, Oishi CS, Gialamas GG: Extreme variations in racial rates of total hip arthroplasty for primary coxarthrosis: a population-based study in San Francisco. Ann Rheum Dis 54(2):107-110, 1995.
163. Lau EM, Lin F, Lam D, et al: Hip osteoarthritis and dysplasia in Chinese men. Ann Rheum Dis 54(12):965-969, 1995.
164. Oishi CS, Hoaglund FT, Gordon L, Ross PD: Total hip replacement rates are higher among Caucasians than Asians in Hawaii. Clin Orthop 353:166-174, 1998.
165. Zhang Y, Xu L, Nevitt MC, et al: Comparison of the prevalence of knee osteoarthritis between the elderly Chinese population in Beijing and whites in the United States: The Beijing Osteoarthritis Study. Arthritis Rheum 44(9):2065-2071, 2001.
166. Ala-Kokko L, Baldwin CT, Moskowitz RW, Prockop DJ: Single base mutation in the type II procollagen gene (COL2A1) as a cause of primary osteoarthritis associated with a mild chondrodysplasia. Proc Natl Acad Sci U S A 87(17):6565-6568, 1990.
167. Palotie A, Vaisanen P, Ott J, et al: Predisposition to familial osteoarthrosis linked to type II collagen gene. Lancet 1(8644):924-927, 1989.
168. MacGregor AJ, Matson M, Spector TD: The genetic contribution to radiographic hip osteoarthritis in women: Results of a classic twin study. Arthritis Rheum 43(7):1450-1455, 2000.
169. Kaprio J, Kujala UM, Peltonen L, Koskenvuo M: Genetic liability to osteoarthritis may be greater in women than men [Letter; Comment]. BMJ (Clinical Research Ed) 313(7051):232, 1996.

170. Chitnavis J, Sinsheimer JS, Clipsham K, et al: Genetic influences in end-stage osteoarthritis. Sibling risks of hip and knee replacement for idiopathic osteoarthritis. J Bone Joint Surg (British) 79(4):660-664, 1997.
171. Spector TD, Cicuttini F, Baker J, et al: Genetic influences on osteoarthritis in women: a twin study. Brit Med J 312(7036): 940-943, 1996.
172. Loughlin J, Dowling B, Mustafa Z, Chapman K: Association of the interleukin-1 gene cluster on chromosome 2q13 with knee osteoarthritis. Arthritis Rheum 46(6):1519-1527, 2002.
173. Chapman K, Mustafa Z, Dowling B, et al: Finer linkage mapping of primary hip osteoarthritis susceptibility on chromosome 11q in a cohort of affected female sibling pairs. Arthritis Rheum 46(7):1780-1783, 2002.
174. Ingvarsson T, Stefansson SE, Hallgrimsdottir IB, et al: The inheritance of hip osteoarthritis in Iceland. Arthritis Rheum 43(12):2785-2792, 2000.
175. Nevitt MC, Cummings SR, Lane NE, et al: Association of estrogen replacement therapy with the risk of osteoarthritis of the hip in elderly white women. Study of Osteoporotic Fractures Research Group. Arch Intern Med 156(18):2073-2080, 1996.
176. Hannan MT, Felson DT, Anderson JJ, et al: Estrogen use and radiographic osteoarthritis of the knee in women. The Framingham Osteoarthritis Study. Arthritis Rheum 33(4):525-532, 1990.
177. Wolfe F, Altman R, Hochberg M, et al: Post menopausal estrogen therapy is associated with improved radiographic scores in OA and RA [Abstract]. Arthritis Rheum 37(Suppl 9):S231, 1994.
178. Samanta A, Jones A, Regan M, et al: Is osteoarthritis in women affected by hormonal changes or smoking? Br J Rheumatol 32(5):366-370, 1993.
179. Spector TD, Nandra D, Hart DJ, Doyle DV: Is hormone replacement therapy protective for hand and knee osteoarthritis in women?: The Chingford Study. Ann Rheum Dis 56(7):432-434, 1997.
180. Vingard E, Alfredsson L, Malchau H: Lifestyle factors and hip arthrosis. A case referent study of body mass index, smoking and hormone therapy in 503 Swedish women. Acta Orthop Scand 68(3):216-220, 1997.
181. Zhang Y, McAlindon TE, Hannan MT, et al: Estrogen replacement therapy and worsening of radiographic knee osteoarthritis: the Framingham Study. Arthritis Rheum 41(10):1867-1873, 1998.
182. Erb A, Brenner H, Gunther KP, Sturmer T: Hormone replacement therapy and patterns of osteoarthritis: Baseline data from the Ulm Osteoarthritis Study. Ann Rheum Dis 59(2):105-109, 2000.
183. Sandmark H, Hogstedt C, Lewold S, Vingard E: Osteoarthrosis of the knee in men and women in association with overweight, smoking, and hormone therapy. Ann Rheum Dis 58(3):151-155, 1999.
184. Oliveria SA, Felson DT, Klein RA, et al: Estrogen replacement therapy and the development of osteoarthritis. Epidemiology 7(4):415-419, 1996.
185. Dequeker J: Inverse relationship of interface between osteoporosis and osteoarthritis. J Rheumatol 24:795-798, 1997.
186. Antoniades L, MacGregor AJ, Matson M, Spector TD: A cotwin control study of the relationship between hip osteoarthritis and bone mineral density. Arthritis Rheum 43(7):1450-1455, 2000.
187. Gevers G, Dequeker J, Martens M, et al: Biomechanical characteristics of iliac crest bone in elderly women according to osteoarthritis grade at the hand joints. J Rheumatol 16(5):660-663, 1989.
188. Dequeker J, Goris P, Uytterhoeven R: Osteoporosis and osteoarthritis (osteoarthrosis). Anthropometric distinctions. JAMA 249(11):1448-1451, 1983.
189. Hannan MT, Anderson JJ, Zhang Y, et al: Bone mineral density and knee osteoarthritis in elderly men and women. The Framingham Study. Arthritis Rheum 36(12):1671-1680, 1993.
190. Nevitt MC, Lane NE, Scott JC, et al: Radiographic osteoarthritis of the hip and bone mineral density. Arthritis Rheum 38(7):907-916, 1995.
191. Sowers M, Lachance L, Jamadar D, et al: The associations of bone mineral density and bone turnover markers with osteoarthritis of the hand and knee in pre- and perimenopausal women. Arthritis Rheum 42(3):483-489, 1999.
192. Zhang Y, Hannan MT, Chaisson CE, et al: Bone mineral density and risk of incident and progressive radiographic knee osteoarthritis in women: the Framingham Study. J Rheumatol 27(4):1032-1037, 2000.
193. Tiku ML, Liesch JB, Robertson FM: Production of hydrogen peroxide by rabbit articular chondrocytes. Enhancement by cytokines. J Immunol 145(2):690-696, 1990.
194. McAlindon TE, Jacques P, Zhang Y, et al: Do antioxidant micronutrients protect against the development and progression of knee osteoarthritis? Arthritis Rheum 39(4):648-656, 1996.
195. Lane NE, Gore LR, Cummings SR, et al: Serum vitamin D levels and incident changes of radiographic hip osteoarthritis: a longitudinal study. Study of Osteoporotic Fractures Research Group. Arthritis Rheum 42(5):854-860, 1999.
196. McAlindon TE, Felson DT, Zhang Y, et al: Relation of dietary intake and serum levels of vitamin D to progression of osteoarthritis of the knee among participants in the Framingham study. Ann Intern Med 125(5):353-359, 1996.
197. Zhang Y, Glynn RJ, Felson DT: Musculoskeletal disease research: should we analyze the joint or the person? J Rheumatol 23:1130-1134, 1996.
198. Cooper C, Snow S, McAlindon TE, et al: Risk factors for the incidence and progression of radiographic knee osteoarthritis. Arthritis Rheum 43(5):995-1000, 2000.
199. Lau EC, Cooper C, Lam D, et al: Factors associated with osteoarthritis of the hip and knee in Hong Kong Chinese: Obesity, joint injury, and occupational activities. Am J Epidemiol 152(9):855-862, 2000.
200. Hadler NM, Gillings DB, Imbus HR, et al: Hand structure and function in an industrial setting. Arthritis Rheum 21(2):210-220, 1978.
201. Kirkeskov LJ, Eenberg W: Occupation as a risk factor for knee disorders. Scand J Work Environ Health 22:165-175, 1996.
202. Felson DT, Hannan MT, Naimark A, et al: Occupational physical demands, knee bending, and knee osteoarthritis: Results from the Framingham Study. J Rheumatol 18(10):1587-1592, 1991.
203. Coggon D, Croft P, Kellingray S, et al: Occupational physical activities and osteoarthritis of the knee. Arthritis Rheum 43(7): 1443-1449, 2000.
204. Jensen LK, Mikkelsen S, Loft IP, et al: Radiographic knee osteoarthritis in floorlayers and carpenters. Scand J Work Environ Health 26(3):257-262, 2000.
205. Sandmark H, Hogstedt C, Vingard E: Primary osteoarthrosis of the knee in men and women as a result of lifelong physical load from work. Scand J Work Environ Health 26(1):20-25, 2000.
206. Croft P, Coggon D, Cruddas M, Cooper C: Osteoarthritis of the hip: an occupational disease in farmers. BMJ 304:1269-1272, 1992.
207. Thelin A: Hip joint arthrosis: an occupational disorder among farmers. Am J Ind Med 18(3):339-343, 1990.
208. Felson DT: Do occupation-related physical factors contribute to arthritis? Baillières Clin Rheumatol 8(1):63-77, 1994.
209. Vingard E, Alfredsson L, Malchau H: Osteoarthrosis of the hip in women and its relation to physical load at work and in the home. Ann Rheum Dis 56(5):293-298, 1997.
210. Yoshimura N, Sasaki S, Iwasaki K, et al: Occupational lifting is associated with hip osteoarthritis: A Japanese case-control study. J Rheumatol 27(2):434-440, 2000.
211. Kujala UM, Kaprio J, Sarna S: Osteoarthritis of weight bearing joints of lower limbs in former elite male athletes. Brit Med J 308(6923):231-234, 1994.
212. Spector TD, Harris PA, Hart DJ, et al: Risk of osteoarthritis associated with long-term weight-bearing sports: A radiologic survey of the hips and knees in female ex-athletes and population controls. Arthritis Rheum 39(6):988-995, 1996.
213. Buckwalter JA, Lane NE: Athletics and osteoarthritis. Am J Sports Med 25(6):873-881, 1997.
214. Sutton AJ, Muir KR, Mockett S, Fentem P: A case-control study to investigate the relation between low and moderate levels of physical activity and osteoarthritis of the knee using data collected as part of the Allied Dunbar National Fitness Survey. Ann Rheum Dis 60(8):756-764, 2001.
215. Felson DT, Zhang Y, Hanna MT, et al: Risk factors for incident radiographic knee osteoarthritis in the elderly: The Framingham Study. Arthritis Rheum 40(4):728-733, 1997.

216. Manninen P, Riihimaki H, Heliovaara M, Makela P: Overweight, gender and knee osteoarthritis. Int J Obes Relat Metab Disord 20(6):595-597, 1996.
217. Spector TD, Hart DJ, Doyle DV: Incidence and progression of osteoarthritis in women with unilateral knee disease in the general population: the effect of obesity. Ann Rheum Dis 53(9):565-568, 1994.
218. Felson DT, Ahange Y, Anthony JM, et al: Weight loss reduces the risk for symptomatic knee osteoarthritis in women. Ann Intern Med 116:535-539, 1992.
219. Schouten JS, van den Ouweland FA, Valkenburg HA: A 12 year follow up study in the general population on prognostic factors of cartilage loss in osteoarthritis of the knee. Ann Rheum Dis 51(8):932-937, 1992.
220. Dougados M, Gueguen A, Nguyen M, et al: Longitudinal radiologic evaluation of osteoarthritis of the knee. J Rheumatol 19(3):378-384, 1992.
221. Oliveria SA, Felson DT, Cirillo PA, et al: Body weight, body mass index, and incident symptomatic osteoarthritis of the hand, hip, and knee. Epidemiology 10(2):161-166, 1999.
222. Carman WJ, Sowers M, Hawthorne VM, Weissfeld LA: Obesity as a risk factor for osteoarthritis of the hand and wrist: a prospective study. Am J Epidemiol 139(2):119-129, 1994.
223. Saville PD, Dickson J: Age and weight in osteoarthritis of the hip. Arthritis Rheum 11(5):635-644, 1968.
224. Tepper S, Hochberg MC: Factors associated with hip osteoarthritis: data from the First National Health and Nutrition Examination Survey (NHANES-I). American J Epidemiol 137(10):1081-1088, 1993.
225. van Saase JL, Vandenbroucke JP, van Romunde LK, Valkenburg HA: Osteoarthritis and obesity in the general population. A relationship calling for an explanation. J Rheumatol 15(7):1152-1158, 1988.
226. Felson DT: Osteoarthritis. Rheum Dis Clin North Am 16(3):499-512, 1990.
227. Uramoto KM, Michet CJJ, Thumboo J, et al: Trends in the incidence and mortality of systemic lupus erythematosus (SLE): 1950-1992. Arthritis Rheum 42(1):46-50, 1999.
228. Michet CJ Jr, McKenna CH, Elveback LR, et al: Epidemiology of systemic lupus erythematosus and other connective tissue diseases in Rochester, Minnesota, 1950 through 1979. Mayo Clin Proc 60:105-113, 1985.
229. Fessel WJ: Systemic lupus erythematosus in the community. Incidence, prevalence, outcome, and first symptoms; the high prevalence in black women. Arch Intern Med 134:1027-1035, 1974.
230. Hochberg MC: Systemic lupus erythematosus. Rheum Dis Clin North Am 16(3):617-639, 1990.
231. Lawrence RC, Helmick CG, Arnett FC, et al: Estimates of the prevalence of arthritis and selected musculoskeletal disorders in the United States. Arthritis Rheum 41(5):778-799, 1998.
232. Hochberg MC, Perlmutter DL, Medsger TA, et al: Prevalence of self-reported physician-diagnosed systemic lupus erythematosus in the USA. Lupus 4(6):454-456, 1995.
233. Lahita RG: Special report: adjusted lupus prevalence. Results of a marketing study by the Lupus Foundation of America. Lupus 4(6):450-453, 1995.
234. Gladman DD: Prognosis and treatment of systemic lupus erythematosus. Curr Opin Rheumatol 8(5):430-437, 1996.
235. Ward MM, Pyun E, Studenski S: Long-term survival in systemic lupus erythematosus. Patient characteristics associated with poorer outcomes. Arthritis Rheum 38:274-283, 1995.
236. Urowitz MB, Gladman DD: How to improve morbidity and mortality in systemic lupus erythematosus. Rheumatology 39(3):238-244, 2000.
237. Ruiz-Irastorza G, Khamashta MA, Castellino G, Hughes GR: Systemic lupus erythematosus. Lancet 357(9261):1027-1032, 2001.
238. Walsh SJ, DeChello LM: Geographical variation in mortality from systemic lupus erythematosus in the United States. Lupus 10(9):637-646, 2001.
239. Wang F, Wang CL, Tan CT, Manivasagar M: Systemic lupus erythematosus in Malaysia: A study of 539 patients and comparison of prevalence and disease expression in different racial and gender groups. Lupus 6(3):248-253, 1997.
240. Xie SK, Feng SF, Fu H: Long term follow-up of patients with systemic lupus erythematosus. J Dermatol 25(6):367-373, 1998.
241. Ka MM, Diallo S, Kane A, et al: Systemic lupus erythematosus and lupus syndromes in Senegal. A retrospective study of 30 patients seen over 10 years. Revue du Rhumatisme (English Edition) 65(7-9):471-476, 1998.
242. Cooper GS, Dooley MA, Treadwell EL, et al: Hormonal, environmental, and infectious risk factors for developing systemic lupus erythematosus. Arthritis Rheum 41(10):1714-1724, 1998.
243. McAlindon T: Update on the epidemiology of systemic lupus erythematosus: New spins on old ideas. Curr Opin Rheumatol 12(2):104-112, 2000.
244. Bengtsson AA, Rylander L, Hagmar L, et al: Risk factors for developing systemic lupus erythematosus: A case-control study in southern Sweden. Rheumatology 41(5):563-571, 2002.
245. Cooper GS, Dooley MA, Treadwell EL, et al: Smoking and use of hair treatments in relation to risk of developing systemic lupus erythematosus. J Rheumatol 28(12):2653-2656, 2001.
246. Ghaussy NO, Sibbitt WL Jr, Qualls CR: Cigarette smoking, alcohol consumption, and the risk of systemic lupus erythematosus: a case-control study. J Rheumatol 28(11):2449-2453, 2001.
247. Strom BL, Reidenberg MM, West S, et al: Shingles, allergies, family medical history, oral contraceptives, and other potential risk factors for systemic lupus erythematosus. Am J Epidemiol 140(7):632-642, 1994.
248. Fessel WJ: Epidemiology of systemic lupus erythematosus. Rheum Dis Clin North Am 14(1):15-23, 1988.
249. Hopkinson ND, Doherty M, Powell RJ: Clinical features and race-specific incidence/prevalence rates of systemic lupus erythematosus in a geographically complete cohort of patients. Ann Rheum Dis 53:676-680, 1994.
250. McCarty DJ, Manzi S, Medsger JTA, et al: Incidence of systemic lupus erythematosus. Race and gender differences. Arthritis Rheum 38(9):1260-1270, 1995.
251. Johnson AE, Gordon C, Palmer RG, Bacon PA: The prevalance and incidence of systemic lupus erythematosus in Birmingham, England: Relationship to ethnicity and country of birth. Arthritis Rheum 38(4):551-558, 1995.
252. Bae SC, Fraser P, Liang MH: The epidemiology of systemic lupus erythematosus in populations of African ancestry: A critical review of the "prevalence gradient hypothesis." Arthritis Rheum 41(12):2091-2099, 1998.
253. Molina JF, Molina J, Garcia C, et al: Ethnic differences in the clinical expression of systemic lupus erythematosus: A comparative study between African-Americans and Latin Americans. Lupus 6(1):63-67, 1997.
254. Gedalia A, Molina JF, Molina J, et al: Childhood-onset systemic lupus erythematosus: A comparative study of African Americans and Latin Americans. J Nat Med Assoc 91(9):497-501, 1999.
255. Thumboo J, Uramoto K, O'Fallon WM, et al: A comparative study of the clinical manifestations of systemic lupus erythematosus in Caucasians in Rochester, Minnesota, and Chinese in Singapore, from 1980 to 1992. Arthritis Rheum 45(6):494-500, 2001.
256. Mayes MD: Epidemiologic studies of environmental agents and systemic autoimmune diseases. Environmental Health Perspectives 107(Suppl 5):743-748, 1999.
257. Sanchez-Guerrero J, Karlson EW, Colditz GA, et al: Hair dye use and the risk of developing systemic lupus erythematosus. Arthritis Rheum 39(4):657-662, 1996.
258. Hardy CJ, Palmer BP, Muir KR, Powell RJ: Systemic lupus erythematosus (SLE) and hair treatment: a large community based case-control study. Lupus 8(7):541-544, 1999.
259. James JA, Neas BR, Moser KL, et al: Systemic lupus erythematosus in adults is associated with previous Epstein-Barr virus exposure. Arthritis Rheum 44(5):1122-1126, 2001.
260. Parks CG, Cooper GS, Nylander-French LA, et al: Occupational exposure to crystalline silica and risk of systemic lupus erythematosus: A population-based, case-control study in the southeastern United States. Arthritis Rheum 46(7):1840-1850, 2002.
261. Sekigawa I, Ogasawara H, Kaneko H, et al: Retroviruses and autoimmunity. Internal Medicine 40(2):80-86, 2001.
262. Tan FK, Arnett FC: The genetics of lupus. Curr Opin Rheumatol 10(5):399-408, 1998.
263. Gaffney PM, Moser KL, Graham RR, Behrens TW: Recent advances in the genetics of systemic lupus erythematosus. Rheum Dis Clin North Am 28(1):111-126, 2002.

264. Molokhia M, McKeigue P: Risk for rheumatic disease in relation to ethnicity and admixture. Arthritis Research 2(2):115-125, 2000.
265. Salvarani C, Cantini F, Boiardi L, Hunder GG: Polymyalgia rheumatica and giant-cell arteritis. N Engl J Med 347(4):261-271, 2002.
266. Baldursson O, Steinsson K, Bjornsson J, Lie JT: Giant cell arteritis in Iceland. An epidemiologic and histopathologic analysis. Arthritis Rheum 37:1007-1012, 1994.
267. Salvarani C, Gabriel SE, O'Fallon WM, Hunder GG: The incidence of giant cell arteritis in Olmsted County, Minnesota: Apparent fluctuations in a cyclic pattern. Ann Intern Med 123:192-194, 1995.
268. Salvarani C, Macchioni P, Zizzi F, et al: Epidemiologic and immunogenetic aspects of polymyalgia rheumatica and giant cell arteritis in northern Italy. Arthritis Rheum 34(3):351-356, 1991.
269. Doran M, Crowson C, O'Fallon W, et al: Trends in the incidence of polymyalgia rheumatica over a 30-year period in Olmsted County, Minnesota. J Rheumatol 29:1694-1697, 2002.
270. Salvarani C, Gabriel SE, O'Fallon WM, Hunder GG: Epidemiology of polymyalgia rheumatica in Olmsted County, Minnesota, 1970-1991. Arthritis Rheum 38(3):369-373, 1995.
271. Boesen P, Sorensen SF: Giant cell arteritis, temporal arteritis, and polymyalgia rheumatica in a Danish county. A prospective investigation, 1982-1985. Arthritis Care Research 30(3):294-299, 1987.
272. Bengtsson BA, Malmvall BE: The epidemiology of giant cell arteritis including temporal arteritis and polymyalgia rheumatica. Incidences of different clinical presentations and eye complications. Arthritis Rheum 24(7):899-904, 1981.
273. Gonzalez-Gay MA, Garcia-Porrua C, Vazquez-Caruncho M, et al: The spectrum of polymyalgia rheumatica in northwestern Spain: Incidence and analysis of variables associated with relapse in a 10 year study. J Rheumatol 26(6):1326-1332, 1999.
274. Nordborg E, Bengtsson B: Epidemiology of biopsy-proven giant cell arteritis (GCA). J Int Med Res 227:233-236, 1990.
275. Machado EBV, Michet CJ Jr, Ballard DJ, et al: Trends in incidence and clinical presentation of temporal arteritis in Olmsted County, Minnesota: 1950-1985. Arthritis Rheum 31:745-749, 1988.
276. Huston KA, Hunder GG, Lie JT, et al: Temporal arteritis. A 25-year epidemiologic, clinical, and pathologic study. Ann Intern Med 88(2):162-167, 1978.
277. O'Brien JP, Regan W: A study of elastic tissue and actinic radiation in "aging," temporal arteritis, polymyalgia rheumatica, and atherosclerosis. The actinic storm in the modern world. J Am Acad Dermatol 24(5 Pt 1):765-776, 1991.
278. Duhaut P, Bosshard S, Calvet A, et al: Giant cell arteritis, polymyalgia rheumatica, and viral hypotheses: A multicenter, prospective case-control study. J Rheumatol 26(2):361-369, 1999.
279. Elling P, Olsson AT, Elling H: Synchronous variations of the incidence of temporal arteritis and polymyalgia rheumatica in different regions of Denmark: Association with epidemics of Mycoplasma pneumoniae infection. J Rheumatol 23(1):112-119, 1996.
280. Gabriel SE, Espy M, Erdman DD, et al: The role of parvovirus B19 in the pathogeneisis of giant cell arteritis: A preliminary evaluation. Arthritis Rheum 42(6):1255-1258, 1999.
281. Hall AP, Barry PE, Dawber TR, McNamara PM: Epidemiology of gout and hyperuricemia. A long-term population study. Am J Med 42(1):27-37, 1967.
282. Currie WJ: Prevalence and incidence of the diagnosis of gout in Great Britain. Ann Rheum Dis 38(2):101-106, 1979.
283. Harris CM, Lloyd DC, Lewis J: The prevalence and prophylaxis of gout in England. J Clin Epidemiol 48(9):1153-1158, 1995.
284. Lawrence RC, Hochberg MC, Kelsey JL, et al: Estimates of the prevalence of selected arthritic and musculoskeletal diseases in the United States. J Rheumatol 16(4):427-441, 1989.
285. Isomaki H, von Essen R, Ruutsalo HM: Gout, particularly diuretics-induced, is one the increase in Finland. Scand J Rheumatol 6(4):213-216, 1977.
286. Klemp P, Stansfield SA, Castle B, Robertson MC: Gout is on the increase in New Zealand. Ann Rheum Dis 56(1):22-26, 1997.
287. Lin KC, Lin HY, Chou P: Community based epidemiological study on hyperuricemia and gout in Kin-Hu, Kinmen. J Rheumatol 27(4):1045-1050, 2000.
288. Chang HY, Pan WH, Yeh WT, Tsai KS: Hyperuricemia and gout in Taiwan: Results from the Nutritional and Health Survey in Taiwan (1993-96). J Rheumatol 28(7):1640-1646, 2001.
289. Roubenoff R, Klag MJ, Mead LA, et al: Incidence and risk factors for gout in white men. JAMA 266(21):3004-3007, 1991.
290. Wortmann RL: Gout and hyperuricemia. Curr Opin Rheumatol 14(3):281-286, 2002.
291. Smythe HA, Moldofsky H: Two contributions to understanding of the "fibrositis" syndrome. Bull Rheum Dis 28(1):928-931, 1977.
292. Schochat T, Croft P, Raspe H: The epidemiology of fibromyalgia. Workshop of the Standing Committee on Epidemiology European League Against Rheumatism (EULAR), Bad Sackingen, 19-21 November 1992. Br J Rheumatol 33(8):783-786, 1994.
293. Wolfe F, Ross K, Anderson J, et al: The prevalence and characteristics of fibromyalgia in the general population. Arthritis Rheum 38:19-28, 1995.
294. White KP, Speechley M, Harth M, Ostbye T: The London Fibromyalgia Epidemiology Study: The prevalence of fibromyalgia syndrome in London, Ontario. J Rheumatol 26(7):1570-1576, 1999.
295. Lindell L, Bergman S, Petersson IF, et al: Prevalence of fibromyalgia and chronic widespread pain. Scand J Prim Health Care18(3):149-153, 2000.
296. Forseth KO, Gran JT, Husby G: A population study of the incidence of fibromyalgia among women aged 26-55 yr. Br J Rheumatol 36(12):1318-1323, 1997.
297. Felson DT: Epidemiologic research in fibromyalgia. J Rheumatol 16(Suppl 19):7-11, 1989.
298. Croft P, Rigby AS, Boswell R, et al: The prevalence of chronic widespread pain in the general population. J Rheumatol 20(4):710-713, 1993.
299. Middleton GD, McFarlin JE, Lipsky PE: The prevalence and clinical impact of fibromyalgia in systemic lupus erythematosus. Arthritis Rheum 37(8):1181-1188, 1994.
300. Pillemer SR, Matteson EL, Jacobsson LT, et al: Incidence of physician-diagnosed primary Sjögren syndrome in residents of Olmsted County, Minnesota. Mayo Clinic Proc 76(6):593-599, 2001.
301. Jacobsson LT, Axell TE, Hansen BU, et al: Dry eyes or mouth–an epidemiological study in Swedish adults, with special reference to primary Sjögren's syndrome. J Autoimmun 2(4):521-527, 1989.
302. Bjerrum KB: Keratoconjunctivitis sicca and primary Sjögren's syndrome in a Danish population aged 30-60 years. Acta Ophthalmologica Scandinavica 75(3):281-286, 1997.
303. Zhang NZ, Shi CS, Yao QP, et al: Prevalence of primary Sjögren's syndrome in China. J Rheumatol 22(4):659-661, 1995.
304. Dafni UG, Tzioufas AG, Staikos P, et al: Prevalence of Sjögren's syndrome in a closed rural community. Ann Rheum Dis 56(9):521-525, 1997.
305. Tomsic M, Logar D, Grmek M, et al: Prevalence of Sjögren's syndrome in Slovenia. Rheumatology 38(2):164-170, 1999.
306. Carbone LD, Cooper C, Michet CJ, et al: Ankylosing spondylitis in Rochester, Minnesota, 1935-1989. Is the epidemiology changing? Arthritis Rheum 35(12):1476-1482, 1992.
307. Kaipiainen-Seppanen O, Aho K, Heliovaara M: Incidence and prevalence of ankylosing spondylitis in Finland. J Rheumatol 24(3):496-499, 1997.
308. Khan MA: Epidemiology of HLA-B27 and Arthritis. Clin Rheumatol 15(Suppl 1):10-12, 1996.
309. Lawrence RC, Everett DF, Benevolenskaya LI, et al: Spondyloarthropathies in circumpolar populations: I. Design and methods of United States and Russian studies. Arctic Medical Research 55(4):187-194, 1996.
310. Benevolenskaya LI, Boyer GS, Erdesz S, et al: Spondylarthropathic diseases in indigenous circumpolar populations of Russia and Alaska. Rev Rhum Engl Ed 63(11):815-822, 1996.
311. Chan K-WA, Felson DT, Yood RA, Walker AM: Incidence of rheumatoid arthritis in central Massachusetts. Arthritis Rheum 36:1691-1696, 1993.

312. Uhlig T, Kvien TK, Glennas A, et al: The incidence and severity of rheumatoid arthritis, results from a county register in Oslo, Norway. J Rheumatol 25(6):1078-1084, 1998.
313. Shichikawa K, Inoue K, Hirota S, et al: Changes in the incidence and prevalence of rheumatoid arthritis in Kamitonda, Wakayama, Japan, 1965-1996. Ann Rheum Dis 58(12):751-756, 1999.
314. Lindqvist E, Eberhardt K: Mortality in rheumatoid arthritis patients with disease onset in the 1980s. Ann Rheum Dis 58(1):11-14, 1999.
315. Petursdottir V, Johansson H, Nordborg E, Nordborg C: The epidemiology of biopsy-positive giant cell arteritis: special reference to cyclic fluctuations. Rheumatology 38(12):1208-1212, 1999.
316. Franzen P, Sutinen S, Von Knorring J: Giant cell arteritis and polymyalgia rheumatica in a region of Finland: An epidemiologic, clinical, and pathologic study, 1984-1988. J Rheumatol 19:273-280, 1992.
317. Noltorp S, Svensson B: High incidence of polymyalgia rheumatica and giant cell arteritis in a Swedish community. Clin Exp Rheumatol 9(4):351-355, 1991.
318. Friedman G, Friedman B, Benbassat J: Epidemiology of temporal arteritis in Israel. Isr J Med Sci 18(2):241-244, 1982.
319. Sonnenblick M, Nesher G, Friedlander Y, Rubinow A: Giant cell arteritis in Jerusalem: A 12-year epidemiological study. Br J Rheumatol 33(10):938-941, 1994.
320. Smith CA, Fidler WJ, Pinals RS: The epidemiology of giant cell arteritis. Report of a ten-year study in Shelby County, Tennessee. Arthritis Rheum 26(10):1214-1219, 1983.
321. Gonzalez-Gay MA, Alonso MD, Aguero JJ, et al: Temporal arteritis in a northwestern area of Spain: Study of 57 biopsy proven patients. J Rheumatol 19(2):277-280, 1992.
322. Gonzalez-Gay MA, Blanco R, Sanchez-Andrade A, Vazquez-Caruncho M: Giant cell arteritis in Lugo, Spain: A more frequent disease with fewer classic features. J Rheumatol 24(11):2166-2170, 1997.
323. Gran JT, Myklebust G. The incidence of polymyalgia rheumatica and temporal arteritis in the county of Aust Agder, south Norway: A prospective study 1987-94. J Rheumatol 24(9):1739-1743, 1997.
324. Haugeberg G, Paulsen PQ, Bie RB: Temporal arteritis in Vest Agder County in southern Norway: Incidence and clinical findings. J Rheumatol 27(11):2624-2627, 2000.
325. Fletcher RH, Fletcher SW, Wagner EH: Clinical Epidemiology: The Essentials. Vol 2. Baltimore, Williams & Wilkins, 1988.

28 Economic Burden of Rheumatic Diseases

ANTHONY D. WOOLF

Musculoskeletal conditions are common and are characterized by pain and physical disability, along with important consequent effects on activities and participation.[1] Their prevalence and impact is increasing worldwide with the aging of the population and changes in risk factors such as physical inactivity and obesity. At present, care is underprovided in most parts of the globe, and priorities do not reflect the increasing need for such care.[2]

The burden of musculoskeletal conditions is one individuals bear as disability and loss of quality of life, as well as an economic burden on them, their family, and their careers in terms of lost income and providing support. In addition, there are the direct costs of care and support borne by the individual and society as a consequence of social and health care.

There must be a better understanding of the health, social, and economic burden of these conditions to develop priorities to inform policy decisions for the provision of appropriate care and to decide on the best approach for management of the clinical problems. This chapter will focus on the economic burden.

Health Economics

Health economics is important in a world where there will always be constraints on the resources for health and social care. They can guide health priorities and decision making about which approach will be most beneficial, overall, to the greatest number of people. Health economics can generate useful information on equity of care, and it can inform the debate as to whether resources should be directed to health care or other activities that influence health-related quality of life. Economic cost studies also help identify information gaps and research needs. Each should have a societal perspective encompassing all, regardless of who incurs them, and all benefits delivered, regardless of who receives them.

THE COSTS OF ILLNESS

The economic impact of any health condition can be considered in terms of the net loss to the economy occasioned by the illness. It can be measured as the societal cost of providing services related to the delivery of health care and social support. It can also be considered as the personal cost to the patient, family, or immediate community. These costs can be estimated within the framework of the direct, indirect, or intangible costs associated with the condition. In economics, the notion of cost is based on the value that would be gained from using resources elsewhere. This is referred to as "opportunity cost." It is usual, in practice, to assume that the price paid reflects the opportunity cost and to adopt a pragmatic approach to costing and use market prices when possible.

Direct Costs

Direct costs are those directly associated with detection, treatment, and prevention of disease. These costs may be disease specific, a direct result of the condition, or disease associated, a consequence of the primary disease or its treatment. Direct costs include costs of physician visits, diagnostic tests, prescription drugs, over-the-counter medications, hospital stays and procedures, aids and devices, and outpatient procedures. These expenditures may be borne solely or in combination by the patients, their health insurer, employers, or a local or national government agency. Direct costs also include other expenditures, generally paid for by the patient, and include transportation to and from the doctor or other allied health worker, higher food bills associated with a special diet, or expenditures to adapt the home environment to make activities of daily living easier. What is included under this heading varies among different forms of economic analyses and depends on the perspective of the study (i.e., who is paying for care and who is receiving it). For example, home care is a direct cost for the patient but an indirect health cost for the funder. Many of the direct costs relate to utilization of available resources and therefore do not reflect burden if the need is unmet. Most are a consequence of treatment and not prevention.

Direct costs are relatively easy to measure. They can be estimated using a "top down" approach (dividing the total health expenditure among different diseases) or a "bottom up" approach in which the number of health care services for individuals who fulfil diagnostic criteria can be counted and costed. The certainty of case definition is better in the bottom up approach. The total costs of disease can then be estimated. The attributable costs give the clearest idea of what potential savings there are; these can be identified by looking for the incremental costs either before or after the onset of disease or the event, such as a fracture. It can also be determined in a case-control study, which compares the total health care costs of individuals with the disease compared to matched controls. The case-control method has the advantage of allowing for comorbidities and associated events.

Indirect Costs

Indirect costs result from the consequences of a condition, such as limitation of usual activities. These include loss of employment due to treatment, sick leave, reduced productivity, early retirement, or death. There are also the losses attributable to the condition preventing the person from having a better paying job or reducing employment opportunities. The additional costs related to self care, maintenance of a home, schooling, or parenting are also included. Both patients and their carers may incur indirect costs. Chronic physical disability has its major impact in indirect costs.

Indirect costs are more difficult to measure. Some can be given a monetary value, although this is dependent on local systems of social support, sickness benefits, and pensions. Lost work productivity is important in chronic musculoskeletal conditions but rarely is included in economic evaluations.[3] It can be estimated in different ways, principally the "human capital approach," which uses the full replacement costs irrespective of whether the worker is replaced, or by the "friction cost" approach in which only the productivity costs during the period needed to restore the individual to his or her initial production level is considered, and the replacement worker is from the labor market. This results in lower estimates of lost productivity costs and is probably more realistic.

Other indirect costs cannot be given a specific value because reduced productivity and lost hours at school or in doing household work are difficult to value and allocate a monetary cost. Methods such as "willingness to pay" that value what individuals are willing to pay (in monetary terms) for a change resulting in improvement in health, such as a reduced probability of morbidity, can be used. This method allows individuals to indicate how they value health, variable degrees of disability, and death. These can be calculated from a societal perspective.

Indirect costs are strongly influenced by people who work, because employment-related costs are easier to quantify. The economic impact on children, women, the elderly, and those unemployed is not adequately captured.

Intangible Costs

Intangible costs are those associated with loss in function, increased pain, and reduced quality of life of patients, families, and careers. These include the costs of lost opportunities. These are very important for musculoskeletal conditions, because disability is a significant outcome with limitations in activities of daily living, reduction in leisure and community activities, chronic pain, psychologic problems including depression and anxiety, and reduced general health. The inverse of the intangible costs of arthritis is the benefit a patient receives from effective treatment. If measurements of the costs of care are to have relevance for clinical decision making, decision makers must also consider the effects of disease and therapy on the patient's health and well-being. Intangible costs are, however, very difficult to quantify and extremely difficult to to assign a monetary value.

Cost Items and Estimates

There are a large number of cost items that can be used in the estimation of the cost of illness. They fall under the categories of direct, indirect, and intangible costs as described previously (Table 28–1). Not all items are considered in health economic evaluations, and such omissions need to be recognized as the value of any evaluation should consider all those cost items that may be influenced by the condition or its treatment. Omissions or different definitions can affect the interpretation and comparability of the data. Attempts are being made to standardize the cost domains for musculoskeletal conditions.[4,5] There also must be some standardization for the way these are costed if there is to be any comparability and meaning to economic evaluations.

COST OF ILLNESS STUDIES

The economics of health can be looked at in different ways depending on the objectives of the analysis. Cost of illness studies and cost analyses[6] examine the resources used in the provision of health care related to the condition and do not relate them to the benefits or outcomes of health care. These costs must relate to the effect of the condition and also its management, including any complications of the disease and treatment or side effects of the therapies. For musculoskeletal diseases with a wide variation of the impact on individuals during their course, information is also required of the different health states of that disease and numbers in those states.

A principal weakness of cost of illness studies is that they are just looking at the supply side. Quantifying expenditures does not mean that money has been spent efficiently. High costs may reflect inefficient use of resources; conversely, low costs may reflect limited availability of health care resources. These do not give information on costs of prevention. Low costs do not mean that a lower priority is appropriate, as it still may be amenable to a very cost-effective intervention.

Cost analysis is not an economic evaluation because it does not measure benefits gained by resources consumed, but rather, it provides an evidence base for such analysis. Its value is in measuring the economic burden and enabling the identification of how it is distributed within the health care system and other parts of the public sector, the patient, the family, and society as a whole. It can facilitate identifying the potential for improvements in care that is provided, showing where change is likely to have greatest effect. It is used to aid policy-making decisions.[7] The value of cost analysis to policy makers for choosing between alternatives is limited. The value of burden of disease and cost of illness studies in guiding policy has been criticized.[8,9] Measures of indirect cost are difficult; not all the same cost domains are included in different studies, and various methods of ascribing cost are used, which limits comparability between studies.

Health economic evaluations require other methods that enable the costs to be measured against health gains achieved by an intervention, but these are not considered within the context of this chapter, which

TABLE 28–1 • DOMAINS OF HEALTH ECONOMIC IMPACT RELEVANT TO MUSCULOSKELETAL CONDITIONS

Category	Domains	How to Identify Costs
Direct Costs		
Health care costs		
Outpatient costs	Visits to physicians (primary care and specialist)	
	Outpatient surgery	Hospital or insurer activity data of visits
	Emergency room	
	Rehabilitation service utilization (physiotherapist, occupational therapist, social worker, etc.)	
	Medication (prescription and nonprescription)	Pharmacy records
	Diagnostic/therapeutic procedures and tests	Radiology activity Laboratory tests
	Devices and aids	Provision of equipment
Inpatient costs	Acute hospital facilities (without surgery)	Hospital or insurer activity, data of admissions, lengths of stay, procedures
	Acute hospital facilities (with surgery)	
	Nonacute hospital facilities	Rehabilitation activity Nursing home activity
Personal costs	Transportation	Transportation distance, frequency, methods
	Patient time	Time spent in health care
	Carer time	Time spent giving care
Other disease related costs	Home health care services	Home health care activity
	Environmental adaptations	Home, work, and transportation adaptations
	Medical equipment (nonprescription)	Equipment provision
	Nonmedical practitioner, alternative therapy	Therapist activity
Indirect Costs		
Change of living status	Nursing home or residential home	Nursing and residential home activity
	Home care services	Formal and informal home care activity
Productivity costs	Loss of productivity in employed patients or their carers	Sick leave, lost wages, work disability benefits, number no longer working, disabilities leading to impaired housekeeping or activities of daily living, loss of productivity
	Opportunity costs—reduced employability at present or higher level	
Out of pocket	Out of pocket expenses	Survey
Intangible costs		
	Deterioration in quality of life of patient, family, carers, friends	Difficult to quantify

Modified from Merkesdal S, Ruof J, Huelsemann JL, et al: Development of a matrix of cost domains in economic evaluation of rheumatoid arthritis. J Rheumatol 28:657-661, 2001.

will principally consider cost of illness and cost analysis data. It will show the breadth of economic impact against which any benefit of an intervention needs to be evaluated.

Cost of Musculoskeletal Conditions

Musculoskeletal problems are very common, affecting up to 20 percent of adults.[1] Their overall economic impact has been measured by utilization of health care and social care resources, as well as by work disability. There are several national cost of illness studies in developed countries within which the costs related to musculoskeletal conditions can be identified. These reflect the expenditure on health care for the management of these conditions, as well as their societal costs. These analyses are not only a measure of the impact the diseases have, but they also include the current provision of health and social care for people with these conditions. Such studies do not measure the costs of unmet need due to lack of provision of adequate services, such as joint arthroplasty in many countries, or because of patients who do not seek medical care because they have a negative attitude about what can be achieved.[10,11]

To understand how the individual with a musculoskeletal disease in any country interacts with health and social care, the normal patterns of care and the local systems of providing support, such as home care and pensions, must be calculated, because these are confounders that will influence costs. Expenditure is influenced by rules of reimbursement of health care and other factors that influence approaches to management of similar conditions in different countries. For example, inpatient care is only available for complicated rheumatoid arthritis in some countries, whereas in other countries such patients commonly receive inpatient rehabilitation. Social care can be provided in different ways, from the extended family and carers to agencies providing homecare, each with different costs—direct, indirect, and intangible. These factors, along with different methods of costing, make it difficult to compare findings in different countries.

In Sweden, musculoskeletal conditions cost SEK52.7 billion (US $5.3 billion) in 1994.[12] The total costs were attributable to back pain (47%), OA (14%), and RA (5.5%). Most of the costs were indirect and related to sick leave (31.5%) and early retirement (59%).

In the Netherlands, musculoskeletal conditions[13] ranked second as a health care cost in 1994,[14] accounting for 6 percent of total health care costs, compared to 8.1 percent for mental retardation. Coronary heart diseases and other circulatory diseases accounted for 4.8 percent. This study only considered medical costs, and the inclusion of the costs informal care would have greatly increased the costs related to chronic disabling conditions such as musculoskeletal diseases. The costs were considerable at all ages, ranking fifth at ages 15 to 44 years, second at ages 45 to 64 years, and third age at ages 65 to 84 years after dementia and stroke.

In Canada, musculoskeletal diseases in 1998 ranked second and accounted for C$16.4 billion of the total costs of illness[15] (Figure 28–1). Direct costs were less (C$2.6 billion) than indirect costs (C$13.7 billion). Musculoskeletal diseases were the leading cause of disability, accounting for about 39 percent of long-term disability costs (C$12.6 billion), followed by diseases of the nervous system (12.9%, C$4.2 billion), cardiovascular diseases (9.8%, C$3.2 billion), and mental disorders (7.0%, C$2.2 billion). Musculoskeletal diseases accounted for 10.3 percent (C$1.0 billion) of total short-term disability costs in 1998. In contrast to this, research expenditure on musculoskeletal diseases was only 1.3 percent of total research costs.

In the United States, the total cost of musculoskeletal conditions was $214.9 billion in 1995,[5] almost 3 percent of the gross domestic product (GDP) compared to estimates of about 0.5 percent in 1963 and 1972. The direct cost amounted to $88.7 billion, of which 38 percent ($33.7 billion) was attributable to hospital admissions, 21 percent to nursing home admissions, and 17 percent to physicians' visits. As in other established economies, the indirect cost was far larger, amounting to 58 percent of the total cost ($126.2 billion). Because musculoskeletal conditions are rarely fatal, 51 percent of the 58 percent of total cost attributable to wage losses arose from morbidity. The costs were greatest in age-groups 18 to 44 years and 45 to 64 years, in which indirect costs were greatest due to work loss, whereas costs in those under 18 years and over 65 years were related to medical care expenditure.

The direct costs of musculoskeletal conditions reflect the fact that musculoskeletal complaints are the second most common reason for consulting a doctor and constitute, in most countries, up to 10 to 20 percent of the primary care practice.[16] There were 44 million ambulatory physician visits in the United States in 1997 for a primary diagnosis of arthritis.[17] Five percent of drug expenditure in Canada was on musculoskeletal conditions in 1998.[18] In the United Kingdom, £276 million was

DIRECT AND INDIRECT COSTS BY DIAGNOSTIC CATEGORY IN CANADA*, 1998

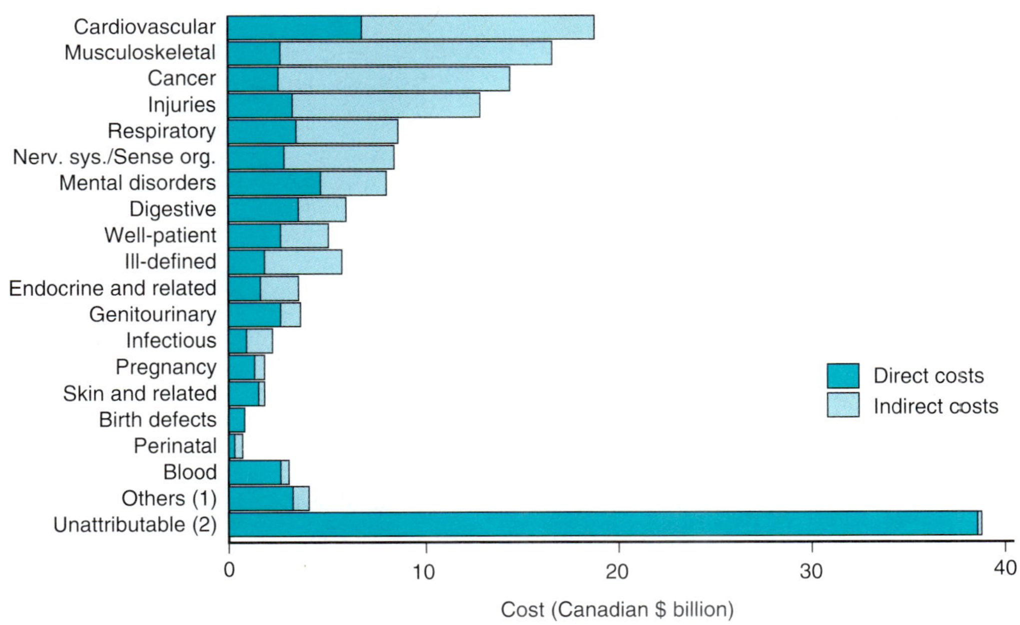

* Based on total cost of illness of $159.4 billion

(1) Refers to data for which coding is not provided (for diagnostic categories), or data that are grouped because of small counts.

(2) Refers to data that could not be coded by ICD-9 code.

FIGURE 28–1 • The direct and indirect costs of illness in Canada (1998) by diagnostic category. (From The Economic Burden of Illness in Canada 1998 (EBIC). Health Canada at URL: *http://www.hc-sc.gc.ca*.)

spent on prescription drugs for musculoskeletal conditions in 1999 (OHE Compendium 2001).

Indirect costs reflect the fact that these conditions are the most common causes of long-term physical disability. Musculoskeletal complaints are a major cause of absence from work in developed countries.[19,20] They are second only to respiratory disorders as a cause of short-term sickness absence (less than weeks).[21] Musculoskeletal complaints are the most common medical causes of long-term absence, accounting for more than half of all sickness absence longer than weeks in Norway.[22] They are also common causes for disability pensions, along with mental disorders and cardiovascular disorders. In Sweden, up to 60 percent of persons on early retirement or long-term disability claim a musculoskeletal problem as the reason.[23]

Cost of Rheumatoid Arthritis

Rheumatoid arthritis (RA) can be a devastating condition with a major impact on the individual, family, and friends, even though modern treatment has significantly improved the prognosis and function of these patients. Understanding the natural history of the disease and the typical health interventions and their outcomes will enable the associated costs to be understood.

The direct costs of RA relate to hospital and primary-care medical consultations to assess disease activity and to monitor treatment for safety and efficacy, drug costs, rehabilitation, and provision of equipment. Arthroplasty may be required. Indirect costs relate to loss of employment by the patient and often by the caregiver. Many with RA and their caregivers do not have the employment opportunities they would have had without the impact of the disease. The intangible costs of RA are great but difficult to quantify.

The direct and indirect costs of illness are twice as high in individuals with RA compared to controls.[24] Two thirds of these costs are a function of comorbidities, although this in part could reflect rules for reimbursement of care for people with RA. In a systematic review of 15 cost of illness studies,[25] it was found that the average direct annual costs were US $5720 per person with RA. These costs are initially high but then usually stabilize at a lower level until joint damage progresses and arthroplasty becomes necessary. A small proportion of patients are responsible for the majority of direct costs,[25] and these costs were highest for younger patients and those with the greatest disease severity. Inpatient care strongly influenced these costs, and admission rates varied in the studies assessed between 12 and 26 percent. The annual number of physician visits per year in the United States averaged between 11 and 12 per patient.[26-28] In France, RA patients use health resources more frequently, more intensively, and in a more diverse manner than nonarthritis subjects in France,[29] and 5.1 percent of all patients had RA-related surgery in the previous year. In a 10-year follow-up of patients with early RA, 17 percent had undergone large-joint replacements.[30] The person's time spent related to their health care is a direct cost often ignored, but it can be considerable in RA.[31] The costs of medication are less than 20 percent of direct costs,[32] but this was before the introduction of anti-TNF therapy.

The indirect costs of RA are typically between 50 and 75 percent of the total costs in developed countries. They are strongly influenced by loss of work, either short term or long term. Days lost from work by those in employment vary in studies from 2.7 to 30 days per year.[25] Employment is 20 percent lower in men and 25 percent lower in women with arthritis compared to those without.[33] Work capacity is restricted in a third within 1 year,[34] and within 3 years about 40 percent will not be working.[35] In the United States, fairly large numbers of patients with RA were found to lose their jobs, were unable to get a job, or retired early due to their illness.[36] Those who do work will often be forced to adjust their work schedules, with loss of potential income; and work-related disability is greatest in those doing manual jobs. Loss of activity days are substantial, with patients reporting 2 to 3 days of restricted activity within the previous 2 weeks.[26] Age and HAQ disability index are predictors of high indirect costs, as well as of acute and nonacute institutional care.[37] Disease activity also is associated with higher costs. The mean indirect costs were US $5822 per person in a systematic review[25] of 15 studies. Sick leave is the predominant cost in the initial phase, but disability increases with duration, and long-term sickness benefits become an increasing cost. Help in the household is often needed, but in the United Kingdom this was provided by family and friends and was seldom paid for directly.[38]

RA also has a considerable impact on all aspects of quality of life, and almost two thirds in a cohort study had restriction of activities of daily living and required help from family or friends, with an adverse effect in many cases on family relations.[39] In addition, the costs of side effects related to treatment must be considered, such as fractures subsequent to steroid-induced osteoporosis, or drugs, hospitalizations, and deaths from nonsteroidal anti-inflammatory drug (NSAID)-induced gastropathy.[40]

Cost of Osteoarthritis

Osteoarthritis (OA) is the most common cause of joint pain, and much of the self-reported burden of arthritis is related to OA. The impact of OA is a function of which joints are affected, as well as the severity and presence of comorbidities.

The socioeconomic impact of OA has not been adequately studied. The top down approach to identifying costs is difficult because diagnostic criteria require radiographs; in many cost analyses, joint pain alone has often been used. It is also difficult to estimate the costs attributable to OA because of the presence of comorbidities.[41]

National studies have largely identified the costs of arthritis as a whole. However, in Sweden, OA was estimated to incur SEK7.4 billion (US $749.4 million) in 1994, of which SEK739 million (US $75 million) was for inpatient care and SEK6.4 billion for productivity losses.[12] In France, estimates of the costs of OA from national data were 0.1 percent of 1991 GNP,[42] equivalent to $51.4 billion in US 2000 dollars. Almost two thirds of this amount was direct costs of medical care. The total medical costs for those with OA under 65 years of age are double that of similar individuals without OA and 50 percent higher in those over 65 years of age.[43] In a case-control study of a large national managed care organization in the United States, of those with an ICD-9 diagnosis of OA, the attributable costs were $2827 per patient year (1993 US$) in those under 65 years; and $1963 per patient year (1993 US$) in those 65 years and older. Two thirds of these costs related to health care facilities. Attributable drug costs were 7 percent ($199) in those under 65 years, but only 2 percent ($30) in those 65 years and older. In the United States, annual physician visits average nine per person and hospitalizations average of 0.3, lasting 8 to 9 days for noninstitutionalized patients with OA.[26]

Health resource utilization also relates to the complications of treatment, most commonly NSAID-induced gastropathy, which results in increased outpatient care, hospitalization, and coprescribing of drugs to prevent gastropathy. It is estimated that the United Kingdom's national health service spends on average £251 million per year (range £166 to 367 million) on NSAID-induced gastric side effects.[44]

Complementary therapy is often used by those with OA, and one study found that nearly half the participants used at least one type of alternative therapy during a 20-week period. The expenditure by users was estimated at US$1127 per year on alternative care providers, compared to US$1148 on ambulatory medical care services.[45]

OA at its end stage is the major indication for hip- and knee-replacement surgery, which are responsible for significant health care resource utilization. These costs reflect supply, not need, and there is a gap between these in all countries. The estimated prevalence of primary total knee replacements was 8.4 joints per 1000 people aged 35 years and over in England, in contrast to an estimated need of 27.4 joint replacements per 1000 people aged 35 years and over based on severity of knee disease.[46] The provision in Sweden is less, but the arthroplasty rate more closely meets needs in the United States.[47]

Total hip replacement rates in OECD countries vary between 50 and 140 procedures per 100,000 people.[48] The reason is predominantly OA, except in the very elderly when it more often follows hip fracture.[49] In the United Kingdom, there were 46,608 total hip replacements performed in 1999 and 2000, 46 percent of which were done in 60- to 74-year-olds and 36 percent of which were done in those older than 75 years. This more closely meets the predicted requirement.[50] The estimated cost was £4076 at 2000 National Health Service (NHS) prices, compared to £641 to 653 for watchful waiting without this treatment.[51] Those with knee disease were more likely than those with hip disease to have sought care from their primary care physician, but they were less likely to have been referred for specialist care or to be awaiting arthroplasty.[46] Patient preference influences resource utilization; 30 to 55 percent of those with severe large-joint OA are not willing to undergo arthroplasty.[10,46]

Indirect costs of OA are difficult to estimate for the reasons stated previously. Estimates from national surveys in the United States revealed that between 0.1 and 0.3 employment days were lost in the last 2 weeks by those with osteoarthritis,[27,28] or 0.8 percent just considering participants in the labor market.[27] More than half of those with symptomatic OA report work disability.[52] Those with OA are more likely to report reduction in working hours or being unable to get a job due to their illness.[36] However, work loss is not as great as with RA because many OA patients are no longer of working age.

In Australia, out-of-pocket expenditure by those with OA increased because of expenditures for medications, special equipment, and assistance from family and friends despite a government-funded health care system.[53]

Loss of mobility is common in those with arthritis, with 18 percent reporting significant loss, most of whom have OA. Limitation of activities, defined as inability to perform the person's major activity, was reported by 25 percent of people with osteoarthritis.[27] Limitation of activities caused by OA increases with age.

Osteoporosis

Osteoporosis manifests clinically as fragility fracture, and its socioeconomic impact relates to these fractures. They occur most commonly at the distal forearm, hip, and spine. The prevalence of osteoporosis and incidence of fragility increase with age. The impact the disease has increases with comorbidity.

The total direct medical expenditure on osteoporotic fractures in the United States in 1995 was estimated at $13.8 billion.[54] In the United Kingdom, the total costs were estimated at £942 million in 1998 for all osteoporotic fractures, of which only 45 percent were estimated to be the direct costs,[55] although treatment costs of antifracture therapy were not fully included. These estimates were revised to £1.7 billion in 2001[56] and are predicted to increase further with the aging population.

In Canada, the cost of hip fracture has been estimated at US$22,292 during the first year, and 58 percent of these costs were related to the initial hospitalization and inpatient rehabilitation. However, there was a wide variation depending on age and care setting before and after the fracture.[57] Estimates of the total yearly cost of hip fractures in the United States have ranged from $24,000 to $33,500 (1995 US$).[58] In the United Kingdom, hip fractures were the most expensive, comprising 87 percent of the total costs of osteoporotic fractures in women. Sixty percent of the cost of osteoporotic fractures is indirect due to the need of many for long-term hospital and community care.[55] The acute hospital cost of a hip fracture was estimated at £4808 in 1998, with a total cost per fracture at £12,124.[55] In the European Community, the total hospital costs of hip fracture in 1998 were estimated to be 3,614,916,079 ECUS, with estimated total care costs of 9,037,290,197 ECUS.[59]

Direct costs of distal forearm fractures are less, but one in five men and women with such a problem were admitted to hospital in a UK study.[60] The proportion requiring admission increased with age from 14.5 percent at ages 50 to 59 years to 26 percent at 80 years or older. Wrist fractures have been estimated to cost £468 (£368 of which is acute costs).[55]

Vertebral fractures only present acutely in about a third of cases, but they were found to be responsible for almost 70,000 hospital admissions in 1997 in the U.S. Nationwide Inpatient Sample, which is about one fourth the number of admissions due primarily to hip fracture. Hospitalization rates increased with age and comorbidity. Hospital stays averaged almost 6 days each and generated charges of US$8000 to 10,000.[61] More than half the patients required post–hospital discharge care. In one year of study,[61] hospitalization for vertebral fracture resulted in almost 400,000 total hospital days and generated charges in excess of US$500 million. In the United Kingdom, vertebral fracture has been estimated to cost £479 (£96 of which are acute costs).[55]

Among the age-group that sustains hip fracture and their associated comorbidities, it is more meaningful to consider the attributable costs. In the United States, the attributable costs for a hip fracture was determined as US$3300 and for other nonvertebral fractures as US$1300, based on Medicaid data.[62] In a case-control study of osteoporotic fractures in Olmsted County, Minnesota, the incremental direct medical costs for the year following an osteoporotic fracture were found to be greatest following distal femur (US$11,756) and hip fractures (US$11,241).[63] Similar figures have been estimated in Europe.[64]

The indirect costs related to social care are a major component of the cost of hip fracture because only about 45 percent of patients are discharged home; 20 percent require long-term residential care after discharge from hospital.[55] Productivity loss is not important because of the age at which fractures occur, although carers may be affected.

Back Pain

Back pain is most often nonspecific in cause and transient, although it may be recurrent. A small number of patients will have chronic back pain with continuous symptoms for more than 3 months, and they account for the largest percentage of costs.[65] In the United States, only 4.6 to 8.8 percent of cases lasted more than a year, but they accounted for 64.9 to 84.7 percent of the costs.[65] In Jersey, Engand, only 3 percent of those with back pain were absent from work for more than 6 months, but they accounted for 33 percent of benefits paid.[66]

The total cost in OECD countries corresponds to 1 to 2 percent of the GNP; about 10 percent of the costs are direct and 90 percent indirect.[67] Most of the costs relate to work loss. The economic impact is dependent on systems of social support and methods used to identify and estimate the costs, and these vary between studies, which makes comparison between studies and countries difficult.

A cost of illness study of low back pain in the United Kingdom estimated direct costs in 1998 at £1.7 billion and estimated that the total costs were between £6.6 billion and £12.3 billion, depending on methods used.[68] In Sweden in 1994 and 1995, back pain was responsible for almost half the economic burden related to musculoskeletal conditions, costing SEK25 to 29 billion (US$2.5 to 3.0 billion), of which SEK24 to 27 billion (US$2.4 to 2.8 billion) were spent on productivity losses.[12] These societal costs of back pain equate to $290 per inhabitant per year (1991 US$) in Sweden, $323 per person per year in the Netherlands, and about 80 to 90 percent of these instances in the United Kingdom.

The health resource utilization varies between countries dependent on clinical practice and the use of inpatient treatment, including investigations such as magnetic resonance imaging (MRI) and frequency of surgery. In general, expenditure is predominately related to ambulatory care and is distributed between physicians and therapists (including osteopaths, chiropractors, and alternative therapists). Physician visits vary from 1.1 per annum in the Netherlands to 3.71 visits in the United Kingdom.[67] Surgery is more common in the United States than in most European countries.[69]

Numbers of sickness days taken varies among countries and speaks to the systems of worker compensation more than it does to differences in severity of disease. In the 1998 US National Health Interview Survey,[70] the prevalence of back pain lasting more than a week was listed at 17.6 percent, and 4.6 percent had low back pain–associated work loss.[71] This amounted to 149 million lost days annually. The annual costs of lost work time associated with chronic low back pain has been estimated at US$1230 for men and US$773 for women. Based on data from the 1987 US National Medical Care Expenditure Survey, this translates into annual productivity losses of about US$28 billion.[72] The annual compensation costs of work loss due to medically certified low back pain in the working population of Jersey, England, was £3.16 million per100,000 people in 1994, or 10.5 percent of the total paid for all claimed absences.[66] Low back disorders are the most common reason for disability pensions in Norway.[23]

The economic impact of musculoskeletal conditions is great. They have a major effect on the indirect costs of health care. The direct costs reflect the supply, rather than the demand, and do not indicate what health gain is achieved. The documented expenditure is clearly an underestimate of need, as there is little priority for these conditions, not much investment in preventive approaches, and many patients who do not present themselves for treatment or do not comply for fear of side effects. Identifying this economic impact can be used to gain priority for these diseases, but it can also help identify the spectrum of cost items that need to be considered in any economic evaluation of strategies to reduce the burden of musculoskeletal conditions.

REFERENCES

1. Woolf AD, Pfleger B: Burden of musculoskeletal conditions. WHO Bulletin, in press.
2. Woolf AD, Akesson KA: How to prevent fractures in an elderly population. BMJ 327:89-95, 2003.

3. Pritchard C, Sculpher M: Productivity Costs: Principles and Practice in Economic Evaluation Office Of Health Economics, 2000.
4. Gabriel S, Drummond M, Maetzel A, et al: OMERACT 6 Economics Working Group Report: A proposal for a reference case for economic evaluation in rheumatoid arthritis. J Rheumatol 30:886-890, 2003.
5. Merkesdal S, Ruof J, Huelsemann JL, et al: Development of a matrix of cost domains in economic evaluation of rheumatoid arthritis. J Rheumatol 28:657-661, 2001.
6. Rice D: The economic burden of musculoskeletal conditions, 1995. *In* Praemer A, Furner S, Rice D (eds): Musculoskeletal Conditions in the United States. Rosemont, Ill, American Academy of Orthopedic Surgeons, 1999, pp 27-33.
7. Murrary CJL, Lopez AD: The Global Burden of Disease. A Comprehensive Assessment of Mortality and Disability from Diseases, Injuries, and Risk Factors in 1990 and Projected to 2020. Cambridge, Mass, Harvard School of Public Health on behalf of the WHO and the World Bank, 1996.
8. Mooney G,Wiseman V: Burden of disease and priority setting. Health Econ 9:369-72, 2000.
9. Byford S, Torgerson DJ, Raftery J: Economic note: cost of illness studies. BMJ 320:1335, 2000.
10. Hawker GA, Wright JG, Coyte PC, et al: Differences between men and women in the rate of use of hip and knee arthroplasty. N Engl J Med 342:1016-1022, 2000.
11. Woolf AD, Zeidler H, Haglund U: Patients' and physicians' perceptions of treatment of musculoskeletal pain: Results of a pan-European study. Ann Rheum Dis, in press.
12. Jonsson D, Husberg M: Socioeconomic costs of rheumatic diseases. Implications for technology assessment. Int J Technol Assess Health Care 16:1193-1200, 2000.
13. World Health Organization: International Classification of Diseases, 9th ed. Geneva, WHO, 1977.
14. Meerding WJ, Bonneux L, Polder JJ, et al: Demographic and epidemiological determinants of healthcare costs in Netherlands: cost of illness study. BMJ 317:111-115, 1998.
15. The Economic Burden of Illness in Canada 1998 (EBIC). Health Canada at URL: http://www.hc-sc.gc.ca/pphb-dgspsp/publicat/ebic-femc 98/pdf/ebic 1998. pdf
16. Rasker JJ: Rheumatology in general practice. Br J Rheumatol 34:494-497, 1995.
17. Impact of arthritis and other rheumatic conditions on the healthcare system–United States, 1997. MMWR Morb Mortal Wkly Rep 48:349-353, 1999.
18. Coyte PC, Asche CV, Croxford R, Chan B: The economic cost of musculoskeletal disorders in Canada. Arthritis Care Res 11:315-325, 1998.
19. Szubert Z, Sobala W, Zycinska Z: [The effect of system restructuring on absenteeism due to sickness in the work place. I. Sickness absenteeism during the period 1989-1994]. Med Pr 48:543-551, 1997.
20. Tellnes G, Bjerkedal T: Epidemiology of sickness certification: A methodological approach based on a study from Buskerud County in Norway. Scand J Soc Med 17:245-251, 1989.
21. Stansfeld SA, North FM, White I, Marmot MG: Work characteristics and psychiatric disorder in civil servants in London. J Epidemiol Community Health 49:48-53, 1995.
22. Brage S, Nygard JF, Tellnes G: The gender gap in musculoskeletal-related long-term sickness absence in Norway. Scand J Soc Med 26:34-43, 1998.
23. National Board of Health and Welfare. Yearbook of Health and Medical Case, 2001. Stockholm: Socialstyrelsen, 2001. Available from URL: http://www.sos.se
24. Birnbaum HG, Barton M, Greenberg PE, et al: Direct and indirect costs of rheumatoid arthritis to an employer. J Occup Environ Med 42:588-596, 2000.
25. Cooper NJ: Economic burden of rheumatoid arthritis: a systematic review. Rheumatology (Oxford) 39:28-33, 2000.
26. Dunlop DD, Manheim LM, Yelin EH, et al: The costs of arthritis. Arthritis Rheum 49:101-113, 2003.
27. Felts W,Yelin E: The economic impact of the rheumatic diseases in the United States. J Rheumatol 16:867-884, 1989.
28. Kramer JS, Yelin EH, Epstein WV: Social and economic impacts of four musculoskeletal conditions. A study using national community-based data. Arthritis Rheum 26:901-907, 1983.
29. Girard F, Guillemin F, Novella JL, et al: Health-care use by rheumatoid arthritis patients compared with non-arthritic subjects. Rheumatology (Oxford) 41:167-175, 2002.
30. Lindqvist E, Saxne T, Geborek P, Eberhardt K: Ten year outcome in a cohort of patients with early rheumatoid arthritis: Health status, disease process, and damage. Ann Rheum Dis 61:1055-1059, 2002.
31. Kuper IH, Prevoo ML, van Leeuwen MA, et al: Disease associated time consumption in early rheumatoid arthritis. J Rheumatol 27:1183-1189, 2000.
32. Fautrel B, Guillemin F: Cost of illness studies in rheumatic diseases. Curr Opin Rheumatol 14:121-126, 2002.
33. Yelin E: The earnings, income, and assets of persons aged 51-61 with and without musculoskeletal conditions. J Rheumatol 24:2024-2030, 1997.
34. Jantti J, Aho K, Kaarela K, Kautiainen H: Work disability in an inception cohort of patients with seropositive rheumatoid arthritis: A 20 year study. Rheumatology (Oxford) 38:1138-1141, 1999.
35. Albers JM, Kuper HH, van Riel PL, et al: Socio-economic consequences of rheumatoid arthritis in the first years of the disease. Rheumatology (Oxford) 38:423-430, 1999.
36. Gabriel SE, Crowson CS, Campion ME, O'Fallon WM: Indirect and nonmedical costs among people with rheumatoid arthritis and osteoarthritis compared with nonarthritic controls. J Rheumatol 24:43-48, 1997.
37. Clarke AE, Zowall H, Levinton C, et al: Direct and indirect medical costs incurred by Canadian patients with rheumatoid arthritis: a 12 year study. J Rheumatol 24:1051-1060, 1997.
38. Cooper NJ, Mugford M, Symmons DP, et al: Total costs and predictors of costs in individuals with early inflammatory polyarthritis: a community-based prospective study. Rheumatology (Oxford) 41:767-774, 2002.
39. Hawley DJ, Wolfe F, Pincus T: Use of combination therapy in the routine care of patients with rheumatoid arthritis: Physician and patient surveys. Clin Exp Rheumatol 17:S78-S82, 1999.
40. Henry D, Lim LL, Garcia Rodriguez LA, et al: Variability in risk of gastrointestinal complications with individual non-steroidal anti-inflammatory drugs: Results of a collaborative meta-analysis. BMJ 312:1563-1566, 1996.
41. March LM, Bachmeier CJ: Economics of osteoarthritis: A global perspective. Baillieres Clin Rheumatol 11:817-834, 1997.
42. Levy E, Ferme A, Perocheau D, Bono I: [Socioeconomic costs of osteoarthritis in France]. Rev Rhum Ed Fr 60:63S-67S, 1993.
43. MacLean CH, Knight K, Paulus H, et al: Costs attributable to osteoarthritis. J Rheumatol 25:2213-2218, 1998.
44. Moore RA: The hidden costs of arthritis treatment and the cost of new therapy: The burden of non-steroidal anti-inflammatory drug gastropathy. Rheumatology (Oxford) 41(Suppl 1):7-15, 2002.
45. Ramsey SD, Spencer AC, Topolski TD, et al: Use of alternative therapies by older adults with osteoarthritis. Arthritis Rheum 45:222-227, 2001.
46. Juni P, Dieppe P, Donovan J, et al: Population requirement for primary knee replacement surgery: A cross-sectional study. Rheumatology (Oxford) 42:516-521, 2003.
47. Holland R, Harvey I: Population needs assessment and knee replacement surgery. Rheumatology (Oxford) 42:503-506, 2003.
48. Merx H, Dreinhofer K, Schrader P, et al: International variation in hip replacement rates. Ann Rheum Dis 62:222-226, 2003.
49. Malchau H, Herberts P, Eisler T, et al: The Swedish total hip replacement register. J Bone Joint Surg Am 84 (Suppl 2):2-20, 2002.
50. Frankel S, Eachus J, Pearson N, et al: Population requirement for primary hip-replacement surgery: A cross-sectional study. Lancet 353:1304-1309, 1999.
51. Vale L, Wyness L, McCormack K, et al: A systematic review of the effectiveness and cost-effectiveness of metal-on-metal hip resurfacing arthroplasty for treatment of hip disease. Health Technol Assess 6:1-109, 2002.
52. Pincus T, Mitchell JM, Burkhauser RV: Substantial work disability and earnings losses in individuals less than age 65 with osteoarthritis: Comparisons with rheumatoid arthritis. J Clin Epidemiol 42:449-457, 1989.
53. Lapsley HM, March LM, Tribe KL, et al: Living with osteoarthritis: patient expenditures, health status, and social impact. Arthritis Rheum 45:301-306, 2001.

54. Ray NF, Chan JK, Thamer M, Melton LJ III: Medical expenditures for the treatment of osteoporotic fractures in the United States in 1995: Report from the National Osteoporosis Foundation. J Bone Miner Res 12:24-35, 1997.
55. Dolan P, Torgerson DJ: The cost of treating osteoporotic fractures in the United Kingdom female population. Osteoporos Int 8:611-617, 1998.
56. Torgerson DJ: Aglesias CP, Reid DM: The economics of fracture prevention. *In* Barlow DH, Francis RM, Miles A (eds): The Effective Management of Osteoporosis. Aesculapiuf Medical Press, 2001.
57. Wiktorowicz ME, Goeree R, Papaioannou A, et al: Economic implications of hip fracture: Health service use, institutional care and cost in Canada. Osteoporos Int 12:271-278, 2001.
58. Tosteson AN: Economic impact of fractures. *In* Orwoll E (ed): The Effects of Gender on Skeletal Health. San Diego, Calif., Academic Press, 1999, pp 15-27.
59. Report on Osteoporosis in the European Community. Luxembourg, European Commission, 1998.
60. O'Neill TW, Cooper C, Finn JD, et al: Incidence of distal forearm fracture in British men and women. Osteoporos Int 12:555-558, 2001.
61. Gehlbach SH, Burge RT, Puleo E, Klar J: Hospital care of osteoporosis-related vertebral fractures. Osteoporos Int 14:53-60, 2003.
62. Martin BC, Chisholm MA, Kotzan JA: Isolating the cost of osteoporosis-related fracture for postmenopausal women. A population-based study. Gerontology 47:21-29, 2001.
63. Gabriel SE, Tosteson AN, Leibson CL, et al: Direct medical costs attributable to osteoporotic fractures. Osteoporos Int 13:323-330, 2002.
64. Autier P, Haentjens P, Bentin J, et al: Costs induced by hip fractures: a prospective controlled study in Belgium. Belgian Hip Fracture Study Group. Osteoporos Int 11:373-380, 2000.
65. Hashemi L, Webster BS, Clancy EA: Trends in disability duration and cost of workers' compensation low back pain claims (1988-1996). J Occup Environ Med 40:1110-1119, 1998.
66. Watson PJ, Main CJ, Waddell G, et al: Medically certified work loss, recurrence and costs of wage compensation for back pain: A follow-up study of the working population of Jersey. Br J Rheumatol 37:82-86, 1998.
67. Norlund AI, Waddell G: Cost of back pain in some OECD countries. *In* Nachemson A, Jonsson E (eds): Neck and Back Pain: The Scientific Evidence of Causes, Diagnosis, and Treatment. Philadelphia, Lippincott Williams & Wilkins, 2000, pp 421-425.
68. Maniadakis N, Gray A: The economic burden of back pain in the UK. Pain 84:95-103, 2000.
69. Deyo RA, Cherkin D, Conrad D, Volinn E: Cost, controversy, crisis: Low back pain and the health of the public. Annu Rev Public Health 12:141-56, 1991.
70. Guo HR, Tanaka S, Cameron LL, et al: Back pain among workers in the United States: National estimates and workers at high risk. Am J Ind Med 28:591-602, 1995.
71. Guo HR, Tanaka S, Halperin WE, Cameron LL: Back pain prevalence in US industry and estimates of lost workdays. Am J Public Health 89:1029-1035, 1999.
72. Rizzo JA, Abbott TA III, Berger ML: The labor productivity effects of chronic backache in the United States. Med Care 36:1471-1488, 1998.

29 Assessment of Health Outcomes

MICHAEL M. WARD

The goal of health care is to improve the health of individuals and populations. For individuals, measures of improved health include fewer signs and symptoms of illness, better functioning, better quality of life, and improved survival. For populations, measures of improved health include lower incidence and prevalence rates of disease, higher levels of functioning across the population, lower morbidity burdens, and lower mortality rates. Accurate measures of health outcomes are needed to identify the aspects of a particular disease most in need of treatment, to assess the effects of treatment, and, in populations, to prioritize the allocation of health care resources.

A given treatment may not affect all health outcomes, or it may benefit some outcomes more than others. Assessment of a particular treatment, therefore, requires careful consideration of the anticipated benefits, and the health outcome measured should match the benefit expected from the treatment. For example, a treatment for Raynaud's phenomenon might be expected to reduce pain, but it might not influence physical functioning. Patients may also differ in the importance they place on the relief of different symptoms, limitations in functioning, or in tradeoffs of suffering and longevity. These differences make it important to consider patients' preferences for particular health outcomes when considering different treatments. In addition, treatments are rarely free of potential toxicities and never free of costs. Balancing the toxicity and expected benefits of treatment choices is done routinely in clinical practice, and balancing the economic costs and expected benefits of treatment choices is most often done for groups of patients or populations.

This chapter will review definitions of common health outcomes and will present several conceptual schemes that provide an overall picture of outcome assessment. Ways of measuring health outcomes and the attributes of good outcome measures will be described. Finally, commonly used outcome measures in rheumatoid arthritis, ankylosing spondylitis, systemic lupus erythematosus, and osteoarthritis will be reviewed.

Terminology and Conceptual Models

DEFINITIONS OF HEALTH OUTCOMES

Health outcomes are all possible results that stem from a disease or condition.[1] This broad definition encompasses effects at multiple levels, ranging from molecular and cellular abnormalities to problems a person may have in social interactions as a result of disease. In common usage, however, health outcomes refer to the results of disease at the level of the individual. Anatomic or physiologic changes that occur with disease may not cause any loss of structural or functional integrity (e.g., a small cerebrovascular accident), or they may result in *impairments*, which are problems with normal body structures or functions.[2] For example, a joint effusion is an anatomic abnormality that may cause the impairment of limited range of motion. Impairments may result from any defect, loss, or deviation from normal in a part of the body. Anatomic or physiologic changes may also cause *symptoms*, somatic sensations that represent the conscious recognition of the abnormality by the individual.

Activity, or functioning, is the execution of a task or action. Conversely, *activity limitation* or *disability* is difficulty in executing tasks.[2] Functioning is often classified into subcategories of physical functioning, mental functioning, social functioning, and role functioning. *Physical functioning* refers to the ability to perform tasks requiring movement, strength, endurance, or dexterity, and includes activities such as dressing, eating, bathing, and mobility. *Mental functioning* refers to one's mood, psychologic distress, and ability to perform tasks requiring memory, thought, and concentration. *Social functioning* refers to the ability to develop and maintain social relationships, and *role functioning* refers to the ability to do work, housework, or schoolwork. Other classification schemes include more narrowly defined subcategories, such as self care, domestic life, recreation, and communication. Activity limitations or functional difficulties may result from either impairments or symptoms.

Health status (sometimes referred to as functional status) and *health-related quality of life* are more global measures of health outcomes that provide an overall assessment of how a person feels and functions.[3-5] These terms are used interchangeably by some authors. Beyond this, definitions of health status often differ among authors, which adds more confusion. However, all definitions of *health status* include, at their core, an assessment of symptom severity, the impact of impairments and symptoms on functioning, and of the impact of impairments, symptoms, and activity limitations on a person's ability to participate in life.[3-5] Health status is a subjective measure and is a measure of how a person perceives his or her symptoms and activity limitations.

Among those who distinguish health status and health-related quality of life as separate concepts, *health-related quality of life* incorporates all aspects of health status, but it is an even broader concept that includes a person's satisfaction with, or emotional response to, his or her current health status.[4-7] This evaluative component is not a feature of health status. For example, being unable to walk one block is an activity limitation and would be a component of a person's health status; the degree to which one was depressed or frustrated by the inability to walk one block is a component of health-related quality of life that is not captured by health status alone. This distinction recognizes that individuals with the same health status (e.g., paraplegics) may have very different self-assessments of their condition and thus very different health-related quality of life. *Patient satisfaction* is a summary evaluation of contentment or displeasure with one's health status, and it is often assessed after an intervention or particular treatment and is colored by expectation and interactions with health care providers.[8]

Quality of life, as defined by the World Health Organization (WHO), is "an individual's perception of their position in life in context of the cultural and value systems in which they live and in relation to their goals, expectations, standards and concerns . . . affected in a complex way by the person's physical health, psychological state, personal beliefs, social relationships and their relationship to salient features of their environment."[9] Because this concept includes aspects of life not directly related to health or amenable to health care interventions, such as financial resources, political freedom, personal security, and spirituality, the subset of health-related aspects of quality of life is usually considered separately.

CONCEPTUAL MODELS OF HEALTH OUTCOMES

Several different schemes for conceptualizing health outcomes have been proposed. The traditional medical model views ill health as a product of impairments or symptoms and seeks to treat these to restore health. Fries presented a scheme in which global health was represented by five D's: death, disability, discomfort, drugs (iatrogenic events), and dollars (costs).[10] By assessing disability or functioning as reported by patients themselves, this model expanded the outcomes of the traditional medical model and incorporated patients' perceptions in health assessment. By including death and costs, this model represents health outcomes more broadly than other models. However, drug side effects are an attribution of the cause of particular symptoms, impairments, or functional limitations, rather than a separate health outcome.

Other models focus selectively on health-related quality of life. The model proposed in 2001 by the WHO replaces the impairment-disability-handicap model with a simplified model of the relationship between a health condition, body structure and function, and activity and participation[2] (Fig. 29–1). This model resolves the difficulty present in the impairment-

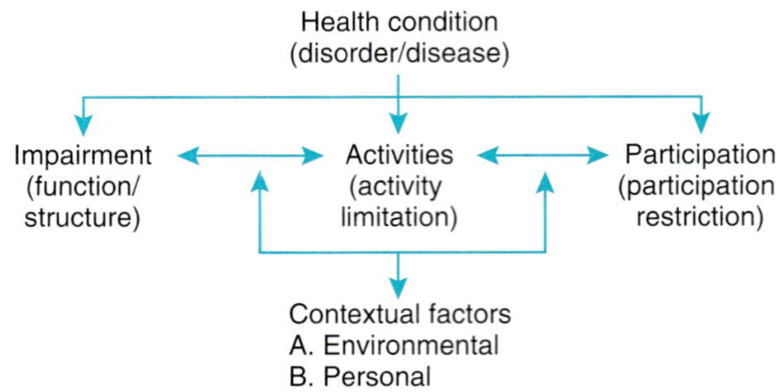

FIGURE 29-1 · World Health Organization Model of Health Outcomes. (Adapted from World Health Organization. ICF: International Classification of Functioning, Disability, and Health. Introduction. World Health Organization, 2001. http://www3.who.int/icf/icftemplate.cfm, accessed on December 2, 2002.)

disability-handicap model of distinguishing functional limitations from their social consequences and uses neutral language (body structure instead of impairment; activity instead of disability) to recognize health-promoting as well as health-depleting effects. The WHO model includes multiple pathways of interactions and does not seek to explain the processes by which health outcomes develop. In contrast, Weiss and Cleary have proposed a model linking the disease, symptoms, function, and health perceptions with overall quality of life in a clinically intuitive way[11] (Fig. 29–2). Both of these models are biopsychosocial models, emphasizing that the characteristics of the patient and the environment have important roles in modifying multiple health outcomes.

The hierarchy of outcomes requires consideration of how one outcome relates to other outcomes. For example, pain is a symptom and a measure of health status, and, therefore, it is also a measure of health-related quality of life. However, only measuring pain would ignore many other aspects of health status and health-related quality of life. Assessment of one or a few components of health-related quality of life should not imply a comprehensive assessment. Also, because the term *health-related quality of life* is used generically to refer to the class of subjective measures of health outcomes and used specifically to refer to the particular outcome of a person's satisfaction with their current state of health, one should be clear on how this term is being applied.

Ways of Measuring Outcomes

CONTENT AND STRUCTURE OF OUTCOME MEASURES

There are several ways of obtaining information about health outcomes, which differ in both content (what is measured) and structure (how the measurement is obtained).[12] The content of an outcome measure includes its level of integration, specificity, station, time window, and method of quantification (Table 29–1). Level of integration refers to whether the measure is a highly integrated summary or global measure, or

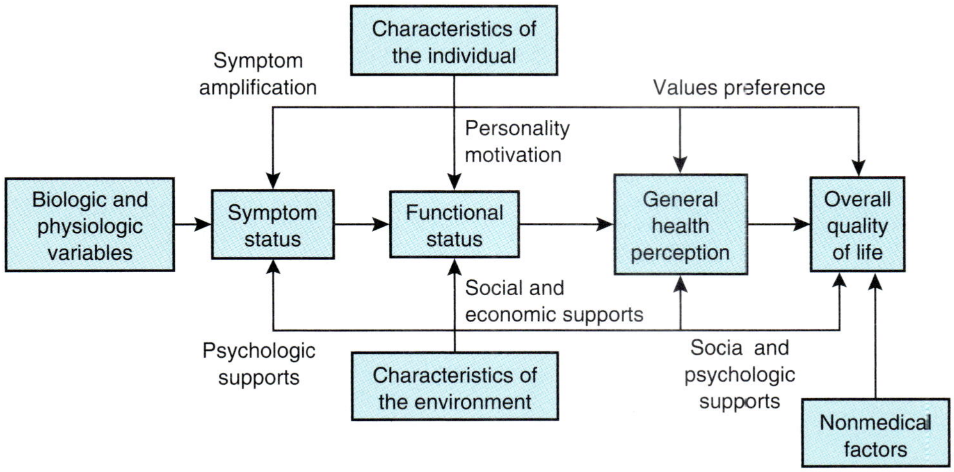

FIGURE 29-2 • Wilson and Cleary's Model of the Relationships between Clinical Characteristics and Health Outcomes. (From Wilson IB, Cleary PD: Linking clinical variables with health-related quality of life. A conceptual model of patient outcomes. JAMA 273:59-65, 1995.)

TABLE 29-1 • CONTENT AND STRUCTURE OF OUTCOME MEASURES

Content	
Level of integration	Global or multidimensional
Specificity	Generic or specific
Station	State or transition
Time window	Current or recalled
Quantification	Amount or quality
Structure	
Action	Observed or reported
Recorder	Clinician/surrogate or patient
Mode of transmission	Oral or written
Format	Narrative or closed-ended
	Single-item or multi-item
	Profile or index
	Uniform or individualized
	Response options
Disclosure	Blinded or disclosed

whether it is multidimensional. *Global* measures, which are often single items, are simple and direct, but they do not provide information about what features contribute most to the summary result. In *multidimensional* measures, each component is identified and measured separately. Specificity refers to whether the measure is *generic* and applicable in diverse settings, or *specific* to a particular disease, setting, population (e.g., children), or function. Because specific measures can be targeted to be more relevant to a particular circumstance, these measures may be better at detecting changes in health over time. Generic measures offer generalizability and the opportunity to compare outcomes among different groups and settings.

Station refers to whether the measure examines the state of the patient at one point in time or if it assesses a transition in health. For example, a measure of pain could ask the patient to report his or her current level of pain (a state) or to report how much better or worse the pain is over some period of time (a transition). Measures of transition are often more sensitive to change than state measures, and they may be particularly useful in assessing the effects of treatment. Time window refers to the period of time during which the outcome is assessed. The measure could assess *current* status, as do most outcomes measures of signs and impairments on physical examination (e.g., number of swollen joints today), or it could assess status over some recent *window* (e.g., level of pain in the past week; degree of functional difficulty over the past month). Longer time windows may provide more stable estimates by assessing the patient's recent average health outcome, but they depend on recalled status and may be subject to problems of memory, saliency, and recall bias. Transition questions always involve recall. Lastly, *quantification* refers to whether the measure attempts to assess the amount of the health outcome (in intensity, severity, or duration) or whether it assesses the quality of the experienced health outcome. For example, pain can be measured by its intensity using a patient self-rated visual analogue scale, or the nature of the pain sensation can be assessed, as with the McGill Pain Questionnaire.[13] Measurement of the amount of an outcome can be a simple dichotomous assessment of present or absent, or it can be counted or rated numerically.

For example, the Health Assessment Questionnaire Disability Index (HAQ-DI) is a multidimensional generic state measure of the severity (amount) of functional disability, on a scale of 0 to 3, with a time window of the past week. The physician global assessment is a global generic state measure of the severity (amount) of arthritis currently present.

The structure of an outcome measure refers to how the measurement is obtained and includes the action, recorder, mode of transmission, format, and disclosure. The action of the measure refers to what happens to allow a measurement to be made and usually consists of either an observation being made or a report being recorded. Observed measures include most measures of impairments, such as joint counts and measures of range of motion and malalignment. Reported measures include most measures of health status. However, functional difficulty or pain behaviors can also be observed measures that are assessed during a physical examination or a prescribed test or "obstacle course." The recorder is the person making the observation or report. The recorder of reports is always the patient. The recorder of observations can be a clinician or a patient surrogate or proxy, such as a spouse or close friend. Surrogates who provide reports for patients are most often basing their responses on observation.

For reports, the mode of transmission of the information can be oral or written, and either narrative, as with a diary, or gathered through use of closed-ended questions. In turn, reports that use closed-ended questions can be single-item or multi-item questionnaires, can be uniform for all patients or individualized, and can use various response options. Multi-item questionnaires can be used to provide a profile of different aspects of a person's health status (e.g., the domains of the Medical Outcomes Study Short-Form 36 (SF-36) of physical functioning, role functioning—physical, pain, general health, vitality, mental health, role functioning—emotional, and social functioning), or it can be summated into an index, which provides a single number to represent the measure (e.g., the HAQ-DI).[14,15] In uniform questionnaires, all respondents answer the same questions. These provide for easy comparisons among patients, but all questions may not be relevant for all persons. Individualized questionnaires, such as the McMaster Toronto Arthritis Patient Preference Disability Questionnaire (MACTAR),[16] allow patients to select and prioritize the functions assessed and may measure aspects of illness that are more relevant and meaningful to the individual. Individualized measures may have greater sensitivity to change than uniform questionnaires.

Response options depend on the quantification scheme used to define the content of the measure. When amount of a health outcome is measured, natural units are used when available (number of tender joints, minutes of morning stiffness). When natural units are not available, as when measuring pain intensity, some options include rating scales (e.g., numbers from 0 to 10 in rank order to represent intensity), visual analogue scales (e.g., a line marked 0 and 100 at the ends to represent gradation in intensity), Likert scales (e.g., "strongly agree," "agree," "no opinion," "disagree," "strongly disagree" with a statement about pain intensity), pictures of faces, and color intensity scales.[17] Lastly, *disclosure* refers to whether observers or reporters are permitted to view their previous responses when making a new assessment. Disclosure makes the assessment similar to use of a transition question, and blinding maintains the assessment of current status.

For example, the HAQ-DI is a reported written measure recorded by the patient, which uses uniform multi-item closed-ended questions about the degree of difficulty doing tasks, usually completed with blinding. The physician global assessment is an observed written measure recorded by the physician that uses a single-item closed-ended question about overall arthritis activity scored on a visual analogue scale, usually completed with blinding.

STRENGTHS AND WEAKNESSES OF SELF-REPORTED AND OBSERVED MEASURES

Many health status and health-related quality of life measures are uniform, multi-item patient self-report profiles that use closed-ended questions. Many measures of impairment are clinician-observed measures. The choice of patient self-report measures or observed measures is often dictated by the purpose of the examination.[5] Observed measures are more appropriate when the goal is to measure a person's ability or capacity to perform a task. Observed measures are not subject to problems with memory or recall and may be less biased than patient self-reported measures when secondary considerations exist (e.g., disability payments, retirement). Observed measures may be the only available measures for patients who are too ill to complete self-report measures or who are cognitively impaired. However, observed measures require skilled observers who are trained to ensure accuracy and consistency. Therefore, observed measures are often more time consuming, effort intensive, and costly than patient self-report measures.

Patient self-report measures are more appropriate when the goal is to measure a person's usual performance of tasks or the perception of difficulty doing tasks, and it is the only way to assess a person's feelings about his or her symptoms or abilities. Patient self-report measures may be subject to response bias. Response bias includes problems of respondents always agreeing with the questioner, avoiding extreme responses, or providing answers that may be viewed as more socially acceptable. Questions may be misinterpreted or answered differently depending on how the question is phrased. Techniques in questionnaire design and analysis can address some of these potential biases.[18] Obtaining patient self-report measures by interview requires training of interviewers and can be costly; however, paper questionnaires provide an often low-cost and efficient way of collecting such information.

Outcome Measures

IMPAIRMENTS AND SYMPTOMS

Most signs on physical examination and laboratory and radiographic measures of the biologic processes of disease are measures of impairment. These include tender and swollen joint counts; assessment of joint range of motion, joint malalignment and deformity, and joint circumferences; assessments of posture and gait; manual muscle strength testing; tests of sensation and deep tendon reflexes and acute phase reactants; and abnormalities in other organ systems. The appropriate measures vary with the disease being assessed and include those usually considered "disease activity" measures. Because most measures of impairment are manifestations of, or direct consequences of, the disease process, they are usually considered highly relevant outcomes. Most are clinician-observed measures, although patient self-reported measures of impairment have been developed, such as the self-reported joint counts of the Rapid Assessment of Disease Activity in Rheumatology (RADAR) instrument.[19,20]

The major symptoms of rheumatic diseases are pain, stiffness, and fatigue. Pain is a completely subjective sensation, and, therefore, it is assessed most accurately by patient self-report. Most pain measures used in rheumatology assess the intensity of pain on single-item or multi-item closed-ended questionnaires. A large number of pain measures are available, which differ in specificity, time window, and response format[5,17,20] (Table 29–2). Among the most commonly used are the numeric rating scale, in which patients select a number from 0 to 10 to estimate the intensity of pain, or the visual analogue scale, in which patients mark the level of pain they experienced on a 10-cm or 15-cm horizontal line labeled at the ends with anchoring descriptors of "no pain" and

TABLE 29–2 • PATIENT SELF-REPORT INSTRUMENTS COMMONLY USED IN RHEUMATOLOGY TO MEASURE SPECIFIC HEALTH OUTCOMES

Impairments
Pain
Numeric rating scale
Visual analogue scale
Health Asssessment Questionnaire Pain scale (visual analog scale)[15]
Arthritis Impact Measurement Scales-Pain subscale[21,22]
Western Ontario and McMaster Universities Osteoarthritis Index-Pain subscale[23]
Australian/Canadian Osteoarthritis Hand Index[24]
McGill Pain Questionnaire[13]
SF-36 pain subscale[14]
Stiffness
Duration of morning stiffness
Visual analogue scale of severity
Western Ontario and McMaster Universities Osteoarthritis Index-Stiffness subscale[23]
Fatigue
Visual analogue scale of severity
Fatigue Severity Scale[27]
SF-36 vitality subscale[14]
Nottingham Health Profile energy subscale[28]
Health Status
Number of work/school days missed
Number of limited activity days
Health Assessment Questionnaire Disability Index[15]
Arthritis Impact Measurement Scales[21,22]
McMaster Toronto Arthritis Patient Preference Disability Questionnaire (MACTAR)[16]
Western Ontario and McMaster Universities Osteoarthritis Index-Physical function subscale[23]
Australian/Canadian Osteoarthritis Hand Index[24]
Childhood Health Assessment Questionnaire[42]
Medical Outcomes Study Short-Form 36 (SF-36)[14]
Nottingham Health Profile[28]
Sickness Impact Profile[43]
Beck Depression Inventory[45]
Centers for Epidemiologic Studies-Depression scale[46]
Health-Related Quality of Life
Global health perception
RAQoL[47]
ASQoL[48]
PedsQL[49]
Numeric rating scale
Time trade-off
Standard gamble
Health Utilities Index[51]
Quality of Well Being Scale[52]
EuroQol[53]
Psychosocial Factors
Arthritis Self-Efficacy Scales[58]
Coping Strategies Questionnaire[59]
Rheumatology Attitudes Index[60]
Interpersonal Evaluation Support List[61]
Social Support Questionnaire[62]

"pain as bad as it could be" or "very severe pain." The pain scale of the HAQ is a 10-cm visual analogue scale that asks patients to report pain intensity over the past week.[15] The pain subscale of the Arthritis Impact Measurement Scales (AIMS) and its revision, the AIMS2, is a composite of several verbal rating scales that asks patients to report pain intensity over the past month.[21,22] The Western Ontario and McMaster Universities Osteoarthritis Index (WOMAC) pain subscale is specifically for patients with knee or hip osteoarthritis and asks patients to report current pain intensity using either visual analogue or Likert (none, mild, moderate, severe, extreme) scales.[23] The Australian/Canadian Osteoarthritis Hand Index takes a similar approach to pain assessment in patients with hand osteoarthritis.[24] The McGill Pain Questionnaire assesses the quality and intensity of pain experienced by asking patients to pick adjectives that best characterize the sensory, affective, and evaluative nature of their pain.[13] Rankings of the severity of words chosen can be collated in a pain rating index, but the absolute number of words chosen can also be used as a pain measure.

In addition to measuring the perception of pain, pain behaviors can also be assessed. An observed method to quantify pain behaviors, such as guarding, grimacing, and rubbing, as patients perform a standard set of maneuvers, has been shown to correlate well with patient-reported pain intensity, independent observers' ratings, and other measures of arthritis activity.[25] The training, complexity, and expense of this technique has limited its use. Analgesic use is another behavioral measure of pain, but it is a poor measure of pain because it is influenced in complex ways by the availability and knowledge of medications, habit and custom, culture, expectation of benefit or relief, and fear of side effects. A dolorimeter is a mechanical device that measures pain threshold, but it does not measure the intensity or experience of pain.

Musculoskeletal stiffness has been assessed by patient self-report of the duration of morning stiffness or stiffness after inactivity, but the severity of stiffness may also be measured. Stiffness may be generalized or limited to particular joints. Part of the difficulty with measuring this symptom is its variable interpretation by patients, who may consider it to mean pain, limited movement, tightness, or functional limitation.[26] Fatigue has been assessed by patient self-report, most often using a visual analogue scale or the Fatigue Severity Scale.[27] Fatigue subscales of general health status instruments, such as the SF-36 or Nottingham Health Profile, have not been commonly used.[14,28]

Pooled indexes that combine ratings of several different impairments, or ratings of impairments and symptoms, have been developed in attempt to provide summary measures of disease activity and damage. Examples include the Disease Activity Score (DAS) in rheumatoid arthritis,[29] the System Lupus Activity Measure (SLAM),[30] the Systemic Lupus Erythematosus Disease Activity Index (SLEDAI),[31] the Systemic Lupus International Collaborating Clinics/American College of Rheumatology Damage Index (SLICC),[32] and the Birmingham Vasculitis Activity Score.[33] The advantages of pooled indexes include conceptual appeal, ease of analyzing a single number, avoidance of multiple testing in clinical trials, and possibly enhanced validity. However, pooled indexes raise questions about which component measures to include, how to weigh these components, and how best to interpret scores that are unfamiliar.

HEALTH STATUS

Measures of health status may include an assessment of symptoms and functioning, or they may focus specifically on functioning. The cause of any difficulty in functioning (e.g., pain, fatigue, deformity, or other specific impairment) is not considered in measures of function. Observed measures of functioning include global measures such as the Steinbrocker and the revised American College of Rheumatology functional classes,[34,35] Karnofsky Performance Index,[36] and the Keitel function index.[37] Performance-based tests of functioning, such as the grip strength, walking time, button test, and timed chair stands, are effort dependent, measure capacity to execute a task rather than performance, and do not directly measure everyday life experiences.

Most measures of health status are patient self-reported because it is important to understand the patient's perception of his or her abilities or symptoms. Single-item measures, such as the number of work days or school days missed or the number of days one's activities were limited by ill health, are simple useful global measures of functioning. Numerous multi-item closed-ended health status indexes and profiles have been developed, and several compendia of these measures are available.[5,18,19,38,39] The most commonly used measures of functioning in rheumatology are the HAQ-DI and the AIMS physical function scale.[15,21,22] The HAQ-DI is a 20-question index that asks respondents to report the degree of difficulty (0 = no difficulty; 1 = some difficulty; 2 = much difficulty; 3 = unable to do) they have had in performing tasks in eight functional areas (dressing, arising, eating, walking, hygiene, reaching, gripping, and errands and chores) in the past week. The highest scores in each functional area are averaged to compute the Disability Index, which is an ordinal scale with increments of 0.125 and a possible range of 0 to 3. Use of aides or help from another person can be incorporated in the scoring. Several shortened versions of the HAQ-DI exist, but these perform less well than the full index. The AIMS2 physical function scale is a 28-question scale that asks respondents to report how often in the past month they have experienced difficulty performing tasks in six functional areas (mobility, walking and bending, hand and finger functions, arm function, self care, and household tasks). Responses can range from 0 (no days) to 5 (all days). Scores in each functional area are summed, normalized to a 0 to 10 scale, and summed across areas to give a possible range of 0 to 60. The reliability and validity of both instruments has been extensively documented.[21,22,40,41] Disease-specific (WOMAC) and population-specific (childhood HAQ) measures of functioning are also available.[23,42]

The most commonly used generic health status profiles are the SF-36, the Nottingham Health Profile, and the Sickness Impact Profile.[14,28,43,44] These instruments include scales of physical functioning, mental functioning, and social interactions. The SF-36 and Nottingham Health Profile also include scales to measure pain and fatigue, and the Nottingham Health Profile and the Sickness Impact Profile measure sleep and rest. In addition, the Sickness Impact Profile includes measures of communication, alertness, work, home management, and recreation. Scales can be used individually to identify particular areas of difficulty or combined to yield summary scores for physical and mental health (SF-36), physical and psychosocial health (Sickness Impact Profile), or an overall score (Sickness Impact Profile). The AIMS includes scales for depression and anxiety.[21,22] Specific measures of depression, such as the Beck Depression Inventory and the Centers for Epidemiologic Studies Depression scale, have also been commonly used.[45,46]

HEALTH-RELATED QUALITY OF LIFE

Measurement of quality implies a value judgment that is not present in a description of a health state. There has been increasing interest in evaluating patients' satisfaction with their health state as another dimension of health outcomes. Specific instruments to measure health-related quality of life in rheumatoid arthritis,[47] ankylosing spondylitis,[48] and pediatric rheumatic diseases[49] have recently been developed.

Preference measures are another way to learn how patients value health. Preferences represent the desirability of a particular health state, compared to some alternative health state such as perfect health or death.[50] Preference measures (or utilities) attempt to incorporate all components that influence a persons' perception of his or her health into this single rating, ranging from 0 (death) to 1 (perfect health). States of health that are preferred or more highly valued should be rated higher than less-preferred states. Interview techniques are used to determine these ratings. These techniques include numeric rating scales, time trade-off, and the standard gamble.[50] Because these techniques are time consuming and can be difficult to apply, simple instruments have been developed that assess several different aspects of the health state of a patient. A prespecified preference rating is then assigned to the patient based on the stratum of health state in which they fall. The prespecified ratings are usually derived from studies of the general population, in which people are asked to rate different health states based on written descriptions. Commonly used instruments that use prespecified ratings of defined health states include the Health Utilities Index, the Quality of Well Being scale, and the EuroQol.[51-53] Preferences are global measures that incorporate the value patients ascribe to their health, but unresolved questions on how best to measure preferences has limited their use.

PATIENT SATISFACTION

Measures of patient satisfaction most often assess a patient's impression of, or pleasure with, the quality of health care he or she has received, rather than measuring health per se.[54] The focus of these measures is, therefore, on the process of health care delivery, and results are usually measured as satisfaction with individual care providers, hospitals, or health plans. Assessment and feedback of this information can be a mechanism to identify problems and improve the delivery of care. However, satisfaction with particular treatments or treatment outcomes can also be measured.

COSTS

Costs of care have been used as an estimate the burden of illness, but costs only measure care that was delivered and resources that were used; it omits care that was needed but not delivered. Costs should be distinguished from charges, which are the amounts paid for a resource or service. Costs and charges for the same item or service may be very different. For example, the cost of manufacturing and distributing a medication may be much lower than its retail charge.

There are three components of total medical costs: direct, indirect, and intangible. Direct costs are the resources used in the provision of care and include costs of visits to physicians and other care providers, hospitalizations, treatments, diagnostic tests, devices, and costs of travel to obtain care. Indirect costs are the costs of lost productivity due to illness, including work days missed or premature retirement. Several alternative methods have been used to estimate indirect costs for persons not in the workforce, but this topic remains controversial. Intangible costs include the costs of suffering, limited activity, and lost opportunity, and they are not usually considered because they cannot be validly measured.

Cost-of-illness studies describe the costs of a group of patients with a particular disease. These studies identify the components that contribute most to the total cost, can be used to identify subsets of patients with high costs, and can be used to compare costs of different diseases. In many rheumatic diseases, indirect costs exceed direct costs, often in a ratio of 3:1 or higher. Cost descriptions also form the basis of cost-effectiveness, cost-benefit, and cost-utility studies, which measure costs relative to a health outcome gained, the amount of money saved or generated, or the health value (utilities) gained, respectively.[55]

MORTALITY

Mortality may be assessed as all-cause mortality or cause-specific mortality. Cause-specific mortality may be a more sensitive and specific measure with which to detect the effects of a treatment. Cause-specific mortality should include deaths due to complications of treatment as well as deaths due to the disease itself to avoid erroneous conclusions. For groups of patients, deaths may be analyzed as mortality rates (number of deaths in a group per unit of time; e.g., deaths per 1000 per year) or as survival rates (time from onset of disease until death).

Measuring survival emphasizes quantity of life, rather than quality. Recognizing that not all years of life are equal in quality, adjustments have been applied to years of life to capture the quality of years lived. The weights used for these adjustments score healthy years higher than years of illness, and the sum of these adjusted years can be used as a measure of both quality and quantity of life. In this way, a person who lived one year in excellent health and then died may have the same quality-adjusted survival as someone who lived 10 years in poor health and then died. When the weights for the quality adjustment are based on preference measures known as utilities, the resulting adjusted survival time is known as quality-adjusted life years (QALYs). When the weights are based on measures of disability, the adjusted survival time is known as disability-adjusted life years (DALYs).[55]

MODIFYING FACTORS OF THE PERSON AND ENVIRONMENT

Characteristics of the patient, including age, sex, ethnicity, socioeconomic status, and response to illness, can modify both the development and expression of health outcomes. Language and culture may affect how health status is assessed, requiring cultural adaptation and not merely translation of existing measures.[56] Psychosocial factors that can affect health status include self-efficacy, pain-coping styles, and learned helplessness.[57] Self-efficacy refers to a patient's confidence in his or her ability to perform specific behaviors (e.g., "I am confident I can reduce my pain").[58] Pain-coping styles include distraction, ignoring pain, reinterpreting pain, and catastrophizing.[59] Learned helplessness is a belief that one's efforts to change one's health will be ineffective.[60] Environmental factors include physical barriers or hazards, access to care and treatment, and social support. Social support includes both the number of people on whom one can rely for material and emotional help and the quality of the support.[61,62]

Properties of Good Outcome Measures

The measures used to assess health outcomes can be judged on how well they do their job. These judgments are based on the measure's reliability, validity, sensitivity to change, and interpretability. Measures should also be feasible and practical. For measures that use questionnaires, respondent burden should be minimized. Lengthy questionnaires may be comprehensive but may cause patients to skip parts or choose not to complete the questionnaire.

RELIABILITY

Reliability refers to the consistency or reproducibility of results. More formally, it is the ratio of the variability in results among patients to the total variability in results, or the proportion of variability in results due to true differences between patients.[18] The reproducibility of results can be assessed by measuring the degree of agreement between different observers who apply the measure at the same time (interobserver reliability), the same observer who applies the measure at different times (intraobserver reliability), or the same patient measured at different times (test-retest reliability). Good reliability is a necessary prerequisite for all other aspects of measurement. The poor reliability of many joint count and range of motion measures can be improved with standardization of techniques and training.[20]

VALIDITY

Validity is the property concerned with whether a questionnaire, laboratory test, or other clinical assessment is a true measure of what it intends to measure.[18] Several types of validity have been described. Face validity and content validity refer to whether the measure appears to be reasonable (face validity) and complete (content validity) to the person using the measure. Criterion validity is used when a gold standard is available and a new measure that is easier or cheaper to obtain than the gold standard is being tested. Criterion validity is a measure of the extent to which the new measure either correlates with or predicts the gold standard. Most often, gold standards exist for diagnoses (e.g., biopsy in vasculitis), rather than for health outcomes. The validity of measures of health outcomes is more often based on construct validity than criterion validity. A construct is a theory of how clinical features may be related. Construct validity tests whether a new measure performs as the theory would predict. For example, a new laboratory test of the construct "rheumatoid arthritis activity" would be expected to correlate with changes over time in other measures thought to represent how active a person's rheumatoid arthritis (RA) is, such as the degree of joint swelling, stiffness, and pain. Construct validity would also be supported if the new test did not correlate with measures that did not represent RA activity. Establishing validity is a cumulative process in which a measure is tested in many different settings and in different constructs.

SENSITIVITY TO CHANGE

Sensitivity to change, or responsiveness, is an important aspect of measures if they are being used to monitor changes in clinical status over time. Sensitivity to change refers to the magnitude of change that occurs in a measure when there is a change in clinical status.[18] Most commonly, this is tested by performing the measurement, such as a joint count or physical functioning questionnaire, before and after patients are treated with a known effective treatment. Measures that are sensitive to change will register large changes with the resultant clinical improvement, but measures that are not sensitive to change will not change much despite clinical improvement. Using measures that are poorly sensitive to change will underestimate the effects of treatment. Measures that have a continuous response format, such as a visual analogue scale, can capture gradations of response and are more sensitive to change than measures that have only a few response categories (e.g., excellent, good, fair, poor). Sensitivity to change also tends to be greater for measures that cover a wide range so that improvement can be detected even in patients who are relatively well (lack of a floor effect), and worsening can be detected even in patients who are relatively ill (lack of a ceiling effect). Disease-specific measures tend to be more sensitive to change than generic measures.

INTERPRETABILITY

Death, inability to work, and being wheelchair-bound are health outcomes known from life experience. Severity of arthritis and other clinical signs and, to some extent, common laboratory tests such as the erythrocyte sedimentation rate, acquire familiarity through repeated use and experience with their typical ranges and variations. However, for other health outcomes, and particularly for quantitative measures of symptoms, health status, and health-related quality of life, there is often little to ground interpretation of results. Descriptions that relate questionnaire scores to familiar benchmarks can greatly aid the interpretation of measures. For example, scores on a fatigue scale can be related to the proportion of patients with that score who need help with household chores or are unable to work. Greater uncertainty arises when attempting to interpret changes in measures over time and in defining how large a change should be to be considered clinically important or clinically meaningful.[63,64] Consensus conferences have begun to address this important issue, but more empiric studies of patients' judgments of what constitutes an important change in health are needed.

Outcome Measures in Clinical Trials

RHEUMATOID ARTHRITIS

Clinical trials in RA have focused on treatments to decrease the activity of RA and to prevent long-term bone and joint damage. Measures of the activity of RA include impairments, symptoms, and health status. Several professional organizations have made recommendations of a minimum "core set" of measures to include as end points in short-term clinical trials, based on reviews of their relevance, reliability, validity, and sensitivity to change[65-67] (Table 29–3). Although the American College of Rheumatology core set recommended specific joint count measures, it did not recommend specific instruments to measure pain, physical function, global assessments, or radiographic changes.[65] In contrast, the European League Against Rheumatism (EULAR) core set included recommendations for specific instruments to be used for each measure.[66] Each core set recommended patient self-reported, rather than observed, health status measures. Other measures in addition to those recommended can be used. Radiographs are recommended for studies of 1 year or longer.

Response criteria define the degree of improvement in measures of disease activity that categorize a patient as improved or not. The American College of Rheumatology preliminary definition of improvement in RA was derived from a review of randomized clinical trials as the set of measures that best discriminated patients who received active treatment from those who received placebo.[68] This definition was at least 20 percent improvement in both the tender joint count and swollen joint count and at least 20 percent improvement in three of five other measures (pain score, patient's global assessment, physician's global assessment, patient's self-reported physical functioning, and acute phase reactant). The EULAR criteria for improvement in RA activity are based on changes in the DAS, a pooled index of the Ritchie Articular Index, swollen joint count, erythrocyte sedimentation rate, and patient global assessment. These criteria define moderate responses and good responses based on both the amount of improvement in the DAS and the final score achieved.[69] Response criteria have been considered benchmarks of clinically important improvement, but they differ in several important conceptual, methodologic, and practical ways from criteria for clinically important improvement.[64]

TABLE 29-3 • RECOMMENDED "CORE SET" MEASURES TO BE INCLUDED IN CLINICAL TRIALS IN RHEUMATOID ARTHRITIS (RA), ANKYLOSING SPONDYLITIS (AS), AND OSTEOARTHRITIS (OA)*

	RA			AS		OA[74]
	ACR[65]	*EULAR[66]*	*WHO[67]*	*Symptom Modifying[70]*	*Disease Controlling[70]*	
Tender joint count	68	28	X		X	
Swollen joint count	66	28	X		X	
Patient reported pain	X	X	X	X	X	X
Patient global	X	X	X	X	X	X
Physician global	X		X			
Physical functioning	X	HAQ-DI	X	X	X	X
Acute-phase reactant	X	X	X			
Imaging	1 year	Larsen score	1 year		X	1 year
Spinal mobility				X	X	
Spinal stiffness				X		

* Specific measure and time points are noted where applicable.

Abbreviations: ACR, American College of Rheumatology; EULAR, European League Against Rheumatism; HAQ-DI, Health Assessment Questionnaire Disability Index.

ANKYLOSING SPONDYLITIS

Using consensus processes similar to those used for RA, a recommended core set of endpoints to be included in clinical trials in ankylosing spondylitis (AS) have been proposed, with an assessment of peripheral joints and entheses, acute-phase reactants, and radiographs included for treatments intended to be disease controlling[70] (see Table 29–3). However, the sensitivity to change of some measures has not been well established. A preliminary definition of improvement in short-term clinical trials of nonsteroidal anti-inflammatory drugs in AS solely recommended patient self-report measures (pain severity, stiffness, physical functioning, and global assessment).[71]

SYSTEMIC LUPUS ERYTHEMATOSUS

Most clinical trials in systemic lupus erythematosus (SLE) have studied treatments of lupus nephritis, which have used organ-specific measures of impairment, end-stage renal disease, or death as end points. Measures of SLE activity have increasingly been used as end points in clinical trials. The SLAM and SLEDAI (or modifications of these) have been used most often, but other valid measures are available, including the British Isles Lupus Assessment Group (BILAG) profile and the European Consensus Lupus Activity Measure (ECLAM).[30,31,72,73] These measures differ in how much weight is given to symptoms, rather than signs and laboratory abnormalities, and in their sensitivity to change. Health status in SLE has most often been assessed using a multidimensional instrument such as the SF-36, rather than individual measures of pain or physical functioning.

OSTEOARTHRITIS

Patient self-reported pain intensity, physical functioning, and global assessment were identified as the core measures to be used as end points in clinical trials in osteoarthritis (OA) (see Table 29–3). At least moderate improvement in two of these measures has been proposed as response criteria.[74] Imaging studies were recommended for trials of one year or longer.

Outcome Measures in Clinical Practice

Evaluation of patients in clinical practice is focused on symptoms and impairments, drawn from the history, physical examination, and laboratory and radiologic tests. Assessment is often not formalized, and few rheumatologists use quantitative measures of symptoms or health status to evaluate patients and their response to treatment.[75] Use of these measures has been advocated to help assess disease activity more accurately and completely, to reveal unrecognized problems patients may be facing, and to elicit the patient's assessment and incorporate his or her perspective in the treatment plan. Barriers to the use of health status measures in clinical practice include unfamiliarity and poor interpretability of some measures, the need for coding and scoring, and the administrative burden associated with collecting these data. Evidence demonstrating that the use of formal measures of health status improved patients' outcomes may spur adoption of these measures in clinical practice.[76]

REFERENCES

1. Last JM: A Dictionary of Epidemiology. New York, Oxford University Press, 1983.
2. World Health Organization. ICF: International Classification of Functioning, Disability, and Health. Introduction. World Health Organization, 2001. http://www.who.int/classification/icif/intros/ICF-Eng-Intro.pdf accessed on December, 2001.
3. Ware JE Jr: The status of health assessment 1994. Annu Rev Public Health 16:327-354, 1995.
4. Patrick DL, Erickson P: Health Status and Health Policy. Quality of Life in Health Care Evaluation and Resource Allocation. New York, Oxford University Press, 1993.
5. Spilker B: Quality of Life and Pharmacoeconomics in Clinical Trials, 2nd ed. Philadelphia, Lippincott-Raven, 1996.
6. Kaplan RM, Anderson JP: A general health policy model: update and applications. Health Serv Res 23:203-235, 1988.
7. Smith KW, Avis NE, Assmann SF: Distinguishing between quality of life and health status in quality of life research: a meta-analysis. Qual Life Res 8:447-459, 1999.
8. Kravitz RL: Measuring patients' expectations and requests. Ann Intern Med 134:881-888, 2001.
9. The World Health Organization Quality of Life Group. The World Health Organization Quality of Life (WHOQOL) Assessment: Development and general psychometric properties. Soc Sci Med 46:1569-1585, 1998.
10. Fries JF: The assessment of disability: From first to future principles. Br J Rheumatol 22 (Suppl):48-58, 1983.
11. Wilson IB, Cleary PD: Linking clinical variables with health-related quality of life: A conceptual model of patient outcomes. JAMA 273:59-65, 1995.
12. Feinstein AR: Clinimetrics. New Haven, Yale University Press, 1987.
13. Melzack R, Katz J: The McGill Pain Questionnaire: appraisal and current status. *In* Turk DC, Melzack R (eds): Handbook of Pain Assessment. New York, Guilford Press, 1992, pp 152-168.
14. Ware JE, Sherbourne CD: The MOS 36-item short-form health survey (SF-36): I. Conceptual framework and item selection. Med Care 30:473-483, 1992.
15. Fries JF, Spitz P, Kraines RG, Holman HR: Measurement of patient outcomes in arthritis. Arthritis Rheum 23:137-145, 1980.
16. Tugwell P, Bombardier C, Buchanan WW, et al: The MACTAR patient preference disability questionnaire: An individualized functional priority approach for assessing improvements in physical disability in clinical trials in rheumatoid arthritis. J Rheumatol 14:446-451, 1987.
17. Bradley LA: Pain measurement in arthritis. Arthritis Care Res 6:178-186, 1993.
18. Streiner DL, Norman GR: Health Measurement Scales: A Practical Guide to Their Development and Use, 2nd ed. New York, Oxford University Press, 1995.
19. Mason JH, Anderson JJ, Meenan RF, et al: The rapid assessment of disease activity in rheumatology (RADAR) questionnaire. Arthritis Rheum 35:156-162, 1992.
20. Bellamy N: Musculoskeletal Clinical Metrology. Dordrecht, Netherlands, Kluwer Academic Publishers, 1993.
21. Meenan RF, Gertman PM, Mason JH: Measuring health status in arthritis. The Arthritis Impact Measurement Scales. Arthritis Rheum 23:146-152, 1980.
22. Meenan RF, Mason JH, Anderson JJ, etal: AIMS2. The content and properties of a revised and expanded Arthritis Impact Measurement Scales health status questionnaire. Arthritis Rheum 35:1-10, 1992.
23. Bellamy N, Buchanan WW, Goldsmith CH, et al: Validation study of WOMAC: a health status instrument for measuring clinically important patient relevant outcomes to antirheumatic drug therapy in patients with osteoarthritis of the hip or knee. J Rheumatol 15:1833-1840, 1988.

24. Bellamy N, Campbell J, Haraoui B, et al: Dimensionality and clinical importance of pain and disability in hand osteoarthritis: Development of the Australian/Canadian (AUSCAN) Osteoarthritis Hand Index. Osteoarthritis Cartilage 10:855-862, 2002.
25. McDaniel LK, Anderson KO, Bradley LA, et al: Development of an observational method for assessing pain behavior in rheumatoid arthritis patients. Pain 24:165-184, 1986.
26. Rhind VM, Unsworth A, Haslock I: Assessment of stiffness in rheumatology: the use of rating scales. Br J Rheumatol 26:126-130, 1987.
27. Krupp LB, LaRocca NG, Muir-Nash J, Steinberg AD: The Fatigue Severity Scale: Application to patients with multiple sclerosis and systemic lupus erythematosus. Arch Neurol 46:1121-1123, 1989.
28. Hunt SM, McEwen J, McKenna SP: Measuring Health Status. London, Croom Helm, 1986.
29. van der Heijde DMFM, van't Hof MA, van Riel PLCM, et al: Judging disease activity in clinical practice in rheumatoid arthritis: first step in the development of a disease activity score. Ann Rheum Dis 49:916-920, 1990.
30. Liang MH, Socher SA, Larson MG, Schur PH: Reliability and validity of six systems for the clinical assessment of disease activity in systemic lupus erythematosus. Arthritis Rheum 32:1107-1118, 1989.
31. Bombardier C, Gladman DD, Urowitz MB, et al: Derivation of the SLEDAI: A disease activity index for lupus patients. Arthritis Rheum 35:630-640, 1992.
32. Gladman D, Ginzler E, Goldsmith C, et al: The development and initial validation of the Systemic Lupus International Collaborating Clinics/American College of Rheumatology damage index for systemic lupus erythematosus. Arthritis Rheum 39:363-369, 1996.
33. Luqmani RA, Bacon PA, Moots RJ, et al: Birmingham Vasculitis Activity Score (BVAS) in systemic necrotizing vasculitis. Q J Med 87:671-867, 1994.
34. Steinbrocker O, Traeger CH, Batterman RC: Therapeutic criteria in rheumatoid arthritis. JAMA 140:659-662, 1949.
35. Hochberg MC, Chang RW, Dwosh I, et al: The American College of Rheumatology 1991 revised criteria for the classification of global functional status in rheumatoid arthritis. Arthritis Rheum 35:498-502, 1992.
36. Karnofsky DA, Burchenal JH: The clinical evaluation of chemotherapeutic agents in cancer. In Macleod CM (ed): Evaluation of Chemotherapeutic Agents in Cancer. New York, Columbia University Press, 1949, pp 191-205.
37. Eberl DR, Fasching V, Rahlfs V, et al: Repeatability and objectivity of various measurements in rheumatoid arthritis: A comparative study. Arthritis Rheum 19:1278-1286, 1976.
38. Spilker B, Molinek FR Jr, Johnston KA, et al: Quality of life bibliography and indexes. Med Care 28 (Suppl):DS1-DS77, 1990.
39. Katz PP (ed). Patient outcomes in rheumotolgy. A review of measures. Arthritis Rheum (Suppl.) 49, 2003.
40. Haavardsholm EA, Kvien TK, Uhlig T, et al: A comparison of agreement and sensitivity to change between AIMS2 and a short form of AIMS2 (AIMS2-SF) in more than 1,000 rheumatoid arthritis patients. J Rheumatol 27:2810-2816, 2000.
41. Ramey DR, Raynauld J-P, Fries JF: The Health Assessment Questionnaire 1992: Status and review. Arthritis Care Res 5:119-129, 1992.
42. Singh G, Athreya BH, Fries JF, Goldsmith DP: Measurement of health status in children with juvenile rheumatoid arthritis. Arthritis Rheum 37:1761-1769, 1994.
43. Bergner M, Bobbit RA, Carter WB, Gilson BS: The Sickness Impact Profile: development and final revision of a health status measure. Med Care 19:787-805, 1981.
44. Coons SJ, Rao S, Keininger DL, Hays RD: A comparative review of generic quality-of-life instruments. Pharmacoeconomics 17:13-35, 2000.
45. Beck AT, Rush AJ, Shaw BF, Emery G: Cognitive Therapy of Depression. New York, Guilford Press, 1979.
46. Radloff LS: The CES-D Scale: a self-report depression scale for research in the general population. Appl Psychol Meas 1:385-401, 1977.
47. DeJong Z, van der Heidje D, McKenna SP, Whalley D: The reliability and construct validity of the RAQoL: a rheumatoid arthritis-specific quality of life instrument. Br J Rheumatol 36:878-883, 1997.
48. Haywood KL, Garratt AM, Jordan K, et al: Disease-specific, patient-assessed measures of health outcome in ankylosing spondylitis: reliability, validity, and responsiveness. Rheumatology 41:1295-1302, 2002.
49. Varni JW, Seid M, Smith Knight T, et al: The PedsQL in pediatric rheumatology. Arthritis Rheum 46:714-725, 2002.
50. Torrance GW: Measurement of health state utilities for economic appraisal. J Health Econ 5:1-30, 1986.
51. Torrance GW, Furlong W, Feeny D, Boyle M: Multi-attribute preference functions. Health Utilities Index. Pharmacoeconomics 7:503-520, 1995.
52. Kaplan RM, Bush JW: Health-related quality of life measurement for evaluation research and policy analysis. Health Psychol 1:61-80, 1982.
53. EuroQol group. EuroQol: A new facility for the measurement of health related quality of life. Health Policy 16:199-208, 1990.
54. Hudak PL, Wright JG: The characteristics of patient satisfaction measures. Spine 25:3167-3177, 2000.
55. Neumann PJ, Goldie SJ, Weinstein MC: Preference-based measures in economic evaluation in health care. Annu Rev Public Health 21:587-611, 2000.
56. Gonzalez VM, Stewart A, Ritter PL, Lorig K: Translation and validation of arthritis outcome measures into Spanish. Arthritis Rheum 38:1429-1446, 1995.
57. Keefe FJ, Smith SJ, Buffington ALH, et al: Recent advances and future directions in the biopsychosocial assessment and treatment of arthritis. J Consult Clin Psychol 70:640-655, 2002.
58. Lorig K, Chastain RL, Ung E, et al: Development and evaluation of a scale to measure perceived self-efficacy in people with arthritis. Arthritis Rheum 32:37-44, 1989.
59. Rosentiel AK, Keefe FJ: The use of coping strategies in chronic low back pain patients: relationship to patient characteristics and current adjustment. Pain 17:33-44, 1983.
60. Callahan LF, Brooks RH, Pincus T: Further analysis of learned helplessness in rheumatoid arthritis using a "Rheumatology Attitudes Index." J Rheumatol 15:418-426, 1988.
61. Cohen S, Mermelstein R, Kamarck T, Hoberman HM: Measuring the functional components of social support. In Sarason BR, Sarason IG (eds): Social Support: Theory, Research and Application. The Hague, Netherlands, Martinus Nijhoff, 1985, pp 73-94.
62. Sarason IG, Levine HM, Basham RB, Sarason BR: Assessing social support. The Social Support Questionnaire. J Personal Social Psychol 44:127-139, 1983.
63. Guyatt GH, Osoba D, Wu AW, et al: Clinical Significance Consensus Meeting Group. Methods to explain the clinical significance of health status measures. Mayo Clin Proc 77:371-383, 2002.
64. Ward MM: Clinical and laboratory measures of rheumatoid arthritis activity. In Haynes BF, Pisetsky DS, St. Clair EW (eds): RA: Textbook of Rheumatoid Arthritis. Philadelphia, Lippincott Williams & Wilkins, in press.
65. Felson DT, Anderson JJ, Boers M, et al: The American College of Rheumatology preliminary core set of disease activity measures for rheumatoid arthritis clinical trials. Arthritis Rheum 36:729-740, 1993.
66. van Riel PLCM. Provisional guidelines for measuring disease activity in clinical trials on rheumatoid arthritis. Br J Rheumatol 31:793-796, 1992.
67. Boers M, Tugwell P, Felson DT, et al: World Health Organization and International League of Associations for Rheumatology Core Endpoints for symptom modifying antirheumatic drugs in rheumatoid arthritis clinical trials. J Rheumatol 21(Suppl 41):86-89, 1994.
68. Felson DT, Anderson JJ, Boers M, et al: American College of Rheumatology preliminary definition of improvement in rheumatoid arthritis. Arthritis Rheum 38:727-735, 1995.
69. van Gestel AM, Prevoo MLL, van't Hof MA, et al: Development and validation of the European League Against Rheumatism response criteria for rheumatoid arthritis. Comparison with the Preliminary American College of Rheumatology and the World Health Organization/International League Against Rheumatism criteria. Arthritis Rheum 39:34-40, 1996.
70. van der Heidje D: Which domains should be included in a core set for endpoints in ankylosing spondylitis? Introduction to the ankylosing spondylitis module of OMERACT IV. J Rheumatol 26:945-947, 1999.

71. Anderson JJ, Baron G, van der Heidje D,et al: Ankylosing Spondylitis Assessment Group preliminary definition of short-term improvement in ankylosing spondylitis. Arthritis Rheum 44:1876-1886, 2001.
72. Symmons DPM, Coppock JS, Bacon PA, et al: Development and assessment of a computerized index of clinical disease activity in systemic lupus erythematosus. Q J Med 69:927-937, 1988.
73. Vitali C, Bencivelli VW, Isenberg DA, et al: Disease activity in systemic lupus erythematosus: report of the Consensus Study Group of the European Workshop for Rheumatology Research. II. Identification of the variables indicative of disease activity and their use in the development of an activity score. Clin Exp Rheumatol 10:541-547, 1992.
74. Dougados M, LeClaire P, van der Heidje D, et al: Response criteria for clinical trials on osteoarthritis of the knee and hip. Osteoarthritis Cartilage 8:395-403, 2000.
75. Wolfe F, Pincus T: Listening to the patient. Arthritis Rheum 42:1797-1808, 1999.
76. Kazis LE, Callahan LF, Meenan RF, Pincus T: Health status reports in the care of patients with rheumatoid arthritis. J Clin Epidemiol 43:1243-1253, 1990.

30 Development, Execution, and Analysis of Clinical Trials

LENORE M. BUCKLEY • BARBARA FINCK

Clinical trials are research studies designed to assess the effectiveness of new drugs or novel combinations of drugs, treatments, devices, or other interventions. The number of clinical trials of novel agents for the treatment of the rheumatic diseases has increased dramatically and has led to refinements and advances in trial design, data analysis, and definitions of disease activity and response criteria. This chapter reviews the basic principles of trial design, execution, and analysis, as well as controversies in these areas. The process for United States Food and Drug Administration (FDA) approval of new drugs and biologic agents is outlined. In addition, the ethical responsibilities of investigators, industry, and academic institutions and protection of human subjects are discussed.

Clinical Trial Design

DEFINING THE RESEARCH OBJECTIVE AND FEASIBILITY

If a research project is to be successful, the design must be feasible (Table 30–1). Given the restrictions of the selection criteria, are subjects available in sufficient numbers? Are the necessary resources (e.g., financial, statistical, support personnel, facilities) present? Are there validated diagnostic criteria and outcome measures? These are critical questions to answer before initiating a clinical trial.[1] It is also important to involve a statistician early in the design of a clinical study for important power and sample size calculations, review of the proposed design and data collection methods, and for a prospective plan for data analysis.

Steps in New Drug Development

There are a number of studies required in the development of new drugs or treatments—from the initial studies to examine pharmacology, safety, and dose range to the large clinical trials designed to demonstrate efficacy for FDA approval. *Phase I* studies are the earliest human trials and are used to determine drug pharmacokinetics, metabolism, distribution, and clinical pharmacology in humans, but they may not determine efficacy.[1] An important goal of Phase I studies is to define a safe dose range and dosing regimen for subsequent Phase II and III studies. The dose range in Phase I studies is based on preclinical (animal) data. Phase I studies may be conducted in healthy volunteers. However, if the drug or treatment has potential serious toxicities, or if the results in healthy volunteers may not reflect the pharmacokinetics of the patient population for whom the treatment is designed (e.g., pregnant women), initial studies may be carried out in patients with the specific disease or condition in question. Standard Phase I trial design includes sequential single-dose escalations until the maximally tolerated dose (MTD) is defined. The MTD is usually defined as the dose level immediately below the dose at which two patients experience dose-limiting toxicity. For drugs with little toxicity and therefore no MTD, surrogate outcome measures can help define the biologic activity or localization of drug to target tissue and may help to determine the dose range for Phase II and III studies. It is important to prospectively define the dose-limiting toxicities that may be used to define the MTD and to exclude those toxicities known to be due to disease progression or previous therapies. Accelerated dose-titration designs for Phase I studies have been evaluated by the National Institute of Health (NIH) Center for Drug Evaluation.[2] These designs attempt to balance the benefits of rapid dose titration (e.g., fewer patients per cohort, shorter trial duration) with possible increased risk to patients.

Phase II trials are larger, longer trials designed to investigate dose effects and toxicity. These trials are usually randomized, parallel-arm trials with different doses and a placebo arm, with or without standard of care background therapies. Data about dose effects and toxicity from phase II trials are used to determine doses for larger Phase III trials. In addition, efficacy end points that are planned for Phase III are evaluated in Phase II, so that the Phase III trials can be appropriately sized and powered. Occasionally, open-labeled Phase II trials are performed to assess the feasibility and likelihood of success before embarking on larger, more expensive, adequately powered Phase II and III studies. Pilot Phase II trial designs may be open or blinded, usually contain no more than 20 patients per treatment arm, and evaluate response. If no response is seen (i.e., fewer than two out of 20 patients respond), the drug may be abandoned for this indication.

Phase III trials are designed to demonstrate efficacy and have prospectively defined primary and secondary end points with prospectively planned statistical analysis. The primary and secondary end points should support the labeling claim if the product is being submitted to the FDA for a new drug approval.

Phase IV studies, or postmarketing surveillance, further delineate common adverse reactions, can identify rare reactions, and further define efficacy in subgroups or special populations. Because there is often no control

TABLE 30–1 • STRUCTURE OF A CLINICAL PROTOCOL

1. Research problem
   a. Background and objectives
   b. Significance
2. Methods
   a. Design
   b. Subjects
   c. Outcomes: primary and secondary
   c. Data collection and measurement procedures
   d. Statistical issues
      i. Power and sample size calculations
      ii. Statistical analysis
   e. Quality control and data management
   f. Timetable and organizational chart
3. Human subjects
   a. Ethical considerations
   b. Informed consent
   c. Gender and racial mix
4. References

group for Phase IV studies, it is more difficult to assess whether the adverse events that occur are greater than would be expected for patients receiving standard therapy. For comparison, large cohorts of patients with similar disease criteria but on different therapies or historical databases can be used to determine the expected frequency of adverse events, including rare events.

Design Considerations

Most clinical trials have *parallel designs* in which treatment assignment is constant throughout the study. In *crossover designs,* each patient receives both treatments.[3] An advantage of a crossover design is that patients can serve as their own controls, and smaller samples sizes are needed. However, this design does not work well if the time to onset of action of the treatment is long or the action continues for a period after the treatment is stopped (i.e., carryover effect). In a *flare design,* the patient's treatment is discontinued and study treatment is started only after a flare in disease is documented. This design maximizes disease activity when the study treatment is initiated. In a *withdrawal design,* the study treatment is administered (with or without a control treatment arm), and after a period of stabilization the treatment is withdrawn to assess and compare the frequency of clinical worsening or disease flare. This can provide further evidence of treatment efficacy. In another type of *withdrawal design,* all subjects are started on active treatment and the responders (by predefined criteria) are then randomized to continue on active treatment or to be withdrawn from treatment, and the rate of flare or disease worsening is compared between groups. This type of trial design has been used in pediatric studies to maximize the number of patients who receive active treatment and to eliminate the need to randomize patients with active disease to placebo prior to demonstrating any effectiveness of the treatment.[4]

Trials can be designed to test a difference (one treatment is superior to another), *noninferiority* (one treatment is not worse than another), or *equivalence* (one treatment is equally effective as another). Equivalency trials are usually undertaken to compare a new product to an older or "standard of care" product and are often performed for ethical reasons; it is on longer ethical to do a placebo-controlled trial if there is a known effective treatment. The disadvantage of equivalency trials is that they require large number of patients because the confidence interval required to rule out a difference between treatments is small. Noninferiority (not worse than) trial design may be more feasible: Fewer subjects are needed because only a one-sided statistical test is performed. When performing equivalency or noninferiority trials, the new treatment should be tested against the best current treatment, and the effect size of the current treatment compared to the placebo should be known.

Ethical and practical considerations have limited the use of placebo-control trials in diseases for which there are known effective treatments, if a period of placebo treatment could lead to permanent loss of function or quality of life. Other alternatives to placebo-controlled trials include add on trials and active control trials. In *active control trials,* the new treatment is compared to a known effective treatment (e.g., a biologic agent compared to methotrexate in rheumatoid arthritis [RA]). In an *add on trial* all the subjects receive a known effective treatment, and the new treatment is given only to the intervention group (e.g., a biologic agent plus methotrexate or methotrexate alone in RA).

The duration of a study is determined by many factors: the expected time for treatment effect to be clinically evident, disease characteristics and relevant end points, and practical limitations on resources. For some indications, the FDA has set standards for the length of a trial designed to support different labeling claims. For instance, studies that demonstrate the efficacy of a new agent to reduce joint inflammation and swelling in RA may be only 3 to 6 months long, but a trial of 2 years or longer may be required to demonstrate improvement in function. The FDA may require long-term follow-up (3 to 5 years) for some new classes of drugs such as biologic response modifiers.

Most clinical trials are conducted at multiple centers allowing the study to enroll greater numbers of subjects, reduce enrollment time, and broaden the racial and socioeconomic mix of patients, thus improving the generalizability of the results. Quality control and uniformity of data collection are more complicated in these trials.[5]

Subjects and Methods

SPECIFYING THE SELECTION CRITERIA

Subjects who are entered into clinical studies should meet accepted diagnostic criteria for the disease or disorder under study. In many trials, patients must also meet certain criteria for disease activity or duration. Some trials require that the patient experience a flare after withdrawal of medication as evidence of active disease. Other studies define disease activity before withdrawal of medication as evidence of lack of response to current treatment. Disease severity can be defined by accepted clinical criteria or by lack of response to previous treatments. For example, RA studies may be limited to patients who have not yet received methotrexate (who presumably have early or mild disease) or to patients who have failed treatment with at least one other disease-modifying antirheumatic drug (DMARD) (more disease severity). Other inclusion criteria may be age, sex, and certain disease subgroups. Evidence of eligibility criteria (documentation of prior drug treatment duration and failure, archives of radiograph results) for each subject should be maintained so that eligibility can be documented at later external review.

Exclusion criteria usually include conditions such as cancer; cardiac, hepatic, or renal disease; hematologic parameters; medication allergies; and pregnancy. Exclusion criteria decrease the background noise or variability due to differences in patient characteristics but can narrow the generalizability of the results as study populations become more homogeneous. The treatment effect or toxicity may be different when the drug is given to patients with other comorbidities in the community setting. Exclusion criteria based on subject safety, contraindications to treatment, or comorbid conditions are generally accepted, but exclusion criteria based on race and gender are discouraged unless the disorder is specific to a certain race or gender.[6]

Decisions must be made about concomitant medications. For example, in RA studies, patients are often allowed to continue nonsteroidal anti-inflammatory drugs and limited doses of oral glucocorticoids. Allowing concomitant therapies can decrease dropout rates. However, concomitant medications should be held stable until the primary end point has been reached, because interpretation of outcomes becomes complicated if concomitant therapies are changing. In contrast, the ability to use lower doses of glucocorticoid is sometimes used as a secondary efficacy end point, adding further evidence of a positive treatment effect. Medications for treatment of acute conditions are generally allowed during studies but must be evaluated if the treatment could confuse the ability of the investigator to evaluate the efficacy or toxicity of the study drug.

Statistical Considerations

TYPE I AND TYPE II ERROR

A *type I error* occurs when the investigator concludes that there is a difference in the effects of two treatments when there is not (i.e., false positive).[7] *Type II error* occurs when the investigator falsely concludes that there is no difference in the effects of two treatments (i.e., false negative). The likelihood of type I and type II errors is less with large sample sizes. The likelihood that a study can detect a difference in outcomes between treatment groups also depends on effect size. If the treatment has a larger effect, it is easier to detect with smaller sample sizes.

The investigator establishes the type I and type II error at the beginning of the study. The probability of a type I error (false positive) is referred to as *alpha*, or the level of statistical significance. The probability of making a type II error (false negative) is *beta*. Power (i.e., 1-beta) is the probability of finding a difference in treatment outcomes if the effect size is as hypothesized or greater. If beta is 10 percent, there is a 90 percent chance of finding a difference between groups of the expected effect or greater. In most studies, alpha, or the p value, is set at .05 or .01, and beta is set at .2 or .1 (power of 80 to 90 percent). If the p value is .05, there is a 1 in 20 chance of a false-positive result. When more than one hypothesis is tested, the chance of a type 1 error (false positive) increases, reinforcing the importance of having a primary outcome variable and limited secondary outcomes.

SAMPLE SIZE

One of the most common causes of an unsuccessful clinical study is inadequate sample size.[3] Sample size is one of the most important determinants of the power of a study to find treatment differences. The sample size is the number of patients who should finish the trial, rather than the number who enter. To determine whether there is an adequate group of patients for participation in a clinical trial, the first step is to assess the number of patients with the diagnosis who are available to participate, using clinical, billing, or other databases. An estimate is made of the proportion of available subjects who can meet entry criteria using a chart review of a subset of subjects identified or a review of clinical information available in databases. This number is then decreased by the proportion who are unlikely to agree to participate (often estimated by participation rates in previous studies at that center) and further decreased by the proportion of expected dropouts due to toxicity or noncompliance. The number left should approximate the proposed sample size.

To determine the appropriate sample size (n) for a study, the investigator needs to have estimates of the effect size of the intervention (i.e., difference in outcome between treatment groups), the variability of the data (i.e., standard deviation), the statistical test to be used, and the alpha (i.e., p value or false-positive rate) and beta (i.e., false-negative rate) level. The effect size is the expected difference in response rate between the treatment and placebo groups. It is important to estimate the placebo effect—the proportion of subjects who meet criteria for improvement in the placebo group (reported as high as 20 to 40 percent in studies of patients with RA). The variability or standard deviation of the outcome measure can be estimated from pilot data or from other published clinical trials. Calculating power (i.e., 1-beta or the power of the study to find a difference at a certain effect size) requires knowing what statistical test will be used, the sample size (n), the variability of the data (e.g., standard deviation), the effect size, and alpha.[3]

Generally, the sample size in each treatment arm is the same; however, unequal but proportional treatment groups are often used (2:1 ratio of treated subjects to control). Equal-size treatment groups have greater power.

However, unequal groups are sometimes used to maximize the number of patients who receive treatment, and patients are sometimes more willing to enter a trial in which they have a greater likelihood of receiving an active treatment.

BIAS AND CONFOUNDING

Random error is an incorrect result due to chance. Bias is a systematic error that enters the clinical trial and distorts the data in one direction.[1] For example, sampling bias occurs when the study population is not representative of the target population. The study group may be healthier than people in the general population with the disorder because the entrance criteria are strict, or the study group may be more ill because they were recruited from a tertiary center and had advanced disease.

Confounding variables are variables associated with disease and with the treatment outcome. For example, if patients in the treatment group have milder disease at baseline than those in the control group, disease severity becomes a possible confounder. If subjects in the treatment arm have a better outcome than those in the control arm, it is difficult to know whether the better outcome is related to the treatment or to less-active disease at entry. The effects of confounders can be sorted out in the statistical analysis at the end of the study, but only with some loss of power. Another way to avoid confounding is to stratify patients at randomization by the possible confounder.

RANDOMIZATION

Randomization is the process by which patients are assigned to treatment to reduce bias. It is usually accomplished by using a randomization code or computer-generated randomization that assigns a patient to treatment. It eliminates the bias that occurs if the investigator assigns treatments to patients. Patients should not be randomized to treatment until they have completed the screening visit or screening period, because many of the patients will not meet eligibility requirements or may refuse to participate in the study. Randomization is often done in "blocks" so that in every block of four or 10, there will be an equal number of patients in the treatment and control groups. Randomizing in blocks ensures that if the sample size is less than expected there will be an equal proportion of patients in each treatment group. However, randomization does not eliminate the possibility that there will be differences between treatment groups in important clinical characteristics.

STRATIFICATION

Even in randomized clinical trials, the treatment groups may not be well matched for all important clinical variables at baseline. This is especially true in smaller studies. Stratification is a way of balancing treatment groups at baseline for characteristics that may have an important influence on outcomes, such as pulmonary or renal involvement in scleroderma trials or sex and previous fractures in osteoporosis trials. Stratification is accomplished by separating patients into groups by the stratifying criteria and then randomizing them separately. For example, treatment assignment is chosen from a different randomization block for men and women to ensure an equal proportion of men and women in each treatment group.

The effects of a variable that is a confounder can be adjusted for in the statistical analysis as a covariate. However, stratification is a more powerful way to control for a possible confounding variable because stratification decreases the variability in the data and therefore increases the statistical power. Only a small number of variables can be used in stratification, or the randomization becomes complex and there are too few subjects in each stratum. Another way to deal with confounding is matched-pair randomization, in which subjects are matched for important and possible confounding characteristics at baseline.

BLINDING

In double-blind studies neither the subject nor the investigator is aware of the treatment group assignment. In single-blind studies, the investigator is aware of the treatment group, but the subject is not. In open-label studies, both the subject and investigator are aware of the treatment assignment. Unblinding may inadvertently occur because of identifiable adverse reactions or minor side effects, lack of efficacy, or changes in laboratory parameters. When possible, the study personnel who prepare the drug should be different from the personnel who administer it and from those who assess efficacy parameters and adverse events.

CHOOSING OUTCOMES

It is important to use the accepted criteria for measuring changes in activity or outcome for a given disease.[8-12] If there are no published criteria, consideration should be given to using the same definitions used in recent important clinical trials in that field. If clinical trials use different outcomes, it is difficult to compare the results across trials.

A single or limited number of primary outcome measures should be chosen, and power and sample size considerations are made using these variables. If too many outcomes are compared, there is a higher chance of making a type I error. Other clinical outcomes of interest are considered secondary efficacy variables, and statistical tests are usually done to test the significance of differences in these variables.

When the effect of treatment on disease course or outcome may not be clear for a number of years, intermediate end points are chosen that have been shown to correlate with the long-term or "gold standard" outcome. Intermediate end points may include changes in laboratory markers of disease activity (e.g., acute-phase reactants, hemoglobin) or in the clinical examination findings (e.g., joint swelling, tenderness in RA trials). Bombardier and Tugwell[13] proposed that the end points for clinical trials meet three criteria:

TABLE 30–2 • OUTCOME MEASURES IN RHEUMATOID ARTHRITIS CLINICAL TRIALS

Criteria*	ACR	ILAR	OMERACT
Swollen joints	+	+	+
Tender joints	+	+	+
Physician's global assessment	+		+
Patient's global assessment	+	+	+
Pain	+	+	+
Functional status or physical disability	+		+
Acute-phase reactant (WESR or CRP)	+	+	+
Radiographs			+

Abbreviations: CRP, C-reactive protein; WESR, erythrocyte sedimentation rate.

*Outcome criteria proposed by the American College of Rheumatology (ACR), International League against Rheumatism (ILAR), and the Outcome Measures in Rheumatoid Arthritis Clinical Trials (OMERACT) committee. The ACR definition of response to treatment is a 20% improvement in swollen and tender joints and 20% improvement in three of the remaining five criteria.

1. *Criterion validity:* The outcome should correlate with death, disability, or radiographic progression (RA trials).
2. *Discriminant validity:* The outcomes are sensitive to change and can detect small changes in clinical trials.
3. *Content validity:* The outcome samples multiple domains.

Multiple outcomes are often assessed in clinical trials in rheumatic diseases because improvement may be difficult to define using one measure. The American College of Rheumatology (ACR), International League of Associations for Rheumatology (ILAR), and the World Health Organization (WHO) have all listed response criteria (different from classification criteria) for RA and other rheumatic diseases.[12]

After outcome criteria are chosen, a decision should be made about the degree of improvement that qualifies as a response.[10,14,15] The current ACR (www.rheumatology.org) and ILAR/WHO RA response criteria, in Table 30-2, define a responder as a subject who has at least a 20 percent improvement in tender and swollen joint count and 20 percent improvement in three of five of the remaining core outcome measures (ACR 20). This type of analysis, referred to as a *responder analysis,* is a dichotomous analysis: Subjects are either classified as responders or nonresponders, and the proportion of responders in the treatment and placebo group at the end of the study are compared. Using the ACR definition of response in RA, only a small proportion of placebo-treated patients are classified as responders. The number of subjects with a 50 or 70 percent improvement is used as a secondary outcome in many RA clinical trials.[15] The responder analysis has been criticized for being insensitive to differences in time of onset of treatment effect and to misclassification of subjects with small treatment effects as "nonresponders."[16]

Another types of analysis is the *Area Under the Curve (AUC)* analysis, which analyzes and compares data measured at multiple time points during the study.[17] This type of analysis is more sensitive to the early onset of treatment effect. The "numeric ACR" (nACR) in RA refers to an analysis that expresses disease activity at every visit as the lowest percent change in number of tender and swollen joints and median improvement in other measures. This analysis is more sensitive to small treatment effects but is also more likely to be affected by a placebo response. Both the nACR and the ACR 20 can be used in an AUC analysis.

QUALITY OF LIFE AND FUNCTIONAL STATUS END POINTS

Changes in disease activity can be measured using process measures and outcome measures. Outcome measures examine the effect of the illness on quality of life, function (disability), and mortality.[18] Process measures are surrogate markers of disease activity such as rheumatoid factor or the number of swollen joints. Although process measures may be relatively sensitive to change in a clinical trial, there is debate about their correlation with long-term outcomes such as quality of life, disability, and death.[19] Clinical trials in rheumatic diseases usually include health status questionnaires to measure change in functional status and disability because these scores have a strong association with later health and functional status of patients with RA.[20] A number of health status measures are available for functional status or disability assessment for patients with RA (e.g., Health Assessment Questionnaire, McMaster Toronto Arthritis Patient Preference Disability Questionnaire, Arthritis Impact Measurement Scales).[21-24] Some health status measures are disease specific, and others are generic.[25] In general, the disease-specific measures are more sensitive to change in clinical trials for RA,[26,27] but both types of measures are often included as outcomes to support a claim of improvement in overall quality of life. A further discussion of these types of measurements can be found in Chapter 29.

DROPOUTS AND NONCOMPLIANCE

Noncompliance with study medication is a serious problem for clinical trials. It can be decreased by carefully screening patients who are entered into the study (excluding patients who are known not to comply with routine medication and office visits) and by explaining the purpose and importance of the study to the subject. Subjects are less likely to be noncompliant with study treatment if they receive clear written instructions and if the treatment regimen is simplified. Noncompliance is generally measured with pill counts, self reports, and urinary or serum tests for the drug or a metabolite.

Patients do not drop out of clinical trials at random. They frequently leave because of lack of treatment effects or toxicity. Patients also may drop out because of disease progression, death or serious illness, lack of interest, relocation, or fears about toxicity. Dropouts can be minimized by using a screening or run-in period in which patients are followed for a time before randomization and administration of study medication to ensure that they are appropriate for the study and likely to return for follow-up. Dropouts due to lack of efficacy can be minimized by allowing more flexibility in treatment options (e.g., joint injections in an RA trial), but these extra treatment options may be a confounder in the statistical analysis. Add on and active control trial designs can minimize dropouts by offering all subjects some type of effective treatment. An attempt should be made to follow all subjects in a clinical trial, including those who have stopped treatment because of noncompliance and toxicity.

The reason for patient dropouts should be carefully documented. Every effort should be made to contact patients and their families to determine whether the patient is alive and the reason for discontinuing study participation. To do this, adequate contact information for the subject and the subject's family and friends must be collected prior to study enrollment.

Conducting a Clinical Trial

STUDY COORDINATORS

An experienced study coordinator is an asset to a smoothly running clinical trial. Appropriate training should be given concerning subject recruitment, maintenance of records, interacting with the coordinating center, data management, sample collections, and human subjects protection.[1] Careful and consistent documentation is essential. Drug logs for dispensing study medication should be considered similar to those required for dispensing narcotics. Good clinical practice (GCP) guidelines are a set of standards with which research sites are expected to comply and are available from the FDA Website (http://www.fda.gov/cber).

SUBJECT RECRUITMENT

Prior to including a site in a multicenter trial there should be an assessment of the center's ability to obtain adequate subjects based on the numbers of patients with a particular diagnosis seen at that center or previous ability to recruit subjects for similar types of studies. Large multicenter trials often use professional study recruiters to maximize enrollment. A recruitment plan should be implemented prior to the start of any study because it can take months to devise and implement such a plan if enrollment is slow. Eligible subjects can be identified at centers from diagnostic, billing, or pharmaceutical databases or by marketing efforts to the public or to health care providers. Subjects can be screened for initial eligibility by phone. Patients who pass initial entry criteria are invited to come for a more complete evaluation, during which all inclusion and exclusion criteria are reviewed. Records should be kept of the number of patients initially identified and the reasons subjects are not enrolled.

MANUAL OF PROCEDURES OR PROTOCOL

The manual of procedures is an expanded version of the protocol and describes each step of how the study is to be conducted. The manual has the inclusion and exclusion criteria, the schedule of visits and testing, the content of the baseline and follow-up visits, instruments and forms needed for each visit, and the instructions on administering questionnaires to ensure uniformity. It also includes forms for assessing compliance, for listing adverse events, and for recording the time of and reason for dropouts.

Data collection forms (case report forms [CRFs]) are tailored to each visit and clearly outline the information to be obtained about efficacy and safety, including elements of the patient's history, physical examination, laboratory testing, and other diagnostic tests such as radiographs, functional status, compliance, and toxicity questionnaires. Questionnaires to assess pain, functional status, or other efficacy or toxicity end points should be validated using instruments that reflect the current state of the art in data collection in that area. If a new instrument is used, it must be tested to assess its reliability and validity. Coding rules or specifications for data collection are established when the data forms are created and should be reviewed by the statistician before use.

General information forms reviewing the purpose of the study, schedule of visits, instructions about how to take study medications, and what medications and materials are to be brought to study visits are given to subjects at the initiation of the study. Subjects should receive information about whom to contact in case of side effects, questions, or a missed appointment.

After the manual of procedures is developed, it is pretested on volunteers or patients who are not eligible for the study. After pretesting, the manual can be revised to improve the clarity of the questions, the procedures, and the flow of the study visit so that corrections can be made before the start of the study. Study diaries are sometimes provided for subjects to record medications and disease flares.

When participating in multicenter trials, CRFs are supplied by the sponsor. Depending on the sponsor, data is sometimes initially collected on source documents that are kept at the site and then transferred to CRFs that are sent to the sponsor. Information on CRFs can then be verified by reviewing the source documents at the time of an audit by a sponsor or the FDA. Electronic data capture (EDC) is becoming more common in large sponsored trials; however, these data still need to be verified by comparison to source documents. Transfer of electronic data requires additional validation to ensure that the data were not changed or corrupted during the electronic transfer.

Data Analysis

DATA QUALITY

It is important for the investigator to review data collection forms as patients are seen to ensure that information is being collected and recorded accurately, that all instances of missing data are recognized, and that an attempt is made to retrieve the data before the study has progressed significantly. After being collected, all data are entered into a database. Ensuring the accuracy of data entry can be increased by double entry: The data are entered twice and compared for inconsistencies. A random sample of files can be chosen and reviewed against the original data sheets for accuracy. Databases can be set up with range checks that only take variables within a certain range (e.g., 1 to 4). It is important to check the data for missing variables and for incorrect values. Statistical and spreadsheet software can be used to look at the frequency distribution of data for each variable to find outliers (i.e., data that do not fit into an expected category or range) that can then be checked against the original data forms, and missing values can be identified.

Imputation is a method of replacing missing data. The most common method of imputation is to average the results of values collected the visit before and after the missing visit, but the validity of this approach may be poor if a long time has elapsed between visits or if the patient did not come for the visit because of illness. A more conservative approach is to replace the missing data with the last data value collected for placebo patients or the worst value for patients in the treatment arm.

DATA ANALYSIS

The statistical analysis should be planned prospectively when the study is designed. The initial part of data analysis is to examine the baseline characteristics of the study groups, including demographic, treatment, and disease characteristics (e.g., severity scales, duration, extent of organ involvement) with descriptive statistics. The frequency distribution of the variables of interest, the type of distribution (are the data normally distributed?), and the associations between pairs of variables can be examined using scatter plots and correlation coefficients. An analysis of the study hypothesis is performed with formal statistical testing.

The mean pretreatment and post-treatment scores for outcome variables should be reported. The outcome usually chosen for statistical analysis is a comparison of mean change from baseline between treatment groups or change from baseline in each treatment group.[28] Patients who stay in clinical trials often improve over time, regardless of treatment or a placebo effect, and improvement in an outcome from baseline to the end of the study does not necessarily imply a positive treatment effect. The change in the outcome measure for the treatment group must be greater than that for the control group.

Decisions must be made about whether the analysis will be "intent to treat" and include data from all patients, regardless of whether they continue on the assigned treatment (relevant terms are defined in Table 30–3). Although this type of analysis has difficulties, it is a conservative one that attempts to deal with the bias introduced when only study completers are included. Completers are often healthier subjects, and dropouts can be caused by lack of efficacy. Excluding data from dropouts makes a treatment appear more effective than it is. In an intent-to-treat analysis, data are included for all patients (including those who are no longer on the assigned study treatment), and each patient is kept in the original treatment group. In a *completer analysis*, the results for the subgroup of patients who continued the study treatment for the duration of the study are analyzed. Often the result of the analysis for the subgroup of subjects who continued the assigned study medication is included as a secondary outcome.

If the treatment groups differ significantly in baseline characteristics, statistical corrections for the baseline differences may be needed in the analysis of the primary and secondary outcome variables if the characteristic

TABLE 30–3 • GLOSSARY OF TERMS

Phase I	Earliest human trials to determine pharmokinetics, metabolism, clinical pharmacology
Phase II	Sequential dose escalations to test safety and tolerability
Phase III	Trials to demonstrate efficacy
Phase IV	Postmarketing testing for toxicity
Type I error	Alpha; false positive: the likelihood of concluding treatments are different when they are not
Type II error	Beta; false negative: the likelihood of falsely concluding that there is no difference between treatment effects
Power	1-Beta; probability of finding a difference in treatment outcomes if the effect size is as large as hypothesized or greater
Confounding	Systematic error; a variable or characteristic that is associated with the treatment and the outcome
Randomization	Random assignment of patients to treatment
Stratification	Balancing treatment groups at baseline for characteristics that may have an important influence on outcomes (potential confounders)
Intermediate or process outcomes	Outcome measures that measure current disease activity and are thought to correlate with long-term outcome (disability, death)
Primary outcome	The main outcome measure of the study with which sample size calculations are made
Secondary outcomes	Outcome measures that support the primary outcome measure
Responder analysis	An analysis of the proportion of subjects in each treatment group who meet criteria for response to treatment
Intent to treat analysis	An analysis of treatment effect, including data from all subjects initially enrolled in the study (including dropouts, subjects off study medication, and those with protocol violations), keeping each subject in his or her original treatment group
Imputation	A method of replacing missing data for missed visits or dropouts

may affect the outcome under study. Occasionally, subgroup analyses are done that were not initially planned. Although valuable information can be obtained from a subgroup analysis, the results should be considered exploratory and should be confirmed in future studies. The FDA often does not allow data from a post hoc analysis to be used to file for an indication, but may allow this information to be used in the clinical section of the package insert. When statistical tests are done on multiple outcomes, statistical corrections should be made to avoid increasing the chances of a type I error.

DATA INTERPRETATION

A statistical analysis determines whether the effects of the treatment effect are statistically significant but not whether the treatment effect is clinically significant. A method of evaluating the quality of a clinical trial is reviewed elsewhere.[29,30] For example, a trial may demonstrate a small improvement in a primary outcome criterion that is statistically significant, but the effect may not have clinical importance because it is not sufficient to impact quality of life or survival, or it does not outweigh the risk or cost of treatment. Similarly, a clinical trial may show a difference between treatment groups that appears to be clinically important (e.g., a 20 percent difference in an outcome variable), but because of small sample size, the results are not statistically significant (i.e., inadequate power). A result may be statistically and clinically significant but have little medical relevance because the benefit does not outweigh the risk or cost of treatment or because the benefit is only seen in a very small subgroup of patients.

Power calculations are particularly important when presenting data suggesting that there are no differences in outcomes between treatments, such as an equivalency study (treatment 1 is as effective as treatment 2), or a placebo-controlled study (treatment 1 is no better than placebo). The power of a study to find a statistically significant treatment effects is strongly determined by sample size. Power calculations should be reported in all studies. An analysis that shows no statistically significant difference in the treatment effect between groups does not demonstrate equivalence or lack of efficacy unless the study had adequate power to find the hypothesized difference.

SAFETY ANALYSIS

A safety assessment system should be devised using standard terminology as defined by the *Medical Dictionary for Regulatory Activities Terminology*.[31] Adverse events are categorized according to the body system using appropriate medical terminology so they are accurately coded. Data about infections should include the body system, severity, and medical importance. Adverse events are graded (1, mild; 2, moderate; 3, severe; 4, serious or life threatening) and the treating physician's assessment of the association to the study treatment (e.g., unrelated, possibly, probably, definitely). Appropriate safety stopping rules should be established. A data safety monitoring board may be required to review adverse events and determine whether the study should be stopped. Serious adverse events and unexpected adverse events must be reported to the FDA by the sponsor or investigator holding an investigational new drug (IND).

Food and Drug Administration Approval of New Drugs

BACKGROUND

The FDA is responsible for the regulation of food, drugs, medical devices, biologics, and veterinary medicines in the United States. Before the FDA approves a new drug, treatment, or device, the manufacturer must demonstrate its safety and efficacy. A new drug is defined as "any drug that is not generally recognized as safe and effective under conditions prescribed, recommended, or suggested in the labeling."[32] The center within the FDA evaluating new treatments for the rheumatic diseases is the Center for Drug Evaluation and Research. Specific guidelines for the development of new treatments for RA, osteoarthritis, and juvenile RA have been published by the FDA (e.g., for RA see http://www.fda.gov/gdlns/rheumcln.pdf).[33-35]

NEW DRUG EVALUATION PROCESS

An IND application is required if a drug that is not approved by the FDA for marketing (no approved indications) will be used for investigation of treatment, an approved (marketed) drug is shipped to be used for an unapproved indication or route of administration, an FDA-approved drug is shipped without FDA-approved labeling, the form of an approved drug is altered in strength or composition or otherwise differs for the approved product, or the safety or efficacy of an approved or unapproved drug is in doubt as planned for use in a study protocol.[32]

Within the Center for Drug Evaluation and Research, the evaluation of new drug products is carried out by the Office of Drug Evaluation I and II.[33] Offices have several drug review divisions with expertise in biometrics, epidemiology, bioequivalence, biopharmaceuticals, and drug advertising, and they have a scientific review staff. Between 1 and 3 years of synthesis and animal testing are required to support safety for a trial in humans. The sponsor then submits an IND exemption application to the FDA, which includes details of the manufacturing process, product testing and product specifications, the preclinical trials that support clinical trials in humans, a clinical development plan, and detailed study protocols for the initial clinical trials. After an IND submission, there is an initial 30-day review to determine whether the clinical trials can proceed, and a complete review is available in 60 days.

Under the FDA Modernization Act (FDAMA) of 1997 (http://www.fda.gov/cder/fdamamtg.htm), a formal mechanism of interaction between the sponsor and the FDA, designated fast track, became available for all applications for marketing claims. The fast track designation is intended for the combination of a product and a claim that address an unmet medical need. The benefits of the fast track include scheduled meetings to seek FDA input into development plans, the option of submitting a new drug application (NDA) in sections rather than all the components simultaneously, and the option of requesting evaluation of studies using surrogate end points (accelerated approval).

As the product proceeds through the developmental process under the IND, the sponsor is required to notify the FDA immediately of serious and unexpected adverse events and to update the FDA at least yearly on the progress of the clinical trials and changes to the clinical plans.

When the Phase I and II studies are completed, data from these studies and from any additional preclinical studies, as well as changes in the chemistry, manufacturing, or formulation of the product, are presented to the FDA. The FDA may provide guidance about whether the phase III plan is sufficient to meet the requirement for approval for specific indications. The FDA publishes guidance documents for the requirements for approval for a specific indication or labeling claims and makes these freely available on the FDA Web site (http://www.fda.gov.cder).

NEW DRUG APPLICATION OR BIOLOGIC LICENSING AGREEMENT

If the phase III trial results demonstrate the efficacy of the new agent, an NDA or a Biologic Licensing Agreement (BLA) is submitted to the FDA. This application contains a summary of the data compiled on the agent to date, including safety, pharmacokinetics, efficacy, manufacturing and formulation data, information about testing and specifications, as well as draft labeling, plans for postmarketing, and additional postmarketing studies. At the time of submission of the NDA or BLA, the sponsor may request priority review. Under the FDAMA, a standard or priority designation is given, a target date is set for completing all aspects of the review, and the time frame for a decision about approval is set (10 months for standard or 6 months for priority). When the NDA or BLA has been accepted by the FDA, the sponsor is put on the agenda for one of the FDA advisory panel meetings. The sponsor and the FDA prepare briefing documents for the panel, and each presents an analysis of the safety and efficacy data. These meetings are open to the public and the schedule is on the FDA Web site (http://www.fda.gov). The FDA generally follows the recommendations of the advisory panel but may request additional premarketing or postmarketing studies.

After a new drug application has been approved, the drug developer is required to report adverse reactions quarterly to the FDA for the first 3 years after approval. Annual reports include drug distribution data, labeling information, manufacturing changes, and the reports of clinical and nonclinical studies carried out with the new drug. Adequate postmarketing surveillance is dependent on physicians' reporting of serious adverse advents that may be associated with a new drug to the drug manufacturer, distributor, the FDA, or all three using the Med-Watch form (http://www.fda.gov/medwatch/).

The FDA has developed specific guidelines for drugs, devices, and biologic products for the treatment of RA, juvenile RA, and osteoarthritis, with specific recommendations about preclinical studies, clinical trial design, and primary and secondary outcomes.[34-36] These include recommendations about concomitant therapy, such as nonsteroidal anti-inflammatory drugs and corticosteroids. Species specificity and immunogenicity, dose responses, toxicity responses, product homogeneity, and the role of antibodies are all important considerations with biologic therapies.

Clinical Trials in Children

There are specific recommendations for the evaluation of drugs in children with rheumatic diseases,[37-39] the informed consent process,[40,41] and outcome measures.[42-43] It is suggested that no drug be tested in children until there has been some safety testing in adults, unless the drug will be limited to use in children. On the other hand, trials in children should not be delayed until adult trials are completed. However, sponsors often do not apply for approval for the use of new treatments in children because of concerns about added expense and the legal ramifications of exposing children to risk.

Informed Consent and Ethical Considerations

RESPONSIBILITIES OF INVESTIGATORS AND INSTITUTIONS

The increasing collaboration of pharmaceutical companies with academic and private clinical investigators raises important ethical questions about financial conflicts of interest, investigator access to data and data analysis for scientific presentations, and criteria for authorship in scientific publications.[44-47] Institutions participating in FDA-sponsored research are required to provide training for investigators in the areas of scientific integrity and human subjects protection.[47] The American Association of Medical Colleges (AAMC) has published guidelines for the management of individual financial interests in biomedical research.[48]

In an effort to ensure investigator access to data collected in industry-sponsored multicenter clinical trials, as well as the involvement of investigators in data analysis and presentation, the International Committee of Medical Journal Editors (ICMJE) updated the "Uniform Requirements for Manuscripts Submitted to Biomedical Journals" (http://www.jcmje.org/).[49] Many biomedical journals now adhere to these guidelines and require information about financial conflict of interest and written statements and about the role of authors in the study design, implementation, statistical analysis, and manuscript preparation.

Contracts between academic medical centers and industry can restrict the investigator's access to data collected in clinical trials and their ability to present that data in peer-reviewed forums. Academic medical centers

TABLE 30–4 • ELEMENTS OF INFORMED CONSENT

Describes the study in detail including risks and benefits
Describes compensation for participation in the study
Explains the participant's rights:
The right to withdraw
The right to refuse participation without jeopardizing care
Specifies whether birth control is required for women and what happens if a subject becomes pregnant
Provides a phone number for the investigator and the IRB
Describes protection of information from stored DNA if such samples are collected

have an important responsibility to negotiate contracts that protect investigator rights.[50]

PATIENTS' RIGHTS AND PROTECTIONS

Federal agencies require that institutions involved in federally supported human research have a local Institutional Review Board (IRB) review all protocols before implementation and monitor ongoing studies at their institution. Using federal guidelines, each local IRB reviews and decides on the ethics and safety of a study. When studies are conducted at multiple institutions, the IRB at each institution must review the protocol and the informed consent document.

An excellent review of the informed consent process is given by Dunn and Chadwick (Table 30–4).[51] The consent form should explain to the study participant the purpose of the study, all potential benefits and risks (including risks to pregnant mother and fetus), alternatives to participation, and who is responsible for conducting the study. Patient confidentiality should be ensured. The consent form should clearly state that participation is completely voluntary and that refusal to participate or withdrawal from the study will not affect future care. If compensation is provided, it must be documented in the consent form. Participants should be given contact information for questions or in case of injury and a statement about whether any medical treatment will be given if injury occurs. Investigators are responsible for ensuring that the risk to subjects is minimized and appropriate for the anticipated benefits (Table 30–5). A recent area of controversy is the use of stored serum or DNA samples for future analyses and how to adequately protect subject privacy and obtain informed consent for unplanned future use of these samples.

TABLE 30–5 • SOURCES OF INFORMATION ABOUT HUMAN SUBJECTS PROTECTION

Office of the Inspector General: Recruiting Human Subjects: Pressures in Industry-Sponsored Clinical Research (OEI-01-97-00195). June 2000, http://www.hhs.gov/oig/reports/a459.pdf
Penslar RL, Porter JP: Institutional Review Board Guide Book. Office for Human Subjects Protection, updated Feb 6, 2001. http://ohrp.osophs.dhhs.gov/irb/irb_guidebook.htm
Code of Federal Regulations. Title 21, Chapter 1 – Food and Drug Administration, – DHHS -Part 50-Protection of Human Subjects. Updated 1 April 1999. www4.law.cornell.edu/cfr/21p56.htm

Conclusions

Clinical trials are used to test the effectiveness of new drugs and devices and to compare efficacy and safety of combinations of drugs. New drug development is a long and expensive process. The choice of clinical trial design and implementation is critically important for safe, efficient, and successful drug development. Because the cost of clinical trials for new drug development has increased substantially, research leading to FDA approval of new treatments is done primarily by the pharmaceutical industry in multicenter clinical trials. However, investigator-initiated clinical trials are important in the studies addressing the effects of combinations of standard drugs, or standard drugs in combination with new treatments, and in the initial studies of the effects of newly approved drugs for other indications.

The clinical trial is only one type of clinical research study. Because subjects are randomized to treatment, confounders are less likely than in case-control or observational studies, and differences in outcomes provide stronger evidence of causality.[52] However, clinical trials are short-term studies and often use intermediate or process measures for outcomes. Longitudinal practice-based studies add important information about the effects of a new treatment when used in a diverse group of patients with other comorbidities. These studies add important information about drug toxicity and the longterm effects of a treatment on functional status, morbidity, and mortality.[19,20]

REFERENCES

1. Spilker B: Guide to Clinical Trials. New York, Raven Press, 1991.
2. Simon R, FreidenB, et al: Accelerated titration designs for Phase I clinical trials in oncology. J National Cancer Inst 89:1138-1147, 1989.
3. Hulley SB, Cummings SR: Designing Clinical Research. Baltimore, Williams & Wilkins, 1988.
4. Lovell D, Giannini EH, Reiff A, et al: Etanercept in children with polyarticular juvenile rheumatoid arthritis. N Engl J Med 342;763-769, 2000.
5. Sylvester RJ, Pinedo HM, DePauw M, et al: Quality of institutional participation in multicenter clinical trials. N Engl J Med 305:852, 1981.
6. Sherman LA, Temple R, Merkatz RB: Women in clinical trials: An FDA perspective. Science 269:793, 1995.
7. Freiman JA, Chalmers TC, Smith H Jr, et al: The importance of beta, the type II error and sample size in the design and interpretation of the randomized control trial. N Engl J Med 299:690, 1978.
8. White B, Bauer EA, Goldsmith LA, et al: Guidelines for clinical trials in systemic sclerosis (scleroderma). I. Disease-modifying interventions. Arthritis Rheum 38:351, 1995.
9. Bellamy N, Kirwan J, Boers M, et al: Recommendations for a core set of outcome measures for future phase III clinical trials in knee, hip, and hand osteoarthritis: Consensus development at OMERACT III. J Rheumatol 24:799, 1997.
10. Felson DT, Anderson JJ, Boers M, et al: The American College of Rheumatology preliminary definition of improvement in rheumatoid arthritis. Arthritis Rheum 38:727, 1995.

11. Graham TB, Lovell DJ: Outcome in pediatric rheumatic disease. Curr Opin Rheumatol 9:434, 1997.
12. Brooks P, Hochberg M: Outcome measures and classification criteria for rheumatic diseases. A compilation of data from OMERACT (Outcome Measures for Arthritis Clinical Trials), ILAR (International League for Associations for Rheumatology), regional leagues and other groups. Rheumatology 40:896-906, 2001.
13. Bombardier C, Tugwell P: A methodological framework to develop and select indices for clinical trials: Statistical and judgmental approaches. J Rheumatol 9:753, 1982.
14. Paulus HE, Egger MJ, Ward JR, et al: Analysis of improvement in individual rheumatoid arthritis patients treated with disease-modifying antirheumatic drugs, based on the findings in patients treated with placebo. Arthritis Rheum 33:477, 1990.
15. Felson DT, Anderson JJ, Lange MLM, et al: Should improvement in rheumatoid arthritis clinical trials be defined as fifty percent or seventy percent improvement in core set measures, rather than twenty percent? Arthritis Rheum 41:1564, 1998.
16. Boers M: Demonstration of response in rheumatoid arthritis patients who are nonresponders according to the American College of Rheumatology 20% criteria: the paradox of beneficial treatment effects in nonresponders in the ATTRACT trial. Arthritis Rheum 44:2703-2704, 2001.
17. van Riel P: Area under the curve for the American College of Rheumatology improvement criteria: A valid addition to existing criteria in rheumatoid arthritis. Arthritis Rheum 44:1719-1720, 2001.
18. Fries JF: Toward an understanding of patient outcome measurement. Arthritis Rheum 26:697, 1983.
19. Pincus T: Limitations of randomized controlled clinical trials to depict accurately long-term outcomes in rheumatoid arthritis. J Rheumatol 57:46, 1998.
20. Wolfe F, Hawley DJ, Cathey MA: Clinical and health status measures over time: Prognosis and outcome assessment in rheumatoid arthritis. J Rheumatol 18:1290, 1991.
21. Bell MJ, Bombardier C, Tugwell P: Measurement of functional status, quality of life, and utility in rheumatoid arthritis. Arthritis Rheum 33:591, 1990.
22. Wolfe F, Kleinheksel SM, Cathey MA, et al: The clinical value of the Stanford Health Assessment Questionnaire Functional Disability Index in patients with rheumatoid arthritis. J Rheumatol 15:1480, 1988.
23. Meenan RF, Mason JH, Anderson JJ, et al: The content and properties of a revised and expanded Arthritis Impact Measurement Scales health status questionnaire. Arthritis Rheum 35:1, 1992.
24. Tugwell P, Bombardier C, Buchanan WW, et al: The MACTAR patient preference disability questionnaire: An individualized functional priority approach for assessing improvement in physical disability in clinical trials in rheumatoid arthritis. J Rheumatol 14:446, 1987.
25. McHorney CA, Ware JE Jr, Raczek AE: The MOS 36-item Short-Form Health Survey (SF-36): II. Psychometric and clinical tests of validity in measuring physical and mental health constructs. Med Care 31:247, 1993.
26. Hawley DJ, Wolfe F: Sensitivity to change of the health assessment questionnaire (HAQ) and other clinical and health status measures in rheumatoid arthritis. Arthritis Care Res 5:130, 1992.
27. Anderson JJ, Firschein HE, Meenan RF: Sensitivity of a health status measure to short-term clinical changes in arthritis. Arthritis Rheum 32:844, 1989.
28. Felson DT, Anderson JJ, Meenan RF: Time for changes in the design, reporting, and analysis of rheumatoid arthritis clinical trials. Arthritis Rheum 33:140, 1990.
29. Chalmers TC, Smith H Jr, Blackburn B, et al: A method for assessing the quality of a randomized control trial. Control Clin Trials 2:31, 1981.
30. DerSimonian R, Charette LJ, McPeek B, et al: Reporting on methods in clinical trials. N Engl J Med 306:1332, 1982.
31. Brown EG, Wood L, Wood S: The medical dictionary for regulatory activities (MedRA). Drug Saf 20:109-117, 1999.
32. Department of Health and Human Services: Food and Drug Administration: New Drugs for Investigational Use. 21 CFR 312:61, 1986.
33. Walters PG: FDA's new drug evaluation process: A general overview. J Public Health Dent 52:333, 1992.
34. Food and Drug Administration: Guidance for Industry: Clinical Development Programs for Drugs, Devices and Biological Products Intended for the Treatment of Osteoarthritis (OA). Rockville, Maryland, Center for Drug Evaluation and Research, February 1998. (www.fda.gov/cder)
35. Food and Drug Administration: Guidance for Industry: Clinical Development Program for Drugs, Devices and Biological Products for the Treatment of Rheumatoid Arthritis (RA). Docket No. 96D-0067 Rockville, Maryland, Center for Drug Evaluation and Research, March 1998.
36. Food and Drug Administration: Clinical Testing for Safe and Effective Drugs. DHEW publication no. (FDA) 74-3015. Rockville, Maryland, Food and Drug Administration, 1974.
37. Food and Drug Administration: Guidelines for the Clinical Evaluation of Anti-inflammatory and Antirheumatic Drugs (adults and children). Docket No. 88D-0050:25–28. Rockville, Maryland, Center for Drug Evaluation and Research, 1988.
38. Food and Drug Administration: Guidance for Industry: General Considerations for the Clinical Evaluation of Drugs in Infants and Children. HEW (FDA) publication no. 77-3041. Rockville, Maryland, Center for Drug Evaluation and Research, September 1977.
39. Giannini EH, Lovell DJ, Hepburn B: FDA draft guidelines for the clinical evaluation of anti-inflammatory and antirheumatic drugs in children: Executive summary. Arthritis Rheum 38:715, 1995.
39. Food and Drug Administration: General considerations for the Clinical Evaluation of Drugs in Infants and Children: Report to the FDA by the Committee on Drugs, American Academy of Pediatrics. FDA publication no. 77-3041, FDA contract no. 223-79-3003 and 223-82-3009. Rockville, Food and Drug Administration, 1982.
40. American Academy of Pediatrics: Informed consent, parental permission, and assent in pediatric practice. Pediatrics 95:314, 1995.
41. Committee on Drugs, American Academy of Pediatrics: Guidelines for the ethical conduct of studies to evaluate drugs in pediatric populations. Pediatrics 95:286, 1995.
42. Giannini EH, Ruperto N, Ravelli A, et al: Preliminary definition of improvement in juvenile arthritis. Arthritis Rheum 40:1202, 1997.
43. Murray KJ, Passo MH: Functional measures in children with rheumatic diseases. Pediatr Clin North Am 42:1127, 1995.
44. Lo B, Wolfe BE, Berkeley A: Conflict-of-interest policies for investigators in clinical trials. N Engl J Med 343:1616-1620, 2000.
45. DeAngelis CD: Conflict of interest and public trust. JAMA 284:2237-2238, 2000.
46. Davidoff F, DeAngelis CD, Drazen JM, et. al.: Sponsorship, authorship, and accountability. N Engl J Med 345:825, 2001.
47. Macrina F: Scientific Integrity: An Introductory Text with References. ASM Press, Washington, DC, 2000.
48. Task Force on Financial Conflicts of Interest in Clinical Research: Protecting Subjects, Preserving Trust, Promoting Progress: Policy and Guidelines for the Oversight of Individual Financial Interests in Human Subjects Research. Washington, DC, Association of American Medical Colleges, December 2001.
49. International Committee of Medical Journal Editors: Uniform Requirements for Manuscripts Submitted to Biomedical Journals. JAMA 277: 927-934, 1997.
50. Drazen JM: Institutions, contracts, and academic freedom. N Engl J Med 347:1362-1363, 2002.
51. McGuire Dunn C, Chadwick G (eds): Protecting Study Volunteers in Research: A Manual for Investigative Sites. Boston, Mass., Center Watch Inc., 1999.
52. Felson DT: Clinical trials in rheumatoid arthritis under attack: Are practice based observational studies the answer? J Rheumatol 18:951, 1991.

31 Occupational and Recreational Musculoskeletal Disorders

RICHARD S. PANUSH

The diseases of persons incident to this craft arise from three causes: first constant sitting, second the perpetual motion of the hand in the same manner, and thirdly the attention and application of the mind. . . . Constant writing also considerably fatigues the hand and whole arm on account of the continual and almost tense tension of the muscles and tendons. I knew a man who, by perpetual writing, began first to complain of an excessive weariness of his whole right arm, which could be removed by no medicines, and which was at last succeeded by a perfect palsy of the whole arm.

Ramazzini (1713)[1]

When job demands . . . repeatedly exceed the biomechanical capacity of the worker, the activities become trauma-inducing. Hence, traumatogens are workplace sources of biomechanical strain that contribute to the onset of injuries affecting the musculoskeletal system.

National Institute for Occupational Safety and Health (NIOSH) (1986)[2]

The notion that "wear and tear" from certain activities can lead to reversible or irreversible damage to the musculoskeletal system has been conventional wisdom.[2-5] This chapter reviews the evidence that occupations or repetitive activities may cause rheumatic and musculoskeletal disorders or soft tissue syndromes. Despite the apparent logic that work or recreational activities might affect the musculoskeletal system, this putative association is controversial, and perhaps seriously flawed. There are confounding aspects to much of the available data, including imprecise diagnostic labels, subjectivity of complaints, anecdotal and survey data, inadequate controls, differing definitions of disease and disability, limited duration of follow-up observations, inadequate epidemiology, inferential observations, difficulty quantifying activities and defining health effects, assuming the validity of claims data, variable quality of reported observations, psychologic factors influencing symptoms, and conflicting data.

Occupation-Related Musculoskeletal Disorders

Many work-related musculoskeletal disorders have been described and are summarized in Table 31–1.[1-11] These have been reported as sprains, strains, inflammations, dislocations, and irritations. The cost of work-related disability from musculoskeletal disorders is equivalent to approximately 1 percent of the United States' gross national product (GNP).[12] Industries with the highest rates of musculoskeletal disorders have been meat packing, knit-underwear manufacture, motor vehicle manufacture, poultry processing, mail and message distribution, health assessment and treatment, construction, butchery, food processing, machine operation, dental hygiene, data entry, hand grinding and polishing, carpentry, industrial truck and tractor operation, nursing assistance, and housecleaning. There have been imprecise associations of age, gender, fitness, and weight with work-related musculoskeletal syndromes.[6,10,11]

A number of work-related regional musculoskeletal syndromes have been described. These include disorders of the neck, shoulder, elbow, hands and wrist, low back, and lower extremities[10] (Table 31–2). (Some of these are presented in greater detail in Chapters 33 to 43.) Neck musculoskeletal disorders are associated with repetition, forceful exertion, and constrained or static postures. Shoulder musculoskeletal disorders occur with work at or above shoulder height, heavy loads, static postures, hand-arm vibration, and repetitive motion. For elbow epicondylitis, risk factors are overexertion of finger and wrist extensions with the elbow in extension and posture. Hand-wrist tendinitis and work-related carpal tunnel syndrome are noted with repetitive work, forceful activities, flexed wrists, and duration of continual effort.[1,10] Hand-arm vibration syndrome (Raynaud's-like phenomenon)[13] has been linked to intensity and duration of vibrating exposure. Work-related low back disorders have been associated with repetition, weight of objects lifted, twisting, and poor biomechanics of lifting.[13,14] Other risk factors for work-related musculoskeletal disorders involving the back have included awkward posture, high static muscle load, high-force exertion at the hands and wrists, sudden applications of force, work with short cycle times, little task variety, frequent tight deadlines, inadequate rest or recovery periods, high cognitive demands, little scope for control over work, cold work environment, localized mechanic stresses to tissues, and poor spinal support.[1]

Development of recommended management (rehabilitation) for these so-called occupational musculoskeletal disorders has included collaboration by workers, employers, insurers, and health professionals. The process has been divided into phases of protection from and resolution of symptoms, restoration of strength and dynamic stability, and return to work. This process includes symptomatic therapies, physical therapy, and ergonomic evaluation.[7] Prognosis for these maladies has not been well studied or defined.[8]

TABLE 31–1 • OCCUPATION (WORK)-RELATED MUSCULOSKELETAL SYNDROMES

Cherry pitter's thumb	Gamekeeper's thumb
Staple gun carpal tunnel syndrome	Espresso maker's wrist
Bricklayer's shoulder	Espresso elbow
Carpenter's elbow	Pizza maker's palsy
Janitor's elbow	Poster presenter's thumb
Stitcher's wrist	Rope maker's clawhand
Cotton twister's hand	Staple gun carpal tunnel syndrome
Telegraphist's cramp	
Writer's cramp	Waiter's shoulder
Bowler's thumb	Ladder shins
Jeweler's thumb	Tobacco primer's wrist
Cherry pitter's thumb	Carpet layer's knee

TABLE 31–2 • SELECTED LITERATURE DESCRIBING REGIONAL OCCUPATION (WORK)-RELATED MUSCULOSKELETAL SYNDROMES

Syndrome	No. of Epidemiologic Studies	Odds Ratio/ Relative Risk
Neck pain	26	0.7–6.9
Shoulder tendinitis	22	0.9–13
Elbow tendinitis	14	0.7–5.5
Hand-wrist tendinitis	16	0.6–31.7
Carpal tunnel syndrome	22	1–34
Hand-arm vibration syndrome	8	0.5–41

Data from references 5 and 6.

The perspective that musculoskeletal disorders are consistantly and predictably work-related was the prevailing view until recently. This understanding has now come under considerable scrutiny and criticism.[2,15-24] The previously cited literature about occupational musculoskeletal disorders is now considered flawed. Despite the quantity of information (see Table 31–2), its quality was uneven, perhaps poor. Definitions of musculoskeletal disorders were imprecise. Diagnoses, by rheumatologic standards, were infrequent. Studies were usually not prospective. There were selection biases. Psychologic influences and secondary gain were often ignored. Questionnaires were often used without validation of subjective complaints. Quantification of putative causative factors was difficult. Indeed, a review of this literature concluded that none of the published studies satisfactorily established a causal relationship between work and distinct medical entities.[20] Certain experiences argued powerfully against the notion of work-related musculoskeletal disorders. In Lithuania, for example, where insurance was limited and disability was not a societal expectation or entitlement, "whiplash" from auto accidents did not exist.[19] In Australia, when legislation for compensability was made more stringent, an epidemic of whiplash and repetitive-strain injuries abated.[21,23] In the United States, too, expressed symptoms have correlated closely with the likelihood of achieving compensation.[25] In other experiences, ergonomic interventions had no effect on alleged work-related symptoms, and close analysis of epidemics of work-related musculoskeletal disorders have revealed serious inconsistencies.[17] These concerns led the American Society for Surgery of the Hand to editorialize that "the current medical literature does not provide the information necessary to establish a causal relationship between specific work activities and the development of well-recognized disease entities. Until scientifically valid studies are conducted, the society urges the government to exercise restraint in considering regulations designed to reduce the incidence of these conditions, as premature regulations could have far-reaching legal and economic effects, and could have an adverse impact on the care of workers."[18]

A review summarized that "most believe scientific data are insufficient to establish a definite causal relationship of these so-called cumulative trauma disorders to the worker's occupation, and many believe the issue has become a sociopolitical problem."[9] Hadler[2,15-17] has written particularly forcefully that popular notions about work-related musculoskeletal disorders have been based on inadequate science. Others, too, have expressed serious reservations about the cumulative trauma disorder hypothesis, including the Industrial Injuries Committee of the American Society for Surgery of the Hands, the Working Group of the British Orthopaedic Association, and the World Health Organization.[2,15-17,20,22] Appreciation of the importance of psychosocial factors influencing work disability has emerged. These factors include lack of job control, fear of layoff, monotony, job dissatisfaction, unsatisfactory performance appraisals, distress and unhappiness with coworkers or supervisors, poor coping abilities, divorce, low income, and less education.[2,15-25] This is reminiscent of the story of silicone breast implants and their putative association with rheumatic disease. In this instance—as seems to be the case with work-related musculoskeletal disorders—there was a coalescence at the same time of naïvely simplistic assumptions, untested hypotheses, confusion of repetition of hypo-theses with scientific validation, media exaggeration, public advocacy intertwined with politics and government regulatory agencies, jackpots of dollars, litigation, and inadequate science. All these confounded and perverted the silicone breast implant story[26,27] and may have confused the interpretation of evidence-based work-related musculoskeletal disorders as well. More needs to be learned about work-related musculoskeletal disorders to clearly identify circumstances in which they occur; they probably do, but they are likely to be less pervasive and less noxious than originally thought.

Occupation-Related Rheumatic Diseases

These, too, have not been consistently well studied, but associations between occupations and well-defined rheumatic disorders are more clear. This topic also recapitulates the simplistic notion that joints, like materials, deteriorate with use. However, this perception is neither necessarily logical nor correct. The discussion focuses largely on osteoarthritis (OA) (see also Chapters 91 and 92).

OSTEOARTHRITIS

Is OA caused, at least in part, by mechanical stress? One analytic approach to determining a possible relationship between activity and joint disease is to consider the epidemiologic evidence that degenerative arthritis may follow repetitive trauma. Most discussions of the pathogenesis of OA include a role for "stress."[28-31] Several studies have suggested an increased prevalence of OA of elbows, knees, and spine in miners[32-34]; of shoulders, elbows, wrists, and metacarpophalangeal joints in pneumatic drill operators[35]; of intervertebral discs, distal interphalangeal joints, elbows, and knees in dockworkers[33]; of hands in cotton workers,[36] diamond cutters,[32,37] seamstresses,[37] and textile workers[38,39]; of knees and hips in farmers; of knees in shipyard workers and a variety of occupations involving knee bending; and of the spine in foundry workers[40-43] (Table 31–3). Population studies have noted increased hip OA in farmers, firefighters, millworkers, dockworkers, female mail carriers, unskilled manual laborers, fishermen, and miners and have reported increased knee OA in farmers, firefighters, construction workers, house and hotel cleaners, craftspeople, laborers, and service workers.[40-43] Activities leading to increased risk for premature OA have been those involving power grip, carrying, lifting, increased physical load, increased static load, kneeling, walking, and bending.[40-43] Studies of skeletons of several populations have suggested that age at onset, frequency, and location of osteoarthritic changes were directly related to the nature and degree of physical activities.[44] However, not all of these studies were carried out with adherence to contemporary standards, nor have they been confirmed. One report, for example, failed to find an increased incidence of OA in pneumatic drill users[34] and criticized inadequate sample sizes, lack of statistical analyses, and omission of appropriate control populations in previous reports. The investigators further commented that earlier work was "frequently misinterpreted" and that studies from their group suggested that "impact, without injury or preceding abnormality of either joint contour or ligaments, is unlikely to produce osteoarthritis."[35]

Do epidemiologic studies of OA implicate physical or mechanical factors pertaining to predisposition or development of disease? The first national Health and Nutrition Examination Survey of 1971 to 1975 (HANES I) and the Framingham studies explored cross-sectional associations between radiologic OA of the knee and possible risk factors.[40-45] Strong associations were noted between knee OA and obesity and those occupations involving stress of knee bending in these and some other studies, but not all habitual physical activities and leisure-time physical activity (running, walking, team sports, racquet sports, and others) were linked with knee OA.[28-30]

OTHER OCCUPATIONAL RHEUMATOLOGIC DISORDERS

Certain rheumatic diseases other than repetitive strain or cumulative trauma disorders have been associated with occupational risks. These include reports of reflex sympathetic dystrophy after trauma; Raynaud's phenomenon with vibration or chemicals (polyvinyl chloride); autoimmune disease from teaching school[43,47]; systemic sclerosis from chemicals and silica; scleroderma-like syndromes from rapeseed oil and L-tryptophan; systemic lupus erythematosus from canavanine, hydrazine, mercury, pesticides, and solvents[48]; lupus, scleroderma, and Paget's disease from pets[49]; perhaps rheumatoid arthritis (Caplan's syndrome) with silica; and gout (saturnine) with lead intoxication[50] (Table 31–4).

TABLE 31–3 • OCCUPATIONAL PHYSICAL ACTIVITY AND POSSIBLE ASSOCIATIONS WITH OSTEOARTHRITIS

Occupation	Involved Joints	Risk of OA	References
Miners	Elbow, knee, spine	Increased	Lawrence[33] (1955), Kellgren and Lawrence[34] (1958), Felson[43,44] (1997, 1998)
Pneumatic drillers	Shoulder, elbow, wrist, MCPs	Increased/none	Jurmain (1977) (cited in 40), Burke et al[35] (1977)
Dockworkers	Intervertebral disks, DIPs, elbow, knee	Increased	Lawrence[33] (1955)
Cotton mill workers	Hand	Increased	Lawrence[36] (1961)
Diamond workers	Hand	Increased	Kellgren and Lawrence[32] (1957), Tempelaar and van Breeman[37] (1932)
Shipyard laborers	Knees	Increased	Goldberg and Montgomery (1987) (cited in 43, 44)
Foundry workers	Lumbar spine	Increased	Lawrence et al (1966) (cited in 43, 44)
Seamstresses Hand		Increased	Tempelaar and Van Breeman[37] (1932)
Textile workers	Hand	Increased	Hadler et al[39] (1978)
Manual laborers	MCPs	Increased	Williams et al (1987) (cited in 43, 44)
Occupations requiring knee bending	Knee	Increased	Felson et al[40-43] (1988, 1991, 1997, 1998)
Farmers	Hip, knee	Increased	Felson[40-43] (1988, 1991, 1997, 1998)

Abbreviations: DIPs, Distal interphalangeal joints; MCPs, metacarpophalangeal joints; OA, osteoarthritis.

Recreation- and Sports-Related Musculoskeletal Disorders

Do recreational or sports-related activities lead to musculoskeletal disorders? Patients with sports injuries (such as downhill skiing and football) to the anterior cruciate and medial collateral ligaments frequently develop the chondromalacia patellae and radiologic abnormalities of OA (20 to 52 percent).[28-30] Retrospective studies have suggested that development of OA may be associated with varus deformity, previous meniscectomy, and relative body weight.[51,52] Both partial and total meniscectomies have been associated with degenerative changes. Early joint stabilization and direct meniscus-repair surgery may decrease the incidence of premature OA. These observations support the concept that abnormal biomechanical forces, either congenital or secondary to joint injury, are important factors in the development of exercise-related OA.[28-30] Other factors considered important in the development of sports-related OA include certain physical characteristics of the participant, biomechanical and biochemical factors, age, gender, hormone influences, nutrition, characteristics of the playing surface, unique features of particular sports, and duration and intensity of exercise participation, as has been reviewed extensively elsewhere.[28-30] It is increasingly recognized that biomechanical factors have an important role in the pathogenesis of OA.

Is regular participation in physical activity associated with degenerative arthritis? Several animal studies have suggested, but not proved, a possible relationship between exercise and OA. It has been stated that the Husky breed of dogs has increased hip and shoulder arthritis associated with pulling sleds, that tigers and lions develop foreleg OA related to sprinting and running, and that racehorses and workhorses develop OA in forelegs and hindlegs, respectively, consistent with their physical stress patterns.[28-30] Rabbits with experimentally induced arthritis in one hind limb did not develop progressive OA when exercised on treadmills,[54-59] but sheep in normal health walking on concrete did.[53] Later studies found that beagle dogs running 4 to 20 km/day did not develop OA.[60] These observations were not entirely consistent, and they suggested, but did not prove, that physical activities in some circumstances might predispose to degenerative joint disease.

There have been some pertinent, largely anecdotal, observations in human studies[28-30] (Table 31–5). Wrestlers were reported to have an increased incidence of OA of the lumbar spine, cervical spine, knees, and elbows; boxers, of the carpometacarpal joints; baseball pitchers, of shoulders and elbows; parachutists, of knees, ankles, and spine; cyclists, of the patella; cricketers, of fingers; and gymnasts, of shoulders, elbows, and wrists.[28-30] Most of these reports were observational, and not all reflected confirmed associations. Soccer players have been reported to have talar joint, ankle, cervical spine, knee, and hip OA.[28-30,61] Few studies of American football players have been reported. There have been suggestions of OA of the knees, particularly in the subgroup of football players who had sustained a knee injury while playing football. Of football players (average age 23 years) competing for a place on a professional team, 90 percent had radiologic abnormalities of the foot or ankle, compared with 4 percent of an age-matched control population; linemen had more changes than ball carriers or linebackers, who in turn had more changes than flankers or defensive backs. All those who had played football for 9 years or longer had abnormal findings on radiography.[28-31] Most of these few studies suffered in several respects: criteria for OA (or "osteoarthrosis" or "degenerative joint disease" or "abnormality") were not always clear, specified, or consistent; duration of follow-up was often not indicated or was inadequate to determine the risk of musculoskeletal problems at a later age; intensity and duration of follow-up were often not indicated or were inadequate to determine the risk of musculoskeletal problems at a later age; intensity and duration of physical activity were variable and difficult to quantify; selection bias toward individuals exercising/participating or not exercising/participating was not weighted; other possible risk factors and predisposition to musculoskeletal disorders were rarely considered; studies were not always properly controlled and examinations not always "blind"; little information regarding the nonprofessional, recreational athlete was available; and little clinical information about functional status was provided.

Several studies have now examined a possible relationship between running and OA. Uncontrolled observations generally suggested that runners without underlying biomechanical problems of the lower-extremity joints did not appear to develop arthritis at a rate different from that of normal populations of nonrunners. However, those individuals who had underlying articular biomechanical abnormalities from a previously injured joint (and perhaps elite athletes, particularly women) did appear to be at greater risk for subsequent development of OA. Early studies showed that groups of long-duration, high-mileage runners and

TABLE 31–4 • OTHER OCCUPATION-RELATED RHEUMATIC DISEASES

Disease or Syndrome	Occupation or Risk Factors
Reflex sympathetic dystrophy	Trauma
Raynaud's phenomenon	Vibration
	Chemicals (polyvinyl chloride)
Autoimmune disease	teaching school
Systemic sclerosis	Chlorinated hydrocarbons
	Organic solvents
	Silica
Scleroderma-like syndromes	Rapeseed oil
	L-Tryptophan
Systemic lupus erythematosus	Canavanine, hydrazine, mercury, pesticides, solvents
lupus, scleroderma, and Paget's disease	pet ownership
Rheumatoid arthritis (Caplan's syndrome)	Silica
Gout (saturnine)	Lead

TABLE 31–5 • SPORTS PARTICIPATION AND ALLEGED ASSOCIATIONS WITH OSTEOARTHRITIS

Sport	Site (Joint)	References*	Risk
Ballet	Talus	Ottani and Betti (1953); Coste et al (1960); Brodelius (1961); Miller et al (1975)	Probably increased
	Ankle, Cervical spine, Hip	Washington (1978); Ende and Wickstrom (1982)	
	Knee, Metatarsophalangeal	Washington (1978)	
Baseball	Elbow	Adams (1965); Hansen (1982)	Probably increased
	Shoulder	Bennett (1941)	
Boxing	Hand (carpometacarpal joints)	Iselin (1960)	
Cricket	Finger	Vere Hodge (1971)	
Cycling	Finger	Bagneres (1967)	
American football	Ankle, Feet, Knee	Vincelette et al (1972) Rall et al (1964)	
	Spine	Ferguson et al (1975); Albright et al (1976); Moretz et al (1984)	
Gymnastics	Elbow, Shoulder, Wrist	Bozdech (1971)	
	Hip	Murray and Duncan (1971)	
Lacrosse	Ankle, Knee	Thomas (1971)	
Martial arts	Spine	Rubens-Duval et al (1960)	
Parachuting	Ankle, Knee	Murray and Duncan (1971)	
	Spine	Murray-Leslie et al (1977a)	
Rugby	Knee	Slocum (1960)	
Running	Knee	McDermott and Freyne (1983); Lane et al (1986, 1987, in press); Panush et al (1986)	Small
	Hip	Puranen et al (1975); de Carvalho and Langfeldt (1977); McDermott and Freyne (1983); Lane et al (1986, 1987, 1998) Panush et al (1986); Konradsen et al (1990)	
	Ankle	Konradsen et al (1990); Marti et al (1990)	
Soccer	Ankle-foot	Pellissier et al (1952); Pellegrini et al (1964) Sortland et al (1982)	Possibly increased
	Hip	Klunder et al (1980)	
	Knee	Pellissier et al (1952); Solonen (1966); Klunder et al (1980)	
	Talus	Brodelius (1961); Solonen (1966)	
	Talofibular	Burel et al (1960)	
Weightlifting	Spine	Aggrawal et al (1965); Muenchow and Albert (1969); Fitzgerald and McLatchie (1980)	Possibly increased
Wrestling	Cervical spine, Elbow, Knee	Layani et al (1960)	

*Cited in Panush RS, Lane NE: Exercise and the musculoskeletal system. Baillieres Clin Rheumatol 8:79, 1994.

Panush RS: Physical activity, fitness, and osteoarthritis. *In* Bouchard C, Shephard RJ, Stephens T (eds): Physical Activity, Fitness, and Health. International Proceedings and Consensus Statement. Champaign, Ill, Human Kinetics Publishers, 1994, pp 712-723.

Panush RS: Does exercise cause arthritis? Long-term consequences of exercise on the musculoskeletal system. Rheum Dis Clin North Am 16:827, 1990.

nonrunning control subjects had comparable (and low) prevalence of OA and suggested that recreational running need not lead inevitably to OA.[54,62] These observations have, in general, now been confirmed by others[55-64] (Table 31–6). Eight- and 9-year follow-up observations were encouraging; most of the original runners were still running, with a prevalence of degenerative joint disease that was comparable with that of the control subjects.[54,56] Perhaps even more significant is the growing evidence that running and other aerobic exercise protects against the development of disability and early mortality.[64] Former college varsity long-distance runners were compared to former college swimmers in another study[65]; there was no association between moderate levels of running or number of years running and the development of symptomatic OA. Other authors concluded that running alone did not cause OA, but rather prior injuries and anatomic variances were directly responsible for some of the changes.[62] Several additional reports have found that runners were not at risk for development of premature OA of knees or ankles.[59,65-67] Studies examining degenerative hip diseases in former athletes[58,68-71] noted that former champion distance runners had no more clinical or radiographic OA than did nonrunners.[66] However, another study found more radiographic changes due to degenerative hip disease in former national team long-distance runners than in bobsled competitors and control subjects.[68] In all these subjects studied, age and mileage run in 1973 were strong predictors of radiographic hip OA; for runners, running pace in 1973 was the strongest predictor of subsequent radiographic hip OA in 1988. These authors concluded that high-intensity, high-mileage running should not be dismissed as a risk factor for premature OA of the hip. Other reports found that former top-level soccer players and weight lifters, but not runners, were at risk for development of knee OA,[61,71] but it was suggested elsewhere that former athletes seemed to be disproportionately represented in hospital admissions for OA of hip, knee, or ankle.[71] A questionnaire of former elite and track and field athletes noted more hip OA.[70] Similarly, radiographic OA of hip and knee was reported in women who were formerly runners and tennis players.[71]

Cross-sectional studies on the effect of weight-bearing exercise on the development of OA of the hip, knee, or ankle and foot, however, must be interpreted with caution. The radiographic scoring methods used by each group of investigators are not the same. Also, the reliability of the different grading methods used in most studies has not been adequately tested. This information is important when the major end points in the studies are radiographic features of OA.

Performing Arts–Related Musculoskeletal Disorders

Musculoskeletal problems are common among performing artists. Performing artists—particularly musicians and dancers—are unique. Each has medical and musculoskeletal problems that deserve special consideration. Injuries that might be trivial to others may be catastrophic to artists. These are usually associated with overuse—the consequences of tissues stressed beyond anatomic or normal physical limits.

INSTRUMENTALISTS

The frequency of musculoskeletal problems seen in musicians rivals the frequency of disability seen in athletes. For example, a report found that 82 percent of orchestral musicians experienced medical problems related to their occupation. Musculoskeletal problems represented the bulk of the difficulties encountered by musicians.[72]

The etiology of, mechanisms of, and therapies for these musculoskeletal problems are unclear (Table 31–7). An editorial suggested that overuse, tendinitis, cumulative trauma disorder, repetitive motion disorder, occupational cervicobrachial disorder, and regional pain syndrome may be critical risk factors in musicians in development of joint laxity.[72] Joint laxity, when it appeared, declined with age and was associated with gender, starting earlier in men but persisting in women through their mid-40s. The presence or absence of hypermobility at certain sites was associated with musicians' complaints of associated symptoms. Hypermobility in musicians was considered to produce advantages and disadvantages, depending on the site of the laxity and the instrument played.[73] Paganini, with his long fingers and reported hyperextensibility, had a wider finger reach on the violin than his contemporaries, but he may have had a predisposition to OA because of this. A review of studies found that 66 percent of professional symphony orchestra members reported severe musculoskeletal problems. Of interest and seemingly unexplained was the high frequency of symptoms among women (68 to 84 percent); perhaps this is related to their higher incidence of hypermobility.[72]

There are a group of disorders that are still not clearly characterized clinically, probably because of overlap of complaints. These include neurologic problems such as carpal tunnel syndrome and ulnar nerve–compression syndromes at the wrist. On occasion, hand and wrist problems are due to cervical or cervicobrachial radiculopathies. Stress is a factor in all performance fields and contributes to problems of motor function, such as occupational cramps; dealing with this problem often requires the best efforts of a team of physicians and therapists.[72-75]

VOCAL ARTISTS

Musculoskeletal problems of singers have not been addressed extensively. In a report from The Royal Theater in Copenhagen, the frequency of musculoskeletal problems was found to be the same in both instrumentalists and opera singers. However, singers had more hip, knee, and foot joint complaints, perhaps reflecting the effects of prolonged standing.[74]

DANCERS

Dance has always been viewed as a demanding art form, but only recently have the athletic rigors of this discipline become widely appreciated. Classic ballet ranked first in activities generating physical and mental stress, followed by professional football and professional hockey. The dancer and athlete have much in common, but there are important differences in training and performance technique that influence the nature of their injuries. Other important sociocultural differences affect their care. Professional dancers (as well as musicians and vocalists) have traditionally been wary of physicians, and their conviction that physicians know little about dance (and music) is still too common. Injured dancers seeking care have often been told that the treatment is to stop dancing. Others, seeking assistance with weight control, have been told to gain weight. Dancers frequently have underreported their injuries and have sought care from nonmedical therapists.

TABLE 31–6 • STUDIES OF RUNNING AND RISK OF DEVELOPING OSTEOARTHRITIS

References	No. of Runners	Mean Age (yr)	Mean No. of Years Run	Miles/Week	Comments
Minor et al (1989) (cited in 28-30)	319	NA	NA	NA	OA noted more frequently in former runners (with underlying anatomic "tilt" abnormality–epiphysiolysis) than in nonathletes
Puranen et al[58] (1975)	74	56	21	NA	Champion distance runners had no more hip OA than did nonrunners in their sixth decade
de Carvalho and Langfeldt[59] (1977)	32	NA	NA	NA	X-ray findings of runners' hips and knees were similar to those of control subjects
Marti et al[69] (1990)	20	35	13	48	OA occurred in those runners with underlying anatomic (biomechanical) abnormality
Sohn and Micheli[65] (1985)	504	57	9–15	18–19	No association between moderate long-distance running and the future development of OA (of hip and knees)
Panush et al[62] (1986)	17	53	12	28	Comparable low prevalence of lower extremity OA in runners and nonrunners
Lane et al[55] (1986)	41	58	9	(5 hr/wk)	No differences between runners and control subjects in cartilage loss, crepitus, joint stability, or symptoms
Lane et al (1987) (cited in 28-30)	498	59	12	27	No differences were found between groups in conditions thought to predispose to OA and musculoskeletal disability
Marti et al[68,69] (1989, 1990)	27	42	NA	61 (in reference years)	More radiologic changes of hip OA in former Swiss national team long-distance runners than in bobsledders and control subjects; few runners had clinical symptoms of OA; Ino difference noted in ankle joints
Konradsen et al[66] (1990)	30	58	40	12–24	No clinical or radiographic differences in hips, knees, and ankles between runners and nonrunners
Vingard et al[70] (1995)	114	50–80	NA	NA	Unvalidated questionnaire reported threefold increase of hip arthrosis in former athletes
Kujala et al[67] (1994)	342	NA	NA	NA	More former athletes hospitalized with hip OA than expected
Kujala et al[61] (1995)	28	60	32	NA	Women soccer players and weight lifters, nonrunners were at risk of premature OA
Panush et al[54] (1995)	16	13	22	22	8-yr follow-up of original observations made in 1986 still found no differences between runners and nonrunners
Lane et al[56] (1998)	35	60	10–13	23–28	Running did not appear to influence the development of radiologic OA (with the possible exception of spur formation in women)

Abbreviations: NA, Not available; OA, osteoarthritis.

TABLE 31–7 • MUSCULOSKELETAL AND RHEUMATIC DISORDERS ASSOCIATED WITH OVERUSE IN PERFORMING ARTISTS

Instrument	Affliction (Common Name)	References*
Pianists, keyboard players	Myalgias	Hochberg et al (1983), Knishkowy and Lederman (1986)
	Tendinitis	Hochberg et al (1983), Caldron et al (1986), Knishkowy and Lederman (1986), Newmark and Hochberg (1987)
	Synovitis	Hochberg et al (1983), Knishkowy and Lederman (1986)
	Contractures	Hochberg et al (1983), Knishkowy and Lederman (1986)
	Nerve entrapment	
	Median nerve (carpal tunnel–pronator syndrome)	Hochberg et al (1983), Knishkowy and Lederman (1986)
	Ulnar nerve	Hochberg et al (1983), Knishkowy and Lederman (1986)
	Brachial plexus	Hochberg et al (1983), Knishkowy and Lederman (1986)
	Posterior interosseous branch of radial nerve	Hochberg et al (1983), Charness et al (1985)
	Thoracic outlet syndrome	Hochberg et al (1983), Knishkowy and Lederman (1986), Lederman (1987)
	Motor palsies	Hochberg et al (1983), Schott (1983), Caldron et al (1986), Knishkowy and Lederman (1986), Merriman et al (1986), Cohen et al (1987), Jankovic and Shale (1989)
	Osteoarthritis	Bard et al (1984)
Strings		
Violin, viola	Myalgias	Fry (1986b), Hiner et al (1987), Bryant (1989)
	Tendinitis	Fry (1986b), Hiner et al (1987)
	Epicondylitis	Fry (1986b), Hiner et al (1987)
	Cervical spondylosis	Fry (1986b), Hiner et al (1987)
	Rotator cuff tears	Fry (1986b), Newmark and Hochberg (1987)
	Thoracic outlet syndrome	Roos (1986), Lederman (1986)
	Temporomandibular joint syndrome	Hirsch et al (1982), Ward (1990), Kovera (1989)
	Motor palsies	Schott (1983), Knishkowy and Lederman (1986), Hiner et al (1987), Jankovic and Shale (1989)
	Garrod's pads	Bird (1987)
	Nerve entrapment	
	Ulnar	Knishkowy and Lederman (1986)
	Interosseous	Maffulli and Maffulli (1991)
Cello	Myalgias	Fry (1986b)
	Tendinitis	Caldron et al (1986), Fry (1986b)
	Epicondylitis	Fry (1986b)
	Low back pain	Fry (1986b)
	Nerve entrapment	Caldron et al (1986), Knishkowy and Lederman (1986)
	Motor palsies	Schott (1983)
	Thoracic outlet syndrome	Lederman (1987), Palmer et al (1991)
Bass	Low back pain	Fry (1986b)
	Myalgias	Fry (1986b)
	Tendinitis	Caldron et al (1986), Fry (1986b), Mandell et al (1986)
	Motor palsies	Caldron et al (1986)
Viola da gamba	Saphenous nerve compression (gamba leg)	Schwartz and Hodson (1980), Howard (1982)
Harp	Tendinitis	Caldron et al (1986)
	Nerve entrapment	Caldron et al (1986)
Woodwinds		
Clarinet and oboe	First web space muscle strain	Fry (1986b), Newmark and Hochberg (1987)
	Tendinitis	Dawson (1986), Fry (1986b)
	Motor palsies	Jankovic and Shale (1989)
Flute	Myalgias	Fry (1986b)
	Spine pain	Fry (1986b)
	Temporomandibular joint syndrome	La France (1985)
	Tendinitis	Patrone et al (1988)
	Nerve entrapment	
	Digital	Cynamon (1981)
	Posterior interosseous	Charness et al (1985)
	Thoracic outlet syndrome	Lederman (1987)
Brass		
Trumpet, cornet	Motor palsies	Turner (1893), Dibbell (1977), Dibbell et al (1979)
	Orbicularis oris rupture (Satchmo's syndrome)	Planas (1982, 1988), Planas and Kaye (1982)

Continued

TABLE 31–7 • MUSCULOSKELETAL AND RHEUMATIC DISORDERS ASSOCIATED WITH OVERUSE IN PERFORMING ARTISTS

Instrument	Affliction (Common Name)	References*
English horn	de Quervain's tenosynovitis	Studman and Milberg (1982)
French horn	Motor palsies	James and Cook (1983), Jankovic and Shale (1989)
Saxophone	Thoracic outlet syndrome	Lederman (1987)
Percussion	Osteoarthritis	Caldron et al (1986)
Drums	Tendinitis	Fry (1986b), Caldron et al (1986)
	Myalgias	Fry (1986b)
	Nerve entrapment	Makin and Brown (1985)
Cymbals	Bicipital tenosynovitis (cymbal player's shoulder)	Huddleston and Pratt (1983)
Miscellaneous		
Guitar	Tendinitis	Newmark and Hochberg (1987)
	Synovitis	Mortanroth (1978), Bird and Wright (1981)
	Motor palsies	Mladinich and De Witt (1974), Cohen et al (1987), Jankovic and Shale (1989)
Congas	Pigmenturia	Fenichel (1974), Furie and Penn (1974)
Spoons	Tibial stress fracture (spoon player's tibia)	O'Donoghue (1984)

*As cited in Greer JM, Panush RS: Musculoskeletal problems of performing artists. Baillieres Clin Rheumatol 8:103, 1994.

It is difficult to generalize about dance injuries because dance is not a monolithic effort. It is a broad-based hierarchic endeavor in which thousands of local school-based and private amateur dance classes supply a much smaller number of university-based dance programs, which lead finally to relatively few professional dance companies. This system of training encompasses many forms of dance that are highly divergent, ranging from classic ballet to breakdancing. Fortunately, the majority of injuries are from overuse and are rarely catastrophic, regardless of the dance style or setting. As with other overuse injuries in sports, they are influenced by a variety of factors that may be classified as intrinsic, such as biomechanical and anatomic variations, or extrinsic, such as those related to occupation or equipment.[72]

There are few reliable data on the epidemiology of amateur dance injuries, but a study of ballet dancers has revealed a high lifetime incidence of a variety of injuries including overuse injuries (reported by 63 percent), stress fractures (26 percent), and major (51 percent) and minor (48 percent) problems throughout a career. In a cumulative study of nine major surveys of dance-related injuries in ballet, modern, jazz, and theatrical dancers, more than 7000 injuries were classified. Not surprisingly, the majority (60 to 80 percent) involved the ankle, foot, or knee. The most common types of overuse injuries include strains of muscles and tendons and tendinitis (particularly of the Achilles and flexor hallucis longus tendons). The distribution of injuries is strongly influenced by the type and style of dance and the age and sex of the population.[73,76]

For example, ballet dancers in companies whose choreography emphasizes bravura technique with big jumps and balances are more likely to develop Achilles tendinitis than are those in companies that do not. Men are more likely to have back injuries because of the required jumping and lifting, whereas women who perform en pointe are more prone to toe, foot, and ankle problems. The surface on which dancers perform is also critically important. Touring companies may encounter nonflexible surfaces, including concrete; this predisposes the dancers to injuries such as shin splints and stress fractures.

Many dance injuries, particularly among nonprofessionals, stem from bodies that are poorly suited to perform the many unphysiologic positions and maneuvers demanded by a variety of dance techniques. For example, in ballet, the most important physical feature is proper turnout (external rotation) of the hip. The extent of a dancer's turnout is determined primarily by anatomic factors as well as by the influence of training before the age of 10 or 11 years. In would-be dancers older than this, attempts to "force" a proper turnout generally result in severe strains to the lower extremity, particularly in the knee and foot. Other anatomic factors are also important, including somatotype, lack of flexibility in general, and particularly lack of ankle-instep flexibility. Occupational factors including long hours of practice and rehearsal, pressures to return to work quickly after an injury, and the "show must go on" mentality must also be considered in the care of dancers.[72]

Physicians caring for dancers, particularly ballet dancers at any level, must be aware of the aesthetic pressures for extreme leanness and their potential consequences. Numerous studies have documented this leanness and also the poor dietary balance and high incidence of disordered eating patterns among dancers.[72,77,78] Dancers, as well as other excessively lean athletes, may suffer serious reproductive and skeletal sequelae as a result of such aberrant dietary practices. The combination of disordered eating, amenorrhea, and osteoporosis has been referred to as the female athletic triad and should be recognized by those caring for athletes, especially dancers. Unfortunately, the dance world is not lacking in other serious medical problems, including mental illness, drug abuse, and human immunodeficiency virus (HIV) infection.[72]

REFERENCES

1. Buckle PW: Work factors and upper limb disorders. BMJ 315:1360, 1997.
2. Hadler NM: Repetitive upper-extremity motions in the workplace are not hazardous. J Hand Surg Am 22:19, 1997.
3. Yassi A: Work-related musculoskeletal disorders. Curr Opin Rheumatol 12:124-130, 2000.
4. Schouten SAG, de Bie RA, Swaen G: An update on the relationship between occupational factors and osteoarthritis of the hip and knee. Curr Opin Rheumatol 14: 89-92, 2002.
5. Mani L, Gerr F: Work-related upper extremity musculoskeletal disorders. Primary Care 27: 845-864, 2000.
6. Colombini D, Occhipinti E, Delleman N, et al: Exposure assessment of upper limb repetitive movements: a consensus document developed by the technical committee on musculoskeletal disorders of international ergonomics association endorsed by international commission on occupation health. G Ital Med Lav Erg 23:129-142, 2000.
7. Straaton KV, Fine PR, White MB, Maisiak RS: Disability caused by work-related musculoskeletal disorders. Curr Opin Rheumatol 10:141, 1998.
8. Cole DC, Hudak PL: Prognosis of nonspecific work-related musculoskeletal disorders of the neck and upper extremity. Am J Ind Med 29:657, 1996.
9. Millender L, Tromanhauser SG, Gaynot S: A team approach to reduce disability in work-related disorders. Orthop Clin 27:669, 1996.
10. Hales TR, Bernard BP: Epidemiology of work-related musculoskeletal disorders. Orthop Clin North Am 27:679, 1996.
11. Malchaire N, Cook N, Vergracht S: Review of the factors associated with musculoskeletal problems in epidemiologic studies. Arch Occup Environ Health 74:79-90, 2001.
12. Harrington JM: Occupational medicine and rheumatic diseases. Br J Rheum 36:153, 1997.
13. Hadler NM: Vibration white finger revisited. J Occup Environ Med 41:772, 1998.
14. Viikari-Juntura ERA: The scientific basis for making guidelines and standards to prevent work-related musculoskeletal disorders. Ergonomics 40:1097, 1997.
15. Hadler NM: Coping with arm pain in the workplace. Clin Orthop 351:57, 1998.
16. Hadler NM: A keyboard for "Daubert." J Occup Environ Med 38:469, 1996.
17. Hadler NM: Occupational Musculosketal Disorders, 2nd ed. Lippincott Williams & Wilkins, Philadelphia, 1999.
18. Lister GD: Ergonomic disorders (editorial). J Hand Surg Am 20:353, 1995.
19. Schrader H, Obelieniene D, Bovim G, et al: Natural evolution of late whiplash syndrome outside the medicolegal context. Lancet 347:1207, 1996.
20. Vender MI, Kasdan ML, Truppa KL: Upper extremity disorders: a literature review to determine work-relatedness. J Hand Surg Am 20:534, 1995.
21. Reilly PA, Travers R, Littlejohn GO: Epidemiology of soft tissue rheumatism: the influence of the law (Editorial). J Rheumatol 18:1448, 1991.
22. Panush RS: Osteoarthritis, regional rheumatic syndromes, fibromyalgia. *In* Sergent JS, LeRoy EC, Meenan RF, et al (eds): Yearbook of Rheumatology. St. Louis, Mosby, 1994, pp 247-249.
23. Bell DS: "Repetition strain injury": an iatrogenic epidemic of simulated injury. Med J Austral 151:280, 1989.
24. Davis TR: Do repetitive tasks give rise to musculoskeletal disorders? Occup Med 49:257-258, 1999.
25. Higgs PE, Edwards D, Martin DS, Weeks PM: Carpal tunnel surgery outcomes in workers: effect of workers' compensation status. J Hand Surg Am 20:354,1995.
26. Panush RS: Introduction to Chapter 1: Health sciences, epidemiology, and economics. *In* Panush RS, Hadler NM, Hellman D, et al (eds): Yearbook of Rheumatology. St. Louis, Mosby, 1999.
27. Angell M: Science on Trial: The Clash of Medical Evidence and the Law in the Breast Implant Case. New York, WW Norton, 1997.
28. Panush RS, Lane NE: Exercise and the musculoskeletal system. Baillieres Clin Rheumatol 8:79, 1994.
29. Panush RS: Physical activity, fitness, and osteoarthritis. *In* Bouchard C, Shephard RJ, Stephens T (eds): Physical Activity, Fitness, and Health: International Proceedings and Consensus Statement. Champaign, Ill, Human Kinetics Publishers, 1994, pp 712-723.
30. Panush RS: Does exercise cause arthritis? Long-term consequences of exercise on the musculoskeletal system. Rheum Dis Clin North Am 16:827, 1990.
31. Callahan LF, Currey SS, Jonas Bl, et al: Osteoarthritis in retired National Football League (NFL) players: the role of injuries and playing position [Abstract]. Arthritis Rheum 46:S415, 2002.
32. Kellgren JH, Lawrence JS: Radiological assessment of osteoarthrosis. Ann Rheum Dis 16:494, 1957.
34. Kellgren JH, Lawrence JS: Osteoarthritis and disc degeneration in an urban population. Ann Rheum Dis 12:5, 1958.
35. Burke MJ, Fear EC, Wright V: Bone and joint changes in pneumatic drillers. Ann Rheum Dis 36:276, 1977.
36. Lawrence JS: Rheumatism in cotton operatives. Br J Ind Med 18:270, 1961.
37. Tempelaar HHG, Van Breeman J: Rheumatism and occupation. Acta Rheumatol 4:36, 1932.
38. Hadler NM: Industrial rheumatology: clinical investigations into the influence of the pattern of usage on the pattern of regional musculoskeletal disease. Arthritis Rheum 21:1019, 1977.
39. Hadler NM, Gillings DB, Imbus HR: Hand structure and function in an industrial setting: the influence of the three patterns of stereotyped, repetitive usage. Arthritis Rheum 21:210, 1978.
40. Anderson J, Felson DT: Factors associated with knee osteoarthritis (OA) in the HANES I survey, evidence for an association with overweight, race and physical demands of work. Am J Epidemiol 128:179, 1988.
41. Felson DT, Hannan MTP, Naimark A, et al: Occupational physical demands, knee bending and knee osteoarthritis. J Rheumatol 18:1587, 1991.
42. Felson DT, Zhang Y, Hannan MT, et al: Risk factors for incident radiographic knee osteoarthritis in the elderly: The Framingham Study. Arthritis Rheum 40:728, 1997.
43. Felson DT, Zhang Y: An update on the epidemiology of knee and hip osteoarthritis with a view to prevention. Arthritis Rheum 41:1343, 1998.
44. Molleson T: The eloquent bones of Abu Hureyra. Sci Am 271:70, 1994.
45. Sutton AJ, Muir KR, Mocket S, et al: A care-control study to investigate the relation between low and moderate levels of physical activity and osteoarthritis of the knee using data collected as part of the allied Dunbar national fitness survey. Ann Rheum Dis 60: 756-764, 2001.
46. Manninen P, Riihimaki H, Heliovaara M, et al: Physical exercise and risk of severe knee osteoarthritis requiring arthroplasty. Rheumatology 40: 432-437, 2001.
47. Walsh SJ, DeChello LM: Excess autoimmune disease mortality among school teachers. J Rheumatol 28:1537-1545, 2001.
48. Cooper GS, Parks CG, Dooley MA, et al: Occupational exposures and risk of systemic lupus erythematosus [Abstract]. Arthritis Rheum 46: S616, 2002.
49. Panush RS, Levine ML, Reichlin M: Dp I need an ANA? Some thoughts about man's best friend and the transmissibility of lupus. J Rheumatol 27:287-291,2000.
50. Morse LH: Unusual occupational rheumatologic and musculoskeletal disorders. Occup Med 7:423, 1992.
51. McDermott M, Freyne P: Osteoarthrosis in runners with knee pain. Br J Sports Med 17:84, 1983.
52. Videman T: The effect of running on the osteoarthritic joint: an experimental matched-pair study with rabbits. Rheumatol Rehabil 21:1, 1982.

53. Radin EL, Evre D, Schiller AL: Effect of prolonged walking on concrete on the joints of sheep (Abstract). Arthritis Rheum 22:649, 1979.
54. Panush RS, Hanson CS, Caldwell JR, et al: Is running associated with osteoarthritis: an eight-year follow-up study. J Clin Rheum 1:35, 1995.
55. Lane NE, Bloch DA, Jones HH, et al: Long-distance running, bone density and osteoarthritis. JAMA 255:1147, 1986.
56. Lane NE, Oehlert JW, Bloch DA, Fries JF: The relationship of running to osteoarthritis of the knee and hip and bone mineral density of the spine: 9 year longitudinal study. J Rheumatol 25:334, 1998.
57. Murry RO, Duncan C: Athletic activity in adolescence as an etiological factor in degenerative hip disease. J Bone Joint Surg Br 53:405, 1971.
58. Puranen J, Ala-Ketola L, Peltokalleo P, Saarela J: Running and primary osteoarthritis of the hip. BMJ 1:424, 1975.
59. De Carvalho A, Langfeldt B: Lobetraeningog arthrosis de formans: en radiologisk vurdering [Running practice and arthrosis deformans: a Radiological assessment]. Ugeskr Laeger 139:2421, 1977.
60. Arokoski J, Kivirantal I, Jirvelin J, et al: Long-distance running causes site-dependent decrease of cartilage glycosaminoglycan content in the knee joints of beagle dogs. Arthritis Rheum 36:1451, 1993.
61. Kujala UM, Kettunen J, Paananen H, et al: Knee osteoarthritis in former runners, soccer players, weight lifters, and shooters. Arthritis Rheum 38:539, 1995.
62. Panush RS, Schmidt C, Caldwell J, et al: Is running associated with degenerative joint disease? JAMA 255:1152, 1986.
63. Wang WE, Ramey DR, Schettler JD, et al: Postponed development of disability in elderly runners: a 13-year longitudinal study. Arch Intern Med 162:2285-2294, 2002.
64. Lane NE, Hochberg MC, Pressman A, et al: Recreational physical activity and the risk of osteoarthritis of the hip in elderly women. J Rheumatol 26:849-854, 1999.
65. Sohn RS, Micheli LJ: The effect of running on the pathogenesis of osteoarthritis of the hips and knees. Clin Orthop Rel Res 198:106, 1985.
66. Konradesen L, Hansen EM, Sondegaard L: Long distance running and osteoarthritis: Am J Sports Med 18:379, 1990.
67. Kujala UM, Kapriio J, Samo S: Osteoarthritis of weight-bearing joints in former elite male atheletes. Br Med J 308:231, 1994.
68. Marti B, Knobloch M, Tschopp A, et al: Is excessive running predictive of degenerative hip disease? Controlled study of former elite athletes. BMJ 229:91, 1989.
69. Marti B, Biedert R, Howald H: Risk of arthrosis of the upper ankle joint in long distance runners: controlled follow-up of former elite athletes. Sportverletz Sportschaden 4:175, 1990.
70. Vingard E, Sandmark H, Alfredsson L: Musculoskeletal disorders in former athletes. Orthop Scand 66:289, 1995.
71. Specter TD, Harris PA, Hart DJ, et al: Risk of osteoarthritis associated with long-term weight-bearing sports. Arthritis Rheum 39:988, 1996.
72. Baum J, Calabrese LH, Greer JM, Panush RS: Performing arts rheumatology. Bull Rheum Dis 44:5, 1995.
73. Larsson L-G, Baum J, Mudholkar GS, Kollia GD: Benefits and disadvantages of joint hypermobility among musicians. N Engl J Med 329:1079, 1993.
74. Greer JM, Panush RS: Musculoskeletal problems of performing artists. Baillieres Clin Rheumatol 8:103, 1994.
75. Hoppman RA: Instrumental musicians' hazards. Occup Med 16:619-631, 2001.
76. Zaza C: Playing-related musculoskeletal disorders in musicians: a systematic review of incidence and prevalence. CMAJ 158:1019, 1998.
77. Hoppmann RA, Reid RR: Musculoskeletal problems of performing artists. Curr Opin Rheumatol 7:147, 1995.
78. Lockwood AH: Medical problems of musicians. N Engl J Med 320:221, 1989.

32 Alternative Care for Arthritis and Related Musculoskeletal Diseases

JAYA K. RAO • DOYT L. CONN

Alternative therapies are usually defined as medical interventions that are neither taught widely in US medical schools nor generally available in US hospitals.[1] Today, alternative medicine might include any of the following practice modalities: herbal medicine, spiritual healing, mega-dose vitamins, imagery, chiropractic, folk remedies, energy healing, homeopathy, chelation therapy, aromatherapy, and acupuncture.[2] However, the boundary between conventional and alternative therapy is a porous one. With data from efficacy studies, some alternative therapies have crossed over this boundary into the mainstream.[3] Modalities that were once considered "alternative" but are now used in mainstream medicine include digitalis, nitroglycerin, colchicine, and, for some pain conditions, acupuncture and chiropractic. Complementary care is often defined as treatments that have been proven to be efficacious and may complement conventional medical care. Examples of complementary therapies include self-help strategies,[4] biofeedback,[5] and various forms of exercise.[6,7]

Most alternative treatments are based on anecdotal experiences and theories rather than on carefully controlled studies. Yet, it is important to remember that many medical treatments and surgical procedures used in conventional medicine have not been rigorously studied either.[8] The medical and scientific community recognizes these gaps in our knowledge and supports the need to rigorously evaluate all medical and surgical treatments to verify their efficacy.[8]

History

Scientific medicine is a relatively recent phenomenon in the history of the healing arts. All ancient and primitive societies held their own beliefs and theories about illnesses and developed healing practices to treat ailments. The earliest attempts to combat illness developed in both empirical and magical directions.[9] When early humans suffered aches, pains, colds, boils, toothaches, rheumatism, or skin disorders, they sought remedies from the natural environment. These treatments included water, sand, steam, poultices, massage, and herbs.[9] Primitive medicine also became inseparable from primitive modes of religious belief. Charms, spells, and psychotherapy were employed to ward off the effects of the supernatural. As primitive societies developed, certain individuals emerged as intermediaries or medicine men—some through their powers of observation and others through their special talents for healing, bone setting, crude surgery, midwifery, and the use of herbs.[10]

Hebrew health practices described in the Old Testament of the Bible contributed to the principles of hygiene and laid the foundation for public health.[9] The ancient Hebrews believed that disease was a punishment for sin, and Jehovah meted out, as well as healed, disease.[9] In ancient Egypt, medical papyri dated approximately 1500 B.C. described traditional therapies to treat disease.[10] These treatments included amulets and talismans, as well as one third of all medical substances known today, including opium, castor oil, and colchicum.[9,10] Different conditions were diagnosed depending on varying degrees of pain, fever, or tumor symptoms manifested by the patient.[9] Practitioners of the healing arts used diets, herbs, enemas, psychotherapy, or purgatives to treat these conditions.[9]

While these healing practices were being developed in ancient Egypt, ancient Indian civilization developed its own system of healing. *Aruyveda* is a Sanskrit term whose literal translation is "knowledge" (*veda*) of "life" (*ayur*).[11] The medical text *Athardaveda* (1500 to 1000 B.C.) described two schools of learning (physicians and surgeons) and eight branches of clinical medicine (internal medicine, surgery, pediatrics, toxicology, psychiatry, ophthalmology and otorhinolaryngology, rejuvenation, sexual vitality).[11] Health depended on the equilibrium of three body elements, or doshas: vata (air + ether), pitta (fire), and kapha (earth + water). Disturbances of the doshas resulted in disease, and treatment was aimed at restoring equilibrium of these elements. Treatments included diet, hygiene, and purgatives,[10] and practitioners prepared medications from vegetable, mineral, or natural products.[11] Ayurvedic medicine is still practiced in India today.

Three legendary emperors are credited with the development of Chinese medicine: Fu Hsi (2800 B.C.), who developed the philosophy of yang and yin in nature; Shen Nung (2700 B.C.), who promoted using herbal medicine and acupuncture for treatment; and Huang Ti (2600 B.C.), author of the ancient medical text *Nei Ching*.[9] The ancient Chinese believed that the two opposing qualities in universe are *yang* (the male element) and *yin* (the female element), and that, as in the universe, a healthy metabolism was dependent on the equilibrium of these two principles.[9] Acupuncture was the basic form of treatment in ancient Chinese medicine. Small needles were introduced into *chin*, or small imaginary canals, in which vital principles circulated (inspired by images of irrigation canals).[9] Puncturing the chin allowed harmful secretions to escape, and thereby reestablished equilibrium.[10]

Skilled observation characterized Greco-Roman medicine. Hippocrates (460 to 370 B.C.) believed that disease was the result of natural causes (environmental, dietary, and lifestyle factors) and that the body possessed its own means to recover from disease.[9] Hippocrates and his students established the existence of many diseases and emphasized exercise, massage, sea baths, diet, and drugs as forms of treatment.[10]

The 19th century marked the emergence of scientific medicine as well as several healing-arts movements. In the early 19th century, Dr. Samuel Hahnemann developed a system of treatment now known as *homeopathy*. Homeopathy emphasizes that "like is cured by like."[3] For example, practitioners of homeopathy believed that a substance such as quinine could cause symptoms in a healthy person and could cure similar symptoms in those who were ill. Hahnemann observed that the potency of a remedy could be retained at high dilutions and believed that these diluted substances worked on the body's energy fields.[10] Today, extensive repertoires of homeopathic medicines serve as sources of treatments for various symptoms. Homeopathic practitioners match the individual's specific symptom with an appropriate remedy, which is prepared from plant and other sources.

The practice of chiropractic originated in the late 19th century when David Daniel Palmer, a grocer and healer in Iowa, supposedly cured a deaf patient by performing cervical spine manipulation. Chiropractic literally means "done by hand."[12] In this system of care, the spine is considered central to maintaining health, and vertebral manipulation forms the basis of treatment.[3,12]

Another alternative health practice, naturopathy, is based on the tradition of the European health spas. Within this system, the philosophy is to take advantage of the body's natural healing capacities.[13] Naturopathic treatments include dietary and lifestyle changes, hydrotherapy, massage, and herbal treatments.[3]

At one time, osteopathic practitioners competed with chiropractors for the same patients.[3] Based on the philosophy of Dr. Andrew T. Still, a doctor in Kirksville, Missouri, osteopathy emphasizes the "unity of body structure and function in health and disease" and includes manipulative techniques as a form of treatment.[3] Today, however, schools of osteopathy have strong ties to conventional medicine and use the same textbooks and materials as allopathic medical schools. Osteopaths enjoy the same status as graduates of schools of medicine.

Approximately 100 years ago, alternative treatment practices dominated the healing arts and were promoted by practitioners in an environment without regulation or medical standards of care. The allure of alternative medicine began to falter with the occurrence of scientific successes in disease prevention and treatment. As significant advancements were made in surgical techniques, medical treatments and devices, and our understanding of disease etiology and pathogenesis, scientific medicine progressed rapidly during the 20th century. The development of standards for medical education and credentials for medical practice[14] were also important factors in the emergence of scientific medicine.

Current Status of Alternative Care

EPIDEMIOLOGY

The use of alternative therapy among people with chronic conditions is well documented.[15-17] Depending on both the population being studied and the definition of what is considered "alternative," the estimates of just how large a percentage of the population uses alternative therapy range from 25 to 90 percent.[1,2,17-22] In 1993, Eisenberg and his colleagues[1] reported that one in three Americans used an alternative therapy in 1990. In a follow-up survey, Eisenberg and his team[2] found that 42 percent of respondents used at least one alternative therapy and 46 percent visited an alternative-medicine practitioner in 1997. Use of alternative therapy is most common among people with neck problems, back pain, anxiety, headaches, and depression. When these data were extrapolated to the U.S. population, these researchers found that Americans spent an estimated $27 billion on alternative therapies and made 629 million visits to alternative practitioners, a figure that far exceeds the total number of visits to primary care providers in 1997.[2] Although most people use alternative therapies concomitantly with conventional therapies, many do so without informing their doctor.[1,2,23,24]

Use of alternative therapy is particularly common among people with musculoskeletal disease. Population- and clinic-based surveys indicate that 28 to 90 percent of people with arthritis and other rheumatologic conditions use alternative therapy, often to supplement conventionally prescribed therapy.[18-20,24-31] Studies of patients with specific conditions, such as rheumatoid arthritis,[32] systemic lupus erythematosus,[33] osteoarthritis,[34] and fibromyalgia[35] reveal a similar degree of use. A wide variety of therapies may be used to treat arthritis symptoms, ranging from self-administered (e.g., prayer, copper bracelets, and liniments) to practitioner-based treatments (e.g., massage therapy, acupuncture, and chiropractic).[18,27,28,30,34]

Racial and ethnic factors may have an important influence on the types of therapies used by arthritis patients.[36-38] For example, several studies indicate that, compared to Caucasians or Hispanics, African Americans have a high degree of reliance on religious prayer and certain self-care strategies (e.g., liniments).[36-38] Use of alternative therapy in general is associated with higher educational level, longer duration of disease, poorer functional status, higher levels of pain, and sleep disturbance.[29-31,33,39,40] In one study, regular use of alternative therapy was more common among patients with a diagnosis of osteoarthritis, severe pain, and a college degree.[30] Although a few studies indicate that patients who are less satisfied with their care may be more likely to use alternative therapy, other investigations show no relationship between patient satisfaction and the use of alternative therapies.[23,28,30,33,41]

WHY PATIENTS USE ALTERNATIVE THERAPIES

Patients' decisions regarding alternative therapies may be based on a combination of factors. Besides the patient-specific factors, external influences may include the recent changes in the delivery of health care, increased public access to health information, and widespread availability of alternative treatments.

During the 1990s, the health care system embarked on a difficult transition from a paternalistic approach to a consumer-driven approach to health care. With the current emphasis on visit efficiency, the physician may not be able to spend enough time addressing the patient's health concerns or treating the patient holistically. At the same time, however, patients are being encouraged to actively participate in decisions regarding their own health. As a consequence, some patients may seek health information from the lay media and the Internet.[42] Some of these sources may provide information that is not scientifically accurate or not easily distinguishable from marketing strategies.

In addition to the increased access to health information about alternative therapies, alternative treatments may be more widely available than in the past. The Dietary Supplemental Health and Education Act of 1994 opened the door to a vast number of "health products" with unknown efficacy, side effects, number and amount of active ingredients, and purity.[43] To qualify as a dietary supplement, products must not be promoted for the prevention or treatment of disease, but manufacturers could claim that their products influence body structure or function (e.g., "maintaining joint health"). The enormous amount of money Americans spend on alternative therapies has attracted the attention of those who typically provide conventional treatments. For example, major pharmaceutical companies have begun to market dietary supplements and herbal products, and some health insurers and managed care plans are offering coverage for certain forms of alternative therapy.[44,45]

Besides these external forces, patients' beliefs about health in general or about their particular condition or current treatment plan may affect their decisions to use alternative therapy. Many Americans who use alternative therapies have a holistic philosophy of health (i.e., they consider the body, mind, and spirit to be important in treating health problems) or are interested in health maintenance.[2,23,46] Some people believe chronic diseases cannot be managed satisfactorily by conventional medicine alone.[41] In a series of focus groups, patients with arthritis reported that conventionally prescribed therapy did not adequately relieve their symptoms and often caused side effects.[47] Other patients may base their decisions on their beliefs about how the alternative therapy might alter disease-related processes. For example, patients with arthritis may believe that certain alternative therapies will help "draw out the swelling" or "dissolve the debris" present in their joints.[47] Finally, there may be some patients who believe that alternative therapies offer fewer risks than do conventional therapies.[48,49]

Undoubtedly, some patients benefit from alternative care. Of those using alternative therapies, many report that these therapies are helpful in relieving their symptoms.[21,30,37,39] In most instances, however, the benefit is probably a result of the placebo response. Placebo is usually defined as an intervention that lacks a specific effect.[50] The placebo response appears to be more frequent when the desired effect is a subjective change in a sensation, such as pain.[51] The response to placebos also commonly occurs in disorders that are mediated by the autonomic nervous system (e.g., nausea, psychoneurosis, phobias, and depression) or neurohormones (e.g., blood pressure and bronchial asthma).[51]

Approach to the Patient

Although many patients use alternative therapy along with conventionally prescribed treatment, most do not disclose this behavior to their doctors.[1,2] These data suggest barriers in patient–physician communication regarding this topic. Some patients may hesitate to raise this issue because they fear being ridiculed by their doctors.[52] Other patients believe their doctor does not need to know or may not mention this information unless they are asked directly.[30] Patients may also perceive that their doctors lack the knowledge to provide effective counseling about alternative therapies.[53] The communication barrier exists on the physician's side as well. Some physicians adopt a "don't ask, don't tell policy."[54] Other physicians may be skeptical about alternative therapies and perhaps convey this belief either directly or indirectly to patients.

Alternative therapy should not be the primary approach when the patient has an ongoing disease-related process that is treatable with effective, proven therapies. Regardless of their particular beliefs about alternative therapy, however, physicians have an ethical obligation to discuss treatment alternatives with their patients.[55] Although physicians should acknowledge their level of knowledge about alternative therapy during these discussions, they should also make sure the patient has received information about the safety (e.g., potency and drug interactions) and efficacy of these treatments.[55] Because patients' use of alternative therapy may change,[56] physicians should periodically review their patients' current regimens.

Because the safety and efficacy of most alternative therapies are unproven, physicians may have legal concerns when they are asked to recommend specific treatments, provide referrals to practitioners, or tolerate continued use of these therapies.[54] As a general rule, the mere referral to an alternative practitioner does not expose the referring physician to liability unless the referral itself deprives the patient of receiving appropriate care (e.g., the referral delays or eliminates the opportunity to receive important care).[45] However, the physician could be held liable if he or she recommends an alternative treatment associated with serious risks or that is known to be ineffective.[54,57] Thus, when recommending specific alternative treatments, physicians should review the literature to determine the level of risk for the treatment, discuss the risks and benefits of this approach with the patient, document this discussion in the medical record, and continue to monitor the patient.[57] When referring patients to alternative practitioners, physicians should also inquire about the practitioner's credentials, competence, and practices.[57]

Confronting this situation is an obligation and opportunity for physicians. What steps should physicians take in providing responsible care to patients in the 21st century (Table 32–1)?

1. Physicians must strive to provide the public—patients, in particular—with reliable information about both health conditions and scientifically tested treatment approaches.
2. Physicians and health plans should provide patients with opportunities for complementary care such as health education, support, self-help strategies, exercise, and, in the case of chronic pain problems, relaxation techniques and biofeedback. The physician should be aware of reputable organizations and individuals who are trained to provide complementary care.
3. Physician should include the patient in decision making related to treatment[44] and acknowledge the importance of quality of life in these decisions.
4. Physicians should be aware that patients frequently use alternative therapies and that they may not disclose this information. Thus, physicians should ask in a supportive manner about the various treatment approaches, including alternative therapies, their patients are using.
5. Physicians should review the safety and efficacy of alternative therapies, just as they review the safety and efficacy of conventional treatments. They should also be aware of the potential interactions between alternative therapies and conventional treatments.
6. Physicians should discourage patients from discontinuing conventionally prescribed medications. Prescribed medications may require adjustment if the patient is using an herbal therapy or dietary supplement.
7. Physicians should volunteer to communicate with their patients' alternative medicine providers.

TABLE 32–1 • PROVIDING RESPONSIBLE CARE TO PATIENTS

1. Provide patients and public with scientific information and tested treatments.
2. Include the patient in discussion and decisions about management.
3. Provide patient with appropriate complementary care: education, support, self help, exercise.
4. Ask about treatments patient is using.
5. Review side effects for conventional and alternative medicine.
6. Emphasize importance of continuing current medicines when using alternative remedies.
7. Communicate with alternative-care practitioner.

Review of Selected Alternative Therapies

DIET THERAPY

Diet has long been considered an important factor in health and disease. Gout attacks, for example, may be influenced by dietary factors. For centuries patients with gout have been depicted as rotund men who eat and consume alcohol lavishly, and we now know that consumption of foods that contain large quantities of purines (such as organ meats) may alter serum uric acid, perhaps causing an elevation of blood uric acid levels.[58] With the emergence of modern medicine, the relationship between nutrition and health has been subjected to scientific scrutiny. Diets containing the proper amounts of minerals, vitamins, protein, fat, and carbohydrates are considered essential to good health. For example, people who chronically consume a diet containing high levels of animal fat and cholesterol are likely to develop coronary artery disease.[59]

For much of the 20th century, rheumatology textbooks have stated that manipulating the diet has no role in the treatment of rheumatoid arthritis or osteoarthritis.[60] Despite the lack of scientific evidence, several books are published each year that advocate particular diets for managing arthritis symptoms. Alternative practitioners may also encourage the use of certain vitamins, minerals, or dietary supplements as treatments for various forms of arthritis.

Several scientific studies examined the role of diet and dietary components in patients with rheumatoid arthritis and osteoarthritis. Patients with rheumatoid arthritis are frequently inactive as a result of their symptoms, and they are often treated with glucocorticoids. These two factors may, in part, explain why rheumatoid arthritis patients have an increased risk of being overweight.[61] Patients with rheumatoid arthritis have lower than average serum levels of pyridoxine and folate[62] and are also deficient in zinc, copper, and magnesium.[63] These deficiencies are likely the result of, rather than the cause for, chronic inflammation. Despite the thousands of people who wear copper bracelets for their arthritis, no evidence has indicated that these bracelets are helpful in alleviating arthritis symptoms. Supplemental zinc has also not been shown to be beneficial for rheumatoid arthritis.[64] On the other hand, patients with osteoarthritis of the knees who consume sufficient amounts of vitamins C and D have less progression of this disease.[65,66]

Questions have arisen about whether allergies to certain foods result in symptoms of inflammatory arthritis, specifically rheumatoid arthritis.[67] Food allergies may account for a small number of rheumatoid arthritis flares,[68] but some diets may have a mildly beneficial effect on inflammatory arthritis. For example, fasting improves the symptoms of pain and stiffness in patients with rheumatoid arthritis,[69] probably because of suppression of the immune system, but this cannot be maintained long-term without causing the patient further health problems.[70] Vegetarian diets, when supplemented with sufficient proteins, vitamins, and minerals, can result in a modest improvement in pain and stiffness. Finally, in controlled studies, researchers have found that diets high in omega-3 polyunsaturated fatty acids reduce joint tenderness and fatigue in patients with rheumatoid arthritis.[67,71] Omega-3 fatty acids, which include eicosapentaenoic acid and docosahexaenoic acid, are derived from marine animals.[67] Fish that contain omega-3 fatty acids include Pacific herring, king mackerel, salmon, and mullet.[72,73]

Diets that minimize the intake of plants in the nightshade family (e.g., tomatoes, potatoes, eggplant, and peppers) have been popularized as having anti-inflammatory effects.[67] Although some practitioners of alternative therapies believe these foods aggravate arthritis, scientific data are lacking to substantiate this claim. Other food components that have been promoted as being beneficial for arthritis include Brewers' yeast, apple cider, honey, wheat germ, cod liver oil, molasses, and garlic, but, again, there is no specific evidence that these substances relieve the symptoms of arthritis.

Epidemiologic data have established the relationship between obesity and the development of osteoarthritis of the knees.[74,75] It is reasonable to suggest that patients with rheumatoid arthritis and osteoarthritis follow a diet that contains mostly polyunsaturated fatty acids and allows for maintaining a reasonable weight. In addition, patients should consume sufficient amounts of vitamins and minerals, including vitamin D, vitamin C, and calcium. A balanced diet helps to maintain joint health as well as overall health.

DIETARY SUPPLEMENTS

Patients often use dietary supplements or herbal remedies to treat their symptoms. An estimated 165 million adults (18.4 percent of all prescription users) used herbal medicines along with conventionally prescribed medications, and they spent $5.1 billion dollars out of pocket on these remedies in 1997.[2] The preponderance of dietary supplements and herbal remedies is a major concern for several reasons. First, because these products are marketed as dietary supplements, they are not subject to regulation by the Food and Drug Administration, and there is no assurance that they contain sufficient quantities of the active ingredient(s) or that they are not adulterated with other substances, such as corticosteroids or benzodiazepines.[76,77] Second, these products are often expensive, which raises the concern that patients will delay necessary treatment. Third, these products may interact adversely with the patient's prescribed medications or have toxicities of their own.[78-80] Because patients may not disclose their use of alternative therapies, physicians should periodically ask patients about their use of these products (Table 32–2).

TABLE 32–2 • APPROACH TO PATIENTS WHO WISH TO USE DIETARY SUPPLEMENTS OR HERBAL REMEDIES

1. Listen to the patient and provide information.
2. Explain that these treatments may help the pain and appear to be safe.
3. Have them obtain the supplement from a reputable company and get advice from the pharmacist.
4. Inform that these treatments are expensive—in the range of $50 per month.
5. Do not stop current medications.
6. Be observant; if there are any untoward effects, which may be due to the supplement or its interaction with currently prescribed medicines, the patient should contact the physician.
7. Do not stop the nonpharmacologic management (e.g., weight reduction, exercise program, or physical therapy).
8. Reassess the situation at 3 months, and if there is no noticeable improvement, the supplements can be stopped.

Glucosamine Sulfate and Chondroitin Sulfate

Glucosamine sulfate and chondroitin sulfate have been used as alternative treatments for osteoarthritis since the early 1980s.[81] Glucosamine is an amino sugar, which is a precursor to the glycosaminoglycan molecule, and chondroitin sulfate is the most abundant glycosaminoglycan found in cartilage. Health food stores and pharmacies in the United States sell preparations containing these substances, either singly or in combined form. These supplements are often advertised as being helpful in "maintaining the health of joints" or "building cartilage and support flexibility or natural joint support." Glucosamine sulfate and chondroitin sulfate received widespread attention with the publication of *The Arthritis Cure* in 1997.[82] The book describes Dr. Jason Theodosakis' experience in using a combination of glucosamine sulfate and chondroitin sulfate to treat osteoarthritis patients and finding that many experienced improvement of their symptoms.

Glucosamine sulfate exists in oral and parenteral forms. Short-term (4 to 6 weeks) controlled studies indicate modest improvements in pain and function among patients treated with glucosamine sulfate compared to those who received placebo.[83] These improvements are similar to those of nonsteroidal anti-inflammatory drugs (NSAIDs).[84] Results from a recent long-term study suggest that glucosamine sulfate could serve as a disease-modifying agent in osteoarthritis.[85] In another study, however, glucosamine was found to be no more effective than placebo.[86] A few studies have examined the treatment of patients with chondroitin sulfate alone or in combination with glucosamine sulfate. In a recent meta-analysis, chondroitin sulfate was associated with larger treatment effects than was glucosamine, but methodologic assessment of the trials indicates that the actual effects of these supplements may be more modest than previously reported.[87] Long-term trials of glucosamine sulfate and chondroitin sulfate are currently under way in the United States and Europe.

Dehydroepiandrosterone

Dehydroepiandrosterone (DHEA) is an androgenic steroid often used as an alternative treatment for arthritis. It is thought to enhance muscle strength, energy, sexual function, and the immune system. Patients with rheumatoid arthritis and systemic lupus erythematosus (SLE) have lower serum DHEA levels than do normal healthy control subjects.[67,88] Increasing the androgen-to-estrogen ratio in the NZB/W mouse model results in clinical improvement of both conditions.[89] For example, NZB/W mice with lupus who were treated with DHEA experienced improvement.[90] In a 3-month, randomized, controlled study of 28 lupus patients with mild to moderately severe symptoms, those treated with DHEA experienced a decline in disease activity, as measured by the SLE-disease acticity index (SLEDAI), and a reduction in their prednisone requirements, but the differences were not statistically significant.[91] In this study, although DHEA was tolerated, the treatment was associated with acne, hirsutism, breast tenderness, and weight gain.[91] Long-term, controlled multi-center trials of DHEA are under way.

The use of DHEA raises several concerns. Long-term use of DHEA may increase the risk of developing hormone-influenced cancers such as prostate, ovarian, or uterine cancers.[67] DHEA may also be associated with other potentially adverse effects, such as liver damage, insulin resistance, and heart disease.[67] Moreover, there is no evidence that DHEA has a beneficial effect on rheumatoid arthritis. Furthermore, the limited information does not indicate that patients with lupus, even those with mild lupus, receive much benefit from DHEA treatment.

S-Adenosyl-*L*-Methionine

S-Adenosyl-*L*-methionine, or SAMe, is a dietary supplement used as an alternative therapy to treat symptoms of depression, osteoarthritis, and liver disease.[92-94] In animal studies, patients treated with SAMe had less cartilage damage than did control subjects.[92] In two randomized studies of patients with osteoarthritis of the hip or knee, researchers found that SAMe was as clinically efficacious as NSAIDs.[84,95] The data, however, are mixed regarding SAMe's usefulness as a treatment for fibromyalgia. In one study fibromyalgia patients randomly treated with SAMe had fewer trigger points and greater improvement in their Hamilton depression scores than did the placebo group, whereas in another study, no significant differences between the placebo and treatment groups were observed.[96,97]

In a recent meta-analysis, researchers found that SAMe was more effective than placebo in relieving symptoms of depression and osteoarthritis.[94] However, SAMe was not more effective than traditional antidepressants or NSAIDs in relieving symptoms of depression and osteoarthritis, respectively.[94]

HERBAL PREPARATIONS

Herbal medicine is a frequently used form of alternative therapy.[2,98] Few patients who use alternative therapies disclose this information to their physicians, so there is an increased likelihood of drug interactions.[2,44,99] For example, gingko may cause bleeding when used concomitantly with warfarin, and St. John's wort decreases blood levels of several medications (e.g., digoxin, cyclosporin, and amitriptyline) and can cause delirium if taken with selective serotonin-reuptake inhibitors.[100] Furthermore, many herbs (e.g., germander, chaparral, skullcap, valerian, comfrey, and the traditional Chinese herbal medicine, jin bu huan) have been associated with hepatitis.[78,101] The potential for adverse interactions or side effects is especially important for the rheumatologist to understand,[99] as many conventionally prescribed arthritis therapies have their own toxicities. Thus, the rheumatologist must ask whether the patient is using these or other herbal preparations.

Patients' use of herbal medicines often reflects their belief in the goodness or healing power of "natural substances," but everything that is natural is not necessarily harmless.[78,102] Indeed, some herbal preparations contain contaminants such as lead, steroids, and other substances.[76,78] These adulterants may be introduced unknowingly but escape detection because of low standards for production.[102] Some herbal preparations may not contain measurable quantities of the herb that is promoted on the label, and the identity of the active ingredient(s) and effective amounts are rarely known. Furthermore, because of the lack of quality control among the makers of herbal remedies, the batch-to-batch content of the promoted herb is not guaranteed.[102]

A few studies describing the efficacy of specific herbal medicines for particular conditions are beginning to appear in the medical literature.[103] Several reports describe the efficacy of two Ayurvedic preparations for the treatment of arthritis.[104-106] RA-1 and RA-11 are ayurvedic plant-mineral formulations that have been used to treat patients with rheumatoid arthritis and osteoarthritis of the knee, respectively. In a randomized, double-blind, placebo-controlled trial, patients with rheumatoid arthritis who were treated with RA-1 experienced modest improvements in pain, joint tenderness, swelling, and the physician's clinical assessment.[106] However, when compared to those receiving placebo, these improvements experienced by those randomized to RA-1 treatment were not statistically significant.[106] The investigators who conducted these trials suggest that long-term studies be performed to evaluate the efficacy of these compounds as treatments for arthritis.

Tripterygium wilfordi, also known as thunder god vine, has been used in China to treat patients with various autoimmune diseases.[107] Plant extracts have shown anti-inflammatory and immunosuppressive activity in vitro and in animal models of autoimmune disease.[108] In a randomized, placebo-controlled, double-blind trial of rheumatoid arthritis patients, a statistically significant number of those treated with an ethanol/ethyl acetate extract of *Tripterygium wilfordi* met the criteria for clinical improvement.[109] In a case report, patients with lupus nephritis who were treated with *T. wilfordi* experienced clinical improvement.[110]

Ginger root extracts have been promoted as alleviating joint discomfort or facilitating joint health.[111] Ginger contains substances that inhibit cyclooxygenase and 5-lipoxygenase in vitro.[112] One randomized, controlled trial showed that a standardized ginger extract was effective in improving symptoms among patients with osteoarthritis of the knee.[113] In another trial among patients with hip or knee osteoarthritis, however, no significant differences in outcome between the treatment or placebo groups were observed.[114] Because ginger is a potent inhibitor of thromboxane synthetase, it should be avoided in patients who are taking warfarin.[99] Long-term trials of ginger are needed before it can be recommended as a treatment for osteoarthritis.

HOMEOPATHY

Homeopathic therapies are among the most widely used forms of alternative medicine. Homeopathy is based on the principle of "similars" and the use of dilutions called "potencies." Because of the low likelihood of side effects, homeopathic therapies appeal to well-educated patients with chronic symptoms who are interested in "natural" remedies.[115] Although one meta-analysis suggested that the clinical effects of homeopathy did not result from a placebo effect, there is no specific disease or condition for which homeopathy is clearly effective.[116] The skepticism concerning homeopathy stems from the lack of scientific basis for its two central tenets. The first tenet, the "principle of similars," states that patients with certain disease manifestations can be cured if they are given a substance that causes the same symptoms in a healthy person. Thus, for example, a person with muscle aching and stiffness would theoretically be expected to respond to alcohol, which is known to produce aching and stiffness in normal individuals. In homeopathy, however, alcohol must be administered in an extremely diluted state to be effective. The use of dilutions, the second tenet of homeopathy, is known as "use of potencies." The remedy is considered to retain biologic effect even if it is repeatedly diluted while shaken or agitated between dilutions. The dilutions are said to produce an effect even when the active substance is diluted to concentrations less than Avogadro's number (10^{24}).[115]

Among patients with rheumatoid arthritis, placebo-controlled studies have yielded conflicting results. Two studies performed by the same investigators showed disparate results.[117,118] Another study conducted with 44 patients with rheumatoid arthritis found no statistically significant differences between the treatment and the placebo groups.[119]

One double-blind, placebo-controlled, crossover study of homeopathy versus fenoprofen was performed in patients with osteoarthritis of the hip and knee.[120] Extracts of poison oak *(Rhus toxicodendron)* produce several toxic effects, a few of which are similar to symptoms experienced by patients with osteoarthritis. The study compared a preparation of *Rhus* toxin to fenoprofen and placebo and found no significant differences between *Rhus* toxin and placebo. Fenoprofen produced highly significant pain relief compared to *Rhus* toxin, however.

A study of 30 patients with primary fibromyalgia demonstrated a positive effect of homeopathic therapy.[121] The "active" preparation contained *R. toxicodendron-6.* A tincture of the leaves of poison oak was diluted 1:99 in ethanol and then vigorously shaken. This process was repeated six times to produce the 6C potency (i.e., a dilution of 10^{-12} of the tincture), and this treatment was administered in pill form. The study outcome measures included the number of tender spots, 10-cm visual analogue scales for pain and sleep, and global assessment of symptoms. Compared to the placebo group, patients receiving "active" treatment had fewer tender points (10.6 versus 14.1, $p < 0.005$) and were more likely to report improvements in pain and sleep (53 versus 27 patients, $p < 0.0052$).[121]

Although homeopathy is appealing, its lack of scientific basis relegates any comment on efficacy to a discussion worthy of "the emperor's new clothes." Although some have called for rigorous clinical studies of homeopathy, the medical and scientific community needs a credible explanation for its mechanism of action before allocating further resources or professional effort towards research in this area.

ADJUNCTIVE THERAPIES

Acupuncture

Acupuncture, an important therapeutic modality in traditional Chinese medicine, may be the complementary therapy most familiar to rheumatologists. In acupuncture, needles are applied transcutaneously, sometimes with ancillary electrical current, heat, or moxibustion (i.e., incense burning), to specific sites on the body. This treatment is intended to restore the patient's balance of vital energy, which is known as *qi* or *chi.*[122] Classic Chinese theory recognizes 365 acupuncture sites located on 14 primary energy channels or meridians within the body.[122] The acupuncturist analyzes the patient's illness and selects the sites for needle insertion. For certain physical complaints, such as joint pain, these sites may be proximal to the area of discomfort; whereas for other problems, such as nausea or drug addiction, needles may be applied to distal sites (e.g., the ear or the scalp). With proper placement of the needle in a therapeutic site, the patient may experience heaviness, numbness, or soreness at the site of needle placement, which is referred to as *teh qi* or *teh chi.*[123] Whether this sensation is required for treatment to be considered successful remains the subject of debate.[123]

Acupuncture is often used to provide pain relief, and, during the past 20 years, investigators have sought to understand its mechanism of action. Acupuncture needling may stimulate the body to release endogenous endorphins (e.g., enkephalin), causing a reduction in pain.[124] This action can be blocked by naloxone and other opiate antagonists.[122] Animals deficient in opiate receptors or endorphins show a poor response to acupuncture. However, acupuncture analgesia can be transferred to a naïve animal through transfer of cerebrospinal fluid.[122] Additional studies have demonstrated that needling induces release of neurohormones or neurotransmitters, such as serotonin, Substance P, or acetylcholine, within the nervous system, thereby resulting in pain relief.[125]

Randomized, controlled trials of acupuncture have highlighted the dilemma of finding the appropriate control to serve as a comparison.[122] Although it would seem most logical to use sham acupuncture as a control, sham treatment may stimulate pain-inhibitory nerve fibers or endorphin release in a manner analogous to real treatment.[122,126] Indeed, careful examination of acupuncture trials demonstrates that the high response rate in sham-treated subjects may complicate the detection of differences between the treatment and placebo groups.[122,126]

Controlled studies have examined acupuncture as a treatment for osteoarthritis and for low back pain.[127-133] In a meta-analysis of low back pain studies, acupuncture was found to perform better than various control interventions, but the evidence was insufficient to indicate that it was superior to placebo (i.e., sham acupuncture).[126] Furthermore, a comparison of findings of the nonblinded studies to those of the blinded studies suggest that patients' and therapists' expectations may influence the clinical outcomes related to acupuncture treatment.[126] A meta-analysis of short-term studies of patients with osteoarthritis of the knee found that acupuncture provided more symptom relief than did sham acupuncture, but when acupuncture was compared to physical therapy, the differences were not significant.[134]

Fibromyalgia is a poorly understood condition that is characterized by diffuse pain. Conventional treatment often provides inadequate relief for this pain, and several studies have examined use of acupuncture in fibromyalgia.[135-138] Sprott and colleagues[137] found improvement in serum levels of serotonin and substance P among 29 fibromyalgia patients who received acupuncture treatment. Deluze and colleagues[136] randomly treated 70 fibromyalgia patients, who met American College of Rheumatology criteria, with either electroacupuncture or sham acupuncture treatment. The study outcomes were pain threshold, number of analgesic tablets used, regional pain score, visual analogue pain scale, sleep quality, morning stiffness, patient's global assessment, and physician's assessment. Seven of these outcomes showed significant improvement among patients randomized to the intervention. However, the study lasted only 3 weeks, and the investigators did not assess the duration of benefit or include a treatment maintenance program. Although acupuncture appears to be promising form of therapy, clinicians should be aware that some patients report exacerbations of fibromyalgia symptoms after treatment.[135]

Although studies have examined the use of acupuncture in treating osteoarthritis, low back pain, and fibromyalgia, few have examined the use of acupuncture to treat rheumatoid arthritis. On balance, these studies have shown conflicting results,[139] and acupuncture has not proved beneficial in stage III or stage IV rheumatoid arthritis.[140] Until further randomized, controlled trials demonstrate acupuncture's efficacy, patients with rheumatoid arthritis should probably not expect benefit from this treatment.[141]

Although acupuncture, when combined with patient education and exercise, may improve the quality of life for patients with osteoarthritis and other noninflammatory musculoskeletal conditions, how this modality should be used over the long term remains unclear. For osteoarthritis in particular, research investigations should examine whether acupuncture delays the need for intra-articular therapies.

CHIROPRACTIC

Chiropractic is an alternative treatment often used by patients with musculoskeletal conditions.[12,30,34] Spinal manipulation may improve symptoms among those with mechanical low back pain, and these treatments are associated with high patient satisfaction.[142,143] Recent controlled studies, however, raise doubts about the cost effectiveness of chiropractic treatment compared to that of other treatments, such as physical therapy or education.[144,145]

Blunt and colleagues[146] randomly treated 21 fibromyalgia patients to either usual standard treatment or a 4-week course of spinal manipulation performed three to five times each week.[146] Compared with those who received standard treatment, the range of motion and self-reported pain improved among those who received chiropractic, but there was no significant improvement in the number of tender points or disability index. Although these preliminary results are promising, the study lacked sufficient sample size to generalize the results to the broader population of fibromyalgia patients.

MAGNETS

Over the years, magnets and various electrical stimulation devices have been promoted as potential treatments for arthritis. Electrical or magnetic fields may have an effect on the "e" pain fibers, resulting in a decreased awareness of pain. Although in vitro experiments suggest that electrical fields modify chondrocyte function, it is not known whether altering the microelectrical environment provides chondroprotective effects in vivo. In two double-blind, controlled studies, pulsed direct current and pulsed electromagnetic treatments were shown to be beneficial in the management of osteoarthritis.[147,148] In one study, Zizic and colleagues[149] treated patients with rheumatoid arthritis with pulsed electrical current and found improvements in pain but not in hand functioning.

Magnetic appliances have received comparatively less scientific investigation than electrical stimulation devices, and the few studies that have been performed show mixed results. In a double-blind study, patients with postpolio syndrome were treated with static magnets applied to their feet; these patients reported subjective pain relief.[150] In another study, patients with knee osteoarthritis were randomly treated either with placebo (magnet off) or with exposure to low-amplitude, low-frequency magnetic fields: The magnet-on group experienced a significantly greater reduction in pain than did the magnet-off group.[151] However, in a study of patients with chronic wrist pain due to carpal tunnel syndrome, patients treated with magnet therapy did not have significantly different outcomes than those treated with the placebo device.[152] Similarly, patients with chronic low back pain who were treated with bipolar magnets did not experience a significant difference in visual analogue pain scores than did patients in the control group.[153] Further investigation should be performed before electric or magnetic therapy can be recommended as adjunctive treatments for arthritis.

MOVEMENT AND MASSAGE THERAPIES

Movement and massage therapies are adjunctive programs that may benefit patients with rheumatic disease. The data supporting their benefit are fairly meager, however, and patients should also be advised that these treatments might not be covered by insurance.

Yoga is a movement and meditation technique that has been studied more rigorously than other movement practices. This ancient practice involves gentle stretches and balancing exercises combined with meditation and relaxation techniques for each individual. Yoga can be taught in a class setting, thereby reducing the cost. Garfinkel and colleagues[154] performed a controlled trial of yoga in patients with osteoarthritis of the hand. The intervention involved eight once-a-week sessions of yoga instruction and daily home practice. Members of the experimental group experienced more improvements in pain, tenderness, and finger range of motion than did members of the control group, who received no therapy. In a group of patients with rheumatoid arthritis of the hand, similar benefits (e.g., improvement in grip strength) occurred, and all patients in the experimental group chose to continue practicing yoga after the study ended.[155] In a recent study of patients with carpal tunnel syndrome, investigators found more improvement in grip strength, pain, and Phelan's sign among patients randomly chosen to participate in the yoga intervention than they found in members of the control group, who received wrist splints.[156] However, no significant differences in sleep disturbance, Tinel's sign, or nerve conduction studies were found between the two groups. Despite this limitation, yoga may be a promising adjunctive therapy for arthritis.

A number of studies indicate that exercise has beneficial effects for patients with rheumatic disease. T'ai chi is based on Chinese martial arts and consists of a series of controlled, rhythmically flowing movements of the upper and lower extremities. These minimal-impact movements are performed while the exerciser stands in place. T'ai chi exercises may be taught in a class format and then practiced at home. For patients with rheumatoid arthritis, these exercises appear to be safe and may serve as an alternative form of exercise therapy.[157] In a randomized, controlled study of older persons, the group performing T'ai chi experienced a 45 percent reduction in falls because of the increase in muscle strength and balance resulting from this program.[158] Older adults with osteoarthritis who received T'ai chi training had significantly more improvements in their ability to manage their arthritis-related symptoms effectively than did members of the control group.[159] This training did not lead to significant changes in lower extremity functioning, however.[159]

Alexander, Feldenkrais, and Trager are different schools of movement re-education named after their founders. Therapists certified in the principles of each of these schools teach people to make subtle changes in their posture and movements to improve function and provide pain relief. Because the safety and efficacy of these schools of movement among those with rheumatic disease have not been studied systematically, patients who use these techniques should maintain contact with their physical therapists to ensure that range of motion is not adversely affected by these movement therapies.

The first written reference to massage has been dated to 2000 B.C., and Hippocrates was known to be a proponent of massage therapy.[12] Some proponents claim that massage restores metabolic balance within the soft tissues by stimulating blood flow and reducing edema, but data are lacking to support these effects.[12] Many patients with arthritis and other pain syndromes use massage therapy for relief of pain.[34] A recent systematic review found that massage therapy may have beneficial effects for those with subacute and chronic low back pain, particularly when this treatment is combined with education.[160]

SPIRITUALITY AND RELIGION

Six Gallup polls conducted over a 35-year period have consistently shown that 95 percent of Americans believe in God or a universal spirit and 75 percent pray regularly.[161] In a 1997 *Newsweek* poll, 79 percent of respondents said God answers prayers for physical healing, 82 percent of respondents to a CNN/*Time* poll believed in the healing power of prayer, and 79 percent of respondents to a *USA Weekend* survey said spiritual faith can help people recover from illness, injury, or disease.[162-164]

Similar attitudes toward religion have been documented in people with health problems. Eighty percent of family practice patients believe their physicians should consider their spiritual needs, 37 percent want their physician to discuss their religious beliefs with them, and 48 percent want their physicians to pray with them.[165] Surveys of patients hospitalized with a variety of conditions, such as gynecologic cancer, end-stage renal disease, and open heart surgery, have shown that religious beliefs are often used to cope with medical illness.[166-168] Spiritual or religious interventions have been shown to improve certain psychologic variables (e.g., coping abilities and depression), which are known to be important in patients with arthritis and other chronic illnesses.[169] Furthermore, frequent attendance at religious services was predictive of lower interleukin-6 levels in a sample of older adults followed for 6 years.[170]

Definitions

The term *religion* often refers to structured religious institutions with prescribed rituals and theology. Spirituality is at the center of religion and represents the personal, individual path to, or relationship with, a sacred or defined transcendent power. Although it is possible to be spiritual without being religious, spirituality and religion are not completely separate concepts. Some people may not wish to follow the structured rituals and relationships associated with a particular religion or religious community, but they can still be spiritual.

Spirituality or religiousness cannot be expressed as a single construct or measure. But, perhaps we can categorize different aspects, or domains, of spirituality so we can measure their effect on health. A National Institute of Aging–Fetzer Institute working group identified 12 domains of spirituality.[171] These domains are daily spiritual experiences, meaning, values, beliefs, forgiveness, private religious practices, religious support, religious or spiritual coping, religious or spiritual history, commitment, religious preferences, and organizational preferences. The working group developed individual scales for measuring these domains in health studies.[171] Because many studies have shown a relationship between spirituality and health in general and specific conditions (e.g., recovery from stroke or cardiac surgery), it seems advisable to include one or more of these measures in studies of clinical interventions.[172]

Sprituality or Religion and Arthritis

Epidemiologic data indicate that a large number of patients with arthritis may rely on spiritual or religious interventions. Cronan and colleagues[18] examined the prevalence of use of unconventional remedies for arthritis and found that respondents most commonly reported use of prayer (44%). In a survey of 235 consecutive patients who attended a rheumatology clinic, 39 percent reported using spiritual modalities such as prayer, meditation, and self relaxation.[27] Bill-Harvey and colleagues[37] interviewed 160 arthritis patients from two urban, low-income, minority communities. African American patients reported that prayer (92%), and equipment (70%) were the most helpful, whereas Hispanics reported prayer (50%) and heat (40%) as being most helpful.[37] In a study of Hispanic women with arthritis, the second most common coping strategy was the use of prayer.[173]

Spirituality or Religion and Other Health Issues

Matthews and Larson[174-177] conducted an exhaustive search of the medical literature to find research studies that examined spiritual or religious interventions in human disease. They found more than 200 studies that considered this link. Approximately 75 percent of the reports indicated that spirituality or religiousness has a beneficial effect on a variety of health conditions, 17 percent of the studies yielded neutral or mixed results, and the remainder demonstrated negative effects. Scholars at the Park Ridge Center for the Study of Faith, Health, and Ethics have chronicled the relationship between faith, beliefs, and health in a 14-volume series.[178,179] Each volume examines the ways in which major religions relate to issues of health, suffering, madness, sexuality, healing, well being, dignity, morality, life passages, caring, and dying.

Perhaps the best-known randomized, controlled trial of spiritual intervention is a study conducted by Byrd and colleagues. Upon admission to the coronary care unit, 393 patients were randomly assigned to an intercessory prayer group, in which others were praying for them, or to a control group.[180] Individuals saying the prayers were outside the hospital and never met the patients in the experimental group, and the doctors and patients were similarly blinded to their study status (i.e., in both the intervention and the control group). All patients were followed for their entire hospitalization. Compared with patients randomized to intercessory prayer, the control patients required significantly more ventilatory assistance, antibiotics, and diuretics, and they had a higher incidence of congestive heart failure ($p < 0.03$) and cardiopulmonary arrest ($p < 0.02$). A recent replication of this study showed a lower rate of overall adverse outcomes for those randomly assigned to the prayer group, but lengths of stay in the coronary care unit and hospital were not affected by the intervention.[181] Another nonrandomized study found clinical improvement among a group of rheumatoid arthritis patients who received intercessory prayer, but the results should be interpreted with caution because the study has significant methodologic limitations.[182] Despite the lack of adequate study, religion and spirituality play a large role in our perception of the healing process.

ACKNOWLEDGMENT

This chapter is a revised and updated version of the chapter entitled, "Alternative Care for Arthritis and Related Musculoskeletal Diseases," written by Doyt L. Conn, J. Roger Hollister, and William J. Arnold and published in Kelly's Textbook of Rheumatology, 6th edition (2001).

REFERENCES

1. Eisenberg DM, Kessler RC, Foster C, et al: Unconventional medicine in the United States: prevalence, costs, and patterns of use. N Engl J Med 328:246, 1993.
2. Eisenberg DM, Davis RB, Ettner SL, et al: Trends in alternative medicine use in the United States, 1990-1997: results from a national survey. JAMA 280:1569, 1998.
3. Kaptchuk TJ, Eisenberg D: Varieties of healing. 2: a taxonomy of unconventional healing practices. Ann Intern Med 135:196, 2002.
4. Lorig KR, Sobel DS, Stewart AL, et al: Evidence suggesting that a chronic disease self-management program can improve health status while reducing hospitalization. Med Care 37:5, 1999.
5. Flor H, Bribaumer N: Comparison of the efficacy of electromyograph biofeedback, cognitive-behavioral therapy, and conservative medical interventions in the treatment of chronic musculoskeletal pain. J Consult Clin Psychol 61:653, 1993.
6. Minor M: Physical activity and management of arthritis. Soc Behav Med 13:117, 1991.
7. Sullivan T, Allegrante JP, Peterson MGE, et al: One-year follow-up of patients with osteoarthritis of the knee who participated in a program of supervised fitness walking and supportive patient education. Arth Care Res 11:228, 1998.
8. Angell M, Kassirer JP: Alternative medicine: the risks of untested and unregulated remedies. N Engl J Med 339:839, 1998.
9. Marti-Ibanez F: Epic of Medicine. New York, Clarkson N. Potter, 1962.
10. Garrison FH: History of Medicine 4th ed. Philadelphia, W. B. Saunders, 1963.
11. Chopra A, Doiphode VV: Ayurvedic medicine. core concept, therapeutic principles, and current relevance. Med Clin North Am 86:75, vii, 2002.
12. Fiechtner JJ, Brodeur RR: Manual and manipulation techniques for rheumatic disease. Rheum Dis Clin North Am 26:83, ix, 2000.

13. Weil A: Spontaneous Healing. New York, Ballantine Books, 1995.
14. Jonas W: Alternative medicine: learning from the past, examining the present, advancing to the future. JAMA 280:1616, 1998.
15. Cassileth BR, Lusk EJ, Guerry D, et al: Survival and quality of life among patients receiving unproven as compared with conventional cancer therapy. N Engl J Med 324:1180, 1991.
16. Krauss HH, Godfrey C, Kirk J, et al: Alternative health care: its use by individuals with physical disabilities. Arch Phys Med Rehab 79:1440, 1999.
17. Nilsson M, Trehn G, Asplund K: Use of complementary and alternative medicine remedies in Sweden. A population-based longitudinal study within the northern Sweden Monica Project. J Intern Med 250:225, 2001.
18. Cronan TA, Kaplan RM, Posner L, et al: Prevalence of the use of unconventional remedies for arthritis in a metropolitan community. Arth Rheum 32:1604, 1989.
19. Kronenfeld JJ, Wasner C: The use of unorthodox therapies and marginal practitioners. Soc Sci Med 16:1119, 1982.
20. Higham C, Ashcroft C, Jayson MI: Non-prescribed treatments in rheumatic diseases. Practitioner 227:1201, 1983.
21. Gray CM, Tan AWH, Pronk NP, et al: Complementary and alternative medicine use among health plan members. Eff Clin Pract 5:17, 2002.
22. Astin JA, Pelletier KR, Marie A, et al: Complementary and alternative medicine use among elderly persons: one-year analysis of a Blue Shield Medicare Supplement. J Gerontol A Biol Med Sci 55A:M4, 2000.
23. Astin JA: Why patients use alternative medicine: results of a National Study. JAMA 279:1548, 1998.
24. Visser GJ, Peters L, Rasker JJ: Rheumatologists, and their patients who seek alternative care: an agreement to disagree. Br J Rheumatol 31:485, 1992.
25. Vecchio PC: Attitudes to alternative medicine by rheumatology outpatient attenders. J Rheumatol 21:145, 1994.
26. Bird HA: Alternative therapy for rheumatic diseases. J R Soc Health 6:27, 1990.
27. Boisset M, Fitzcharles M-A: Alternative medicine use by rheumatology patients in a universal health care setting. J Rheumatol 21:148, 1994.
28. Chandola A, Young Y, McAlister J, et al: Use of complementary therapies by patients attending musculoskeletal clinics. J Soc Med 92:13, 1999.
29. Ramos-Remus C, Gamez-Nava JI, Gonzalez-Lopez L, et al: Use of alternative therapies by patients with rheumatic disease in Guadalajara, Mexico: prevalence, beliefs, and expectations. Arthritis Care Res 11:411, 1998.
30. Rao JK, Mihaliak K, Kroenke K, et al: Use of complementary therapies for arthritis among patients of rheumatologists. Ann Intern Med 131:409, 1999.
31. Kaboli PJ, Doebbeling BN, Saag KG, et al: Use of complementary and alternative medicine by older patients with arthritis: a population-based study. Arthritis Rheum 45:398, 2001.
32. Kestin M, Miller L, Littlejohn G, et al: The use of unproven remedies for rheumatoid arthritis in Australia. Med J Aust 143:516, 1985.
33. Moore AD, Petri MA, Manzi S, et al: The use of alternative medical therapies in patients with systemic lupus erythematosus. Arthritis Rheum 43:1410, 2000.
34. Ramsey SD, Spencer AC, Topolski TD, et al: Use of alternative therapies by older adults with osteoarthritis. Arthritis Rheum 45:222, 2001.
35. Pioro-Boisset M, Esdaile JM, Fitzcharles M-A: Alternative medicine use in fibromyalgia syndrome. Arthritis Care Res 9:13, 1996.
36. Arcury TA, Bernard SL, Jordan JM, et al: Gender and ethnic differences in alternative and conventional arthritis remedy use among community dwelling rural adults with arthritis. Arthritis Care Res 9:384, 1996.
37. Bill-Harvey D, Rippey RM, Abeles M, et al: Methods used by urban, low-income minorities to care for their arthritis. Arthritis Care Res 2:60, 1989.
38. Ibrahim SA, Siminoff LA, Burant CJ, et al: Variation in perceptions of treatment and self-care practices in elderly with osteoarthritis: a comparison between African American and white patients. Arthritis Rheum 45:340, 2001.
39. Cronan TA, Kaplan RM, Kozin F: Factors affecting unprescribed remedy use among people with self-reported arthritis. Arthritis Care Res 6:149, 1993.
40. Jordan JM, Bernard SL, Callahan LF, et al: Self-reported arthritis-related disruptions in sleep and daily life and the use of medical, complementary, and self-care strategies for arthritis. Arch Family Med 9:143, 2000.
41. Eisenberg DM, Kessler RC, Van Rompey MI, et al: Perceptions about complementary therapies relative to conventional therapies among adults who use both: results from a national survey. Ann Intern Med 135:344, 2001.
42. Suarez-Almazor ME, Kendall CJ, et al: Surfing the Net: information on the World Wide Web for persons with arthritis: patient empowerment or patient deceit? J Rheumatol 28:185, 2001.
43. The Dietary Supplemental Health and Education Act of 1994, Public Law 103-417. 103rd Congress (25 October 1994).
44. Eisenberg D: Advising patients who seek alternative therapies. Ann Intern Med 127:61-69, 1997.
45. Studdert DM, Eisenberg DM, Miller FH, et al: Medical malpractice implications of alternative medicine. JAMA 280:1610, 1998.
46. Furnham A, Bhagrath R: A comparison of health beliefs and behaviours of clients of orthodox and complementary medicine. Br J Clin Psychol 32:237, 1993.
47. Rao JK, Arick R, Mihaliak K, et al: Using focus groups to understand arthritis patients' perceptions about unconventional therapy. Arthritis Care Res 11:253, 1998.
48. Klepser TB, Doucette WR, Horton MR, et al: Assessment of patients' perceptions and beliefs regarding herbal therapies. Pharmacotherapy 20:83, 2000.
49. Povar GJ, Mantell M, Morris LA: Patients' therapeutic preferences in an ambulatory care setting. Am J Public Health 74:1395, 1984.
50. Getzche PC: Placebos in medicine: is there logic in the placebo? Lancet 344:925, 1994.
51. de Saintonge DMC, Herxheimer A:. Placebos in medicine: harnessing placebo effects in health care. Lancet 344:995, 1994.
52. Perlman AI, Eisenberg DM, Panush RS: Talking with patients about alternative and complementary medicine. Rheum Dis Clin North Am 25:815, 1999.
53. Lazar JS, O'Connor BB: Talking with patients about their use of alternative therapies. Prim Care 24:699, 1997.
54. Adams KE, Cohen MH, Eisenberg DM, et al: Ethical considerations of complementary and alternative medical therapies in conventional medical settings. Ann Intern Med 137:660, 2002.
55. Sugarman J, Burk L: Physicians' ethical obligations regarding alternative medicine. JAMA 280:1623, 1998.
56. Rao JK, Kroenke K, Mihaliak KA, et al: Rheumatology patients' use of complementary therapies: results from a one-year longitudinal study. Arthritis Care Res, in press.
57. Cohen MH, Eisenberg DM: Potential physician malpractice liability associated with complementary and integrative therapies. Ann Intern Med 136:596, 2002.
58. Rodman GP: Early theories concerning the etiology and pathogenesis of gout. Arthritis Rheum 8:599, 1965.
59. Keyes A: Diet and development of coronary artery disease. Chron Dis 4:364, 1956.
60. Lamont-Havers R: Diet in rheumatoid arthritis. *In* Hollander JL (ed): Arthritis and Allied Conditions.. Philadelphia, Lea & Febiger, 1966.
61. Morgan SL, Anderson AM, Hood SM, et al: Nutrient intake, patterns of body mass index, and vitamin levels in patients with rheumatoid arthritis. Arthritis Care Res 10:9, 1997.
62. Kremer JM, Bigaquett J: Nutrient intake of patients with rheumatoid arthritis is deficient in pyridoxine, zinc, copper, and magnesium. J Rheumatol 23:990, 1996.
63. Stone J, Doube A, Dudson D, et al: Inadequate calcium, folic acid, vitamin E, zinc, and selenium intake in rheumatoid arthritis patients: results of a dietary survey. Semin Arthritis Rheum 27:180, 1997.
64. Simkin PA: Zinc, again [Editorial]. J Rheumatol 24:626, 1997.
65. McAlindon TE, Felson DT, Zhang Y, et al: Relation of dietary intake and serum levels of vitamin D to progression of osteoarthritis of the knee among participants in the Framingham Study. Ann Intern Med 125:353, 1996.
66. McAlindon TE, Jacques P, Zhang Y, et al: Do antioxidant micronutrients protect against the development and progression of knee osteoarthritis? Arthritis Rheum 39:648, 1996.
67. Henderson CJ, Panush RS: Diets, dietary supplements, and nutritional therapies in rheumatic diseases. Rheum Dis Clin North Am 25:937, ix, 1999.

68. Panush RS, Webster EM: Food allergies and other adverse reactions to foods. Med Clin North Am 69:533, 1985.
69. Palmblad J, Hafstrom I, Ringertz B: Antirheumatic effects of fasting. Rheum Dis Clin North Am 17:3512, 1991.
70. Kjelsen-Hragh J, Haugen M, Brochgrevink CF, et al: Controlled trial of fasting and one year vegetarian diet in rheumatoid arthritis. Lancet 338:899, 1991.
71. Volker D, Fitzgerald P, Major G, et al : Efficacy of fish oil concentrate in the treatment of rheumatoid arthritis. J Rheumatol 27:2343, 2000.
72. Kremer JM, Lawrence DA, Petrillo GF, et al: Effects of high-dose fish oil on rheumatoid arthritis after stopping nonsteroidal anti-inflammatory drugs. Arthritis Rheum 38:107, 1995.
73. Aariza-Ariza R, Mstanza-Peralta M, Cardiel MH: Omega-3 fatty acids in rheumatoid arthritis: an overview. SeminArthritis Rheum 27:366, 1998.
74. Felson DT, Anderson JJ, Naimark A, et al: Obesity and knee osteoarthritis: The Framingham Study. Ann Intern Med 109:18, 1988.
75. Felson DT, Zhang Y, Anthony JM, et al: Weight loss reduces the risk for symptomatic knee osteoarthritis in women: The Framingham study. Ann Intern Med 116:535, 1992.
76. Gertner E, Marshall PS, Filandrinos D, et al: Complications resulting from the use of Chinese herbal medications containing undeclared prescription drugs. Arthritis Rheum 38:614, 1995.
77. Slifman NR, Obermeyer WR, Musser SM, et al: Contamination of botanical dietary supplements by Digitalis lanata. New Engl J Med 339:806, 1998.
78. Ernst E: Harmless herbs? A review of the recent literature. Am J Med 104:170, 1998.
79. Weisbord SD, Soule JB, Kimmel PL: Poison on line: acute renal failure caused by oil of wormwood purchased through the internet. New Engl J Med 337:825, 1997.
80. Brooks PM, Lowenthal RM: Chinese herbal arthritis cure and agranulocytosis. Med J Aust 2:860, 1977.
81. Hungerford DS: Treating osteoarthritis with chondroprotective agents. Orthopedic Special edition, vol. 4, no. 1, 1998.
82. Theodosakis J, Adderly B, Fox B: The Arthritis Cure. New York, St. Martin's Press, 1997.
83. Noack W, Fischer M, Forster KK, et al: Glucosamine sulfate in osteoarthritis of the knee. Osteoarthritis Cartilage 2:51, 1994.
84. Mueller-FasBender H, Bach GL, Haase W, et al: Glucosamine sulfate compared to ibuprofen in osteoarthritis of the knee. Osteoarthritis Cartilage 2:61, 1994.
85. Reginster JY, Gillot V, Bruyere O, et al: Evidence of nutriceutical effectiveness in the treatment of osteoarthritis. Curr Rheumatol Rep 2:472, 2000.
86. Hughes R, Carr A: A randomized, double-blind, placebo-controlled trial of glucosamine sulfate as an analgesic in osteoarthritis of the knee. Rheumatology 41:279, 2002.
87. McAlindon TE, LaValley MP, Gulin JP, et al: Glucosamine and Chondroitin for the treatment of osteoarthritis: a systematic quality assessment and meta-analysis. JAMA 283:1469, 2000.
88. Lahita RF, Bradlow HL, Ginzler E, et al: Low plasma androgens in women with systemic lupus erythematosus. Arthritis Rheum 30:241, 1987.
89. Roubinian JR, Papoian R, Talal N: Androgenic hormones modulate autoantibody responses and improve survival in murine lupus. J Clin Invest 59:1066, 1977.
90. Lucas JA, Ahmed AA, Casey ML, et al: Prevention of autoantibody formation and prolonged survival in New Zealand black/New Zealand white F1 mice fed dehydroisoandosterone. J Clin Invest 75:2091, 1985.
91. Vollenhoven RFV, Engleman EG, McGuire JL: Dehydroepiandosterone (DHEA) in systemic lupus erythematosus: results of a double-blind, placebo-controlled, randomized clinical trial. Arthritis Rheum 38:1826, 1995.
92. Massey PB: Dietary supplements. Med Clin North Am 86:127, 2002.
93. Horowitz S: SAMe for depression, arthritis, cirrhosis, and other disorders. Alternative Complement Ther 10:266, 1999.
94. Southern California Evidence-Based Practice Center: S-Adenosyl-L-methionine for treatment of depression, osteoarthritis, and liver disease. (http://www.ahrq.gov/clinic/epcsums/samesum.htm Summary, Evidence Report/Technology Assessment: Number 64, AHRQ Publication No. 02-E033, August 2002. Agency for Healthcare Research and Quality, Rockville, MD.), accessed December 10, 2002.
95. Caruso I, Pietrogrande V: Italian double-blind multicenter study comparing S-adenosylmethionine, naproxen, and placebo in the treatment of degenerative joint disease. Am J Med 83:66, 1987.
96. Tavoni A, Vitali C, Bombardieri S, et al: Evaluation of S-adenosylmethionine in primary fibromyalgia. Am J Med 83:107, 1987.
97. Volkmann H, Norregaard J, Jacobsen S, et al: Double-blind, placebo-controlled cross-over study of intravenous S-adenosyl-L-methionine in patients with fibromyalgia. Scan J Rheumatol 26:206, 1997.
98. Landmark Healthcare: The Landmark Report on Public Perceptions of Alternative Care. Sacramento, Calif., Landmark Healthcare, 1998.
99. Miller LG: Herbal medicinals: selected considerations focusing on known or potential drug-herb interactions. Arch Intern Med 158:2200, 1998.
100. Izzo AA, Ernst E: Interactions between herbal medicines and prescribed drugs: a systematic review. Drugs 61:2163, 2001.
101. Anderson IB, Mullen WH, Meeker JE, et al: Pennyroyal toxicity: measurement of toxic metabolic levels in two cases and review of the literature. Ann Intern Med 124:726, 1996.
102. Winslow LC, Kroll DJ: Herbs as medicines. Arch Intern Med 158:2192-2199, 1998.
103. Ernst E: The risk-benefit profile of commonly used herbal therapies: gingko, St. John's wort, ginseng, echinacea, saw palmetto, and kava. Ann Intern Med 136:42-53, 2002.
104. Chopra A, Patwardhan B, Lavin P, et al: A clinical study of a herbal formulation in RA. Arthritis Rheum 39:S283, 1996.
105. Chopra A, Lavin P, Chitre D, et al: A clinical study of an ayurvedic medicine in OA of the knee. Arthritis Rheum 26:713, 1997.
106. Chopra A, Lavin P, Patwardhan B, et al: Randomized double blind trial of an ayurvedic plant derived formulation for treatment of rheumatoid arthritis. J Rheumatol 27:1365-1372, 2000.
107. Lipsky PE, Tao XL: A potential new treatment for rheumatoid arthritis: thunder god vine. Sem Arthritis Rheum 26:713, 1997.
108. Tao X, Schulze-Koops H, Ma L, et al: Effects of Tripterygium wilfodii Hook F extracts on induction of cyclooxygenase 2 activity and prostaglandin E2 production. Arthritis Rheum 41:130, 1998.
109. Tao X, Younger J, Fan FZ, et al: Benefit of an extract of Tripterygium wilfordii Hook F in patients with rheumatoid arthritis: a double-blind, placebo-controlled study. Arthritis Rheum 46:1735-1743, 2002.
110. Kao NL: Resolution of severe lupus nephritis associated with Tripterygium wilfordii Hook F ingestion. Arthritis Rheum 36:1751, 1993.
111. Srivastava KC, Mustafa T: Ginger (Zingiber officianale) and rheumatic disorders. Med Hypotheses 19:25, 1989.
112. Kiuchi F, Iwakami S, Shibuya M, et al: Inhibition of prostaglandin and leukotriene biosynthesis by gingerols and diarylheptanoids. Chem Pharm Bull 40:387, 1992.
113. Altman RD, Marcussen KC: Effects of a ginger extract on knee pain in patients with osteoarthritis. Arthritis Rheum 44:2531-2538, 2001.
114. Bliddal H, Rosetzsky A, Schlichting P, et al: A randomized, placebo-controlled, cross-over study of ginger extracts and ibuprofen in osteoarthritis. Osteoarthritis Cartilage 8:9-12, 2000.
115. Goldstein MS, Glik D: Use of and satisfaction wtih homeopathy in a patient population. Altern Ther 4:60, 1997.
116. Leride K, Clausius N, Ramirez G, et al: Are the clinical effects of homeopathy placebo effects? A meta-analysis of placebo-controlled trials. Lancet 350:834, 1997.
117. Gibson RG, Gibson SLM, MacNeil AD, et al: Salicylates and homeopathy in rheumatoid arthritis: preliminary observations. Br J Clin Pharmacol 6:391, 1978.
118. Gibson RG, Gibson SLM, MacNeil AD, et al: Homeopathic therapy in rheumatoid arthritis: evaluations by double-blind clinical therapeutic trial. Br J Clin Pharmacol 9:453, 1980.
119. Andrade LEC, Ferraz MB, Atra E, et al: A randomized controlled trial to evaluate the effectiveness of homeopathy in rheumatoid arthritis. Scan J Rheumatol 20:204, 1991.
120. Shipley M, Berry H, Broster G, et al: Controlled trial of homeopathic treatment of osteoarthritis. Lancet 1:96, 1983.

121. Fisher P, Greenwood A, Huskisson EC, et al: Effect of homeopathic treatment on fibrositis (primary fibromyalgia). BMJ 299:365, 1989.
122. Kaptchuk TJ: Acupuncture: theory, efficacy, practice. Ann Intern Med 136:374, 2002.
123. Riet Gt, Kleijnen J, Knipschild P: Acupuncture and chronic pain: a criteria-based meta-analysis. J Clin Epidemiol 43:1191, 1990.
124. Pomeranz B: Scientific research into acupuncture for the relief of pain. J Altern Compl Med 2:53, 1996.
125. van Tulder M, Cherkin DC, Berman B, et al: Acupuncture for low back pain (Cochrane Review). In the Cochrane Library, Issue 1, 2003. Oxford Update Software.
126. Ernst E, White AR: Acupuncture for back pain: a meta-analysis of randomized controlled trials. Arch Intern Med 158:2235, 1998.
127. Gaw AC, Chang LW, Shaw LC: Efficacy of acupuncture on osteoarthritic pain: a controlled, double-blind study. New Engl J Med 293:357, 1975.
128. Dickens W, Lewith GT: A single-blind controlled and randomized clinical trial to evaluate the effect of acupuncture in the treatment of trapezio-metacarpal osteoarthritis. Comp Med Res 3:508, 1989.
129. Lundberg T, Eriksson SV, Lundberg S, et al: Effect of acupuncture and naloxone in patients with osteoarthritis pain: a sham acupuncture controlled study. Pain Clin 4:155, 1991.
130. Thomas M, Eriksson SV, Lundberg T: A comparative study of diazepam and acupuncture in patients with osteoarthritic pain: a placebo-controlled study. Am J Clin Med 19:95, 1991.
131. Takeda W, Wessel J: Acupuncture for the treatment of pain of osteoarthritic knees. Arthritis Care Res 7:118, 1991.
132. Christensen BV, Iuhl IU, Vilbek H, et al: Acupuncture treatment of severe knee osteoarthritis: a long-term study. Acta Anaesthesiol Scand 36:519, 1992.
133. Mendelson G, Selwood TS, Kranz H, et al: Acupuncture treatment of chronic back pain: a double-blind placebo-controlled trial. Am J Med 74:49, 1983.
134. Ezzo J, Hadhazy V, Birch S, et al: Acupuncture for osteoarthritis of the knee: a systematic review. Arthritis Rheum 44:819, 2001.
135. Berman BM, Swyers JP: Complementary medicine treatments for fibromyalgia syndrome. Ballieres Clin Rheumatol 13:487, 1999.
136. Deluze C, Bosia L, Zirbs A, et al: Electroacupuncture in fibromyalgia: results of a controlled trial. BMJ 305:1249, 1992.
137. Sprott H, Kluge FS, Hein G: Pain treatment of fibromyalgia by acupuncture. Rheumatol Int 18:35, 1998.
138. Waylonis GW: Long-term follow-up on patients with fibrositis treated with acupuncture. Ohio State Med J 73:399, 1977.
139. Man SC, Bargar FD: Preliminary clinical study of acupuncture in rheumatoid arthritis. J Rheumatology 1:126, 1974.
140. Camberlain M, Leung CY, Santerre A, et al: Evaluation del acupuncture dans l'arthrite rheumatoide. Union Med Can 110:1041, 1981.
141. Bhatt-Sanders D: Acupuncture for rheumatoid arthritis: an analysis of the literature. Sem Arthritis Rheum 14:225, 1985.
142. Peterson JR: A focused view of the AHCPR guidelines on acute low back pain problems. I. Clinical care recommendations. J Clin Outcomes Manage 3:51, 1996.
143. Bigos SJ, Bowyer OR, Braen GR, et al: Acute Low Back Problems in Adults: Clinical Practice Guideline Number 14. Rockville, Agency for Health Care Policy and Research, Public Health Service, U. S. Department of Health and Human Services, 1994.
144. Meade TW, Dyer S, Browne W, et al: Low back pain of mechanical origin: randomized comparison of chiropractic and hospital outpatient treatment. BMJ 300:1431, 1990.
145. Cherkin DC, Deyo RA, Battie M, et al: A comparison of physical therapy, chiropractic manipulation, and provision of an educational booklet for the treatment of patients with low back pain. New Engl J Med 339:1021, 1998.
146. Blunt KL, Rajwani MH, Gurerriero RC: The effectiveness of chiropractic management of fibromyalgia patients: a pilot study. J Manipulative Physiol Ther 20:389, 1997.
147. Trock DH, Bollet AJ, Markoll R: The effect of pulsed electromagnetic fields in the treatment of osteoarthritis of the knee and cervical spine: report of randomized double-blind, placebo controlled trials. J Rheumatol 21:1903, 1994.
148. Zizic TM, Hoffman KC, Holt PA, et al: The treatment of osteoarthritis of the knee with pulsed electrical stimulation. J Rheumatol 22:1757, 1995.
149. Zizic TM, Hoffman KC, Caldwell J, et al: Effectiveness of treating rheumatoid arthritis of the hand with pulsed electrical stimulation. Arthritis Rheum 39:S283, 1996.
150. Vallbona C, Hazelwood CF, Jurida G: Response of pain to static magnetic fields in post-polio patients: a double-blind pilot study. Arch Phys Med Rehab 78:1200, 1997.
151. Jacobsen J, Gorman R, Yamanashi WS, et al: Low-amplitude, extremely low frequency magnetic fields for the treatment of osteoarthritic knees: a double-blind clinical study. Altern Ther Health Med 7:54, 66, 2001.
152. Carter R, Hall T, Aspy CB, et al: The effectiveness of magnet therapy for treatment of wrist pain attributed to carpal tunnel syndrome. J Fam Pract 51:38, 2002.
153. Collacott EA, Zimmerman JT, White DW, et al: Bipolar permanent magnets for the treatment of chronic low back pain: a pilot study. JAMA 283:1322, 2000.
154. Garfinkel MS, Shumacher HR, Husain A, et al: Evaluation of a yoga-based program for the treatment of osteoarthritis of the hands. J Rheumatology 21:2341, 1994.
155. Haslock I, Monro R, Nagrathna R, et al: Measuring the effects of yoga in rheumatoid arthritis. J Rheumatol 33:787, 1994.
156. Garfinkel MS, Singhal A, Katz WA, et al: Yoga-based intervention for carpal tunnel syndrome: a randomized trial. JAMA 280:1601, 1998.
157. Kirsteins AE, Dietz F, Hwang SM: Evaluating the safety and potential use of a weight-bearing exercise, Tai-Chi Chuan, for rheumatoid arthritis patients. Am J Phys Med Rehabil 70:136, 1991.
158. Wolf SL, Barnhart HX, Kutner NG, et al: Reducing frailty and falls in older persons: an investigation of Tai Chi and computerized balance training. J Am Geriatr Soc 44:489, 1996.
159. Hartman CA, Manos TM, Winter C, et al: Effects of T'ai Chi training on function and quality of life indicators in older adults with osteoarthritis. J Am Geriatr Soc 48:1553, 2000.
160. Furlan AD, Brosseau L, Imamura M, et al: Massage for low back pain: a systematic review within the framework of the Cochrane Collaboration Back Review Group. Spine 27:1896, 2002.
161. G. Gallup Jr, Lindsey DM: Surveying the Religious Landscape: Trends in U. S. Beliefs. Harrisburg, Morehouse Publishing, 1999.
162. The mystery of prayer: Does God play favorites? Newsweek, May 20, 1998:56.
163. Faith and healing: Can prayer, faith, and spirituality really improve your physical health? Time June 24, 1996:58..
164. The new faith in medicine: believing in God may be good for your health according to the latest research. USA Weekend. April 5-7, 1996.
165. King DE, Bushwick B: Beliefs and attitudes of hospital inpatients about faith, healing and prayer. Fam Pract 39:349, 1994.
166. Roberts JA, Brian D, Elkins T, et al: Factors influencing views of patients with gynecologic cancer about end-of-life decisions. Am J Obstet Gynecol 176:166, 1997.
167. O'Brien ME: Religious faith and adjustment to long-term hemodialysis. J Religion Health 21:68, 1982.
168. O'Connor BB: Healing Traditions: Alternative Medicine and the Health Professions. Philadelphia, University of Pennsylvania Press, 1995.
169. Koenig HG: Use of religion by patients with severe medical illness. Mind Body Med 2:31, 1997.
170. Koenig HG, Cohen JH, George LK, et al: Attendance at religious services, interleukin-6 and other biological indicators of immune function in older adults. Int J Psychosom Med 27:233, 1997.
171. National Institute on Aging–Fetzer Institute Working Group. Multidimensional Measurement of Religiousness/Spirituality for Use in Health Care Research. Bethesda, MD: John L. Fetzer Institute Publishers, 1999.
172. Matthews DA: Religion and spirituality in primary care. Mind Body Med 2:9, 1997.
173. Abraodo-Lanza AF, Guerier C, Revenson TA: Coping and social support resources among Latinos with arthritis. Arthritis Care Res 9:501, 1996.
174. Matthews DA, Larson DB, Barry CB: The Faith Factor. Vol. 1. An Annotated Bibliography of Clinical Research on Spiritual Subjects. Rockville, MD, National Institute for Healthcare Research, 1993.

175. Matthews DA, Larson DB, Barry CB: The Faith Factor. Vol. 2. An Annotated Bibliography of Clinical Research on Spiritual Subjects. Rockville, MD, National Institute for Healthcare Research;,1993.
176. Matthews DA, Larson DB: The Faith Factor. Vol. 3. Enhancing Life Satisfaction. Rockville, MD, National Institute for Healthcare Research, 1995.
177. Matthews DA, Saunders DM: The Faith Factor. Vol. 4. Prevention and Treatment of Illness. Rockville, MD, National Institute for Healthcare Research, 1997.
178. Park Ridge Center for the Study of Faith, Health, and Ethics: Health/Medicine and the Faith Traditions. Vols. 1-12. Chicago, Crossroad, 1983-1993.
179. Park Ridge Center for the Study of Faith, Health, and Ethics: Health/Medicine and the Faith Traditions. Vols. 13-14. Chicago,Trinity Press International, 1993-1995.
180. Byrd RC: Positive effects of intercessory prayer in a coronary care unit population. South Med J 81:826, 1988.
181. Harris WS, Gowda M, Kolb JW, et al: A randomized, controlled trial of the effects of remote, intercessory prayer on outcomes in patients admitted to the coronary care unit. Arch Intern Med 159:2273, 1999.
182. Matthews DA, Marlowe SM, MacNutt FS: Effects of intercessory prayer on patients with rheumatoid arthritis. South Med J 93:1177, 2000.

SECTION V

Evaluation of Generalized and Localized Symptoms

33 History and Physical Examination of the Musculoskeletal System

KEVIN G. MODER • GENE G. HUNDER

History in the Patient with Musculoskeletal Disease

A detailed description of musculoskeletal symptoms often provides much of the information needed for making a diagnosis. The goal of the interview is to understand precisely what the patient means when describing symptoms. In taking a history of the patient's illness, the physician must probe for details regarding the sequence and severity of symptoms and the patterns of progression, exacerbation, or remission. The effects of associated diseases and other life stressors must be elucidated. The functional impact of the disease on the patient should be assessed.

The effects of current or previous therapy on the course of the illness are helpful in understanding current symptoms. Assessment of compliance is extremely important; even an ideal therapeutic regimen will fail if the patient does not comply with the outlined program. Therefore, communication with the patient is essential in regard to the anticipated effect and the timing of this effect when a new medication is introduced. Sometimes, patients describe a medication as a failure when they have not had an adequate course of therapy. This is especially true in trying to assess the efficacy of slow-acting agents.

The patient's behavior often provides clues to the nature of the illness and the response to it. It is important to determine whether the patient is reacting appropriately to an illness. On occasion, a patient either will be overly concerned or will inappropriately ignore the symptoms. In addition, it is important to recognize that the patient's understanding of the illness affects the response to it.

PAIN

Pain is the complaint that most commonly brings the patient with musculoskeletal disease to the physician. Pain is a complex, subjective sensation that is difficult to define, qualify, or measure. The patient's response to pain is affected by current emotional state as well as by previous experiences.

The examiner must elicit the distribution of the patient's pain and determine if it fits with an anatomic structure. Sometimes patients use terms in a nonanatomic manner. For example, the patient may complain of hip pain when actually the patient is describing pain in the buttock or thigh. To clarify this, it is often helpful to ask the patient to point to the area of pain with a finger. If the pain is in a joint, an articular disorder is likely to be present. Pain between joints may suggest bone or muscle disease or referred pain. Pain in bursal areas, in fascial planes, or along tendons, ligaments, or nerve distributions suggests disease in these structures. Pain arising from deeper structures is often less focal than pain originating from superficial tissues. Pain in small joints of the hands or feet tends to be localized more accurately than pain in larger, more proximal joints such as the shoulder, hip, or spine. When pain is diffuse, variable, poorly described, or unrelated to anatomic structures, fibromyalgia, malingering, or psychologic problems should be considered.

The character of pain is helpful in understanding the patient's illness. For example, "aching" in a joint area suggests an arthritic disorder, whereas "burning" or "numbness" in an extremity may indicate a neuropathy. It is important to ask about the severity of pain. Many physicians find it helpful to ask the patient to describe pain on a numeric scale from 1 to 10. Description of "intolerable" or "excruciating" pain in a patient who is otherwise able to perform normal activities provides a clue that emotional factors may be playing a role in amplifying symptoms.

It is useful to determine whether pain is present at rest. Joint pain present at rest but worse with movement is more suggestive of an inflammatory process, whereas pain mainly during or after activity can indicate a mechanical disorder such as degenerative arthritis. As discussed in the next section, the time of day when the pain or stiffness occurs can yield valuable information.

STIFFNESS

Stiffness has different meanings to different patients. Some equate it with pain or fatigue and others to soreness, weakness, or restrictions of movement. Most rheumatologists define stiffness as discomfort perceived by the patient attempting to move joints after a period of inactivity. When it occurs, stiffness or "gelling" usually develops after 1 or more hours of inactivity. Mild stiffness may resolve within a few minutes. When severe, as in rheumatoid arthritis or polymyalgia rheumatica, the stiffness may persist for hours.

Morning stiffness can be a prodromal symptom of rheumatoid arthritis or other inflammatory arthritis, and it is a criterion of the American College of Rheumatology for the diagnosis of rheumatoid arthritis (see Chapter 66). Morning stiffness associated with noninflammatory joint diseases is almost always of short duration (usually less than half an hour) and less severe than stiffness of inflammatory joint disease. In addition, in mechanical or degenerative joint disease, the degree of stiffness is related to the extent of use of the damaged joint. After excessive use it is worse, and it generally improves within a few days with rest. Although the absence of stiffness does not exclude the possibility of a systemic inflammatory disease such as rheumatoid arthritis, its absence is uncommon. Stiffness from neurologic disorders such as Parkinson's disease also occurs, although the "limbering up" component is usually lacking.

LIMITATION OF MOTION

Patients with rheumatic disorders frequently complain of limitation of motion. This complaint must be distinguished from stiffness; stiffness is usually transient and variable, whereas true limitation in motion is more fixed and varies less over time. Determination of the extent of disability resulting from lack of motion is important. The duration of restriction of motion often predicts the likelihood of recovery with interventions such as medications and physical therapy. Whether the limitation of motion in a joint exists with active *and* passive motion should be ascertained. This can usually be determined by the physician at the physical examination. It is helpful to know whether the limitation of motion began abruptly, which would be more suggestive of a mechanic derangement, such as a tendon rupture, or if the onset was gradual, as is more common with inflammatory joint disease.

SWELLING

Joint swelling is an important finding in patients with rheumatic disease. The presence of true joint swelling (true arthritis) helps to narrow the differential diagnosis in a patient who complains of arthralgias. The interviewer needs to determine where and when the swelling occurs. It is often difficult for the patient to recognize swelling, and, not infrequently, the patient describes a feeling of swelling when an actual effusion is not present. Description of the exact location of the swelling helps in understanding whether the swelling conforms to an anatomically discrete area, such as a particular joint, bursa, or other specific extra-articular area. An obese person may interpret normal collections of adipose tissue over the medial aspect of the elbow or knee and lateral aspect of the ankle as joint swelling.

It is useful to gain information about the onset and persistence of the swelling and the factors that influence it. Discomfort with use of the swollen part may indicate synovitis or bursitis because of tension on these tissues during motion of a joint. On the other hand, if swollen, inflamed tissues are not put under stress during joint movement, pain is minimal; for example, movement of the knee is generally painless in cases of prepatellar bursitis. Swelling in a confined area, such as a synovial sac or bursa, is most painful when it has developed acutely, whereas a similar degree of swelling that has developed slowly is often much more tolerable.

WEAKNESS

Many patients complain of weakness, but the physician needs to ascertain exactly what is meant by this. Often patients will use the term *weakness* to describe other entities, most commonly fatigue. Weakness is the true loss of muscle power. When present, it should be demonstrable on examination.

Weakness may occur secondary to dysfunction of muscle, neurologic disorders, or as part of a systemic illness. It is important to question the patient about the timing of the symptom. Sudden onset of weakness is more often seen with a neurologic disorder, such as an acute cerebrovascular event. These events often result in a deficit that is fixed but not progressive. Insidious onset of weakness is more suggestive of a muscular disorder such as an inflammatory myopathy (polymyositis or dermatomyositis). These conditions tend to be ongoing and progressive. Therefore, the patient should be questioned about whether or not the weakness is worsening. Intermittent weakness could be suggestive of a disorder of the neuromuscular junction, such as myasthenia gravis. Patients with this disorder may describe easy fatigue of the muscles rather than true weakness.

The distribution of the weakness should also be ascertained. Proximal weakness can be more suggestive of an inflammatory myopathy. Generally, inflammatory myopathies also tend to be bilateral with symmetric weakness. This is in contrast to inclusion body myositis, which can cause an asymmetric and more distal weakness. The description of unilateral or isolated deficits would be more suggestive of neurologic etiology.

Neurologic disorders such as peripheral neuropathies more commonly cause distal symptoms. In addition, patients with peripheral neuropathies usually complain of pain and describe sensory symptoms such as paresthesias. This is in contrast to patients with inflammatory myopathies, who usually present with painless weakness.

It is important to inquire about the patient's family. If other family members have had similar symptoms, a hereditary disorder such as muscular dystrophy or a familial neuropathy may need to be considered. The patient should also be questioned about prior episodes of weakness. For example, in a patient with a history of polio who has developed a postpolio syndrome, more prominent weakness in the same distribution develops years later.

It is important to question the patient about any medications taken currently or recently. Many common medications, including corticosteroids and lipid-lowering agents, can cause myopathy. Less commonly, environmental exposures could lead to symptoms of weakness. For example, heavy metal poisoning causes a peripheral neuropathy. In terms of diet, patients should be questioned about the eating of undercooked pork as a risk for trichinosis. Excessive alcohol intake has also been associated with both neuropathy and myopathy.

A complete review of systems is also helpful in evaluating the patient with weakness. Significant weight loss may suggest another systemic process, such as a malignancy, that may produce symptoms of generalized weakness. Rash, arthralgias, or Raynaud's syndrome may prompt further evaluation for an underlying connective tissue disease

FATIGUE

Fatigue is a common complaint of patients with musculoskeletal disease. Fatigue can be defined as an inclination to rest even though pain and weakness are not limiting factors. Fatigue is a normal phenomenon after variable degrees of activity but should resolve after rest. In rheumatic diseases, fatigue may be prominent even when the patient has not been active. Typically, if the systemic rheumatic disease improves, so does the degree of fatigue. Malaise often occurs with fatigue but is not a synonymous term. Malaise is an indefinite feeling of lack of health that frequently occurs at the onset of an illness. Both fatigue and malaise can be seen in the absence of identifiable organic disease, and anxiety, tension, stress, and emotional factors can play a role.

Patients with inflammatory arthritis may use the terms *fatigue* and *weakness* interchangeably and often confuse stiffness with these. The differentiation of fatigue from stiffness and weakness may be facilitated by remembering that stiffness is a discomfort during movement, and weakness is an inability to move normally, especially against resistance. Fatigue is an inclination to rest because of a sense of exhaustion, not because of muscle weakness or pain.

Systematic Method of Examination

As with other parts of the general physical examination, a systematic method of examining joints is the best way to obtain a thorough assessment of the status of the joints. Many rheumatologists begin with the joints of the upper extremities and proceed to the joints of the trunk and lower extremity, but each examiner should establish his or her own routine. Gentle handling of tender and painful joints enhances cooperation by the patient and allows an accurate evaluation of the joints.[1-5]

IMPORTANT PHYSICAL SIGNS OF ARTHRITIS

The general aim of the examination of the joints is to detect abnormalities in structure and function.[6] The common signs of articular disease are swelling, tenderness, limitation of motion, crepitation, deformity, and instability.

Swelling

Swelling around a joint may be caused by intra-articular effusion, synovial thickening, or periarticular subcutaneous tissue inflammation; it may be expressed as bursitis, tendinitis, bony enlargement, or extra-articular fat pads. Familiarity with the anatomic configuration of the synovial membrane in various joints aids in differentiating soft tissue swelling due to synovitis (true articular effusion or synovial thickening) from swelling of the periarticular tissues. A joint effusion is often visible on observation of a joint. It is helpful to compare joints of one side of the body with those of the other for evidence of symmetry (or asymmetry). The presence of palpable fluid in a joint in the absence of recent trauma usually indicates synovitis.

The normal synovial membrane is too thin to palpate, whereas the thickened synovial membrane in many chronic inflammatory arthritides such as rheumatoid arthritis may have a "doughy" or "boggy" consistency. In some joints, such as the knee, the extent of the synovial cavity can be delineated on physical examination by compressing the fluid into one of the extreme limits of synovial reflection. The edge of the resulting bulge may thus be palpated more easily. If this palpable edge is within the anatomic confines of the synovial membrane and disappears on release of the compression, the distention usually represents synovial effusion; if it persists, it is an indication of a thickened synovial membrane. However, reliable differentiation between synovial membrane thickening and effusion is not always possible by physical examination. Occasionally, intrasynovial loose bodies or plicae may be palpated.

Tenderness

Tenderness is an unusual sensitivity to touch or pressure. Localization of tenderness to palpation may help to determine whether the pathologic condition is in an articular or periarticular structure, such as a fat pad, tendon attachment, ligament, bursa, muscle, or skin. Palpation of noninvolved structures helps assess the significance of tenderness. For example, the finding of a tender joint in a patient who also has numerous other extra-articular tender points is less suggestive of arthritis than the finding the tender joint in the absence of other nonarticular tender tissues.

Limitation of Motion

Because limitation of motion is a common manifestation of articular disease, it is important to know the normal type and range of motion of each joint. Comparison of an unaffected joint of the opposite extremity helps evaluate individual variations. Restriction in joint motion may be related to changes in the joint itself or in periarticular structures. In many patients, passive range of motion is often greater than active motion; this may be the result of pain, weakness, or the state of the articular or periarticular structures. It is important that the patient be relaxed during the examination, because increased muscle tension may result in what appears to be significantly decreased range of motion. Stressing passive joint motion at the extremes of flexion and extension is sometimes helpful in assessing joint tenderness. Pain in the joint with attempted active motion usually indicates an abnormality in the joint or periarticular tissues.

Crepitation

Crepitation is a palpable, audible, or both grating or crunching sensation produced by motion. It may or may not be accompanied by pain. Crepitation occurs when roughened articular or extra-articular surfaces are rubbed together by active motion or by manual compression. Fine crepitation is often palpable over joints involved in chronic inflammatory arthritis and usually indicates roughening of the opposing cartilage surfaces as a result of erosion or the presence of granulation tissue. Coarse crepitation may be caused by inflammatory or noninflammatory arthritis. Bone-on-bone crepitus produces a higher-frequency, palpable, and audible squeak. Crepitation from within a joint should be differentiated from cracking or popping sounds caused by the slipping of ligaments or tendons over bony surfaces during motion, which are usually less significant to the diagnosis of joint disease and may be heard over normal joints. In scleroderma, a distinct, coarse, creaking, leathery crepitation may be palpable, audible, or both, especially over tendon sheaths.

Deformity

Deformity is the malalignment of joints and may manifest as a bony enlargement, articular subluxation, contracture, or ankylosis in nonanatomic positions. Deformed joints do not function normally, frequently restrict activities, and may be associated with pain, especially when put to stressful use. On occasion, a deformed joint may retain good functional use but be more of a cosmetic concern. In these cases, surgical correction should be approached with caution because a deformed joint that functions satisfactorily has more utility than a cosmetically altered joint that does not.

Instability

Joint instability is present when the joint has greater-than-normal movement in any plane. Subluxation refers to a joint in which there is partial displacement of the articular surfaces but still some joint surface-to-surface contact. A dislocated joint has lost all cartilage surface-to-surface contact. Instability is best determined by supporting the joint between the examiner's hands and stressing the adjacent bones in directions in which the normal joint does not move. The patient must be relaxed during the examination, because muscle tension may serve to stabilize an otherwise unstable joint. For example, a knee with a deficient ligament might appear stable if the patient contracts the quadriceps muscles during evaluation.

OTHER ASPECTS OF THE EXAMINATION

Examinations of the cervical spine and low back are discussed in Chapters 37 and 39, respectively.

Recording the Joint Examination

A permanent record of the joint examination is important in evaluating the extent and activity of arthritic disease and in determining the efficacy of interventions. Many recording methods have been described. Abbreviations for each joint can be used, such as PIP for the proximal interphalangeal joints. A simple system called the S-T-L system records the degree of swelling (S), tenderness (T), and limitation of motion (L) of each joint based on a quantitative estimate of gradation.[7] The system of grades ranges from 0 (normal) to 4 (highly abnormal). The scoring of the degree of swelling and tenderness is semiqualitative, but the examiner should endeavor to be consistent from patient to patient and over time. A score of 1 indicates a small effusion or mild tenderness, whereas a 3 indicates a large effusion or significant tenderness. In the case of limitation of motion, grade 1 may be used to indicate about 25 percent loss of motion; grade 2, about 50 percent loss; grade 3, about 75 percent loss; and grade 4, ankylosis. For example, a moderately swollen, mildly tender but unlimited second right metacarpophalangeal joint would have an abbreviated score of R_2MCP: $S_2T_1L_0$. If many joints are abnormal, a table can be constructed with a column for S, T, and L and the findings recorded for each joint.

In a patient with limited disease, it is easier to record only the joints that are abnormal in narrative form. Examiners with more experience may add additional degrees to the scoring system after each numeral (e.g., 1− or 1+) to give a wider scale. Alternatively, one may use intermediate scores, such as 1 to 2, to further widen the scale. However, use of the aforementioned system will suffice in most instances. When more accuracy is desired, one can estimate and record the degrees of motion in a joint or measure the motion in joints by using a goniometer.

An attractive alternative method of recording the joint examination findings, especially useful in patients with multiple joint involvement, is a schematic skeleton with marked articulations that may be used to record the status of individual joints (Fig. 33–1).

Assessment of the degree of disease activity can involve calculation of the total number of tender or swollen joints, or both, and the use of this number as a joint count or joint index. Other systems, which may be inefficient and cumbersome for daily office use but may

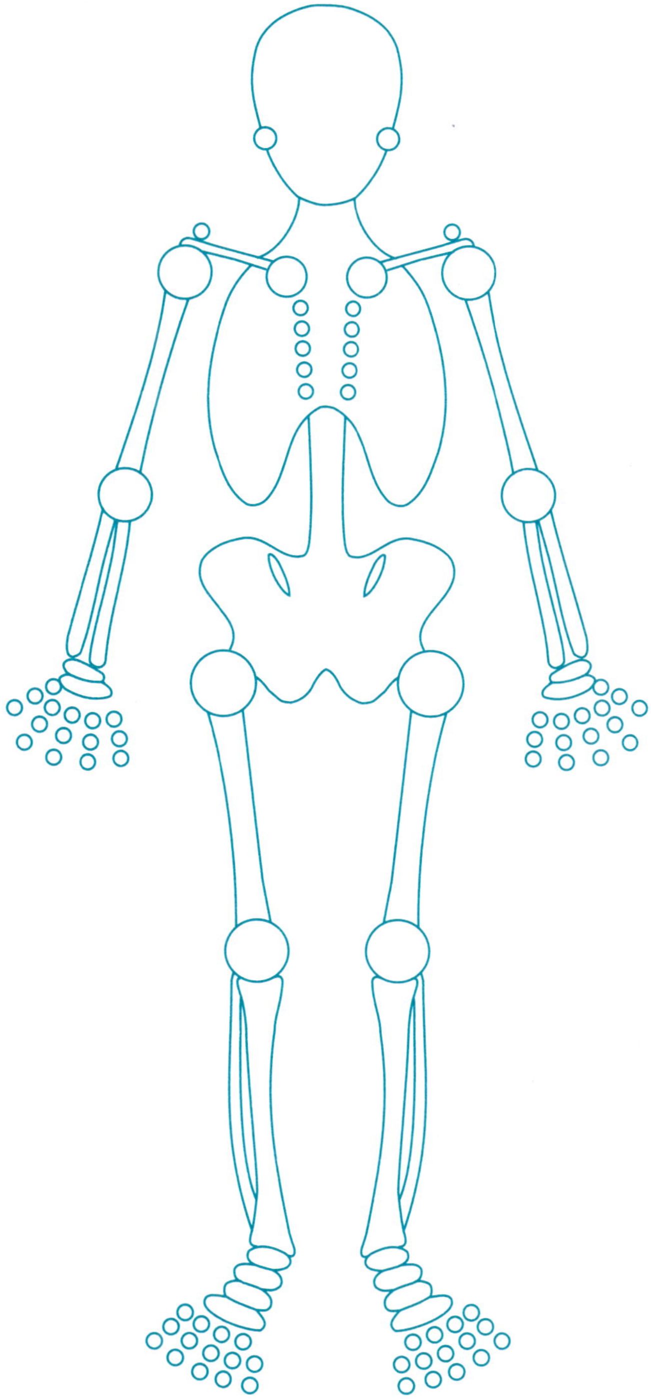

FIGURE 33–1 · Skeleton diagram for recording joint examination findings. (From Polley HF, Hunder GG: Rheumatologic Interviewing and Physical Examination of the Joints, 2nd ed. Philadelphia, WB Saunders, 1978, p 43.)

have value in academic studies, include measurement of the size of joints by use of a tape measure or jeweler's rings, determination of the degree of warmth by use of thermography, and measurement of the amount of tenderness by use of a dolorimeter.

Although the previously described tests and examinations can give a physical description of the joints, they do not necessarily measure function. A sense of joint function can be assessed in part by use of grip strength testing. The patient's grip strength can be measured by asking a patient to squeeze a partially inflated (20 mmHg) sphygmomanometer cuff or through use of a dynamometer. Other tests are available that attempt to measure functional use of joints by determining the ability to perform and the speed of other specified coordinated functions (e.g., measuring the 50-foot walk time). All of these functional tests, however, have an inherent tendency toward variability of results. For observations such as joint tenderness or grip strength, interobserver variability is often greater than intraobserver variability. There may be significant intraobserver variability in observations of the same patient, even over a short interval. Furthermore, biologic factors contribute to variability, such as the circadian changes in joint size and grip strength among rheumatoid patients observed during a 24-hour interval. These tests are best suited for research studies and tend to be less useful in observing individual patients.

Examination of Specific Joints

TEMPOROMANDIBULAR JOINT

The temporomandibular joint is formed by the condyle of the mandible and the fossa of the temporal bone just anterior to the external auditory canal. It is difficult to visibly note swelling in this joint. The joint is palpated by placing a finger just anterior to the external auditory canal and asking the patient to open and close the mouth and to move the mandible from side to side. Because of normal differences in soft tissue thickness, the presence of synovial thickness or swelling of minimal or moderate degree can be detected most easily if the synovitis is unilateral or asymmetric by comparison with the other side. Vertical movement of the temporomandibular joint can be measured by determining the space between the upper and lower incisor teeth with the patient's mouth open maximally. This distance is normally 3 to 6 cm. Lateral movement can be determined by using incisor teeth as landmarks. Audible or palpable crepitus or clicking may be noted in patients with and without evidence of severe arthritis.

Many forms of arthritis can affect the temporomandibular joints, including juvenile and adult rheumatoid arthritis. In children, if these joints are affected, there may be an arrest of bone growth of the mandible with resultant micrognathia. Some patients without inflammatory arthritis describe arthralgias of the temporomandibular joint, and many of these fit the temporomandibular joint syndrome. This syndrome is thought by some to result from bruxism and is likely to be a form of myofascial pain. This syndrome may often be seen in patients with other types of myofascial pain, such as fibromyalgia.

CRICOARYTENOID JOINTS

The paired cricoarytenoid joints are formed by the articulation of the base of the small pyramidal arytenoid cartilage and the upper posterolateral border of the cricoid cartilage. The vocal ligaments (true vocal cords) are attached to the arytenoid cartilages. The cricoarytenoid joints are normally mobile diarthrodial joints that move medially and laterally and rotate during the opening and closing of the vocal cords. Examination of these joints is performed by direct or indirect laryngoscopy. Erythema, swelling, and lack of mobility during phonation may result from inflammation of the joints. The cricoarytenoid joints may be affected in rheumatoid arthritis, trauma, and infection. Involvement in rheumatoid arthritis is more common than clinically apparent. Symptoms may include hoarseness or a sense of fullness or discomfort in the throat, which is worse when speaking or swallowing. Significant airway obstruction has been reported infrequently.

STERNOCLAVICULAR, MANUBRIOSTERNAL, AND STERNOCOSTAL JOINTS

The medial ends of the clavicles articulate on each side of the sternum at its upper end to form the sternoclavicular joints. The articulations of the first ribs and the sternum (sternocostal joints) are immediately caudad. The articulation of the manubrium and body of the sternum is at the level of the attachment of the second costal cartilage to the sternum. The third through seventh sternocostal joints articulate distally along the lateral borders of the sternum. The sternoclavicular joints are the only articulations in this group that are always diarthrodial; the others are amphiarthroses or synchondroses. The sternoclavicular joints are the only true points of articulation of the shoulder girdle with the trunk. These joints are just beneath the skin; therefore, synovitis is usually visible and palpable. These joints have only slight movement, which cannot be accurately measured.

Involvement of the sternoclavicular joints is common in ankylosing spondylitis, rheumatoid arthritis, and degenerative arthritis but is frequently not recognized. The sternoclavicular joint may be the site of septic arthritis, especially in intravenous drug abusers. Tenderness of the manubriosternal or costosternal joints is much more frequent than actual swelling. Tenderness of these joints without actual swelling has been termed costochondritis; Tietze's syndrome may be the term used if there is actual swelling observed or palpable.

ACROMIOCLAVICULAR JOINT

The acromioclavicular joint is formed by the lateral end of the clavicle and medial margin of the acromion process of the scapula. Bony enlargement of this joint, secondary to degenerative arthritis, may be seen in middle-aged or older persons, but soft tissue swelling is not usually visible or palpable. Tenderness over the joint and pain with adduction of the arm across the chest suggest involvement of this joint. Arthritis of the acromioclavicular joint is usually secondary to trauma leading to degenerative disease. It is not usually significantly affected by rheumatoid arthritis. Movement occurs at this joint during shoulder motion, but the extent of motion is difficult to measure accurately.

SHOULDER

See Chapter 38.

ELBOW

The elbow joint is composed of three bony articulations. The principal articulation is the humeroulnar joint, which is a hinge joint. The radiohumeral and proximal radioulnar articulations allow rotation of the forearm (Fig. 33–2).

To examine the elbow joint, the examiner's thumb is placed between the lateral epicondyle and the olecranon process in the lateral paraolecranon groove, and one or two fingers are placed in the corresponding groove medial to the olecranon. The elbow should be relaxed and moved passively through flexion, extension, and rotation. One should carefully examine the skin about the elbow joint. In rheumatoid arthritis patients, the examiner may be able to palpate or visually observe nodules. In patients with psoriasis, plaques are often present over the extensor surface of the elbow.

Limitation of motion and crepitus may be noted. Synovial swelling is most easily palpated as it bulges under the examiner's thumb when the elbow is passively extended. Synovial membrane sometimes can be palpated over the posterior aspect of the joint between the olecranon process and distal humerus. Synovitis is frequently associated with limitation of joint extension.

The olecranon bursa overlies the olecranon process of the ulna. Olecranon bursitis is common after

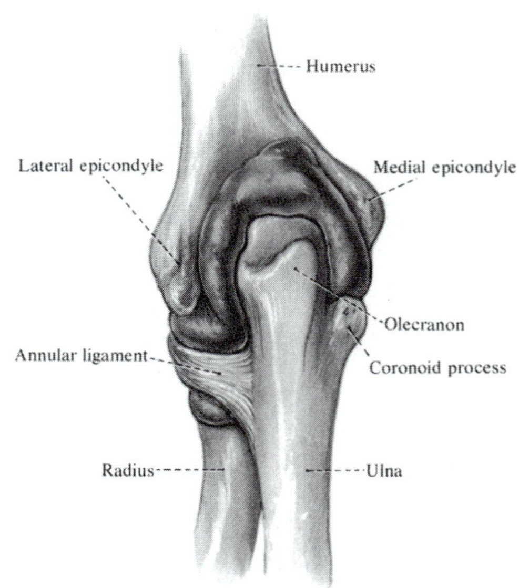

FIGURE 33–2 • Posterior aspect of the elbow joint showing radius and ulna in extension and distribution of synovial membrane in distention. (From Polley HF, Hunder GG: Rheumatologic Interviewing and Physical Examination of the Joints, 2nd ed. Philadelphia, WB Saunders, 1978, p 82.)

chronic local trauma and in rheumatic diseases, including rheumatoid arthritis and gout. A septic olecranon bursitis may occur. A patient who has olecranon bursitis usually presents with a swelling over the olecranon process, which is often tender and may be erythematous. Sometimes there is a large collection of fluid over the area, which is palpable as a cystic mass and often requires aspiration and drainage. There is generally no pain with elbow movement.

The medial and lateral epicondyles of the humerus are tendinous attachment sites. These areas may be tender without other objective signs of inflammation in conditions thought to result from overuse, such as tennis elbow (lateral epicondylitis) and golfer's elbow (medial epicondylitis). In addition to localized tenderness on palpation, discomfort can be elicited in medial epicondylitis by resisted flexion of the supinated wrist. In lateral epicondylitis, supination of the forearm or extension of the pronated wrist against resistance elicits pain localized to the lateral epicondyle. Treatment with ice, use of forearm splints, anti-inflammatory medications, rest, and occasionally local injection of the painful tendon are usually helpful.

Muscle function of the elbow can be assessed by testing flexion and extension. The prime movers of flexion are the biceps brachii (nerve roots C5 and C6), brachialis (C5 and C6), and brachioradialis (C5 and C6) muscles. The prime mover of extension is the triceps brachii muscle (C7 and C8). On occasion, a patient may rupture the attachment site of one of the heads of the biceps. This results in a visible and palpable muscle swelling on the anterior upper arm.

WRIST AND CARPAL JOINTS

The wrist is a complex joint formed by several articulations between the radius, ulna, and carpal bones. The true wrist or radiocarpal articulation (see also Chapter 42) is a biaxial ellipsoid joint formed proximally by the distal end of the radius and the triangular fibrocartilage and distally by a row of three carpal bones: scaphoid (navicular), lunate, and triquetrum (triangular). The distal radioulnar joint is a uniaxial pivot joint. The midcarpal joints are formed by the junction of the proximal and distal rows of the carpal bones. The midcarpal and carpometacarpal articular cavities often communicate. The intercarpal joints refer to the articulations between the individual carpal bones.

Movements of the wrist include palmar flexion (flexion), dorsiflexion (extension), radial deviation, ulnar deviation, and circumduction. Pronation and supination of the hand and forearm occur primarily at the proximal and distal radioulnar joints. The only carpometacarpal joint that moves to a significant degree is the carpometacarpal joint of the thumb. This joint is saddle shaped (sella) and possesses 3 degrees of freedom. Crepitus at this joint is common because it is frequently involved in degenerative arthritis.

The wrist can normally be extended to about 70 or 80 degrees and flexed to 80 or 90 degrees. Ulnar and radial deviation should allow 50 degrees and 20 to 30 degrees of movement, respectively. Loss of dorsiflexion is the most incapacitating functional impairment of wrist motion.

The long flexor tendons of the forearm musculature cross the palmar surface of the wrist and are enclosed in the flexor tendon sheath under the flexor retinaculum (transverse carpal ligament). The flexor retinaculum and the underlying carpal bones form the carpal tunnel. The median nerve passes through the carpal tunnel superficial to the flexor tendons. The extensor tendons of the forearm pass under the extensor retinaculum and are enclosed in a synovial sheath.

The palmar aponeurosis (fascia) spreads out into the palm from the flexor retinaculum. Dupuytren's contracture is a fibrosing condition affecting the palmar aponeurosis, which becomes thickened and contracted and may draw one or more fingers into flexion at the metacarpophalangeal joint. The fourth finger is frequently affected first.

Swelling of the wrist may be due to inflammation involving the sheaths of the tendons crossing the wrist or the wrist joint itself, or both. When swelling is due to tenosynovitis, the outpouching tends to be more localized and is altered by flexing and extending the fingers. Articular swelling tends to be more diffuse and protrudes anteriorly and posteriorly from under the tendons.

Synovitis of the wrist joint is more reliably detected by palpation over the dorsal surface. Because of the structures overlying both surfaces of the wrist, accurate localization of the synovial margins is difficult. To examine the wrist, the physician should palpate the joint gently between the thumb and fingers. Prominence or thickening of the synovium may be noted; if significant, it will have the characteristics of true synovitis.

A ganglion is a cystic enlargement arising from a joint capsule; it characteristically occurs on the dorsum of the wrist between the extensor tendons.

Subluxation of the ulna may occur secondary to chronic inflammatory arthritis. The subluxed ulna appears as a prominence on the dorsolateral wrist and may press against the extensor tendons, especially those of the fourth and fifth digits. Potentially, these tendons can rupture (Fig. 33–3).

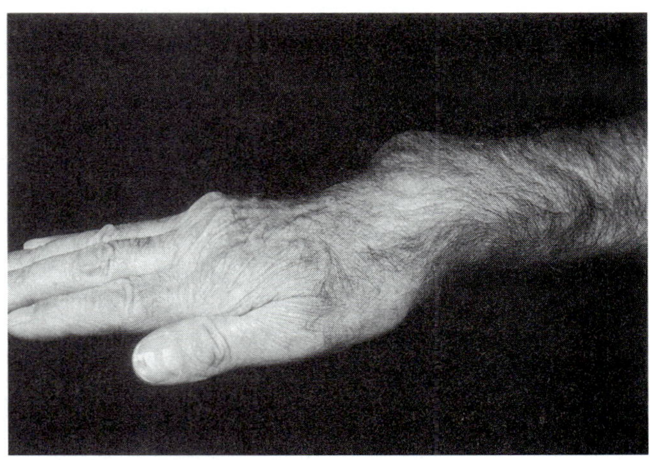

FIGURE 33–3 · Subluxation of the Wrist. Side view of the wrist of a patient with rheumatoid arthritis. Note the prominence of the ulna.

Trigger fingers can be detected by palpating crepitus or nodules along the tendons in the palm while the patient slowly flexes and extends the fingers. The patient usually gives a history of the affected finger's catching or locking with movement.

Stenosing tenosynovitis occurs commonly at the radial styloid process (de Quervain's tenosynovitis) and characteristically involves the long abductor and short extensor tendons of the thumb. Patients usually localize pain to the radial side of the wrist, and tenderness is often elicited by palpation near the radial styloid process. The Finkelstein test for de Quervain's tenosynovitis is done by having the patient make a fist with the thumb in the palm of the hand. The examiner then moves the patient's wrist into ulnar deviation. The development of severe pain over the radial styloid is a positive finding and is caused by the stretching of thumb tendons in the stenosed tendon sheath.

Carpal tunnel syndrome results from pressure on the median nerve in the carpal tunnel and is discussed in detail in Chapter 42.

Muscle function of the wrist can be measured by testing flexion and extension as well as supination and pronation of the forearm. Prime movers in wrist flexion are the flexor carpi radialis (C6 and C7) and flexor carpi ulnaris (C8 and T1) muscles. Each of these muscles can be tested separately. This can be accomplished if the examiner provides resistance to flexion at the base of the second metacarpal bone in the direction of extension, ulnar deviation in the case of the flexor carpi radialis and resistance at the base of the fifth metacarpal in the direction of extension, and radial deviation in the case of the flexor carpi ulnaris. The prime extensors of the wrist are the extensor carpi radialis longus (C6 and C7), extensor carpi radialis brevis (C6 and C7), and extensor carpi ulnaris (C7 and C8) muscles. The radial and ulnar extensor muscles can be tested separately. Prime movers in supination of the forearm are the biceps brachii (C5 and C6) and supinator (C6). Prime movers in pronation are the pronator teres (C6 and C7) and pronator quadratus (C8 and T1).

METACARPOPHALANGEAL AND PROXIMAL AND DISTAL INTERPHALANGEAL JOINTS

The metacarpophalangeal joints are hinge joints. Lateral collateral ligaments that are loose in extension tighten in flexion, thereby preventing lateral movement of the digits. The extensor tendons that cross the dorsum of each joint strengthen the articular capsule. When the extensor tendon of the digit reaches the distal end of the metacarpal head, it is joined by fibers of the interossei and lumbricales and expands over the entire dorsum of the metacarpophalangeal joint and onto the dorsum of the adjacent phalanx. This expansion of the extensor mechanism is known as the extensor hood.

The proximal and distal interphalangeal joints are also hinge joints. The ligaments of the interphalangeal joints resemble those of the metacarpophalangeal joints. When the fingers are flexed, the bases of the proximal phalanges slide toward the palmar side of the heads of the metacarpal bones. The metacarpal heads form the rounded prominences of the knuckle, with the metacarpal joint spaces situated about 1 cm distal to the apex of the prominences.

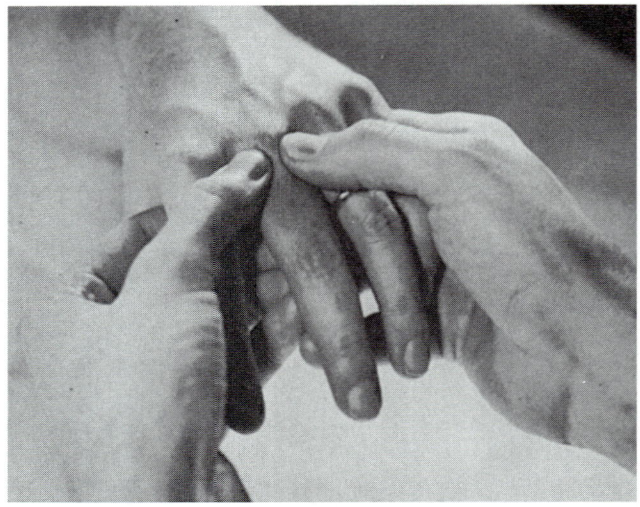

FIGURE 33–4 · Palpation of the metacarpophalangeal joints is done with the examiner's thumbs palpating the dorsal aspect of the joint while the forefingers are palpating the volar aspect of the metacarpal head. The joints should be examined while held in a relaxed position of partial flexion. (From Polley HF, Hunder GG: Rheumatologic Interviewing and Physical Examination of the Joints, 2nd ed. Philadelphia, WB Saunders, 1978, p 128.)

The skin on the palmar surface of the hand is relatively thick and covers a fat pad between it and the metacarpophalangeal joint. This makes palpation of the palmar surface of the joint difficult.

To examine the metacarpophalangeal joints, one should palpate over the dorsal aspect and sides of each joint, with the more proximal joints in 20 to 30 degrees of flexion (Fig. 33–4). It is especially helpful in examining the small joints to compare one with another to detect subtle synovitis. Gentle lateral compression with force applied at the base of the second and fifth metacarpophalangeal joints often elicits tenderness if synovitis is present. This is termed the *squeeze test* by some.

The proximal and distal interphalangeal joints are best examined by palpating gently over the lateral and medial aspects of the joint where the flexor and extensor tendons do not interfere with assessment of the synovial membrane. Alternatively, the joint can be compressed anteroposteriorly by the thumb and index finger of one of the examiner's hands, while the other thumb and index finger palpate for synovial distention medially and laterally.

The Bunnell test is useful to differentiate synovitis of the proximal interphalangeal joints from spasm of the intrinsic muscles (see Chapter 42).

Swelling of the fingers may result from articular or periarticular causes. Synovial swelling usually produces symmetric enlargement of the joint itself, whereas extra-articular swelling may be diffuse and extend beyond the joint space. Asymmetric enlargement, involving only one side of the digit or joint, is less common and usually indicates an extra-articular process. Diffuse swelling of an entire digit may result from a tenosynovitis and is seen more commonly in the spondyloarthropathies, such as Reiter's syndrome or psoriatic arthritis. The term *sausage digit* applies to this type of dactylitis. Chronic swelling and distention of the metacarpophalangeal joints tend to produce stretching and laxity of the articular capsule and ligaments. This laxity, combined with muscle imbalance and other forces, eventually results in the extensor tendons of the digits slipping off the metacarpal heads to the ulnar sides of the joints. The abnormal pull of the displaced tendons is one of the factors that causes ulnar deviation of the fingers in chronic inflammatory arthritis (Fig. 33–5).

Swan neck deformity describes the appearance of a finger in which there is a flexion contracture of the metacarpophalangeal joint, hyperextension of the proximal interphalangeal joint, and flexion of the distal interphalangeal joint. These changes are produced by contraction of the interossei and other muscles that flex the metacarpophalangeal joints and extend the proximal interphalangeal joints. This deformity is characteristic of rheumatoid arthritis but may be seen in other chronic arthritides (Fig. 33–6).

Boutonnière deformity describes a finger with a flexion contracture of the proximal interphalangeal joint associated with hyperextension of the distal interphalangeal joint. The deformity is relatively common in rheumatoid arthritis and results when the central slip of the extensor tendon of the proximal interphalangeal joint becomes detached from the base of the middle phalanx, allowing palmar dislocation of the lateral bands. The dislocated bands cross the fulcrum of the joint and then act as flexors instead of extensors of the joint.

Another abnormality is telescoping or shortening of the digits produced by resorption of the ends of the phalanges secondary to destructive arthropathy. This may be seen in the arthritis mutilans form of psoriatic arthritis. Shortening of the fingers is associated with wrinkling of the skin over involved joints and is also called opera-glass hand or la main en lorgnette.

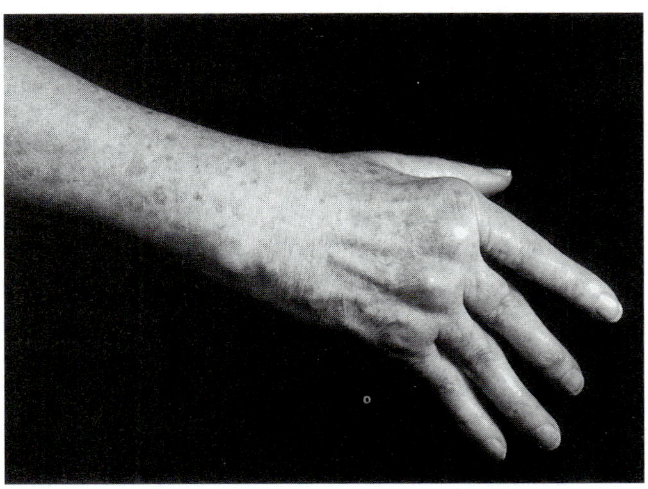

FIGURE 33–5 · **Ulnar Deviation at the Metacarpophalangeal (MCP) Joints.** This is a common deformity seen in patients with inflammatory arthritis, as in this patient with rheumatoid arthritis.

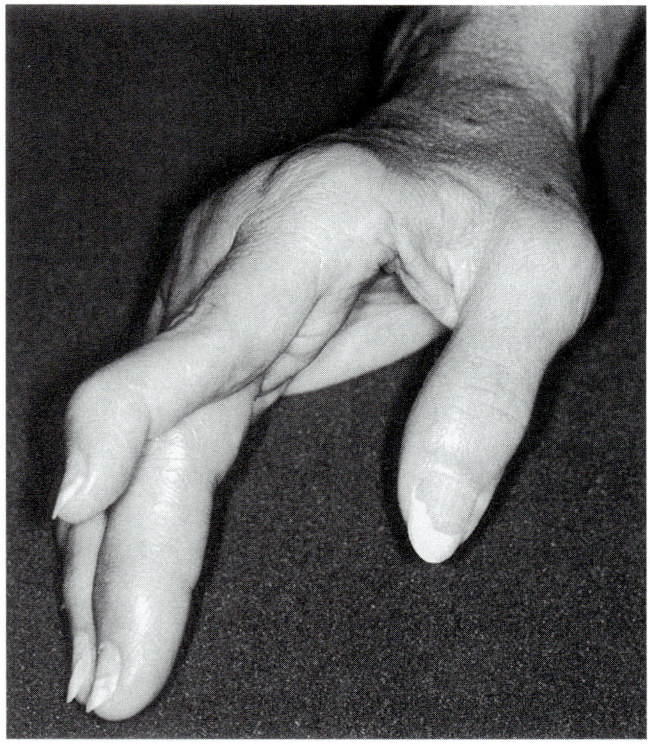

FIGURE 33–6 · **Swan Neck Deformity.** Note the hyperextension at the proximal interphalangeal joint (PIP) and hyperflexion at the distal interphalangeal joint (DIP) of the second digit in this patient with rheumatoid arthritis.

A mallet finger results from avulsion or rupture of the extensor tendon at the level of the distal interphalangeal joint. With this deformity, the patient is unable to extend the distal phalanx, which remains in a flexed position. This deformity frequently results from traumatic injuries.

Murphy's sign is a test for lunate dislocation. The patient is asked to make a fist. The third metacarpal head is usually more prominent than the second and fourth. If the third metacarpal is level with the second and fourth, the finding is positive for lunate dislocation.

Involvement of the distal interphalangeal joints in rheumatoid arthritis is uncommon. However, bony hypertrophy or osteophytic changes are commonly seen at both the distal and proximal interphalangeal joints in patients with osteoarthritis. Enlarged, bony, hypertrophic distal interphalangeal joints are called Heberden nodes, whereas similar changes at the proximal interphalangeal joints are called Bouchard nodes. These are usually easily differentiated from the synovitis of inflammatory arthritis because on palpation the enlargement is hard or bony. In addition, signs of inflammation are minimal. Furthermore, Heberden and Bouchard nodes should be easily distinguished from rheumatoid nodules, but patients will occasionally confuse these when describing swellings over joints. One should be aware of other causes of nodules on the hands, including tophaceous gout and, rarely, multicentric reticulohistiocytosis (Fig. 33–7). The

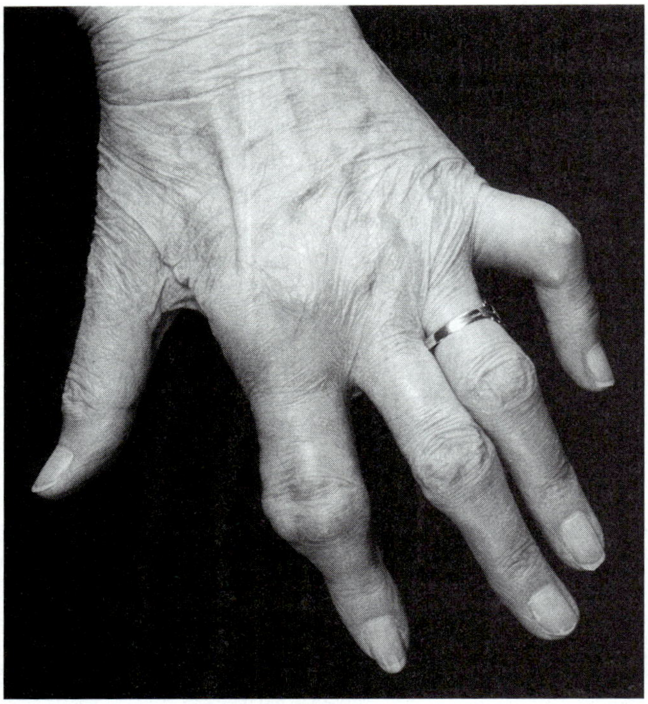

FIGURE 33–7 · This patient has gout, and aspiration of this joint has confirmed the presence of uric acid crystals. Note the enlargement and deformity of the left second PIP joint.

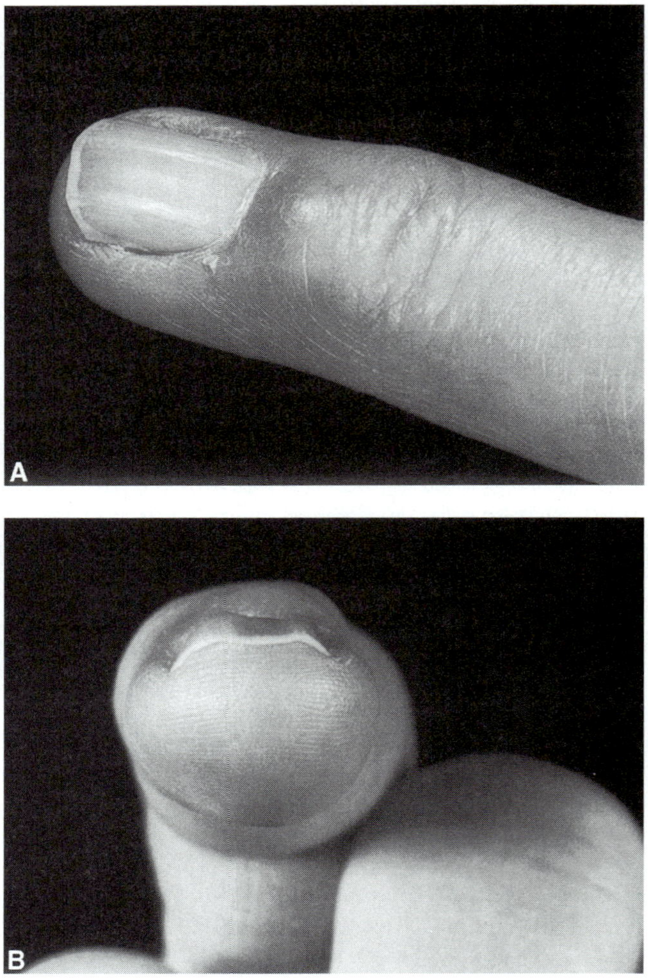

FIGURE 33–8 · Heberden's Node Nail. Note the groove that has developed in the fingernail of this patient with osteoarthritis and a Heberden's node in the DIP joint.

first carpometacarpal joint is also often affected in osteoarthritis.

The patient's fingernails should be inspected for evidence of clubbing or other abnormalities. Often in patients with psoriatic arthritis, ridging, onycholysis, or nail pitting is present. On occasion, patients with osteoarthritis will develop a deformity of the nail on a digit with a Heberden's node (Fig. 33–8). This nail deformity has been called a Heberden's node nail.[8] The abnormality is felt to occur secondary to the synovial cyst encroachment on the nailbed by the evolving osteoarthritis process. With time the nail may return to normal.

A crude but sometimes useful assessment of hand function can be made by asking the patient to make a fist. An estimate of the patient's ability to form a full fist can be recorded as a percentage, with 100 percent being a complete fist. A fist of 75 percent indicates that the patient can touch the palm with the fingertips. The ability to oppose fingers, especially the thumb, is critical to hand function because of the necessity to grasp or at least pinch objects. If the patient is unable to form a full fist, a demonstration of the ability or inability to pinch or oppose fingers can be made by asking the patient to pick up a small object.

Strength of the hands can be assessed crudely by asking the patient to firmly grip two or more of the examiner's fingers. More accurate measures of grip strength can be made by using a dynamometer or having the patient squeeze a partially inflated sphygmomanometer (at 20 mmHg). It is sometimes useful to test the strength of the fingers separately. The prime movers of flexion of the second through fifth metacarpophalangeal joints are the dorsal and palmar interosseus muscles (C8 and T1). The lumbrical muscles (C6, C7, and C8) flex the metacarpophalangeal joints when the proximal phalangeal joints are extended. The flexors of the proximal interphalangeal joints are the flexor digitorum superficialis muscles (C7 and C8, T1), and the flexor of the distal interphalangeal joints is the flexor digitorum profundus muscle (C7 and C8, T1).

The prime extensors of the metacarpophalangeal joints and interphalangeal joints of the second through fifth fingers are the extensor digitorum communis (C6, C7, and C8), the extensor indicis proprius (C6, C7, and C8), and the extensor digiti minimi (C7) muscles. The interosseous and lumbric muscles simultaneously flex the metacarpophalangeal joints and extend the interphalangeal joints. The dorsal interosseous muscles (C8 and T1) and abductor digiti minimi (C8) abduct the fingers, whereas the palmar interosseous muscles adduct the fingers.

The thumb is moved by several muscles. The prime flexor of the first metacarpophalangeal joint is the flexor pollicis brevis muscle (C6, C7, and C8, T1). The prime flexor of the interphalangeal joint is the flexor pollicis longus muscle (C8 and T1). The metacarpophalangeal joint of the thumb is extended by the extensor pollicis brevis muscle, and the prime extensor of the interphalangeal joint is the extensor pollicis longus muscle (C6, C7, C8, and C9).

The prime abductors of the thumb are the abductor pollicis longus (C6 and C7) and the abductor pollicis brevis (C6 and C7) muscles. Motion takes place primarily at the carpometacarpal joint. The prime mover in thumb adduction is the adductor pollicis muscle (C8 and T1). Motion takes place primarily at the carpophalangeal joint. The prime movers in opposition of the thumb and fifth fingers are the opponens pollicis muscle (C6 and C7) and opponens digiti minimi muscle (C8 and T1).

Sensation and nerve injuries in the upper extremity are discussed in Chapters 37 and 42.

HIP

The hip is a spheroidal or ball-and-socket joint formed by the rounded head of the femur and the cup-shaped acetabulum (see also Chapter 40). Stability of the joint is ensured by the fibrocartilaginous rim of the glenoid labrum and the dense articular capsule and surrounding ligaments, including the iliofemoral, pubofemoral, and ischiocapsular ligaments that reinforce the capsule. Support is also supplied by the powerful muscle groups that surround the hip. The primary hip flexor is the iliopsoas muscle assisted by the sartorius and the rectus femoris muscles. Hip adduction is accomplished by the three adductors (the longus, brevis, and magnus) plus the gracilis and pectineus muscles. The gluteus medius is the major hip abductor, whereas the gluteus maximus and hamstrings extend the hip. There are several clinically important bursae about the hip joint. Anteriorly, the iliopsoas bursa lies between the psoas muscle and the joint surface. The trochanteric bursa lies between the gluteus maximus muscle and the posterolateral greater trochanter, and the ischiogluteal bursa overlies the ischial tuberosity.

Examination of the hip should begin by observing the patient's stance and gait. The patient should stand in front of the examiner so that the anterior iliac spines are visible. Pelvic tilt or obliquity may be present and related to a structural scoliosis, anatomic leg length discrepancy, or hip disease. Hip contractures may result in abduction or adduction deformities. To compensate for an adduction contracture, the pelvis is tilted upward on the side of the contracture. This allows the legs to be parallel during walking and weight bearing. With a fixed abduction deformity, the pelvis becomes elevated on the normal side during standing or walking. This causes an apparent shortening of the normal leg and forces the patient to stand or walk on the toes of the normal side or to flex the knee on the abnormal leg.

Viewed from behind with the legs parallel, the patient with hip disease and an adducted hip contracture may have asymmetric gluteal folds due to pelvic tilt, with the diseased side elevated. In this situation, the patient is unable to stand with the foot of the involved leg flat on the floor. In abduction contracture, the findings are reversed; with both legs extended and parallel, the uninvolved side is elevated.

A hip flexion deformity commonly occurs in diseases of the hip. Unilateral flexion of the hip in the standing position reduces weight bearing on the involved side and relaxes the joint capsule, causing less pain. This posture is best noted by observing the patient from the side. There is a hyperlordotic curve of the lumbar spine to compensate for lack of full hip extension.

The patient with possible hip disease should be observed walking. With a normal gait, the abductors of the weight-bearing leg contract to hold the pelvis level or elevate the non–weight-bearing side slightly. Two abnormalities of gait may be commonly observed in patients with hip disease. The most common abnormality seen with a painful hip is the antalgic (limping) gait. In this gait, the person leans over the diseased hip during the phase of weight bearing on that hip, placing the body weight directly over the joint to avoid painful contraction of the hip abductors. In a Trendelenburg gait, with weight bearing on the affected side, the pelvis drops and the trunk shifts to the normal side. Although the antalgic gait is frequently seen with painful hips and the Trendelenburg gait is seen in patients with weak hip abductors, neither gait is specific and either may accompany a painful hip. A mild Trendelenburg gait is seen often in normal persons.

The Trendelenburg test assesses the stability of the hip together with the hip abductor's ability to stabilize the pelvis on the femur. It is a measure of the gluteus medius hip abductor strength. The patient is asked to stand bearing weight on only one leg. Normally, the abductors will hold the pelvis level or the nonsupported side slightly elevated. If the non–weight-bearing side drops, the test is positive for weakness of the weight-bearing side hip abductors, especially the gluteus medius. This test is nonspecific and may be observed in primary neurologic or muscle disorders and in hip diseases that lead to weakness of the hip abductors.

In the supine position, the presence of a hip flexion contracture is suggested by persistence of lumbar lordosis and pelvic tilt masking the contracture by allowing the involved leg to remain in contact with the examination table. The Thomas test demonstrates the flexion contracture. In this test, the opposite hip is fully flexed to flatten the lumbar lordosis and fix the pelvis. The involved leg should then be extended toward the table as far as possible. The diseased hip's flexion contracture will become more obvious and can be estimated in degrees from full extension. Measurement for leg length discrepancy is performed with the patient supine and the legs fully extended. Each leg is measured from the anterior superior iliac spine to the medial malleolus. A difference of 1 cm or less is unlikely to cause any abnormality of gait and may be considered normal. In addition to true leg length asymmetries, apparent leg length discrepancies may result from pelvic tilt or abduction or adduction contractures of the hip.

The range of motion of the hip includes flexion, extension, abduction, adduction, internal and external rotation, and circumduction. The degree of flexion permitted varies with the manner with which it is assessed. When the knee is held flexed at 90 degrees, the hip normally flexes to an angle of 120 degrees between the thigh and long axis of the body. If the knee is held in extension, the hamstrings limit the hip flexion to about 90 degrees.

Abduction is measured with the patient supine and the leg in an extended position perpendicular to the pelvis. Pelvic stabilization is achieved by placing an arm across the pelvis with the hand on the opposite anterior iliac spine. With the other hand, the examiner grasps the patient's ankle and abducts the leg until the pelvis is noted to begin moving. Abduction to about 45 degrees is normal. It is helpful to compare one side with the other because the normal range of motion may vary. Alternatively, the examiner could stand at the foot of the table, grasp both ankles, and simultaneously abduct both legs. Abduction is commonly limited in hip joint disease. Adduction is tested by grasping the ankle and raising the leg off the examination table by flexing the hip enough to allow the tested leg to cross over the opposite leg. Normal adduction is about 20 to 30 degrees. Hip rotation may be tested with both hip and knee flexed to 90 degrees or with the leg extended. Normal hip external rotation and internal rotation are to 45 degrees and 40 degrees, respectively. There is also a difference in rotation between the flexed and extended hip owing to the increased stabilization of the joint by the surrounding ligaments in the extended position. Rotation decreases with extension. To test hip rotation, the extended leg is grasped above the ankle and rotated externally and internally from the neutral position. Limitation of internal rotation of the hip is a sensitive indicator of hip joint disease.

Extension is tested with the patient in the prone position. Estimating hip extension can be difficult because some of the apparent motion arises from hyperextension of the lumbar spine, pelvis rotation, motion of the buttock soft tissue, and flexion of the opposite hip. The pelvis and lumbar spine can be partially immobilized by placing an arm across the posterior iliac crest and lower lumbar spine. The examiner places the other hand under the thigh with the knee flexed and hyperextends the thigh. Normal extension ranges from 10 to 20 degrees. Limitation of extension is often secondary to a hip flexion contracture.

Swelling about the hip rarely can be discerned on examination.

The Patrick test or fabere maneuver is a commonly used test to screen for pathologic conditions of the hip. In this test, the patient lies supine, and the examiner flexes, abducts, and externally rotates the patient's test leg so that the foot of the test leg is on top of the opposite knee. The examiner then slowly lowers the test leg toward the examining table. For a negative test result, the test leg falls at least parallel to the opposite leg. A positive test result occurs when the test leg remains above the opposite leg. A positive result of the Patrick test may indicate hip disease, iliopsoas spasm, or sacroiliac abnormality.

Two useful screening tests in the pediatric population for congenital hip disease are the Ortolani maneuver and the Galeazzi sign. In the Ortolani maneuver, the examiner flexes the hips and grasps the legs of a supine infant so that the examiner's thumbs are against the inner thighs and fingers are draped over the outer (lateral) side of the thighs. With gentle traction, the hips are abducted and laterally rotated. Resistance is usually felt at 30 to 40 degrees of lateral rotation and abduction. In a positive result of the Ortolani test, a click is felt before abduction to the normal 70 degrees can be attained. The Ortolani test should not be done repeatedly because it can lead to damage of the articular cartilage on the femoral head. The Galeazzi sign is useful for assessing unilateral congenital hip dislocation in children younger than 18 months. The child is instructed to lie supine with the knees and hips flexed to 90 degrees. Both knees should normally reside at the same level, and a positive test result is indicated if one knee is higher than the other.

The iliotibial band is a part of the fascia lata extending from the iliac crest, sacrum, and ischium over the greater trochanter to the lateral femoral condyle, tibial condyle, and fibular head and along the lateral intermuscular system, separating the hamstrings from the vastus lateralis. The tensor fascia lata may cause an audible snap as it slips over the greater trochanter if the weight-bearing leg moves from hip flexion and adduction to a neutral position, as in climbing stairs. Most commonly observed in young women, the snapping hip usually does not cause any significant degree of pain. The Ober test evaluates the iliotibial band for contracture. The patient lies on the side with the lower leg flexed at the hip and knee. The examiner abducts and extends the upper leg with the knee flexed at 90 degrees. The hips should be slightly extended to allow the iliotibial band to pass over the greater trochanter. The examiner slowly lowers the limb with the muscles relaxed. A positive test result indicative of an iliotibial band contracture occurs if the leg does not fall back to the level of the table top.

A common cause of lateral hip pain is trochanteric bursitis. Patients with this condition often complain of pain and tenderness when they attempt to lie on the affected side or ambulate stairs. The greater trochanter should be palpated for tenderness and compared with the opposite side. In trochanteric bursitis, this area is usually exquisitely tender. The pain of trochanteric bursitis is aggravated by actively resisted abduction of the hip. Aching and tenderness over the buttock area may be secondary to an ischial bursitis. Other causes of lateral and posterior hip (buttock) discomfort include pain at muscle and tendon insertion sites.

Anterior hip and groin pain may be secondary to hip abnormality, most commonly degenerative arthritis. Decreased range of motion should be noted in these cases. Other causes include iliopsoas bursitis in which swelling and tenderness may be noted in the middle third of the inguinal ligament lateral to the femoral pulse. This pain is aggravated by hip extension and reduced by flexion. The bursitis may be a localized problem or represent extension of hip synovitis or even a synovial cyst to the bursa. It is not possible to make this distinction from physical examination. If the patient is tender in the region of the iliopsoas bursa but no swelling is palpable, one should also consider tendinitis of the iliopsoas muscle. The inguinal region should be palpated for other abnormalities such as hernias, femoral aneurysms, adenopathy, tumor, and psoas abscess or masses.

Muscle strength testing should include the hip flexors, extensors, abductors, and adductors. The primary hip flexor is the iliopsoas muscle (L2 and L3). Flexion may be tested with the patient sitting at the edge of a table. The examiner exerts downward pressure against the thigh proximal to the knee while the patient attempts to flex the hip. The pelvis may be stabilized by the examiner's other hand placed on the ipsilateral iliac crest. Alternatively, with the patient supine and holding the leg in 90 degrees of flexion at the hip, the examiner may attempt to straighten the hip. Hip extension is tested with the patient lying prone.

The primary hip extensor is the gluteus maximus muscle (L5 and S1). With the knee flexed to remove hamstring action, the patient is instructed to extend the hip and thigh off the surface of the table as the examiner places a forearm across the posterior iliac crest to stabilize the pelvis and applies downward pressure to prevent the lateral trunk muscles from elevating the pelvis and leg off the table.

Abduction may be tested with the patient prone or supine. The patient should abduct the thigh and leg against resistance from the examiner applied at the midthigh level.

The primary adductor is the adductor longus (L3 and L4). The examiner holds the upper leg proximal to the knee in slight abduction while the patient resists and attempts to adduct the leg. Testing for abduction and adduction may also be done in the two legs simultaneously. The patient lies supine with the legs fully extended and the hips moderately abducted. To test abduction, the patient actively pushes out against the examiner's resistance against the lateral malleoli. Adduction is tested by movement against resistance at the medial malleoli.

KNEE

The knee is a compound condylar joint with three articulations: the patellofemoral and the lateral and medial tibiofemoral condyles with their fibrocartilaginous menisci.[9,10] The knee is stabilized by its articular capsule, the ligamentum patella, medial and lateral collateral ligaments, and anterior and posterior cruciate ligaments. The collateral ligaments provide medial and lateral stability, whereas the cruciates provide anteroposterior support and rotatory stability. Normal knee motion is a combination of flexion or extension and rotation. With flexion, the tibia internally rotates, and with extension, it externally rotates on the femur. The surrounding synovial membrane is the largest of the body's joints; it extends up to 6 cm proximal to the joint as the suprapatellar pouch beneath the quadriceps femoris muscle. There are several clinically significant bursae about the knee, including the superficial prepatellar bursa, the superficial and deep infrapatellar bursae, the pes anserine bursa distal to the medial tibial plateau, and the posterior medial semimembranous and posterolateral gastrocnemius bursae.

Knee extension is primarily provided by the quadriceps femoris muscle, flexion by the hamstrings. The biceps femoris externally rotates the lower leg on the femur, whereas the popliteus and semitendinous muscles are involved with internal rotation. Examination of the knees should always include observation of the patient while standing and walking. Deviation of the knees, including genu varum (lateral deviation of the knee joint with medial deviation of the lower leg), genu valgum (medial deviation of the knee with lateral deviation of the lower leg), and genu recurvatum, is most easily appreciated in the standing patient (Fig. 33–9). The patient should also be observed ambulating for evidence of gait abnormalities.

The patient should be asked about symptoms of locking, catching, or give way. Locking is the sudden loss of ability to extend the knee; it is usually painful and may be associated with an audible noise, such as a click or pop. It often implies significant intra-articular abnormality, including loose bodies or cartilaginous tears. Catching refers to a subjective sensation of the patient that the knee might lock; the patient may experience a momentary interruption in the smooth range of motion of the joint but is able to continue with normal

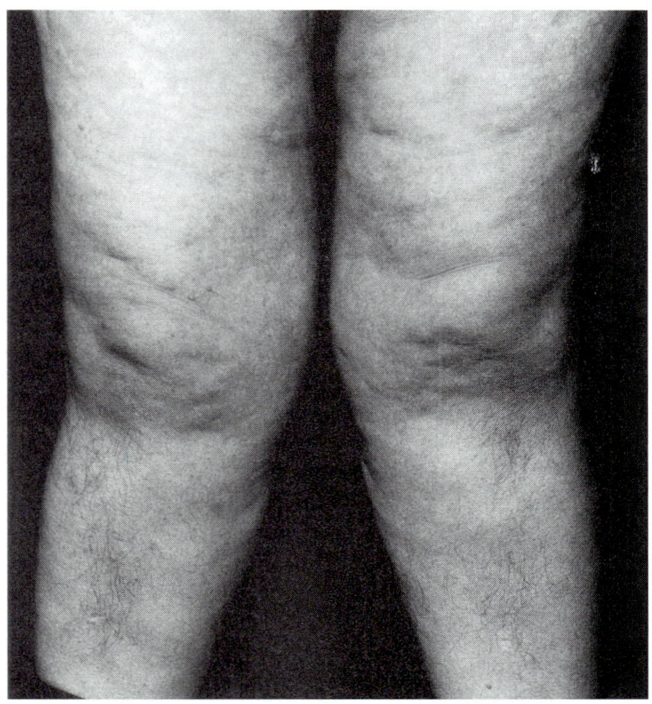

FIGURE 33–9 · Valgus Deformity of the Knees. This a common knee deformity that develops in patients with osteoarthritis of the lateral compartment. (From Polley HF, Hunder GG: Rheumatologic Interviewing and Physical Examination of the Joints, 2nd ed. Philadelphia, WB Saunders, 1978, p 214.)

motion after this brief catch. Catching usually implies less significant abnormality than true locking, and it may occur because of various pathologic conditions. True give way implies that the knee actually buckles and gives out in certain positions or with certain activities. Many patients state that their leg gives out, but it is important to question them to ascertain exactly what they mean by this. Patients often experience a sensation that their knee will give out or is unstable, but it actually is not. Other patients may use this term to describe severe pain that occurs and necessitates their stopping an activity. True give way implies significant intra-articular abnormality, such as an unstable joint from ligamentous injury or incompetence.

Asymmetry from swelling or muscle atrophy may be noted on inspection. Patellar alignment should be noted, including high-riding or laterally displaced patellae. The examiner should inspect the knee from behind to identify popliteal swelling due to a popliteal or Baker cyst, which is most commonly a medial semimembranous bursal swelling. If the calves appear asymmetric, calf circumference should be measured and compared bilaterally. Popliteal cysts may rupture and dissect down into the calf muscles, producing enlargement and palpable fullness. Edema may be present if the cyst causes secondary venous or lymphatic obstruction. Acute rupture or dissection (or both) of a popliteal cyst can mimic thrombophlebitis, with local pain, heat, redness, and swelling. This is probably a more common cause of unilateral calf swelling in patients with rheumatoid arthritis than is deep venous thrombosis. The two conditions may not be distinguishable on physical examination alone.

In the supine position, inability to extend the knee fully may be related to a flexion contracture or a large synovial effusion. Suprapatellar swelling with fullness of the distal anterior thigh that obliterates the normal depressed contours along the side of the patella usually indicates a knee joint effusion or synovitis. Localized swelling over the surface of the patella is generally secondary to prepatellar bursitis.

Quadriceps femoris muscle atrophy often develops in chronic arthritis of the knee. Atrophy of the vastus medialis is the earliest change and may be appreciated by comparing the two thighs for medial asymmetry and circumference. Measurement of the thigh circumference should be performed at 15 cm above the knee to avoid spurious results due to suprapatellar effusions.

Palpation of the knee should be performed with the joint relaxed. This is usually best accomplished with the patient supine and the knees fully extended and not touching. Palpation should begin over the anterior thigh approximately 10 cm above the patella. To identify the superior margin of the suprapatellar pouch, which is an extension of the knee joint cavity, the examiner should palpate the tissues, moving distally toward the knee. Swelling, warmth, thickness, nodules, loose bodies, and tenderness should be noted. A thickened synovial membrane has a boggy, doughy consistency, which differs from the surrounding soft tissue and muscle. It is usually palpated earlier over the medial aspect of the suprapatellar pouch and medial tibiofemoral joint. To enhance detection of knee fluid, any fluid in the suprapatellar pouch is compressed with the palm of the hand placed just proximal to the patella. The synovial fluid forced into the inferior distal articular cavity is then palpated with the opposite thumb and index finger laterally and medially to the patella. If the examiner alternates compression and release of the suprapatellar pouch, the synovial thickening can be differentiated from a synovial effusion. An effusion will intermittently distend the joint capsule under the thumb and index finger of the opposite hand, whereas synovial thickening will not. The examiner should not compress the suprapatellar pouch too firmly or push the tissues distally because the patella or normal soft tissue, including the fat pads, will fill the palpated space and could be misinterpreted as synovitis or joint swelling. With a large effusion, the patella can be ballotted by pushing it posteriorly against the femur with the right forefinger while maintaining suprapatellar compression with the left hand.

At the other extreme, effusions as small as 4 to 8 ml can be detected by eliciting the bulge sign. This test is performed with the knee extended and relaxed. The examiner strokes or compresses the medial aspect of the knee proximally and laterally with the palm of a hand to move the fluid from the area. The lateral aspect of the knee is then tapped or stroked, and a fluid wave or bulge appears medially (Fig. 33–10). A so-called spontaneous bulge sign occurs if, on compression along the medial side of the joint space, fluid reaccumulates without any pressure or compression along the lateral side of the joint.

The medial and lateral tibiofemoral joint margins are palpated for tenderness and bony lipping or exostosis, as can be seen in degenerative joint disease. Palpating the joint margins can be done easily with the hip flexed to 45 degrees, the knee flexed to 90 degrees, and the foot resting on the examining table. Tenderness localized over the medial or lateral joint margins may represent articular cartilage disease, medial or lateral meniscal abnormality, or medial or lateral collateral ligament injury. Other causes of tenderness include pathologic conditions in the underlying bony structures.

Bursitis can be another cause for localized tenderness about the knee, and the two most common sites involved are the pes anserine and prepatellar bursae. Exquisite local tenderness can usually be elicited if bursitis is present. On occasion, mild swelling will also be appreciated. The prepatellar bursa can become quite swollen. It is important not to mistakenly interpret this swelling as knee joint synovitis. The two can usually be differentiated because the bursal margins can be outlined by palpation, and other features of true joint effusion, such as the bulge sign, will be absent.

Patellofemoral articulation abnormality is another common cause of knee pain. It is more common in female patients because of the wider Q angle caused by the broader female pelvis. The Q angle is the angle formed between the quadriceps and the patellar tendon. Patients with patellofemoral disease may complain of stiffness in the knee after a period of flexion (the

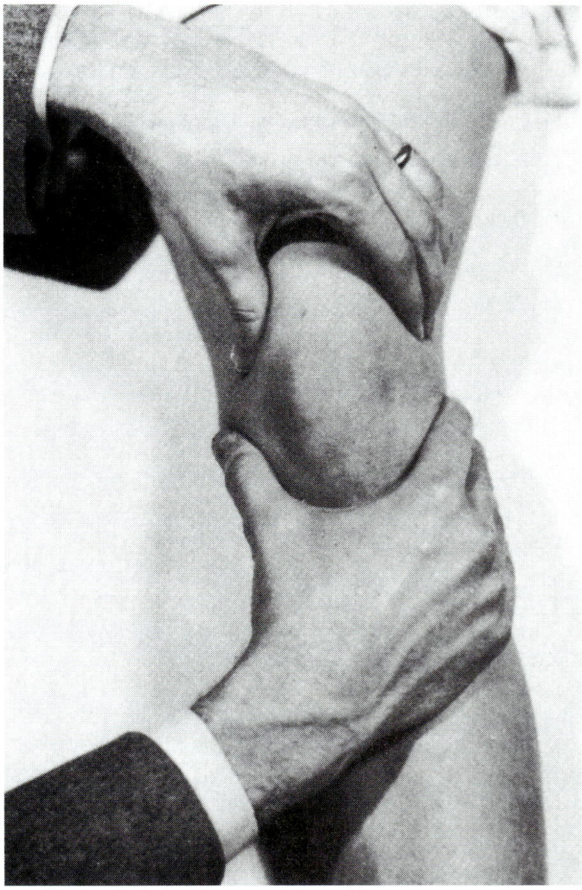

FIGURE 33–10 · Demonstration of the Bulge Sign for a Small Synovial Knee Effusion. *A*, The medial aspect of the knee has been shaded to move the synovial fluid from this area. *B*, Bulge in previously shaded area after lateral aspect of the knee has been tapped. (From Polley HF, Hunder GG: Rheumatologic Interviewing and Physical Examination of the Joints, 2nd ed. Philadelphia, WB Saunders, 1978, p 227.)

moviegoer sign) or have particular difficulty when ambulating stairs. Some patients may experience a sensation of catching as the patella moves over the distal femur.

Patellar palpation is best performed with the knee extended and relaxed. The patella is compressed and moved so that its entire articular surface will come into contact with the underlying femur. Slight crepitation may be observed in many normally functioning knees. Pain with crepitation may suggest patellofemoral degenerative arthritis or chondromalacia patellae. Retropatellar pain occurring with active knee flexion and extension and secondary to patellofemoral disease may be differentiated from tibiofemoral articular pain. To test this, the examiner should attempt to lift the patella away from the knee while passively moving the knee through the range of motion. Painless motion during this maneuver indicates that the patellofemoral joint is the likely source. In addition, the "patellar grind" test is useful in patients with significant patellofemoral abnormality. In this test, the examiner compresses the patella distally away from the femoral condyles while instructing the patient to isometrically contract the quadriceps. Sudden patellar pain and quadriceps relaxation indicate a positive test result. However, this test does have frequent false-positive results.

The patellar stability should be assessed. The Fairbanks apprehension test is done with the patient supine, the quadriceps relaxed, and the knee in 30 degrees of flexion. The examiner slowly pushes the patella laterally. A sudden contraction of the quadriceps and a distressed reaction from the patient constitute a positive apprehension test result. A patient who has had previous patella dislocations usually has a positive apprehension test result. The patella can also be examined for subluxation while the knee is moved through a range of motion from full flexion to extension.

The plica syndrome also occasionally causes symptoms suggestive of patellofemoral disease. Plicae are bands of synovial tissue, most often located on the medial side of the knee. If present, a tender bandlike structure may be palpated parallel to the medial border of the patella. During flexion and extension, a palpable or audible snapping may be heard and the patient may experience symptoms of catching. Many plicae are, however, asymptomatic and are common, so they may be considered a normal variant.

The normal knee range of motion should be from full extension (0 degrees) to full flexion of 120 to 150 degrees. Some normal persons may be able to hyperextend to up to 15 degrees. Loss of full extension due to a flexion contracture is a common finding that accompanies chronic arthritis of the knee. In advanced arthritis, such as in some cases of rheumatoid arthritis, a posterior subluxation of the tibia on the femur may be observed.

Ligamentous instability is tested by applying valgus and varus stress to the knee and by using the drawer test. The knee should be extended and relaxed. The abduction or valgus test is performed by stabilizing the lower femur while placing a valgus stress on the knee by abducting the lower leg with the other hand placed proximal to the ankle. A medial joint line separation with the knee fully extended indicates a tear of the medial compartment ligaments plus the posterior cruciate ligament. The test is then performed with the knee in 30 degrees of flexion. If the test is negative at 0 degrees but positive at 30 degrees, the instability represents a tear of the medial compartment ligaments with the posterior cruciate ligament remaining intact. The adduction or varus test is then performed with the knee extended and again at 30 degrees of flexion. Separation of the lateral joint line indicates a lateral compartment ligament tear, again either associated or not associated with a posterior cruciate ligament tear.

The degree of ligamentous laxity observed during testing can be graded on a scale of 1 to 3. A mild or grade 1 instability indicates that the joint surfaces separate 5 mm or less; for moderate grade 2 instability, a separation of 5 to 10 mm is seen. Grade 3 instability is a separation greater than 10 mm. In cases of trauma, opening of the joint space indicates ligamentous instability secondary to rupture or stretching of the ligaments. However, in cases of chronic arthritis of the tibiofemoral compartment, there may be apparent medial or lateral separation due to the "pseudolaxity" created by loss of cartilage and bone. If the ligaments are intact, the resulting degree of valgus or varus displacement with stressing will not be any greater than in the normal knee.

The drawer test is performed with the hip flexed to 45 degrees and the knee flexed to 90 degrees. To stabilize the knee, the examiner either sits on the foot while grasping the posterior calf with both hands or supports the lower leg between his or her lateral chest wall and forearm. The anterior drawer test is performed by pulling the tibia forward. More than 6 mm of movement is abnormal and may indicate an anterior cruciate tear or laxity. However, anterior subluxation may represent more complex instability. Rotatory instability of the knee may also exist. A positive result of the anterior drawer test, in which the lateral tibial plateau subluxes forward while the medial stays in normal position, can represent anterolateral rotatory instability. If both plateaus sublux, tears of the middle third of the medial lateral capsular ligaments may be present. If the subluxation is not present with the tibia internally rotated, the posterior cruciate ligament is intact. A positive result of the anterior drawer test with the leg in external rotation represents a tear of the medial capsular ligament.

The Lachman test is a modification of the anterior drawer sign and tests for one-plane anterior instability. At least six variations of this test have been described. In the test as originally described, the patient lies supine with the tested knee between full extension and 30 degrees of flexion. The femur is stabilized with a hand of the examiner while the hand pulls the proximal aspect of the tibia forward. A positive test result is indicated by a soft feel rather than a firm end point when the tibia moves forward on the femur. A positive result of the Lachman test may indicate an anterior cruciate injury or abnormality in the posterior oblique ligament or arcuate popliteus complex. A posterior drawer test may be done with the patient positioned as for an anterior drawer test, but the examiner pushes the tibia toward the patient. A positive test result suggests damage to the posterior cruciate ligament.

During the complete joint examination, tests for meniscal injury should be included. Symptoms suggestive of a meniscal tear include locking during joint extension, clicking or popping during motion, and localized tenderness along the medial or lateral joint line. To examine the menisci, the medial and lateral joint line should be palpated with the lower leg internally rotated and the knee flexed to 90 degrees. Localized tenderness over the medial or lateral joint line suggests involvement of the medial or lateral meniscus, respectively. The McMurray test evaluates for evidence of meniscal tear, especially in the posterior half of the menisci. The patient's knee is placed in full flexion, and the examiner places a hand over the knee with the fingers along the side of the knee over the joint line and the thumb along the other side. The other hand holds the leg at the ankle and is used to rotate the lower leg medially and apply varus stress. This test can be done repeatedly, with the knee in gradually decreasing degrees of flexion. A palpable or audible snap suggests a tear of the medial meniscus. The test can be done in a similar fashion by laterally rotating the tibia and applying valgus stress to test for a lateral meniscal injury. A positive result of a lateral test may also represent a tear of the popliteus tendon, which can accompany a lateral meniscal tear.

The Apley grind test also evaluates for a torn meniscus. With the patient lying prone and the knee flexed to 90 degrees, the examiner places downward compression on the foot while medially and then laterally rotating the tibia on the femur. Pain elicited during this maneuver suggests a meniscal tear.

The distraction test is then performed by the examiner's placing his or her knee on the patient's posterior thigh to stabilize the leg while applying an upward distractive force on the foot. Pain from rotating the tibia suggests ligament damage.

A simple hyperflexion test is a useful screening test for meniscal damage. If the examiner is able to hyperflex the knee to more than 135 degrees without eliciting pain, it is unlikely that significant cartilaginous injury is present. If pain occurs with hyperflexion, the patient sometimes is able to localize it medially or laterally, which often correlates with the location of the meniscal injury. However, although helpful, none of these tests for meniscal injury is completely reliable when verified by arthroscopy. Tenderness along the joint line is most sensitive but not as specific as manipulative tests such as the McMurray test.

Muscle strength testing includes testing flexion supplied by the hamstrings (i.e., the biceps femoris, semitendinosus, and semimembranosus) (L5 to S3) and extension supplied by the quadriceps femori (L2, L3, and L4). The hamstrings are tested best with the patient prone and attempting to flex the knee from 90 degrees to beyond. The ankle should be kept in neutral position or dorsiflexed to remove gastrocnemius action. With the leg externally rotated, the biceps femoris, which inserts on the fibula and lateral tibia, is primarily tested, whereas flexion with internal rotation tests the semitendinosus and semimembranosus muscles, which insert on the medial side of the tibia. Extension is tested with the patient sitting upright with the knee fully extended. The examiner stabilizes the thigh with downward pressure just proximal to the knee and places downward pressure at the ankle to test the knee extensors.

ANKLE

The true ankle is a hinged joint, and movement is limited to plantar flexion and dorsiflexion. It is formed by the distal ends of the tibia and fibula and proximal aspect of the body of the talus (Fig. 33–11). Inversion and eversion occur at the subtalar joint (see Chapter 41). The tibia forms the weight-bearing portion of the ankle joint, whereas the fibula articulates on the side of the tibia. The malleoli of the tibia and fibula extend downward beyond the weight-bearing part of the joint and articulate with the sides of the talus. The malleoli

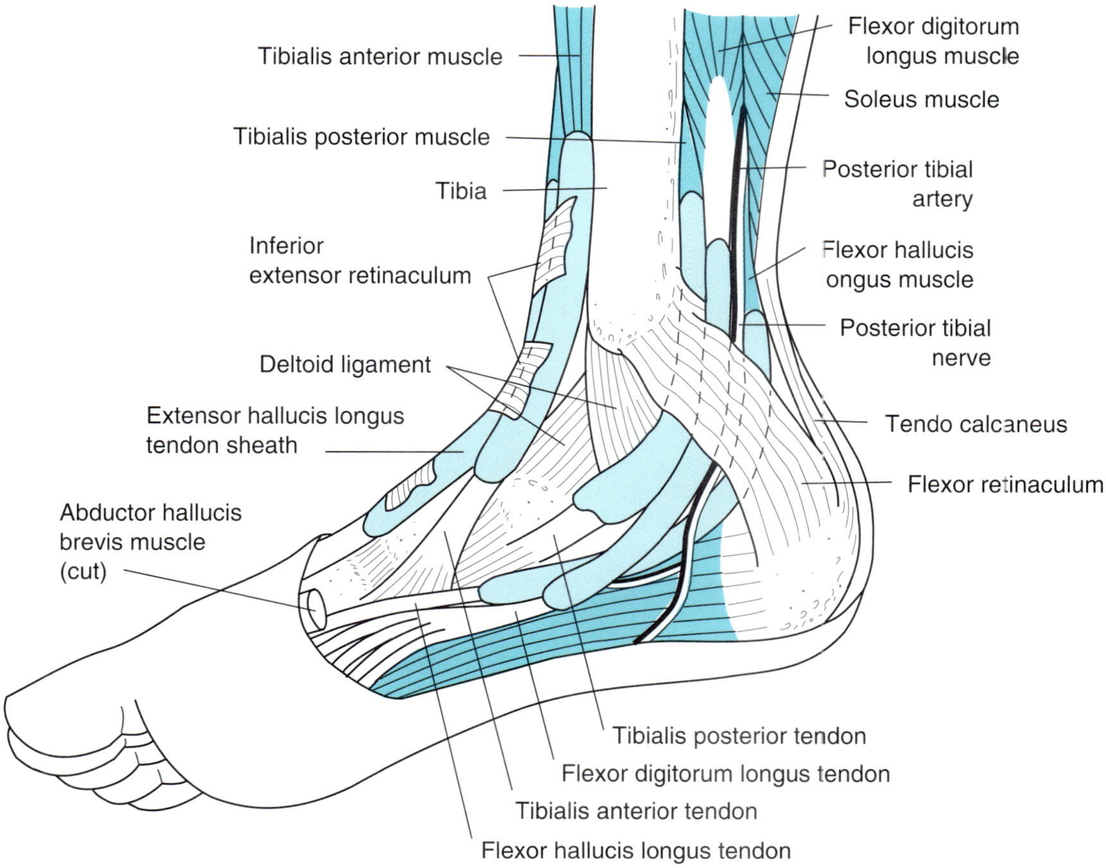

FIGURE 33–11 · Medial aspect of the ankle demonstrates the relationship between the tendons, ligaments, artery, and nerve. (From Polley HF, Hunder GG: Rheumatologic Interviewing and Physical Examination of the Joints, 2nd ed. Philadelphia, WB Saunders, 1978, p 242.)

provide medial and lateral stability by enveloping the talus in a mortise-like fashion.

The articular capsule of the ankle is lax on the anterior and posterior aspects of the joint, allowing extension and flexion, but it is tightly bound bilaterally by ligaments. The synovial membrane of the ankle on the inside of the capsule usually does not communicate with any other joints, bursae, or tendon sheaths.

The medial and lateral ligaments surrounding the ankle contribute to medial and lateral stability of the joint. The deltoid ligament, the only ligament on the medial side of the ankle, is a triangle-shaped fibrous band that tends to resist eversion of the foot. It may be torn in eversion sprains of the ankle. The lateral ligaments of the foot consist of three distinct bands forming the posterior talofibular, the calcaneofibular, and the anterior talofibular ligaments. These ligaments may be injured in inversion sprains of the ankle.

All tendons crossing the ankle joint lie superficial to the articular capsule and are enclosed in synovial sheaths for part of their course across the ankle. On the anterior aspect of the ankle, the tendons and synovial tendon sheaths of the tibialis anterior, extensor digitorum longus, peroneus tertius, and extensor hallucis longus overlie the articular capsule and synovial membrane. On the medial side of the ankle, posteriorly and inferiorly to the medial malleolus, lie the flexor tendons and tendon sheaths of the tibialis posterior, flexor digitorum longus, and flexor hallucis longus (see Fig. 33–10). All three of these muscles plantar flex and supinate the foot. The tendon of the flexor hallucis longus is located more posteriorly than the other flexor tendons and lies beneath the Achilles tendon for part of its course. The calcaneus tendon (Achilles tendon) is the common tendon of the gastrocnemius and soleus muscles and inserts into the posterior surface of the calcaneus, where it is subject to external trauma, various inflammatory reactions, and irritations from bone spurs beneath it. On the lateral aspect of the ankle, posteriorly and inferiorly to the lateral malleolus, a synovial sheath encloses the tendons of the peroneus longus and peroneus brevis. These muscles extend the ankle (plantar flex) and evert (pronate) the foot. Each of the tendons adjacent to the ankle may be involved separately in traumatic or disease processes.

Three sets of fibrous bands or retinacula hold down the tendons that cross the ankle in their passage to the foot. The extensor retinaculum consists of a superior part (transverse crural ligament) in the anterior and inferior portions of the leg and an inferior part in the proximal portion of the dorsum of the foot. The flexor retinaculum is a thickened fibrous band on the medial side of the ankle. On the lateral side of the ankle, the peroneal retinaculum forms a superior and an inferior fibrous band. These bands bind down tendons of the peroneus longus and peroneus brevis as they cross the lateral aspect of the ankle.

Synovial swelling of the ankle joint is most likely to cause fullness over the anterior or anterolateral aspect of the joint, because the capsule is more lax in this area. Mild swelling of the joint may not be apparent on inspection because of the many structures crossing the joint superficially. Efforts should be made to differentiate superficial linear swelling localized to the distribution of the tendon sheaths from more diffuse fullness and swelling due to involvement of the ankle joint. Similarly, it is difficult to observe synovitis of the intertarsal joints. Intertarsal joint synovitis may produce an erythematous puffiness or fullness over the dorsum of the foot.

From the normal position of rest in which there is a right angle between the leg and foot, labeled 0 degrees, the ankle normally allows about 20 degrees of dorsiflexion and about 45 degrees of plantar flexion. Inversion and eversion of the foot occur mainly at the subtalar and other intertarsal joints. From the normal position of the foot, the subtalar joint normally permits about 20 degrees of eversion and 30 degrees of inversion. To test the subtalar joint, the examiner grasps the calcaneus with a hand and attempts to invert and evert it, holding the ankle motionless.

A general assessment of muscular strength of the ankle can be obtained by asking the patient to walk on toes and on heels. If the patient can satisfactorily walk on the toes and on the heels, the muscle strength of the flexors and extensors of the ankle can be considered normal. Many entities can, however, prevent the patient from satisfactorily doing this, including pain. In these cases, it is desirable to test muscles individually.

Prime movers in plantar flexion of the ankle are the gastrocnemius (S1 and S2) and the soleus (S1 and S2) muscles. The prime mover in dorsiflexion is the tibialis anterior muscle (L4 and L5, S1). The tibialis posterior muscle (L5 and S1) is the prime mover in inversion. To test the tibialis posterior muscle, the foot should be in plantar flexion. The examiner applies graded resistance on the medial border of the forefoot while the patient attempts to invert the foot. The prime movers in eversion of the foot are the peroneus longus (L4 and L5, S1) and peroneus brevis (L4 and L5, S1) muscles.

FOOT

See Chapter 41.

Muscle Examination

A general examination of the patient should be carried out looking for any signs of systemic illness. This should include a skin examination in which signs of pallor (suggestive of anemia) and any rashes suggestive of lupus, vasculitis, and dermatomyositis are noted.

The patient should be appropriately disrobed for muscle examination. The patient should be assessed for appearance of the muscles including bulk, tone, and tenderness.

Muscle bulk should be compared on one side of the body to the other to look for any assymmetry, hypertrophy, or atrophy. The distribution of the atrophy should be noted as this maybe indicative of the underlying cause. For example, distal atrophy can be seen in patients with motor neuron disease. Fasciculations are also seen more commonly in this condition. Muscle tone should also be evaluated. Increased muscle tone and spasticity can be seen with demyelinating conditions. Muscle rigidity maybe an indication of Parkinson's disease. Muscle tenderness maybe noted in patients with true weakness, such as infectious myopathies. Other conditions that do not cause true weakness, such as fibromyalgia, can also be associated with tender muscles.

Strength testing should be carried out on both distal and proximal muscle groups. Commonly tested areas include plantar and dorsiflexion of the foot; hip abduction, adduction, and flexion; finger abduction; arm flexion; shoulder abduction; and neck flexion and extension. The patient should be seated and both sides of the body compared for asymmetric weakness. Typically, resistance will be noted against a force applied by the examiner. The examiner should attempt to confirm whether or not true weakness is present and if it is, in what distribution.[11]

A neurologic examination should also be done. This should include reflex testing and testing for sensory loss.[12] Typically, patients with inflammatory myopathies should not have significant abnormalities on neurologic examination.

REFERENCES

1. Polley HF, Hunder GG: Rheumatologic Interviewing and Physical Examination of the Joints, 2nd ed. Philadelphia, WB Saunders, 1978.
2. Hoppenfeld S: Physical Examination of the Spine and Extremities. New York, Appleton-Century-Crofts, 1976.
3. Magee DJ: Orthopedic Physical Assessment, 2nd ed. Philadelphia, WB Saunders, 1992.
4. Buchanan WW, de Ceulaer K, Bálint GP: Clinical Examination of the Musculoskeletal System: Assessing Rheumatic Conditions. Baltimore, Williams & Wilkins, 1997.
5. Musculoskeletal examination. *In* Seidel Henry M, Ball JW, Dains JE, et al (eds): Mosby Guide to Physical Examination, 4th ed. St. Louis, Mosby, 1999. pp. 689-755.
6. American College of Rheumatology Ad Hoc Committee on Clinical Guidelines: Guidelines for the initial evaluation of the adult patient with acute musculoskeletal symptoms. Arthritis Rheum 39:1, 1996.
7. Moder KG: A working guide to joint examination in rheumatoid arthritis. J Musculoskel Med 12:17, 1995.
8. Alarcon-Segovia S, Vega-Ortiz JM: Heberden's nodes' nails. J Rheumatol 8(3):509-511, 1981.
9. Press JM, Casazza BA, Young JL: Knee ligament injuries: Making the diagnosis, restoring use. J Musculoskel Med 13:14, 1996.
10. Swenson EJ Jr: Diagnosing and managing meniscal injuries in athletes. J Musculoskel Med 12:35, 1995.
11. Miller, Marc L: Weakness. *In* Kelley WN, Harris ED, Ruddy S, et al (eds): Kelley's Textbook of Rheumatology, 4th ed. Philadelphia, WB Saunders, 1993. pp.389-397.
12. Medical Research Council: Aids to the Examination of the Peripheral Nervous System. Memorandum 45. London, Her Majesty's Stationary Office, 1981.

34 Monarticular Arthritis

W. JOSEPH MCCUNE • JOSEPH GOLBUS

With rare exceptions, any joint disorder is capable of presenting initially as monarthritis. Monarthritis, therefore, represents a diagnostic challenge to even the most experienced clinician. It often remains incompletely understood after the initial evaluation. Nonetheless, it is almost always possible to identify patients who require vigorous evaluation and treatment to prevent rapid disease progression, such as those with suspected septic arthritis. The physician can then proceed in a measured and systematic manner with the remainder of patients, in whom the short-term clinical course and response to simple therapeutic measures may provide additional useful information. This chapter is intended to aid the clinician in distinguishing true arthritis from syndromes that also manifest with pain in the surrounding joint structures, in narrowing the list of diagnostic possibilities based on the clinical presentation, and in using diagnostic tests effectively. Special attention is given to common entities that present as acute inflammatory arthritis suggesting joint sepsis.

Differential Diagnosis

Confronted with a patient complaining of pain or swelling in the region of a single joint, the physician must first attempt to localize the anatomic site of the abnormality (Fig. 34–1). Joint pain can be the result of abnormalities in the joint itself, adjacent bone, surrounding ligaments, tendons, bursae, or soft tissues. It can also be referred, resulting from nerve root impingement, an entrapment neuropathy, or even pathology in another joint. Pain from hip arthritis, for example, can be referred entirely or partially to the knee. It is also important to remember that the differential diagnosis of an acute monarthritis includes most causes of polyarticular arthritis, as many forms of polyarthritis can present with a single painful or swollen joint.

Arthritis involving a diarthrodial joint causes stiffness, reduced range of motion, and pain during normal use. With few exceptions (e.g., the patellofemoral joint in chondromalacia[1]), intra-articular abnormalities can be detected during passive and active range of motion. The patient history and physical examination are essential in determining the cause of the arthritis. Inflammatory forms of arthritis are characterized by stiffness of the joint that is most noticeable in the morning (i.e., morning stiffness) or after a period of inactivity (i.e., gelling) and that improves with motion. Inflammatory arthritis is often associated with systemic symptoms, such as fever or malaise. Joint pain due to mechanical factors usually worsens with activities, improves with rest, and is not associated with systemic symptoms (Table 34–1).

During physical examination, it is important to compare the abnormalities (e.g., swelling, warmth, redness) with findings in the contralateral joint. Although most inflamed joints show signs of inflammation, deeper-seated articulations, such as the shoulders, hips, and sacroiliac joints, may not. Effusions almost always result from intra-articular pathology, although they may accompany osteomyelitis, fractures, or tumors.[2] The presence of excess synovial fluid does not specifically indicate joint inflammation unless the white blood cell count is elevated. The range of disorders causing monarthritis is listed in Table 34–2. The conditions discussed in the following sections may be confused with arthritis (Table 34–3).

INTERNAL DERANGEMENTS

Torn menisci or ligaments or loose bodies may episodically wedge into the joint, producing clicking, locking, or "giving way." These conditions may precede or accompany degenerative arthritis and can be a consequence of inflammatory arthritis when fronds of proliferative synovium become lodged within the joint. Symptoms are frequently intermittent. They can often be elicited on physical examination by repeatedly flexing and extending the joint in various degrees of internal and external rotation.[3] Internal derangements of the hip, particularly tears of the acetabular labrum, are easily overlooked. Such tears may be treated arthroscopically by an orthopedic surgeon with sufficient experience in hip arthroscopy.

BONE PAIN

Pain in bone usually results from involvement by a disease process of the periosteum or the marrow space as the result of sensory nerves located in these areas. Bone pain is commonly caused by fractures, osteomyelitis, or periostitis, such as occurs in pulmonary hypertrophic osteoarthropathy, hemoglobinopathies, hematologic malignancy,[4] primary or metastatic bone tumors, and occasionally with infiltrative processes such as Paget's disease. Characteristically, bone pain is accompanied by tenderness to pressures over involved periosteum or pain on weight bearing. When symptoms are long standing, radiographic findings are typically abnormal. Earlier disease may be identified by radionuclide scanning,

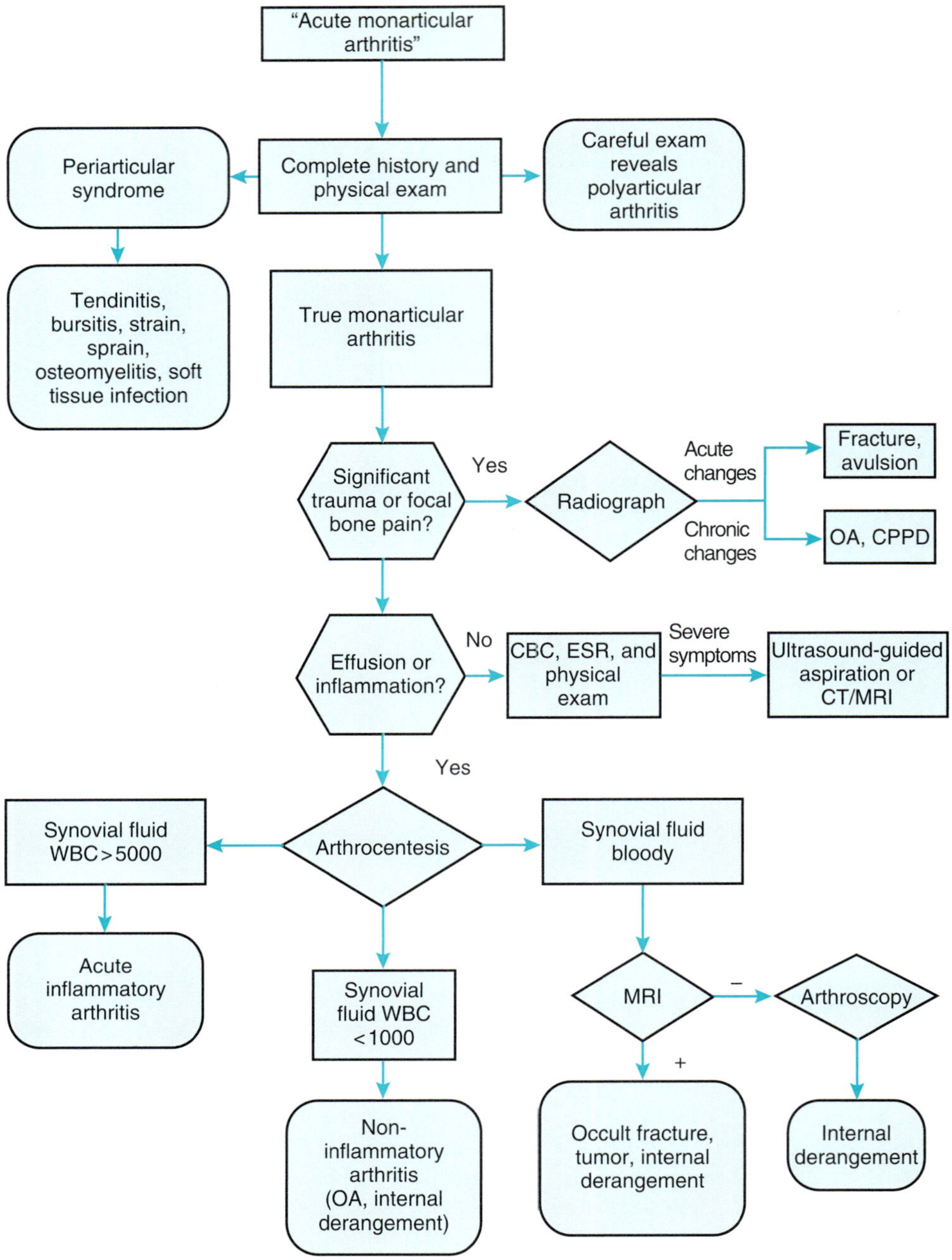

FIGURE 34–1 · **Initial Approach to Acute Monarticular Arthritis.** CBC, complete blood count; CPPD, calcium pyrophosphate deposition disease; CT, computed tomography; ESR, erythrocyte sedimentation rate; MRI, magnetic resonance imaging; OA, osteoarthritis; WBC, white blood cell count.

computed tomography (CT), or magnetic resonance imaging (MRI). Paget's disease may be associated with both bone pain and arthritic symptoms as the result of expansion and deformity of subchondral bone and cartilage, particularly in the hips and knees.[5]

TENDINITIS OR BURSITIS

Findings of tendinitis or bursitis are usually localized to one area around the joint.[6] Local tenderness and pain often increase with active motion more than with passive motion of the joint, because active motion stresses the involved periarticular structures more than does passive motion. An exception to this rule is supraspinatus tendinitis of the shoulder, in which passive and active motion may produce similar pain, and there may be no localized tenderness. The clinical findings seen with tendinitis or bursitis can usually be reduced or eliminated by local instillation of lidocaine. The presence of a puncture site, a history of glucocorticoid injection, an adjacent source of infection, such as an ulcerated rheumatoid nodule,[7] or severe inflammation may signify infectious bursitis.[8] Isolated tendinitis less commonly results from hematogenous spread of infection, except in disseminated gonococcal disease, which commonly manifests with dorsal tenosynovitis of the wrists,[9] and similar septic tenosynovitis may complicate brucellosis.[10] Infected olecranon or prepatellar bursae commonly mimic septic arthritis. These conditions may often be identified by high-resolution ultrasound.[11]

TABLE 34–1 • USEFUL CLINICAL FEATURES IN THE INITIAL EVALUATION OF THE PATIENT WITH ACUTE MONOARTICULAR PAIN

	Tendinitis	Noninflammatory Joint Pain (osteoarthritis, internal derangement)	Systemic Rheumatic Disease
Symptoms			
Morning stiffness	Localized, brief	Localized, brief	Often greater than 15 minutes
Constitutional symptoms	None	None	Present (fever, malaise)
Peak period of discomfort	With use	After prolonged use	After prolonged inactivity
Locking or Instability	Unusual, except with rotator cuff tears or trigger fingers	Suggests internal derangement or loose body	None
Signs			
Tenderness	Localized, periarticular	Mild, over joint line	Diffuse over exposed joint space
Inflammation	Over tendon or bursa	Unusual	Common
Instability	Uncommon	Occasional	Uncommon
Multisystem disease	No (occasionally with GC)	No	Often

Modified from American College of Rheumatology Ad Hoc Committee on Clinical Guidelines.Guidelines for the initial evaluation of the adult patient with acute musculoskeletal symptoms. Arthritis Rheum 39:1-8, 1996.

NEUROPATHIC PAIN

Compression or irritation of peripheral nerves may produce pain referred to the region of joints, such as pain radiating from the wrist to the palmar surface of the first four digits in carpal tunnel syndrome,[12] pain in the hip region in lumbosacral radiculopathies, or shoulder pain with brachial plexopathies. Such symptoms are usually in the distribution of a peripheral nerve and tend to follow an irregular time course with sudden exacerbations, particularly at night. Maneuvers that compress the affected nerve at the site of injury, such as straight leg raising or percussion of the median nerve at the wrist, are helpful when they exactly reproduce the patient's pain in the distribution of a peripheral nerve. Diffuse polyneuropathies may produce pain that is poorly localized and that superficially resembles joint pain in a stocking-glove distribution. Pain that localizes exactly to a joint in the setting of a polyneuropathy may be related to neuropathic joint disease or reflex sympathetic dystrophy, or it may have an unrelated cause.[13]

SOFT TISSUE INFECTIONS

Soft tissue infections may simulate arthritis, particularly when they occur in the region of deeply buried joints that are difficult to examine. Hip pain may result from cellulitis, pyomyositis, psoas or retroperitoneal abscesses, or intrapelvic pathology, such as diverticulitis. Fever and the acute onset of hip pain and stiffness with normal radiographic and synovial fluid findings suggest soft tissue or bone infection. Pain referred to the sacroiliac joint may result from a variety of soft tissue infections, including perirectal abscesses. Infectious processes in these locations manifest with unremitting severe pain, marked elevation of the erythrocyte sedimentation rate, and variably severe systemic toxicity.[14,15] Physical examination may reveal muscular rigidity and guarding, local tenderness, increased girth of the affected limb, or draining sinuses. Imaging studies such as radionuclide scanning, ultrasound, CT, or MRI may be essential in identifying deep infections.

MUSCULAR PAIN SYNDROMES

Muscular pain syndromes (e.g., myofascial pain, fibromyalgia) consist of local or diffuse tenderness in muscles, which causes pain in characteristic regional zones. These can result in a variety of complaints, including headache; jaw, neck, or low back pain; and occasionally joint pain, particularly in the shoulder. They tend to be diffuse, symmetric, and often associated with complaints outside of the musculoskeletal system, such as fatigue, intermittent diffuse paresthesias, and irritable bowel syndrome (see Chapter 36). Trigger points represent specific sites of exaggerated sensitivity to pressure and are often seen in patients with fibromyalgia. Myofascial syndromes rarely cause monarticular pain but may be associated with exaggerated distress associated with benign causes of monarticular pain.

Patient History

IS THE ARTHRITIS ACUTE OR CHRONIC?

Extremely rapid onset of pain (over seconds or minutes) suggests an internal derangement, fracture, trauma, or loose body. Acute onset over several hours to 2 days is typical of most forms of inflammatory arthritis, particularly bacterial infection and crystal-induced synovitis. When a careful history reveals marked worsening

TABLE 34-2 • DIFFERENTIAL DIAGNOSIS OF MONARTICULAR ARTHRITIS

Usually Monarticular	Often Polyarticular
Common	
Septic arthritis	Rheumatoid arthritis
Bacterial	Osteoarthritis
Tuberculous	Psoriatic arthritis
Fungal	Reiter's syndrome (idiopathic and human immunodeficiency virus)
Lyme disease	Calcium pyrophosphate deposition disease
Crystal disease	Chronic articular hemorrhage
Gout	Most juvenile rheumatoid arthritis and juvenile spondylitis
Pseudogout	Erythema nodosum/sarcoid
Internal derangement	Serum sickness
Ischemic necrosis	Acute hepatitis B
Hemarthrosis	Rubella
Coagulopathy	Henoch-Schönlein purpura
Warfarin (Coumadin)	Systemic lupus erythematosus
Trauma or overuse	Lyme disease
Pauciarticular juvenile rheumatoid arthritis	Parvovirus
Neuropathic	Dialysis arthropathy
Congenital hip dysplasia	Other crystal-induced arthropathies
Osteochondritis dissecans	Undifferentiated connective tissue disease
Reflex sympathetic dystrophy	
Hydroxyapatite deposition	
Hemoglobinopathies	
Loose body	
Palindromic rheumatism	
Paget's disease involving joint	
Stress fracture	
Osteomyelitis	
Osteogenic sarcoma	
Metastatic tumor	
Synovial osteochondromatosis	
Rare	
Pigmented villonodular synovitis	Relapsing polychondritis
Plant thorn synovitis	Enteropathic disease
Familial Mediterranean fever	Ulcerative colitis
Synovioma	Regional enteritis
Synovial metastasis	Bypass arthritis
Intermittent hydrarthrosis	Whipple's disease
Pancreatic fat necrosis	Chronic sarcoidosis
Gaucher's disease	Hyperlipidemia types II and IV
Behçet's disease	Still's disease
Regional migratory osteoporosis	Pyoderma gangrenosum
Giant cell arteritis or	Pulmonary hypertrophic osteoarthropathy
Sea urchin spine	Chondrocalcinosis-like syndromes
Amyloidosis (myeloma)	polymyalgia rheumatica
	due to ochronosis,
	hemochromatosis,
	Wilson's disease
	Rheumatic fever
	Paraneoplastic syndromes

of long-standing symptoms in a joint, it is important to distinguish exacerbations of preexisting disease (e.g., worsening of degenerative joint disease with excessive use) from a second superimposed process (e.g., infection).[16]

IS THE ARTHRITIS MECHANICAL OR INFLAMMATORY?

The question of an inflammatory versus a mechanical process is most reliably answered by the synovial fluid white blood cell count (Table 34–4). Waxing and waning of disease activity unrelated to patterns of use, including fluctuations of pain and swelling, protracted morning stiffness, and gelling, suggest inflammation. Pain that occurs only after use, improves with rest, and involves weight-bearing joints suggests mechanical disease.

IS THE ARTHRITIS TRULY MONARTICULAR?

Careful inquiry may elicit evidence of antecedent or coincident involvement of additional joints. A history of inflammatory symptoms in multiple joints for more than a month suggests a chronic, noninfectious inflammatory condition. Diffuse arthralgias of shorter duration may accompany the onset of many illnesses, especially systemic infections. Truly migratory disease, in which there is only one inflamed joint but a clear-cut history of recent inflammatory arthritis of other joints occurring sequentially, suggests gonococcal arthritis or rheumatic fever. Coexistence of symptoms in the axial skeleton may provide a clue to presence of a spondyloarthropathy.[16-18] A careful physical examination may reveal involvement of additional joints at the time of presentation.

Approach to the Patient with Acute Inflammatory Monarthritis

Evaluation of an acute inflammatory monarthritis deserves special emphasis, because immediate benefit may result from identification and treatment of the underlying disease (Fig. 34–2). Although the differential diagnosis of an acute inflammatory arthritis is long, the three most common considerations are infection, crystal-induced arthritis, or the onset of a potentially chronic inflammatory arthropathy. Each of these disorders is capable of manifesting with an explosive onset of inflammation over a few hours, but the "hyperacute" presentation is most typical of infection or crystal-induced disease. As a rule, the most important diagnostic study in the evaluation of an acute monarthritis is synovial fluid analysis, especially when infection or crystal disease is suspected (see Chapter 46).

In most cases, the diagnosis of gout can be made immediately by aspirating joint fluid and examining it with the use of polarizing microscopy. Calcium pyrophosphate crystals can sometimes be more difficult to identify. The diagnosis of pseudogout is often uncertain until repeated aspirations are performed and culture results are negative. The finding of chondrocalcinosis on radiography, however, can increase the examiner's clinical suspicion. Infectious arthritis can be diagnosed by Gram stain in some patients and can be proved by culture in most within 48 hours. The presence of other conditions may be suggested by extra-articular disease features, but laboratory testing and continued observation often are

TABLE 34–3 • REGIONAL PERIARTICULAR SYNDROMES

Region	Periarticular Syndrome	Monarticular Syndrome
Jaw	Temporomandibular joint dysfunction (myofascial pain syndrome) Preauricular lymphadenitis	Temporal arteritis Molar dental problems Parotid swelling
Shoulder	Subacromial bursitis Long-head bicipital tendinitis Rotator cuff tear	Pancoast tumor Brachial plexopathy Cervical nerve root injury
Elbow	Olecranon bursitis Epicondylitis	Ulnar nerve entrapment
Wrist	Extensor tendinitis (including deQuervain's tenosynovitis) Gonococcal tenosynovitis	Carpal tunnel syndrome
Hand	Palmar fasciitis (Dupuytren's contracture) Ligamentous or capsular injury	
Hip	Greater trochanteric bursitis Adductor syndrome Ischial bursitis Fascia lata syndrome	Meralgia paresthetica Deep infection Paget's disease Neoplasm
Knee	Anserine bursitis Prepatellar bursitis Meniscal injury Ligamentous tear-laxity Baker's cyst	Neoplasm Osteomyelitis
Ankle	Peroneal tendinitis Achilles tendinitis Retrocalcaneal bursitis Calcaneal fasciitis Sprain Erythema nodosum	Hypertrophic pulmonary osteoarthropathy Tarsal tunnel syndrome
Foot	Plantar fasciitis Pes planus ("fallen arches")	Morton's neuroma Vascular insufficiency Cellulitis

needed before the diagnosis can be made with certainty. The following observations are intended to aid in the differential diagnosis of these entities.

INFECTIOUS ARTHRITIS

In evaluating an acutely inflamed joint, the physician must first ask whether the likelihood of septic arthritis is sufficient to hospitalize the patient and intervene immediately.[19] Joint sepsis produces dramatic inflammation followed quickly by irreversible destruction of cartilage and bone (see Chapter 98). It may also be the initial sign of a life-threatening systemic infection. In healthy adults, the signs are usually obvious. The patient complains of intense local pain and may resist attempts to examine the affected joint. Infected peripheral joints are swollen, warm, very tender, and sometimes red, and they have markedly restricted range of motion. As a general rule, large joints are more frequently affected than small ones in the absence of local trauma or peripheral vascular disease.[8] Unfortunately, persons at highest risk for joint sepsis are those in whom confounding factors obscure symptoms or blunt the inflammatory response. Infection should be strongly suspected in less sick-appearing patients when systemic risk factors (e.g., corticosteroid therapy; immunodeficiency or immunosuppression; diabetes; intravenous drug abuse; pulmonary, cardiac, or genitourinary focus of infection) and local pathology (e.g., inflammatory arthritis, effusions, penetrating trauma, previous injection of corticosteroids, prosthetic joint) are present.

Although the clinical picture is never diagnostic of a particular infectious agent, certain presentations are characteristic: Gonococcal infection rarely escapes attention, because it tends to manifest as an inordinately painful monarthritis or polyarthritis and a painful, diffuse tenosynovitis in an otherwise healthy individual.[20] Skin lesions ranging from macules to pustules and vesicles are well described[15,21] but may be subtle. Meningococcal arthritis occasionally presents with clinical and Gram-stain findings identical to those of gonococcal disease. The diagnosis of gonococcal arthritis is typically based on the history, physical examination, synovial fluid cultures, and cultures of any skin lesions, as well as the pharynx,and anogenital area.

The large increase in intravenous drug abuse in the past few decades has resulted in a dramatic increase in associated septic arthritis through the introduction of infectious material into the intravascular space with subsequent hematogenous spread to the joints. Under unusual conditions, direct inoculation can also occur. These infections are most commonly caused by *Staphylococcus aureus* and gram-negative organisms, especially *Pseudomonas*. They commonly occur in unusual locations compared to septic arthritis in other populations. There is a marked predilection for infections in the fibrocartilaginous joints of the skeleton, such as the sternoclavicular joints, sacroiliac joints, and intervertebral disk spaces.

Lyme arthritis manifests as a true inflammatory arthritis—most commonly in the knee—weeks to months after initial exposure and after the development of the early

TABLE 34–4 • SYNOVIAL FLUID AND ASSOCIATED LABORATORY FINDINGS IN MONARTICULAR ARTHRITIS

Synovial Fluid White Blood Cell Count	Predominant Cell	Appearance	Viscosity	Micro-Organisms	Crystals	RBC	Glucose	Protein	Complement	Cartilage Debris	Other
0-200 Normal	M	Clear	↑	–	–	–	90%	1.5-2	–	–	Small amount not demonstrable on physical examination
0-2000 Osteoarthritis	M	Clear	↑	–	+/– Occasional CPPD	–	–	–/↑	–	+	Radiographs positive in advanced disease; synovial fluid findings variable
Structural	M	Clear	↑	–	–	+/–	–	–/↑		+	
Internal derangement						+/–					MR scan, arthrogram, (knee) arthroscopy
Neuropathic						+++/–					Marked radiographic changes
Osteochondritis dissecans							–				MR scan, CT scan
Ischemic necrosis							–				MR scan, bone scan, radiograph in advanced cases
Traumatic	RBC	Cloudy, bloody	↑	–	–	+++	–	↑/↑↑↑			Radiograph
2000-10,000											
Pigmented villonodular synovitis	RBC	Brown, bloody	↓	–	–	+–	↓	↑↑↑		–	Synovial biopsy
Amyloid	M	Slightly turbid		–	–						Congo red: synovial fluid Monoclonal gammopathy
Enteropathic arthritis	M/P	Slightly turbid		–	–	–					Positive stool occult blood
Systemic lupus erythematosus	M	Slightly turbid	↑	–	–	–			↓		LE cells Serum autoantibodies
5000-50,000											
Juvenile rheumatoid arthritis	P	Slightly turbid	↓	–	–	–	↓	↑/↑↑	–/↓		Synovial fluid leukocytes may be ≥100,000 Serum: + ANA (50%) + rheumatoid factor (<20%)
Sarcoidosis		Slightly turbid	↓	–	–	–					Chest radiographs, slit-lamp examination
Reiter's syndrome	P	Slightly turbid	↓	–	–	–	↓	↑/↑↑	↑		
Psoriatic arthritis	P	Slightly turbid	↓	–	–	–	↓				Negative rheumatoid factor, ANA positive sign
Rheumatoid arthritis	P	Turbid	↓↓	–	–	–	↓↓	↑/↑↑↑	↓		Serum (+) rheumatoid factor (50-80%) + ANA
Tuberculous arthritis	M	Turbid	↓↓	+/–	–	–	↓↓↓	↑↑/↑↑↑			PPD usually positive unless anergic Synovial biopsy essential

10,000-150,000											
CPPD pseudogout	P	Turbid	↑↓	–	CPPD (approximately 60%)	–	↓	↑↑		+/–	Repeated crystal examinations Radiographs: chondrocalcinosis
Gout	P	Turbid	↑	–	Monosodium urate (>90%)	–	↓	↑↑			Serum uric acid unreliable
Gonococcal infection	P	Turbid to pus	↓↓	+/–		–	↓↓	↑↑↑			Synovial fluid culture 20-50% positive Culture portals of entry Urogenital Gram stain
Nongonococcal bacteria	P	Turbid to pus	↓↓↓	+		–	↓↓↓	↑↑↑			Gram stain—gram-positive organisms Synovial fluid, blood cultures

Abbreviations: ANA, Antinuclear antibodies; CPPD, calcium pyrophosphate dihydrate; CT, computed tomography; LE, lupus erythematosus; M, mononuclear; MR, magnetic resonance; P, polynuclear, PPD, purified protein derivative; RBC, red blood cells.

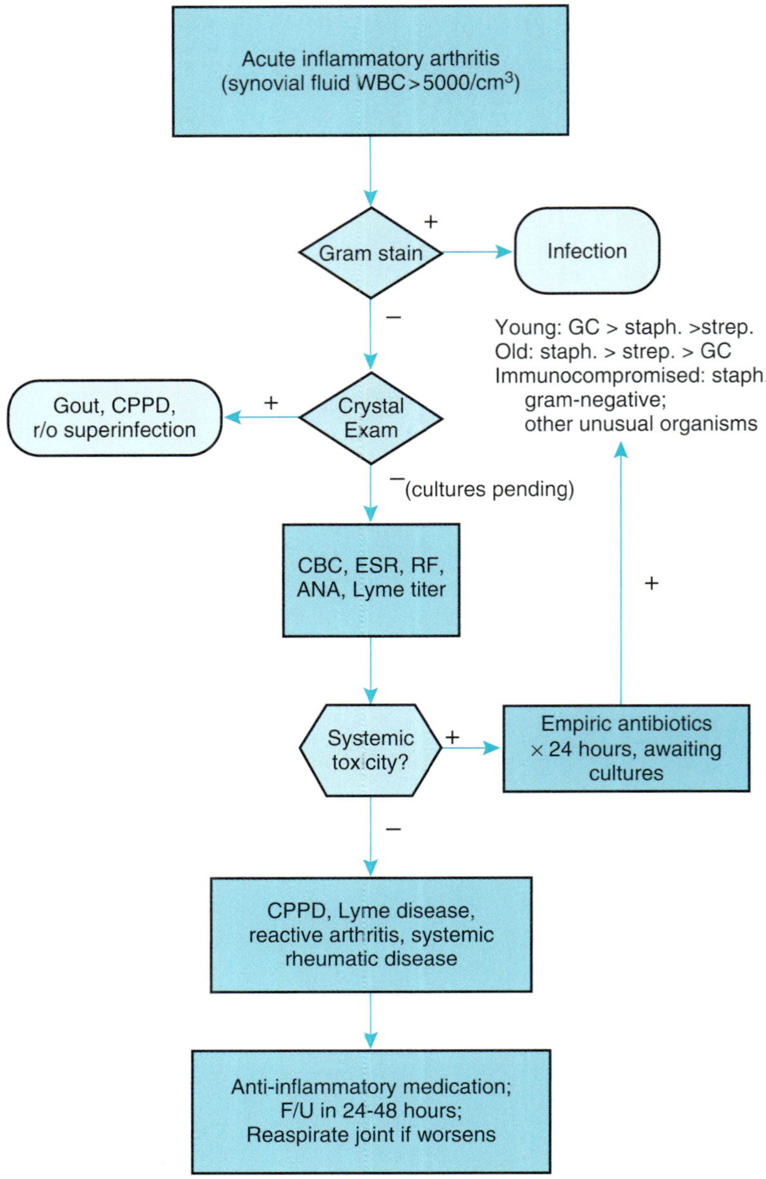

FIGURE 34–2 • **Approach to Acute Inflammatory Arthritis.** ANA, antinuclear antibody test; CBC, complete blood count; CPPD, calcium pyrophosphate deposition disease; ESR, erythrocyte sedimentation rate; F/U, follow-up; GC, gonococcal infection; RF, rheumatoid factor; r/o, rule out; staph., staphylococcal infection; strep., streptococcal infection; WBC, white blood count.

syndrome of fevers, arthralgias, lymphadenopathy, and rash. This curable infection should be suspected in patients with compatible symptoms, a history of travel to endemic areas, or coexistent neurologic or cardiac abnormalities. The diagnosis can be difficult, however, as many affected individuals may not recall a tick bite or antecedant rash. If infection is suspected, serum antibodies to *Borrelia burgdorferi* should be obtained. Viral illnesses, including hepatitis B, infectious mononucleosis, parvovirus, rubella, and rubella vaccination, rarely present as monarticular synovitis.

A number of arthritic syndromes that closely mimic known rheumatic diseases have now been described in association with human immunodeficiency virus (HIV) infection.[22] Most of these are polyarticular and appear as arthralgias rather than true arthritis. Opportunistic infections in individuals infected with HIV can develop within one joint and in contiguous bone. In addition to the more typical organisms, such as *S. aureus*, less common microorganisms have been cultured from fluids of septic joints in patients with HIV infection, including *Sporothrix schenkii*, *Cryptococcus neoformans*, several *Salmonella* species, *Ureaplasma urealyticum*, and *Campylobacter fetus*. HIV-infected individuals can also experience an extremely painful, noninflammatory monarthritis. Although the mechanism of this syndrome is unknown, it usually resolves spontaneously in 24 to 28 hours (see Chapter 101).

CRYSTAL-INDUCED ARTHRITIS

Crystal-induced arthritis commonly manifests as acute monarticular arthritis. It is particularly likely when there is a history of recurrent, self-limited attacks of inflammation of the same joint. Fortunately, the most fulminant arthropathy, gout, is also the most easily and reliably diagnosed. Monosodium urate crystals can be identified in at least 95 percent of acute joint effusions by polarized microscopy and even in some asymptomatic joints.[23] Calcium pyrophosphate crystals are often not identified initially in patients who are later diagnosed as having pseudogout.[24] Hydroxyapatite crystals present a particular problem in diagnosis, because they are reliably identified only by electron microscopy or alizarin red stain.[25] Occasionally, in patients with renal failure and an acute monarthritis, calcium oxalate crystals can be identified in joint fluid aspirates. As a general rule, identification of crystals in joint fluid does not prove the absence of coexistent infection. Crystal-induced arthropathies are particularly common and difficult to manage in patients who are uremic or undergoing dialysis.

Gouty arthritis is definitely present when intracellular birefringent, needle-shaped crystals (sodium urate) are identified in synovial fluid or confirmed by documentation of urate crystals in a tophus, and it is probably present if the crystals are extracellular. The most characteristic clinical features are extremely rapid onset of severe pain and inflammation with extension of the inflammatory process into the surrounding tissues, producing the appearance of cellulitis. Desquamation of overlying skin may occur as the attack subsides. In the ankle, the initial phases visually resemble the periarthritis of erythema nodosum, but the pain is much more severe.[26]

Podagra is characteristic but not pathognomonic of gout.[27] First attacks of gout can occur in other large joints or in the small joints of the upper extremities (see Chapter 87).

Calcium pyrophosphate dihydrate (CPPD) deposition is associated with acute or chronic inflammatory arthritis and may be superimposed on osteoarthritis.[24] Pseudogout can be diagnosed by the finding of weakly positive, rhomboid-shaped birefringent crystals in the white blood cells of synovial fluid aspirates (see Chapter 88). These are identified in one half of effusions from patients presenting with monarthritis due to CPPD. Their presence does not exclude infection in a patient with a first episode of monarticular arthritis. The physician can also suspect the diagnosis in an elderly person with an acute monarthritis of the knee or wrist and chondrocalcinosis on radiographs in whom there are no obvious reasons to suspect infection. Less common forms of crystal-induced arthritis may result from deposition of hydroxyapatite (often in the shoulder) or calcium oxalate (especially in patients with renal failure).

OTHER CAUSES OF ACUTE INFLAMMATORY ARTHRITIS

Patients without Systemic Manifestations

If a patient does not have one of the previously mentioned disorders, there is a significant likelihood that the cause will remain elusive for a time, and the physician will be obliged to make a practical decision about how aggressively to pursue a diagnosis. The initial workup under these circumstances should be as focused as possible so that a satisfactory result can be achieved with the greatest possible economy of patient discomfort and medical resources.

Juvenile Rheumatoid Arthritis

Although most children with juvenile rheumatoid arthritis presenting with monarticular disease eventually experience involvement of additional joints, about 25 percent have isolated monarthritis that may recur intermittently into adulthood. Antinuclear antibodies are more common than rheumatoid factor; monarticular disease and antinuclear antibodies correlate with the development of iritis.[28]

Rheumatoid Arthritis

Rheumatoid arthritis may manifest with acute or insidious onset of monarthritis. A detailed history often reveals gradual onset of fatigue or arthralgias. Physical examination may reveal unsuspected involvement of other joints, particularly the metatarsophalangeal joints.

Seronegative Spondyloarthropathies

The spondyloarthropathies were mentioned previously in the context of monarthritis accompanied by axial skeleton stiffness or pain. Joints most typically involved are those of the lower extremities. There may also be extra-articular clues to the diagnosis, such as urethritis, diarrhea, inflammatory eye disease, nail pitting, or a psoriasiform rash. Joint swelling may be fusiform, creating "sausage digits."

Neuropathic Arthropathy

Neuropathic arthropathy (Charcot joints) should be suspected in patients with diabetes who present with a subacute or chronic monarthritis of the knee, ankle, or foot, usually with swelling and effusion but with little pain. The arthritis develops most commonly in those with peripheral neuropathy and sensory loss. The radiographic picture is usually pathognomonic.

Hemarthroses

Hemarthroses may result from trauma, synovial hemangiomas, pigmented villonodular synovitis, excessive anticoagulation, or inherited coagulopathies.

Lyme Arthritis

Lyme arthritis should be suspected in endemic areas, especially if there is a history of rash, tick bite, or exposure.

Patients with Signs of Systemic Illness

Enteropathic Arthritis

Whipple's disease, which is rare, can appear with a monarticular arthritis when the bowel disease is not evident. Regional enteritis and ulcerative colitis are more likely to be symptomatic when arthritis develops[29] (see Chapter 73). Celiac disease (sprue) is associated with rheumatic diseases, including rheumatoid arthritis and lupus.

Systemic Autoimmune Disease

Systemic lupus erythematosus occasionally manifests with monarticular arthritis, although small joint polyarthritis is more common. Marked swelling of the wrist accompanied by tenosynovitis may also be accompanied by fever and severe systemic signs. Monarticular or large joint pain in a steroid-treated lupus patient suggests avascular necrosis[30] or infection. Sarcoidosis often manifests as arthritis of the ankles, wrists, or knees, usually bilateral, which may be associated with erythema nodosum or hilar adenopathy.[31] Henoch-Schönlein purpura,[32] Takayasu's disease,[33] overlap syndromes,[34] polymyalgia rheumatica,[35] and giant cell arteritis[36] can all manifest with monarticular or polyarticular arthritis, although polyarthritis is the rule in many of these disorders.

Familial Mediterranean fever typically causes exquisitely painful monarthritis with moderately impressive physical findings.[37,38] The combination of fever and evanescent rash suggests Still's disease[39] or rheumatic fever.[40]

Chronic Inflammatory Monarticular Arthritis

Many disorders that can manifest as acute monarticular inflammation progress to polyarticular involvement, remit and relapse, or spontaneously resolve. Persistent monarticular inflammation raises special concern that a more narrow spectrum of disorders is present, particularly chronic infections or tumors. Synovial biopsy and arthroscopy may be useful in identifying the cause of chronic monarthritis (Fig. 34–3) (see Chapter 46).

Chronic infections result from slow-growing organisms or the presence of foreign bodies in the joint. Typically, there are persistent signs of inflammation, including stiffness, pain, and warmth, and characteristically there is synovial thickening, regardless of whether an effusion is present.

Tuberculosis, which is undergoing a resurgence in the United States, almost always affects a single diarthrodial joint[41] (see Chapter 100). A positive tuberculin test may be the only clue. Infection with atypical mycobacteria or

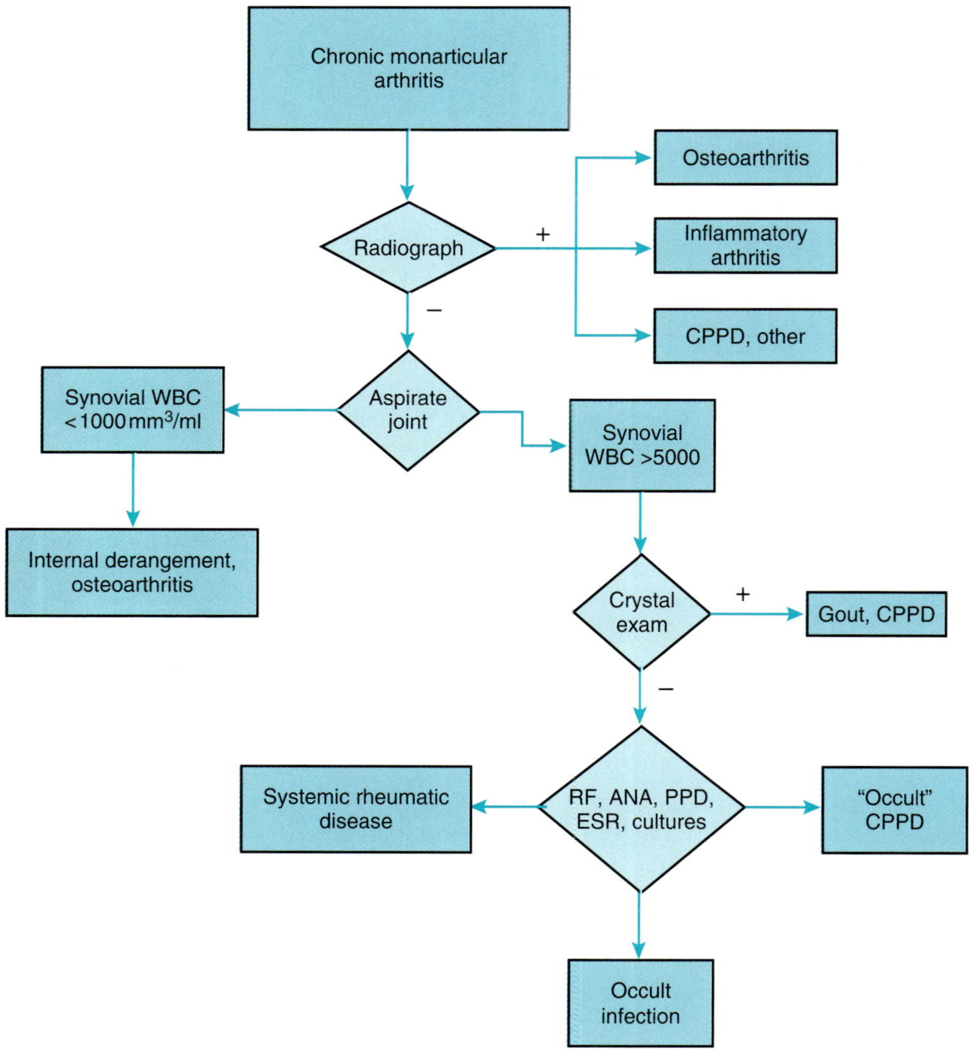

FIGURE 34–3 · Approach to Chronic Monarticular Arthritis. ANA, antinuclear antibody test; CPPD, calcium pyrophosphate deposition disease; ESR, erythrocyte sedimentation rate; PPD, purified protein derivative test for tuberculosis; RF, rheumatoid factor test; WBC, white blood cell count.

Candida, coccidioidomycosis, histoplasmosis, and blastomycosis can produce similar syndromes.

Chronic infections may also result from penetrating wounds or the introduction of foreign bodies. Superficially located joints on the hands and the feet are most likely to be penetrated during normal activity, often without awareness on the part of the individual. Sporotrichosis should be suspected in a gardener with involvement of a hand joint, especially if there is surrounding soft tissue reaction.[42]

Tumors, particularly pigmented villonodular synovitis,[43] should be suspected when there is chronic monarticular inflammation in conjunction with a bloody effusion. Metastasis to synovium from solid tumors or joint involvement by hematologic malignancies is rare. Tumors involving periarticular structures can mimic arthritis.

Noninflammatory Monarticular Arthritis

Structural joint disease should be suspected when there is little synovial inflammation in proportion to the degree of destruction of bone and cartilage and when the synovial fluid white blood cell count is less than 1000 to 2000 cells/mm^3. Truly noninflammatory fluid, however, contains fewer than 200 cells/mm^3. An internal derangement of the knee is suggested by a history of trauma, episodes of joint locking or "giving way," and tenderness at the joint margin; physical examination reveals locking or episodic pain during range of motion. It may be confirmed by MRI or arthroscopy, which demonstrates meniscal or ligamentous tears.

Osteoarthritis frequently manifests as monarthritis, particularly in the knee, hip, acromioclavicular joint, first radiocarpal joint, or first metatarsophalangeal joint (i.e., hallux rigidus). Elderly patients with osteoarthritis may have inflammatory joint effusions that contain CPPD crystals.[26] In monarticular disease, a predisposing factor, such as congenital dysplasia of the hip, trauma to or prior surgical removal of ligaments or fibrocartilage from the knee, prior inflammatory arthritis or infection, occupational stress, or obesity, should be sought.

Hip symptoms in a young patient suggest congenital dysplasia of the hip or a slipped capital femoral epiphysis.[44,45] Spontaneous osteonecrosis may occur in the hip (Legg-Calvé-Perthes disease), metatarsal bones (Freiberg's disease), capitellum of the humerus, or carpal lunate. Osteochondritis dessicans should be suspected in a child or teenager who, after minor trauma, has relatively severe knee pain followed by mechanical dysfunction.[46] There is now considerable experience, especially in pediatric patients, using ultrasound to identify hip effusions and periarticular abnormalities.[47]

Rapid development of "osteoarthritis" should lead to consideration of the possibility of fracture related to osteopenia, an adjacent destructive process such as metastatic tumor, or avascular necrosis.

Osteonecrosis is a common cause of monarthritis of the hip, shoulders, and knees in young people with systemic diseases who require corticosteroid therapy. It also occurs in a variety of other conditions, such as alcoholism, barotrauma, hemoglobinopathies, diabetes, hyperlipidemia, hyperuricemia, and systemic lupus erythematosus.

Diagnostic Studies

SYNOVIAL FLUID ANALYSIS

The most important laboratory test in the evaluation of an acute monoarthritis is synovial fluid analysis.[25] The primary purpose of synovial fluid analysis is to answer the following questions:

Is the effusion inflammatory?
Is it infected?
Does it contain intracellular or extracellular crystals?

Even a few drops of fluid can be sufficient to obtain a white blood cell count and differential cell count, crystal analysis, and culture. No other tests are needed (see Chapter 46). If fluid is difficult to obtain, ultrasound-guided aspiration may yield fluid even, in the authors' experience, from proximal interphalangeal joints.

CULTURES

If septic arthritis is a possibility, blood, synovial fluid, and urine cultures are indicated. If gonococcal arthritis is a consideration, cervicourethral, rectal, and pharyngeal samples should be placed on Thayer-Martin medium. Culture specimens from normally sterile sites, including the synovial cavity, tenosynovial space, and intracutaneous lesions, should be placed on chocolate agar without added preservative. Synovial fluid cultures are usually negative in gonococcal arthritis (see Chapter 98).

LABORATORY STUDIES

In the initial evaluation of monarthritis, diagnostic laboratory testing for rheumatic diseases should only be undertaken after a careful history and physical examination.[4] A complete blood count with differential, Westergren sedimentation rate, C-reactive protein, tests of renal and liver function, and a urinalysis can be useful if infection or a multisystem disease is suspected. In the appropriate clinical setting, studies that may be of value include a uric acid level, rheumatoid factor, and certain serologic studies such as an ANA, antineutrophil cytoplasmic antibodies, Lyme disease, hepatitis, or parvovirus serologies. Routinely ordered serology studies, especially if bundled into "arthritis panels," in the wrong clinical setting may cause confusion and lead to further unnecessary testing.

RADIOGRAPHY

Plain radiographs of the affected and contralateral joints should almost always be obtained in patients with symptoms of more than several weeks' duration. They may also be helpful for patients with an acute arthritis in whom infection or crystal disease is suspected. For those with no prior joint complaints, common findings are soft tissue calcification and evidence of intra-articular pathology not known to the patient, such as osteoarthritis, chondrocalcinosis, or loose bodies. Occasionally, an unsuspected bony lesion (e.g., a fracture) or evidence of osseous or hematologic malignancy, osteomyelitis, or Paget's disease may be detected. Care should be taken to include enough surrounding bone in the radiograph to identify such lesions.

NUCLEAR MEDICINE

Radionuclide scans are useful primarily because of their sensitivity. They are used when it is important to search for a site of infection that cannot be detected or localized by other means, such as in deeply buried joints that are difficult to examine, fibrocartilaginous joints in which range of motion is poorly tested, and the spine (see Chapter 51).

MAGNETIC RESONANCE IMAGING

Magnetic resonance imaging has been shown to be superior to other imaging modalities in the diagnosis of ischemic necrosis of bone[49] and possibly Legg-Calvé-Perthes disease,[50] particularly in early cases. In addition, MRI is the study of choice to detect radiographically occult fractures, especially in the hip and pelvis.[51] In the knee, MRI provides a more accurate and noninvasive alternative to arthrography for detection of meniscal and cruciate ligament injuries.[52] Because of their superior definition of soft tissue pathology, both MRI and ultrasound are useful in investigating deep infections about the hip, such as psoas abscesses, which may mimic arthritis.[53,54] Although superior in most cases to CT in detecting subchondral bone and marrow involvement by tumor or osteomyelitis, MRI does not provide the ability to survey the entire body that is characteristic of radionuclide scans.

ULTRASOUND

Musculoskeletal ultrasound has advanced rapidly in the past decade. It is possible to aspirate almost any joint under ultrasonic control, no matter how inaccessible or small. This facilitates the workup for infection. Evaluation for the presence of fluid in joints, bursae, and periarticular structures is greatly facilitated by ultrasound. It is possible to use "power Doppler" to identify areas of increased tissue perfusion.[54] This may be helpful in localizing inflammation. Identification of lesions in tendons such as an inflamed Achilles or patellar tendon, as well as compromise of smaller tendons by rheumatoid nodules, can also be done by ultrasound. Evaluation of structural abnormalities of joints, such as osteoarthritis or internal derangements is more difficult.

SYNOVIAL AND BONE BIOPSY

Although rarely needed, synovial biopsy may play a role in the diagnosis of chronic, unexplained monarticular arthritis.[55] Tuberculous or fungal synovitis is more frequently identified by staining and culture of open biopsy material than by similar studies of synovial fluid. Closed-needle biopsy or arthroscopic biopsy of the knee is preferable to open biopsy because of reduced morbidity. In acute inflammatory arthritis, a surgical biopsy is indicated in the diagnosis of infection of fibrocartilaginous joints, such as the sacroiliac and sternoclavicular joints, and probably the symphysis pubis if an initial attempt at aspiration is not diagnostic.[56] General anesthesia may be required for pain control. If osteomyelitis is suspected, the physician should consider obtaining a bone biopsy specimen before initiating antibiotic therapy.

REFERENCES

1. Radin EL: Chondromalacia of the patella. Bull Rheum Dis 34(1):1, 1984.
2. Lagier R: Synovial reaction caused by adjacent malignant tumors: Anatomico-pathological study of three cases. J Rheumatol 4:65, 1997.
3. Feagin JA Jr: The office diagnosis and documentation of common knee problems. Clin Sports Med 8:453, 1989.
4. Isenberg DA, Schoenfield Y: The rheumatologic complications of hematologic disorders. Semin Arthritis Rheum 12:348, 1983.
5. Hadjipavlou AG, Gaintanis IN, Kontalis GM: Paget's disease of bone and its management. J Bone Joint Surg Am 84: 160, 2002.
6. Larsson LG, Baum J: The syndromes of bursitis. Bull Rheum Dis 36(1):1, 1986.
7. Viggiano DA, Garrett JC, Clayton ML: Septic arthritis presenting as olecranon bursitis in patients with rheumatoid arthritis. J Bone Joint Surg Am 62:1011, 1980.
8. Ho O Jr, Su EY: Antibiotic therapy of septic bursitis. Arthritis Rheum 24:905, 1981.
9. Cucurull E, Espinoza LR: Gonococcal arthritis (review). Rheum Dis Clin North Am 24: 305-322, 1998.
10. Gotuzzo E, Alarcon GS, Bocanegra TS, et al: Articular involvement in human brucellosis: A retrospective analysis of 304 cases. Semin Arthritis Rheum 12:245, 1982.
11. Grassi W, Tittarelli E, Blasetti P, et al: Finger tendon involvement in rheumatoid arthritis: Evaluation with high-frequency sonography. Arthritis Rheum 38:786, 1995.
12. Dowart BB: Carpal tunnel syndrome: A review. Semin Arthritis Rheum 14:134, 1984.
13. Putten J: Neurological Differential Diagnosis. New York, Springer-Verlag, 1980.
14. Gibson RK, Rosenthal SJ, Lukert BP: Pyomyositis. Am J Med 11:421, 1982.
15. Kallen PS, Louie JS, Nies KM, et al: Infectious myositis and related syndromes. Am J Med 11:421, 1982.
16. Goldenberg DL: Infectious arthritis complicating rheumatoid arthritis and other chronic rheumatic disorders. Arthritis Rheum 32:496, 1989.
17. Resnick D, Niwayana G: Reiter's disease. *In* Diagnosis of Bone and Joint Disorders, 2nd ed. Philadelphia, WB Saunders, 1988.
18. Resnick D, Niwayana G: Psoriatic arthritis. *In* Diagnosis of Bone and Joint Disorders, 2nd ed. Philadelphia, WB Saunders, 1988, pp 1218-1251.
19. Cimmino, MA: Recognition and management of bacterial arthritis. Drugs 54:50-60, 1997.
20. Seifert MH, Warin AP, Miller A: Articular and cutaneous manifestations of gonorrhea: Review of sixteen cases. Ann Rheum Dis 33:140, 1974.
21. Goldenberg DL: Septic arthritis. Lancet 351:197-202, 1998.
22. Rynes RI, Goldenberg DL, DiGiacomo R, et al: Acquired-immunodeficiency syndrome–associated arthritis. Am J Med 84:810-816, 1988.
23. Bomalaski JS, Lluberas G, Schumacher HR Jr: Monosodium urate crystals in the knee joint of patients with asymptomatic nontophaceous gout. Arthritis Rheum 29:1480, 1986.
24. Masuda I, Ishikawa K: Clinical features of pseudogout attack: A review of fifty cases. Clin Orthop Rel Res 229:123, 1988.
25. Gatter RA, Schumacher HR Jr: A Practical Handbook of Synovial Fluid Analysis. Philadelphia, Lea and Febiger, 1991.

26. Yu T: Diversity of clinical features in gouty arthritis. Semin Arthritis Rheum 13:360, 1984.
27. McCarty DJ: Calcium pyrophosphate dihydrate crystal deposition disease—1975. Arthritis Rheum 19:275, 1976.
28. Chylack LT Jr: The ocular manifestations of juvenile rheumatoid arthritis. Arthritis Rheum 20 (Supp):224, 1976.
29. Weiner SR, Utsinger P: Whipple disease. Semin Arthritis Rheum 15:157, 1986.
30. Zizic TM, Hungerford DS, Stevens MB: Ischemic bone necrosis in systemic lupus erythematosus. Medicine (Baltimore) 59:134, 1980.
31. Spilberg I, Siltzbach LE, McEwen C: The arthritis of sarcoidosis. Arthritis Rheum 12:126, 1969.
32. Cream JJ, Gumpel JM, Peachey RDG: Schönlein-Henoch purpura in the adult. Q J Med 39:461, 1940.
33. Hall S, Barr W, Lie JT, et al: Takayasu arthritis. Medicine 64:89, 1985.
34. Bennett RM, O'Connell DJ: Mixed connective tissue disease: A clinicopathologic study of 20 cases. Semin Arthritis Rheum 10:25, 1980.
35. Healey L: Long-term follow-up of polymyalgia rheumatica: Evidence for synovitis. Semin Arthritis Rheum 23:322, 1984.
36. Ginsberg WW, Cohen MD, Hall SB, et al: Seronegative polyarthritis in giant cell arthritis. Arthritis Rheum 28:1362, 1985.
37. Meyerhoff J: Familial Mediterranean fever: Report of a large family, review of the literature, and discussion of the frequency of amyloidosis. Medicine (Baltimore) 59:66, 1980.
38. Sohar E, Pras M, Gafni J: Familial Mediterranean fever and its articular manifestations. Clin Rheum Dis 1:195, 1975.
39. van de Putte LB, Wouters JM: Adult-onset Still's disease. Ballieres Clinic Rheumatol 5:263, 1991.
40. Ben-Dov I, Berry E: Acute rheumatic fever in adults over the age of 45 years: An analysis of 23 patients together with a review of the literature. Semin Arthritis Rheum 10:100, 1980.
41. Nathanson L, Cohen W: A statistical and roentgen analysis of two hundred cases of bone and joint tuberculosis. Radiology 36:550, 1940.
42. Wilson DE, Mann JJ, Bennett JE, Utz P: Clinical features of extracutaneous sporotrichosis. Medicine (Baltimore) 63:25, 1984.
43. Docken WP: Pigmented villonodular synovitis. Semin Arthritis Rheum 9:1, 1979.
44. Wilson PD, Jacobs B, Schecter L: Slipped capital femoral epiphysis. J Bone Joint Surg Am 14:549, 1967.
45. Ponseti IV, McClintock R: The pathology of slipping of the upper femoral epiphysis. J Bone Joint Surg Am 38:71, 1956.
46. Pappa AM: The osteochondroses. Pediatr Clin North Am 14:549, 1967.
47. Harcke HT, Mandell GA, Cassell IL: Imaging techniques in childhood arthritis. Rheum Dis Clin North Am 23:523, 1997.
48. American College of Rheumatology Ad Hoc Committee on Cllinical Guidelines. Guidelines for the initial evaluation of the adult patient with acute musculoskeletal symptoms. Arthritis Rheum 39:1-8, 1996.
49. Imhof H, BreitenseherM, Trattnig S, et al: Imaging of avascular necrosis of bone. European Radiology 7:160-166, 1997.
50. Lamer S, Dorgeret S, Khairouni A, et al: Femoral head vascularization in Legg-Calve-Perthes disease: comparison of dynamic gadolinium-enhanced subtraction MRI with bone scintigraphy. Pediatric Radiology 32:580-585, 2002.
51. Sadro C: Current concepts in magnetic resonance imaging of the adult hip and pelvis. Seminars in Roentgenology 35:231-248, 2000.
52. Crotty JM, Monu JU, Pope TL: Magnetic resonance imaging of the musculoskeletal system. Part 4. The knee. Clin Orthoped Rel Res 330:288-303, 1996.
53. Strouse PJ, DiPietro MA, Adler RS: Pediatric hip effusions: Evaluation with power Doppler sonography. Radiology 206:731, 1998.
54. Weintraub JC, Cohen JM, Maravilla KR: Iliopsoas muscles: MR study of normal anatomy and disease. Radiology 156:435, 1985.
55. Schumacher HR: Joint pathology in infectious arthritis. Clin Rheum Dis 4:33, 1978.
56. Gordon G, Kabins SA: Pyogenic sacroiliitis. Am J Med 69:50, 1980.

35 Polyarticular Arthritis

JOHN S. SERGENT

Joint pain is extremely common and is almost always referred to as "arthritis" by the lay public. Because the majority of people who believe they have arthritis actually have some other cause for their pain, the initial challenge for the physician is to learn to differentiate between true arthritis and other causes of pain in and around joints.[1,2] Then, for those whose polyarticular pain does appear to represent polyarthritis, the challenge is to use the history, physical examination, and ancillary tests first to develop a differential diagnosis and then to establish a probable or, in most cases, a definitive diagnosis. Because polyarticular pain is the most frequent complaint bringing patients to rheumatologists, it is imperative that students of the field become proficient in this area.

History, Physical Examination, and Laboratory Tests

HISTORY

As Mackenzie[3] and others have pointed out, the clinical history is "by far the most important diagnostic tool" in the evaluation of polyarticular disorders. Many clinicians augment their histories with the use of self-report patient questionnaires that may be especially beneficial in following patients over time.[4] A number of items deserve special attention.

Onset

The physician should direct attention early to the nature of the first symptoms. This is not always easy, especially if months or years have passed, because most patients prefer to talk about their current symptoms. It is also difficult because most patients think of arthritis as a disease, rather than a symptom or finding, and, in their histories, they may discuss all the joint problems of a lifetime, even obviously traumatic ones.

Course

The physician must determine what has occurred since the onset of symptoms and at what rate. Chronic arthritis may be relentlessly progressive from the onset, or it may be intermittent, with periods of partial or complete remission. As individual joints become involved, the process may be migratory or additive. The term *migratory polyarthritis* implies that previously involved joints become asymptomatic as new joints become inflamed; the disease appears to migrate from joint to joint.

Specific Joint Symptoms

These features include locking, localized pain, "giving way" without warning, palpable or audible crepitation, warmth, and swelling.

Systemic Symptoms

Patients who seek a physician's help because of joint pain often do not perceive, unless asked, relationships between joint pain and other complaints, such as fever, night sweats, weight loss, and generalized muscle stiffness. The history of these symptoms should be sought specifically and, when possible, quantified.

Rheumatic Disease Systems Review

In addition to systemic symptoms, patients with arthritis must be asked specifically about conditions associated with various forms of arthritis, including rash (i.e., photosensitive, psoriatic, purpuric, or petechial), areas of alopecia, Raynaud's phenomenon, sicca syndrome, uveitis, scleritis, oral and genital ulcers, urethritis or cervicitis, symptoms of inflammatory bowel disease, and pleuropericardial symptoms.

Past History

Previous diagnoses are not always correct. A childhood history of rheumatic fever, for example, needs to be explored, because a number of children who were labeled as having rheumatic fever in fact had Still's disease or another form of juvenile chronic polyarthritis; the reverse is also true. Special emphasis should be given to events of the immediate weeks or months preceding the onset of joint disease, including sore throats, febrile illnesses, venereal disease, sexual contacts, diarrhea, rashes, and uveitis.

Family History

In addition to asking about any type of arthritis, the examiner should inquire about a family history of any associated condition, such as psoriasis, uveitis, or inflammatory bowel disease. In patients suspected of having ankylosing spondylitis, it is important to obtain the history of any family members with chronic back pain and then to attempt to determine the nature of that condition.

PHYSICAL EXAMINATION

A complete physical examination is essential. Special consideration must be given to searching for features such as small patches of psoriasis, psoriatic nails, oral and genital ulcers, funduscopic changes, murmurs, rubs, bruits, and peripheral pulses. A careful neurologic examination is also warranted.

The details of a complete musculoskeletal examination are reviewed in Chapter 33. Each joint should be examined for warmth, synovial thickening, effusions, crepitation, deformity, and tenderness. Active and passive ranges of motion should be tested. The spinal examination should include the range of motion of the cervical and lumbar regions, chest expansion, tenderness of the spinous processes and sacroiliac joints, abnormal curves, and muscle spasm.

LABORATORY TESTS

Nonspecific tests of inflammation include hematocrit, erythrocyte sedimentation rate, C-reactive protein, and white blood cell count. Tests sometimes helpful in specific diseases are shown in Table 35–1. They must be ordered wisely because the background false-positive rate can be quite high.

If obtainable, synovial fluid should be examined as described in Chapter 46. The primary benefit of synovial fluid examination is to differentiate among osteoarthritis, inflammatory arthritis, and infection. Rarely are tests indicated other than appearance, total white blood cell count and differential, crystal examination, and culture.

TABLE 35–1 • LABORATORY TESTS FOR POLYARTHRITIS

Antistreptolysin O
Helpful in young
If repeated levels

Test	Significance: Positive	Significance: Negative
Rheumatoid factor	Helpful in young persons, in whom background positivity is low	Prognostic significance only, not helpful in individual cases
Antinuclear antibody	High titer, suggestive of a rheumatic disease	Virtually rules out active systemic lupus
Uric acid	Elevated levels, indicating that gout is possible	If repeated levels are normal, gout unlikely
Antistreptolysin O	Recent streptococcal exposure	Rheumatic fever unlikely
HLA-B27	Possibly marginally useful in early-onset ankylosing spondylitis	No benefit
Anti-*Borrelia*	Only helpful if pretest probability is high	Chronic Lyme disease unlikely

RADIOGRAPHIC FEATURES

Important radiographic features that may help in patient evaluation include cartilage loss, erosions, periarticular osteoporosis, osteophytes, periostitis, and soft tissue changes. In many cases, properly chosen radiographs may be virtually diagnostic or may eliminate certain diseases from further consideration.

Principles of Diagnosis

Physicians are expert in pattern recognition, and in no area is this more important than in rheumatology, where the specific joints involved, the sequence of events, and associated features—as opposed to specific diagnostic tests—define most diseases. Of course, being competent in pattern recognition can sometimes be a two-edged sword if the clinician settles too quickly on a diagnosis or is inflexible about changing the presumed diagnosis as new data become available.

After other causes of joint pain have been eliminated and it appears that the patient does in fact have polyarticular arthritis, there are a number of classification schemes that may aid in determining the correct diagnosis. One might, for example, consider the size of the involved joints (small [digits] vs large), the age of onset, or other features. We have chosen a system based on the presence or absence of inflammation and the number and pattern of joint involvement.

In most situations the best determinant of inflammation is the synovial fluid examination (see Chapter 46) and especially the synovial fluid white blood cell count, which will be less than 1000 in most noninflammatory conditions and significantly greater in inflammatory disease. However, there are also clinical features that suggest the arthritis is inflammatory in nature. These include prolonged and severe morning stiffness, fever, night sweats, weight loss, and spontaneous (not activity-related) joint swelling. Physical examination in inflammatory arthritis often reveals local warmth, synovial thickening, and large effusions. In addition to inflammatory synovial fluid, other features suggesting inflammation include anemia, thrombocytosis, an increased erythrocyte sedimentation rate, and increased acute-phase reactants such as C-reactive protein and ferritin.

Table 35–2 shows a classification of polyarthritis based on two features: the presence or absence of inflammation and the number and pattern of joint involvement.

Polyarticular Peripheral Arthritis

RHEUMATOID ARTHRITIS

This condition is the prototype of this group of diseases (see Chapter 66). Rheumatoid arthritis accounts for about one fourth of all patients referred to rheumatologists,[1] and other forms of peripheral joint disease are often defined in part by how they differ from rheumatoid arthritis.

TABLE 35–2 • CLASSIFICATION OF POLYARTHRITIS

Inflammatory

Peripheral polyarticular
- Rheumatoid arthritis
- Systemic lupus erythematosus
- Viral arthritis
- Psoriatic arthritis (occasionally)

Peripheral pauciarticular
- Psoriatic arthritis
- Reiter's syndrome
- Rheumatic fever
- Polyarticular gout
- Enteropathic arthritis
- Behçet's disease
- Bacterial endocarditis

Peripheral with axial involvement
- Ankylosing spondylitis (especially juvenile onset)
- Reiter's syndrome
- Enteropathic arthritis
- Psoriatic arthritis

Noninflammatory (osteoarthritis)

Hereditary
- Osteoarthritis of the hands
- Primary generalized osteoarthritis

Traumatic osteoarthritis
- Osteoarthritis following local injury
- Osteoarthritis of the knees in obese people
- Chondromalacia following aggressive exercise programs
- Osteoarthritis in the elderly

Metabolic diseases (may have an unusual pattern)
- Hemochromatosis
- Ochronosis
- Acromegaly

Idiopathic

Typically beginning in multiple small joints of the hands and feet in a symmetric fashion, rheumatoid arthritis has many variations, including months or years of recurrent monarthritis (palindromic rheumatism)[5] before a typical pattern evolves. Disease duration of 12 weeks or more is strongly predictive of persistent rheumatoid arthritis.[6] The symmetry of rheumatoid arthritis is sometimes overemphasized, and it must be appreciated that this is a general, rough symmetry. It is rare for rheumatoid arthritis to cause extensive damage to one hand and completely spare the other.

The arthritis of rheumatoid arthritis is typically additive, with sequential involvement of groups of joints. Most joints remain more or less symptomatic as new joints are involved. The earliest joints involved are usually small joints of the hands and feet, but the distal interphalangeal joints are spared until late in the course.

Although arthritis is usually the presenting feature of rheumatoid arthritis, occasional patients have extra-articular features of the disease at roughly the same time or even earlier. Episcleritis, subcutaneous nodules, and pleural effusions are the most frequent early extra-articular features of the disease.

SYSTEMIC LUPUS ERYTHEMATOSUS

Systemic lupus erythematosus (SLE) (see Chapter 75) often presents as chronic polyarthritis and may be confused with rheumatoid arthritis in such patients. The arthritis is typically intermittent, may be extremely painful, and is almost never erosive. Mixed connective tissue disease may cause an identical arthritis.

SCLERODERMA

Scleroderma (see Chapter 79) typically begins as painful swollen hands, with early contractures as prominent features. Indeed, the combination of puffy hands and Raynaud's phenomenon is often called *undifferentiated connective tissue disease* in recognition of the fact that the condition of such patients may evolve into SLE, scleroderma, mixed connective tissue disease, or rheumatoid arthritis. Some individuals may remain in the undifferentiated state for many years. Rarely, patients are seen with characteristic features of both scleroderma and rheumatoid arthritis.[7]

PSORIATIC ARTHRITIS

Although typically pauciarticular at onset, psoriatic arthritis may evolve into a polyarticular disease that resembles rheumatoid arthritis (see Chapter 72). This presents particular diagnostic problems in children, whose disease may resemble pauciarticular juvenile chronic arthritis at onset and may then evolve into a pattern resembling polyarticular juvenile or adult rheumatoid arthritis.[8]

GONOCOCCAL ARTHRITIS

Unlike the monarthritis typical of most septic joint diseases, gonococcal arthritis usually presents with fever, tenosynovitis, and papular or pustular skin lesions. As it evolves over several days, it may gradually involve one or more joints in a frankly purulent arthritis (see Chapter 98).

VIRAL ARTHRITIS

Viral arthritis, including that caused by the human immunodeficiency virus (HIV), can cause impressive polyarticular pain, often lasting for weeks or months (see Chapter 102). Parvovirus B19 is the prototype,[9] but similar symptoms have been reported with rubella,[10] mumps,[11] hepatitis B,[12] and other viruses. Acquired immunodeficiency syndrome (AIDS), Reiter's syndrome, psoriatic arthritis, and a painful polyarthritis possibly specific for HIV have been described. In such patients, the arthritis is frequently the presenting manifestation of HIV infection.[13] Another presentation of HIV infection resembles SLE, with fever, rash, polyarthritis, proteinuria, and hematologic abnormalities.[14] Infectious polyarthritis may complicate HIV infection.

PAUCIARTICULAR PERIPHERAL ARTHRITIS

In general, the term *pauciarticular* is used to describe arthritis that affects four or fewer joints, although certain latitude may be taken, such as counting the midfoot or wrist as a single joint. This term is usually limited to the early phase of the disease, because many of these conditions gradually become polyarticular as the course progresses.

PSORIATIC ARTHRITIS

This condition may precede skin disease in a minority of patients and usually begins as asymmetric pauciarticular disease, often including distal interphalangeal joints. In many cases, entire digits are involved with arthritis and periostitis, producing the "sausage digit" appearance. The arthritis is typically asymmetric (Fig. 35–1), and occasional patients show severe damage to one group of joints with no involvement of the contralateral side (see Chapter 72).

REACTIVE ARTHRITIS

Previously known as Reiter's syndrome (i.e., arthritis, conjunctivitis, and skin or mucosal lesions), this process may become manifest in a manner similar to that of psoriatic arthritis but with a greater predilection for the lower extremity. The arthritis is often asymmetric and is frequently associated with involvement of the heel, other enthuses, or the sacroiliac joints (see Chapter 71).

ADULT RHEUMATIC FEVER

Apparently increasing in frequency of occurrence, adult rheumatic fever often causes a painful pauciarticular disease, which is most prominent in the larger joints of the lower extremities. The typical migratory pattern of childhood rheumatic fever is uncommon in adults,[15] and the response to aspirin is less dramatic. Although some fever is usually present, carditis is uncommon, and other features, such as chorea, rash, and subcutaneous nodules, are rare. The presentation in adults may be less acute, with a more insidious arthritis developing over several days or 1 to 2 weeks.

GOUT

Unfortunately, gout all too often presents to the rheumatologist as undiagnosed chronic polyarthritis (see Chapter 87). Particularly confusing can be the syndrome of acute and chronic gouty arthritis superimposed on osteoarthritis of the finger joints.[16] Examination of synovial fluid or material draining from a tophus yields the diagnosis.

CALCIUM PYROPHOSPHATE DEPOSITION DISEASE

This disease is most easily recognized when it manifests as an acute monarthritis (pseudogout). It has many forms, however, including a chronic polyarthritis (see Chapter 88).

BEHÇET'S DISEASE

Uncommon in the United States, Behçet's disease almost invariably causes chronic polyarthritis limited to a few joints. It is characterized by painful acute flare-ups associated with oral, genital, and ophthalmologic manifestations (see Chapter 86).

ENTEROPATHIC ARTHRITIS

This is the arthritis associated with inflammatory bowel disease and characteristically involves large joints of the lower extremity or the lumbosacral spine (see Chapter 73).

RELAPSING POLYCHONDRITIS

This condition usually causes severe inflammation of the ears, nose, and sclera and is associated with a pauciarticular arthritis of the knees or wrists (see Chapter 94).

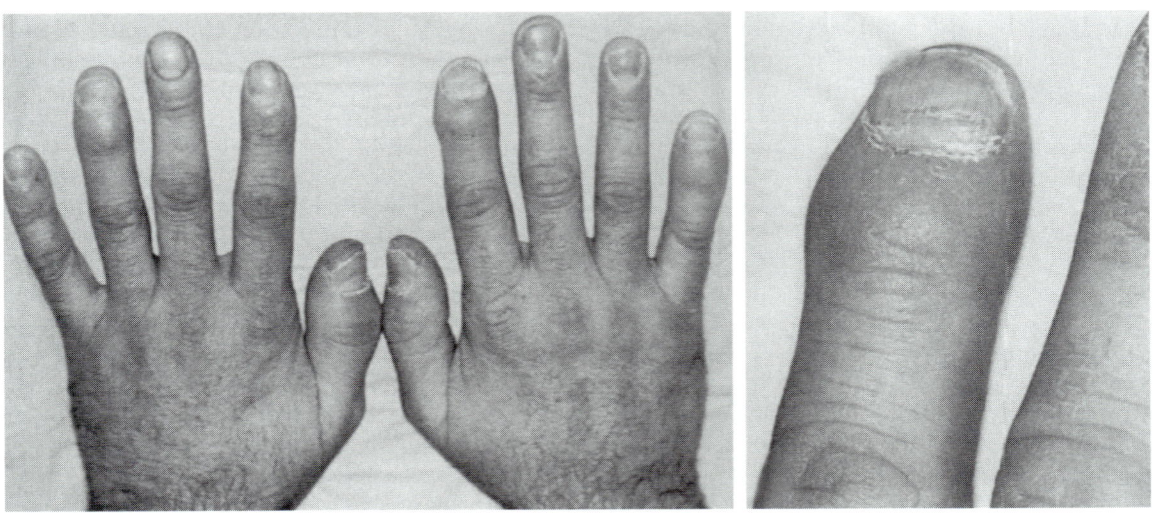

FIGURE 35–1 • **Psoriatic Arthritis.** Note the asymmetry of the distal interphalangeal joint involvement and the associated psoriatic nail disease.

SARCOIDOSIS

Sarcoidosis causes a number of articular problems. The most frequent is an oligoarthritis of the knees or ankles in association with erythema nodosum and bilateral hilar adenopathy. Joint effusions are rare. Occasionally, in patients with long-standing sarcoidosis, a chronic, destructive polyarthritis resembling rheumatoid arthritis may develop (see Chapter 105). In many of these patients, lytic bone disease is visible on radiographs.

LYME DISEASE

The arthritis of Lyme disease is usually monarticular or oligoarticular, but a chronic symmetric polyarthritis has also been described[17] (see Chapter 99).

BACTERIAL ENDOCARDITIS

The arthritis of bacterial endocarditis is also typically monarticular or oligoarticular, usually in the lower extremities. Polyarthralgias are common, however, and the frequent association of positive rheumatoid-factor test results can add to the diagnostic difficulties.[18]

AMYLOID ARTHROPATHY

Amyloid arthropathy may include virtually all joints, but pauciarticular involvement of the upper extremities is most frequent. Bilateral shoulder disease may cause joint enlargement known as the "shoulder pad" sign. This finding, especially in association with carpal tunnel syndrome and purpura in skin folds, should always prompt the examiner to suspect primary amyloidosis. The amyloidosis caused by β_2-microglobulin deposition in chronic dialysis patients may present with an impressive destructive arthritis of large joints, especially the knees, shoulders, and hips[19] (see Chapter 104).

Inflammatory Polyarthritis with Axial Involvement

Early involvement of the axial skeleton can be an extremely important clue to the correct diagnosis of inflammatory polyarthritis. For that reason, it may be very helpful to question the patient carefully about neck and lumbar spine pain and prolonged stiffness to rule out unusual presentations of ankylosing spondylitis, Reiter's syndrome, or other spondyloarthropathies (see Chapters 70 and 71).

ANKYLOSING SPONDYLITIS

This disease is the prototype of this group of diseases. Although it typically begins in the patient's late teens or early twenties with back pain and stiffness, when it begins in juveniles or young teenagers, peripheral arthritis is common and may precede back symptoms by months or years. The arthritis involves predominantly the lower extremities and includes knees, ankles, and feet in most patients.[20]

REITER'S SYNDROME

Although only one fourth to one third of patients with Reiter's syndrome have overt back symptoms on presentation, most of these patients have unilateral or bilateral sacroiliitis and spine disease during the course of the disease.[21]

ENTEROPATHIC ARTHRITIS

The arthritis of inflammatory bowel disease, enteropathic arthritis may present as either axial or peripheral arthritis, or the two may coexist.[22] The axial arthritis is identical to ankylosing spondylitis and is strongly associated with HLA-B27. Once present, the spondylitis runs a progressive course regardless of the activity of the bowel disease.[23] Spondylitis typically develops at around the same time as the bowel disease, but may precede it by years.

PSORIATIC ARTHRITIS

This condition may cause both an axial and a peripheral arthritis, but the axial disease is rarely an important presenting manifestation.

WHIPPLE'S DISEASE

Whipple's disease typically causes a polyarthritis similar to Reiter's syndrome, with sacroiliitis plus a peripheral arthritis usually involving only a few joints at a time.

Noninflammatory Polyarthritis

Many of the features that support the diagnosis of noninflammatory polyarthritis (i.e., osteoarthritis) are simply the absence of features that suggest inflammation. A number of specific findings, however, are helpful in establishing a diagnosis of osteoarthritis (see Chapter 92).

The patient usually describes a history of pain primarily during and after use of the affected joints, with minimal pain at rest and only minimal morning stiffness. Physical examination often reveals coarse crepitation, and loose bodies and other debris may be palpable while the joint is moved through its range of motion. Bony osteophytes may be palpable, especially in the fingers.

Results of routine tests of inflammation are normal unless another disease is present. Because osteoarthritis increases in frequency with advancing age, positive test results for rheumatoid factor become less valuable in older people. In a French study, nearly half of the patients seeking care for osteoarthritis had polyarticular arthritis.[24]

The ultimate diagnostic test for osteoarthritis is the radiograph. A number of important biochemical changes in cartilage precede radiographic changes, but for all practical purposes, symptomatic osteoarthritis is nearly always accompanied by radiographic changes (see Chapter 51) and presents as specific syndromes.

OSTEOARTHRITIS OF THE HANDS

A hereditary disease much more prevalent in women, this form of osteoarthritis typically develops within a few years of menopause and is often associated with mild inflammation for the first year or two that a particular joint is involved. The joints may intermittently be warm and tender. After 1 or 2 years, the evidence of inflammation, if any, gradually subsides, and the typical osteophytes of Heberden's and Bouchard's nodes develop in the distal and proximal interphalangeal joints, respectively. The disease is strikingly symmetric, although the degree of involvement may vary somewhat[25] (Fig. 35–2).

PRIMARY GENERALIZED OSTEOARTHRITIS

A rare, hereditary disease with osteoarthritis of multiple joints, primary generalized osteoarthritis usually begins in middle age and involves "typical" joints, such as the hips, knees, and hands.[26]

OSTEOARTHRITIS SECONDARY TO METABOLIC DISEASES

This type of osteoarthritis is increasingly recognized as particular patterns of osteoarthritis have been described in association with several disorders, which are discussed in the following sections.

Hemochromatosis

Hemochromatosis, an underdiagnosed but relatively common disorder,[27] may present with osteoarthritis involving the metacarpophalangeal joints, especially the second and third. Early-onset osteoarthritis of weight-bearing and large non–weight-bearing joints also is seen (see Chapter 106).

Calcium Pyrophosphate Deposition Disease

This disease may be associated with generalized osteoarthritis, including severe involvement of unusual joints, such as the wrist and patellofemoral joint (see Chapter 88).

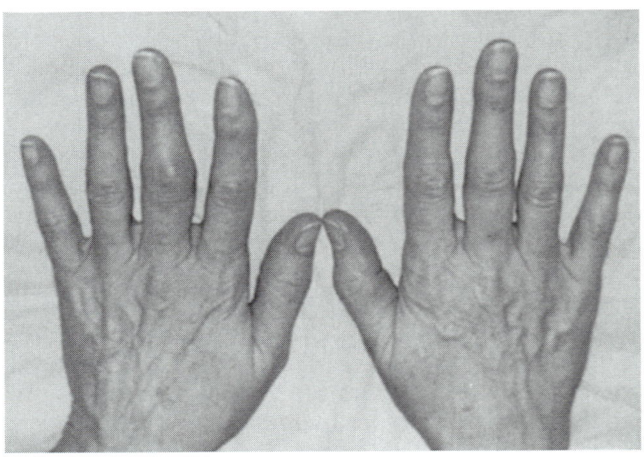

FIGURE 35–2 · Osteoarthritis. Although the left third proximal interphalangeal joint is involved most severely, the right is also involved, and there are several early Heberden's nodes. The patient is a 60-year-old secretary who has moderate soreness in these joints at the end of the day.

Hypothyroidism

Hypothyroidism is associated with symmetric, noninflammatory, highly viscous effusions, frequently in joints with preexisting osteoarthritis (see Chapter 109).

Acromegaly

Acromegaly causes polyarthritis as a result of cartilage overgrowth, with the most severe involvement occurring in the hips and spine (see Chapter 109).

CHONDROMALACIA

Chondromalacia of the patella has multiple causes, but, as a clinical presentation, it is usually seen in physically active young and middle-aged women. Physical findings include small effusions, laxity of the patellar ligaments, and patellofemoral crepitation (see Chapters 40 and 92).

OTHER

Obesity causes a number of joint problems, the most common of which is bilateral osteoarthritis of the knees, especially in women.[28] Various developmental defects, such as congenitally shallow acetabulae, are often asymptomatic until osteoarthritis develops later in life.

Differential Diagnosis

ARTHRITIS VERSUS ARTHRALGIA

Table 35–3 lists the major nonarticular considerations in patients with chronic polyarticular pain. The first challenge to the physician is to differentiate among arthritis, arthralgia, and periarticular inflammation.

TENDINITIS AND RELATED DISORDERS

These include painful shoulder syndromes, tennis elbow (lateral epicondylitis), golfer's elbow (medial epicondylitis), trochanteric bursitis, prepatellar bursitis, Achilles tendinitis, and tendinitis along the radial aspect of the

TABLE 35–3 · DIFFERENTIAL DIAGNOSIS OF POLYARTICULAR PAIN

Polyarthritis	Neuropathies
Tendinitis	Diseases of the spine
Muscle disorders	Primary bone diseases
Polymyalgia rheumatica	Periostitis
Vasculitis	Fibrositis
Vaso-occlusive disease	Malingering

wrist (de Quervain's disease). In these syndromes, pain is often maximal at the beginning of an activity and then starts to subside as the activity is continued. A thorough history, including a description of job and sports activities, is essential. In many cases, physical examination reveals areas of local tenderness near, but distinct from, the joint. Pain may be exacerbated by movement of the affected structures against resistance. In tendinitis, swelling, if present, is usually minimal and limited to tendon sheaths and bursae, rather than joints.

Thickening of tendons and subcutaneous tissues in patients with diabetes can cause a variety of clinical features, including Dupuytren's contractures and, especially in patients with juvenile-onset diabetes, the diabetic stiff hand syndrome[29] (Fig. 35–3) (see Chapter 109).

MUSCLE DISORDERS

Although weakness predominates in most of these conditions, and arthritis, therefore, is not a serious consideration, occasional patients present with periarticular pain as a primary complaint (see Chapter 80).

POLYMYALGIA RHEUMATICA

Because many patients with polymyalgia rheumatica (see Chapter 82) have preexisting polyarticular disorders such as osteoarthritis and tendinitis, it may require skill and experience to differentiate among these problems. Several investigators[30-32] have pointed out the difficulty of distinguishing polymyalgia rheumatica from older-onset rheumatoid arthritis and have stressed that in the early stages it may be impossible to tell them apart.

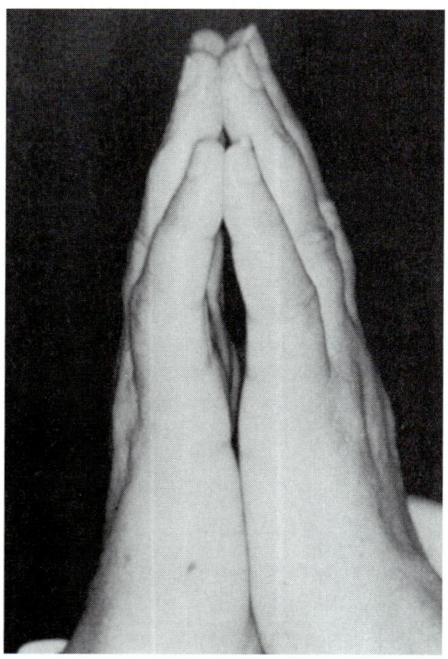

FIGURE 35–3 · The "Prayer Sign" in the Diabetic Stiff Hand Syndrome. As a result of progressive thickening of tendons, joint capsules, and subcutaneous tissues, progressive stiffness and flexion contractures develop in these patients.

VASCULITIS

Frank arthritis is an uncommon manifestation of systemic vasculitis. Joint pain, however, may be deep, aching, and constant.

VASO-OCCLUSIVE DISEASES

The vaso-occlusive diseases include atherosclerosis; cholesterol emboli; emboli from cardiac sources such as a myxoma, diabetes, Raynaud's disease, Buerger's disease, and the antiphospholipid syndrome, which rarely are manifest with polyarticular pain without some other manifestations of disease. Patients with cholesterol emboli may present with polyarthralgias, myalgias, renal disease, elevated erythrocyte sedimentation rates, eosinophilia, and positive test results for rheumatoid factor and antinuclear antibody.[33]

NEUROLOGIC DISEASES

The neurologic diseases include peripheral neuropathies, compression neuropathies such as carpal tunnel syndrome, and infiltrative diseases such as amyloidosis and Waldenström's macroglobulinemia. Pain is usually associated with paresthesias and is usually worse at night. Although patients may have pain localized to joints, it is more typically diffuse, and examination reveals no objective joint abnormalities.

DISEASES OF THE SPINE

A variety of diseases of the neck and spine, including spinal stenosis (congenital or acquired), spondylolisthesis, and tumors of the lower cord and cauda equina, may present in a similar fashion. The pain is usually primarily in the buttocks and is worse with certain postures or activities. In spinal stenosis, for example, pain is typically that of neurogenic claudication, with aching in the buttocks and thighs brought on by certain activities and that is often worse going down hills or steps (see Chapter 39).

PRIMARY BONE DISEASES AND MALIGNANCY

Metastatic tumors and myeloproliferative disorders may masquerade as polyarticular arthritis. In childhood, sickle cell crises and leukemia are especially likely to present as widespread joint pain, and any large series of children with the initial diagnosis of juvenile rheumatoid arthritis contains a small percentage who ultimately are found to have leukemia.[34] In adults, myeloma and a variety of widely metastatic cancers manifest as bone and joint pain. In childhood leukemia, joint effusions, warmth, and tenderness may be present (see Chapter 111). These objective findings are rare in adults.

Other widespread bone diseases, especially osteonecrosis (see Chapter 114), may occasionally resemble polyarticular arthritis. When osteonecrosis involves peripheral joints, such as the knee and ankle, swelling and tenderness may be impressive.[35]

It is not uncommon to see stress fractures in runners or weekend athletes mimicking polyarthritis in the feet and ankles.

PERIOSTITIS

Periostitis, especially as part of the syndrome of hypertrophic pulmonary osteoarthropathy, may cause severe widespread joint pain, tenderness, and warmth. Careful examination reveals tenderness around joint structures and along the shafts of the involved long bones (see Chapter 110) and often a related "clubbing" of fingertips.

FIBROMYALGIA AND PSYCHOGENIC PAIN SYNDROMES

Objective examination of these patients reveals nothing other than areas of tenderness, often in typical trigger points (see Chapter 36).

Summary

Polyarticular arthritis, the most common indication for rheumatologic consultation, represents a challenge to the skills and experience of the clinician. However, by careful history taking and physical examination, along with appropriate tests, the physician can almost always establish the correct diagnosis and institute appropriate therapy. In an era of increasing demand that medicine demonstrate that it is cost-effective, the bedside skills required to evaluate these patients prove valuable indeed.

ACKNOWLEDGEMENT

The author wishes to acknowledge the assistance of Dr. John S. Johnson in the preparation of this chapter.

REFERENCES

1. Hooker RS, Brown JB: Rheumatology referral patterns. HMO Practice 4:61, 1990.
2. Pauker SG, Kassirer JP: Medical progress: Decision analysis. N Engl J Med 316:250, 1987.
3. Mackenzie AH: Differential diagnosis of rheumatoid arthritis. Am J Med 85(Suppl 4):2, 1985.
4. Wolfe F, Pincus T: Listening to the patient: A practical guide to self-report questionnaires in clinical care. Arthritis Rheum 42:1797, 1999.
5. Hannonen P, Mottonen T, Oka M: Palindromic rheumatism: A clinical survey of sixty patients. Scand J Rheumatol 16:413, 1987.
6. Green M, Marzo-Ortega H, McGonagle D, et al: Persistence of mild, early inflammatory arthritis: The importance of disease duration, rheumatoid factor, and the shared epitope. Arthritis Rheum 42:2184, 1999.
7. Zimmerman C, Steiner G, Skriner K, et al: The concurrence of rheumatoid arthritis and limited systemic sclerosis: Clinical and serologic characteristics of an overlap syndrome. Arthritis Rheum 41:1938, 1998.
8. Southwood TR, Petty RE, Malleson PN, et al: Psoriatic arthritis in children. Arthritis Rheum 32:1007, 1989.
9. Moore TL: parvovirus-associated arthritis. Curr Opinion Rheum 12:289, 2000.
10. Chambers RJ, Bywaters EG: Rubella synovitis. Ann Rheum Dis 22:263, 1963.
11. Gordon SC, Lauter CB: Mumps arthritis: A review of the literature. Rev Infect Dis 6:338, 1984.
12. Sergent JS: Extrahepatic manifestations of hepatitis B infection. Bull Rheum Dis 33:1, 1983.
13. Winchester R: AIDS and the rheumatic diseases. Bull Rheum Dis 39:1, 1990.
14. Kopelman RH, Zolla-Pazner S: Association of human immunodeficiency virus infection and autoimmune phenomenon. Am J Med 84:82, 1988.
15. Wallace MR, Garst PD, Papadimos TJ, et al: The return of acute rheumatic fever in young adults. JAMA 262:2557, 1989.
16. Lally EV, Zimmerman B, Ho G Jr, et al: Urate-mediated inflammation in nodal osteoarthritis: Clinical and roentgenographic correlations. Arthritis Rheum 32:86, 1989.
17. Steere AC, Schoen RT. Taylor E: The clinical evolution of Lyme arthritis. Ann Intern Med 107:725, 1987.
18. Churchill MA, Geraci JE, Hunder GG: Musculoskeletal manifestations of bacterial endocarditis. Ann Intern Med 87:754, 1977.
19. Alfrey AC: Beta$_2$-microglobulin amyloidosis. Nephrol Lett 6:27, 1989.
20. Khan MA: Editorial comment. J Rheumatol 16:634, 1989.
21. Lionarons RJ, van Zoeren M, Verhagen JN, et al: HLA-B27–associated reactive spondyloarthropathies in a Dutch military hospital. Ann Rheum Dis 45:141, 1986.
22. Gravallese EM, Kantrowitz FG: Arthritic manifestations of inflammatory bowel disease. Am J Gastroenterol 83:703, 1987.
23. Burgos-Vargas R, Clark P: Axial involvement in the seronegative enteropathy and arthropathy syndrome and its progression to ankylosing spondylitis. J Rheumatol 16:192, 1989.
24. Fautrel B, Hilliquiin P. Allaert F-A, et al: Who are the patients who consult for osteoarthritis? [Abstract] Arthritis Rheum 44:5237, 2001.
25. Cushnaghan J, Dieppe P: Study of 500 patients with limb joint osteoarthritis. I. Analysis by age, sex, and distribution of symptomatic joint sites. Ann Rheum Dis 50:8, 1991.
26. Ala-Kokko L, Baldwin CT, Moskowitz RW, Prockop DJ: Single base mutation in the type II procollagen gene (COL2A1) as a cause of primary osteoarthritis associated with a mild chondrodysplasia. Proc Natl Acad Sci U S A 87:6565, 1990.
27. Edwards CQ, Griffen LM, Goldgar D, et al: Prevalence of hemochromatosis among 11,065 presumably healthy blood donors. N Engl J Med 318:1355, 1988.
28. Felson DT, Anderson JJ, Naimark A, et al: Obesity and knee osteoarthritis: The Framingham Study. Ann Intern Med 109:18, 1988.
29. Kapoor A, Sibbitt WL Jr: Contractures in diabetes mellitus: The syndrome of limited joint mobility. Semin Arthritis Rheum 18:168, 1989.
30. Healey LA: Late-onset rheumatoid arthritis vs. polymyalgia rheumatica: Making the diagnosis. Geriatrics 43:65, 1988.
31. Deal CL, Meenan RF, Goldenberg DL, et al: The clinical features of elderly-onset rheumatoid arthritis. Arthritis Rheum 28:987, 1985.
32. Healy LA: Polymyalgia rheumatica and seronegative RA may be the same entity. J Rheumatol 19:270, 1991.
33. Cappiello RA, Espinoza LR, Adelman, H, et al: Cholesterol embolism: A pseudovasculitic syndrome. Semin Arthritis Rheum 18:240, 1989.
34. Kunnamo I, Kallio P, Pelkonen P, et al: Clinical signs and laboratory tests in the differential diagnosis of arthritis in children. Am J Dis Child 141:34, 1987.
35. Lotke PA, Steinberg ME: Osteonecrosis of the hip and knee. Bull Rheum Dis 35:1, 1985.

36 Fibromyalgia: A Chronic Pain Syndrome

JENNIFER BURKHAM • EDWARD D. HARRIS, JR.

The syndrome of fibromyalgia (FMS) has been defined as a constellation of complaints including diffuse chronic pain and the presence of tender points.[1] The syndrome is often debilitating, frustrating physicians and patients alike. The frustration stems from the chronic nature of the symptoms, the multiplicity of possible etiologies, the vague boundaries of definitions, and the lack of treatments that reliably and completely treat the symptoms.

History of Chronic Pain and Fatigue Syndromes

The first references to patients who have chronic pain, an "aching, stiffness, a readiness to feel muscular fatigue, interference with free muscular movement, and very often a want of energy and vigour," was made by Ralph Stockman, an Edinburgh pathologist, in 1904.[2] William Osler,[3] in the third edition of his text *The Principles and Practice of Medicine*, published just a few years earlier, defined *myalgia* in similar terms but added that "as a rule, myalgia is a transient affection, lasting from a few hours to a few days."

Because of wide variability in symptoms in patients with pain, and no apparent reason for discomfort, there was little enthusiasm among clinical investigators to examine these patients more closely until 1939 when Lewis and Kellgren enlisted volunteers and subjected them to injections of muscles and ligaments with hypertonic saline.[4-6] These deep injections caused discomfort in a myotomal, or referred, pattern, as opposed to a dermatomal, or radicular, pattern. Bennett[7] has emphasized that these concepts and observations were relevant to understanding the fibrositis syndrome in which myotomal origins of discomfort often can be traced.

It is noteworthy that chronic pain and fatigue with normal physical examinations has approached epidemic proportions during times of war. Comroe,[8] in his text *Arthritis and Allied Conditions*, noted in 1944 that "a large percentage of our soldiers entering the medical service of an Army General Hospital with symptoms simulating fibrositis have developed these on a psychogenic basis and that these symptoms cannot be relieved by heat, massage and exercise, but are abolished by discharge from the army . . ." The Persian Gulf syndrome may be another example of this, because 45 percent of deployed veterans, compared to 15 percent of those not deployed to the first Persian Gulf War, developed a constellation of symptoms including muscle and joint pain, fatigue, memory problems, headaches, and gastrointestinal complaints.[9]

A resurgence of interest in this vague symptomatology was introduced in the 1980s when several groups of investigators published data showing that patients with fibrositis or fibromyalgia had particular tenderness in at least 11 of 18 defined "tender points" not shared by asymptomatic control patients.[10-12] During the 1990s, however, it has become apparent that normal people have tender points, that FMS patients are often tender all over their bodies and could best be characterized as having a low pain threshold, and that FMS, the chronic fatigue syndrome, exposure syndromes, and somatoform disorders have considerable overlap in their clinical manifestations.[13]

Definition, Epidemiology, and Diagnostic Criteria

FIBROMYALGIA (A.K.A. FIBROSITIES AND FIBROMYOSITIS)

The diagnosis of FMS is currently made by history of chronic pain and a physical examination exhibiting tender points[1] (Table 36–1). The history must include the presence of at least 3 months of widespread pain that is bilateral, is both above and below the waist, and includes axial skeletal pain. The physical examination must exhibit pain to palpation with approximately 4 kg of pressure at a minimum of 11 of 18 predefined tender points.[1] The diagnosis of FMS is not excluded by the presence of other diseases. The sensitivity and specificity of the criteria are quite high,[1] even when FMS

TABLE 36–1 • 1990 AMERICAN COLLEGE OF RHEUMATOLOGY CRITERIA FOR DIAGNOSIS OF FIBROMYALGIA[1]

Criteria for Diagnosis of Fibromyalgia Syndrome
At least 3 months of widespread pain defined as: Bilateral Above and below the waist, including axial skeletal pain AND Pain to palpation with 4-kg pressure at a minimum of 11 out of 18 predefined tender points
Exclusions
The diagnosis of other diseases does not exclude the diagnosis of fibromyalgia

patients are compared to other rheumatology patients who have chronic painful conditions.

The tender points are located as follows (each on both sides of the body):

1. The insertion of the suboccipital muscles
2. The anterior aspects of the intertransverse spaces at C5-C7
3. The midpoint of the upper border of the trapezius
4. The origin of the supraspinatus, above the scapula spine near the medial border
5. The second rib, just lateral to the costochondral junction
6. Two centimeters distal to the lateral epicondyle
7. The upper outer quadrant of the buttocks in the anterior fold of muscle
8. Just posterior to the greater trochanteric prominence
9. The medial fat pad proximal to the knee joint line[1]

These areas have been proposed to be relatively specific for the diagnosis of FMS. The use of control points, which should be less tender even in FMS patients, has been advocated for increasing the specificity of the trigger points.[14] However, good arguments can be generated to support the hypothesis that the presence of tender points is a marker of patient distress rather than a marker specifically for FMS.

FMS is a generalized chronic pain syndrome that affects eight times more women than men and has an overall prevalence in the society of 1 to 5 percent, making it second only to osteoarthritis (OA) as the most common rheumatologic diagnosis. The complex has been described in children, but symptoms usually begin in a broad age range, from 25 to 65 years (Table 36–2).

In addition to the defining symptomatology for FMS, there are many related symptoms. Fatigue, depression, sleep disorders, paresthesias, migraine headaches, anxiety, sicca symptoms, and Raynaud's phenomenon are each more prevalent in patients with FMS than in the general population. Many patients with chronic illnesses ranging from rheumatoid arthritis (RA) to inflammatory bowel disease develop concurrent symptoms that resemble those found in classic fibromyalgia, making their treatment even more difficult.

TABLE 36–2 • EPIDEMIOLOGY OF FIBROMYALGIA SYNDROME (FMS)[10,11,15-38]

Prevalence	0.7-4.8%
Patient Characteristics	
Female predominance	8-9:1
Predominant age	50-69
Increasing prevalence with age	Yes
Described in children	Yes
Overlap with Other Diagnoses	
Chronic fatigue syndrome	21-70%
Irritable bowel syndrome	32-80%
Multiple chemical sensitivity	33-55%
Psychiatric diagnoses	75%
	Varies between primary and tertiary care

FIBROMYALGIA AND CHRONIC FATIGUE IN THE SAME PATIENT

Underscoring the difficulty in diagnosis and classification of patients with somatic complaints of diffuse body pain and constant fatigue, numerous physicians end their evaluations of patients by giving them two diagnoses: fibromyalgia and chronic fatigue (Fig. 36–1). Chronic fatigue is a syndrome defined by unexplained, persistent, or relapsing fatigue with a definite onset that is not thought to be caused by another medical condition, is not the result of ongoing exertion, is not alleviated by rest, and that causes significant reduction in previous levels of activity.[39,40] More often than not, the patients presenting with both diagnoses are women who have had moderate to severe stress in their life and have, relatively suddenly, become morbidly fatigued and consumed with diffuse and generalized pain not limited to the classic "tender points." Depression and dysthymia are not unusual in these individuals. As in the more differentiated individual syndromes, abnormalities on physical examination are limited to tenderness to the physician's touch and the absence of abnormal laboratory findings.

Controversial Aspects of Fibromyalgia Syndrome

Due to the nonspecific and subjective nature of FMS, there has been controversy focusing on three primary issues: 1) whether fibromyalgia is a "garbage-bin" diagnosis for all unexplained chronic complaints, 2) whether fibromyalgia is primarily a psychiatric disease, and 3) whether fibromyalgia is a nondisease of malingerers or hypochondriacs[41] (see Table 36–1).

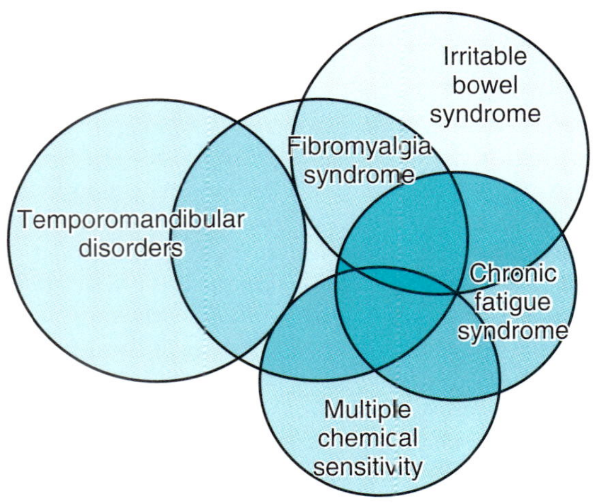

FIGURE 36–1 • Overlap between syndromes with unexplained etiologies such as fibromyalgia, chronic fatigue syndrome (CFS), irritable bowel syndrome, temporomandibular disorder, and multiple chemical sensitivity.

THE "GARBAGE-BIN" DIAGNOSIS?

A comment often heard by nonspecialists with regard to the syndrome of fibromyalgia is that it is a so-called "garbage-bin" diagnosis that serves as a "catch-all" for patients with otherwise unexplained chronic complaints. This comment is not surprising, given that FMS is defined as a syndrome, or constellation of symptoms, rather than a disease with a known etiology. Given the overlap in the symptomatology of FMS with other syndromes,[42] many people believe the definitions are not precise enough to be describing a single entity (see Fig. 36–1). Indeed, although many researchers have searched for a single etiology as the cause of one of the syndromes, none of the currently proposed etiologies for FMS provides an adequate explanation for symptoms in all patients. In addition, it has been demonstrated that the symptom constellation of FMS can develop secondarily in people suffering from other chronically painful diseases, including RA and OA. However, despite the considerable overlap and nonspecific complaints, FMS usually can be differentiated from other forms of chronic, widespread pain based on the American College of Rheumatology (ACR) criteria.[1] Although FMS may eventually be attributed to several etiologies, people presenting with these complaints demand help in present, real time, and our best treatment regimens are based on studies utilizing our current definitions.

PSYCHIATRIC DISEASE?

It is generally accepted that there is an increased incidence of psychiatric disease in FMS patients. This association potentially may be explained in three ways. First, preexisting psychiatric disorders may put patients at risk of developing FMS through an abnormal stress response.[43] Thus, a person without good cognitive, emotional, and behavioral skills could develop maladaptive coping strategies that increase stress and aggravate normally occurring distress, pain, and tenderness.[44] Second, the chronic pain itself affects the hormonal balances and the psyche.[45,46] Thus, people suffering from FMS may suffer a deterioration of their psychologic health secondary to the pain. Indeed, improved psychologic function has been reported in patients who have had their chronic pain effectively treated.[47] Third, the association between FMS and psychologic dysfunction may be in part due to a selection bias in the studies of FMS. Specialty referral clinics where FMS research is carried out have a disproportionately high number of patients with above-average health care–seeking habits compared to FMS patients in general medical clinics. Individuals with above-average health care–seeking habits have been shown to score highly for psychosocial and psychiatric dysfunction.[48,49]

As will be discussed subsequently, the concept of central pain pathways plays an increasingly important role in the discussion of FMS, and, therefore, the vague myotomal distribution of pain need not be evidence for an emotional point of genesis. There is evidence that chronic activation of local pain pathways can cause hypertrophy or hyperactivity of geographically distant pain pathways, resulting in the chronic perception of widespread pain.[50-54]

A NONDISEASE OF MALINGERERS OR HYPOCHONDRIACS?

The suspicion that FMS may be a nondisease exploited by malingerers stems from the observation of the high rates of disability claims for FMS patients[55,56] despite very little objective diagnostic data. FMS is diagnosed based on symptoms and physical examination; there is no objective diagnostic test for FMS. It is highly unlikely that many patients with FMS are malingering.

Diagnosis

In the present era, most patients that have musculoskeletal pain without objective evidence of disease arrive at the rheumatologist's office either by primary care physician referral with diagnosis of FMS (with or without a concurrent diagnosis of chronic fatigue syndrome) or by self-referral after having friends or fellow sufferers suggest this diagnosis. The rheumatologist is, therefore, confronted with two challenges: 1) selecting patients with localized or systemic illness that would be amenable to specific therapy; and 2) designing a reasonable treatment and management plan for those who fit best into the diagnostic categories of FMS or chronic fatigue syndrome (CFS).

The algorithm shown in Figure 36–2 is a useful tool for analyzing these patients. The typical patient is a woman, often one who has been productive and a useful contributor to her family and society. Most will be in the 30-year age bracket that spans menopause. Older men and women (late sixties and older) rarely present with a new onset of diffuse pain and fatigue that cannot be related to a systemic disease or to localized inflammation or a degenerative process in the neurologic or musculoskeletal systems. A sad, and fortunately rare, patient is the adolescent brought in by her mother; shortly into the interviews it becomes apparent to the doctor that the pathology lies primarily with the parent, and the child's somatic complaints are a derivative of this.

Often, the patient will be able to describe a specific day and time when symptoms first appeared. One woman wrote, "On November 17, 1990, I was struck suddenly with what I later found out was CFS and fibromyalgia." This trigger may be an event such as whiplash from being rear-ended in an automobile, a flu-like illness, excessive fatigue from strenuous exercise (sometimes, paradoxically, on vacations), or a psychologic stress that has crescendoed as personal and professional troubles combine. Following this event, the patient develops symptoms that take her into one of several pathways.

FIBROMYALGIA SYNDROME PATHWAY

This is chronic, diffuse pain that interferes with performance of the simplest daily tasks (e.g., brushing teeth and combing hair, cooking and cleaning, shopping). The pain is most often generated from the axial skeleton and rarely involves the hands and feet; an

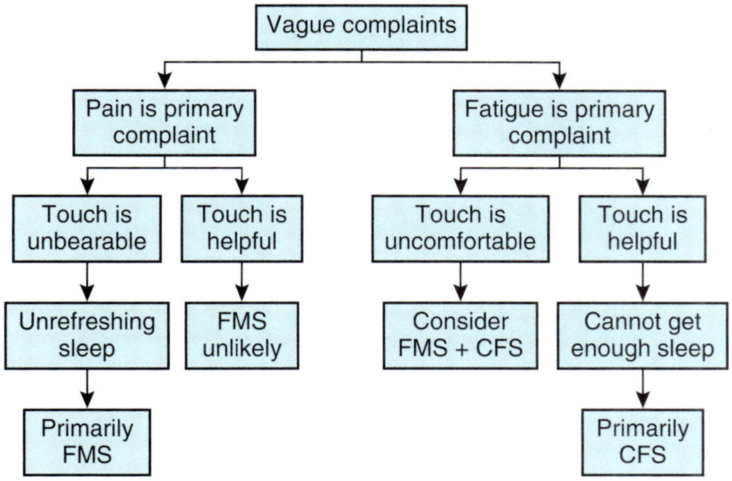

FIGURE 36–2 · Algorithm for the diagnosis of chronic fatigue syndrome (CFS) and fibromyalgia syndrome (FMS).

exception to this is the atypical Raynaud's phenomenon that some describe: cold hands, purplish discoloration, but no blanching or severe pain. Sufferers will often complain of diffuse headache, small and frequent painful bowel movements, diminished libido, and a remarkable inability to focus on anything other than their discomfort in life. One astute rheumatologist has noted, "They have no trouble walking. They just can't stop talking about their pain." This is important: There is no mild to moderate activity that they cannot perform; it is the pain in performing it that limits them. One woman, now a successful vocalist, wrote ". . . it felt like I was moving through quicksand. Just walking down the hallway was a challenge, and painful." This subset of patients rarely awakes in the morning feeling refreshed and eager to start the day. Their sleep has been interrupted many times, and their analogy is often that "I feel like I have been run over by a truck." Patients may become fearful of being touched by another person anywhere on their body, a symptom that often generates marital discord. For the same reason, massage therapy is often intolerable. They will admit to being depressed, but deny that their emotional distress is related to any source other than their pain and poor sleep. Using tact, and after an initial good relationship has been established with the patient, it is important for the physician to inquire and get a satisfactory history about any and all abuse—verbal, physical, or sexual—the patient may have been exposed to earlier in life, long before the present symptom complex evolved. This also applies to patients who present with more fatigue than pain, the next topic. Many FMS patients have failed trials of glucocorticoids, which almost always improve entities associated with inflammation of connective tissue.

CHRONIC FATIGUE SYNDROME PATHWAY

The similarities of this presentation are greater than differences when compared to the FMS symptom complex, and this is the reason many patients arrive carrying both diagnoses. The major difference is that whereas those in the FMS group have trouble getting restorative sleep, CFS patients cannot seem to get enough sleep. If they ever feel good, it is just after wakening from sleep; they arise, begin moving, and quickly are overwhelmed with fatigue, loss of initiative, and a sense of generalized inanition. These are the patients who often relate the beginnings of their problem to a flu-like illness that included fever, fatigue, headache, and swollen glands in the neck or a sore throat. They have musculoskeletal discomfort, but it is more diffuse, and being touched (or massaged) is often pleasant and therapeutic. It is important to realize that there are no physical limitations of joint motion or muscle function in these patients; they can perform well (e.g., Michelle Akers, the world-class soccer player who carries this diagnosis), but after exertion they may not be able to rise from their bed for many days.

Physical Examination

While anticipating that there will be no physical findings to explain symptoms, it is crucial for the physician to perform a detailed physical examination to rule out both localized and systemic abnormalities. The quantification of pressure point sensitivity is worth performing, but many patients will complain of pain wherever they are touched, negating the usefulness of comparing the designated pain areas from the homunculus with control sites. As emphasized in the following section, the absence of bursitis, tendinitis, myofascial pain, excessive joint mobility, adenopathy, splenomegaly, true synovitis, thyromegaly, and abnormal deep-tendon reflexes are among important negatives to register in the medical record.

Routine Laboratory Examinations

In requesting laboratory tests for patients in whom FMS has been suggested as a possible diagnosis, it is important first to follow up on any abnormalities found on physical examination or brought out from the history that could implicate specific organ or tissue pathology. FMS is a diagnosis of exclusion. As examples, a young, completely fatigued, and occasionally febrile woman with some adenopathy should have a human immunodeficiency virus (HIV) test, a screen for hepatitis viruses, and a "rule-out" of Hodgkin's disease. A middle-aged man with a diffuse pain syndrome who smokes several packs of cigarettes each day warrants a careful screen for lung cancer.

In the patient with no historic or physical leads to other diagnoses, the following tests should be performed if not available from a referring physician:

- Complete blood count with smear review
- Urinalysis
- C-reactive protein/erythrocyte sedimentation rate
- Liver function tests (including alkaline phosphatase)
- Creatinine
- Thyroid function tests
- Creatine kinase
- Fasting serum calcium and phosphorus

Any abnormalities in any of these should be followed up with more focused and special tests. Specific abnormal laboratory tests have been noted in FMS but are not diagnostic of FMS. (See Table 36-3.)

Differential Diagnoses

As mentioned, there is considerable overlap among patients with FMS and CFS.[20-24,32,36] Patients with fibromyalgia are also more likely than the general population to have concurrent diagnoses of chronic, unexplained symptoms, such as irritable bowel syndrome,[10,11,16,23-32,37] multiple chemical sensitivity,[33,38] tempomandibular disorder,[34,35] interstitial cystitis,[57] and psychiatric diagnoses (Table 36–2). In addition to the overlap with other diseases of unknown etiologies, both CFS and FMS have been associated with infectious diseases. CFS was originally thought to be strongly associated with chronic Epstein-Barr virus infection,[58] although it is not exclusively associated with this virus.[59] FMS has been found at increased incidence in persons with chronic hepatitis C infection, with 2 to 16 percent of persons with chronic hepatitis C meeting the criteria for FMS and 15 percent of FMS patients testing positive for antibodies against the hepatitis C virus.[60] Other entities that must be considered in these patients are shown in Table 36–4.

TABLE 36-3 • LABORATORY STUDIES IN FIBROMYALGIA SYNDROME (FMS)

Normal Studies
Complete blood count (CBC)
Chemistries
Sedimentation rate
Thyroid function tests
Liver function tests (except with chronic hepatitis C infection)
Rheumatologic serologies
Abnormal Studies in FMS (not diagnostic and not necessarily useful in patient evaluation)
Cerebral spinal fluid (CSF) levels of substance P
Serum somatomedin C levels
Serum and CSF tryptophan levels
CSF biogenic amino acids
Hypothalamic-pituitary-adrenal axis
Thalamic and caudate blood flow
Sleep studies
Neurogenic flare studies with infrared thermography
Electrodermal and microcirculartory activity
Orthostatics

Prognosis and Natural History of Fibromyalgia

Patients with FMS should be reassured that the syndrome need not be progressive. In addition, no long-term organ damage has been noted with FMS at any level of involvement. Despite this reassurance, clinical remission is rare for fibromyalgia.[60,61] As will be emphasized in subsequent sections, the best opportunities for successful management include an up-beat, optimistic approach by the physician; good therapy must be instituted early in the patient's course if there is to be any chance of achieving substantial improvement or a remission.

Despite the lack of organic pathology, patients with FMS often suffer disruption of their social structure in ways that potentiate their symptoms. For example, an executive in a corporation may, secondary to severe stress, have an emotional breakdown that evolves into a chronic pain syndrome. This may, in turn, lead to a loss of employment, disability, separation or divorce, and maladaptive illness behavior.

Proposed Etiologies and Pathophysiology

Many etiologies have been proposed for FMS, but neither the etiology nor the pathophysiologic mechanism for this diffuse pain syndrome is known. It is possible that several phenomena may play overlapping roles in the development of the syndromes (Table 36–5).

MICROTRAUMA TO MUSCLES OR TENDONS WITH REFERRED PAIN

Because FMS is characterized by stiff and painful muscles with tender points that are primarily at the insertion points of tendons, it has been proposed that persons who develop FMS may be predisposed to microtrauma of the muscles or tendons with exertion. The microtrauma would then cause the pain seen in FMS by the same referred pain pathways reported by Lewis and Kellgren[6] after deep injections of hypertonic saline. Although no muscle-biopsy studies have supported this hypothesis, even a small amount of trauma could hypothetically set off a cycle of increased sensitivity to pain through reactive changes in the nervous system.

Several nonspecific changes in muscle biopsies have been reported for FMS patients. The abnormalities of the muscle are structural, metabolic, and functional in nature but do not typically include inflammatory changes.[62,63] Changes have been reported in the membranes, mitochondria, and fibers of muscle biopsies. Specifically reported are atrophy of type II muscle fibers;[64] moth-eaten appearance of type I fibers;[64,65] ragged, red fibers,[65] lipid accumulation,[64,66] glycogen accumulation,[64] subsarcolemmal mitochondrial accumulation,[64] and decreased capillaries per millimeter.[67] These changes are consistent with many types of muscle damage, ranging from ischemia to simple deconditioning. There is disagreement about whether the differ-

TABLE 36–4 • DIFFERENTIAL DIAGNOSES FOR FIBROMYALGIA SYNDROME

Affective disorders (dysthymia, seasonal affective disorders, and melancholic major depression) – Dysthymia represents a more mild and more chronic variant of major depression. The melancholic depressed patients have a marked lack of reactivity to any pleasurable stimuli that often is associated with early morning awakening, psychomotor retardation, and anorexia with weight loss. When present along with symptoms of fibromyalgia syndrome (FMS), the physician must come to a decision about which causes what. In the patient with long-standing chronic pain, depression is an almost inevitable result.

Celiac sprue – When undiagnosed and untreated, celiac sprue can cause both pain and fatigue in addition to gastrointestinal complaints. Diagnosis is made by evidence of malabsorption, flattening of villi on small bowel biopsy, and clinical improvement to the institution of a gluten-free diet.

Costochondritis – The inflamed and tender areas on the chest wall that mark the junction of bony rib and the cartilaginous part of the rib are similarly located to some of the positive pressure points in FMS.

Hepatitis C – In the stages preceding liver dysfunction, up to 15% of patients with this viral infection have been reported to meet criteria for FMS.[62,63]

Hyperparathyroidism – Although ruled out by serum calcium and phosphorus levels, this entity can produce diffuse aching in muscles and bones and (if calcium levels are >12 mg/dl), confusion, and altered consciousness.

Hypophosphatemia – Induced by laxatives, antacids, or both, this causes muscle weakness, but rarely pain in muscles.

Hypothyroidism – This is an untenable diagnosis without an elevated thyroid simulating hormone (TSH) level in blood. Interestingly, these patients may have an elevated creatine kinase.

Lumbar nerve root compression – Symptoms are isolated to the lower extremity and are often worse during coughing, sneezing, or Valsalva maneuver.

Nonviral meningoencephalitis – Possible chronic sequelae, with diffuse pain syndromes and headaches, can include leptospirosis, *Mycoplasma* infections, sarcoidosis, granulomatous arteritis, Whipple's disease, Behçet's disease, and Lyme disease. Once of the diagnosis is considered, specific testing (including imaging) can be done to rule them out.

Obstructive sleep apnea and other sleep disorders – Alteration in sleep patterns can cause pain and fatigue that mimic FMS. If a patient or partner gives a history of severe snoring, apnea, or severe daytime sleepiness, a formal sleep study should be pursued.

Paraneoplastic disorders – Tumors of the lung are particularly likely to produce diffuse neurologic syndromes, with or without hypercalcemia. The relatively sudden onset (in older patients who have been smokers) of fatigue, anorexia, and weight loss have been inappropriately designated as FMS patients while their lung cancer was expanding, undiagnosed.

Polymyalgia rheumatica – With or without an associated biopsy-proven giantcell arteritis, this is rare in anyone under 50 years of age, is marked by anemia and a high C-reactive protein (CRP) and erythrocyte sedimentation rate (ESR), and is exquisitely responsive to glucocorticoid therapy.

Polymyositis – This inflammation of muscle is marked by proximal muscle weakness out of proportion to pain.

Postviral encephalitis and meningitis – This is a difficult diagnosis to make, particularly if the antecedent viral infection was symptomatically mild, and if the CNS was not examined for cells and culture during the acute attack. Close questioning about possible epidemics of a viral encephalitis in months preceding FMS symptoms is needed.

Reflex sympathetic dystrophy – Continuous pain in one extremity, exacerbated by stress, associated with hyperpathia and with findings of glazed and swollen skin and vasomotor changes can readily be separated out from FMS by unilimb involvement with physical findings.

Seronegative spondyloarthropathy – Because these entities usually affect the axial skeleton, the symptoms may resemble those seen in FMS. Concurrent inflammatory bowel disease, uveitis, psoriasis, or skin and mucous membrane lesions suggestive of Reiter's syndrome may lead to the correct diagnoses, as can a limitation of motion of the lumbar spine (Schober test) or cervical spine.

Spinal stenosis – With similar symptomatology to FMS, this entity is associated with increased pain on walking, but it rarely is associated with pain above the waist and is characterized by worsening discomfort on spinal hyperextension and improvement with spine flexion.

Temporomandibular joint pain – This joint, either because of an unbalanced bite, degenerative arthritis, or bruxism, can generate sustained pain syndromes that begin with headaches but spread to the axial skeleton.

ences between FMS and normal muscle could withstand a blinded examination.[66,68,69]

TABLE 36–5 • PROPOSED ETIOLOGIES FOR FIBROMYALGIA

Central nervous system
- Neuroplasticity or remodeling from chronic pain
- Dysfunction of pain processing
- Genetic abnormalities of serotonin metabolism

Autonomic nervous system dysfunction
- Neuroendocrine dysfunction
- Disordered stress response

Hormonal axis dysfunction
Sleep disorder
Microtrauma to muscles and tendons
Post-traumatic
Psychiatric or psychological disorder
Biopsychosocial factors (combination)

Patients with fibromyalgia report decreased strength and endurance. Most objective measures of the mechanical performance of muscles in FMS patients have shown normal contraction strength.[70] Magnetic resonance studies of fibromyalgia muscles have been normal.[71] Studies of P-31 magnetic resonance spectroscopy (MRS) calculations of work/energy-cost ratios have not shown an alteration in energy metabolism in fibromyalgia.[72,73] Twitch-interpolation techniques, however, demonstrated a 35-percent reduction in estimated muscle strength per area unit in muscles of patients with FMS.[74] Muscle oxygen tension and levels of high-energy phosphate compounds have been reported to be low in fibromyalgia patients in comparison to healthy controls.[75,76] There has also been findings in FMS of an inability to relax between contractions.[70] Both normal[77-79] and abnormal[80] aerobic functioning have been demonstrated in FMS. Effort measures in these studies appear lower in fibromyalgia patients than in healthy controls.[79]

NEUROPLASTICITY OR CENTRAL NERVOUS SYSTEM PAIN-PROCESSING PATHWAY DYSFUNCTION

Research in both animals and humans has shown that the presence of chronically painful stimuli can be a cause of neuroplasticity and dysfunction of the central nervous system (CNS) pain-processing pathways that permits "spreading" of localized pain to the sensation of generalized discomfort. The major centers involved include descending and ascending spinal cord tracts, the thalamus, and the somatosensory insular and anterior cingulate cortices. Animal studies suggest that dorsal descending spinal tracts (antinocioceptive tracts) decrease the activity of pain neurons, raise the mechanical threshold for the pain neurons to fire, and decrease the degree of response these pain neurons have to stimuli.[81,82] These descending tracts have a larger degree of control over deep-tissue pain than cutaneous pain. This allows one to speculate that the deep-tissue pain associated with fibromyalgia could be experienced because of damage or underactivity of these descending tracts. Of note, placebo analgesia has been shown to depend on the activity of the pain-processing centers of the CNS and on descending tracts modulating spinal nociceptors.[83]

If FMS is thought to be due to an alteration in the presence or activity of CNS pain pathways, one needs to ask what causes these changes. One hypothesis is that the neurochemical changes in FMS and related syndromes are a result of intermittent stimuli such as drugs, chemicals, infections, endogenous mediators, or stressors.[84,85] The hypothesis is enticing because of the anecdotes of FMS onset following an exposure or emotional trauma and the increased incidence of FMS in patients with histories of childhood stress (including abuse). Although it is controversial, it has been proposed that the Chiari I malformation, a crowding of the brainstem and spinal cord at the outlet of the skull, is more common in people with FMS than in normal controls or other patient populations.[86]

There has been discussion about the possibility that fibromyalgia is caused by an inborn hypersensitivity to all stimuli, resulting in more stimuli than usual seeming unpleasant or painful. Some studies support this idea, finding "hypervigilance" in FMS patients,[87,88] whereas another study found that FMS patients, although more sensitive to pain, are no more sensitive to nonpainful stimuli than normal controls.[89] Surveys have shown that FMS patients are more likely to prefer less-stimulating environments compared to controls.[88]

Several endocrine and neurologic differences have been found between persons with fibromyalgia and healthy controls. One of the most striking and reproducible differences is an increase in the amount of substance P, a neuromodulator of pain, in the Cerebral spinal fluid (CSF) of persons with fibromyalgia.[90-92] This elevation is not specific to FMS, however, and has been demonstrated in people suffering from other types of pain as well. Additionally, it has been shown that molecules released by the action of substance P are present at higher levels in the serum and peripheral blood mononuclear cells of fibromyalgia patients than in healthy controls. These downstream effectors of substance P (i.e., interleukin-8 [IL-8] and IL-6) can cause sympathetic pain (IL-8), and hyperalgesia, fatigue, and depression (IL-6).[93] Similarly, a molecule responsible for the degradation of substance P through the breakdown of the peptide prolyl endopeptidase (PEP) has been shown to be present at decreased levels in fibromyalgia patients compared to healthy controls.[94] Increasing levels of substance P in the serum have been associated with sleep disturbance and are correlated with low levels of tryptophan, a precursor of serotonin.[95]

Abnormal edematous response of the skin to mechanical stimulation has been noted in fibromyalgia patients.[96] The decrease in threshold for, and increase in size of, the neurogenic flare reaction known as *dermatographia*. In patients with fibromyalgia, it is thought to be due to the release of substance P, neurokinin A, and CGRP by the C-fiber nociceptors.[97,98] The reaction may be modulated by the central nervous system (CNS) because increased CNS activation has been noted just prior to the eruption of the erythematous, edematous flare.[99]

In addition, magnetic resonance imaging (MRI) studies of the brains of patients with fibromyalgia have shown abnormal blood flow to the thalamus and caudate, areas of the brain that are thought to function in the filtering of somatic input and the suppression of nocioception.[100] Position emission tomography (PET) scans of patients with fibromyalgia have shown decreased cerebral blood flow to the thalamus and pontine tegmentum.[52,101,102] Bell and colleagues have proposed that these changes in the activity of hypothalamus and mesolimbic dopaminergic pathways may be elicited by a number of various sensitizers, from chemicals to hormones to neurobehavioral patterns.[85]

ALLELIC ABNORMALITIES IN SEROTONIN RECEPTORS AND PROCESSING GENES

It has been hypothesized that polymorphisms of serotonin receptors could play a role in the etiology of fibromyalgia. Some differences in genotype distribution between FMS patients and healthy controls have been noted that appear to correlate with self-reported pain scores.[103,104] Although they may exacerbate an otherwise painful experience and make the diagnosis of FMS more likely, allelic polymorphisms of serotonin receptors do not currently explain why certain individuals develop FMS.[105,106]

Fibromyalgia patients have been shown to have decreased levels of tryptophan and other biogenic amino acids in the serum and CSF.[107-111] The metabolite of serotonin, 5-hydroxyindoleacetic acid (5-HIAA), has also been shown to be decreased in fibromyalgia patients.[95] Serotonin levels measured in the plasma of FMS patients have been reported as low.[112] This observation is particularly interesting because serotonin is thought to play a role in pain reactivity through changes in sleep patterns and through modulation of neuron excitability and pain signaling in the CNS. Drugs that alter the metabolism or action of serotonin have been studied in the treatment of fibromyalgia. Antibodies against serotonin have been reported in approximately four times as many FMS patients as healthy controls.[113-116] In summary, serotonin studies in FMS are enticing but have had mixed results.

DISORDERED STRESS RESPONSE AND ENDOCRINE OR HORMONAL FACTORS

Many stress responses and endocrine axes are disturbed in FMS, but many of these changes are commonly seen in patients that have known external sources of chronic pain. Thus, it is not clear whether these endocrine disturbances in FMS are primary to the disease or are secondary to the pain associated with FMS.

Studies have shown that several hormonal axes controlled by the hypothalamus are disrupted in FMS patients.[100,117] Although the results among studies are not always consistent, it does appear that plasma-cortisol response is abnormal in fibromyalgia.[118-129] Furthermore, hormones downstream of the hypothalamic-pituitary-adrenal axis (HPA) have been shown to be abnormal in FMS. A summary of the studies on the HPA in FMS has reported that approximately one third of the studies show baseline cortisol to be low in approximately one third of the patients.[130] Most studies, however, show abnormally low HPA responses and enhanced 5-HT (serotonin) function on neuroendocrine challenge tests.[131] The resulting hormonal changes may affect nocioception, possibly worsening the response to the pain by "spreading" to other dermatomes or deep pain area distributions.

Serum levels of somatomedin C (insulin-like growth factor I [IGF-I]) have been studied in fibromyalgia. The studies were performed because somatomedin C is a modulator of growth hormone's actions and a neuromediator of chronic stress. It is secreted along with growth hormone during stage-4 sleep, the stage that is disrupted in fibromyalgia. Although the levels of somatomedin C and growth hormone have often been reported as abnormal in fibromyalgia, the results have been inconsistent,[131-141] and it is difficult to make valid conclusions about the interaction between the growth factor pathway and symptomatology in FMS.

AUTONOMIC NERVOUS SYSTEM DYSFUNCTION

It has been proposed that fibromyalgia is a generalized form of reflex-sympathetic dystrophy.[142] Abnormal autonomic balance has also been implicated in altered visceral perception,[143] which could contribute to the pain syndrome of fibromyalgia. In addition, it has been proposed that a process dubbed "neurogenic switching" could be contributing to fibromyalgia. Neurogenic switching or "spreading" is a proposed process by which noxious stimuli at one site can cause an inflammatory reaction at a distant site via neuronal activity.[144]

Studies have shown functionally elevated,[145-151] functionally depressed,[152] and no abnormality[153] in sympathetic function of FMS patients. There appears to be a derangement of the sympathetic tone and reaction in some FMS patients, but whether it is too high or too low depends on the situation. Some studies indicate that reactions previously characterized as Raynaud's syndrome in fibromyalgia patients may be a decreased vasoconstriction response secondary to an altered sympathetic nervous system response.[154,155]

One of the clearest indications that there is autonomic nervous system dysfunction in fibromyalgia patients is the study done using sympathetic blocks in patients and controls. In a well-controlled study by Bengtsson and Bengtsson,[156] it was shown that FMS resting pain and tender points can be reduced by a complete sympathetic blockade. The authors suggest that the improvement may be due to an increase in the microcirculation following the sympathetic block.[156] In another study, peripheral sympathetic blockade increased an abnormally slow relaxation rate of the muscles of FMS patients but did not increase muscle strength.[157] The converse was also shown to be true in a study examining norepinephrine-induced pain.[158] In this study, fibromyalgia patients were more than twice as likely to have pain from the injection of norepinephrine than were RA patients or normal controls; this difference was not present for saline injections.[158] This sensitivity to pain with injection of norepinephrine may implicate the nascent sympathetic neurotransmitter in the maintenance of the pain syndrome. This was supported by a recent study by Malt and colleagues,[159] which showed that high pain scores were associated with a drop in systolic blood pressure after buspirone challenge. Patients with FMS have been shown to be more likely than healthy controls (60% vs. 0%[160] and 64.7% vs. 21.3%)[161] to have orthostatic hypotension during an upright tilt–table test. An upright tilt has been shown to result in a paradoxical lowering of sympathetic tone in FMS patients.[162] Further-more the abnormal autonomic response to upright stress seen in FMS patients was also associated with a worsening of pain symptoms.[160] A controlled tilt–table study by Cohen and coworkers on men with fibromyalgia showed a baseline sympathetic hyperactivity and abnormal sympathovagal response to the orthostatic stress.[150] A tilt-table study comparing FMS patients to CFS patients showed different reactions of the two groups of patients to the test,[163] calling into question the assumed related nature of the two syndromes.[164]

SLEEP DISORDER

Patients with fibromyalgia usually report unrefreshing and nonrestorative sleep.[165-168] They have an abnormality of the deepest stage of sleep, delta-wave sleep. The usual low-frequency, high-amplitude electroencephalogram (EEG) tracings of delta-wave sleep are overlaid with high-frequency, low-amplitude waves (alpha waves) that are usually seen in only the waking state and the rapid eye movement (REM) stage of sleep.[165-168] Alpha waves are tracings on the EEG with 8 to 13 cycles per second (cps) that are usually associated with relaxed wakefulness. Intrusion of alpha waves into slow-wave sleep is associated with the sensation of nonrefreshing sleep.[169]

Of utmost importance in the study of fibromyalgia is the question of whether sleep abnormalities cause or contribute to the symptoms of fibromyalgia or whether the pain associated with fibromyalgia causes the sleep abnormalities. There is no easy answer to this question, and it has been suggested that the relationship between pain and poor sleep may be bidirectional.[170] Pain is associated with anxiety and depression, both of which are themselves associated with sleep disturbances, and intense focus on one's own pain has been shown to adversely affect the quality of sleep.[170] The interrelationships have been studied in many ways. In healthy volunteers, a given day's mood and musculoskeletal pain scores correlated better with the previous night's sleep than the following night's sleep quality,[171] indicating that less sleep can cause increased pain. However, in a long-term study of patients with RA, baseline pain levels predicted future sleep disorders, but baseline sleep disorders did not predict future pain.[172] When one examines the specific sleep abnormality in FMS (i.e., the alpha-wave intrusion into delta-wave sleep), no clear answer to the cause-and-effect conundrum is evident. Pain seems to be both a cause of this sleep disorder and its effect. In healthy volunteers, deep pain has been shown to cause an increase in alpha activity during slow-wave sleep,[173] whereas three out of four studies of slow-wave sleep deprivation and musculoskeletal pain have demonstrated a decreased pain threshold with slow-wave sleep deprivation.[134,165,174,175]

In adults, growth hormone is secreted primarily during slow-wave sleep,[176] and it has been suggested that impaired slow-wave sleep causes the decreased growth hormone levels noted in fibromyalgia.[131] Serotonin, endorphins, and substance P are known to be altered in FMS, and each is associated with sleep and pain.[109] Melatonin is a sleep-associated hormone that is a downstream metabolite of serotonin. FMS patients have been shown to have 31-percent less melatonin secretion than healthy controls during sleep hours.[177] Finally, experimental studies with normal control patients who undergo sleep deprivation have shown that disruption of delta-wave sleep can result in fibromyalgia-like symptoms, including an increase in the size of and a decrease in the threshold for a neurogenic flare.[175] The etiologic significance of the relationship between sleep and fibromyalgia, as well as possible sleep-centric treatments for fibromyaglia, are discussed later.

POST-TRAUMATIC FIBROMYALGIA SYNDROME

There has been a fair amount of discussion about the association between fibromyalgia and trauma. A study examining people who sustained neck injuries found that they had a 10-times-higher risk of developing fibromyalgia in the year after their injury than did people who had experienced non-neck injuries of approximately equal severity.[178] There have not been good physiologic follow-up studies to these observations.

BIOPSYCHOSOCIAL MODELS ALLOW FOR COMBINATIONS OF COMPETING PATHOPHYSIOLOGY

It has been demonstrated in a study of persons with chronic pain that the proportion of "adaptive copers" decreased and the proportion of "interpersonally distressed" people increased linearly with increased duration of pain.[179] Malt and colleagues[159] created a model for the variance in pain in fibromyalgia patients that demonstrated that psychologic, neuroendocrine, and autonomic factors all play a role in pain perception in fibromyalgia. Their study showed that high pain scores were associated with high neuroses, low baseline cortisol levels, and a drop in blood pressure after a buspirone challenge, all indicating mild autonomic dysfunction.[159] It may be that there are psychiatric or psychologic predispositions to fibromyalgia, as well as physiologic predispositions. In people with one or both factors, environmental factors could trigger the syndrome of fibromyalgia.

Treatments

The treatment of fibromyalgia has been an area of frustration for patients and practitioners alike. No more than modest benefits have been demonstrated with any technique. At present, the ideal treatment goal is to manage the symptoms, with a continual emphasis by the treating physician that this is a chronic illness. This goal, although currently the best option we have, remains unsatisfactory for patients whose pain and fatigue has altered their physical and social functioning. For these patients, it is imperative from the outset to include psychologic- and coping-skills treatments in their care plans. The major treatment modalities for FMS are outlined in Table 36–6, and a recommendation for a treatment algorithm is shown in Figure 36–3.

EXERCISE

Aerobic exercise is one of the best validated treatments for fibromyalgia and CFS.[180-182] Unfortunately, it is a difficult task to get patients to agree to exercise training when they are experiencing severe pain, fatigue, or both. It is advisable to reassure them that exercise is safe and effective for patients with their condition and to advise them to start slowly and increase duration or intensity only slowly. It is important to acknowledge the difficulty patients will have following the exercise program while expressing the hope that they will benefit from perseverance.

TABLE 36–6 • TREATMENTS FOR FIBROMYALGIA SYNDROME (FMS)

Effective in Clinical Trials
Exercise
Tricyclics, especially amitripiline
Cognitive behavioral therapy
Not Effective in Clinical Trials
Nonsteroidal anti-inflammatory drugs (NSAIDs)
Glucocorticoids
Equivocal or Insufficient Evidence
Opiates (no long-term studies)
Alpha-adrenergic blockade
Alternative medicine
Selective Serotonin reuptake inhibitors (SSRIs) (except for mild response in combination with other antidepressants)
Likely Harmful
Prolonged rest

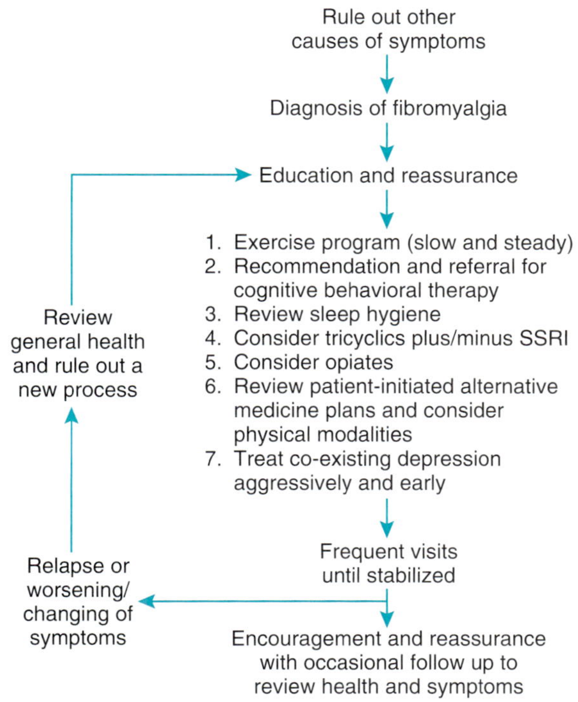

FIGURE 36–3 · Treatment algorithm for fibromyalgia.

Patients should begin slowly, at a level that is tolerable. Then, while keeping a detailed daily log of duration and intensity of effort, they should gradually increase the duration of effort. A reasonable objective, for example, would be to have a FMS patient walk briskly 15 minutes each day for a week, then increase slowly up to an hour as tolerated, and then move on to a stationary bicycle or vigorous aquatic workouts.

COGNITIVE BEHAVIORAL THERAPY

Cognitive behavioral therapy (CBT) is a process that examines a patient's way of reacting to experiences and attempts to restructure maladaptive coping habits into effective coping skills. CBT has been shown to be effective in reducing disability and increasing function in patients with OA, RA, and CFS.[183-187] A few studies of CBT in fibromyalgia have been done, with most showing an improvement.[188] Most experts suggest that CBT works by allowing patients to experience a greater locus of control over their symptoms and their illness. It has been shown to improve patients' compliance with other aspects of their care, such as exercise programs.

SYMPATHETIC BLOCKADE

Regional sympathetic blockade through stellate ganglion blockade with local bupivacaine injection has been shown to decrease trigger points and resting pain in the affected area in fibromyalgia patients.[156] Intravenous regional sympathetic blockade with guanethidine decreased trigger points.[156] Although these findings are interesting from a pathophysiologic point of view, they do not offer a practical therapeutic option for FMS patients.

GROWTH HORMONE

Growth hormone (GH) administration has been studied in both FMS and CFS, but this practice has not gained widespread acceptance. In a 9-month study, FMS patients injecting GH twice daily were shown to have more improvement in symptoms than FMS patients injecting placebo.[189] In this study, the GH group experienced more carpal tunnel syndrome that the placebo group.[189] GH seems not to improve quality of life in CFS patients assessed by questionnaires.[190]

NONSTEROIDAL ANTI-INFLAMMATORY DRUGS AND GLUCOCORTICOIDS

NSAIDs are of limited use in FMS. Although a trial should be initiated at the beginning of treatment for any FMS patient complaining of pain, NSAIDs do not hold much hope for the long-term treatment of people suffering chronic pain associated with fibromyalgia.[191] Similarly, glucocorticoids are ineffective in the treatment of FMS. Another good reason for not using these drugs in FMS is that the syndrome of glucocorticoid withdrawal that is initiated when tapering dosage often mimics that of the underlying fibromyalgia.

ANTIDEPRESSANTS

Tricyclic antidepressants, amytriptiline in particular, are among the best studied and most effective pharmaceutical interventions in FMS. Selective serotonin reuptake inhibitors (SSRIs) have for the most part been less effective than tricyclic medications, but newer studies demonstrate some efficacy of SSRIs.[192] A randomized, double-blind crossover trial of fluoxetine (an SSRI), amitriptyline, and placebo in FMS patients[193] showed that both amitriptyline and fluoxetine were effective in decreasing FMS symptoms and that the two drugs given simultaneously were more effective than either drug alone. A meta-analysis of the treatment of fibromyalgia with antidepressants showed that antidepressants tended to improve sleep, fatigue, pain, and well-being, but not trigger points, and that FMS patients treated with antidepressants were more than four times as likely to report improvements as patients treated with placebo.[194]

SLEEP

Because abnormal sleep patterns are a hallmark of fibromyalgia, sleep-restoring interventions have been studied in the treatment of FMS. Tricyclic antidepressants such as amitriptyline are able to reduce alpha-wave intrusion into slow-wave sleep and improve sleep quality in patients with fibromyalgia,[195] and their use is associated with improved symptomatology.[194] Chlorpromazine was shown to increase slow-wave sleep and improve both mood and pain scores in patients with fibromyalgia, but L-tryptophan had no effect.[196] A preliminary study with γ-hydroxybutyrate in fibromyalgia patients showed an increase in slow-wave sleep, a decrease in alpha intrusion into slow-wave sleep, and improvement of fatigue and pain scores.[197] Many of the treatments reported to be beneficial for fibromyalgia, such as exercise, are associated with improved sleep quality.[198] It is crucial to take a history for obstructive sleep apnea, as this sleep disorder may masquerade as FMS but has a vastly different treatment pathway.

OPIATES

Opiates have not been studied as well as other pharmaceutical interventions for FMS. Double-blinded trials of intravenous injections of morphine, lidocaine, ketamine, and placebo have shown mixed results, with most studies showing some decrease in pain with opiate administration.[199-201] Of note, it appears that not all FMS patients respond to opiates. Thus, an individualized approach to the use of opiates for the treatment of FMS is recommended, and it should not be initiated without the direct supervision of an experienced expert in pain therapy.

ALTERNATIVE MEDICINE

Alternative forms of medicine are used by many FMS patients. A reasonable open-communication strategy toward these practices has been recommended by Clauw.[202] He recommends first assessing the safety of the proposed therapy, then determining if the proposed therapy will be counterproductive for patient. If the treatment is safe and is not deemed to be counterproductive, he recommends having the patient do an "experiment" with the treatment under an otherwise controlled situation to determine personal efficacy.

REFERENCES

1. Wolfe F, Smythe HA, Yunus MB, et al: The American College of Rheumatology 1990 Criteria for the Classification of Fibromyalgia: Report of the Multicenter Criteria Committee. Arthritis Rheum 33:160-172, 1990.
2. Stockman R: The causes, pathology, and treatment of chronic rheumatism. Edinburgh Med J 134:107, 1904.
3. Osler W: The Principles and Practice of Medicine. New York, D. Appleton, 1900, p 406.
4. Kellgren JH: Observations on referred pain arising from muscles. Clin Sci 3:42-46, 1938.
5. Kellgren JH: On distribution of pain arising from deep somatic structures, with charts of segmental pain areas. Clin Sci 4: 126-130,1939.
6. Lewis T, Kellgren JH: Observations relating to referred pain, visceromotor reflexes, and other associated phenomena. Clin Sci 4: 131-135, 1939.
7. Bennett RM: Fibrositis. *In* Kelley WN, Harris ED Jr, Ruddy S, Sledge CB (eds): Textbook of Rheumatology. Philadelphia, W.B. Saunders, 1989, pp 541-553.
8. Comroe: Fibrositis. Arthritis and Allied Conditions. Philadelphia, Lea & Febiger, 1944, pp 679-701.
9. Fukuda K, Nisenbaum R, Stewart G, et al: Chronic multisymptom illness affecting Air Force veterans of the Gulf War. JAMA 280: 981-988, 1998.
10. Yunus M, Masi AT, Calabro JJ, et al: Primary fibromyalgia (fibrositis): clinical study of 50 patients with matched normal controls. Semin Arthritis Rheum 11:151-71, 1981.
11. Campbell SM, Clark S, Tindall EA, et al: Clinical characteristics of fibrositis. I. A "blinded," controlled study of symptoms and tender points. Arthritis Rheum 26:817-824, 1983.
12. Wolfe F, Hawley DJ, Cathey MA, et al: Fibrositis: Symptom frequency and criteria for diagnosis: An evaluation of 291 rheumatic disease patients and 58 normal individuals. J Rheumatol 12:1159-1163, 1985.
13. Clauw DJ, Chrousos GP: Chronic pain and fatigue syndromes: overlapping clinical and neuroendocrine features and potential pathogenic mechanisms. Neuroimmunomodulation 4:134-153, 1997.
14. White KP, Harth M, Speechley M, Ostbye T: A general population study of fibromyalgia tender points in noninstitutionalized adults with chronic widespread pain. J Rheumatol 27:2677-682, 2000.
15. Gowin KM: Diffuse pain syndromes in the elderly. Rheum Dis Clin North Am 26:673-682, 2000.
16. Wolfe F, Ross K, Anderson J, et al: The prevalence and characteristics of fibromyalgia in the general population. Arthritis Rheum 38:19-28, 1995.
17. White KP, Speechley M, Harth M, Ostbye T: The London Fibromyalgia Epidemiology Study: The prevalence of fibromyalgia syndrome in London, Ontario. J Rheumatol 26:1570-1576, 1999.
18. Wessely S, Chalder T, Hirsch S, et al: The prevalence and morbidity of chronic fatigue and chronic fatigue syndrome: A prospective primary care study. Am J Public Health 87:1449-1455, 1997.
19. Steele L, Dobbins JG, Fukuda K, et al: The epidemiology of chronic fatigue in San Francisco. Am J Med 105:83S-90S, 1998.
20. Buchwald D, Garrity D: Comparison of patients with chronic fatigue syndrome, fibromyalgia, and multiple chemical sensitivities. Arch Intern Med 154:2049-2053, 1994.
21. White KP, Speechley M, Harth M, Ostbye T: Co-existence of chronic fatigue syndrome with fibromyalgia syndrome in the general population: A controlled study. Scand J Rheumatol 29:44-51, 2000.
22. Wysenbeek AJ, Shapira Y, Leibovici L: Primary fibromyalgia and the chronic fatigue syndrome. Rheumatol Int 10:227-229, 1991.
23. Aaron LA, Burke MM, Buchwald D: Overlapping conditions among patients with chronic fatigue syndrome, fibromyalgia, and temporomandibular disorder. Arch Intern Med 160:221-227, 2000.
24. Hudson JI, Goldenberg DL, Pope HG Jr, et al: Comorbidity of fibromyalgia with medical and psychiatric disorders. Am J Med 92:363-367, 1992.
25. Yunus MB, Inanici F, Aldag JC, Mangold RF: Fibromyalgia in men: comparison of clinical features with women. J Rheumatol 27:485-490, 2000.
26. Sivri A, Cindas A, Dincer F, Sivri B: Bowel dysfunction and irritable bowel syndrome in fibromyalgia patients. Clin Rheumatol 15:283-286, 1996.
27. Gomborone JE, Gorard DA, Dewsnap PA, et al: Prevalence of irritable bowel syndrome in chronic fatigue. J R Coll Physicians Lond 30:512-513, 1996.
28. Triadafilopoulos G, Simms RW, Goldenberg DL: Bowel dysfunction in fibromyalgia syndrome. Dig Dis Sci 36:59-64, 1991.
29. Goldenberg DL, Simms RW, Geiger A, Komaroff AL: High frequency of fibromyalgia in patients with chronic fatigue seen in a primary care practice. Arthritis Rheum 33:381-387, 1990.
30. Romano TJ: Coexistence of irritable bowel syndrome and fibromyalgia. W V Med J 84:16-18, 1988.
31. Sperber AD, Atzmon Y, Neumann L, et al: Fibromyalgia in the irritable bowel syndrome: Studies of prevalence and clinical implications. Am J Gastroenterol 94:3541-3546, 1999.
32. Veale D, Kavanagh G, Fielding JF, Fitzgerald O: Primary fibromyalgia and the irritable bowel syndrome: Different expressions of a common pathogenetic process. Br J Rheumatol 30: 220-222, 1991.
33. Slotkoff AT, Radulovic DA, Clauw DJ: The relationship between fibromyalgia and the multiple chemical sensitivity syndrome. Scand J Rheumatol 26:364-367, 1997.
34. Eriksson PO, Lindman R, Stal P, Bengtsson A: Symptoms and signs of mandibular dysfunction in primary fibromyalgia syndrome (PSF) patients. Swed Dent J 12:141-149, 1988.
35. Plesh O, Wolfe F, Lane N: The relationship between fibromyalgia and temporomandibular disorders: Prevalence and symptom severity. J Rheumatol 23:1948-1952, 1996.
36. Buchwald D, Pearlman T, Kith P, Schmaling K: Gender differences in patients with chronic fatigue syndrome. J Gen Intern Med 9:397-401, 1994.
37. Morriss RK, Ahmed M, Wearden AJ, et al: The role of depression in pain, psychophysiological syndromes and medically unex-

plained symptoms associated with chronic fatigue syndrome. J Affect Disord 55:143-148, 1999.
38. Jason LA, Taylor RR, Kennedy CL: Chronic fatigue syndrome, fibromyalgia, and multiple chemical sensitivities in a community-based sample of persons with chronic fatigue syndrome-like symptoms. Psychosom Med 62:655-663, 2000.
39. Holmes GP, Kaplan JE, Gantz NM, et al: Chronic fatigue syndrome: a working case definition. Ann Intern Med 108:387-389, 1988.
40. Komaroff AL, Buchwald DS: Chronic fatigue syndrome: an update. Annu Rev Med 49:1-13, 1998.
41. Rau CL, Russell IJ: Is fibromyalgia a distinct clinical syndrome? Curr Rev Pain 4:287-294, 2000.
42. Aaron LA, Buchwald D: A review of the evidence for overlap among unexplained clinical conditions. Ann Intern Med 134: 868-881, 2001.
43. McBeth J, Silman AJ: The role of psychiatric disorders in fibromyalgia. Curr Rheumatol Rep 3:157-164, 2001.
44. Winfield JB: Pain in fibromyalgia. Rheum Dis Clin North Am 25:55-79, 1999.
45. Monti DA, Herring CL, Schwartzman RJ, Marchese M: Personality assessment of patients with complex regional pain syndrome type I. Clin J Pain 14:295-302, 1998.
46. Zagari MJ, Mazonson PD, Longton WC: Pharmacoeconomics of chronic nonmalignant pain. Pharmacoeconomics 10:356-377, 1996.
47. Skevington SM, Carse MS, Williams AC: Validation of the WHO-QOL-100: Pain management improves quality of life for chronic pain patients. Clin J Pain 17:264-275, 2001.
48. Aaron LA, Bradley LA, Alarcon GS, et al: Psychiatric diagnoses in patients with fibromyalgia are related to health care-seeking behavior rather than to illness. Arthritis Rheum 39:436-445, 1996.
49. Kersh BC, Bradley LA, Alarcon GS, et al: Psychosocial and health status variables independently predict health care seeking in fibromyalgia. Arthritis Rheum 45:362-371, 2001.
50. Sotgui ML: Descending influence on dorsal horn neuronal hyperactivity in a rat model of neuropathic pain. Neuroreport 4:21-24, 1993.
51. Honore P, Rogers SD, Schwei MJ, et al: Murine models of inflammatory, neuropathic and cancer pain each generates a unique set of neurochemical changes in the spinal cord and sensory neurons. Neuroscience 98:585-598, 2000.
52. Apkarian AV, Gelnar PA, Krauss BR, Szeverenyi NM: Cortical responses to thermal pain depend on stimulus size: A functional MRI study. J Neurophysiol 83:3113-3122, 2000.
53. Kwiatek R, Barnden L, Tedman R, et al: Regional cerebral blood flow in fibromyalgia: single-photon-emission computed tomography evidence of reduction in the pontine tegmentum and thalami. Arthritis Rheum 43:2823-2833, 2000.
54. Mountz JM, Bradley LA, Modell JG, et al: Fibromyalgia in women. Abnormalities of regional cerebral blood flow in the thalamus and the caudate nucleus are associated with low pain threshold levels. Arthritis Rheum 38:926-938, 1995.
55. Wolfe F, Anderson J, Harkness D, et al: A prospective, longitudinal, multicenter study of service utilization and costs in fibromyalgia. Arthritis Rheum 40:1560-1570, 1997.
56. Wolfe F, Anderson J, Harkness D, et al: Work and disability status of persons with fibromyalgia. J Rheumatol 24:1171-1178, 1997.
57. Alagiri M, Chottiner S, Ratner V, et al: Interstitial cystitis: Unexplained associations with other chronic disease and pain syndromes. Urology 49:52-57, 1997.
58. Holmes GP, Kaplan JE, Stewart JA, et al: A cluster of patients with a chronic mononucleosis-like syndrome: Is Epstein-Barr virus the cause? JAMA 257:2297-2302, 1987.
59. Hellinger WC, Smith TF, Van Scoy RE, et al: Chronic fatigue syndrome and the diagnostic utility of antibody to Epstein-Barr virus early antigen. JAMA 260:971-973, 1988.
60. Rivera J, de Diego A, Trinchet M, Garcia Monforte A: Fibromyalgia-associated hepatitis C virus infection. Br J Rheumatol 36:981-985, 1997.
61. Kennedy M, Felson DT: A prospective long-term study of fibromyalgia syndrome. Arthritis Rheum 39:682-685, 1996.
62. Park JH, Niermann KJ, Olsen N: Evidence for metabolic abnormalities in the muscles of patients with fibromyalgia. Curr Rheumatol Rep 2:131-140, 2000.
63. Henriksson KG: Muscle pain in neuromuscular disorders and primary fibromyalgia. Eur J Appl Physiol Occup Physiol 57:348-352, 1988.
64. Kalyan-Raman UP, Kalyan-Raman K, Yunus MB, Masi AT: Muscle pathology in primary fibromyalgia syndrome: a light microscopic, histochemical and ultrastructural study. J Rheumatol 11:808-813, 1984.
65. Bengtsson A, Henriksson KG, Larsson J: Muscle biopsy in primary fibromyalgia: Light-microscopical and histochemical findings. Scand J Rheumatol 15:1-6, 1986.
66. Drewes AM, Andreasen A, Schroder HD, et al: Pathology of skeletal muscle in fibromyalgia: A histo-immuno-chemical and ultrastructural study. Br J Rheumatol 32:479-483, 1993.
67. Lindh M, Johansson G, Hedberg M, et al: Muscle fiber characteristics, capillaries and enzymes in patients with fibromyalgia and controls. Scand J Rheumatol 24:34-37, 1995.
68. Yunus MB, Kalyan-Raman UP, Masi AT, Aldag JC: Electron microscopic studies of muscle biopsy in primary fibromyalgia syndrome: A controlled and blinded study. J Rheumatol 16:97-101, 1989.
69. Jacobsen S, Bartels EM, Danneskiold-Samsoe B: Single cell morphology of muscle in patients with chronic muscle pain. Scand J Rheumatol 20:336-343, 1991.
70. Elert JE, Rantapaa-Dahlqvist SB, Henriksson-Larsen K, et al: Muscle performance, electromyography and fibre type composition in fibromyalgia and work-related myalgia. Scand J Rheumatol 21:28-34, 1992.
71. Kravis MM, Munk PL, McCain GA, et al: MR imaging of muscle and tender points in fibromyalgia. J Magn Reson Imaging 3:669-670, 1993.
72. de Blecourt AC, Wolf RF, van Rijswijk MH, et al: In vivo 31P magnetic resonance spectroscopy (MRS) of tender points in patients with primary fibromyalgia syndrome. Rheumatol Int 11:51-54, 1991.
73. Jacobsen S, Jensen KE, Thomsen C, et al: 31P magnetic resonance spectroscopy of skeletal muscle in patients with fibromyalgia. J Rheumatol 19:1600-1603, 1992.
74. Norregaard J, Bulow PM, Danneskiold-Samsoe B: Muscle strength, voluntary activation, twitch properties, and endurance in patients with fibromyalgia. J Neurol Neurosurg Psychiatry 57:1106-1111, 1994.
75. Lund N, Bengtsson A, Thorborg P: Muscle tissue oxygen pressure in primary fibromyalgia. Scand J Rheumatol 15:165-173, 1986.
76. Bengtsson A, Henriksson KG, Larsson J: Reduced high-energy phosphate levels in the painful muscles of patients with primary fibromyalgia. Arthritis Rheum 29:817-821. 1986.
77. Mengshoel AM, Forre O, Komnaes HB: Muscle strength and aerobic capacity in primary fibromyalgia. Clin Exp Rheumatol 8:475-479, 1990.
78. Sietsema KE, Cooper DM, Caro X, et al: Oxygen uptake during exercise in patients with primary fibromyalgia syndrome. J Rheumatol 20:860-865, 1993.
79. Norregaard J, Bulow PM, Lykkegaard JJ, et al: Muscle strength, working capacity and effort in patients with fibromyalgia. Scand J Rehabil Med 29:97-102, 1997.
80. Bennett RM, Clark SR, Goldberg L, et al: Aerobic fitness in patients with fibrositis: A controlled study of respiratory gas exchange and 133xenon clearance from exercising muscle. Arthritis Rheum 32:454-460, 1989.
81. Mense S: Descending antinociception and fibromyalgia. Z Rheumatol 57(Suppl 2):23-26, 1998.
82. Mense S: Neurobiological concepts of fibromyalgia: the possible role of descending spinal tracts. Scand J Rheumatol Suppl 113:24-29, 2000.
83. Rainville P, Bushnell MC, Duncan GH: Representation of acute and persistent pain in the human CNS: Potential implications for chemical intolerance. Ann N Y Acad Sci 933:130-141, 2001.
84. Bell IR, Baldwin CM, Russek LG, et al: Early life stress, negative paternal relationships, and chemical intolerance in middle-aged women: Support for a neural sensitization model. J Womens Health 7:1135-1147, 1998.
85. Bell IR, Baldwin CM, Schwartz GE: Illness from low levels of environmental chemicals: Relevance to chronic fatigue syndrome and fibromyalgia. Am J Med 105:74S-82S, 1998.

86. Garland EM, Robertson D: Chiari I malformation as a cause of orthostatic intolerance symptoms: a media myth? Am J Med 111:546-552, 2001.
87. Kosek E, Ekholm J, Hansson P: Sensory dysfunction in fibromyalgia patients with implications for pathogenic mechanisms. Pain 68:375-83, 1996.
88. McDermid AJ, Rollman GB, McCain GA: Generalized hypervigilance in fibromyalgia: Evidence of perceptual amplification. Pain 66:133-144, 1996.
89. Lorenz J: Hyperalgesia or hypervigilance? An evoked potential approach to the study of fibromyalgia syndrome. Z Rheumatol 57(Suppl 2):19-22, 1998.
90. Russell IJ, Orr MD, Littman B, et al: Elevated cerebrospinal fluid levels of substance P in patients with the fibromyalgia syndrome. Arthritis Rheum 37:1593-1601, 1994.
91. Vaeroy H, Sakurada T, Forre O, et al: Modulation of pain in fibromyalgia (fibrositis syndrome): Cerebrospinal fluid (CSF) investigation of pain related neuropeptides with special reference to calcitonin gene related peptide (CGRP). J Rheumatol Suppl 19:94-97, 1989.
92. Vaeroy H, Helle R, Forre O, et al: Elevated CSF levels of substance P and high incidence of Raynaud phenomenon in patients with fibromyalgia: New features for diagnosis. Pain 32:21-26, 1988.
93. Wallace DJ, Linker-Israeli M, Hallegua D, et al: Cytokines play an aetiopathogenetic role in fibromyalgia: A hypothesis and pilot study. Rheumatology (Oxford) 40:743-749, 2001.
94. Maes M, Libbrecht I, Van Hunsel F, et al: Lower serum activity of prolyl endopeptidase in fibromyalgia is related to severity of depressive symptoms and pressure hyperalgesia. Psychol Med 28:957-965, 1998.
95. Schwarz MJ, Spath M, Muller-Bardorff H, et al: Relationship of substance P, 5-hydroxyindole acetic acid and tryptophan in serum of fibromyalgia patients. Neurosci Lett 259:196-198, 1999.
96. Helme RD, Littlejohn GO, Weinstein C: Neurogenic flare responses in chronic rheumatic pain syndromes. Clin Exp Neurol 23:91-94, 1987.
97. Littlejohn GO, Weinstein C, Helme RD: Increased neurogenic inflammation in fibrositis syndrome. J Rheumatol 14:1022-1025, 1987.
98. Sann H, Pierau FK: Efferent functions of C-fiber nociceptors. Z Rheumatol 57(Suppl 2):8-13, 1998.
99. Gibson SJ, Littlejohn GO, Gorman MM, et al: Altered heat pain thresholds and cerebral event-related potentials following painful CO2 laser stimulation in subjects with fibromyalgia syndrome. Pain 58:185-193, 1994.
100. Neeck G, Crofford LJ: Neuroendocrine perturbations in fibromyalgia and chronic fatigue syndrome. Rheum Dis Clin North Am 26:989-1002, 2000.
101. Bradley LA, McKendree-Smith NL, Alberts KR, et al: Use of neuroimaging to understand abnormal pain sensitivity in fibromyalgia. Curr Rheumatol Rep 2:141-148, 2000.
102. Lekander M, Fredrikson M, Wik G: Neuroimmune relations in patients with fibromyalgia: a positron emission tomography study. Neurosci Lett 282:193-196, 2000.
103. Offenbaecher M, Bondy B, de Jonge S, et al: Possible association of fibromyalgia with a polymorphism in the serotonin transporter gene regulatory region. Arthritis Rheum 42:2482-2488, 1999.
104. Bondy B, Spaeth M, Offenbaecher M, et al: The T102C polymorphism of the 5-HT2A-receptor gene in fibromyalgia. Neurobiol Dis 6:433-439, 1999.
105. Gursoy S, Erdal E, Herken H, et al: Association of T102C polymorphism of the 5-HT2A receptor gene with psychiatric status in fibromyalgia syndrome. Rheumatol Int 21:58-61, 2001.
106. Skeith KJ, Hussain MS, Coutts RT, et al: Adverse drug reactions and debrisoquine/sparteine (P450IID6) polymorphism in patients with fibromyalgia. Clin Rheumatol 16:291-295, 1997.
107. Moldofsky H, Warsh JJ: Plasma tryptophan and musculoskeletal pain in non-articular rheumatism ("fibrositis syndrome"). Pain 5:65-71, 1978.
108. Russell IJ, Michalek JE, Vipraio GA, et al: Platelet 3H-imipramine uptake receptor density and serum serotonin levels in patients with fibromyalgia/fibrositis syndrome. J Rheumatol 19:104-109, 1992.
109. Russell IJ, Michalek JE, Vipraio GA, et al: Serum amino acids in fibrositis/fibromyalgia syndrome. J Rheumatol Suppl 19:158-163, 1989.
110. Yunus MB, Dailey JW, Aldag JC, et al: Plasma tryptophan and other amino acids in primary fibromyalgia: a controlled study. J Rheumatol 19:90-94, 1992.
111. Russell IJ, Vaeroy H, Javors M, Nyberg F: Cerebrospinal fluid biogenic amine metabolites in fibromyalgia/fibrositis syndrome and rheumatoid arthritis. Arthritis Rheum 35:550-556, 1992.
112. Wolfe F, Russell IJ, Vipraio G, et al: Serotonin levels, pain threshold, and fibromyalgia symptoms in the general population. J Rheumatol 24:555-559, 1997.
113. Klein R, Bansch M, Berg PA: Clinical relevance of antibodies against serotonin and gangliosides in patients with primary fibromyalgia syndrome. Psychoneuroendocrinology 17:593-598, 1992.
114. Klein R, Berg PA: A comparative study on antibodies to nucleoli and 5-hydroxytryptamine in patients with fibromyalgia syndrome and tryptophan-induced eosinophilia-myalgia syndrome. Clin Investig 72:541-549, 1994.
115. Klein R, Berg PA: High incidence of antibodies to 5-hydroxytryptamine, gangliosides and phospholipids in patients with chronic fatigue and fibromyalgia syndrome and their relatives: Evidence for a clinical entity of both disorders. Eur J Med Res 1:21-26, 1995.
116. Werle E, Fischer HP, Muller A, et al: Antibodies against serotonin have no diagnostic relevance in patients with fibromyalgia syndrome. J Rheumatol 28:595-600, 2001.
117. Neeck G: Neuroendocrine and hormonal perturbations and relations to the serotonergic system in fibromyalgia patients. Scand J Rheumatol Suppl 113:8-12, 2000.
118. McCain GA, Tilbe KS: Diurnal hormone variation in fibromyalgia syndrome: A comparison with rheumatoid arthritis. J Rheumatol Suppl 19:154-157, 1989.
119. Griep EN, Boersma JW, de Kloet ER: Altered reactivity of the hypothalamic-pituitary-adrenal axis in the primary fibromyalgia syndrome. J Rheumatol 20:469-474, 1993.
120. Crofford LJ, Pillemer SR, Kalogeras KT, et al: Hypothalamic-pituitary-adrenal axis perturbations in patients with fibromyalgia. Arthritis Rheum 37:1583-1592, 1994.
121. Griep EN, Boersma JW, Lentjes EG, et al: Function of the hypothalamic-pituitary-adrenal axis in patients with fibromyalgia and low back pain. J Rheumatol 25:1374-1381, 1998.
122. Maes M, Lin A, Bonaccorso S, et al: Increased 24-hour urinary cortisol excretion in patients with post-traumatic stress disorder and patients with major depression, but not in patients with fibromyalgia. Acta Psychiatr Scand 98:328-335, 1998.
123. Riedel W, Layka H, Neeck G: Secretory pattern of GH, TSH, thyroid hormones, ACTH, cortisol, FSH, and LH in patients with fibromyalgia syndrome following systemic injection of the relevant hypothalamic-releasing hormones. Z Rheumatol 57(Suppl 2): 81-87, 1998.
124. Adler GK, Kinsley BT, Hurwitz S, et al: Reduced hypothalamic-pituitary and sympathoadrenal responses to hypoglycemia in women with fibromyalgia syndrome. Am J Med 106:534-543, 1999.
125. Torpy DJ, Papanicolaou DA, Lotsikas AJ, et al: Responses of the sympathetic nervous system and the hypothalamic-pituitary-adrenal axis to interleukin-6: A pilot study in fibromyalgia. Arthritis Rheum 43:872-880, 2000.
126. Korszun A, Young EA, Engleberg NC, et al: Follicular phase hypothalamic-pituitary-gonadal axis function in women with fibromyalgia and chronic fatigue syndrome. J Rheumatol 27:1526-1530, 2000.
127. Catley D, Kaell AT, Kirschbaum C, Stone AA: A naturalistic evaluation of cortisol secretion in persons with fibromyalgia and rheumatoid arthritis. Arthritis Care Res 13:51-61, 2000.
128. Lentjes EG, Griep EN, Boersma JW, et al: Glucocorticoid receptors, fibromyalgia and low back pain. Psychoneuroendocrinology 22:603-614, 1997.
129. Kirnap M, Colak R, Eser C, et al: A comparison between low-dose (1 microg), standard-dose (250 microg) ACTH stimulation tests and insulin tolerance test in the evaluation of hypothalamo-pituitary-adrenal axis in primary fibromyalgia syndrome. Clin Endocrinol (Oxf) 55:455-459, 2001.

130. Parker AJ, Wessely S, Cleare AJ: The neuroendocrinology of chronic fatigue syndrome and fibromyalgia. Psychol Med 31:1331-1345, 2001.
131. Bennett RM, Clark SR, Campbell SM, Burckhardt CS: Low levels of somatomedin C in patients with the fibromyalgia syndrome: A possible link between sleep and muscle pain. Arthritis Rheum 35:1113-1116, 1992.
132. Bennett RM, Cook DM, Clark SR, et al: Hypothalamic-pituitary-insulin-like growth factor-I axis dysfunction in patients with fibromyalgia. J Rheumatol 24:1384-1389, 1997.
133. Bagge E, Bengtsson BA, Carlsson L, Carlsson J: Low growth hormone secretion in patients with fibromyalgia: A preliminary report on 10 patients and 10 controls. J Rheumatol 25:145-148, 1998.
134. Older SA, Battafarano DF, Danning CL, et al: The effects of delta wave sleep interruption on pain thresholds and fibromyalgia-like symptoms in healthy subjects: Correlations with insulin-like growth factor I. J Rheumatol 25:1180-1186, 1998.
135. Leal-Cerro A, Povedano J, Astorga R, et al: The growth hormone (GH)-releasing hormone-GH-insulin-like growth factor-1 axis in patients with fibromyalgia syndrome. J Clin Endocrinol Metab 84:3378-81, 1999.
136. Jacobsen S, Main K, Danneskiold-Samsoe B, Skakkebaek NE: A controlled study on serum insulin-like growth factor-I and urinary excretion of growth hormone in fibromyalgia. J Rheumatol 22:1138-1140, 1995.
137. Buchwald D, Umali J, Stene M: Insulin-like growth factor-I (somatomedin C) levels in chronic fatigue syndrome and fibromyalgia. J Rheumatol 23:739-742, 1996.
138. Griep EN, Boersma JW, de Kloet ER: Pituitary release of growth hormone and prolactin in the primary fibromyalgia syndrome. J Rheumatol 21:2125-2130, 1994.
139. Dinser R, Halama T, Hoffmann A: Stringent endocrinological testing reveals subnormal growth hormone secretion in some patients with fibromyalgia syndrome but rarely severe growth hormone deficiency. J Rheumatol 27:2482-2488, 2000.
140. Gursel Y, Ergin S, Ulus Y, et al: Hormonal responses to exercise stress test in patients with fibromyalgia syndrome. Clin Rheumatol 20:401-405, 2001.
141. Bennett RM: Disordered growth hormone secretion in fibromyalgia: a review of recent findings and a hypothesized etiology. Z Rheumatol 57(Suppl 2):72-76, 1998.
142. Martinez-Lavin M: Is fibromyalgia a generalized reflex sympathetic dystrophy? Clin Exp Rheumatol 19:1-3, 2001.
143. Tougas G: The autonomic nervous system in functional bowel disorders. Can J Gastroenterol 13(Suppl A):15A-17A, 1999.
144. Meggs WJ: Neurogenic switching: A hypothesis for a mechanism for shifting the site of inflammation in allergy and chemical sensitivity. Environ Health Perspect 103:54-56, 1995.
145. Visuri T, Lindholm H, Lindqvist A, et al: Cardiovascular functional disorder in primary fibromyalgia: a noninvasive study in 17 young men. Arthritis Care Res 5:210-215, 1992.
146. Hubbard DR, Berkoff GM: Myofascial trigger points show spontaneous needle EMG activity. Spine 18:1803-1807, 1993.
147. Martinez-Lavin M, Hermosillo AG, Rosas M, Soto ME: Circadian studies of autonomic nervous balance in patients with fibromyalgia: A heart rate variability analysis. Arthritis Rheum 41:1966-1971, 1998.
148. Anderberg UM, Liu Z, Berglund L, Nyberg F: Elevated plasma levels of neuropeptide Y in female fibromyalgia patients. Eur J Pain 3:19-30, 1999.
149. Wachter KC, Kaeser HE, Guhring H, et al: Muscle damping measured with a modified pendulum test in patients with fibromyalgia, lumbago, and cervical syndrome. Spine 21:2137-2142, 1996.
150. Cohen H, Neumann L, Alhosshle A, et al: Abnormal sympathovagal balance in men with fibromyalgia. J Rheumatol 28: 581-589, 2001.
151. Cohen H, Neumann L, Shore M, et al: Autonomic dysfunction in patients with fibromyalgia: Application of power spectral analysis of heart rate variability. Semin Arthritis Rheum 29: 217-227, 2000.
152. van Denderen JC, Boersma JW, Zeinstra P, et al: Physiological effects of exhaustive physical exercise in primary fibromyalgia syndrome (PFS): Is PFS a disorder of neuroendocrine reactivity? Scand J Rheumatol 21:35-37, 1992.
153. Elam M, Johansson G, Wallin BG: Do patients with primary fibromyalgia have an altered muscle sympathetic nerve activity? Pain 48:371-375, 1992.
154. Vaeroy H, Qiao ZG, Morkrid L, Forre O: Altered sympathetic nervous system response in patients with fibromyalgia (fibrositis syndrome). J Rheumatol 16:1460-1465, 1989.
155. Qiao ZG, Vaeroy H, Morkrid L: Electrodermal and microcirculatory activity in patients with fibromyalgia during baseline, acoustic stimulation and cold pressor tests. J Rheumatol 18:1383-1389, 1991.
156. Bengtsson A, Bengtsson M: Regional sympathetic blockade in primary fibromyalgia. Pain 33:161-167, 1988.
157. Backman E, Bengtsson A, Bengtsson M, et al: Skeletal muscle function in primary fibromyalgia: Effect of regional sympathetic blockade with guanethidine. Acta Neurol Scand 77:187-191, 1988.
158. Martinez-Lavin M, Vidal M, Barbosa RE, et al: Norepinephrine-evoked pain in fibromyalgia: A randomized pilot study [ISRCTN70707830]. BMC Musculoskelet Disord 3:2, 2002.
159. Malt E, Olafsson S, Lund A, Ursin H: Factors explaining variance in perceived pain in women with fibromyalgia. BMC Musculoskelet Disord 3:12. 2002.
160. Bou-Holaigah I, Calkins H, Flynn JA, et al: Provocation of hypotension and pain during upright tilt table testing in adults with fibromyalgia. Clin Exp Rheumatol 15 239-246, 1997.
161. Raj SR, Brouillard D, Simpson CS, et al: Dysautonomia among patients with fibromyalgia: A noninvasive assessment. J Rheumatol 27:2660-2665, 2000.
162. Martinez-Lavin M, Hermosillo AG, Mendoza C, et al: Orthostatic sympathetic derangement in subjects with fibromyalgia. J Rheumatol 24:714-718, 1997.
163. Naschitz JE, Rozenbaum M, Rosner I, et al: Cardiovascular response to upright tilt in fibromyalgia differs from that in chronic fatigue syndrome. J Rheumatol 28:1356-1360, 2001.
164. Buskila D, Press J: Neuroendocrine mechanisms in fibromyalgia-chronic fatigue. Best Pract Res Clin Rheumatol 15:747-758, 2001.
165. Moldofsky H, Scarisbrick P, England R, Smythe H: Musculoskeletal symptoms and non-REM sleep disturbance in patients with "fibrositis syndrome" and healthy subjects. Psychosom Med 37:341-351, 1975.
166. Smythe HA, Moldofsky H: Two contributions to understanding of the "fibrositis" syndrome. Bull Rheum Dis 28:928-931, 1977.
167. Branco J, Atalaia A, Faiva T: Sleep cycles and alpha-delta sleep in fibromyalgia syndrome. J Rheumatol 21:1113-1117, 1994.
168. Roizenblatt S, Moldofsky H, Benedito-Silva AA, Tufik S: Alpha sleep characteristics in fibromyalgia. Arthritis Rheum 44:222-230, 2001.
169. Anch AM, Lue FA, MacLean AW, Moldofsky H: Sleep physiology and psychological aspects of the fibrositis (fibromyalgia) syndrome. Can J Psychol 45:179-184, 1991.
170. Affleck G, Urrows S, Tennen H, et al: Sequential daily relations of sleep, pain intensity, and attention to pain among women with fibromyalgia. Pain 68:363-368, 1996.
171. Totterdell P, Reynolds S, Parkinson B, Briner RB: Associations of sleep with everyday mood, minor symptoms and social interaction experience. Sleep 17:466-475, 1994.
172. Nicassio PM, Wallston KA: Longitudinal relationships among pain, sleep problems, and depression in rheumatoid arthritis. J Abnorm Psychol 101:514-520, 1992.
173. Drewes AM, Nielsen KD, Arendt-Nielsen L, et al: The effect of cutaneous and deep pain on the electroencephalogram during sleep: An experimental study. Sleep 20:632-640, 1997.
174. Perlis ML, Giles DE, Bootzin RR, et al: Alpha sleep and information processing, perception of sleep, pain, and arousability in fibromyalgia. Int J Neurosci 89:265-280, 1997.
175. Lentz MJ, Landis CA, Rothermel J, Shaver JL: Effects of selective slow wave sleep disruption on musculoskeletal pain and fatigue in middle aged women. J Rheumatol 26:1586-1592, 1999.
176. Van Cauter E, Copinschi G: Interrelationships between growth hormone and sleep. Growth Horm IGF Res 10(Suppl B): S57-S62, 2000.
177. Wikner J, Hirsch U, Wetterberg L, Rojdmark S: Fibromyalgia: A syndrome associated with decreased nocturnal melatonin secretion. Clin Endocrinol (Oxf) 49:179-183, 1998.

178. Buskila D, Neumann L, Vaisberg G, et al: Increased rates of fibromyalgia following cervical spine injury: A controlled study of 161 cases of traumatic injury. Arthritis Rheum 40:446-452, 1997.
179. Hellstrom C, Jansson B, Carlsson SG: Perceived future in chronic pain: The relationship between outlook on future and empirically derived psychological patient profiles. Eur J Pain 4:283-290, 2000.
180. Richards SC, Scott DL: Prescribed exercise in people with fibromyalgia: Parallel group randomised controlled trial. BMJ 325:185, 2002.
181. Mannerkorpi K, Ahlmen M, Ekdahl C: Six- and 24-month follow-up of pool exercise therapy and education for patients with fibromyalgia. Scand J Rheumatol 31:306-310, 2002.
182. Busch A, Schachter CL, Peloso PM, Bombardier C: Exercise for treating fibromyalgia syndrome. Cochrane Database Syst Rev CD003786, 2002.
183. Sharpe M, Hawton K, Simkin S, et al: Cognitive behaviour therapy for the chronic fatigue syndrome: A randomized controlled trial. BMJ 312:22-26, 1996.
184. Deale A, Chalder T, Wessely S: Illness beliefs and treatment outcome in chronic fatigue syndrome. J Psychosom Res 45:77-83, 1998.
185. Deale A, Husain K, Chalder T, Wessely S: Long-term outcome of cognitive behavior therapy versus relaxation therapy for chronic fatigue syndrome: A 5-year follow-up study. Am J Psychiatry 158:2038-2042, 2001.
186. Price JR, Couper J: Cognitive behaviour therapy for adults with chronic fatigue syndrome. Cochrane Database Syst Rev CD001027, 2000.
187. Akagi H, Klimes I, Bass C: Cognitive behavioral therapy for chronic fatigue syndrome in a general hospital: Feasible and effective. Gen Hosp Psychiatry 23:254-260, 2001.
188. Williams DA, Cary MA, Groner KH, et al: Improving physical functional status in patients with fibromyalgia: A brief cognitive behavioral intervention. J Rheumatol 29:1280-1286, 2002.
189. Bennett RM, Clark SC, Walczyk J: A randomized, double-blind, placebo-controlled study of growth hormone in the treatment of fibromyalgia. Am J Med 104:227-231, 1998.
190. Moorkens G, Wynants H, Abs R: Effect of growth hormone treatment in patients with chronic fatigue syndrome: A preliminary study. Growth Horm IGF Res 8(Suppl B):131-133, 1998.
191. Moulin DE: Systemic drug treatment for chronic musculoskeletal pain. Clin J Pain17:S86-S93, 2001.
192. Arnold LM, Hess EV, Hudson JI, et al: A randomized, placebo-controlled, double-blind, flexible-dose study of fluoxetine in the treatment of women with fibromyalgia. Am J Med 112:191-197, 2002.
193. Goldenberg D, Mayskiy M, Mossey C, et al: A randomized, double-blind crossover trial of fluoxetine and amitriptyline in the treatment of fibromyalgia. Arthritis Rheum 39:1852-1859, 1996.
194. O'Malley PG, Balden E, Tomkins G, et al: Treatment of fibromyalgia with antidepressants: A meta-analysis. J Gen Intern Med 15:659-666, 2000.
195. Carette S, McCain GA, Bell DA, Fam AG: Evaluation of amitriptyline in primary fibrositis: A double-blind, placebo-controlled study. Arthritis Rheum 29:655-659, 1986.
196. Moldofsky H, Lue FA: The relationship of alpha and delta EEG frequencies to pain and mood in 'fibrositis' patients treated with chlorpromazine and L-tryptophan. Electroencephalogr Clin Neurophysiol 50:71-80, 1980.
197. Scharf MB, Hauck M, Stover R, et al: Effect of gamma-hydroxybutyrate on pain, fatigue, and the alpha sleep anomaly in patients with fibromyalgia: Preliminary report. J Rheumatol 25:1986-1990, 1998.
198. Granges G, Littlejohn GO: A comparative study of clinical signs in fibromyalgia/fibrositis syndrome, healthy and exercising subjects. J Rheumatol 20:344-351, 1993.
199. Sorensen J, Bengtsson A, Backman E, et al: Pain analysis in patients with fibromyalgia: Effects of intravenous morphine, lidocaine, and ketamine. Scand J Rheumatol 24:360-365, 1995.
200. Sorensen J, Bengtsson A, Ahlner J, et al: Fibromyalgia: Are there different mechanisms in the processing of pain? A double blind crossover comparison of analgesic drugs. J Rheumatol 24:1615-1621, 1997.
201. Biasi G, Manca S, Manganelli S, Marcolongo R: Tramadol in the fibromyalgia syndrome: A controlled clinical trial versus placebo. Int J Clin Pharmacol Res 18:13-19, 1998.
202. Clauw DJ: Fibromyalgia. *In* Ruddy S, Harris Ed Jr, Sledge CB, et al (eds): Textbook of Rheumatology. Philadelphia, WB Saunders, 2001, pp 717-728.

37 Neck Pain

KENNETH K. NAKANO

By creating anxiety and limiting activity, pain serves to forewarn of physiologic excess and to prevent tissue damage and organ dysfunction; thus, pain is an evolutionary protective mechanism. Pain exists in at least two types: neuropathic and nociceptive. Neuropathic pain arises from abnormal neural activity due to injury or disease of the nervous system, and it remains persistent even in the absence of ongoing disease processes (e.g., thalamic pain, trigeminal neuralgia, and diabetic neuropathy). Furthermore, neuropathic pain may be central, mediated sympathetically, or conveyed nonsympathetically. Nociceptive pain can be subdivided into visceral and somatic pain. Visceral pain originates from the viscera, mediated by stretch receptors, and will be poorly localized, cramping, and dull (e.g., pleurisy, appendicitis, or cholecystitis). On the other hand, somatic pain arises from injury or damage to body tissues and will be well localized and variably manifested in experience and description. An alternative means to divide pain is according to its duration: acute versus chronic. Nociceptive pain is typically acute pain; it results from the temporary effects of trauma, injury, surgery, or acute exacerbation of chronic disease processes. On the other hand, chronic pain will generally be at least partially neuropathic. Generally, chronic pain is that which persists beyond the period of time it would normally take the body to heal following an injury or insult.

Epidemiology

Neck pain exists as a common complaint, especially in middle age; it occurs slightly less frequently than low back pain and has a lifetime prevalence of at least one significant neck pain in the 40 to 70 percent range.[1-3] In certain general populations, the point prevalences of neck pain have been in the 10 to 15 percent range.[4-6] Commonly the peak prevalence of neck pain occurs around 50 years of age and appears more often in women than men.[4,5,7-9] Although less disabling and relatively not as costly as low back pain, neck pain can result in disability and prove expensive to society.[10-12] In the Netherlands, neck pain constitutes up to 2 percent of general practitioners' consultations,[13] in the United Kingdom approximately 15 percent of hospital-based physical therapy,[14] and in Canada 30 percent of chiropractic referrals.[15]

Neck stiffness is a common disorder; for the age-group 25 to 29 years in the U.S. working population, there is up to a 30-percent frequency of one or more attacks of stiff neck.[16] For the same work population over 45 years of age, this figure rises to 50 percent. Episodes of "simple" stiff neck last 1 to 4 days and seldom require medical care in the vast majority of people. Radicular pain to the shoulder and arm occurs later in life than does stiff neck; it has a frequency of up to 10 percent in the 25 to 29 age-group, subsequently rising to 25 to 40 percent after age 45 years. Overall, 45 percent of working men experience at least one attack of stiff neck, 23 percent report at least one attack of radiculopathy, and 51 percent suffer both these symptoms at some time during their working career.

Pain in the neck exists in all occupational groups. Stiffness of the neck appears first, followed by headache and shoulder-arm/hand pain (brachial neuralgia).[16] Investigations have reported that, at any time, as many as 12 percent of women and 9 percent of men experience pain in the neck with or without associated arm pain, and 35 percent of the population can recall an episode of neck pain.[2]

Functional Anatomy

The pain-sensitive structures of the neck include the ligaments, nerve roots, articular facets and capsules, muscle, and dura. Pain in the neck region can originate from many tissue sites (Tables 37–1 and 37–2) and can result from a number of mechanisms (Table 37–3). The cervical zygapophyseal joints (C0/1 to C7/T1) and the cervical dorsal rami (C3 to C7) are sources of referred pain.[17] Pain in the occipital region will be referred from C2/3 and C3, whereas pain in the upper posterolateral cervical region will be referred from C0/1, C1/2, and C2/3. Pain in the upper posterior cervical region will be referred

TABLE 37–1 • CERVICAL PAIN REFERRAL PATHWAYS

Location of Pain	Source
Upper posterolateral cervical region	C0-1,C1-2,C2-3
Occipital region	C2-3,C3
Upper posterior cervical region	C2-3,C3-4,C3
Middle posterior cervical region	C3-4,C4-5,C4
Lower posterior cervical region	C4-5,C5-6,C4,C5
Suprascapular region	C4-5,C5-6,C4
Superior angle of scapula	C6-7,C6,C7
Midscapular region	C7-T1,C7

From Nakano KK: Neck pain. *In* Kelley WN, Harris ED Jr, Ruddy S, Sledge CB (eds): Textbook of Rheumatology, 5th ed. Philadelphia, WB Saunders, 1997, p 394.

TABLE 37–2 • STRUCTURES THAT CAUSE NECK PAIN

Acromioclavicular joint
Heart and coronary artery disease
Apex of lung, Pancoast's tumor, bronchogenic cancer (C3, C4, C5 nerve roots in common)
Diaphragm muscle (C3, C4, C5 innervation)
Gallbladder
Spinal cord tumor
Temporomandibular joint
Fibrositis and fibromyositis syndromes (upper thoracic spine, proximal arm, and proximal shoulder)
Aorta
Pancreas
Disorders of any somatic or visceral structure (produces cervical nerve root irritation)
Peripheral nerves
Central nervous system (posterior fossa lesions)
Hiatus hernia (C3, C4, C5)
Gastric ulcer

From Nakano KK: Neck pain. *In* Kelley WN, Harris ED Jr, Ruddy S, Sledge CB (eds): Textbook of Rheumatology, 5th ed. Philadelphia, WB Saunders, 1997, p 395.

from C2/3, C3/4, and C3, which in the middle posterior cervical region form C3/4, C4/5, and C4, and which in the lower posterior cervical region form C4/5, C5/6, C4, and C5. Additionally, pain in the suprascapular region will be referred from C4/5, C5/6, and C4, which in the superior angle of the scapula from C6/7, C6, and C7, and which in the midscapular region from C7/T1 and C7.[17]

Normal function of the cervical spine requires physiologic movements of the joints, bones, spinal cord, nerve roots (through the intervertebral foramina), muscles, ligaments, tendons, fascia, sympathetic nervous system, and the vascular supply to all these structures. The neck is the most complicated articular system in the body and the most mobile segment of the spine. Through a cylinder that connects the head to the thorax pass structures that require the greatest protection and possess the least: the vertebral and carotid arteries, the spinal cord, and the spinal nerve roots. The head, weighing 6 to 8 pounds, balances on the seven cervical vertebrae in a flexible chain held together by 14 apophyseal joints; five intervertebral disks; 12 joints of Luschka; and a system of ligaments (anterior longitudinal [AL], posterior longitudinal [PL], ligamentum flavum, interspinous, and ligamentum nuchae) and muscles (14 paired anterior, lateral, and posterior) (Figs. 37–1 and 37–2). Thirty-seven separate joints enable the myriad movements of the head and neck in relation to the trunk.

The shape and mode of articulation of the joints influence the axes and range of movement of the neck. The neck normally moves more than 600 times each hour, whether one is asleep or awake. The cervical spine is subject to stress and strain from daily activities such as sitting, lying in the supine or prone position, speaking, rising, walking, turning, and gesturing. The articular surfaces of the vertebral bodies are covered by plates of avascular hyaline cartilage and united by intervertebral disks. The intervertebral disks increase in area from below the axis (C2) downward, and the normal cervical lordosis results from their wedge shape (see Figs. 37–1 and 37–2). The thickness of the intervertebral disks varies; the two deepest disks lie below the sixth and fifth vertebrae, respectively. Each intervertebral disk consists of fibrocartilage and contains a nucleus pulposus, which changes in shape but cannot be compressed in the normal state.[18]

TABLE 37–3 • CERVICAL SPINE SYNDROMES

Localized Neck Disorders
Osteoarthritis (apophyseal joints, C1–3 levels most often)
Rheumatoid arthritis (atlantoaxial)
Juvenile rheumatoid arthritis
Sternocleidomastoid tendinitis
Acute posterior cervical strain
Pharyngeal infections
Cervical lymphadenitis
Osteomyelitis (staphylococcal, tuberculosis)
Meningitis
Ankylosing spondylitis
Paget's disease
Torticollis (congenital, spasmodic, drug involved, hysterical)
Neoplasms (primary or metastatic)
Occipital neuralgia (greater and lesser occipital nerves)
Diffuse idiopathic skeletal hyperostosis
Rheumatic fever (infrequently)
Gout (infrequently)
Lesions Producing Neck and Shoulder Pain
Postural disorders
Rheumatoid arthritis
Fibrositis syndromes
Musculoligamentous injuries to neck and shoulder
Osteoarthritis (apophyseal and Luschka)
Cervical spondylosis
Intervertebral osteoarthritis
Thoracic outlet syndrome
Nerve injuries (serratus anterior, C3–4 nerve root, long thoracic nerve)
Lesions Producing Predominantly Shoulder Pain
Rotator cuff tears and tendinitis
Calcareous tendinitis
Subacromial bursitis
Bicipital tendinitis
Adhesive capsulitis
Reflex sympathetic dystrophy
Frozen shoulder syndromes
Acromioclavicular secondary osteoarthritis
Glenohumeral arthritis
Septic arthritis
Tumors of the shoulder
Lesions Producing Neck and Head Pain with Radiation
Cervical spondylosis
Rheumatoid arthritis
Intervertebral disk protrusion
Osteoarthritis (apophyseal and Luschka joints; intervertebral disk; osteoarthritis)
Spinal cord tumors
Cervical neurovascular syndromes
Cervical rib
Scalene muscle
Hyperabduction syndrome
Rib-clavicle compression

From Nakano KK: Neck pain. *In* Kelley WN, Harris ED Jr, Ruddy S, Sledge CB (eds): Textbook of Rheumatology, 5th ed. Philadelphia, WB Saunders, 1997, p 395.

PL and AL ligaments extend upward to the occipital bone and downward into the sacrum, joining the verte-

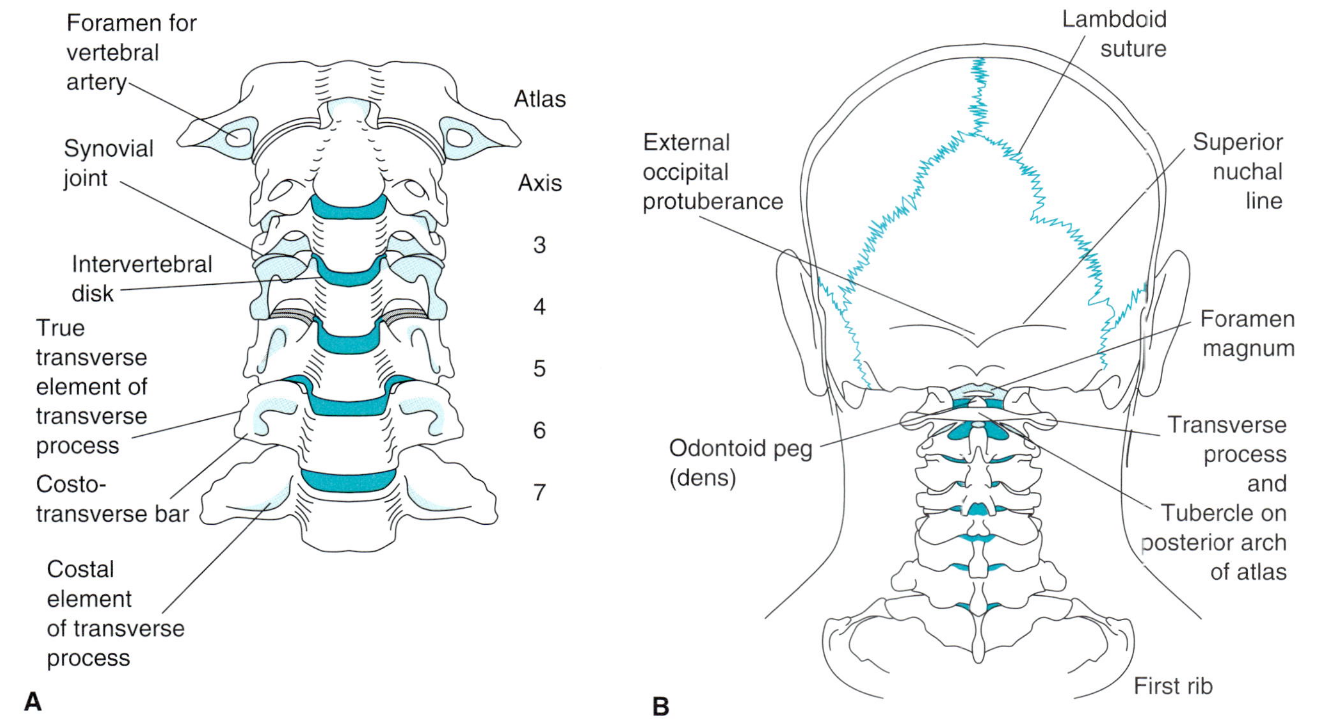

FIGURE 37–1 · *A*, Cervical spine. Anterior view of articulated cervical vertebrae. *B*, Posterior view of the skull, seven cervical vertebrae, and first thoracic vertebra. (Taken from Nakano KK: Neck pain. In Ruddy S, Harris ED Jr, Sledge CB (eds): Kelley's Textbook of Rheumatology, 6th ed. Philadelphia, WB Saunders, 2001, p 458 [Figs. 34-1A, 34-1B].)

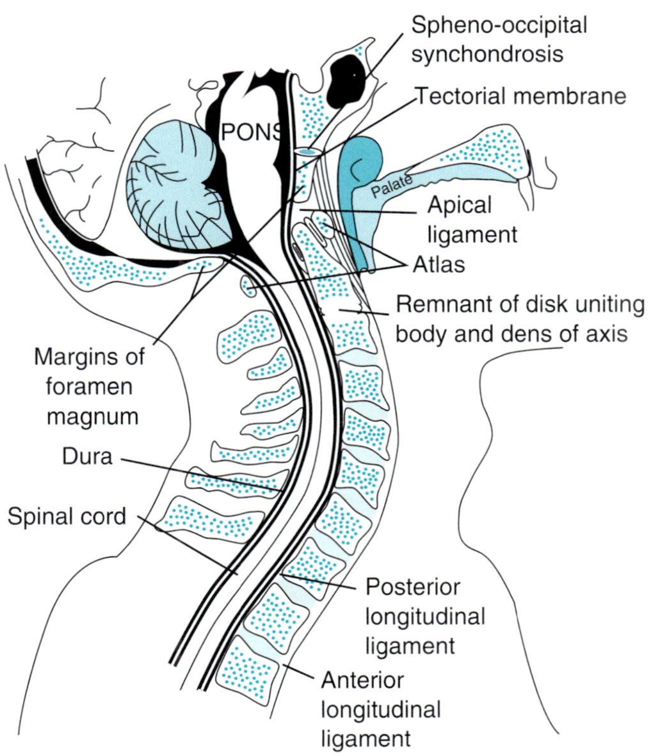

FIGURE 37–2 · Sagittal view of the lower head and neck to show the relationship of the spinal cord and brain stem to the bones, ligaments, and joints between the bodies of the cervical vertebrae. The cervical lordosis can be seen, as well as the relationship of the anterior and posterior longitudinal ligaments to intervertebral disks and the ligaments at the craniovertebral junction. (Taken from Nakano KK: Neck pain. In Ruddy S, Harris ED Jr, Sledge CB (eds): Kelley's Textbook of Rheumatology, 6th ed. Philadelphia, WB Saunders, 2001, p 459 [Fig. 34-2].)

bral bodies. The AL ligament attaches to the bodies and becomes tightly fixed at the disks (see Fig. 37–2). A sudden extending force may rupture it and lead to severe hyperextension associated with damage to the spinal cord. The PL ligament attaches to the disks and adjacent bones but not to the center of the vertebral bodies.

The specialized atlanto-occipital and atlantoaxial joints are controlled by intersegmental muscles. The head and atlas (C1) move together around the odontoid peg (C2) and the upper articular facets of the axis (C2) (see Fig. 37–1) with the long transverse processes of the atlas providing the levers used in rotation. The anterior surface of the odontoid articulates with the posterior surface of the anterior arch of the atlas. The total excursion of the head can be measured in flexion, extension, rotation, and lateral flexion (Table 37–4). The overall range of movement in the sagittal plane (flexion and extension) approximates 90 degrees, with about three fourths due to extension. About 10 degrees of flexion and 25 degrees of extension occur at the atlanto-occipital joints. In this range of movement, the ligaments help protect the spinal cord from damage by the normal, fractured, or dislocated odontoid process. The lower parts of the cervical spine contribute to the remainder of full range in this plane. The maximal range of movement between individual vertebrae occurs between the fourth and fifth vertebrae in young children and between the fifth and sixth vertebrae in teenagers and adults. The total range of rotation of the head and neck encompasses 80 to 90 degrees. Approximately 35 to 45 degrees occurs at the atlantoaxial joint and is associated with a screwing movement of the upper vertebra on the lower vertebra, a movement that reduces the cross-sectional area of the spinal canal.

TABLE 37–4 • AGE AND NORMAL CERVICAL MOVEMENT

Age (yrs)	Flexion-Extension (degrees)	Lateral Rotation (degrees)	Lateral Flexion (degrees)
<30	90	90	45
31–50	70	90	45
>50	60	90	30

From Nakano KK: Neck pain. *In* Kelley WN, Harris ED Jr, Ruddy S, Sledge CB (eds): Textbook of Rheumatology, 5th ed. Philadelphia, WB Saunders, 1997, p 396.

Lateral flexion does not occur in isolation but accompanies some rotation. There usually is about 30 degrees of lateral mobility on both sides in the lower cervical spine. The spinal canal shortens on the side of the concavity of the spine and lengthens on the side of the convexity.

With age, the nucleus pulposus becomes vulnerable to acute and chronic trauma. With loss of disk substance, the annulus fibrosus may bulge into the spinal canal, and because of its eccentric position, the nucleus pulposus tends to prolapse backward if any tear develops in the annulus fibrosus. The most common sites for both types of herniation are the mobile regions (i.e., C5-6 and C6-7). With degenerative changes, the disk space narrows and the spinal column shortens. The intervertebral foramina become narrowed, movements become restricted, and unusual mechanical strains on the synovial joints result. These changes may be confined to a localized area or may become widespread in generalized degenerative disease. The formation of osteophytes leads to encroachment on the spinal canal and intervertebral foramina. The canal may also be further narrowed by bulging of the ligamentum flavum. Changes in the caliber of the vertebral arteries can result because of the degenerative changes in the joints of the cervical spine. Arterial branches that supply joints and nervous tissue can be distorted at rest and further obstructed with movement. With severe vertebral artery stenosis, syncope occasionally results from rotation of the head.

The lower six cervical vertebrae articulate with each other at five points: two zygapophyseal joints, two uncovertebral (neurocentral) joints, and one intervertebral disk. The upper two cervical vertebrae articulate at the odontoid peg, the two zygapophyseal joints and the intervertebral joint. The former are synovial joints and can be affected by various arthritic diseases and by the natural forces of the aging process. The articular cartilage may suffer from a synovitis that thins the articular cartilage and exposes the underlying bone to the disease process. If the repair process can outpace the destruction, normal bone will be laid down. If the destruction prevents this, disordered articular bone will be laid down in the form of osteophytes. The uncovertebral joints have no articular cartilage or synovial membrane and are pseudoarthroses. They are not affected by arthritis in the true sense, but their reaction to attrition ultimately leads to osteophyte formation without synovitis. All the joints are supplied with sensory nerves and nutrient vessels on the segmental basis, as well as with sympathetic pain fibers. Pain from these joints is non-neuralgic and felt locally; it is derived mostly from the joint capsule rather than the synovium or bone. Articular cartilage in all joints is avascular and aneural and cannot give rise to pain. The PL ligament is sensitive to stretch through the fibers of the recurrent meningeal nerve of Luschka and can give rise to midline non-neuralgic pain. The AL ligament is pain sensitive, but the nerve supply is still not fully defined.

The emerging nerve root is invested in dura to the outer border of the intervertebral foramina and is also supplied by the recurrent meningeal nerve (Figs. 37–3 and 37–4). If the dura and its nerve are stretched, the

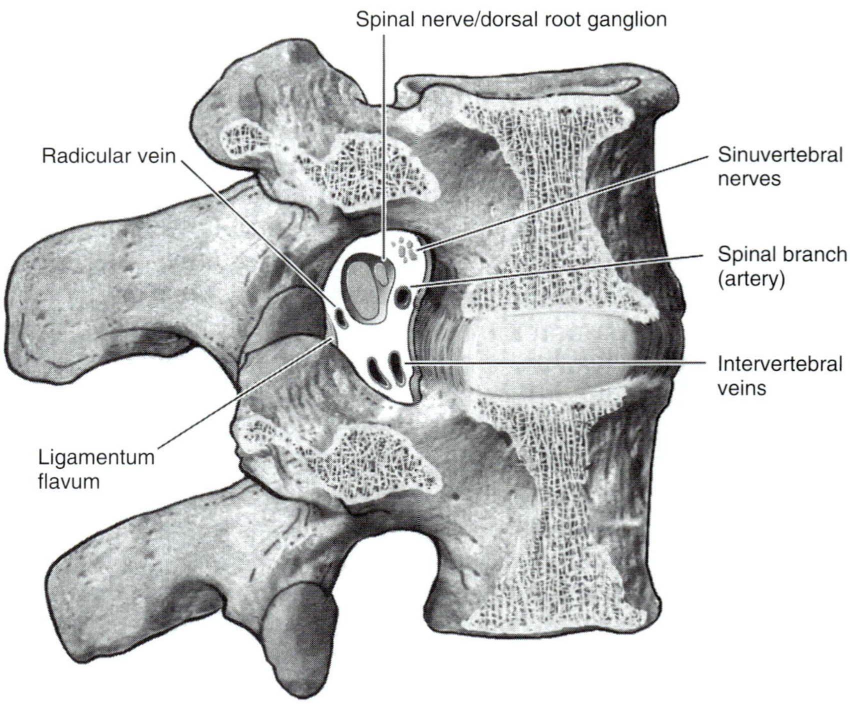

FIGURE 37–3 • View of a vertebra, composed of a body, two pedicles, two lamina, four articular facets, and a spinous process. Between each pair of vertebrae are two openings: the foramina through which pass a spinal nerve, radicular blood vessels, and the recurrent meningeal nerves (sinuvertebral nerves). (Taken from Levin KH (ed): Neck and Back Pain. Continuum 7 (no. 1), Philadelphia, Lippincott Williams & Wilkins, 2002, p 9 [Fig. 1].)

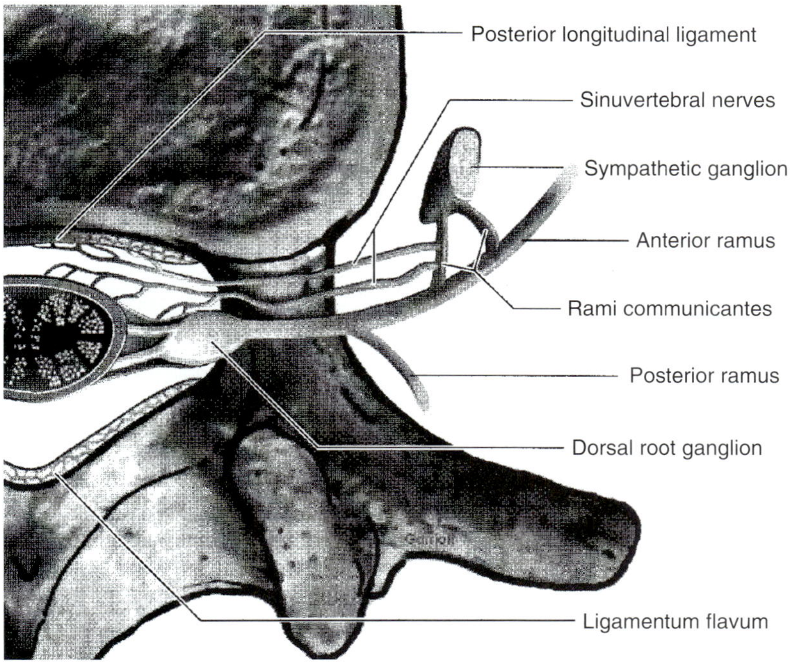

FIGURE 37–4 • Localized cervical pain is mediated primarily through the posterior primary ramus and the recurrent meningeal (sinuvertebral) nerves, which supply structures within the spinal canal. The recurrent meningeal nerves arise from rami communicantes and enter the spinal canal via intervertebral foramina; branches ascend and descend one or more levels, interconnecting with the recurrent meningeal nerves from other levels, and innervating, among other structures, the anterior and posterior longitudinal ligaments, the anterior and posterior portion of the dura, and blood vessels. (Taken from Levin KH (ed): Neck and Back Pain. Continuum 7 (no. 1), Philadelphia, Lippincott Williams & Wilkins, 2002, p 9 [Fig. 3].)

accompanying nutrient vessels can be narrowed and promptly cause ischemic neuralgic pain. The production of upper-limb neuralgia, with or without paresthesias, by stretching the arm at the shoulder can lead to an incorrect diagnosis of local joint or soft tissue pain. The nerve root is anchored firmly to the intervertebral foramina by the dura and does not glide in or out of the dura or the intervertebral foramina during movement of the neck. The dura accordions on extension and unfolds as well as tightens on flexion, placing traction on the nerve root and blood supply. Because the nerve root fills only about one fifth of the intervertebral foramina, it follows that cervicobrachial neuralgia is more commonly due to irritation, inflammation, and ischemia than to physical compression. As it leaves the intervertebral foramina, the nerve root is bounded above and below by the two vertebra pedicles, medially by the uncovertebral joint and laterally by the zygapophyseal joint. Involvement of these joints is the most common cause of cervicobrachial neuralgia.

The main load-bearing structure of the neck is the intervertebral disk, whereas the uncovertebral and zygapophyseal joints evolved as limiters of cervical movement to protect the spinal cord, rather than as load bearers. The intervertebral disk consists of a tough fibroelastic envelope that has a blood supply and can therefore undergo repair. It has a nerve supply that is highly sensitive to stretching, and diskogenic pain is non-neuralgic and felt locally. The nucleus pulposus has no nerve supply; thus, desiccation is painless. As it dries out, it loses volume; as it loses volume, it loses height. Because the nucleus pulposus is incompressible, the annulus fibrosis bulges under pressure from the head above. These changes are physiologic and not necessarily pathologic. As the disk loses height, it places increased pressure on the uncovertebral and zygapophyseal joints, which are now converted into load-bearing joints, a function for which they are not designed. Because these joints have a surface area inadequate for the imposed pressure, they become irritated. The irritation can lead to joint damage, and attempts to repair the joints can cause the formation of osteophytes. The emerging roots get caught up in the process, which can also cause perineural fibrosis and microvascular obliteration.

Pathophysiology

Mere bony changes do not necessarily correspond with the segmental level of neurologic damage. Two reasons exist for this: 1) The disproportionate growth of the spinal column and cord; the first thoracic segment of the spinal cord lies opposite the seventh cervical vertebra (see Fig. 37–2), and upper rootlets of the lower cervical and first thoracic nerves cross over two intervertebral disks, whereas the lower rootlets of these two nerves normally cross over only one disk. 2) Severe degeneration of the disks may shorten the vertebral canal to such an extent that the spinal cord, which remains unaltered in length, drops down relative to the bones. The spinal nerve roots may then become acutely folded as they travel toward the intervertebral foramina, with the lowest roots becoming the most severely affected.

Familiarity with the distribution of sensory, motor, and autonomic components in segmental nerves becomes necessary for localization of neurologic segments during the clinical examination (Fig. 37–5; Table 37–5). For practical purposes, the lower fibers of the cervical plexus supply the top of the shoulder; C5 and C6 nerve roots supply the lateral side of the arm and forearm; C6, C7, and C8 nerve roots innervate the hand; and C8 extends into the forearm. The T1 segment innervates the medial side of the arm and forearm. Visceral pain can be referred in some instances to well-defined segmental areas (Fig. 37–6); for example,

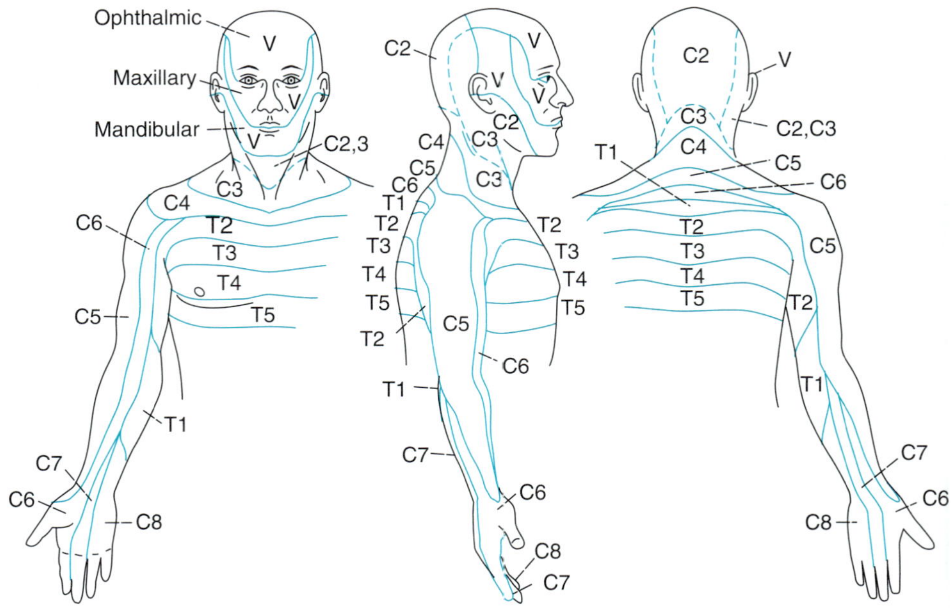

FIGURE 37–5 • Dermatome distribution of nerve fibers from C1 through T5, carrying senses of pain, heat, cold, vibration, and touch to the head, neck, arm, hand, and thoracic area. The sclerotomes and myotomes are similar but with some overlap. Pain arising from structures deep to the deep fascia (myotome and sclerotome) do not precisely follow the dermatome distribution. (Taken from Nakano KK: Neck pain. In Ruddy S, Harris ED Jr, Sledge CB (eds): Kelley's Textbook of Rheumatology, 6th ed. Philadelphia, WB Saunders, 2001, p 461 [Fig. 34-3].)

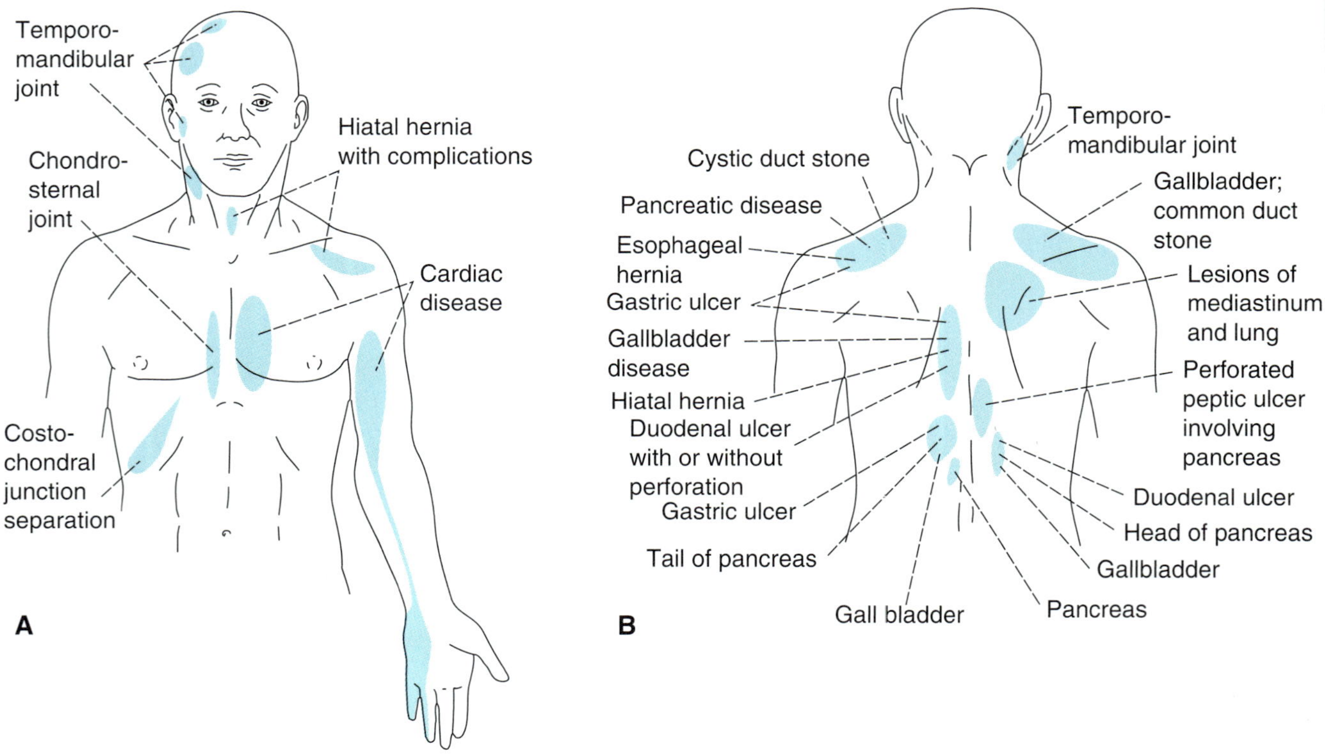

FIGURE 37–6 • Patterns of Reflex-Referred Pain from Visceral and Somatic Structures. *A*, Anterior distribution. *B*, Posterior distribution. (Taken from Nakano KK: Neck pain. In Ruddy S, Harris ED Jr, Sledge CB (eds): Kelley's Textbook of Rheumatology, 6th ed. Philadelphia, WB Saunders, 2001, p 463 [Fig. 34-4].)

pain at the point of the shoulder (C3-4) may be associated with cholecystitis. The segmental supplies of individual muscles are listed in Table 37–5.

NERVE ROOT COMPRESSION

A cervical radicular nerve normally occupies 20 to 25 percent of the intervertebral foramen (see Figs. 37–3 and 37–4). There may be considerable variation in the anatomy of the lower cervical nerves and their root pouches, and with increasing age, they become relatively fixed and vulnerable to injury. Two types of disk lesions cause pressure on the radicular nerves or nerve roots: 1) a dorsolateral protrusion that does not invade the intervertebral foramina but compresses the intrameningeal nerve roots against the vertebral laminae; and 2) an

TABLE 37–5 • NERVES AND TESTS OF PRINCIPAL MUSCLES

Nerve	Nerve Roots	Muscle	Test
Accessory	Spinal	Trapezius	Elevation of shoulders Abduction of scapula
	Spinal	Sternocleidomastoid	Tilting of head to same side with rotation to opposite side
Brachial plexus		Pectoralis major	
	C5, C6	Clavicular part	Adduction of arm
	C7, C8, T1	Sternocostal part	Adduction, forward depression of arm
	C5, C6, C7	Serratus anterior	Fixation of scapula during forward thrusting of the arm
	C4, C5	Rhomboid	Elevation and fixation of scapula
	C4, C5, C6	Supraspinatus	Initiate abduction of arm
	(C4), C5, C6	Infraspinatus	External rotation of arm
	C6, C7, C8	Latissimus dorsi	Adduction of horizontal, externally rotated arm, coughing
Axillary	C5, C6	Deltoid	Lateral and forward elevation of arm to horizontal
Musculocutaneous	C5, C6	Biceps Brachialis	Flexion of supinated forearm
Radial	C6, C7, C8	Triceps	Extension of forearm
	C5, C6	Brachioradialis	Flexion of semiprone forearm
	C6, C7	Extensor carpi radialis longus	Extension of wrist to radial side
Posterior interosseous	C5, C6	Supinator	Supination of extended forearm
	C7, C8	Extensor digitorum	Extension of proximal phalanges
	C7, C8	Extensor carpi ulnaris	Extension of wrist to ulnar side
	C7, C8	Extensor indicis	Extension of proximal phalanx of index finger
	C7, C8	Abductor pollicis longus	Abduction of first metacarpal in plane at right angle to palm
	C7, C8	Extensor pollicis longus	Extension of first interphalangeal joint
	C7, C8	Extensor pollicis brevis	Extension of first metacarpophalangeal joint
Median	C6, C7	Pronator teres	Pronation of extended forearm
	C6, C7	Flexor carpi radialis	Flexion of wrist to radial side
	C7, C8, T1	Flexor digitorum superficialis	Flexion of middle phalanges
	C8, T1	Flexor digitorum profundus (lateral part)	Flexion of terminal phalanges, index and middle fingers
	C8, T1	Flexor pollicis longus (anterior interosseous nerve)	Flexion of distal phalanx, thumb
	C8, T1	Abductor pollicis brevis	Abduction of first metacarpal in plane at right angle to palm
	C8, T1	Flexor pollicis brevis	Flexion of proximal phalanx, thumb
	C8, T1	Opponens pollicis	Opposition of thumb against 5th finger
	C8, T1	1st and 2nd lumbricals	Extension of middle phalanges while proximal phalanges are fixed in extension
Ulnar	C7, C8	Flexor carpi ulnaris	Observation of tendons while testing abductor digiti minimi
	C8, T1	Flexor digitorum profundus (medial part)	Flexion of distal phalanges of ring and little fingers
	C8, T1	Hypothenar muscles	Abduction and opposition of little finger
	C8, T1	3rd and 4th lumbricals	Extension of middle phalanges while proximal phalanges are fixed in extension
	C8, T1	Adductor pollicis	Adduction of thumb against palmar surface of index finger
	C8, T1	Flexor pollicis brevis	Flexion of proximal phalanx, thumb
	C8, T1	Interossei	Abduction and adduction of fingers

From Nakano KK: Neck pain. *In* Kelley WN, Harris ED Jr, Ruddy S, Sledge CB (eds): Textbook of Rheumatology, 5th ed. Philadelphia, WB Saunders, 1997, p 399.

intraforaminal protrusion from the uncinate part of the disk that compresses the cervical radicular nerve against the articular process. The extent of nerve root compression depends on the angulation of the cervical radicular nerve and its location in the foramen, as well as the size and position of the protrusion. Marginal lipping of the vertebrae and narrowing of the disks lead to secondary osteophyte formation of the articular processes and consequent posterolateral narrowing of the foramen.

BLOOD SUPPLY

Variations in the pattern of blood vessels in the cervical spinal cord exist, but the main blood supply comes through a few major articular arteries. The anterior and posterior spinal arteries act more as connecting links than as main channels of blood. The blood supply to the spinal cord may be impaired in individuals with cervical spondylosis when one or more radicular arteries become compressed. The resultant ischemia may be either continuous or intermittent, and sometimes the maximal impairment occurs only when the head is in a certain position (usually extension). The vertebral arteries vary in size, and one (usually the left side) may be larger than the other. The vertebral arteries lie within the vertebral canal, on their medial aspect closely related to the neurocentral joint, and pass immediately anterior to the emerging cervical nerve roots. Each nerve root receives a small arterial branch (see Fig. 37–3). Spondylotic changes of the cervical vertebrae may displace the artery laterally and, in severe cases, posteriorly as well. The degree of displacement depends on the size and position of the bony prominence that arises as a result of spondylosis.

Atheroma of the vertebral artery also may be important in the production of neurologic symptoms. Cerebel-lar infarction may result from a critical reduction of blood flow to the vertebral artery in the neck. When the obstruction occurs in the cervical part of the vertebral artery, the cerebellar infarcts tend to be bilateral, approximately symmetric, and in the territory of the superior cerebellar artery. Most often, the blockage is incomplete, and blood flow is reduced only when the patient turns or extends his or her head. Rotation and extension of the head to one side can obstruct the contralateral vertebral artery, and in patients with atherosclerosis, rotation and extension of the head can produce posterior circulation signs such as nystagmus, vertigo, weakness, dysarthria, drop attacks, and a Babinski response. An anterior spinal artery spinal cord syndrome results from either compromise of the anterior spinal artery or compression of one of the main radicular arteries by osteophytes or adhesions associated with nerve root sleeve fibrosis. In diseases that involve the major blood vessels (e.g., arteriosclerosis, diabetes, syphilis), the blood supply of the spinal cord may be impaired, especially if the condition is associated with spondylosis.

Clinical Evaluation

The essential means in the diagnosis and management of neck pain include the patient history and the general physical and neurologic/orthopedic examinations. Neuroimaging studies (cervical radiographs, computed tomograph [CT], CT myelography, nuclear bone scan with single photon emission computerized tomography [SPECT], and magnetic resonance imaging [MRI]) and neurophysiologic procedures (electromyography [EMG], nerve conduction studies [NCS], and somatosensory evoked responses [SER]) assist in confirming the clinical formulation. Optimally the clinician will find it useful to group the clinical symptoms into functional units (i.e., pain, paresthesias, weakness, articular symptoms, vascular symptoms, headache and occipital neuralgia, pseudoangina pectoris, eye and ear symptoms, throat symptoms, and miscellaneous symptoms).

PAIN

Pain will be the most common symptom of a cervical spine disorder. Clinically, the approach to pain is to define it in terms of type of onset, distribution, frequency, constancy versus intermittency, duration, quality, association with neurologic symptoms and signs, localization, and various associated features. Cervical nerve root irritation causes well-localized areas of pain (see Fig. 37–5), whereas poorly defined areas of pain arise from irritation of deep connective tissue structures including muscle, joint, bone, or disk. The patient's ability to describe his or her pain provides the examiner with essential clues to diagnosis. Retro-orbital, temporal, and occipital pain reflects a referral pattern from the atlas, axis, C3, and their surrounding structures. In cervical spine disorders, pain may radiate to the upper thoracic spine, shoulder, or scapular regions or into one or both upper limbs. Additionally, this pain may be produced, relieved, or exaggerated by various normal movements of the cervical spine. The areas of pain designation may be tender to palpation (i.e., transverse spinous process, apophyseal joints, or anterior vertebral bodies).

Sensory symptoms can be classified as somatic and autonomic, with the somatic complaints being the most common. Somatic pain due to cervical nerve root irritation is appreciated by the sufferer in two distinct forms, which often coexist. Neuralgic pain is caused by irritation of the dorsal sensory root. It is experienced as a "lightning" or "electric" sensation and is referred to dermatomal areas. It is felt mainly in the upper limb, scapula, and the trapezius ridge and is often associated with numbness or paresthesias. It is common for the pain to be felt more proximally and the paresthesias to be felt more distally, but the two usually overlap. Myalgic pain is caused by irritation of the ventral motor root. It is experienced as a deep, boring, unpleasant sensation, which is frequently poorly localized because it is referred to sclerotomal areas. The sensory topography of the ventral root myalgic pain therefore conforms somewhat to the muscle supplied by that root, whereas dorsal root neuralgic pain conforms more with the territory of the peripheral nerves supplied by that root. Neuralgic and myalgic pains are not always felt in precise anatomic zones, because muscle groups and bordering areas of skin have overlapping sensory supplies; also, pain can radiate up or down a spinal segment by recruitment within the spinal column.

PARESTHESIAS

Numbness and tingling follow the segmental distribution of the nerve roots (see Fig. 37–5) in cervical spine disorders; however, these symptoms often occur without demonstrable sensory changes. Paresthesias that involve the face, head, or tongue suggest involvement of the upper three nerve roots of the cervical plexus, whereas numbness of the neck, shoulders, arm, forearms, and fingers indicates involvement of the C5 to T1 nerve roots. Sensory root involvement can also produce numbness, which is usually incomplete and often experienced as a feeling of swelling or soddenness that can inadvertently be accepted and then misinterpreted as soft tissue swelling. Compete numbness is more likely to be accompanied by signs of sensory loss and indicates a more serious nerve or root lesion.

WEAKNESS

Muscular weakness, hypotonia, and fasciculation indicate a lower motor neuron disorder secondary to an anterior radiculopathy. More than one cervical nerve root innervates a given muscle, and the appearance of muscle weakness and atrophy suggests dysfunction of several roots. Pain and guarding produce functional weakness. On the other hand, a motor deficit may elicit sensory symptoms (such as a feeling of heaviness of the limbs). Motor symptoms are usually vague and consist of complaints of clumsiness or unexpectedly dropping objects, early fatigue, or a sensation of insufficient power or gripping. A pseudomotor symptom is loss of coordination of power, and in this instance, the problem often is sensory and due to disordered proprioception with partial numbness.

ARTICULAR SYMPTOMS

Articular complaints are felt in the joints and can be grouped as articular or pseudoarticular. Articular symptoms arise from the neck owing to the underlying pathology and include local pain, stiffness made worse with disuse and in bed, grating, clicking, and a feeling of "sand" in the neck. Pseudoarticular symptoms are felt in the shoulder and elbow as the result of referred pain and of the gelling effect of muscles that accompanies myalgic sensory pain. Stiffness with consequent limitation of motion of the neck, shoulder, elbow, wrist, and even fingers may occur subsequent to injury response, articular involvement, nerve root irritation, or reflex sympathetic dystrophy. Tenosynovitis and tendinitis often accompany syndromes of the cervical spine and may involve the rotator cuff, tendons about the wrist or hand with stenosis or fibrosis of tendon sheaths, and palmar fascia. To further complicate matters, these symptoms are often accompanied by trigger points over the affected joints, which give rise to the false impression of local pathology in the joints, ligaments, tendons, or muscles.

VASCULAR SYMPTOMS

Vascular symptoms are related to the underlying cause and not specifically to the cervical nerve root irritation. Compression of the vertebral arteries by osteophytes or a prolapsed disk in the bony vertebral canals can intensify the symptoms on neck movement and also in certain sleep postures.

HEADACHE AND OCCIPITAL NEURALGIA

Head pain appears commonly and is characteristic of cervical spine disorders; it results from nerve root or sympathetic nerve compression, vertebral artery pressure, autonomic dysfunction, and posterior occipital muscle spasm, as well as osteoarthritic changes of the apophyseal joints of the upper three cervical vertebrae. Occipital headache occurs commonly in the age-group in which spondylosis appears and becomes associated with pain in the neck and upper limbs. The pain may, in turn, spread to the eye region and become dull rather than pulsating. It is aggravated by strain, sneeze, and cough, as well as by movements of the head and neck. Opinions remain divided on the use of the term cervicogenic headache (CGH) in cases with no evidence of cervical damage.[19]

Migraines with and without aura often are accompanied by tension headache–like symptoms, such as neck pain.[20] Conversely, tension-type headaches are often accompanied by migraine-like symptoms, such as phonophobia or photophobia and aggravation by activity. The clinician caring for patients with headache as well as neck pain should be cognizant of these overlaps and their implications in the management of his or her patient.

PSEUDOANGINA PECTORIS

A lesion at C6 and C7 may produce neurologic or myalgic pain with tenderness in the precordium or scapular region, causing confusion with angina pectoris. Pain from C6 and C7 may be associated with the sensation of pressure in the chest, may increase with exercise, may refer down the arm, may be aggravated by neck movement, or may be associated with torticollis or muscle spasm in the neck. Differentiation of heart disease from radiculopathy can be made in the presence of other neurologic signs of C6 and C7 dysfunction (e.g., muscle weakness, fasciculations, sensory, or reflex changes). Difficulty will arise in clinical situations in which true angina and pseudoangina coexist, however.

EYE AND EAR SYMPTOMS

Blurring of vision relieved by changing neck position, increased tearing, pain in one or both eyes, retro-orbital pain, and descriptions of eyes being "pulled backward" or "pushed forward" may be reported by patients with cervical spine disorders. These symptoms result from irritation of the cervical sympathetic nerve supply to eye structures through the plexuses that surround the vertebral and internal carotid arteries and their branches.

Changes in equilibrium develop with irritation of surrounding sympathetic plexuses, vertebral artery vascular insufficiency, or both. Gait disturbances with or without associated tinnitus and altered auditory acuity result from vascular insufficiency secondary to vasospasm or compression of the vertebral arteries by cervical structures.

THROAT SYMPTOMS

Dysphagia results from muscle spasm, anterior osteophyte compression of the pharynx and esophagus, or abnormalities of cervical cranial nerve and sympathetic communications.

MISCELLANEOUS SYMPTOMS

Occasionally, bizarre symptoms appear in patients with cervical spine disorders. Dyspnea results from a deficit in C3 to C5 innervation of respiratory muscles. Cardiac palpitations and tachycardia associated with unusual positions or hyperextension of the neck appear with irritation of the C4 nerve root, which innervates the diaphragm and pericardium, or of the cardiac sympathetic nerve supply. Nausea and emesis, ill-defined pain, and paresthesias may accompany spinal cord compression. Drop attacks with abrupt loss of proprioception and collapse without loss of consciousness may suggest posterior circulation insufficiency.

Clinical Examination

Identifying the origin of the neck pain is the first essential step in the diagnostic process. To do this, the physician must have a detailed knowledge of the anatomy and physiology and of the nature and distribution of the pain from each structure.[21,22] An attempt must then be made to correlate the type of neck pain with the clinical signs.

A general physical and neurologic examination yields objective information from the precise identification of the pain-sensitive structure and the mechanism of pain production. Systematic examination of patients with cervical spine syndromes includes the head, neck, upper thoracic spine, shoulders, arms, forearms, wrists, and hands with the patient fully undressed. The clinician should observe the patient's posture, movements, facial expression, gait, and various positions (e.g., standing, sitting, supine). As the patient walks into the office, the clinician should observe the patient's head position and how naturally and rhythmically the head and neck move with body movement.

The neck should be inspected for normal anatomic positions of the hyoid bone, thyroid cartilage, thyroid gland, and presence of the normal cervical lordosis as well as identifying skin markings (e.g., scars, unusual skin pigmentation, or neurocutaneous lesions). Palpation of bony structures in the neck should be done with the patient supine to relax the overlying muscles. To palpate the anterior neck, the examiner should stand at the patient's side and support the neck from behind with one hand, palpating with the other, relaxing the spine as much as possible.

The horseshoe-shaped hyoid bone lies above the thyroid cartilage and is at the level of the C3 vertebra. With the index finger and thumb (pincer-like), the examiner should feel the stem of the horseshoe; as the patient swallows, the hyoid bone moves up and then down. The thyroid cartilage possesses a superior notch and a flaring upper portion (at the C4 level), whereas the lower border lies at the C5 level. Below the lower border of the thyroid cartilage, the examiner should palpate the first cricoid ring (opposite the C6 vertebra); this is the upper border of the trachea and is just superior to the site for an emergency tracheotomy. The cricoid ring moves with swallowing. About 2 to 3 cm lateral to the first cricoid ring, the carotid tubercle, the anterior tubercle of the transverse process of C6, can be felt. The carotid arteries lie adjacent to the tubercle, and their pulsation can be appreciated. The transverse process of C1 lies between the angle of the jaw and the styloid process of the skull. Because it is the broadest transverse process of the cervical spine, palpation is facilitated. Normal anatomic movements of the atlanto-occipital and atlantoaxial joints and bony structures can be appreciated by a lateral sliding movement, holding the atlas between the thumb and index finger by the transverse processes.

The posterior landmarks of the cervical spine include the occiput, inion, superior nuchal line, mastoid process, spinous processes of each vertebra, and apophyseal joints. The examiner palpates the occiput, then the inion, marking the center point of the superior nuchal line (the line feels like a transverse ridge extending outward on both sides of the inion). The round mastoid process sits at the lateral edge of the superior nuchal line (see Fig. 37–1). The spinous process of the axis (C2) can be palpated below the indented area immediately under the occiput. As each spinous process from C2 to T1 is palpated, the examiner notes the cervical lordosis. The C7 and T1 spinous processes are larger than the others. Alignment of the spinous processes should be recorded. The apophyseal joints can be felt as small, rounded domes, deep to the trapezius muscles and about 2.5 cm lateral to the spinous processes. To palpate these joints, the patient must be relaxed, because spasm and tension preclude access on examination. The joint involved can be determined by lining up with the hyoid bone at C3, the thyroid cartilage at C4 and C5, and the first cricoid ring at C6. These joints often become tender with osteoarthritis, especially in the upper cervical spine, whereas the C5-6, C6-7 level is most often involved in cervical spondylosis.

Examination of the soft tissues in the neck should be divided into two anatomic areas: anterior and posterior. The anterior portion is bordered laterally by the two sternocleidomastoid (SCM) muscles, superiorly by the mandible, and inferiorly by the suprasternal notch (an inverted triangle). The posterior aspect includes the entire area posterior to the lateral border of the SCM muscle. The SCM muscle can be examined anteriorly by asking the patient to turn the head to the opposite side; the muscle then stands out and can be palpated from origin to insertion. The opposite muscle can be compared for any discrepancies in size, bulges, or strength. Hyperextension injuries overstretch the SCM muscle with resultant hemorrhage into the tissue. Localized swelling may be due to hematomas. In torticollis, the SCM muscles will be involved. The lymph node chain resides along the medial border of the SCM muscle and normally cannot be palpated. Small, tender lymph nodes can be palpated if enlarged secondary to infections (throat, ear structures), metastases, or lymphoma. Enlarged lymph nodes may, in turn, produce torticollis. The thyroid gland overlies the thyroid cartilage in an H pattern, the bar being the isthmus with the two lobes situated laterally. Normally, the thyroid gland is smooth and palpable without enlargement. Diffuse enlargement of the thyroid gland, cysts, or nodules or tenderness from thyroiditis should be recorded. The carotid arteries, best felt near the carotid tubercle on C6, should be examined separately because of the carotid reflex secondary to simultaneous palpation.

Posteriorly, with the patient sitting, the clinician should examine the trapezius muscle, lymph nodes, greater occipital nerves, and superior nuchal ligament. The trapezius muscle extends from the inion to the spinous process of T12 and inserts laterally in a continuous arc into the clavicle, the acromion, and the spine of the scapula. The trapezius should be felt from the origin to insertion, beginning high on the neck. Flexion injuries may traumatize the trapezius, and hematomas in the muscle occur frequently. Furthermore, the trapezius is the site of focal points of pain and tenderness in fibrositis syndromes (see Chapter 36). The two trapezius muscles should be palpated bilaterally and simultaneously while assessing for tenderness, lumps, swelling, or asymmetry of the two muscles. The lymph node chain lies at the anterolateral border of the trapezius and normally cannot be palpated. The greater occipital nerves sit laterally to the inion, extending upward in the scalp, and be easily palpated when tender and inflamed. A flexion-extension injury of the spine commonly produces traumatic inflammation and swelling of the occipital nerves with resultant painful occipital neuralgia, a frequent cause of headache. The superior nuchal ligament arises from the inion and extends to the C7 and T1 spinous processes. It is under the examining finger when the spinous processes are felt and may become tender, irregular, and lumpy if overstretched or injured.

As with the symptoms, the physical signs can be grouped by range of cervical motion, motor, sensory, autonomic, and articular findings. This grouping often assists in establishing an ordered approach to the diagnostic process.

RANGE OF CERVICAL SPINE MOTION

The cervical spine has a large range of motion (see Table 37–4), which in turn provides a wide scope of vision and remains essential to the sense of balance. The basic movements of the neck are flexion, extension, lateral flexion to the right and left, and rotation to the right and left. About half of the total flexion and extension of the neck occurs at the occiput-C1 level, the other half being equally distributed among the other six cervical vertebrae, with a slight increase at the C5-6 level. About half the rotation occurs at the atlantoaxial joint; the other half distributes equally among the other five vertebrae. All vertebrae share in lateral flexion. A decrease in specific motion may occur in the presence of locking of a joint, pain, fibrous contractures, bony ankylosis, muscle spasm, mechanical alteration in joint and skeletal structures, or a tense and uncooperative patient. Other causes of muscle spasm include injury to muscle, involuntary splinting over painful joints or skeletal structures, and irritation or compression of cervical nerve roots of the spinal cord.

Because of the risk of neurologic trauma to an unstable spine or spinal cord, range-of-motion testing of the cervical spine should not be performed in cases of acute head or cervical injury or in cases of suspected spinal cord compression. When range-of-motion testing is performed in a patient without these contraindications, it should be done in the following manner: 1) actively and to the extreme of motion (to assess muscle function and strength), as observed by the examiner; 2) passively (to assess non-mobile structures, ligaments, capsules, and fascia), as the examiner moves the relaxed cervical spine through all its motions; 3) against resistance (to study origin and insertions of tendon and ligaments and to assess motor strength), with each motion maximally attempted against force of the examiner's hand.

Flexion and Extension

The patient should nod his or her head forward and touch the chin to the sternum. If one of the examiner's fingers can be placed between the patient's chin and sternum, there is 10 degrees limitation of flexion; this limitation is 30 degrees if three fingers can be inserted within this area. Observation of the cervical spine curve should be done as the examiner instructs the patient to look from floor to ceiling. The arc of neck motion normally remains smooth and is not halting or irregular. In full hyperextension, the base of the occiput normally touches the spinous process of T1.

Lateral Flexion

The patient should attempt to touch his or her ear to the shoulder without rotation or shoulder shrugging. Clinically normal people can laterally flex to this degree in either direction.

Rotation

The patient should rotate the head maximally and will usually be able to bring the chin into alignment with the shoulder. Normally, the motion remains smooth, whereas torticollis restricts motion.

Passive Range of Motion

The examiner should ask for complete relaxation and take the patient's head firmly in his or her hands, putting the spine through maximal flexion, extension, lateral flexion, and rotation. Passive motion may be more extensive than active motion if muscles remain stiff and painful or exhibit involuntary spasm.

Motion Against Resistance

All testing of the range of neck motion can be done with the examiner offering firm resistance to each movement. The anchorage of muscle, tendon insertion and origin, muscle strength, and muscular function should be assessed. This phase of the examination should be done with the patient seated. The primary (SCM muscles) and the secondary (three scalenes and small prevertebral muscles) flexors of the neck can be assessed by the examiner's placing his or her left hand flat on the patient's upper sternum and placing the right (resisting) hand with the palm cupped on the patient's forehead; the patient should then flex his or her neck, slowly increasing the power to maximal pressure. The primary (paravertebral extensor mass, splenius and semispinalis capitis, and trapezius) and secondary (small intrinsic neck) extensor muscles should be assessed by the examiner's placing his or her left hand over the patient's shoulder (for stability) and placing the right palm (fingers extended against the side of the patient's head); the patient then laterally flexes against the examiner's resistance. The rotators of the neck (SCM and intrinsic neck muscles) can be tested to right lateral rotation by placing the examiner's stabilizing left hand on the patient's left shoulder and the examiner's right hand along the right side of the patient's mandible while the patient rotates against resistance. Left rotations will be tested in the reverse fashion. Either SCM muscle functioning alone provides the main pull to the side being tested.

MOTOR SIGNS

If weakness, hypotonia, and fasciculations coexist, the clinician should suspect a lower motor neuron disease, whereas weakness, hyperreflexia, and spasticity suggest an upper motor neuron disorder. Weakness of the muscles may be difficult to assess because innervation of the shoulder girdle, arm, forearm, and muscles occurs by two or more nerve roots (see Table 37–5). Wasting of muscles is uncommonly due to nerve root irritation and usually indicates either a nerve lesion or disuse atrophy. The distribution of the localized wasting and abnormal reflexes indicates the structure and the level in which the lesion reside. Wasting with vasomotor changes indicates an autonomic dystrophy. Muscular weakness has many possible causes; to narrow the choice down to one or a few, the physician must ascertain the anatomic localization of the patient's complaints.

REFLEXES

Reflexes indicate the state of the nervous system and its afferent pathways (Table 37–6). Certain abnormal reflexes appear only with spasticity and paralysis; these indicate injury to the corticospinal tract. The primary deep tendon reflexes, abdominal reflexes, and plantar responses should be routinely examined; bulbocavernosus and anal reflexes should be tested in all suspected lower spinal cord (conus or cauda equina) lesions and in cases of sphincter disturbances. In eliciting the deep tendon reflexes, adequate relaxation of the patient and a mild degree of passive tension on the muscle become essential, especially in the radial (supinator) and ankle reflexes. The examiner varies the tension on the muscle by manipulating the joint, and reinforcement procedures enable the patient to relax completely, as by pulling one of his or her hands with the other (Jendrassik's maneuver). The tendon jerk normally occurs in only a part of each muscle, and in a myopathy, the reflex jerk may be lost in the quadriceps through wasting in the vastus internus, although the power of contraction of the remainder persists to a fair degree. Some clinically normal people show reduced reflexes, and before the examiner completes the assessment, he or she should ascertain whether other evidence of peripheral nerve (e.g., sensory loss, atrophy) or muscle disease exists.

SENSORY SIGNS

Sensory signs include numbness, hyperalgesia, hyperpathia, and pain produced by compression, percussion, or stretching an involved nerve. Hyperalgesia is a heightened appreciation of pain, and hyperpathia is an appreciation of pain in response to a non-noxious stimulus. The physician should test both the entire upper limbs and the neck and be prepared to test and reexamine any nonanatomic distributions of sensory loss and to match the findings with known areas of neuroanatomy. In the presence of nerve root irritation, the entire peripheral nerve supplied by that nerve root can be hyperirritable. It is therefore not surprising that (for example) nerve root irritation at the level of C6 or C7 can cause a positive brachial plexus stretch test result and a positive carpal tunnel compression test result, giving rise to the "double crush" syndrome.[23] From this, it follows that it is imperative to locate the upper level of the likely site of pathology.

AUTONOMIC SIGNS

Autonomic signs are infrequent and can be grouped as vascular and dystrophic. To diagnose reflex sympathetic dystrophy (RSD) in the absence of signs of dystrophy will be inappropriate and will lead to erroneous and excessive treatment and an unduly glum prognosis. Vascular changes produce a local maldistribution of tissue perfusion that causes the skin first to become mottled blue or red. The skin will be either unduly warm or cold, and autonomic changes produce excessive sweating or dryness. Dystrophic signs herald the next stage, with loss of hair over the site followed by glazing and thinning of the skin and loss of subcutaneous tissue. With time, and in extreme cases, the underlying joints become stiff and sore; very rarely, the entire area becomes atrophic leading to contractures.

ARTICULAR SIGNS

Articular signs are found relating to the underlying disease and to RSD, if present. The most common neck findings are restriction of movement, which may be painless, followed by pain on movement and local tenderness. The examiner may feel or even hear crepitus. A loud click may occur just once and indicate either a facet malalignment or an obstructing osteophyte. In degenerative diseases, lateral flexion is the earliest and most impaired movement; in rheumatoid arthritis (RA), however, the first motion impaired is rotation as a result of early involvement of the synovium around the odontoid peg. A uniformly stiff neck should raise suspicion of diffuse idiopathic skeletal hyperostosis (DISH), ankylosing spondylosis (AS), or recent trauma to the neck. The rest of the vertebral column and peripheral joints must be examined for evidence of further arthritis, and a search for extra-articular manifestations should complete the clinical assessment.

Diagnostic Evaluation

The clinical investigation of patients experiencing neck pain is constructed to evaluate the origin of the symptoms and signs, the extent of the lesion, and whether medical or surgical treatment is required. If the clinical history or general physical and neurologic/orthopedic examinations suggest an abnormality, then appropriate laboratory studies, neurophysiologic evaluation (i.e., EMG, NCS, SER), and neuroimaging procedures (radiographs, CT, MRI, CT myelography, nuclear bone scan) may be required for an accurate diagnosis and appropriate therapy (Fig. 37–7).

TABLE 37–6 • RELATION OF REFLEXES TO PERIPHERAL NERVES AND SPINAL CORD SEGMENTS

Reflex	Site and Mode of Elicitation	Response	Muscle(s)	Peripheral Nerve(s)	Cord Segment
Scapulohumeral reflex	Tap on lower end of medial border of scapula	Adduction and lateral rotation of dependent arm	Infraspinatus and teres minor	Suprascapular (axillary)	C4 to C6
Biceps jerk	Tap on tendon of biceps brachii	Flexion at elbow	Biceps brachii	Musculocutanecus	C5 and C6
Supinator jerk (also called radial reflex)	Tap on distal end of radius	Flexion at elbow	Brachioradialis (and biceps brachii and brachialis)	Radial (musculocutaneous)	C5 and C6
Triceps jerk	Tap on tendon of triceps brachii above olecranon, with elbow flexed	Extension at elbow	Triceps brachii	Radial	C7 and C8
Thumb reflex	Tap on tendon of flexor pollicis longus in distal third of forearm	Flexion of terminal phalanx of thumb	Flexor pollicis longus	Median	C6 to C8
Extensor finger and hand jerk	Tap on posterior aspect of wrist just proximal to radiocarpal joint	Extension of hand and fingers (inconstant)	Extensor of hand and fingers	Radial	C6 to C8
Flexor finger jerk	Tap on examiner's thumb placed on palm of hand; sharp tap on tips of flexed fingers (Trömner's sign)	Flexion of fingers	Flexor digitorum superficialis (and profundus)	Median	C7 and C8 (T1)
Epigastric reflex (exteroceptive)	Brisk stroking of skin downward from nipple in mamillary line	Retraction of epigastrium	Transversus abdominis	Intercostal	T5 and T6
Abdominal skin reflex (exteroceptive)	Brisk stroking of skin on abdominal wall in lateromedial direction	Shift of skin of abdomen and displacement of umbilicus	Muscles of abdominal wall	Intercostal, hypogastric, and ilioinguinal	T6 and T12
Cremasteric reflex (exteroceptive)	Stroking skin on medial aspect of thigh (pinching adductor muscles)	Elevation of testis	Cremaster	Genital branch of genitofemoral	L2 and L3 (L1)
Adductor reflex	Tap on medial condyle of femur	Adduction of leg	Adductors of thigh	Obturator	L2, L3, and L4
Knee jerk	Tap on tendon of quadriceps femoris below patella	Extension at knee	Quadriceps femoris	Femoral	(L2), L3, and L4
Gluteal reflex (exteroceptive)	Stroking skin over gluteal region	Tightening of buttock (inconstant)	Gluteus medius and gluteus maximus	Superior and inferior gluteal	L4, L5, and S1
Posterior tibial reflex	Tap on tendon of tibialis posterior behind medial malleolus	Supination of foot (inconstant)	Tibialis posterior	Tibial	L5
Semimembranosus and semitendinosus reflex	Tap on medial hamstring tendons (patient prone and knee slightly flexed)	Contraction of semimembranosus and semitendinosus muscles	Semimembranosus and semitendinosus	Sciatic	S1
Biceps femoris reflex	Tap on lateral hamstring tendon (patient prone and knee slightly flexed)	Contraction of biceps femoris	Biceps femoris	Sciatic	S1 and S2
Ankle jerk	Tap on tendon calcaneus	Plantar flexion of foot	Triceps surae and other flexors of foot	Tibial	S1 and S2
Bulbocavernosus reflex (exteroceptive)	Gentle squeezing of glans penis or pinching of skin of dorsum of penis	Contraction of bulbocavernosus muscle, palpable at root of penis	Bulbocavernosus	Pudendal	S3 and S4
Anal reflex (exteroceptive)	Scratch or prick of perianal skin (patient lying on side)	Visible contraction of anus	Sphincter ani externus	Pudendal	S5

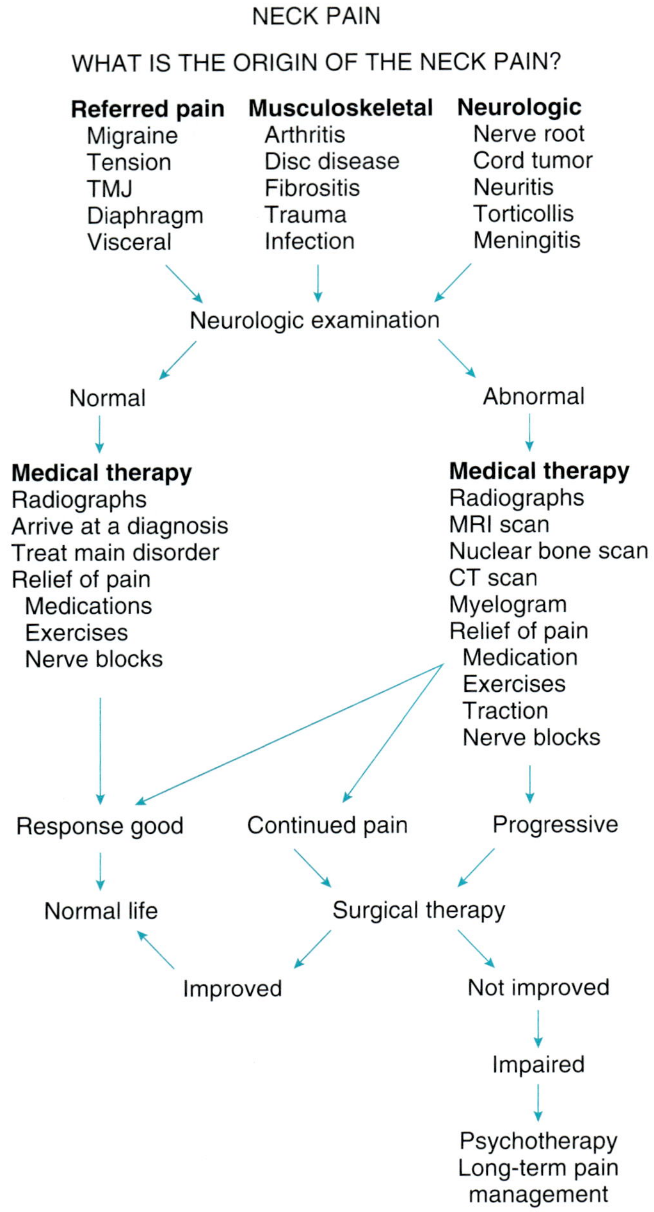

FIGURE 37–7 · Neck Pain Algorithm for Diagnosis and Treatment. CT, computed tomography; MRI, magnetic resonance imaging; TMJ, temporomandibular joint. (Taken from Nakano KK: Neck and back pain. In Stein JH (ed): Internal Medicine, 5th ed. St. Louis, Mosby, 1998, pp 963-971.)

NEUROIMAGING EXAMINATION

When ordering cervical spine radiography, the physician should not rely solely on the radiologist. Clinical correlation is necessary because gross radiologic signs and abnormalities may be associated with minimal or no clinical disturbance,[24] whereas the reverse situation (minimal radiographic change in the presence neurologic signs) may also occur. Routine cervical spine radiographic views include: 1) anteroposterior (AP) view of the atlas and axis through the open mouth; 2) AP view of the lower five vertebrae; 3) lateral views in flexion, neutral position, and extension; and 4) both right and left oblique views. Unless the junction of C7-T1 can be adequately visualized on the cross-table lateral view, a swimmer's view is often performed. After fractures and subluxations have been excluded in patients with trauma who have these nonstressed views, spinal stability may be evaluated with stressed-view radiographs in a flexion-extension series.[25] The bones should be examined for lytic lesions, fractures, and osteoporosis. The joints might reveal osteophytes with or without encroachment of the foramina or even the erosions of systemic arthritis. One must not neglect to look for congenital abnormalities, such as vertebral fusion. Ligamentous calcification might indicate degeneration, trauma, AS, or DISH. Instability in the action views might be due to trauma (such as an athletic injury) but is far more often due to constitutional ligament laxity in an unfit individual. Signs of previous surgery might give a clue to the nature of the clinical problem at hand.

Neuroimaging studies include CT, MRI, and radionuclide bone scan with SPECT. MRI combines the best features of these conventional techniques; it can display vertebrae, intervertebral disks, the thecal space, neural elements, blood vessels, and paraspinal structures without the use of radiographic or intravenous or intrathecal contrast agents.[26-28] Patients who undergo spinal MRI should be evaluated with at least two pulse sequences, a combination of T1- and a T2-weighted technique.[29] Sagittal images are supplemented with axial slices through the level of clinical interest. MRI is the preferred method for evaluation of suspected cervical radiculopathy, spinal stenosis, congenital anomalies (particularly Chiari malformations), syringomyelia, spinal cord neoplasm, multiple sclerosis, and early disk degeneration. CT and MRI are about equivalent in the evaluation of extramedullary spinal tumors and trauma.[30,31] In an unstable patient, CT remains the imaging test of choice, given MRI's limitations in terms of examination length and lack of adequate patient access. CT also assesses the specific details of osseous injuries better than does MRI. Although injury to supporting ligaments of the cervical spine can often be inferred by mechanism of injury, MRI can directly demonstrate avulsion, stripping, or disruption of ligamentous structures.[29]

Cervical discography as a diagnostic method using reproduced pain appears to be unreliable for diagnosing symptomatic disk levels.[31,32] Moreover, the investigation of neck pain by diskography alone or by zygapophyseal blocks alone constitutes an inadequate approach to neck pain that fails to identify most patients whose symptoms stem from multiple elements in the three-joint complexes of the neck.[32]

NEUROPHYSIOLOGY (ELECTRODIAGNOSTIC STUDIES)

Neurophysiology can be used to distinguish sensory and motor dysfunction of the peripheral nerves.[33-35] It can also be used to distinguish a lesion in the periphery from a nerve root lesion, by combining EMG, NCS, and somatosensory-evoked responses (SER).[35,36] Additionally, EMG and NCS can be used to differentiate normal conditions from a diffuse polyneuropathy, focal entrapment neuropathy, radiculopathy, myopathy, disorder of the neuromuscular junction (e.g., myasthenia gravis), and anterior horn cell disease (e.g., amyotrophic lateral sclerosis [ALS]). No single feature of the EMG provides a diagnosis (except true myotonia); rather, it requires the combined information of needle EMG coupled with NCS and SER, as well as the clinical examination as performed by an experienced physician. Continuous intraoperative SER monitoring appears to be a practical tool for monitoring scoliosis and cervical surgery.[37]

Dynamic posturography is a neurophysiologic tool to assess the presence of vertigo of cervical origin.[38] Dynamic posturography on the sway-referenced forceplate demonstrated lower equilibrium scores in patients with vertigo or unsteadiness than in controls when recorded in neutral position of the head, in rotation, and in lateral flexion.[38] In addition, the patients with vertigo also show lower equilibrium scores in the position most prone to elicit vertigo or unsteadiness as compared with patients with only neck pain.

LABORATORY STUDIES

The clinical laboratory offers some assistance in the diagnosis and management of neck pain in specific diseases (e.g., RA, hyperparathyroidism, infection with human immunodeficiency virus [HIV], multiple myeloma, AS, and certain metastatic malignant cancers). Cerebrospinal fluid (CSF) evaluation should be performed in patients with neck pain who are suspected of having infection (meningitis) or subarachnoid hemorrhage (SAH).

Differential Diagnosis

Major rheumatologic conditions may be a source of neck pain (Table 37–7). Occipital and neck pain occur in more than 80 percent of patients with long-standing RA, whether or not they possess disease of the C1-C2 joint.[39,40] In a clinical outpatient setting neck and shoulder complaints or signs can be appreciated in more than 20 percent of patients with RA.[41] When neck pain or headache appear concomitantly with structural cervical spine abnormalities in a patient with RA, this is commonly associated with disease of the C1-2 lateral facet joints.[42] RA patients with lateral facet joint disease often lose range of rotary cervical motion; when the lateral facet mass collapses, the head tilts permanently toward the side of the collapse. Many patients with RA, however, demonstrate limited cervical range of motion without evident C1-2 subluxation.[43] Cervical myelopathy from RA occurs infrequently.[44]

Many clinical conditions that arise outside the cervical spine, but that are perceived in or about the neck area, mimic cervical nerve root irritation, muscle spasm, ligament strain, bone disease, or a joint disorder (see Table 37–2). Disorders of somatic or visceral structures that have cervical nerve root innervation (same embryologic origin) cause pain that is felt in the neck. Because these areas constitute reflexively referred pain along the segmental distribution of the nerve roots, such areas of referral are not tender on deep palpation.

TABLE 37–6 • RHEUMATOLOGIC DISORDERS CAUSING NECK PAIN

Rheumatologic Disorder or Condition
Rheumatoid arthritis
without disease of the C1-C2 joint
with structural cervical abnormalities
C1-C2 subluxation
C1-C2 facet involvement
Spondyloarthropathies
ankylosing spondylitis
Reiter's syndrome and reactive arthritis
psoriatic arthritis
enteropathic arthritis
Polymyalgia rheumatica
Osteoarthritis
Fibromyalgia
Nonspecific musculoskeletal pain
Miscellaneous spondyloarthropathies
Whipple's disease
Behçet's disease
Paget's disease
Acromegaly
Ossification of the posterior longitudinal ligament (OPLL)
diffuse idiopathic skeletal hyperostosis (DISH)

Areas of superficial peripheral tenderness develop because of reflex or direct sympathetic irritation secondary to vasomotor changes. Referred painful areas do not have muscle spasm and often are described as experiencing a burning or cramping sensation. Nausea, emesis, and pallor may accompany this type of pain. The visceral causes of neck and arm pain can be often suggested by the history. For example, esophageal pain is usually related to food and can be promptly relieved by a liquid antacid. Cardiac pain is usually exertional and should respond to sublingual nitroglycerin. Shoulder pain radiates to the deltoid area; in severe cases, however, the brachial plexus can be irritated as it passes in proximity to the joint and may cause pain in the arm, with paresthesias. This pain does not radiate into the neck, and examination of the shoulder usually reveals the lesion. Neck pain can cause secondary shoulder muscle tension, which can give a false impression of a local arthritis or capsulitis. An important clinical fact in the differential diagnosis of neck pain is that compression or irritation of cervical nerve roots with radiation of pain is associated with deep tenderness at the site of pain. Segmental areas of deep tenderness that are not painful until palpated indicate nerve root involvement. A 1 percent injection of lidocaine into the painful area results in transient reproduction of the radicular pain, followed by relief of pain for days or weeks in the patient with nerve root involvement. If local anesthetic injection fails to reproduce (and relieve) the pain, one then looks at potential visceral or somatic structures that have the same segmental neural supply.

Peripheral neuropathy may produce pain both proximal and distal to the irritative site. With peripheral neuropathy, there is no muscle spasm. Spinal cord tumor produces a poorly localized and ill-defined neck pain, hyperreflexia, and spasticity; immobilization does not relieve the pain, and deep tenderness and local muscle spasms are absent. Furthermore, in spinal cord lesions, paralysis or weakness exists below the cord level (not dermatome) associated with sensory changes and Babinski's signs.

Neck pain may occur in malingerers, depressed persons, individuals seeking compensation, psychoneurotic patients, and victims of motor vehicle accidents (MVA).[45-53] If these patients possess no concomitant nerve root irritation, they derive no relief from local anesthesia injected into the painful areas. Absence of muscle spasm, an antalgic position, and feigning limitation of motion should arouse the examiner's suspicion.

Skilled clinical elicitation of historic data and the physical and neurologic/orthopedic examination constitute the principal and most reproducible means of differential diagnosis (see Fig. 37–7). In evaluating a patient with neck pain, the examiner will soon realize there may be a syndrome of neck pain alone; head and neck pain; neck and shoulder pain; shoulder pain alone; shoulder and arm pain; or just arm, forearm, hand, or finger pain. When the examiner observes muscle weakness in a patient with neck pain, he or she must differentiate among nerve root compromise, myelopathy, peripheral neuropathy,[54,55] and a primary muscle disease.[56]

Headaches may be associated with a Chiari type I malformation.[57] The various types of headaches include "cough headache" attacks that last less than 5 minutes, relatively long-lasting attacks that last 3 hours to several days, and continuous headache. Unlike the short-lasting cough headache attacks, long-lasting attacks are usually not precipitated by a Valsalva-like maneuver. Dizziness was the most distinguishing feature in the patients with Chiari type I malformations. It has been postulated that the Chiari type I malformation may cause long-lasting headache attacks or continuous head pain by compression of the brain stem, by central spinal cord degeneration, or by intracranial hypertension. In some cases, neurosurgical treatment provided a beneficial effect on the symptoms.[57] The neck appears to play an important, but largely ignored, role in the manifestations of adult benign headaches. Both patients with tension (muscle contraction) headaches and those with migraines have high occurrences of occipital and neck pain during their headache, tender points in the upper cervical region, greatly reduced or absent cervical curve, and radiographic evidence of joint dysfunction in the upper and lower cervical spine.[20,58,59]

Treatment

The goals of treatment will be to provide pain relief, to improve range of neck movement, and to prevent long-term disability. In any therapeutic regimen, the clinician must consider the severity of the symptoms, the presence or absence of neurologic findings, and the severity of the condition as seen by the clinical examination, the neurophysiologic assessment, and neuroimaging procedures.

Nontraumatic neck pain will be either soft tissue disorders (e.g., acute neck strain, posture-related problems, occupation-related problems, sports activity, "fibrositis/fibromyalgia" and pain amplification syndromes and psychologic conditions [anxiety, depression, "tension"]) or degenerative and mechanical disorders (e.g., cervical spondylosis and cervical disk prolapse/herniation). When nontraumatic neck pain presents acutely (less than 3 days duration) early mobilization (defined as any manual treatment to improve joint function that does not involve high-velocity movement, anesthesia, or instrumentation) and manipulation (defined as the use of short- or long-lever high velocity thrusts directed at one or more of the cervical spine joints that does not involve anesthesia or instrumentation) of the cervical spine may provide benefit.[60-64]

For relief of neck pain, there exists insufficient scientific evidence on the effects of any drug treatments, although medications are widely used as a first-line intervention.[65,66] A systematic review compared 1) analgesics and cervical collar; 2) analgesics, cervical collar, and transcutaneous nerve stimulation (TNS) for 1 week (3 treatments); and 3) analgesics, cervical collar, and mobilization (1 week, 3 treatments).[63] This review found no significant difference in pain or range of movement at 1 week, 6 weeks, or 3 months among the various forms of treatments. Several studies include the use of analgesics or nonsteroidal anti-inflammatory drugs (NSAIDs) as adjunctive treatments, but they do not allow for subgroup analysis.[37,42,67-71]

Approximately 15 percent of hospital-based physical therapy and 30 percent of chiropractic referrals are for neck pain.[63] A systematic review of these treatment modalities highlighted the poor quality of available research.[62] Many patients with acute nontraumatic neck pain appreciate physical therapy modalities,[72] whereas "active physiotherapy was at least as effective as passive physiotherapy."[73] However, the significance of this from the point of view of symptom relief remains obscure because the effects of both types of treatment were of short duration. Furthermore, a substantial part of manual therapy and physiotherapy may appear to be due to nonspecific (placebo) effects.[74] In a pilot study on 52 patients in general practice with pain or stiffness in the neck and pain/paresthesia in the shoulder, as well as the arm or hand, manipulation produced an increase in measured rotation that was maintained for 3 weeks and an immediate improvement in lateral flexion that was not maintained.[75] In another study of 100 consecutive outpatients suffering from unilateral neck pain with referral into the trapezius muscle, a single manipulation was found to be more effective than mobilization in decreasing pain in patients with mechanical neck pain.[76] Both single manipulation and mobilization increased range of motion in the neck to a similar degree in these patients. In a randomized, control trial of 183 patients, 18 to 70 years of age, who had had nonspecific neck pain for at least 2 weeks, manual therapy–specific mobilization techniques proved a favorable treatment option for patients with neck pain compared to physical therapy (exercise therapy) or continued care by a general practitioner (analgesics, counseling, and education).[77] From a meta-analysis of the literature over a 30-year period it was found that cervical spine manipulation and mobilization probably provide at least short-term benefits for some patients with neck pain and headaches.[63] In North America today, manual therapy (use of hands to manipulate, mobilize, apply traction to, or massage the tissues) is widely utilized by physical therapists, osteopaths, massage therapists, and, most notably, chiropractors.[78] Although the complication rate appeared low in these forms of therapy, the potential for manipulation to cause permanent neurologic disability or even death must be considered.[79,80]

When nontraumatic neck pain becomes subacute or chronic (lasting more than 3 months) various treatment modalities have been advocated. In a study of 63 patients comparing three weeks' treatment with 1) aspirin only; 2) aspirin coupled with massage, electrical stimulation, traction, and patient education ("cervical school"); and 3) aspirin plus "cervical school" and added passive mobilization, the last group showed significant improvement in self report one week after the end of treatment (83 percent with no or slight pain vs. 61 percent and 59 percent).[81] Range of movement was greater in group 3 at three weeks (65 percent vs. 30 percent and 35 percent) but not at four weeks. Two studies compared muscle relaxant alone versus muscle relaxant plus rotational cervical spine manipulations (1 to 3 treatments)[75,82]; there was no significant difference between the groups, though there was a trend toward improved pain, range of movement, and patient satisfaction at 1 and 3 weeks with manipulation. In another study comparing manipulation, mobilization, or both vs. physical therapies, shortwave diathermy, or continued treatment by a general practitioner, there was no significant difference at 3 or 12 weeks, but a modest benefit favoring manual therapy at 12 months.[74] A randomized, prospective clinical study conducted on 119 patients with chronic neck pain of more than 3 months' duration compared the relative effectiveness of intensive training of the cervical musculature, a physiotherapy treatment regimen, and chiropractic treatment.[83] There was no clinical difference among the three treatments. All three treatment interventions demonstrated meaningful improvement in all primary effect parameters. Improvements were maintained at 4- and 12-month follow-up; however, whether this was a result of the treatments or simply the result of time remained unknown. Future studies will be needed to delineate optimal treatment strategies in chronic neck pain patients. In an uncontrolled study to evaluate the effectiveness of acupuncture as compared with physiotherapy in the management of chronic neck pain, both acupuncture and physiotherapy were effective forms of treatment.[84] However, because an untreated control group was not part of the study design, the magnitude of this improvement could not be quantified. Previously, a controlled study of acupuncture in chronic neck pain versus placebo transcutaneous nerve stimulation indicated no significant difference between the two treatments either post-treatment or at follow-up, suggesting that acupuncture might have no greater effect than that of a powerful placebo.[85]

Traumatic soft tissue disorders include "whiplash" syndrome and musculoligamentous injury. Immediate management remains controversial in these cases. Rest in a cervical collar has been advocated, with physical therapy being started as soon as the acute spasm has settled, but there exists little evidence to support such an approach. There exists some evidence to support immediate resumption of normal activities rather than immobilization and rest.[60] In comparing analgesics, mobilization, or advice on mobilization versus analgesics, rest, and immobilization, groups receiving mobilization experienced less pain and greater mobility (follow-up ranging from 4 weeks to 2 years). In 201 patients with acute whiplash injuries, investigators compared resuming normal activities in the first 2 weeks to being off work and immobilized in a cervical collar.[86] There was better pain reduction at 6 months for patients asked to resume normal activities immediately when compared to those immobilized for the first 2 weeks. However, active mobilization is not always tolerated by patients in the acute stage following traumatic soft tissue injuries.

Approximately 40 percent of patients with whiplash injuries will suffer long-term symptoms, irrespective of therapy.[87] Of 40 patients followed for 15 years, 70 percent were reported to have continuing symptoms, with 52 percent of these also having evidence of psychogenic disturbance. Although 18 percent of these patients had improved between 10 and 15 years of follow-up, 28 percent had deteriorated. Poorer outcome could be predicted by assessment at 3 months[88] and was associated with older age, neck stiffness, referred symptoms, abnormal neurologic findings, degenerative changes on radiographs, and symptoms persisting for more than 2 months. It remains uncertain if whiplash injury accelerates the progression of degenerative change.[89]

Surgery appears to be appropriate for two groups of patients.[90,91] In the first group, symptoms relate principally to the nerve roots emerging from the cervical spine, and the condition presents itself with either neck or arm pain. In the second group, a slowly progressive spinal cord syndrome involves the legs first and then the arms. One of the primary factors in the pathogenesis of radiculopathy and myelopathy is compression. Treatment is aimed at the elimination of this pressure. The most clear-cut indication for surgery is the presence of a neurologic deficit related to compression that is unrelieved by medical treatment. Recent data indicate that cervical spine surgery for neck pain is an increasingly common procedure with wide geographic variability.[92] Rational treatment of neck pain requires further definition of indications for cervical spine surgery, preferably based on firm data about the outcomes of surgical and nonsurgical care. In the management of cervical radiculopathy, serial periradicular epidural corticosteroid injection techniques provided satisfactory recovery without the need for surgical intervention in 68 patients.[93] There were several case reports of infection after this procedure; lack of a control group thus limited the value of this study.

Radicular symptoms may respond readily to surgical treatment. In the past, the initial surgical approach was from the posterior midline, but many surgeons have recently advocated an anterior approach. In patients with defined neurologic deficits, results have been excellent in 80 to 90 percent of cases, regardless of surgical approach. This appears especially the case with a centrally herniated disk.[94–96] In cases of myelopathy, the surgical approach may be either anterior or posterior.[97,98] However, surgical repair of cervical myelopathies is less effective than in cases of acute radiculopathy, with approximately 60 to 70 percent of treated patients remaining stable or improving. In patients with cervical bony-canal diameter of 11 mm or less at several levels, a long posterior decompression may become necessary.[99] In patients with a diffuse bulging disk or an osteophytic ridge, and in whom the bony elements are normal (or slightly small), the site of compression and approach may be anterior (several levels may be operated on at the same time). In patients with a large, centrally herniated cervical disk, the surgeon may have difficulty deciding on the appropriate approach; opinions differ as to the optimal surgical technique in these cases.[100-101]

In RA, when severe posterior neck pain, occipital headaches, or both are caused by lateral facet disease or by subluxations of the C1-2 joint, pain may improve after surgical stabilization of the C1-2 joint.[41,102,103] Potential clinical indications for cervical spine surgery for RA patients include head pain, neck pain, or both; progressive instability; or progressive neurologic deterioration. Those RA patients who develop progressive brain stem dysfunction or a myelopathy from cervical spine involvement will usually become candidates for surgery if their general medical health permits. The surgical operative approach will depend on the RA patient's pathologic anatomy.[104] C1-C2 fusion will be the most common surgery in RA patients with anterior C1-C2 subluxation but without significant vertical subluxation. Some patients with RA will require laminectomies, subaxial fusions, or anterior vertebrectomy. In the presence of a pannus or soft tissue mass contributing to the cord compression, the pannus may require excision.[105] Pachymeningitis or rheumatoid inflammatory changes may completely surround the dura at the C1-C2 level and demand excision.[106] In RA patients who have vertical subluxation, fusion of the occiput to some level of the upper cervical spine may be required.[107] Certain surgeons preoperatively place patients in a halo cervical traction for initial and intraoperative stabilization.[108] After surgical fusion, RA patients require 3 or more months of cervical halo stabilization or cervical-thoracic orthosis.[104,109] Other surgeons recommend use of wires and methylmethacrylate at the time of surgery to facilitate rapid mobilization of the patient without prolonged dependency on external stabilizing devices.[110,111]

BOTULINUM TOXIN TYPE A IN THE TREATMENT OF CERVICOTHORACIC PAIN

Botulinium toxin type A (BTX-A), used successfully for years to treat cervical dystonia,[112-114] may have a place in the treatment of chronic upper back and neck pain.[115] It appears that BTX-A's mechanism of action includes muscle relaxation, and preliminary data in animal models suggest BTX-A inhibits the release of inflammatory neuropeptides and interferes with peripheral pain-sensitization pathways. After BTX-A injections for neck pain, aftercare includes a home exercise program that stresses pectoral stretching, midback strengthening and cervical spine stretching. Further randomized controlled clinical trials will be needed to determine the true efficacy of this treatment modality in patients with neck pain.

Patient Education

An important aspect in the treatment of patients with neck pain entails patient education, occupation, and some lifestyle factors.[116,117] The clinician should define the medical problem, instruct the patient in the rationale of treatment, and teach the patient how to care for his or her neck in standing, sitting, driving, occupational tasks, and other activities of daily living.[118] With the availability of computers and the Internet, patients may find it both beneficial and convenient to visit medically designated Web sites (e.g., http://www.aan.com; http://www.rheumatology.org; http://www.aaos.org; http://www.neuohub.net; http://www.merckmedicus.com; http://www.nih.gov).

REFERENCES

1. Hult L: The Munkfors investigation: A study of the frequency and causes of stiff neck-brachialgia and lumbago-sciatic syndromes, as well as observations on certain signs and symptoms from the dorsal spine and the joints of the extremities in industrial and forest workers. Acta Orthop Scand 16(Suppl):1, 1954.
2. Hult L: Cervical, dorsal and lumbar spinal syndromes. Acta Orthop Scand 17(Suppl):175, 1954.
3. Anderson G: The epidemiology of spinal disorders. *In* Frymoyer JW(ed): The Adult Spine: Principles and Practice. New York, Raven Press, 1999, pp 107-146.
4. Makela M, Heliovaara M, Sievers K, et al: Prevalence, determinants, and consequences of chronic neck pain in Finland. Am J Epidemiol 134:1356, 1991.
5. Andersson HI, Ejlertsson G, Leden I, et al: Chronic pain in a geographically defined general population: studies of differences in age, gender, social class, and pain localization. Clin J Pain 9:174, 1993.
6. Brattberg G, Thorslund M, Wikman A: The prevalence of pain in a general population. The results of a postal survey in a county of Sweden. Pain 37:215, 1989.
7. Takala EP, Viikari-Juntura E, Tynkkynen EM: Does group gymnastics at the workplace help in neck pain? A controlled study. Scan J Rehabil Med 26:17, 1994.
8. Bovim G. Schrader H, Sand T: Neck pain in the general population. Spine 19:1307, 1994.
9. Jacobsson L, Lindgarde F, Manthorpe R: The commonest rheumatic complaints of over six weeks' duration in a twelve-month period in a defined Swedish population. Prevalences and relationships. Scan J Rheumatol 18:353, 1989.
10. Cot'e P, Cassidy JD, Carroll L: The Saskatchewan Health and Back Pain Survey. The prevalence of neck pain and related disability in Saskatchewan adults. Spine 23:1689, 1998.
11. Borghouts JA, Koes BW, Vondeling H, et al: Cost-of-illness of neck pain in the Netherlands in 1996. Pain 80:629, 1999.
12. Borghouts JA, Koes BW, Bouter LM: The clinical course and prognostic factors of non-specific neck pain: a systematic review. Pain 77:1, 1998.
13. Lamberts H, Brouwer H, Groen AJM, et al: Het transitiemodel in de huisartspraktijk. Huisart Wet 30:105, 1987.
14. Haackett GI, Hudson MF, Wylie JB, et al: Evaluation of the efficacy and acceptability to patients of a physiotherapist working in a health centre. BMJ 294:24, 1987.
15. Waalen D, White P, Waalen J: Demographic and clinical characteristics of chiropractic patients: a 5-year study of patients treated at the Canadian Memorial Chiropractic College. J Can Chiropract Assoc 38:75, 1994.

16. Hult L: Frequency of symptoms for different age groups and professions. *In* Hirsch C, Sotterman Y (eds): Cervical Pain. New York, Pergamon Press, 1971, pp 17-20.
17. Fukui S, Ohseto K, Shiotani M, et al: Referred pain distribution of the cervical zygapophyseal and cervical dorsal rami. Pain 68:79, 1996.
18. Cassaday JJ, Hiltner A, Baer E: Hierarchical structure of the intervertebral disc. Clin Rheumatol 8:282, 1989.
19. Leone M, D'Amico D, Grazzi L, et al: Cervicogenic headache: a critical review of the current diagnostic criteria. Pain 78:1, 1998.
20. Kaniecki RG: Migraine and tension-type headache: An assessment of challenges in diagnosis. Neurology 58(9):(Suppl 6)15, 2002.
21. Nakano KK: Neurology of Musculoskeletal and Rheumatic Disorders. Boston, Houghton Mifflin, 1979.
22. Nakano KK: Neck and back pain. *In* Stein JH (ed): Internal Medicine, 5th ed. St. Louis, Mosby, 1998, pp 963-971.
23. Upton ARM, McComas AJ: The double crush in nerve entrapment syndromes. Lancet 2:359, 1973.
24. Gore DR, Sepic SB, Gardner GM: Roentgenographic findings of the cervical spine in asymptomatic people. Spine 11:521, 1986.
25. Davidorf J, Hoyt D, Rosen P: Distal cervical spine evaluation using swimmer's flexion-extension radiographs. J Emerg Med 11:55, 1993.
26. Bradley WG, Waluch V, Yadley RA, et al: Comparison of CT and NMR in 400 patients with suspected disease of the brain and spinal cord. Radiology 152:695, 1984.
27. Murayama S, Numaguchi Y, Robinson AE: The diagnosis of herniated intervertebral discs with MR imaging: A comparison of gradient-refocused-echo pulse sequences. AJNR 11:19, 1990.
28. Davis SJ, Teresi LM, Bradley WG Jr, et al: Cervical spine hyperextension injuries: MR findings. Radiology 180:245, 1991.
29. Mirvis SE, Wolf AL: MRI of acute cervical spine trauma. Appl Radiol 21:15,1992.
30. Yasuyuki Y, Matsumasa T, Matsuno Y, et al: Acute spinal cord injury: Magnetic resonance imaging correlated with myelopathy. Br J Radiol 64:201, 1991.
31. Shinomiya K, Nakao K, Shidoh S, et al: Evaluation of cervical diskography in pain origin and provocation. J Spinal Disord 6:422, 1993.
32. Bogduk N, Aprill C: On the nature of neck pain, discography and cervical zygapophyseal joint blocks. Pain 54:213, 1993.
33. Kimura J: Electrodiagnosis in Diseases of Nerve and Muscle: Principles and Practices, 2nd ed. Philadelphia, FA Davis, 1989.
34. Harg A, Tseng H, LeBreck D: The value of electrodiagnostic consultation for patients with upper extremity nerve complaints: A prospective comparison with the history and physical examination. Arch Phys Med Rehabil 80:1273, 1999.
35. Narden RA, Rutkove SB, Raynor EM: Diagnostic accuracy of electrodiagnostic testing in the evaluation of weakness. Muscle Nerve 26:201, 2002.
36. Chiappa KH: Evoked Potentials in Clinical Medicine, 2nd ed. New York, Raven Press, 1990.
37. Epstein NE, Danto J, Nardi D: Evaluation of intraoperative somatosensory-evoked potential monitoring during 100 cervical operations. Spine 18:737, 1993.
38. Alund M, Ledin T, Odkvist L, et al: Dynamic posturography among patients with common neck disorder: A study of 15 cases with suspected cervical vertigo. J Vestib Res 3:383, 1993.
39. Rosa C, Alves M, Queir'os MV, et al: Neurologic involvement in patients with rheumatoid arthritis with atlantoaxial subluxation: a clinical and neurophysiological study. J Rheumatol 20:248, 1993.
40. Conlon PW, Isdale IC, Rose BS: Rheumatoid arthritis of the cervical spine: an analysis of 333 cases. Ann Rheum Dis 25:120, 1966.
41. Halla JT, Hardin JG Jr: The spectrum of atlantoaxial facet joint involvement in rheumatoid arthritis. Arthritis Rheum 33:325, 1990.
42. Rosenbaum RB, Campbell SM, Rosenbaum JT: Clinical Neurology of Rheumatic Diseases. Boston, Butterworth-Heinemann, 1996.
43. Stevens JC, Cartlidge NEF, Saunders M, et al: Atlanto-axial subluxation and cervical myelopathy in rheumatoid arthritis Q J Med 40:391, 1971.
44. Nakano KK, Schoene WC, Baker RA, et al: The cervical myelopathy associated with rheumatoid arthritis: analysis of 32 patients, with 2 postmortem cases. Ann Neurol 3:144, 1978.
45. Sturzenegger M, DiStefano G, Radanov BP, et al: Presenting symptoms and signs after whiplash injury: The influence of accident mechanisms. Neurology 44:688, 1994.
46. Barnsley L, Lord SM, Wallis BJ, et al: Lack of effect of intraarticular corticosteroids for chronic pain in the cervical zygapophyseal joints. N Engl J Med 330:1047, 1994.
47. Carette S: Whiplash injury and chronic neck pain. N Engl J Med 330:1083, 1994.
48. Leino P, Magni G: Depressive and distress symptoms as predictors of low back pain, neck-shoulder pain, and other musculoskeletal morbidity: A 10-year follow-up of metal industry employees. Pain 53:89, 1993.
49. Ketoser DB: Whiplash, chronic neck pain, and zygapophyseal joint disorders. A selective review. Minn Med 83:51, 2000.
50. Hamer AJ, Gargan MF, Bannister GC, et al: Whiplash injury and surgically treated cervical disc disease. Injury 24:549, 1993.
51. Gargan M, Bannister G, Main C, et al: The behavioral response to whiplash injury. J Bone Joint Surg 79B:523, 1997.
52. Borchgrevink GE, Kaasa A, McDonagh D, et al: Acute treatment of whiplash neck sprain injuries. Spine 23:25, 1998.
53. Bourbeau R, Desjardins D, Maag U, et al: Neck injuries among belted and unbelted occupants of the front seat of cars. J Trauma 35:794, 1993.
54. Schaumburg HH, Berger AR, Thomas PK: Disorders of Peripheral Nerves, 2nd ed. Philadelphia, FA Davis, 1992.
55. Katz JN, Simmons BP: Carpal tunnel syndrome. New Engl JMed 346:1807, 2002.
56. Emery AEH: Population frequencies of inherited neuromuscular diseases: A world survey. Neuromuscul Disord 1:19, 1991.
57. Stovner LJ: Headache associated with Chiari type I malformation. Headache 33:175, 1993.
58. Vernon H, Steiman I, Hagino C: Cervicogenic dysfunction in muscle contraction headache and migraine: A descriptive study. J Manipulative Physiol Ther 15:418, 1992.
59. Blau JN, MacGregor EA: Migraine and the neck. Headache 34:88, 1994.
60. McKinney LA: Early mobilization and outcome in acute sprains of the neck. BMJ 299:1006, 1989.
61. Koes BW, Assendelft WJ, Van Der Heijden GJ, et al: Spinal manipulation and mobilization for back and neck pain: a blinded review. BMJ 303:1298, 1992.
62. Aker PD, Gross AR, Goldsmith CH, et al: Conservative management of mechanical neck pain: systematic overview and meta-analysis. BMJ 313:1291, 1996.
63. Hurwitz EL, Aker PD, Adams AH, et al: Manipulation and mobilization of the cervical spine: A systematic review of the literature. Spine 24:1746, 1996.
64: Kjellman GV, Skargren EI, Oberg BE: A critical analysis of randomized clinical trials on neck pain and treatment efficacy. A review of the literature. Scan J Rehabil Med 31:139, 1999.
65. Spitzer WO, Skovron ML, Salmi LR, et al: Scientific monograph of the Quebec Task Force on whiplash associated disorders: redefining "whiplash" and its management. Spine 20(Suppl 8):1, 1995.
66. Suissa S, Harder S, Veilleux M: The Quebec whiplash-associated disorders cohort study. Spine 20(Suppl 8):12S, 1995.
67. Koes BW, Bouter LM, van Mameren H, et al: Randomized clinical trial of manipulative therapy and physiotherapy for persistent back and neck complaints: results of one year follow up. BMJ 304:601, 1992.
68. Trock DH, Bollet AJ, Markoll R: The effect of pulsed electromagnetic fields in the treatment of osteoarthritis of the knee and cervical spine. Report of randomized double-blind placebo controlled trials. J Rheumatol 21:1903, 1994.
69. Nordemar R, Thorner C: Treatment of acute cervical pain: a comparative group study. Pain 10:93, 1981.
70. Howe DH, Newcombe RG, Wade MT: Manipulation of the cervical spine: a pilot study. J R Coll Gen Pract 33:574, 1983.
71. Jordan A, Bendix T, Nielsen H, et al: Intensive training, physiotherapy, or manipulation for patients with chronic neck pain. A prospective, sing-blinded, randomized clinical trial. Spine 23:311, 1998.
72. Hackett GI, Hudson MF, Wylie JB, et al: Evaluation of the efficacy and acceptability to patients of a physiotherapist working in a health centre. BMJ 294:24, 1987.

73. Levoska S, Keinanen-Kiukaanniemi S: Active or passive physiotherapy for occupational cervicobrachial disorders? A comparison of two treatment methods with a 1-year follow-up. Arch Phys Med Rehabil 74:425, 1993.
74. Koes BW, Bouter LM, van Mameren H, et al: The effectiveness of manual therapy, physiotherapy, and treatment by the general practitioner for nonspecific back and neck complaints: A randomized clinical trial. Spine 17:28, 1992.
75. Howe DH, Newcombe RG, Wade MT: Manipulation of the cervical spine-a pilot study. J Royal Coll Gen Pract 33:574, 1983.
76. Cassidy JD, Lopes AA, Yong-Hing K: The immediate effect of manipulation versus mobilization of pain and range of motion in the cervical spine: A randomized controlled trial. J Manipulative Physiol Ther 15:570, 1992.
77. Hoving JL, Koes BW, Henrica CW, et al: Manual therapy, physical therapy, or continued care by a general practitioner for patients with neck pain. Ann Int Med 136:713, 2002.
78. Posner J, Glew C: Neck pain [Editorial]. Ann Int Med 136:758, 2002.
79. Miller RG, Burton R: Stroke following chiropractic manipulation of the spine. JAMA 229:189, 1974.
80. Powell FC, Hanigan WC, Olivero WC: A risk/benefit analysis of spinal manipulation therapy for relief of lumbar or cervical pain. Neurosurgery 33:73, 1993.
81. Brodin H: Cervical pain and mobilization. Manual Med 2:18, 1985.
82. Sloop PR, Smith DS, Goldenberg E, et al: Manipulation for chronic neck pain: A double-blind controlled study. Spine 7:532, 1982.
83. Bendix JA, Nielsen H, Hansen FR, et al: Intensive training, physiotherapy, or manipulation for patients with chronic neck pain. A prospective, single-blinded, randomized clinical trial. Spine 23:311, 1998.
84. David J, Modi S, Aluko AA, et al: Chronic neck pain: a comparison of acupuncture treatment and physiotherapy. Br J Rheumatol 37:1118, 1998.
85. Petric JP, Hazleman BL: A controlled study of acupuncture in neck pain. Br J Rheumatol 3:271, 1986.
86. Borchgrevink GE, Kaasa A, McDonagh D, et al: Acute treatment of whiplash neck sprain injuries. A randomized trial of treatment during the first 14 days after a car accident. Spine 23:25, 1998.
87. Squires B, Gargan MF, Bannister GC: Soft-tissue injuries of the cervical spine: 15-year follow-up. J Bone Joint Surg Br 78:955, 1996.
88. Gargan M, Bannister G, Main C, et al: The behavioral response to whiplash injury. J Bone Joint Surg Br 79:53, 1997.
89. Hamer AJ, Gargan MF, Bannister GC, et al: Whiplash injury and surgically treated cervical disc disease. Injury 24:549, 1993.
90. Dunsker SB: Cervical spondylosis. *In* Seminars in Neurological Surgery. New York, Raven Press, 1981.
91. Jacchia GE, Innocenti M, Pavolini B, et al: Indications and results of surgical treatment of cervical disc disease by anterior and posterior approach. Chir Organi Mov 77:111, 1992.
92. Einstadter D, Kent DL, Fihn SD, et al: Variation in the rate of cervical spine surgery in Washington State. Med Care 31:711, 1993.
93. Bush K, Hillier S: Outcome of cervical radiculopathy treated with periradicular/epidural corticosteroid injections: A prospective study with independent clinical review. Eur Spine J 5:319, 1996.
94. Lunsford LN, Bassonette DJ, Jannetta PJ, et al: Anterior surgery for cervical disc disease. J Neurosurg 53:1, 1980.
95. Laus M, Pignatti G, Alfonso C, et al: Anterior surgery for the treatment of soft cervical disc herniation, Chir Organi Mov 77:101, 1992.
96. Figueiredo SR, Vital JP, Dominguez ML, et al: Cervical discectomies by anterior approach. Acta Med Port 6:249, 1993.
97. Cooper PR: Posterior stabilization of the cervical spine. Clin Neurosur 40:286, 1993.
98. Epstein N: The surgical management of ossification of the posterior longitudinal ligament in 51 patients. J Spinal Disord 6:432, 1993.
99. Kohno K, Kumon Y, Oka Y, et al: Evaluation of prognostic factors following expansive laminoplasty for cervical spinal stenotic myelopathy. Surg Neurol 48:237, 1997.
100. Murphy KP, Opitz JL, Cabanela ME, et al: Cervical fractures and spinal cord injury: Outcome of surgical and nonsurgical management. Mayo Clin Proc 65:949, 1990.
101. Snyder GM, Berhardt M: Anterior cervical fractional interspace decompression for treatment of cervical radiculopathy: A review of the first 66 cases. Clin Orthop Rel Res 246:92, 1989.
102. Santavirta S, Konttinen Y, Lindquist C, et al: Occipital headache in rheumatoid cervical facet joint arthritis. Lancet 2:695, 1986.
103. Chan DPK, Ngian KS, Cohen L: Posterior upper cervical fusion in rheumatoid arthritis. Spine 17:268, 1992.
104. Clark CR, Goetz DD, Menezes AH: Arthrodesis of the cervical spine in rheumatoid arthritis. J Bone Joint Surg Am 71:381, 1989.
105. Crockard HA, Pozo JL, Ransford AO, et al: Transoral decompression and posterior fusion for rheumatoid atlanto-axial subluxation. J Bone Joint Surg Br 68:350, 1986.
106. Hotta Y, Katoh H, Watanabe J, et al: Non-osseous dural compression in rheumatoid atlanto-axial subluxation. Spine 14:236, 1989.
107. Menezes AH, van Gilder JC, Clark CR, et al: Odontoid upward migration in rheumatoid arthritis. J Neurosurg 63:500, 1985.
108. Stirrat AAN, Fyfe IS: Surgery of the rheumatoid cervical spine. Clin Orthop 293:135, 1993.
109. Papadopoulos SM, Dickman CA, Sonntaag VKH: Atlantoaxial stabilization in rheumatoid arthritis. J Neurosurg 74:1, 1991.
110. Toolanen G: Cutaneous sensory impairment in rheumatoid atlanto-axial subluxation assessed quantitatively by electrical stimulation. Scan J Rheumatol 16:27, 1987.
111. Bryan WJ, Inglis AE, Sculco TP, et al: Methylmethacrylate stabilization for enhancement of posterior cervical arthrodesis in rheumatoid arthritis. J Bone Joint Surg 64A:1045, 1982.
112. Figgitt DP, Noble S: Botulinum toxin B: a review of its therapeutic potential in management of cervical dystonia. Drugs 62:705, 2002.
113. Hilker R, Schischniaschvili M, Ghaemi M, et al: Health related quality of life is improved by botulinum neurotoxin type A in long term treated patients with focal dystonia. J Neurol Neurosurg Psychiatry 71:193, 2001.
114. Wissel J, Kanovsky P, Ruzicka E, et al: Efficacy and safety of a standardized 500 unit dose of Dysport (clostridium botulinum toxin type A haemaglutinin complex) in a heterogeneous cervical dystonia population: results of a prospective, multicentre, randomized, double-blind, placebo-controlled, parallel group study. J Neurol 248:1073, 2001.
115. Kjellman G, Skargren E, Oberg B: Prognostic factors for perceived pain and function at one-year follow-up in primary care patients with neck pain. Disabil Rehabil 24:364, 2002.
116. Jacobsson L, Lindgarde F, Manthorpe R, et al: Effect of education, occupation and some lifestyle factors on common rheumatic complaints in a Swedish group aged 50-70 years. Ann Rheum Dis 51:835, 1992.
117. Hellsing AL, Linton SJ, Kalvemark M: A prospective study of patients with acute back and neck pain in Sweden. Phys Ther 74:116, 1994.
118. Ariens GAM, van Mechelen W, Bongers PM, et al: Physical risk factors for neck pain. Scand J Work Environ Health 26:7, 2000.

38 Shoulder Pain

SCOTT DAVID MARTIN • THOMAS S. THORNHILL

The shoulder joint is an extremely mobile and complex joint. What makes accurate diagnosis of shoulder pain so difficult is the unique anatomy and position of the shoulder as a link between the upper extremity and thorax. Traversed by muscle, tendon, and bone, the shoulder is surrounded by major neurovascular structures, all of which may serve as potential sources of local and referred pain.

Because of this complexity, shoulder pain is one of the most common musculoskeletal complaints that may require evaluation in the office setting. The examining physician must be able to differentiate the occurrence of shoulder pain caused by intrinsic or local factors, extrinsic or remote factors, or a combination of the two. Intrinsic factors originate from the shoulder girdle and include glenohumeral and periarticular disorders, whereas extrinsic factors occur outside of the shoulder girdle with secondary referral pain to the shoulder (Table 38–1). Examples of extrinsic factors include left shoulder pain as the initial presentation of coronary artery disease. Hepatic or splenic disease may also initally manifest as shoulder pain.

Accurate evaluation, diagnosis, and treatment requires a thorough understanding of shoulder anatomy, including pain referral patterns. A complete and systematic physical examination is critical to an accurate diagnosis. During the initial evaluation, care must be taken to discern all possible causes of the shoulder pain. Final diagnosis may require repeated office examinations and correlation of diagnostic tests with symptoms and response to selective injections. Improvements in diagnostic tests such as magnetic resonance imaging (MRI), arthrography-computed tomography (arthro-CT), sonography, and electromyography (EMG) have facilitated early diagnosis of shoulder pain and have provided a better understanding of shoulder pathology.

This chapter provides practical guidelines for the diagnosis and treatment of painful shoulder disorders that may be encountered in a rheumatology or general practice. A detailed analysis of shoulder problems and the treatment of major trauma are beyond the scope of this chapter and have been covered by other physicians.[1-5] However, a useful algorithm has been included that can direct the clinician in the initial treatment of traumatic and nontraumatic causes of shoulder pain (Fig. 38–1).

Anatomy and Function

Because of its complexity, an understanding of the structural and functional anatomy of the shoulder is requisite for the clinician treating shoulder pain. The shoulder joint is the most mobile joint of the body, although mobility is gained at the sacrifice of stability. Only 25 percent of the humeral head surface has contact with the glenoid at any time. The labrum increases the contact area of the articular surface and confers stability to the joint.[6] Lesions of the labrum may result from instability, and the type of lesion may indicate the type of instability. Labral tears may also be a source of pain from internal derangement of the shoulder.[7] Joint stability is also provided by a thin capsule and the glenohumeral ligaments, which are thickenings of the capsule anteriorly, posteriorly, and inferiorly.[6] Anterior stability is predominantly conferred by the anterior band of the inferior glenohumeral ligament. The rotator cuff provides dynamic stability of the joint. It is composed of three musculotendinous units posteriorly—the supraspinatus, infraspinatus, and teres minor—and the subscapularis anteriorly. The shoulder consists of three joints—acromioclavicular (AC), sternoclavicular, and glenohumeral—and two gliding planes—the scapulothoracic and subacromial surfaces.

Figure 38–2 shows the musculoskeletal and topographic localization of pain associated with common shoulder disorders. Figure 38–3 demonstrates the relationship of the three posterior rotator cuff muscles coursing anteriorly underneath the acromion to insert on the greater tuberosity. The only anterior rotator cuff muscle, the subscapularis, inserts on the lesser tuberosity. By understanding the relationship between the rotator cuff and the subacromial region, bounded inferiorly by the humeral head and superiorly by the undersurface of the acromion, the clinician can visualize the problems of impingement syndrome and can accurately aspirate and inject this space. Knowledge of the route of the tendon of the long head of the biceps through the bicipital groove and onto the superior aspect of the glenoid helps in understanding bicipital tendinitis. Before attempting to diagnose and treat shoulder pain, the clinician should review in some detail one of the many sources describing the structural and functional relationships of the shoulder girdle.[2,3]

Diagnosis

CLINICAL EVALUATION OF THE SHOULDER

Accurate diagnosis and successful treatment of a shoulder disorder begins with a thorough history and physical examination. Most of the information needed to make a correct diagnosis can be elicited with basic clinical skills,

TABLE 38–1 • COMMON CAUSES OF SHOULDER PAIN

Intrinsic Causes
Periarticular Disorders
Rotator cuff tendinitis or impingment syndrome
Calcific tendinitis
Rotator cuff tear
Bicipital tendinitis
Acromioclavicular arthritis
Glenohumeral Disorders
Inflammatory arthritis
Osteoarthritis
Osteonecrosis
Cuff arthropathy
Septic arthritis
Glenoid labral tears
Adhesive capsulitis
Glenohumeral instability
Extrinsic Causes
Regional Disorders
Cervical radiculopathy
Brachial neuritis
Nerve entrapment syndromes
Sternoclavicular arthritis
Reflex sympathetic dystrophy
Fibrositis
Neoplasms
Miscellaneous
Gallbladder disease
Splenic trauma
Subphrenic abscess
Myocardial infarction
Thyroid disease
Diabetes mellitus
Renal osteodystrophy

rather than relying on expensive and highly technologic investigative aids. Diagnostic tests should be used only to confirm an established diagnosis or to assist in cases with a challenging presentation.

HISTORY

In establishing a diagnosis, it is important to consider the patient's age and chief complaint. The differential diagnosis of shoulder pain in a 70-year-old person is entirely different from shoulder pain in a 20-year-old pitcher. Did the pain occur slowly over time or suddenly with a particular event? The gradual onset of pain over the anterolateral or deltoid region that is increased with forward elevation of the shoulder suggests impingement with rotator cuff tendinitis. The presence of significant weakness with pain on overhead activities suggests impingement with rotator cuff tear. Initiating factors relative to the onset of the symptoms should be elicited, and any history of shoulder pain or trauma should be carefully documented.

Pain intensity, character, location, and periodicity and aggravating or alleviating factors should be assessed. Pain should be graded on a visual analogue score of 0 to 10; 0 indicates no pain, and 10 indicates the worst pain the patient has ever experienced. Another indication of the severity of pain is disruption of sleep. The patient should be asked whether the pain prevents sleep, if pain awakens the patient, and whether he or she can lie on the affected shoulder. Is the pain sharp or dull? Sharp, burning pain indicates neurogenic origin, whereas a dull, aching pain suggests rotator cuff pathology with impingement. Location or distribution of the pain should be identified. Is it local around the shoulder girdle, or does the pain radiate down the arm? Is there concomitant sensory loss or weakness? Periodicity of the pain as constant or intermittent should be determined, as should factors that aggravate or alleviate the pain. Pain caused by rotator cuff tendinopathy is usually exacerbated by repetitive activities that involve the elbow away from the side of the body. Any history of neck pain should be considered, along with any history of radicular pain. Radicular-type pain frequently extends below the elbow and is associated with sensory loss and weakness. Pain located in the paracervical region may indicate a cervical origin, or it can be localized to the trapezius. Trapezial pain is often associated with shoulder pain and results from the patient trying to favor the shoulder. Assuming a military brace position may produce fatiguing and spasm of the trapezius.

Any pertinent medical history, such as a history of malignancy, should be considered. Neurologic, visceral, and vascular disease can produce referred pain to the shoulder and should always be kept in mind, especially in a patient with a painless range of motion.

PHYSICAL EXAMINATION

Proper physical examination of the shoulder includes close inspection of the shoulder girdle from the front and back (see Chapter 33). The evaluation is started by standing behind the patient, who has both shoulders exposed. The normal shoulder is always inspected and compared with the injured shoulder. Examination can be started with the patient in the sitting or standing position. Contour and symmetry are observed and compared between shoulders, assessing any atrophy or asymmetry in shoulder position or level. Spinatus muscle atrophy may result from disuse, chronic cuff tear, or from suprascapular or brachial neuropathy.[8] If evidence of scapular winging is evident, the patient should be asked to do a wall push-up, which accentuates winging.

Range of motion should be carefully recorded while noticing any absence of rhythmic shoulder motion or excessive scapulothoracic motion that may compensate for the lack of glenohumeral motion. Internal rotation of the shoulder is checked by having the patient reach behind the back with the thumb while the examiner notices the vertebral level. Loss of internal rotation is seen quite early with shoulder pain and usually indicates some tightness of the posterior shoulder capsule. Palpation of the biceps tendon, coracoid, lesser and greater tuberosities, and posterior cuff is carried out, and any tenderness is gauged (Fig. 38–4*A*). Tenderness on palpation of the long head of the biceps frequently is associated with rotator cuff tendinopathy and tenderness of the greater tuberosity. Any spasm or tenderness of the trapezius or levator scapulae may be associated with rotator cuff disease or cervical spine disease. Cervical range

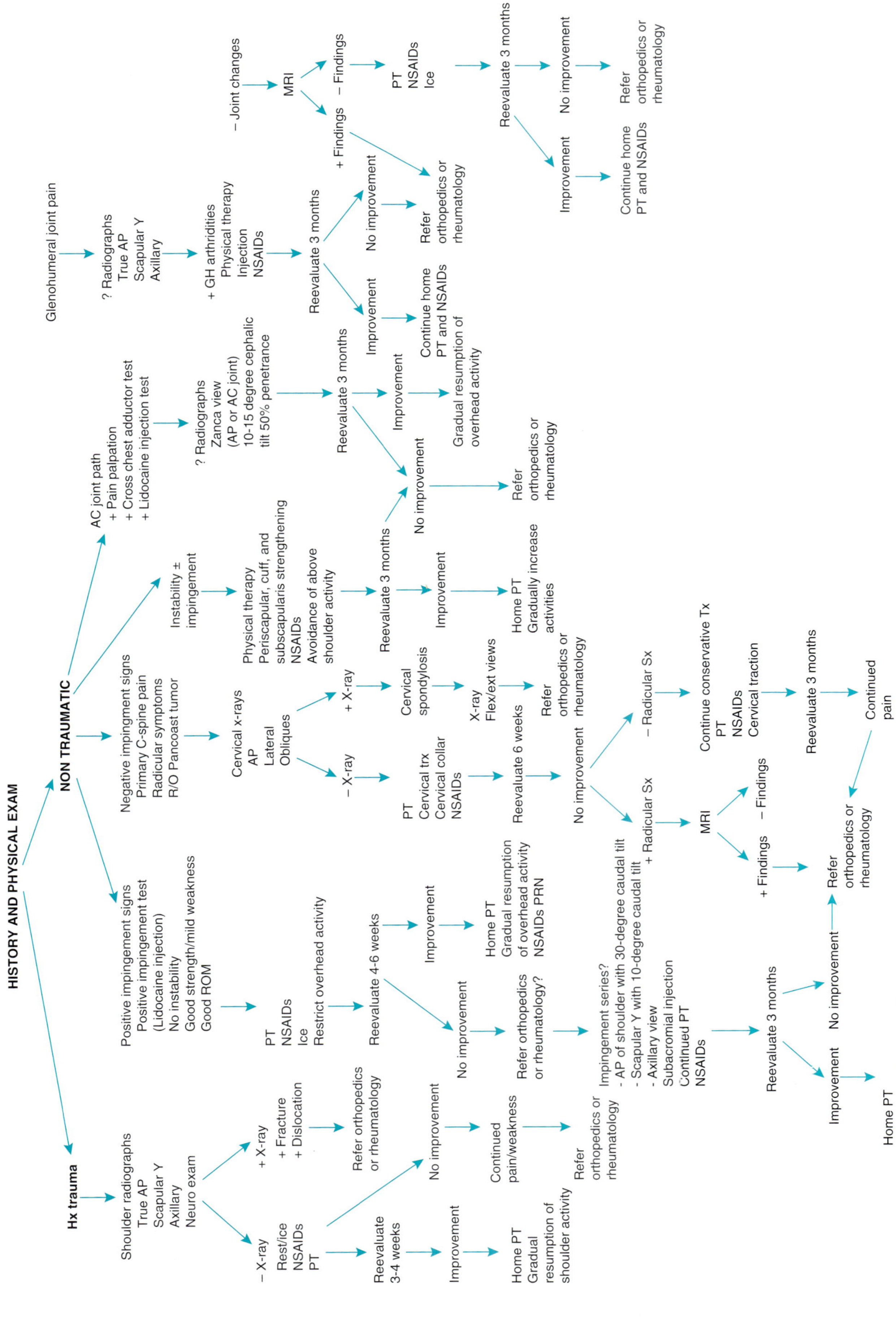

FIGURE 38–1 · **Algorithmic Evaluation of Shoulder Pain.** AC, acromioclavicular; AP, anteroposterior; GH, glenohumeral; Hx, history; MRI, magnetic resonance imaging; NSAID, nonsteroidal anti-inflammatory drug; PRN, as required; PT, physical therapy; R/O, rule out; ROM, range of motion; Sx, symptoms; trx, traction; Tx, therapy.

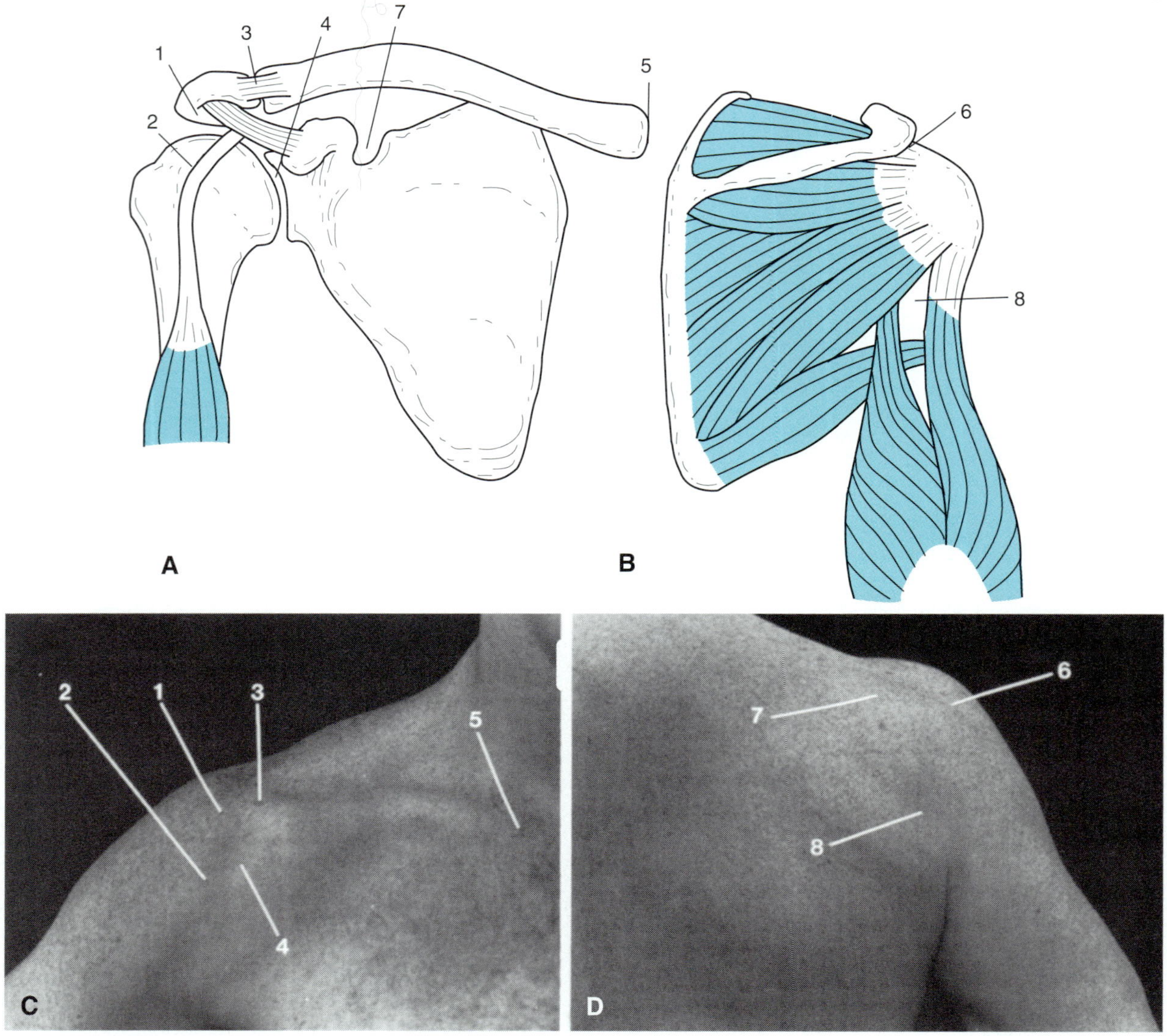

FIGURE 38–2 · Musculoskeletal (*A* and *B*) and topographic (*C* and *D*) areas localizing pain and tenderness associated with specific shoulder problems. 1, Subacromial space (rotator cuff tendinitis/impingement syndrome, calcific tendinitis, rotator cuff tear). 2, Bicipital groove (bicipital tendinitis, biceps tendon subluxation and tear). 3, Acromioclavicular joint. 4, Anterior glenohumeral joint (glenohumeral arthritis, osteonecrosis, glenoid labrum tears, adhesive capsulitis). 5, Sternoclavicular joint. 6, Posterior edge of acromion (rotator cuff tendinitis, calcific tendinitis, rotator cuff tear). 7, Suprascapular notch (suprascapular nerve entrapment). 8, Quadrilateral space (axillary nerve entrapment). These areas of pain and tenderness frequently overlap.

of motion and palpation of the paracervical muscles are carried out. Paracervical tenderness and limited range of motion of the neck may indicate cervical spondylosis or neurogenic disease. A Spurling test is performed by flexing the neck laterally while applying axial compression to the skull. The production of pain that radiates to the ipsilateral shoulder is considered a positive test result and indicates radiculopathy.

To elicit the impingement sign, the shoulder is elevated passively in forward flexion while depressing the scapula with the opposite hand, forcing the greater tuberosity against the anterior acromion and producing pain in cases of impingement[9] (see Fig. 38–4*B*). This manuever may also be painful in conditions such as adhesive capsulitis, glenohumeral and acromioclavicular arthritis, glenohumeral instability, and calcific tendinitis. A new dynamic impingement test, the circumduction-adduction shoulder manuever, also called the Clancy test, is 95-percent sensitive and 95-percent specific for diagnosing rotator cuff tendinopathy, including partial tears.[10] The test is performed with the patient in the standing position and with the head turned to the contralateral shoulder. The affected shoulder is circumducted and adducted across the body to shoulder level, keeping the elbow in extension, the shoulder in internal rotation, and the thumb pointing toward the floor (see Fig. 38–4*C*). In this position, the patient is instructed to maximally resist as a uniform downward force is applied to the extended arm by the examiner. The test result is considered positive if pain or weakness is elicited during the manuever, with pain being localized to the anterolateral aspect of the shoul-

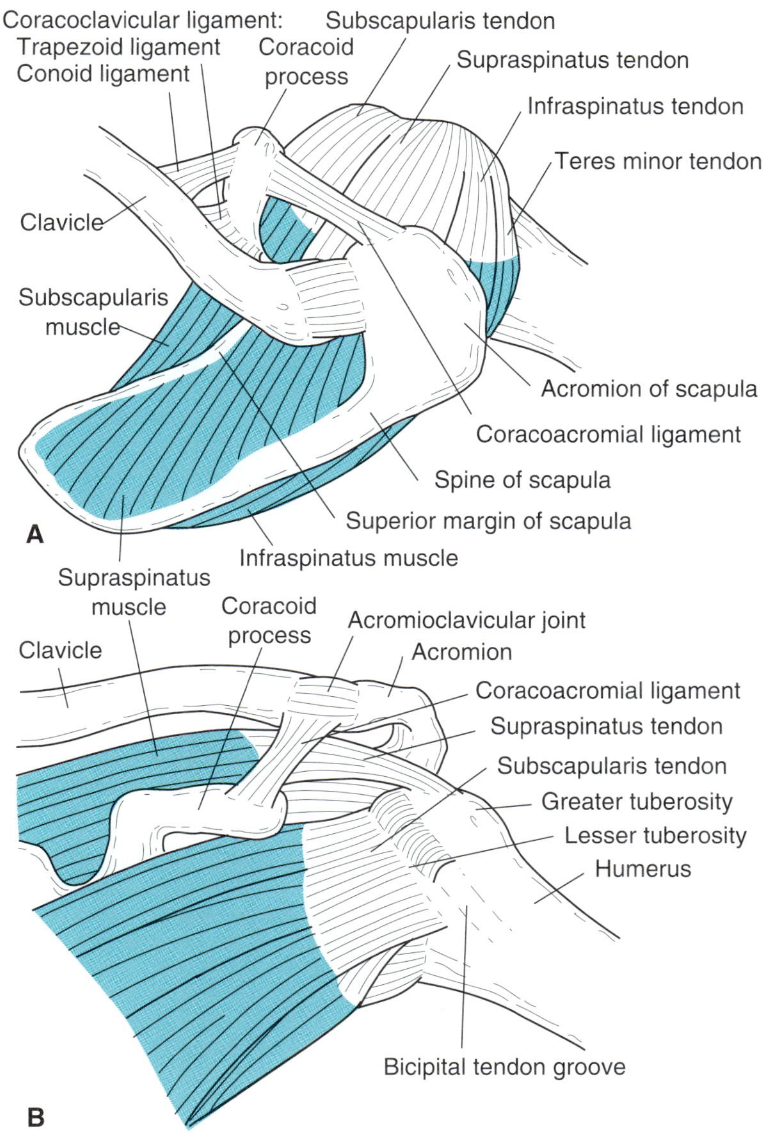

FIGURE 38–3 · *A*, Superior view of the rotator cuff musculature as it courses anteriorly underneath the coracoacromial arch to insert on the greater tuberosity. (Reproduced by permission of Ciba-Geigy. From The Ciba Collection of Medical Illustrations, Volume 8, Part I.) *B*, Anterior view of the shoulder reveals the subscapularis, which is the only anterior rotator cuff muscle inserting on the lesser tuberosity. It internally rotates the humerus and provides dynamic anterior stability to the shoulder. (From Martin TL, Martin SD: Rotator cuff tendinopathy. Hosp Med, 12:23-31)

der. There is a strong positive correlation of pain and weakness with complete cuff tear.[10]

The sternoclavicular and AC joints should be observed for prominences and palpated for stability and tenderness. Many patients with impingement have tenderness on direct downward palpation of the AC joint from impingement on the cuff from undersurface osteophytes of the distal clavicle.[2,8]

AC joint tenderness may also result from primary AC joint arthrosis and should be differentiated by physical examination, including the cross-chest adduction test and O'Brien's test.[11] Radiographic evidence of AC joint arthrosis is common in patients older than 40 years but is not usually painful.[12]

The cross-chest adduction test or horizontal adduction test is performed by forward flexion of the arm 90 degrees with subsequent cross-chest adduction of the arm (see Fig. 38–4*D*). Pain localized to the AC joint is considered a positive test result. If pain occurs posteriorly over the shoulder, a tight posterior capsule with impingement is suspected. O'Brien's test is performed by forward flexing the arm 90 degrees and adducting the arm 10 degrees out of the sagittal plane of the body. The first part of the test is performed with the hand maximally pronated with the thumb pointed down. In this position, the patient is asked to resist as the examiner applies a downward force on the arm. If the test elicits pain, the patient is asked if the pain is on top of the shoulder or deep inside. Pain localized to the top of the shoulder indicates AC joint pain, and pain deep inside the shoulder indicates a superior labrum anterior posterior (SLAP) lesion. In the second part of the test the patient is asked to maximally supinate the hand while the examiner applies a downward force to the arm. If the patient notices significantly less pain, the test result is positive for a SLAP lesion. If the pain is unchanged and located on top of the shoulder, the test result is positive for AC joint pathology.[11]

If the cause of AC joint tenderness is still in question, a lidocaine injection should be carried out, carefully avoiding injecting the subacromial space by advancing the needle too far inferiorly through the AC joint, which

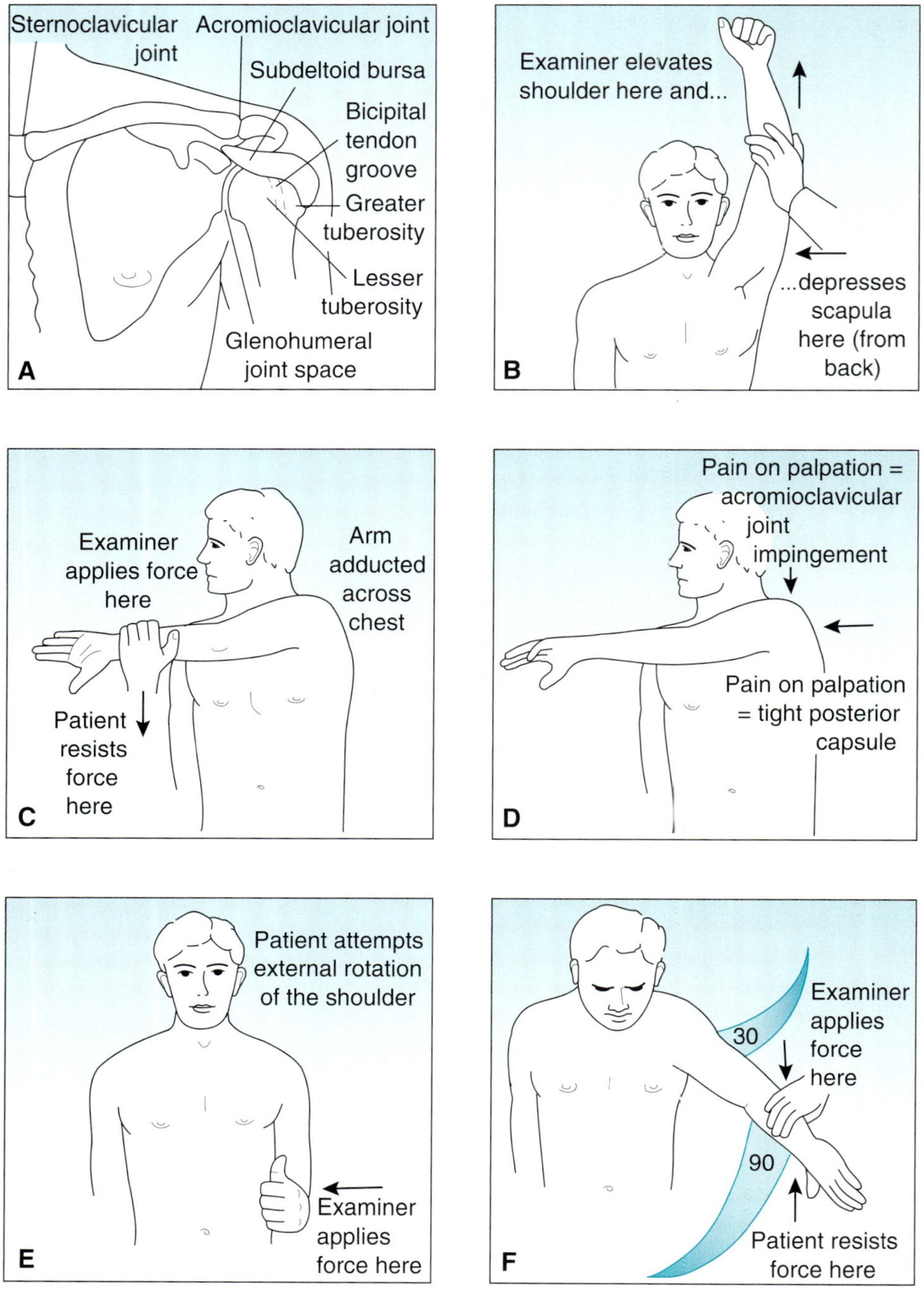

FIGURE 38–4 • *A*, Tenderness on palpation of trigger points may help localize the site of pathology. Tenderness on palpation of the long head of the biceps and greater tuberosity suggests impingement with possible cuff tendinopathy. *B*, To elicit the impingement sign, the shoulder is elevated in forward flexion while the scapula is depressed with the opposite hand, forcing the greater tuberosity and rotator cuff against the anterior acromion and producing pain when impingement exists. Relief of pain after injection of local anesthetics (i.e., impingement test) provides additional evidence of subacromial pathology. *C*, The Clancy test is performed with the patient standing and with the head turned toward the contralateral shoulder. The affected shoulder is then circumducted and adducted across the body to shoulder level, keeping the elbow in extension with the arm internally rotated with the thumb pointed toward the floor. In this position, the patient is asked to maximally resist as a uniform downward force is applied to the extended arm by the examiner. The production of pain or weakness localized to the anterior lateral portion of the shoulder is considered a positive test result. *D*, The test is performed by forward flexion of the arm at 90 degrees and subsequent cross-chest adduction of the arm. Pain localized to the acromioclavicular joint is considered a positive test result. *E*, The test is performed with the patient's elbow flexed at 90 degrees and held at the patient's side by the examiner. The patient is asked to attempt external rotation of the shoulder from a neutral position (0 degrees of adduction) as the examiner applies resistance to the forearm. Strength is compared with that of the contralateral arm. *F*, Abduction strength testing is performed with the patient's shoulder in 30 degrees of forward flexion and 90 degrees of abduction and with the thumb pointed toward the floor. The patient is asked to resist as the examiner exerts a downward force on the abducted arm. Strength is compared with the contralateral shoulder. (From Martin TL, Martin SD: Rotator cuff tendinopathy. Hosp Med 12:23-31.)

can lead to false interpretation. Painful degenerative changes of the AC joint may exist concomitantly with subacromial impingement and should be evaluated thoroughly when surgical treatment (i.e., distal clavicle excision) is being considered.[13]

In patients with pain out of proportion to objective findings, other causes of shoulder pain should be sought, including calcific tendinitis, infection, reflex sympathetic dystrophy, and fracture. Patients with significant wasting of the supraspinatus and infraspinatus muscles and posterior shoulder pain, especially younger patients, may have suprascapular neuropathy or brachial plexopathy.[8,14]

Patients with chronic cuff disease frequently have variable disuse atrophy of the supraspinatus and infraspinatus fossae; in cases of chronic massive cuff tears, atrophy and weakness can be severe. Strength testing of external rotation should be carried out with the elbow at the side and supported by the examiner; the patient is asked to attempt external rotation of the shoulder from a neutral position (0 degrees of adduction) while the examiner applies resistance (see Fig. 38–4*E*).[15] Weakness in this position may suggest a tear of the infraspinatus tendon. Abduction strength testing against resistance is carried out with the shoulder in 30 degrees of forward flexion, 90 degrees of abduction, and the thumb pointed toward the floor (see Fig. 38–4*F*).[16,17] Weakness in this position may sugggest a tear of the supraspinatus tendon. A lift-off test should be performed with the shoulder in internal rotation; the patient is asked to try and hold the hand away from the back. Inability to do so indicates a subscapularis tear.

If after a thorough physical examination impingement is suspected, an impingement test should be performed with injection of 5 ml of local anesthetic into the subacromial space.[18,19] Before performing the test, the patient is asked to grade the pain during the impingement signs on a visual analogue scale of 0 to 10, with 0 equal to no pain and 10 equal to the most severe pain the patient has ever experienced. The injection may be carried out anteriorly or posteriorly, depending on physician's preference. Ten minutes after injection of local anesthetic into the subacromial space, the patient should be reexamined and asked to regrade the pain on the same visual analogue scale. A 50 percent or more reduction in pain is thought to be a positive test result for impingement; otherwise, an alternative cause of shoulder pain should be sought, or inadequate placement of the anesthetic suspected. If the AC joint is thought to be contributing to the shoulder pain, 1 to 2 ml of local anesthetic should be injected into the joint and the shoulder reexamined. When both subacromial impingement and the AC joint are thought to be contributing to shoulder pain, serial injections during separate office visits may be needed to evaluate the shoulder while minimizing discomfort to the patient.[12]

In cases of suspected bicipital tendinitis, Speed's test is performed by having the patient flex the shoulder and extend the elbow while a downward force is applied to the arm. The production of pain over the long head of the biceps is a positive test result and suggests bicipital tendinitis.

Upper extremity strength testing should be performed and compared with the contralateral side so any atrophy is detected. Grip strength is checked, and the hands are carefully examined for evidence of intrinsic atrophy. The biceps (C5), triceps (C7), and brachioradialis (C6) reflexes are checked for symmetry and briskness.

Light touch sensory testing should be carried out and the dermatomal distribution of any deficits that may suggest cervical radiculopathy identified. The crevical, supraclavicular, axillary, and epitrochlear regions should be palpated for enlarged lymph nodes, which may suggest malignancy.

RADIOGRAPHIC ASSESSMENT

For nontraumatic painful shoulder evaluation, standard radiographic profiles are used. An impingement series should be obtained, which includes anteroposterior views with a 30-degree caudal tilt (Rockwood view), outlet view (scapular Y with 10- to 15-degree caudal tilt), and axillary view. Internal and external rotational views may be obtained if calcific tendinitis or instability are suspected. The Rockwood view can reveal any osteophytes off the anterior acromion and AC joint.[20] In cases of traumatic injury, a trauma series is obtained that includes a true anteroposterior view, scapular Y view, and an axillary view. The axillary view is useful in assessing posterior or anterior subluxation of the humeral head. Additional views such as the West Point view, which evaluates the glenoid for evidene of a bony Bankart lesion, or the Styker notch view, which assesses the humeral head for a Hill-Sachs lesion, may be obtained to assist the evaluation if the diagnosis of instability is in doubt. Secondary impingement-type rotator cuff tendinitis may be caused by increased anterior translation with subluxation of the humeral head. In such cases, an axillary view or fluoroscopy can help demonstrate the subluxation.[21,22]

When AC joint pathology is suspected, a 15-degree cephalic-tilt view of the AC joint at 50 percent penetrance, as described by Zanca,[23] should be obtained (Fig. 38–5). Stress views of the AC joint may be obtained by strapping 5 to 10 pounds of weight to the patient's forearms and determining AC separation. Comparing the coracoclavicular distance of both shoulders may be helpful. When clinically indicated, cervical spine radiographs should be obtained to exclude cervical spondylosis as a cause of shoulder pain.

SCINTIGRAPHY

Technetium methyldiphosphonate (99mTc-MDP) or gallium may be of diagnostic help in evaluating skeletal lesions about the shoulder joint. Bone scans are generally not helpful in the diagnosis of non-neoplastic or noninfectious shoulder disease.

Scintigraphy may have a role in identifying patients with complete rotator cuff tears that proceed to cuff-tear arthropathy. This is an important distinction, because patients with complete rotator cuff tears may do well, whereas those who develop progressive changes of

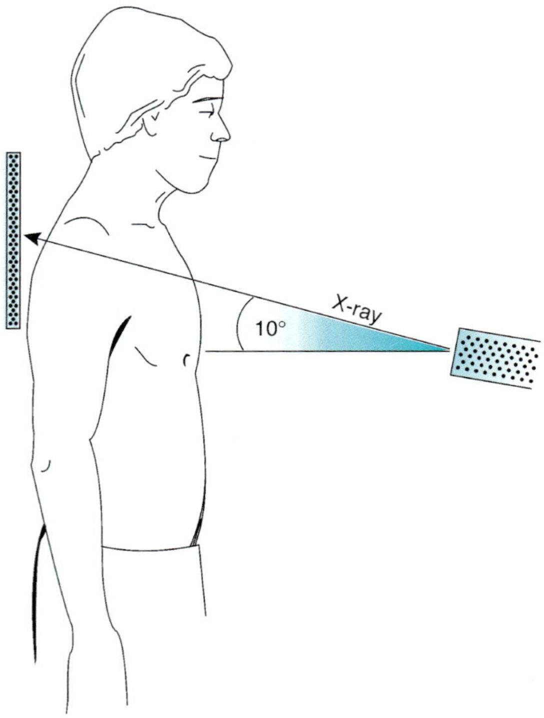

FIGURE 38–5 • Zanca view of the acromioclavicular joint is obtained with a 15-degree cephalic tilt and 50-percent penetrance. (From Rockwood CA Jr, Young DC: Disorders of the acromioclavicular joint. *In* Rockwood CA Jr, Matsen TA III: The Shoulder. Philadelphia, WB Saunders, 1985, pp 413-476.)

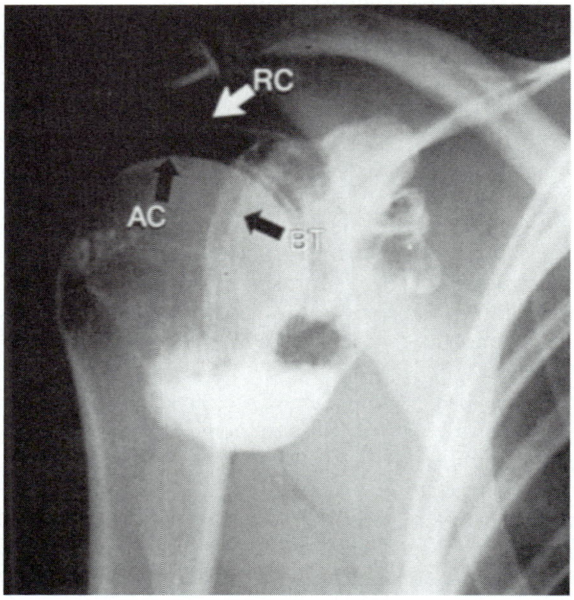

FIGURE 38–6 • Normal double-contrast arthrogram shows the inferior edge of the rotator cuff *(RC)* as it courses through the subacromial space to the greater tuberosity, the tendon of the long head of the biceps *(BT)*, and the articular cartilage of the humeral head *(AC)*.

cuff-tear arthropathy have progressive arthritis, pain, and significant functional impairment. Synovitis or calcium pyrophosphate deposition disease may be an important factor in the pathogensis of cuff-tear arthropathy. In such cases, scintigraphy may demonstrate the increased blood flow and blood pooling associated with the chronic synovitis.

ARTHROGRAPHY

Single-contrast arthrography, double-contrast arthrography, and double-contrast arthrotomography (DCAT) are valuable tools in evaluating problems of the rotator cuff, glenoid labrum, biceps tendon, and shoulder capsule.[24-27] Figure 38–6 shows a normal double-contrast arthrogram of the shoulder. Rotator cuff tears can be demonstrated by single-contrast or double-contrast studies. The proponents of double-contrast arthrography believe that the extent of the tear, the preferred surgical approach, and the quality of the rotator cuff tissue are best determined by double-contrast studies.[25-29] Figure 38–7 demonstrates extravasation of contrast material into the subacromial space from a rotator cuff tear. Arthrography can be misleading and result in underestimating the extent of a rotator cuff tear.

Tears of the glenoid labrum without shoulder dislocation are sources of anterior shoulder pain in athletes.[7] Glenoid labrum tears (Fig. 38–8), with or without associated glenohumeral subluxation, frequently can be identified by DCAT.[27,28] Kneisl and colleagues[30] described 55 patients who underwent DCAT followed by diagnostic shoulder arthroscopy. DCAT predicted the arthroscopic findings in 76 percent of anterior labra and 96 percent of posterior labra. This test was 100-percent sensitive and 94-percent specific in diagnosing complete rotator cuff tears. Partial rotator cuff tears identified at arthroscopy were missed in 83 percent of patients undergoing DCAT. The investigators believed DCAT was better in diagnos-

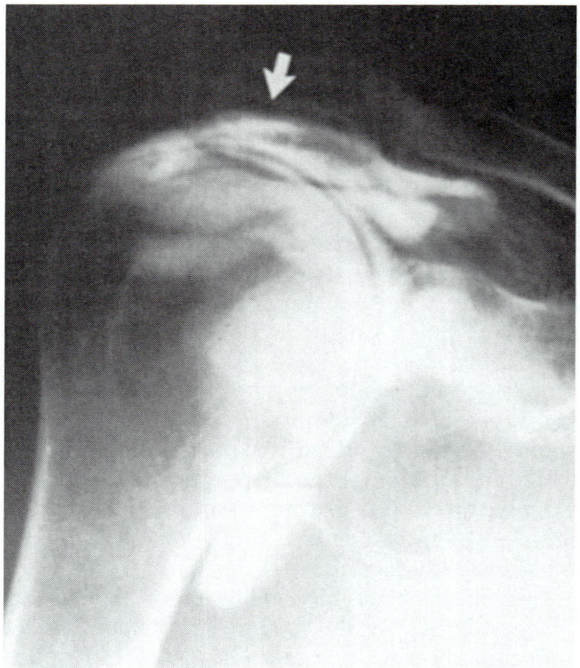

FIGURE 38–7 • Single-contrast arthrogram demonstrates a massive rotator cuff tear with extravasation of contrast into the subacromial space *(arrow)*.

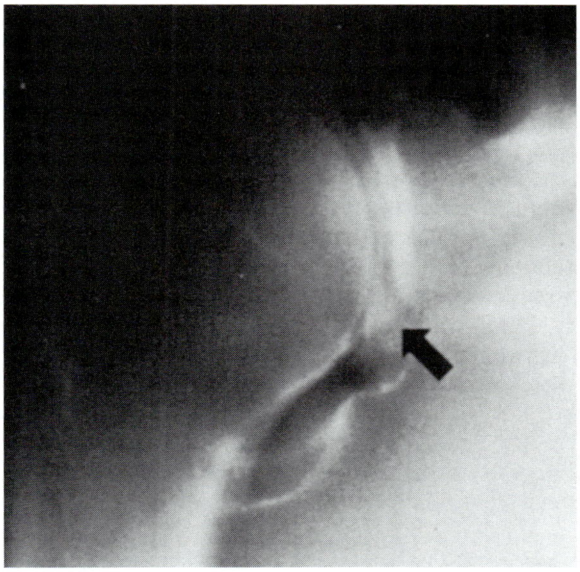

FIGURE 38–8 · A double-contrast arthrotomogram demonstrates a tear of the anteroinferior portion of the glenoid labrum *(arrow)*.

ing intra-articular and cuff pathology in cases of instability than when pain alone was the presenting diagnosis.[30]

Shoulder arthrography can confirm a diagnosis of adhesive capsulitis by showing a contracted capsule with an obliterated axillary recess (Fig. 38–9). The use of subacromial bursography has been beneficial in visualizing the outer surface of the rotator cuff and the subacromial space in cases of impingement.[31,32] Fukuda and associates[33] reported a small series of younger patients (average age, 41.8 years) who underwent subacromial bursography after a negative glenohumeral arthrographic result. These patients demonstrated pooling of contrast medium on the bursal side of a tear, which was confirmed at the time of surgery. Subacromial bursography is not routinely used diagnostically, and in our opinion, it is of little value in planning surgical procedures.

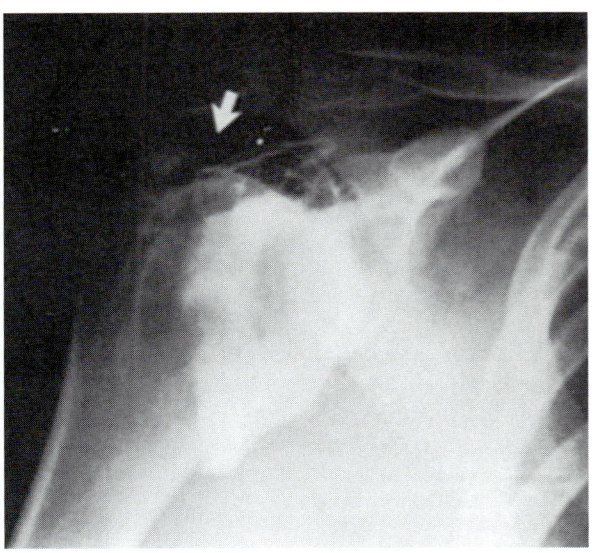

FIGURE 38–9 · Double-contrast Arthrogram of a Patient with Calcific Tendinitis *(arrow)* and Adhesive Capsulitis. Notice the contracted capsule with diminution of the synovial space and obliteration of the axillary recess.

COMPUTED TOMOGRAPHY

Computed tomography (CT) is helpful in the evaluation of the musculoskeletal system, and CT combined with contrast arthrography (arthro-CT) has become a major diagnostic tool for the evaluation of glenoid labrum tears, loose bodies, and chondral lesions (Fig. 38–10). Rafii and coworkers[34] reported using arthro-CT in the evaluation of shoulder derangement. This study found a 95-percent accuracy of arthro-CT for investigating lesions of the labrum and articular surface.[34] More recently, multidetector arthro-CT scans have been used to evaluate partial cuff tears (Fig. 38–11*A*), cystic lesions (see Fig. 38–11*B*), and calcific tendinopathy (see Fig. 38–11*C*).

ULTRASONOGRAPHY

The technologic improvement of sonographic equipment has allowed improved ultrasonographic study of the rotor cuff. The technique is noninvasive, rapid, and involves no radiation exposure.[30-32,35] The cuff is examined in the horizontal and transverse planes with the arm in different positions to visualize various areas of the cuff. These techniques generally provide visualization of the distal cuff, where most rotator cuff tears are located. Figure 38–12 shows normal and abnormal ultrasound images of the rotator cuff in longitudinal and transverse planes.

Several studies report a high sensitivity and specificity for the ultrasonographic diagnosis of a rotator cuff tear.[32-35] The specificity and sensitivity of the procedure are reported to be greater than 90 percent as determined by arthrographic and surgical correlations.[34,35] This technique has also been used for the postoperative evaluation of a rotator cuff repair and for evaluation of abnormalities of the biceps tendon.[36-40]

Gardelin and Perin[41] reported ultrasound to be 96-percent sensitive in determining rotator cuff and biceps tendon pathology. Mack and associates[36] found ultrasound to be valuable in evaluating the postoperative paient with recurrent shoulder symptoms. In a prospective study, Hodler and colleagues[39] compared ultrasound with MRI and arthrography in evaluating rotator cuff lesions in 24 shoulders. Ultrasound identified 14 of 15 torn cuffs, MRI 10 of 15, and arthrography 15 of 15.[39] Ultrasound identified seven of nine intact rotator cuffs, whereas MRI was accurate in eight of nine intact cuffs.[39] Vestring and colleagues[42] found ultrasound to be as accurate as MRI in the diagnosis of humeral head defects and joint effusions but inferior to MRI in the diagnosis of labrum lesions, rotator cuff lesions, subacromial spurs, and synovial inflammatory disease.

In the hands of an experienced sonographer, ultrasound may be the most cost-effective test for the initial evaluation of a rotator cuff injury, but most surgeons require arthro-CT or MRI confirmation before surgical exploration.[36,39,41-43]

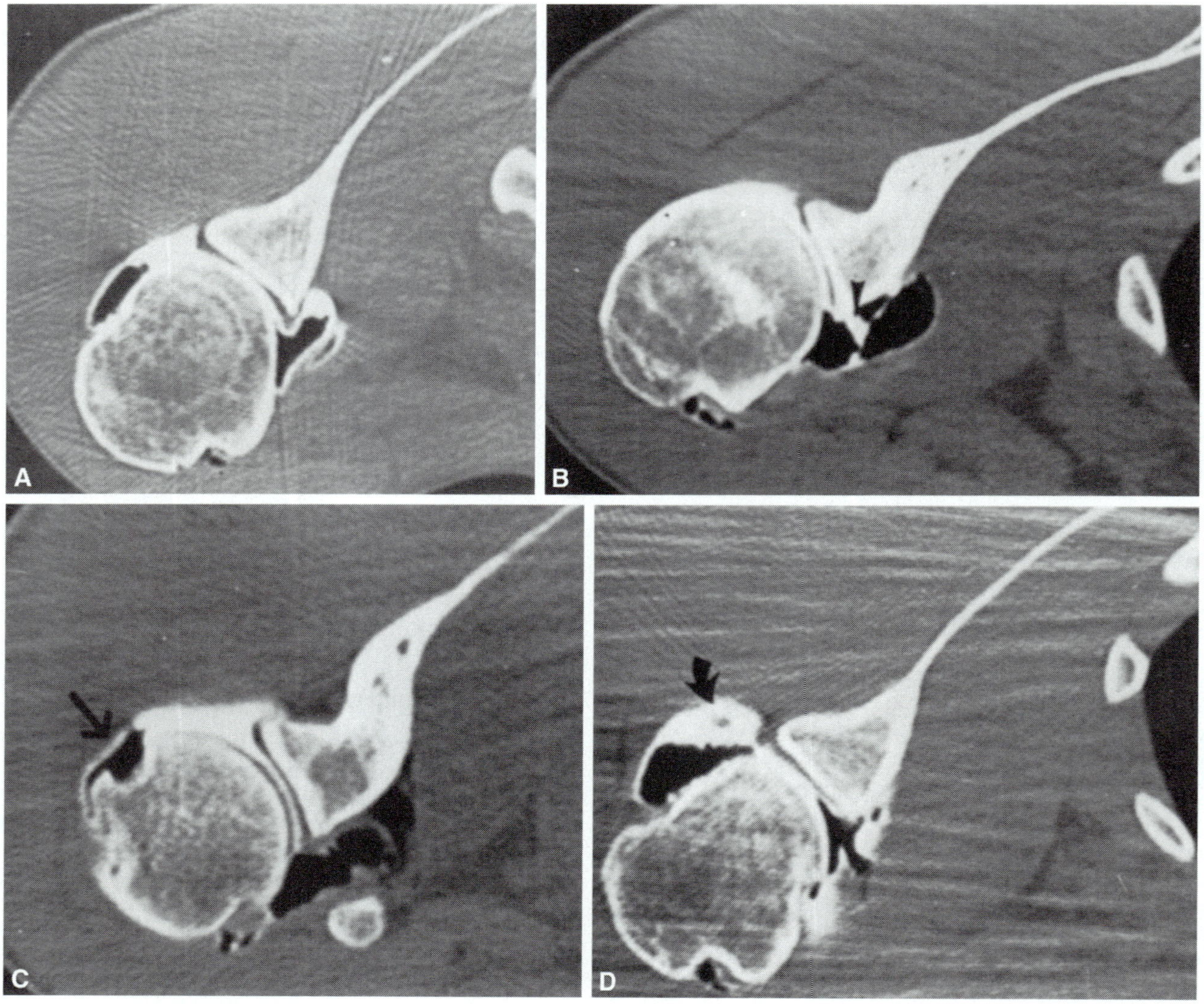

FIGURE 38–10 · Arthrographic Computed Tomography (CT) Scan of Shoulder Shows: *A,* Normal findings; *B,* Tear of the anterior glenoid labrum; *C,* A large defect of the articular surface of the posterior portion of the humeral head (Hill-Sachs lesion) *(arrow); D,* Loose body in the posterior recess *(arrow).*

ARTHROSCOPY

The use of arthroscopy for the diagnosis of shoulder pathology increased in the 1980s, partially because of its accuracy, which was far greater than clinical examination and better than other diagnostic modalities of the time. With technologic advances of fiber optics, video output, and arthroscopic instrumentation, the use of arthroscopy to diagnose and treat shoulder problems exponentially increased to include procedures once considered reserved only for open techniques.[44]

Compared with DCAT, arthroscopy is more accurate in the diagnosis of intra-articular lesions associated with a painful shoulder.[30] An additional benefit is that arthroscopy can be used to diagnose and treat shoulder problems of the glenohumeral joint and the subacromial region. With the increased accuracy of MRI arthrograms in detecting partial cuff tears and labral lesions, diagnostic shoulder arthroscopy has become less common in the absence of clear indications and specific treatment plans. In combination with a detailed history and physical examination, and along with examination under anesthesia, shoulder arthroscopy has been helpful in the diagnosis of chronic instability patterns of the glenohumeral joint.[44-47]

The indications and usefulness of shoulder arthroscopy in the treament of common pathologic conditions have continued to increase as the technology improves and the understanding of the pathophysiology of shoulder problems grows. Shoulder arthroscopy has been routinely used to confirm and treat SLAP lesions, labral tears, partial cuff tears, refractory adhesive capsulitis, partial biceps tendon tears, and multidirectional instability. Other conditions that are routinely treated arthroscopically are rotator cuff tears, glenohumeral instability, AC joint pathology, loose bodies, sepsis, osteochondritis dissecans, synovitis, chondral lesions, subacromial impingement, and calcific tendinitis.[7,13,44,47]

MAGNETIC RESONANCE IMAGING

MRI has been used to diagnose partial-thickness and full-thickness rotator cuff tears, biceps tendon tears, impingement of the rotator cuff, synovitis, articular cartilage

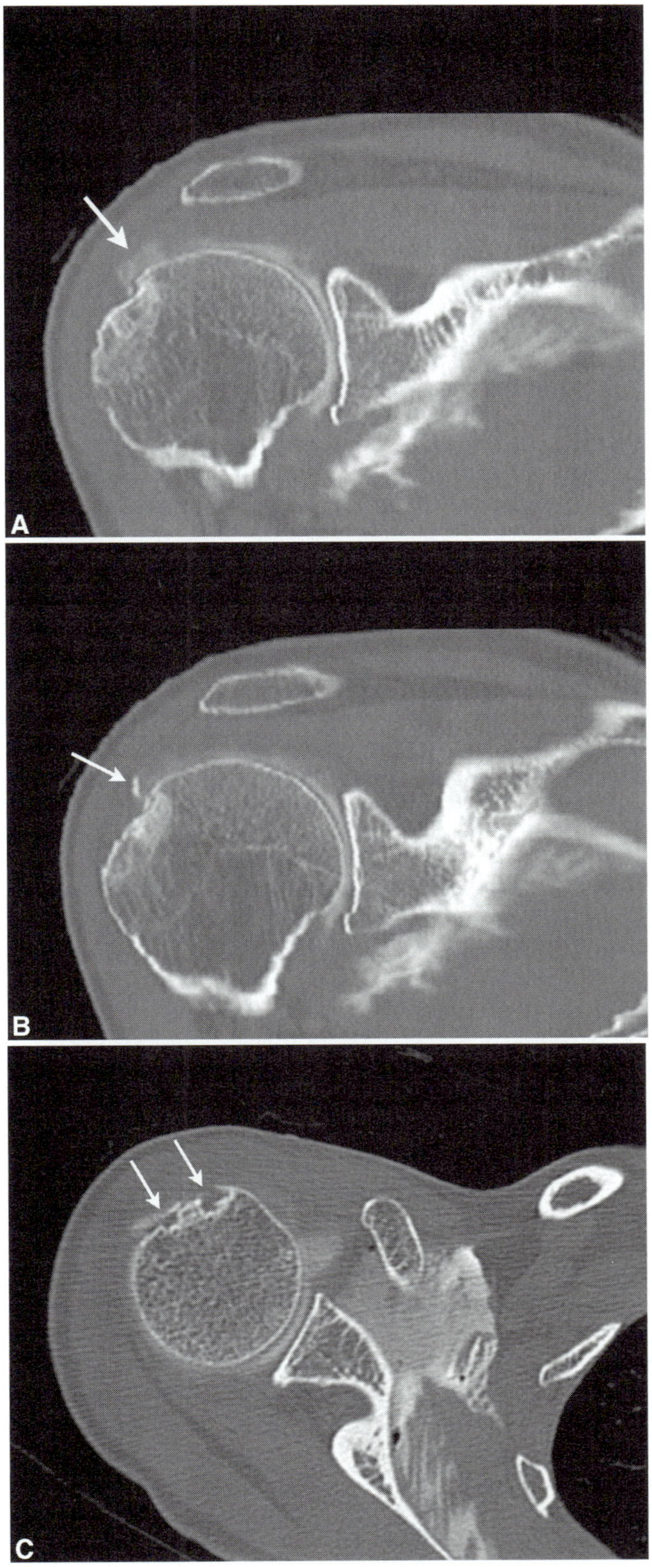

FIGURE 38–11 • Multidetector arthrogram computer tomography revealing: *A*, Partial rotator cuff tear (coronal view); *B*, Cystic humeral head erosions with calicification (axial view); *C*, calcification within rotator cuff tendon (coronal view).

damage, and labral pathology associated with glenohumeral instability.[48-50] In rheumatoid arthritis, MRI is reported to be more sensitive than plain radiographs in determining soft tissue abnormalities and osseous abnormalities of the glenoid and humeral head.[51]

One of the most useful diagnostic uses of the MRI is for rotator cuff pathology. Morrison and Offstein[52] studied 100 patients with chronic subacromial impingement syndrome using arthrography and MRI. MRI was 100-percent sensitive but only 88-percent specific in confirming arthrography-proven rotator cuff tears. Nelson and associates[53] studied 21 patients with shoulder pain and found MRI to be more accurate than arthro-CT or ultrasound in identifying partial-thickness cuff tears. These investigators also reported MRI to be as accurate as arthro-CT in the diagnosis of abnormalities of the glenoid labrum.[53]

The characteristic MRI findings in rotator cuff tears include a hypointense gap within the supraspinatus muscle tendon complex on T1-weighted films, absence of a demonstrable supraspinatus tendon with narrowing of the subacromial space, and an increased signal within the supraspinatus tendon on T2-weighted images.[54] Seeger and colleagues,[55] reporting the results of 170 MRI scans, found that T1-weighted images were highly sensitive for identifying abnormalities within the supraspinatus tendon, but T2-weighted images were required to differentiate tendinitis from a small supraspinatus tendon tear. Large full-thickness tears, however, could be identified on T1- and T2-weighted images. Figure 38–13 depicts common shoulder pathology as seen by MRI. MRI is nearly as sensitive and certainly more specific than scintigraphy in the diagnosis of osteonecrosis and neoplastic lesions about the shoulder.

ELECTROMYOGRAPHY AND NERVE CONDUCTION VELOCITY STUDIES

EMG and nerve conduction velocity studies can be helpful in differentiating shoulder pain from pain of neurogenic origin. They may also be beneficial in determining the localization of neurogenic pain to a particular cervical root, the brachial plexus, or a peripheral nerve.[56,57]

INJECTION

Injection of local anesthetics and glucocorticoids is a useful technique for the diagnosis and treatment of shoulder pain. However, the physician must have a thorough understanding of the anatomy of the shoulder girdle and a presumptive diagnosis to direct the injection properly. Injection of referred pain areas may be misleading. For example, in the patient with lateral arm pain due to deltoid bursal involvement from calcific tendinitis of the supraspinatus tendon, injection should be in the subacromial space rather than the area of referred pain in the deltoid muscle.

It is often better to use a posterior subacromial approach when injecting a rotator cuff tendinitis in a patient with anterior impingement symptoms because it is easier to enter the subacromial region posteriorly, and this approach is less traumatic to contracted anterior structures.

The instillation of rapidly acting local anesthetics can be beneficial in determining the source of shoulder pain. Obliteration of pain, for instance, by injection of a local anesthetic along the bicipital groove can confirm a diagnosis of bicipital tendinitis. The use of local

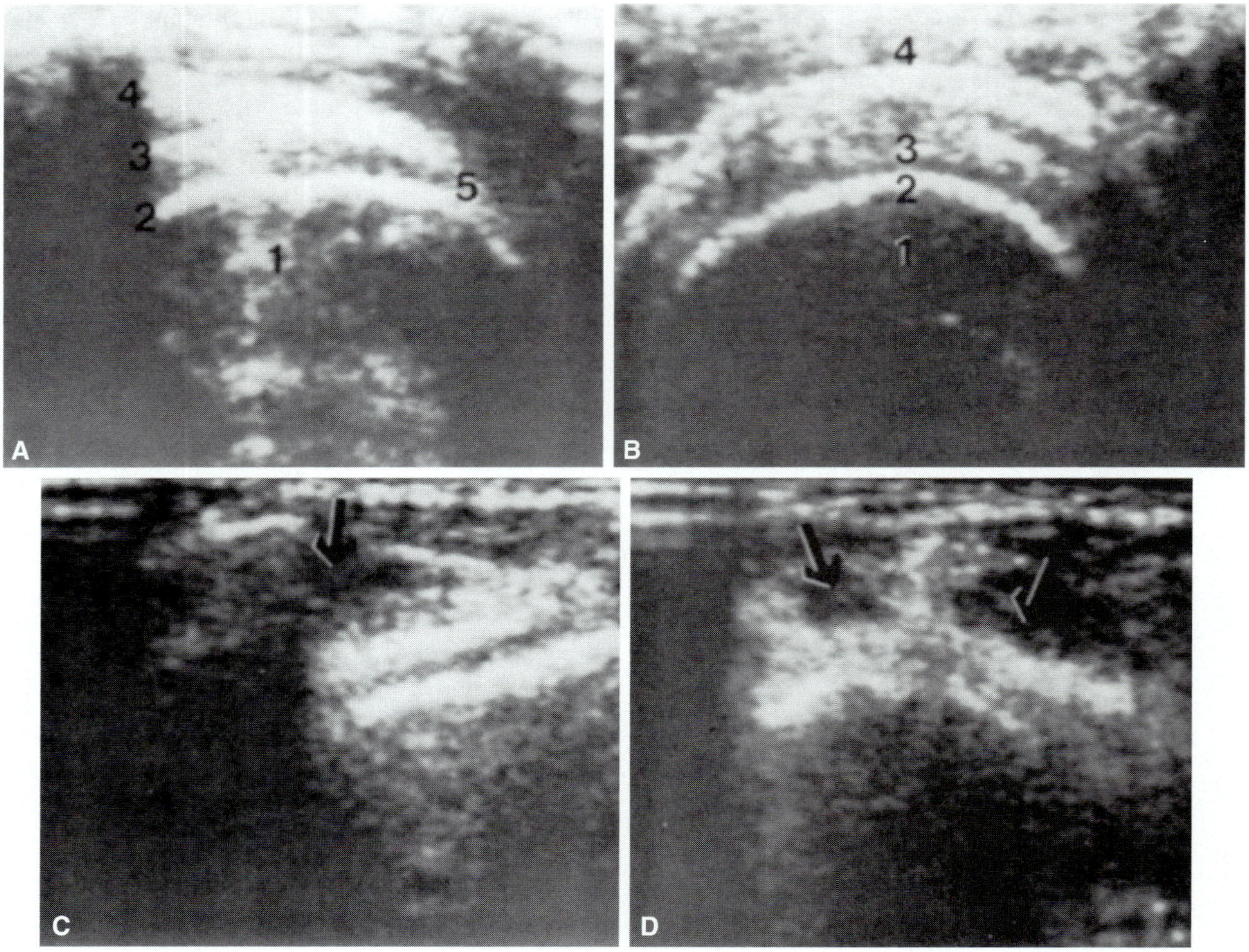

FIGURE 38–12 • *A*, Normal longitudinal view of rotator cuff by ultrasound shows (1) the humeral head, (2) the superior articular surface, (3) the rotator cuff, (4) the deltoid tendon, and (5) tapering of the cuff to its insertion on the greater tuberosity. *B*, Transverse view of a normal intact rotator cuff covering the humeral head. *C*, Rotator cuff tear, showing a hypoechoic area *(arrow)* on a longitudinal view. *D*, Rotator cuff tear, demonstrating hypoechoic area *(arrows)* on a transverse view.

anesthetics is somewhat less helpful when injecting the subacromial space because of its extensive communication with the rest of the shoulder girdle, but relief of symptoms by such an injection can exclude pain from conditions such as cervical radiculopathy or entrapment neuropathy.

AUTHORS' PREFERRED DIAGNOSTIC TESTS

Table 38–2 lists the reimbursement and charges for various shoulder diagnostic tests based on 2003 Medicare fee schedules and 2003 charges at a single institution. Choice of a specific test depends on its sensitivity, specificity, and cost-benefit analysis. History and physical examination are the most important factors in establishing diagnosis of the painful shoulder. Plain radiographs (three views) should be the first radiographic test performed. Although not as sensitive as the more sophisticated tests, plain radiographs can identify arthritic change, calcific tendinitis, established osteonecrosis, and most neoplasms. If intra-articular pathology (e.g., labrum tear, capsular tear, loose body, or chondral defect) is suspected, arthro-MRI is preferable to arthro-CT. In diagnosing acute rotator cuff tears in the younger patient, ultrasound is the most cost-effective test to confirm a clinical suspicion. In cases of impingement syndrome, MRI is sensitive, but it is difficult to differentiate tendinitis, partial tears, and small complete tears without arthro-MRI. The orthopedic surgeons prefer an arthro-MRI for verification of labral tears or partial rotator cuff tears. In the case of a suspected rotator cuff tear, MRI is preferred over an arthrogram to determine the size of the tear, amount of retraction, and quality of the remaining tissue for repair.

Intrinsic Factors Causing Shoulder Pain

PERIARTICULAR DISORDERS

Shoulder Impingement and Rotator Cuff Tendinopathy

One of the most common nontraumatic causes of shoulder pain is impingement with rotator cuff tendinopathy. In 1972, Neer described his results of 100 anatomic shoulder dissections and coined the term *impingement*

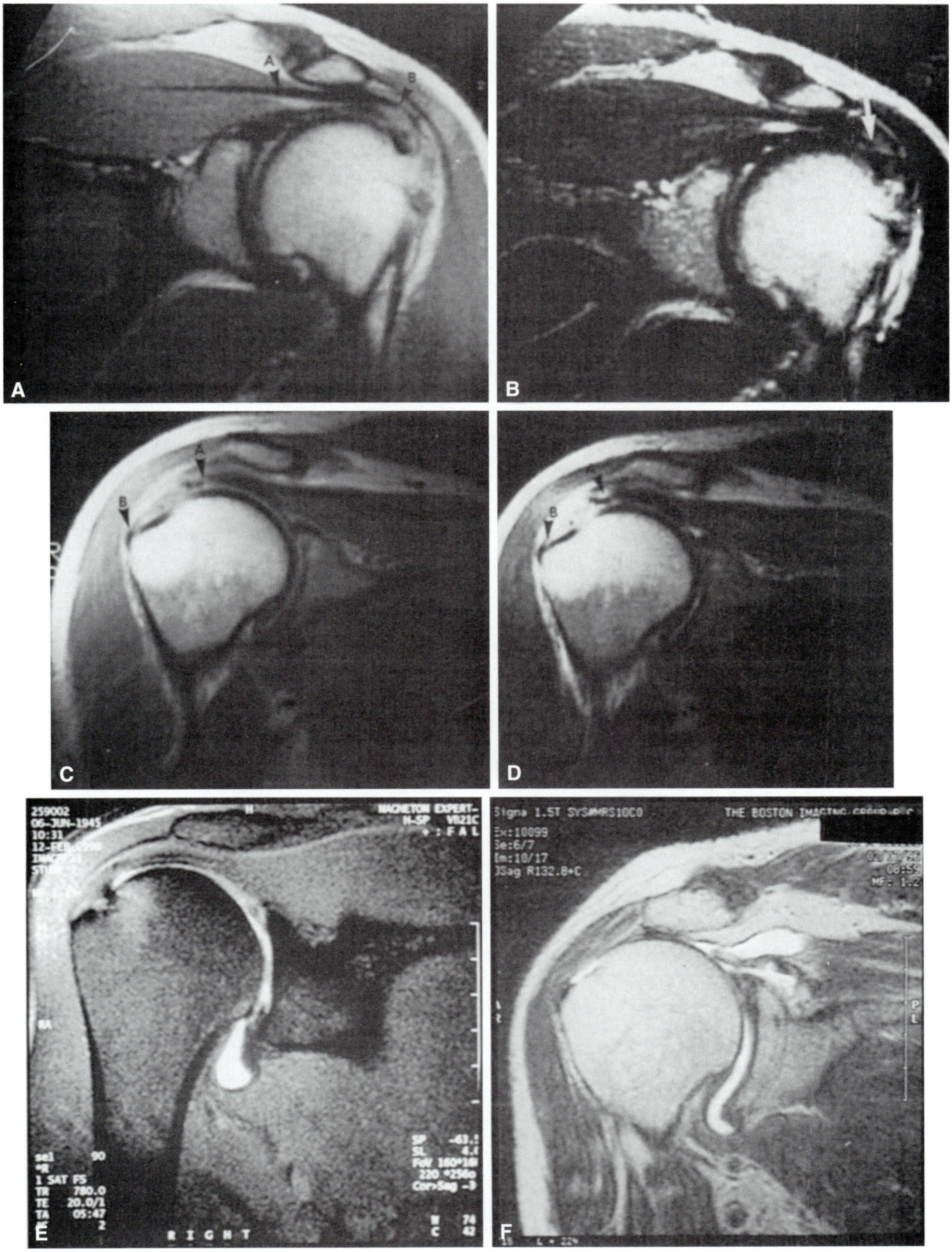

FIGURE 38–13 · *A*, Magnetic resonance imaging (MRI) proton density-weighted coronal view shows (A) supraspinatus tendon as a black band that has an increased signal (B) as it nears insertion on the greater tuberosity. *B*, Similar view in a T2-weighted image shows increased signal as gray *(arrow)*, indicating partial-thickness tear or tendinitis. *C*, MRI proton density-weighted coronal view shows (A) abrupt end of supraspinatus tendon as it courses right to left. From (A) to (B) is area of increased signal followed by a short portion of tendon (B) inserting at greater tuberosity. *D*, Similar view in a T2-weighted image shows increased signal as white (fluid density), indicating fluid in the gap of a complete rotator cuff tear. *E*, MRI arthrography shows normal rotator cuff. *F*, MRI arthrography shows a chronic cuff tear with retraction.

syndrome.[9] Impingement may be defined as the encroachment of the acromion, coracoacromial ligament, coracoid process, or AC joint on the rotator cuff as it passes beneath them during glenohumeral motion. The function of the posterior rotator cuff is to abduct and externally rotate the humerus. The cuff with the biceps tendon serves as a humeral head depressor to maintain the head centered within the glenoid fossa as the cuff and deltoid elevate the arm.[58-60] Controversy continues, however, as to the exact cause of impingement—whether it is a primary, intrinsic, degenerative event within the tendon with superior migration of the head on arm elevation and secondary impingment on the acromion or a purely mechanical attrition of the tendon with primary impingement against the acromion. The mechanical impingement of the rotator cuff may be influenced by variations in the shape and slope of the acromion.[61,62] The supraspinatus outlet may become narrowed from proliferative spur formation of the acromion or degenerative changes of the AC joint. These changes, along with intrinsic degenerative changes of the rotator cuff, may lead to rotator cuff tear, but the exact pathogenesis remains controversial. Many studies have found a strong correlation between degenerative hypertrophic spur formation, with its resulting narrowing of the supraspinatus outlet, and the presence of full-thickness cuff tears,[9,19,63-70] but clinical studies have failed to resolve whether the hypertrophic changes of the coracoacromial arch are caused by the cuff lesions or are a cause of the lesions themselves.

Neer[9] developed a staging system for description of impingement lesions of the shoulder. A stage I lesion involves edema and hemorrhage of the rotator cuff and is typically found in individuals younger than 25 years of age who are active in overhead athletics. The condition usually reponds to conservative treatment of rest, anti-inflammatory medication, and physical therapy. Stage II lesions usually occur in the third or fourth decade of life and represent the biologic response of fibrosis and thickening of the tendon after repeated episodes of mechanical impingement over time. The lesion is also treated conservatively, as in stage I, but attacks may recur. If symptoms persist despite adequate conservative management for more than 6 to 12 months, surgical intervention is warranted. Stage III lesions involve rotator cuff tears, biceps tendon rupture, and bone changes, and they rarely occur before age 40. Patients may present with pain, weakness, or supraspinatus atrophy, depending on the chronicity of the tear. Surgical treatment is contingent on the patient's age, loss of function, weakness, and pain.

Patients usually present to the clinician with a complaint of pain that has failed to resolve after a variable period. Pain can be sudden and incapacitating in cases of traumatic cuff tears, or more commonly it manifests as a dull ache in cases of chronic impingement. Pain is usually located over the anterior and lateral aspects of the shoulder and may radiate into the lateral deltoid. The pain may worsen with sleeping on the affected extremity and is exacerbated by overhead activity. Tenderness on palpation may be elicited over the greater tuberosity and long head of the biceps within the bicipital groove, indicating an associated biceps tendinitis. In cases with concomitant degenerative changes of the AC joint, there may be tenderness on palpation over the AC joint as an offending osteophyte impinges on the rotator cuff beneath.

The impingement sign as described by Neer[9] (Fig. 38–14) is useful in the diagnosis of rotator cuff tendinopathy. The patient often describes a catch as the arm is brought into the overhead position. The patient may be observed to raise the arm by abduction and external rotation to clear the greater tuberosity of the acromion, bypassing the painful area. A typical painful arc usually occurs between 70 and 110 degrees of abduction. Neer also described an impingement test that involves injection of lidocaine into the subacromial bursa.[9] Relief of pain is indicative of a positive impingement test result and usually indicates rotator cuff orign of the shoulder pain.

TABLE 38–2 • RELATIVE COSTS OF SHOULDER DIAGNOSTIC PROCEDURE IN 2003

Procedure	Initial Fee ($)	Technical Fee ($)	Interpretation Fee ($)
Medicare B Fee Schedule			
Initial office visit (30 minutes)	156.00		
Plain radiography (3 views)		25.25	10.07
Arthrography		150.05	30.09
Ultrasonography		62.80	32.83
Magnetic resonance imaging		494.73	73.44
Computed tomography		219.00	59.78
Tomography		62.80	32.37
Institutional Charges			
Initial office visit (30 minutes)	190.00		
Plain radiography (3 views)		160.00	61.00
Arthrography		437.00	180.00
Ultrasonography		375.00	121.00
Magnetic resonance imaging		1,410.00	206.00
Computed tomography		761.00	155.00
Tomography		Not offered	Not offered

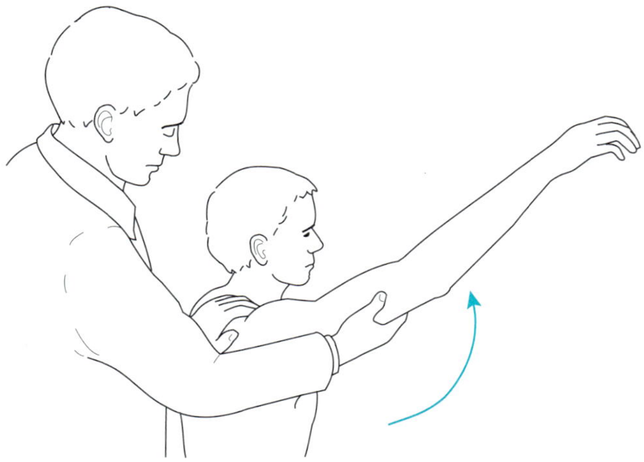

FIGURE 38–14 · The Impingement Sign Is Elicited by Forced Forward Elevation of the Arm. Pain results as the greater tuberosity impinges on the acromion. The examiner's hand prevents scapular rotation. This maneuver may be positive in other periarticular disorders. (From Neer CS II: Impingement lesions. Clin Orthop 173:70, 1983.)

Radiographs in the early stages of cuff tendinopathy may be normal or may reveal a hooked acromion. As the disease progresses, there may be some sclerosis, cyst formation, and sclerosis of the anterior third of the acromion and the greater tuberosity. An anterior acromial traction spur may appear on the undersurface of the acromion lateral to the AC joint and represents contracture of the coracoacromial ligament. Late radiographic findings include narrowing of the acromiohumeral gap, superior subluxation of the humeral head in relation to the glenoid, and erosive changes of the anterior acromion.[70] Arthrography, MRI, and ultrasound may be helpful in diagnosing a full-thickness tear of the rotator cuff in association with stage III disease. In some cases of chronic large rotator cuff tears, proximal migration of the humeral head leads to a pattern of degenerative arthritis known as cuff-tear arthropathy.

The choice of treatment and frequently its result are functions of the stage of the impingement and response to pain. In stage I disease, in which there is little mechanical impingement, most patients respond to rest. It is important not to immobilize the shoulder for any period because contraction of the shoulder capsule and periarticular structures can produce an adhesive capsulitis. After a period of rest, a progressive program of stretching and strengthening exercises generally restores the shoulder to normal function. Use of aspirin and other nonsteroidal anti-inflammatory drugs (NSAIDs) may shorten the symptomatic period. Modalities such as ultrasound, neuroprobe, and transcutaneous electric nerve stimulation (TENS) are generally not helpful. Patients with stage I and II disease may have a dramatic response to local injection of glucocorticosteroids and local anesthetic agents. For stage II disease in which there is fibrosis and thickening anteriorly, it is frequently better to inject through a posterior approach. We prefer a combination of 3 ml of 1-percent lidocaine (Xylocaine), 3 ml of 0.5-percent bupivacaine, and 20 mg of triamcinolone. This combines a short-acting anesthetic to help confirm the diagnosis, a longer-acting anesthetic for analgesic purposes, and a steroid preparation in a depot form.

An integrated program of occupational and physical therapy often precludes the need for surgery in patients with stage II disease. Job modification for individuals with impingement syndrome caused by overuse may alleviate symptoms. More businesses are becoming aware of the cost savings associated with proper job ergonomics.[71,72]

The initial rehabilitation in stage II impingement is the cessation of repetitive overhand activity. Ice, NSAIDs, and local injections also may be beneficial. The initial physical therapy includes passive, active assisted, and active range of motion combined with stretching and mobilization exercises to prevent contracture. As pain and inflammation subside, isometric or isotonic exercises are used to strengthen the rotator cuff musculature. Isokinetic training at variable speeds and in variable positions is instituted before returning the patient to full activity. For patients with a job-related injury, it is critical to review and modify job mechanics to prevent recurrent episodes that can cause further disability and may precipitate the need for surgery.[71]

Neer[19] suggested that the patient with refractory stage II disease may respond to division of the coracoacromial ligament and bursectomy of the subacromial bursa. Neer's description of open anterior acromioplasty has become accepted as the procedure of choice for stage II and III impingement lesion, with many investigators reporting high success rates in treating impingement syndrome and rotator cuff tears.[73-76] Reported results show good and excellent relief of symptoms in 71 to 87 percent of patients treated by the open surgical procedure.[77-80]

In 1985, Ellman[45] described the technique of arthroscopic subacromial decompression. His initial results[46] and the results of others are comparable to those of open surgical techniques.[47,81] Arthroscopic subacromial decompression has become a widely accepted treatment for refractory stage II and III impingement lesions. The procedure can be performed as outpatient surgery, and because no deltoid is detached as with the open technique, the procedure facilitates rehabilitation and overall recovery rates.

Calcific Tendinitis

Calcific tendinitis is a painful condition about the rotator cuff and is associated with deposition of calcium salts, primarily hydroxyapatite.[82-84] The cause of calcific tendinitis is unknown. The commonly accepted cause is degeneration of the tendon, which leads to calcification through a dystrophic process.[84] A common clinicopathologic correlation is three distinct phases of the disease process: the precalcific or formative phase, which can be relatively painless; the calcific phase, which tends to be quiescent and may last from months to years; and the resorptive or postcalcific phase, which tends to be painful, as calcium crystals are resorbed.[82] Although it is more common in the right shoulder, there is at least a 6 percent incidence of bilaterality. Patients with bilateral shoulder involvement often have the syndrome of calcific periarthritis, in which calcium hydroxyapatite crystals are found at multiple sites.[85] The patients usually present with impingement-type pain in the affected shoulder during overhead activity. The pain may seem to be out of proportion to any objective physical findings. There may be difficulty sleeping on the shoulder and in falling asleep. The symptoms may last for a few weeks or a few months.

The incidence of calcific tendinitis varies in the literature among asymptomatic individuals from 2.7 to 20 percent. Most calcification occurs in the supraspinatus tendon, and 57 to 76.7 percent of patients are female. The average age of patients with this disease is between 40 and 50 years.[82,86]

Codman[1] pointed out the localization of calcification within the tendon of the supraspinatus. He provided a detailed description of the symptoms and the natural history of this condition. In describing the phases of pain, spasm, limitation of motion, and atrophy, he noted the lack of correlation between symptoms and the size of the calcific deposit. According to Codman, the natural history includes degeneration of the supraspinatus tendon, calcification, and eventual rupture into the subacromial bursa. During the latter phase, pain and decreased motion can lead to adhesive capsulitis (see Fig. 38–9).

Several factors may affect localization of the calcium within the supraspinatus. Many of these patients have an early stage of impingement, compressing the supraspinatus tendon on the anterior portion of the acromion.[9,19] This long-standing impingement may lead to local degeneration of the tendon fibers. In patients without impingement, localization of the calcium within the supraspinatus may be related to the blood supply of the rotator cuff, which normally is derived from an anastomotic network of vessels from the greater tuberosity or the bellies of the short rotator muscles.[83] The watershed of these sources is just medial to the tendinous attachment of the supraspinatus.[87] Rathburn and Macnab[88] referred to this watershed as the critical zone and pointed out that during abduction this area was rendered ischemic.

Treatment of calcific tendinitis depends on the clinical presentation and the presence of associated impingement. These patients can have an acute inflammatory reaction that may resemble gout. The acute inflammation can be treated with local glucocorticoid injection, NSAIDs, or both. Ultrasound may be of some benefit. If there is associated impingement, treatment depends on the stage at presentation. The radiographic appearance of the calcification can direct and perhaps predict the response to therapy. In the resorptive state, the deposits appear floccular, suggesting that the process is in the phase of repair and that a conservative program is indicated. Patients with discrete calcification and perhaps associated adhesive capsulitis (see Fig. 38–9) may be at a stable phase in which the calcium produces a mechanical block and is unlikely to be resorbed. For these patients, mechanical removal of the calcific deposits and correction of associated pathologic lesions may be necessary.[89-91] Percutaneous disruption of the calcified areas may be performed using a needle directed by fluoroscopy. This technique allows lavage and injection but does not treat associated impingement. Subacromial arthroscopy allows the mechanical débridement of calcific deposits under direct visualization. Moreover, this technique can be combined with arthroscopic removal of the inflamed bursa and decompression of associated impingement. In many cases of refractory calcific tendinitis associated with impingement, open or arthroscopic acromioplasty, subacromial bursectomy, and decompression are indicated.

ROTATOR CUFF TEAR

Pathophysiology

Spontaneous tear of the rotator cuff in an otherwise normal individual is rare.[19] It can occur in patients with rheumatoid arthritis or lupus as part of the pathologic process with invasion from underlying pannus. Metabolic conditions such as renal osteodystrophy or agents such as glucocorticoids are occassionally associated with cuff tears. Most patients report a traumatic episode such as falling on an outstretched arm or lifting a heavy object. The usual presenting symptoms are pain and weakness of abduction and external rotation. There may be associated crepitus and even a palpable defect. Long-standing tears are generally associated with atrophy of the supraspinatus and infraspinatus muscles. It may be difficult to differentiate a painful tendinitis from a partial- or small full-thickness cuff tear.

Controversy exists about the exact cause of cuff tendinopathy.[87,91-93] Most likely, the pathophysiology involves a combination of factors including decreased vascularity and cellularity of the tendon along with changes in the collagen fibers of the tendon that occur with aging.

Loss of motion with subsequent capsular tightness, particularly the posterior capsule, may lead to cephalad migration of the humeral head, with subsequent impingement of the cuff under the coracoacromial arch.[94] Rehabilitation exercises stress regaining a normal range of motion. To achieve full, painless motion, the normal relationship of glenohumeral to scapulothoracic motion must be achieved.[16,17,95]

Diagnosis

History

Patients with nontraumatic tears of the rotator cuff report symptoms of chronic impingement. There is often a loss of motion and feeling of stiffness with extremes of motion and difficulty during activities of daily living such as combing the hair, hooking a bra strap, putting on a shirt or coat, and reaching into the back pocket. In chronic cases of cuff tendinopathy, there is usually a loss of motion. Limitation of internal rotation occurs initially, is caused by posterior capsular contracture, and is often associated with posterior shoulder pain with adduction of the ipsilateral shoulder. This leads to further shoulder impingement with forward flexion because of superior migration of the humeral head against the anterior inferior acromion. This upward translation is analogous to the action of a yo-yo climbing on a string.[94,96] In time, loss of forward flexion, abduction, and external rotation occurs with passive and active motion of the shoulder.

Diagnostic Imaging

In acute cases, there may be a history of trauma, such as a fall onto the affected shoulder. In cases involving an anterior shoulder dislocation with subsequent profound weakness of the rotator cuff, a large tear on greater tuberosity avulsion should be suspected in addition to axillary nerve palsy. In younger patients, traumatic failure of the cuff under tensile overload may result in cuff failure because of forced adduction of the affected shoulder or active abduction against resistance, and it may also occur with traumatic dislocation. Repetitive tensile overload can also result in partial rotator cuff tears in the overhead athlete.

Initial evaluation of impingement-type shoulder pain with cuff tendinopathy includes plain radiographs (see Chapter 43). An impingement series should be ordered, including an anteroposterior radiograph with a 30-degree cephalic tilt (Rockwood view), which can reveal osteophytes off the anterior os acromion and AC joint, a scapular Y view with a 10-degree cephalic tilt (supraspinatus outlet view), which can evaluate the type of acromion and reveal anterior and AC osteophytes, and an axillary view, which can evaluate the acromion for possible os acromionale. Calcific deposits within the rotator cuff tendon can best be viewed with rotational anteroposterior radiographs. Cuff arthropathy should be suspected if the acromial-humeral distance is less than 7 mm or there is cyst formation within the greater tuberosity, humeral head osteopenia, sclerosis about the greater tuberosity, or humeral head collapse. In advanced stages of cuff arthropathy, there may be complete loss of glenohumeral joint space with superior migration and abutment of the humeral head against the undersurface of the acromion.[58]

In the past, shoulder arthrography was considered the gold standard for diagnosing full-thickness rotator cuff tears, with sensitivity and specificity of more than 90 percent. Some authorities also feel arthrography is accurate in the diagnosis of partial-thickness tears.[33,97] Double-contrast arthrography with injection of contrast and air is considered to be more accurate in evaluating tear size, whereas single-contrast arthrography is better for evaluating partial-thickness cuff tears.[28,29]

Ultrasonography has been accurate in the diagnosis of full-thickness rotator cuff tears.[39,98-101] Ultrasonography does have advantages of being relatively inexpensive and noninvasive, but disadvantages include unproven effectiveness in determining subacromial impingement, capsular and labral abnormalities, and partial cuff tears. The procedure and its results are technician dependent. Ultrasonography may have a useful role in determining postoperative integrity of the cuff.[38]

MRI has been invaluable in evaluating rotator cuff tears. The sensitivity and specificity for diagnosing full-thickness cuff tears are 100 and 95 percent, respectively.[102] Through the use of gadolinium or saline, partial tears that are otherwise difficult to detect with conventional imaging can also be detected.

Diagnosing cuff tears with MRI is usually based on discontinuity of the tendon on T1-weighted images and consistent with fluid signal on T2-weighted images. Ancillary findings include fluid in the subacromial space on T2 images, loss of the subacromial fat plane on T1-weighted images, and proliferative spur formation of the acromion or AC joint. Large, chronic cuff tears may also be associated with cephalad migration of the humeral head and fatty atrophy of the spinatus muscle. Periarticular soft tissues, including the capsulolabral complex and biceps tendon, and the rotator cuff can be thoroughly examined. The degree of tear, tendon retraction, and evidence of muscle atrophy can be evaluated, all of which is critical in preoperative planning for possible cuff repair.

Nonsurgical Treatment

Codman and Akerson[63] recommended early operative repair for acute full-thickness rotator cuff tears and reported the first documented repair in 1911. McLaughlin recommended early repair on cases of grossly displaced tuberosity fractures or massive tears.[65] Several other clinical studies also supported the concept that a full-thickness tear does not preclude good shoulder function. DePalma[103] reported that 90 percent of patients with rotator cuff tears responded to conservative measures such as rest, analgesics, anti-inflammatory agents, and physiotherapy.

The reported percentage of patients responding to nonsurgical treatment in the literature varies from 33 percent to 90 percent.[3,18,104] Conservative treatment includes pain control with NSAIDs, ultrasound, heat before shoulder stretching and exercise, and ice after overhead activity. Deep massage therapy is employed to reduce trigger point tenderness within the trapezius, levator scapulae, and periscapular muscles. Patients on long-term anti-inflammatory medications are monitored periodically for evidence of gastrointestinal bleeding and for hepatic or renal toxicity. Opiate-based drugs are only used in the acute setting, such as after a fall or in the perioperative period.

Steroid and local anesthetic injections are used when the patient has significant pain that prohibits rehabilitation. Injections may be repeated once every 3 months if needed, and injection into the cuff tendon is to be avoided. If the patient fails to improve after 3 months of conservative treatment or does not continue to improve after three sequential injections, surgical options should be discussed.

The mainstay of conservative therapy is exercise. The rehabilitation stresses pain relief with exercises aimed at restoring shoulder motion, strengthening the remaining cuff muscles, deltoid, and scapular stabilizers. Therapy can be divided into three phases.

The goals of the initial phase of therapy are to relieve pain and restore shoulder motion. Motion therapy includes pendulum exercises, passive motion with use of a wand with the assistance of the uninvolved shoulder, an overhead pulley system, and posterior capsular stretching. The arc of motion is gradually increased and is guided by the patient's discomfort to avoid painful impingement arcs.

The second phase of therapy is entered after the patient has return of motion and little discomfort with overhead activity. Emphasis is placed on strengthening the remaining rotator cuff musculature, deltoid, and periscapular muscles. Strengthening is carried out with elastic surgical tubing that provides variable degrees of resistance, depending on size of the tubing. Initial strengthening is performed out of the impingement arc (70 to 120 degrees of shoulder flexion). The goal of this phase is to strengthen the shoulder to prevent dynamic proximal humeral migration with impingement during active shoulder elevation.[58,60] Normal shoulder kinematics relies on combined and synchronous glenohumeral flexion and scapular rotation.[59,91] In addition to strengthening the cuff and deltoid, the scapular rotators, including the trapezius and serratus anterior muscles, are emphasized.[105] After the patient has successfully completed phase two of the rehabilitation program with minimal symptoms and good shoulder function, the final phase is entered.

Phase three is characterized by a gradual return to normal overhead activities, including work and sporting activities. This part of the rehabilitation program should be tailored to the individual patient's needs and the demands placed on the shoulder.

Surgical Treatment

Severity and duration of pain remains one of the primary indications for surgical intervention in a rotator cuff tear. Other factors important in surgical decision making include shoulder dominance, activity level, physiologic age, acuteness of the tear, degree of tear, loss of function, amount of tendon retraction, and fatty atrophy of the remaining cuff musculature.

Acute Tears

Acute tears of the rotator cuff can be treated with conservative measures of periscapular and cuff strengthening along with capsular stretching to restore motion. However, in the young patient, especially the overhead athlete, early surgical intervention should be considered. Conservative shoulder rehabilitation should be maintained for 3 to 6 months before deciding on surgery for the older sedentary patient in whom functional results without surgery may be quite acceptable. Many older patients may function well with chronic cuff tears, but they may become debilitated if an acute tear is superimposed on chronic changes. Surgical intervention may be required in these cases to return the patient to baseline function by repairing the acute tear and attempting to repair the chronic tear if possible.

Chronic Tears

For elderly patients whose pain and weakness do not create a functional problem, a conservative program is preferable. Pain unresponsive to conservative management is the main indication for surgery in the older patient with a chronic rotator cuff tear. In these cases, surgery should be considered on an individual basis after at least 3 months of conservative treatment, including subacromial steroid injection. If the cuff tear is massive and irreparable, débridement and subacromial decompression may provide good pain relief without extensive surgery and prolonged immobilization.[46,81,106-110] In the younger patient with a chronic tear and weakness, surgery to repair the cuff may be indicated to improve strength and prevent further extension of the tear.[108]

In cases of rotator cuff arthropathy with glenohumeral joint degeneration, humeral head hemiarthroplasty is carried out with a slightly oversized head and increased offset to avoid impingement against the acromion while increasing the mechanical advantage of the deltoid and remaining cuff.

BICIPITAL TENDINITIS AND RUPTURE

The long head of the biceps passes through the bicipital groove, crosses over the head of the humeral, and inserts on the superior rim of the glenoid[111] (see Fig. 38–2*A*). The biceps tendon aids in flexion of the forearm, supination of the pronated forearm if the elbow is flexed, and forward elevation of the shoulder.[3] Bicipital tendinitis, subluxation or dislocation of the biceps tendon within the bicipital groove, and rupture of the long head of the biceps are generally associated with anterior shoulder pain.

Bicipital tendinitis is sometimes an associated feature of a rotator cuff tear. The rotator cuff tear compromises centering of the humeral head on the glenoid. This results in increased mechanical loading of the long head of the biceps, which initiates a hypertrophic tendinitis.[112]

Dislocation of the long head of the biceps is usually combined with a lesion of the subscapularis tendon.[12] Isolated rupture of the long head of the biceps tendon is rare when the rotator cuff is intact. However, rupture of the long head of the biceps is common when there is a coexisting rotator cuff tear.[113] The effect of rotator cuff tear and concomitant biceps tendon rupture on strength can be substantial.[12]

The early phases of bicipital tendinitis are associated with hypervascularity, edema of the tendon, and tenosynovitis.[114] Persistence of this process leads to adhesions between the tendon and its sheath, with impairment of the normal gliding mechanism in the groove. Stretching of the adhesions may be associated with chronic bicipital tendinitis.[115] The diagnosis of bicipital tendinitis is based on the localization of tenderness. It is often confused with impingement symptoms and is frequently seen with an impingement syndrome.[24] Isolated bicipital tendinitis can be differentiated by the fact that the tender area migrates with the bicipital groove as the arm is abducted and externally rotated. Many eponyms are associated with tests to identify bicipital tendinitis.[3] Yergason's supination sign refers to pain in the bicipital groove when the examiner resists supination of the pronated forearm with the elbow at 90 degrees. Ludington's sign refers to pain in the bicipital groove when the patient interlocks the fingers on top of the head and actively abducts the arms.

Biceps tendon ruptures can occur in some patients who report no history of shoulder pain. The patients often complain of an acute onset of pain and ecchymosis around the anterior shoulder and sagging of the biceps muscle belly. In these cases, a concomitant rotator cuff injury should be excluded by clinical examination. More often, the biceps tendon rupture is preceded by painful shoulder symptoms that often improve or disappear after the rupture.[115,116]

Treatment is generally conservative and consists of rest, analgesics, NSAIDs, and local injection of glucocorticoids. The use of ultrasound and neuroprobe is more beneficial in this condition than in isolated rotator cuff tendinitis. Patients with refractory bicipital tendinitis and recurrent symptoms of subluxation are treated by opening the bicipital groove and resecting the proximal portion of the tendon with tenodesis of the distal portion into the groove or transfer to the coracoid process. The proponents of tenodesis believe it prevents proximal migration of the humeral head, whereas those who advocate transfer to the coracoid think that the procedure maintains biceps power.

ACROMIOCLAVICULAR DISORDERS

The AC joint is a common source of shoulder pain. Acute causes of AC joint pain are often related to direct trauma of the affected shoulder that may result in a distal clavicle injury with an intra-articular chondral fracture or in AC joint instability from ligamentous disruption.[117]

Post-traumatic distal clavicle osteolysis, with resorption of the distal clavicle, may ensue as soon as 4 weeks after a shoulder injury, leading to AC joint pain.[118,119] Osteolysis may be caused by microfractures of the subchondral bone and subsequent attempts at repair.[120] Others believe the cause to be an autonomic nerve dysfunction affecting the blood supply to the clavicle. The increased blood supply leads to resorption of bone from the distal clavicle.[118,121] More commonly, chronic osteolysis results from repetitive microtrauma to the AC joint from activities such as weightlifting, gymnastics, and swimming.[120,122,123]

The underlying pathophysiology is believed to be an inflammatory process from stress fractures of the subchondral bone with hyperemic resorption of the distal clavicle.[120, 124] Other causes of osteolysis include rheumatoid arthrosis, hyperparathyroidism, and sarcoidosis, which should be considered in the differential diagnosis, especially in bilateral cases.[118,119] Patients with atraumatic osteolysis of the distal clavicle should be forewarned that bilateral involvement may occur, with an incidence of 70 percent reported for one long-term follow-up.[125] Other chronic causes of AC pain include idiopathic, intra-articular disk pathology, post-traumatic degenerative arthrosis from joint incongruity, primary degenerative arthrosis, and rheumatoid arthrosis.

Evaluation should always include a detailed history, physical examination, and radiographic evaluation. There may be a history of trauma to the AC joint from a direct fall or blow to the ipsilateral shoulder. Less commonly, the AC joint may be injured indirectly, such as during a fall on the outstretched arm with the forces being transmitted through the arm to the AC joint.[117,126] Patients with osteolysis of the distal clavicle sometimes give a history of acute trauma, although the more common cause is repetitive microtrauma to the AC joint from activities such as weightlifting or gymnastics.[118,119,122,123]

Patients frequently complain of pain over the AC joint when adducting the ipsilateral shoulder, such as during a golf swing or when buckling a seat belt. Often, there is pain when sleeping on the affected shoulder. Athletes may experience AC joint pain on bench pressing, push-ups, and dips.[125,127,128] Pain and weakness of the affected shoulder may also be experienced with forward flexion and adduction of the arm.[118]

On physical examination, there may be a visible stepoff between the medial acromion and the distal clavicle, indicating a probable AC separation. Pain can usually be elicited on direct palpation of the AC joint and is made worse by a cross-arm adduction maneuver. This test is performed by internally rotating the arm, which is then maximally adducted across the chest and is considered positive if pain is produced in the AC joint (see Fig. 38–4*D*). Pain may also be elicited by moving the arm from a horizontally abducted position to the extended position and on maximum internal rotation of the shoulder.[127,129] These tests cause rotation and compression of the AC joint and are sensitive but less specific. They may also be positive with other disorders of the shoulder such as posterior capsular stiffness.[130]

Frequently, AC joint pain coexists with subacromial impingement and rotator cuff pathology. In these cases, impingement signs are positive, and rotator cuff weakness may be present. Otherwise, there should be no detectable muscle weakness on manual resistance testing and no evidence of muscle atrophy.[125,130,131] The AC joint and subacromial space may have to be injected on separate occasions to determine the true source of the symptoms. Some physicians have noticed an association of AC joint symptoms with shoulder instability.[125] Glenohumeral motion can be variable, depending on the chronicity and isolation of the problem to the AC joint. In isolated cases, there may be some loss of internal rotation of the affected shoulder because of pain.

Radiographs should include anteroposterior views of the shoulder in the scapular plane in neutral, internal, and external rotation, a transcapular Y view, axillary view, and a 15-degree cephalic tilt view of the AC joint at 50 percent penetrance as described by Zanca[23] (see Fig. 38–5). Stress views may be obtained by strapping 5 to 10 pounds of weight to the forearms and determining acromioclavicular separation. Comparing the coracoclavicular distance of both shoulders also may be helpful. When clinically indicated, cervical spine radiographs should be obtained to exclude cervical spondylosis.

Radiographic evaluation may reveal AC joint arthrosis with microcystic changes in the subchondral bone, sclerosis, osteophytic lipping, and joint space narrowing.[132] In cases of osteolysis, radiographs may reveal a loss of subchondral bone detail with microcystic appearances in the subchondral region of the distal clavicle and osteopenia of the lateral one third of the clavicle.[119,120,122,123] In the late stages of osteolysis, resorption of the distal end of the clavicle results in marked widening of the AC joint and, at times, complete resorption of the distal clavicle. There may be evidence of AC separation with widening of the coracoclavicular distance and post-traumatic ossification of the coracoclavicular ligaments.

The AC symptoms do not always correlate with the radiographic appearance of the joint. DePalma found AC joint degeneration to be an age-related process, with symptoms not always correlating with radiographic findings of AC joint arthrosis.[23,133] AC joint pain may occur despite normal radiographs.[134]

A technetium 99m phosphate bone scan may assist in the diagnosis, revealing increased uptake in the distal clavicle and medial acromion.[120] In cases of atraumatic osteolysis of the distal clavicle, increased uptake may be isolated to the distal clavicle, but in approximately 50 percent of cases, there is increased scintigraphic activity of the adjacent medial acromion.[125] The bone scan may reveal pathologic changes of the AC joint when plain radiographs appear normal.

In selected cases, MRI scans can be valuable in determining a diagnosis and evaluating the glenohumeral and subacromial regions for coexisting pathology (Fig. 38–15). AC joint involvement may reveal increased fluid with synovitis, soft tissue enlargement, and periarticular ossifications with encroachment on the underlying bursal and cuff tissue.

Patients with AC joint pain usually respond well to nonoperative treatment; however, complete relief of symptoms may take an extended period. Conservative therapy includes heat, NSAIDs, steroid injections, shoulder rehabilitation, and avoidance of painful positions and activities. Steroid injections are repeated at 3-month intervals if painful conditions persist.

Open resection of the distal clavicle for chronic AC joint pain was initially reported by Gurd and by Mumford, both with good results.[135,136] Since then, other surgeons have reported similar good results with open resection, but significant morbidity, such as disruption of the deltotrapezial fascia and anterior deltoid rupture, can occur.[118,119,132,134,137] Arthroscopic resection of the distal clavicle has been described with results similar to open resection.[13,124,129-131,138-141]

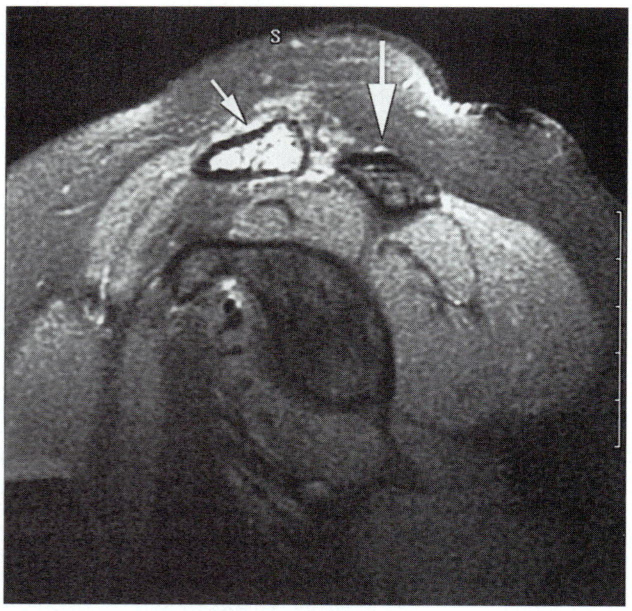

FIGURE 38–15 · Sagittal Section MRI of Shoulder in 32-Year-Old Weightlifter Complaining of Shoulder Pain. Fat-suppressed proton density fast-spin echo images of distal clavicle and acromion reveal distal clavicle osteolysis, with increased signal observed in the distal clavicle *(small arrow)* compared with the acromion *(large arrow)*.

GLENOHUMERAL DISORDERS

The various arthritides that affect the shoulder joint are discussed in detail in other chapters. They are presented here to address aspects that are unique to the glenohumeral joint. The usual presentation of intra-articular disorders is pain with motion and symptoms of internal derangement such as locking and clicking. The pain is generalized throughout the shoulder girdle and sometimes referred to the neck, back, and upper arm. The usual response to pain is to decrease glenohumeral motion and substitution with increased scapulothoracic mobility. Patients with adequate elbow and scapulothoracic motion require little glenohumeral motion for activities of daily living; patients with glenohumeral arthrodesis can achieve adequate function.[142,143] The response to pain is therefore diminution of motion and secondary soft tissue contractures with muscle atrophy. With increasing weakness and involvement of adjacent joints, pain, limitation of motion, and weakness cause a substantial functional deficit.

INFLAMMATORY ARTHRITIS

Although the most common inflammatory arthritis involving the shoulder joint is rheumatoid arthritis, other systemic disorders such as lupus erythematosus (SLE), psoriatic arthritis, ankylosing spondylitis, Reiter's syndrome, and scleroderma may cause glenohumeral degeneration. Motion is limited by splinting of the joint with secondary soft tissue contractures or by primary soft tissue involvement with scarring or rupture. Plain radiographs confirm glenohumeral involvement (Fig. 38–16A). There is narrowing of the glenohumeral joint space, with erosion and cyst formation without significant sclerosis or osteophytes. As the disease progresses, superior and posterior erosion of the glenoid with proximal subluxation of the humeral head may occur. Eventually, there may be secondary degenerative changes and even osteonecrosis of the humeral head.

Treatment is initially conservative and directed toward controlling pain, inducing a systemic remission, and maintaining joint motion by physical therapy. The use of intra-articular glucocorticoids may be beneficial in controlling local synovitis. In rheumatoid arthritis, the involvement of periarticular structures with subacromial bursitis and rupture of the rotator cuff magnifies the functional deficit. When the synovial cartilage interactions produce significant symptoms and radiographic

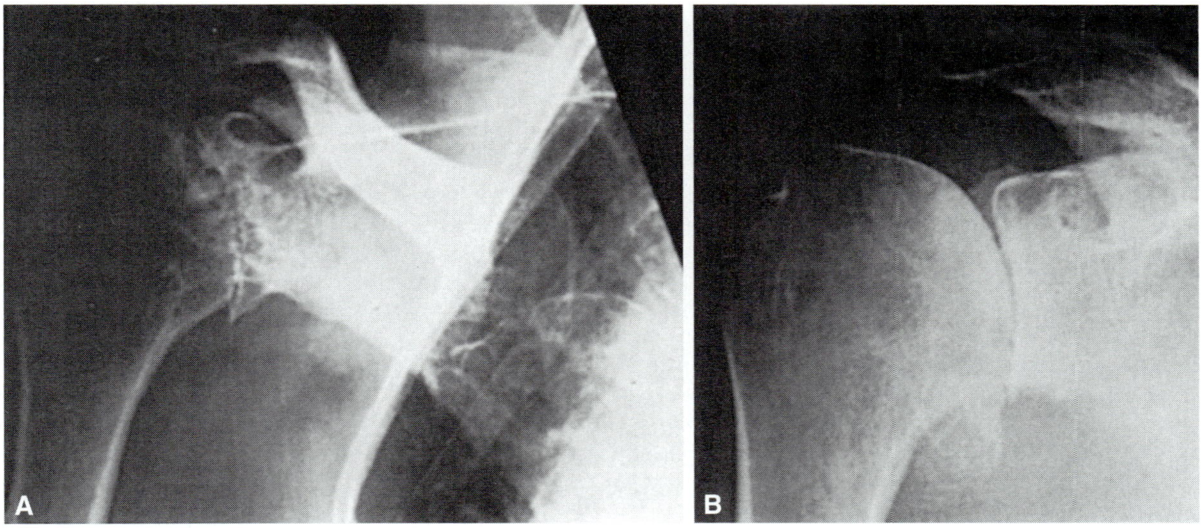

FIGURE 38–16 • Plain Radiographs. *A*, Rheumatoid arthritis with loss of joint space, cyst formation, glenohumeral erosion, and early proximal subluxation of the humerus, indicating a rotator cuff tear. *B*, Osteoarthritis with narrowing of the glenohumeral joint space, sclerosis, and osteophyte formation. Notice the preservation of the subacromial space, suggesting an intact rotator cuff.

changes that cannot be controlled by conventional therapy, glenohumeral resurfacing should be considered.

When following a rheumatoid patient with shoulder involvement, the rheumatologist should carefully assess range of motion and obtain periodic radiographs. Patients with progressive loss of motion or radiographic destruction should be referred for evaluation for possible surgical treatment. The treatment of choice is an unconstrained shoulder arthroplasty of the type reported in Chapters 115 and 116.[144,145] Total shoulder arthroplasty is best performed in patients with rheumatoid arthritis before end-stage bony erosion and soft tissue contractions have occurred.[146,147] Acute inflammatory arthritis of the glenohumeral joint may also be associated with gout, pseudogout, hydroxyapatite deposition of renal osteodystrophy, and recurrent hemophiliac hemarthrosis.

OSTEOARTHRITIS

Osteoarthritis of the glenohumeral joint is less common than that in the hip, its counterpart in the lower extremity. This is the result of the non–weight-bearing characteristics of the shoulder joint and the distribution of forces throughout the shoulder girdle. Osteoarthritis is divided into conditions associated with high unit loading of articular cartilage and those in which there is an intrinsic abnormality within the cartilage that causes abnormal wear at normal loads. Because the shoulder is normally a non–weight-bearing joint and is less susceptible to repeated high loading, the presence of osteoarthritis of the glenohumeral joint should alert the physician to consider other factors. Has the patient engaged in unusual activities such as boxing, heavy construction, or chronic use of a pneumatic hammer? Is there some disorder such as epiphyseal dysplasia that has created joint incongruity with high unit loading of the articular cartilage? Is this a neuropathic process caused by diabetes, syringomyelia, or leprosy? Is there associated hemochromatosis, hemophilia, or gout that may have altered the ability of articular cartilage to withstand normal loading? Is unrecognized chronic dislocation responsible?

Pain is the usual presentation, but it is generally not as acute or associated with the spasm seen in inflammatory conditions. Plain radiographs show narrowing of the glenohumeral joint, osteophyte formation, sclerosis, and some cyst formation (see Fig. 38–16*B*). Because the rotator cuff usually is intact, there is less bone erosion of the glenoid and proximal subluxation of the humerus. Patients with osteoarthritis of the glenohumeral joint frequently do well by functional adjustments and conservative therapy. Analgesics and NSAIDs may provide symptomatic relief. The use of glucocorticoid injections is less beneficial unless there is evidence of synovitis. Patients with severe involvement who fail to respond are best treated by shoulder arthroplasty[144-147] (see Chapters 115 and 116).

OSTEONECROSIS

Osteonecrosis of the shoulder refers to necrosis of the humeral head seen in association with a variety of conditions. Symptoms are due to synovitis and joint incongruity resulting from resorption, repair, and remodeling. The pathogenesis and various causes are discussed in Chapter 114.

The most common cause of osteonecrosis of the shoulder is avascularity resulting from a fracture through the anatomic neck of the humerus.[148] Fracture through this area disrupts the intramedullary and capsular blood supplies to the humeral head.[149] Another common cause of osteonecrosis of the shoulder is steroid therapy in conjunction with organ transplantation, SLE, or asthma. Other conditions associated with osteonecrosis of the humeral head include hemoglobinopathies, pancreatitis, and hyperbarism.

Early diagnosis is difficult because there is frequently a considerable delay until symptoms are present. Bone scans may be helpful in early cases before radiographic changes are evident. MRI is highly sensitive and more specific than scintigraphy. Plain radiographs demonstrate progressive phases of necrosis and repair (as discussed in Chapter 114). In the early stages, the films may be normal or show osteopenia or bone sclerosis. A crescent sign representing subchondral fracture or demarcation of the necrotic segment appears during the reparative process. Patients who fail to remodel show collapse of the humeral head with secondary degenerative changes. There is often a considerable discrepancy between symptoms and radiographic involvement. Patients with extensive bone changes may be asymptomatic. Treatment should be directed by the patient's symptoms rather than the radiographs and is similar to that for osteoarthritis. Arthroscopy occasionally is helpful by removing loose chondral fragments and débriding chondral incongruities.[150] Patients with severe symptoms that cannot be controlled by conservative means are best treated with an unconstrained shoulder arthroplasty or hemiarthroplasty.[144]

CUFF-TEAR ARTHROPATHY

In 1873, Adams described the pathologic changes in rheumatoid arthritis of the shoulder and a condition that has since been referred to as Milwaukee shoulder or cuff-tear arthropathy.[151] McCarty called the condition *Milwaukee shoulder* and reported that the factors predisposing to this syndrome included deposition of calcium pyrophosphate dihydrate crystals, direct trauma, chronic joint overuse, chronic renal failure, and denervation.[152] Patients with Milwaukee shoulder have elevated levels of synovial fluid 5-nucleotidase activity and elevated levels of synovial fluid inorganic pyrophosphate and nucleotide pyrophosphohydrolase activity.[153]

Neer and colleagues[154] reported a similar condition in which untreated massive tears of the rotator cuff with proximal migration of the humeral head are associated with erosion of the humeral head. The erosion of the humeral head is different from that seen in other arthritides and is presumed to be caused by a combination of mechanical and nutritional factors acting on the superior glenohumeral cartilage.

Patients with cuff-tear arthropathy present a difficult therapeutic problem because the bone erosion and disruption of the cuff jeopardize the functional result from an unconstrained prosthesis.[146] Hemiarthroplasty or a constrained total shoulder arthroplasty may be indicated.[155,156]

The major question in treating cuff-tear arthropathy is to determine which patients with massive rotator cuff tears will proceed to the syndrome of cuff-tear arthropathy. Patients with massive rotator cuff tears who develop localized calcium pyrophosphate disease may be predisposed to further proximal migration and further joint destruction. This situation poses a dilemma for the treating physician. Many patients with massive rotator cuff tears remain stable and require little or no treatment. Occasionally, symptomatic patients can be treated by arthroscopic débridement of the cuff tear. It is critical to define the patient who will proceed to the syndrome of cuff-tear arthropathy. If crystal deposition disease predisposes patients to proximal migration and joint destruction, joint aspiration with crystal analysis or scintigraphy to determine synovial reaction may be helpful diagnostic tools.

Hamada and coworkers[157] followed 22 patients with massive rotator cuff tears treated conservatively. The radiographic findings included narrowing of the acromiohumeral interval and degenerative changes of the humeral head, tuberosities, acromion, AC joint, and glenohumeral joint. Five of seven patients followed for more than 8 years progressed to cuff-tear arthropathy. The investigators concluded that progressive radiographic changes were associated with repetitive use of the arm in elevation, rupture of the long head of the biceps, impingement of the humeral head against the acromion, and weakness of external rotation.[157]

SEPTIC ARTHRITIS

Septic arthritis can masquerade as any of the conditions classified as periarticular or glenohumeral disorders (see Chapters 96 and 98). Sepsis must be included in any differential diagnosis of shoulder pain because early recognition amd prompt treatment are necessary to achieve a good functional result. The diagnosis is confirmed by joint aspiration with synovial fluid analysis and culture. Cultures should include aerobic, anaerobic, mycobacterial, and fungal studies.

LABRAL TEARS

The glenoid labrum increases the depth of the glenoid and serves as an anchor for the attachment of the glenohumeral ligaments. Historically, labral tears have been difficult to diagnose. Findings on physical examination can be confused with impingement and rotator cuff tendinopathy and bicipital tendinitis. Diagnosis can be confirmed with arthro-MRI, arthro-CT, and double-contrast arthrotomography.[27] Arthroscopy has greatly increased the knowledge of the glenoid labrum in normal and pathologic situations and has aided the diagnosis and treatment of labral lesions.

Labral tears can be divided into those associated with symptoms of internal derangement and those associated with anterior or posterior instability. A soft tissue Bankart lesion is associated with a tear of the anterior band of the inferior glenohumeral ligament and is associated with anterior instability. Isolated labral tears that do not involve detachment of the ligaments can cause internal derangement and may have an arthroscopic appearance similar to a meniscal tear of the knee.

Andrews first described lesions of the anterosuperior labrum in throwing athletes; these lesions were often associated with biceps tendon tears (10 percent).[7] These tears result from traction of the biceps tendon. Snyder and coworkers[158] introduced the term *SLAP lesion* in 1990 to describe an injury involving the long head of the biceps tendon and the superior portion of the glenoid labrum.

The long head of the biceps tendon originates at the supraglenoid tubercle and glenoid labrum in the superior-most portion of the glenoid. The major portion of the tendon blends with the posterosuperior aspect of the labrum. The most common mechanism of a SLAP injury is a fall onto the outstretched arm with the shoulder in abduction and slight forward flexion.[158] The lesion can also result from an acute traction on the arm and from abduction and external rotation mechanism.[160]

Patients usually complain of pain with overhead activities and frequent catching or popping sensation in the shoulder. The most reliable diagnostic test is the O'Brien test. The test is performed against resistance with the arm in forward flexion with the elbow extended and the forearm pronated. In the second part of the test, the arm is supinated. If less pain occurs during the latter part of the test, it suggests a SLAP lesion.[158] The most accurate diagnostic test is an MRI arthrogram with gadolinium.[161] Treatment for symptomatic SLAP lesions is surgical.

ADHESIVE CAPSULITIS

Adhesive capsulitis, or frozen shoulder syndrome (FSS), is a condition characterized by limitation of motion of the shoulder joint with pain at the extremes of motion. It was first described by Putman[162] in 1882 and later by Codman.[1] The initial presentation is pain, which is generalized and referred to the upper arm, back, and neck. As the pain increases, loss of joint motion ensues. The process is generally self-limiting and in most cases resolves spontaneously within 10 months unless there is an underlying problem.

The exact cause of FSS is unknown.[91,163] It is frequently associated with conditions such as diabetes mellitus, parkinsonism, thyroid disorders, and cardiovascular disease. When one of these conditions exists, there is often a history of some mild trauma that initiated the frozen shoulder. Major skeletal trauma and soft tissue injury may coexist with FSS. It may also be seen with a variety of other conditions, including apical lung tumors, pulmonary tuberculosis, cervical radiculopathy, and postmyocardial infarction.[164-166] In one review of FSS, 3 of 140 patients with this syndrome had local primary invasive neoplasms.[167] Another study reviewed three patients with adhesive capsulitis who subsequently were found to have neoplastic lesion of the midshaft of the humerus.[168] In the high-risk patient with an underlying disorder, even minor surgery or trauma in a remote location such as the hand can precipitate FSS.[91,169,170]

The pathophysiology involves a diffuse inflammatory synovitis with subsequent adherence of the capsule and a loss of the normal axillary pouch and joint volume, which leads to a significant loss of motion. Capsular contracture is thought to result from adhesion of the capsular surfaces or fibroblastic proliferation in response to cytokine production.[163,169,171] The condition is more common in women in their fourth or fifth decade. Typically, the patient relays a history of diffuse, dull aching about the shoulder, with weakness and loss of motion occurring over a period of a few months.

Usually, there are three distinct clinical stages of the syndrome. Stage one is the painful or freezing phase. During this stage, the pain is severe, exacerbated by any attempts at movement, and usually lasts for a few weeks or months. The patient usually feels most comfortable with the arm at the side in an adducted and internally rotated position. Phase two is the adhesive or stiffening phase and generally lasts 4 to 12 months. Pain is usually minimal during this phase, although periscapular symptoms may develop from compensatory motion to achieve elevation of the arm. The third phase of the syndrome is the resolution or thawing phase and may last 5 to 26 months. During this time, the pain eases and motion slowly improves, although some patients may dramatically improve over a short period.[172]

In the early stages, any attempts at motion may produce severe pain and associated weakness. The syndrome is usually associated with a prolonged period of immobilization.[173] Night pain is common, with an inability to sleep on the associated shoulder, which is similar to findings of impingement syndrome.

In patients with a history of minimal or no trauma and FSS, a metabolic cause should be excluded. A complete blood cell count, sedimentation rate, serum chemistry, and thyroid function tests are done as a screening panel. Further testing is done if the results suggest the possibility the patient may have a systemic illness. Plain radiographs should include a true anteroposterior, axillary, and scapular Y views of the shoulder. In patients with no underlying detectable illnesses and a negative workup result, a technetium-99m pertechnetate scan may show increased uptake in FSS, but more importantly, it is used to exclude occult lesions or metastasis.[174]

Treatment of FSS is mainly conservative using intra-articular injections, heat, gentle stretching, NSAIDs, and modalities such as TENS. The disease is usually self-limited and, after the painful phase, is not severely disabling. Communication between the physician and the patient, with a thorough explanation of the condition, is essential because resolution of the syndrome occurs slowly over time. Closed manipulation and surgery (open and arthroscopic) are reserved for the patient whose condition is recalcitrant to conservative measures or for whom the diagnosis is in question. Paramount in the prevention of FSS is avoiding overimmobilization in a minor shoulder injury in addition to careful identification of the patient at risk for FSS.

Fareed and Gallivan[175] reported good results with hydraulic distention of the glenohumeral joint using local anesthetic agents. Rizk and associates[176] performed a prospective, randomized study to assess the effect of steroid or local anesthetic injection in 48 patients with FSS. There was no significant difference in outcome between individuals who received intrabursal or intra-articular injection. Moreover, steroid with lidocaine had no advantage over lidocaine alone in restoring shoulder motion. Transient pain relief, however, occurred in two thirds of the steroid-treated patients.[176]

General anesthesia occasionally is indicated for closed manipulation. Hill and Bogumill[177] reported the results of manipulation of 17 frozen shoulders in 15 patients who did not respond to physical therapy. Seventy-eight percent of the individuals working before their shoulder problems returned to work an average of 2.6 months after manipulation. The investigators concluded that manipulation allowed patients to return to a normal lifestyle and to work sooner than the reported natural history of the condition.[177] Surgical intervention for adhesive capsulitis should be limited to treatment of an underlying problem such as calcific tendinitis or an impingement syndrome.

GLENOHUMERAL INSTABILITY

Glenohumeral instability is a pathologic condition that presents as pain associated with excessive translation of the humeral head on the glenoid during shoulder motion. Instability can range from excessive laxity with episodes of subluxation to frank dislocation of the joint. Traumatic dislocation of the glenohumeral joint has characteristic clinical and radiographic findings that are beyond the scope of this chapter and have been reviewed in detail elsewhere.[178] The most common type of instability is anterior, although posterior and multidirectional laxity of the shoulder are increasingly recognized as causes of shoulder pain. Anterior dislocation usually occurs with the arm in an abducted and externally rotated position, and the diagnosis is usually obvious. Posterior dislocation is frequently associated with convulsive disorders or unusual trauma with the arm in a forward flexed and internally rotated position. The diagnosis is often missed and should always be suspected in the patient who is unable to externally rotate the arm after trauma.

Recurrent subluxation without dislocation may be difficult to diagnose and may be mistakenly identified as impingement with chronic cuff tendinitis. The overhead athlete may experience repetitive stresses to the shoulder, causing microtrauma to the static stabilizers. Jobe and colleagues[21] described the syndrome of shoulder pain in overhead or throwing athletes that presents as impingement but is caused by anterior subluxation of the joint with the humeral head impinging on the anterior aspect of the coracoacromial arch. Fu and coworkers[179] underscored this distinction by dividing the cause of rotator cuff tendinitis into primary impingement of the tendon on the coracoacromial arch and anterior subluxation with secondary impingement in young athletes performing overhead movements. Walch and colleagues[180] described intra-articular impingement between the undersurface of the rotator cuff (supraspinatus and infraspinatus) and the posterosuperior glenoid rim and labrum. This "internal impingement" is usually observed in overhead athletes with subtle anterior glenohumeral instability and results in tendinitis or partial tears of the rotator cuff (Fig. 38–17).

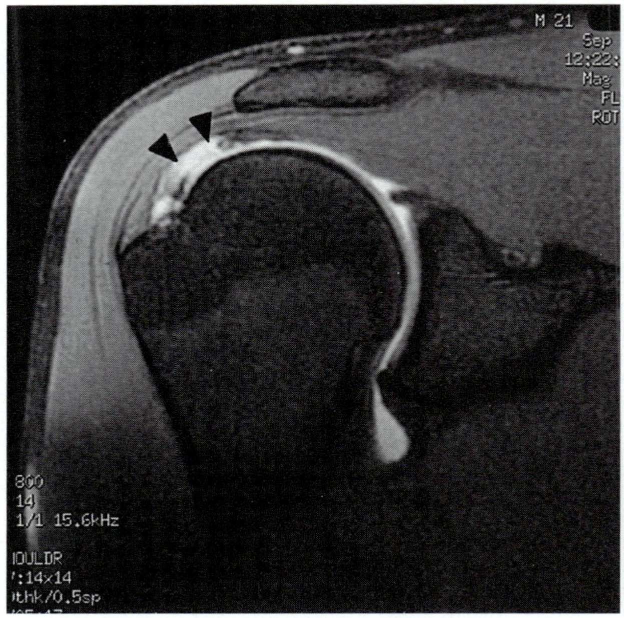

FIGURE 38–17 · MRI arthrogram using gadolinium in a 21-year-old professional pitcher with right shoulder pain and internal impingement. T2 sequencing reveals a large, partial rotator cuff tear affecting more than 50 percent of the cuff thickness *(black arrows)*.

The diagnosis of glenohumeral instability with subluxation in one or multiple directions is made by the combination of a detailed history and physical examination and the use of adjuncts such as arthrography, CT, MRI, and arthroscopy with examination under anesthesia. The syndrome of multidirectional instability (MDI) has been recognized in patients with symptomatic inferior instability in addition to anterior or posterior instability. Approximately 50 percent of the affected patients have evidence of generalized laxity. Frequently, the syndrome occurs in young athletic patients who are loose jointed, in particular in the dominant arm of pitchers, racket sports players, and swimmers. In this type of athlete, repetitive microtrauma may cause stretching of the shoulder, resulting in a large capsular pouch without labral detachment. A traumatic event may damage the shoulder, resulting in the MDI and a Bankart lesion.[181]

The most common manifestation in these individuals is pain, often mistakenly considered to be rotator cuff tendinitis. The patient may relate a history of minor trauma causing acute pain and a "dead arm" syndrome lasting for minutes or hours. Other associated symptoms include a sense of instability, weakness, and even radicular symptoms suggestive of neuropathy. There may be few or no positive physical findings associated with chronic subluxation or multidirectional instability. The patient may have signs of generalized ligamentous laxity, and pain may be reproduced by subluxating the glenohumeral joint in multiple directions. One particularly helpful sign for inferior laxity is the sulcus sign, which refers to the subacromial indentation that occurs when longitudinal traction is applied to the humerus with the arm at the side. The sign occurs with inferior translation of the humeral head. Because this syndrome frequently occurs in athletes with highly developed musculature about the shoulder girdle, these physical findings of subluxation may be difficult to reproduce in the office setting.

Plain radiographs are generally normal, although some inferior subluxation may be demonstrated by obtaining stress radiographs with weights. Special radiographs, as discussed previously, may demonstrate a Bankart lesion (i.e., avulsion of the anterior inferior glenoid rim) or a Hill-Sachs lesion (i.e., osteochondral defect of the posterior humeral head) occurring with subluxation of the humeral head in front of the anterior glenoid rim. Arthro-CT scan or arthro-MRI may demonstrate increased capsular volume, a labral detachment, o a Hill-Sachs lesion (see Fig. 38–10). When surgery is indicated, examination under anesthesia and shoulder arthroscopy may assist in diagnosing the primary direction of instability in MDI. In selected patients with traumatic anterior dislocation without a history of MDI, arthroscopic stabilization may be carried out with stabilization of the capsulolabral complex.

Treatment of chronic subluxation or MDI is first directed toward prolonged rehabilitation. Activities that stress the shoulder and produce symptoms are avoided. Strengthening exercises of the shoulder girdle may control symptoms, dynamically stabilizing the glenohumeral joint, and obviate the need for surgical intervention. If a conservative treatment program fails, surgery is performed on the side associated with the greatest amount of clinical instability. Stabilization is directed toward tightening of the capsular structures to stabilize the glenohumeral joint.[181,182] A new arthroscopic technique of capsular shrinkage using a thermal probe is being investigated in patients with MDI and overhead athletes with symptomatic microinstability without labral detachment.

Extrinsic or Regional Factors Causing Shoulder Pain

Because the shoulder girdle connects the thorax with the upper extremity and the major neurovascular structures pass in proximity to the joint, shoulder pain is a hallmark of many nonarticular conditions.

CERVICAL RADICULOPATHY

Cervical pathology may manifest with associated shoulder pain. The area of referred pain is along a dermatomal pattern consistent with the distribution of the dermatomal nerve roots. Isolation of the pain usually defines the exact location of the associated cervical pathology. It can be differentiated from shoulder pain on the basis of history, physical examination, EMG, cervical radiographs, and myelography or MRI when indicated. Because conditions causing cervical neck pain and those causing shoulder pain, such as calcific tendinitis and cervical radiculopathy, may coexist, it is often difficult to distinguish which lesion is responsible for the symptoms. These conditions can often be differentiated by injection of local anesthetics to block certain components of the pain.

The thoracic outlet is an interval created by the anterior and middle scalene muscles and the first rib through which the brachial plexus and vessels pass to the arm. In thoracic outlet syndrome, compression of these nerves and vessels often manifests as a vague shoulder pain with numbness of the ipsilateral fourth and fifth digits. Cervical rib or hypertrophy of the scalene muscles can be related to the onset of pain.[183-185] Its occurrence has also been related to scapular ptosis, poor posture, and clavicular fracture with malunion or copious callus formation.

BRACHIAL NEURITIS

In the 1940s, Spillane[186] and Parsonage and Turner[187,188] described a painful condition of the shoulder associated with limitation of motion. As the pain subsided and motion improved, muscle weakness and atrophy became apparent. The deltoid, supraspinatus, infraspinatus, biceps, and triceps are the most frequently involved muscles,[189] although diaphragmatic paralysis has also been reported.[188,190] The cause remains unclear, but the clustering of cases suggests a viral or postviral syndrome.[187,188] Occasionally, an associated influenza-like syndrome or previous vaccination has been reported.[189]

Hershman and colleagues[191] described acute brachial neuropathy in athletes. The findings that suggest an acute brachial neuropathy include acute onset of pain without trauma, persistent severe pain that continues despite rest, and patchy neurologic signs. The diagnosis is confirmed by EMG and nerve conduction studies.[191]

The prognosis for recovery is excellent, although full recovery may take 2 to 3 years. Tsairis and associates[192] reported 80 percent recovery within 2 years and more than 90 percent recovery by the end of 3 years.

NERVE ENTRAPMENT SYNDROMES

Peripheral compression neuropathies of the upper extremities may also produce referral pain to the shoulder. Distant compression neuropathies such as carpal tunnel (median nerve) and cubital tunnel (ulnar nerve) syndromes may manifest with concomitant and separate shoulder impingement with rotator cuff disease. Associated numbness and paresthesias with mapping of the dermatomal distribution and with peripheral neuropathy often directs the examiner to the appropriate diagnosis. Patients often give a history of dropping objects and a feeling of clumsiness with the affected hand. A Tinel sign may be elicited over the region of entrapment at the elbow or wrist. Provocative maneuvers such as Phalen's test may be positive and usually indicate median nerve compression at the wrist. Diminished vibratory sensation is an early finding in the disease and is easily reproducible,[193,194] whereas decreased two-point discrimination and intrinsic atrophy are relatively late findings of peripheral compression neuropathy.[193]

The diagnosis can usually be made by clinical examination with exclusion of other possible causes. EMG and nerve conduction velocity tests may reveal slowed conduction and latency at the appropriate compression points to aid in diagnosis. *Spinal accessory nerve* injury with subsequent denervation of the trapezius may cause weakness and pain in the shoulder consistent with impingement. The injury can occur from traction injury to the neck or a direct blow or pressure to the base of the neck. Iatrogenic nerve injury may occur from surgical procedures on the neck such as lymph node biopsy.[195] The injury produces weakness in shoulder abduction with associated pain that radiates from the neck into the trapezius and shoulder. Subsequent atrophy of the trapezius may lead to dysymmetry and ptosis of the involved shoulder, with narrowing of the supraspinatus outlet and secondary impingement with shoulder pain.

Definitive diagnosis can be made by EMG examination. Early treatment is conservative; however, if return of function is not evident at 6 months, surgical exploration of the nerve with possible tendon transfers may be indicated.[196]

Injury to the *long thoracic nerve* (cervical fifth, sixth, and seventh roots) can lead to scapular winging. The resultant scapular dysrhythmia and weakness can lead to a painful shoulder that may mimic rotator cuff disease.[195] Patients also complain of pain and discomfort with active forward flexion of the shoulder. Patients who remain symptomatic after conservative treatment may require surgery for scapulothoracic fusion or tendon transfer using the pectoralis major or minor to stabilize the scapula.[197,198]

In *quadrilateral space syndrome*, the axillary nerve is compressed by fibrous bands in the quadrilateral space.[195,199,200] This typically occurs when the arm is held in abduction and external rotation, with subsequent tightening of the fibrous bands across the nerve.[201] It is most commonly seen in the dominant shoulder of young athletic individuals such as pitchers, tennis players, and swimmers who function with excessive overhead activity. The pain may occur throughout the shoulder girdle and radiate down the arm in a nondermatomal pattern. Neurologic and EMG testing may be normal. Diagnosis is often made by an arteriogram of the subclavian artery. A positive arteriogram reveals compression of the posterior humeral circumflex artery as it traverses the quadrangular space when the arm is in the abducted and externally rotated position. Surgical intervention may be required to release the fibrotic bands or tendon of the teres minor if the patient fails conservative treatment.[195,202]

Suprascapular nerve entrapment syndrome can result from a traction lesion, compression lesion, or both to the nerve caused by tethering of the nerve at the suprascapular notch by the suprascapular ligament or the spinoglenoid notch by the transverse ligament. It can also result from direct compression of a space-occupying lesion such as a ganglion or lipoma. Rengachary and coworkers[203] described variations in the size and shape of the suprascapular notch that may predispose the nerve to entrapment.

The resulting suprascapular neuropathy produces pain in the posterolateral aspect of the shoulder that may radiate into the ipsilateral extremity, shoulder, or side of the neck. Although uncommon, undiagnosed, it can have a prolonged and disabling course. Because the suprascapular nerve has no cutaneous innervation, there is no associated numbness, tingling, or paresthesias. There is usually weakness in abduction and external rotation, and significant atrophy is often noticed at diagnosis. The pain is frequently described as a deep burning or aching that can be well localized and can often be elicited by palpation over the region of the suprascapular notch. Any activity that brings the scapula forward, such as reaching across the chest, may aggravate the pain.[204] The location of the pain and other symptoms can mimic those of more common entities such as impingement, rotator cuff disease, cervical disk disease, brachial neuropathy, biceps tendinitis, thoracic outlet syndrome, acromioclavicular disease, and instability of the shoulder.[205]

Fritz and colleagues[206] reported the efficacy of MRI in the diagnosis of suprascapular nerve entrapment secondary to space-occupying lesions. Definitive diagnosis is made with EMG and nerve conduction studies. EMG changes usually reveal spontaneous activity in the muscle at rest and fibrillations indicating motor atrophy and denervation. Nerve conduction studies may reveal slowing across the site of entrapment. As with axillary nerve entrapment, the syndrome is often associated with young, athletic individuals with excessive overhead activity.[207] However, it has also been associated with trauma.[205,208,209]

There has been a lack of consensus regarding the optimal treatment of suprascapular neuropathy.[6,205,207,210,211] Post and Grinblat[210] reported 25 of 26 cases to have good-to-excellent results with surgical treatment. However, no difference in residual atrophy and strength deficits has been demonstrated for operative and nonoperative treaments. Ferretti and coworkers[207] evaluated 96 top-level volleyball players from the 1985 European Champion-ships and found that 12 had isolated suprascapular neuropathy with atrophy of the infraspinatus of the dominant shoulder. However, all the players were unaware of any impairments and played without limitations. After a space-occupying lesion has been excluded, a 6-month trial of conservative treatment may be indicated for some individuals. If the entrapment does not improve or symptoms worsen with conservative treatment, surgical decompression is warranted for pain relief; however, resolution of atrophy and strength gains can be variable.[205]

STERNOCLAVICULAR ARTHRITIS

Occasionally, traumatic, nontraumatic, or infectious conditions can cause pain about the sternoclavicular joint (see Fig. 38–2). The most common problem is ligamentous injury and painful subluxation or dislocation. This can be diagnosed by palpable instability and crepitus over the sternoclavicular joint. Sternoclavicular views may radiographically demonstrate dislocation.[212]

Inflammatory arthritis of the sternoclavicular joint has been associated with rheumatoid arthritis, ankylosing spondylitis, and septic arthritis. The association of palmoplantar pustulosis and sternoclavicular arthritis has been reported.[213] Seven of the 15 patients who underwent biopsies for this condition had cultures positive for *Propionibacterium acnes*, suggesting an infectious origin of the condition.[213]

Two other conditions involving the sternoclavicular joint are Tietze's syndrome, a painful, nonsuppurative swelling of the joint and adjacent sternochondral junctions, and Friedrich's syndrome, a painful osteonecrosis of the sternal end of the clavicle.[3] Condensing osteitis of the clavicle is a rare benign idiopathic lesion of the medial one third of the clavicle. This condition, better described as aseptic enlarging osteosclerosis of the clavicle, is most commonly seen in middle-aged women and manifests as a tender swelling over the medial one third of the clavicle.[214]

REFLEX SYMPATHETIC DYSTROPHY

Since its original description by Mitchell[215] in 1864, reflex sympathetic dystrophy (RSD) has remained a poorly understood and frequently overlooked condition. Its cause is unknown but may be related to sympathetic overflow or short-circuiting of impulses through the sympathetic system. Any clinician dealing with painful disorders must be familar with the diagnosis and treatment of this condition. Bonica[216] has provided an excellent review, which covers the clinical presentation, various stages of the disease, and importance of early intervention to ensure a successful outcome.

RSD has been confusingly called causalgia, shoulder-hand syndrome, and Sudeck's atrophy. It is generally associated with minor trauma and is to be differentiated from causalgia that involves trauma to major nerve roots.[215] RSD is divided into three phases, which are important in determining treatment.[216] Phase one is characterized by sympathetic overflow with diffuse swelling, pain, increased vascularity, and radiographic evidence of demineralization. If left untreated for 3 to 6 months, this may progress to phase two, which is characterized by atrophy. The extremity may now be cold and shiny, with atrophy of the skin and muscles. Phase three refers to progression of the tropic changes, with irreversible flexion contracture and a pale, cold, painful extremity. It has been speculated that phase one is related to a peripheral short-circuiting of nerve impulses, phase two represents short-circuiting through the internuncial pool in the spinal cord, and phase three is controlled by higher thalamic centers.[216,217]

Steinbrocker[218] reported that recovery is possible as long as there is evidence of vasomotor activity with swelling and hyperemia. After trophic phase two or three is established, the prognosis for recovery is poor. Prompt recognition of the syndrome is important because early intervention to control pain is mandatory. Careful supervision and reassurance are critical because many of these patients are emotionally labile as a result of the pain or an underlying problem. The syndrome may be remarkably reversed by a sympathetic block. Patients who receive transient relief from sympathetic blockade may be helped by surgical sympathectomy.

NEOPLASMS

Primary and metastatic neoplasms may cause shoulder pain by direct invasion of the musculoskeletal system or by compression with referred pain.[2,219] Primary tumors are more likely to occur in younger individuals. The more common lesions have a typical distribution, such as the predilection of a chondroblastoma for the proximal humeral epiphysis or an osteogenic sarcoma for the metaphysis.[220] The differential diagnosis of spontaneous onset of shoulder pain in older individuals should include metastatic lesions and myeloma. Neoplasms are best identified by plain radiographs, MRI, 99mTc-MDP scintigraphy, and CT.

Neoplasms may also involve the shoulder region by metastases to the region. An associated history of carcinomas should alert the examiner to the possibility of a bone tumor, especially those who had malignancies with a predilection for metastasis to bone (e.g., thyroid, renal, lung, prostate, breast). Pain is often present at rest and exacerbated at night. Atypical pain distribution that is not relieved by injection without specific dermatomal distribution should also alert the examiner to the other underlying possibilities. Plain radiographs should be thoroughly evaluated for any cortical destruction or lytic lesions.

Pancoast syndrome or apical lung tumor may present as shoulder pain or cervical radiculitis because of invasion of the brachial plexus or invasion of the C8 or T1 roots.[221-223] With invasion of the cervical sympathetic chain, the patient may also develop Horner's syndrome.

MISCELLANEOUS CONDITIONS

With the increasing numbers of patients undergoing long-term maintainence hemodialysis, a shoulder pain syndrome known as *dialysis shoulder arthropathy* has been described. It consists of shoulder pain, weakness, loss of motion, and functional limitation. The cause and pathogenesis of this syndrome are unclear, although rotator cuff disease, pathologic fracture, bursitis, and local amyloid deposition have been implicated as causative factors.[224] There are insufficient surgical or necropsy data to confirm a specific diagnosis. These patients generally respond poorly to local measures of injection, heat, and NSAIDS, but they may improve with correction of underlying metabolic disorders such as osteomalacia and secondary hyperthyroidism.

REFERENCES

1. Codman EA: The Shoulder: Rupture of the Supraspinatus Tendon and Other Lesions in or About the Subacromial Bursa. Boston, Thomas Todd, 1934.
2. Bateman E: The Shoulder and Neck, 2nd ed. Philadelphia, WB Saunders, 1978.
3. Post M: The Shoulder. Surgical and Non-Surgical Management. Philadelphia, Lea & Febiger, 1988.
4. Caillet R: Shoulder Pain, 2nd ed. Philadelphia, FA Davis, 1981.
5. Greep JM, Lemmens HAJ, Roos DB, Urschel HC: Pain in the Shoulder and Arm: An Integrated View. The Hague, Martinus Nijhoff, 1979.
6. O'Brien SJ, Arnoczky SP, Warren RF: Developmental anatomy of the shoulder and anatomy of the glenohumeral joint. *In* Rockwood CA, Matsen FA III (eds): The Shoulder. Philadelphia, WB Saunders, 1990.
7. Andrews JR, Carson W, McLeod W: Glenoid labrum tears related to the long head of the biceps. Am J Sports Med 13:337, 1985.
8. Martin SD, Warren RF, Martin TL, et al: The non-operative management of suprascapular neuropathy. J Bone Joint Surg Am 79:1159, 1997.
9. Neer CS II: Anterior acromioplasty for the chronic impingement syndrome in the shoulder: A preliminary report. J Bone Joint Surg Am 54:41, 1972.
10. Martin SD, Al-Zahrani SM, Andrews JR, Clancy WG: The circumduction adduction shoulder test. Sixty-third Annual Meeting of the American Academy of Orthopedic Surgeons, Atlanta, Georgia, February 22, 1996.
11. O'Brien SJ, Pagnani MJ, McGlynn SR, et al: A new and effective test for diagnosing labral tears and AC joint pathology. Sixty-third Annual Meeting of the American Academy of Orthopedic Surgeons, Atlanta, Georgia, February 22, 1996.
12. DePalma AF: Surgical anatomy of the acromioclavicular and sternoclavicular joints. Surg Clin North Am 43:1540, 1963.

13. Martin SD, Baumgarten T, Andrews JR: Arthroscopic subacromial decompression with concomitant distal clavicle resection. J Bone Joint Surg Am 85:328, 2001.
14. Dillin L, Hoaglund FT, Scheck M: Brachial neuritis. J Bone Joint Surg Am 67:878, 1985.
15. Kelly BT, Kadrmas WR, Speer KP: The manual muscle examination for rotator cuff strength. Am J Sports Med 24:581, 1996.
16. Saha AK: Theory of Shoulder Mechanism. Springfield, Ill, Charles C Thomas, 1961, p 54.
17. Saha AK: Mechanics of elevation of glenohumeral joint: Its application in rehabilitation of flail shoulder in upper brachial plexus injuries and poliomyelitis and in replacement of the upper humerus by prosthesis. Acta Orthop Scand 44:668, 1973.
18. Brown JT: Early assessment of supraspinatus tears: Procaine infiltration as a guide to treatment. J Bone Joint Surg Br 31:423, 1949.
19. Neer CS: Impingement lesions. Clin Orthop 173:70, 1983.
20. Rockwood CA: The role of anterior impingement in lesions of the rotator cuff. J Bone Joint Surg 62:274, 1980.
21. Jobe FW, Kvitne RS, Giangarra CE: Shoulder pain in the overhead or throwing athlete: The relationship of anterior instability and rotator cuff impingment. Orthop Rev 18:963, 1989.
22. Dalton SE, Snyder SJ: Glenohumeral instability. Baillieres Clin Rheumatol 3:511, 1989.
23. Zanca P: Shoulder pain: Involvement of the acromioclavicular joint (analysis of 1000 cases). AJR Am J Roentgenol 112:493, 1971.
24. Goldman AB: Shoulder Arthrography. Boston, Little, Brown, 1982.
25. Goldman AB, Ghelman B: The double contrast shoulder arthrogram: A review of 158 studies. Radiology 127:655, 1978.
26. Mink J, Harris E: Double contrast shoulder arthrography: Its use in evaluation of rotator cuff tears. Orthop Trans 7:71, 1983.
27. Braunstein EM, O'Connor G: Double-contrast arthrotomography of the shoulder. J Bone Joint Surg Am 64:192, 1982.
28. Ghelman B, Goldman AB: The double contrast shoulder arthrogram: Evaluation of rotator cuff tears. Radiology 124:251, 1977.
29. Goldman AB, Ghelman B: The double contrast shoulder arthrogram. Cardiology 127:665, 1978.
30. Kneisl JS, Sweeney HJ, Paige ML: Correlation of pathology observed in double contrast arthrotomography. Arthroscopy 4:21, 1988.
31. Strizak AM, Danzig L, Jackson DW, et al: Subacromial bursography. J Bone Joint Surg 64:196, 1982.
32. Lie S: Subacromial bursography. Radiology 144:626, 1982.
33. Fukuda H, Mikasa M, Yamanaka K: Incomplete thickness rotator cuff tears diagnosed by subacromial bursography. Clin Orthop 223:51, 1987.
34. Rafii M, Minkoff J, Bonana J, et al: Computed tomography (CT) arthrography of shoulder instabilities in athletes. Am J Sports Med 16:352, 1988.
35. el-Khoury GY, Kathol MH, Chandler JB, Albright JP: Shoulder instability: Impact of glenohumeral arthrotomography on treatment. Radiology 160:669, 1986.
36. Mack LA, Matsen FA, Kilcoyne RF, et al: US evaluation of the rotator cuff. Radiology 157:206, 1985.
37. Crass JR, Craig EV, Bretzke C, Feinberg SB: Ultrasonography of the rotator cuff. Radiographics 5:941, 1985.
38. Harryman DT, Mack LA, Wang KA, et al: Integrity of the postoperative cuff: Ultrasonography and function. Fifty-seventh Annual Meeting of the American Academy of Orthopedic Surgeons, New Orleans, February 9, 1990.
39. Hodler J, Fretz CJ, Terrier F, et al: Rotator cuff tears: Correlation of sonic and surgical findings. Radiology 169:791, 1988.
40. Middleton WD, Edelstein G, Reinus WR, et al: Ultrasonography of the rotator cuff: Technique and normal anatomy. J Ultrasound Med 3:549, 1984.
41. Gardelin G, Perin B: Ultrasonics of the shoulder: Diagnostic possibilities in lesions of the rotator cuff. Radiol Med (Torino) 74:404, 1987.
42. Vestring T, Bongartz G, Konermann W, et al: The place of magnetic resonance tomography in the diagnosis of diseases of the shoulder joint. ROFO. Fortschr Geb Rontgenstr Neuen Bildgeb Verfahr 154:143, 1991.
43. Ahovuo J, Paavolainen P, Slatis P: Diagnostic value of sonography in lesions of the biceps tendon. Clin Orthop 202:184, 1986.
44. Ogilvie-Harris DJ, D'Angelo G: Arthroscopic surgery of the shoulder. Sports Med 9:120, 1990.
45. Ellman H: Arthroscopic subacromial decompression. Orthop Trans 9:49, 1985.
46. Ellman H: Arthroscopic subacromial decompression: Analysis of one- to three-year results. Arthroscopy 3:173, 1987.
47. Paulos LE, Franklin JL: Arthroscopic shoulder decompression development and application: A five year experience. Am J Sports Med 17:235, 1990.
48. Zlatkin MB, Reicher MA, Kellerhouse LE, et al: The painful shoulder: MRI imaging of the glenohumeral joint. J Comput Assist Tomogr 12:995, 1988.
49. Meyer SJ, Dalinka MK: Magnetic resonance imaging of the shoulder. Orthop Clin North Am 21:497, 1990.
50. Seeger LL, Gold RH, Bassett LW: Shoulder instability: Evaluation with MR imaging. Radiology 168:696, 1988.
51. Kieft GJ, Dijkmans BA, Bioem JL, Kroon HM: Magnetic resonance imaging of the shoulder in patients with rheumatoid arthritis. Ann Rheum Dis 49:7, 1990.
52. Morrison DS, Offstein R: The use of magnetic resonance imaging in the diagnosis of rotator cuff tears. Orthopedics 13:633, 1990.
53. Nelson MC, Leather GP, Nirschl RP, el al: Evaluation of the painful shoulder: A prospective comparision of magnetic resonance imaging, computerized tomographic arthrography. J Bone Joint Surg Am 73:707, 1991.
54. Reeder JD, Andelman S: The rotator cuff tear: MR evaluation. Magn Reson Imaging 5:331, 1987.
55. Seeger LL, Gold RH, Bassett LW, Ellman H: Shoulder impingement syndrome: MR findings in 53 shoulders. AJR Am J Roentgenol 150:343, 1988.
56. Nakano KK: Neurology of Musculoskeletal and Rheumatic Disorders. Boston, Houghton Mifflin, 1979.
57. Leffert RD: Brachial plexus injuries. N Engl J Med 291:1059, 1974.
58. Altchek DW, Schwartz E, Warren RF, et al: Radiologic measurement of superior migration of the humeral head in impingement syndrome. Sixth Open Meeting of the American Shoulder and Elbow Surgeons, New Orleans, February 11, 1990.
59. Inman VT, Saunders JB, Abbott LC: Observations on the functions of the shoulder joint. J Bone Joint Surg 26:1, 1944.
60. Poppen NK, Walker PS: Normal and abnormal motion of the shoulder. J Bone Joint Surg Am 58:195, 1976.
61. Bigliani LU, Morrison D, April EW: The morphology of the acromion and its relationship to rotator cuff tears. Orthop Trans 10:228, 1986.
62. Morrison DS, Bigliani LU: The clinical significance of variations in acromial morphology. Orthop Trans 11:234, 1987.
63. Codman E, Akerson TB: The pathology associated with rupture of the supraspinatus tendon. Ann Surg 93:354, 1911.
64. Fukuda H, Hamada K, Yamanaka K: Pathology and pathogenisis of bursal side rotator cuff tears: Views from en-bloc histological sections. Clin Orthop 254:75, 1990.
65. McLaughlin HL: Lesions of the musculotendinous cuff of the shoulder. I. The exposure and treatment of tears with retraction. J Bone Joint Surg 26:31, 1944.
66. Neer CS II, Flatow EL, Lech O: Tears of the rotator cuff: Long term results of anterior acromioplasty and repair. Fourth Open Meeting of the American Shoulder and Elbow Surgeons, Atlanta, February 1988.
67. Ogata S, Uhthoff HK: Acromial enthesopathy and rotator cuff tears: A radiographic and histiologic postmortem investigation of the coracoacromial arch. Clin Orthop 254:39, 1990.
68. Olsson O: Degenerative changes in the shoulder joint and their connection with shoulder pain: A morphological and clinical investigation with special attention to the cuff and biceps tendon. Acta Chir Scand 181(Suppl):1, 1953.
69. Ozaki J, Fujimoto S, Nakagawa Y, et al: Tears of the rotator cuff of the shoulder associated with pathologic changes of the acromion: A study in cadavers. J Bone Joint Surg 70:1224, 1988.
70. Skinner HA: Anatomical consideration relative to ruptures of the supraspinatus tendon. J Bone Joint Surg Br 19:137, 1937.
71. Ellman H: Occupational supraspinatus tendinitis: The rotator cuff syndrome. Ugeskr Laeger 151:2355, 1989.
72. Scheib JS: Diagnosis and rehabilitation of the shoulder impingement syndrome in the overhand and throwing athlete. Rheum Dis Clin North Am 16:971, 1990.

73. Jackson DW: Chronic rotator cuff impingement in the throwing athlete. Am J Sports Med 4:231, 1976.
74. Hawkins RJ, Kennedy JC: Impingement syndrome in athletes. Am J Sports Med 8:151, 1980.
75. McShane RB, Leinberry CF, Fenlin JM: Conservative open anterior acromioplasty. Clin Orthop 223:137, 1987.
76. Rockwood CA, Lyons FA: Shoulder impingement syndrome: Diagnosis, radiographic evaluation, and treatment with a modified Neer acromioplasty. J Bone Joint Surg Am 75:1593, 1993.
77. Hawkins RJ, Brock RM, Abrams JS, Hobeika P: Acromioplasty for impingement with an intact rotator cuff. J Bone Joint Surg Br 70:797, 1988.
78. Stuart MJ, Azevedo AJ, Cofield RH: Anterior acromioplasty for treatment of the shoulder impingement syndrome. Clin Orthop 260:195, 1990.
79. Bigliani LU, D'Alesandro DF, Dduralde XA, McLveen SJ: Anterior acromioplasty for subacromial impingement in patients younger than 40 years of age. Clin Orthop 246:111, 1988.
80. Bjorkheim JM, Paavolainen P, Ahovuo J, Slatis P: Surgical repair of the rotator cuff and the surrounding tissues: Factors influencing the results. Clin Orthop 236:148, 1988.
81. Levy HJ, Gardner RD, Lemak LJ: Arthroscopic subacromial decompression in the treatment of full-thickness rotator cuff tears. Arthroscopy 7:8, 1991.
82. McKendry RJR, Uhthoff HK, Sarkar K, Hyslop P: Calcifying tendinitis of the shoulder: Prognostic value of clinical, histologic, and radiographic features in 57 surgically treated cases. J Rheumatol 9:75, 1982.
83. Uhthoff HK, Sarkar K, Maynard JA: Calcifying tendinitis, a new concept of its pathogenesis. Clin Orthop 118:164, 1976.
84. Sarkar K, Uhthoff HK: Ultrastructure localization of calcium in calcifying tendinitis. Arch Pathol Lab Med 102:266, 1978.
85. Hayes CW, Conway WF: Calcium hydroxyapatite deposition disease. Radiographics 10:1031, 1990.
86. Vebostad A: Calcific tendinitis in the shoulder region: A review of 43 operated shoulders. Acta Orthop Scand 46:205, 1975.
87. Moseley HF, Goldie I: The arterial pattern of the rotator cuff of the shoulder. J Bone Joint Surg Br 45:780, 1963.
88. Rathburn JB, Macnab I: The microvascular pattern of the rotator cuff. J Bone Joint Surg Br 52:540, 1970.
89. Bosworth BM: Calcium deposits in the shoulder and subacromial bursitis: A survey of 12,122 shoulders. JAMA 116:2477, 1941.
90. Bosworth BM: Examination of the shoulder for calcium deposits. J Bone Joint Surg 23:567, 1941.
91. DePalma AF, Kruper JS: Long term study of shoulder joints afflicted with and treated for calcified tendonitis. Clin Orthop 20:61, 1961.
92. Linblom K: Arthrography and roentgenography in ruptures of the tendon of the shoulder joint. Acta Radiol 20:548, 1939.
93. Swiontkowski M, Iannotti JP, Herrmann HJ, et al: Intraoperative assessment of rotator cuff vascularity using laser Doppler flowmetry. *In* Post M, Morrey BE, Hawkins RJ (eds): Surgery of the Shoulder. St. Louis, Mosby, 1990, pp 208-212.
94. Matsen FA III, Arntz CT: Subacromial impingment. *In* Rockwood CA Jr, Matsen FA III (eds): The Shoulder. Philadelphia, WB Saunders, 1990, pp 623-646.
95. Neer CS II, Poppen NK: Supraspinatus outlet. Orthop Trans 11:234, 1987.
96. Clark J, Sidles JA, Matsen FA: The relationship of the glenohumeral joint capsule to the rotator cuff. Clin Orthop 254:29, 1990.
97. Samilson RL, Raphael RL, Post L, et al: Arthrography of the shoulder. Clin Orthop 20:21, 1961.
98. Collins RA, Gristina AG, Carter RE, et al: Ultrasonography of the shoulder. Orthop Clin North Am 18:351, 1987.
99. Crass JR, Craig EV, Feinberg SB: Ultrasonography of rotator cuff tears: A review of 500 diagnostic studies. J Clin Ultrasound 16:313, 1988.
100. Crass JR, Craig EV, Feinberg SB: The hyperextended internal rotation view in rotator cuff ultrasonography. J Clin Ultrasound 15:415, 1987.
101. Mack LA, Gannon MK, Kilcoyne RF, et al: Sonographic evaluation of the rotator cuff: Accuracy in patients without prior surgery. Clin Orthop 234:21, 1988.
102. Iannotti JP, Zlatkin MB, Esterhai JL, et al: Magnetic resonance imaging of the shoulder: Sensitivity, specificity, and predictive value. J Bone Joint Surg Am 73:17, 1991.
103. DePalma AF: Surgery of the Shoulder, 2nd ed. Philadelphia, JB Lippincott, 1973.
104. Wolfgang GL: Surgical repair of tears of the rotator cuff of the shoulder: Factors influencing the result. J Bone Joint Surg Am 56:14, 1974.
105. Jobe FW, Moynes DR: Delineation of diagnostic criteria and a rehabilitation program for rotator cuff injuries. Am J Sports Med 10:336, 1982.
106. Earnshaw P, Desjardins D, Sakar K, Uhthoff HK: Rotator cuff tears: The role of surgery. Can J Surg 25:60, 1982.
107. Rockwood CA, Williams GR, Burkhead WZ: Debridement of massive, degenerative lesions of the rotator cuff. Seventh open meeting of the American Shoulder and Elbow Society Surgeons, Anaheim, California, March 10, 1991.
108. Martin SD, Andrews JR: The rotator cuff: Open and mini-open repairs. American Orthopaedic Society for Sports Medicine 20th Annual Meeting, Palm Desert, June 26, 1994.
109. Rockwood CA Jr: The shoulder: Facts, confusion and myths. Int Orthop 15:401, 1991.
110. Steffens K, Konermann H: Rupture of the rotator cuff in the elderly. Z Gerontol 20:95, 1987.
111. Goss CM: Gray's Anatomy of the Human Body, 28th ed. Philadelphia, Lea & Febiger, 1966.
112. Neer CS, Craig EV, Fukuda H: Cuff tear arthropathy. J Bone Joint Surg Am 65:1232, 1983.
113. Neer CS II, Bigliani LU, Hawkins RJ: Rupture of the long head of the biceps related to subacromial impingement. Orthop Trans 1:111, 1977.
114. Crenshaw AH, Kilgore WE: Surgical treatment of bicipital tendonitis. J Bone Joint Surg Am 48:1496, 1966.
115. Hitchcock HH, Bechtol CO: Painful shoulder: Observations on the role of the tendon of the long head of the biceps brachii in its causation. J Bone Joint Surg Am 30:263, 1948.
116. Meyer AW: Spontaneous dislocation and destruction of the tendon of the long head of the biceps brachii, fifty-nine instances. Arch Surg 17:493, 1928.
117. Rockwood RA Jr, Williams GR, Young CD: Injuries to the acromioclavicular joint. *In* Rockwood CA Jr, Green DP, Bucholz RW (eds): Fractures in Adults. Philadelphia, JB Lippincott, 1991, pp 1181-1251.
118. Jacobs P: Post-traumatic osteolysis of the outer end of the clavicle. J Bone Joint Surg Br 46:705, 1964.
119. Murphy OB, Bellamy R, Wheeler W, Brower TD: Post-traumatic osteolysis of the distal clavicle. Clin Orthop 109:108, 1975.
120. Cahill RB: Osteolysis of the distal part of the clavicle in male athletes. J Bone Joint Surg Am 64:1053, 1982.
121. Maden B: Osteolysis of the acromial end of the clavicle following trauma. Br J Radiol 36:822, 1963.
122. Scavenius M, Iversen BF: Nontraumatic clavicular osteolysis in weight lifters. Am J Sports Med 20:463, 1992.
123. Slawski DP, Cahill BR Atraumatic osteolysis of the distal clavicle. Am J Sports Med 22:267, 1994.
124. Meyers JF: Arthroscopic debridement of the acromioclavicular joint and distal clavicle resection. *In* McGinty JB, Caspari RB, Jackson RW, et al (eds): Operative Arthroscopy. New York, Raven Press, 1991, pp 557-560.
125. Cahill BR, Lee MT: Atraumatic osteolysis of the distal clavicle. *In* Torg JS, Shephard RJ (eds): Current Therapy in Sports Medicine. St. Louis, Mosby, 1995, pp 177-181.
126. Rockwood CA Jr: Disorders of the acromioclavicular joint. *In* Rockwood CA Jr, Matsen FA III (eds): The Shoulder. Philadelphia, WB Saunders, 1985, p 449.
127. Gartsman GM, Combs AH, Davis PF, Tullos HS: Arthroscopic acromioclavicular joint resection: An anatomic study. Am J Sports Med 19:2-5, 1991.
128. Fink EP: Injuries to the acromioclavicular joint. *In* Torg JS, Shephard RJ (eds): Current Therapy in Sports Medicine. St. Louis, Mosby, 1995, pp 174-177.
129. Gartsman GM: Arthroscopic resection of the acromioclavicular joint. Am J Sports Med 21:71, 1993.
130. Flatow EL, Cordasco FA, Bigliani LU: Arthroscopic resection of the outer end of the clavicle from a superior approach: A

critical, quantitative, radiographic assessment of bone removal. Arthroscopy 8:55, 1992.
131. Flatow EL, Duralde XA, Nicholson GP, et al: Arthroscopic resection of the distal clavicle with a superior approach. J Shoulder Elbow Surg 4:41, 1995.
132. Worcester JN, Green DP: Osteoarthritis of the acromioclavicular joint. Clin Orthop 58:69, 1987.
133. DePalma AF: The role of the disks of the sternoclavicular and acromioclavicular joints. Clin Orthop 13:222, 1959.
134. Novack PJ, Bach BB, Romeo AA, Hager CA: Surgical resection of the distal clavicle. J Shoulder Elbow Surg 4:35, 1995.
135. Gurd FB: The treatment of complete dislocation of the outer end of the clavicle. A hitherto undescribed operation. Ann Surg 63:1094, 1941.
136. Mumford EB: Acromioclavicular dislocation: A new operative treatment. J Bone Joint Surg Am 23:799, 1941.
137. Cook FF, Tibone JE: The Mumford procedure in athletes: An objective analysis of function. Am J Sports Med 16:97, 1988.
138. Bigliani LU, Nicholson GP, Flatow EL: Arthroscopic resection of the distal clavicle. Orthop Clin North Am 24:133, 1993.
139. Gartsman GM, Combs AH, Davis PF, Tullos HS: Arthroscopic acromioclavicular joint resection: An anatomic study. Am J Sports Med 19:2, 1991.
140. Kay SP, Ellman H, Harris E: Arthroscopic distal clavicle resection: Technique and early results. Clin Orthop 301:181, 1994.
141. Tolin BS, Snyder SJ: Our technique for the arthroscopic Mumford procedure. Orthop Clin North Am 24:143, 1993.
142. Cofield RH, Briggs BT: Glenohumeral arthrodesis. J Bone Joint Surg Am 61:668, 1979.
143. Rowe CR: Arthrodesis of the shoulder used in treating painful conditions. Clin Orthop 173:92, 1983.
144. Neer CS II, Watson KC, Stanton FJ: Recent experience in total shoulder replacement. J Bone Joint Surg Am 64:319, 1982.
145. Cofield RH: Unconstrained total shoulder prosthesis. Clin Orthop 173:97, 1983.
146. Thornhill TS, Karr MJ, Averill RM, et al: Total shoulder arthroplasty, the Brigham experience. Fiftieth Annual Meeting of the American Academy of Orthopedic Surgeons, Anaheim, 1983.
147. Thornhill TS, Barrett WP: Total shoulder arthroplasty. *In* Rowe CR (ed): The Shoulder. New York, Churchill Livingstone, 1988.
148. Neer CS II: Fractures and dislocations of the shoulder. *In* Rockwood CA, Green DP (eds): Fractures. Philadelphia, JB Lippincott, 1975.
149. Ficat RP, Arlet J: Ischemia and Necrosis of the Bone. Baltimore, Williams & Wilkins, 1980.
150. Hayes JM: Arthroscopic treatment of steroid-induced osteonecrosis of the humeral head. Arthroscopy 5:218, 1989.
151. McCarty DJ: Robert Adams' rheumatic arthritis of the shoulder: "Milwaukee shoulder" revisited. J Rheumatol 32:668, 1989.
152. Halverson PB, Carrera GF, McCarty DJ: Milwaukee shoulder syndrome: Fifteen additional cases and a description of contributing factors. Arch Intern Med 150:677, 1990.
153. Wortmann RL, Veum JA, Rachow JW: Synovial fluid 5-nucleotidase activity: Relationship to other purine catabolic enzymes and to arthropathies associated to calcium deposition disease. Arthritis Rheum 34:1014, 1991.
154. Neer CS II, Craig EV, Fukada H, Mendoza FX: Cuff tear arthropathy. Exhibit at the Annual Meeting of the American Academy of Orthopedic Surgeons, New Orleans, 1982.
155. Post M, Haskell SS, Jablon M: Total shoulder replacement with a constrained prosthesis. J Bone Joint Surg Am 62:327, 1980.
156. Post M, Jablon M: Constrained total shoulder arthroplasty: Long term follow-up observations. Clin Orthop 173:109, 1983.
157. Hamada K, Fukuda H, Mikasa M, Kobayashi Y: Roentgenographic findings in rotator cuff tears: A long-term observation. Clin Orthop 254:92, 1990.
158. Snyder SJ, Karzel RP, Del Pizzo W, et al: SLAP lesions of the shoulder. Arthroscopy 6:274, 1990.
159. Burkhart SS, Fox DL: SLAP lesions in association with complete tears of the long head of the biceps tendon: A report of two cases. Arthroscopy 8:31, 1992.
160. Maffet MW, Gartsman GM, Moseley B: Superior labrum-biceps tendon complex lesions of the shoulder. Am J Sports Med 23:93, 1995.
161. Grauer JD, Paulos LE, Smutz WP: Biceps tendon and superior labral injuries. Arthroscopy 8:488, 1992.
162. Putman JJ: The treatment of a form of painful periarthritis of the shoulder. Boston Med Surg J 107:536, 1882.
163. Neviaser JS: Adhesive capsulitis of the shoulder: Study of the pathologic findings in periarthritis of the shoulder. J Bone Joint Surg 27:211, 1945.
164. McLaughlin HL: The "frozen shoulder." Clin Orthop 20:126, 1961.
165. Johnson JTH: Frozen shoulder syndrome in patients with pulmonary tuberculosis. J Bone Joint Surg Am 41:877, 1959.
166. Dee PE, Smith RG, Gullickson MJ, Ballinger CS: The orthopedist and apical lung carcinoma. J Bone Joint Surg Am 42:605, 1960.
167. Demaziere A, Wiley AM: Primary chest wall tumor appearing as frozen shoulder: Review and case presentations. J Rheumatol 18:911, 1991.
168. Smith CR, Binder AI, Paice EW: Lesions of the mid-shaft of the humerus presenting as shoulder capsulitis. Br J Rheumatol 29:386, 1990.
169. Dickson JA, Crosby EH: Periarthritis of the shoulder: An analysis of two hundred cases. JAMA 99:2252, 1932.
170. McLaughlin HL: On the frozen shoulder. Bull Hosp Joint Dis 12:383, 1951.
171. Lundberg BJ: The frozen shoulder. Acta Orthop Scand 119:59, 1969.
172. Rowe CR, Leffert RD: Idiopathic chronic adhesive capsulitis. *In* Rowe CR (ed): The Shoulder. New York, Churchhill Livingstone, 1988, pp 155-163.
173. Coventry MB: Problem of the painful shoulder. JAMA 151:177, 1953.
174. Waldburger M, Meier JL, Gobelet C: The frozen shoulder: Diagnosis and treatment. Clin Rheumatol 11:364, 1992.
175. Fareed DO, Gallivan WR Jr: Office management of frozen shoulder syndrome: Treatment with hydraulic distention under local anesthesia. Clin Orthop 242:177, 1989.
176. Rizk TE, Pinalls RA, Talaiver AS: Corticosteroid injections in adhesive capsulitis: Investigation of their value and site. Arch Phys Med Rehabil 72:20, 1991.
177. Hill JJ Jr, Bogumill H: Manipulation in the treatment of frozen shoulder. Orthopedics 11:1255, 1988.
178. Rowe CR: Dislocations of the shoulder. *In* Rowe CR (ed): The Shoulder. New York, Churchill Livingstone, 1988.
179. Fu FH, Harner CD, Klein AH: Shoulder impingement syndrome: A clinical review. Clin Orthop 269:162, 1991.
180. Walch G, Bioleau P, Noel E: Impingement of the deep surface of the supraspinatus tendon on the posterosuperior glenoid rim: An arthroscopic study. J Shoulder Elbow Surg 1:238, 1992.
181. Altchek DW, Warren RF, Ortiz G: T-plasty: A technique for treating multidirectional instability in the athlete. Orthop Trans 13:560, 1989.
182. Neer CS, Foster CR: Inferior capsular shift for involuntary and multidirectional instability of the shoulder: A preliminary report. J Bone Joint Surg Am 62:897, 1980.
183. Roos DB: Congenitial anomalies associated with thoracic outlet syndrome: Anatomy, symptoms, diagnosis and treatment. Am J Surg 132:771, 1976.
184. Leffert RD: Thoracic outlet syndrome. *In* Gelberman RH (ed): Operative Nerve Repair and Reconstruction. New York, JB Lippincott, 1991, pp 1177-1195.
185. Urschel HC, Paulson DL, MacNamara JJ: Thoracic outlet syndrome. Ann Thorac Surg 6:1, 1968.
186. Spillane JD: Localized neuritis of the shoulder girdle: A report of 46 cases in the MEF. Lancet 2:532, 1943.
187. Parsonage MJ, Turner JWA: Neurologic amyotrophy: The shoulder girdle syndrome. Lancet 1:1973, 1948.
188. Turner JWA, Parsonage MJ: Neurologic amyotrophy (paralytic brachial neuritis): With special reference to prognosis. Lancet 2:209, 1957.
189. Bacevich BB: Paralytic brachial neuritis. J Bone Joint Surg Am 58:262, 1976.
190. Walsh NE, Dumitru D, Kalantri A, Roman AM Jr: Brachial neuritis involving the bilateral phrenic nerves. Arch Phys Med Rehabil 68:46, 1987.
191. Hershman EB, Wilbourn AJ, Bergfield JA: Acute brachial neuropathy in athletes. Am J Sports Med 17:655, 1989.
192. Tsairis P, Dyck PJ, Mulder DW: Natural history of brachial plexus neuropathy. Arch Neurol 27:109, 1972.

193. Szabo RM: Carpal tunnel syndromeÆgeneral. *In* Gelberman RH (ed): Operative Nerve Repair and Reconstruction. New York, JB Lippincott, 1991, pp 869-888.
194. Slater RR, Bynum DK: Diagnosis and treatment of carpal tunnel syndrome. Orthop Rev 22:1095, 1993.
195. Narakas AO: Compression and traction neuropathies about the shoulder and arm. *In* Gelberman RH (ed): Operative Nerve Repair and Reconstruction. New York, JB Lippincott, 1991, pp 1147-1175.
196. Bigliani L, Perez-Sanz JR, Wolfe IN: Treatment of trapezius paralysis. J Bone Joint Surg 67:871, 1985.
197. Chavez JP: Pectoralis minor transplanted for paralysis of the serratus anterior. J Bone Joint Surg Br 33:21, 1951.
198. Marmor L, Bechtal CO: Paralysis of the serratus anterior due to electric shock relieved by transplantation of the pectoralis major muscle: A case report. J Bone Joint Surg 45:156, 1983.
199. Cahill BR, Palmer RE: Quadrilateral space syndrome. J Hand Surg 8:65, 1983.
200. Jobe FW, Tibone JE: The shoulder in sports. *In* Rockwood CA, Matsen FA (eds): The Shoulder. Philadelphia, WB Saunders, 1990, pp 961-990.
201. Cahill BR: Quadrilateral space syndrome. *In* Omer GE Jr, Spinner MD (eds): Management of Peripheral Nerve Problems. Philadelphia, WB Saunders, 1980, pp 56-65.
202. Bretzke CA, Crass JR, Craig EV, Feinberg SB: Ultrasonography of the rotator cuff: Normal and pathologic anatomy. Invest Radiol 20:311, 1985.
203. Rengachary SS, Neft JP, Singer PA, Brackett CE: Suprascapular entrapement neuropathy: A clinical, anatomical and comparative study. Neurosurgery 5:441, 1979.
204. Habermeyer P, Rappaport D, Wiedermann E, Wilhelm K: Incisura scapulae syndrome. Handchir Mikrochir Plast Chir 22:120, 1990.
205. Martin SD, Warren RF, Martin TL, et al: Suprascapular neuropathy. J Bone Joint Surg Am 79:1159, 1997.
206. Fritz RC, Helms CA, Steinbach LS, Genant HK: Suprascapular nerve entrapment: Evaluation with MR imaging. Radiology 182:437, 1992.
207. Ferretti A, Cerullo G, Russo G: Suprascapular neuropathy in volleyball players. J Bone Joint Surg Am 69:260, 1987.
208. Rask MR: Suprascapular nerve entrapment: A report of two cases treated with suprascapular notch resection. Clin Orthop 123:73, 1977.
209. Solheim LF, Roaas A: Compression of the suprascapular nerve after fracture of the suprascapular notch. Acta Orthop Scand 49:338, 1978.
210. Post M, Grinblat E: Suprascapular nerve entrapment: Diagnosis and results of treatment. J Shoulder Elbow Surg 2:197, 1993.
211. Hadley MN, Sonntag VK, Pittman HW: Suprascapular nerve entrapment: A summary of seven cases. J Neurosurg 64:843, 1986.
212. Rockwood CA Jr: Fractures and dislocations of the shoulder. Part II. *In* Rockwood CA Jr, Green DP (eds): Fractures. Philadelphia, JB Lippincott, 1975, pp 262-270.
213. Edlund E, Johnsson U, Lidgren L, et al: Palmoplantar pustulosis and sternocostoclavicular arthro-osteitis. Ann Rheum Dis 47:809, 1988.
214. Lissens M, Bruyninckx F, Rossele N: Condensing osteitis of the clavicle: Report of two cases and review of the literature. Acta Belg Med Phys 13:235, 1990.
215. Mitchell SW: Phantom limbs. Lippincott 8:563, 1871.
216. Bonica JJ: Causalgia and other reflex dystrophies. *In* Bonica JJ (ed): Management of Pain. Philadelphia, Lea & Febiger, 1979, pp 139-142.
217. Evans JA: Reflex sympathetic dystrophy. Surg Gynecol Obstet 82:36, 1946.
218. Steinbrocker O: The shoulder-hand syndrome: Present perspective. Arch Phys Med 49:388, 1968.
219. Brown C: Compressive invasive referred pain to the shoulder. Clin Orthop 173:55, 1983.
220. Dahlin DC: Bone Tumors. Springfield, Ill, Charles C, Thomas, 1978.
221. DePalma AF: Loss of scapulohumeral motion. Ann Surg 135:193, 1952.
222. Pancoast HK: Importance of careful roentgen ray investigation of apical chest tumors. JAMA 83:1407, 1923.
223. Vargo MM, Flood KM: Pancoast tumor presenting as cervical radiculopathy. Arch Phys Med Rehabil 71:606, 1990.
224. Brown EA, Arnold LR, Gower PE: Dialysis arthropathy: Complication of long term treatment with haemodialysis. BMJ 292:163, 1986.

39 Low Back Pain

DEVIN DATTA • SOHAIL K. MIRZA • AUGUSTUS A. WHITE III

Idiopathic low back pain is a classic example of a disorder with a large burden of illness; it accounts for a large share of our society's health problems.[1] Low back pain ranks second only to upper respiratory infection as the ailment prompting the most visits to physicians.[2] A precise diagnosis cannot be determined for up to 80 percent of patients presenting with low back pain.[3] A person presenting to a primary care setting with acute low back pain has a 0.2-percent probability of the pain having a specific, treatable cause.[4] There is little consensus among physicians about the effectiveness of commonly used treatments for low back pain. Correlation between treatments physicians believe are effective and those that have been found effective by well-designed studies is poor.[5] It must be emphasized that the direct and indirect costs attributable to chronic back pain each year are very large.

Epidemiology

PREVALENCE

Lifetime incidence for low back pain in the general population is 60 to 70 percent.[6] Low back pain results in an average of 2.8 office visits per affected person.[7] Eighty-four percent of patients with low back symptoms seek consultation with a physician, and 31 percent consult a chiropractor.[8] Using strict diagnostic criteria for radicular pain, lifetime prevalence of sciatica is 5 percent for men and 4 percent for women. Twelve percent of patients with low back pain have sciatica.

RISK FACTORS

Risk factors for low back pain have been studied by Frymoyer and colleagues[9] and Pope and coworkers.[10] They noted that heavy lifting, use of jack hammers, driving motor vehicles, jogging, crosscountry skiing, weaker trunk strength, and smoking were associated with an increased risk of back pain. They found no association with height, weight, body-mass index, lumbar lordosis, or leg-length inequality. In an evidence-based review, an association was noted between some types of "whole body vibrations" for prolonged periods, frequent bending and twisting of the trunk, frequent heavy lifting, and poor psychosocial conditions, including poor job satisfaction, with low back pain.[11] A 1.7 higher prevalence has been found in comparisons of the highest quintile with lowest quintile of body-mass index.[12] This supports the popular notion that obesity is related to back pain. Cigarette smoking, in addition to all the other pathology it induces or accentuates, is also a risk factor for back pain.[13]

Relative risk of men to women is 5.6 at age 20 years and decreases to 1.8 at age 60 years.[14] Frequent lifting of heavy objects or or children weighing more than 25 pounds was associated with a relative risk of 3.95 for lumbar disk herniation.[15] Spinal stenosis is a risk factor for low back pain, particularly when the space available for the cauda equina is diminished by 50 percent (to approximately 70 mm^2).[16,17] Numerous studies have implicated other risk factors. Many are difficult to interpret due to the high prevalence of back pain in the general population. An historic review by Allan and Waddell concluded that human beings have had back pain all through history, and it is currently no more common or severe than it has always been.[18]

Sports

Bowling, golf, baseball, and skiing have been associated with increased risk of low back pain.[19] Jogging and crosscountry skiing have also been associated with low back pain.[9,10] Flexibility or lack of flexibility is not a risk factor.[19] Unfortunately, and somewhat surprisingly, physical fitness may not change the prevalence of back pain, but it has been identified as an adjunct to improve recovery from back pain.[19]

Industrial Injuries

Back injuries account for 15 to 22 percent of all industrial injuries.[19] Seventy-five percent of all compensation payments in the United States go to patients with low back pain, who constitute only 3 percent of all individuals receiving those benefits.[20] In aircraft-industry workers,[21-24] it has been calculated that back injuries were reported by 2 percent of all employees and represented 19 percent of all worker's compensation claims.[24] In a prospective study of 3020 workers over 4 years, the factors most predictive of a future report of a back injury were history of current or recent back problems, work perceptions, and certain responses on the Minnesota Multiphasic Personality Inventory (MMPI), an assessment of psychologic profile.[22]

A study of work-related back injuries in the United Kingdom showed that mining was associated with the highest prevalence of back-injury reports.[25] Overall incidence of back injury claims was 1.8 per 1000 people per year, compared to 28.3 per 1000 people for those in mining. Construction workers reported an average of 7.7 injuries per 1000 people, and transportation workers reported 7.5 per 1000. The Quebec Task Force on Spinal Disorders reported an incidence rate of 4.9 percent per year in forestry workers, compared to 2 percent for transportation workers and less than 0.5 percent for insurance workers.[14]

Frymoyer[26] reviewed work-related back pain and noted that 70.9 percent of worker's compensation patients associated the onset of their symptoms with a specific event, compared to 35.5 percent of patients not on worker's compensation.

Biology

The pathophysiology of back pain remains unclear. Substance P, a known chemical mediator of pain, has been identified in the posterior longitudinal ligament nerve endings, and it has been postulated that substance P is involved in the primary transmission of pain in low back pain syndromes.[27] A review of the pathophysiology of low back pain has led to the conclusion[28] that some chemical event in the course of disk degeneration and herniation is necessary to produce low back pain and sciatica. Olmarker and Rydevik[29] also concluded that pain may be produced by a combination of mechanic deformation and chemical irritation by agents from surrounding structures, and in particular, from the intervertebral disk. The chemical mediators involved in the transmission of spinal pain, and presumably involved in back pain,[30] are listed in Table 39–1.

An increased intraosseous pressure in vertebral bodies, lower pH, and increased Pco_2 in patients with low back pain has been linked with abnormal magnetic resonance imaging (MRI) signal in the sampled vertebrae, and it has been concluded that abnormalities of intraosseous pressure or blood gas concentrations may be related to mechanisms of pain production in some patients with low back pain.[31]

Hypertonic saline injection of the interspinous ligaments produces low back pain in healthy volunteers.[32] Others have noted that saline injection of the facet joints in the lumbar spine produced sclerotomal back pain and hamstring spasm, both of which are relieved by local-anesthetic injection of the facet joint.[33] Kuslich and colleagues[34] attempted to identify pain generators in the lumbar spine by sequentially stimulating structures during lumbar surgery under progressive local anesthesia. They concluded that the outer annulus is the tissue of origin in most cases of low back pain. The frequency of pain provocation by location of stimulus in that study is listed in Table 39–2.

The disk is commonly considered to be a pain generator in idiopathic low back pain.[35] An animal model for disk injury as an initiating event leading to pain and disk degeneration has been developed.[36] Segmental lumbar instability is thought to provide the stimulus for disk degeneration and irritation.[37] Pain reproduced by injection of contrast material into the disk in diskography is considered to confirm a diskogenic pain source in patients with back pain.[38] This issue, however, continues to be the focus of intense investigation, and diskography as a diagnostic procedure remains controversial.[39,40]

TABLE 39–1 • CHEMICAL MEDIATORS IN SPINAL PAIN

Chemical Mediators of Pain		Mechanisms for Central Modulation of Pain
Neurogenic	*Nonneurogenic*	
Substance P Somatostatin Cholecystokinin Vasoactive intestinal peptide Calcitonin gene-related peptide Gastrin-releasing peptide Dynorphin Enkephalin Galanin B4	Bradykinin Serotonin Histamine Acetylcholine Prostaglandins E1 (blocked by NSAIDs) E2 Leukotrienes diHETE (not blocked by NSAIDS)	Dorsal horn → thalamus → post-central gyrus Frontal lobe → affect input Temporal lobe → memory input β-endorphins → μ receptors Dynorphins → κ receptors

Abbreviation: NSAIDs, nonsteroidal anti-inflammatory drugs.

Back pain has also been attributed to sacroiliac joint pathology. Back pain symptoms have been reproduced by sacroiliac joint contrast injection, and these pains have been relieved by subsequent injection of local anesthetic.[41] Clinicians concluded that the sacroiliac joint–related pain was present in 13 to 30 percent of patients with low back pain.

TABLE 39–2 • SOURCE OF PAIN IN LOW BACK SYNDROMES

Frequency of Pain Production with Stimulation
Always Produced Pain
Skin Compressed nerve root
Often Produced Pain
Outer annulus fibrosus Vertebral end plate Tissues in anterior epidural space (anterior dura and posterior longitudinal ligament [PLL])
Rarely Produced Pain
Supra and interspinous ligament Facet capsule Muscle attachment at bone or neurovascular bundle
Never Produced Pain
Ligamentum flavum Lumbar fascia Lamina bone Spinous process bone Facet synovium Uncompressed nerve root Uninflamed dura Facet cartilage
Location of Pain with Stimulation
Nerve root → buttock and leg pain Facet capsule → occasional cause of back pain Outer annulus → the site of back pain

A pain-spasm-pain cycle in which pain initiates muscle spasm, which in turn increases tissue strain and exacerbates pain, also has been proposed as a mechanism of chronic back pain.[42] In a review of the evidence for this hypothesis, it was concluded that although this cycle of pain generation and maintenance may exist in some patients, the occurrence and significance of muscle spasm has been poorly quantified. Pain was observed to occur without spasm, and spasm occurred without pain.[42]

The exact pathophysiology of low back pain remains elusive. It is complex, multifactorial, and requires considerable basic science and clinical study to be resolved. Considering all data, the intervertebral disk seems the most probable pain generator. In the majority of patients with low back pain, a definitive treatable cause cannot be identified. A differential diagnosis of low back pain is listed in Table 39–3.

The following discussion reviews key studies and includes guidelines for the useful application of available knowledge to help low back pain patients. This will enable the clinician to effectively diagnose, treat, and educate the patient with low back pain. Future research may identify a genetic predisposition for degenerative disk disease and increased sensitivity to pain.[16]

Clinical Presentation

HISTORY

A few key questions in the history can ensure that a serious underlying condition such as fracture, infection, tumor, or cauda equina syndrome is not missed.[43] Important points in the history that indicate a possible serious underlying condition as a source for low back pain were labeled as "red flags" in the Agency for Health Care Policy and Research (AHCPR) guidelines on acute low back pain.[44] These red flags are summarized in Table 39–4. Presence of any of these symptoms is an indication for obtaining special diagnostic studies[44] (see Table 39–9 for some of the recommended studies and tests).

Self-administered questionnaires are a reproducible method of gathering historic data.[45] Roland and Morris[46] developed a questionnaire by selecting items from the Sickness Impact Profile to reliably assess disability related to back pain. They found that the questionnaire was more sensitive than a physician examination in assessing disability and compared well to the self-rated measure of disability. The questionnaire is simple to use, requires 5 minutes for completion, and provides an objective method for following the severity of the patient's symptoms and predicting outcome.[47]

To quantitatively assess pain, a visual rating (acuity) scale has been recommended.[46,48] The physical characteristics that provide the best explanation of subjective disability are the anatomic and time pattern of pain, lumbar flexion measurement, nerve-root compression signs such as weakness or absent reflex, and straight leg raise (SLR).[49,50] A history of previous spinal fracture and previous lumbar surgery also correlated with subjective disability. Nine activity-related questions reproducibly quantify the severity of low back disorders, and these are listed in Table 39–5. These factors were noted to be present in 13 percent of normal people and had more than 73 percent agreement between examiners.

TABLE 39–3 • DIFFERENTIAL DIAGNOSIS OF LOW BACK PAIN

Idiopathic low back pain (80%)
Disk herniation
Degenerative disk disease
Intervertebral disk annular tears
Spinal stenosis
Fracture
Spondylolisthesis
Spondyloarthropathies
Sacroiliac dysfunction
Infection
Malignancy
Cauda equina syndrome
Renal disease
Vascular disease
Psychosocial issues

TABLE 39–4 • RED FLAGS

Red Flags for Spinal Fracture
History of Significant Trauma
Moving-vehicle accident, fall, or direct blow in a young person Minor fall or heavy lift in a potentially osteoporotic person
Prolonged use of Steroids
Age > 70 y
Red Flags for Cancer or Infection
History of Cancer
Unexplained weight loss Immunosuppression
Intravenous Drug use
History of urinary infection
Pain Increased by Rest
Fever Age >50 y
Red Flags for Cauda Equina Syndrome
Bladder Dysfunction
Urinary retention Overflow incontinence
Bowel Dysfunction
Loss of anal sphincter tone Fecal incontinence
Saddle Anesthesia
Global or Progressive Motor Weakness

Data from Bigos et al.[44]

TABLE 39–5 • DISABILITY FACTORS FOR LOW BACK PAIN

Lifting limited to < 30–40 pounds
Sitting limited to < 30 min
Traveling limited to < 30 min
Standing limited to < 30 min
Walking limited to < 30 min
Sleep disturbance
Limited social activities (excluding sports)
Diminished sexual activity
Help required with footwear

EXAMINATION

Twenty-one test items to be observed during a logical sequence of patient positioning are listed in Table 39–6 and comprise an examination requiring 12 to 13 minutes to complete.[51] Another approach is an abbreviated neurologic examination for patients presenting with leg symptoms in the primary care setting[52] (Table 39–7). This examination is also endorsed by the AHCPR.[44]

The reproducibility of physical signs in low back pain has been well studied. Palpation for bony tenderness, measurement of lordosis and flexion, SLR, and femoral stretch test were found to be reliable and reproducible. Posture, heel and toe standing for weakness, buttock wasting for atrophy, and the bowstring test for root tension were less reproducible.[53] Stress tests for examination of the sacroiliac joints have been shown to have poor discriminatory value in the assessment of low back pain.[54] In addition, the physician must always be aware of psychologic components that may be additive or even causative of back pain.[55]

TABLE 39–6 • EXAMINATION FOR LOW BACK DISORDERS

Tests in Standing Position
Single trunk flexion Single trunk extension Repeated trunk flexion Repeated trunk extension Trunk twist* Head compression*
Tests in Seated Position
Seated SLR-left Seated SLR-right
Tests in Supine Position
Single Williams knee pull Repeated Williams knee pull Supine SLR-left Supine SLR-right Bilateral active SLR
Tests in Prone Position
Skin tenderness* Single partial push-up Repeated partial push-up Back tenderness Instability test Femoral stretch-left Femoral stretch-right
Test of Consistency
Incongruence (between sitting and supine SLR)

*Test of nonorganic pain behavior (Waddell's signs).

Abbreviations: SLR, straight leg vaise.

TABLE 39–7 • ABBREVIATED NEUROLOGIC EXAMINATION

Strength
Dorsiflexion of ankle → L4 Dorsiflexion of great toe → L5 Ankle reflexes → S1
Light Touch in the Foot
Medial → L4 Dorsal → L5 Lateral → S1
Straight Leg Raise (SLR)

Pain behavior is defined as behavior that signals to others that pain is being experienced.[56] It can be expressed in the pattern of ambulation, activity avoidance, use of facial expressions, and affect. Five observations during physical examination to objectively assess pain behavior in patients with low back pain may be useful. They include looking for behavior indicating guarding, rubbing, grimacing, sighing, and verbalization of pain.[57] Exhibition of pain behavior is believed to correlate with a poor prognosis for pain relief and return to work.

DIAGNOSTIC STUDIES

The AHCPR guidelines state that for more than 95 percent of patients with acute low back problems, no special interventions or diagnostic tests are required within the first month of symptoms.[44] The guidelines indicate that an abbreviated neurologic examination will allow detection of most clinically significant neurologic compromise. They recommend a complete blood count (CBC) and an erythrocyte sedimentation rate (ESR) if any red flags for tumor or infection are present.[58] Recommendations for further special studies as proposed by the AHCPR panel are summarized in Tables 39–8 and 39–9.

It must be emphasized that anatomic changes may be unrelated to symptoms, and anatomic diagnoses can be identified in 10 to 30 percent of normal populations.[59] It is of particular note that MRI will reveal a high incidence of abnormal findings in asymptomatic individuals. In one study, a 20-percent incidence of disk herniation and 1-percent incidence of spinal stenosis in patients younger than 50 years of age was found.[60] A 35-percent incidence

TABLE 39–8 • SPECIAL STUDIES AND DIAGNOSTIC CONSIDERATIONS

Special Studies: Tests for Physiologic Dysfunction	
Electromyography (EMG)	
Needle EMG and H-reflex	Useful for patients with leg symptoms > 4 weeks Not recommended if radiculopathy is present
Surface EMG and F-wave	Not recommended
Somatosensory evoked potentials (SEP)	Useful in spinal stenosis and spinal cord myelopathy
Bone scan	Recommended if red flags are present
Thermography	Not recommended
Special Studies: Tests to Provide Anatomic Definition	
Plain radiographs	Not recommended unless a red flag is present Recommended for patients with red flags for fracture Recommended in combina tion with CBC and erythrocytes sedimentation rate (ESR) for patients with red flags for tumor or infection Other imaging indicated if radiographs are negative in the presence of red flags
Oblique Views	Not Recommended

TABLE 39–9 • INDICATIONS FOR IMAGING STUDIES

Red flags for cauda equina syndrome	Prompt CT, MRI, myelography, or CT-myelography and surgical consultation
Red flags for tumor, infection, or fracture	Prompt CT, MRI, myelography, or CT-myelography and surgical consultation
Symptoms for <1 mo without red flags	Spinal imaging tests not recommended
Symptoms for >1 mo	Imaging test acceptable when surgery is being considered
Prior back surgery	MRI with contrast imaging test of choice
CT-myelography and myelography	Invasive, indicated only in special situations for preoperative planning

Abbreviations: CT, computed tomography; MRI, magnetic resonance imaging.

of disk herniation and a 21-percent incidence of spinal stenosis were seen in asymptomatic patients older than age 60.[61] These patients were reexamined after 7 years and did not develop sciatica or a more-than-expected amount of back pain.[62] Physicians are encouraged to consider the predictive values of particular test before its application to specific individuals, because diagnostic tests can be misleading when they are applied to patients who are very unlikely to have the target condition. Erroneous inferences from diagnostic tests can lead to a cascade of ill-advised clinical interventions resulting in increased iatrogenic complications and increased cost in the management of patients with low back pain.

RADIOGRAPHS

Plain radiography of the spine is of little use in determining the causes of low back pain.[62] This consideration is particularly significant in view of the radiation exposure involved in standard lumbar radiographs. Radiation exposure to the gonads for five views of the lumbar spine is 382 mrads for women and 82 mrads for men.[63] For women, this is equivalent to a daily chest radiograph for 6, 16, or 96 years depending on the machine.[64] In terms of adverse consequences of lumbar radiography, it has been estimated that 1 million lumbar radiographs produced 20 excess deaths from leukemia, and studies in 1 million prospective parents resulted in 400 excess cases of genetic diseases.[58] Oblique views and cone-down lateral views double the radiation exposure and are unnecessary.

There appears to be no association between back pain and transitional vertebrae, Schmorl's nodes, the disk vacuum sign, disk-space narrowing at L3-L4 interspace and L5-S1 interspace, and claw-type spur formation.[62] The same studies found an association of severe back pain with disk-space narrowing or traction-type spur formation at the L4-L5 level. The findings on spine radiographs for low back pain and their classification in relation to their significance for back pain are shown in Table 39–10.[65]

ADDITIONAL DIAGNOSTIC STUDIES

The sensitivity and specificity of common laboratory screening tests for patients with low back pain has been

TABLE 39–10 • SIGNIFICANCE OF RADIOGRAPH FINDINGS FOR LOW BACK PAIN

Irrelevant
Disk space narrowing Spondylosis Facet arthrosis, subluxation, tropism Disk calcification Lumbarization, sacralization Intraspongy disk hernation (Schmorl) Spina bifida occulta Accessory ossicles Mid-moderate scoliosis
Questionable Association
Spondylolysis Retrolisthesis Severe lumbar scoliosis (>80°) Severe lordosis
Definite Association
Spondylolisthesis Lumbar osteochondrosis (Scheuermann) Congenital or traumatic kyphosis Osteoporosis Marked multiple disk narrowing Ankylosing spondylitis

calculated.[58] Prevalence of malignancy, infection, or spondyloarthropathy in patients presenting with low back pain was less than 2 percent. A CBC and ESR were sufficient for screening for these conditions. A list of nine indications for considering spine radiographs and laboratory studies on initial evaluation of patients presenting with low back pain are in Table 39–11.[58]

Some physicians advocate having the patient create a pain drawing indicating the location and character of the pain and correlating this with an MMPI evaluation.[66] It has been noted that characteristics of the pain drawing indicating emphasis on severity and location of the pain, magnification of the pain, and unreal pain drawings correlated with increases on the hysteria and hypochondriasis scales of the MMPI. Such findings are thought to be associated with a guarded prognosis for pain relief.

Imaging studies are indicated for patients with a possible underlying serious medical condition who present with low back pain. Patients at risk for a possible neoplastic or metastatic process or infection should be evaluated with a bone scan or MRI and appropriate screening laboratory studies. Patients with a neurologic deficit, cauda equina syndrome, or radicular symptoms unresponsive to nonoperative measures for 4 to 6 weeks should be evaluated with MRI scan to assess the neural anatomy. Computed tomography (CT) scan is an alternative for patients who cannot have an MRI study. Myelography or CT-myelography may be helpful in delineating nerve-root pathology in patients with radicular symptoms and history of prior back surgery. MRI with gadolinium can be of use in evaluating patients with previous lumbar disk surgery without hardware present to help differentiate scar tissue from recurrent disk herniation. These neuroimaging studies are appropriate at the time of consultation for evaluation of patients unresponsive to initial nonoperative treatments and preoperatively for patients anticipating surgery.

Classification

Classification schemes for low back pain have not been standardized sufficiently to provide reliable prognostic information or to guide therapeutic intervention. A familiarity with the classification systems, however, is important for accurate communication of clinical information and determination of the applicability of clinical studies to relevant patient populations.

TABLE 39–11 • INDICATIONS FOR RADIOGRAPHS ON INITIAL EVALUATION FOR LOW BACK PAIN

Age >50 years
Fever
Ankylosing spondylitis
History of malignancy
Weight loss
Trauma
Motor deficit
Litigation or compensation
Steroids
Drug abuse

Nachemson and Bigos[67] have proposed four categories for classifying low back pain (Table 39–12). This classification is simple to use but it has limitations. Specifically, patients with acute exacerbations of low chronic baseline pain do not fit into this classification.

An alternative classification based on consideration of back pain as a condition occurring in phases (Table 39–13) has been proposed.[68] Changing symptoms are recorded as a transition between the classification categories. This classification has the advantage of time specific and mutually exclusive categories for clearly identifying the patient's current status.

Another system has classified low back syndromes into four groups, ranging from a purely organic to a purely psychiatric disorder. Using this system it was found that even the purely organic category was marked by extensive clinical diversity.[70]

Natural History

Studies on natural history of low back pain are limited by methodologic deficiencies and the variable course of the condition itself. Assessment of patient recall indicates that subjective responses should be taken with caution and the method of data collection influences response.[71] The natural history of back pain is extremely variable: Some patients are better within days, and others complain of back pain for years; the tendency to improve is universal and absence from work may be influenced by factors other than pain and disability experienced by the patient.

TABLE 39–12 • CLASSIFICATION OF LOW BACK PAIN

Acute	0-3 mo duration with immediate onset
Subacute	0-3 mo duration with slow onset
Chronic	>3 mo duration
Recurrent	Recurring after a pain-free Interval

Data from Nachemson and Bigos.[67]

TABLE 39–13 • CLASSIFICATION OF LOW BACK PAIN

Transient	< 90 consecutive days, does not recur over a 12-mo period
Recurrent	Less than half the days in a 12-mo period, occurring in multiple episodes
Chronic	At least half the days in a 12-mo period in a single or multiple episodes
Acute	Not recurrent or chronic; onset is recent and sudden
First onset	First occurrence in a person's lifetime
Flare-up	A period when back pain is more than usual; the patient meets the criteria for recurrent or chronic categories and is able to identify the beginning of a period when the back pain was substantially more intense than usually experienced

Data from Von Korff.[68]

One study reported that acute low back pain episodes lasted less than 4 weeks in one third, less than 6 months in one third, and more than 6 months in one third of the patients.[7] In another group of patients followed for four months, only 28 percent were pain free; 47 percent were unchanged, and 25 percent were worse 1 month after treatment.[72] In a longitudinal study[73] it was shown that 40 percent of patients with acute back injury continued to report back pain at 6 months. In a prospective study,[74] 62 percent of patients with acute back pain had one or more relapses during a 1-year follow-up. Median time to relapse was 2 months, and median number of days of back pain was 60 days.

Outcome at 1 year has been reviewed in a more recent outcome study.[74] The authors noted that 69 percent of recent-onset and 82 percent of non–recent-onset patients reported experiencing an episode of back pain within the month before the 1-year follow-up. In a 2-year follow-up, 44 percent of all patients were noted to be in a chronic phase of back pain.[76] The course of back pain is typically recurrent and more often chronic than believed.

As mentioned previously, one useful suggestion has been to view low back pain as a disorder occurring in phases changing over time. Physicians should counsel patients that pain is likely to improve. Function may be restored even though pain continues. The large majority of patients return to work quickly whether the pain has resolved or not. Back pain is usually a recurrent condition and often enters a chronic stage. The large majority of patients with chronic back pain continue working.

Management

The randomized control trial is the best study design for determining treatment effect.[78-80] Unfortunately, very few randomized controlled trials have been conducted to assess the various treatment options currently available. The Quebec Task Force on Spinal Disorders and Deyo have reviewed treatment options for low back pain with regard to their efficacy as reported in the literature.[14,81] Bigos and colleagues[44] elegantly summarized the literature on the management of acute low back pain. Their report is a very thorough critical assessment of the published literature. Their recommendations are summarized in Table 39–14.

PATIENT EDUCATION

Insufficient explanation is the most frequent reason for dissatisfaction among patients receiving medical care for low back pain.[82] Patients who thought they did not receive an adequate explanation wanted more diagnostic tests, were less satisfied, and were less likely to return to the same doctor. Information booklets are an efficient means of providing information to patients. In a randomized study, it was found that patients receiving education booklets on low back pain were less likely to consult physicians again for low back pain in a 1-year follow-up period.

TABLE 39–14 • MANAGEMENT OF ACUTE LOW BACK PAIN (AHCPR GUIDELINES)

Patient Information	
Patient education back school	Booklets effective May be effective for worksite-specific education Nonoccupational setting: efficacy not shown
Symptom Control: Medications	
Acetaminophen	Safe and acceptable
NSAIDs	Acceptable but have potential side effects
Muscle relaxants	Option; not more effective than NSAIDs
Opioid analgesics	Option; side effects and dependence a concern
Phenylbutazone	Not recommended
Oral steroids	Not recommended
Antidepressant medication	Not recommended
Colchicine	Not recommended
Physical Treatments	
Spinal Manipulation	
Acute low back pain without radiculopathy	Effective
Low back pain >1 mo	Inconclusive
Radiculopathy	Inconclusive
Physical Agents and Modalities	
Heat	(Option: self-application of heator cold)
Massage	Insufficiently proven
Ultrasound	Insufficiently proven
Cutaneous laser treatment	Insufficiently proven
Electrical stimulation (not TENS)	Insufficiently proven
TENS	*Not recommended*
Shoe insoles	Option
Shoe lifts	Not recommended for leg length inequality ≤2 cm
Lumbar corsets and back belts	Not proven beneficial for treatment May reduce time lost from workin individuals required to do frequent lifting
Traction	Not recommended
Biofeedback	*Not recommended*
Injection treatments	
Trigger point	Not recommended
Ligamentous	Not recommended
Facet joint	Not recommended
Epidural	No evidence for back pain without radiculopathy Option for short-term relief of radicular pain
Acupuncture	*Not recommended*

Abbreviation: NSAIDS, nonsteroidal anti-inflammatory drugs.

"Back school" is a structured patient-education program on low back pain and ergonomics of lifting and other activities. Back school has been noted to decrease the duration of initial work absence in industrial low back pain; however, it had no difference in preventing further episodes at 1-year follow-up.[74] Bigos[84] noted that back school may be effective for worksite-specific patient education but has not been shown to be effective in nonoccupational settings.

ACTIVITY

In a study comparing 2 days of bed rest with 7 days of bed rest, it was concluded that 2 days of bed rest was preferable to longer periods.[85] In a randomized prospective study comparing bed rest, exercise program under the direction of physiotherapist, and ordinary activity, Malmivaara and coworkers[86] found that continuing ordinary activities within the limits permitted by pain lead to a more rapid recovery than either bed rest or back-mobilizing exercises. A randomized study comparing exercises as recommended by physiotherapist to usual information and analgesics given by a general practitioner found that exercise therapy under supervision of a physiotherapist offered no advantage.[87] This study, however, has been criticized for not prescribing diagnosis-specific exercise to the exercise-treatment group.[88,89]

For patients who have recovered from acute attacks of low back pain, many practitioners believe that abdominal-strengthening exercises that result in a decrease of lordotic tendencies will yield a decrease in back pain and radicular symptoms and less recurrence of acute attacks.

Dynamic mechanic assessment may be helpful in identifying the direction of beneficial exercise.[90] Back-specific exercise machines, however, have not been shown to provide added benefit over traditional exercise in improving back strength and flexibility in patients with low back pain.[91] Proponents of exercise therapy have argued that exercise should include progressive resistance, stabilization, and emphasis on patient empowerment and patient activity.[92]

Lindstrom and colleagues performed a randomized study of aerobic and back-strengthening exercises in auto workers out of work for more than 6 weeks because of back problems[93] and concluded that for patients who had had their symptoms for fewer than 3 months, a program of gradually increased aerobic and back-strengthening exercises was superior to no exercise. The exercise group lost less time from work and achieved a higher level of fitness compared to the control group. In a study of hospital workers, it was found that, compared to a control group, the exercise group had fewer days lost from work, fewer days with back pain complaints, lower average duration of low back pain complaints, and also achieved greater average trunk strength (not different from control at the start of the study). In a randomized study in kitchen cabinet manufacturing workers with current or prior back pain, results showed that the treatment group receiving weekly aerobic exercise sessions and educational lectures on proper lifting techniques had a decreased incidence of back pain and days lost from work. They noted, however, that the cardiovascular fitness was not different between the treated and control groups before and after the study.[95] The observed effect may have been the result of patient education or other factors.

Physical and psychosocial training programs may also improve physical disability in patients with chronic low back pain.[96] Patients should be advised about the debilitating aspects of excessively restricted activity, too much medication, and unwarranted surgery, with emphasis on "reactivation" of the patient and avoidance of the fault-oriented injury model by counseling patients with the following points:

1. Back pain is part of life.
2. The vast majority of patients improve quickly.
3. Activity tolerance at age 50 years is not expected to be the same as at age 18 years.
4. Cost of being labeled a "low back loser" is avoidable.
5. Trying to prove that the back problem is someone else's fault is loaded with pitfalls.[97]

There is strong evidence that advice to continue ordinary activity as normally as possible can foster equivalent or faster symptomatic recovery from the acute attack of low back pain and can lead to less chronic disability and less time lost from work than "traditional" medical treatment with analgesics as required and advice to rest and "let pain be your guide" for return to normal activity.[98]

MEDICATIONS

Based on Nachemson's review of the literature, there is strong evidence that nonsteroidal anti-inflammatory drugs (NSAIDs) prescribed at regular intervals provide effective pain relief for simple acute low back pain, but they do not affect return to work, natural history, or chronicity. Different types of NSAIDs appear to be equally effective.[98] NSAIDs carry a 20- to 30-percent risk of gastrointestinal bleeding in patients with a history of peptic ulcer disease and are associated with 20,000 hospitalizations and 2000 deaths each year because of this complication.[99,100] Newer cyclooxygenase-2 (COX-2)–specific inhibitors are associated with significantly fewer gastrointestinal side effects than traditional NSAIDs and may be an acceptable alternative[101]. The AHCPR guidelines state that acetaminophen is safe and acceptable for initial treatment of low back pain.[84]

There also is evidence that muscle relaxants effectively reduce acute low back pain and that the different types of muscle relaxants are equally effective.[98] Colchicine has also been used for treatment of low back pain and has been proven both ineffective and toxic.[102] Oral steroids have been shown not to be effective in the management of sciatica.[84,103] Steroids are associated with numerous serious systemic side effects and are not recommended in the management of low back problems. A blinded randomized study showed that trazodone was no more effective than placebo in patients with chronic back pain.[104] Patients with long-standing, chronic, debilitating low back pain without an identified cause may have to be managed in consultation with experts in pain clinics.

PHYSICAL TREATMENTS

Braces

Custom-molded corsets have been shown to have no significant influence on back injury rates or time lost from work because of back problems.[105] A lumbar corset with a back support may, however, improve symptoms in patients with low back pain of fewer than 6 months.[106] Shoe insoles may be effective in relieving symptoms in 44 percent of the patients with mild back pain who spend more than 75 percent of each day standing.[107]

Manipulation

Koes and colleagues[108] conducted a randomized study comparing manual therapy, physiotherapy, placebo to detuned ultrasound and diathermy, and continued treatment by a general practitioner. The group treated by the general practitioner included prescriptions, advice, and home exercises as instructed by the physician. They concluded that both manual therapy and physiotherapy decreased the severity of symptoms more than continued treatment by the general practitioner. They noted, however, that the effect of manual therapy and physiotherapy appeared to be caused by nonspecific placebo effects. This study has been criticized for its methods of data interpretation.[109] In a meta-analysis of spinal manipulation for back pain reviewing 29 studies, short-term benefits of manipulation in decreasing the duration of low back symptoms have been reported,[110] particularly when treated within 2 to 4 weeks of the onset of symptoms, not before nor after.[111]

Traction

Traction has been proven not to be effective in a randomized study.[112] Because of the disability and complications associated with the bed rest inherent in traction treatments, this modality is not recommended.[84]

Acupuncture

A meta-analysis of the literature on acupuncture for the treatment of chronic pain, including back pain, has been published; the conclusions were that the quality of studies was mediocre and efficacy could not be shown.[113]

Ultrasound, Massage, and Biofeedback

Diathermy, ultrasound, massage, electrotherapy, and transcutaneous electrical nerve stimulation (TENS) unit treatments have not been shown to be effective in treatment of chronic back pain.[114] Biofeedback also has been shown not to be effective in the management of back pain in a randomized blinded study.[115]

INJECTION TREATMENTS

Local Injections

Local injections and facet-joint injections with anesthetic agents or steroids are not effective in relieving symptoms of back pain.[116,117]

Epidural Injection

Epidural injections may be an option for patients with radicular symptoms who have been unresponsive to noninvasive options of management. They may also be an option for patients in whom surgery is contraindicated for other medical reasons. Patients should undergo a consultation with a spine specialist before instituting epidural steroid treatment to provide a complete evaluation of the underlying spinal pathology. White and coworkers[118] studied epidural injections in 304 patients in a prospective study with up to 2 years of follow-up. They noted short-term improvement in 87 percent and improvement lasting longer than 6 months in 36 percent of patients with diskogenic pain, annulus tear, and disk herniations. Complication rate was 0.4 percent. No patient had a "cure" from injection therapy, but the epidural injections provided temporary relief and appeared to shorten the clinical course.

One evidence-based review found limited evidence that epidural steroid injections are more effective than placebo or bed rest for acute low back pain without nerve root pain.[98]

Special Considerations

CHRONIC PAIN AND DISABILITY RELATED TO BACK PROBLEMS

Functional restoration programs or pain management clinic evaluations are options for patients with chronic back pain and related disability. Patients should be evaluated by a spine specialist before referral for the management options to exclude specifically treatable underlying pathology.

FUNCTIONAL RESTORATION

A 1-year follow-up study of a program of functional restoration with behavioral modification (New England Back Center [NEBC] program) for patients with chronic low back pain reported a success rate of 81 percent for graduates of the program compared to 29 percent for patients not in the program.[119] One prospective study of a comprehensive functional restoration program (the PRIDE program) has been reported.[120] Eighty-six percent of the graduates of this program were working at 1-year follow-up evaluation, compared to 45 percent of the controls. At 2 years of follow-up, 86 percent of the graduates were still working, compared to 41 percent of the controls.[121] Of note, 9 percent of the graduates from the program had undergone further surgery, compared to 50 percent of the patients who dropped out of the program. This comparison is difficult to interpret, however, because the two groups were not randomized and may not have been comparable at the start of the PRIDE program.

PAIN CLINICS

Pain clinics are designed to provide comprehensive management of medical issues, physical deactivation, belief systems, vocational issues, and support.[122] The results of studies on pain clinic management of low back pain have been reviewed.[123,124] They reported an overall success rate of 50% to 80%. In a retrospective review of 40 patients with 1 to 5 years follow-up, 60% of the treatment group had a successful outcome, compared with 0% of the comparison group[125]. Successful outcome was defined as patients who returned to work, were not receiving compensation, had no pain-related hospitalization or operations, and were not using prescription medications.

PREGNANCY

Back pain is common in pregnancy. In the ninth month, 49 percent of pregnant women complain of back pain and 1 percent complain of sciatica. Point prevalence throughout pregnancy is 25 percent. Pain usually starts before the 12th week.[126] Pain localizes to the lumbar region and rarely progresses during pregnancy. Pain initially localized to the S1 area increases during pregnancy. Risk factors for back pain pregnancy are listed in Table 39–15.[126] Back pain occurs twice as often in patients with history of prior back pain. Patients with history of prior back pain also have longer duration and increased intensity of pain during pregnancy compared to patients with no prior back problems.

During pregnancy, abdominal muscles become weak, accentuating a tendency for lordosis.[128] Back pain in pregnancy, however, cannot be explained by biomechanic factors alone.[129] Hormonal effects of estrogen and ligamentous laxity associated with relaxin may be contributing factors. Preexisting pain is often increased during the menstrual period.[130]

Back pain can be difficult to treat in pregnancy, but good physical fitness has been shown to reduce the risk of back pain in subsequent pregnancy.[131] Patients with back problems anticipating pregnancy in the future should be advised of this association. It should be noted that use of an inelastic low sacroiliac belt that does not compress the abdomen decreased symptoms in 82 percent of pregnant patients who experienced posterior pelvic pain.[132] An individually designed approach is necessary for patients who develop back pain in pregnancy.

A history of back pain is an important factor for predicting the occurrence of back pain and the intensity of back pain in future pregnancy. However, the severity of back pain is not such that women with a history of back pain should be advised against becoming pregnant.[127]

TABLE 39–15 • FACTORS ASSOCIATED WITH INCREASED RISK OF LOW BACK PAIN IN PREGNANCY

- Back problems before pregnancy
- Young age
- Multiparity
- Work factors
  - Physical, heavy work
  - Lifting, twisting, bending
  - Poor satisfaction
  - Constrained work postures
  - Inability to take breaks
  - Postwork fatigue

Outcome

Patient perspectives are essential in judging the results of treatment.[132] Therapeutic trials for low back pain are lacking, particularly in terms of treatment endpoints that matter to patients.[78,132,133] Changing physician practice with regard to management of back problems is difficult. Simple education about scientifically proven methods of treatment appears not to be sufficient to change active patient care or patient outcome.[134]

NONOPERATIVE TREATMENTS

As noted by Von Korff and coworkers,[75] the course of back pain is typically recurrent and more often chronic than believed (Table 39–16). At 2-year follow-up, 44 percent of all patients were in a chronic phase of back pain.[76]

Surgery

Surgery is not a treatment option for idiopathic acute low back pain. The only exception is acute low back pain combined with radicular symptoms secondary to disk herniation that fails at least 6 to 8 weeks of conservative therapy. This situation may be helped by laminotomy and diskectomy. Lumbar spinal stenosis is a common cause of low back and leg pain in patients over age 50. Decompressive lumbar laminectomy with or without fusion for lumbar spinal stenosis is highly successful in improving chronic back and leg pain.

Lumbar fusion may be considered in patients with severe chronic low back pain. Results of fusion for chronic low back pain are variable. In general, satisfactory results are reported in 40 to 65 percent of patients. Diskography can be a useful tool in patient selection. A recent randomized controlled study by the Swedish Lumbar Spine Study Group showed statistic improvement in pain and disability in patients undergoing lumbar fusion for chronic severe low back pain compared to patients treated nonsurgically.[141] Hagg and colleagues[142] found that improved selection of successful surgical candidates with chronic low back pain seems to be promoted by attention to severe disk degeneration, evaluation of personality traits and shorter preoperative sick leave. Several methods can be used to achieve spinal fusion,

TABLE 39–16 • OUTCOME OF BACK PAIN AT 1 YEAR

Duration of Low Back Pain	Fair to poor Outcome at 1 year	>30 Days of Low Back Pain in the Prior 6 Months	>1 Episode of Low Back Pain in the Prior Month
Recent onset	24%	36%	69%
Nonrecent onset	36%	46%	82%

including posterolateral lumbar fusion, posterior lumbar interbody fusion, anterior interbody fusion, or a combination of methods.[143] Intradiskal electrothermal annuloplasty (IDET) has gained some popularity as a minimally invasive treatment for chronic diskogenic pain confirmed by positive diskography. A catheter is inserted into the disk and heated to a targeted temperature. Theoretically, the heat shrinks collagen fibrils and cauterizes granulation and nerve tissue of the posterior annulus. A 23 to 60 percent success rate has been reported, depending on criteria used at 12 months follow up.[136] Further long-term studies are needed.

Recently, trials of artificial disks in the lumbar spine have begun in the United States as an alternative to fusion surgery for degenerative disk disease causing chronic low back pain. The artificial disk is inserted through an anterior lumbar exposure. The theoretical advantages are quicker recovery time and less risk of adjacent-level degenerative disk disease often seen after lumbar fusion surgery. Early results in Europe are encouraging, but long-term studies are needed.

Work

Nonphysical factors such as education level, perception of job characteristics, and perception of fault concerning the back problem are strong predictors of outcome with regard to return to work for patients with low back pain.[137] The large majority of patients with worker's compensation back pain return to work within 3 months.[14] Those patients not back to work within 3 months are more likely to remain disabled. Waddell reported a return-to-work rate of 50 percent after an injury-related work absence of 6 months, 25 percent after 1 year, and almost 0 percent after 2 years of work absence.[138] These numbers underscore the importance of getting patients back to an active functional environment. Interestingly and ironically, one study showed that patients with work-related back injuries represented by counsel had a 9 percent return-to-work rate compared to 77 percent of those not represented by counsel,[139] but some recent studies have contradicted this association.[140]

The general message about low back pain for rheumatologists and primary care physicians is that conservative therapy works, invasive treatment is rarely needed, and that a good attitude, assiduous attention to exercise, and minimal reliance on medications are the keys to effective management and return to good function.

REFERENCES

1. Bombardier C, Kerr MS, Shannon HS, et al: A guide to interpreting epidemiologic studies on the etiology of back pain. Spine 19(Suppl 18): 2047S-2056S, 1994.
2. Andersson GBJ: Epidemiology features of chronic low-back pain. Lancer 354: 581-585, 1999.
3. White AA, Gordon SL: Synopsis: Workshop on idiopathic low back pain. Spine 7:141-149, 1982.
4. Liang M, Komaroff AL: Roentgenograms in primary care patients with acute low back pain. Arch Intern Med 142:1108-1112, 1982.
5. Cherkin DC, Deyn RA, Wheeler K, et al: Physician views about treating low back pain: The results of a national survey. Spine 20:1-8, 1995.
6. Nacheinson AL, Waddell G, Norlund AI: Epidemiology of neck and low back pain. *In* Nachemson AI, Jonsson E (eds): Neck and Back Pain: The Scientific Evidence of Causes, Diagnosis and Treatment. Philadelphia, Lippincott Williams and Wilkins, 2000, pp 165-187.
7. Deyo RA, Tsui-Wu Y-J: Descriptive epidemiology of low back pain and its related medical care in the United States. Spine 12:264-268, 1987.
8. Deyo RA, Bass JF: Lifestyle and low back pain. Spine 14:501-506, 1989.
9. Frymoyer JW, Pope MH, Clements JH, et al: Risk factors in low back pain: An epidemiological survey. J Bone Joint Surg Am 65:213, 1983.
10. Pope MH, Bevins T, Wilder DG, et al: The relationship between anthropometric, postural, muscular, and mobility characteristics of males, ages 18-55. Spine 10:644-648, 1985.
11. Vingard L, Nachemson AL: Work-related influences on neck and low back pain. *In* Nachemson AL, Jonsson E (eds): Neck and Back Pain: The Scientific Evidence of Causes, Diagnosis and Treatment. Philadelphia, Lippincott Williams & Wilkins, 2000, pp 97-126.
12. Deyo RA, Bass JE: Lifestyle and low back pain. Spine 14:501-506, 1989.
13. Boshuizen HC, Verbeck JH, Broersen JP, et al: Do smokers get more back pain? Spine 18:35-40, 1993.
14. Spitzer WO, LeBlanc FE, Dupuis M: Scientific approach to the assessment and management of activity related spinal disorders. A monograph for physicians: Report of the Quebec Task Force on Spinal Disorders. Spine 12(Suppl 7):S1-S59, 1987.
15. Mundt DJ, Kelsey JL, Golden AL, et al: An epidemiologic study of non-occupational lifting as a risk factor for herniated lumbar intervertebral disc. The Northcast Collaborative Group on Low Back Pain. Spine 18:595-602, 1993.
16. Carlsson CA, Nachemson A: Neurophysiology of back pain: Current knowledge. *In* Nachemson AL, Jonsson E (eds): Neck and Back Pain: The Scientific Evidence of Causes, Diagnosis and Treatment. Philadelphia, Lippincott Williams & Wilkins, 2000, pp 149-163.
17. Porter RW, Bewley B: A ten year prospective study of vertebral canal size as a predictor of back pain. Spine 19:173-175, 1994.
18. Allan DB, Waddell G: An historical perspective on low back pain and disability. Acta Orthop Scand 60(Suppl 234):1-23, 1989.
19. Andersson GBJ: Epidemiology of spinal disorders. *In* Frymoyer JW (ed): The Adult Spine. New York, Raven, 1991, pp 109-146.
20. Hart LG, Deyo RA, Cherkin DL: Physician office visits for low back pain: Frequency, clinical evaluation, and treatment patterns from a U.S. national survey. Spine 20:11-19, 1995.
21. Bigos SJ, Battie MC, Fisher LD, et al: A prospective evaluation of preemployment screening methods for acute industrial back pain. Spine 17:922-926, 1992.
22. Bigos SJ, Battie MC, Spengler DM, et al: A prospective study of work perceptions and psychosocial factors affecting the report of back injury. Spine 16:1-6, 1991.
23. Battie MC, Bigos SJ, Fisher LD, et al: The role of spinal flexibility in back pain complaints within industry. A prospective study. Spine 15:768-773, 1990.
24. Spengler DM, Bigos SJ, Martin NA, et al: Back injuries in industry: A retrospective study. Spine 11:241-245, 1986.
25. David GC: UK statistics on handling accidents and lumbar injuries at work. Ergonomics 28:9-16, 1985.
26. Frymoyer JW: Back pain and sciatica. N Engl J Med 318:291-300, 1988.
27. Liesi P, Gronblad M, Korkala O, et al: Substance P: A neuropeptide in low back pain. Lancet Jun 1328-1329, 1983.
28. Brown M: The source of low back pain and sciatica. Semin Arthritis Rheuml 18(Suppl 2):67-72, 1989.
29. Olmarker K, Rydevil B: Pathophysiology of sciatica. Orthop Clin North Am 22:223-234, 1991.
30. Weinstein J: Neurogenic and nonneurogenic pain and inflammatory mediators. Orthop Clin North Am 22:235-246, 1991.
31. Moore MR, Brown CW, Brugman JL, et al: Relationship between vertebral intraosseons pressure, pH, PO_2, PCO_2, and magnetic resonance imaging signal inhomogeneity in patients with back pain. An in vivo study, Spine 16(Suppl 6):S239-S2343, 1991.
32. Hirsch C, Ingelmark BE, Miller M: The anatomical basis for low back pain: Studies on the presence of sensory nerve endings in

ligamentous, capsular and intervertebral disc structures in the human lumbar spine. Acta Orthop Scand 33:1-17, 1963.
33. Mooney V, Robertson J: The facet syndrome. Clin Orthop 115:149-156, 1976.
34. Kuslich SD, Ulstrom CL, Michael CJ: The tissue origin of low back pain and sciatica: A report of pain response to tissue stimulation during operations on the lumbar spine using local anesthesia. Orthop Clin North Am 22:181-187, 1991.
35. Goldner JL, Urbaniak JR, McCullom DE: Anterior disc excision and interbody fusion for chronic low back pain. Orthop Clin North Am: 2:543-568, 1971.
36. Weinstein JN, Claveric W, Gibson S: The pain of discography. Spine 13:1344-1348, 1988.
37. Morgan FP, King T: Primary instability of the lumbar vertebrae as a common cause of low back pain. J Bone Joint Surg Br 69(B):6-22, 1957.
38. Executive committee of the North American Spine Society: Position statement on discography: Spine 13:1343, 1988.
39. Esses SI, Botsford DJ, Kostuik JP: The role of external spinal fixation in the assessment of low-back disorders. Spine 14:594-601, 1989.
40. Nachemson A: Lumbar discography—where are we today? Spine 14:555-557, 1989.
41. Schwarzer AC, Aprill CN, Bogduk N: The sacroiliac joint in chronic low back pain. Spine 20:31-37, 1995.
42. Roland MO: A critical review of the evidence for a pain-spasm-pain cycle in spinal disorders. Clin Biomech 1:102-109, 1986.
43. Deyo RA, Diehl AK: Cancer as a cause of back pain: Frequency, clinical presentation, and diagnostic strategies. J Gen Intern Med 3:230-238, 1988.
44. Bigos S, Bowyer O, Braen G, et al: Acute Low Back Problems in Adults. Clinical practice Guideline No. 14. AHCPR Publication No. 95-062. Rockville, MD, Agency for Health Care Policy Research, Public Health Service, US Department of Health and Human Services, December 1994.
45. Walsh K, Coggon D: Reproducibility of histories of low-back pain obtained by self-administered questionnaire. Spine 16:1075-1077, 1991.
46. Roland M, Morris R: A study of the natural history of back pain. Part I: Development of a reliable and sensitive measure of disability in low-back pain. Spine 8:141-144, 1983.
47. Roland M, Morris R: A study of the natural history of back pain. Part II: Development of guidelines for trials of treatment in primary care. Spine 8:145-150, 1983.
48. Waddell G: Clinical assessment of lumbar impairment. Clin Orthop 221:110-120, 1987.
49. Waddell G, Main CJ: Assessment of severity in low back disorders. Spine 9:204-208, 1984.
50. Waddell G, Main CJ, Morris EW, et al: Normality and reliability in the clinical assessment of backache. Br Med J Clin Res 284:1519-1523, 1982.
51. Spratt KE, Lehmann TR, Weinstein JN, et al: A new approach to the low-back physical examination. Behavioral assessment of mechanical signs. Spine 15:96-102, 1990.
52. Deyo RA, Rainville J, Kent DL: What can history and physical examination tell us about back pain? JAMA 268:760-765, 1992.
53. McCombe PF, Fairbank JCT, Cockersole BC, et al: Reproducibility of physical signs in low-back pain. Spine 14:908-918, 1989.
54. Russel AS, Maksymowych W, LeClercq S: Clinical examination of the sacroiliac joints: A prospective study. Arthritis Rheum 24:1575-1577, 1981.
55. Waddell G, McCulloch JA, Kummel E, et al: Non-organic physical signs in low back pain. Spine 5:117-125, 1980.
56. Keefe FJ: Psychology of chronic back pain. *In* Frymoyer JW (ed): The Adult Spine. New York, Raven, 1991, pp 109-146.
57. Keefe FJ, Wilkins RH, Cook WA: Direct observation of pain behavior in low back pain patients during physical examination. Pain 20:59-68, 1984.
58. Deyo RA: Early diagnostic evaluation of low back pain. J Gen Intern Med 1:328-338, 1986.
59. Deyo RA, Haselkorn J, Hoffman R, et al: Designing studies of diagnostic tests for low back pain or radiculopathy. Spine 19:2057S-2065S, 1994.
60. Boden SD, Davis DO, Dina TS, et al: Abnormal magnetic resonance scans of the lumbar spine in asymptomatic subjects: A prospective investigation. J Bone Joint Surg Am 72:403-408, 1990.
61. Borenstein DG, O'Mara JW, Boden SD, et al: A 7-year follow up study of the value of lumbar spine MR to predict the development of low back pain in asymptomatic individuals [abst]. *In*: Abstracts of the ISSLS Meeting, Brussels, ISSI S, 1998, p 112.
62. Frymoyer JW, Newberg A, Pope MH, et al: Spine radiographs in patients with low back pain: An epidemiological study in men. J Bone Joint Surg Am 66:1048-1055, 1984.
63. Liang MH: Clinical evaluation of patients with a suspected spine problem. *In* Frymoyer JW (ed): The Adult Spine. New York, Raven, 1991, pp 296-298.
64. Hali FM: Back pain and the radiologist. Radiology 137:861-863, 1980.
65. Nachemson A: The lumbar spine: An orthopaedic challenge. Spine 1:59-71, 1976.
66. Ransford AO, Cairns D, Mooney V: The pain drawing as an aid to the psychological evaluation of patients with low back pain. Spine 1:127-134, 1976.
67. Nachemson A, Bigos SJ: The low back. *In* Creuss J, Remie WRJ (eds): Adult Orthopaedics. New York, Churchill Livingstone, 1984, pp 843-937.
68. Von Korff M: Studying the natural history of back pain. Spine 19(Suppl 18):2041S-2046S, 1994.
69. Coste J, Paolaggi JR, Spira A: Classification of nonspecific low back pain. I. Psychological involvement in low back pain. A clinical, descriptive approach. Spine 17:1028-1037, 1993.
70. Coste J, Paolaggi JB, Spira A: Classification of nonspecific low back pain. II. Clinical diversity of organic forms. Spine 17:1038-1042, 1992.
71. Biering-Sorenson F, Hilden J: Reproducibility of history of low-back trouble. Spine 9:280-286, 1984.
72. Chavennes AW, Gubbels I, Post D, et al: Acute low back pain: Patients' perceptions of pain four weeks after initial diagnosis and treatment in general practice. J R Coll Gen Pract 36:271-273, 1986.
73. Philips HC, Grant L: The evolution of chronic back problems: A longitudinal study. Behav Res Ther 29:435-441, 1991.
74. Bergquist-Ullman M, Larsson U: Acute low back pain in industry: A controlled prospective study with special reference to therapy and confounding factors. Acta Orthop Scand 170:1-117, 1977.
75. Von Korff M, Deyo RA, Cherkin D, et al: Back pain in primary care. Outcomes at 1 year. Spine 18:855-862, 1993.
76. Von Korff M, Barlow W, Cherkin D, et al: Effects of practice style on managing back pain. Ann Intern Med 121:187-195, 1994.
77. Von Korff M: Studying the natural history of back pain. Spine 19(Suppl 18):2041S-2046S, 1994.
78. Andersson GB, Bombardier C, Cherkin DC, et al: An introduction to therapeutic trials for low back pain. Spine 19(Suppl 18):2066S-2067S, 1994.
79. Andersson GB, Weinstein JN: Health outcomes related to low back pain. Spine 19(suppl 18):2026S-2027S, 1994.
80. Liang MH, Andersson G, Bombardier C, et al: Strategies for outcome research in spinal disorders. An introduction. Spine 19(Suppl 18):2037S-2040S, 1994.
81. Deyo RA: Conservative treatment for low back pain: Distinguishing useful from useless therapy. JAMA 250:1057-1062, 1983.
82. Deyo RA, Diehl AK: Patient satisfaction with medical care for low back pain. Spine 11:28-30, 1986.
83. Roland M, Dixon M: Randomized controlled trial of an educational booklet for patients, presenting with back pain in general practice. J R Coll Gen Pract 39:244-246, 1989.
84. Bigos SJ: Acute Low Back Problems in Adults. AHCPR Publication No. 95-0642 1994 Dec: Clinical Practice Guideline Number 14.
85. Deyo RA, Diehl AK, Rosenthal M: How many days of bedrest for acute low back pain? N Engl J Med 315:1064-1070, 1986.
86. Malmivaara A, Hakkinen U, Aro T, et al: The treatment of acute low back pain–Bed rest, exercises, or ordinary activity? N Engl J Med 332:351-355, 1995.
87. Faas A, Chavannes AW, van Fijk JT, et al: A randomized, placebo-controlled trial of exercise therapy in patients with acute low back pain. Spine 18:1388-1395, 1993.
88. Mooney V: A randomized, placebo-controlled trial of exercise therapy in patients with acute low back pain [letter; comment]. Spine 19:1101; discussion 1103-1104, 1994.
89. Bunch RW: A randomized, placebo-controlled trial of exercise therapy in patients with acute low back pain [letter; comment]. Spine 19:1101-1103; discussion 1103-1104, 1994.

90. Donelson R, Grant W, Kamps C, et al: Pain response to sagittal end-range spinal motion. A prospective, randomized, multicentered trial. Spine 16(Suppl 6):S206-S212, 1991.
91. Sachs BL, Ahmad SS, LaCroix M, et al: Objective assessment for exercise treatment on the B-200 isostation as part of work tolerance rehabilitation. A random prospective blind evaluation with comparison control population. Spine 19:49-52, 1994.
92. Van Dyke M: A randomized, placebo-controlled trial of exercise therapy in patients with acute low back pain [letter; comment]. Spine 19:1101; discussion 1103-1104, 1994.
93. Lindstrom I, Ohlund C, Eck C, et al: The effect of graded activity on patients with subacute low back pain: A randomized prospective study with an operant-conditioning behavioral approach. Phys Ther 72:279-293, 1992.
94. Gundewall B, Liljeqvist M, Hansson T: Primary prevention of back symptoms and absence from work. A prospective randomized study among hospital employees. Spine 18:587-594, 1993.
95. Kellet KM, Kellet DA, Nordhholm JA: Effects of an exercise program on sick leave due to back pain. Phys Ther 71:283-291, 1991.
96. Ajaranta H, Rytokoski U, Rissanen A, et al: Intensive physical and psychosocial training program for patients with chronic low back pain. A controlled clinical trial. Spine 19:1339-1349, 1994.
97. Bigos SJ: *In* Frymoyer JW (ed): The Adult Spine. New York, Raven, 1991.
98. Van Tulder MW, Waddell G: Conservative treatment of acute and subacute low back pain. *In* Nachemson AL, Jonsson E (eds): Neck and Back Pain: The Scientific Evidence of Causes, Diagnosis and Treatment. Philadelphia, Lippincott Williams & Wilkins, 2000, pp 241-269.
99. Brooks PM, Day RO: Nonsteroidal antiinflammatory drugs—differences and similarities. N Engl J Med 324:1716-1725, 1991.
100. Goodman TA, Simon LS: Minimizing the complications of NSAID therapy. J Musculoskeletal Med 11:33-46, 1994.
101. Bombardier C, Laine L, Reiem A, et al: Comparison of upper gastrointestinal toxicity of rofecoxib and naproxen in patients with rheumatoid arthritis. N Engl J Med 343:1520-1528, 2000.
102. Schnebel BE, Simmons JW: The use of oral colchicine for low back pain. A double-blind study. Spine 13:354-357, 1988.
103. Haimovic IC, Beresford HR: Dexamethasone is not superior to placebo for treating lumbosacral radicular pain. Neurology 36:1593-1594, 1986.
104. Goodkin K, Gullion CM, Agras WS: A randomized, double-blind, placebo-controlled trial of trazadone hydrochloride in chronic low back pain syndrome. J Clin Psychopharmacol 10:269-278, 1990.
105. Walsh NE, Schwartz RK: The influence of prophylactic orthoses on abdominal strength and low back injury in the workplace. Am J Phys Med Rehabil 69:245-250, 1990.
106. Million R, Haavik NK, Jayson MIV, et al: Evaluation of low back pain and assessment of lumbar corsets with and without back supports. Ann Rheum Dis 40:449-454, 1981.
107. Basford JR, Smith MA: Shoe insoles in the workplace. Orthopedics 11:285-288, 1988.
108. Koes BW, Bouter LM, van Mameren H, et al: The effectiveness of manual therapy, physiotherapy, and treatment by the general practitioner for nonspecific back and neck complaints. A randomized clinical trial. Spine 17:28-35, 1992.
109. Ebrall PS: A blinded randomized clinical trial of manual therapy and physiotherapy for chronic back and neck complaints: Physical outcome measures [letter; comment]. Spine 18:169-170, 1993.
110. Shekelle PG, Phillips RB, Morris EK: Spinal manipulation for back pain. Ann Intern Med 117:590-598, 1992.
111. MacDonald RS, Bell CM: An open controlled assessment of osteopathic manipulation in nonspecific low-back pain [published erratum appears in Spine 16:104, 1991]. Spine 364-370, 1990.
112. Mathews JA, Hickling J: Lumbar traction: A double-blind controlled study for sciatica. Rheumatol Rehabil 14:422-425, 1975.
113. Riet G, Kleijnen J, Knipschild P: Acupuncture and chronic pain: A criteria-based meta-analysis. J Clin Epidemiol 43:1191-1199, 1990.
114. Deyo RA, Walsh NE, Martin DC, et al: A controlled trial of transcutaneous electrical nerve stimulation (TENS) and exercise for chronic low back pain. N Engl J Med 322:1627-1634, 1990.
115. Bush C, Ditto B, Feuerstein M: A controlled evaluation of paraspinal EMG biofeedback in the treatment of chronic back pain. Health Psychol 4:307-321, 1985.
116. Lilius G, Laasonen EM, Myllynen P, et al: Lumbar facet joint syndrome. A randomized clinical trial. J Bone Joint Surg Br 71:681-684, 1989.
117. Garvey TA, Marks MR, Wiesel SW: A prospective, randomized, double-blind evaluation of trigger-point injection therapy for low back pain. Spine 14:962-964, 1989.
118. White AH, Derby R, Wynne G: Epidural injections for the diagnosis and treatment of low back pain. Spine 5:78-86, 1980.
119. Hazard RG, Fenwick JW, Kalisch SM, et al: Functional restoration with behavioral support: A one year prospective study of patients with chronic low back pain. Spine 14:157-161, 1989.
120. Mayer TG, Gatchel RJ, Kishino N, et al: Objective assessment of spine injury following an injury: A prospective study with comparison group and one-year follow-up. Spine 10:482-493, 1985.
121. Mayer TG, Gatchel RJ, Mayer H, et al: A prospective two-year study of functional restoration in industrial low back injury. An objective assessment procedure. JAMA 258:1763-1767, 1987.
122. Loeser J: The role of pain clinics in managing chronic back pain. *In* Frymoyer JW (ed): The Adult Spine. New York, Raven, 1991, pp 211-219.
123. Linton SJ: Behavioral remediation of chronic pain: A status report. Pain 24:125-141, 1986.
124. Aronoff GM, Evans WO, Erders PL: A review of follow-up studies of multidisciplinary pain units. Pain 16:1-11, 1983.
125. Guck TP, Skultety FM, Meilman PW, et al: Multidisciplinary pain center follow-up study: Evaluation with a no treatment control group. Pain 21:295-306, 1985.
126. Ostergaard HC, Andersson GB, Karlsson K: Prevalence of back pain in pregnancy. Spine 16:549-552, 1991.
127. Ostergaard HC, Andersson GB: Previous back pain and risk of developing back pain in a future pregnancy. Spine 16:432-436, 1991.
128. Fast A, Weiss L, Ducommun EJ, et al: Low-back pain in pregnancy. Abdominal muscles, sit-up performance, and back pain. Spine 15:28-30, 1990.
129. Ostergaard HC, Andersson GB, Schultz AB, et al: Influence of some biomechanical factors on low-back pain in pregnancy. Spine 18:61-65, 1993.
130. Svensson HO, Andersson GB, Hagstad A, et al: The relationship of low-back pain to pregnancy and gynecologic factors. Spine 15:371-375, 1990.
131. Ostergaard HC, Zetherstrom G, Roos-Hansson E, et al: Reduction of back and posterior pelvic pain in pregnancy. Spine 19:894-900, 1994.
132. Deyo RA, Andersson G, Bombardier C, et al: Outcome measures for studying patients with low back pain. Spine 19(Suppl 18): 2032S-2036S, 1994.
133. Shekelle PG, Andersson G, Bombardier C, et al: A brief introduction to the critical reading of the clinical literature. Spine 19(Suppl 18):2028S-2031S, 1994.
134. Cherkin D, Deyo RA, Berg AO: Evaluation of a physician education intervention to improve primary care for low-back pain. II. Impact on patients. Spine 16:1173-1178, 1991.
135. Karasek M, Bogduk N: Twelve-month follow-up of a controlled trial of intradiscal thermal anuloplasty for back pain due to internal disc disruption. Spine 25:2601-2607, 2000.
136. Cats-Baril WL, Frymoyer JW: Identifying patients at risk of becoming disabled because of low-back pain. The Vermont Rehabilitation Engineering Center predictive model. Spine 16:605-607, 1991.
137. Weinstein JN, Wiesel SW (eds): The Lumbar Spine. Philadelphia, WB Saunders, 1990, p 39.
138. Haddad GH: Analysis of 2,932 worker's compensation back injury cases. Spine 12:765-769, 1987.
139. Schofferman J, Wasserman S: Successful treatment of low back pain and neck pain after a motor vehicle accident despite litigation. Spine 19:1007-1010, 1994.
140. Fritzell P, Hagg O, Wessberg P, Nordwall A: 2001 Volvo Award Winner in Clinical Studies: Lumbar fusion versus nonsurgical treatment for chronic low back pain: a multicenter randomized controlled trial from the Swedish Lumbar Spine study Group. Spine 26(23):2521-2532, 2001.
141. Hagg O, Fritzell P, Ekselius L, Nordwall A: Predictors of outcome in fusion surgery for chronic low back pain. A report from the Swedish Lumbar Spine Study. Eur Spine J 12(1):22-33, 2003.
142. Fritzell P, Hagg O, Wessberg P, Nordwall A: Chronic low back pain and fusion: a comparison of three surgical techniques: a prospective multicenter randomized study from the Swedish lumbar spine study group. Spine 27(11):1131-1141, 2002.

40 Hip and Knee Pain

MICHAEL F. DILLINGHAM • N. NICHOLE BARRY • ANTHONY J. ABENE

Pressures on the cost of health care have mandated an emphasis on nonsurgical care for orthopedic and musculoskeletal conditions. This limits resources for patients' medical visits, diagnostics, and treatment. The physician is beset not only with decreasing resources but also with patients' expectations of a speedy return to high activity levels. For the efficient evaluation of hip and knee pain in this setting, the internist's algorithmic approach to diagnosis must be coupled with the orthopedist's and physiatrist's specific knowledge. The differential diagnosis of such pain entails a subset analysis of the disorders affecting the lower limb and of systemic disease manifestations.

Knee Pain

RELEVANT ANATOMIC FEATURES

Knowledge of topographic anatomy remains the key to diagnosis of pain in the knee. Pain in a knee joint or the surrounding soft tissue is only infrequently referred. Rather, the painful area usually correlates with local pathology. Information on intra-articular anatomy can be obtained by arthroscopy. For example, Figure 40–1 shows the relation of a normal medial meniscus to the femur and tibia; Figure 40–2 shows the patella in relation to the femoral trochlea; and Figure 40–3 shows an osteoarthritic medial compartment with a meniscal tear. Arthroscopy has enhanced our understanding of the intra-articular environment and patterns of injury secondary to overload and trauma. Moreover, this procedure has expanded our knowledge of the natural history of knee pathology, improved the correlation between topographic findings and intra-articular anatomy, and provided the diagnosis of knee pain generators through direct observation. Pain is directly related to the structure involved and can often localize to one portion of the knee.[1]

Some knowledge of the mechanics of joint load is necessary for the diagnosis of knee pain. The knee can be conceptually separated into the medial and lateral tibiofemoral compartments and the patellofemoral compartment. An abnormal articular surface, whether the result of a destructive process from inflammatory disease, advancing age, overuse, repetitive microtrauma, macrotrauma, or a combination of these factors, does not distribute load normally, and the abnormal focus of load in the joint and subchondral bone is painful.[2] The physician must be aware of the factors that influence joint load and, thus, the development of symptoms. Among these diverse factors are ligament competence, muscular strength and coordination, and type and volume of activity and exercise. Weight and limb alignment should also be taken into account. Exercise and rehabilitation programs are more aggressive, precise, and effective when based on knowledge of these factors.[3]

HISTORY AND PHYSICAL EXAMINATION

A well-taken history can help guide the physical examination. Important questions include whether or not the pain was caused by a specific injury versus a gradual onset. Characterization and localization of the pain can help narrow the differential. Important clues such as hearing a loud pop or symptoms of "catching" alert the examiner to perform specific maneuvers during the examination. The physical examination of the knee should be conducted with the patient as comfortable and relaxed as possible, or else reflex guarding or postural muscle activation can impede the evaluation.

Acute trauma, tense effusion, mechanical derangement, or localized acute areas of articular inflammation may all inhibit complete relaxation. A pillow placed under the knee for support often contributes to relaxation. In some cases, aspiration of a tense effusion or hematoma is required for comfort. Examination of the normal knee first allows for comparison and often helps the patient anticipate what will be done on the painful knee.

With the patient standing, the physician can evaluate for any gross abnormalities in alignment. Once the patient is lying down and comfortable, the knee and surrounding structures should be examined for any abnormality, effusion, or deformity. Palpation should be performed with a secure knowledge of topographic anatomy and the relevant underlying structures. Withdrawal of the fat pad in knee flexion facilitates palpation of the condyles. The lateral joint line is best palpated in varus flexion, or the "figure-four" position. Methodical palpation of the patellar tendon and parapatellar area is vital. Small variations in the sites exhibiting tenderness may have significant diagnostic implications.

The range of motion must be checked actively and, if necessary, passively (gently). During the range-of-motion examination, palpation for crepitus of the articular surfaces, the snapping or catching of a scar or plica (i.e., a redundant fold of the synovium), and tenderness of the hamstring tendons and iliotibial band may also be performed. The location of any finding should be noted.

Special attention should be paid to the patella. An abnormal tilt, lateralization, and an alta (high-riding) or baja (low-riding) position should be noted, and the

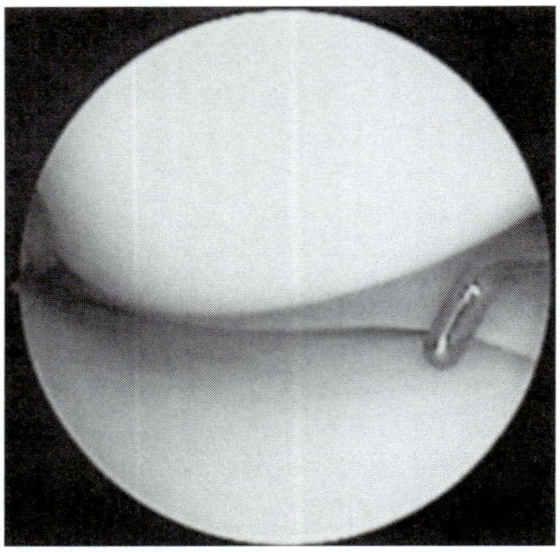

FIGURE 40–1 · Normal meniscus as seen by arthroscopy, with the surface of the femoral condyle above and the tibial plateau below.

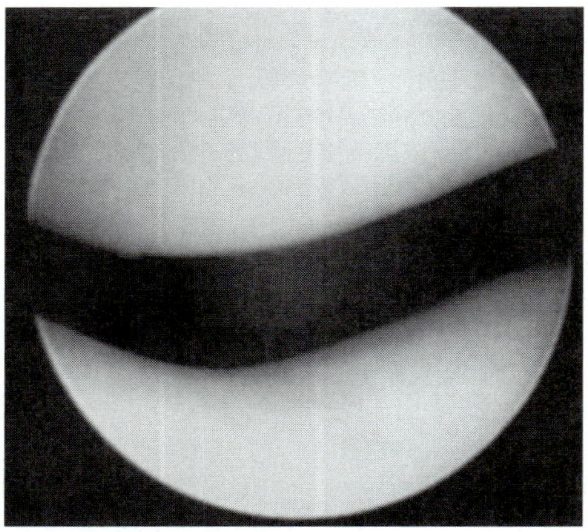

FIGURE 40–2 · Articular surface of the patella (above) in relation to the trochlea (below), as seen by arthroscopy.

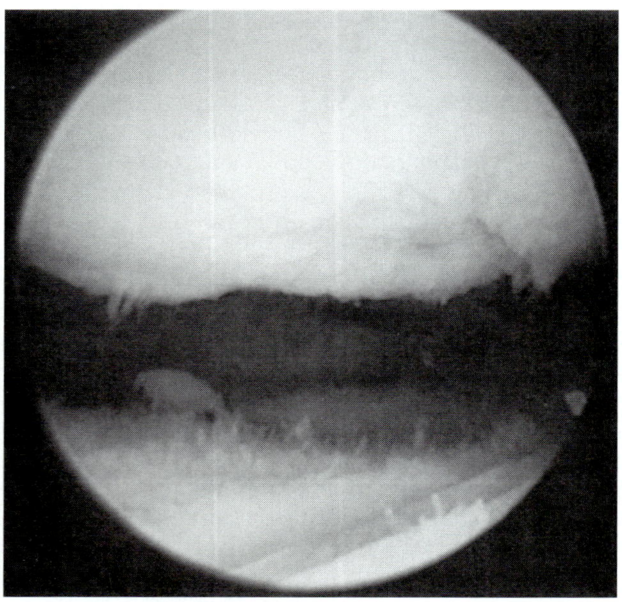

FIGURE 40–3 · Arthroscopic view of osteoarthritis of the medial compartment of the knee, with the surface of the femoral condyle above and the tibial plateau below.

patella should be tracked through the range of motion. The relative tension of the medial and lateral structures of the patella should be assessed by mobilization. Vigorous patellar compression is painful to even a normal patient and is therefore relatively worthless in establishing a diagnosis of patellofemoral overload or degenerative arthritis or in implicating the patella as a pain generator.

An assessment of the stability of the knee is a crucial part of the basic examination. Application of valgus and varus stress to the knee in a 30-degree flexed position and in full extension stretches the medial and lateral collateral ligaments, respectively. Some laxity will be evident in the 30-degree position but should diminish as the knee is brought to full extension. A comparison with the opposite knee should always be made. The competence of the anterior cruciate ligament can be assessed by anterior displacement of the tibia on the femur with the knee in 20 to 30 degrees of flexion (i.e., Lachman maneuver). The lack of solid resistance to anterior displacement beyond 2 to 3 mm, especially when compared with the resistance of the opposite knee, strongly suggests compromise of the anterior cruciate ligament. A posterior stress in the same position tests the posterior cruciate ligament. More sophisticated maneuvers exist for the assessment of instabilities, some of which involve rotary manipulation.[4] Learning the advanced aspects of knee-ligament examination requires repetition and coaching and may be hampered by the limited number of appropriate patients.

Hamstring flexibility should be assessed by a straight leg raise, which also stretches the sciatic nerve and its branches. Neurologic examination should include palpation of the tibial nerve in the popliteal space with the knee extended, the peroneal nerve, and any other area of neurogenic discomfort.

IMAGING AND DIAGNOSTIC TESTS

Some type of imaging should be included in the evaluation of most patients with significant knee complaints.

Plain Radiography

A series of simple non–weight-bearing anteroposterior (AP) and lateral radiographs can evaluate gross fracture changes, excessively superior or inferior patellar position, severe arthritic changes, spurring, some loose bodies, gross bone-density changes, and calcifications. The inclusion of weight bearing on the AP view adds valuable information regarding articular surface abnormalities, which are seen as the joint collapses. These views are best obtained in 30 degrees of flexion, a position that allows maximal contact between the femoral condyles and the tibia.[5] A notch view may be added for evaluation of osteochondral defects.

A modified axial patellar view, or Merchant's view (Fig. 40–4), allows an approximation of patellar alignment and a reasonable estimate of arthritic changes.[6] The alignment shown on these views is approximate because the patient is relaxed and static, and the position of the patella is not being influenced by muscle activity. A complete knee

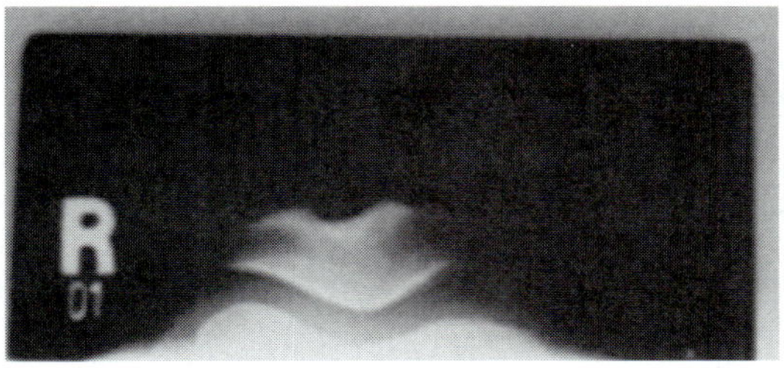

FIGURE 40–4 · Merchant's view (modified axial view of the patella).

series typically includes a standing AP, a lateral, a notch, and a Merchant's view, but the series can be modified on an individual basis to include other useful views. For example, an oblique projection of the tibial plateaus may reveal plateau fractures not seen on an AP view.

A long cassette view, including the hip, knee, and ankle, allows simple calculation of the mechanical axis and the weight-bearing line. This information is valuable in diagnosis and treatment and especially in the evaluation of a patient as a candidate for osteotomy,[7] an underused procedure for osteoarthritis and traumatic arthritis associated with angular deformity (Figs. 40–5 and 40–6).

Scintigraphy

Technetium-99m scans have traditionally been used for load analysis. A positive scan result reflects an increase in blood flow in reaction to acute or chronic overload in a given area[8] (Fig. 40–7). Some studies have shown resolution of abnormal overload following ligamentous reconstruction.[9] Although relatively inexpensive and sensitive, this method is not very specific. The specificity of the bone scan can be greatly surpassed by the use of short tau inversion recovery (STIR) or fat-suppression sequences on magnetic resonance imaging (MRI), which dramatically reveal areas of subchondral overload as defined by fluid in bone.[10,11]

Arthrography and Arthroscopy

MRI has supplanted arthrography for nonsurgical, noninvasive evaluation except when MRI is contraindicated. Arthroscopy, particularly when performed by the rheumatologist, is reviewed extensively in Chapter 48.

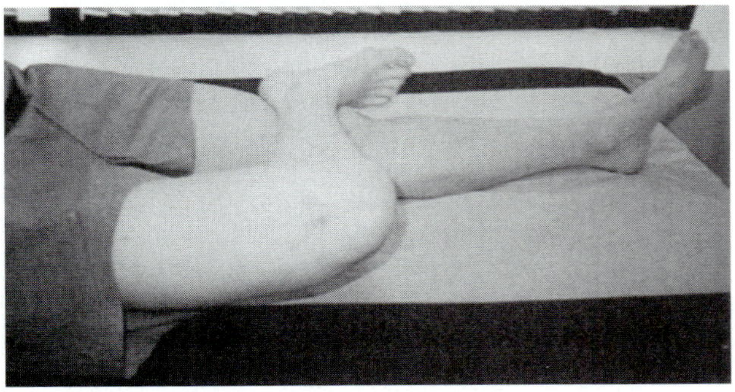

FIGURE 40–5 · Knee in the "figure-four" position (varus flexion).

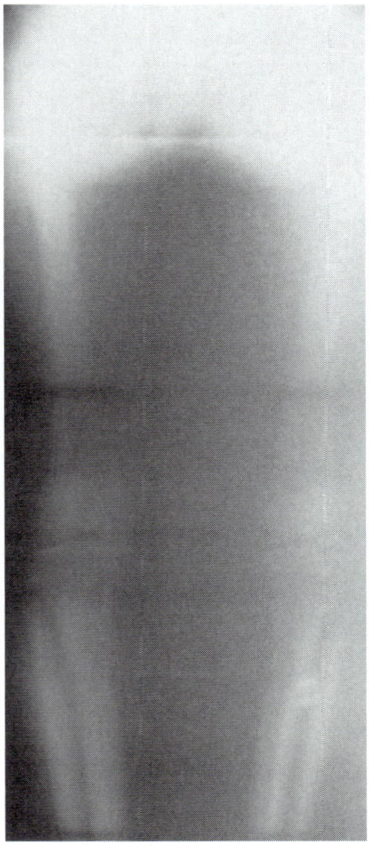

FIGURE 40–6 · Fifty-one-inch cassette view illustrating axial alignment and calculation of the mechanical varus-valgus angle of the knees and the weight-bearing line.

Computed Tomography

Computed tomography (CT) is rarely used in the evaluation of knee pain, except for the specific examination of bone, as in a fracture or a tumor.

Ultrasonography

Ultrasonography of the lower limb is used primarily to evaluate fluid-filled spaces. It is also employed to detect thrombi in phlebitis. Post-traumatic hematomas and seromas and popliteal cysts can be identified and, if necessary, aspirated under direct ultrasonographic control[12] (Fig. 40–8).

Magnetic Resonance Imaging

A noninvasive modality of unprecedented precision and scope, MRI, which postdates the revolution in arthroscopic technique, has changed the algorithm for the diagnosis of pain in peripheral joints. Its development continues, with increasing technical capacity, broader application, and better understanding of which particular images are useful in a given case. The pictures are software-derived re-formations, and the type and number of cuts is operator dependent. Use of the "standard series" in every case is not required and can be quite costly. The application of new technology and the use of the most appropriate or of modified studies, or both, can help

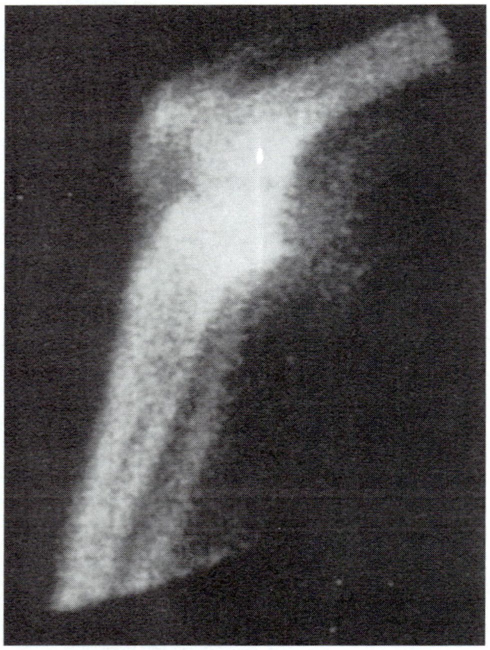

FIGURE 40–7 · Technetium-99m bone scan (medial view) illustrating increased uptake in the knee of a patient with osteoarthritis.

contain cost while retaining precision. Close consultation with the radiologist can help guide the appropriate study.

MRI has proved useful in imaging the articular cartilage surface, subchondral bone changes, and edema in arthritis and in post-traumatic and postoverload bone stress reactions, effusions, synovial abnormalities, menisci, plicae, intra-articular and extra-articular ligaments, medial and lateral retinacular changes, patellar position, meniscal and popliteal cysts, intra-articular ganglions, ganglions of tendons, and intraosseous cysts.[13,14] It reveals edema in tendons as a result of inflammation or trauma and tears of menisci, muscles, tendons, and ligaments[15] (Fig. 40–9). MRI elucidates neurogenic postexercise and post-traumatic changes or fluid collections[16] and is used to assess nerves and tumors.[17] This technique so precisely depicts the intra-articular, subchondral, and periarticular structures that it is often a major factor in decisions regarding medical and surgical treatments. MRI is an invaluable teaching aid for the patient and the physician, providing a picture of the pathology. One must always be aware, for example, that MRI can show meniscal tears in up to 5 percent of asymptomatic individuals. History and physical still remain the most important components of diagnosis.[18]

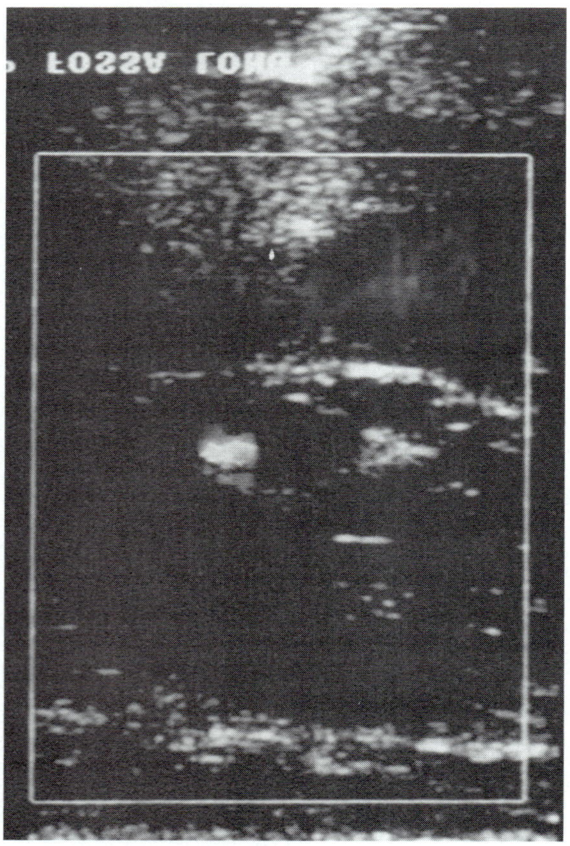

FIGURE 40–8 · Ultrasound of Baker's cyst.

In general, T_1 images offer the best anatomic detail, and T_2 images permit better evaluation of fluid.[19] Fat-suppression images show marrow fluid or edema very well, with good anatomic detail.[19] STIR images show muscle, tendon, joint, and marrow fluid best and are quite useful for the detection of bone trauma or overload (Figs. 40–10). Some loss of detail in the bone is encountered with STIR.[20]

Contrast Magnetic Resonance Imaging

Contrast MRI is extremely valuable in several settings. The injection of intra-articular solution may facilitate the visualization of certain intra-articular structures, such as a plica or medial shelf. The plica tissue sits on subchondral bone in the axial view and is not easily differentiated from the sclerotic subchondral bone of the femoral condyle unless it is "floated" up by contrast in the axial view (Fig. 40–11). Articular surface defects and osteochrondral lesions are also best defined by contrast MRI.[21]

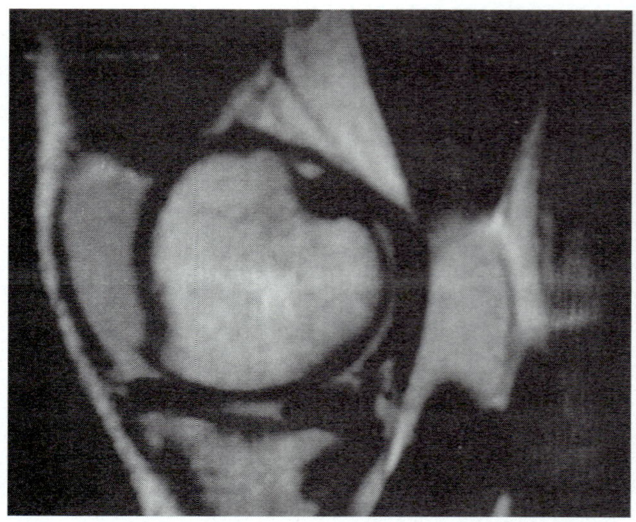

FIGURE 40–9 · Magnetic resonance imaging (MRI) (sagittal view) revealing a tear of the posterior medial meniscus as a line of increased uptake through the meniscus.

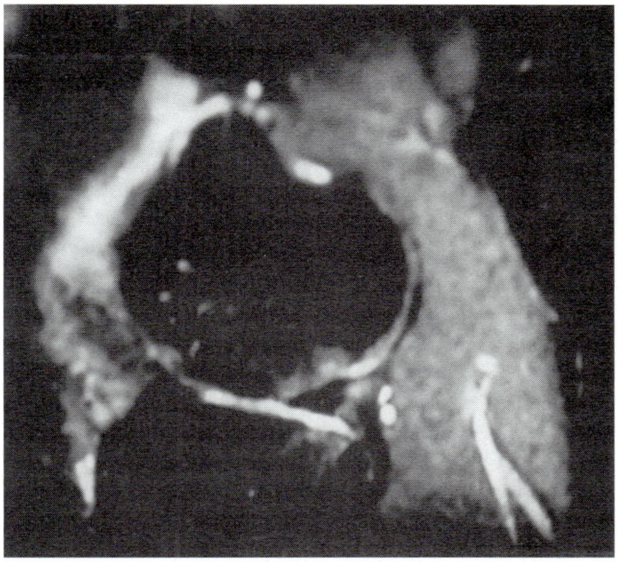

FIGURE 40–10 · Short Tau Inversion Recovery (STIR) Image of the Knee (sagittal view). High signal intensity from bone edema in the femoral condyle indicates an area of force overload.

Simple saline solution is a satisfactory and inexpensive contrast agent, especially when used with T_2 imaging (HC, personal communication). The use of gadolinium is controversial and is certainly not necessary in all cases. It may be most useful in detecting retears of menisci.[22]

Diagnostic Injection

Diagnostic injection is most frequently performed to delineate local nerve irritation, to determine whether pain is extra-articular in origin (e.g., referable to the tibiofibular joint), or to identify specific periarticular soft tissue sites or bursae as the source of pain. Occasionally, fluoroscopy is used to enhance precision. One recent study demonstrated increased intra-articular accuracy when using a lateral parapatellar approach for knee injection.[23]

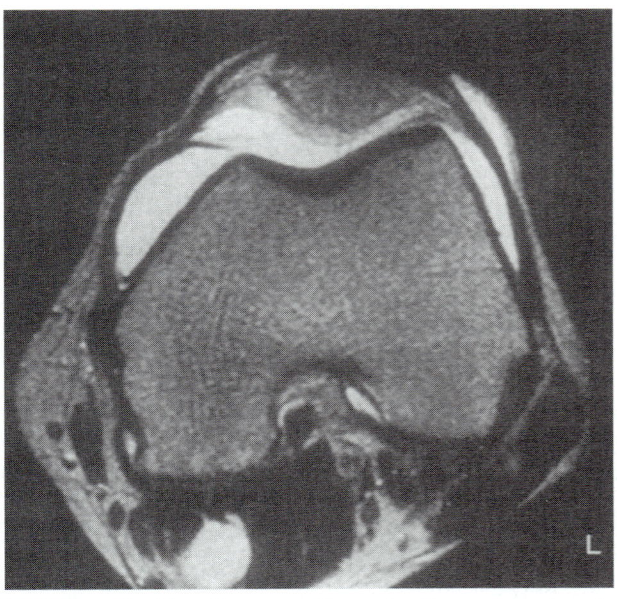

FIGURE 40–11 · Contrast Magnetic Resonance Imaging (MRI) Scan of the Knee (axial view) Illustrating a Plica or Medial Shelf. The redundant fold of synovium is seen to the left of the patella as a line of low uptake outlined by contrast within the joint space.

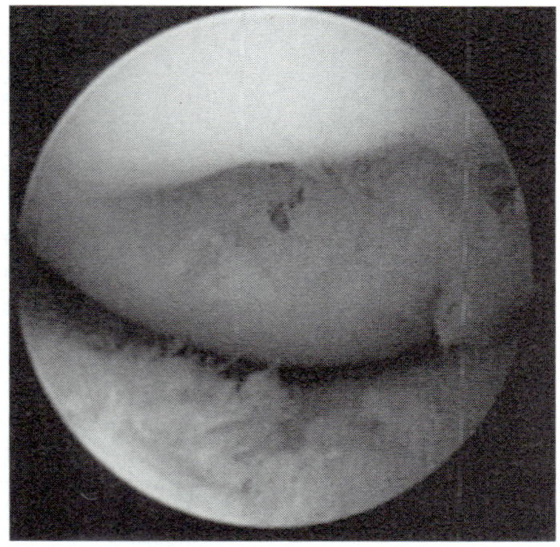

FIGURE 40–12 · Osteochondritis dissecans of the femoral condyle as seen by arthroscopy.

DISORDERS GENERATING KNEE PAIN

Anterior Knee Pain

Bursitis

The prepatellar bursa normally covers the patella and portions of the patellar tendon. With macrotrauma (e.g., a blow) or repetitive microtrauma (e.g., repeated kneeling), the bursa can become inflamed, fill with fluid, and enlarge in volume and area. Eventually, if this condition is not treated, bands and "loose bodies" of scar tissue may develop. The patient with prepatellar bursitis presents with pain on flexion or direct pressure and reports pain with walking or running. On physical examination, a soft tissue enlargement—sometimes warm, tender, and erythematous—is found anterior to the patella. Signs of acute inflammation require aspiration and fluid analysis to exclude septic bursitis. Cultures of bursal fluid may need review before glucocorticoids are administered. Treatment usually is nonsurgical, consisting of measures to prevent repetitive trauma, compression, use of oral nonsteroidal anti-inflammatory drugs (NSAIDs) or a steroid dose pack, and rest. If this conservative treatment fails, aspiration and glucocorticoid injection may be considered. Rarely, surgical excision is necessary.[24]

Disorders of the Patellar Tendon and Related Structures

Similar to all tendons, the patellar tendon is subject to inflammation (tendinitis), degeneration (microtears, tendinosis), and macrotears (partial or complete). The patellar tendon serves as a site of attachment for the patella and is subject to large tension loads, especially with high-impact activities such as jumping or running. Overload of the patellar tendon may also result from simple activities of daily living if the quadriceps muscle is weak or inhibited.[25] The patient presents with anterior knee pain that is exacerbated by jumping, cutting, running, squatting, and sometimes even walking. Inflammation or tearing is most common at the tendon's point of origin at the distal pole of the patella; damage and pain at this site are commonly referred to as *jumper's knee.*[26] Bone tension overload (stress fracture or reaction) commonly occurs distally at the point of the tendon's insertion on the tibia in adolescents (Osgood-Schlatter disease),[27] and proximally at its origin on the patella in highly active individuals. Rarely, a complete tendon rupture or fracture at the distal pole of the patella occurs.

Information on the inciting activity is useful in diagnosis and treatment. Careful palpation serves to determine the site of maximal pain, which is usually along the tendon or at its origin on the patella. MRI reveals tendon changes consistent with inflammation or tears and bone stress reactions.[28]

Initial treatment targets symptoms and includes rest, compressive bracing, use of NSAIDs, and muscle strengthening, with an emphasis on eccentric quadriceps work to shield the involved structures from stress.[25] Because glucocorticoid injection may weaken the tendon and predispose it to rupture, this mode of treatment should be used only rarely, with injection of the peritendinous sheath alone, after the patient is advised of the risks.[29] The risk of injury increases for several weeks after injection.

Surgical repair and debridement are sometimes necessary for chronic tendinitis or tendinosis. Incomplete tears that do not heal or that remain symptomatic may require surgical repair. MRI performed early in cases that start with a specific event, and in refractory cases, identifies partial tears that are not likely to improve with the passage of time and physical therapy.[29]

Plicae

During development of the fetus, the knee is divided into compartments by tissue septa that eventually disappear in humans. In some people, remnants of these septa, or plicae, remain in one of three areas: the medial parapatellar area, the infrapatellar area of the fat pad, and the suprapatellar area underneath the quadriceps tendon. Because the plica runs along the knee capsule, the patient generally presents with medial or inferomedial parapatellar pain. Other symptoms may include snapping, catching, or giving way as the plica moves across the medial condyle during flexion and extension. Anterior knee pain is sometimes more diffuse, and an effusion sometimes develops.[30] Plicae often begin to cause symptoms in the second decade of life.[31] Plicae also may become symptomatic in patients who are physically active and in those who have experienced a trauma.[30]

In many cases, physical examination reveals tenderness to palpation in the medial parapatellar and medial fat pad areas. Occasionally, a snap can be felt medially during flexion.[30] In the differential diagnosis, medial patellofemoral degenerative arthritis is most commonly considered; also considered are medial capsular fibrosis, anteromedial meniscal tears and ganglion cysts of the anterior knee, and tibiofemoral arthritis.[31] MRI with contrast or with saline solution injected intra-articularly can differentiate the plica from other conditions on the axial view.[31] Treatment consists of arthroscopic resection.[32] Nonsurgical therapy generally gives only temporary relief.

Patellofemoral Arthritis or Overload

A common source of anterior knee pain is patellofemoral arthritis. This condition is often described as *chondromalacia*—a broad, nonspecific term that conveys neither the importance of mechanics in its development nor its significance to the patient.[33]

Patellar biomechanics are highly specific. The patella absorbs load across approximately one fourth of its surface area at any time, the exact site varying with the degree of flexion of the knee.[34] The same is true of the femoral groove (trochlea). With the knee in full extension, the patella sits above the femoral joint surface on the suprapatellar fat. The load on the patella increases with increasing flexion. Accordingly, symptoms tend to arise from activities of daily life that involve flexion, such as squatting, rising from a seated position, climbing stairs or hills, and running. Exercises involving knee flexion impose the maximum load near full flexion and, therefore, tend to cause pain at that point. Rehabilitation for patellofemoral arthritis emphasizes the use of knee flexion or press (closed chain) exercises, or both, rather than knee extension (open chain) exercises.[35]

Factors predisposing to patellofemoral arthritis include repetitive flexion in work or sports (e.g., alpine skiing), congenital or traumatic malalignment, malpositioning (baja or alta), and malformation (flattening of the trochlea or patellar maldevelopment). All of these conditions reduce the contact surface area, resulting in increased stress and osteoarthritis.[36] Any factor that significantly weakens the quadriceps muscle (especially the vastus medialis oblique [VMO]) may result in malalignment of the patella and predispose to patellofemoral arthritis.[35] Inflammatory arthritis can also affect the patellofemoral joint.

Physical examination can reveal lateral tilt of the patella, tightness of lateral or medial retinacular tissues, lateral tracking, patella alta or baja, parapatellar tenderness, or subpatellar crepitus on extension or flexion.[37] Vigorous compression of the patella against resistance may cause pain; however, this pain may not reflect patellar pathology. Patellar pain is local and does not usually radiate to other areas of the knee.

Options for treatment are similar to those for any osteoarthritic joint. The focus should be on the modification of abnormal patterns or degrees of load and stress. One option is relative rest, which implies the modification of lifestyle in a way that minimizes the inciting or overload activity. A second option is shock absorption, with specific physical therapy and strengthening exercises to shield the joint from stress during flexion activity.[35] The patient should be counseled on how to maintain a personal exercise program after physical therapy has been completed. Third, surgical realignment or local manipulation of the articular surface, with drilling or burring, results in relocation or wider distribution of the patellar load. Multiple surgical techniques exist for this purpose.[38] Fourth, biologic resurfacing—a relatively new approach—uses chondrocyte reimplantation after growth and tissue culture or osteochondral auto- or allograft to fill in defects.[39] Fifth, total joint replacement is an option, but specific replacement of only the patellofemoral joint has a very narrow range of indications.[40,41]

All of these techniques directly address the issue of force per area, or overload. Arthroscopic débridement and treatment with oral or injectable medications focus on pain relief or reduction of synovitis, enhancing comfort, increasing function, and, in some cases, providing an opportunity for rehabilitation. They do not, however, address the fundamentals of abnormal load distribution, except by facilitation of strength, shock absorption, and coordination.

Arthrofibrosis

Knees that lack a full range of motion after surgery, trauma, or inflammation or as the result of osteoarthritis have two specific generators of fog. First, the fibrous tissue itself can be painful during an inflammatory phase that, depending on an individual's genetics, may last for many months. Treatment consists of anti-inflammatory medication including NSAIDS, steroids, and physical therapy. If this approach fails to relieve pain and increase range of motion to a satisfactory degree, surgical release may be necessary. Although it is preferable to perform surgery after the inflammatory phase, it is not always possible to wait.

Second, the techniques of physical therapy, especially aggressive use of passive range of motion, may lead to compressive joint overload, bone stress, and pain. It is critical that therapists be aware of this possibility. Distraction of the joint, with extension and careful compression at the end range of flexion, is an important component of therapy. MRI may show the stress reaction on fat suppression or STIR.

Mediolateral Knee Pain

Specificity in categorizing mediolateral knee pain according to the topographic anatomy of the knee is critical. For example, joint-line pain should refer to pain on palpation on what is confidently felt to be the joint line. A 1-cm difference in any direction can change the differential diagnosis.

Meniscal Abnormalities

Both menisci are subject to abnormalities that can create joint-line pain on palpation and with manipulation. Occasionally, the patient describes catching or locking of the knee that, at times, can be elicited on examination. An effusion often can be identified. Although the patient may describe more diffuse knee pain, the hallmark of a meniscal tear—and often the only finding on examination—is tenderness along the joint line. Physical examination has been shown in some studies to be more accurate than MRI in diagnosing meniscal tears.[42]

In the younger population, meniscal tears are related to activity and are therefore traumatic in origin. With increasing age, degenerative tears predominate as the internal architecture of the meniscus fails. Not all degenerative tears are symptomatic. The treatment for a symptomatic tear, regardless of its cause, is generally surgical. Certain degenerative tears manifest as pain and a palpable mass at the joint line, most frequently involving the lateral meniscus. The mass may be a ganglion cyst that connects directly to the meniscus.[43] Treatment consists of arthroscopic débridement of the meniscus and cyst.[44]

Chondrocalcinosis can increase the likelihood of meniscal tears as the calcific deposits make the meniscus brittle. The liberation of calcium pyrophosphate in the knee at the time of arthroscopy often generates troublesome significant postoperative synovitis.[45,46]

One of the most important functions of the menisci is load distribution. The removal of menisci may reduce the area of forced distribution at the posterior tibia by more than half.[47] Multiple studies from 1948 onward[48] have demonstrated that meniscectomy, especially in a young population, correlates with an earlier-than-anticipated appearance of degenerative arthritis, which is aggravated in knees with significant valgus or varus alignment.[49-53] If possible, menisci should be repaired in persons who have not yet reached middle age[54]; if the meniscus is not degenerative it can often be repaired.[55] When repair is not feasible, the smallest possible portion of the meniscus should be removed to alleviate symptoms and prevent further tears. The utility of meniscal allograft is not yet clear.[56-58]

Tibiofemoral Arthritis

Degenerative or traumatic arthritis of the medial or the lateral compartment manifests itself as joint-line pain, effusion, stiffness, or an insidious impairment of flexion or extension. Often, more than one compartment is involved, and the result is diffuse pain.

Moderate to severe changes can be diagnosed by examination and by standing AP radiography, which often is best done at 30 degrees of flexion to reveal the area of greatest loss of articular cartilage.[5] MRI shows articular cartilage defects (particularly if an effusion is present) and bone edema of overloaded subchondral bone on fat suppression or STIR sequences.[19]

Options for treatment include those described for patellofemoral arthritis; however, rehabilitation and arthroscopic débridement can delay—or in some cases eliminate—the need for other interventions if adequate shock-absorbing strength is developed.[59] The efficacy of arthroscopy and joint "irrigation" in the face of osteoarthritis has recently been called into question.[60] Tibial or femoral osteotomy is significantly underused and may delay for years or eliminate the need for joint replacement. Osteotomy can be done on patients as old as their early 70s if they are fit enough to undergo rehabilitation, and it allows a much wider range of function than joint replacement. Certain conditions that may cause presenting symptoms similar to those of osteoarthritis or post-traumatic arthritis include osteochondritis dissecans, osteonecrosis, and chondrolysis.

Osteochondritis dissecans is a developmental abnormality in which a fragment of subchondral bone and the overlying articular material spontaneously detach. This abnormality can involve any joint surface of the knee and generally affects relatively young patients. It may be painless and be manifested only by locking as the fragment of subchondral bone catches. More commonly, it causes pain, often along the joint line or in the patellofemoral area, depending on the location of the lesion[61] (Fig. 40–12). The diagnosis is frequently made by routine radiography but may require MRI. Treatment in the early phases is variable, but an attempt should be made to repair lesions that are loose or have nearly come loose.[61]

Posterior Knee Pain

Any affliction of the joint in its posterior recesses, including arthritis, synovitis, meniscal abnormalities, and inflammation of any of the posterior tendons, can cause posterior knee pain. Posterior cruciate trauma and posterior capsular trauma are also possible sources of such pain. Tibial neuritis can cause posterior pain.

One source of knee pain deserves specific mention. The most common is the popliteal or Baker's cyst (see Fig. 40–8). Rising off the posteromedial capsule, this type of cyst is oftenassociated with synovitis and the subsequent effusion of any etiology. Symptoms result from compression of the fluid-filled cyst as the knee is flexed or from inflammation in the cyst itself. MRI has permitted the recognition of other cysts in the area (often of gastrocnemius origin) that produce symptoms locally by inflammation or compression.[19] Cysts may be treated with aspiration or, more definitively, with surgical excision.

Neurogenic Pain

Pain from tibial, peroneal, or saphenous nerve entrapment or pathology is often misinterpreted as knee pain or radiculopathy. Local nerve tenderness, with reproduction of symptoms with nerve stretch, is common.

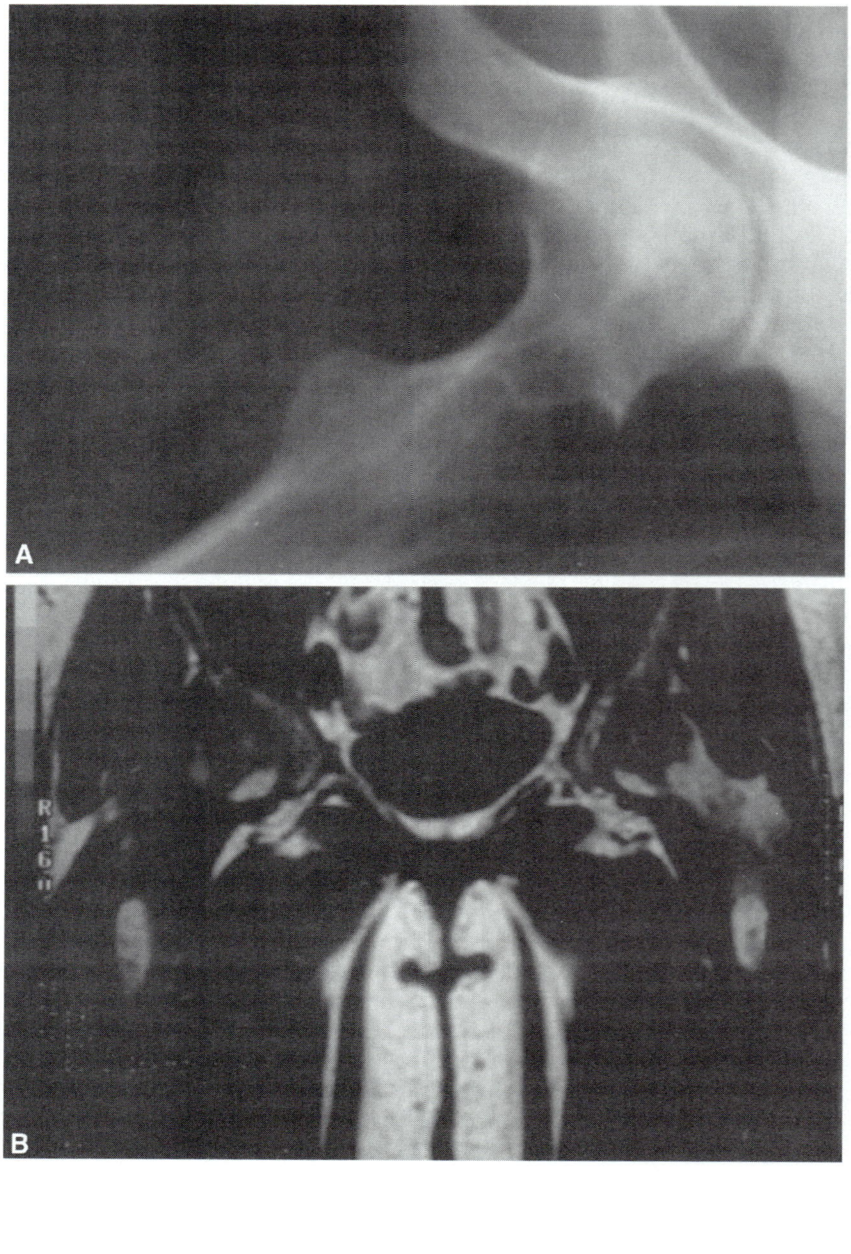

FIGURE 40–13 · Aseptic Necrosis of the Femoral Head. *A*, Plain film. *B*, Magnetic resonance imaging (MRI) scan.

The history often includes local deep aching or paresthesias with radiation of discomfort.

Hip Pain

The diagnosis of hip pain is a problem commonly encountered by musculoskeletal experts such as rheumatologists and orthopedists and more frequently by family practitioners and internists who initially see the patient. Identification of the cause of this discomfort is complicated by the fact that different patients mean different things by "hip pain." Referred pain patterns are common with hip pathology such as sciatica or bursitis. The anatomic source of an ache in the distal thigh or knee may be the hip joint. The hip joint and its periarticular structures are relatively deep and therefore relatively inaccessible to evaluation by manual elicitation of tenderness.

RELEVANT ANATOMIC FEATURES

The practitioner evaluating a patient with hip pain should attempt to find the anatomic source of the pain by eliciting a history and conducting a physical examination. Having tentatively identified the source, the physician should then define the pathophysiologic condition responsible for the pain.

Pathology in four general anatomic areas should be considered. The first category is intra-articular hip joint pathology, which includes processes that affect the articular cartilage (e.g., osteoarthritis), the synovium (e.g., rheumatoid arthritis, pigmented villonodular synovitis), the intra-articular soft tissue structures (e.g., tearing or infolding of the labrum), and the bones forming the joints (e.g., avascular necrosis affecting the femoral head and trauma). The second category is pathology of the extra-articular bony structures around the hip joint, including any process of the femoral shaft (e.g., fracture or tumor) and any process affecting the pelvic bones (including pelvic fracture, stress fracture, and osteitis pubis). The third category is pathology of the extra-articular soft tissues, which includes muscular pathology, soft tissue overuse syndromes (e.g., tendinitis, bursitis), and local nerve processes (e.g., meralgia paresthetica). The fourth category is pathology outside the hip area that can refer to the hip, which includes lumbosacral radiculopathy, femoral and inguinal hernias, and intrapelvic pathology (e.g., endometriosis, lymphoma).

The broad categories of entities to be considered after the anatomic source of pain has been identified include the following:

- Infections, such as septic arthritis and osteomyelitis
- Degenerative conditions, such as osteoarthritis
- Metabolic conditions, such as Paget's disease of the femur or pelvis
- Inflammatory conditions, such as rheumatoid arthritis, synovial chondromatosis, and pigmented villonodular synovitis
- Neurogenic conditions, such as radiculopathy and local nerve entrapment
- Traumas, such as femoral neck fractures and stress or insufficiency fractures
- Overuse syndromes, such as tendinitis and osteitis pubis
- Tumors, such as metastatic disease to the femoral neck or pelvis
- Vascular conditions, such as avascular necrosis of the femoral head and claudications with pain referred to the hip and leg

HISTORY

The history of the patient with hip pain is the key to determining the source of the pain. Questions such as time of onset, location, and whether or not trauma was involved point the physician toward a diagnosis. For example, time of onset can determine whether or not the pain came on gradually (osteoarthritis) or acutely (fracture). The location of the pain allows the diagnosis to be narrowed. Hip pain beginning in the low back and radiating down the buttock and back of the leg to the side of the calf and lateral side of the foot is more likely to be referred radiculopathy than an arthritic hip joint. Pain deep in the groin or the front of the hip that radiates down the thigh to the knee, accompanied by hip stiffness and pain with weight bearing, is more likely to be an arthritic hip than high lumbar radiculopathy. Range of motion and limited activities should also be elicited. In addition to these specific points, a general medical history may assist in the diagnosis. A patient with a history of prolonged oral steroid treatment who has groin pain or limitation of motion of the hip may have avascular necrosis of the femoral head. A thin runner with menstrual irregularities or amenorrhea and who now has hip or pelvic pain may have insufficiency stress fractures.

PHYSICAL EXAMINATION

The physical examination of the hip contributes important diagnostic information. The patient's gait should be assessed for signs of antalgic limp, Trendelenburg's weakness, steppage gait, footdrop, and other abnormalities. Range-of-motion examination of the hip in the supine position is revealing. Lack of internal rotation or pain with internal rotation is frequently a sign of hip joint pathology (e.g., osteoarthritis, avascular necrosis, inflammatory synovitis). A patient who has neither pain nor limitation of internal rotation but who has tenderness to palpation posterior to the trochanter is much more likely to have trochanteric bursitis than hip osteoarthritis. "Hip-irritability signs" are informative. A patient who cannot raise a straight leg off the table against gravity, who cannot hold the leg straight against resistance, or who is experiencing pain in the groin or thigh during the maneuver is likely to have primary hip joint pathology.

The results of local palpation are somewhat difficult to interpret. Palpation of the inguinal region is frequently uncomfortable even when the hip is normal. However, gentle palpation should be attempted and may be helpful in distinguishing among osteitis pubis;

pubic ramus fractures; ischial tendinitis, bursitis, or fractures; posterior trochanteric bursitis or abductor tendinitis; and iliac crest tensor fascia lata tendinitis. Palpation of the groin or inguinal region may reveal a femoral or inguinal hernia. Significant lymphadenopathy may indicate infection or lymphoma.

A thorough neurologic examination is helpful. As in most musculoskeletal conditions, examination of the opposite (uninvolved) side may be valuable for comparison.

DIAGNOSTIC TESTING

Plain Radiography

Plain radiographs of the hip and pelvis are frequently helpful. An AP pelvic radiograph and a "frog-leg" lateral-hip film may reveal fractures, joint-space narrowing indicative of articular cartilage loss, spurs or osteophytes indicative of arthritic change, segmental radiolucency or sclerotic changes of the femoral head indicative of avascular necrosis, calcifications indicative of synovial chondromatosis, or soft tissue calcification indicative of calcific tendinitis.

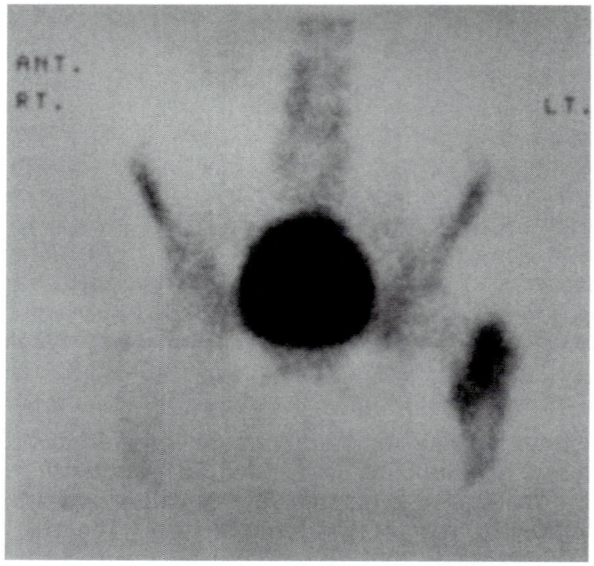

FIGURE 40–14 · Technetium bone scan of an occult hip fracture.

Arthrography

Arthrography may be valuable in the demonstration of labral pathology, especially when done in conjunction with an MRI.[62] It is certainly useful in confirming the intra-articular localization of an injection when differential injections are being administered, and it continues to have a role in the diagnosis of infection and loosening of the prosthesis in the patient with a painful total joint.[63]

Computed Tomography

CT of the hip and pelvis is probably most useful in the assessment of fractures, particularly complex acetabular and pelvic fractures.

Magnetic Resonance Imaging

MRI has dramatically facilitated the diagnosis of hip pain, and the indications for its use continue to expand, replacing scintigraphy in most cases.[64] Although its value depends on the quality of the image and the skill of the interpreter, MRI has become the standard technique for the diagnosis of several hip conditions.

The diagnosis of aseptic necrosis of the femoral head is made earlier by MRI than by any other technique, including bone scan, CT, and plain films[65] (Fig. 40–13). As information gained by MRI accumulates, new staging classifications of avascular necrosis are being developed.[66,67] MRI is the method of choice for the diagnosis of occult hip fracture in the elderly and, despite its expense, can be cost effective for this purpose. MRI is the best test for the diagnosis of transient osteonecrosis of the hip.[68] It is also the most valuable test for the staging of bony and soft tissue tumors around the hip.[69] MRI is frequently helpful in documenting synovitis of the hip joint by revealing effusion and sometimes (e.g., in pigmented villonodular synovitis) accurately shows synovial change.[70] MRI is the most accurate method for the diagnosis of stress fractures around the hip and pelvis.[71] MR arthrogram is useful in defining labral pathology.

Electromyography and Nerve Conduction Velocity Studies

Electromyography (EMG) and nerve conduction velocity (NCV) studies are used in the differential diagnosis of hip pain to evaluate referred lumbosacral plexopathies and to assess local nerve entrapment or nerve damage from trauma, surgery, or other disease states.

Injections

Differential block of the hip joint can be a valuable adjunct in differentiating intra-articular hip joint pain generated from other sources. This procedure is best undertaken in the fluoroscopy suite, with arthrography used to confirm the location of the injection. The technique may be particularly useful in distinguishing intra-articular hip pathology from referred lumbosacral radiculopathy and possible soft tissue conditions.[72,73] Dye injection along the iliopsoas tendon sheath under fluoroscopy sometimes reveals the snapping of the iliopsoas tendon over the pelvic brim and, when accompanied by lidocaine or corticosteroid injection, may help prove that the tendon condition is the pain generator.

DISORDERS CAUSING HIP PAIN

Intra-articular Disorders

Intra-articular disorders of the femoral head of the acetabular joint account for a significant portion of cases of hip pain. Manifestations of these disorders vary but frequently include pain deep in the groin or thigh and involve the anterior hip more than the posterior. Hip pain is often worse with weight bearing and associated with true passive loss of motion, with internal rotation and extension particularly affected. There may also be pain on forced internal rotation and with straight leg raising against resistance. Plain radiography is generally helpful in this situation, sometimes revealing narrowing and osteophytes associated with osteoarthritis, fractures of the femoral neck, and mottling or even collapse with the crescent sign of avascular necrosis.

Osteoarthritis of the hip joint, inflammatory arthritis, avascular necrosis of the femoral head, and septic hip joint are covered extensively in other portions of this book and are not discussed here. The other prominent causes of intra-articular hip disease are discussed briefly.

Labral Pathology

Hip pain accompanied by a painful mechanical snap can have a number of causes (see "Snapping Hip" section later in this chapter). One intra-articular cause of hip pain with snapping is a tear of the acetabular labrum.[62,74] The patient with acetabular labral tear is frequently a young, active adult with a history of trauma ranging from relatively minor twists, slips, and falls to more violent injuries, such as those incurred in an automobile accident. Most patients present with pain or discomfort deep in the anterior groin, and pivoting or twisting frequently exacerbates these symptoms. Most patients describe a click or mechanical catch associated with their discomfort.

On physical examination, patients most commonly have a normal range of motion or only mild limitation. Special maneuvers, such as a click seen in acute flexion with external rotation and full abduction followed by extension with internal rotation and adduction accompanied by pain, may point to the diagnosis.[74] Routine radiography is usually normal. MR arthrography has become the diagnostic procedure of choice.[75] Initial treatment of the patient with a labral tear may be nonsurgical, with activities restricted and NSAIDs administered in an effort to reduce or eliminate the inflammation of the hip. However, given the mechanical nature of the problem, this effort may fail, and surgery may be required. Interestingly, there may be a link between labral tears and the development of early osteoarthritis.[76] Advances in hip arthroscopy have given orthopedic surgeons the tools to perform partial resections with minimal trauma.[77]

Fractures

Hip fractures are a common source of hip pain. They can result in substantial morbidity or even death. Surgical and medical management techniques of hip fractures are beyond the scope of this chapter. We simply reiterate that aggressive management, with an emphasis on stabilization and early mobilization (aimed at reducing the problems associated with prolonged recumbency), is recommended.

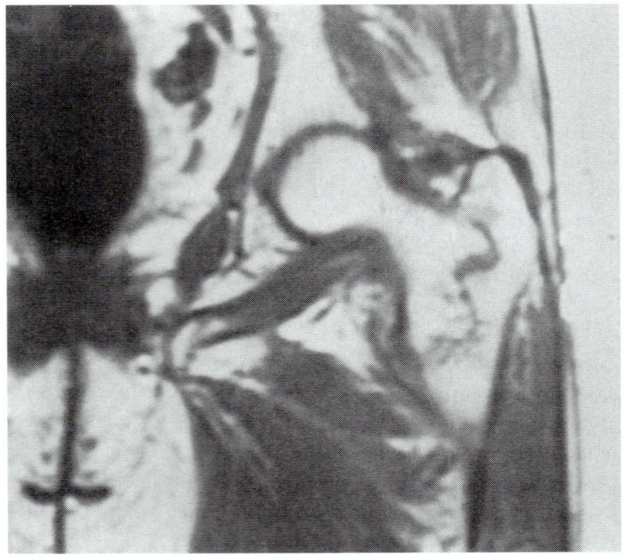

FIGURE 40–15 · Short tau inversion recovery (STIR) image of an occult fracture of the hip; note areas of increased intensity.

Most hip fractures are easily diagnosed. More difficult, however, is the diagnosis of an occult fracture in a patient with normal plain films. Although technetium bone scanning has been used to detect occult hip fractures (Fig. 40–14),[78] it may delay the diagnosis. MRI has become the method of choice for diagnosing occult hip fractures (Fig. 40–15).[79] Nondisplaced hip fractures can often be treated with minimally invasive procedures, such as percutaneous screw fixation. A missed occult fracture in a patient who continues to bear weight can lead to displacement, resulting in more extensive surgery. Displaced hip fractures are usually treated with replacement, especially in elderly patients.[80]

Stress Fractures

Another cause of hip pain can be a stress fracture of the bone. Two types of stress fractures exist. *Insufficiency fractures* occur in diseased bone that is involved in routine activity, and these typically affect older persons with osteopenic bone.[81] *Fatigue fractures* occur in normal healthy bones repeatedly subjected to high-level stress that is not great enough on any individual occasion to cause acute traumatic fracture but that cumulatively causes fatigue failure of the bone. The latter fractures are most likely to occur in young healthy persons involved in new activities (e.g., military recruits participating in training, athletes intensifying their training regimens). The popularity of competitive athletics in the United States has resulted in an increased rate of fatigue stress fractures among young patients.[82] Around the hip, such fractures can occur in the femoral neck and pelvic rami. Similar to occult fractures in the elderly, stress fractures in young athletes can be hard to diagnose and are commonly missed, occasionally with disastrous consequences.[83] Because a displaced femoral neck fracture in a young person often results in nonunion or avascular necrosis, it is important to maintain a high index of suspicion and to detect these fractures before they become displaced. MRI can generally make the diagnosis.

Stress fractures of the femoral neck can be categorized as being either on the compression (inferior) side or on the stress (superior) side of the neck.[84] This distinction is important as the latter type has a higher propensity for displacement and often requires prophylactic screw fixation.[85]

Transient Osteoporosis

Transient osteoporosis of the hip has been described in numerous reports and by various names, including *regional migratory osteoporosis* and *transient regional osteoporosis*.[86–94] The causes of this syndrome are unknown, and it is unclear whether it represents a single clinical entity or a group of entities with similar clinical presentations. Most cases have affected young and middle-aged men or pregnant women in the third trimester. The presentation frequently consists of the sudden or gradual onset of dull, aching pain in the region of the hip joint, typically including the groin and thigh and sometimes accompanied by minor trauma. Patients are not likely to have risk factors for avascular necrosis. Physical examination generally shows some hip irritability with pain on passive range of motion, particularly rotational maneuvers. Weight bearing typically exacerbates the condition. Radiographs characteristically show demineralization of the femoral head and neck, although no radiologic abnormalities may be seen early on. Findings on routine laboratory examination are frequently normal. Technetium isotope studies characteristically demonstrate increased uptake within the femoral head. MRI typically shows decreased signal intensity on T_1-weighted images and increased signal intensity on T_2-weighted images, with a so-called bone marrow edema pattern[94] There may be effusion in the joint, but there is usually no erosion or cartilage involvement. In most cases, the problem is self-limiting; generally, pain resolves and function returns within 2 to 6 months. With resolution of symptoms, plain radiographs show gradual remineralization of bone.

To a certain extent, the diagnosis is one of exclusion, because more serious problems need to be excluded. In its early stages, osteonecrosis can produce similar MRI findings; ultimately, however, in osteonecrosis MRI shows the T_2-weighted double-line sign.[95] The possibility of hip infection, inflammatory arthritis, tumor, and trauma needs to be considered. An aspirate of synovial fluid is occasionally evaluated; although in transient osteoporosis of the hip, the aspirate may be sterile. Inflammatory arthritis, infiltrative tumors, and trauma should also be considered.

Treatment is basically supportive, entailing activity modification; occasional protective weight bearing during the active phase of the disease; maintenance of range of motion, with gradual ambulation as comfort allows and as the process progresses; and use of NSAIDs or other mild analgesics for pain relief. It has not been demonstrated that the use of glucocorticoids speeds resolution.[89]

Snapping Hip

Not uncommonly, patients present with hip pain accompanied by a biomechanical snapping sensation. These patients are usually relatively young, are frequently athletes or dancers, and may give a history of trauma or repetitive overuse activity, such as running. The numerous causes of this problem fall into three categories: external, internal, and intra-articular.[96] External causes are thought to be most common and involve thickening of the posterior part of the iliotibial band or of the anterior border or the gluteus maximus, with snapping over the greater trochanter. The thickened band lies posterior to the greater trochanter when the hip is in extension and snaps forward over the greater trochanter with flexion. Patients report that the hip pops out of place or dislocates; they generally perceive the problem to be in the area of the greater trochanter—a description that helps to distinguish this type of snapping from the internal and intra-articular types. The snapping is frequently detectable when the examiner places a hand over the greater trochanter and walks along with the patient. The iliotibial band can often be felt to pop over the greater trochanter if the patient lies on the unaffected side with the affected hip adducted, keeps the knee in extension (keeping the fascia lata tight), and then actively flexes and extends the hip.

Diagnostic testing usually is not helpful or necessary, although dynamic ultrasound may be of use.[97] Treatment is initially nonsurgical, consisting of stretching of the iliotibial band, reduction of inflammation (e.g., ice, NSAIDs), occasional injection of glucocorticoids, and short-term modification of activity. If the pain remains significant, surgical treatment can be undertaken.[98,99] Internal causes are usually related to the iliopsoas tendon snapping back and forth over the femoral head.[96] Patients presenting with this problem frequently report a painful snapping sensation that they perceive to be in the anterior hip and groin. An examiner can sometimes reproduce the snap by having the patient lie supine, flex and abduct the hip, and then bring it back into a position of extension and abduction.

Diagnostic testing may be helpful in the evaluation of internal snapping. Iliopsoas bursography or iliopsoas tenography is most useful.[100] This technique can help visualize the iliopsoas tendon snapping over the femoral head. Initial treatment is nonsurgical, with stretching of the iliopsoas in extension, use of NSAIDs, and modification of activities until symptoms diminish. If symptoms persist, surgical treatment can be undertaken.[100] Intra-articular snapping may be caused by tearing of the acetabular labrum, as described earlier in this chapter (see "Labral Pathology"). Other causes include traumatic loose body, synovial chondromatosis, and post-traumatic femoral head defects.[96]

Bursitis

Frequently, patients present to the clinician's office with pain on the side of the hip over or posterior to the greater trochanteric area. Although this symptom could have numerous causes, three major entities are commonly seen in this setting in clinical practice: referred pain from the low back with sciatica; referred pain from intra-articular hip pathology, most often osteoarthritis; and local soft tissue inflammation, frequently called *trochanteric bursitis*. Because no findings are pathognomonic for trochanteric bursitis, the diagnosis is generally based on clinical impression.

The patient is most often middle-aged, female, and heavy. Pain is typically located along the lateral side of the upper thigh, frequently radiates from the buttock down toward the knee, is characteristically aggravated by activity such as walking or stair climbing, is typically worse at night, and prevents patients from lying on the affected side. Physical examination reveals localized tenderness over the greater trochanter that is best elicited by palpation with the patient lying on the unaffected side. Plain radiographs may show peritrochanteric calcification. MRI occasionally shows trochanteric bursitis, but these results may not alter clinical recommendations, and MRI may not be warranted except to exclude other pathologic conditions.[101]

The differential diagnosis of hip bursitis includes lymphadenopathy, tumors, hernias, and vascular malformations. CT with arthrography can demonstrate communication between the hip joint and the bursa, and the lesion can be well defined on MRI.[102] Treatment depends on the nature of the symptoms and of the underlying or associated conditions. Aspiration of the bursa with corticosteroid injection is sometimes effective. Occasionally, resection of the bursa is indicated.

Osteitis Pubis

Osteitis pubis is an inflammatory condition of unknown origin affecting the pubic symphysis and surrounding muscular attachments. Osteitis pubis has been associated with complications of suprapubic surgery and with peripartum urinary tract infections.[103] However, most reports have described its occurrence in athletes.[104] An athlete's variety of symptoms at presentation may lead to a delay in the diagnosis of osteitis pubis. These symptoms include pain in the groin, medial thigh, testicles, hips, or lower abdomen. It may well be that a number of underlying conditions initiate the process and that compensatory mechanisms (e.g., an adductor strain) then increase the shear stress across the symphysis pubis, leading to mechanical irritation, inflammation, and (ultimately) bony resorption.

Patients may have tenderness at the symphysis or pubic rami, but associated tenderness of other adjacent muscle groups may confuse the issue. Plain radiographs may show changes typical of osteitis pubis, with osteolysis at the joint; however, these radiologic changes may not be evident early on. Technetium bone scanning is likely to give positive results.[105] MRI—particularly fat-suppression sequences—may document stress around the symphysis but may also detect adjacent areas of pathology or help identify other conditions (e.g., pubic stress fracture). Limited STIR sequences may be economical for the monitoring of changes in the stress reaction with treatment.[16]

The initial focus of treatment is the reduction of inflammation. Rest from the inciting activity is required, with cross training used to maintain aerobic fitness. NSAIDs or even oral corticosteroids may be used. Intra-articular cortisone injection may be of value when other methods are not working. After the stress has been reduced across the symphysis and the inflammation diminished, a stretching and strengthening program emphasizing abdominal, hip, and short-arc closed-chain exercises should be instituted.[104] The use of bisphosphonates is being examined.[106] Unfortunately, recurrence is not uncommon. Surgical intervention can be considered for the recalcitrant cases.[107]

A differential diagnosis must be undertaken in evaluating groin pain in an athlete and should include osteitis pubis, stress fracture to the pubic or ischial rami or femoral neck, hernias, isolated muscle tears or strains in the adductor abdominal muscles, apophysitis or bony avulsion injuries, genitourinary infection, or urolithiasis. In rare cases, seronegative spondyloarthropathy, such as ankylosing spondylitis or Reiter's syndrome, may be associated.[104]

Regional Disorders

The source of hip pain commonly is the hip joint or the immediate periarticular structures. Only a high index of suspicion may prompt a thorough examination of other areas of anatomy. Nevertheless, such an examination can be crucial in the evaluation of hip pain.

Lumbosacral Radiculopathy

The need for a regional approach is illustrated by hip pain arising from lumbosacral pathology. Posterior buttock and lateral hip pain is most likely attributable to lumbosacral radiculopathy from local soft tissue inflammation (e.g., trochanteric bursitis) or is referred from intra-articular hip pathology (e.g., osteoarthritis). Certain features of the patient's history may help to distinguish among the choices. Referred radicular pain is frequently worsened by prolonged sitting and sometimes by lying flat, whereas rest and lack of weight bearing usually relieve intra-articular hip pathology. The neurologic nature of the referred pain may be apparent in the patient's description of its character: Burning and tingling symptoms are uncharacteristic of intra-articular discomfort. Pain that radiates from the hip all the way into the foot and is accompanied by tingling or weakness is more frequently neurogenic than of hip joint origin. Comprehensive physical and neurologic evaluations are frequently helpful; if a patient has a true flexion or external rotation contracture of the hip joint, with limitation of internal rotation and hip irritability on these maneuvers, the pain is more likely to be attributable to intra-articular hip pathology than referred from the lumbar area. True motor loss and reflex changes are more likely signs of lumbar radiculopathy. Local tenderness over the trochanter and the lumbar area and relief of pain by anesthetic and cortisone injection are hallmarks of trochanteric bursitis; their absence warrants consideration of other referred sources of pain. The situation may include the presence of more than one disorder; an elderly patient with an osteoarthritic hip may have concomitant lumbosacral spinal stenosis, with mixed symptoms and signs.

An EMG can be included in the workup to look for signs of radiculopathy or nerve entrapment. MRI frequently reveals disk herniation, nerve impingement, and bony spinal stenosis impingement. Differential injections can be extremely helpful in distinguishing referred lumbar radicular pain from hip joint or periarticular pain. Particularly valuable are selective nerve root blocks, epidural glucocorticoid injection, local soft tissue bursal injection, and intra-articular hip injection.

Miscellaneous Disorders

A variety of miscellaneous disorders can cause pain referred to the hip. Local nerve entrapments may cause referred pain. For example, entrapment of lateral cutaneous branches of the iliohypogastric nerve and the subcostal nerves can produce pain in the upper lateral thigh. Meralgia paresthetica is anterolateral thigh pain caused by entrapment of the lateral femoral cutaneous nerve.[108] Femoral and inguinal hernias can produce pain in the inguinal and hip areas and can be diagnosed by history and physical examination. Tumors, particularly lymphomas, can manifest in the hip and inguinal regions. The proximal femur and the pelvis are common sites of metastatic bone disease. Low intrapelvic pathology (e.g., ovarian pathology, intrapelvic or extrapelvic endometriosis) sometimes presents as hip pain.[109]

REFERENCES

1. Dye SF, Vaupel GL, Dye CC: Conscious neurosensory mapping of the internal structures of the human knee without intraarticular anesthesia. Am J Sports Med 6:773-777, 1998.
2. Radin EL, Rose RM: Role of subchondral bone in the initiation and progression of cartilage damage. Clin Orthop 213:34, 1986.
3. Saal J, Dillingham MF: Nonoperative treatment and rehabilitation of disc, facet, and soft-tissue injuries in athletes. *In* Hershman E (ed): The Lower Extremity and Spine in Sports Medicine, 2nd ed. St. Louis, Mosby, 1994.
4. Feagin JA: The office diagnosis and documentation of common knee problems. Clin Sports Med 8:453, 1989.
5. Messieh SS, Fowler PJ, Munro T: Anteroposterior radiographs of the osteoarthritic knee. J Bone Joint Surg Br 72:639, 1990.
6. Merchant AC: Classification of patellofemoral disorders. Arthroscopy 4:235, 1988.
7. Moreland JR, Bassett LW, Hanker GJ: Radiographic analysis of the axial alignment of the lower extremity. J Bone Joint Surg Am 69:745, 1987.
8. McCrae F, Shouls J, Dieppe P, et al: Scintographic assessment of osteoarthritis of the knee joint. Ann Rheum Dis 51:938, 1992.
9. Dye SF, Chew MH: Restoration of osseous homeostasis after anterior cruciate ligament reconstruction. Am J Sports Med 5:748-750, 1993.
10. Schietzer ME, Mandel S, Schwartzman RJ, et al: Reflex sympathetic dystrophy revisited: MR imaging findings before and after infusion of contrast material. Radiology 195:211, 1995.
11. Rankine JJ, Smith FW, Scotland TR: Case report: Short tau inversion recovery (STIR) sequence MRI appearances of reflex sympathetic dystrophy. Clin Radiol 50:188, 1995.
12. Ostergaard M, Court-Payen M, Weislander S, et al: Ultrasonography in arthritis of the knee: A comparison with MR imaging. Acta Radiol 36:19, 1995.
13. Burk DL, Mitchell DG, Rifkin MD, et al: Recent advances in magnetic resonance imaging of the knee. Radiol Clin North Am 28:379, 1990.
14. Leunig M, Werlen S, Ungersbock A, et al: Evaluation of the acetabular labrum by MR arthrography [published erratum appears in J Bone Joint Surg Br 79:693, 1997]. J Bone Joint Surg Br 79:230, 1997.
15. Tehrazadeh J, Kerr R, Amster J: Magnetic resonance imaging of tendon and ligament abnormalities. Skeletal Radiol 21:79, 1992.
16. Tuite MJ, DeSmet AA: MRI of selected sports injuries: Muscle tears, groin pain, and osteochondritis dissecans. Semin Ultrasound CT MR 15:318, 1994.
17. Stoller D: Magnetic Resonance Imaging in Orthopedics and Rheumatology. Philadelphia, JB Lippincott, 1989.
18. LaPrade RF, Burnett QM II, Veenstra MA, Hodgman CG: The prevalence of abnormal magnetic resonance imaging findings in asymptomatic knees with correlation of magnetic resonance imaging to arthroscopic findings in symptomatic knees. Am J Sports Med 6: 739-745,1994.
19. Stoller D: Magnetic Resonance Imaging in Orthopedics and Rheumatology. Philadelphia, JB Lippincott, 1989.
20. Newberg AH, Wetzner SM: Bone bruises: Their patterns and significance. Semin Ultrasound CT MR 15:396, 1994.
21. Chandnani VP, Ho CH, Chu P, et al: Knee hyaline cartilage evaluated with MR imaging: A cadaveric study involving multiple imaging sequences and intra-articular injection of gadolinium and saline solution. Radiology 178:557, 1991.
22. Sciulli RL, Boutin RD, Brown RR, et al: Evaluation of the postoperative meniscus of the knee: a study comparing conventional arthrography, conventional MR imaging, MR arthrography with iodinated contrast material, and MR arthrography with gadolinium-based contrast material. Skeletal Radiol 9: 508-514, 1999.
23. Jackson DW, Evans NA, Thomas BM: Accuracy of needle placement into the intra-articular space of the knee. J Bone Joint Surg Am 84:1522-1527, 2002.
24. Kerr DR: Prepatellar and olecranon arthroscopic bursectomy. Clin Sports Med 12:137, 1993.
25. Mangine-Eifert M, Brewster C, Wong M, et al: Patellar tendonitis in the recreational athlete. Orthopedics 15:1359, 1992.
26. Nichols CE: Patellar tendon injuries. Clin Sports Med 11:807, 1992.
27. Tachdjian OM: Pediatric Orthopedics, 2nd ed. Philadelphia, WB Saunders, 1990, p 1010.
28. Davies SG, Baudouin CJ, King JB, et al: Ultrasound, computed tomography, and magnetic resonance imaging in patellar tendonitis. Clin Radiol 43:52, 1991.
29. Leadbetter WB, Pekka PA, Lane GJ, et al: The surgical treatment of tendinitis. Clin Sports Med 11:679, 1992.
30. Tindel NL, Nisonson B: The plica syndrome. Orthop Clin North Am 23:613, 1992.
31. Johnson DP, Eastwood DM, Witherow PJ: Symptomatic synovial plica of the knee. J Bone Joint Surg Am 75:1485, 1993.
32. Dorchak JD, Barrack RL, Kneisl JS, et al: Arthroscopic treatment of symptomatic synovial plica of the knee. Am J Sports Med 19:503, 1991.
33. Kelly MA, Insall JN: Historical perspectives of chondromalacia patellae. Orthop Clin North Am 4:517, 1992.
34. Reilly D, Martens M: Experimental analysis of the quadriceps muscle force and patellofemoral joint reaction force for various activities. Acta Orthop Scand 43:126, 1972.
35. Zappala FG, Taffel CB, Scuderi GR: Rehabilitation of patellofemoral disorders. Orthop Clin North Am 23:555, 1992.
36. Tria AJ, Palumbo RC, Alicea JA: Conservative care for patellofemoral pain. Orthop Clin North Am 23:545, 1992.
37. Fu FH, Maday MG: Arthroscopic lateral release and the lateral compression syndrome. Orthop Clin North Am 23:601, 1992.
38. Fulkerson JP, Schutzer SF: After failure of conservative treatment for painful patellofemoral malalignment: Lateral release or realignment? Orthop Clin North Am 17:283, 1986.
39. Kolettis GT, Stern SH: Patellar resurfacing for patellofemoral arthritis. Orthop Clin North Am 23:665, 1992.
40. Mont MA, Haas S, Mullick T, Hungerford DS: Total knee arthroplasty for patellofemoral arthritis. J Bone Joint Surg Am 84: 1977-1981, 2002.
41. Smith AM, Peckett WR, Butler-Manuel PA, et al: Treatment of patello-femoral arthritis using the Lubinus patello-femoral arthroplasty: a retrospective review. Knee 9:27-30,2002.

42. Miller GK: A prospective study comparing the accuracy of the clinical diagnosis of meniscal tear with magnetic resonance imaging and its effect on clinical outcome. Arthroscopy 12:406-413, 1996.
43. Glasgow MM, Allen PW, Blakeway C: Arthroscopic treatment of cysts of the lateral meniscus. J Bone Joint Surg Br 75:299, 1993.
44. Mills CA, Henderson IJ: Cysts of the medial meniscus: Arthroscopic diagnosis and management. J Bone Joint Surg Br 75:293, 1993.
45. Fisseler-Eckhoff A, Muller KM: Arthroscopy and chondrocalcinosis. Arthroscopy 8:98, 1992.
46. Zarins B, McInerney VK: Calcium pyrophosphate and pseudogout. Arthroscopy 1:8, 1985.
47. Baratz ME, Fu FH, Mengato R: Meniscal tears: The effect of meniscectomy and of repair on intra-articular contact areas and stress on the human knee. Am J Sports Med 14:270, 1986.
48. Fairbank TJ: Knee joint changes after meniscectomy. J Bone Joint Surg Br 30:664, 1948.
49. Allen PR, Denham RA, Swan AV: Late degenerative changes after meniscectomy. J Bone Joint Surg 66:666, 1984.
50. Lynch MA, Henning CE, Glick KR: Knee joint surface changes, long-term follow-up meniscus tear treatment in stable anterior cruciate ligament reconstruction. Clin Orthop 172:148, 1983.
51. McGinty JB, Guess LF, Marvin RA: Partial or total meniscectomy, a comparative analysis. J Bone Joint Surg Am 59:763, 1977.
52. Tapper EM, Hoover NW: Late results after meniscectomy. J Bone Joint Surg Am 51:517, 1969.
53. Yocum LA, Kerlan RK, Jobe FW, et al: Isolated lateral meniscectomy. J Bone Joint Surg Am 61:338, 1979.
54. Noyes FR, Barber-Westin SD: Arthroscopic repair of meniscal tears extending into the avascular zone in patients younger than twenty years of age. Am J Sports Med 30:589-600, 2002.
55. Scott GA, Jolly BL, Henning CE: Combined posterior incision and arthroscopic intra-articular repair of the meniscus. J Bone Joint Surg Am 68:847, 1986.
56. Veltri DM, Warren RF, Wickiewicz TL, et al: Current status of allograft transplantation. Clin Orthop 303:44,1994.
57. Wirth CJ, Peters G, Milachowski KA, et al: Long-term results of meniscal allograft transplantation. Am J Sports Med 30:174-181, 2002.
58. Ryu RK, Dunbar V WH, Morse GG: Meniscal allograft replacement: a 1-year to 6-year experience. Arthroscopy 18:989-994, 2002.
59. Rand JA: Role of arthroscopy in osteoarthritis of the knee. Arthroscopy 7:358, 1991.
60. Moseley JB, O'Malley K, Petersen NJ, et al: A controlled trial of arthroscopic surgery for osteoarthritis of the knee. N Engl J Med 347:81-88, 2002.
61. Garrett JC: Osteochondritis dissecans. Clin Sports Med 10:569, 1991.
62. Fitzgerald RH: Acetabular labrum tears. Clin Orthop 311:60, 1995.
63. Kraemer WJ, Saplys R, Waddel JP, et al: Bone scan, gallium scan, and hip aspiration in the diagnosis of infected total hip arthroplasty. J Arthroplasty 8:611, 1993.
64. Pitt MJ, Lund PJ, Speer DP: Imaging of the pelvis and hip. Orthop Clin North Am 21:545, 1990.
65. Fordyce MJ, Solomon L: Early detection of avascular necrosis of the femoral head by MRI. J Bone Joint Surg Br 75:365, 1993.
66. Sugano N, Ohzono K, Masuhara K, et al: Prognostication of osteonecrosis of the femoral head in patients with systemic lupus erythematosus by magnetic resonance imaging. Clin Orthop 305:190, 1994.
67. Lafforgue P, Dahan E, Chanaud C, et al: Early-stage avascular necrosis of the femoral head: MR imaging for prognosis in 31 cases with at least 2 years of follow-up. Radiology 187:199, 1993.
68. Rhodes I, Matzinger MA: Residents' corner: Answer to case of the month: Transient osteonecrosis of the hip. Can Assoc Radiol J 44:399, 1993.
69. Aboulfia AJ, Malawer M: Surgical management of pelvic and extremity osteosarcoma. Cancer 71(Suppl):3358, 1993.
70. Boyd AD, Sledge CB: Evaluation of the hip with pigmented villonodular synovitis: A case report. Clin Orthop 275:180, 1992.
71. Bencardino JT, Palmer WE.: Imaging of hip disorders in athletes. Radiol Clin North Am 40: 267-287, 2002.
72. Traycoff RB: "Pseudotrochanteric bursitis": The differential diagnosis of lateral hip pain. J Rheumatol 18:1810, 1991.
73. Alcock P: Diagnostic value of intra-articular anaesthetic in primary osteoarthritis of the hip [letter, comment]. J Bone Joint Surg Br 80:934, 1998.
74. Byrd JW: Labral lesions: An elusive source of hip pain: case reports and literature review. Arthroscopy 12:603, 1996.
75. Czerny C, Hofmann S, Urban M, et al: MR arthrography of the adult acetabular capsular-labral complex: correlation with surgery and anatomy. AJR 173:345-349, 1999.
76. McCarthy JC, Noble PC, Schuck MR, et al: The Otto E. Aufranc Award: The role of labral lesions to development of early degenerative hip disease. Clin Orthop 393:25-37, 2001.
77. Farjo LA, Glick JM, Sampson TG: Hip arthroscopy for acetabular labral tears. Arthroscopy 15:132-137, 1999.
78. Geslien GE, Thrall JH, Espinosa JL, et al: Early detection of stress fractures using 99m-Tc-polyphosphate. Radiology 121:683, 1976.
79. Perron AD, Miller MD, Brady WJ: Orthopedic pitfalls in the ED: radiographically occult hip fracture. Am J Emerg Med 20: 234-237, 2002.
80. Parker MJ, Khan RJ, Crawford J, Pryor GA: Hemiarthroplasty versus internal fixation for displaced intracapsular hip fractures in the elderly: A randomised trial of 455 patients. J Bone Joint Surg Br 84:1150-1155, 2002.
81. Tountas AA: Insufficiency stress fractures of the femoral neck in elderly women. Clin Orthop 292:202, 1993.
82. Matheson GO, Clement DC, McKenzie JE, et al: Stress fractures in athletes: a case study of 320 cases. Am J Sports Med 15:46, 1987.
83. Johansson C, Ekenman I, Tornkvist H, et al: Stress fractures in the femoral neck in athletes. Am J Sports Med 18:524, 1990.
84. Shin AY, Gillingham BL: Fatigue fractures of the femoral neck in athletes. J Am Acad Orthop Surg 5:293-302, 1997.
85. Boden BP, Osbahr DC: High-risk stress fractures: evaluation and treatment. J Am Acad Orthop Surg 8:344-353, 2000.
86. Rhodes I, Matzinger MA: Residents' corner: Answer to case of the month: Transient osteonecrosis of the hip. Can Assoc Radiol J 44:399, 1993.
87. Potter H, Moran M, Schneider R, et al: Magnetic resonance imaging in diagnosis of transient osteoporosis of the hip. Clin Orthop 280:223, 1992.
88. Urbanski SR, deLange EE, Eschenroeder HC: Magnetic resonance imaging of transient osteoporosis of the hip. J Bone Joint Surg Am 73:451, 1991.
89. Lakhanpal S, Ginsburg WW, Luthra HS, et al: Transient regional osteoporosis: A study of 56 cases and review of the literature. Ann Intern Med 106:444, 1987.
90. Grimm J, Higer HP, Benning R, et al: MRI of transient osteoporosis of the hip. Arch Orthop Trauma Surg 110:98, 1991.
91. Ben-David Y, Bornstein J, Sorokin Y, et al: Transient osteoporosis of the hip during pregnancy: A case report. J Reprod Med 36:672, 1991.
92. Daniel WW, Sanders PC, Alarcon GS: The early diagnosis of transient osteoporosis by magnetic imaging: A case report. J Bone Joint Surg Am 74:1262, 1992.
93. Schapira D: Transient osteoporosis of the hip. Semin Arthritis Rheum 22:98, 1992.
94. Hayes CW, Conway WF, Daniel WW: MR imaging of bone marrow edema pattern: Transient osteoporosis, transient bone marrow edema syndrome, or osteonecrosis. Radiographics 13: 1001, 1993.
95. Guerra JJ, Steinberg ME: Distinguishing transient osteoporosis from avascular necrosis of the hip. J Bone Joint Surg Am 77: 616-624,1995.
96. Allen WC, Cope R: Coxa saltans: The snapping hip revisited. J Am Acad Orthop Surg 3:303, 1995.
97. Choi YS, Lee SM, Song BY, et al: Dynamic sonography of external snapping hip syndrome. J Ultrasound Med 21:753-758, 2002.
98. Brignall CG, Stainsby GD: The snapping hip: Treatment by Z-plasty. J Bone Joint Surg Br 73:253, 1991.
99. Gruen GS, Scioscia TN, Lowenstein JE: The surgical treatment of internal snapping hip. Am J Sports Med 30:607-613, 2002.
100. Jacobson T, Allen WC: Surgical correction of the snapping iliopsoas tendon. Am J Sports Med 18:470, 1990.
101. Caruso FA, Toney MA: Trochanteric bursitis: A case report of plain film, scintographic, and MRI correlation. Clin Nucl Med 19:393, 1994.

102. Wunderbaldinger P, Bremer C, Schellenberger E, et al: Imaging features of iliopsoas bursitis. Eur Radiol 12:409-415, 2002.
103. Lentz SS: Osteitis pubis: A review. Obstet Gynecol Surv 50:310, 1995.
104. Batt ME, McShane JM, Dillingham MF: Osteitis pubis in collegiate football players. Med Sci Sports Exerc 27:629, 1995.
105. Burke G, Joe C, Levine M, et al: Tc-99m bone scan in unilateral osteitis pubis. Clin Nucl Med 19:535, 1994.
106. Maksymowych WP, Aaron SL, Russell AS: Treatment of refractory symphysitis pubis with intravenous pamidronate. J Rheumatol 28:2754-2757, 2001.
107. Williams PR, Thomas DP, Downes EM: Osteitis pubis and instability of the pubic symphysis: When nonoperative measures fail. Am J Sports Med 28:350-355, 2000.
108. Macnicol MF, Thompson WJ: Idiopathic meralgia paresthetica. Clin Orthop 254:270, 1990.
109. Moeser P, Donofrio P, Karstaedt N, et al: MRI findings of sciatic endometriosis. Clin Imaging 14:64, 1990.

41 Ankle and Foot Pain

TIMOTHY M. SPIEGEL

Understanding the anatomy of the foot, associated rheumatologic problems, skeletal alignment, and techniques to overcome these problems contribute substantially to the improvement of a patient's life and function. The foot and ankle often are overlooked as significant contributors to disease and decreased function because the focus of the rheumatologic examination is on available anatomy such as hands, wrists, and elbows. Examination of the feet requires a setting that comfortably lets patients remove cumbersome shoes, tights, or socks and enables the physician to carefully focus on the inflammation and structural anatomy of the foot. Substantial clinical symptoms, progressive deformity, and functional limitations result from active and progressive arthritis of the feet.[1] Clinical studies infrequently focus on the foot because measurement of foot abnormalities is difficult, radiographs have confounding problems, such as osteoarthritis (OA), and functional tests include problems associated with knee and hip problems.

TABLE 41–1 • LOCATION OF PAIN

	Fore foot	Mid foot	Hind foot	Ankle	Diffuse
Rheumatoid arthritis	X		X	X	
Osteoarthritis	X		X		
Fasciitis/tendinitis		X	X		
Gout/pseudogout	X			X	
Spondyloarthropathy	X		X		
Infection	X			X	
Bone Injury	X			X	
Nerve Injury					X
RSDS					X
Vascular					X
Tumor				X	

Abbreviations: RSDS, reflex sympathetic dystrophy syndrome.

Anatomy

The functional anatomic unit of the foot is divided into three components: the forefoot, midfoot, and hindfoot. These divisions are somewhat arbitrary because ligaments, tendons, and muscles may contribute to mechanical stress in one area and altered anatomy in another area. The pathomechanics in the rheumatoid foot result from synovitis and mechanical stress.

The benefit of dividing the foot into the three regions is that specific diseases are more common in a region. For example, rheumatoid arthritis (RA) results in early synovitis of the metatarsalphalangeals (MTPs). OA occurs in the first MTP and results in a bone spur, bunion, and hallux valgus. Gout may occur in the great toe.

Midfoot pain may result from plantar fasciitis and tendinitis. With pronation of the foot and chronic alignment changes, secondary OA occurs.

Hindfoot pain occurs in spondyloarthropathies and RA. Calcaneal pain can occur at the insertion of the inferior plantar fascial insertion. Table 41–1 identifies the location of pain in specific rheumatologic diseases. With chronic alignment changes, pain symptoms become more diffuse.

FOREFOOT

The forefoot consists of the five MTP joints, the first interphalangeal (IP) joint, four proximal interphalangeal (PIP) joints, and four distal interphalangeal (DIP) joints. Rheumatologic pain syndromes occur in the MTPs and first IP. The PIPs and DIPs are difficult to individually examine. Traumatic OA of the digits results in fusion. "Sausage" toe refers to swelling of the entire digit and may be seen with HLA B-27–related diseases such as reactive arthritis. Nail pitting is present with psoriatic arthritis. Onychomycosis (fungal infection) occurs with thickened nails and can be painful without proper nail care.

A rheumatoid patient's symptoms include morning pain and stiffness with difficulty arising in the morning and beginning ambulation. Patients may describe "walking on glass" or a "bruised" metatarsal region. Because RA is a symmetric polyarthritis, most MTPs are affected and symptoms are worse with weight bearing and toe-off (Fig. 41-1). Palpation of the MTP region may reveal synovitis and bursal swelling on the inferior MTP region. Confusion with a Morton's neuroma may be present, and some patients will have previously had surgery to correct a Morton's neuroma.

In elderly patients, the inferior metatarsal pad may be atrophied and have no subcutaneous fat. Symptoms are chronic metatarsal pain when standing.

The hammertoe alignment refers to superior subluxation of the MTPs, and then plantar flexion of the proximal and distal joint of the toes. When synovitis is present in all joints, the periarticular structures, ligaments, aponeuroses, and tendons are weakened, which results in forefoot abnormalities.

MIDFOOT

The midfoot consists of the five tarsal bones and the adjacent articulations. The midfoot provides horizontal

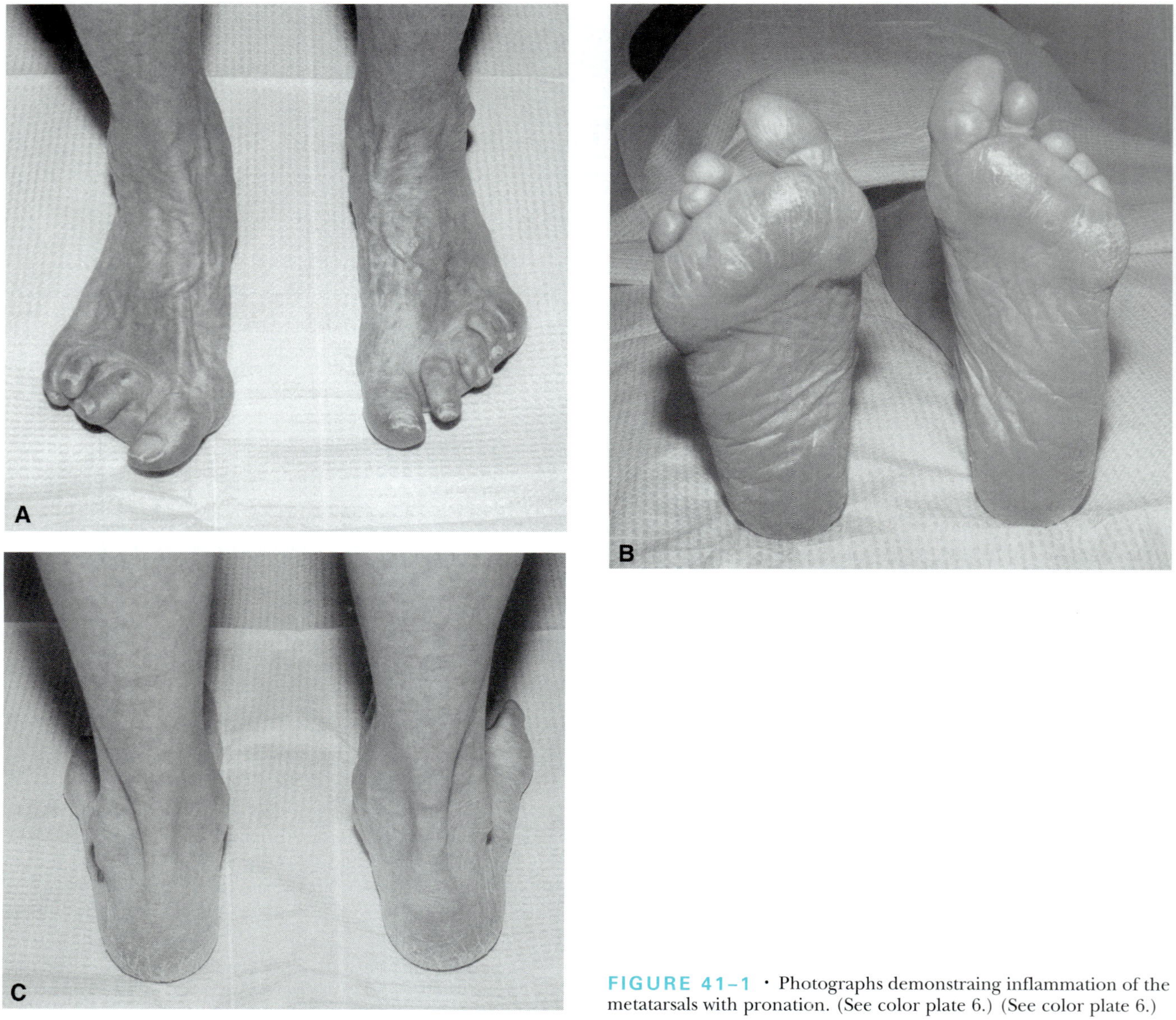

FIGURE 41–1 • Photographs demonstraing inflammation of the metatarsals with pronation. (See color plate 6.) (See color plate 6.)

and longitudinal arches that distribute weight during ambulation. Palpation rarely reveals active synovitis. Radiographs may reveal joint space narrowing, but erosions are uncommon. Radiographs may reveal secondary bone spurs associated with OA. Midfoot inflammation can result in tendinitis, plantar fasciitis, pronation, and chronic weight-bearing pain.[2]

HINDFOOT

The hindfoot consists of the talus, calcaneus, and the navicular with their common subtalar joint. Synovitis may be difficult to palpate, but tendinitis is common. Significant alignment abnormalities rarely occur early in the disease, but changes in the hindfoot result in progressive pronation, flatfoot, tendinitis, and tendon ruptures. With weight-bearing, mechanical changes result in hindfoot valgus. A weight-bearing examination is best to demonstrate midfoot pronation and hindfoot valgus.

Two other hindfoot areas that result in localized pain are the Achilles tendon insertion in the posterior calcaneus and the plantar fascial insertion in the inferior calcaneus. Achilles tendinitis is more common in HLA B27-related spondyloarthropathies.

ANKLE

The ankle is an amazing structure because it helps transfer vertical to horizontal weight-bearing and rarely deteriorates over the course of a lifetime. Trauma-induced OA is the most common rheumatologic presentation. The true ankle mortise consists of the tibiotalar joint with the fibular component. Palpation of synovitis is difficult because of overlying soft tissue, ligaments, and tendons, but warmth and erythema suggests synovitis. Pedal edema may be difficult to separate from synovial swelling. An important clue is whether there is swelling over the medial or lateral malleolus. Any swelling in this region is due to pedal edema and not synovitis, because there is no synovium over the malleolus.

Radiographic Imaging

Radiographs of the foot help to confirm the diagnosis and progression of rheumatoid disease.

Radiographic examinations may include the anterior, posterior, lateral, and oblique radiographs of the feet. Radiographic joint scores demonstrate joint-space narrowing, erosive disease, and correlate with progressive active RA. However, in most clinical studies, hand radiographs are the preferred technique because foot radiographs are more difficult to evaluate and the foot has more associated OA and structural damage due to walking and previous traumatic injury.

Radiographic scoring systems have been developed and modified by Sharp, Larsen, and Kellgren.[3] In one study van der Heijde and colleagues[4,5] report 147 RA patients followed for 2 years with radiographs of the hands and feet. At the beginning of the study, more foot joints were affected than hand joints. Over the course of the study, radiographic joint scores progressed at the same rate for both hands and feet. Therefore, at the conclusion of the study the feet still exhibited the predominance of radiographic damage.

Hand magnetic resonance imaging (MRI) is currently being studied to determine whether it is beneficial to evaluate for early RA. Foot MRIs are not only helpful to identify joint-space narrowing and erosions but also are helpful in identifying a tendon injury and tendon rupture (Fig. 41-2).[6] MRIs of the hindfoot and midfoot frequently demonstrate joint-space narrowing and tendon injury.

Specific Diseases

RA often presents with inflammatory synovitis of the MTPs.

A joint alignment and motion scale (JAMS) has been developed, which is a simple measurement of joint deformity in rheumatoid patients.[7] It is a five-point scale that has been correlated to measures of joint pain, swelling, sedimentation rate, and functional activity. Inflammation, ligament instability, tendinitis, and capsular contractures can cause changes in foot alignment and motion.

The frequency of ankle and foot problems in RA patients depends on disease duration and success of treatment. In a nonselected sample of 955 adult RA patients seen in an orthopedic hospital in Finland, Vainio reports 89 percent of patients had foot problems. We have reported RA foot pathology in 50 patients selected because of progressive functional limitations.[8] Patients were analyzed by disease duration and measurement included synovitis and deformity of each joint on the forefoot, midfoot, and hindfoot. Sixty-five percent of patients with disease duration of 1 to 3 years had synovitis at the MTPs, 32 percent with 3 to 5 years, 55 percent with 5 to 10 years, and 18 percent with more than 10 years. Clinical synovitis was equally distributed among all MTP heads.

Alignment changes of the forefoot are most pronounced at the first MTP with hallux valgus and may occur in 80 percent of patients. Hallux valgus, however, is common in the general population due to age, gait,

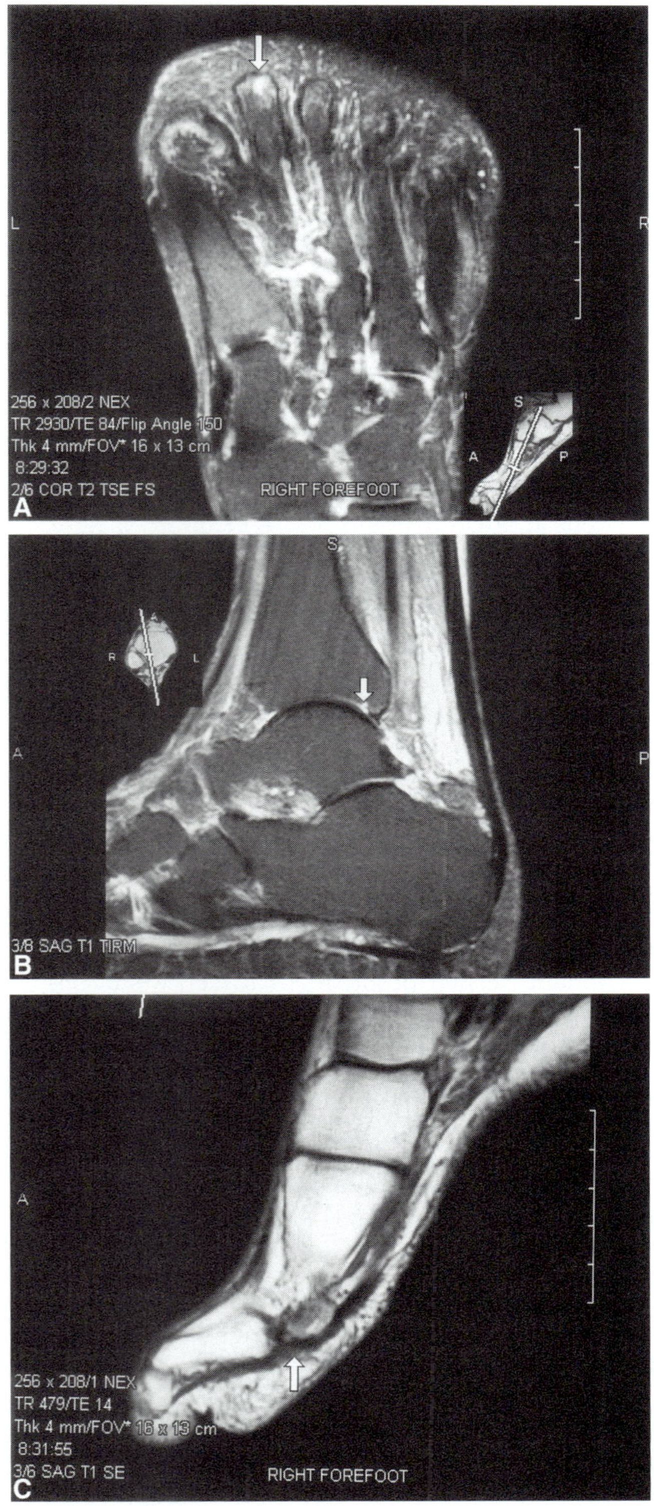

FIGURE 41–2 · Magnetic resonance imaging (MRI) of the forefoot demonstrating synovial proliferation and periarticular erosions.

trauma, shoes, and OA. We found that 39 percent of patients with greater than 10 years of disease duration had moderate to severe deformity of the first MTP, whereas this degree of change was present in only 6 percent of patients with 1 to 3 years of disease duration.

With chronic RA, inflammation of the subtalar joint and ankle result in hindfoot valgus and pronation of the foot.[9,10]

The foot and ankle may also be associated with multiple abnormalities not associated with specific joint problems. Table 41-2 includes multiple changes that can occur and cause difficulties for the RA patient.

Tendinitis and tendon injury are frequent complications in patients with rheumatoid disease. With inflammation and structural alignment, increased stretching and injury to tendons occurs. As individuals walk and place pressure across joint space, progressive injury to the tendons and tendon sheaths of the peroneal and posterior tibialis tendon occur. Patients with substantial pronation typically will have pain associated with tendinitis.

Rheumatoid nodules may occur at any portion of the foot (Fig. 41-3). Typically, they are associated in areas of repeated trauma. Hammertoe deformities resulting in persistent pressure are sites of rheumatoid nodules. The nodules result in pain secondary to ongoing pressure and inability to find appropriate shoes. Injection in the nodules can help reduce the local extent of nodules, but nodules may be very difficult to treat.

Rheumatoid vasculitis may be associated with foot pain because of injury to nerves. With rheumatoid vasculitis the pain is less distinct, does not have as clear association with walking, and may result in ulcers if associated breakdown of skin.

Rheumatoid ulcerations typically occur at signs of repeated trauma and may involve the plantar surface as well as areas of the foot with repeated contact to shoes (Fig. 41-4). Rheumatoid ulcerations may result from vascular changes, but also may be associated with local and repeated trauma.

OA of the foot and ankle progresses slowly and is inevitably present in the elderly patient. Forefoot pain and hallux valgus result in part because of shoe wear. A common related problem is flat feet, which results from ligamentous laxity in association with a hypermobility syndrome such as benign Ehlers-Danlos syndrome. Chronic tendon stretching and ligament injury result in chronic pain. Secondary midfoot bone spurs are present in the superior midtarsal bones.

TABLE 41–2 • ASSOCIATED PATHOLOGY OF RHEUMATOID FEET

Tendinitis and tendon rupture
Nodules
Vasculitis
Mononeuritis
Ulceration
Achilles tendinitis
Vascular disease
Infection
Osteoarthritis
Osteoporosis

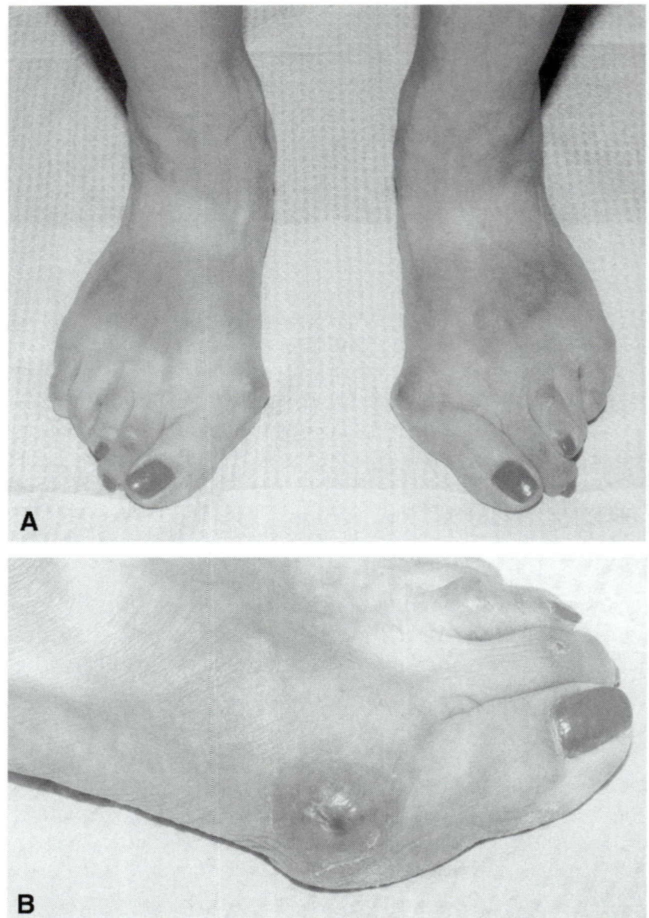

FIGURE 41–3 • Photographs demonstrating alignment changes with nodules. (See color plate 7.)

Gout and pseudogout may present with acute pain in the great toe or ankle. Aspiration and examination under polarized microscopy is important to confirm the diagnosis. Particularly difficult at times is the separation of traumatic OA, crystal-induced disease or infection. If synovial fluid is obtained, polarizing microscopy and culture will direct therapy. To obtain fluid, the needle may be placed between the extensor tendon and the MTP joint.

Miscellaneous Syndromes

Bone injury may result from fractures, stress fractures or avascular necrosis. Because of decreased ambulatory ability and associated inflammation, osteoporosis of the foot is a common occurrence. Measurement has not been carefully studied, but many patients with RA will have decreased bone density and pain associated with osteoporosis. Osteopenia and microfractures may be present. Avascular necrosis and joint collapse occur with glucocorticoids. Radiographs may be used as a first diagnostic test, but frequently MRI or nuclear bone scan is necessary to confirm the diagnosis of a microfracture or avascular necrosis.

Tarsal tunnel syndrome results from inflammation, alignment changes, and entrapment of the posterior

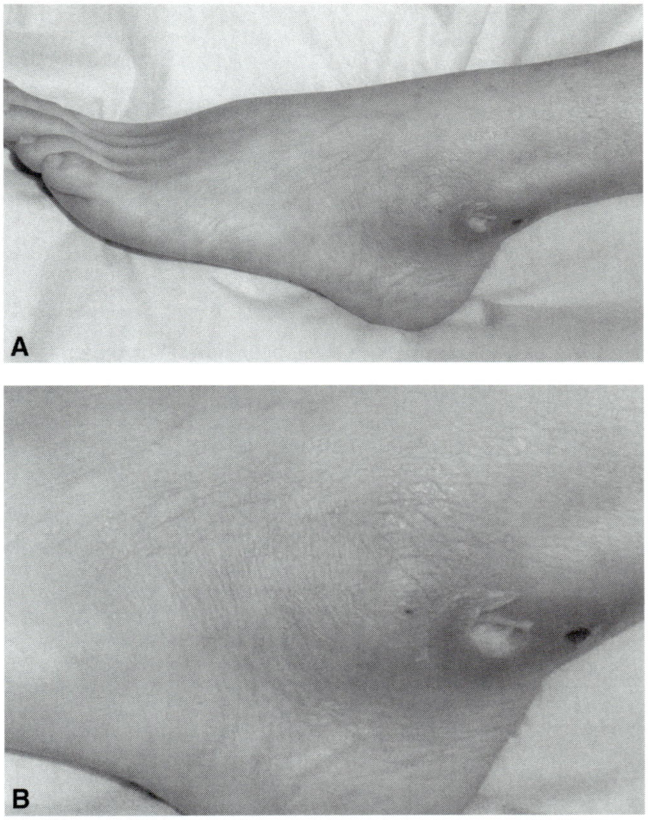

FIGURE 41–4 · Photographs demonstrating small vasculitis on lateral ankle. (See color plate 8.)

tibial nerve in the area posterior and inferior to the medial malleolus. Compression of the nerve results in poorly localized symptoms in the midfoot and hindfoot. Entrapment neuropathies typically result in burning neuralgia pain rather than ambulatory pain.

Morton's neuroma can at times be difficult to separate from early rheumatoid disease. The pain occurs in the metatarsal region and is frequently worse when pressing between the distal metatarsals. At times, one can separate inflammatory RA because of bunions and swelling on the inferior metatarsal surface as opposed to pain between the metatarsal bones.

Nerve injury may be an isolated problem such as tarsal tunnel syndrome, but is more commonly a diffuse peripheral neuropathy. The location of pain is diffuse, and patients describe burning, dysesthesia, and numbness. Diabetes, renal failure, and vasculitis result in nerve damage that can result in a Charcot joint in the ankle and foot.

Arterial insufficiency results in diffuse ankle and foot pain that worsens with activity. Examination reveals coolness of the foot with a mottled discoloration of the entire foot. Venous insufficiency creates pedal edema and chronic, diffuse pain.

Reflex sympathetic dystrophy syndrome (RSDS) is a neurovascular disorder with diffuse pain, particularly with weight-bearing. Radiographs may reveal osteoporosis, and a nuclear bone scan may be necessary to confirm the diagnosis.

Infection is an ongoing problem in the rheumatoid foot. Ulcerations secondary to skin breakdown occur commonly at repeatedly traumatized sites. The issues for patients with rheumatoid disease include poor hygiene and difficulty cleaning feet properly.

Nonsurgical Treatment

The treatment of rheumatoid foot and ankle pain is consistent with the general treatment for RA using nonsteroidal anti-inflammatory drugs (NSAIDS), analgesics, disease-modifying medication, and biologics to reduce the inflammation and thereby reduce structural changes.

Special attention to the foot and ankle involve those problems associated with adaptive shoe requirements to reduce the pain as a result of the structural alignments. Specifically, shoes that have a wider and deeper toe box, support of the midfoot, design that reduces ankle valgus are helpful in reducing pain in the RA foot and ankle. Because of hand abnormalities, adaptive shoelaces or Velcro latches may be necessary. A long-handled shoe horn can help the patients place feet in shoes without needing help from others.[11]

To prevent ulcers and pain of metatarsalgia, orthotic inserts with metatarsal pads can provide relief with some patients. The typical cost of an individually manufactured orthotic can at times be prohibitive for the patient with rheumatoid disease and, therefore, existing soft-soled athletic shoes can often provide appropriate pain control.

Occasionally, a local injection of the metatarsal region, particularly of the inferior bursa are very helpful. Typically, a Kenalog (20 mg) and lidocaine (0.25cc) injection in the inferior bursal space will reduce the bursal inflammation and reduce pain in the metatarsal region.

Surgical Treatment

Surgical reconstruction has been available for many years for patients with rheumatoid disease. Forefoot surgery with metatarsalgia replacements and reconstruction of the supporting structures is recommended in those patients with advanced changes who have persistent pain even with shoe modification. Synovectomy may also help reduce pain. However, the long-term effects of surgical reconstruction typically involve problems with ongoing structural changes, dislocation, or breaking of the plastic prosthesis. Therefore, only selected patients with rheumatoid disease should undergo forefoot reconstruction.[12]

With advanced hindfoot disease, a subtalar fusion offers an excellent technique to stabilize the hindfoot, reduce pain, and provide more normal gait.[13,14]

With destructive ankle disease, fusion of the ankle may be necessary in some individuals.[15] Ankle fusion, however, prevents substantial motion, requiring special shoe adaptation, and is rarely necessary. Current orthopedic studies involve a total ankle prosthesis. Cemented total ankle replacement may offer benefits in some individuals.[16] Ankle replacement is potentially more beneficial in a patient with rheumatoid disease. With advanced RA, activity will be substantially reduced, and the total ankle prosthesis may not have as great a trauma as with a person who has a degenerative or traumatic OA and has otherwise normal joints. With substantial osteoporosis, however, ankle fusion and total ankle replacement are more difficult.

Ankle arthrodesis and arthroplasty fail in patients with RA because of multiple factors including underlying inflammatory disease, osteoporosis, change in gait, decreased vasculature, skin ulcers and infection, and abnormalities of the tendon and ligament reconstruction necessary with foot surgery.[17] However, foot and ankle surgery should be considered on selected patients with rheumatoid disease who do not respond to more conservative treatment.

Conclusions

Control of foot and ankle pain is an integral part of the overall care of patients with rheumatoid diseases. Special considerations for the foot include provision for the long-term weight-bearing and attention to the structural changes caused by inflammation, capsular and ligament instability, and generalized pain. Medication treatment is similar. Special attention to foot care, ulceration, and infection will prevent many problems. Importantly, inflammation may be controlled with disease-modifying antirheumatic drugs (DMARDs) and biologic agents, but patients with rheumatoid disease may have persistent pain because of the structural abnormalities that have occurred. Physiotherapists with special interests, podiatrists, and orthopedic surgeons can contribute to the overall reduction in pain and improvement in function, but these individuals should be carefully selected and have substantial knowledge in reducing the symptoms without causing resultant pain or progressive disability. The enhanced function with reduction in foot symptoms permits a patient to have a more active and complete life.

REFERENCES

1. Tillman K: The rheumatoid foot: Diagnosis, pathomechanics and treatment. Stuttgart, Thieme (Littletone) Mass, 1979.
2. Mandracchia VJ, Buddecke DE, Haverstock BD, Pendarvis JA: Evaluation and surgical management of the arthritic midfoot secondary to rheumatic disease. Clin Podiatr Med Surg 16(2):303, 1999.
3. Drossaers-Bakker KW, Amesz E, Zwinderman AH, et al: A comparison of three radiologic scoring systems for the long-term assessment of rheumatoid arthritis: findings of an ongoing prospective inception cohort study of 132 women followed up for a median of twelve years. Arthritis Rheum 43(7):1465, 2000.
4. Van der Heijde DM, van Leeuwen MA, van Riel PL, et al: Biannual radiographic assessments of hands and feet in a three-year prospective follow-up of patients with early rheumatoid arthritis. Arthritis Rheum 35(1):26, 1992.
5. Van der Heijde DM, van Leeuwen MA, van Riel PL, van de Putte LB: Radiographic progression on radiographs of hands and feet during the first three years of rheumatoid arthritis measured according to Sharp's modification (van der Heijde modification). J Rheum 22(9):1792, 1995.
6. Morrison WB, Ledermann HP, Schweitzer ME: MR imaging of inflammatory conditions of the ankle and foot. Magn Reson Imaging Clin North Am 9(3):615, 2001.
7. Spiegel TM, Spiegel JS, Paulus HE: The joint alignment and motion scale: a simple measure of joint deformity in patients with rheumatoid arthritis. J Rheum 14(5):1987.
8. Spiegel TM, Spiegel JS: Rheumatoid arthritis in the foot and ankle: diagnosis, pathology, and treatment. The relationship between foot and ankle deformity and disease duration in 50 patients. Foot Ankle 2(6):318, 1982.
9. Cimino WG, O'Malley MJ: Rheumatoid arthritis of the ankle and hindfoot. Rheum Dis Clin North Am 24(1):157, 1998.
10. Shi K, Tomita T, Hayashida K, et al: Foot deformities in rheumatoid arthritis and relevance of disease severity. J Rheumatol 27(1):84, 2000.
11. Shrader JA: Nonsurgical management of the foot and ankle affected by rheumatoid arthritis. J Orthop Sports Physiotherapy Ther 29(12):703, 1999.
12. Nassar J, Cracchiolo A III: Complications in surgery of the foot and ankle in patients with rheumatoid arthritis. Clin Orthop 391:140, 2001.
13. Belt EA, Kaarela K, Maenpas H, et al: Relationship of ankle joint involvement with subtalar destruction in patients with rheumatoid arthritis: a 20-year follow-up study. Joint Bone Spine 68(2): 154, 2001.
14. Steinberg JS, Hadi SA: Surgical correction of the rearfoot in rheumatoid arthritis. Clin Podiatr Med Surg 16(2):327, 1999.
15. Caron M, Kron E, Saltrick KR: Tibiotalar joint arthrodesis for the treatment of severe ankle joint degeneration secondary to rheumatoid arthritis. Clin Podiatr Med Surg 16(2):337, 1999.
16. Voutilainen N, Patiala H, Juutilainen T, et al: Long-term results of ankle and triple arthrodeses fixed with self-reinforced polylevolactic acid implants in patients with rheumatoid arthritis. Rheum Int 20(6):229, 2001.
17. Maenpas H, Lehto MU, Belt EA: Why do ankle arthrodeses fail in patients with rheumatic disease? Foot Ankle Int 22(5):403, 2001.

42 Hand and Wrist Pain

CARRIE R. SWIGART • SCOTT W. WOLFE

The multiple functions the hand performs in daily life are usually taken for granted until they become affected by disease or injury. Depending on the nature of the disorder, patients will have different capacities to adapt. Patients presenting with pain and dysfunction of the hand, wrist, or both will represent a wide spectrum, diverse in their age, occupations, and avocations. They will have a broad range of medical conditions that may or may not be related to their current problem. Each person will have a different story to tell about the hand and wrist and why they are seeking treatment. It is up to the clinician to sort out these various factors, some of which may appear confounding, and determine the most appropriate diagnosis and course of treatment.

This chapter will present guidelines that will be useful in the evaluation of patients presenting with hand and wrist pain. Complete coverage of all of the various conditions that can affect the hand and wrist are beyond the scope of this chapter. Instead, the conditions discussed include the most common pathologies seen by both general practitioners and hand surgeons. They are grouped by their anatomic area to include pain localized to the volar, dorsal, radial, or ulnar wrist; the base of the thumb; and the palm and digits.

Patient Evaluation

ANATOMY

The complex anatomy of the hand and wrist demonstrates many structures interacting in close proximity to one another. Several different diagnoses can present with similar symptom patterns despite varying pathologies. A precise knowledge of the anatomy of the hand and wrist will often eliminate several diagnostic considerations on the basis of the physical examination alone. The history of the illness and the examination will also help to narrow further investigation by enabling the physician to better choose appropriate diagnostic tests. Several common sites of pain in the hand and wrist and their corresponding leading diagnoses are illustrated in Figure 42–1. It is evident that pain in one location can have multiple etiologies depending on the patient profile and the history of the problem. A thorough review of the pertinent regional anatomy will be important to help successfully differentiate the many possible causes of hand and wrist pain.

HISTORY

Important patient factors include age, sex, hand dominance, occupation, and hobbies or sports participation. When determining the history of the problem, a history of recent or distant trauma should be sought and an estimation of the severity of the trauma noted. Next, questions as to the duration and frequency of the pain, as well as the intensity and quality, should be addressed. The pain of degenerative arthritis is often described as a localized, "toothache"-type pain, which is always present at a low level and increases with activity, whereas the pain of tendinitis may be sharp, poorly localized, and present only with activity. Rheumatoid arthritis has initial hand and wrist involvement in up to 25 percent of patients and is characterized by joint effusion with bilateral hand and wrist involvement and morning stiffness. Nighttime symptom of a burning pain in the hand and wrist that is exacerbated by arm position is often associated with nerve entrapment syndromes. Specific activities that either cause pain or alleviate it should also be noted. Arthritis at the base of the thumb, or first carpometacarpal joint, is often aggravated by such things as opening jars, turning doorknobs, and needlework or hobbies.

PHYSICAL EXAMINATION

A thorough examination of the involved extremity, as well as comparison to the uninvolved extremity, is essential. Attention should be paid to abnormalities of the more proximal joints of the elbow and shoulder as well as the cervical spine. As the differential narrows, the examination should be tailored as needed to include or eliminate any possible systemic etiologies. As with other musculoskeletal examinations, a complete record of the range of motion of the involved joints should be made, as well as comparison measurements of the opposite side. Any difference between active and passive motion should be noted. Careful palpation for the site of maximal tenderness is important in differentiating the source of pain and is particularly important when trying to exclude possible factors of secondary gain. Measurements of both grip and pinch strength are also helpful in many situations as a diagnostic aid as well as a baseline measurement to follow for improvement. There are many provocative maneuvers useful in differentiating etiologies that will be discussed in the section for the specific pathology with which they are associated.

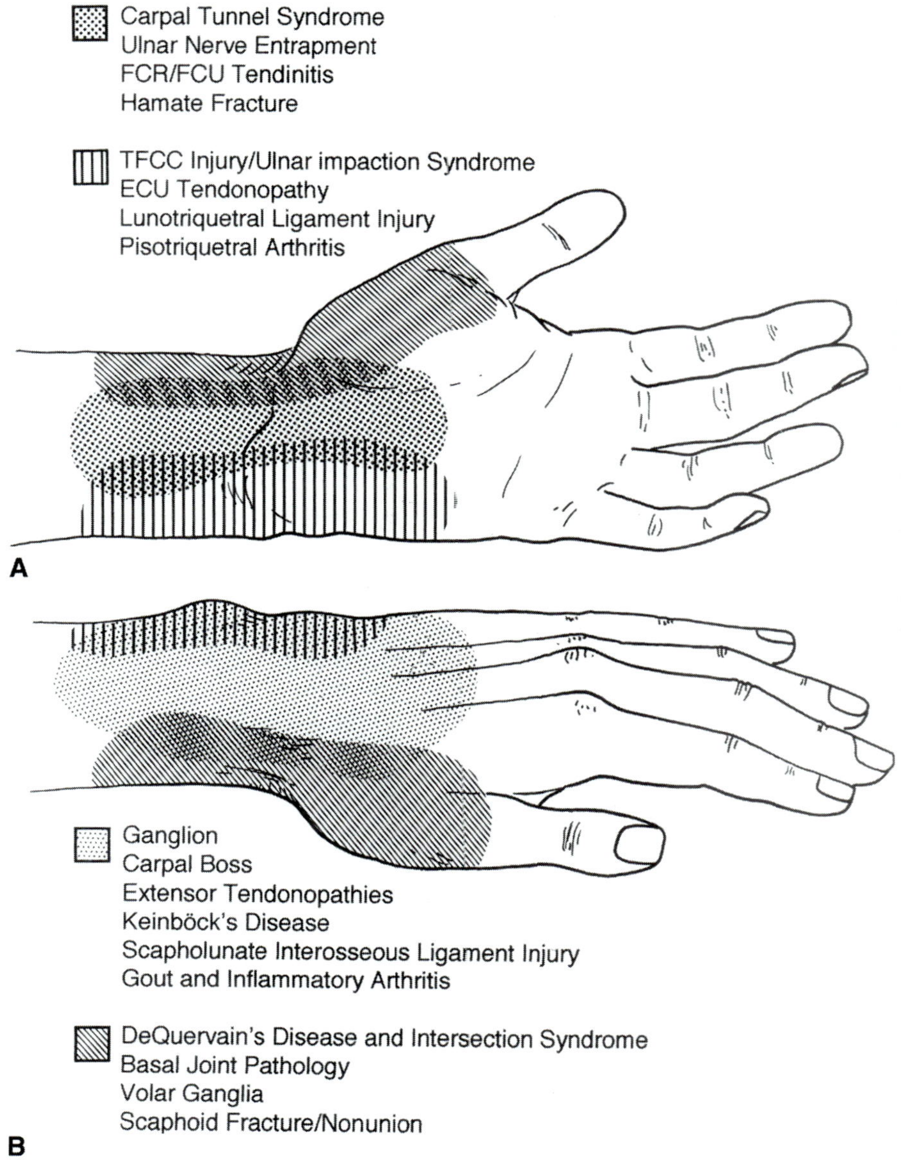

FIGURE 42–1 • *A*, Palmar and ulnar view of the hand and wrist with areas of pain and tenderness marked with their corresponding leading differential diagnoses. *B*, Dorsal and radial view of the hand and wrist with areas of pain and tenderness marked with their corresponding leading differential diagnoses.

IMAGING STUDIES

Recent technologic advances have increased the availability of imaging studies for the hand and wrist. Improvements in magnetic resonance resolution using small joint coils allow more precise imaging of small structures in the hand and wrist. Advancements in ultrasound technology have allowed this tool to be increasingly utilized in the diagnosis of musculoskeletal complaints. With the multitude of ancillary studies at our disposal, it becomes critical to be selective in using these to establish or refute diagnostic possibilities. In this era of cost containment, imaging studies should be used most often to confirm a diagnosis rather than to find one. An understanding of the advantages and limitations of each study is necessary to enable using them to their fullest potential.

Plain radiographs are the easiest and most readily available study that can be obtained in most offices. A routine hand or wrist series, including an anteroposterior (AP), lateral, and an oblique view is a useful screening tool, but it often lacks the specificity required. Depending on the suspected diagnosis, there are many available special views. These will be discussed with the specific diagnoses to which they pertain later in this chapter.

If further detail of the bony anatomy is required, computed tomography (CT) is the best available tool today. The most common uses for CT in the hand and wrist include evaluation of intra-articular fractures of the distal radius and metacarpals, scaphoid fractures and nonunions, and intraosseous cysts or tumors.[1,2]

Advances in both ultrasound and magnetic resonance imaging (MRI) technology have enhanced our ability to evaluate the soft tissue structures of the hand and wrist. Smaller ultrasound probes with higher resolution have made it possible to visualize and differentiate structures such as flexor tendons, ganglion cysts, and ligaments. Doppler ultrasound can help to differentiate among vascular disorders of the hand. MRI technology is constantly improving and allowing for new uses in the hand and wrist. By altering the parameters of this test, information about both anatomy and physiology can be obtained.[3] Specific uses of these tests, as well as others such as arthrography and bone scans, will be addressed with the diagnoses for which they are most useful.

ADDITIONAL DIAGNOSTIC TESTS

Neurodiagnositc Tests

Neurodiagnostic tests, including both nerve conduction studies (NCS) and electromyography (EMG), are very useful in the diagnosis of suspected neurologic disorders of the upper extremity. Specifying the type and nature of examination required will enhance the information gained by these studies. If there is the suspicion of a nerve compression syndrome such as carpal or cubital tunnel syndrome, NCS may be sufficient without the added cost and patient discomfort of formal EMG testing. Nerve conduction testing evaluates the speed of conduction of nerves, both motor and sensory, across a set distance at a specific location and compares this to established normal values. A decrease in the speed of nerve conduction, as evidenced by an increase in the latency, is seen with localized nerve compression and will be demonstrated in several different nerves concomitantly in demyelinating diseases such as multiple sclerosis. When more severe nerve injuries are suspected, or if there is clinical evidence of muscle weakness or atrophy, an EMG can be useful to better delineate the extent of the process or to rule out a myopathic process.[4]

Injections and Aspirations

The use of injections and aspirations can be both therapeutic and diagnostic. A so-called "lidocaine challenge" can be useful to discriminate between different diagnoses when it is placed precisely in one joint or painful area. Corticosteroids can be given selectively in conjunction with the local anesthetic for more lasting relief, and in some cases they can be curative.[5-11] Some of the most common sites for injection are the A1 pulley region of the finger for trigger finger, the carpal canal for carpal tunnel syndrome, and the first dorsal compartment of the wrist for de Quervain's disease.

Aspiration of joints, or other fluid collections such as ganglions, can yield vital diagnostic information and can be therapeutic. If infection is suspected, aspiration should be used to get a sample of joint fluid for Gram stain, cell count, and culture. Diagnoses such as gout and pseudogout can be confirmed by crystal analysis under polarized light. Many ganglions and retinacular cysts can be temporarily or permanently treated with simple aspiration.[12,13]

Arthroscopy

Direct visualization of a joint via arthroscopy can be an invaluable diagnostic tool. Despite the increasing sensitivity of imaging techniques such as MRI, arthroscopy provides a dynamic evaluation that static imaging cannot provide.[14] Since the first published report of a series of cases by Roth in 1988,[15] it has become the "gold standard" for evaluation of chronic wrist pain.[16-18] With new surgical techniques being developed, surgeons can often proceed directly to the definitive treatment using arthroscopy entirely or in part.[19-24]

Common Etiologies for Hand and Wrist Pain

PALMAR WRIST PAIN

Carpal Tunnel Syndrome

Carpal tunnel syndrome is the most commonly diagnosed compression neuropathy in the upper extremity. It usually begins as an isolated phenomenon, but symptoms of carpal tunnel syndrome can accompany many systemic diseases, such as congestive heart failure, multiple myeloma, and tuberculosis.[25-28] More commonly, carpal tunnel syndrome is associated with conditions such as pregnancy, diabetes, obesity, rheumatoid arthritis, and gout.[29-39]

The classic constellation of symptoms consists of weakness or clumsiness of the hand; parathesias or hypesthesias in the thumb, index, and long fingers; and nocturnal parasthesias in the affected digits. Patients may often complain of forearm and elbow pain that is aggravated by activities but is poorly localized and aching in nature. Occasionally, more proximal symptoms, such as shoulder pain, will be the main initial complaint.[40] Past reports have indicated a three to one prevalence of the condition in women. Approximately half of the patients will be between 40 and 60 years of age, although carpal tunnel syndrome has been occasionally diagnosed in children.[41,42]

The diagnosis of carpal tunnel syndrome is usually clinical. Tinel's sign, demonstrated by radiating parasthesias in the median nerve distribution with gentle percussion over the volar wrist, is indicative of nerve irritation. A reproduction of symptoms with wrist flexion, as described by Phalen,[43] and with the carpal compression test, as described by Durkan,[44] have been shown to be more specific.[45] Decreased sensation and thenar atrophy are late signs seen in advanced median nerve entrapment. Bilateral electrodiagnostic tests should be used to confirm the diagnosis, particularly in patients claiming a compensable injury or in patients with atypical signs or symptoms. Prolonged motor or sensory latencies across the carpal canal confirm pathologic compression of the median nerve.[46-48] With classic clinical findings, a recent study found that carpal tunnel syndrome could be diagnosed with a high degree of accuracy on clinical grounds alone and that the addition of electrodiagnostic tests did not increase the accuracy.[49] When attempting to differentiate carpal tunnel syndrome from more proximal nerve entrapments such as cervical root compression or thoracic outlet syndrome, the addition of electromyography of the cervical paraspinal muscles and proximal conduction tests (H reflex, f-waves) can be useful.[50]

Conservative treatment for carpal tunnel syndrome consists of splinting the wrist in neutral position and possibly oral nonsteroidal anti-inflammatory drugs (NSAIDs) for pain control. Splinting should be used sparingly during the workday to prevent secondary muscle weakness and fatigue and is best prescribed to prevent provocative wrist positioning at night. The splint should not hold the wrist in extension beyond 10 degrees. Although splinting may be beneficial for relief of symptoms in cases of mild compression, its long-term effectiveness is limited.[51] The use of vitamin B_6 (100 to 200 mg/day) has been helpful in some patients, but its efficacy has not been confirmed in a randomized trial. The popularity of injections of corticosteroid in the treatment of carpal tunnel syndrome has waxed and waned over the last half century. Although it has been shown to be quite effective in the short term, the long-term efficacy is mixed.[52,53] Also, injections have been associated with exacerbation of the condition and permanent median nerve injury if performed incorrectly.[54,55] For these reasons, injections are most often indicated in cases in which the condition is thought to be temporary, such as with pregnancy, or if surgery has to be deferred due to a medical condition or major life event.

Surgical release is indicated for patients with confirmed carpal tunnel syndrome who have failed a course of conservative treatment. In patients who demonstrate late findings of objective sensory loss or thenar atrophy, early surgery should be recommended.

Ulnar Nerve Entrapment

Cubital Tunnel Syndrome

Entrapment of the ulnar nerve as it passes through the cubital tunnel just posterior to the medial epicondyle of the elbow can be noted by symptoms localized to the ulnar border of the hand. There may also be associated medial forearm pain and irritability of the ulnar nerve at the elbow. Initial symptoms usually consist of parasthesias, numbness, or both in the small and ring fingers. Percussion of the nerve in the cubital tunnel will elicit a Tinel's sign. Prolonged elbow flexion will reproduce the symptoms. Unlike carpal tunnel syndrome, it is not unusual for patients to present with early atrophy of the intrinsics, most easily appreciated in the first dorsal interosseous muscle.

Electrodiagnostic studies can help to confirm the diagnosis and diferentiate cubital tunnel syndrome from more distal compression of the ulnar nerve in Guyon's canal (see following). If malalignment of the elbow is present or the patient relates a history of childhood trauma, radiographs should be obtained to rule out a supracondylar or epicondylar malunion. So-called "tardy" ulnar nerve palsy can develop years after a supracondylar fracture of the elbow.[56]

Conservative treatment includes strategies to help the patient avoid having the elbow flexed for prolonged periods of time, particularly at night. Soft, or semirigid, elbow splints prevent elbow flexion beyond 50 to 70 degrees. Medial elbow pads can be used if the patient's job or hobbies require resting the medial elbow on a hard surface. NSAIDs can be of benefit in acute or traumatic cases. Surgical decompression of the nerve is indicated if a patient fails to obtain relief from splinting and activity modification or if there is clinical or electrodiagnostic evidence of muscle denervation.

Guyon's Canal

Felix Guyon, in 1861, published a description of the contents of an anatomic canal at the wrist.[58] Through this space pass the distal branch of the ulnar nerve and the ulnar artery. As it exits the canal, the ulnar nerve divides into its sensory and motor branches. Compression of the nerve within or proximal to the canal usually creates a combination of sensory and motor symptoms in the ulnar nerve distribution. Patients will complain of numbness and parasthesias of the palmar aspect of the ring and small fingers. Motor symptoms usually are described as a cramping weakness with grasping and pinching. As with median neuropathy, atrophy of the intrinsics and objective sensory loss are late findings.

Unlike carpal tunnel syndrome, in which patients usually have an ill-defined onset of symptoms, ulnar nerve compression in the canal of Guyon is often of more acute onset. It can be associated with repeated blunt trauma,[58-60] a fracture of the hamate or the metacarpal bases, or occasionally a fracture of the distal radius.[61,62] Space-occupying lesions, such as a ganglion or lipoma, can also cause compression.[63-67] Because of the difference in etiology, this nerve entrapment syndrome is often not amenable to conservative treatment. If there is an anatomic lesion such as a fracture or a mass, this must be addressed. If repetitive blunt trauma is the cause, without associated fracture or arterial thrombosis, splinting and activity modification can alleviate the symptoms.

Flexor Carpi Radialis or Flexor Carpi Ulnaris Tendinitis

Like other tendonopathies about the wrist, irritation of the wrist flexors occurs with stress of the wrist in a particular position. Activities that require forced wrist flexion for prolonged periods of time, or with repetition, put patients at risk for inflammation about the flexor carpi radialis (FCR) tendon,[68] the flexor carpi ulnaris (FCU) tendon, or both. The condition is manifested by tenderness along the course of the tendon, especially near its insertion. Wrist flexion against resistance with radial or ulnar deviation will reproduce the symptoms. Treatment consists of splinting and rest, elimination of the activities that cause pain, and oral NSAIDs. Injection of corticosteroid into the FCR or FCU sheath may be curative. Sharp pain associated with an intense inflammatory localized reaction is suggestive of calcific tendinitis and is most commonly seen about the FCU tendon.[69,70]

Hamate Fracture

A relatively uncommon and underdiagnosed etiology of palmar pain in young, active individuals is a fracture of the hook of the hamate. These fractures can occur from a fall on an extended wrist, a "dubbed" golf shot, or from forcefully striking a ball with a club or bat. Plain radiographs of the wrist are usually read as normal. The condition should be established and treated expeditiously, as it may lead to ulnar nerve entrapment, ulnar artery thrombosis, or rupture of flexor tendons.[71] Pain in the base of the palm overlying the hamate is the most common initial symptom. Often, the pain will only be present during the activity that caused the fracture, such as driving a golf ball or swinging a bat. Because of the proximity of the ulnar nerve, patients can also have both sensory and motor symptoms of distal ulnar neuropathy. Occasionally, in the acute setting, vascular complaints such as cold intolerance or frank ischemia from ulnar artery thrombosis can be the initial condition.

A carpal tunnel view, obtained with the wrist in a hyperextended position, may demonstrate the fracture (Fig. 42–2). Alternatively, a selective CT scan through the hamate is a more accurate way to confirm the diagnosis.[72] If diagnosed within 2 to 3 weeks of injury, casting should be attempted to allow the fracture to heal.[73] If this fails, or if the condition is diagnosed late, surgical treatment is indicated, and most authors favor excision of the hook followed by a gradual return to activities.[74-77]

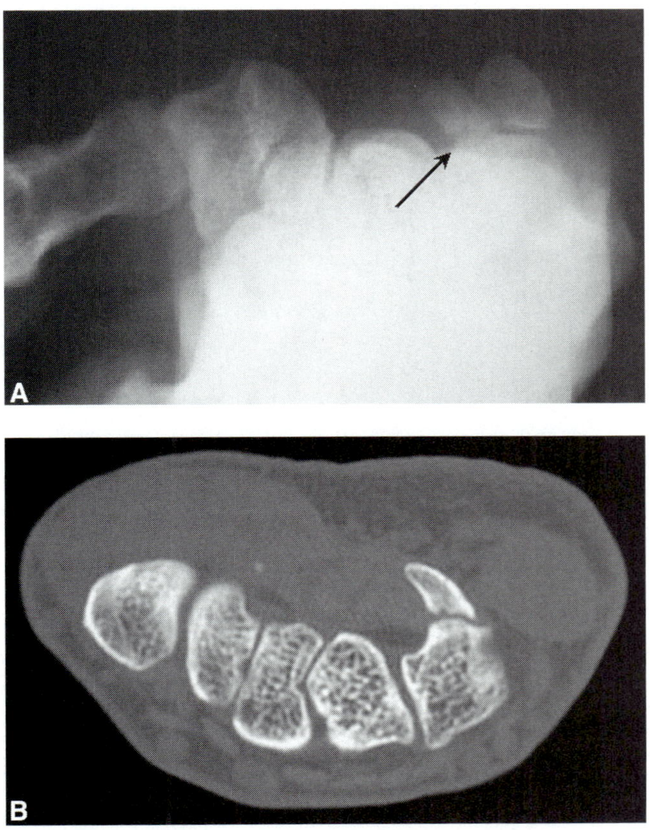

FIGURE 42–2 • *A*, A carpal tunnel view radiograph showing a hamate hook fracture (arrow). *B*, A coronal computed tomography (CT) scan showing the same hamate hook fracture.

DORSAL WRIST PAIN

Ganglion

Ganglions account for between 50 and 70 percent of all soft tissue tumors of the hand and wrist. Of these, 60 to 70 percent occur about the dorsal wrist. These mucin-filled cysts usually arise from an adjacent joint capsule or tendon sheath. The most common site of origin is the scapholunate ligament, and the main body of the cyst may be located elsewhere on the dorsum of the wrist and attached to this ligament by a long pedicle. Although most ganglions present as a well-circumscribed and obvious soft mass, some are more subtle and are only evident with the wrist in marked volar flexion. Due to their characteristic appearance, ganglions are not often misdiagnosed, but they should be differentiated from the less well-demarcated swelling of extensor tenosynovitis, lipomas, and other hand tumors. Plain radiographs are usually normal, but occasionally they show an intraosseous cyst or an osteoarthritic joint. Some ganglions may not be clinically apparent and are know as "occult" ganglions. Both ultrasound and MRI are useful in the diagnosis of these ganglia.[78,79]

Not all ganglions are painful, but the tendency is for the smaller ganglions to be more painful. Patients may present with complaints of wrist weakness or may seek treatment simply because of the cosmetic appearance of the cyst. In approximately 10 percent of cases, there is evidence of associated trauma to the wrist. The ganglions may appear suddenly or develop over many months. Intermittent complete resorption followed by reappearance months or years later is not uncommon.

Most conservative measures, such as splinting and rest, have only a temporary effect on ganglions. They tend to diminish in size with rest and enlarge with increased activity. Spontaneous rupture is common and, at one time, attempting to rupture the cyst with a heavy object such as a Bible was recommended as treatment. Aspiration can be performed but has mixed results due to the thick, gelatinous nature of the fluid within the cyst. Even if adequate decompression of the cyst can be achieved, reaccumulation of the fluid usually occurs. Aspiration in conjunction with irrigation or injection of corticosteroid can be effective in alleviating the symptoms for varying periods of time.[12,13,80]

Occasionally a ganglion can become so large that it interferes with the function of the wrist by limiting the motion, especially in extension. Pressure of the mass on the terminal branches of the posterior interosseous nerve may be painful. Excision is generally curative but may result in short-term stiffness and some loss of terminal flexion due to surgical scarring. Occasionally, a patient will desire excision of the cyst for cosmetic reasons. With proper excision, recurrence is less than 10 percent,[81-83] but if the dissection is incomplete and fails to identify the origin of the cyst, recurrence rates can be as high as 50 percent. Recently, arthroscopic resection has been shown to be a safe and effective method of treating dorsal wrist ganglions.[23,24]

Carpal Boss

Often confused with a dorsal ganglion, the carpal boss is a bony, nonmobile prominence on the dorsum of the wrist. It is an osteoarthritic spur that forms at the second or third carpometacarpal joints.[84] The boss is most evident with the wrist in volar flexion. Patients usually present with pain and localized tenderness over the prominence. The condition is twice as common in women as in men, and most patients are in their third or fourth decades of life. It is not unusual for a small ganglion to be associated with the boss. Radiographs are best taken with the hand and wrist in 30 to 40 degrees of supination and 20 to 30 degrees of ulnar deviation to put the bony prominence on profile (the "carpal boss view").[85] Conservative treatment consists of rest, immobilization, NSAIDs, and occasionally, injection with corticosteroids. If the boss is persistently painful despite these measures, surgical excision may be necessary; however, surgery is associated with a prolonged recovery and continued symptoms in a high percentage of patients.

Extensor Tendinopathies

The extensor pollicis longus (EPL) tendon can be irritated as it passes around Lister's tubercle. This condition, unlike other tendinopathies about the wrist, carries a significant risk of tendon rupture. Early diagnosis and sometimes even urgent operative treatment are necessary to prevent this complication. Localized pain, swelling, and tenderness are the hallmarks of this condition, and like other tendinopathies, initial treatment consists of decreased activity and splinting. A short course of oral anti-inflammatory medication can be useful in decreasing symptoms. Diagnostic injections with lidocaine can help to differentiate the condition from other causes of wrist pain, but corticosteroids are not routinely used in this condition because of a propensity for the EPL to rupture in chronic cases.

It is not unusual for a patient to present with a rupture of the EPL without antecedent pain or swelling. There is a well-known association of EPL rupture with fractures of the distal radius, which likely occurs due to a relative "watershed zone" of vascular supply within its tight retinacular sheath. Tendon rupture most often occurs with minimally or nondisplaced fractures and can occur several weeks or months after the original injury.[86-89]

Kienböck's Disease

Keinböck's disease is so named for Robert Kienböck who first described, in 1910, what he postulated were avascular changes in the lunate.[90] Nearly a century later, the cause of this disease remains unclear and is likely multifactorial. Kienböck's should be suspected when a young adult presents with pain and stiffness of the wrist as well as swelling and tenderness about the region of the dorsal lunate. There is an increased propensity of the disease among patients with an ulna that is anatomically shorter than the radius ("ulnar negative variance"). Radiographs are needed to confirm and stage the process. Kienböck's is staged by the degree of fragmentation and collapse of the lunate, associated osteoarthritis, and carpal collapse in a system originally proposed by Stahl.[91] In this system, the earliest sign of the disease is a linear or compression fracture in the lunate. Later stages show sclerosis of the lunate, followed by lunate collapse, and a loss of carpal height. In the final stage, the carpus shows signs of diffuse osteoarthritis with complete collapse and fragmentation of the lunate (Fig. 42–3). With the increased sensitivity of MRI, it is possible to identify avascular changes within the lunate before they become evident on plain radiographs. This is referred to as "stage zero" Kienböck's disease.

The treatment for Kienböck's is largely surgical. Depending on the stage of the disease and the postulated etiology, there are several surgical procedures that have been described. In early stages of the disease, when there is little lunate collapse and no osteoarthritis, the goal of surgery is to "unload" the lunate by redistributing articular contact forces and allow it to revascularize.[92-95] The most common procedure is a radial shortening osteotomy, performed to neutralize ulnar variance. In later stages, various intercarpal arthrodeses have been used to readjust and maintain carpal height and alignment.[96-98] Microsurgical techniques have been used recently to revascularize the lunate with promising early results.[99]

Scapholunate Interosseous Ligament Injury

The interosseous ligament between the scaphoid and the lunate is a stout structure, especially dorsally, and usually requires a significant force to cause disruption.

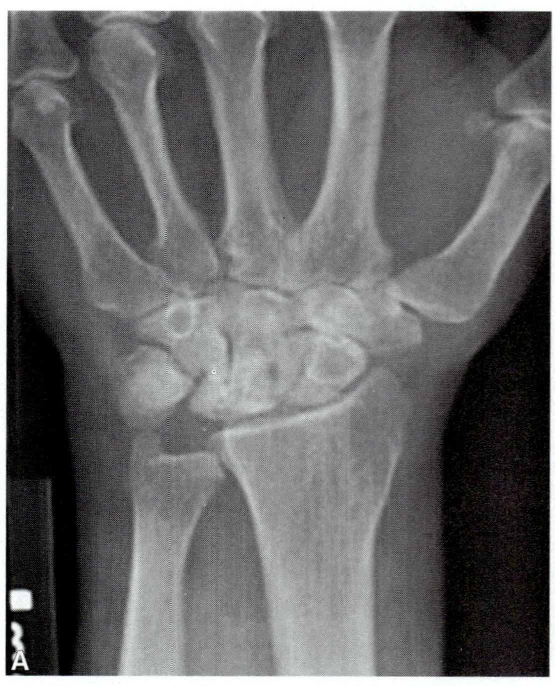

FIGURE 42–3 · Advanced Kienböck's disease, showing carpal collapse, intercarpal and radiocarpal arthrosis, and fragmentation of the lunate. *A*, posteroanterior (PA) view.

Continued

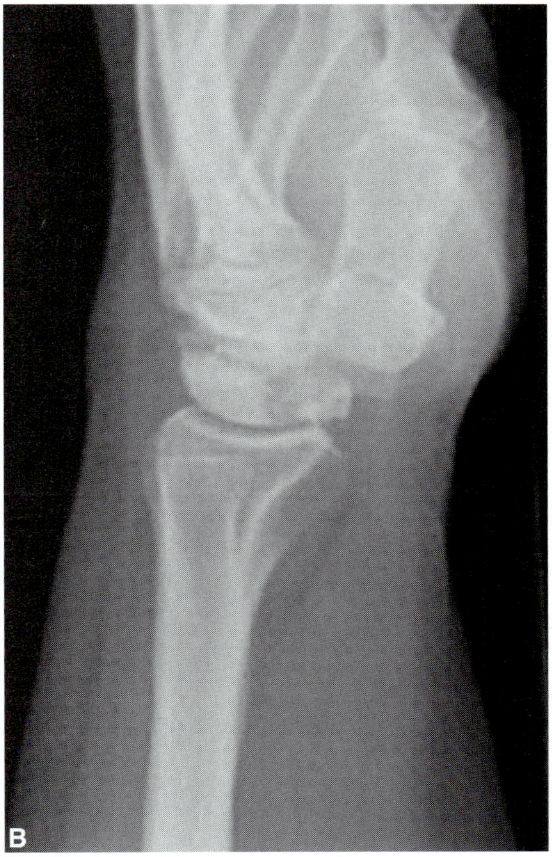

FIGURE 42–3, CONT'D · *B*, lateral view.

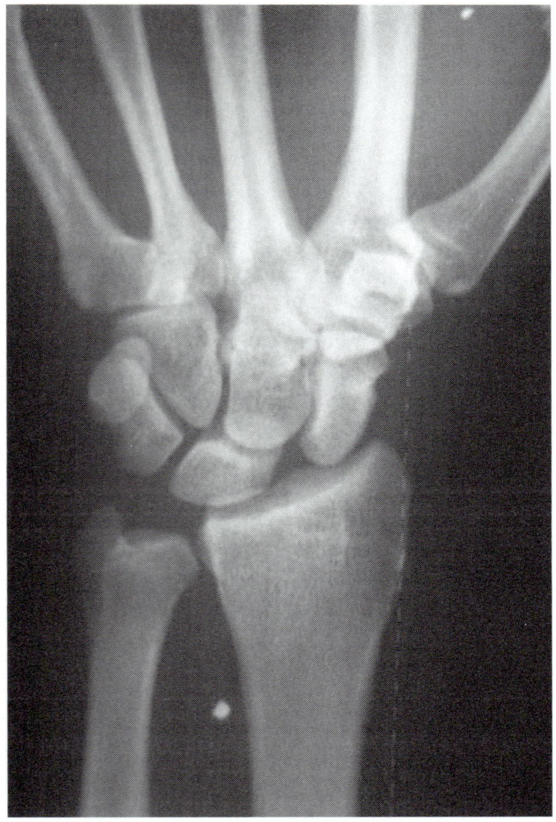

FIGURE 42–4 · Anteroposterior (AP) radiograph of the wrist showing scapholunate interosseous space widening, scaphoid foreshortening, and the "cortical ring" sign associated with scapholunate interosseous ligament disruption.

The typical mechanism of injury is a fall onto the outstretched hand with the wrist extended. Early diagnosis is essential to prevent the late sequelae of carpal collapse. The key radiographic features of scapholunate dissociation (scapholunate interval widening) are demonstrated in Figure 42–4. The AP, rather than the posteroanterior (PA), view has been shown to better demonstrate the scapholunate interval.[100] Early surgical intervention is recommended with the goal of maintaining carpal alignment and prevention of an otherwise inevitable progression to carpal collapse and degenerative arthritis.

Gout and Inflammatory Arthritis

All the inflammatory arthritidies, including the crystalline arthropathies, can present as dorsal wrist pain. Approximately 25 percent of patients with a diagnosis of rheumatoid arthritis will present initially with hand and wrist symptoms. The reader is referred to Chapters 66 and 87 of this text for further details on these conditions.

ULNAR WRIST PAIN

Triangular Fibrocartilage Complex Injury and Ulnocarpal Impaction Syndrome

One of the most complex and confusing areas of the wrist from a diagnostic standpoint is the articulation of the ulna with the carpus. The triangular fibrocartilage complex (TFCC), so named by Palmer and Werner,[101] comprises the articular disk itself, as well as the immediately surrounding ulnocarpal ligaments. It can be injured by a variety of mechanisms, both acute and chronic. Hyperpronation or hypersupination of the carpus during forceful activities are the usual causes of acute injuries, whereas repetitive pronation and supination more often cause attritional changes in the TFCC. Careful physical examination is important to determine the origin of the pain and to try to discover the maneuver or wrist position that most closely reproduces the symptoms.

The radius and ulna must remain congruent through a 190-degree arc.[102] Limitation of motion and pain with pronation and supination are consistent with a tear of the supporting ligaments and resultant distal radioulnar joint (DRUJ) instability. If a sufficient portion of the stability has been lost, the ulna will appear clinically dislocated or subluxated, and there will be severe limitation of forearm rotation. Lateral radiographs of the wrist in neutral as well as full pronation and supination are not generally specific enough to confirm ulnar subluxation. To better evaluate the congruency of the DRUJ through its range of motion, and to assess for subtle subluxations, CT scan can be performed on both wrists simultaneously in neutral position, as well as full pronation and full supination.[103-106]

Tears of the TFCC may present with painful clicking during wrist rotation. Patients generally demonstrate localized tenderness on the midaxial border of the wrist and directly beneath the extensor carpi ulnaris (ECU) tendon. If forced ulnar deviation of the wrist or gripping reproduces the patient's symptoms, a degenerative tear of the central portion of the TFCC is more likely. The degenerative tear is frequently a component of the ulnocarpal impaction syndrome, a condition associated with higher-than-normal loads on the ulnar carpus due to a congenitally positive ulnar variance.

Plain radiographs are most useful in determining ulnar variance and for ruling out fractures or arthritis as a cause of ulnar wrist pain. Because of the variable relationship of the radius and ulna, depending upon forearm rotation, it is important to take standardized films when measuring ulnar variance.[107,108] A PA view of the wrist with the shoulder abducted to 90 degrees and the elbow flexed to 90 degrees shows the DRUJ in neutral forearm rotation and is easily reproducible (Fig. 42–5). Because the ulna lengthens relative to the radius during power grip, a radiograph in the same position during maximal grip will best demonstrate impaction of the ulna on the carpus.

Ancillary studies for TFCC tears include three-compartmental arthrography and MRI. In arthrography, sequential injections of radio-opaque dye are performed into the carpal, midcarpal, and distal radioulnar joints.

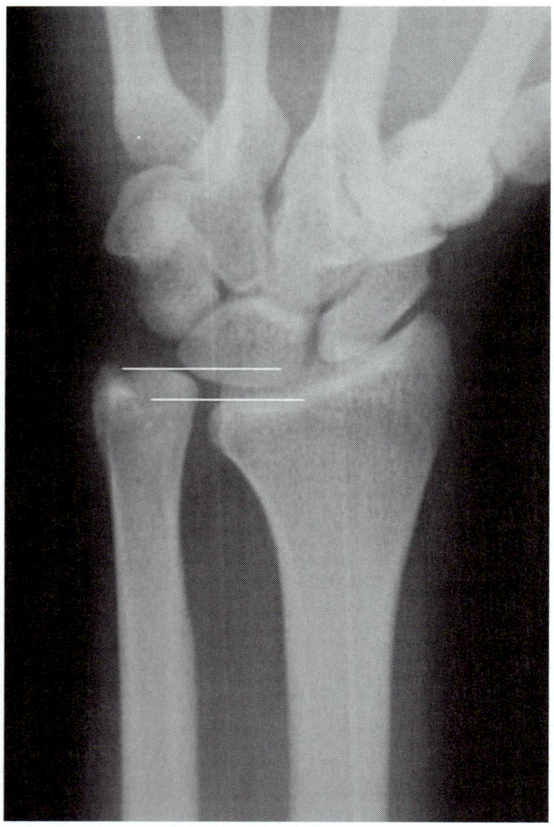

FIGURE 42–5 · Posteroanterior (PA) radiograph of the wrist in neutral forearm rotation showing the method of measuring ulnar variance by drawing tangential lines to the distal ulna and distal radius. The space between these lines in millimeters is the ulnar variance. Positive value indicates the ulnar length is greater than the radial length.

The test is considered positive when the dye is seen leaking from one compartment to another. The site of the leak determines the location of the torn structure.[109] Several studies have shown, however, that there are age-related attritional tears that occur in the TFCC as well as other ligamentous structures of the wrist.[110-112] Recent technologic advancements in MRI have improved the ability to visualize and diagnose abnormalities in the triangular fibrocartilage. Both peripheral detachments and central degenerative tears can be visualized. MRI effectiveness remains highly operator and technique dependent, and the studies should be interpreted in the context of the findings on physical examination.[113]

Patients presenting with pain localized to the ulnar side of the wrist often respond to simple splinting and rest. This conservative treatment, as well as NSAIDs, can be used effectively while a workup is in progress. A course of rest and splinting, followed by a gradual return to activities, may completely alleviate ulnar-sided symptoms.

Despite the recent advancements in imaging techniques, there is often no substitute for direct visualization of the ulnocarpal joint, the DRUJ, or both. Arthroscopy has become an invaluable diagnostic as well as surgical tool; tears of the TFCC can be visualized and their clinical significance better determined. Arthroscopy, done in conjunction with fluoroscopy, can assess for instability of the DRUJ or intercarpal joints. Several surgical procedures can now be performed either entirely or in part through the arthroscope.[114,115]

Extensor Carpi Ulnaris Tendinitis and Subluxation

The ECU tendon can become irritated with forced pronation and supination activities such as putting topspin on a tennis ball. In severe cases, the tendon can begin to sublux about the ulnar head as its compartment becomes increasingly lax. Patients will complain of pain with forceful rotation of the forearm, and sometimes there will be an associated snapping of the ECU tendon. Early treatment consists of immobilization of the wrist and forearm to prevent rotation. Anti-inflammatory medication can help decrease the inflammation more quickly. If after an adequate period of rest the acute inflammation resolves but the ECU tendon continues to be unstable, surgery may be indicated to reconstruct or release the sheath at the wrist.

Lunotriquetral Ligament Injury

Tears in the short, stout intraosseous ligament connecting the lunate and the triquetrum are uncommon and often difficult to diagnosis. As with the previously mentioned diagnoses, patients present with ulnar-sided wrist pain usually made worse by either pronation or supination. Forceful translation of the triquetrum against the lunate will cause pain in affected individuals. If diagnosed within 3 to 4 weeks of injury, a short arm cast will allow healing and eliminate symptoms. Chronic tears may lead to advanced carpal instability and collapse. MRI, wrist arthroscopy, or both may be necessary to make the diagnosis. Treatment is predicated on the staging of instability and ranges from simple casting for acute instability to ligament reconstruction or intercarpal fusion for more advanced cases.

Pisotriquetral Arthritis

Degenerative changes in the pisotriquetral articulation usually are post-traumatic in nature. Patients may recall a fall onto the extended wrist with direct trauma to ulnar side of the palm. Affected patients present with pain during passive wrist hyperextension and exacerbation with flexion against resistance. With palpation of the pisotriquetral joint there will be tenderness and often crepitus. As with many joints, splinting, NSAIDS, and occasionally injection with corticosteroid and lidocaine are the mainstays of conservative treatment. If this is inadequate to control the symptoms, surgical resection of the pisiform is indicated.

RADIAL WRIST AND BASE OF THUMB PAIN

de Quervain's Disease and Intersection Syndrome

One of the most common sites of tendon irritation about the wrist is in the first dorsal extensor compartment, a phenomenon known as de Quervain's disease. The tendons involved are the extensor pollicis brevis (EPB) and the abductor pollicis longus (APL). At the level of the radial styloid, these two tendons pass through an osteoligamentous tunnel comprised of a shallow groove in the radius and an overlying ligament. Anatomic studies have shown that a high percentage of patients have a divided first dorsal compartment, and this can account for failure of conservative treatment and injections.[116-118]

Patients with de Quervain's are typically women in their 4th and 5th decades, although men and women can develop the condition at any age. Any activity requiring repeated thumb abduction and extension in combination with wrist radial and ulnar deviation can aggravate this problem. Patients will complain of pain along the course of these tendons with grasping activities. Clinically there will be tenderness along the affected compartment, and there may be swelling over the radial styloid. In severe cases, a creaking sound can be elicited with movement of the involved tendons. Finklestein's test of forced ulnar deviation of the wrist with the thumb clasped in the fisted palm is pathognomonic of the condition.[119,120]

A less-common condition that may occur in the same general location in the wrist is intersection syndrome. Although initially attributed to friction between the first and second dorsal compartment tendons, Grundberg and Reagan[121] subsequently demonstrated that the condition represents a tendonopathy of the radial wrist extensors within the second dorsal compartment.

The primary treatment for both de Quervain's disease and intersection syndrome is rest with splinting. For de Quervain's, the wrist should be held in slight extension and the thumb abducted in a thumb spica splint to the level of interphalangeal joint. Immobilization of the wrist alone, in approximately 15 degrees of extension, is usually adequate for intersection syndrome. The addition of a 2- to 4-week course of anti-inflammatory medication can be helpful as well. Phonophoresis with a corticosteroid cream, injection of the compartment with corticosteroid, or both are second-line treatments if immobilization alone fails to give adequate relief. Injection of corticosteroid into the affected first dorsal compartment is curative for de Quervain's disease in approximately 75 percent of patients.[122] If a patient does not respond to a course of conservative treatment, surgery may be indicated. For both de Quervain's disease and intersection syndrome, surgery consists of releasing the stenotic retinacular sheath of the involved compartment.

Basal Joint Arthropathy

Inflammation and pain related to the carpometacarpal (CMC) joint of the thumb are very common and can present at any age. In younger patients, instability due to ligamentous laxity is associated with joint subluxation and abnormal cartilage wear and may lead to pain with mechanical activities. In women over 45 years of age, studies show that 25 percent have radiographic evidence of degeneration of the basal joint.[123,124] Patients generally present with pain at the base of the thumb, worsened by pinch such as opening jars and bottles, turning doorknobs and keys, and other activities of daily living. The thumb CMC joint may be swollen and subluxed and is generally tender to palpation. The joint should be assessed for the presence of increased laxity by manual subluxation of the base of the metacarpal out of the trapezial "saddle" with radial and volar force. With advanced degenerative disease, crepitus is sometimes appreciated.

Radiographs should be obtained to determine the stage of the disease. The addition of a basal joint PA stress film, in which the patient presses the tips of the thumbs together firmly with the nail plates facing up, is helpful in assessing joint subluxation (Fig. 42–6). The most commonly used staging system was developed by Eaton and Glickel[125] and is based on the degree of involvement of the trapeziometacarpal (TM) joint and whether or not the scaphotrapezial (ST) joint is involved. Advancing stages show increased subluxation of the basal joint, with development of joint-space narrowing, osteophytes, and subchondral cysts. Stage four implies the presence of pantrapezial degenerative disease.

Regardless of the stage of the disease, the first line of treatment is immobilization of the thumb metacarpal, leaving the interphalangeal joint free. Splinting has been shown to alleviate the symptoms of CMC joint inflammation in more than 50 percent of patients.[126] NSAIDs can be a useful adjunct. Injections of corticosteroid and local anesthetic mixture are quite effective, but usually for a limited time. Although therapy for thenar muscle strengthening has been advocated,

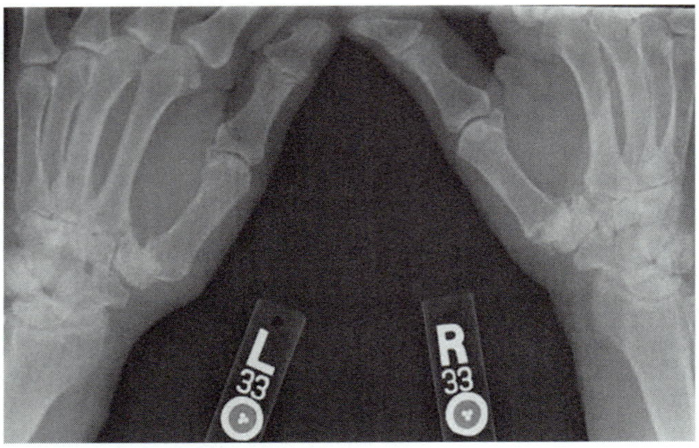

FIGURE 42–6 • A "basal joint stress" radiograph showing stage-three degeneration of the left thumb and stage-four degeneration of the right thumb.

especially in early stages, its benefits are minimal and can occasionally aggravate the problem.

Many patients will be able to manage their symptoms with a combination of splinting, medications, corticosteroid injections, and activity modification. If this is not sufficient, surgery may be indicated in young patients to reconstruct the ligaments that stabilize the metacarpal base. In patients with advanced degenerative changes, excision of the trapezium with or without soft tissue interposition arthroplasty may be required.

Volar Ganglion

Another common location for a ganglion is the radial side of the volar wrist. They typically originate from the ST joint but become superficial and are clinically evident at or near the distal wrist crease over the flexor carpi radialis tendon. Volar ganglions can present in close proximity to the radial artery and should be differentiated from a radial artery aneurysm. Aspiration, if attempted, should be performed carefully to avoid vascular injury, and surgery should be preceded by an Allen's test to document patent ulnar arterial flow. Volar ganglions are associated with a higher recurrence rate and a higher complication rate than their dorsal counterparts.[127]

Scaphoid Fracture or Nonunion

Occasionally a young or middle-aged patient will present with a nonunited scaphoid fracture without recollection of a traumatic incident. When evaluating a relatively young patient with pain at the base of the thumb, wrist swelling in the region of the anatomic snuffbox, and a decreased range of motion of the wrist, plain radiographs and a specialized ulnar-deviation "navicular" radiograph should be obtained to rule out scaphoid pathology. If a scaphoid nonunion has been present for a significant period of time, secondary changes in carpal alignment and joint degeneration have usually occurred. Although splint or cast immobilization can be tried, surgical repair of the scaphoid, or some other wrist salvage procedure, is usually required.

PALM PAIN

Trigger Finger

Painful clicking and locking of the digits in flexion is one of the most common causes of pain in the hand. This condition, caused by a thickening of the A1 retinacular pulley in the palm, is commonly known as *trigger finger.* The thumb is the most commonly affected digit, followed by the ring and long fingers.[128] Patients may present with isolated activity-related pain in the proximal interphalangeal (PIP) joint without frank clicking or locking. Early clicking is felt as a snapping sensation during digital motion and is frequently worst upon awakening. As the condition progresses, the digital range of motion can be reduced and secondary PIP joint contractures develop. The final stage is a locked trigger finger that cannot be straightened actively.

Primary trigger finger is the most common type and is found most often in middle-aged individuals. Triggering of the thumb is up to four times more frequent in women than in men.[5] Secondary triggering is seen in association with such diseases as rheumatoid arthritis, diabetes, and gout. In this type, trigger fingers are often multiple and can also coexist with other stenosing tendinopathies such as de Quervain's or carpal tunnel syndrome. Congenital or developmental triggering can be identified in children and is much less common. As in adults, the thumb is most commonly affected; but unlike adults, this condition often includes the IP joint locked in flexion.

Nonoperative treatment of this condition consists primarily of splinting and local steroid injections. In adults, injection of steroid into the tendon sheath has been shown to be quite effective.[5,6,129] Injection is used infrequently in infants or children. When nonoperative treatments fail to give lasting relief, surgical treatment consists of longitudinal division of the A1 pulley at the level of the metacarpal head. It is a simple procedure that yields reliable and permanent results with few complications.

Retinacular Cysts

Retinacular ganglion cysts can occur in conjunction with a triggering digit or in isolation. They are located at the base of the digit over the A1 pulley as a discrete, pea-sized nodule. They originate from the flexor tendon sheath or annular pulleys and contain synovial fluid. Patients usually complain of pain on gripping objects or with direct pressure over the cyst. A retinacular cyst is most easily treated initially by needle decompression, with care to avoid injury to the sensory nerves that lie immediately adjacent to the flexor tendon and associated cyst. Approximately 50 percent of cysts will recur following aspiration, and surgical resection may be required.

PAIN IN DIGITS

Mallet Finger

Mallet finger refers to a loss of terminal extension of the distal interphalangeal (DIP) joint of the digit and can be classified as either bony or soft tissue depending on where the disruption in the extensor mechanism occurred. Mallet fingers can occur with minimal trauma, such as tucking in bed sheets, and may not be recalled by the patient. This sometimes leads to a delay in diagnosis and treatment. When presented with a digit that droops at the DIP joint and cannot be actively extended, but that has full passive motion, a radiograph should be obtained to determine whether there is an associated fracture of the distal phalanx. An extension splint is the treatment of choice for both bony and soft tissue mallet fingers. The DIP joint should be held in full extension and care should be taken not to force the DIP joint into hyperextension to prevent dorsal skin ischemia and necrosis. Splinting is employed full time for 6 weeks. The patient should not remove the splint for showering or any other activity, but he or she may carefully change the splint for skin care, provided the joint is maintained in extension throughout. PIP flexion exercises are initiated from the outset and are important to help reset the tension in the extensor mechanism. Gentle DIP flexion exercises are begun at 6 weeks and splinting is decreased to nighttime after 6 to 8 weeks. Patients can usually expect a small extension lag, on the order of 5 degrees, and a return of most of their flexion.

Osteoarthritis of the Digits

Osteoarthritis of the interphalangeal joints is extremely common in the older patient and is most often manifested as Heberden's nodes of the DIP joint. Despite gross deformities, pain and dysfunction may be minimal. A mucous cyst may appear in association with degenerative arthritis. These appear on the dorsum of the joint and can cause nail growth deformities due to pressure on the germinal matrix (Fig. 42–7). The changes in nail growth may even precede clinical detection of the cyst. These cysts should not be aspirated with a needle due to the close proximity of the DIP joint and the risk of secondary joint infection. Treatment consists of surgical excision of the cyst and, in particular, the underlying osteophytic spurs.

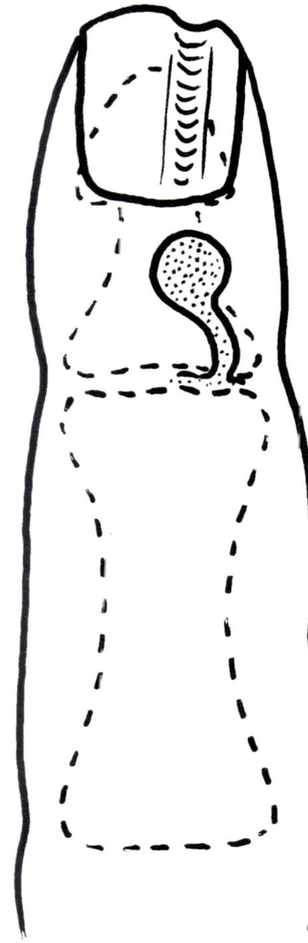

FIGURE 42–7 • Dorsal view of a digit with an as-yet clinically unapparent mucous cyst and the corresponding groove deformity of the nail plate.

Tumors

Benign bone tumors such as simple bone cysts and enchondromas are not uncommon in the phalanges. These usually cause no symptoms and are frequently diagnosed as incidental findings on routine hand radiographs. Enchondromas are most commonly located in the metaphysis of the proximal phalanx and may lead to fracture with minimal trauma due to weakening of the bone structure. If a pathologic fracture occurs, nonoperative treatment is indicated until the fracture heals. The bone tumor can subsequently be addressed with curettage and bone grafting. Occasionally, because of malalignment, earlier surgical intervention will be necessary.

There are many soft tissue tumors that can occur in the hand and digits. Some of the more common benign tumors are giant cell tumor of the tendon sheath (GCTS), lipomas[SWW6], and glomus tumors. Both lipomas and GCTS present clinically as painless, slow-growing masses in the palm and digits. Surgical excision is necessary for diagnosis. Glomus tumors arise from the pericytes in the fingertip or subungual area and typically present with intermittent sharp pain in the fingertip. These vascular tumors become intensely symptomatic when the hand is exposed to cold temperatures, due to abnormal arteriovenous shunting through the hypertrophic glomus system. Surgical excision is generally curative and should be preceded by MRI to rule out multifocal sites.

Infection

The most common infection in the hand is the paronychia. It involves the fold of tissue surrounding the fingernail. *Staphylococcus aureus* is the usual pathogen, introduced by a hangnail, a manicure instrument, or nail biting. Patients will present with an exquisitely painful and erythematous swelling involving a part of the nail fold. Occasionally, the infection can progress to surround the nail in a horseshoe fashion and undermine the nail plate. If seen early, within the first 24 to 48 hours, oral antibiotics and local treatment of the finger with warm soaks can be effective. Superficial abscesses can be drained with a sharp blade through the thin skin without requiring local anesthesia. Larger or more chronic infections require surgical drainage.

An infection of the distal pulp of the fingertip, known as a felon, is a particular problem in diabetic patients. This infection differs from other subcutaneous infections because of the vertical fibrous septa that divide and stabilize the pulp of the fingertip. Often patients will have had some recent penetrating injury in the area. Because of the tightly constrained area of the infection, patients will present with an intensely painful fingertip. There may be an area of "pointing" over the abscess. Surgical drainage is required followed by soaks and oral antibiotics, and intravenous antibiotics are generally recommended in diabetic patients.

Although similar in appearance to a paronychia, herpetic whitlow is caused by the herpes simplex virus, and must be differentiated from other fingertip infections because of a radically different treatment protocol.[130,131] Whitlow was common among dental hygienists prior to the widespread use of gloves for all health care workers. As with bacterial infections, the area becomes painful and erythematous, but local tenderness is much less severe. Diagnosis is by clinical presentation and history. If seen early, vesicles can be ruptured for fluid analysis and viral culture. Nonoperative treatment with oral antiviral agents is recommended.

Other hand and digit infections such as suppurative flexor tenosynovitis, deep space infections of the palm, pyogenic arthritis, infections from bite wounds, and osteomyelitis should be evaluated initially with radiographs of the hand and appropriate blood work. If possible, antibiotics should be withheld until definitive cultures are obtained from the affected area. Antibiotics should then be administrated intravenously and the hand and wrist should be immobilized. Most of these infections will require surgical drainage for definitive treatment.

REFERENCES

1. Metz VM, Gilula LA: Imaging techniques for distal radius fractures and related injuries. Orthop Clin North Am 24:217-228, 1993.
2. Larsen CF, Brondum V, Wienholtz G, et al: An algorithm for acute wrist trauma. A systematic approach to diagnosis. J Hand Surg 18:207-212, 1993.
3. Schreibman KL, Freeland A, Gilula LA, Yin L: Imaging of the hand and wrist. Orthop Clin North Am 28:537-582, 1997.
4. Kaufman MA: Differential diagnosis and pitfalls in electrodiagnostic studies and special tests for diagnosing compressive neuropathies. Orthop Clin North Am 27:245-252, 1996.
5. Marks MR, Gunther SF: Efficacy of cortisone injection in treatment of trigger fingers and thumbs. J Hand Surg 14:722-727, 1989.
6. Newport ML, Lane LB, Stuchin SA: Treatment of trigger finger by steroid injection. J Hand Surg 15:748-750, 1990.
7. Freiberg A, Mulholland RS, Levine R: Nonoperative treatment of trigger fingers and thumbs. J Hand Surg 14:553-558, 1989.
8. Gelberman RH, Aronson D, Weisman MH: Carpal tunnel syndrome: Results of a prospective trial of steroid injection and splinting. J Bone Joint Surg 62:1181-1184,1980.
9. Avci S, Yilmaz C, Sayli U: Comparison of nonsurgical treatment measures for de Quervain's disease of pregnancy and lactation. J Hand Surg 27:322-324, 2002.
10. Lane LB, Boretz RS, Stuchin SA: Treatment of de Quervain's disease: Role of conservative management. J Hand Surg 26:258-260, 2001.
11. Taras JS, Raphael JS, Pan WT, et al: Corticosteroid injections for trigger digits: is intrasheath injection necessary? J Hand Surg 23:717-722, 1998.
12. Esteban JM, Oertel YC, Mendoza M, Knoll SM: Fine needle aspiration in the treatment of ganglion cysts. South Med J 79:691-693, 1986.
13. Richman JA, Gelberman RH, Engber WD, et al: Ganglions of the wrist and digits: Results of treatment by aspiration and cyst wall puncture. J Hand Surg 12:1041-1043, 1987.
14. Ruby LK, Cooney WP III, An KN, et al: Relative motion of selected carpal bones: A kinematic analysis of the normal wrist. J Hand Surg 13:1-10, 1988.
15. Roth JH, Poehling GG, Whipple TL: Arthroscopic surgery of the wrist. Instr Course Lect 37:183-194, 1988.
16. Adolfsson L: Arthroscopy for the diagnosis of post-traumatic wrist pain. J Hand Surg 17:46-50, 1992.
17. Koman LA, Poehling GG, Toby EB, Kammire G: Chronic wrist pain: Indications for wrist arthroscopy. Arthroscopy 6:116-119, 1990.
18. Terrill RQ: Use of arthroscopy in the evaluation and treatment of chronic wrist pain. Hand Clin 10:593-603, 1994.
19. DeSmet L, Dauwe D, Fortems Y, et al: The value of wrist arthroscopy. An evaluation of 129 cases. J Hand Surg 21:210-212, 1996.
20. Kelly EP, Stanley JK: Arthroscopy of the wrist. J Hand Surg 15:236-242, 1990.
21. Poehling GP, Chabon SJ, Siegel DB: Diagnostic and operative arthroscopy. *In* Gelberman RH (ed): The Wrist: Master Techniques in Orthopedic Surgery. New York, Raven Press, 1994.
22. Bienz T, Raphael JS: Arthroscopic resection of the dorsal ganglia of the wrist. Hand Clin 15:429-434, 1999.
23. Luchetti R, Badia A, Alfarano M, et al: Arthroscopic resection of dorsal wrist ganglia and treatment of recurrences. J Hand Surg 25B:38-40, 2000.
24. Ho PC, Griffiths J, Lo WN, et al: Current treatment of ganglion of the wrist. Hand Surg 6:49-58, 2001.
25. Arnold AG: The carpal tunnel syndrome in congestive cardiac failure. Postgrad Med J 53:623, 1977.
26. Doll DC, Weiss RB: Unusual presentations of multiple myeloma. Postgrad Med 61:116-121, 1977.
27. Klofkorn RW, Steigerwald JC: Carpal tunnel syndrome as the initial manifestation of tuberculosis. Am J Med 60:583, 1976.
28. Mayers LB: Carpal tunnel syndrome secondary to tuberculosis. Arch Neurol 10:426, 1964.
29. Champion D: Gouty tenosynovitis and the carpal tunnel syndrome. Med J Aust 1:1030, 1969.
30. Gould JS, Wissinger HA: Carpal tunnel syndrome in pregnancy. South Med J 71:144-145, 1978.
31. Green EJ, Dilworth JH, Levitin PM: Tophacceous gout. An unusual cause of bilateral carpal tunnel syndrome. JAMA 237:2747-2748, 1977.
32. Leach RE, Odom JA: Systemic causes of the carpal tunnel syndrome. Postgrad Med 44:127-131, 1968.
33. Massey EW: Carpal tunnel syndrome in pregnancy. Obstet Gynecol Surg 33:145, 1978.
34. Michaelis LS: Stenosis of carpal tunnel, compression of median nerve, and flexor tendon sheaths, combines with rheumatoid arthritis elsewhere. Proc R Soc Med 43:414, 1950.
35. O'Hara LJ, Levin M: Carpal tunnel syndrome and gout. Arch Intern Med 120:180, 1967.
36. Phillips RS: Carpal tunnel syndrome as manifestation of systemic disease. Ann Rheum Dis 26:59, 1967.
37. Stallings SP, Kasdan ML, Soergel TM, Corwin HM: A case-control study of obesity as a risk factor for carpal tunnel syndrome in a population of 600 patients presenting for independent medical examination. J Hand Surg 22:211-215, 1997.

38. Karpitskaya Y, Novak CB, Mackinnon SE: Prevalence of smoking, obesity, diabetes mellitus, and thyroid disease in patients with carpal tunnel syndrome. Ann Plastic Surg 48:269-273, 2002.
39. Mondelli M, Giannini F, Giacchi M: Carpal tunnel syndrome incidence in a general population. Neurology 58:289-294, 2002.
40. Kummel BM, Zazanis GA: Shoulder pain as the presenting complaint in carpal tunnel syndrome. Clin Orthop 83:41-47, 1972.
41. Lettin AWF: Carpal tunnel syndrome in childhood. J Bone Joint Surg 47:556-559, 1965.
42. al-Qattan MM, Thomson HG, Clarke HM: Carpal tunnel syndrome in children and adolescents with no history of trauma. J Hand Surg 21B:108-111, 1996.
43. Phalen GS: Spontaneous compression of the median nerve at the wrist. JAMA 145:1128, 1951.
44. Durkan JA: A new diagnostic test for carpal tunnel syndrome. J Bone Joint Surg Am 73:535-538, 1991.
45. Gonzalez del Pino J, Delgado-Martinez AD, Gonzalez Gonzalez I, Lovic A: Value of the carpal compression test in the diagnosis of carpal tunnel syndrome. J Hand Surg 22:38-41, 1997.
46. Kemble F: Electrodiagnosis of the carpal tunnel syndrome. J Neurol Neurosurg Psychiatry 31:23, 1968.
47. Ludin HP, Lutschg J, Valsangiacomo F: Comparison of orthodromic and antidromic sensory nerve conduction. I. Normals and patients with carpal tunnel syndrome. EEG EMG 8:173, 1977.
48. Richier HP, Thoden U: Early electroneurographic diagnosis of carpal tunnel syndrome. EEG, EMG 8:187, 1977.
49. Szabo RM, Slater RR Jr, Farver TB, et al: The value of diagnostic testing in carpal tunnel syndrome. J Hand Surg 24:704-714, 1999.
50. Melvin JL, Schuckmann JA, Lanese RR: Diagnostic specificity of motor and sensory nerve conduction variables in the carpal tunnel syndrome. Arch Phys Med Rehabil 54:69, 1973.
51. Gerritsen AAM, deVet HCW, Scholten RJPM, et al: Splinting vs. surgery in the treatment of carpal tunnel syndrome: A randomized controlled trial. JAMA 288:1245-1251, 2002.
52. Gonzalez MH, Bylak J: Steroid injection and splinting in the treatment of carpal tunnel syndrome. Orthopedics 24:479-481, 2001.
53. Irwin LR, Beckett R, Suman RK: Steroid injection for carpal tunnel syndrome. J Hand Surg 21B:355-357, 1996.
54. Linskey ME, Segal R: Median nerve injury from local steroid injection for carpal tunnel syndrome. Neurosurgery 26:512-515, 1990.
55. Tavares SP, Giddins GE: Nerve injury following steroid injection for carpal tunnel syndrome. A report of two cases. J Hand Surg 21:208-209, 1996.
56. Ogino T, Minami A, Fukada K: Tardy ulnar nerve palsy caused by cubitus varus deformity. J Hand Surg 11:352-356, 1986.
57. Guyon F: Note sur une disposition anatomique proper a la face anterieure do la region du poignet et non encores decritie par la docteur. Bull Soc Anat Paris 36:184-186, 1861.
58. Blunden R: Neuritis of deep branch of the ulnar nerve. J Bone Joint Surg Br 40:354, 1958.
59. Eckman PB, Perlstein G, Altrocchi PH: Ulnar neuropathy in bicycle riders. Arch Neurol 32:130-131, 1975.
60. Uriburu IJF, Morchio FJ, Marin JC: Compression syndrome of the deep branch of the ulnar nerve (Piso-hamate hiatus syndrome). J Bone Joint Surg Am 58:145-147, 1976.
61. Poppi M, Padovani R, Martinelli P, Pozzati E: Fractures of the distal radius with ulnar nerve palsy. J Trauma 18:278-279, 1978.
62. Vance RM, Gelberman RH: Acute ulnar neuropathy with fractures at the wrist. J Bone Joint Surg Am 60:962-965, 1978.
63. Jeffery AK: Compression of the deep palmar branch of the ulnar nerve by an anomalous muscle. J Bone Joint Surg Br 53:718-723, 1971.
64. Kalisman M, Laborde K, Wolff TW: Ulnar nerve compression secondary to ulnar artery false aneurysm at the Guyon's canal. J Hand Surg 7:137-139, 1982.
65. McFarland GB, Hoffer MM: Paralysis of the intrinsic muscles of the hand secondary to lipoma in Guyon's canal. J Bone Joint Surg Am 53:375-376, 1971.
66. Richmond DA: Carpal ganglion with ulnar nerve compression. J Bone Joint Surg 45:513-515, 1963.
67. Toshima Y, Kimata Y: A case of ganglion causing paralysis of intrinsic muscles innervated by the ulnar nerve. J Bone Joint Surg 43:153, 1961.
68. Bishop AT, Gabel G, Carmichael SW: Flexor carpi radialis tendinitis. Part I: Operative anatomy. J Bone Joint Surg Am 76: 1009-1014, 1994.
69. Carroll RE, Sinton W, Garcia A: Acute calcuim deposits in the hand. JAMA 157:422-426, 1955.
70. Moyer RA, Bush DC, Harrington TM: Acute calcific tendonitis of the hand and wrist: a report of 12 cases and a review of the literature. J Rheum 16:198-202, 1989.
71. Yang SS, Kalainov DM, Weiland AJ: Fracture of the hook of hamate with rupture of the flexor tendons of the small finger in a rheumatoid patient: a case report. J Hand Surg 21:916-917, 1996.
72. Kato H, Nakamura R, Horii E, et al: Diagnostic imaging for fracture of the hook of the hamate. Hand Surg 5:19-24, 2000.
73. Whalen JL, Bishop AT, Linscheid RL: Nonoperative treatment of acute hamate hook fractures. J Hand Surg 17:507-511, 1992.
74. Bishop AT, Bechenbaugh RD: Fracture of the hamate hook. J Hand Surg 13:863-868, 1988.
75. Carter PR, Eaton RG, Littler JW: Ununited fracture of the hook of the hamate. J Bone Joint Surg Am 59:583-588, 1977.
76. Stark HH, Chao EK, Zemel NP, et al: Fracture of the hook of the hamate. J Bone Joint Surg Am 71:1202-1207, 1989.
77. Stark HH, Jobe FW, Boyes JH, Ashworth CR: Fracture of the hook of the hamate in athletes. J Bone Joint Surg Am 59: 575-582, 1977.
78. Cardinal E, Buckwalter KA, Braunstein EM, Mih AD: Occult dorsal carpal ganglion: comparison of US and MR imaging. Radiology 193:259-262, 1994.
79. Vo P, Wright T, Hayden F, et al: Evaluating dorsal wrist pain: MRI diagnosis of occult dorsal wrist ganglion. J Hand Surg 20:667-670, 1995.
80. Zubowicz VN, Ishii CH: Management of ganglion cysts of the hand by simple aspiration. J Hand Surg 12:618-620, 1987.
81. Angelides AC, Wallace PF: The dorsal ganglion of the wrist: Its pathogenesis, gross and microscopic anatomy, and surgical treatment. J Hand Surg 1:228-235, 1976.
82. Clay NR, Clement DA: The treatment of dorsal wrist ganglia by radical excision. J Hand Surg 13:187-191, 1988.
83. Janzon L, Niechajev IA: Wrist ganglia. Incidence and recurrence rate after operation. Scand J Plast Reconstr Surg 15:53-56, 1981.
84. Angelides AC: Ganglions of the hand and wrist. *In* Green DP (ed): Operative Hand Surgery. New York, Churchill Livingstone, 1993.
85. Cuono CB, Watson HK: The carpal boss: Surgical treatment and etiological considerations. Plast Reconstr Surg 63:88-93, 1979.
86. Bonatz E, Dramer TD, Masear VR: Rupture of the extensor pollicis longus tendon. Am J Orthop 25:118-122, 1996.
87. Stahl S, Wolff TW: Delayed rupture of the extensor pollicis longus tendon after nonunion of a fracture of the dorsal radial tubercle. J Hand Surg 13:338-341, 1988.
88. Hove LM: Delayed rupture of the thumb extensor tendon. A 5-year study of 18 consecutive cases. Acta Ortho Scand 65:199-203, 1994.
89. Dawson WJ: Sports-induced spontaneous rupture of the extensor pollicis longus tendon. J Hand Surg 17:457-458, 1992.
90. Keinbock R: Uber Traumatische Malazie des Mondbeins und Kompression Fracturen. Fortschr Roentgenstrahlen 16:77-103, 1910.
91. Stahl F: On lunatomalacia (Keinböck's disease): Clinical and rentgenological study, especially on its pathogenesis and late results of immobilization treatment. Acta Chir Scand 126(suppl): 1-133, 1947.
92. Wada A, Miura H, Kubota H, et al: Radial closing wedge osteotomy for Kienböck's disease: an over 10 year clinical and radiographic follow-up. J Hand Surg 27B:175-179, 2002.
93. Wintman BI, Imbriglia JE, Buterbaugh GA, Hagberg WC: Operative treatment with radial shortening in Kienbock's disease. Orthopedics 24:365-371, 2001.
94. Quenzer DE, Dobyns JH, Linscheid RL, et al: Radial recession osteotomy for Kienböck's disease. J Hand Surg 22:386-395, 1997.
95. Nakamura R, Imaeda T, Miura T: Radial shortening for Kienbock's disease: Factors affecting the operative result. J Hand Surg 15:40-45, 1990.

96. Oishi SN, Muzaffar AR, Carter PR: Treatment of Kienböck's disease with capitohamate arthrodesis: pain relief with minimal morbidity. Plast Recon Surg 109:1293-1300, 2002.
97. Watson HK, Monacelli DM, Milford RS, Ashmead DIV: Treatment of Kienböck's disease with scaphotrapezio-trapezoid arthrodesis. J Hand Surg 21:9-15, 1996.
98. Chuinard RG, Zeman SC: Keinbock's disease: An analysis and rationale for treatment by capitate-hamate fusion. Orthop Trans 4:18, 1980.
99. Kakinoki R, Matsumoto T, Suzuki T, et al: Lunate plasty for Kienböck's disease: use of a pedicled vascularised radial bone graft combined with shortening of the capitate and radius. Hand Surg 6:145-156, 2001.
100. Thompson TC, Campbell RD Jr, Arnold WD: Primary and secondary dislocation of the scaphoid bone. J Bone Joint Surg 46:73-82, 1964.
101. Palmer AK, Werner FW: The triangular fibrocartilage complex of the wrist: Anatomy and function. J Hand Surg 6:153-161, 1981.
102. King GJ, McMurtry RY, Rubenstein JD, Gertzbein SD: Kinematics of the distal radioulnar joint. J Hand Surg 11:798-804, 1986.
103. Burk DL Jr, Karasick D, Wechsler RJ: Imaging of the distal radioulnar joint. Hand Clinics 7:263-275, 1991.
104. King GJ, McMurtry RY, Rubenstein JD, Ogston NG: Computerized tomography of the distal radioulnar joint: Correlation with ligamentous pathology in a cadaveric model. J Hand Surg 11:711-717, 1986.
105. Mino DE, Palmer AK, Levinsohn EM: The role of radiography and computerized tomography in the diagnosis of subluxation and dislocation of the distal radioulnar joint. J Hand Surg 8:23-31, 1983.
106. Mino DE, Palmer AK, Levinsohn EM: Radiography and computerized tomography in the diagnosis of incongruity of the distal radio-ulnar joint. A prospective study. J Bone Joint Surg Br 67:247-252, 1985.
107. Steyers CM, Blair WF: Measuring ulnar variance: A comparison of techniques. J Hand Surg 14:607-612, 1989.
108. Epner RA, Bowers WH, Guilford WB: Ulnar variance: The effect of wrist positioning and roentgen filming technique. J Hand Surg 7:298-305, 1982.
109. Gilula LA, Hardy DC, Totty WG: Distal radioulnar joint arthrography. Am J Roeutgenol 150:180-189, 1988.
110. Mikic ZD: Age changes in the triangular fibrocartilage of the wrist joint. J Anat 126:367-384, 1978.
111. Mikic ZD: Arthrography of the wrist joint. An experimental study. J Bone Joint Surg Am 66:371-378, 1984.
112. Palmer AK, Levinsohn EM, Kuzma GR: Arthrography of the wrist. J Hand Surg 8:18-23, 1983.
113. Potter HG, Asnis-Ernberg L, Weiland AJ, et al: The utility of high-resolution magnetic resonance imaging in the evaluation of the triangular fibrocartilage complex of the wrist. J Bone Joint Surg Am 79:1675-1684, 1997.
114. Feldon P, Terronon AL, Belsky MR: The wafer procedure. Partial distal ulnar resection. Clin Orthop 275:124-129, 1992.
115. de Araujo W, Poehling GG, Kuzma GR: New Tuohy needle technique for triangular fibrocartilage complex repair: preliminary studies. Arthroscopy 12:699-703, 1996.
116. Lacey T II, Goldstein LA, Tobin CE: Anatomical and clinical study of the variations in the insertions of the abductor pollicus longus tendon, associated with stenosing tendovaginitis. J Bone Joint Surg Am 33:347-350, 1951.
117. Leao L: De Quervain's disease; A clinical and anatomical study. J Bone Joint Surg Am 40:1063-1070, 1958.
118. Strandell G: Variations of the anatomy in stenosing tenosynovitis at the radial styloid process. Acta Chir Scand 113:234-240, 1957.
119. Finkelstein H: Stenosing tendovaginitis at the radial styloid process. J Bone Joint Surg Am 12:509-540, 1930.
120. Pick RY: De Quervain's disease: A clinical triad. Clin Orthop 143:165-166, 1979.
121. Grundberg AB, Reagan DS: Pathologic anatomy of the forearm: Intersection syndrome. J Hand Surg 10:299-302, 1985.
122. Weiss AP, Akelman E, Tabatabai M: Treatment of de Quervain's disease. J Hand Surg 19:595-598, 1994.
123. Kelsey JL, Pastides H, Kreiger N, et al: Arthritic Disorders, Upper Extremity Disorders: A Survey of Their Frequency and Cost in the United States. St. Louis, Mosby, 1980, pp 19-22.
124. Armstrong AL, Hunter JB, Davis TRC: The prevalence of degenerative arthritis of the base of the thumb in post-menopausal women. J Hand Surg 19:340-341, 1994.
125. Eaton RG, Glickel SZ: Trapeziometacarpal osteoarthritis: Staging as a rationale for treatment. Hand Clin 3:455-469, 1987.
126. Swigart CR, Eaton RG, Glickel SZ, Johnson C: Splinting in the treatment of trapeziometacarpal joint arthritis. J Hand Surg 24:86-91, 1999.
127. Gundes H, Cirpici Y, Sarlak A, Muezzinoglu S: Prognosis of wrist ganglion operations. Acta Ortho Belg 66:363-367, 2000.
128. Bonnici AV, Spencer JD: A survey of "trigger finger" in adults. J Hand Surg 13:202-203, 1988.
129. Murphy D, Failla JM, Koniuch MP: Steroid versus placebo injection for trigger finger. J Hand Surg 20:628-631, 1995.
130. Fowler JR: Viral infections. Hand Clin 5:533-552, 1989.
131. LaRossa D, Hamilton R: Herpes simplex infections of the digits. Arch Surg 102:600-603, 1971.

43 Temporomandibular Joint Pain

DANIEL M. LASKIN

Pain in the temporomandibular joint (TMJ) region, a commonly encountered symptom, affects more than 10 million Americans. However, because of its diverse etiology, there is often considerable difficulty in proper diagnosis and treatment. Owing to the proximity of the ear and parotid gland and the similar nature of pain in these areas, pathologic conditions involving these structures are often confused with those arising in the TMJ. Moreover, pain occurring in the adjacent muscles of mastication, also a frequently encountered situation, not only is similar to TMJ pain in character and location, but it is also associated with jaw dysfunction, a common finding with painful conditions directly involving the TMJ. For these reasons, a knowledge of the various painful conditions occurring in the TMJ region is essential in establishing a correct diagnosis.

Because patients with primary TMJ disease often have secondary myofascial pain, and patients with primary myofascial pain problems can develop secondary TMJ disease, the generally accepted term used to describe this overlapping group of conditions is *temporomandibular disorders*. These conditions are then subdivided for purposes of diagnosis and treatment into those that primarily involve the TMJ (TMJ problems) and those that primarily involve the muscles of mastication (myofascial pain and dysfunction, masticatory myalgia). However, from a diagnostic standpoint, it is also important to consider the numerous conditions that mimic the temporomandibular disorders by producing similar signs and symptoms (Tables 43–1 and 43–2).

The various pathologic entities that commonly involve the TMJ are listed in Table 43–3. Although there are a variety of conditions, only three types are commonly considered to produce pain. They include the various arthritides, derangements of the intra-articular disk, and certain neoplasms.

Arthritis of the Temporomandibular Joint

Arthritis is the most common condition affecting the TMJ, just as it is in other joints. Although degenerative arthritis and rheumatoid arthritis are most frequently encountered, cases of infectious arthritis, metabolic arthritis, and the spondyloarthropathies have also been reported. Traumatic arthritis is also a common occurrence.

DEGENERATIVE ARTHRITIS (OSTEOARTHRITIS)

Degenerative arthritis is the most common type of arthritis involving the TMJ and the most frequent cause of pain in that region. Clinical symptoms of the disease have been reported in up to 16 percent of the general population,[1] but radiographic evidence has been found in up to 44 percent of asymptomatic persons.[2] Although the TMJ is not a weight-bearing joint in the same sense as those of the long bones, the stresses associated with such parafunctional habits as clenching and grinding of the teeth are sufficient to contribute to similar degenerative changes in some patients.[3] Acute and chronic trauma and derangements of the intra-articular disk are also common causes of secondary degenerative arthritis.

Clinical Findings

Primary degenerative arthritis, which is usually seen in older people, is insidious in its onset; it generally produces only mild discomfort, and persons rarely complain about the condition. On the other hand, secondary degenerative arthritis usually occurs in younger patients (20 to 40 years old) and tends to be painful. In contrast to primary degenerative joint disease and rheumatoid arthritis, it is often limited to only one TMJ, although it may become bilateral in the late stages, and involvement of other joints is uncommon. The condition is characterized by TMJ pain that is increased by function, joint tenderness, limitation of mouth opening, and occasional clicking and popping sounds. In the late stages, there may be crepitation in the joint.

Imaging Findings

The earliest radiologic feature of degenerative arthritis of the TMJ, whether primary or secondary, is subchondral sclerosis in the mandibular condyle. If the condition progresses, condylar flattening and marginal lipping may be noted. In the later stages, erosion of the cortical plate, osteophyte formation, or both may occur. There may also occasionally be breakdown of the subcortical bone resulting in the formation of bone cysts. Although the changes in the articular fossa are generally not as severe as those in the condyle, cortical erosion can sometimes be seen. Narrowing of the joint space also occurs in the late stages, and this is indicative of concomitant degenerative changes in the intra-articular disk. Although the changes in the TMJ can usually be seen on plain radiographs, sagittal and coronal computed tomographic

TABLE 43–1 • DIFFERENTIAL DIAGNOSIS OF NONARTICULAR CONDITIONS MIMICKING PAIN OF MYOFASCIAL PAIN-DYSFUNCTION SYNDROME

Disorder	Limitation	Muscle Tenderness	Diagnostic Features
Pulpitis	No	No	Mild to severe ache or throbbing; intermittent or constant; aggravated by thermal change; eliminated by dental anesthesia; positive radiographic findings
Pericoronitis	Yes	Possible	Persistent mild to severe ache; difficulty swallowing; possible fever; local inflammation; relieved with dental anesthesia
Otitis media	No	No	Moderate to severe earache; pain constant; fever; usually history of upper respiratory infection; no relief with dental anesthesia
Parotitis	Yes	No	Constant aching pain, worse when eating; pressure feeling; absent salivary flow; ear lobe elevated; ductal suppuration
Sinusitis	No	No	Constant aching or throbbing; worse with change of head position; nasal discharge; often molar pain not relieved by dental anesthesia
Trigeminal neuralgia	No	No	Sharp stabbing pain of short duration; trigger zone; pain follows nerve pathway; older age-group; often relieved by dental anesthesia
Atypical (vascular) neuralgia	No	No	Diffuse throbbing or burning pain of long duration; often associated autonomic symptoms; no relief with dental anesthesia
Temporal arteritis	No	No	Constant throbbing preauricular pain; artery prominent and tender; low-grade fever, may have visual problems; elevated sedimentation rate
Trotter's syndrome (nasopharyngeal carcinoma)	Yes	No	Aching pain in ear, side of face, lower jaw; deafness; nasal obstruction; cervical lymphadenopathy
Eagle's syndrome (elongated styloid process)	No	No	Mild to sharp stabbing pain in ear, throat, retromandible; provoked by swallowing, turning head, carotid compression; usually post-tonsillectomy; styloid process longer than 2.5 cm

From Laskin DM, Block S: Diagnosis and treatment of myofascial pain dysfunction (MPD) syndrome. J Prosthet Dent 56:75-84, 1986.

TABLE 43–2 • DIFFERENTIAL DIAGNOSIS OF NONARTICULAR CONDITIONS PRODUCING LIMITATION OF MANDIBULAR MOVEMENT

Disorder	Pain	Muscle Tenderness	Diagnostic Features
Odontogenic infection	Yes	Yes	Fever; swelling; positive radiographic findings; tooth tender to percussion; pain relieved and movement improved with dental anesthesia
Nonodontogenic infection	Yes	Yes	Fever; swelling; negative dental findings on radiograph; dental anesthesia may not relieve pain or improve jaw movement
Myositis	Yes	Yes	Sudden onset; movement associated with pain; areas of muscle tenderness; usually no fever
Myositis ossificans	No	No	Palpable nodules seen as radiopaque areas on radiograph; involvement of nonmasticatory muscles
Neoplasia	Possible	Possible	Palpable mass; regional nodes may be enlarged; may have paresthesia; radiograph may show bone involvement
Scleroderma	No	No	Skin hard and atrophic; mask-like facies; paresthesias: arthritic joint pain; widening of periodontal ligament
Hysteria	No	No	Sudden onset after psychologic trauma; no physical findings; jaw opens easily under general anesthesia
Tetanus	Yes	No	Recent wound; stiffness of neck; difficulty swallowing; spasm of facial muscles; headache
Extrapyramidal reaction	No	No	Patient on antipsychotic drug or phenothiazine tranquilizer; hypertonic movement; lip smacking; spontaneous chewing motions
Depressed zygomatic arch	Possible	No	History of trauma; facial depression; positive radiographic findings
Osteochondroma coronoid process	No	No	Gradual limitation; jaw may deviate to unaffected side; possible clicking sound on jaw movement; positive radiograph findings

From Laskin DM, Block S: Diagnosis and treatment of myofascial pain dysfunction (MPD) syndrome. J Prosthet Dent 56:75-84, 1986.

TABLE 43–3 • DIFFERENTIAL DIAGNOSIS OF TEMPOROMANDIBULAR JOINT DISEASE

Disorder	Pain	Limitation	Diagnostic Features
Agenesis	No	Yes	Congenital; usually unilateral; mandible deviates to affected side; unaffected side long and flat; severe malocclusion; often ear abnormalities; radiograph shows condylar deficiency
Condylar hypoplasia	No	No	Congenital or acquired; affected side has short mandibular body and ramus, fullness of face, deviation of chin; body of mandible elongated and face flat on unaffected side; malocclusion; radiograph shows condylar deformity, antegonial notching
Condylar hyperplasia	No	No	Facial asymmetry with deviation of chin to unaffected side; cross-bite malocclusion; prognathic appearance; lower border of mandible often convex on affected side; radiograph shows symmetric enlargement of condyle
Neoplasia	Possible	Yes	Mandible may deviate to affected side; radiographs show enlarged, irregularly shaped condyle or bone destruction, depending on type of tumor; unilateral condition
Infectious arthritis	Yes	No	Signs of infection; may be part of systemic disease; radiograph may be normal early, later can show bone destruction; fluctuance may be present; pus may be obtained on aspiration; usually unilateral
Rheumatoid arthritis	Yes	Yes	Signs of inflammation; findings in other joints (hands, wrists, feet, elbows, ankles); positive laboratory test results; retarded mandibular growth in children; anterior open bite in adults; radiograph shows bone destruction; usually bilateral
Spondyloarthropathies Psoriatic arthritis	Yes	Yes	Presence of cutaneous psoriasis; nail dystrophy; involvement of distal interphalangeal joints; radiograph shows condylar erosion; negative for rheumatoid factor
Ankylosing spondylitis	Yes	Yes	Frequent involvement of the spine and sacroiliac joint; extra-articular manifestations include iritis, anterior uveitis, aortic insufficiency, and conduction defects; erosive condylar changes; TMJ ankylosis may occur
Metabolic arthritis Gout	Yes	Yes	Usually sudden onset; often monoarticular; commonly involves great toe, ankle, and wrist; joint swollen, red, and tender; increased serum uric acid; late radiographic changes
Pseudogout	Yes	Yes	Generally unilateral; TMJ may be only joint involved; joint frequently swollen; presence of intra-articular calcification; may be a history of trauma
Traumatic arthritis	Yes	Yes	History of trauma; radiograph normal except for possible widening of joint space; local tenderness; usually unilateral
Degenerative arthritis	Yes	Yes	Unilateral joint tenderness; often crepitus; TMJ may be only joint involved; radiograph may be normal or show condylar flattening, lipping, spurring, or erosion
Ankylosis	No	Yes	Usually unilateral but can be bilateral; may be history of trauma; young patient may show retarded mandibular growth; radiographs show loss of normal joint architecture
Internal disk derangement	Yes	Yes	Pain exacerbated by function; clicking on opening, or opening limited to less than 25 mm with no click; positive arthrographic or magnetic resonance imaging findings; may be history of trauma; usually unilateral

Modified from Laskin DM, Block S: Diagnosis and treatment of myofascial pain dysfunction (MPD) syndrome. J Prosthet Dent 56:75-84, 1986.

scans are the preferred way of imaging the bony structures.

Diagnosis

The diagnosis of degenerative arthritis is based on the patient's history and clinical and radiographic findings. There is often a history of trauma or parafunctional oral habits. The involvement is frequently unilateral, and there are no significant changes in any of the other joints. The pain tends to be well localized, and the TMJ is often tender to palpation.

Treatment

The treatment of degenerative arthritis of the TMJ is generally medical, just as in other joints in the body. It involves the use of nonsteroidal anti-inflammatory drugs, application of heat, eating a soft diet, limitation of jaw function, and use of a bite appliance if the patient has a chronic habit of clenching or grinding the teeth. Physical therapy with thermal agents, ultrasonography, and iontophoresis can also be beneficial, and isotonic and isometric exercises improve joint stability once the acute symptoms have subsided. The use of intra-articular steroid injections is controversial, and they should be limited to those patients with acute symptoms that do not respond to other forms of medical management. Because of the potential damaging effects of long-acting steroids, they should be limited to no more than three or four single injections given at 3-month intervals. Intra-articular injection of high-molecular-weight sodium hyaluronate given twice, 2 weeks apart, has been shown to have essentially the same therapeutic effect as a steroid injection, without the potential adverse side effects.[4]

Once the acute symptoms have been controlled, therapy is directed toward control of the factors possibly contributing to the degenerative process. Unfavorable loading of the joint is eliminated by replacement of missing teeth to establish a good, functional occlusion; by correction of any severe dental malrelationships through orthodontics or orthognathic surgery; and by continued use of a bite appliance at night to control any teeth-clenching or -grinding habits.[5]

In those patients in whom medical management for 3 to 6 months fails to relieve the symptoms, surgical management may be indicated. This involves removal of only the minimal amount of bone necessary to produce a smooth articular surface. The unnecessary removal of the entire cortical plate, as occurs with the so-called condylar shave procedure or high condylotomy, can lead to a continuation of the resorptive process in some instances and should be avoided if possible.

RHEUMATOID ARTHRITIS

As many as 50 percent of patients with rheumatoid arthritis have involvement of the TMJ. Although the TMJ may be affected early in the course of the disease, other joints in the body are usually involved first. Both children and adults are affected, with a female-to-male ratio of 3:1. In the child, destruction of the mandibular condyle by the disease process results in growth retardation and facial deformity characterized by a severely retruded chin. Fibrous or bony ankylosis is a possible sequelae at all ages.

Clinical Findings

Patients with rheumatoid arthritis of the TMJ have bilateral pain, tenderness, and swelling in the preauricular region as well as limitation of mandibular movement. These symptoms are characterized by periods of exacerbation and remission. Joint stiffness and pain are usually worse in the morning and decrease during the day. The limitation in mandibular movement becomes worse as the disease progresses, and the patient may also develop an anterior open bite.

Imaging Findings

Although there may not be any radiographic changes in the early stages of the disease, about 50 to 80 percent of the patients show bilateral evidence of demineralization, condylar flattening, and bone erosion as the disease progresses, so the articular surface appears irregular and ragged. Erosion of the glenoid fossa is also sometimes seen. With continued destruction of the condyle, the loss of ramus height can lead to contact of only the posterior teeth and an anterior open bite.

Diagnosis

The diagnosis of rheumatoid arthritis is made on the basis of the clinical and radiographic findings and confirmatory laboratory tests. The distinguishing features for rheumatoid arthritis and degenerative arthritis of the TMJ are shown in Table 43–3.

Treatment

The treatment of rheumatoid arthritis of the TMJ is similar to that for other joints.[6] Anti-inflammatory drugs are used during the acute phases, and mild jaw exercises are used to prevent excessive loss of motion when the acute symptoms subside. In severe cases, drugs such as hydroxychloroquine, gold, methotrexate, etanercept, and lefunomide are also used. Surgery may be necessary if ankylosis develops.

SPONDYLOARTHROPATHIES

In addition to the adult and juvenile forms of rheumatoid arthritis, psoriatic arthritis and ankylosing spondylitis can also involve the TMJ.[7,8]

Psoriatic Arthritis

This condition occurs in a small percentage of patients who have long-standing cutaneous psoriasis. It can have a sudden onset, can be episodic in nature, and may show spontaneous remission.[8] Often only one TMJ is involved. Symptoms include TMJ pain and tenderness, restricted jaw movement, and crepitation, mimicking the symptoms of rheumatoid arthritis.[8] The radiographic changes are nonspecific and cannot be distinguished easily from other types of arthritis, particularly rheumatoid arthritis and ankylosing spondylitis.[9] They usually involve erosive changes in the condyle and glenoid fossa associated with extreme narrowing of the joint space.[10] The diagnosis is usually based on the triad of psoriasis, radiographic evidence of erosive arthritis, and a negative serologic test for rheumatoid factor. However, even in the presence of a rash, the diagnosis cannot be absolutely confirmed. The differential diagnosis should always include rheumatoid arthritis, Reiter's syndrome, ankylosing spondylitis, and gout.

Ankylosing Spondylitis

About one third of the patients with ankylosing spondylitis develop TMJ involvement several years after the onset of the disease. Pain and limitation of jaw movement are the most common symptoms, and ankylosis can develop in advanced cases.[7,11] On radiographic examination, about 30 percent of the patients show erosive changes in the condyle and fossa and narrowing of the joint space.[12] However, in long-standing cases, there is sometimes a more florid osteophytic response during quiescent periods. The severity of the changes appears to be related to the severity of the disease.

Treatment

The treatment of psoriatic arthritis and ankylosing spondylitis of the TMJ is medical and generally is part of the total management of the patient. Physical therapy is used to improve jaw mobility, and bite appliances are used, when indicated, to reduce parafunctional stress on the joint.

TRAUMATIC ARTHRITIS

Acute trauma to the mandible that does not result in a fracture can still produce injury to the TMJ. When this occurs in a child, it is essential to warn the parents about the possibility of future retardation of mandibular growth and associated facial deformity resulting from damage to the articular cartilage, which is an important growth site.[13]

Traumatic arthritis is characterized by TMJ pain and tenderness and limitation of jaw movement. The resultant inflammation and occasional hemarthrosis can also result in loss of tooth contact on the affected side. Frequently, there are bruises or lacerations at the site of the initial injury. There may be no radiographic changes seen, or there may be widening of the joint space due to intra-articular edema or hemorrhage. In some instances, the radiographs may show an intracapsular fracture that was not recognized on clinical examination.

The treatment of traumatic arthritis consists of the use of nonsteroidal anti-inflammatory drugs, application of heat, a soft diet, and initial restriction of jaw movement. When the acute symptoms subside, range-of-motion exercises should be used to avoid fibrous ankylosis.

INFECTIOUS ARTHRITIS

This condition rarely involves the TMJ. Although it can affect the joint as part of such systemic diseases as gonorrhea, syphilis, tuberculosis, and Lyme disease, the most common way is by direct extension of an adjacent infection of dental, parotid gland, or otic origin.[14] On occasion, it may also occur from the localization of blood-borne organisms in the joint after a traumatic injury or by direct involvement through a penetrating wound.

Clinical Findings

Infectious arthritis generally results in unilateral pain, tenderness, swelling, and redness in the region of the TMJ. This is usually accompanied by chills, fever, and sweating, as well as by the systemic findings characteristic of the specific type of infection. There is often an inability to occlude the teeth because of the swelling within the joint. In the pyogenic forms of infectious arthritis, fluctuation may be present in the joint region.

Imaging Findings

The radiographic findings are usually normal in the early stages of the disease because of the lack of bony involvement, but the intra-articular accumulation of pus or inflammatory exudate may cause separation of the articulating surfaces that can be detected on magnetic resonance imaging. Later, depending on the severity and chronicity of the infection, varying degrees of bony destruction, ranging from damage to the articular surface of the mandibular condyle to extensive osteomyelitis, may be seen. In the late stages, fibrous or bony ankylosis may occur. In a child, infectious arthritis can affect the growth of the condyle and result in facial asymmetry.

Treatment

The treatment of infectious arthritis includes the use of the appropriate antibiotics, proper hydration, control of the pain, and limitation of jaw movement. Suppurative infections may require aspiration, incision and drainage, or sequestrectomy. When there has been extensive bone loss, reconstructive procedures may be necessary. In children in whom mandibular growth has been affected, a costochondral graft can be used to correct the facial asymmetry and reestablish growth of the mandible.

METABOLIC ARTHRITIS

Metabolic arthritis, which can accompany gout or pseudogout (calcium pyrophosphate dehydrate arthropathy) is rare in the TMJ.[15]

Gout

Gouty arthritis of the TMJ occurs most frequently in men older than 40 years and is usually preceded by involvement of one or more joints of the feet or hands. The attack usually occurs suddenly, and the joint becomes swollen, painful, red, and tender. Recovery may occur in a few days, and remission can last for months to years.

When the attacks are infrequent, there may not be any radiographic changes for a long period. Because there have been so few cases reported, the precise radiographic changes that occur have not been well documented. Calcified areas in the disk, destruction of the hard tissues of the joint, exostoses, spurring, and the presence of tophi have been described.[15]

The initial approach to treatment of gout involving the TMJ is medical. However, if the symptoms are not controlled, surgical débridement of the joint and arthroplasty may be indicated.

Pseudogout

Calcium pyrophosphate dehydrate arthropathy (pseudogout) in the TMJ clinically mimics gout, and the mandibular condyle may show degenerative and erosive changes radiographically. In the primary form, which is usually seen in older patients, there is intra-articular calcification (chondrocalcinosis), and diffuse calcification also occurs in the intra-articular disk.[15-19] Similar changes are seen in the secondary form, but it occurs in younger patients and is frequently preceded by a history of trauma. Just as in gout of the TMJ, the initial treatment of pseudogout is medical, and surgery is reserved for patients in whom such treatment is ineffective.

Internal Derangements

Internal derangements are a common cause of pain in the TMJ. They represent a disturbance in the normal anatomic relationship between the intra-articular disk and the condyle, resulting in an interference with the smooth movement of the joint.

CLINICAL FINDINGS

There are three stages of internal derangement: a painless incoordination phase in which there is a momentary catching sensation during mouth opening; anterior disk displacement with reduction into the normal position during mouth opening, which is characterized by a clicking or popping sound (Fig. 43–1); and anterior disk displacement without reduction on attempted mouth opening, which is characterized by a restriction of jaw movement, or locking (Fig. 43–2). The joint pain in patients with anterior disk displacement, with or without reduction, is caused by condylar compression of the highly innervated retrodiskal tissue that occupies the glenoid fossa as the intra-articular disk assumes a more forward position, as well as by the accompanying inflammation.

ETIOLOGY

The three main causes of internal derangement of the intra-articular disk are trauma, abnormal functional loading of the joint, and degenerative joint disease.[20] It has also been suggested that spasm in the lateral pterygoid muscle, a portion of which attaches to the anterior aspect of the disk, can lead to a disk derangement, but the evidence for this theory is circumstantial. Although some clinicians believe that occlusal factors also play a role in causing internal derangements, there have been no conclusive studies that show such a relationship.

Acute macrotrauma is probably the most common cause of internal derangement. Among the incidents that have been implicated are a blow to the jaw, endotracheal intubation, cervical traction, and iatrogenic stretching of the joint during dental or oral surgical procedures. Although whiplash injuries have frequently been implicated in the etiology of internal derangement, a study of 155 patients with this type of injury showed that only one developed clicking in the TMJ immediately after the automobile accident.[21] At 1 month of follow-up, two additional patients of the 129 contacted experienced clicking, but at 1 year, no additional patients of the 104 contacted had developed clicking. Thus, although internal derangements of the TMJ can be due to whiplash injury, the incidence appears to be low.

Whether a patient develops merely alterations in the articular surface leading to a catching or binding sensation, anterior disk displacement with reduction on mouth opening (clicking or popping), or anterior disk displacement without reduction during mouth opening (locking) after trauma to the TMJ depends on the severity of the injury. Although the associated traumatic arthritis causes pain during function in each of these instances, the pain is more severe in the last two conditions because of compression of the retrodiskal tissue, which is now located in the articular zone.

The functional overloading of the TMJ associated with a chronic teeth-clenching habit is another frequent cause of internal derangements. Although the TMJ is constructed for eccentric movements, it is not constructed for the constant isometric loading and unloading that occurs during this activity. Such parafunction affects the lubrication of the joint, introducing friction between the disk and the condyle that leads to degenerative changes in the articular surfaces and results in gradual anterior displacement of the disk.[20,22]

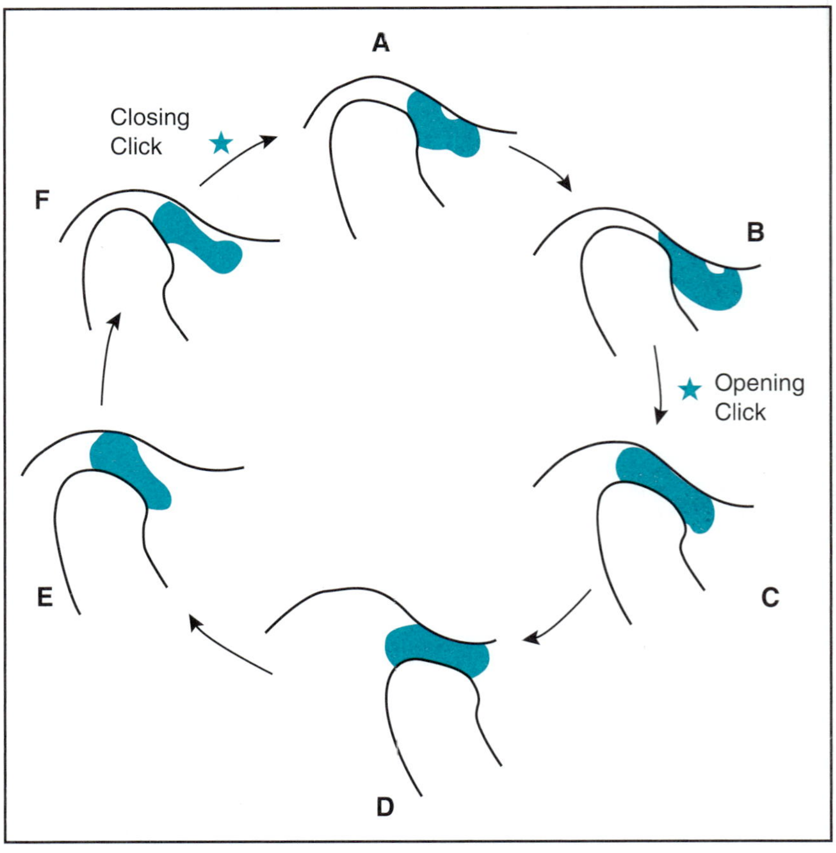

FIGURE 43-1 · **Anterior Displacement of the Intra-Articular Disk with Reduction on Opening of the Mouth.** A clicking or popping sound occurs as the disk returns to its normal position in relation to the condyle. During closure, the disk again becomes anteriorly displaced, sometimes accompanied by a second sound (reciprocal click). (Modified and reprinted with permission from McCarty W: Diagnosis and treatment of internal derangements of the articular disc and mandibular condyle. *In* Solberg WK, Clark GT [eds]: Temporomandibular Joint Problems: Biologic Diagnosis and Treatment. Chicago, Quintessence, 1980, p 155.)

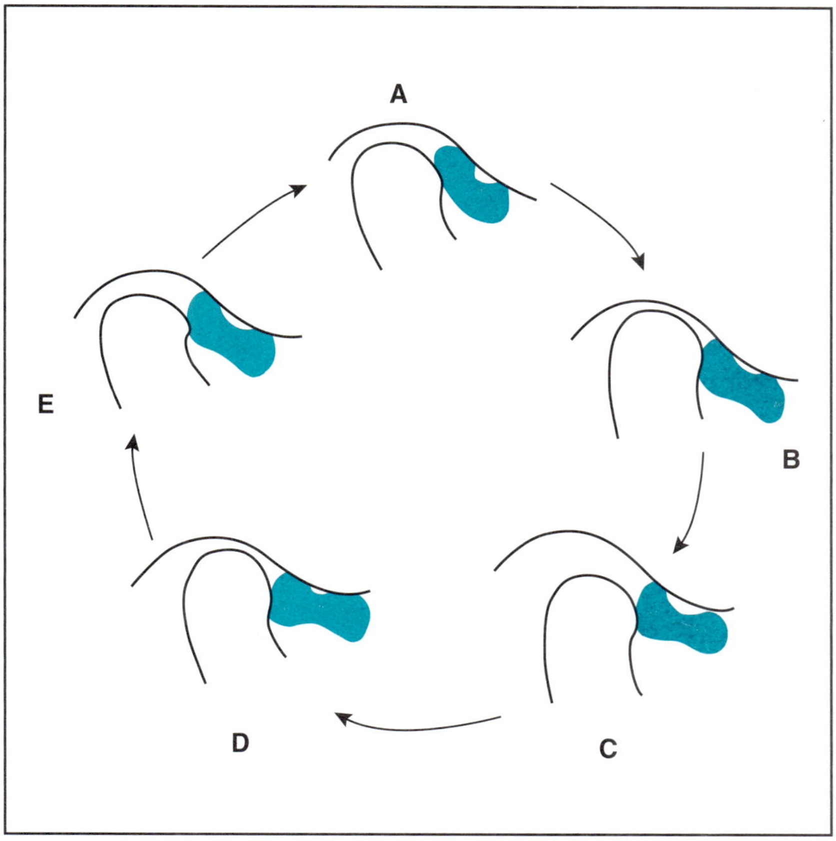

FIGURE 43-2 · Anterior Displacement of the Intra-Articular Disk Without Reduction on Attempted Mouth Opening. The displaced disk acts as a barrier and prevents full translation of the condyle. (Modified and reprinted with permission from McCarty W: Diagnosis and treatment of internal derangements of the articular disc and mandibular condyle. *In* Solberg WK, Clark GT [eds]: Temporomandibular Joint Problems: Biologic Diagnosis and Treatment. Chicago, Quintessence, 1980, p 151.)

Degenerative joint disease may precede the development of an internal derangement, or it may occur after the development of an internal derangement due to other causes. In the first instance, the changes in the character of the articulating surfaces result in an inability of the parts to glide smoothly over each other, gradually leading to a forward displacement of the disk, which normally rotates posteriorly during mouth opening. In the second instance, the displaced disk results in an altered relationship between the articulating components of the joint, which then leads to the degenerative changes in these structures. In patients in whom the condition causing the degenerative joint disease is still active, whether primarily or secondarily, it—as well as the disk derangement—must be treated to completely resolve the problem.

IMAGING FINDINGS

Depending on the cause of the internal derangement and its duration, the radiographs may or may not show any evidence of degenerative joint disease. However, magnetic resonance imaging shows anterior disk displacement in the closed mouth position and a return to a normal disk relationship in patients with clicking and popping; in those patients with locking, the disk remains in the anterior position, and there is limited movement of the condyle. There is also a small group of patients with locking who show the intra-articular disk in normal position when the teeth are in occlusion, rather than anteriorly displaced, and there is no change in disk position when the person attempts to open the mouth.[23] In such cases there is adhesion of the disk to the articular eminence preventing translation of the condyle. These patients differ from those with anteriorly displaced, nonreducing disks in that they do not have a history of TMJ clicking preceding the sudden onset of locking.

TREATMENT

The initial treatment of patients with painful clicking or popping in the TMJ consists of a nonsteroidal anti-inflammatory drug and the use of a bite-opening appliance made by a dentist to reduce compression of the retrodiskal tissue. A muscle relaxant drug can be added to the regimen if the patient has associated myofascial pain. Once the pain has stopped, no further treatment is necessary, even though the joint noise may still be present. A long-term follow-up study (1 to 15 years) of 190 patients with a history of clicking treated by such conservative nonsurgical modalities, which are not directed specifically to the problems of joint noise or disk displacement, showed that the condition became worse in only 1 percent, indicating that it is permissible to observe people with painless clicking as long as they remain otherwise asymptomatic.[24] However, in patients with pain and clicking in the TMJ that is unresponsive to nonsurgical management, the disk should be repositioned arthroscopically or by open surgery (diskoplasty).

In patients with locking (anterior disk displacement without reduction), whether painful or not, treatment is urgent because if the condition is left untreated for a long period, the subsequent management can be complicated by further degenerative changes in the disk and condyle that make disk salvage (diskoplasty) impossible. The initial treatment involves joint lavage and lysis of adhesions either arthroscopically or by arthrocentesis. The latter involves establishing inlet and outlet portals in the upper joint space with hypodermic needles, irrigation with lactated Ringer's solution to remove inflammatory breakdown products and cytokines, and lysis of adhesions by hydrolic distention and manual manipulation of the joint. The results of arthrocentesis parallel those achieved with arthroscopic lysis and lavage, but the procedure is less invasive.[25] Although neither of these procedures restore the disk to its normal position,[26] they do restore disk and joint mobility and, thus, reduce the pain and improve function in most patients.[27,28]

In patients who do not respond favorably to arthroscopy or arthrocentesis, repositioning of the displaced disk by an open operation should be attempted. However, if the disk is extremely deformed and cannot be repositioned, or if there is a large, nonreparable perforation in the disk or retrodiskal tissue, it should be removed. Although some patients seem to tolerate a diskless joint,[29] most surgeons prefer to replace the disk with an autogenous auricular cartilage or dermal graft or a temporal muscle flap. Currently, there are no acceptable alloplastic substitutes for the disk.

Neoplasms

Although primary neoplasms involving the TMJ are uncommon, they still need to be considered in the differential diagnosis of painful conditions affecting this region. Chondroma,[30] osteochondroma, and osteoma are the most frequently encountered benign tumors, but isolated cases of fibro-osteoma, myxoma, fibrous dysplasia, giant-cell reparative granuloma, aneurysmal bone cyst, synovialoma, synovial chondromatosis, chondroblastoma, osteoblastoma, glomus tumor, and synovial hemangioma have been reported.[31] Malignant tumors of the TMJ are even rarer, with infrequent reports of fibrosarcoma, chondrosarcoma, synovial fibrosarcoma, osteosarcoma, malignant fibrous histiocytoma, malignant schwannoma, leiomyosarcoma, and multiple myeloma. The TMJ can also be invaded by neoplasms from the cheek, the parotid gland, the external auditory canal,[32] and the adjacent ramus of the mandible. Metastasis to the condyle from distant neoplasms in the breast, lung, prostate, colon, and thyroid gland has also been described.[33]

Tumors of the TMJ can cause pain, limitation of jaw movement, deviation of the mandible to the affected side on attempted mouth opening, and difficulty in occluding the teeth. Depending on the nature of the condition, the radiographs may show bony deformation, apposition, or resorption. A biopsy is necessary to establish the definitive diagnosis.

Myofascial Pain and Dysfunction

Myofascial pain and dysfunction (MPD), or masticatory myalgia, is a psychophysiologic disease that primarily involves the muscles of mastication and not the TMJ. Women are affected more frequently than men; the ratio in various reports ranges from 2:1 to 5:1. Although the condition can occur in children, the greatest incidence appears to be in the 20- to 40-year-old age-group. MPD is frequently confused with painful conditions affecting the TMJ such as degenerative arthritis or internal derangements because patients with primary MPD can develop these diseases secondarily and patients with primary joint disease can develop secondary MPD. However, a better understanding of the causes and pathogenesis of this condition now makes its diagnosis easier and its treatment more effective.[34]

ETIOLOGY

MPD is believed to be a stress-related disorder.[35] It is hypothesized that centrally induced increases in muscle tension, frequently combined with the presence of parafunctional habits such as clenching or grinding of the teeth, result in muscle fatigue and spasm that produce the pain and dysfunction. Similar symptoms, however, can also occasionally result from muscle overextension, muscle overcontraction, or trauma (Fig. 43–3).

CLINICAL FINDINGS

Pain of unilateral origin is the most common symptom of MPD. In contrast to the pain associated with joint disease, which is well localized, the pain of muscle origin is more diffuse and the patient is generally unable to identify the specific site involved. This can serve as an important diagnostic criterion in distinguishing between muscle and joint disorders.

Depending on the muscle involved, the pain associated with MPD may be described by the patient in a variety of ways. The masseter is the most frequent muscle involved, and the patient usually refers to the pain as a jaw ache. The temporalis is the next most commonly involved muscle, and it produces pain on the side of the head and is interpreted by the patient as a headache. Involvement of the lateral pterygoid muscle produces earache or a deep pain behind the eye, whereas medial pterygoid involvement causes discomfort on swallowing and the feeling of a painful, swollen gland beneath the angle of the mandible. Patients who complain of stuffiness or a full feeling in the ear may also have medial pterygoid involvement.

The pain associated with MPD is usually constant, but it is often more severe on arising in the morning or may gradually worsen as the day progresses. It is generally exacerbated by use of the mandible, especially during such activities as eating and excessive talking. Myofascial pain tends to be regional rather than local, and patients with a long-standing problem may complain that the pain in the facial region has spread to the cervical area and later to the shoulders and back.

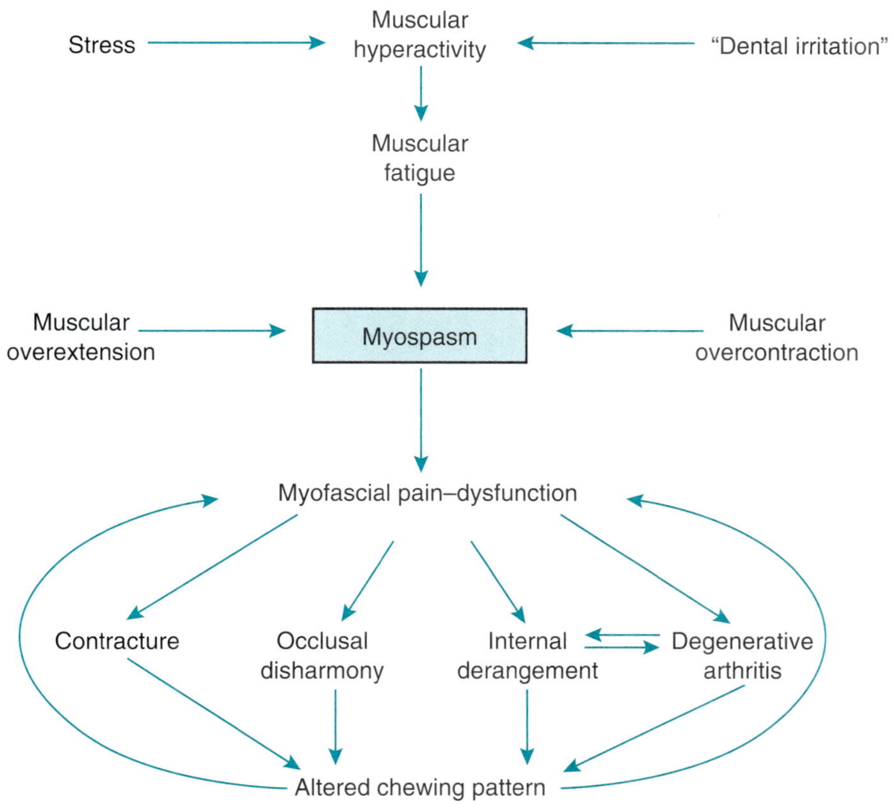

FIGURE 43-3 · Causes of Myofascial Pain and Dysfunction (MPD). Although the diagram shows three pathways, the one involving psychologic stress is most common. The mechanism by which stress leads to myospasm is termed the *psychophysiologic theory of MPD.* (Modified from Laskin DM: Etiology of the pain-dysfunction syndrome. J Am Dent Assoc 79:147-153, 1969. Copyright © 1969 American Dental Association. Reprinted by permission of ADA Publishing Co., Inc.)

Tenderness in the muscles of mastication is another common finding, and its presence can be used to confirm the source of the pain in those muscles that are accessible to palpation (masseter, temporalis, and medial pterygoid). Although muscle tenderness is usually not reported by the patient, this symptom can be elicited easily by the examiner. The most frequent sites of tenderness are near the angle of the mandible, in the belly and posterosuperior aspect of the masseter, in the anterior temporal region, and over the temporal crest on the anterior aspect of the coronoid process. The location of some of the tender areas suggests that the tendons, as well as the muscles, may be the source of the pain and tenderness.

Limitation of mandibular movement is the third cardinal symptom of MPD. It manifests itself as an inability to open the mouth as wide as usual and as a deviation of the mandible to the affected side when mouth opening is attempted. Lateral excursion to the unaffected side is also reduced. The limitation of mandibular movement is usually correlated with the amount of pain present.

A clicking or popping sound in the TMJ is another finding in some patients with MPD. Although intermittent clicking may accompany the lateral pterygoid spasm that occurs in some of these patients, the frictional changes introduced by a chronic teeth-clenching habit are a more common causative factor.[20] Therefore, although clicking and popping sounds are not always an early cardinal sign, they can be a later finding in some patients with MPD. The presence of joint sounds alone, however, is not sufficient to make a diagnosis of MPD. They must be accompanied by myofascial pain and tenderness in the masticatory muscles that began before the onset of the joint noise. Such patients must be distinguished from those with a primary internal derangement, in whom muscle splinting produces myofascial pain and tenderness after the onset of the joint noise. The history and the difference in physical findings are helpful in making this distinction.

In addition to having the three cardinal symptoms of pain, muscle tenderness, and limitation of mouth opening, patients with MPD usually have an absence of clinical and radiographic evidence of pathologic changes in the TMJ. These negative characteristics are important in establishing the diagnosis because they confirm that the primary site of the problem is not the articular structures.

DIAGNOSIS

Because the cardinal signs and symptoms of MPD are similar to those produced by such organic problems involving the TMJ as degenerative joint disease and internal disk derangement, as well as by a variety of nonarticular conditions (see Tables 43–1 and 43–2), the diagnosis of this condition can be difficult, requiring a careful history and a thorough clinical evaluation. Periapical radiographs of the teeth and screening views (transcranial, transpharyngeal, or panoramic) of the TMJs can be helpful in eliminating dental or joint disease. If the screening views of the TMJs show some abnormality, tomographic views or computed tomographic scans are usually advisable. Magnetic resonance imaging can also be useful in determining the position of the disk when an internal derangement of the TMJ is being considered. Depending on the suspected condition, other radiographic views of the head and neck and scintigraphy may be needed to establish a final diagnosis. In addition, certain laboratory tests may be helpful in some instances. These include a complete blood cell count if an infection is suspected; serum calcium, phosphorus, and alkaline phosphatase measurements for possible bone disease; serum uric acid determination for gout; serum creatinine and creatinine kinase levels as indicators of muscle disease; and erythrocyte sedimentation rate, rheumatoid factor, latex fixation, and antinuclear antibody tests for suspected rheumatoid arthritis. Electromyography can be used to evaluate muscle function. Psychologic evaluation and psychometric testing are good research tools but have little diagnostic value other than for determining the presence of any associated abnormal behavioral characteristics.

A condition that is sometimes confused with myofascial pain is fibromyalgia, particularly when MPD involves several regions in addition to the face. Although a small subset of patients with MPD may eventually develop fibromyalgia, they are probably distinct conditions.[36] The distinguishing characteristics are listed in Table 43–4.

TREATMENT

The treatment of MPD is divided into four phases.[37] Once a definitive diagnosis is made, phase I therapy should be started (Fig. 43–4). This initially involves providing the patient with some understanding of the problem. Because patients often have difficulty accepting a psychophysiologic explanation for their condition, the discussion should deal with the issue of muscle fatigue and spasm as the cause of the pain and dysfunction, delaying consideration of the role of stress and psychologic factors until the symptoms have improved and the patient's confidence has been gained. Relating the symptoms to the specific masticatory muscles from which they arise helps the patient understand the reason for the type and location of the pain; for example, headache from the temporalis muscle, jaw ache from the masseter muscle, discomfort on swallowing and stuffiness in the ear from the medial pterygoid muscle, and earache and pain behind the eye from the lateral pterygoid muscle.

In addition to the initial explanation, the patient should be counseled regarding home therapy. This includes recommendations about avoidance of clenching and grinding of the teeth, eating a soft diet, use of moist heat and massage on the masticatory muscles, and limitation of jaw motion. Because the patient has muscle spasm and pain, a muscle relaxant and a nonsteroidal anti-inflammatory drug should be prescribed.

About 50 percent of these patients have a resolution of their symptoms within 2 to 4 weeks with phase I therapy. For those whose symptoms persist, however, phase II therapy is initiated. Home therapy and medications are continued, but a bite appliance is also made for the patient. Although numerous types have been used, the Hawley-type maxillary appliance is probably most effective because it prevents contact of the posterior teeth and thereby also prevents most forms of parafunctional activity. The appliance is generally worn at night, but it can be worn for 5 to 6 hours during the day, if necessary. However, it should not be worn continuously because the posterior teeth may supraerupt in some patients.

With phase II therapy, another 20 to 25 percent of the patients become free of symptoms in 2 to 4 weeks. When this occurs, the medications are stopped first, and wearing the bite appliance is discontinued next. If the patient has a return of symptoms and the appliance is worn only at night, its use can be continued indefinitely.

Patients who do not respond to the use of a bite appliance are entered into phase III treatment for 4 to 6 weeks. In this phase, either physical therapy (ultrasonography, electrogalvanic stimulation) or relaxation therapy (electromyographic biofeedback, conditioned relaxation) is added to the regimen.[38] There is no evidence to show that one form of treatment is better than the other, and either can be used first. If one is not successful, the other can then be tried. Phase III therapy usually helps another 10 to 15 percent of the patients.

If all of these approaches fail and there is no question about the correctness of the diagnosis, psychologic counseling is recommended. This involves helping patients identify possible stresses in their lives and learn to cope with such situations. If there is a doubt about the diagnosis, the patient should first be referred for appropriate dental and neurologic consultation and reevaluation. Another alternative is to refer patients with recalcitrant MPD to a TMJ center or pain clinic, because such patients generally require a multidisciplinary approach for successful treatment.

TABLE 43–4 • FEATURES OF MYOFASCIAL PAIN AND FIBROMYALGIA

	Myofascial Pain	Fibromyalgia
Age distribution	20-40 yr old	20-50 yr old
Gender distribution	Mainly women	Mainly women
Distribution of the pain	Localized; usually unilateral	Generalized; bilaterally symmetric
Tender points	Few	Multiple
Trigger points	Uncommon	Common
Fatigue	Localized muscle fatigue	Generalized fatigue
Sleep disturbance	Common	Common

Summary

The successful management of patients with temporomandibular disorders is dependent on establishing an accurate diagnosis and using proper therapy based on an understanding of the etiology of the condition being treated. Of particular importance is separating those patients with MPD, who constitute the major group encountered and who are not surgical candidates,

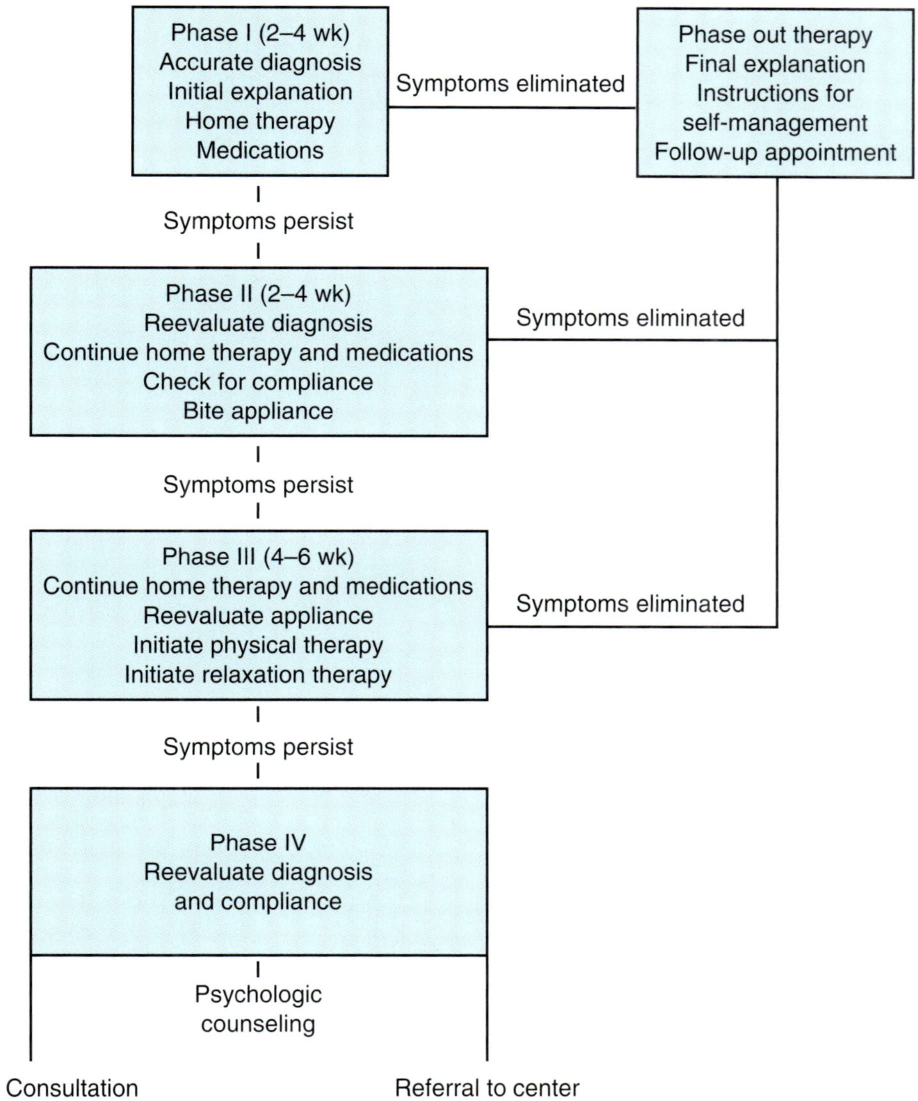

FIGURE 43-4 · Management of Myofascial Pain-Dysfunction (MPD) The treatments are divided into four phases. If the symptoms are eliminated in any of the first three phases, the ongoing therapy is gradually phased out and the patient is instructed in continued self-management of the condition. (From Laskin DM, Block S: Diagnosis and treatment of myofascial pain dysfunction [MPD] syndrome. J Prosthet Dent 56:75-84, 1986.)

from those with TMJ disease, who frequently require surgical treatment. However, even in the latter group, many of the commonly encountered conditions, such as arthritis and internal disk derangements, often respond to nonsurgical therapy, and this type of treatment should be given a fair trial before more aggressive management is considered.

REFERENCES

1. Merjersjo C: Therapeutic and prognostic considerations in TMJ osteoarthrosis: a literature review and a long-term study in 11 subjects. J Craniomandib Pract 5:70, 1987.
2. Madsen B: Normal variations in anatomy, condylar movements and arthrosis frequency of the TMJs. Acta Radiol 4:273, 1966.
3. Milam SB, Zardeneta G, Schmitz JP: Oxidative stress and degenerative temporomandibular joint disease. J Oral Maxillofac Surg 56:214, 1998.
4. Kopp S, Wenneberg B, Haraldson T, et al: The short-term effect of intra-articular injections of sodium hyaluronate and corticosteroid on temporomandibular joint dysfunction. J Oral Maxillofac Surg 43:429, 1985.
5. Abubaker AO, Laskin DM: Nonsurgical management of arthritis of the temporomandibular joint. Oral Maxillofac Surg Clin North Am 7:1, 1995.
6. Zide MF, Carlton D, Kent JH: Rheumatoid arthritis and related arthropathies: systemic findings, medical therapy, and peripheral joint surgery. Oral Surg Oral Med Oral Pathol 61:119, 1986.
7. Davidson C, Wojtulewsky JA, Bacon PA, et al: Temporomandibular joint disease in ankylosing spondylitis. Ann Rheum Dis 34:87, 1975.
8. Wilson A, Braunwald E, Issilbacker KJ: Psoriatic arthropathy of the temporomandibular joint. Oral Surg Oral Med Oral Pathol 70:555, 1990.
9. Kononen M: Radiographic changes in the condyle of the temporomandibular joint in psoriatic arthritis. Acta Radiol 28:185, 1987.
10. Koorbusch GF, Zeitler DL, Fotos PG, et al: Psoriatic arthritis of the temporomandibular joint with ankylosis. Oral Surg Oral Med Oral Pathol 71:267, 1991.
11. Wenneberg B: Inflammatory involvement of the temporomandibular joint: diagnostic and therapeutic aspects and a study of individuals with ankylosing spondylitis. Swed Dent J Suppl 20:1, 1983.
12. Wenneberg B, Hollender L, Kopp S: Radiographic changes in the temporomandibular joint in ankylosing spondylitis. Dentomaxillofac Radiol 12:25, 1983.

13. Harris S, Rood JP, Testa HJ: Post-traumatic changes of the temporomandibular joint by bone scintigraphy. Int J Oral Maxillofac Surg 17:173, 1988.
14. Moses JJ, Lange CR, Arredondo A: Septic arthritis of the temporomandibular joint after the removal of third molars. J Oral Maxillofac Surg 56:510, 1998.
15. Gross BD, Williams RB, DiCosimo CT, et al: Gout and pseudogout of the temporomandibular joint. Oral Surg Oral Med Oral Pathol 63:551, 1987.
16. Nakagawa Y, Ishibashi K, Kobayoshi K, et al: Calcium phosphate deposition disease in the temporomandibular joint: report of two cases. J Oral Maxillofac Surg 57:1357, 1999.
17. Chuong R, Piper MA: Bilateral pseudogout of the temporomandibular joint: report of a case and review of the literature. J Oral Maxillofac Surg 53:691, 1995.
18. Pynn BR, Weinberg S, Irish J: Calcium pyrophosphate dihydrate deposition disease of the temporomandibular joint. Oral Surg Oral Med Oral Pathol Endod 79:278, 1995.
19. Aoyama S, Kino K, Amagosa T, et al: Differential diagnosis of calcium pyrophosphate dihydrate deposition of the temporomandibular joint. Br J Oral Maxillofac Surg 38:550, 2000.
20. Laskin DM: Etiology and pathogenesis of internal derangements of the temporomandibular joint. Oral Maxillofac Surg Clin North Am 6:217, 1994.
21. Heise AP, Laskin DM, Gervin AS: Incidence of temporomandibular joint symptoms following whiplash injury. J Oral Maxillofac Surg 50:825, 1992.
22. Nitzan DW: The process of lubrication impairment and its involvement in temporomandibular disk displacement: a theoretical concept. J Oral Maxillofac Surg 59:36, 2001.
23. Nitzan DW, Samson B, Better H: Long-term outcome of arthrocentesis for sudden-onset persistent, severe closed lock of the temporomandibular joint. J Oral Maxillofac Surg 55:151, 1997.
24. Greene CS, Laskin DM: Long-term status of TMJ clicking in patients with myofascial pain and dysfunction. J Am Dent Assoc 117:461, 1988.
25. Nitzan DW: Arthrocentesis for management of severe closed lock of the temporomandibular joint. Oral Maxillofac Surg Clin North Am 6:245, 1994.
26. Gabler MJ, Greene CS, Palacios E, et al: Effect of arthroscopic temporomandibular joint surgery on articular disk position. J Craniomandib Disord 3:191, 1989.
27. Dimitroulis G: A review of 55 cases of chronic closed lock treated with temporomandibular joint arthroscopy. J Oral Maxillofac Surg 60:519, 2002.
28. Carvajal W, Laskin DM: Long-term evaluation of arthrocentesis for treatment of internal derangement of the temporomandibular joint. J Oral Maxillofac Surg 58:852, 2000.
29. Eriksson L, Westesson PL: Discectomy as an effective treatment for painful temporomandibular joint internal derangement: a 5 year clinical and radiographic follow-up. J Oral Maxillofac Surg 59:750,2001.
30. Lazow SK, Pihlstrom RT, Solomon MP, et al: Condylar chondroma: report of a case. J Oral Maxillofac Surg 56:373, 1998.
31. Keith DA: Tumors of the temporomandibular joint. *In* Keith DA (ed): Surgery of the Temporomandibular Joint, 2nd ed. Boston, Blackwell Scientific Publications, 248, 1992.
32. Treasure T: External auditory canal carcinoma involving the temporomandibular joint: two cases presenting as temporomandibular disorders. J Oral Maxillofac Surg 60:465, 2002.
33. DeBoom GW, Jensen JL, Siegal W, et al: Metastatic tumors of the mandibular condyle. Oral Surg Oral Med Oral Pathol 60:512, 1985.
34. Laskin DM: Diagnosis and etiology of myofascial pain and dysfunction. Oral Maxillofac Surg Clin North Am 7:73, 1995.
35. Laskin DM: Etiology of the pain-dysfunction syndrome. J Am Dent Assoc 59:147, 1969.
36. Cimino R, Michelotti A, Stradi R, et al: Comparison of the clinical and psychologic features of fibromyalgia and masticatory myofascial pain. J Orofac Pain 12:35, 1998.
37. Laskin DM, Block S: Diagnosis and treatment of myofascial pain-dysfunction (MPD) syndrome. J Prosthet Dent 56:75, 1986.
38. Adler RC, Adachi NY: Physical medicine in the management of myofascial pain and dysfunction. Oral Maxillofac Surg Clin North Am 7:99, 1995.

INTERNET LINKS

1. www.nicdr.nih.gov: General information, clinical trials and sponsored research in TMJ and related areas
2. www.aaoms.org: General information about TMJ surgery
3. www.tmj.org: Advocate group that provides general information for patients

44 The Eye and Rheumatic Disease

DENIS M. O'DAY • JEFFREY D. HORN

The patient with rheumatic disease frequently stands at the interface between ophthalmology and internal medicine. Although the joint and systemic manifestations of the illness are naturally central to the management of these patients, ocular involvement is often an important consideration and requires careful attention to optimize vision and function and to avoid the devastating complications, including blindness.

Many patients with rheumatic diseases are best managed via a collaborative effort between the rheumatologist and the ophthalmologist in which the informed patient has a pivotal role. Ocular tissues, including the ocular adnexa, that are critical to the health, and therefore the function, of the eye may become involved. The actual degree of involvement to a great extent depends on the nature of the underlying disorder.

The Eye as a Sentinel for Rheumatologic Disease

Although ocular involvement is viewed as a complication of systemic rheumatic disease, an ocular or visual system complaint may be the first indication of a rheumatologic disorder. This places a burden on the ophthalmologist and, in these days of managed care, on family practitioners, internists, and nonphysician providers, particularly the nurse practitioners and optometrists who may be confronted with patients whose ocular disease is difficult to diagnose and whose systemic disease is not immediately obvious. Clinical features are frequently ill defined and easily confused with purely ophthalmic disease, but they may have grave prognostic implications for visual function in the long term. In this chapter, we use the approach of describing the major ophthalmic manifestations of rheumatologic disease (i.e., keratoconjunctivitis sicca, scleritis, episcleritis, and uveitis), and we outline the likely presentation of various syndromes as well as complications, disease course, and impact on visual function. We hope to provide a perspective that is helpful to nonophthalmically trained physicians by alerting them to the diagnostic significance of ophthalmic symptoms and signs in the otherwise apparently healthy patient and in the patient with overt rheumatologic disease.

Ophthalmic Manifestations

KERATOCONJUNCTIVITIS SICCA

Keratoconjunctivitis sicca, also known as *dry eye disease*, is a term used to indicate the presence of markedly reduced or absent tear production. It has many causes and may arise independent of any systemic disorder. When associated with certain immunologic features, it is known as Sjögren's syndrome. Regardless of the cause, the patient's symptoms, arising from the effects of dryness of the underlying conjunctiva and cornea, are remarkably consistent.

The tear film is composed of three layers. The aqueous layer is secreted by the lacrimal glands and accessory lacrimal glands of Wolfring and Krause. It floats on a mucin layer secreted mainly by goblet cells in the conjunctiva. This layer of mucin functions as a surface wetting agent. By facilitating spreading of the aqueous layer, it helps coat the hydrophobic corneal epithelial cells after each blink of the eyelids. Floating on this aqueous layer is a superficial lipid layer composed of oily secretions from the meibomian glands along the margin of the eyelid. The lipid retards evaporation from the corneal surface. If any part of these layers is missing, dry eye symptoms result.[1]

Dry eye disease can be classified as tear deficient when aqueous secretion is deficient or evaporative when there is excessive evaporation. Evaporative disease is most commonly a result of Meibomian gland dysfunction, whereas tear deficiency is associated with lacrimal gland and systemic diseases. However, features of the two overlap and both may occur in the same patient.[2]

Ophthalmic disease may affect any of the three layers, but patients with connective tissue disease are most likely to experience a decrease in aqueous tear production. The difficulty in resolving the cause arises from the fact that dry eye also occurs most frequently in patients without any evidence of systemic disease and is more likely to be present in older, otherwise healthy patients. In younger individuals, the condition is associated with pregnancy and the use of certain medications, including oral contraceptives and antihistamines. Refractive corneal surgery is now recognized as a cause of dry eye in both young and older individuals, presumably as a result of corneal sensory denervation.[3]

An adequate supply of tears is vital to the health of the cornea. The tear film has an important effect on the optical function of the anterior refracting surface of the cornea, and tears are a vital component of the host defenses to the eye. They remove foreign bodies and potential infectious agents from the surface of the cornea mechanically. Tears also carry vital soluble components of the host defense that protect the cornea from attack. The cornea, deprived of an adequate tear layer, has its optical efficiency degraded, and it is open to complications as a result of minor trauma and infections that may then lead to corneal ulceration, scarring, and corneal perforation.

From the rheumatologic perspective, the importance of keratoconjunctivitis sicca lies in the fact that it may be the first evidence of an underlying systemic disorder. Patients with Sjögren's syndrome have dry eyes and a dry mouth. There are three subsets of the syndrome: patients with systemic immune dysfunction but no defined connective tissue disease, patients who lack evidence of either, and patients with a defined connective tissue disease. Primary Sjögren's syndrome refers to the first two types, and patients in the third group are classified as having secondary Sjögren's syndrome. Rheumatoid arthritis is the disorder most frequently associated with Sjögren's syndrome[1,4] (Table 44–1).

Patients with dry eye, regardless of the underlying etiology, present with an important cluster of symptoms all related to the effects of tear deficiency on the cornea and external eye (Table 44–2). The eye may appear normal on external examination, or there may be moderate to severe diffuse conjunctival injection. Depending on the severity of the disease, the light reflex from the corneal surface may appear normal or may be dulled. Only with the slit-lamp biomicroscope can discreet pathologic changes be discerned in the cornea and conjunctiva. The diagnostic dilemma, however, is whether these findings arise from dry eye without other organ involvement or from Sjögren's syndrome and therefore have an underlying systemic disorder that would justify more extensive investigation.

The diagnosis of Sjögren's syndrome can be difficult. The current definition requires at least two components of the clinical triad: dry eyes, dry mouth, and an autoimmune disease.[4] Despite considerable investigation, there is still controversy about how best to make the diagnosis.[5] The combination of ocular and oral symptoms and signs is helpful, particularly symptoms suggestive of reduced production of saliva. In addition to evidence of oral dryness, especially at night or while eating, patients with salivary gland deficiency may also have poor oral hygiene, a tendency to dental caries, and may easily become infected with oral *Candida albicans*. Recently, women with Sjögren's syndrome have been shown to be androgen deficient, and a linkage with regulation of Meibomian gland function has been postulated.[6]

TABLE 44–1 • RHEUMATOLOGIC DISEASES IN SJÖGREN'S SYNDROME

- Rheumatoid arthritis
- Systemic lupus erythematosus
- Polyarteritis nodosa
- Scleroderma

TABLE 44–2 • SYMPTOMS OF KERATOCONJUNCTIVITIS SICCA

- Foreign body sensation
- Red eye
- Ocular burning sensation
- Ocular pain
- Photophobia
- Inability to tear
- Ocular mucus production

Adapted from Whitcher JP, Gritz DC, Daniels TE: The dry eye: A diagnostic dilemma. *In* Smolin G (ed): Infections and Immunologic Diseases of the Cornea. Philadelphia, Lippincott, Williams & Wilkins, 1998, pp 23–37.

The evidence of a highly significant association between focal lymphocytic sialadenitis in labial salivary gland biopsies and the presence of keratoconjunctivitis sicca suggests that labial salivary gland biopsy may be helpful in such cases.[7] To complete the triad, serologic evidence of a systemic autoimmune disorder is required.[1] A more precise definition of Sjögren's syndrome awaits the results of further research.

Disease Course, Complications, and Management

Both eyes are involved, although tear reduction may be worse in one eye than in the other. Reduced tear production in keratoconjunctivitis sicca is permanent, and the reduction is likely to become more severe over time. This has important implications for the health of the eye.

Management options include artificial tear preparations, punctal plugs, punctal occlusion, topical cyclosporine in some instances, and tarsorrhaphy in advanced cases. Although the focus of treatment should be amelioration of the truly distressing symptoms of dry eye, it is important to remember that visual function and even the eye itself may be threatened by the pathologic consequence of absent or reduced tear production. In the otherwise healthy patient, the cornea heals rapidly after minor trauma. Vision-threatening complications are rare. The consequences are far more serious in the patient with dry eye because of the unfavorable effect of reduced tear function. For this reason, any untoward event that may seem trivial in a patient with normal tear production must be treated with the utmost seriousness. Severe visual loss occurring in a patient already functionally disabled by rheumatologic disease can be devastating to overall quality of life and survival.

EPISCLERITIS AND SCLERITIS

Episcleritis and scleritis are ophthalmologic diagnoses. They can be difficult to recognize in the absence of a detailed ophthalmic examination. The sclera, the opaque covering of the eyeball continuous with the cornea, is composed of three layers: episcleral tissue, the sclera proper, and the lamina fusca. The episclera is a loose structure of fibrous and elastic tissue continuous superficially with overlying Tenon's capsule that surrounds the globe. The episclera merges with the sclera, but unlike the sclera, which is relatively avascular, it has many small blood vessels. When inflamed, the episcleral and scleral vessels become markedly injected, and the patient presents with a red eye. The diagnostic dilemma for the clinician is how to differentiate scleritis from episcleritis and to differentiate these conditions from other causes of red eye, particularly conjunctivitis or keratoconjunctivitis, uveitis, and acute glaucoma.

In patients with episcleritis, pain is usually minimal or absent. Although the eye appears red, the distribution of the redness is usually sectorial, often in the exposed areas of the globe, and may be unilateral or bilateral (Fig. 44–1). The patient usually complains more of the redness of the eye rather than of pain or visual loss. The individual with scleritis typically presents with pain, often described as boring, and complains of the red appearance of the eye (Fig. 44–2). Pain can be severe, and involvement tends to be bilateral. A characteristic feature is nocturnal worsening of the pain, which at times can be so severe as to be disabling. With more severe manifestations, vision can be affected.

Scleritis may present in several different forms: diffuse anterior scleritis, nodular anterior scleritis,

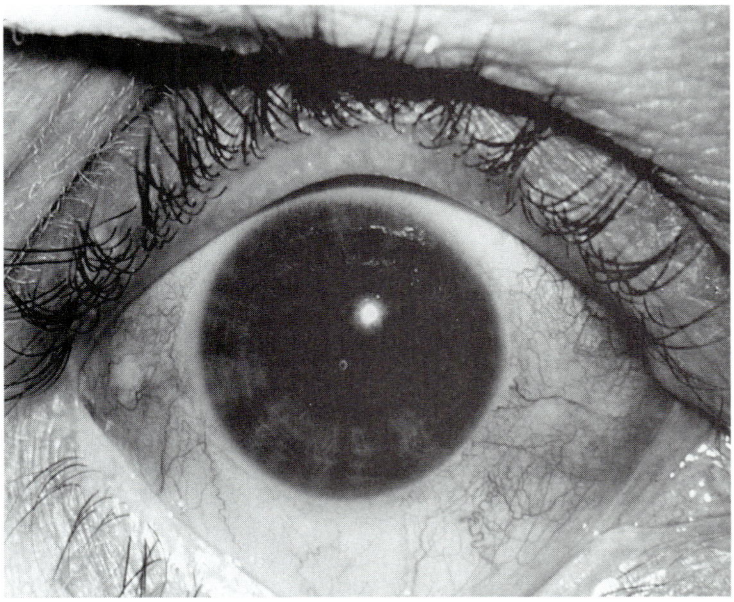

FIGURE 44–1 · Episcleritis, Occurring Nasally and Temporally in Palpebral Fissure. Remainder of episclera not involved. Lesions may be mistaken for pterygium or pinguecula.

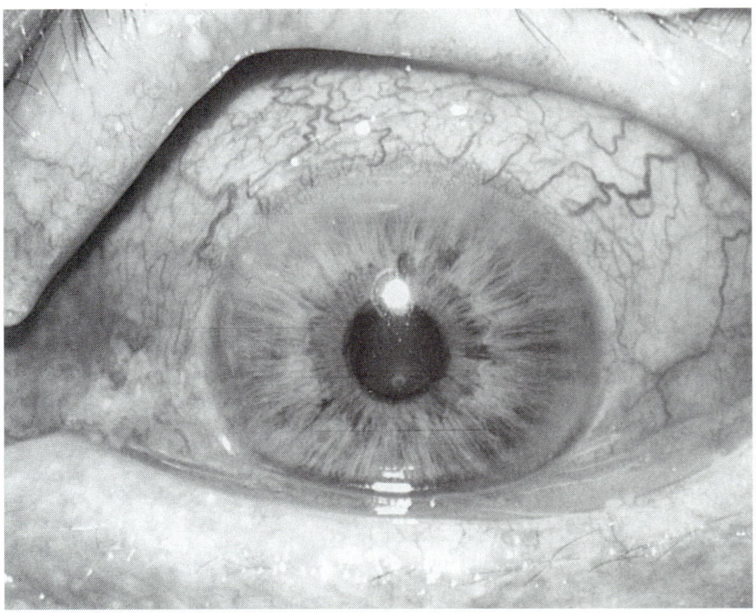

FIGURE 44–2 · Mild Diffuse Scleritis. Appearance mimics conjunctivitis, but note lack of purulent discharge.

necrotizing scleritis with inflammation, scleromalacia perforans (scleritis without inflammation), and posterior scleritis (Table 44–3). Diffuse anterior scleritis is the most common and least severe manifestation. Patients tend to be younger, and there is no gender predilection. As the name implies, the entire visible sclera is involved in the inflammatory process.[8]

Nodular anterior scleritis, the second most common presentation, occurs more frequently in women than in men. These patients are subject to recurrent attacks characterized by painful localized inflammatory nodules in the sclera with overlying episcleritis. About one fifth of patients may have progression to necrotizing scleritis.[8]

The most severe form of scleritis is known as necrotizing scleritis. It may present with or without inflammation. The disease tends to occur in older women. It has a higher association with systemic disease than the other forms of scleritis.[8] In necrotizing scleritis with inflammation, episodes start with severe, boring pain that often worsens in the early morning. On examination, the eye is exquisitely tender. Scleral inflammation with edema is apparent and surrounds a focal area of acute necrosis. Necrotizing scleritis without inflammation (or scleromalacia perforans) is most likely to occur in females and is the least common form of the disease. Unlike other manifestations of scleritis, it is relatively asymptomatic. In scleromalacia perforans, there is progressive thinning and atrophy of the episclera without evidence of active inflammation, and it is accompanied by the development of localized areas of scleral infarction. In time, these lead to the typical appearance of dark, exposed areas of choroid covered by conjunctiva.

When the sclera is involved posterior to the ora serrata, the condition is known as posterior scleritis. The pain is similar to that occurring in patients with anterior scleritis, but ocular movement may exacerbate it. The diagnosis may be difficult because of the lack of external evidence of scleral inflammation. Vision is likely to be affected early because of the consequences of scleral inflammation spreading to contiguous structures in the posterior globe. The disease is more common in women and may be unilateral or bilateral.

Disease Course, Complications, and Management

Episcleritis

Episcleritis may run a protracted course with intermittent episodes over many years, but patients rarely experience other complications. Patients may be bothered more by the appearance than by ocular discomfort or pain. In some instances, episcleritis may merge into scleritis as the underlying disease progresses. The patients tend to be young adults. In about 30 percent, there is an associated underlying disease, but only in 5 percent can a connective tissue disorder be identified. A study of referred patients with episcleritis emphasizes the importance of considering the presence of systemic disease. In this selected series, 36 percent of patients had evidence of a systemic disorder.[9]

Treatment is best accomplished with topical nonsteroidal agents in courses related to exacerbations. However, spontaneous resolution is common, and patients may elect to avoid treatment. In cases refractory to treatment, topical corticosteroid is effective, but prolonged use should be avoided because of the attendant complications.

Scleritis

Scleritis is a serious disease that carries considerable morbidity. In addition to pain, which can be severe, other ocular tissues can become involved in the inflammation in the form of sclerokeratitis, uveitis, and macular edema. Secondary cataract may also develop. Overall, scleritis is a vision-threatening disease, and there may be long-lasting and permanent functional visual impairment. Necrotizing scleritis itself may lead to scleral thinning and staphyloma formation, particularly in patients with rheumatoid arthritis. Ultimately, the sclera may be essentially destroyed without treatment.

Scleritis is a disease distinct from episcleritis, with a serious prognostic significance. For example, necrotizing scleritis has an associated 5-year mortality rate of 29 percent.[10] The association of scleritis with an underlying disease is high[11] (Table 44–4).

In one randomized study, only 7 percent of patients with scleritis failed to show evidence of systemic dis-

TABLE 44–3 • SCLERITIS

Type	Gender	Onset
Diffuse	Males and females equally affected	Younger adults
Nodular	More common in females	Older adults
Necrotizing with inflammation	More common in females	Older adults
Scleromalacia perforans	More common in females	Older adults
Posterior	More common in females	Young to middle aged

TABLE 44–4 • SCLERAL INVOLVEMENT IN RHEUMATOLOGIC DISEASE

- Systemic lupus erythematosus
- Rheumatoid arthritis
- Systemic lupus erythematosus
- Wegener's granulomatosis
- Polyarteritis nodosa
- Relapsing polychondritis
- Ankylosing spondylitis
- Reiter's syndrome
- Psoriatic arthritis
- Crohn's disease
- Ulcerative colitis
- Uveitis

ease.[12] In another series, an associated systemic disorder (usually rheumatoid arthritis) was found in all patients with scleromalacia perforans, in half of those with severe necrotizing scleritis, and in one third of patients with anterior scleritis. Only about 10 percent of patients with posterior scleritis had evidence of accompanying disease.[12]

For patients with scleritis, collaboration between the ophthalmologist and the rheumatologist is appropriate to diagnose the underlying systemic disease and, after the diagnosis is established, to coordinate management. The approach should be to reduce patient discomfort with effective local or systemic treatment. When complications develop, they should be treated promptly to minimize effects on vision. Surgical intervention may be required for the consequences of scleral inflammation and the corneal and intraocular complications. In the early stages of scleritis, therapy with topical and systemic nonsteroidal agents is appropriate. If this strategy fails to ameliorate the condition, systemic therapy with immunosuppressive agents under the direction of the rheumatologist and in collaboration with the ophthalmologist is indicated. Systemic treatment with corticosteroids is reserved for cases with severe necrotizing scleritis.[8,12] Once acquired, scleritis is a lifelong disease, but with careful and appropriate care, many of the complications can be successfully managed so as to optimize patient comfort and preserve vision.

UVEITIS

Inflammation of the uveal tract, or uveitis, is a relatively common ophthalmic manifestation of rheumatologic disease. Uveitis of the anterior part of the eye, also known as iritis or iridocyclitis, is the more common manifestation, but posterior uveitis also occurs. As is the case with other forms of ocular inflammation related to rheumatologic disease, the patient usually presents with a red eye. Differentiating the patient with uveitis from other causes of this presentation can be difficult. Added to this difficulty is the fact that the uveitis may occur in conjunction with scleritis. Ocular pain, photophobia, and redness are the usual presenting symptoms of anterior uveitis, but other unrelated forms of ocular inflammation may have a similar presentation. In patients with posterior uveitis, blurred vision and floaters are more likely to be the complaints. Careful observation by penlight should reveal the ciliary flush (i.e., ring of injected vessels around the limbus) that helps distinguish uveal inflammation from scleritis or conjunctivitis, in which the vascular injection has a more diffuse appearance (Fig. 44–3). The presence of this sign in conjunction with symptoms of photophobia should alert the physician to the possibility of anterior uveitis. However, important exceptions to this presentation of uveitis associated with rheumatic disease are juvenile rheumatoid arthritis, sarcoidosis, and Behçet's disease. Patients with the pauciarticular form of juvenile rheumatoid arthritis may have few symptoms but exhibit marked intraocular inflammation without any external evidence of a red eye. Sarcoidosis and Behçet's disease can cause uveitis involving the entire uveal tract. Because any part of the eye may be involved, symptoms may vary widely.

Disease Course, Complications, and Management

Inflammation of the uveal tract has numerous causes, but in many patients, the precise cause remains elusive. Because evaluation depends on the slit-lamp biomicroscope, an ophthalmologist best manages it. Treatment with topical corticosteroids is the mainstay of most uveitis therapy. However, intraocular inflammation may subside or may be more easily controllable in response to therapy directed toward the underlying systemic disease. Uveal inflammation can lead to serious

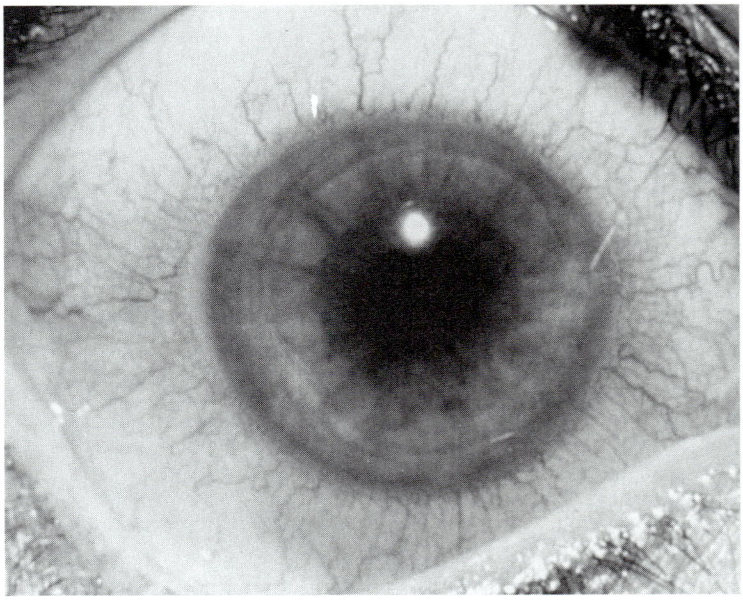

FIGURE 44–3 · Ciliary Infection in Patient with Uveitis. Remainder of sclera is relatively uninflamed.

consequences for vision and the eye, including the development of cataract, secondary glaucoma, and edema of the macula. The cornea, in long-standing cases and particularly in juvenile rheumatoid arthritis, may develop band keratopathy, a condition in which calcium is deposited in the cornea. All of these complications lead to visual loss that may significantly impair overall function. Careful collaborative management between the rheumatologist and the ophthalmologist can help minimize the effect on the overall function of the patient.

Syndromes

RHEUMATOID ARTHRITIS

The incidence of scleritis in patients with rheumatoid arthritis varies from 0.15 to 6.3 percent.[13] Although it may manifest predominantly in one eye, bilateral disease eventually occurs in at least two thirds of patients with rheumatoid disease.[14] Ocular involvement tends to be seen in patients in whom the disease is of long duration. Patients with rheumatoid arthritis who develop scleritis or episcleritis usually have more widespread systemic disease, particularly of the cardiovascular and respiratory systems, and radiologic evidence of more advanced joint disease than patients without scleral involvement. Subcutaneous granulomatous nodules and atrophy of the skin are more common in patients with rheumatoid arthritis and scleritis or episcleritis compared to those without ocular involvement.

Disease Course, Complications, and Management

The disease tends to be relapsing with progressive damage from the necrotizing scleritis over time. The end result may be development of scleromalacia perforans, the condition in which the sclera becomes progressively thinned and rarely may perforate. Because scleral thinning may occur adjacent to the cornea, there may be distortion of the corneal surface, producing an astigmatism that degrades vision. Patients with rheumatoid arthritis are also prone to develop spontaneous noninfectious ulcers in the periphery of the cornea that may rapidly deepen and perforate over a few days (Fig. 44–4).

Management of scleritis and episcleritis in patients with rheumatoid arthritis is further complicated by associated dry eye as a result of tear deficiency. Close cooperation between the treating rheumatologist and the ophthalmologist is needed to deal with the underlying disease and the complications of agents used to treat the ocular and rheumatologic manifestations of this disease.

JUVENILE RHEUMATOID ARTHRITIS

Ocular involvement in juvenile rheumatoid arthritis (JRA) differs from the adult disease. Anterior uveitis, band keratopathy, and secondary cataract are the principal features of JRA. Scleritis is rare, and tear dysfunction is unusual. Females are predominantly affected. In most children, the joint involvement is pauciarticular or oligoarticular. Rheumatoid factor serology is negative, but test results for antinuclear antibody tend to be positive. The uveitis usually involves the anterior segment of the eye in the form of an iritis or iridocyclitis.[15] The incidence of anterior uveitis in oligoarticular JRA is about 20 percent and is about 5 percent in polyarticular JRA. Children with systemic-onset JRA usually do not develop uveitis.[15] Band keratopathy is prone to develop in children with JRA, but it is not pathognomic of the disease because it occurs in a variety of other conditions.

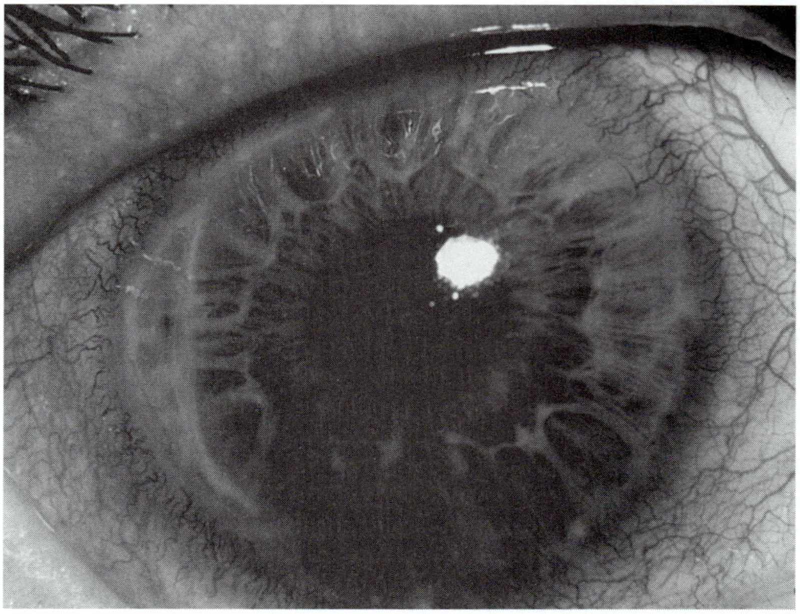

FIGURE 44–4 · Corneal Perforation in Area of Keratolysis. The black dot in the ulcer at 9 o'clock is a button of iris prolapse through the perforation. Patient has severe rheumatoid arthritis.

Disease Course, Complications, and Management

Ocular involvement in JRA is a serious threat to vision. In children, vision loss is a particularly devastating complication with far-reaching consequences for overall development and function. The prolonged inflammatory course in these patients leads to cataract formation and to the development of adhesions between the iris and the lens that may cause a secondary angle-closure glaucoma and further visual loss.[16] Band keratopathy causes eye pain and, by interfering with the optical function of the cornea, leads to a further decrease in vision and can be a serious problem in management. Appropriate medical therapy is critical in children with JRA, but surgical intervention may be required for complications.

SYSTEMIC LUPUS ERYTHEMATOSUS

Severe tear deficiency, scleral inflammation, and retinal vasculitis are hallmarks of ophthalmic involvement in this disease. Dry eye is often the presenting sign. Scleral involvement in the form of scleritis or episcleritis is similar to that seen in other forms of connective tissue disease. Retinal cotton-wool spots seen in systemic lupus erythematosus (SLE) are a manifestation of retinal vasculitis. They are grayish white, soft, and fluffy in appearance, resembling exudate, but they are actually areas of inner retinal ischemia caused by precapillary arteriole closure. The spots are small, usually about one third of an optic disk diameter, and most frequently are situated in the posterior part of the retina where they can easily be seen with a direct ophthalmoscope. Pathologically, cotton-wool spots are a fusiform thickening of the retinal nerve fiber layer.[17] Cotton-wool spots in the retina also occur in other conditions such as anemia, diabetes, human immunodeficiency virus retinopathy, other connective tissue diseases, hypertension, disproteinemia, and leukemia. Thus, they are not pathognomic of SLE.

Disease Course, Complications, and Management

The ocular manifestations of SLE often tend to progress over time despite therapy. Particularly troublesome are the consequences of the tear deficiency. However, as the disease advances, other manifestations of the underlying disorder occur, including a corneal surface disorder unrelated to the dry eye, deep keratitis, iritis, and peripheral keratitis.[18] The vasculitis can involve the retina and optic nerve. Ocular complications require specific ophthalmic therapy. As in patients affected with other rheumatologic diseases, the long-term consequences of the disease and the complications of treatment can wreak havoc on vision.

WEGENER'S GRANULOMATOSIS

Ocular involvement may be the initial symptom in up to 50 percent of patients with Wegener's granulomatosis.[11] As a result, the patient may first visit the ophthalmologist. Ocular findings include conjunctivitis, episcleritis, scleritis, keratitis, uveitis, retinal vasculitis, and proptosis secondary to retrobulbar granulomatous inflammation.[19] Ulceration in the peripheral cornea adjacent to the limbus in the form of a ring also occurs as an initial sign, sometimes preceded by localized conjunctivitis or scleritis.[18] Wegener's granulomatosis is another condition sometimes presenting with nonspecific red eye complaints that may be the harbinger of a grave prognosis for the patient.

Disease Course, Complications, and Management

What appears at first to be a benign conjunctivitis or episcleritis may progress inexorably to a scleritis or ulcerative keratitis. After peripheral corneal ulceration develops, the likelihood of perforation is high. The treating physician should be alert to Wegener's granulomatosis as part of the differential diagnosis in such cases.

Managing the systemic disease is key to treatment of the ocular component. Close collaboration between the rheumatologist and the ophthalmologist is essential. With the advent of the antineutrophil cytoplasmic antibody test (ANCA), the diagnosis can be made relatively rapidly so that more effective systemic treatment with immunosuppressive agents can be instituted.[20,21] As a result, the prognosis for salvaging vision has improved along with the dramatically improved overall prognosis.

POLYARTERITIS NODOSA

The ophthalmic manifestations of polyarteritis nodosa and microscopic polyarteritis are protean, including episcleritis, scleritis, keratitis, ptosis, and extraocular muscle palsies. This is hardly surprising given that the underlying pathology is a systemic necrotizing vasculitis involving small and medium-sized muscular arteries. Particularly destructive is the scleral and corneal disease, usually in the form of a peripheral sclerokeratitis. As the inflammation progresses, peripheral corneal ulceration develops that then can expand rapidly to the central cornea.[18]

Disease Course, Complications, and Management

Untreated the 5-year mortality rate of polyarteritis nodosa is 85 percent.[22] Treatment with corticosteroids and immunosuppressive agents can reduce this rate substantially (see Chapter 84). Systemic treatment is also effective in treating ophthalmic manifestations, although additive local therapy and surgery may be required.

SERONEGATIVE SPONDYLOARTHROPATHIES

Patients with ankylosing spondylitis, psoriatic arthritis, Reiter's disease, and inflammatory bowel disease may develop ocular inflammation. Episodes usually involve one eye. In most instances, the manifestation is an acute anterior uveitis. Patients with Reiter's syndrome often present with conjunctivitis alone. Scleritis and episcleritis can occur but are much less common.

Disease Course, Complications, and Management

It is common for patients with seronegative spondyloarthropathies, and particularly those with ankylosing spondylitis and Reiter's disease, to first notice ocular symptoms. The episode may be severe, but it usually responds to corticosteroid administration. When scleritis occurs, systemic therapy is indicated.

BEHÇET'S DISEASE

Behçet's disease is a chronic, multisystem occlusive vasculitis with dermatologic findings that include ophthalmic and cutaneous lesions.[23] Although Behçet's disease is not usually considered a primary rheumatic disorder, it is appropriately discussed here because rheumatologists are usually involved in the management of immunosuppressive therapy for these patients.

The hallmark of ocular involvement is an acute, recurrent, severe iridocyclitis. However, episcleritis, scleritis, retinal and choroidal vasculitis, optic neuritis, retina edema and hemorrhages, and central retinal artery or vein occlusion can also occur. These myriad conditions make diagnosis without expert help extremely difficult; the presentation may mimic other more benign ophthalmic conditions such as conjunctivitis or nonspecific episcleritis.

Red eye and associated symptoms may be the initial presentation of a patient with Behcet's disease. Hypopyon is a common feature of the iridocyclitis and may be visible with the direct ophthalmoscope. However, as is the case with other diseases causing uveitis, precise diagnosis requires the use of a slit-lamp biomicroscope.

Disease Course, Complications, and Management

Over time and despite rigorous treatment, recurrent episodes of panuveitis lead to the development of inflammation in the vitreous, retinal vasculitis, and retinal ischemia. In such patients, visual loss can be profound. Inflammatory glaucoma can ensue. These patients, because of the severe intraocular inflammation, are prone to develop cataracts. Blindness, multiple neurologic deficits, and a fatal vasculitis are possible outcomes of prolonged episodes of this disease. Patients with Behçet's disease are best managed by a combination of local and topical corticosteroids, systemic corticosteroids, and systemic cytotoxic agents[24] (see Chapter 6).

RELAPSING POLYCHONDRITIS

At least one half of the patients in one series with a firm diagnosis of relapsing polychondritis had evidence of ocular involvement. In one fifth, ocular symptoms were the intial manifestations. Scleritis is the most frequent ocular manifestation, but keratitis and retinal vasculitis may also occur. The symptoms are usually fairly nonspecific, with red eye being the most outstanding sign. However, on detailed ophthalmologic examination, the patient is observed to have a necrotizing scleritis sometimes associated with peripheral ulceration in the cornea.[22]

Disease Course and Complications

Because relapsing episodes occur over many years, management can be difficult. Rapid diagnosis to allow treatment of the scleritis is necessary to reduce the risk of corneal ulceration and preserve the eye and vision. Patients who develop scleritis and peripheral ulcerative keratitis seem to have more severe underlying disease. In mild cases, local and systemic treatment with nonsteroidal anti-inflammatory agents is appropriate, but patients with severe disease and repeated relapses are best treated with systemic immunosuppressive therapy. Results of a retrospective study suggest that immunosuppressive agents such as azathioprine and cyclophosphamide are more effective than systemic corticosteroids alone or in combination with dapsone in controlling the inflammatory episodes.[25]

Conclusions

Rheumatologic diseases with ocular involvement present an extraordinary challenge in management. Patients ravaged by systemic manifestations of these diseases also have to contend with what, at times, are severe ocular symptoms and the threat or the reality of diminished visual function. Early recognition of the possible significance of nonspecific ocular symptoms offers the best opportunity for prompt diagnosis and the institution of appropriate therapy. Evaluation of the ophthalmic findings can be difficult and requires close collaboration between the ophthalmologist and the rheumatologist. Because most of these diseases run protracted chronic courses, every effort should be made to minimize ocular tissue damage in the eye to preserve visual function in the patient already compromised by rheumatologic dysfunction.

REFERENCES

1. Whitcher JP, Gritz DC, Daniels TE: The dry eye: a diagnostic dilemma. *In* Smolin G (ed): Infections and Immunologic Diseases of the Cornea. Philadelphia, Lippincott, Williams & Wilkins, 1998, pp 23-37.
2. Bron AJ: Diagnosis of dry eye. Surv Ophthalmol 45(Suppl 2):S221-226, 2001.
3. Battat L, Macri A, Dursun D, Pflugfelder SC: Effects of laser in situ keratomileusis on tear production, clearance, and the ocular surface. Ophthalmology 108(7):1230-1235, 2001.
4. Pflugfelder SC, Whitcher JP, Daniels TE: Sjögren syndrome. *In* Pepose JS, Holland CN, Wilhelmus KR (eds): Ocular Infection and Immunity. St. Louis, Mosby, 1996, p 313.
5. Nelson JD: Diagnosis of keratoconjunctivitis sicca. Int Ophthalmol Clin 34:37, 1994.
6. Sullivan DA, Sullivan BD, Evans JE, et al: Androgen deficiency, Meibomian gland dysfunction, and evaporative dry eye. Ann N Y Acad Sci 966:211-222, 2002.

7. Daniels TE, Whitcher JP: Associations of patterns of labial salivary gland inflammation with keratoconjunctivitis sicca. Arthritis Rheum 37:869, 1994.
8. McClusky PJ, Wakefield D: Scleritis and episcleritis. *In* Pepose JS, Holland CN, Wilhelmus KR (eds): Ocular Infection and Immunity. St. Louis, Mosby, 1996, p 642.
9. Alpek EK, Uy HS, Christen W, et al: Severity of episcleritis and systemic disease association. Ophthalmology 106:729, 1999.
10. Foster CS, Forster SL, Wilson LA: Mortality rate in rheumatoid arthritis patients developing necrotizing scleritis on peripheral ulcerative keratitis: effects of systemic immunosuppression. Ophthalmology 91:1253, 1984.
11. Hakin KN, Watson PG: Systemic associations of scleritis. Int Ophthalmol Clin 31:111, 130, 1991.
12. Watson P: Diseases of the sclera and episclera. *In* Tasman W, Jaeger E (eds): Clinical Ophthalmology. Philadelphia, Lippincott-Raven, 1995, pp 1-45.
13. Watson PG, Hazleman BL: The Sclera and Systemic Disorders. London, WB Saunders, 1976, p 220.
14. McGavin DD, Williamson J, Forrester JV, et al: Episcleritis and scleritis: a study of their clinical manifestations and association with rheumatoid arthritis. Br J Ophthalmol 60:192, 1976.
15. Kanski JJ, Petty RE: Chronic childhood arthritis and uveitis. *In* Pepose JS, Holland GN, Wilhelmus KR (eds): Ocular Infection and Immunity. St. Louis, Mosby, 1996, p 485.
16. Wolf MD, Lichter HR, Ragsdale CG: Prognostic factors in the uveitis of juvenile rheumatoid arthritis. Ophthalmology 94:1242, 1987.
17. Ferry AP: Retinal cotton-wool spots and cytoid bodies. Mt Sinai J Med 39:604, 1972.
18. Robin SB, Robin JB, Mondino BJ: Peripheral corneal disorders associated with systemic immune-related disease. *In* Pepose J, Holland G, Wilhelmus K (eds): Ocular Infection and Immunology. St. Louis, Mosby, 1996, pp 460-470.
19. Haynes BF, Fishman ML, Fauci AS, Wolff SM: The ocular manifestations of Wegener's granulomatosis: fifteen years' experience and review of the literature. Am J Med 63:131, 1977.
20. Soukiasian SH, Foster CS, Niles JL, Raizman MB: Diagnostic value of antineutrophil cytoplasmic antibodies in scleritis associated with Wegener's granulomatosis. Ophthalmology 99:125, 1992.
21. Pulido JS, Goeken JA, Nerad JA, et al: Ocular manifestations of patients with circulating antineutrophil cytoplasmic antibodies. Arch Ophthalmol 108:845, 1990.
22. Power WJ, Foster CS: Immunologic diseases of the cornea. *In* Liebowitz HM, Waring GO (eds): Corneal Disorders: Clinical Diagnosis and Management, 2nd ed. Philadelphia, WB Saunders, 1998, p 560.
23. Rosen WJ: Behçet disease. *In* Mannis MJ, Macsai MS, Huntley AG (eds): Eye and Skin Disease. Philadelphia, Lippincott-Raven, 1996, p 279.
24. Mochizuku M, Akduhan L, Nussenblatt RB: Behçet disease. *In* Pepose JS, Holland GN, Wilhelmus KR (eds): Ocular Infection and Immunity. St. Louis, Mosby, 1996, p 671.
25. Hoang-Xuan T, Foster CS, Rice BA: Scleritis in relapsing polychondritis. Ophthalmology 97:892, 1990.

45 The Skin and Rheumatic Diseases

NICHOLAS A. SOTER • ANDREW G. FRANKS, JR.

The skin may be involved in many rheumatic diseases, and its participation often reflects the pathophysiology of the underlying systemic process. Thus, it should be assessed with the same diligence and precision that is devoted to the examination of the joints and musculoskeletal system.

Rheumatoid Arthritis

The most frequently recognized cutaneous lesion in patients with rheumatoid arthritis is the *rheumatoid nodule*. This lesion occurs over areas subjected to trauma or pressure, such as the ulnar aspect of the forearm and the lumbosacral area. Rheumatoid nodules vary in size, are firm in consistency, may be movable or fixed to underlying structures, and may ulcerate after trauma. They occur in 20 percent of patients with rheumatoid arthritis; affected individuals have severe forms of the disease and high titers of rheumatoid factor. Multiple rheumatoid nodules of the fingers with little or no articular disease is a rare variant that is termed *rheumatoid nodulosis*.[1] Accelerated development of rheumatoid nodules, which involve the hands and feet, has been reported in patients receiving methotrexate therapy.[2]

The skin over the fingers and toes is often pale, translucent, and atrophic. The swelling of the proximal interphalangeal joints with atrophic skin may mimic sclerodactyly. Other features include palmar erythema, telangiectases of the nail folds, and Raynaud's phenomenon. Longitudinal ridges of the nails are often found.[3] Occasionally, rheumatoid neutrophilic dermatitis appears as erythematous papules and plaques on the extremities; biopsy specimens contain neutrophilic infiltrates without vasculitis.[4] Pyoderma gangrenosum and other netrophilic dermatoses may occur in individuals with severe rheumatoid arthritis.[5,6]

Necrotizing vasculitis in patients with rheumatoid arthritis appears as a variety of syndromes.[7] Frequently involved are the small arteries, such as the vasa nervorum and the digital arteries, and there are cutaneous features, including digital gangrene and nail fold infarcts. Patients with nodular and erosive disease and high titers of rheumatoid factor are particularly susceptible to arteritis. Some patients experience involvement of the medium, rather than the small, arteries. The nodular lesions in these instances resemble those of polyarteritis nodosa.

The most common form of necrotizing vasculitis in the skin of patients with rheumatoid arthritis involves the venules and is recognized as purpuric papules.[8] The venular lesions are associated with severe articular disease, which is generally but not invariably seropositive. Arteritic, arteriolar, and venular lesions may coexist in the same patient. Cutaneous lesions of necrotizing vasculitis also may be induced by therapy with methotrexate[9] and etanercept.[10] Pigmentary disturbances of skin, nails, and teeth may occur with minocycline therapy.[11]

Sjögren's Syndrome

The dermatologic manifestations in patients with Sjögren's syndrome reflect glandular dysfunction, with desiccation of the skin and mucous membranes, or represent involvement of blood vessels. Dry skin (i.e., xerosis) affects approximately 50 percent of these individuals. Annular erythema of Sjögren's syndrome is considered to be the Asian counterpart of subacute cutaneous lupus erythematosus (SCLE) in Caucasians.[12,13] Anti-Ro (SS-A) and anti-La (SS-B) autoantibodies, with anti-Ro (SS-A) antibody against the 60-kD but not the 52-kD epitope, are a pattern observed in both Asians with annular erythema of Sjögren's syndrome and in white patients with SCLE.[14] The mucous membranes of the eyes, oral cavity, and vagina are involved in the sicca complex. A burning sensation of the eyes may occur with erythema, pruritus, decreased ability to form tears, and the accumulation of inspissated, rope-like material at the inner canthus. The oral cavity and tongue may be red and dry, with oral erosions and decreased amounts of saliva. Scale of the lips and fissures at the angles of the mouth may occur; the teeth readily decay. Vaginal involvement results in burning, pruritus, and dyspareunia. Enlargement of lacrimal, parotid, and accessory salivary glands is common. Raynaud's phenomenon may be present with nailfold capillary disturbances similar to those observed in systemic lupus erythematosus (SLE).

Necrotizing vasculitis of venules occurs in patients with Sjögren's syndrome and appears as episodes of palpable purpura or urticaria. The venular lesions are present over the lower extremities, appear after exercise, and are associated with hyperpigmentation and cutaneous ulcers. Anti-Ro (SS-A) antibodies occur in most individuals with primary Sjögren's syndrome, especially when it is associated with systemic or cutaneous necrotizing vasculitis. Antineutrophil cytoplasmic antibodies (ANCAs) can be found in patients with primary Sjögren's syndrome, and their presence is associated with clinical manifestations that are attributable to vascular involvement, such as cutaneous vasculitis, peripheral neuropathy, and Raynaud's phenomenon.[15] Although hepatitis C virus infection is considered an exclusion criterion in classifying Sjögren's syndrome, up to 25 percent of patients with hepatitis C virus infection may also have positive SS-A or SS-B antibodies, and there is an increased incidence of cryoglobulinemia and purpura.[16,17] Features of Sjögren's syndrome without SS-A or SS-B antibodies also occur in association with hypergammaglobulinemic purpura, SLE, rheumatoid arthritis, scleroderma, biliary cirrhosis, and lymphoproliferative disorders; the dermatologic manifestations may reflect the presence of the coexistent disorder.

Reiter's Syndrome

Reiter's syndrome occurs primarily in men and consists of a tetrad of features: conjunctivitis, urethritis, arthritis, and skin lesions. Postdysenteric forms of Reiter's syndrome often are not diagnosed because the classic tetrad of features is lacking. An association between human immunodeficiency virus (HIV) infection and Reiter's syndrome has been noted.[18,19]

The conjunctivitis and urethritis tend to be transient, in contrast to the more persistent arthritis and skin manifestations. Approximately 50 to 80 percent of patients experience mucocutaneous alterations with involvement of the acral regions, especially the soles, toes, and fingers. Confusion with Kawasaki's disease in children has occurred.[20] The most characteristic skin lesions, which are rare, begin as vesicles on erythematous bases, become sterile pustules, and evolve to manifest scale; these lesions are known as *keratoderma blennorrhagica* (Fig. 45–1). In addition, papules and plaques with scale, which are reminiscent of psoriasis, occur on the scalp and elsewhere on the skin. There have been patients reported with Reiter's syndrome *and* psoriasis, but the skin lesions in these two disorders are often difficult or impossible to distinguish clinically and histologically. Sterile pustules may develop beneath the nail plate; onychodystrophy frequently is identified, although the characteristic discrete pits of psoriasis are absent.

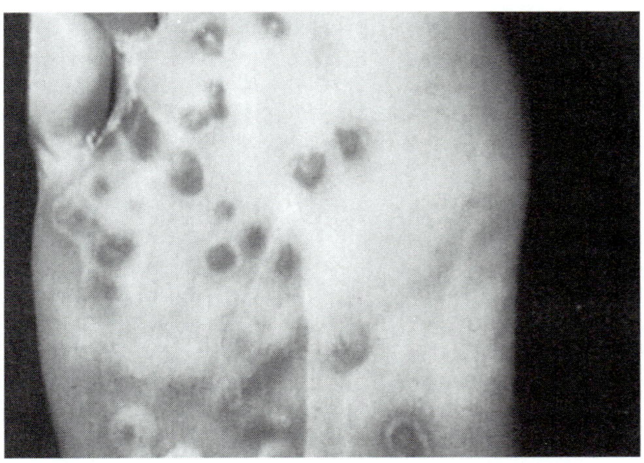

FIGURE 45–1 · Keratoderma Blennorrhagica. Vesicles and pustules of the sole in a patient with Reiter's syndrome. (From Soter NA, Franks AG Jr: Cutaneous manifestations of rheumatic diseases: An update. *In* Kelley WN, Harris ED Jr, Ruddy S, Sledge CB [eds]: Textbook of Rheumatology, 4th ed. Update 15. Philadelphia, WB Saunders, 1995, p 3.)

Conjunctivitis, which occurs in 50 percent of patients with Sjögren's syndrome, is usually bilateral. Balanitis occurs in 25 percent of individuals with Sjögren's syndrome and appears as papules and plaques with scale over the glans penis. Mouth erosions similar to aphthous stomatitis have been described.[21,22]

Psoriatic Arthritis

Psoriasis appears as erythematous papules and plaques with layers of silver-white scale that are sharply demarcated from adjacent uninvolved skin. Individual lesions may heal with transient hyperpigmentation or hypopigmentation.

Psoriasis occurs in two distinct forms; one form is hereditary with human leukocyte antigen (HLA) associations and an onset in the second and third decades, and the other is sporadic with an onset in the sixth decade.[23] Psoriasis may occur over any portion of the integument, especially the scalp, elbows, knees, lumbosacral area, gluteal cleft, and glans penis. The oral mucosa and tongue are infrequently involved. Flexural or *inverse* psoriasis is a clinical variant that affects the intertriginous areas; involvement of the axillary folds, inframmary areas, groin, and antecubital and popliteal fossae may be overlooked or mistaken for other dermatologic conditions, such as seborrheic dermatitis or moniliasis. Considerable numbers of small, drop-like plaques, designated as *guttate psoriasis,* may occur after streptococcal and viral infections.[24] Sometimes, fissures and scale of the distal portions of the fingers may be a prominent manifestation. The skin lesions often appear at sites of trauma (i.e., Koebner reaction or isomorphic phenomenon). Although the stimulus is usually mechanical, excess exposure to sunlight and allergic reactions to the administration of drugs are other causes. β-Adrenergic receptor antagonists, calcium channel blockers, terbinafine, and lithium may exacerbate psoriasis.[25-27]

The nails are frequently affected; the extent of involvement varies in severity and may include one or several nails. The nail plate has a translucent quality with a yellow or brown coloration. There may be subungual accumulations of keratotic material, which frequently contains *Candida* or *Pseudomonas* species; however, dermatophyte infections are rare. The most widely recognized alteration of the nail plate is discrete pits (Fig. 45–2). In addition to pits, other commonly recognized findings include onycholysis, the "oil-droplet" appearance at the proximal junction of the nailbed, and transverse ridges (i.e., Beau's lines).

Generalized erythroderma or exfoliative dermatitis may develop spontaneously or occur after systemic illness, the administration of medications, or prolonged exposure to the sun.

Pustular types of psoriasis are uncommon; they may occur in a generalized form or in a form localized to the palms and soles.

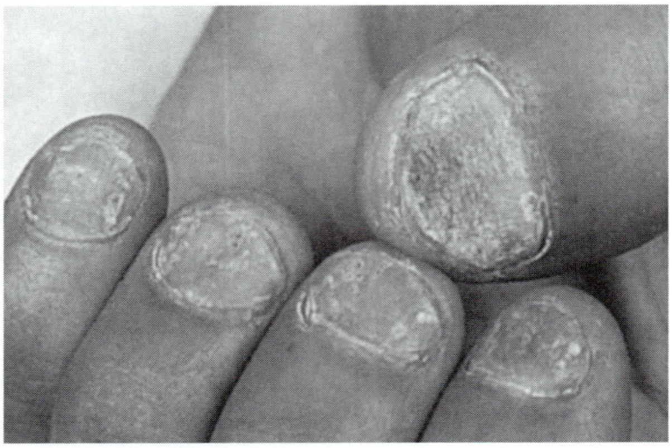

FIGURE 45–2 · Psoriasis. Onychodystrophy of the nail plate with pits. (From Soter NA, Franks AG Jr: Cutaneous manifestations of rheumatic diseases: An update. *In* Kelley WN, Harris ED Jr, Ruddy S, Sledge CB [eds]: Textbook of Rheumatology, 4th ed. Update 15. Philadelphia, WB Saunders, 1995, p 5.)

In patients with *generalized pustular psoriasis* (Fig. 45–3), the onset is sudden, with pyrexia, myalgia, and arthralgia. The skin lesions consist of superficial pustules that may evolve into larger purulent areas; existing psoriatic plaques may also contain sterile pustules. The episodes of pustules may continue to appear over intervals of days to weeks. It has been suggested that patients with psoriatic arthritis are more susceptible to generalized pustular psoriasis than are patients without arthritis.

Localized pustular psoriasis of the palms and soles is bilateral and often recalcitrant to standard treatment. Onychodystrophy is common, and the plaques of ordinary psoriasis may be found elsewhere on the body.

There are increased numbers of *Staphylococcus aureus* organisms on the lesional skin of patients with psoriasis. Scale has been suggested as a source of hospital infection. Surgical intervention through psoriatic plaques, such as in prosthetic joint replacement, also has been associated with increased risk of local infection.[28]

Arthritis represents the most common complication of psoriasis and affects as many as 20 percent of patients[29] (see Chapter ***). The clinical manifestations of psoriatic arthritis fall into several subtypes that may overlap,[30] including asymmetric oligoarthritis, symmetric polyarthritis, spondyloarthritis, distal interphalangeal arthritis, and arthritis mutilans. Mild, monosymptomatic forms of psoriatic arthritis may be difficult to diagnose and frequently mimic soft tissue rheumatism that includes recurrent bouts of bursitis, tendinitis, or both.[31,32] The presence of psoriasis in patients with rheumatoid arthritis is considered to be the coincidental association of two common disorders. Onychodystrophy in patients with symmetric psoriatic arthritis may help to differentiate them from patients with rheumatoid arthritis. Nail psoriasis is much more common than is psoriasis of the skin alone in patients with psoriatic arthritis, and it occurs in more than 80 percent of these patients.

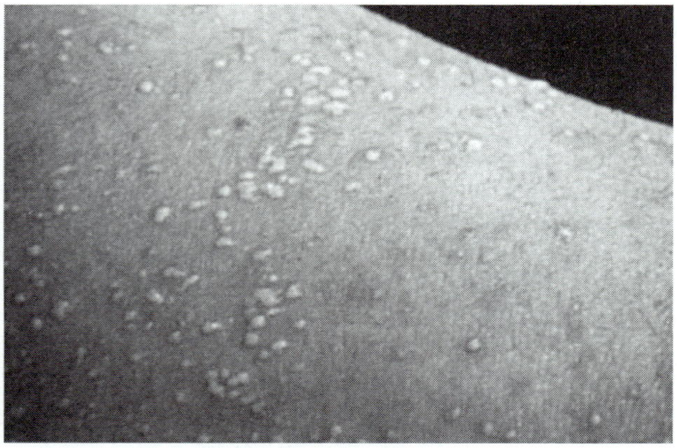

FIGURE 45–3 · Psoriasis. Generalized pustules. (From Soter NA, Franks AG Jr: Cutaneous manifestations of rheumatic diseases: An update. *In* Kelley WN, Harris ED Jr, Ruddy S, Sledge CB [eds]: Textbook of Rheumatology, 4th ed. Update 15. Philadelphia, WB Saunders, 1995, p 5.)

Although no distinctive pattern of skin involvement suggests a particular form of psoriatic arthritis, certain features can be helpful.[33] As many as one third of patients with generalized pustular psoriasis have arthritis, which is usually severe and predominantly affects the spine. Localized pustular psoriasis of the fingertips (i.e., acrodermatitis continua) may be associated with severe peripheral arthritis. Pustular psoriasis of the palms and soles (i.e., pustulosis palmoplantaris) may be associated with an increased incidence of the anterior chest wall syndrome (Synovitis, ache, pustulosis, hyperostosis, osteitis [SAPHO]) with arthritis and sclerosis of the sternum.

In individuals with acquired immunodeficiency syndrome (AIDS), psoriasis and psoriatic arthritis were frequently more extensive and recalcitrant[18,34] before the introduction of treatment with protease inhibitors.

Relapsing Polychondritis

Relapsing polychondritis involves the cartilaginous portions of the joints, respiratory tract, and external ear; the eyes; the inner ears; and the cardiovascular system. The chondritis is characterized by the sudden onset of redness, swelling, and tenderness, which are limited to the cartilaginous portions of the affected sites, and by resolution of symptoms in 1 to 2 weeks. There may be recurrences over weeks or months.[35] This inflammatory process results in floppy ears and nasal deformities and is associated with HLA-DR4. Less-frequent skin manifestations include aphthae, urticaria, angioedema, vasculitis, livedo reticularis, erythema elevatum diutinum, and panniculitis[36]. Other dermatologic manifestations occur frequently in patients with relapsing polychondritis, especially in association with myelodysplasia[37]; they are nonspecific and sometimes resemble those observed in Behçet's disease or inflammatory bowel diseases. Other features of the disease include uveitis, optic neuritis, and aortic insufficiency.

Lupus Erythematosus

Lupus erythematosus may occur as a systemic disease or as a disorder in which the lesions are restricted to the skin. The term *discoid lupus erythematosus* has been used to refer to disease limited to the skin and to the gross appearance of the atrophic skin lesions, regardless of whether systemic disease is present. A useful classification of cutaneous lupus is divided into chronic cutaneous, subacute cutaneous, and acute cutaneous disease.[38] When lupus erythematosus initially is restricted to the skin, particularly involving only the head and neck, available data suggest that patients are at low risk for the development of systemic disease. However, widespread cutaneous involvement is more likely to be associated with extracutaneous manifestations.

In approximately 80 percent of patients with lupus erythematosus, the skin is involved at some time during the course of disease. The most widely recognized manifestation is an erythematous eruption (i.e., butterfly rash) over the malar areas of the face, usually sparing the nasolabial folds, which occurs in patients with systemic lupus erythematosus (SLE) (Fig. 45–4). Rarely, bullous skin lesions (Fig. 45–5) that contain infiltrates of neutrophils occur in the superficial dermis.[39]

The discoid skin lesions in patients with lupus erythematosus are identified by their characteristic features—follicular *p*lugs, *a*trophy, *s*cale, *t*elangiectases, and *e*rythema (PASTE features). The pigmentary alterations are especially prominent in black patients, in whom the cosmetic alterations may be disfiguring. The cutaneous lesions are usually multiple and can occur over any portion of the body. In some individuals, there is a predilection for sun-exposed areas. The skin lesions are usually asymptomatic, but pruritus may occur.

The term *SCLE* defines a systemic form of disease with symmetric, nonscarring skin lesions.[40] The skin lesions in SCLE predominantly affect the neck, the

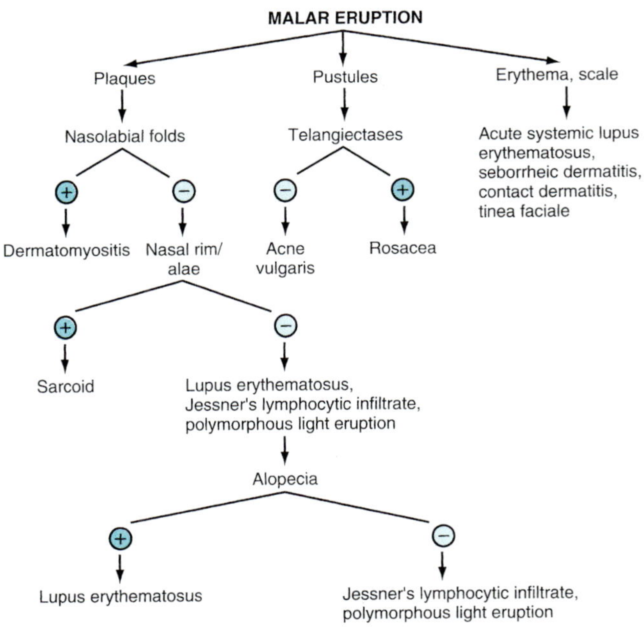

FIGURE 45–4 · Clinical algorithm for diagnosis of a malar eruption, which must be confirmed by appropriate cultures, serology, and biopsy. (From Soter NA, Franks AG Jr: The skin. *In* Ruddy S, Harris ED Jr, Sledge CB, et al [eds]: Kelley's Textbook of Rheumatology, 6th ed. Philadelphia, WB Saunders, 2001, p 404.)

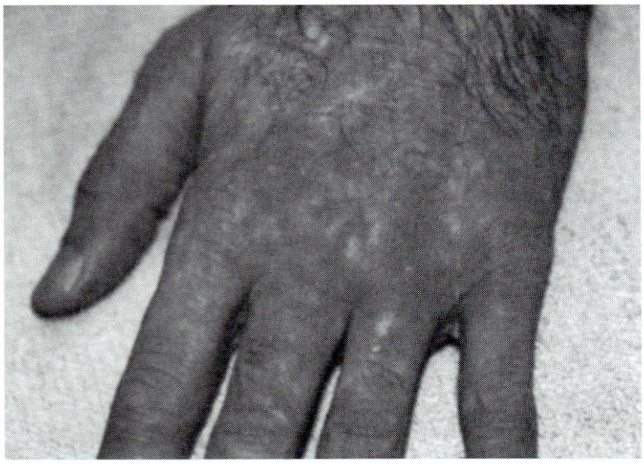

FIGURE 45–5 · Systemic Lupus Erythematosus. Note the bulla over the dorsum of the hand. (From Soter NA, Franks AG Jr: Cutaneous manifestations of rheumatic diseases: An update. *In* Kelley WN, Harris ED Jr, Ruddy S, Sledge CB [eds]: Textbook of Rheumatology, 4th ed. Update 15. Philadelphia, WB Saunders, 1995, p 6.)

extensor surfaces of the arms, and the upper portions of the trunk.[41] The cutaneous lesions may resemble psoriasis or may appear as annular and polycyclic configurations. Although SCLE originally was thought to be associated with mild systemic features, one study suggests that the prevalence of severe systemic disease in SCLE may be similar to that in SLE. There is a strong association with SS-A and SS-B antibodies. SCLE is arguably the most common presentation of drug-induced lupus erythematosus. It is associated with the use of many common drugs, which include thiazides, calcium channel blockers, angiotensin converting enzyme inhibitors, terbinafine, statins, and interferons.[42-45] This form of the disease is frequently SS-A or SS-B positive and may also be antihistone antibody positive without extracutaneous components. Histopathologic features include an interface dermatitis and a positive lupus band test.[46]

A variant of chronic cutaneous lupus erythematosus, *tumid lupus erythematosus* (Fig. 45–6), appears as erythematous, indurated papules, plaques, and nodules without surface changes. Systemic features are usually absent. It is often confused with polymorphous light eruption or pseudolymphomas. It may be difficult to diagnose histologically because basement-membrane zone changes are sparse or absent, and the direct immunofluorescence test is frequently negative[47]; however, it is characterized by an abundance of dermal mucin. *Hypertrophic lupus erythematosus* is a rare variant that resembles warts or seborrheic keratoses.

Alopecia is common in patients with lupus erythematosus; it occurs in both scarring and nonscarring forms.[48] Recession of the frontal hairline that progresses to diffuse hair loss without scars may occur, especially in individuals with SCLE or with SLE.

Although telangiectases tend to develop over the nail folds in many patients with SCLE or SLE, this sign also occurs in patients with rheumatoid arthritis, dermatomyositis, and scleroderma. Whereas these telangiectases usually are linear in patients with SLE and rheumatoid arthritis, polygonal mats with areas of vascular

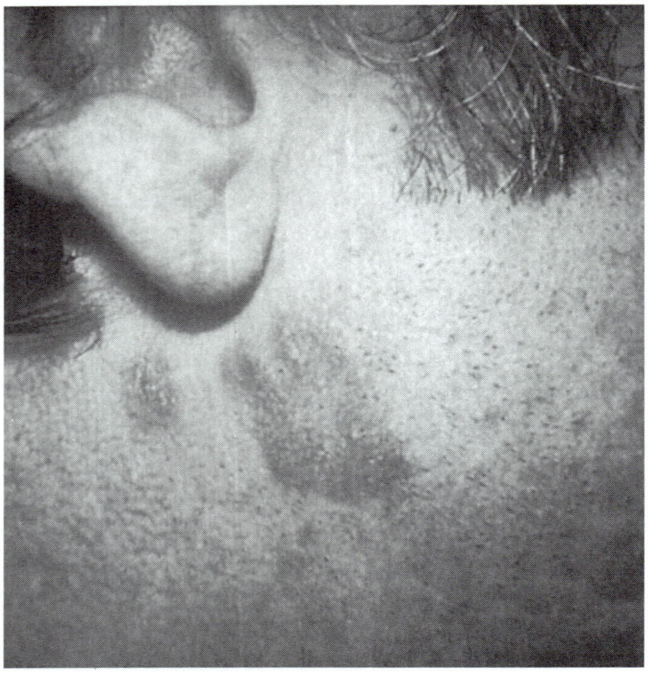

FIGURE 45–6 · Tumid lupus erythematosus, showing erythematous, indurated plaques. (From Soter NA, Franks AG Jr: Cutaneous manifestations of rheumatic diseases: An update. *In* Kelley WN, Harris ED Jr, Ruddy S, Sledge CB [eds]: Textbook of Rheumatology, 4th ed. Update 15. Philadelphia, WB Saunders, 1995, p 7.)

dropout develop in patients with dermatomyositis and scleroderma.

Necrotizing vasculitis of venules may occur during exacerbations of systemic disease and may appear as either palpable purpura or urticaria. Involvement of larger arterial blood vessels may manifest as peripheral gangrene. Flat purpura and petechiae may occur as manifestations of thrombocytopenia or of the administration of glucocorticoid preparations. Raynaud's phenomenon is reported to occur in 10 to 30 percent of patients with lupus erythematosus. Livedo reticularis appears as a reticulate, erythematous mottling of the skin.

Photosensitivity occurs in at least one third of patients with SLE and may be associated with flares of the cutaneous and the systemic manifestations of the disease. Both ultraviolet B and ultraviolet A radiation are thought to play a role.

Oral and lingual lesions are more common in patients with SLE and consist of erythematous patches, dilated blood vessels, and erosions that are frequently painful. Ulcers of the nasal septum and palate may occur.

A rare skin manifestation is panniculitis (i.e., lupus profundus),[49] which appears as firm, deep nodules that have a predilection for the face, upper arms, and buttocks. The overlying skin may be normal, erythematous, atrophic, or ulcerated. Healing results in a depressed scar.[50]

Focal and generalized mucin deposition may occur in lupus erythematosus, which may mimic sclerodermatous changes clinically. Histologic confirmation is usually required.[51,52] The association of lupus erythematosus with porphria cutanea tarda,[53] with polymorphous light eruption,[54] and with lichen planus has been reported. Parvovirus B-19 infection in adults may resemble SLE.[55]

Alterations in the integument are prominent features that aid in the classification of patients with SLE. Noteworthy features include the presence of an erythematous, macular eruption, atrophic plaques with follicular plugs, photosensitivity, and oral or nasopharyngeal ulcers. Alopecia and Raynaud's phenomenon are excluded as discriminating factors because of their lack of specificity and sensitivity.

Direct immunofluorescence techniques have been applied to the study of the skin of patients with lupus erythematosus as an aid in diagnosis and prognosis.[56,57] This procedure is known as the *lupus band test* (Fig. 45–7). In the skin lesions of systemic and cutaneous lupus erythematosus, immunoglobulins and complement proteins are deposited in a granular pattern along the dermoepidermal junction in 90 to 95 percent of patients, whereas these immunoreactants are detected in uninvolved, non–sun-exposed skin of approximately 50 percent of patients with systemic, but not cutaneous, lupus erythematosus, which is an important distinguishing feature. When uninvolved sun-exposed skin is examined, the lupus band test is usually negative in those with the cutaneous form of the disease, but it is positive in about 80 percent of those with the systemic form.

The types of immunoglobulins (Ig) detected in the deposited materials include mainly IgG and IgM. Complement proteins from both the classic activation and the amplification pathways are deposited at the same site, notably Clq, C4, C3, properdin, and B, as well as those of the terminal membrane attack complex, C5b-C9.

It has been suggested that the deposition of immunoreactants in uninvolved, non–sun-exposed skin of patients

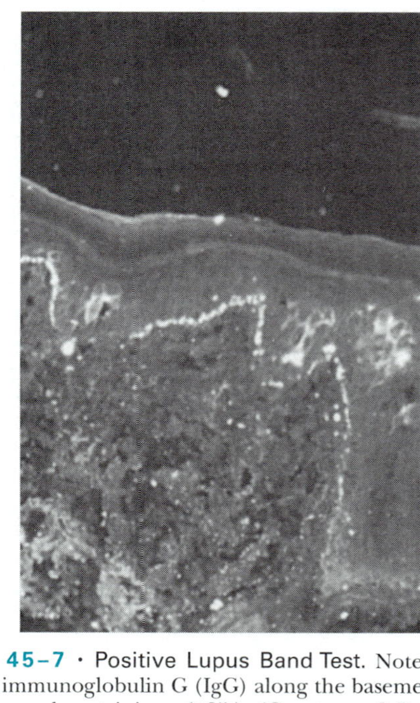

FIGURE 45–7 · Positive Lupus Band Test. Note the granular deposits of immunoglobulin G (IgG) along the basement membrane zone and vascular staining. (×25.) (Courtesy of Dr. Jean-Claude Bystryn, New York University School of Medicine, New York.)

with SLE can be correlated with renal disease. In a longitudinal analysis of 10 years' duration that attempted to assess the relation between the deposition of cutaneous immunoreactants and renal disease in SLE, an initial positive lupus band test identified patients with renal disease and a decreased survival rate. It appears that the specificity and predictive value of the lupus band test depend, at least in part, on the nature and number of the immunoreactants detected at the dermoepidermal junction.

Mixed Connective Tissue Disease

Mixed connective tissue disease is an overlap disorder with clinical features of SLE, scleroderma, and polymyositis in association with a circulating antibody to a soluble ribonuclear protein (anti-RNP). When the onset occurs before age 16 years, the dermatologic features tend to resemble SLE; when the onset is after age 16, scleroderma-like features are more frequent.[58] The inflammation and swelling of the fingers and hands, which leads to "sausage-shaped" digits and progresses to sclerodactyly, is characteristic, as is the associated Raynaud's phenomenon with periungual suffusion. There may be dilated and tortuous, corkscrew periungual telangiectases with alternating avascular areas or dropout. Hair loss may be gradual but leads to nonscarring alopecia. Pigmentary disturbances with hyperpigmentation and hypopigmentation are similar to those observed in scleroderma.

Cutaneous vasculitis includes initial symptoms of livedoid vasculitis, palpable purpura, tender nodules along blood vessels, and ulcers. Erosions of the lips, tongue, and buccal area may be observed. Prominent polygonal telangiectases may be found on the face, along with swelling of the eyelids; these changes sometimes suggest the heliotrope alteration of dermatomyositis. Calcinosis cutis and subcutaneous nodules are less severe than are those associated with dermatomyositis.

Necrotizing Vasculitides

Necrotizing angiitis or vasculitis refers to disorders in which there is segmental inflammation with fibrinoid necrosis of the blood vessels. Clinical syndromes are based on criteria that include the gross and histologic appearance of the vascular lesions, the caliber of the affected blood vessels, the frequency of involvement of specific organs, and the presence of hematologic, serologic, and immunologic abnormalities. Systemic involvement of the small blood vessels with cutaneous vascular lesions has been classified as hypersensitivity angiitis or vasculitis, systemic polyangiitis, and microscopic polyangiitis. Although all sizes of blood vessels may be affected, necrotizing vasculitis of the skin in most instances involves venules and has been called cutaneous necrotizing venulitis and leukocytoclastic vasculitis. The cutaneous vascular lesions may occur with coexistent chronic diseases, may be precipitated by infections or drugs, or may develop for unknown reasons[59] (Table 45–1). The

TABLE 45–1 • CUTANEOUS NECROTIZING VENULITIS

Associated Chronic Disorders
Rheumatoid arthritis
Sjögren's syndrome
Systemic lupus erythematosus
Hypergammaglobulinemic purpura
Paraneoplastic vasculitis
Cryoglobulinemia
Antineutrophil cytoplasmic or antiphospholipic antibody syndromes
Precipating Events
Infections
Therapeutic and diagnostic agents
Idiopathic Disorders
Henoch-Schönlein syndrome
Acute hemorrhagic edema of childhood
Urticarial vasculitis and variants
Erythema elevatum diutinum
Nodular vasculitis
Livedoid vasculitis

most characteristic lesion is an erythematous papule, in which the erythema does not blanch when the skin is pressed (i.e., palpable purpura) (Fig. 45–8). Urticaria or angioedema, nodules, pustules, vesicles, ulcers, necrosis, and livedo reticularis may occur. Occasionally, subcutaneous edema may be present in the area of the vascular lesions.

The vascular eruption most often appears on the lower extremities and frequently occurs over the dependent portions of the body or areas under local pressure. The lesions may appear anywhere on the skin but are uncommon on the face, palms, soles, and mucous membranes.

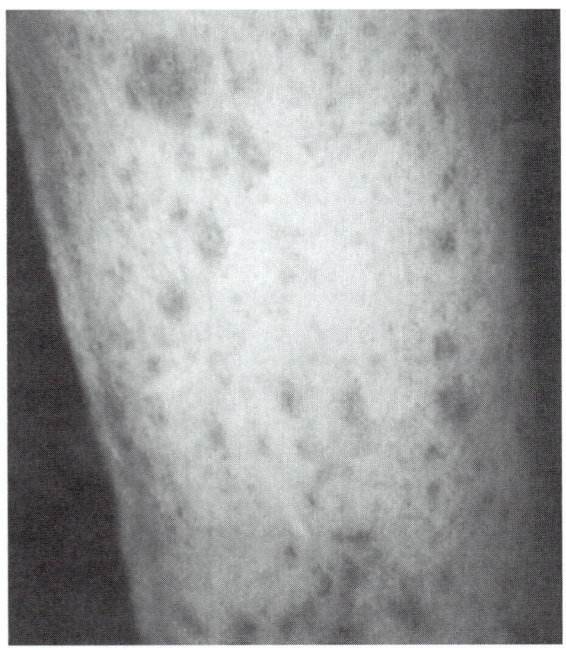

FIGURE 45–8 • Necrotizing Venulitis. Palpable purpura is distributed over the lower extremities.

The skin lesions occur in episodes that may recur for various periods ranging from weeks to years. Palpable purpuric lesions persist for 1 to 4 weeks and then resolve with hyperpigmentation, atrophic scars, or both. An episode of cutaneous vascular lesions may be attended by pyrexia, malaise, arthralgias, or myalgias. When present, associated systemic involvement of the small blood vessels most commonly occurs in joints, muscles, peripheral nerves, gastrointestinal tract, and kidneys.

Involvement of arteries occurs in polyarteritis nodosa, which is recognized in the skin as nodular lesions and ulcers over an artery and in giant-cell (temporal) arteritis, which is present as erythema, edema, or eschars overlying the affected vessel. Both Wegener's granulomatosis[60] and allergic angiitis and granulomatosis (i.e., Churg-Strauss syndrome) affect large and small vessels; the skin lesions in both disorders are erythematous nodules with or without necrosis and a variety of less specific erythematous, edematous, purpuric, papular, pustular, and necrotic lesions.

Cutaneous necrotizing venulitis has been associated with certain connective tissue disorders, notably rheumatoid arthritis, Sjögren's syndrome, SLE, and hypergammaglobulinemic purpura. It rarely occurs in mixed connective disease, relapsing polychondritis, and scleroderma.

The term *paraneoplastic vasculitis* has been used to describe patients with cutaneous necrotizing venulitis associated with malignant conditions, which include Hodgkin's disease, lymphosarcoma, adult T cell leukemia, myelofibrosis, mycosis fungoides, acute and chronic myelogenous forms of leukemia, IgA myeloma, diffuse large cell leukemia, hairy cell leukemia, squamous cell bronchiogenic carcinoma, prostate carcinoma, and colon carcinoma.

Cryoglobulins[61] may occur in patients with cutaneous necrotizing venulitis, with and without concomitant connective tissue and lymphoproliferative disorders; in patients with hepatitis A, B, and C virus infections; and idiopathically. Cutaneous necrotizing venulitis has been noted in patients with cystic fibrosis, inflammatory bowel diseases, and Behçet's disease.

Both ANCAs and antiphospholipid antibodies have been associated with various forms of necrotizing vasculitis.[62] ANCAs have been noted in patients with microscopic polyangiitis, polyarteritis nodosa, Churg-Strauss syndrome, systemic polyangiitis, Wegner's granulomatosis, and cutaneous vasculitis associated with hepatitis C virus infection.[63] The most common cutaneous feature in patients with antineutrophil cytoplasmic antibodies is palpable purpura. Microscopic polyangiitis is associated with small-vessel systemic vasculitis that also involves the skin, in which venules and arterioles are involved.[64] It is associated with necrotizing and crescentic glomerulonephritis and with peripheral ANCAs with antimyeloperoxidase specificity.[65]

Antiphospholipid antibodies (i.e., anticardiolipin antibodies and lupus anticoagulant) occur in patients with autoimmune and connective tissue diseases and as an idiopathic disorder. Livedo reticularis is the most frequently recognized cutaneous finding. Antiphospholipid antibodies of the IgA class were detected in 6 of 10 patients with idiopathic cutaneous necrotizing vasculitis,[66] and antiphospholipid antibodies have been detected in some individuals with livedoid vasculitis.

The most commonly recognized infectious agents are hepatitis B and C viruses, group A streptococci, *Staphylococcus aureus*, and *Mycobacterium leprae*. In hepatitis B virus infection, transient urticaria may occur early in the course and represents vasculitis. HIV infection has been associated, in a limited number of patients, with cutaneous vasculitis. Necrotizing vasculitis caused by the direct invasion of the blood vessels occurs with a variety of microorganisms, such as *Neisseria meningitidis* and Rocky Mountain spotted fever.

The most commonly incriminated medications are sulfonamides, allopurinol, phenytoins, thiazides, penicillin, and nonsteroidal anti-inflammatory agents. Propylthiouracil and hydralazine may cause vasculitis in association with ANCAs. Cutaneous vasculitis has developed after the administration of granulocyte colony-stimulating factor, streptokinase, monoclonal antibodies, staphylococcal protein A column immunoadsorption therapy, drug additives, radiocontrast media, and etanercept.[67]

In perhaps 50 percent of instances, the cause of cutaneous necrotizing venulitis remains unknown. The Henoch-Schönlein syndrome is the most widely recognized subgroup. A history of upper respiratory tract symptoms and signs is often obtained. The syndrome, which occurs predominantly in children and less frequently in adults, includes involvement of the skin, joints, gastrointestinal tract, and kidneys. IgA is deposited around blood vessels in the skin, synovium, kidneys, and gastrointestinal tract.[68]

Acute hemorrhagic edema of childhood[69] occurs in children and appears as painful, edematous areas with petechiae and ecchymoses on the head and distal aspects of the extremities. Infection, drugs, or immunization may be triggering factors. Systemic features usually are absent. This form of vasculitis must be differentiated from Henoch-Schönlein syndrome, with which it has been confused in the past.

Urticarial vasculitis[70] occurs in serum sickness, connective tissue disorders, and infections; in association with an IgM_K M component (i.e., Schnitzler's syndrome)[71]; after the administration of potassium iodide and nonsteroidal anti-inflammatory agents; and as an idiopathic disorder.

Urticarial vasculitis affects mainly women. The skin lesions, which appear as wheals that may have foci of purpura, often last 3 to 5 days. Episodic arthralgias are a major clinical manifestation and affect the wrists, fingers, knees, ankles, and toes. Jaccoud's syndrome may be associated.[72] General features of the syndrome include fever, malaise, myalgia, and enlargement of the lymph nodes, liver, and spleen. Specific organ manifestations may involve the kidneys, in the form of glomerulitis or glomerulonephritis; the gastrointestinal tract as nausea, vomiting, diarrhea, and pain; the respiratory tract as laryngeal edema and chronic obstructive or restrictive pulmonary disease; the eyes as conjunctivitis, episcleritis, and uveitis; and the central nervous system as headaches and benign intracranial hypertension (i.e., pseudotumor cerebri). The term *hypocomplementemic urticarial vasculitis syndrome* has been used to describe patients with more severe systemic manifestations, hypocomplementemia, and an autoantibody to C1q.

Schnitzler's syndrome consists of episodes of urticarial vasculitis with an IgM_K M component. Associated features include fever, lymphadenopathy, hepatosplenomegaly, bone pain with osteosclerosis, and a sensorimotor neuropathy. Evolution into a lymphoplasmacytic malignant condition has been reported in 15 percent of patients.[73]

Erythema elevatum diutinum[74] consists of erythematous papules, plaques, and nodules that are predominantly disposed over the buttocks and extensor surfaces and are often accompanied by arthralgias. Associated conditions include IgA monoclonal gammopathy, multiple myeloma, myelodysplasia, celiac disease, relapsing polychondritis, and HIV infection.[75]

Nodular vasculitis occurs as painful, red nodules over the lower extremities, especially the calves. Recurrent episodes are common, and ulcers sometimes occur. Erythema induratum, which has been associated with tuberculosis, as demonstrated by polymerase chain reaction amplification for *Mycobacterium tuberculosis* DNA in skin-biopsy specimens,[76] represents a form of nodular vasculitis.

Livedoid vasculitis[77] occurs in women as recurrent, painful ulcers of the lower legs, which are associated with a persistent livedo reticularis that often is deep purple in color. Healing results in sclerotic, pale areas surrounded by telangiectases that have been called *atrophie blanche*. Livedoid vasculitis may be idiopathic, or it may occur in patients with SLE who develop central nervous system involvement; antiphospholipid antibodies have been detected in both groups of patients. Livedoid vasculitis has been reported in protein C deficiency[78] and in factor V Leiden mutation.[79] Some investigators consider this condition to be a thrombogenic vasculopathy rather than a small-vessel vasculitis. Sneddon's syndrome is a clinical syndrome of livedo reticularis and livedoid vasculitis with transient cerebral ischemia, hypotension, and extracerebral arterial and venous thromboses. Circulating antiphospholipid and antiendothelial cell antibodies have been reported.[80]

Dermatomyositis and Polymyositis

Patients with classic dermatomyositis usually have skin involvement several months before the onset of overt proximal muscular weakness.[81,82] The early skin lesions are often nonspecific, but may mimic allergic contact dermatitis of the eyelids or eczematous dermatitis.[83] The cutaneous lesions appear as transient macular erythema, which is the more common presentation, or as persistent violaceous plaques. The violaceous erythema of dermatomyositis is often accompanied by scale or atrophy. *Amyopathic dermatomyositis* is the preferred term used to describe individuals who have typical cutaneous features but no apparent myositis during 2 years of continual observation. *Hypomyopathic dermatomyositis* is the term used to identify those patients without evidence of muscle involvement for up to 2 years of observation. Some patients with amyopathic dermatomyositis can slowly progress to develop symptomatic muscle weakness over a period of years, whereas other patients are without apparent muscle disease for 10 to 20 years. However, despite lack of muscle involvement, these patients experience the same risk for the development of potentially life-threatening complications of classic dermatomyositis, such as interstitial fibrotic lung disease and internal malignant conditions.[84]

Sun-exposed areas and extensor surfaces are frequently involved. Photosensitivity[85] (Fig. 45–9) is prominent over the malar region of the face and the V area of the neck and chest. The lesions are initially flat, but they may become raised and edematous with a purple-red hue. In contradistinction to lupus erythematosus, the malar eruption usually also involves the nasolabial folds. As the disease progresses, the intensity of the eruption diminishes and may be replaced by a reticulated, hyperpigmented, and hypopigmented atrophy and a network of fine telangiectases known as *poikiloderma*.

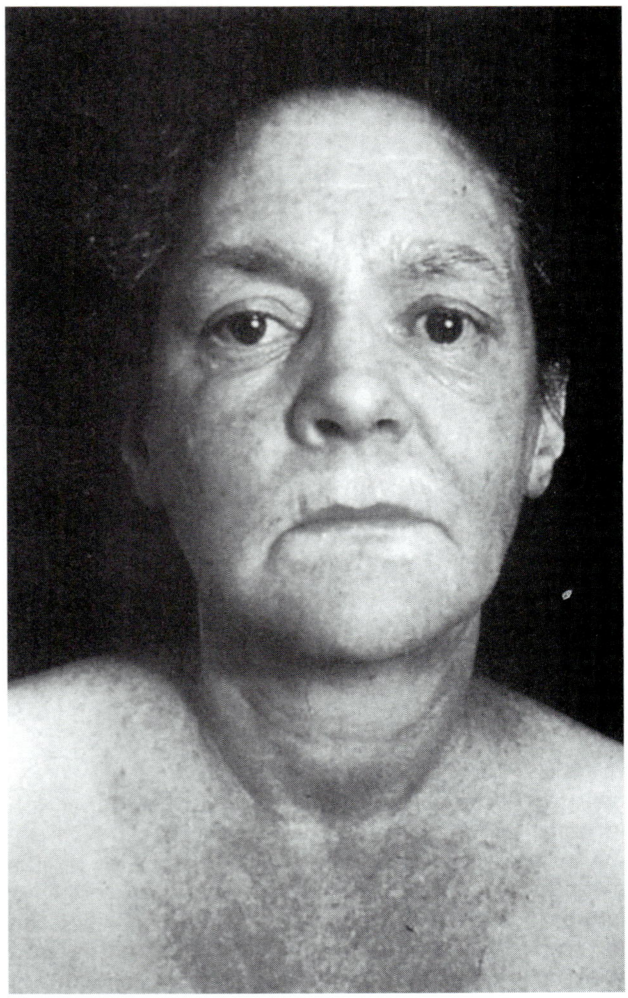

FIGURE 45–9 · Dermatomyositis. Photosensitivity is prominent. (From Soter NA, Franks AG Jr: Cutaneous manifestations of rheumatic diseases: An update. *In* Kelley WN, Harris ED Jr, Ruddy S, Sledge CB [eds]: Textbook of Rheumatology, 4th ed. Update 15. Philadelphia, WB Saunders, 1995, p 11.)

Poikiloderma is rarely found in other connective tissue diseases. Raynaud's phenomenon may be associated with sclerodactyly in about one third of patients. Mucous membrane changes with erythema, scars, and ulcers may mimic SLE; however, nasal or palatal perforation is rare.[86]

The heliotrope eruption is a lilac or erythematous coloration of and around the eyelids, with or without periorbital edema. The edema can occur independently. Gottron's sign is a flat or raised purple-red area over the interphalangeal joints of the hands, olecranons, patellae, and malleoli that evolves into atrophic plaques with telangiectases and pigmentary alterations (Fig. 45–10). Linear extensor erythema characteristically follows the course of the extensor tendons or body surfaces alone. A distinctive shawl pattern of erythema on the upper back and shoulders also is characteristic (Fig. 45–11). Mechanic's hand, with scale and fissures of the lateral aspects of the fingers, may be found in up to one third of patients and resembles contact dermatitis. Periungual suffusion with dilated, corkscrew vessels alternating with areas of avascularity may be prominent and is often associated with cuticular overgrowth.

Calcinosis cutis (Fig. 45–12) is rarely observed in connective tissue diseases other than dermatomyositis and scleroderma. The calcinosis in dermatomyositis is usually more extensive than it is in scleroderma and extends into both muscle and subcutaneous tissues. These changes are observed more frequently when the disease begins in childhood. Calcification occurs, especially over the shoulders, elbows, and buttocks, and, in contrast to scleroderma, is rare over the fingers. Cutaneous ulcers and sinuses may develop after the extrusion of deposited calcium. Raynaud's phenomenon is rare in children, although they may have facial erythema and necrotizing vasculitis involving the gastrointestinal tract that may lead to intestinal perforation.

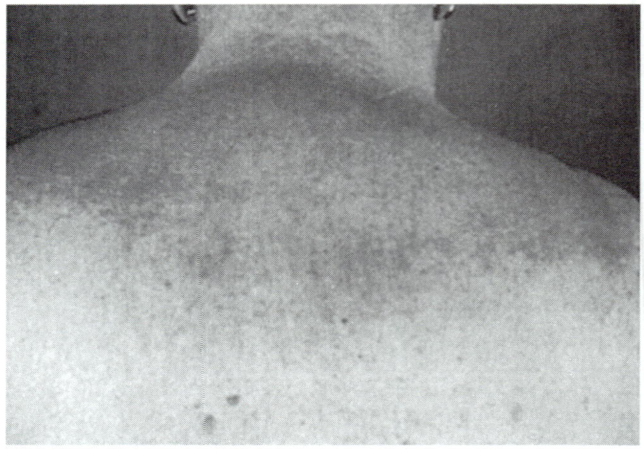

FIGURE 45–11 · Dermatomyositis. Shawl pattern of erythema on the upper back. (From Soter NA, Franks AG Jr: Cutaneous manifestations of rheumatic diseases: An update. *In* Kelley WN, Harris ED Jr, Ruddy S, Sledge CB [eds]: Textbook of Rheumatology, 4th ed. Update 15. Philadelphia, WB Saunders, 1995, p 12.)

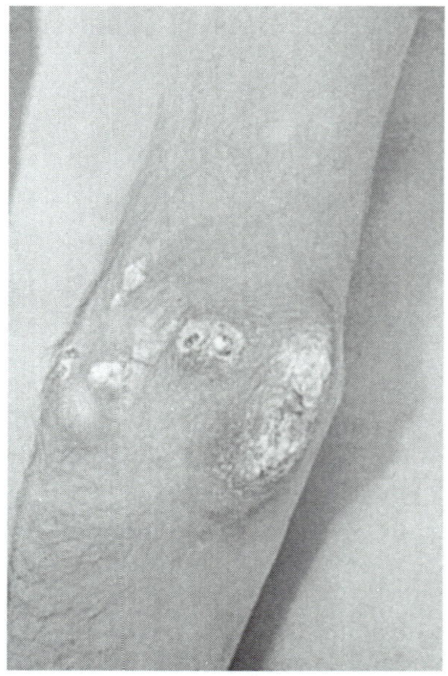

FIGURE 45–12 · Dermatomyositis. Calcinosis cutis can extend into muscle and subcutaneous tissues. (From Soter NA, Franks AG Jr: Cutaneous manifestations of rheumatic diseases: An update. *In* Kelley WN, Harris ED Jr, Ruddy S, Sledge CB [eds]: Textbook of Rheumatology, 4th ed. Update 15. Philadelphia, WB Saunders, 1995, p 13.)

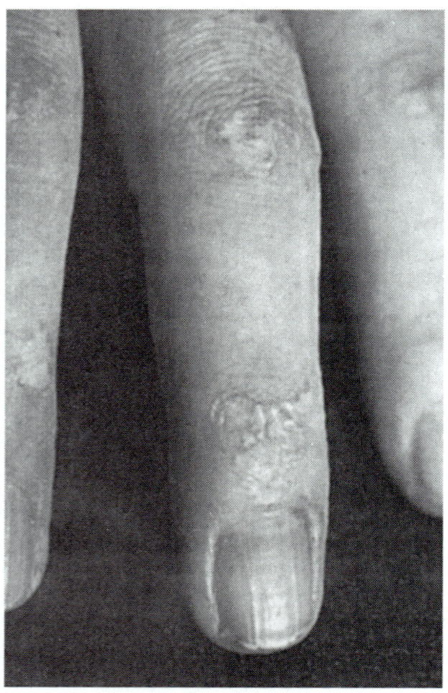

FIGURE 45–10 · Dermatomyositis. Atrophic plaques with telangiectases and pigmentary alterations occur over the intephalangeal joints of the fingers. (From Soter NA: Cutaneous manifestations of rheumatic disorders. *In* Kelley WN, Harris ED Jr, Ruddy S, Sledge CB [eds]: Textbook of Rheumatology, 1st ed. Philadelphia, WB Saunders, 1981, p 543.)

Some patients with dermatomyositis or polymyositis may have associated connective tissue disorders, such as mixed connective tissue disease, SLE, rheumatoid arthritis, Sjögren's syndrome, scleroderma, and polyarteritis nodosa. Most of these individuals have polymyositis rather than dermatomyositis.[87]

Certain patterns of dermatomyositis or polymyositis may be associated with myositis-specific autoantibodies. Anti-Jo-1 is associated with Raynaud's phenomenon, myositis, arthritis, interstitial lung disease, and mechanic's hand. Anti-Mi-2 antibodies are associated with classic dermatomyositis with the V sign, shawl sign, and cuticular overgrowth.

When contemplating antimalarial therapy for dermatomyositis, both the physician and patient should recognize that cutaneous reactions consonant with drug hypersensitivity may occur in approximately one third of patients and that antimalarial therapy may not be so effective as it is in lupus erythematosus.[88]

Scleroderma

Scleroderma may be broadly divided into systemic sclerosis and localized scleroderma. Systemic sclerosis is a multisystem disease with two major subsets: limited (formerly known as calcinosis, Reynauds's phenomenom, esophageal dysfunction, sclerodactyly, and telangiectasia (CREST) syndrome) and diffuse. Limited scleroderma is distinguished clinically by a long history of Raynaud's phenomenon before other symptoms, such as sclerodactyly (i.e., skin thickening limited to the hands), digital ulcers, and esophageal dysmotility, develop. Although limited scleroderma is considered to be milder than diffuse scleroderma, intestinal hypomotility, pulmonary hypertension, and cor pulmonale may occur with considerable morbidity. Diffuse scleroderma is often rapid in onset with early widespread proximal skin thickening associated with cardiopulmonary and renal involvement.[89]

Localized scleroderma of various forms primarily affects the skin. The most common type is morphea, in which the skin lesions are circumscribed areas of atrophy with an ivory color in the center and a violet hue at the periphery. The lesions of morphea commonly persist for years; however, they may disappear spontaneously and heal with or without residual pigmentary alterations. Some forms of morphea have been causally related to *Borrelia* infection (discussed later).[90,91]

Linear scleroderma appears in a band-like distribution. The lower extremities are most frequently affected. In addition to the skin, underlying muscles and bones may be involved. Linear scleroderma begins most frequently during the first 2 decades of life. It has been associated with abnormalities of the axial skeleton, especially occult spina bifida. Melorheostosis, a dense, linear cortical hyperostosis underlying the sclerotic plaques, can be observed on radiographs.[92] Other variants of scleroderma include frontal or frontoparietal involvement of the head, known as *en coup de sabre*, which is characterized by an atrophic furrow that extends below the plane of the skin and progressive facial hemiatrophy (i.e., Parry-Romberg syndrome).

Although proximal cutaneous involvement is characteristic in systemic scleroderma, cutaneous alterations of the face and hands may be especially prominent. Features include a mask-like, expressionless face with a fixed stare, inability to wrinkle the forehead, tightening of the skin over the nose with a beak-like appearance, and restriction of the mouth with radial folds and loss of tissue such that the teeth are prominent. An early sign is indolent, nonpitting edema over the dorsa of the fingers, hands, and forearms. Sclerodactyly occurs with tapered fingers over which the skin is atrophic; flexion contractures of the fingers, elbows, and knees may be present.[93]

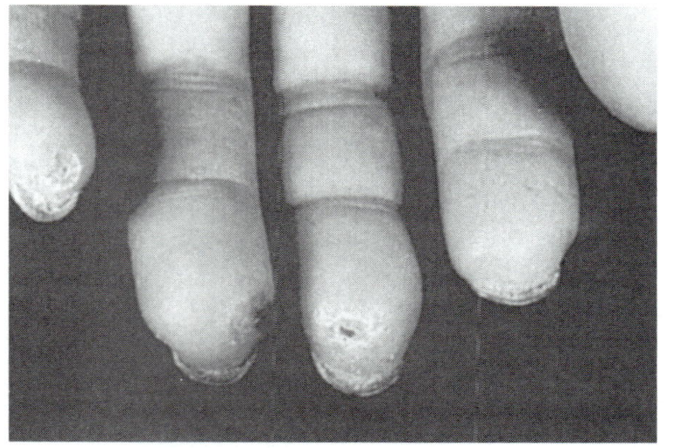

FIGURE 45–13 · Scleroderma. Ulcers and scars occur on the tips of the digits in an individual with Raynaud's phenomenon. (From Soter NA: Cutaneous manifestations of rheumatic disorders. *In* Kelley WN, Harris ED Jr, Ruddy S, Sledge CB [eds]: Textbook of Rheumatology, 1st ed. Philadelphia, WB Saunders, 1981, p 544.)

Corkscrew telangiectases with areas of dropout occur commonly on the nail folds and may correlate with pulmonary hypertension.[94] Square or polygonal telangiectatic macules may involve the face, lips, tongue, and hands. Other features include generalized hyperpigmentation and alopecia. Various outcome measures, which include the severity of Raynaud's phenomenon and the presence of digital ulcers, have been utilized to measure disease activity and the functional status in patients with scleroderma.[95] In limited scleroderma, calcification may eventually occur with Raynaud's phenomenon (Fig. 45–13), esophageal abnormalities, sclerodactyly, and telangiectases.

Disorders with cutaneous sclerosis that should be considered in the differential diagnosis of scleroderma or systemic sclerosis include eosinophilic fasciitis; scleromyxedema (papular mucinosis); scleredema of diabetes mellitus; porphyria cutanea tarda; lichen sclerosus et atrophicus and other variants of localized scleroderma, lipodermatosclerosis, or stasis panniculitis; chronic graft-versus-host disease; and eosinophilia-myalgia syndrome related to *L*-tryptophan ingestion.[96] In addition, a fibrosing disorder that clinically mimics scleroderma, scleromyxedema, or both has been described in patients with renal disease who were treated with dialysis or who received kidney transplants.[97] The cutaneous changes were indurated papules and plaques on the extremities and trunk, which resembled scleromyxedema and resulted in contractures and limited mobility. The IgG λ paraprotein detected in scleromyxedema was not found, although the histologic features were similar to those of scleromyxedema, with thick collagen bundles and increased amounts of dermal mucin. The term *nephrogenic fibrosing dermopathy* has been proposed for this entity until a specific cause has been identified.[98]

Juvenile Rheumatoid Arthritis

Cutaneous eruptions occur in association with juvenile rheumatoid arthritis (i.e., Still's disease).[99,100] The most frequently recognized form is an evanescent,

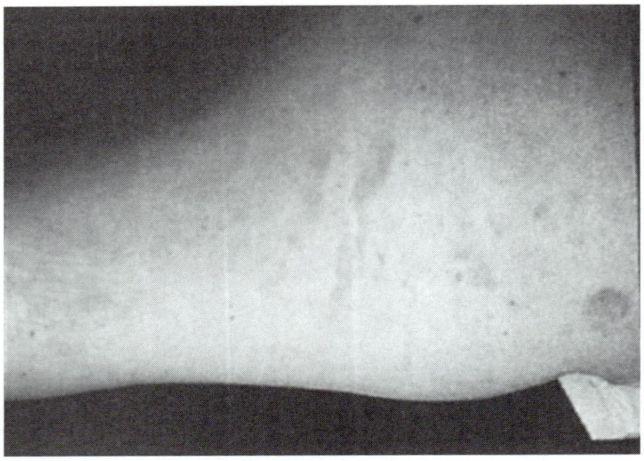

FIGURE 45–14 · Juvenile Rheumatoid Arthritis. Salmon-colored lesions occur on the arm. (From Soter NA, Franks AG Jr: Cutaneous manifestations of rheumatic diseases: An update. *In* Kelley WN, Harris ED Jr, Ruddy S, Sledge CB [eds]: Textbook of Rheumatology, 4th ed. Update 15. Philadelphia, WB Saunders, 1995, p 15.)

erythematous eruption that accompanies the late-afternoon temperature rise in 25 to 40 percent of patients, especially boys. The skin lesions (Fig. 45–14) appear as small, erythematous or salmon-colored macules and papules that are distributed over the face, trunk, and extremities. They are usually not pruritic and, once formed, do not move or enlarge. The lesions occur when the disease is active, subside with remission, heal without residua, and are not related to prognosis. An eruption may appear in the neonatal period in association with elevated body temperatures and increased C-reactive protein levels. The eruption may be evanescent, recur on a daily basis, and antedate joint involvement. Early-onset, systemic juvenile rheumatoid arthritis can mimic congenital infections and should be considered in the differential diagnosis of neonatal exanthems.[101] Subcutaneous nodules may also occur and must be differentiated from the subcutaneous form of granuloma annulare.

Rheumatic Fever

A variety of erythematous eruptions has been detected in patients with rheumatic fever. The most specific eruption is erythema marginatum, which occurs in 5 to 13 percent of patients. It appears as transient, erythematous rings, usually with raised margins, that rapidly spread peripherally to form polycyclic or geographic outlines and that leave a pale or pigmented center. The essential feature is the rapid spread, which may be 2 to 10 mm in 12 hours. The lesions occur on the trunk and proximal portions of the extremities; they are rarely pruritic. The flat or macular form is known as erythema circinatum. Erythema marginatum and circinatum are usually associated with carditis and are unaffected by treatment of the underlying disease. Small, multiple, subcutaneous nodules may develop, especially in patients with carditis. A rare manifestation is erythema papulatum, which appears as indolent, asymptomatic papules, especially over the elbows and knees.

Poststreptococcal reactive arthritis is an inflammatory articular syndrome that occurs after a group A streptococcal infection in persons not fulfilling the Jones criteria for the diagnosis of acute rheumatic fever. Characteristic features include nonmigratory arthritis, lack of response to aspirin or nonsteroidal anti-inflammatory agents, and extra-articular manifestations, which include vasculitis and glomerulonephritis. Whether or not patients with poststreptoccal reactive arthritis develop carditis is not yet established.[102]

Lyme Borreliosis

Lyme borreliosis is a multisystem disorder caused by the spirochete *Borrelia burgdorferi* and transmitted by the tick *Ixodes dammini.* The clinical manifestations occur in three stages. Early infection consists of regional lymphadenopathy, mild constitutional features, and cutaneous lesions. Although the skin lesions are most often described as a bull's-eye, red area with central clearing—the characteristic erythema migrans (Fig. 45–15)—they

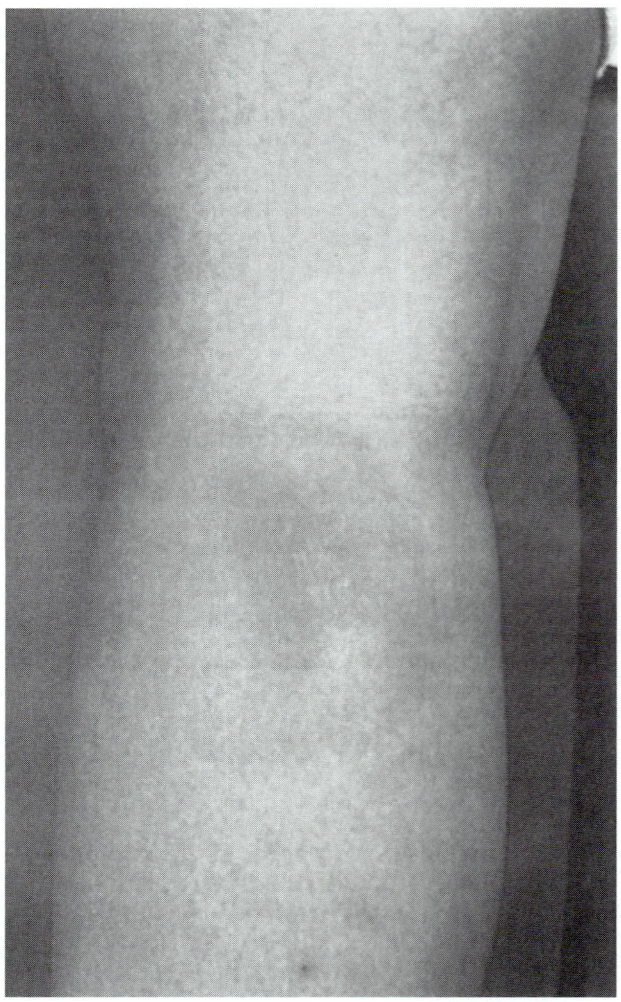

FIGURE 45–15 · Lyme Borreliosis. Erythema migrans is a characteristic lesion. (From Soter NA, Franks AG Jr: Cutaneous manifestations of rheumatic diseases: An update. *In* Kelley WN, Harris ED Jr, Ruddy S, Sledge CB [eds]: Textbook of Rheumatology, 4th ed. Update 15. Philadelphia, WB Saunders, 1995, p 16.)

may be uniform in color and vary from red to dark purple or may be bruise-like. Lesions are usually neither painful nor pruritic and are best recognized by an expanding margin, which radiates from the site of the bite with borders expanding daily. About the time the eruption appears, other symptoms, such as chills, fever, headache, and generalized myalgias, may occur. The lesion may enlarge to up to 20 to 60 cm over days to weeks and then begins to fade within 3 to 6 weeks. The skin manifestations of this early stage usually resolve without treatment. Erythema migrans is the most common manifestation of early Lyme borreliosis and occurs in a high percentage of cases. Because this phase of infection with *B. burgdorferi* offers an opportunity for treatment, its variations need prompt recognition. In addition to lesions of uniform color, those with necrotic or vesicular centers and with shapes that are not circular or oval are not uncommon. Serologic tests and histologic evaluation at this phase of the illness are potentially misleading. Diagnosis is clinical, and prompt initiation of appropriate antibiotic therapy may cure most patients at this early stage of the disease. Up to 15 percent of patients may have concomitant infections with a second tick-borne pathogen, which could alter the clinical manifestations and response to treatment.[103]

The early disseminated or second stage disease develops within days to weeks. The cutaneous features include erythema migrans, one or more annular lesions, morbilliform eruptions, lymphocytoma cutis, urticaria, and macular erythema in up to 50 percent of patients. These cutaneous lesions are associated with other systemic manifestations that include arthralgias, stiff neck, Bell's palsy, palpitations, and visual disturbances.

Late cutaneous features include atrophic or scleroderma-like lesions (i.e., acrodermatitis chronica atrophicans), particularly in Europe, which may be associated with neuropathy of the extremities. Other manifestations of the chronic stage include arthritis, central nervous system involvement, and uveitis.[104]

In skin-biopsy specimens obtained from erythema migrans, spirochetes may be detected in the epidermis, upper dermis, and follicular epithelium with a Warthin-Starry stain, and molecular detection of *B. burgdorferi* can be achieved with the polymerase chain reaction technique. The existence of more than a single strain of *B. burgdorferi sensu stricto* in a single patient has been documented.[105] Peripheral blood mononuclear cells obtained from individuals with erythema migrans underwent lymphoproliferative responses when stimulated with sonicated extracts of *B.burgdorferi*.[91,106] Some forms of localized scleroderma (morphea) may be due to *B. burgdorferi* species unrelated to Lyme disease.[107]

Amyloid

Amyloid may be present as a primary cutaneous disease, may occur with multiple myeloma or genetic disorders, may be associated in a secondary fashion with chronic inflammatory conditions (such as rheumatoid arthritis), or may be restricted to a single tissue site, which includes forms localized to the skin. Skin lesions occur in primary amyloid; secondary amyloid is rarely accompanied by skin lesions. However, clinically uninvolved skin may contain amyloid deposits in both primary and secondary types, which suggests that a skin biopsy of such uninvolved skin can have a high diagnostic yield.[108] Amyloid fat deposits are not uncommon in adult rheumatoid arthritis. In the majority of these patients, the deposits do not indicate clinical organ dysfunction, even after several years of follow-up. Patients with more extensive fat deposits may have a higher risk of developing amyloidosis.[109]

The skin lesions of primary amyloidosis appear as firm, translucent papules that occur on the face, especially about the eyes, neck, intertriginous areas, and extremities, especially on the palms and volar aspects of the fingers. They vary in color from rose to yellow to brown; pruritus is absent. A conspicuous feature is hemorrhage; the tendency for the development of purpura is the basis for a diagnostic maneuver, in which purpura occurs after a blunt instrument is used to traumatize the lesions. Ecchymoses may occur in the absence of papules. Macroglossia is present in 25 to 40 percent of patients; the surface of the tongue may be smooth, contain papules or nodules, or manifest ulcers and purpura (Fig. 45–16).

Localized cutaneous amyloidosis may be present as macules, papules, or nodules. Macular amyloidosis, which consists of pruritic, brown macules that are distributed over the upper back and extremities, has been related to friction.[110] Lichen amyloidosis, which appears as pruritic, discrete, multiple papules and plaques distributed over the anterior aspects of the lower legs, has been related to scratching and lichen simplex chronicus.[111] Some individuals have the lesions of macular and lichen amyloidosis, which is known as biphasic amyloidosis. Localized nodular amyloidosis presents as single or multiple nodules on the face, trunk, or genitalia. These lesions are indistinguishable from those lesions associated with systemic amyloidosis. These patients should be followed carefully, because systemic

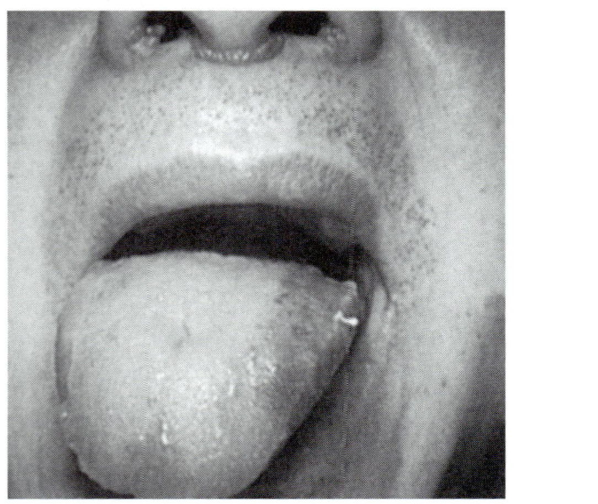

FIGURE 45–16 · **Amyloid.** Macroglossia with purpura affects 25 to 40 percent of these patients. (From Soter NA, Franks AG Jr: Cutaneous manifestations of rheumatic diseases: An update. *In* Kelley WN, Harris ED Jr, Ruddy S, Sledge CB [eds]: Textbook of Rheumatology, 4th ed. Update 15. Philadelphia, WB Saunders, 1995, p 16.)

amyloidosis develops in 7 percent,[112] and paraproteinemia occasionally occurs.

Epstein-Barr virus DNA was detected by in situ hybridization dinucleotide probes in the lesional skin of 40 percent of Chinese individuals with primary cutaneous amyloidosis.[113]

In lesional skin of Japanese individuals with nodular localized cutaneous amyloidosis,[114] monoclonal plasma cells were detected by non-nested polymerase chain amplification for the VDJ region of the immunoglobulin heavy chain. β-Microglobulin and advanced glycation end products,[115] immunoglobulin light chains,[115] and apolipoprotein E[116] also have been detected. Keratin epitopes were detected in macular and lichen amyloidosis but not in nodular primary cutaneous amyloidosis.[117]

Sarcoid

Cutaneous involvement is divided into specific and nonspecific categories. Specific skin lesions[118] occur in 25 percent of patients with sarcoid, and erythema nodosum occurs in 30 percent. Specific lesions include nodules, plaques, lupus pernio, subcutaneous nodules, as well as infiltrates within scars. The most characteristic lesions observed in the United States are yellow-brown to violaceous macules and papules with a predilection for the face, especially the alae nasi and the periocular areas.[119] Similar lesions may be widely distributed over the trunk and extremities.

Macules and papules are associated with erythema nodosum and a good prognosis; the most frequent extracutaneous features include bilateral pulmonary infiltrates and uveitis. Subcutaneous nodules are less common, appear late in the course of the disease, and are associated with systemic features. Purple plaques have been described on the nose (i.e., nasal rim lesions), cheeks, and lobes of the ears; these lesions are known as lupus pernio, which is associated with pulmonary fibrosis, uveitis, and bone cysts. Erythema nodosum is the hallmark of acute and benign disease and is more common in women.[120] Infiltration of scars is associated with long-standing pulmonary and mediastinal involvement, uveitis, peripheral lymphadenopathy, bone cysts, and parotid enlargement. Other nonspecific skin manifestations include acquired ichthyosis over the lower legs, ulcers, generalized pruritus, subcutaneous calcification, and hypopigmentation.[121] Cutaneous sarcoid has developed in patients with hepatitis C virus infection, who were treated with interferon α.[122]

Panniculitis

Panniculitis[123,124] is the term used to describe disorders in which inflammation occurs in the subcutaneous tissue. Panniculitis of all types is recognized as erythematous or violaceous nodules that may or may not ulcerate. When the inflammation is more prominent in septa, it is designated septal panniculitis; inflammation, that is more prominent in the fat lobules that is classified as lobular panniculitis.

Erythema nodosum is the most widely recognized form of panniculitis (Fig. 45–17). Erythema nodosum is more common in women,[125] and its incidence peaks between 20 and 30 years of age. The age and sex distributions vary throughout the world and depend on the eliciting etiologic agents, which include a variety of infections, medications, and systemic diseases. Streptococcal infections are the most frequent associations in children, whereas medications, sarcoid, and inflammatory bowel diseases are the most common associations in adults.

The clinical eruption appears as the sudden onset of tender, erythematous nodules over the extensor aspects of the lower extremities, which may be accompanied by fever, chills, malaise, and leukocytosis. The erythema evolves into a violet-blue color and contused appearance during the second week. Individual nodules usually resolve spontaneously in 3 to 6 weeks without ulcers or scars. Patients with erythema nodosum often experience arthralgias, which may persist after the cutaneous lesions have resolved. Episcleral lesions also may occur. Erythema nodosum has been reported in three patients with elevated levels of anticardiolipin antibodies.[126]

Weber-Christian disease is the term applied to a relapsing form of idiopathic panniculitis associated with systemic manifestations. The cutaneous lesions occur as recurrent episodes of erythematous, sometimes tender, subcutaneous nodules that appear at intervals of weeks

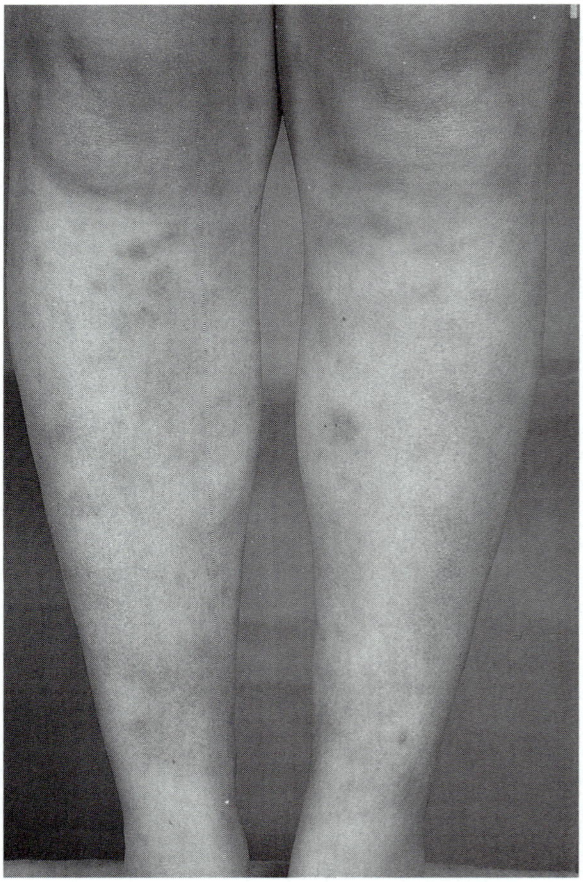

FIGURE 45–17 · Erythema Nodosum.

to months. The lesions are symmetric in distribution, and the thighs and lower legs usually are affected. Occasionally, necrosis of the overlying skin occurs, and an oily, yellow-brown liquid is discharged. Individual nodules, which involute over the course of a few weeks, result in hyperpigmented and atrophic scars. When an underlying cause of panniculitis is identified, the term *Weber-Christian disease* should not be used, and a more specific diagnosis should be made on the basis of pathogenesis.[127] Physical trauma can result in panniculitis. The most common physical factors are exposure to cold or direct physical or chemical trauma; sometimes these traumatic factors are factitious, and the lesions are self-induced.

Lipodermatosclerosis[128] is a painful induration that begins on the medial aspects of the lower extremities, may progress to encirclement of the ankles and pretibial areas, and results in an inverted bottle-shaped leg. Other clinical features include erythema, edema, ulcers, hyperpigmentation, and varicosities.[129] This condition is more common in women with a high body mass. Lipomembranous fat necrosis may also be stasis related and is clinically indicated by chronic sclerotic plaques on the lower extremities in obese women.[130]

Lobular panniculitis may be associated with pancreatic carcinoma or pancreatitis.[131] Painful, erythematous nodules may appear in any location, but there is a predilection for the legs. The nodules occasionally drain an oily substance. Arthritis occurs in about 60 percent of the cases, and a polyserositis can occur as pleuritis, pericarditis, or synovitis.

Panniculitis may be a sign of underlying systemic diseases, such as SLE, lymphomas, leukemias, sarcoidosis, gout, α_1-antitrypsin deficiency, and fungal and bacterial infections. Panniculitis occurring after jejunoileal bypass surgery has been reported. Cytophagic histiocytic panniculitis[132,133] occurs as tender, erythematous nodules or plaques with ulcers. The hemophagocytic features include a consumptive coagulopathy, peripheral cytopenias, and hepatosplenomegaly. This condition has tumor cells that pursue a lineage of cytotoxic T cells and represents a lymphoid malignant condition or subcutaneous T cell lymphoma. The term *panniculitis-like syndrome with cytophagocytosis*[134,135] has been suggested.

Parvovirus Arthropathy

Parvovirus B19 infection in children is a viral disorder with cutaneous features known as *erythema infectiosum* (i.e., fifth disease) and arthritis. The eruption begins with confluent, erythematous, and edematous plaques over the malar eminences (i.e., slapped cheeks). The facial eruption fades over 1 to 4 days; erythematous macules or papules with a lace-like or reticulated appearance then develop on the trunk and extensor surfaces of the extremities.

Rheumatologic manifestations of human parvovirus B19 infection in adults have been described as polyarthralgia and polyarthritis, with a chronic disease pattern sometimes suggesting seronegative rheumatoid arthritis.[136] Arterial occlusive disease and digital ischemia have been associated with acute parvovirus B19 infection.[137] It has also been implicated in a number of other rheumatic diseases, which include giant-cell arteritis,[138] dermatomyositis,[139] juvenile rheumatoid arthritis,[140] Henoch-Schönlein syndrome, and SLE.[141] Although the dermatologic features of parvovirus B19 in children are not found in adults, a malar eruption mimicking lupus erythematosus, as well as a morbilliform eruption, have been described.[142]

Parvovirus B19 is responsible for the papular-purpuric "gloves and socks syndrome" that affects young adults during the spring and summer. Features include fever, oral erosions, lymphadenopathy, myalgia, arthralgia, or arthritis.[143] The sudden onset of pruritic or painful symmetric erythema and edema occurs on the palms, soles, and dorsal surfaces of the hands and feet. Confluent papules and purpura develop with sharply demarcated margins at the wrists and ankles. Erythema, petechiae, and erosions may appear on the hard and soft palates. Atypical clinical presentations include an asymptomatic papular eruption, an eruption that resembles Sweet's syndrome, and palpable purpura on the lower extremities. Skin biopsy specimens may show an interstitial infiltrate of histiocytes with fragmentation of collagen, a mononuclear cell-predominant vascular injury pattern, an interface dermatitis, and papillary dermal edema.[144]

REFERENCES

1. Lagier R, Gerster JC: Palmar rheumatoid nodulosis of the fingers. Clin Rheumatol 14:592, 1995.
2. Williams FM, Cohen PR, Arnett FC: Accelerated cutaneous nodulosis during methotrexate therapy in a patient with rheumatoid arthritis. J Am Acad Dermatol 39:359, 1998.
3. Michel C, Cribier B, Sibilia J, et al: Nail abnormalities in rheumatoid arthritis. Br J Dermatol 137:958, 1997.
4. Mashek HA, Pham CT, Helm TN, Klaus M: Rheumatoid neutrophilic dermatitis. Arch Dermatol 133:757, 1997.
5. von den Driesch: Pyoderma gangrenosum: a report of 44 cases with follow-up. Br J Dermatol 137:1000, 1997.
6. Weenig RH, David MD, Dahl PR, Su WP: Skin ulcers misdiagnosed as pyoderma gangrenosum. N Engl J Med 347:1412, 2002.
7. Voskuyl AE, Zwinderman AH, Westedt ML, et al: The mortality of rheumatoid vasculitis compared with rheumatoid arthritis. Arthritis Rheum 39:266, 1996.
8. Chen K-R, Toyohara A, Suzuki A, Miyakawa S: Clinical and histopathological spectrum of cutaneous vasculitis in rheumatoid arthritis. Br J Dermatol 147:905, 2002.
9. Simonart T, Durez P, Margaux J, et al: Cutaneous necrotizing vasculitis after low dose methotrexate therapy for rheumatoid arthritis: a possible manifestation of methotrexate hypersensitivity. Clin Rheumatol[16]:623, 1997.
10. Brion PH, Mittal-Henkle A, Kalunian KC: Autoimmune skin rashes associated with etanercept for rheumatoid arthritis. Ann Intern Med 131:634, 1999.
11. Kaplan H: Clinical images: skin hyperpigmentation associated with minocycline therapy. Arthritis Rheum 40:1353, 1997.
12. Watanabe T, Tsuchida T, Ito Y, et al: Annular erythema associated with lupus erythematosus/Sjögren's syndrome. J Am Acad Dermatol 36: 214, 1997.
13. Higuchi T, Taniguchi H, Katayama I, Nishioka K: Spongiotic annular erythema in SS-A/SS-B antibody negative Sjögren's syndrome. J Dermatol 25:90, 1998.
14. Haimowitz JE, McCauliffe DP, Seykora J, Werth VP: Annular erythema of Sjögren's syndrome in a white woman. J Am Acad Dermatol 42:1069, 2000.

15. Font J, Ramos-Casals M, Cervera R, et al: Antineutrophil cytoplasmic antibodies in primary Sjögren's syndrome: Prevalence and clinical significance. Br J Rheumatol 37:1287, 1998.
16. Garcia-Carrasco M, Ramos M, Cervera R, et al: Hepatitis C virus infection in 'primary' Sjögren's syndrome: Prevalence and clinical significance in a series of 90 patients. Ann Rheum Dis 56:173, 1997.
17. De Vita S, Damato R, De Marchi G, et al: True primary Sjögren's syndrome in a subset of patients with hepatitis C infection: A model linking chronic infection to chronic sialadenitis. Isr Med Assoc J 4:1101, 2002.
18. Weitzul S, Duvic M: HIV-related psoriasis and Reiter's syndrome. Semin Cutan Med Surg 16:213, 1997.
19. Khan MA: Update on spondyloarthropathies. Ann Intern Med 18:896, 2002.
20. Bauman C, Cron RQ, Sherry DD, Francis JS: Reiter syndrome initially misdiagnosed as Kawasaki disease. J Pediatr 128:366, 1996.
21. Gladman DD: Clinical aspects of the spondyloarthropathies. Am J Med Sci 316:234, 1998.
22. Livneh A, Zaks N, Katz J, et al: Increased prevalence of joint manifestations in patients with recurrent aphthous stomatitis (RAS). Clin Exp Rheumatol 14:407, 1996.
23. Gladman DD, Farewell VT: HLA studies in psoriatic arthritis: Current situation and future needs. J Rheumatol 30:4, 2003.
24. Leung DY, Travers JB, Giomo R, et al: Evidence for a streptococcal superantigen-driven process in acute guttate psoriasis. J Clin Invest 96:2106, 1995.
25. Kitamura K, Kanasashi M, Suga C, et al: Cutaneous reactions induced by calcium channel blocker: High frequency of psoriasiform eruptions. J Dermatol 20:279, 1993.
26. Gupta AK, Sibbald RG, Knowles SR, et al: Terbinafine therapy may be associated with the development of psoriasis de novo or its exacerbation: Four case reports and a review of drug-induced psoriasis. J Am Acad Dermatol 36:858, 1997.
27. Tsankov N, Angelova I, Kazandjieva J: Drug-induced psoriasis: Recognition and management. Am J Clin Dermatol 1:159, 2000.
28. Stern SH, Insall JN, Windsor RE, et al: Total knee arthroplasty in patients with psoriasis. Clin Orthopedics 248:108, 1989.
29. Ruzicka T: Psoriatic arthritis: New types, new treatments. Arch Dermatol 132:215, 1999.
30. Kammer GM, Soter NA, Gibson DJ, Schur PH: Psoriatic arthritis: A clinical, immunologic and HLA study of 100 patients. Semin Arthritis Rheum 9:75, 1979.
31. Dougados M, van der Linden S, Juhlin R, et al: The European Spondylarthropathy Study Group preliminary criteria for the classification of spondylarthropathy. Arthritis Rheum 34:1218, 1991.
32. Sieper J, Rudwaleit M, Braun J, van der Heijde D: Diagnosing reactive arthritis: Role of clinical setting in the value of serologic and microbiologic assays. Arthritis Rheum 46:319, 2002.
33. Franks AG Jr: Psoriatic arthritis. *In* Sontheimer RD, Provost TT (eds): Cutaneous Manifestations of Rheumatic Diseases. Baltimore, Williams & Wilkins, 1996, p 233.
34. Bruce IN, Silman AJ: The aetiology of psoriatic arthritis. Rheumatology 40:363, 2001.
35. Mark KA, Franks AG Jr: Colchicine and indomethacin for the treatment of relapsing polychondritis. J Am Acad Dermatol 46:S22, 2002.
36. Trentham DE, Le CH: Relapsing polychrondritis. Ann Intern Med 15:114, 1998.
37. Frances C, el Rassi R, Laporte JL, et al: Dermatologic manifestations of relapsing polychondritis: A study of 200 cases in a single center. Medicine (Baltimore) 80:173, 2001.
38. Sontheimer RD: The lexicon of cutaneous lupus erythematosus -a review and personal perspective on the nomenclature and classification of the cutaneous manifestations of lupus erythematosus. Lupus 6:84, 1997.
39. Shirahama S, Furukawa F, Yagi H, et al: Bullous systemic lupus erythematosus: Detection of antibodies against noncollagenous domain of type VII collagen. J Am Acad Dermatol 38:844, 1998.
40. B lack DR, Hornung CA, Schneider PD, Callen JP: Frequency and severity of systemic disease in patients with subacute cutaneous lupus erythematosus. Arch Dermatol 138:1175, 2002.
41. Chlebus E, Wolska H, Blaszczyk M, Jablonska S: Subacute cutaneous lupus erythematosus versus systemic lupus erythematosus: Diagnostic criteria and therapeutic implications. J Am Acad Dermatol 38:405, 1998.
42. Crowson AN, Magro CM: Subacute cutaneous lupus erythematosus arising in the setting of calcium channel blocker therapy. Hum Pathol 28:67, 1997.
43. Brooke R, Coulson IH, Al-Dawoud A: Terbinafine-induced subacute cutaneous lupus erythematosus. Br J Dermatol 139:1132, 1998.
44. Nousari HC, Kimyai-Asadi A, Tausk FA: Subacute cutaneous lupus erythematosus associated with interferon beta-1a. Lancet 352:1825, 1998.
45. Callen JP: Drug-induced cutaneous lupus erythematosus: A distinct syndrome that is frequently unrecognized. J Am Acad Dermatol 45:315, 2001.
46. Srivastava M, Rencic A, Diglio G, et al: Drug-induced, Ro/SSA-positive cutaneous lupus erythematosus. Arch Dermatol 139:45, 2003.
47. Alexiades-Armenakas MR, Baldassano M, Bince B, et al: Tumid lupus erythematosus: Criteria for classification with immunohistochemical analysis. Arthritis Rheum 49:494, 2003.
48. Headington JT: Cicatricial alopecia. Dermatol Clin 14:773, 1996.
49. Peters SM, Su DWP: Lupus erythematosus panniculitis. Med Clin North Am 73:1113, 1989.
50. Martens PB, Moder KG, Ahmed I: Lupus panniculitis: Clinical perspectives from a case series. J Rheumatol 26:68, 1999.
51. Maruyama M, Miyauchis T, Hashimoro K: Massive cutaneous mucinosis associated with systemic lupus erythematosus. Br J Dermatol 137:450, 1997.
52. Kanda N, Tsuchida T, Watanabe T, Tamaki K: Cutaneous lupus mucinosis: A review of our cases and the possible pathogenesis. J Cutan Pathol 24:553, 1997.
53. Gibson GE, McEvoy MT: Coexistence of lupus erythematosus and porphyria cutanea tarda in fifteen patients. J Am Acad Dermatol 38:569, 1998.
54. Nyberg F, Hasan T, Pushka P, et al: Occurrence of polymorphous light eruption in lupus erythematosus. Br J Dermatol 136:217, 1997.
55. Tanaka A, Sugawara A, Sawai K, Kuwahara T: Human parvovirus B19 infection resembling systemic lupus erythematosus. Intern Med 37:708, 1998.
56. Cardinali C, Caproni M, Fabbri P: The utility of the lupus band test on sun-protected non-lesional skin for the diagnosis of systemic lupus erythematosus. Clin Exp Rheumatol 17:427, 1999.
57. George R, Kurian S, Jacob M, Thomas K: Diagnostic evaluation of the lupus band test in discoid and systemic lupus erythematosus. Int J Dermatol 34:170, 1995.
58. Kotajima L, Aotsuka Sumiya M, Yokohari R, et al: Clinical features of patients with juvenile onset mixed connective tissue disease: Analysis of data collected in a nationwide collaborative study in Japan. J Rheumatol 23:1088, 1996.
59. Soter NA: Cutaneous necrotizing venulitis. *In* Freedberg IM, Eisen AZ, Wolff K, et al (eds): Fitzpatrick's Dermatology in General Medicine, 6th ed. New York, McGraw-Hill,2003, p. 177.
60. Francès C, Du LTH, Piette J-C, et al: Wegener's granulomatosis: Dermatological manifestations in 75 cases with clinicopathologic correlation. Arch Dermatol 130:861, 1994.
61. Trejo O, Ramos-Casals M, Garcia-Carrasco M, et al: Cryoglobulinemia: Study of etiologic factors and clinical immunologic factors in 443 patients from a single center. Medicine (Baltimore) 80:252, 2001.
62. Burrows NP, Lockwood CM: Antineutrophil cytoplasmic antibodies and their relevance to the dermatologist. Br J Dermatol 132:173, 1995.
63. Romani J, Puig L, de Moragas JM: Detection of antineutrophil cytoplasmic antibodies in patients with hepatitis C virus-induced cutaneous vasculitis with mixed cryoglobulinemia. Arch Dermatol 132:974, 1996.
64. Peñas PF, Porras JI, Fraga J, et al: Microscopic polyangiitis: A systemic vasculitis with a positive P-ANCA. Br J Dermatol 134:542, 1996.
65. Irvine AD, Bruce IN, Walsh MY, Bingham AB: Microscopic polyangiitis: Delineation of a cutaneous-limited variant associated with antimyeloperoxidase autoantibody. Arch Dermatol 133:474, 1997.

66. Burden AD, Tiliman DM, Foley P, Holme B: IgA class anticardiolipin antibodies in cutaneous leukocytoclastic vasculitis. J Am Acad Dermatol 35:411, 1996.
67. Galaria NA, Werth VP, Schumacher MR: Leukocytoclastic vasculitis due to etanercept. J Rheumatol 27:2041, 2000.
68. Tancrede-Bohin E, Ochonisky S, Vignon-Pennamen M-D, et al: Schönlein-Henoch purpura in adult patients: predictive factors for IgA glomerulonephritis in a retrospective study of 57 cases. Arch Dermatol 133:438, 1997.
69. Tomac N, Saraclar Y, Turrktas I, Kalayei O: Acute haemorrhagic oedema of infancy: a case report. Clin Exp Dermatol 21:217, 1996.
70. Soter NA: Urticarial venulitis. Derm Therapy 13:400, 2000.
71. Baty V, Hoen B, Hudziak H, et al: Schnitzler's syndrome: two case reports and review of the literature. Mayo Clin Proc 70:570, 1995.
72. Ishikawa O, Miyachi Y, Watanabe H: Hypocomplementaemic urticarial vasculitis associated with Jaccoud's syndrome. Br J Dermatol 137:804, 1997.
73. Lipsker D, Veran Y, Grunenberger F, et al: The Schnitzler syndrome: four new cases and review of the literature. Medicine (Baltimore) 80:37, 2001.
74. Sangueza OP, Pilcher B, Sangueza JM: Erythema elevatum diutinum: a clinicopathological study of eight cases. Am J Dermatopathol 19:214, 1997.
75. Dronda F, Gonzales-Lopez A, Lecona M, Barros C: Erythema elevatum diutinum in human immunodeficiency virus-infected patients: report of a case and review of the literature. Clin Exp Dermatol 21:222, 1996.
76. Baselga E, Margall N, Barnadas MA, et al: Detection of *Mycobacterium tuberculosis* DNA in lobular granulomatosus panniculitis (erythema induratum-nodular vasculitis). Arch Dermatol 133:457, 1997.
77. Acland KM, Darvay A, Wakelin SH, Russell-Jones R: Livedoid vasculitis: a manifestation of the antiphospholipid syndrome? Br J Dermatol 140:131, 1999.
78. Boyvat A, Jundakçi N, Babikir MD, Gürgey E: Livedoid vasculopathy associated with heterozygous protein C deficiency. Br J Dermatol 143:840, 2000.
79. Calamia KT, Balabanova M, Perniciaro C, Walsh JS: Livedo (livedoid) vasculitis and the factor V Leiden mutation: additional evidence for abnormal coagulation. J Am Acad Dermatol 46:133, 2002.
80. Francès C, Le Tonguèze M, Salohzin KV, et al: Prevalence of antiendothelial cell antibodies in patients with Sneddon's syndrome. J Am Acad Dermatol 33:64, 1995.
81. Dawkins MA, Jorizzo JL, Walker FO, et al: Dermatomyositis: a dermatology-based case series. J Am Acad Dermatol 38:397, 1998.
82. Kovacs SO, Kovacs SC: Dermatomyositis. J Am Acad Dermatol 39:899, 1998.
83. Guin JD: Eyelid dermatitis: experience in 203 cases. J Am Acad Dermatol 47:755, 2002.
84. Sontheimer RD: Dermatomyositis: an overview of recent progress with emphasis on dermatologic aspects. Dermatol Clin 20:387, 2002.
85. Cheong WK, Hughes GR, Norris PG, Hawk JL: Cutaneous photosensitivity in dermatomyositis. Br J Dermatol 131:205, 1994.
86. Martinez-Cordero E, Lasky D, Katona G: Nasal septal perforation. J Rheumatol 13: 231, 1986.
87. Sontheimer RD: Cutaneous features of classic dermatomyositis and amyopathic dermatomyositis. Curr Opin Rheumatol 11:475, 1999.
88. Pelle MT, Callen JP: Adverse reactions to hydroxychloroquine are more common in patients with dermatomyositis than in patients with cutaneous lupus erythematous. Arch Dermatol 138:1231,2002.
89. Steen V: Clinical manifestations of systemic sclerosis. Semin Cutan Med Surg 17:48, 1997.
90. Fujiwara H, Fujiwara K, Hashimoto K, et al: Detection of *Borrelia burgdorferi* DNA (*B garinii* or *B afzelii*) in morphea and lichen sclerosis et atrophicus tissues of German and Japanese but not of US patients. Arch Dermatol 133:41, 1997.
91. Buechner SA, Lautenschlager S, Itin P, et al: Lymphoproliferative responses to *Borrelia burgdorferi* in patients with erythema migrans, acrodermatitis chronica atrophicans, lymphadenosis benigna cutis, and morphea. Arch Dermatol 131:673, 1995.
92. Birtane M, Eryavuz M, Unalan H, Tuzun F: Melorheostosis: Report of a new case with linear scleroderma. Clin Rheumatol 17:543, 1998.
93. Seibold JR, McCloskey DA: Skin involvement as a relevant outcome measure in clinical trials of systemic sclerosis. Curr Opin Rheumatol 6:571, 1997.
94. Ohtsuka T, Hasegawa A, Nakano A, et al: Nailfold capillary abnormality and pulmonary hypertension in systemic sclerosis. Int J Dermatol 2:116, 1997.
95. Merkel PA, Herlyn K, Martin RW, et al: Measuring disease activity and functional status in patients with scleroderma and Raynaud's phenomenon. Arthritis Rheum 46:2410, 2002.
96. Mori Y, Kahari VM, Varga J: Scleroderma-like cutaneous syndromes. Curr Rheumatol Rep 22:113, 2002.
97. Fibrosing skin condition among patients with renal disease-United States and Europe. MMWR Morb Mortal Wkly Rep 18:25, 2002.
98. Cowper SE, Su LD, Bhawan J, et al: Nephrogenic fibrosing dermopathy. Am J Dermatopathol 23:383, 2001.
99. Dressler F: Juvenile rheumatoid arthritis and spondyloarthropathies. Curr Opin Rheumatol 5:468, 1998.
100. Woo P, Wedderburn LR: Juvenile chronic arthritis. Lancet 351:969, 1998.
101. Hoeger PH, Veelken N, Foeldvari I, et al: Neonatal onset of rash in Still's disease. J Pediatr 137:128, 2000.
102. Iglesias-Gamarra A, Mendez EA, Cuellar ML, et al: Poststreptococcal reactive arthritis in adults: long-term follow-up. Am J Med Sci 321:173, 2001.
103. Edlow JA: Erythema migrans. Med Clin North Am 86:239, 2002.
104. Donta ST: Late and chronic Lyme disease. Med Clin North Am 86:341, 2002.
105. Seinost G, Golde WT, Berger BW, et al: Infection with multiple strains of *Borrelia burgdorferi* sensu stricto in patients with Lyme disease. Arch Dermatol 135:1329, 1999.
106. Breier F, Klade H, Stanek G, et al: Lymphoproliferative responses to *Borrelia burgdorferi* in circumscribed scleroderma. Br J Dermatol 134:285, 1996.
107. Aberer E, Kersten A, Klade H,et al: Heterogeneity of *Borrelia burgdorferi* in the skin. Am J Dermatopathol 18:571, 1996.
108. Huang CY, Wang WJ, Wong CK: Skin biopsy gives the potential benefit in the diagnosis of systemic amyloidosis associated with cardiac involvement. Arch Dermatol 134:643, 1998.
109. Gomez-Casanovas E, Sanmarti R, Sole M, et al: The clinical significance of amyloid fat deposits in rheumatoid arthritis: a systematic long-term follow-up study using abdominal fat aspiration. Arthritis Rheum 44:66, 2001.
110. Siragusi M, Ferri R, Cavallari V, Schepis C: Friction melanosis, friction amyloidosis, macular amyloidosis, towel melanosis: many names for the same clinical entity. Eur J Dermatol 11:545, 2001.
111. Weyers W: Lichen amyloidosis: a consequence of scratching? [Reply]. J Am Acad Dermatol 41:501, 1999.
112. Woollons A, Black MM: Nodular localized primary cutaneous amyloidosis: a long-term follow-up study. Br J Dermatol 145:400, 2002.
113. Chang YT, Liu HN, Wong CK, et al: Detection of Epstein-Barr virus in primary cutaneous amyloidosis. Br J Dermatol 136:823, 1997.
114. Hagari Y, Mihara M, Konohana I, et al: Nodular localized cutaneous amyloidosis: further demonstration of monoclonality of infiltrating plasma cells in four additional Japanese patients. Br J Dermatol 138:652, 1998.
115. Fujimoto N, Yajima M, Ohnishi Y, et al: Advanced glycation end product-modified β_2 microglobulin is a component of amyloid fibrils of primary localized cutaneous nodular amyloidosis. J Invest Dermatol 118:479, 2002.
116. Furumoto H, Shimizu T, Asagami C, et al: Apolipoprotein E is present in primary localized cutaneous amyloidosis. J Invest Dermatol 111:417, 1998.
117. Huilgol SC, Ramnarian N, Carrington P, et al: Cytokeratins in primary cutaneous amyloidosis. Australas J Dermatol 39:81, 1998.
118. Giuffrida TJ, Kerdel FA: Sarcoidosis. Dermatol Clin 20:435, 2002.

119. Maña J, Marcoval J, Graells J, et al: Cutaneous involvement in sarcoidosis: relationship to systemic disease. Arch Dermatol 133:882, 1997.
120. Baughman RP, Teirstein AS, Judson MA, et al: Clinical characteristics of patients in a case control study of sarcoidosis. Am J Respir Crit Care Med 164:1885, 2001.
121. Mashek H, Kalb R: Hypopigmentation of the extremities: sarcoidosis. Arch Dermatol 134:743, 1998.
122. Neglia V, Sookoians S, Herrea M, et al: Development of cutaneous sarcoidosis in a patient with chronic hepatitis C treated with interferon alpha 2b. J Cutan Med Surg 5:406, 2001.
123. Raquena L, Yus ES: Panniculitis. I. Mostly septal panniculitis. J Am Acad Dermatol 45:163, 2001.
124. Raquena L, Yus ES: Panniculitis. II. Mostly lobular panniculitis. J Am Acad Dermatol 45:325, 2001.
125. Psychos DN, Voulgari PV, Skopouli FN, et al: Erythema nodosum: The underlying conditions. Clin Rheumatol 19:212, 2000.
126. Nekhlyudov L, Gradzka M, Conti-Kelly AM, Greco TP: Erythema nodosum associated with antiphospholipid antibodies: a report of three cases. Lupus 9:641, 2000.
127. White JW Jr, Winkelmann RK: Weber-Christian panniculitis: a review of 30 cases with this diagnosis. J Am Acad Dermatol 39:56, 1998.
128. White L, Wieselthier JS, Hitchcock MG: Panniculitis: recent developments and observations. Semin Cutan Med Surg 4:278, 1998.
129. Bruce AJ, Bennett DD, Lohse CM, et al: Lipodermatosclerosis: Review of cases evaluated at Mayo Clinic. J Am Acad Dermatol 46:187, 2002.
130. Snow JL, Su WPD: Lipomembranous (membranocystic) fat necrosis: clinicopathologic correlation of 38 cases. Am J Dermatopathol 18:151, 1996.
131. Brown R, Buckley R, Kelley M: Pancreatic panniculitis. J Clin Oncol 15:3418, 1997.
132. Craig AJ, Cualing H, Thomas G, et al: Cytophagic histiocytic panniculitis: a syndrome associated with benign and malignant panniculitis: case comparison and review of the literature. J Am Acad Dermatol 39:721, 1998.
133. Marzano AV, Berti E, Paulli M, Caputo R: Cytophagic histiocytic panniculitis and subcutaneous panniculitis-like T-cell lymphoma. Arch Dermatol 136:889, 2000.
134. Wick MR, Patterson JW: Cytophagic histiocytic panniculitis: critical reappraisal. Arch Dermatol 136:922, 2000.
135. Weenig RH, Ng CS, Perniciaro C: Subcutaneous panniculitis-like T-cell lymphoma: an elusive case presenting as lipomembranous panniculitis and a review of 72 cases in the literature. Am J Dermatopathol 23:206, 2001.
136. Naides SJ: Rheumatologic manifestations of parvovirus B19 infection. Rheum Dis Clin N Am 24:375, 1998.
137. Dingli D, Pfizenmaier DH, Arromdee E, et al: Severe digital arterial occlusive disease and acute parvovirus B19 infection. Lancet 356:312, 2000.
138. Gabriel SE, Espy M, Erdman DD, et al: The role of parvovirus B19 in the pathogenesis of giant cell arteritis: a preliminary evaluation. Arthritis Rheum 42:1255, 1999.
139. Chevrel G, Calvet A, Belin V, Miossec P: Dermatomyositis associated with the presence of parvovirus B19 DNA in muscle. Rheumatology (Oxford) 39:1037, 2000.
140. Oguz F, Adkeniz C, Unuvar E, et al: Parvovirus B19 in the acute arthropathies and juvenile rheumatoid arthritis. J Paediatr Child Health 38:358, 2002.
141. Hsu TC, Tsay GJ: Human parvovirus B19 infection in patients with systemic lupus erythematosus. Rheumatology 40:152, 2001.
142. Kalish RA, Knopf AN, Gary, GW, et al: Lupus-like presentation of human parvovirus B19 infection. J Rheumatol 19:169, 1992.
143. Vargas-Diéz B, Buezo GF, Aragües M, et al: Papular-purpuric gloves-and-socks syndrome. Int J Dermatol 35:626, 1996.
144. Magro CM, Dawood MR, Crowson AN: The cutaneous manifestations of human parvovirus B19 infection. Human Pathol 31:488, 2000.

S E C T I O N

VI

Diagnostic Tests and Procedures in Rheumatic Diseases

46 Synovial Fluid Analyses, Synovial Biopsy, and Synovial Pathology

DANIELLE M. GERLAG • PAUL P. TAK

Analysis of synovial fluid (SF) and synovial tissue can provide insight into both the diagnosis and response to therapy in patients with rheumatic diseases. The former is especially important in the case of an acute (mono)arthritis, such as a suspected bacterial or crystal-induced arthritis, when initiating immediate treatment is warranted. Also, the efficacy of treatment and the prognosis can be assessed by analysis of fluid or tissue from an arthritic joint. Finally, evaluation of these clinical samples can help us understand the pathophysiology and pathogenesis of joint diseases, because the etiology of many forms of inflammatory arthritis still remains uncertain (Table 46-1).

Synovial Fluid Analysis

Analysis of synovial fluid (SF) remains a routine diagnostic procedure to differentiate various causes of arthritis. Several aspects of SF, including gross examination (color, viscosity), leukocyte counts, biochemical tests, and microscopy, can provide key information that can distinguish between noninflammatory and inflammatory forms of arthritis. This is especially important in the case of an acute monoarthritis, when an infectious cause needs to be ruled out. Septic arthritis is a disease with a high morbidity and mortality rate, which calls for immediate treatment.[1,2]

TABLE 46–1 • CHARACTERISTICS OF SYNOVIAL FLUID

	Appearance	Viscosity	Cells per mm³	% PMN	Crystals	Culture
Normal	Transparent	High	< 180	<10%	Negative	Negative
Osteoarthritis	Transparent	High	200-2000	<10%	Occasional calcium pyrophospate and hydroxyapatite crystals	Negative
Rheumatoid arthritis	Translucent	Low	2000-50,000	variable	Negative	Negative
Psoriatic arthritis	Translucent	Low	2000-50,000	variable	Negative	Negative
Reactive arthritis	Translucent	Low	2000-50,000	variable	Negative	Negative
Spondylarthropathy	Translucent	Low	2000-50,000	variable	Negative	Negative
Gout	Translucent to cloudy	Low	200 to >50,000	>90%	Needle-shaped, positive birefringent monosodium urate monohydrate crystals	Negative
Pseudogout	Translucent to cloudy	Low	200-50,000	>90%	Rhomboid, negative birefringent calcium pyrophosphate crystals	Negative
Bacterial arthritis	Cloudy	Variable	2000 to >50,000	>90%	Negative	Positive
PVNS	Hemorrhagic or brown	Low			Negative	Negative
Hemarthrosis	Hemorrhagic	Low			Negative	Negative

Abbreviations: PVNS, pigmented villonodular synovitis; PMN, polymorphic nuclear cell.

In 1994, a critical reappraisal of SF analysis[3] mentioned two main reasons for SF analysis: to identify septic arthritis by Gram stain and culture and to diagnose crystal-induced arthritis by polarizing microscopy. Biochemical tests, such as glucose, protein, and lactic dehydrogenase concentrations, were not felt to be useful as diagnostic tools for SF analysis. The value of SF assays for differential diagnosis was also critically evaluated in a more recent report.[4] The authors found little support for the use of SF analysis in the literature, except in the case of acute monoarthritis when a crystal arthropathy or septic arthritis is suspected, as well as in the case of intercritical gout (i.e., when SF is taken from asymptomatic joints). These reports clearly show that many tests currently used for SF analysis need more evidence to justify their routine use. In addition, standardization of assays and guidelines for their use should be developed.

ARTHROCENTESIS

SF can usually be obtained safely and easily in the clinic by simple aspiration guided by physical landmarks. In some cases of arthritis, for instance in the hip and sacroiliac joints, imaging techniques are necessary to be certain that the joint space has been identified. The techniques used and the routes for arthrocentesis are described in Chapter 47.

Fluid may be difficult to aspirate due to fibrin or "rice bodies" clogging the needle. Rice bodies occur in many rheumatic diseases, most commonly in rheumatoid arthritis (RA). They consist of fibrin, debris, cells, and calcium apatite crystals[5] and are thought to be a result of synovial inflammation and ischemia.[6] Their clinical significance remains unclear. Furthermore, SF can be loculated, and fluid may therefore be difficult to obtain. Continued suction when withdrawing the needle from the joint space may sometimes help to obtain a drop of fluid in the needle. When it is difficult to obtain SF, a small amount of nonbacteriostatic normal saline can be used to irrigate the joint for culture in case of suspected septic arthritis.

NORMAL SYNOVIAL FLUID AND PERFUSION

Normally, the SF contains solutes, such as urea, urate, and creatinine, which are in stable equilibrium with those in plasma. Most of these small solutes freely diffuse in and out of the joint through the highly permeable fenestrae in the synovial microvessels.

The protein concentration in SF is, under normal conditions, somewhat lower than plasma, but it can increase with articular inflammation. The proteins enter the joint by size-specific diffusion from the synovial microvessels and clear the joint through the lymphatics. This process of clearance is relatively independent of size.[7] There is also local, intra-articular synthesis and release of proteins, such as lubricin, immunoglobulins, components of the complement system, hyaluronan, and cytokines. The levels of these proteins measured in SF reflect a balance between production and release, on the one hand, and clearance on the other. Of interest, the rate of lymphatic drainage from a joint may vary among different diseases.[8] Ideally, one should combine SF levels with clearance values from the joints to provide insight into the events that take place in the synovial compartment and to evaluate the effects of therapeutic interventions in various arthritides.

ACCUMULATION OF SYNOVIAL FLUID IN ARTHRITIS

The SF volume depends on fluid production, fluid transport out of the joint cavity into the periarticular tissue, and transport from the periarticular tissue into the lymphatic vessels. In the case of synovitis, the lymphatic system fails to drain the transsynovial effusion, leading to accumulation of SF even though the inflamed synovial tissue contains an increased number of lymphatic vessels.

Increased metabolic demands of the hyperplastic synovium create a circulatory-metabolic imbalance, in which the vascular response is functionally inadequate. This leads to microinfarctions and ischemia of the synovium, resulting in increased oxygen radical activity and lactate levels and decreased intra-articular pH in the synovial fluid[9,10] (Fig. 46–1).

MEASUREMENT OF FLOW

Flow of synovial fluids can be measured by laser doppler, ultrasound, and magnetic resonance imaging (MRI) techniques. These methods are convenient, but sampling and positioning error and lack of a validated outcome measure are major problems.[11]

Methods that give absolute values of flow (in ml/min) are better for use in chronic conditions and for interindividual comparison. The clearance of a γ-emitting isotope injected intra-articularly, by measuring counts serially over the joint, is an example of this method. Arterial perfusion of radiolabeled microspheres, another well-described technique, is recognized as the "gold standard" of blood perfusion measures in vivo. This method, however, cannot be used in humans because it requires substantial amounts of tissue for quantification.

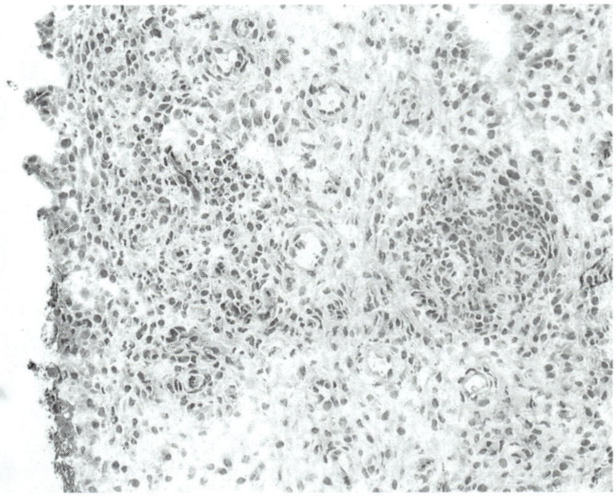

FIGURE 46–1 • Rheumatoid synovial tissue, showing hyperplasia of the intimal lining layer and infiltration of mononuclear cells in the sublining layer. (H&E, ×200.) (See color plate 9.)

GROSS EXAMINATION

Normal SF is clear, colorless to pale yellow, and viscous. It is in stable equilibrium with plasma and consists of extravasated plasma and a high-molecular-mass component, in particular hyaluronan. When the effusion is cloudy, this typically suggests the presence of inflammatory cells. Fibrin, crystals, lipids, or amyloid can also interfere with the transparency of SF.

Pigmented villonodular synovitis, trauma, tumors, and hematologic disorders (such as VonWillebrand's disease) need to be excluded if, after nontraumatic puncture, the SF color is orange-brown, red, or bloody. If streaks of blood appear into the syringe or fluid during the procedure, this is probably due to the puncture itself.

The viscosity can be judged by watching the SF being slowly expressed out of the syringe or needle. The synovial fluid should form a "string," stretching approximately 10 cm before surface tension is broken due to hyaluronan. Enzymes that digest hyaluronan, produced by inflammatory cells, can markedly decrease viscosity. In former days, the mucine clot test was used to assess hyaluronan content and was included in the criteria for the diagnosis of RA proposed by the American College of Rheumatism.[12] A few drops of SF placed into 2-percent acetic acid would normally lead to a stable clump of hyaluronate-protein complex, or mucin. In inflammatory fluid, the clump fragments easily, reflecting the loss of integrity of hyaluronan. The viscosity and mucin clot test have no additive value in the differential diagnosis, the latter test having low specificity and low positive predictive value (52%) for the diagnosis of RA.[13] Therefore, this test has no place in the routine diagnostic analysis of SF.

CELL COUNT

Measurement of total white cell counts and the percentage of polymorphonuclear leukocytes is generally recommended as a simple way to differentiate between inflammatory and noninflammatory arthritis. Based on cell counts in SF, different subsets of joint diseases can be recognized.[14] SF normally contains fewer then 180 cells/mm^3, and a leukocyte count of 200 to 2000 cells/mm^3 is generally termed *noninflammatory*. This can be found, for instance, in osteoarthritis or after a trauma. Cell counts between 2000 and 50,000 cells/mm^3 are usually called *inflammatory* and can be found in all forms of (active) inflammatory synovitis. In certain acute conditions, such as septic arthritis or gout, counts can rise above 50,000 cells/mm^3. Using cell counts to separate SF into these different groups should be done with care because of significant overlap. Thus, low cell counts never exclude a possible infection. In septic arthritis, however, at least 95 percent of SF leukocytes are polymophonuclear cells,[15] but this result is not specific for infection.

The interpretation of the SF leukocyte determinations may be complicated by the wide variability between different laboratories and observers.[16] One factor relevant for the interpretation of the results is the stability of cells in the SF, which may cause a decrease in white blood cell counts over time. Therefore, SF should be examined without delay whenever possible. If it is difficult to perform direct microscopic analysis, one might consider the use of reagent strips, originally designed for semiquantification of leukocytes in urine, which could be used to assess the inflammatory character of SF.[17] Alternatively, the results of counting cells can still be accurate after 24 or even 48 hours of storage when the sample is stored at 4°C or when preserved in ethylenecliamine tetra-acetic acid (EDTA) and kept at room temperature.[18]

SPECIAL BIOCHEMICAL TESTS

Biochemical tests and immunologic assays have been used as research tools and are not widely recommended for diagnostic purposes. Glucose, lactic dehydrogenase, and protein concentration are highly inaccurate markers of inflammation and are of little or no value as part of the diagnostic evaluation of SF.[15] Of interest, in the field of forensic medicine, measurement of small molecules in the postmortem SF, such as sodium, potassium, calcium, chloride, urea, creatinine, and glucose, can be of help in establishing the antemortem metabolic state, because most solutes in SF are stable after death.[19]

Immunologic assays of SF, such as rheumatoid factor (RF) and complement, have also been evaluated. Detection of RF in SF has sensitivity, specificity, and predictive values that are essentially equal to the values for serum RF and are therefore of little additional diagnostic value.[20] Increased levels of complement proteins or metabolites have been found in the SF of patients with RA. Recently, in situ hybridization, immunohistochemistry, and Western blot techniques have shown that complement components and receptors are produced in the inflamed synovium.[21,22] However, measurements of complement components in SF to date have no proven diagnostic value.

CYTOPATHOLOGY

Microscopic analysis of a drop of synovial fluid on a slide, covered with a glass coverslip, also called "wet preparation," can yield valuable information about the cellular and crystalline contents of SF. Different cell types can be recognized in SF. "Ragocytes," cells containing immune complexes and complement, can be found in SF of patients with RA and other arthritides. Furthermore, so-called Reiter cells or cytophagocytic mononuclear cells (CPMs) can be found in SF. These tissue macrophages with ingested apoptotic polymorphonuclear leukocytes are commonly found in reactive arthritis and other spondylarthropathies, as well as in crystal arthritides, but only rarely in RA. In case of synovial metastasis or malignancy, which is rare, malignant cells can be found in the SF.

The use of stained cytocentrifuged preparations could facilitate the ability to recognize a range of cells with possible diagnostic implications, such as eosinophils, mast cells, apoptotic or nonapoptotic polymorphonuclear leukocytes, and CPMs.[23] Data showing the potential of this approach for differential diagnosis are limited, and due to the significant overlap of the results, differentiation of various diseases based on cytology is not possible.

POLARIZED LIGHT MICROSCOPY

One of the primary reasons to perform SF analysis is to diagnose crystal-induced arthritis by polarized light microscopy.[24] If birefringent (crystalline) material is placed between the two polarizing filters in the light bundle, light rays are rotated in such a way that they can pass through the second filter. The material appears bright on a dark field. Birefringent materials are characterized by the ability to split light into fast and slow waves, vibrating in axes perpendicular to each other. If a first-order red compensator (that filters green from the background) is placed between the filters, the field becomes red, and birefringent crystal becomes yellow or blue, depending on the orientation to the direction of the slow-vibration axis of the compensator and its identity. A crystal that is yellow when oriented parallel to the slow-vibration axis of the compensator is considered negatively birefringent. In this case, the fast wave vibrates along the axis of the crystal. When a crystal shows a blue color in this situation, the slow wave vibrates parallel to the slow-vibration axis of the compensator. This is called positive birefringence.

Monosodium urate monohydrate (MSUM) crystals are long, needle shaped, and show strongly negative birefringence. They are often found within cells during acute attacks of gout. If a tophus is examined, many long, needle-shaped crystals are seen outside cells.

Calcium pyrophosphate dihydrate (CPPD) crystals are typically rhomboid and only weakly positive or sometimes even nonbirefringent. Because of these characteristics, the use of ordinary light microscopy to examine the SF sample can be useful when CPPD deposition disease is suspected.[25]

MSUM and CPPD crystals are known to be pathogenic. Other crystals, including basic calcium phosphates (hydroxyapatite, octacalcium phosphate, and tricalcium phosphate), cholesterol, and other lipid particles, are of uncertain significance.[26] However, in the pediatric setting, these crystals can give clues to systemic diseases, such as primary hyperoxaluria and cystinosis.[27]

Hydroxyapatite crystals have been identified in miscellaneous forms of arthritis, including osteoarthritis. Their appearance varies greatly, mostly they are seen as clumps, either round or irregular, and are usually nonbirefringent.[28] A simple, rapid screening method using alizarin red S stain and ordinary light microscopy can be used to detect microcrystalline or noncrystalline calcium phosphate salts. Apatite crystal clumps and small CPPD crystals are more readily detected using this method.[29]

Octacalcium and tricalcium phosphate crystals form clumps as well and are seen as nonbirefringent chunks or coins. Individual crystals cannot be seen with ordinary light microscopy.

Cholesterol crystals can be detected in several joint diseases, and they appear as flat rectangular plates with notched corners outside the cells. They can also occasionally have a long, needle-shaped appearance. They exhibit strong positive and negative birefringence.

Lipid liquid crystals appear like Maltese crosses, with intense double birefringence. Furthermore, contamination with dust on the slide or coverslip, powder from rubber gloves, and crystals after an intra-articular corticosteroid injection, can be seen as birefringent material.

Reliability of Crystal Identification

Although the identification of MSUM and CPPD crystals seems simple, previous studies suggest otherwise. Quality control studies have shown that the correlation between different laboratories and observers is poor. The results for identifying MSUM crystals are a bit better than for CPPD crystals, probably because CPPD crystals are only weakly and sometimes nonbirefringent. These results can often be explained by lack of experience and skill of the investigator, the small size of the crystals, and the low concentration of crystals in the SF. Reliable identification requires 10 μg/ml or higher levels of crystals in SF.[30] The clinician should, therefore, keep in mind that that there is a threshold for crystal identification, and a negative report can be a false negative. A second sample, or an SF sample from another joint or taken the next day, might reveal the diagnosis. MUSM and CPPD crystals can sometimes also be detected in SF from asymptomatic joints.[31] After a recent evaluation, the value of SF analysis in intercritical gout appears to be established as a reliable method for this diagnosis.[32] Although prompt examination of SF is preferred, postponement of this procedure in the case of diagnosing crystals does not seem to influence the accuracy. Studies have been published showing results of microscopic examination of SF that was refrigerated or deep frozen for many hours to months.[33] It was still possible to find crystals in 81 to 100 percent of the cases when samples were examined after 72 hours, if kept refrigerated, or stored at −80°C for more than months. Also, using a fast, alcoholic staining method originally designed for cytology (Diff Quick), MSUM and CPPD crystals could still be detected after 12 months. In this method, SF smears are air dried, stained, and coverslipped with a nonaqueous mounting medium. When compared to wet slide preparations, an overall sensitivity and specificity for both MSUM and CCPD crystal confirmation of 94.4 percent and 87.5 percent, respectively, was found.[34]

DETECTION OF BACTERIA BY CULTURE, GRAM STAINING, AND POLYMERASE CHAIN REACTION

Diagnosis of infectious arthritis is one of the main reasons to sample SF. The mainstay of this diagnosis is a positive culture, but unfortunately this can take days or even weeks for slow-growing pathogens. Cultures can also be negative when the pathogen is difficult to culture, because inappropriate culture media have been used, or due to logistic problems, such as prior exposure to antibiotics or bacteriostatic solutions, when aspirating the fluid. Sensitivity and specificity for culture are estimated to be 75 to 95 percent and more than 90 percent, respectively, in the case of nongonococcal infections without prior antibiotic treatment.[3] When antibiotics are used prior to culture, 30 to 80 percent of SF cultures give negative results.[35] Recently, BACTEC Peds Plus/F bottles (Becton Dickinson Diagnostic Instrument Systems, Sparks, MD) were compared with conventional methods (agar plates) for SF analysis, showing that the former system revealed more pathogens and contained fewer contaminants.[36] Because bacterial arthritis needs to be treated without delay, antibiotics must be administered as soon as possible, even while awaiting the results of the culture. Gram stain has the advantage of being rapidly available and easy to perform and interpret. The sensitivity was estimated to be 50 to 75 percent, but the specificity is quite high, especially for nongonococcal infection. For gonoccocal arthritis, it is less than 10 percent.[3]

Recently, the use of the polymerase chain reaction (PCR) has been evaluated in detecting bacterial DNA in the diagnosis and in monitoring therapy of infectious arthritis. By applying broad-range bacterial primers to analyze and amplify gene coding for ribosomal RNA (16S rRNA), most bacterial species can be detected. This method could be used successfully even when culture failed.[37,38] PCR might especially be helpful when antibiotic treatment has been initiated before SF was obtained for culture[39]; in case of slow-growing micro-organisms like mycobacteria[39]; or when *Borrelia*, *Chlamydia*, or *Neisseria* species is suspected.[40-42] Very stringent conditions are required because of the risk of false-positive results caused by contamination.[37] In addition, a positive result does not necessarily proof the presence of a viable or proliferating organism.

SYNOVIAL FLUID ANALYSIS FOR RESEARCH

With growing knowledge about potential factors influencing both inflammatory and noninflammatory joint diseases, many new assays are being developed. These assays are used as research tools, and their clinical value still needs to be defined.

Bone Degradation Markers

Increasing evidence suggests that bone and cartilage degradation markers in SF could predict the degree of bone and cartilage destruction in patients with inflammatory joint disease and osteoarthritis (see Chapter 50). Comparing such markers in SF of different patient groups might lead to a better understanding of the process of bone destruction in various conditions.[43] However, more studies are needed to assess the value of measuring biomarkers of bone and cartilage degradation in clinical practice.

Cytokine and Chemokine Levels

Assays measuring pro- and anti-inflammatory cytokine levels in SF have been of increasing interest. A variety of cytokines, mostly proinflammatory types such as interleukin (IL)-1, IL-6, IL-8, and tumor necrosis factor (TNF)-α, are present at higher levels in SF of patients with different arthritides. The value of these assays to provide diagnostic and prognostic markers still needs be determined. The same is true for chemokine and chemokine-receptor levels in SF. Several of the chemokines and their receptors, such as macrophage inflammatory protein-1 alpha (MIP-1 α) and macrophage inflammatory protein-1 beta (MIP-1 β) and regulated upon activation normal T cell expressed and secreted (RANTES), have been reported to be present in the SF in inflamed joints.

Other Tests

Measurement of soluble granzyme A and B, produced by cytotoxic T cells and natural killer (NK) cells, is significantly elevated in serum and SF of patients with RA compared with osteoarthritis (OA) and reactive arthritis.[44] Larger studies in early arthritis cohorts need to be performed to determine a possible role in differential diagnosis.

Synovial Biopsy

In the clinical setting, obtaining SF is preferred for rapid crystal and bacteriologic analysis. However, when SF cannot be aspirated, or in case of suspicion of neoplastic or granulomatous disease, deposition disease, or infection in spite of negative SF culture, synovial tissue (ST) examination can be of additional value.[45,46] Another reason for examining ST is to investigate the pathologic changes of the synovium for research purposes. Examination of ST samples has provided insight into the pathogenesis of various forms of arthritis by studies of the cell infiltrate and various mediators known to play a role in the inflammatory process. Of interest, synovial biopsies taken at an early stage of osteoarthritis also exhibit signs of inflammation, changing our view on disease mechanisms and possible targets for therapy in this disease.[47,48] Possible diagnostic and prognostic features are being identified in the synovium of patients with various arthritides and at different stages of disease. For instance, diagnosis of RA can be predicted with an accuracy of 85 percent when there is massive infiltration of plasma cells and macrophages in the synovial sublining. When there is only minimal infiltration of these cells, a diagnosis other than RA can be found in 97 percent of the cases.[46]

The discovery of specific characteristics of synovial inflammation has led to the identification of new therapeutic targets, such as TNF-α, IL-1, and chemokines and chemokine receptors for RA and spondylarthropathies. Also, studies of the changes in the synovium observed after targeted interventions have provided useful information about clinical efficacy, pharmacologic effect, and disease pathogenesis.[49,50] Examination of serial synovial biopsy samples might be useful as markers to determine the potential efficacy of new therapies (see Chapter 50). The highly significant correlation between macrophage infiltration and expression of macrophage-derived mediators of inflammation, on the one hand, and clinical signs and symptoms on the other, supports the view that the features of synovial inflammation might be used as alternative endpoints in early-phase clinical studies.[51]

METHODS TO OBTAIN SYNOVIAL BIOPSY SAMPLES

Early studies have used blind needle-biopsy techniques, for instance the Parker-Pearson needle, which is a simplified 14-gauge biopsy needle that does not require a skin incision.[52] Many investigators have used this method to obtain ST samples, mostly for diagnostic reasons. It is a well-tolerated, safe, inexpensive, and technically easy method that yields adequate tissue samples in most of the cases. It is important to note that measures of inflammation in tissue samples taken from clinically inflamed joints with the blind needle technique are generally similar to samples obtained by arthroscopy under vision.[53]

There are also limitations and disadvantages of the use of blind needle biopsy. It is usually restricted to larger joints, such as the knee joint; the operator is not able to visually select the tissue, causing potential sampling error; and it is not always possible to obtain adequate tissue samples. This is especially true when clinically quiescent joints are investigated(e.g., after successful therapy).

During the 1970s arthroscopy made its entrance in rheumatology (see also Chapter 48). Since then, technology has considerably improved, and the use of local and regional anesthetics have made this a safe, office-based procedure. A recent survey showed a rapid increase in the numbers of arthroscopies performed by rheumatologists in an outpatient setting.[54]

Although the technique is more complicated and more expensive than the blind needle biopsy, there are several advantages. First, arthroscopy allows macroscopic evaluation of the synovium. A positive correlation between the macroscopic signs of inflammation at the biopsy site and the immunohistologic features of inflammatory activity in the corresponding tissue sample has been observed.[55] However, it is not possible to predict in a reliable way the microscopic features of the inflamed synovium on the basis of the macroscopic appearance at arthroscopy. Previous reports have also suggested that macroscopic scoring systems could be used to distinguish different patient groups,[56,57] but these visual scoring systems still need to be validated. In addition, the evaluation of the articular cartilage by arthroscopy could potentially be used for the evaluation of the effects of treatment.[58]

A second advantage of arthroscopy over blind needle biopsy is that it is always possible to obtain tissue in adequate amounts, even when the ST volume has decreased as a result of effective treatment. Third, using narrow-diameter arthroscopes, small joints, such as ankles, wrists, and even metacarpophalangeal and proximal interphalangeal joints, can also be evaluated. This allows one to study the synovium in an early stage of disease because RA and other arthritides often begin in small joints.

Arthroscopy has also been used therapeutically. Various investigators have suggested a beneficial effect of arthroscopic joint lavage in arthritis.[59-61] However, a recent randomized, placebo-controlled trial revealed that this approach is not successful for treatment of osteoarthritis without clinical signs of inflammation.[62]

The arthroscopic procedure is well tolerated and has a low complication rate. Thirty-five percent of patients reported minimal pain or discomfort during the procedure.[59] Minor complications, such as vasovagal reactions and temporary swelling of the joint, were mentioned in 5 to 10 percent of cases. In a recent survey, in which information on 15,682 arthroscopies performed by rheumatologists was collected, the complication rate of hemarthrosis was 0.9 percent, deep vein thrombosis 0.2 percent, and wound and joint infection 0.1 percent. The total of complications reported was 15.1 per 1000 arthroscopies, which is comparable to the figures reported in the orthopedic literature.[54] The irrigation volume of the knee joint was positively correlated with the rate of wound infection and the total complication rate. A possible explanation for this is the extended length of the procedure.

HANDLING OF TISSUE

Depending on the reason for the biopsy procedure, diagnostic or for research, the tissue must be handled differently. For routine pathologic examination by light microscopy, the tissue samples should be fixed in 4-pecent formalin and embedded in paraffin. This can be used for hematoxylin and eosin staining and certain immunohistochemical stainings. When gout is suspected, the ST should be conserved in absolute alcohol because the monosodium urate crystals will dissolve in most other fixatives. Unstained sections can be examined with the polarization microscope, but using DeGolanthal stain for urate is also possible.

In the case of a suspected infection, the tissue should be kept in suitable culture media. Recent progress has been made in the use of PCR on synovial biopsies for detection of bacterial DNA (see previous discussion of this technique). DNA contamination needs be avoided, and the samples should be snap frozen in liquid nitrogen.

For research purposes ST can be processed for histology, immunohistochemical staining, immunofluorescense, in situ hybridization, PCR, microarray, and cell or tissue culture. Immunohistochemistry can be performed on formalin-fixed, paraffin-embedded material or on samples that were snap frozen in optical cutting temperature (OCT) embedding medium and stored in liquid nitrogen. Detection of mRNA is possible in samples that are snap frozen immediately after the tissue is obtained. It is also possible to culture synovial cell populations and whole biopsy samples[63] in tissue culture media.

TISSUE HETEROGENEITY AND BIOPSY SAMPLES

Several studies have suggested a degree of morphologic heterogeneity in ST samples taken from one joint.[55] Still, it is possible to quantify several markers of inflammation in a reliable way when examining a limited area of tissue.[64-66] For T cell infiltration and expression of activation antigens in RA synovium, a variance of less than 10 percent can be reached when at least six biopsy specimens are examined,[67] suggesting that representative data can be obtained when a limited number of biopsy samples from different areas within one joint are investigated. When the biopsies are taken from an actively inflamed joint, there is—on average—no difference in the features of synovial inflammation at the pannus-cartilage junction (the site of invasion of the inflamed ST into the cartilage and underlying bone) compared to other regions away from the pannus-cartilage junction.[68,69]

The signs of inflammation in tissue samples taken from inflamed small joints are generally comparable to those taken from larger joints, such as the knee,[70] indicating that the inflammation in one inflamed joint is representative of that in other inflamed joints. In contrast, there is large variability of synovial inflammation between different patients in all phases of the disease.[51,71,72] It is, therefore, important that the number of patients is sufficient when different conditions are being compared. In addition, patient cohorts should be stratified for disease activity and use of medication to allow meaningful conclusions based on analysis of synovial biopsies.

MEASURING SYNOVIAL INFLAMMATION

There are several methods to quantify the features of inflammation of ST. Conventional quantitative analysis by counting cells is a reliable, but time-consuming method, making it less suitable to evaluate large series of synovial tissue sections. Semiquantitative scoring of the tissue is reliable, more time efficient, and has been validated in several clinical studies.[51,53] Compared to cell counting, this method might be less sensitive in detection of small changes in mononuclear cell infiltration.[73] A third method, computerized image analysis, has the advantage of both being sensitive and time efficient.[74,75] It allows reliable analysis of the cell infiltrate and expression of adhesion molecules, matrix metalloproteinases, and cytokines in the synovium. With further refinement of computer systems and software, this method will be of increasing importance in evaluating the features of inflamed synovium.

Synovial Pathology

The synovium normally is comprised of a synovial lining layer (or intimal lining) that contains one to three layers of cells without an underlying basal membrane, which overlays the synovial stroma, also called the synovial sublining or subsynovium. The intimal lining layer lacks tight junctions and is discontinuous in some regions, resulting in direct contact between SF and synovial sublining. The intimal lining layer is formed by two types of cells: the intimal macrophages (also called macrophage-like synoviocytes or type A synoviocytes) and the fibroblast-like synoviocytes (also called type B synoviocytes).[76] The synovial sublining is formed by a loose collagen-fiber network with fibroblasts, fat cells, and scattered blood vessels.

Increased interest in the architecture and characteristics of inflamed synovium, especially in RA and OA, has lead to new insights into the pathology and function of cells involved in the disease process. Most of the data describe the changes of the synovium in RA, and tissue samples of other diseases, such as reactive arthritis and psoriatic arthritis, are typically used as controls. In general, the characteristics of synovium in patients with arthritis are highly variable.

RHEUMATOID ARTHRITIS

Hypertrophy and edema characterize the ST in RA. The intimal lining layer is hyperplastic, forming villi that protrude into the joint cavity. The inflamed synovium overgrows and invades the underlying cartilage and bone. At the junction between cartilage and synovium, the proliferating synovium is often referred as pannus. Here, specialized cell types have been identified, such as pannocytes and cells functionally resembling osteoclasts.[77] Pannocytes are rhomboid-shaped cells that show functional and morphologic characteristics of both fibroblast-like synoviocytes and chondrocytes, but it is still unclear whether these cells represent a separate lineage.[78,79]

The increased cellularity of the RA synovium is likely a result of enhanced migration of inflammatory cells into the synovium and local retention and proliferation of these cells, combined with impaired apoptosis. Little is known about the dynamics of cell migration in the rheumatoid synovium, but it appears that the continuous influx of inflammatory cells plays an important role in cell accumulation. In situ proliferation of fibroblast-like synoviocytes also contributes to some extent, although rates of cell division within the synovium are relatively low.[80,81] Various factors could be involved in defective apoptosis,[82] such as overexpression of anti-apoptotic proteins like sentrin, which could contribute to the modulation of Fas- and TNF-receptor (TNF-R)-mediated apoptosis in RA synovium and thereby extend the life span of invasive, cartilage-destructive fibroblast-like synoviocytes.[83] The antiapoptotic FLIP (FLICE-like inhibitory protein), expressed at high levels by macrophages in the RA synovium,[84,85] and IL-15[86] could also be involved in inhibition of apoptosis in the synovium. Additionally, it has been suggested that genotoxic changes due to the toxic microenvironment[87] and a deficient Fas-Fas ligand mechanism[88] could play a role.

Synovial histology in "early" RA (i.e., within the first few months of symptoms) is essentially the same as in long-standing RA.[89] Intimal lining layer hyperplasia, marked infiltration of the synovial sublining by inflammatory cells, increased vascularity, and edema are observed in all stages of the disease process. Of importance, systematic comparison of the features of the synovium in patients with (very) early RA to synovial tissue from patients with long-standing disease revealed that the characteristics were, on average, the same.[51,57] This could be explained by the observation that asymptomatic synovial inflammation may precede the development of RA.[90] The differences in cell infiltrate and in the expression of mediators of inflammation between early RA and long-standing disease, which are sometimes reported, can often be explained by differences in disease activity and medication.

Intimal Lining Layer

Intimal Macrophages

In RA two thirds of the intimal lining layer is formed by macrophages. These macrophages are activated, expressing a variety of cytokines, such as IL-1, TNF-α, granulocyte macrophage colony-stimulating factor (GM-CSF), IL-15, and IL-18,[91,92] adhesion molecules,[93,94] and matrix metalloproteinases.[95,96] They exhibit phagocytic capacity and carry lysosomes, granular structures called residual bodies, and vacuoles. Specific markers, such as CD68, CD97, FcRIIIa, myeloid-related proteins (MRP)-8 and -14, and nonspecific esterase, are strongly expressed by (subsets of) these cells in RA[97-99] (Fig. 46–2). Recently, high mobility group box chromosomal protein-1 (HMGB-1), a ubiquitous chromatin component expressed in nucleated mammalian cells, was found to be expressed intracellularly as well as in the extracellular matrix by cells with a macrophage phenotype in the ST of RA patients. HMGB 1 is expressed by stimulated mononuclear phagocytes and acts as a potent factor that causes inflammation and protease activation.[100] In addition to these markers, macrophages also express human leukocyte antigen (HLA) class II molecules and intercellular adhesion molecule (ICAM)-1,[101] again reflecting their highly activated state and suggesting a role in cell–cell interaction. Intimal lining macrophages express CD14, although the cellular expression is reduced in association with activation.[102]

The accumulation of intimal macrophages is thought to be the result of recruitment of bone marrow–derived monocytes from the blood stream, which enter the synovial sublining through endothelial cells.[103,104] Chemotactic factors are produced by activated macrophages, fibroblast-like synoviocytes, and other cells in the inflamed ST and contribute to further cell recruitment. Of the chemokine family, monocyte chemoattractant protein (MCP)-1, RANTES, MIP-1α and -2α, and epithelial neutrophil activator (ENA)-78 have been associated with monocyte recruitment.[105,106] Also, C5a and C3a and their receptors (C5aR, C3aR) show chemoattractive capacities and are present in the ST and SF of RA patients. In a model of experimental arthritis, genetic deletion of C5aR completely protected mice from arthritis, indicating a pivotal role for this complement receptor in cell recruitment in this model.[107]

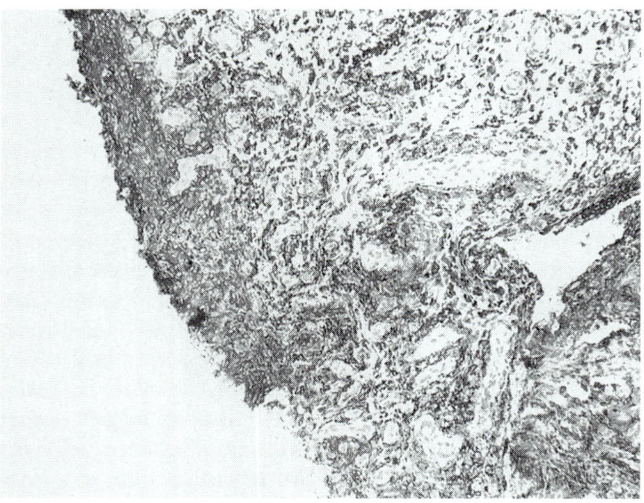

FIGURE 46–2 · Activated macrophages expressing CD68 (red-brown) in the intimal lining layer and in the sublining layer of rheumatoid synovial tissue. (×100.) (See color plate 10.)

Fibroblast-like Synoviocytes

The fibroblast-like synoviocyte is very specific to the intimal lining layer. This cell type, presumably derived from mesenchymal origin,[76] appears to be in a highly activated state, producing a variety of cytokines, matrix metalloproteinases, cysteine proteinases, proteoglycans, and arachidonic acid metabolites.[108] The marked expression of CD55 and vascular cell adhesion molecule (VCAM)-1 differentiates them from other fibroblasts.[109,110] The accumulation of these cells in the intimal lining layer is thought to be caused by a combination of impaired apoptosis, some in situ proliferation, and possible migration and differentiation of mesenchymal cells from the synovial sublining into the intimal lining layer.[84,108,111] The fibroblast-like synoviocytes could invade the cartilage and possibly bone, promoting joint degradation.[108] Somatic mutations in the p53 suppressor gene might explain, in part, the aggressive behavior of fibroblast-like synoviocytes, although the relative contribution to the disease process remains to be clarified.[87] Other cells occasionally found in the RA intimal lining layer include multinucleated or polynuclear synovio-genous giant cells, derived from ST monocytes,[112] and rare T cells, especially when synovial hyperplasia is severe.

Synovial Sublining Layer

Although normally there are only a few cells present in the tissue underlying the intimal lining layer, excessive cell infiltration, proliferation of blood vessels, and edema cause the synovial sublining to be markedly thickened in RA. The cells found in this layer are mainly T cells, plasma cells, and macrophages. Mast cells, NK cells, dendritic cells, and neutrophils are also found, but not in large quantities.

T Cells

Although not pathognomic for RA, T lymphocytes are found in aggregates in 50 to 60 percent of RA patients. These aggregates resemble germinal centers, as found in lymphoid tissue, containing mainly CD4+ T cells in association with B cells, a few CD8+ T cells, and large interdigitating dendritic cells. It has recently been suggested that the CD8+ T cells are involved in the structural integrity and functional activity of the lymphocyte aggregates[113] (Fig. 46–3).

Adjacent to the aggregates, the endothelial cells of the postcapillary venules are larger and resemble high endothelial venules. The microarchitecture suggests that this is an area where antigen presentation and

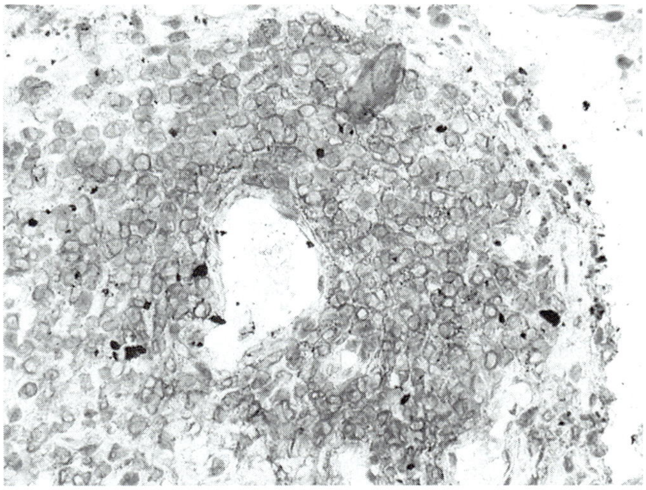

FIGURE 46–3 • CD4+ T cells in a lymphocytic aggregate in the sublining layer of rheumatoid synovial tissue. (×400.) (See color plate 11.)

local synovial B cell maturation takes place.[114] The CD4+ T cells found in these areas are of the CD45RA-CD45RO+ memory subtype, suggesting earlier antigen exposure either in the periphery or in the ST. These memory T cells have greater migratory capacity and accumulate at sites of inflammation.[115] The close relationship of the T cells with interdigitating cells suggests (mutual) interaction between these two cell types, which may lead to activation and cytokine production. In addition, membrane contact between synovial T cells and synovial macrophages could enhance proinflammatory cytokine production, such as TNF-α,[116,117] in these regions.

The CD4+CD45RO+ memory T cells may also express CD27, which, together with its ligand CD70, plays a role in T cell proliferation,[118] the generation of T cell memory,[119] and B cell help.[120] Interestingly, the majority of the CD4+ T cells found in the lymphocyte aggregates are predominantly CD27+.[121] These cells are thought to be attracted from the peripheral blood into the rheumatoid ST, where further activation and differentiation into CD4+CD45RO+CD27 cells follows.[121] Their close relationship with B cells and interdigitating dendritic cells suggests a role in the activation and maturation of lymphocytes in the aggregates.

T cells can also be found diffusely scattered throughout the ST of patients with RA. Many of these are CD8+ T cells, with a relative increase in the percentage of CD27– cells,[121] suggesting that these cells are antigen-induced cytotoxic effector cells.[122] Previous work has shown that there is an increase in cytototoxic effector cells in the synovial compartment of RA of patients, which may be involved in promoting synovial inflammation and joint damage.[44,123]

B Cells and Plasma Cells

Less than 5 percent of synovial lymphocytes in RA are B cells. They are mainly found in close relation with the CD4+ cells when lymphocytic aggregates are present.[124] This spatial relationship might be a reflection of their role (i.e., giving B cell help, leading to production of immunoglobulins).[125,126] T cell activation in RA ST may be, in part, dependent on B cells.[127] When CD4+ T cells from RA ST were adoptively transferred in the severe combined immune deficient (SCID) mouse model to ST with CD20+ B cell clusters, the T cells became activated, whereas this was not the case in tissues lacking B cells.[127] Furthermore, elimination of B cells from the RA ST abrogated T cell activation and the production of proinflammatory cytokines. Particularly RF-positive B cells are able to act like antigen-presenting cells, and they might be able to activate T cells by capturing antigens with their immunoglobulin (Ig) receptors.[128,129]

Plasma cells may surround the lymphocyte aggregates in large numbers in so-called coronas, but they are also found scattered throughout the synovium[51,130] (Fig. 46–4). The detection of clonally related plasma cells within single infiltrates suggests that these cells underwent terminal differentiation within the synovium.[131] The plasma cells are probably mainly derived from B cells that have migrated from the circulation. They may be long lived and, thus, accumulate in the synovial tissue where they are a major source of autoantibodies.[132,133]

Sublining Macrophages

The macrophages found in the synovial sublining can form the majority of the inflammatory cells in the rheumatoid ST[51,68] and can be distinguished by high expression of CD68 and CD163.[134] CD163 could be a more specific macrophage marker, with the exception of the cells near the lymphocyte aggregates, where downregulation of CD163 has been observed.[134] The sublining macrophages are derived from circulating monocytes and are found in areas adjacent to the articular cartilage, as well as a distance from the cartilage-pannus junction[53,68] (Fig. 46–5). The migration to these specific areas is probably the result of chemotactic fac-

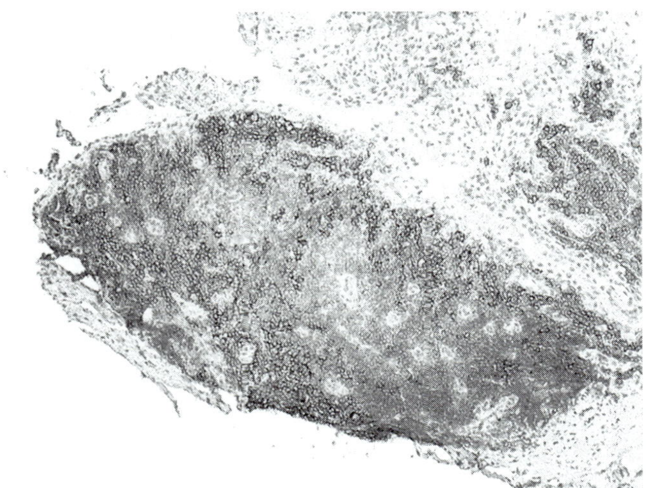

FIGURE 46–4 • Plasma cells, expressing CD38 (red-brown), surrounding a lymphocyte aggregate in the sublining layer of rheumatoid synovial tissue. This architecture is also called corona. (×100.) (See color plate 12.)

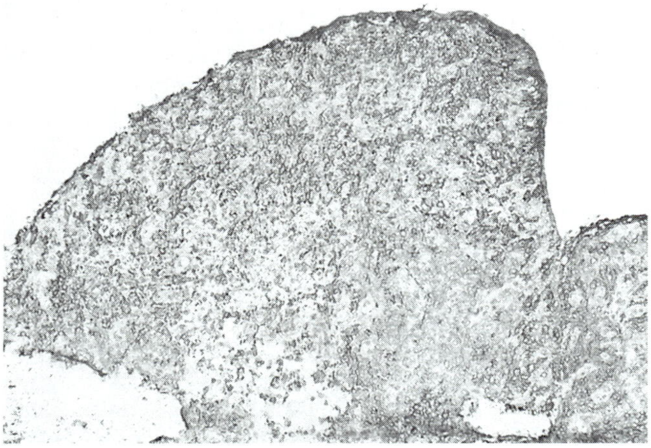

FIGURE 46–5 · CD163+ macrophages in the intimal lining and sublining layer of rheumatoid synovial tissue. (×100.) (See color plate 13.)

tors, such as chemokines and adhesion molecules, that are highly expressed in the RA synovium. The synovial macrophages display an activated phenotype, expressing several activation markers and secreting a variety of proinflammatory mediators.[103] Of interest is the recent observation that the majority of the CD68+ macrophages in rheumatoid ST, but not in synovium of OA or trauma patients, may express the recently described dendritic cell marker dendritic cell specific I-CAM3 grabbing nonintegrin (DC-SIGN).[135] These cells are found in close association with ICAM-3–positive T cells, which are able to bind to DC-SIGN–positive cells and might be involved in the production of degrading enzymes. The importance of synovial macrophages in the disease process is supported by the clinical observation that macrophage numbers in the synovium are associated with clinical signs of disease activity.[51]

Mast Cells

The rheumatoid synovium contains an increased number of mast cells, compared to normal synovium and ST of patients with other rheumatic diseases.[51,136,137] These cells are found in perivascular regions, around the lymphocytic aggregates, at the cartilage-pannus junction, and perhaps in contact with nerves.[138,139] ST mast cells are in an activated state, expressing cell surface antigens, cytokine receptors, and adhesion molecules, and they produce potent mediators, including histamine; proteinases, such as tryptase and chymase; cytokines; and growth factors.[140,141] Their localized accumulation at cartilage erosion sites in combination with the expression of potent mediators of inflammation suggests that mast cells contribute to the inflammatory process in the rheumatoid lesion.[142]

Natural Killer Cells

NK cells are found in increased numbers the RA ST. Because of the abundance of different cell surface markers expressed by various subpopulations, characterizing these cells morphologically and functionally has been difficult. There are, however, functional markers carried by all activated NK subtypes (e.g., granzymes, which can be detected in specialized granules in NK cells and cytotoxic T cells).[143-145] Compared to other forms of arthritis, granzyme-positive cells are found in increased numbers in the RA ST in both the intimal lining layer and in the synovial sublining, as well as at the pannus-cartilage junction.[68,146-148] Furthermore, a special subset of CD4+T cells carrying receptors that regulate NK cells is present in the ST.[149] These T cells could bridge functions of the innate and adaptive immune systems, such as responsiveness to specific antigens, rapid release of interferon-γ, and cytotoxicity.

Dendritic Cells

Two types of dendritic cells, the interdigitating and follicular dendritic cell, are found in the synovial sublining of RA patients. The interdigitating dendritic cells (IDC), known as the most potent antigen-presenting cells, are found close to CD4+ T cells in the perivascular lymphocytic aggregates.[150-152] Mature and immature IDCs migrate from the blood, and possibly through the intimal lining layer, into the synovial sublining, attracted by chemokines.[153] Under influence of cytokines, such as GM-CSF and TNF-α, IDCs differentiate from precursor cells of the myeloid and probably lymphoid lineage into mature IDCs.[154-156] They have an activated phenotype, expressing HLA class II molecules, adhesion molecules, CC-chemokine receptor (CCR)7, and costimulatory molecules, such as CD80 and CD86. CD86 is a costimulatory molecule that plays an important role in antigen presentation.[157,158] Recently, the expression of nuclear RelB by differentiated IDCs was demonstrated.[159] These data suggest that, after differentiation in the RA ST, the activated IDCs may present antigen to CD4+ T cells in the perivascular lymphocyte aggregates. Although it still remains unclear what kind of antigens are being presented, potential candidates include exogenous antigens, such as bacterial[160,161] or viral,[162] and endogenous autoantigens.[156,163,164]

The second type of dendritic cells in the synovium is the follicular dendritic cells (FDC). The FDCs may be derived from fibroblastic reticulum cells rather than from bone marrow–derived cells.[165] Of interest, when fibroblast-like synoviocytes are cultured in vitro, some cell lines may be induced to express the FDC phenotype.[166,167] The FDCs are mainly present in the proximity of B cells in the lymphocyte aggregates and close to the intimal lining layer.[155,168,169] They can be found in close association with CD4+ T cells and B cells, especially when the perivascular lymphocytic aggregates are large. As noted previously, the aggregates are surrounded by large fields of plasma cells. FDCs are thought to play an important role in the accumulation and differentiation of B cells into plasma cells.

Neutrophils

Although the neutrophils constitute the majority of inflammatory cells in the SF, only a few neutrophils are present in the ST, mainly in fibrin depositions.[51] Little is known about the dynamics of neutrophil migration through the synovium into the SF compartment.

SPONDYLARTHROPATHIES

The synovia of patients with spondylarthropathies share many features with RA tissue.[170] Still, some differences in the architecture and types of inflammatory cells and their products can be found. These might reflect a difference in the etiology of synovitis of these disease entities.

Ankylosing Spondylitis

Information about the features of synovial tissue in various forms of seronegative spondylarthropathy is limited compared to RA. One issue complicating the interpretation of the literature is the fact that many reports describe different spondylarthropathies as one group despite differences in their respective pathogeneses.

Early studies of ankylosing spondylitis (AS) ST suggested that the changes were indistinguishable from those seen in RA. Clear intimal cell hyperplasia with largely macrophage, as well as diffuse lymphocyte and plasma cell infiltration, and occasionally formation of lymphocyte aggregates, can be found. However, compared to RA ST, the intimal lining layer hyperplasia is less pronounced, with an average cell depth of only three.[171] Also, mononuclear cell infiltration even more intense than in RA and psoriatic arthritis has been observed in the ST of patients with peripheral arthritis in AS.[171] Large fields of plasma cells can be detected in AS ST,[171] although the percentage of IgM-containing cells appears to be lower in AS than in RA.[172] CD4+ cells clearly outnumber CD8+ T cells in RA, but apparently not in AS. In contrast, the CD4:CD8 ratio was reportedly 1:6 in a small group of AS patients with peripheral arthritis.[171]

T cells appear to play a pivotal role in the pathogenesis of AS and other spondylarthropathies, but their role might be different than that in RA.[173] In several studies, the expression of T helper type 1 (Th1)-like cytokines, such as interferon-γ (IFN-γ) and IL-2, and T helper type 2 (Th2) cytokines such as IL-4, IL-5, and IL-10, has been examined. These studies have shown a decreased Th1:Th2 ratio in seronegative spondylarthropathies compared to RA.[174]

The synovium of the inflamed sacroiliac joint of patients with AS contains infiltrating T cells and macrophages.[175] Also, diffuse expression of mRNA for TNF-α was found, whereas mRNA for transforming growth factor (TGF-β), a cytokine with mainly anti-inflammatory properties, was absent in these same areas.[176] TGF-β was found near the bone, where it could play a role in the formation of new bone formation.

Reactive Arthritis

Compared to RA tissue, the changes in the ST of patients with reactive arthritis show significantly less infiltration by T and B lymphocytes, CD 38+ plasma cells, and granzyme B + cytotoxic cells, regardless of disease duration.[147] Analysis of the cytokine profile has shown that the expression of IFN-γ–positive T cells is lower in ST of reactive arthritis patients, whereas IL-2, IL-10, and IL-4 expression do not differ significantly, resulting in a decreased Th1:Th2 ratio compared to RA.[147,177] Conceivably, this might be explained in part by the lower IL-15 levels in the reactive arthritis ST, because this cytokine plays a pivotal role in migration and activation of T cells.[178,179] The fact that fewer granzyme B+ cytotoxic cells are present in reactive arthritis, compared to RA, seems to be a specific feature.[44,147] Because granzyme B is capable of degrading the extracellular matrix of cartilage,[180,181] this could be one of the explanations why reactive arthritis is not as destructive as RA.

The role of arthritogenic bacteria and their interaction with the host is of fundamental importance in the pathogenesis of reactive arthritis. The synovial cavity is accessible to (fragments of) micro-organisms, either by bacteremia or by transport within monocytes or lymphoid cells. Bacterial DNA, messenger and ribosomal RNA, and bacterial cell wall fragments have been demonstrated with PCR and immunohistochemical techniques in arthritic joints of reactive arthritis patients.[37,182] These intra-articular microbial components may trigger a sterile acute inflammatory reaction or give rise to a chronic inflammatory process, probably depending on the host defense and specific bacterial characteristics.

Psoriatic Arthritis

Previous work has suggested that the appearance of the ST of patients with psoriatic arthritis differs from RA ST macroscopically. Higher intensity of villous vascularization with typical morphology, described as tortuosity, has been reported by macroscopic evaluation of the ST in psoriatic arthritis.[56,57] Although these vascular changes may be prominent in some patients with psoriatic arthritis, they are also seen in RA to a lesser degree. Endothelial cell swelling and marked thickening of the vessel walls has already been observed in the ST of psoriatic arthritis patients by both light and electron microscopy,[183] and this was later confirmed by immunohistochemical techniques.[184] However, another study could not detect significant differences in vascularity between RA, reactive arthritis, and psoriatic arthritis ST.[185]

Intimal lining layer hyperplasia in psoriatic arthritis may be less pronounced compared to RA. Conflicting results have been published about cell infiltration in the synovial sublining of psoriatic arthritis patients,[184,186,187] perhaps due to patient selection or the differences in microscopic evaluation of the tissue. T lymphocytes, thought to play an important role in the pathogenesis of psoriasis, are present in similar numbers in psoriatic arthritis as in RA ST.[187] In another study, CD3+, CD4+, CD20+ cells, and lymphocyte aggregates were reportedly less abundant in psoriatic arthritis than in RA ST.[57] The fact that novel T cell–specific therapies have a beneficial effect on synovial inflammation in psoriatic arthritis clearly supports the hypothesis that T cell activation plays an important role in this disease.[188] Interestingly, treatment with alefacept, a T cell–specific agent inhibiting the CD2–lymphocyte function associated antigen (CD2–LFA) interaction, led to decre-ased macrophage infiltration in the ST of psoriatic arthritis patients,[188] supporting the view that macro-phage infiltration and activation is T cell dependent in this condition.

The expression of TNF-α and IL-15 appears to be lower in psoriatic synovium than in RA, even after correction for the number of macrophages.[187] This could suggest that these proinflammatory cytokines are perhaps less important in psoriatic arthritis than in RA. In contrast with these observations are the results of studies with infliximab and eternacept, TNF-α-directed therapies that are effective in psoriatic arthritis patients. Examination of the ST before and after treatment with infliximab showed decreased intimal lining layer hyperplasia, reduced vascularity, and inhibition of neutrophil and macrophage infiltration of the psoriatic arthritis ST.[189]

Inflammatory Osteoarthritis

Although OA is traditionally considered a noninflammatory arthropathy, synovial inflammation is a well-known feature of this disease.[47] Inflammatory osteoarthritis refers to the situation of marked synovial inflammation in OA, commonly associated with more destructive disease; elevated C-reactive protein (CRP); and the presence of morning stiffness. Intimal lining layer hyperplasia, increased numbers of inflammatory cells in the synovial sublining, and increased vascularity are all found in the osteoarthritic ST, but these changes are less prominent than in RA.[48,190] These changes are not only seen in patients with advanced osteoarthritis, but also in early stages of the disease.[47] This inflammatory reaction of the ST is believed to be secondary to the release of breakdown products of cartilage and bone, perpetuating inflammation and leading to progression of the structural changes. Production of proinflammatory cytokines, in particular IL-1β and TNF-α, growth factors, and matrix metalloproteinases, has an important role in the pathogenesis of OA.[191] These factors are produced by macrophages, T lymphocytes, and other cells in the synovium, as well as by chondrocytes.[192,193] Taken together, these results strongly suggest that OA is in part an inflammatory disease.

SYNOVIAL PATHOLOGY OF OTHER DISEASES

Little has been published about the specific pathology of the synovium in other autoimmune diseases, such as systemic lupus erythematosus (SLE). The histopathologic changes found in ST of patients with SLE arthritis are not specific, but there is generally less intimal lining layer hyperplasia and less infiltration by inflammatory cells in the synovial sublining layer compared to other forms of arthritis.[194,195]

Two patients with polyarteritis and arthritis of the knee joint associated with cutaneous polyarteritis have been described.[196] Necrotizing inflammation was not seen in the small vessels observed in the ST.

In bacterial arthritis, Gram stain of the ST can sometimes reveal bacteria. Culture of ST biopsies can sometimes be of importance in the diagnostic workup, when blood and SF cultures are negative. Especially in the case of chronic infections, such as tuberculosis and fungal infections, the possibility of culturing synovial biopsy specimens should be considered. The histologic changes found in tuberculosis show nonspecific intimal lining layer hyperplasia, and sometimes granulomas. The use of mycobacterial genus-specific PCR applied on DNA extracts isolated directly from joint samples may be employed as an additional diagnostic tool in the case of clinical suspicion of a mycobacterial infection.

In gout and pseudogout, tophus-like deposits can be found in the synovial membrane and cartilage.[197] This may reveal the diagnosis in occasional cases when SF analysis is negative. As described previously, urate crystals will dissolve in formalin, and special precautions should be taken to demonstrate these crystals.

In amyloidosis, often associated with long-term hemodialysis and RA, amyloid deposits may be found in synovial biopsy samples. Amyloid appears pink on hematoxylin-eosin staining and red with Congo red. The amyloid deposits can be surrounded by macrophages, multinucleated giant cells, and granulation tissue. In cases with marked inflammation, phagocytosis and degradation of amyloid deposits by multinucleated giant cells can be observed.[198] Amyloid can promote cartilage and bone destruction, causing irregularities in the articular surface, bone cysts, and cortical erosions.[199]

The ST in ochronosis exhibits granular or shard-shaped pigment in the ST, articular cartilage, and subchondral tissue. The dispersed pigment can also be seen in the SF; occasionally black fragments of ochronotic cartilage are seen floating in the fluid.[200] Macrophages adjacent to the cartilage fragments often show pigment granules.[201] Erosions near shards and fibrosis of the cartilage edge may be observed. Chondrocytes and the intracellular matrix also contain pigment. The collagen fibrils are altered and appear wavy or fragmented with loss of periodicity. They are always mixed with the dispersed pigment.[202,203] In hemochromatosis, hemosiderin pigment deposited in the intimal lining layer, as well as in the macrophages of the sublining layer, can be detected.[204,205] Similar abnormalities can also be found after recurrent hemarthrosis.

Of the proliferative disorders originating from the joint tissues, pigmented villonodular synovitis (PVNS) and synovial chondromatosis are the most common. Other neoplasms arising in the joint are very rare. They include synovial chondrosarcomas, synovial hemangiomas, lipoma aborescens, and intracapsular chondromas.

Three forms of PVNS have been described: with localization in the tendon sheaths (also called giant cell tumor of the tendon sheath), as a solitary intra-articular nodule, and a diffuse villous and pigmented lesion of the synovial membrane. Histologically, all three forms are characterized by hypercellular subsynovial connective tissue protruding into the joint cavity, forming nodules and villi (Fig. 46–6). No hyperplasia of the intimal lining layer is seen in this condition. The synovial sublining contains a dense infiltrate of polygonal or spindle cells with abundant cytoplasm and vesicular nuclei. Multinucleated giant cells are sometimes

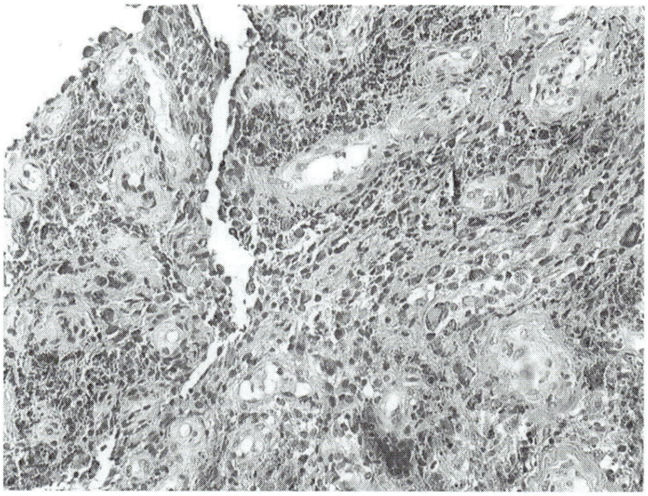

FIGURE 46–6 · Synovial tissue showing pigmented villonodularis synovitis. (H&E, ×200.) (See color plate 14.)

present, either scarcely distributed or in large numbers. Aggregation of foamy cells can also be seen. Abundant production of collagen, fibrosis, and hyalinization may be evident in patients with long-standing disease.[206] Hemosiderin-laden macrophages cause the rusty brown color of the ST, which is more commonly observed in the diffuse form.

Synovial chondromatosis can be primary or secondary—associated with an underlying joint disease, such as osteoarthritis. Mesenchymal cells from the synovial sublining differentiate into chondroblasts and form islands of cartilage that can be seen on gross examination of the synovium. Microscopically, cartilage nodules in different sizes and stages of maturation can be found. The nodules may undergo ossification and become detached from the synovial membrane, forming loose bodies in the joint cavity.

Synovial metastases from distant neoplasms are very uncommon. Of the patients reported in the literature, the knee is the most common joint involved, and the lung the most common site of the primary tumor. Joint metastases carries a poor prognosis with a mean survival of less than 5 months.[207] Synovial involvement of lymphoreticular malignancy is also rare.

REFERENCES

1. Goldenberg DL: Septic arthritis. Lancet 351(9097):197-202, 1998.
2. Weston VC, Jones AC, Bradbury N, et al: Clinical features and outcome of septic arthritis in a single UK Health District 1982-1991. Ann Rheum Dis 58(4):214-219, 1999.
3. Shmerling RH: Synovial fluid analysis: a critical reappraisal. Rheum Dis Clin North Am 20(2):503-512, 1994.
4. Swan A, Amer H, Dieppe P: The value of synovial fluid assays in the diagnosis of joint disease: a literature survey. Ann Rheum Dis 61(6):493-498, 2002.
5. Li-Yu J, Clayburne GM, Sieck MS, et al: Calcium apatite crystals in synovial fluid rice bodies. Ann Rheum Dis 61(5):387-390, 2002.
6. McCarthy DJ, Cheung HS: Origin and significance of rice bodies in synovial fluid. Lancet 2(8300):715-716, 1982.
7. Simkin PA: Synovial perfusion and synovial fluid solutes. Ann Rheum Dis 54(5):424-428, 1995.
8. Wallis WJ, Simkin PA, Nelp WB: Protein traffic in human synovial effusions. Arthritis Rheum 30(1):57-63, 1987.
9. Blake DR, Merry P, Unsworth J, et al: Hypoxic-reperfusion injury in the inflamed human joint. Lancet 1(8633):289-293, 1989.
10. Geborek P, Forslind K, Wollheim FA: Direct assessment of synovial blood flow and its relation to induced hydrostatic pressure changes. Ann Rheum Dis 48(4):281-286, 1989.
11. Simkin PA, Bassett JE, Koh EM: Synovial perfusion in the human knee: a methodologic analysis. Semin Arthritis Rheum 25(1): 56-66,1995.
12. Hasselbacher P: Measuring synovial fluid viscosity with a white blood cell diluting pipette: a simple, rapid,and reproducible method. Arthritis Rheum 19(6):1358-1362, 1976.
13. Sibley JT, Harth M, Burns DE: The mucin clot test and the synovial fluid rheumatoid factor as diagnostic criteria in rheumatoid arthritis. J Rheumatol 10(6):889-893, 1983.
14. Ropes MWBW: Synovial fluid Changes in Joint Disease. Cambridge, Mass., Harvard University Press, 1953.
15. Shmerling RH, Delbanco TL, Tosteson AN, Trentham DE: Synovial fluid tests: what should be ordered? JAMA 264(8): 1009-1014, 1990.
16. Hasselbacher P: Variation in synovial fluid analysis by hospital laboratories. Arthritis Rheum 30(6):637-642, 1987.
17. Ravaud P, Hudry C, Giraudeau B, et al: Rapid diagnosis of inflammatory synovial fluid with reagent strips. Rheumatology (Oxford) 41(7):815-818, 2002.
18. Salinas M, Rosas J, Iborra J, et al: Comparison of manual and automated cell counts in EDTA preserved synovial fluids: storage has little influence on the results. Ann Rheum Dis 56(10): 622-626, 1997.
19. Madea B, Kreuser C, Banaschak S: Postmortem biochemical examination of synovial fluid: a preliminary study. Forensic Sci Int 118(1):29-35, 2001.
20. MacSween RN, Dalakcs TK, Jasani MK, Buchanan WW: Rheumatoid factor in serum and synovial fluid. Scand J Rheumatol 1(4):177-180, 1972.
21. Neumann E, Barnum SR, Tarner IH, et al: Local production of complement proteins in rheumatoid arthritis synovium. Arthritis Rheum 46(4):934-945, 2002.
22. Guc D, Gulati P, Lemercier C, et al: Expression of the components and regulatory proteins of the alternative complement pathway and the membrane attack complex in normal and diseased synovium. Rheumatol Int 13(4):139-146, 1993.
23. Freemont AJ, Denton J: Atlas of Synovial Fluid Cytopathology: Current Histopathology. Dordrecht, Kluwer Academic, 1991.
24. Phelps P, Steele AD, McCarty DJ Jr: Compensated polarized light microscopy: identification of crystals in synovial fluids from gout and pseudogout. JAMA 203(7):508-512, 1968.
25. Ivorra J, Rosas J, Pascual E: Most calcium pyrophosphate crystals appear as non-birefringent. Ann Rheum Dis 58(9):582-584, 1999.
26. Dieppe P, Swan A: Identification of crystals in synovial fluid. Ann Rheum Dis 58(5):261-263, 1999.
27. Reginato AJ, Falasca GF Usmani Q: Do we really need to pay attention to the less common crystals? Curr Opin Rheumatol 11(5):446-452, 1999.
28. Schumacher HR, Reginato AJ: Atlas of Synovial Fluid Analysis and Crystal Identification. Philadelphia, London, Lea and Febiger, 1991.
29. Paul H, Reginato AJ, Schumacher HR: Alizarin red S staining as a screening test to detect calcium compounds in synovial fluid. Arthritis Rheum 26(2):191-200, 1983.
30. Gordon C, Swan A, Dieppe P: Detection of crystals in synovial fluids by light microscopy: sensitivity and reliability. Ann Rheum Dis 48(9):737-742, 1989.
31. Pascual E, Jovani V: A quantitative study of the phagocytosis of urate crystals in the synovial fluid of asymptomatic joints of patients with gout. Br J Rheumatol 34(8):724-726, 1995.
32. Pascual E, Batlle-Gualda E, Martinez A, et al: Synovial fluid analysis for diagnosis of intercritical gout. Ann Intern Med 131(10):756-759, 1999.
33. Galvez J, Saiz E, Linares LF, et al: Delayed examination of synovial fluid by ordinary and polarised light microscopy to detect and identify crystals. Ann Rheum Dis 61(5):444-447, 2002.
34. Selvi E, Manganelli S, Catenaccio M, et al Diff Quik staining method for detection and identification of monosodium urate and

calcium pyrophosphate crystals in synovial fluids. Ann Rheum Dis 60(3):194-198, 2001.

35. Freemont AJ: Synovial fluid analysis: its place, usefulness, indications, and potential relevant findings. Rheumato Eur 24:69-71, 1995.
36. Hughes JG, Vetter EA, Patel R, et al: Culture with BACTEC Peds Plus/F bottle compared with conventional methods for detection of bacteria in synovial fluid. J Clin Microbiol 39(12):4468-4471, 2001.
37. Wilbrink B, van der Heijden, I, Schouls LM, et al: Detection of bacterial DNA in joint samples from patients with undifferentiated arthritis and reactive arthritis, using polymerase chain reaction with universal 16S ribosomal RNA primers. Arthritis Rheum 41(3):535-543, 1998.
38. Jalava J, Skurnik M, Toivanen A, et al: Bacterial PCR in the diagnosis of joint infection. Ann Rheum Dis 60(3):287-289, 2001.
39. van der Heijden, I, Wilbrink B, Vije AE, et al: Detection of bacterial DNA in serial synovial samples obtained during antibiotic treatment from patients with septic arthritis. Arthritis Rheum 42(10):2198-2203, 1999.
40. Nikkari S, Puolakkainen M, Yli-Kerttula U, et al: Ligase chain reaction in detection of Chlamydia DNA in synovial fluid cells. Br J Rheumatol 36(7):763-765, 1997.
41. Muralidhar B, Rumore PM, Steinman CR: Use of the polymerase chain reaction to study arthritis due to Neisseria gonorrhoeae. Arthritis Rheum 37(5):710-717, 1994.
42. van der Heijden, I, Wilbrink B, Rijpkema SG, et al: Detection of Borrelia burgdorferi sensu stricto by reverse line blot in the joints of Dutch patients with Lyme arthritis. Arthritis Rheum 42(7):1473-1480, 1999.
43. Mansson B, Gulfe A, Geborek P, et al: Release of cartilage and bone macromolecules into synovial fluid: differences between psoriatic arthritis and rheumatoid arthritis. Ann Rheum Dis 60(1):27-31, 2001.
44. Tak PP, Spaeny-Dekking L, Kraan MC, et al: The levels of soluble granzyme A and B are elevated in plasma and synovial fluid of patients with rheumatoid arthritis (RA). Clin Exp Immunol 116(2):366-370, 1999.
45. Johnson JS, Freemont AJ: A 10 year retrospective comparison of the diagnostic usefulness of synovial fluid and synovial biopsy examination. J Clin Pathol 54(8):605-607, 2001.
46. Kraan MC, Haringman JJ, Post WJ, et al: Immunohistological analysis of synovial tissue for differential diagnosis in early arthritis. Rheumatology (Oxford) 38(11):1074-1080, 1999.
47. Smith MD, Triantafillou S, Parker A, et al: Synovial membrane inflammation and cytokine production in patients with early osteoarthritis. J Rheumatol 24(2):365-371, 1997.
48. Haraoui B, Pelletier JP, Cloutier JM, et al: Synovial membrane histology and immunopathology in rheumatoid arthritis and osteoarthritis: in vivo effects of antirheumatic drugs. Arthritis Rheum 34(2):153-163, 1991.
49. Bresnihan B, Tak PP, Emery P, et al: Synovial biopsy in arthritis research: five years of concerted European collaboration. Ann Rheum Dis 59(7):506-511, 2000.
50. Tak PP: Lessons learnt from the synovial tissue response to antirheumatic treatment. Rheumatology (Oxford) 39(8):817-820, 2000.
51. Tak PP, Smeets TJ, Daha MR, et al: Analysis of the synovial cell infiltrate in early rheumatoid synovial tissue in relation to local disease activity. Arthritis Rheum 40(2):217-225, 1997.
52. Parker HR, Pearson CM: A simplified synovial biopsy needle. Arthritis Rheum 6:172-176, 1963.
53. Youssef PP, Kraan M, Breedveld F, et al: Quantitative microscopic analysis of inflammation in rheumatoid arthritis synovial membrane samples selected at arthroscopy compared with samples obtained blindly by needle biopsy. Arthritis Rheum 41(4):663-669, 1998.
54. Kane D, Veale DJ, Fitzgerald O, Reece R: Survey of arthroscopy performed by rheumatologists. Rheumatology (Oxford) 41(2): 210-215, 2002.
55. Lindblad S, Hedfors E: Intraarticular variation in synovitis: local macroscopic and microscopic signs of inflammatory activity are significantly correlated. Arthritis Rheum 28(9):977-986, 1985.
56. Reece RJ, Canete JD, Parsons WJ, et al: Distinct vascular patterns of early synovitis in psoriatic, reactive, and rheumatoid arthritis. Arthritis Rheum 42(7):1481-1484, 1999.
57. Baeten D, Demetter P, Cuvelier C, et al: Comparative study of the synovial histology in rheumatoid arthritis, spondyloarthropathy, and osteoarthritis: influence of disease duration and activity. Ann Rheum Dis 59(12):945-953, 2000.
58. Ayral X, Ravaud P, Bonvarlet JP, et al: Arthroscopic evaluation of post-traumatic patellofemoral chondropathy. J Rheumatol 26(5): 1140-1147, 1999.
59. Baeten D, Van den BF, Elewaut D, et al: Needle arthroscopy of the knee with synovial biopsy sampling: technical experience in 150 patients. Clin Rheumatol 18(6):434-441, 1999.
60. Ike RW, Arnold WJ, Rothschild EW, Shaw HL: Tidal irrigation versus conservative medical management in patients with osteoarthritis of the knee: a prospective randomized study—Tidal Irrigation Cooperating Group. J Rheumatol 19(5):772-779, 1992.
61. Van Oosterhout M, Sont JK, Van Laar JM: Superior effect of arthroscopic lavage compared with needle aspiration in the treatment of inflammatory arthritis of the knee. Rheumatology (Oxford) 42(1):102-107, 2003.
62. Moseley JB, O'Malley K, Petersen NJ, et al: A controlled trial of arthroscopic surgery for osteoarthritis of the knee. N Engl J Med 347(2):81-88, 2002;
63. Miossec P, Briolay J, Dechanet J, et al: Inhibition of the production of proinflammatory cytokines and immunoglobulins by interleukin-4 in an ex vivo model of rheumatoid synovitis. Arthritis Rheum 35(8):874-883, 1992.
64. Bresnihan B, Cunnane G, Youssef P, et al: Microscopic measurement of synovial membrane inflammation in rheumatoid arthritis: proposals for the evaluation of tissue samples by quantitative analysis. Br J Rheumatol 37(6):636-642, 1998.
65. Youssef PP, Triantafillou S, Parker A, et al: Variability in cytokine and cell adhesion molecule staining in arthroscopic synovial biopsies: quantification using color video image analysis. J Rheumatol 24(12):2291-2298, 1997.
66. Kraan MC, Smith MD, Weedon H, et al: Measurement of cytokine and adhesion molecule expression in synovial tissue by digital image analysis. Ann Rheum Dis 60(3):296-298, 2001.
67. Dolhain RJ, Ter Haar NT, De Kuiper R, et al: Distribution of T cells and signs of T-cell activation in the rheumatoid joint: implications for semiquantitative comparative histology. Br J Rheumatol 37(3):324-330, 1998.
68. Smeets TJ, Kraan MC, Galjaard S, et al: Analysis of the cell infiltrate and expression of matrix metalloproteinases and granzyme B in paired synovial biopsy specimens from the cartilage-pannus junction in patients with RA. Ann Rheum Dis 60(6):561-565, 2001.
69. Kirkham B, Portek I, Lee CS, et al: Intraarticular variability of synovial membrane histology, immunohistology, and cytokine mRNA expression in patients with rheumatoid arthritis. J Rheumatol 26(4):777-784, 1999.
70. Kraan MC, Reece RJ, Smeets TJ, et al: Comparison of synovial tissues from the knee joints and the small joints of rheumatoid arthritis patients: implications for pathogenesis and evaluation of treatment. Arthritis Rheum 46(8):2034-2038, 2002.
71. Ulfgren AK, Grondal L, Lindblad S, et al: Interindividual and intra-articular variation of proinflammatory cytokines in patients with rheumatoid arthritis: potential implications for treatment. Ann Rheum Dis 59(6):439-447, 2000.
72. Klimiuk PA, Goronzy JJ, Bjorn J, et al: Tissue cytokine patterns distinguish variants of rheumatoid synovitis. Am J Pathol 151(5): 1311-1319, 1997.
73. Youssef PP, Smeets TJ, Bresnihan B, et al: Microscopic measurement of cellular infiltration in the rheumatoid arthritis synovial membrane: a comparison of semiquantitative and quantitative analysis. Br J Rheumatol 37(9):1003-1007, 1998.
74. Kraan MC, Haringman JJ, Ahern MJ, et al: Quantification of the cell infiltrate in synovial tissue by digital image analysis. Rheumatology (Oxford) 39(1):43-49, 2000.
75. Cunnane G, Bjork L, Ulfgren AK, et al: Quantitative analysis of synovial membrane inflammation: a comparison between automated and conventional microscopic measurements. Ann Rheum Dis 58(8):493-499, 1999.
76. Edwards JC, Willoughby DA: Demonstration of bone marrow derived cells in synovial lining by means of giant intracellular granules as genetic markers. Ann Rheum Dis 41(2):177-182, 1982.

77. Gravallese EM, Harada Y, Wang JT, et al: Identification of cell types responsible for bone resorption in rheumatoid arthritis and juvenile rheumatoid arthritis. Am J Pathol 152(4):943-951, 1998.
78. Zvaifler NJ, Tsai V, Alsalameh S, et al: Pannocytes: distinctive cells found in rheumatoid arthritis articular cartilage erosions. Am J Pathol 150(3):1125-1138, 1997.
79. Xue C, Takahashi M, Hasunuma T, et al: Characterisation of fibroblast-like cells in pannus lesions of patients with rheumatoid arthritis sharing properties of fibroblasts and chondrocytes. Ann Rheum Dis 56(4):262-267, 1997.
80. Lalor PA, Mapp PI, Hall PA, Revell PA: Proliferative activity of cells in the synovium as demonstrated by a monoclonal antibody, Ki67. Rheumatol Int 7(5):183-186, 1987.
81. Qu Z, Garcia CH, O'Rourke LM, et al: Local proliferation of fibroblast-like synoviocytes contributes to synovial hyperplasia: results of proliferating cell nuclear antigen/cyclin, c-myc, and nucleolar organizer region staining. Arthritis Rheum 37(2): 212-220, 1994.
82. Firestein GS, Yeo M, Zvaifler NJ: Apoptosis in rheumatoid arthritis synovium. J Clin Invest 96(3):1631-1638, 1995.
83. Franz JK, Pap T, Hummel KM, et al: Expression of sentrin, a novel antiapoptotic molecule, at sites of synovial invasion in rheumatoid arthritis. Arthritis Rheum 43(3):599-607, 2000.
84. Schedel J, Gay RE, Kuenzler P, et al: FLICE-inhibitory protein expression in synovial fibroblasts and at sites of cartilage and bone erosion in rheumatoid arthritis. Arthritis Rheum 46(6): 1512-1518, 2002.
85. Perlman H, Pagliari LJ, Liu H, et al: Rheumatoid arthritis synovial macrophages express the Fas-associated death domain-like interleukin-1beta-converting enzyme-inhibitory protein and are refractory to Fas-mediated apoptosis. Arthritis Rheum 44(1): 21-30, 2001.
86. Salmon M, Scheel-Toellner D, Huissoon AP, et al: Inhibition of T cell apoptosis in the rheumatoid synovium. J Clin Invest 99(3):439-446, 1997.
87. Tak PP, Zvaifler NJ, Green DR, Firestein GS: Rheumatoid arthritis and p53: how oxidative stress might alter the course of inflammatory diseases. Immunol Today 21(2):78-82, 2000.
88. Cantwell MJ, Hua T, Zvaifler NJ, Kipps TJ: Deficient Fas ligand expression by synovial lymphocytes from patients with rheumatoid arthritis. Arthritis Rheum 40(9):1644-1652, 1997.
89. Tak PP: Is early rheumatoid arthritis the same disease process as late rheumatoid arthritis? Best Pract Res Clin Rheumatol 15(1):17-26, 2001.
90. Kraan MC, Versendaal H, Jonker M, et al: Asymptomatic synovitis precedes clinically manifest arthritis. Arthritis Rheum 41(8):1481-1488, 1998.
91. Vervoordeldonk MJ, Tak PP: Cytokines in rheumatoid arthritis. Curr Rheumatol Rep 4(3):208-217, 2002.
92. Liew FY, McInnes IB: The role of innate mediators in inflammatory response. Mol Immunol 38(12-13):887-890, 2002.
93. Oppenheimer-Marks N, Lipsky PE: Adhesion molecules in rheumatoid arthritis. Springer Semin Immunopathol 20(1-2): 95-114, 1998.
94. Szekanecz Z, Koch AE: Update on synovitis. Curr Rheumatol Rep 3(1):53-63, 2001.
95. Tak PP, Bresnihan B: The pathogenesis and prevention of joint damage in rheumatoid arthritis: advances from synovial biopsy and tissue analysis. Arthritis Rheum 43(12):2619-2633, 2000.
96. Martel-Pelletier J, Welsch DJ, Pelletier JP: Metalloproteases and inhibitors in arthritic diseases. Best Pract Res Clin Rheumatol 15(5):805-829, 2001.
97. Hamann J, Wishaupt JO, van Lier RA, et al: Expression of the activation antigen CD97 and its ligand CD55 in rheumatoid synovial tissue. Arthritis Rheum 42(4):650-658, 1999.
98. Broker BM, Edwards JC, Fanger MW, Lydyard PM: The prevalence and distribution of macrophages bearing Fc gamma R I, Fc gamma R II, and Fc gamma R III in synovium. Scand J Rheumatol 19(2):123-135, 1990.
99. Youssef P, Roth J, Frosch M, et al: Expression of myeloid related proteins (MRP) 8 and 14 and the MRP8/14 heterodimer in rheumatoid arthritis synovial membrane. J Rheumatol 26(12): 2523-2528, 1999.
100. Kokkola R, Sundberg E, Ulfgren AK, et al: High mobility group box chromosomal protein 1: a novel proinflammatory mediator in synovitis. Arthritis Rheum 46(10):2598-2603, 2002.
101. Hale LP, Martin ME, McCollum DE, et al: Immunohistologic analysis of the distribution of cell adhesion molecules within the inflammatory synovial microenvironment. Arthritis Rheum 32(1):22-30, 1989.
102. Danks L, Sabokbar A, Gundle R, Athanasou NA: Synovial macrophage-osteoclast differentiation in inflammatory arthritis. Ann Rheum Dis 61(10):916-921, 2002.
103. Kinne RW, Brauer R, Stuhlmuller B, et al: Macrophages in rheumatoid arthritis. Arthritis Res 2(3):189-202, 2000.
104. Kawanaka N, Yamamura M, Aita T, et al: CD14+, CD16+ blood monocytes and joint inflammation in rheumatoid arthritis. Arthritis Rheum 46(10):2578-2586, 2002.
105. Katschke KJ Jr, Rottman JB, Ruth JH, et al: Differential expression of chemokine receptors on peripheral blood, synovial fluid, and synovial tissue monocytes/macrophages in rheumatoid arthritis. Arthritis Rheum 44(5):1022-1032, 2001.
106. Walz A, Schmutz P, Mueller C, Schnyder-Candrian S: Regulation and function of the CXC chemokine ENA-78 in monocytes and its role in disease. J Leukoc Biol 62(5):604-611, 1997.
107. Grant EP, Picarella D, Burwell T, et al. Essential role for the c5a receptor in regulating the effector phase of synovial infiltration and joint destruction in experimental arthritis. J Exp Med 196(11):1461-1471, 2002.
108. Firestein GS: Invasive fibroblast-like synoviocytes in rheumatoid arthritis: passive responders or transformed aggressors? Arthritis Rheum 39(11):1781-1790, 1996.
109. Stevens CR, Mapp PI, Revell PA: A monoclonal antibody (Mab 67) marks type B synoviocytes. Rheumatol Int 10(3):103-106, 1990.
110. Morales-Ducret J, Wayner E, Elices MJ, et al: Alpha 4/beta 1 integrin (VLA-4) ligands in arthritis: vascular cell adhesion molecule-1 expression in synovium and on fibroblast-like synoviocytes. J Immunol 149(4):1424-1431, 1992.
111. Perlman H, Pagliari LJ, Volin MV: Regulation of apoptosis and cell cycle activity in rheumatoid arthritis. Curr Mol Med 1(5): 597-608, 2001.
112. Toyosaki-Maeda T, Takano H, Tomita T, et al: Differentiation of monocytes into multinucleated giant bone-resorbing cells: two-step differentiation induced by nurse-like cells and cytokines. Arthritis Res 3(5):306-310, 2001.
113. Kang YM, Zhang X, Wagner UG, et al: CD8 T cells are required for the formation of ectopic germinal centers in rheumatoid synovitis. J Exp Med 195(10):1325-1336, 2002.
114. Magalhaes R, Stiehl P, Morawietz L, et al: Morphological and molecular pathology of the B cell response in synovitis of rheumatoid arthritis. Virchows Arch 441(5):415-427, 2002.
115. Cush JJ, Pietschmann P, Oppenheimer-Marks N, Lipsky PE: The intrinsic migratory capacity of memory T cells contributes to their accumulation in rheumatoid synovium. Arthritis Rheum 35(12):1434-1444, 1992.
116. Vey E, Burger D, Dayer JM: Expression and cleavage of tumor necrosis factor-alpha and tumor necrosis factor receptors by human monocytic cell lines upon direct contact with stimulated T cells. Eur J Immunol 26(10):2404-2409, 1996.
117. McInnes IB, Leung BP, Sturrock RD, et al: Interleukin-15 mediates T cell-dependent regulation of tumor necrosis factor-alpha production in rheumatoid arthritis. Nat Med 3(2):189-195, 1997.
118. Bigler RD, Bushkin Y, Chiorazzi N: S152 (CD27). A modulating disulfide-linked T cell activation antigen. J Immunol 141(1): 21-28, 1988.
119. Hendriks J, Gravestein LA, Tesselaar K, et al: CD27 is required for generation and long-term maintenance of T cell immunity. Nat Immunol 1(5):433-440, 2000.
120. van Lier RA, Pool MO, Kabel P, et al: Anti-CD27 monoclonal antibodies identify two functionally distinct subpopulations within the CD4+ T cell subset. Eur J Immunol 18(5):811-816, 1988.
121. Tak PP, Hintzen RQ, Teunissen JJ, et al: Expression of the activation antigen CD27 in rheumatoid arthritis. Clin Immunol Immunopathol 80(2):129-138, 1996.

122. Hamann D, Kostense S, Wolthers KC, et al: Evidence that human CD8+CD45RA+. Int Immunol 11(7):1027-1033, 1999.
123. Gulan G, Ravlic-Gulan J, Strbo N, et al: Systemic and local expression of perforin in lymphocyte subsets in acute and chronic rheumatoid arthritis. J Rheumatol 30(4):660-670, 2003.
124. Kim HJ, Berek C: B cells in rheumatoid arthritis. Arthritis Res 2(2):126-131, 2000.
125. Williams DG, Taylor PC: Clonal analysis of immunoglobulin mRNA in rheumatoid arthritis synovium: characterization of expanded IgG3 populations. Eur J Immunol 27(2):476-485, 1997.
126. Schroder AE, Greiner A, Seyfert C, Berek C: Differentiation of B cells in the nonlymphoid tissue of the synovial membrane of patients with rheumatoid arthritis. Proc Natl Acad Sci U S A 93(1):221-225, 1996.
127. Takemura S, Klimiuk PA, Braun A, et al: T cell activation in rheumatoid synovium is B cell dependent. J Immunol 167(8): 4710-4718, 2001.
128. Carson DA, Chen PP, Kipps TJ: New roles for rheumatoid factor. J Clin Invest 87(2):379-383, 1991.
129. Roosnek E, Lanzavecchia A: Efficient and selective presentation of antigen-antibody complexes by rheumatoid factor B cells. J Exp Med 173(2):487-489, 1991.
130. Brown KA, Perry ME, Mustafa Y, et al: The distribution and abnormal morphology of plasma cells in rheumatoid synovium. Scand J Immunol41(5):509-517, 1995.
131. Kim HJ, Krenn V, Steinhauser G, Berek C: Plasma cell development in synovial germinal centers in patients with rheumatoid and reactive arthritis. J Immunol 162(5):3053-3062, 1999.
132. Mellbye OJ, Vartdal F, Pahle J, Mollnes TE: IgG and IgA subclass distribution of total immunoglobulin and rheumatoid factors in rheumatoid tissue plasma cells. Scand J Rheumatol 19(5): 333-340, 1990.
133. Masson-Bessiere C, Sebbag M, Durieux JJ, et al: In the rheumatoid pannus, anti-filaggrin autoantibodies are produced by local plasma cells and constitute a higher proportion of IgG than in synovial fluid and serum. Clin Exp Immunol 119(3):544-552, 2000.
134. Fonseca JE, Edwards JC, Blades S, Goulding NJ: Macrophage subpopulations in rheumatoid synovium: reduced CD163 expression in CD4+ T lymphocyte-rich microenvironments. Arthritis Rheum 46(5):1210-1216, 2002.
135. van Lent PL, Figdor CG, Barrera P, et al: Expression of the dendritic cell-associated C-type lectin DC-SIGN by inflammatory matrix metalloproteinase-producing macrophages in rheumatoid arthritis synovium and interaction with intercellular adhesion molecule 3-positive T cells. Arthritis Rheum 48(2):360-369, 2003.
136. Godfrey HP, Ilardi C, Engber W, Graziano FM: Quantitation of human synovial mast cells in rheumatoid arthritis and other rheumatic diseases. Arthritis Rheum 27(8):852-856, 1984.
137. Crisp AJ, Chapman CM, Kirkham SE, et al: Articular mastocytosis in rheumatoid arthritis. Arthritis Rheum 27(8):845-851, 1984.
138. Gruber B, Poznansky M, Boss E, et al: Characterization and functional studies of rheumatoid synovial mast cells: activation by secretagogues, anti-IgE, and a histamine-releasing lymphokine. Arthritis Rheum 29(8):944-955, 1986.
139. Tetlow LC, Woolley DE: Distribution, activation and tryptase/chymase phenotype of mast cells in the rheumatoid lesion. Ann Rheum Dis 54(7):549-555, 1995.
140. Tetlow LC, Woolley DE: Mast cells, cytokines, and metalloproteinases at the rheumatoid lesion: dual immunolocalisation studies. Ann Rheum Dis 54(11):896-903, 1995.
141. Gotis-Graham I, McNeil HP: Mast cell responses in rheumatoid synovium: association of the MCTC subset with matrix turnover and clinical progression. Arthritis Rheum 40(3):479-489, 1997.
142. Woolley DE, Tetlow LC: Mast cell activation and its relation to proinflammatory cytokine production in the rheumatoid lesion. Arthritis Res 2(1):65-74, 2000.
143. Griffiths GM, Isaaz S: Granzymes A and B are targeted to the lytic granules of lymphocytes by the mannose-6-phosphate receptor. J Cell Biol 120(4):885-896, 1993.
144. Liu CC, Young LH, Young JD: Lymphocyte-mediated cytolysis and disease. N Engl J Med 335(22):1651-1659, 1996.
145. Froelich CJ, Dixit VM, Yang X: Lymphocyte granule-mediated apoptosis: matters of viral mimicry and deadly proteases. Immunol Today 19(1):30-36, 1998.
146. Tak PP, Kummer JA, Hack CE, et al: Granzyme-positive cytotoxic cells are specifically increased in early rheumatoid synovial tissue. Arthritis Rheum 37(12):1735-1743, 1994.
147. Smeets TJ, Dolhain RJ, Breedveld FC, Tak PP: Analysis of the cellular infiltrates and expression of cytokines in synovial tissue from patients with rheumatoid arthritis and reactive arthritis. J Pathol 186(1):75-81, 1998.
148. Muller-Ladner U, Kriegsmann J, Tschopp J, et al: Demonstration of granzyme A and perforin messenger RNA in the synovium of patients with rheumatoid arthritis. Arthritis Rheum 38(4): 477-484, 1995.
149. Warrington KJ, Takemura S, Goronzy JJ, Weyand CM: CD4+. Arthritis Rheum 44(1):13-20, 2001.
150. Klareskog L, Forsum U, Scheynius A, et al: Evidence in support of a self-perpetuating HLA-DR-dependent delayed-type cell reaction in rheumatoid arthritis. Proc Natl Acad Sci U S A 79(11):3632-3636, 1982.
151. Janossy G, Panayi G, Duke O, et al: Rheumatoid arthritis: a disease of T-lymphocyte/macrophage immunoregulation. Lancet 2(8251):839-842, 1981.
152. Duke O, Panayi GS, Janossy G, Poulter LW: An immunohistological analysis of lymphocyte subpopulations and their microenvironment in the synovial membranes of patients with rheumatoid arthritis using monoclonal antibodies. Clin Exp Immunol 49(1):22-30, 1982.
153. Page G, Lebecque S, Miossec P: Anatomic localization of immature and mature dendritic cells in an ectopic lymphoid organ: correlation with selective chemokine expression in rheumatoid synovium. J Immunol 168(10):5333-5341, 2002.
154. Witmer-Pack MD, Olivier W, Valinsky J, et al: Granulocyte/macrophage colony-stimulating factor is essential for the viability and function of cultured murine epidermal Langerhans cells. J Exp Med 166(5):1484-1498, 1987.
155. Thomas R, Lipsky PE: Dendritic cells: origin and differentiation. Stem Cells 14(2):196-206, 1996.
156. Pettit AR, Thomas R: Dendritic cells: the driving force behind autoimmunity in rheumatoid arthritis? Immunol Cell Biol 77(5):420-427, 1999.
157. Balanescu A, Radu E, Nat R, et al: Co-stimulatory and adhesion molecules of dendritic cells in rheumatoid arthritis. J Cell Mol Med 6(3):415-425, 2002.
158. Thomas R, Quinn C: Functional differentiation of dendritic cells in rheumatoid arthritis: role of CD86 in the synovium. J Immunol 156(8):3074-3086, 1996.
159. Pettit AR, MacDonald KP, O'Sullivan B, Thomas R: Differentiated dendritic cells expressing nuclear RelB are predominantly located in rheumatoid synovial tissue perivascular mononuclear cell aggregates. Arthritis Rheum 43(4):791-800, 2000.
160. van der Heijden, I, Wilbrink B, Tchetverikov I, et al: Presence of bacterial DNA and bacterial peptidoglycans in joints of patients with rheumatoid arthritis and other arthritides. Arthritis Rheum 43(3):593-598, 2000.
161. Schrijver IA, Melief MJ, Tak PP, et al: Antigen-presenting cells containing bacterial peptidoglycan in synovial tissues of rheumatoid arthritis patients coexpress costimulatory molecules and cytokines. Arthritis Rheum 43(10):2160-2168, 2000.
162. Nakagawa K, Brusic V, McColl G, Harrison LC: Direct evidence for the expression of multiple endogenous retroviruses in the synovial compartment in rheumatoid arthritis. Arthritis Rheum 40(4):627-638, 1997.
163. Thomas R, Lipsky PE: Could endogenous self-peptides presented by dendritic cells initiate rheumatoid arthritis? Immunol Today 17(12):559-564, 1996.
164. Tsark EC, Wang W, Teng YC, et al: Differential MHC class II-mediated presentation of rheumatoid arthritis autoantigens by human dendritic cells and macrophages. J Immunol169(11):6625-6633, 2002.
165. Imal Y, Yamakawa M: Morphology, function and pathology of follicular dendritic cells. Pathol Int 46(11):807-833, 1996.
166. Lindhout E, van Eijk M, van Pel M, et al: Fibroblast-like synoviocytes from rheumatoid arthritis patients have intrinsic properties of follicular dendritic cells. J Immunol 162(10):5949-5956, 1999.
167. Bofill M, Akbar AN, Amlot PL: Follicular dendritic cells share a membrane-bound protein with fibroblasts. J Pathol 191(2): 217-226, 2000.

168. Krenn V, Schalhorn N, Greiner A, et al: Immunohistochemical analysis of proliferating and antigen-presenting cells in rheumatoid synovial tissue. Rheumatol Int 15(6):239-247, 1996.
169. Takemura S, Braun A, Crowson C, et al: Lymphoid neogenesis in rheumatoid synovitis. J Immunol 167(2):1072-1080, 2001.
170. Wagner T: The microscopic appearance of synovial membranes in peripheral joints in ankylosing spondylitis. Reumatologia 8(3):209-215, 1970.
171. Cunnane G, Bresnihan B, Fitzgerald O: Immunohistologic analysis of peripheral joint disease in ankylosing spondylitis. Arthritis Rheum 41(1):180-182, 1998.
172. Revell PA, Mayston V: Histopathology of the synovial membrane of peripheral joints in ankylosing spondylitis. Ann Rheum Dis 41(6):579-586, 1982.
173. Burmester GR, Daser A, Kamradt T, et al: Immunology of reactive arthritides. Annu Rev Immunol 13:229-250, 1995.
174. Canete JD, Martinez SE, Farres J, et al: Differential Th1/Th2 cytokine patterns in chronic arthritis: interferon gamma is highly expressed in synovium of rheumatoid arthritis compared with seronegative spondyloarthropathies. Ann Rheum Dis59(4): 263-268, 2000.
175. Bollow M, Fischer T, Reisshauer H, et al: Quantitative analyses of sacroiliac biopsies in spondyloarthropathies: T cells and macrophages predominate in early and active sacroiliitis-cellularity correlates with the degree of enhancement detected by magnetic resonance imaging. Ann Rheum Dis 59(2):135-140, 2000.
176. Braun J, Bollow M, Neure L, et al: Use of immunohistologic and in situ hybridization techniques in the examination of sacroiliac joint biopsy specimens from patients with ankylosing spondylitis. Arthritis Rheum 38(4):499-505, 1995.
177. Simon AK, Seipelt E, Sieper J: Divergent T-cell cytokine patterns in inflammatory arthritis. Proc Natl Acad Sci U S A 91(18):8562-8566, 1994.
178. McInnes IB, al Mughales J, Field M, et al: The role of interleukin-15 in T-cell migration and activation in rheumatoid arthritis. Nat Med 2(2):175-182, 1996.
179. Thurkow EW, van dH, I, Breedveld FC, et al: Increased expression of IL-15 in the synovium of patients with rheumatoid arthritis compared with patients with Yersinia-induced arthritis and osteoarthritis. J Pathol 181(4):444-450, 1997.
180. Froelich CJ, Zhang X, Turbov J, et al: Human granzyme B degrades aggrecan proteoglycan in matrix synthesized by chondrocytes. J Immunol 151(12):7161-7171, 1993.
181. Ronday HK, van der Laan WH, Tak PP, et al: Human granzyme B mediates cartilage proteoglycan degradation and is expressed at the invasive front of the synovium in rheumatoid arthritis. Rheumatology (Oxford) 40(1):55-61, 2001.
182. Li F, Bulbul R, Schumacher HR Jr, et al: Molecular detection of bacterial DNA in venereal-associated arthritis. Arthritis Rheum 39(6):950-958, 1996.
183. Espinoza LR, Vasey FB, Espinoza CG, et al: Vascular changes in psoriatic synovium: a light and electron microscopic study. Arthritis Rheum 25(6):677-684, 1982.
184. Veale D, Yanni G, Rogers S, et al: Reduced synovial membrane macrophage numbers, ELAM-1 expression, and lining layer hyperplasia in psoriatic arthritis as compared with rheumatoid arthritis. Arthritis Rheum 36(7):893-900, 1993.
185. Ceponis A, Konttinen YT, Imai S, et al: Synovial lining, endothelial and inflammatory mononuclear cell proliferation in synovial membranes in psoriatic and reactive arthritis: a comparative quantitative morphometric study. Br J Rheumatol 37(2):170-178, 1998.
186. Konig A, Krenn V, Toksoy A, et al: Mig, GRO alpha and RANTES messenger RNA expression in lining layer, infiltrates and different leucocyte populations of synovial tissue from patients with rheumatoid arthritis, psoriatic arthritis and osteoarthritis. Virchows Arch 436(5):449-458, 2000.
187. Danning CL, Illei GG, Hitchon C, et al: Macrophage-derived cytokine and nuclear factor kappaB p65 expression in synovial membrane and skin of patients with psoriatic arthritis. Arthritis Rheum 43(6):1244-1256, 2000.
188. Kraan MC, van Kuijk AW, Dinant HJ, et al: Alefacept treatment in psoriatic arthritis: reduction of the effector T cell population in peripheral blood and synovial tissue is associated with improvement of clinical signs of arthritis. Arthritis Rheum 46(10):2776-2784, 2002.
189. Baeten D, Kruithof E, Van den BF, et al: Immunomodulatory effects of anti-tumor necrosis factor alpha therapy on synovium in spondylarthropathy: histologic findings in eight patients from an open-label pilot study. Arthritis Rheum 44(1):186-195, 2001.
190. Farahat MN, Yanni G, Poston R, Panayi GS: Cytokine expression in synovial membranes of patients with rheumatoid arthritis and osteoarthritis. Ann Rheum Dis 52(12):870-875, 1993.
191. Fernandes JC, Martel-Pelletier J, Pelletier JP: The role of cytokines in osteoarthritis pathophysiology. Biorheology 39(1-2):237-246, 2002.
192. Sakkas LI, Scanzello C, Johanson N, et al: T cells and T-cell cytokine transcripts in the synovial membrane in patients with osteoarthritis. Clin Diagn Lab Immunol 5(4):430-437, 1998.
193. Sakkas LI, Platsoucas CD: Role of T cells in the pathogenesis of osteoarthritis. Arthritis Rheum 46(11):3112-3113, 2002.
194. Goldenberg DL, Cohen AS: Synovial membrane histopathology in the differential diagnosis of rheumatoid arthritis, gout, pseudogout, systemic lupus erythematosus, infectious arthritis and degenerative joint disease. Medicine (Baltimore) 57(3):239-252, 1978.
195. Natour J, Montezzo LC, Moura LA, Atra E: A study of synovial membrane of patients with systemic lupus erythematosus (SLE). Clin Exp Rheumatol 9(3):221-225, 1991.
196. Smukler NM, Schumacher HR Jr: Chronic nondestructive arthritis associated with cutaneous polyarteritis. Arthritis Rheum 20(5):1114-1120, 1977
197. Schumacher HR: Ultrastructural findings in chondrocalcinosis and pseudogout. Arthritis Rheum 19(Suppl 3):413-425, 1976.
198. Ohashi K: Pathogenesis of beta2-microglobulin amyloidosis. Pathol Int 51(1):1-10, 2001.
199. Sole M, Munoz-Gomez J, Campistol JM: Role of amyloid in dialysis-related arthropathies: a morphological analysis of 23 cases. Virchows Arch A Pathol Anat Histopathol 417(6):523-52, 1990.
200. Stiehl P, Kluger KM: [Joint effusion findings in alkaptonuric arthropathy (ochronosis)]. Z Rheumatol 53(3):150-154, 1994.
201. Schumacher HR, Holdsworth DE: Ochronotic arthropathy. I. Clinicopathologic studies. Semin Arthritis Rheum 6(3):207-246, 1977.
202. Gaines JJ Jr: The pathology of alkaptonuric ochronosis. Hum Pathol 20(1):40-46, 1989.
203. Melis M, Onori P, Aliberti G, et al: Ochronotic arthropathy: structural and ultrastructural features. Ultrastruct Pathol 18(5):467-471, 1994.
204. Walker RJ, Dymock IW, Ansell ID, et al: Synovial biopsy in haemochromatosis arthropathy: histological findings and iron deposition in relation to total body iron overload. Ann Rheum Dis 31(2):98-102, 1972.
205. Schumacher HR Jr: Ultrastructural characteristics of the synovial membrane in idiopathic haemochromatosis. Ann Rheum Dis 31(6):465-473, 1972.
206. Schwartz HS, Unni KK, Pritchard DJ: Pigmented villonodular synovitis: a retrospective review of affected large joints. Clin Orthop (247):243-255, 1989.
207. Younes M, Hayem G, Brissaud P, et al: Monoarthritis secondary to joint metastasis: two case reports and literature review. Joint Bone Spine 69(5):495-498, 2002.

47 Arthrocentesis and Injection of Joints and Soft Tissues

CHRISTOPHER WISE

Arthrocentesis and injection of joints are safe and relatively simple procedures that can be performed routinely in the setting of an outpatient visit. With analysis of synovial fluid, few procedures in medical practice have the potential to be as diagnostically definitive as arthrocentesis, and few modalities can be as effective in achieving symptomatic relief of painful or swollen articular structures as the injection of corticosteroids. For these reasons, it is not surprising that one out of five visits to a rheumatology practice include aspiration or injection of a joint or periarticular structure.[1] In spite of this, surveys have estimated that 60 to 70 percent of internists finishing their residency training feel they need more training in these important, safe, and effective procedures.[2]

Paracelsus is credited with the first descriptions, in the early 16th century, of the viscous fluid present within synovial cavities, but aspiration of synovial fluid for analysis and aid in diagnosis did not become a topic of increasing interest until the first half of the 20th century. A number of studies of synovial fluid components and techniques used to obtain this fluid appear in a 1935 textbook by Pemberton.[3] An early description of arthrocentesis technique can be found in Ropes' classic book on synovial fluid analysis, published in 1953, which used data collected over a 20-year period.[4] During this era, swollen, distended joints were often aspirated for relief of discomfort. However, in most instances, the prompt reaccumulation of fluid and concerns about infection from repeated aspirations limited the usefulness of aspiration for the relief of symptoms of arthritis. A wide variety of substances were injected into joints throughout the early 20th century, including formalin and glycerin, lipiodol, lactic acid, petroleum jelly, and liquified oil prepared from the patient's own subcutaneous fat.[5,6] However, most of these therapies were apparently abandoned, and the most therapeutic injections discussed in arthritis textbooks from the 1940s related to temporary relief via injections of procaine for osteoarthritic knees and bursitis of the shoulder.[7]

In 1950, after observations on the efficacy of topical cortisone for ocular inflammation, Hollander first reported a minimal, transient improvement in 25 knees of patients with rheumatoid arthritis when injected with cortisone. In subsequent years, he injected hydrocortisone acetate with a much better response, providing further evidence that this was the active anti-inflammatory metabolite of cortisone.[8] Further reports of benefit from injectable corticosteroids appeared during the 1950s. During this period, studies showed that more stable and less soluble compounds in the form of esterified crystalline hydoxycortisone and its analogs were even more effective and had longer duration of anti-inflammatory effects.[9] By the early 1960s, Hollander had reported a series of more than 100,000 injections of joints, bursae, and tendon sheaths in 4000 patients with a variety of conditions.[10] During the 40 years since then, the aspiration and therapeutic injection of joints and periarticular tissues has become a common and essential part of rheumatology practice.

Indications and Clinical Evidence

ARTHROCENTESIS

Aspiration of synovial fluid may be indicated in any joint with detectable effusion or may be attempted in joints without detectable effusions when diagnosis is in doubt (Table 47–1). In patients in whom a diagnosis is uncertain, synovial fluid analysis usually provides important information regarding the inflammatory or noninflammatory nature of the process within the affected joint and may be definitive in patients with crystal-induced or infectious arthritis. In patients with recently diagnosed bacterial arthritis, repeated aspiration of accumulated fluid is often an important adjunct to antibiotic therapy. Joints with detectable effusions may be aspirated for relief of discomfort, with or without a subsequent injection of corticosteroid. In some patients, aspiration alone, without steroid injection, may be particularly effective for noninflammatory effusions or self-limited conditions.

THERAPEUTIC INJECTION

Inflammatory Arthritis

Therapeutic injection of corticosteroids is generally felt to be most effective in joints affected by inflammatory arthritis (Table 47–2). Most of the experience in this area has been with more common conditions, such as rheumatoid arthritis, juvenile rheumatoid arthritis, crystal-induced arthritis, psoriatic arthritis, and reactive arthritis. In addition, anecdotal experience has been reported in less-common conditions such as systemic lupus and sarcoidosis. In self-limited conditions, such as gout, injections generally lead to more prompt resolution of exacerbations.

In rheumatoid arthritis, injections are used frequently to suppress inflammation in individual joints. Such injections are generally considered to be adjunc-

TABLE 47–1 • INDICATIONS FOR ARTHROCENTESIS

Undiagnosed Arthritis with Effusion
Characterize type of arthritis Noninflammatory (WBC <2000/mm³) Inflammatory (WBC >2000/mm³) Septic (WBC > 50,000/mm³) Definitive diagnosis Gout (urate crystals) Pseudogout (CPPD crystals) Septic arthritis (Gram stain [rare] or culture)
Undiagnosed Arthritis without Effusion
May be definitive in gout (knee, 1st MTP joint)
Patient with Known Diagnosis
Septic arthritis (repeated taps for adequate drainage) Other types of arthritis for symptomatic relief (with or without injection) (most studies show improved effect if fluid aspirated before injection)

Abbreviations: CPPD, calcium pyrophosphate dihydrate; MTP, metarsal = phalangeal; WBC, white blood cells.

tive to disease-modifying drug therapy and are not felt to affect overall outcomes. The efficacy of individual joint injections in rheumatoid arthritis is supported by a number of large, uncontrolled case series dating back to the 1950s. Most of Hollander's early reports suggested long-lasting relief in a vast majority of joints injected, with improvement lasting several months in most patients.[10,11] This has been confirmed in several series of patients in subsequent years. In 1972, McCarty reported that 88 percent of patients attained remission for an average of 22 months in small joints of the hands and wrists, much better than comparable joints not injected in the opposite hands of the same patients.[12] In a subsequent report on 956 injections in 140 patients followed for an average of 7 years, 75 percent of injected joints remained in remission.[13] In this series, patients received about two injections during the first year of treatment and averaged 0. 6 injections per patient-year for the next 15 years. The authors of this report used a regimen that emphasized 3 weeks of splinting for upper extremity joints and 6 weeks of crutch walking for lower extremity joints. Removal of fluid prior to aspiration will increase the efficacy of steroid injections in most patients with inflammatory arthritis. One study of 191 knee injections in patients with rheumatoid arthritis showed that aspiration of fluid reduced the rate of relapse from 47 percent to 23 percent within a 6-month period after injection compared to joints not aspirated.[14]

Corticosteroid injection is considered to be a safe and effective option for prompt relief of acute crystal-induced arthritis, both in gout and pseudogout. Steroid injections are so widely accepted as an effective treatment that few reports have attempted to address the degree or duration of efficacy for injections in these conditions. Many of the patients described in early reports of steroid injections were being treated for acute crystal-induced arthritis, with prompt relief being almost uniform. In a recent report, small doses of intra-articular steroids were successful in relieving pain and swelling completely in all patients within 48 hours, and no relapses were noted in 20 patients over a 3-month period of time.[15]

In patients with recent onset of inflammatory oligoarthritis, without definitive diagnosis, corticosteroids can be used to relieve symptoms of swelling in individual joints, and the response to these injections can be used as a prognostic marker. This was demonstrated in a series of 51 patients with recent-onset inflammatory arthritis involving five or fewer joints. In this study, a strategy of injecting all joints with clinical synovitis resulted in improvement in all patients, and a complete resolution of synovitis after 2 weeks in 57 percent of patients. The response at 2 weeks was the best predictor of continued improvement persisting for 26 and 52 weeks.[16] Thus, a trial of steroid injection may be used for symptomatic relief in such patients, and a complete response at 2 weeks can be used as a prognostic indicator for a better outcome.

Patients with refractory sacroiliac joint pain related to ankylosing spondylitis or other spondyloarthropathies may benefit from injection of the sacroiliac joints.[17-20] Because of the anatomy of this joint, such injections often require radiographic confirmation of needle placement in the joint space, and use of fluoroscopic-, computerized tomography–, and magnetic resonance–guided injections has been reported. In uncontrolled studies, a good response has been reported in roughly 80 percent of injections, with an average time of improvement of 6 to 9 months. At least one controlled study in a small number of patients has shown slight benefit of steroid compared to placebo injection. However, the degree of improvement seen after sacroiliac injections has not been consistent among studies to date, probably because of a lack of uniformity of patient selection and outcomes assessed.

Joint injection has been utilized with increasing frequency in recent years in patients with juvenile rheumatoid arthritis.[21,22] The use of injections has become more common, particularly in the pauciarticular variant of the disease, in which a limited number of joints are involved and potentially toxic systemic therapy can be avoided. Complete remission lasting more than 6 months has been reported in roughly 65 to 80 percent of joints injected in this condition, most commonly in the knees. Benefit has also been demonstrated in smaller numbers of ankles, wrists, shoulders, and elbows, with a majority of children being able to stop oral medications, and correction of joint contracture noted in most as well.[23,24] A median duration of improvement of approximately 74 weeks has been documented in another large study.[25] One study demonstrated a significant decrease in leg-length discrepancy in a population of children treated with repeated injections (average of 3.25 injections per child over 42 months), compared to a population in another center who were not injected.[26] A recent study specifically addressed the efficacy and safety of steroid injections in the hip in juvenile rheumatoid arthritis.[27] In this prospective study of 67 hip injections, 58 percent of hips remained in remission for 2 years after a single injection, and another 18 percent required a second

TABLE 47–2 • INDICATIONS FOR THERAPEUTIC INJECTION

Inflammatory Arthritis

Rheumatoid arthritis: almost always effective, duration varies, should be used as an adjunct to an overall regimen of disease modifying therapy
Crystal-induced arthritis: few published studies, effective in 24 to 48 hours
Undiagnosed early inflammatory oligoarthritis: complete response in 2 weeks in 57%; predictor of good outcome
Spondyloarthropathies:
  peripheral joints respond as in RA
  sacroiliac joint injections under fluoroscopy
Juvenile rheumatoid arthritis: particularly useful in oligoarticular form; may be "disease modifying"
Miscellaneous diseases (anecdotal):
  sarcoidosis, lupus, etc.

Noninflammatory Arthritis

Osteoarthritis:
  Knees: 60 to 80% response in 1 to 6 wks vs. placebo; no difference at 12 wks
  Hips: anecdotal reports, require fluoroscopy, usually avoided
  Hyaluronic acid derivatives (Hyalgan, Synvisc) weekly for 3 to 5 weeks, moderately better than placebo
Hemophilic arthropathy: reported, but rarely used

Nonarticular Conditions (tendinitis, bursitis, myofascial pain, etc.)

Trigger point injections: done frequently, not supported by studies
Painful shoulder (rotator cuff tendinitis, frozen shoulder, etc.): efficacy compared to placebo, lasting 4 to 6 months
Lateral epidondylitis (tennis elbow): efficacy for 1 to 2 mos vs. placebo
Carpal tunnel syndrome: 90% short-term response, variable at 6 to 12 mos; good response to injection may be predictor of surgical response
de Quervain's tenosynovitis: 70 to 90% improved with 1 or 2 injections, relapse in 30% at 1 year
Trochanteric pain of hip (bursitis, tendinitis): 60 to 70% at 6 mos (uncontrolled)
Knee pain syndromes:
  anserine bursitis
  patellofemoral pain syndromes
  synovial plica
  popliteal cyst (usually treated with intra-articular knee injection)
Plantar fasciitis: variable, but probably better for 1 to 3 months
Morton's neuroma: response often prolonged (no controls)
Tarsal tunnel syndrome: rarely reported, usually only temporary
Achilles tendinitis, bursitis: usually avoided
Cervical girdle, lumbar areas, posterior hip: uncertain what structure(s) injected (without fluoroscopic facet block); efficacy not proven

injection to maintain remission. Only two cases of avascular necrosis were seen in this group, and both of these were in patients on systemic steroids, suggesting no role for local steroid injections in the development of avascular necrosis in this population.

Noninflammatory Arthritis

Corticosteroid injection is used frequently in common noninflammatory articular conditions, such as osteoarthritis, internal derangements, and post-traumatic arthritis. Clinical studies that support efficacy are less convincing and suggest a less predictable and smaller degree of response in these conditions than is seen in inflammatory arthritis.[28] Most studies of steroid injections in osteoarthritis have studied patients undergoing knee injections.[29] Early uncontrolled studies suggested improvement in approximately 60 to 80 percent of patients.[9,11] In controlled studies, most benefit, compared to placebo, seems to last 1 to 6 weeks, with return to the same pain levels seen in placebo groups by around 12 weeks after injection.[30-36] Factors associated with a better response to steroid injections have included less-severe radiographic changes, the presence of effusion at the time of injection, and successful aspiration of fluid at the time of injection. The theoretic concern about the potential for negative effects of injected steroids on cartilage (discussed in following section) is often sited as a reason to limit injections in osteoarthritis and other forms of noninflammatory arthritis.

Injections are not usually performed in patients with osteoarthritis of the hip, in part due to the technical difficulty of accurate needle placement. However, some relief can be obtained in patients with less-severe disease or in a rare patient with more severe involvement. A prospective, open study of intra-articular steroid in 45 patients with hip arthritis, 27 of whom had osteoarthritis (OA), found a significant reduction in pain at 2 and 12 weeks, although the effect was lost by 26 weeks.[37] In a report of 510 patients treated with a single injection done under fluoroscopic guidance, pain relief that persisted 8 weeks was seen in 90 percent of patients with mild disease, 58 percent of those with moderate disease, and 9 percent of those with severe hip osteoarthritis, and improved range of motion was demonstrated in most of those responding.[38]

Local steroid injection may be a useful adjunct in managing patients with hemophilic arthropathy.[39] In an open trial of 19 injections, 79 percent of joints improved within 24 hours, and this improvement persisted for up to 8 weeks in 58 percent of joints. A decrease in need for clotting factor was demonstrated in this small group.

Injectable hyaluronic acid derivatives have been studied extensively in recent years and are now approved for use in the United States and Canada for injection into osteoarthritic knees. A series of three to five weekly injections has been shown to provide more pain relief than placebo in most studies. However, the degree and duration of improvement in these studies has varied, and the optimal role for hyaluronic acid injections in the management of arthritis has yet to be determined[40] (see Chapter 93).

Nonarticular Conditions

Patients with various forms of tendinitis, bursitis, myofascial pain, and nerve entrapment syndromes are frequently treated with local injections of corticosteroids.[41] In many of these conditions, uncontrolled clinical experience suggests a high response rate, and in many others, controlled trials show variable levels of benefit, often depending on whether short-term or long-term outcomes are considered. The injection of "trigger points" for pain relief has been utilized by many practitioners over the past several decades, but few controlled studies to support efficacy have been published. Cummings and White[42] reviewed 23 papers dealing with trigger-point injections and concluded that none of the trials were of sufficient quality to demonstrate or refute the efficacy of any needling technique beyond placebo in the treatment of myofascial pain.

Steroid injections are frequently utilized in the management of rotator cuff tendinitis, frozen shoulder, and other causes of shoulder pain. Most controlled studies have demonstrated significant short-term improvement from steroid injection compared to placebo injection, usually lasting up to 4 to 6 months.[43,44] In most such trials, short-term treatment success of 75 to 80 percent is usually reported in steroid-treated groups, compared to 40 to 50 percent in placebo or other treatment groups.

Lateral epicondylitis is also commonly treated by local injections. Controlled studies typically document improvement of 90 percent compared to 50 percent in placebo treatment in the first month or two after injection, but outcomes at 6 to 12 months are usually not affected.[45,46]

In femoral trochanteric pain syndromes (i.e., bursitis), the response rate to locally injected steroids has been reported to be in the 60 to 100 percent range, but no placebo-controlled studies have been done. A recent prospective study reported significant improvement after a single injection in 77 percent of patients at 1 week; this number decreased to 69 percent at 6 weeks and 61 percent at 26 weeks.[47] Patients receiving larger amounts of locally injected steroid (24 mg of betamethasone) were more likely to have sustained improvement.

Around the knee, anecdotal and retrospective studies have shown that a majority of patients with anserine bursitis respond to local steroid injection.[48]

Local steroid injection may be a useful nonsurgical therapy for carpal tunnel syndrome. Most studies report up to 90 percent short-term relief of symptoms from a single injection; longer-term relief ranges from 20 to 90 percent, and surgery is eventually required in about half of patients treated with injection. A good response to local injection is sometimes useful as a diagnostic test and is a predictor of good surgical response. As noted later in this chapter, care should be taken to avoid injection into the body of the median nerve.[49,50]

Most patients with de Quervain's tenosynovitis involving the tendons at the base of the thumb will respond to local steroid injection.[51] In three prospective studies, 60 to 76 percent of patients with this condition had their symptoms adequately controlled with a single injection, and another 10 to 33 percent required a second injection.[52-54] About 30 percent had exacerbations an average of 1 year later, but overall, only 10 to 17 percent of patients were not controlled and required surgical release. Another small controlled study demonstrated that injection was much better than splinting.[55] Similar success rates have been reported in patients with flexor tenosynovitis,[56,57] and ganglion cysts.[58]

In the ankle and foot area, injection therapy has been used to treat plantar fasciitis, tarsal tunnel syndrome, Achilles tendinitis or bursitis, and interdigital neuroma (Morton's neuroma). Most of the data about efficacy for these conditions is anecdotal and uncontrolled. In general, the response in tarsal tunnel syndrome is usually temporary, whereas that in Morton's neuroma is more often prolonged.[59,60] Reported response rates for plantar fasciitis are variable, but one controlled trial has shown a significant improvement at 1 month compared to placebo, but results no different from placebo at 3 months.[61]

Local injections for neck pain and low back pain have been used for a number of years, with anecdotal reports of improvement, but controlled or prospective studies have shown variable results, depending on patient selection and methodology. Few controlled studies have assessed local "trigger point" or other soft tissue injections in the paracervical or paralumbar areas. Most studies of radiographically assisted facet joint injection of steroids in the lumbar or cervical areas show no difference compared to placebo, facet block, or local paraspinous injections.[62-66] Injections of the sacroiliac joint in patients with noninflammatory pain have shown a slight benefit from steroids compared to lidocaine alone.[67]

Preparations

CORTICOSTEROIDS

All hydroxycorticosteroid preparations are effective for intra-articular and periarticular injections (Table 47–3). The originally injected hydroxycortisone acetate is still available, widely used, and inexpensive. Triamcinolone hexacetonide is one of the least soluble agents with the presumed most-prolonged effect. Not all preparations are equivalent in efficacy or duration of effect, but few studies have been done to compare the efficacy of the various preparations. One recent report suggested a more prolonged response from triamcinolone hexacetonide compared to triamcinolone

TABLE 47–3 • INJECTABLE PREPARATIONS FOR INTRA-ARTICULAR INJECTION

Corticosteroids	Prednisone Equivalent
Betamethasone sodium phosphate (6 mg/ml)	50 mg
Dexamethasone sodium (4 mg/ml)	40 mg
Dexamethasone acetate (8 mg/ml)	80 mg
Hydrocortisone acetate (24 mg/ml)	5 mg
Methylprednisolone acetate (40 mg/ml)	50 mg
Prednisolone terbutate (20 mg/ml)	20 mg
Triamcinolone acetonide (40 mg/ml)	50 mg
Triamcinolone hexacetonide (20 mg/ml)	25 mg
Hyaluronic Acid (weekly for 3 to 5 weeks, indicated in osteoarthritis of knee)	
Hyalgan (20 mg/2 ml)	
Synvisc (16 mg/2 ml)	

acetonide, and both of these were more effective than hydrocortisone.[68] Most clinicians have developed familiarity with certain preparations and have continued to use these with efficacy for years. Some prefer to inject combinations of short-acting and long-acting preparations. Steroid preparations are often mixed with local anaesthetics, particularly for injecting small joints, tendon sheaths, and periarticular structures. This serves to reduce the local discomfort of injection into a confined space and also dilutes the concentration of the locally injected steroid and reduces the risk of soft tissue atrophy. Guidelines for the dosage of steroid injected into given joints is based roughly on the size of the joint injected. Although no consensus exists regarding these amounts, most experts suggest injecting 1 cc of steroid preparation into large joints, with smaller amounts into smaller joints.

OTHER INJECTABLE PRODUCTS

Over the years, a number of other agents have been injected into joints, including salicylates, phenylbutazone, gold, orgotein, progesterone, glycosaminoglycan polysulfate, and various antibiotics, but most have been abandoned due to lack of efficacy or local reactions. Various cytotoxic agents have been used sporadically or in small numbers of patients for intrasynovial tumors and refractory proliferative synovitis, including nitrogen mustard, osmic acid, methotrexate, and radioactive prepartions (yttrium-90, colloidal P32 chromic phosphate, dysprosium-165-ferric hydroxide). Intra-articular hyaluronic acid preparations have been in use for many years in Europe and have been approved for clinical use in Canada and the United States in the past decade. Currently two preparations of hyaluronic acid (Hyalgan and Synvisc) are approved for the treatment of osteoarthritis of the knee and appear to be superior to placebo injections in most clinical trials, although no evidence for long-term efficacy or disease modification has been demonstrated.[40,69,70] These preparations are given weekly in a series of three to five injections. Studies of hyaluronic acid preparations in other types of arthritis are inconclusive or small.

Contraindications

Contraindications to diagnostic arthrocentesis are few (Table 47–4). Established infection, such as a cellulitis, in periarticular structures is generally considered to be an absolute contraindication to inserting a needle into a joint. However, if inflammation in an underlying joint or bursa is felt to be the cause of the appearance of infection, then aspiration of the joint or bursa should be attempted. Septicemia carries the theoretic risk of introducing blood-borne bacteria into a joint, but such complications are not well documented, and joints suspected of being infected should be aspirated regardless of the presence of septicemia. Arthrocentesis through an area of irregular or disrupted skin, as seen in psoriasis, should be avoided due to the increased numbers of colonizing bacteria in these areas. Caution should be exercised in patients with bleeding disorders or those taking anticoagulants, due to the theoretic risk of inducing hemarthrosis. However, the risk of significant hemarthrosis after arthrocentesis is quite low, even in patients on regular warfarin therapy with international normalized ratio (INR) levels up to as high as 4.5.[71]

Complications

Iatrogenic infection is the most serious, but least common, complication of arthrocentesis and joint injection. In Hollander's large series, an incidence of infection of 0.005 percent was reported in a series of 400,000 injections.[11] Gray and colleague,[72] reported an incidence of 0.001 percent several years later. A more recent publication noted an infection ratio of 1:2000 to 10,000 in patients with rheumatoid arthritis.[73] In this series, infections occurred almost exclusively in debilitated patients on immunosuppressive therapy. Few other prospective or systematic studies of infection after arthrocentesis have been published, but most reported anecdotal experience has noted a similar rare incidence of this serious complication. A recent arthroscopic study showed that a small fragment of skin stained with surgical marking pen could be identified within the joint space after most percutaneous insertions of a needle into the joint space, with identifications of bacterial nucleic acid by polymerase chain reaction in about one third of these.[74] Considering the rarity of joint infection after arthrocentesis, these findings suggest that bacteria introduced at the time of arthrocentesis are either not viable or are quickly cleared in almost all cases.

The most common complications of local steroid injections are related to local irritation of synovial and subcutaneous tissues and atrophy of soft tissues. Postinjection "flare" may develop in 1 to 6 percent of patients a few hours after injection and may last up to 48 hours, sometimes mimicking iatrogenic infection.[11,13,75] These flares are reportedly more common with needle-shaped crystals and are felt to be similar to the acute arthritis related to other crystals phagocytosed by leukocytes, but they may also be caused by preservatives in some steroid suspensions.

TABLE 47–4 • CONTRAINDICATIONS TO ARTHROCENTESIS AND JOINT INJECTION

Established infection in nearby structures (e.g., cellulitis, septic bursitis)	Sometimes gout will mimic cellulitis, creating confusing picture
Septicemia (theoretic risk of introducing organism into joint)	Need to tap suspected septic joints in septic patients
Disrupted skin barrier (e.g., psoriasis)	Do not tap through lesions
Bleeding disorder (not absolute, but use more care)	Risk of bleeding very low, even in patients on warfarin
Septic joint	Steroid injection contraindicated
Prior lack of response	Relative contraindication
Difficult-to-access joint	Relative contraindication without imaging aid

TABLE 47–5 • POTENTIAL COMPLICATIONS OF ARTHROCENTESIS AND JOINT INJECTION

Iatrogenic infection	<1/10,000, may be higher in RA patients
Post-injection "flare"	1 to 6%, lasting up to 48 hr, may be related to preparation
Local soft tissue atrophy or pigment change	May occur 1 to 6 months later
Local nerve damage	In structures near prominent nerves (e.g., carpal tunnel syndrome)
Tendon rupture or weakening	Case reports, animal studies show highest risk in Achilles tendon and plantar fascia
Systemic steroid absorption	Inevitable, usually subclinical Hypothalmic-pituitary suppression 2 to 7 days; changes in bone formation 14 days Flushing, facial warmth, diaphoresis Transient elevation of blood glucose, lymphopenia, eosinopenia
A vascular necrosis of bone (ischemic necrosis)	Controversial; reported but usually explained by underlying disease or systemic steroids in same patient
Negative effects on cartilage	Controversial; found in animal models of normal cartilage, but not in primates case reports in humans receiving multiple injections some animal models of arthritis are better with steroid injections large human observational studies have not documented more problems than expected (OA, RA, juvenile RA)

Abbreviations: OA, osteoarthritis; RA, rheumatoid arthritis.

Weakening of tendons and tendon rupture have also been reported as a result of locally injected steroids,[76,77] emphasizing the importance of avoiding direct injection of steroids into the body of tendons. Most reports of tendon rupture have been anecdotal and described in patients involved in athletic activities or with rheumatoid arthritis. The risk of tendon rupture has not been adequately determined, but it appears be quite low in the hands and wrists, where no ruptures were seen in a series of more than 200 injections,[78] and only two were seen in another series of 956 injections.[13] Areas felt to be at highest risk for rupture include the Achilles tendon, bicipital tendon, and plantar fascia, where the risk of rupture has been estimated as high as 10 percent.[79,80] Systemic absorption occurs with locally injected depot corticosteroids. Since the earliest intra-articular injections of steroids, an anti-inflammatory effect has been demonstrated not only in the injected joint, but also in other joints in the same patient.[8] Subsequent studies have documented decrease in plasma cortisol and suppression of the hypothalamic-pituitary axis lasting from 2 to 7 days after a single injection.[81] The degree and duration of adrenal suppression from a single intra-articular dose of depot steroid is less pronounced than that seen from an equal intramuscular dose.[82] The effect of the systemic absorption of locally injected steroid on bone metabolism has also been studied. In a study of markers of bone turnover, a single injection of triamcinolone in knees of rheumatoid arthritis patients resulted in no change in bone resorption markers, but yielded a drastic reduction in markers of bone formation within a day, which returned to normal levels in 14 days.[83] Some patients experience prominent erythema, warmth, and diaphoresis of the face and torso within minutes to hours after steroid injections.[77,81] This is most likely related to systemic absorption, but idiosyncratic reaction to preservatives in steroid preparations has also been implicated. Similarly, some patients may experience other typical metabolic effects of systemic steroids, such as transient rises in blood glucose or decreases in peripheral blood eosinophil or lymphocyte counts.

Avascular necrosis of bone (ischemic necrosis) has long been considered a potential complication of intra-articular steroids, with a reported prevalence of this complication in injected joints ranging from less than 0.1 percent to 3 percent.[11,22,27] However, most studies have suggested that the occurrence of this complication is more related to the severity of the associated disease or systemic steroid therapy and is unrelated to local injections.

The potential for negative effects of locally injected corticosteroids on cartilage metabolism has been a controversial area of study for several decades. Anecdotal reports of Charcot-like arthropathy attributed to intra-articular steroids first appeared in the late 1950s and 1960s, often occurring in patients having more than 10 (and sometimes hundreds) joint injections over many months or years.[84-86] Several studies in the 1960s and 1970s demonstrated that locally injected steroids caused destructive changes, catabolic effects, or both in normal animal cartilage.[87-89] These included findings of decreased protein and matrix synthesis with degenerative cellular changes in chondrocytes, and fissures and decreased proteoglycan content in cartilage matrix. However, similar studies done in primate joints failed to show any negative effects from intra-articular corticosteroids.[90] In addition, studies done in subsequent years have demonstrated protective effects on cartilage lesions and reduction in osteophyte development in animal models of experimentally induced osteoarthritis, and associated reduction in metalloprotease levels in cartilage and increase in lubricating synovial surfactant.[91-94] In humans with osteoarthritis, intra-articular steroids have been shown to decrease macrophage infiltration of the synovial lining, but no change was noted in metalloprotease levels.[95] Observations on humans treated with frequent corticosteroid injections have yielded conflicting information regarding changes in articular cartilage. More recent observations in patients with oligoarticular juvenile rheumatoid arthritis, noted previously, suggest that frequent steroid injections have the potential to help protect cartilage from the destructive process of the underlying disease process and are not associated with negative effects on articular cartilage. [23-27] In addition, a study of patients with rheumatoid arthritis has shown no increase in the need for subsequent joint replacement surgery in the joints receiving four or more injections in a 1-year period of time.[96]

General Arthrocentesis Techniques

MATERIALS

Most practitioners find that an arthrocentesis tray containing needed items allows more flexibility in preparing for aspirating or injecting joints or other articular structures. Syringes greater than 20 cc are not needed for most procedures, but a swollen knee may occasionally contain 60 cc of fluid or more, and it is reasonable to have at least one syringe of this size in a tray, with others available for the rare patient with effusions greater than 100 to 200 cc in volume. Heparinized or citrated tubes to prevent coagulation of inflammatory fluids for accurate cell counts and crystal analysis, plain tubes for chemistry evaluations, and sterile tubes for transporting fluid to a microbiology lab for culture should be included. In joints being aspirated for the presence of bacteria and crystals, small amounts of fluid or debris may be present in the bore of the needle, even when no obvious fluid is obtained. In such situations, it is best to have clean microscope slides and coverslips available at the bedside for microscopic examination for cellularity, Gram stain, and crystals. A hemostat is helpful for changing syringes after aspiration in order to inject corticosteroid. The size and length of needles used will depend on anticipated amount of fluid to be obtained from a joint and the size of the involved joint. A 20- to 22-gauge needle is usually sufficient to aspirate most detectable effusions, but large effusions with large amounts of debris, as seen in septic joints, may require larger-bore needles. In small joints, a 23- to 27-gauge needle may be used, particularly when no fluid appears to be present and only therapeutic injection is being considered. A needle 1. 5 inches in length is adequate for almost all procedures, but a 3-inch spinal needle may be needed occasionally for a large knee or hip.

SITE PREPARATION AND TECHNIQUE

Sterile technique designed to avoid the introduction of skin bacteria into the joint should be observed in all procedures. After careful examination and identification of the specific point of aspiration, this point may be marked by the end of a ballpoint pen with writing point retracted. The area should be carefully cleaned with one or two layers of iodine followed by alcohol. These precautions are sufficient to minimize the risk of infection to no more than 1 in 10,000 in most studies, although a single "swipe" of isopropyl alcohol has been shown to provide a similar level of protection.[97] A physician experienced in arthrocentesis may elect not to use topical anesthesia in many patients because the amount of pain is often no more than that experienced from phlebotomy. In an anxious patient or when small joints or those with minimal fluid are being aspirated, topical anesthesia may be attained by the use of spray coolant (ethyl chloride) or an intradermal wheal and subcutaneous infiltration of lidocaine. The application of spray coolant may be done after sterile preparation and has been shown not to contaminate the field.[98] In pediatric patients, particularly when multiple joints are injected, sedation or general anesthesia may be required for safe and accurate injections.[99] Nonsterile gloves should be worn by the operator to avoid contamination with the patient's synovial fluid or blood. Drapes and sterile gloves are not necessary, but the gloved hand should not touch the prepared site. A joint is usually entered at a 90-degree angle to the skin, slowly and evenly, and negative pressure should be applied to the syringe once the needle has been advanced ½ to 1 inch (in a large joint). If the needle's course is obstructed by bone, the needle should be withdrawn slightly and redirected at a slightly different angle. If no fluid is obtained, the needle should be slowly advanced and negative pressure continued. If fluid flows initially and then stops, the needle may be advanced or retracted slightly or rotated in case it is blocked by an intra-articular structure or synovial tissue. After an adequate amount of fluid is obtained, a hemostat may be used to secure the needle, the syringe removed, and a new syringe with injectable steroid attached if injection is indicated. After injection, the needle and syringe should be removed and pressure applied over the site until a bandage is applied. When synovial fluid is to be examined for crystals, care should be taken not to replace the needle used for steroid injection on the syringe with synovial fluid because the contamination of fluid with steroid crystals will make accurate identification of urate and calcium pyrophosphate crystals more difficult.

POSTPROCEDURE INSTRUCTIONS AND CARE

After the procedure, patients should be reminded about the risk for postinjection "flare" within 24 to 48 hours after local steroid injection. If pain, redness, or swelling progress after this, are particularly severe, or are accompanied by fever, the patient should be instructed to call and be reevaluated for the remote possibility of iatrogenic infection. Patients should also be reminded about the soft tissue atrophy and hypopigmentation that may occur weeks to months after the procedure, particularly when structures close to the skin are injected. For patients in whom tendon sheaths are injected, heavy activities using the involved tendons should be avoided for several days.

After injection of joints, particularly weight-bearing joints, activities should be limited due to evidence that this will prolong the effect of the injected steroid. In a large series reported in 1995, McCarty and colleagues [13] used a regimen that emphasized 3 weeks of splinting for upper extremity joints and 6 weeks of crutch walking for lower extremity joints, suggesting that rest after the injection was important in prolonging the effect of injections. Several other retrospective studies and anecdotal observations have suggested a role for strict rest or non–weight bearing after injection to improve duration of efficacy.[100,31] One small controlled study showed that rest provided no advantage over regular activities in regard to short- or long-term outcomes.[101] However, in a larger prospective controlled trial of knees in patients with rheumatoid arthritis, a 24-hour period of strict bed rest after injection resulted in a more prolonged improvement compared to patients that were not restricted.[102] Most practitioners advise restricted activities after steroid injections, particularly in weight-bearing joints, but opinions on the relative importance of rest after injections still vary, and no specific regimen of rest would be considered standard practice among physicians.[103]

Specific Regional Arthrocentesis Techniques

CERVICAL SPINE AREA

Most injections in the region of the cervical spine, trapezius, and scapular areas are best considered to be myofascial or "trigger point" injections. The point of injection is usually determined by palpating for the areas of most tenderness, and few reliable landmarks are available for localization of anatomic structures. Using a 22- to 25-gauge needle, a combination of 0.5 cc of steroid and 0.5 to 2 cc of lidocaine can be injected into areas in the paracervical muscles or other areas where tenderness can be elicited. Some of the injections performed in these areas are likely to be close enough to the posterior cervical facet joints to reduce inflammation in the joints themselves, whereas others are probably reducing inflammation in ligaments, tendons, or bursal structures. More precise injection of posterior cervical facet joints may be accomplished under fluoroscopic visualization.[66]

ANTERIOR CHEST WALL

The anterior chest area may occasionally be the site of inflammatory disease of the sternoclavicular joints. It is usually difficult to obtain much fluid for diagnostic purposes from this joint, but a few drops for microscopic analysis and culture may be available in some patients. The point of aspiration should be dictated by the point of maximal swelling near the surface. Aspiration should be attempted with caution, using as short and small a needle as possible to avoid damage to nearby vascular structures, lung, or airway. A small amount of steroid (0.1 to 0.5 cc) may be injected in this joint, as long as the suspicion of infection is low. In Tietze's syndrome, one or more of the anterior costochondral junctions may be swollen, but such areas do not contain fluid for analysis and should be approached with caution for injection of small amounts of steroid and lidocaine.

TEMPOROMANDIBULAR JOINT

The temporomandibular joint may be involved in patients with rheumatoid arthritis, spondyloarthropathies, or osteoarthritis, and internal derangement of this joint may be a source of discomfort usually treated by oral surgeons.[104] This joint is palpated as a depression just below the zygomatic arch about 1 to 2 cm anterior to the targus. The depression is usually more easily palpated by having the patient open and close the mouth. After a mark is made over the area, a 22- to 25-gauge needle is inserted perpendicular to the skin and directed slightly posteriorly and superiorly; then, 0.1 to 0.25 mg of steroid preparation can be injected. This joint seldom has enough fluid for diagnostic aspiration.

SHOULDER

A number of structures in and around the shoulder may be involved in systemic processes, injury, or overuse syndromes, and each has the potential to benefit from local steroid injection. Ideally, injections should be directed toward specific anatomic sites based on clinical findings. However, for practical purposes, injections into the glenohumeral joint or subacromial bursal space are often beneficial for pain related to other nearby structures, such as the rotator cuff tendons or bicipital tendon.

Glenohumeral Joint

The glenohumeral joint may be entered from an anterior or posterior approach. From the anterior, the patient should be in a sitting position with the shoulder externally rotated (Fig. 47–1). A mark is made just medial to the head of the humerus and slightly inferiorly and laterally to the coracoid process. A 20- to 22-gauge, 1.5-inch needle is directed posteriorly and slightly upward and laterally. For a posterior approach, the upper arm should be against the lateral chest and forearm across the chest. A mark should be made about 2 inches inferior to the acromion. One should be able to feel the needle enter the joint space, but if bone is hit, the needle should be pulled back and redirected at a slightly different angle. Once the joint is entered, fluid should be aspirated, if present, and the joint injected

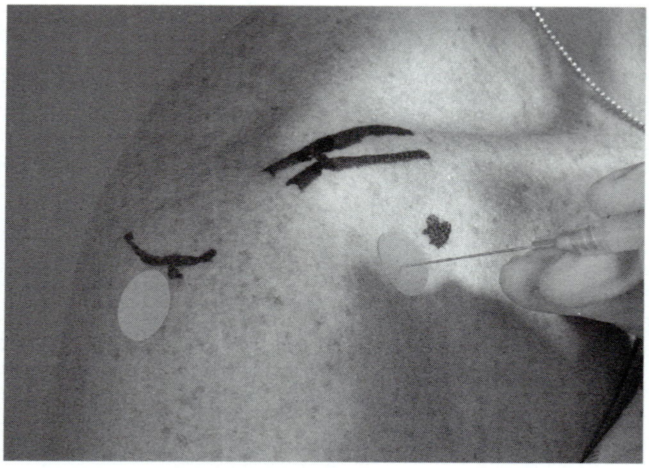

FIGURE 47–1 · Shoulder (Glenohumeral) Joint Arthrocentesis: Anterior Approach. With the shoulder externally rotated, the needle is inserted at a point just medial to the head of the humerus, slightly inferior and lateral to the coracoid process *(marked in black)*, which is just inferior to the lateral aspect of the clavicle *(marked in black above)*. (See color plate 15.)

with 1 cc of steroid preparation, with or without 1 to 3 cc of lidocaine.

Acromioclavicular Joint

This joint, like the sternoclavicular joint, is made of fibrocartilage and rarely contains fluid. The joint is palpated as a groove at the lateral end of the clavicle, just medial to the tip of the acromion, and may display some degree of soft tissue swelling or bony prominence, depending on the underlying disease process. To enter the joint with a needle, a mark should be made over the groove, and a 22- to 25-gauge needle introduced 1 inch or less. After an attempt to obtain fluid, 0.25 to 0.5 cc of steroid preparation may be injected.

Rotator Cuff Tendon and Subacromial Bursa

This area may be entered using a 22- to 25-gauge needle, usually 1.5 inches in length (Fig. 47–2). Over the lateral or posterolateral aspect of the shoulder, the groove between the acromion and humerus should be palpated and marked. The needle is inserted at this point and advanced in a horizontal plane medially, usually 1 to 1.5 inches. It is unusual to obtain fluid from this space. Thus, in most cases, the area is injected without aspiration; usually 1 cc of steroid preparation with 1 to 3 cc of lidocaine is injected to allow wider distribution of medication in this area.

Bicipital Tendon

Bicipital tendinitis may be treated by injecting the shoulder joint or the tendon sheath itself. If the tendon is to be injected, it can be palpated over the anterior aspect of the shoulder in the bicipital groove of the shoulder; it is usually tender and can be rolled under the examiner's finger. A 22-gauge, 1.5-inch needle should be inserted in the sheath and portions of the steroid and lidocaine preparation injected directly, and

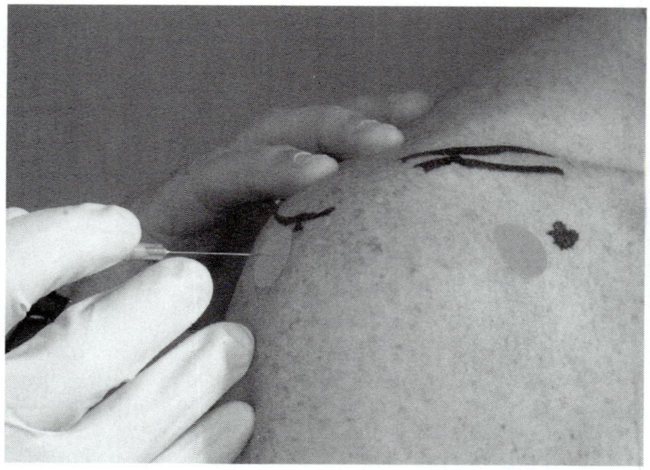

FIGURE 47–2 · Rotator Cuff Tendon/Subacromial Bursa Injection: Lateral Approach. Over the lateral aspect of the shoulder, the groove between the acromion (*marked in black*) and humerus is palpated and marked (*spot*). The needle is inserted at this point and advanced in a horizontal plane medially. (See color plate 16.)

then superiorly and inferiorly, along the course of the tendon after redirecting the needle in each direction. Discretion, however, is advised when considering injection of this tendon sheath as there may be increased risk of tendon rupture in this area.

ELBOW

Elbow Joint

The elbow is best entered by insertion of the needle into the area over the lateral elbow where a bulge can be palpated if fluid is present within the joint (Fig. 47–3). This is best determined with the elbow flexed at 90 degrees. A mark should be made just below the lateral epicondyle in the groove just proximal to the head of the radius and above the olecranon process of the ulna. After preparation, a 20- to 22-gauge needle held perpendicular to the skin is inserted approximately 1 inch and the joint is aspirated, followed by injection if indicated.

Medial and Lateral Epicondyle

These areas are commonly affected by overuse syndromes involving the origins of muscle groups of the forearm, particularly the lateral epicondyle, which is the area of inflammation in tennis elbow (Fig. 47–4). With the elbow flexed, the area of tenderness over the anterolateral surface of the external condyle of the humerus should be marked. After preparation, a 22- to 25-gauge needle 1 to 1.5 inches long should be inserted about 1 to 2 cm distal to the mark, and 0.5 cc of steroid preparation mixed with 1 to 3 cc of lidocaine administered in several small doses after partially withdrawing and redirecting the needle and reinjecting in two to three passes of the needle in the area. Injections in this area often deliver steroids to subcutaneous tissues very close to the skin, and patients should be advised about

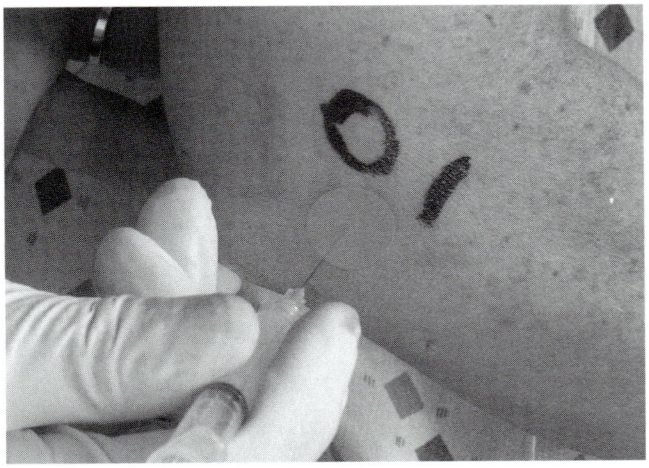

FIGURE 47–3 · Elbow Arthrocentesis. With the elbow flexed 90 degrees, the needle is inserted into the recess just below the lateral epicondyle *(black circle)* and radial head *(black line)* and is directed parallel to the shaft of the radius. (See color plate 17.)

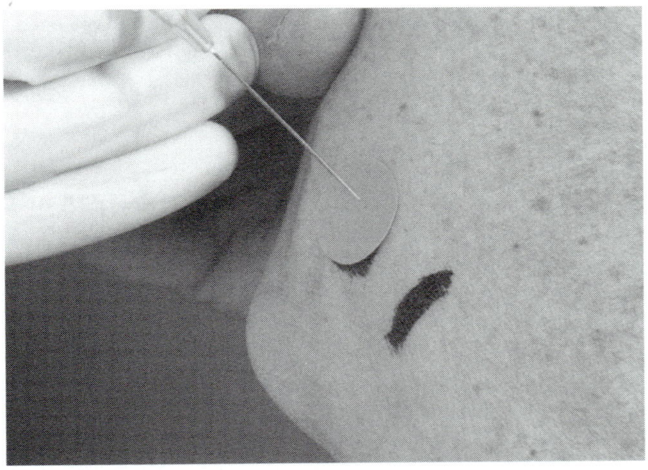

FIGURE 47–4 · Lateral Epicondyle (Tennis Elbow) Injection. With the elbow flexed and pronated, the needle is inserted at the most tender area over the bony prominence on the anterolateral aspect of the lateral humerus, which is proximal to radial head *(black line)*. A combination of steroid and local anesthetic is then injected into the subcutaneous tissues at the attachment of the extensor muscles to the epicondyle. (See color plate 18.)

the likelihood of subcutaneous atrophy and pigment changes that may occur weeks or months after the injection. The medial epicondyle is injected in a similar fashion, with more care required to avoid inadvertent injection of steroids into the area of the ulnar groove just behind the bony prominence of the epicondyle.

Olecranon Bursa and Nodules

This area is located just under the skin over the tip of the olecranon process at the posterior aspect of the elbow. Swelling in this area is easily detected as a localized collection of fluid and can be easily aspirated and injected if fluid is present. A smaller gauge needle (22- to 23-gauge) may be used for noninflammatory processes, but a larger gauge (20 gauge) is often needed for bursal effusions related to rheumatoid arthritis or gout. After preparation, the needle should be inserted under the skin into the easily palpable area of fluid and as much fluid as possible aspirated. For noninfectious processes, 0.5 to 1 cc of steroid can be injected into the space. Subcutaneous nodules in this area, or at other locations around the body, may be aspirated for diagnostic purposes, usually to differentiate rheumatoid nodules from tophi. For this type of aspiration, an 18- to 20-gauge needle is inserted into the nodule and rotated, retracted to near the surface, and then reinserted and rotated, with negative pressure applied on the syringe. After removal, the contents of the syringe should be expelled onto a microscope slide and may be examined for cellular content and crystals.

WRIST AND HAND

Radiocarpal Joint

The wrist joint is complex, but most of the intercarpal spaces communicate with the radiocarpal joint, which may be entered from a dorsal approach. A mark should be made just distal to the radius and just ulnar to the "anatomic snuff box" (Fig. 47–5). A 22- to 25-gauge needle, 0.5 to 1 inch long is usually adequate. Occasionally, up to 3 to 5 cc of fluid may be obtained from the wrist by aspiration, and if indicated, 0.5 cc of steroid may be injected into the space.

Dorsal Wrist Tendons

The extensor tendon sheaths over the dorsal wrist may become inflamed and swollen due to a number of inflammatory process, most commonly rheumatoid arthritis, but occasionally crystal-induced arthritis or infectious processes. The areas of swelling are well defined and close to the surface, and they are easily entered with a direct aspiration, usually at a 30- to 45-degree angle, with needle directed along the course of the swollen tendon. Fluid is often easily obtained,

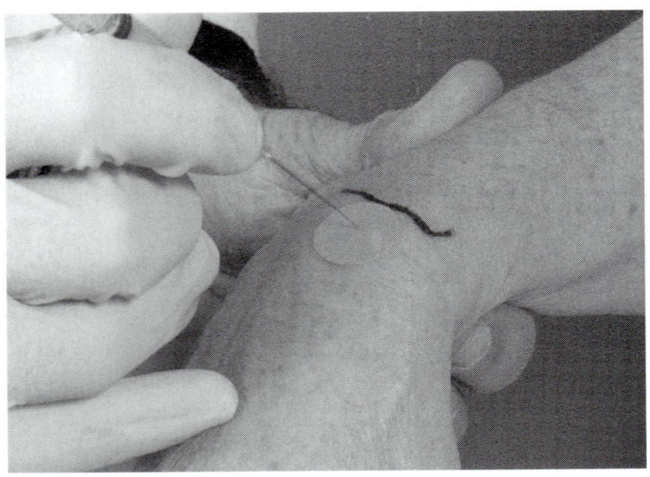

FIGURE 47–5 · Wrist (Radiocarpal) Arthrocentesis. The needle is inserted just distal to the radius *(marked in black)* at a point just ulnar to the anatomic snuffbox. It is directed perpendicular to the skin and advanced until fluid is obtained or the needle is advanced 1 to 1.5 inches. (See color plate 19.)

but in some patients, those with rheumatoid arthritis in particular, proliferative synovial tissue limits the amount of fluid that can be aspirated. After aspiration, the area can be injected with 0.5 cc of corticosteroid mixed with 0.5 to 1 cc of lidocaine, if indicated.

de Quervain's Tenosynovitis

This common overuse syndrome involving the tendons at the radial aspect of the "anatomic snuff box" is often helped by local injection of the tendon sheath. After examination, the area of most tenderness along the course of the tendon should be marked and the needle inserted directed almost parallel to the skin, either proximally or distally (Fig. 47–6). As the needle is advanced, 0.5 cc of steroid with 0.5 to 2 cc of lidocaine can be injected along the sheath of the tendon, and a palpable bulge is usually felt along the tendon. Care should be taken to avoid injection of steroid into the body of the tendon by moving the needle slightly if resistance to injection is noted.

Carpal Tunnel Syndrome

Inflammation with swelling in the many flexor tendons in the carpal tunnel area may result in median nerve compression, and injection in this area has the potential to relieve symptoms by reducing this inflammation (Fig. 47–7). This area should be injected by making a mark on the volar aspect of the wrist along the flexor tendons, on the ulnar side of the long palmar tendon, approximately 1 inch proximal to the distal wrist crease.[105] A 22- to 26-gauge needle may be introduced perpendicular to the skin, or alternatively at a 30- to 45-degree angle, directing the needle proximally or distally along the course of the tendon. The needle should be introduced about ½ to 1 inch and the area injected with 0.5 cc of steroid with 0.5 to 1 cc of lidocaine. If the needle meets obstruction, or if the patient experiences paresthesias, the needle should be withdrawn and redirected slightly to avoid injecting into the body of a tendon or into the median nerve itself.

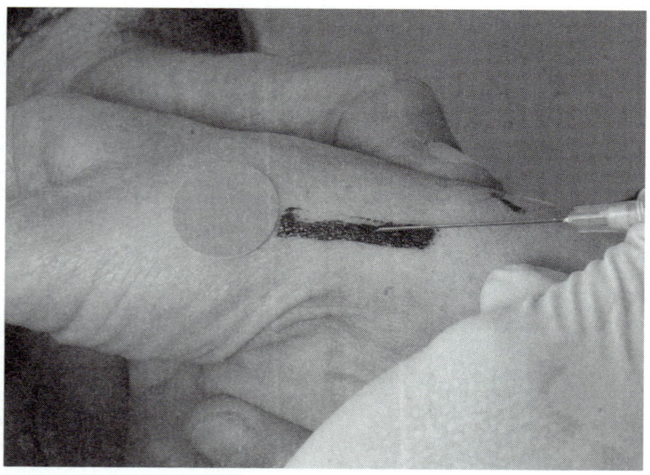

FIGURE 47–6 · Injection for de Quervain's Tenosynovitis. The needle is inserted along the course of the tendons *(black line)*, proximal to the thumb carpometacarpal joint *(spot)*, at the radial aspect of the anatomic snuffbox. The needle is directed almost parallel to the skin either proximally or distally. As the needle is advanced, a mixture of steroid and anesthetic is injected along the sheath of the tendon, and a palpable bulge is usually felt along the tendon. Care should be taken to avoid injection of steroid into the body of the tendon. (See color plate 20.)

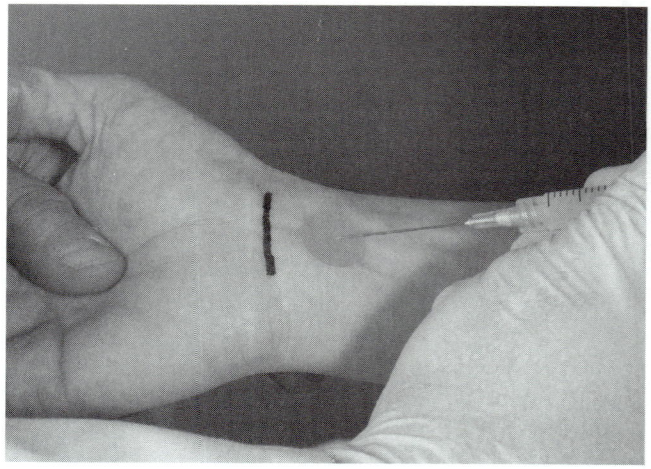

FIGURE 47–7 · Injection for Carpal Tunnel Syndrome. To begin an injection in this area, the clinician should make a mark on the volar aspect of the wrist along the flexor tendons, on the ulnar side of the long palmar tendon, and approximately 1 inch proximal to the distal volar skin crease at the wrist *(black)*. A 22- to 26-gauge needle is introduced at a 30- to 45-degree angle and is directed proximally or distally along the course of the tendon. The needle should be introduced about ½ to 1 inch. If the needle meets obstruction, or if the patient experiences paresthesias, the needle should be withdrawn and redirected slightly to avoid injecting into the body of a tendon or into the median nerve itself. (See color plate 21.)

Ganglia

Small, often hard, nodular structures known as ganglia are frequently present around the hands and wrists, and they may occur in many other areas near joints or tendons. These structures usually contain a thick, gelatinous substance that is difficult to aspirate. In cases in which pain, tendon dysfunction, or nerve entrapment symptoms are bothersome to the patient, aspiration may be attempted, usually with an 18- to 20-gauge needle. Even if no fluid is obtained, the process of puncture will occasionally cause the structure to dissipate its contents, and symptoms will be relieved. A small amount (0.2 to 0.5 cc) of steroid with lidocaine may be injected in an attempt to prevent reaccumulation of fluid.

Thumb Carpometacarpal Joint

Aspiration of fluid from this joint is seldom possible and rarely indicated. However, this joint is commonly involved in osteoarthritis and may be a source of localized pain amenable to local injection (Fig. 47–8). The joint space is narrowed and often surrounded by osteophytes, but it may be entered by flexing the thumb across the palm and making a mark at the base of the thumb metacarpal away from the border of the snuffbox. A 22- to 25-gauge needle should then be inserted ½ to 1 inch at this mark and directed away from the radial artery; 0.2 to 0.5 cc of steroid may be injected.

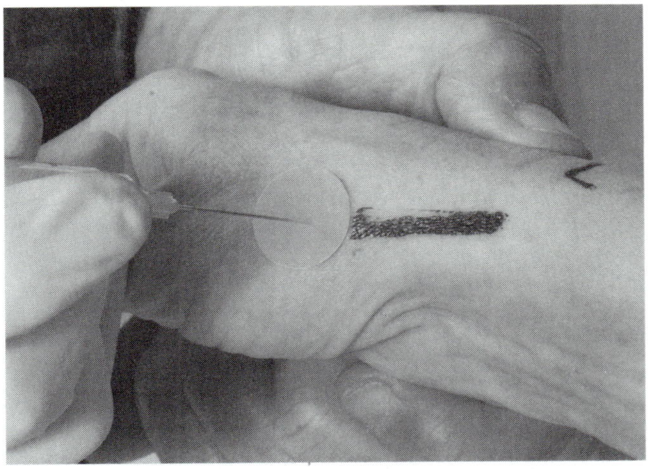

FIGURE 47–8 · Injection of the Thumb Carpometacarpal Joint. The procedure begins by flexing the thumb across the palm and making a mark at the base of the thumb metacarpal distal to the radial tendons of the snuffbox *(black)*. A 22- to 25-gauge needle is inserted ½ to 1 inch at this mark and directed away from the radial artery; 0.2 to 0.5 cc of steroid may then be injected. (See color plate 22.)

Metacarpal-Phalangeal and Interphalangeal Joints

Inflammation in the small joints of the hands usually causes the synovium to bulge dorsally. Occasionally, these small joints may have enough swelling for a drop or two of fluid to be obtained for crystal analysis, culture, or both. In most cases, however, arthrocentesis is performed for symptom relief, which may be done by injecting 0.1 to 0.2 cc of corticosteroid, with or without local anesthetic. A 24- to 27-gauge, 0.5- to 1-inch needle can be inserted on either side of the joint at a mark made at the joint line, just under the extensor tendon mechanism. Some physicians prefer to have the joint slightly flexed to improve the chances for entry into the joint space itself.

Flexor Tenosynovitis (Trigger Fingers)

The pathologic process in this condition usually involves the tendon at the level of the metacarpal-phalangeal joint in the palm. Usually, a localized swelling that moves with the tendon sheath may be palpated in this area. After a mark has been made at this area, a 22- to 27-gauge needle may be introduced at a 30- to 45-degree angle, directing the needle proximally or distally along the course of the tendon. The needle should be introduced about ½ inch and the area injected with 0.5 cc of steroid with 0.5 cc of lidocaine. Lack of resistance during injection indicates proper needle placement, as is the case with other tendon sheath injections.

LUMBOSACRAL SPINE AREA

Back pain is difficult to explain anatomically in most patients, but many patients with back pain have areas tender to deep palpation, particularly in the presacral area and paraspinous muscles. As is the case in the cervical spine area, most injections in this region are best considered to be myofascial or "trigger point" injections. The point of injection is usually determined by palpating for the areas of most tenderness, with few reliable landmarks available for localization of anatomic structures. Using a 22- to 25-gauge needle, a combination of 0.5 to 1 cc of steroid and 0.5 to 2 cc of lidocaine can be injected into areas of the paraspinous muscles or other tender areas. Some of the injections performed in these areas are likely to be close enough to the posterior lumbar facet or upper sacroiliac joints to reduce inflammation in the joints themselves, whereas others are probably reducing inflammation in ligaments, tendons, or bursal structures. More precise injection of posterior lumbar facet or sacroiliac joints requires radiographic guidance, either with fluoroscopy, computerized tomography, or magnetic resonance imaging.[17,19,62,63]

PELVIC GIRDLE

Ischiogluteal Bursitis

The bursa over the ischial tuberosity is located by direct palpation in the buttock while the patient lies on the opposite side with knees fully flexed. The prominence is more easily palpated as the gluteus muscles are displaced from the area. After marking the area of tenderness over the prominence, a 3-inch needle should be inserted horizontally until bone is hit and 1 cc of steroid with 1 to 2 cc of lidocaine are instilled. Care should be taken to avoid the sciatic notch medially.

Trochanteric Pain Syndrome (Bursitis)

This common pain syndrome is diagnosed by physical findings of normal hip joint motion and a reproducible tender area in the region of the greater trochanter where the gluteal muscles insert (Fig. 47–9). This area can be easily injected after marking the area of tenderness with the patient lying on the opposite side. A 1- to

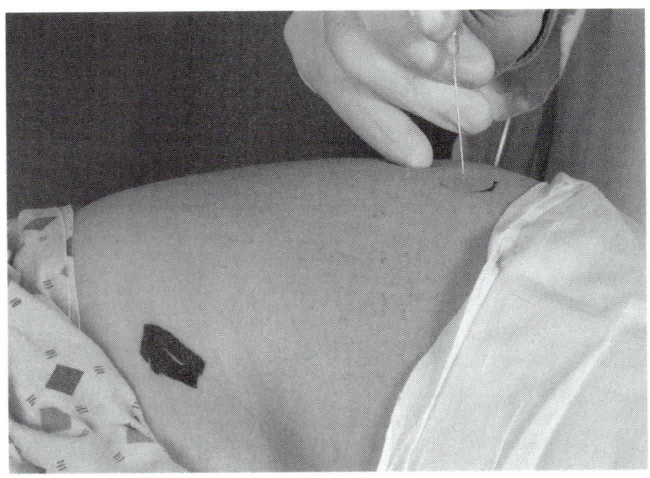

FIGURE 47–9 · Injection for Trochanteric Pain Syndrome. This area is easily injected after marking the area of tenderness over bony prominence of the lateral hip with the patient lying on the opposite side. A 1- to 3-inch needle is inserted perpendicular to the skin over the bony prominence, and 1 cc of steroid with 2 to 4 cc of local anesthetic are injected into the area. (Anterior superior iliac spine is marked for reference.) (See color plate 23.)

3-inch needle should be inserted perpendicular to the skin of the bony prominence and 1 cc of steroid with 2 to 4 cc of local anesthetic injected into the area.

Hip (Acetabular) Joint

The hip is a difficult joint to aspirate and inject, and synovial fluid is seldom obtained from the hip in clinical practice. Two approaches can be attempted, either an anterior or lateral approach, but accuracy of each is variable. A recent cadaver study found the rate of correct needle placement was only 60 percent with the anterior approach and 80 percent with the lateral approach, and the anterior approach frequently resulted in needle placement in the vicinity of the femoral nerve.[106] Thus, in situations where synovial fluid analysis is essential to patient management, particularly when infection is suspected, fluoroscopic guidance is necessary to obtain fluid for culture and other studies.

If aspiration without fluroscopic guidance is attempted, a 20-gauge, 3-inch needle should be used. For the anterior approach, the patient should be supine with the hip fully extended and externally rotated. A mark should be made 2 to 3 cm below the anterior superior iliac spine and 2 to 3 cm lateral to the femoral pulse. The needle is inserted at a 60-degree angle and directed posteriorly and medially until bone is hit. The needle is then withdrawn slightly, and an attempt should made to aspirate fluid. Injection of 1 cc of steroid with lidocaine may follow if indicated. For a lateral approach (Fig. 47–10), the patient should be supine and the hips rotated internally with knees apart and toes touching. A mark should be made just anterior to the greater trochanter and the needle inserted and directed medially and slightly cephalad toward a point slightly below the middle of the inguinal ligament. Often, the clinician can feel the tip of the needle slide into the joint, and aspiration can be attempted.

KNEE

Knee Joint

The knee is the easiest joint to enter with certainty by arthrocentesis, and is, thus, the joint most frequently aspirated for synovial fluid analysis in clinical practice. The knee may be aspirated with the patient in the supine or sitting position and from medial, lateral, or anterior aspects. Aspiration is usually considered to be easiest with the patient in the supine position with the knee almost fully extended. A mark should be made just posterior to the medial or lateral aspect of the patella in the recess behind the patella, where a bulge or "fluid wave" can be detected on physical examination if fluid is present (Figs. 47–11 and 47–12). An 18- to 22-gauge needle should be directed posteriorly and slightly inferiorly, and fluid can be aspirated after advancing the needle 0.5 to 1.5 inches into the joint space. A lateral approach is preferred by some clinicians because more fluid can be removed from this side in many patients.[107] In patients with rheumatoid arthritis or septic arthritis, synovial debris or proliferative synovial tissue may occlude the needle, and it may be necessary to rotate the needle to facilitate aspiration. In some patients, the knee can be aspirated and injected with the patient in a sitting position with the knee flexed. A mark can be made just below the distal border of the patella in the recess on either side of the infrapatellar tendon. One recent study demonstrated that a lateral midpatellar approach had a higher accuracy rate than the anteromedial or anterolateral approaches done in a sitting position.[108] In some patients, the suprapatellar bursa may become distended with fluid. Because this space is an extension of the knee joint, either the knee joint or the suprapatellar bursa may be aspirated directly to remove fluid from this area. In some patients with large effusions, compression of the suprapatellar area will allow more fluid to obtained by arthrocentesis from the knee joint itself. In other patients, a popliteal cyst may form in the area behind the

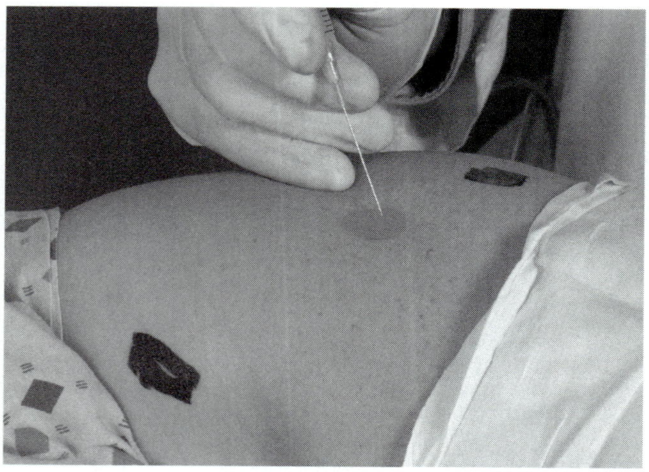

FIGURE 47–10 · Hip Arthrocentesis: Lateral Approach. With the hip internally rotated, the needle is inserted just anterior to the greater trochanter *(black)* and directed toward a point slightly below the inguinal ligament (anterior superior iliac spine is marked for reference). As noted in the text, accuracy of any approach to the hip joint is limited, and radiographic guidance should be considered unless synovial fluid is easily obtained using this approach. (See color plate 24.)

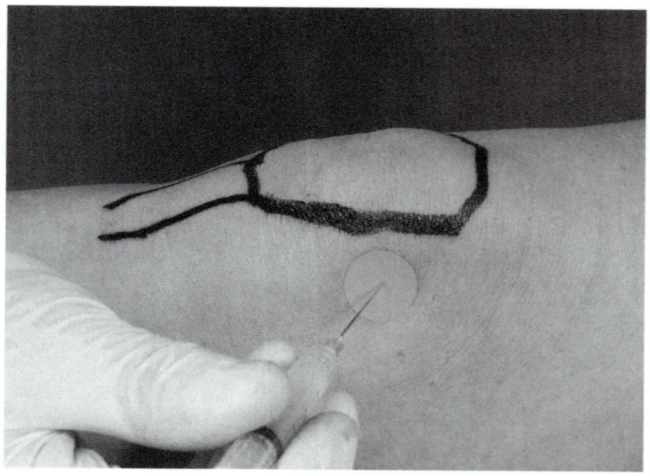

FIGURE 47–11 · Knee Arthrocentesis: Medial Approach. With the patient supine, a mark is made in the recess (or where there is a fluid bulge) behind the medial portion of the patella *(black)*, approximately at the midline. The needle should be advanced 1.5 inches or more until fluid is obtained (patellar tendon marked for reference). (See color plate 25.)

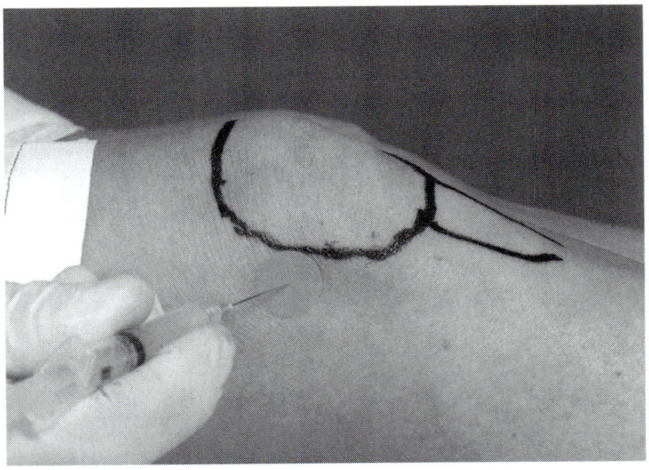

FIGURE 47–12 · Knee Arthrocentesis: Lateral Approach. With the patient supine, a mark is made in the recess (or where there is a fluid bulge) behind the lateral portion of the patella *(black)*, approximately at the midline. The needle should be advanced 1.5 inches or more until fluid is obtained (patellar tendon marked for reference). (See color plate 26.)

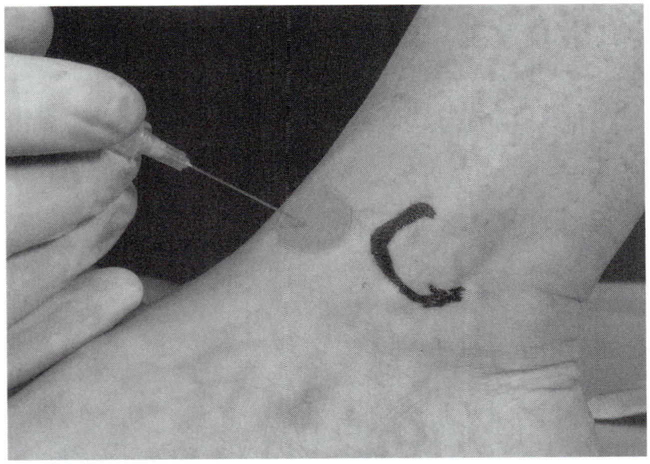

FIGURE 47–13 · Ankle Arthrocentesis: Anterior Approach (Tibiotalar Joint). With ankle at a 90-degree angle to the lower leg, the needle is inserted at a point just lateral to the medial malleolus *(black)* and just medial to the tibialis anterior tendon. The needle is then directed posteriorly, perpendicular to the shaft of the tibia. (See color plate 27.)

knee joint, and there may often be a ball-valve leakage of fluid from the knee joint.[109] The cyst may sometimes be difficult to aspirate due to its location or lack of distinct borders. Fortunately, injection of corticosteroid into the knee joint will usually result in the passage of medication into the cyst with a therapeutic effect.

Periarticular Knee Pain Syndromes

Pain related to the anserine bursa, located over the medial aspect of the tibia just below the joint line, can be treated with a local injection into this area. In addition, some patients may have an area of localized soft tissue tenderness above the joint line over the medial and lateral condyles, often felt to be related to an irritated iliotibial band (lateral) or infrapatellar plica (medial). In each of these conditions, the area of tenderness should be marked, and a 22-gauge needle introduced to the bone, withdrawn slightly, and the area injected with 0.5 cc of steroid with 1 to 3 cc of local anesthetic. Prepatellar bursitis may result in swelling in the soft tissues anterior to the patella and should be distinguishable from a knee effusion. Like olecranon bursitis at the elbow, this area may be aspirated directly at the point of maximal swelling, and the area may be injected with 0.5 cc of corticosteroid preparation if indicated.

ANKLE AND FOOT

Tibiotalar Joint

This joint is best aspirated with the patient in a supine position with the leg-foot angle at 90 degrees (Fig. 47–13). A mark is made just medial to the tibialis anterior tendon and lateral to the medial malleolus. A 20- to 22-gauge, 1.5-inch needle is directed posteriorly and should enter the joint space without striking bone. If resistance is felt and no fluid obtained, the needle should be withdrawn to close to the surface and redirected slightly while aspirating for fluid. After aspiration, the area may be injected with 0.5 cc of corticosteroid, with or without lidocaine.

Subtalar Joint

Swelling from this joint is usually detected by swelling beneath the lateral malleolus. A mark is made just inferior to the tip of the lateral malleolus, usually over the area of swelling. A 20- to 22-gauge needle should be directed perpendicular to the skin and the area aspirated as the needle is advanced (Fig. 47–14). The needle may be partially withdrawn and readvanced if no fluid is obtained with the first pass, and 0.5 cc of corticosteroid may be injected after fluid is aspirated, if indicated.

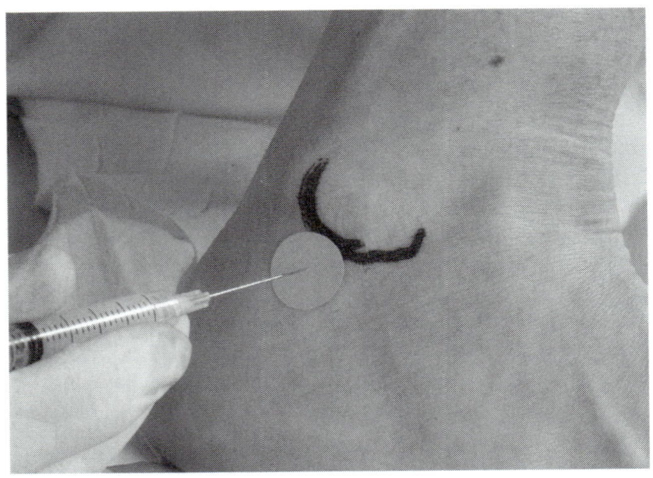

FIGURE 47–14 · Subtalar (Lateral) Ankle Arthrocentesis. The needle is inserted into the recess just inferior to the tip of the lateral malleolus *(black)* and directed perpendicularly. A bulge is often easily palpated here if fluid is present in this joint. (See color plate 28.)

Achilles Tendon Area

In general, the area around the insertion of the Achilles tendon on the calcaneus should not be approached with a needle. In some patients, however, an area of swelling may be detected in the subcutaneous Achilles bursa between the skin and tendon or in the retrocalcaneal bursa between the tendon and calcaneus. In either case, the area may be aspirated for fluid analysis, using a lateral or medial approach for the deeper area, to avoid inserting needle through the Achilles tendon. In rare patients, these areas or the sheath of the Achilles tendon itself may be injected with 0.25 to 0.5 cc of steroid preparation with lidocaine. As noted previously, any injection in this area should be undertaken with extreme care to avoid injection within the body of the Achilles tendon, due to the risk and potential consequences of rupture.

Tarsal Tunnel Syndrome

This uncommon condition is sometimes amenable to local steroid injection, although the optimal approach to therapy in this condition is uncertain. The skin should be marked just inferior and posterior to the medial malleolus. The tendon sheaths in this area may be injected with a 22- to 25-gauge needle with 0.5 cc of steroid and 0.5 to 1 cc of lidocaine. Care should be taken not to inject the nerve.

Plantar Fascia

In this condition, tenderness is usually elicited along the course of the plantar fascia and at its insertion at the calcaneus. This area may be injected by inserting a 22- to 25-gauge, 1.5-inch needle from the lateral or medial aspect of the heel and directing it through the tissues of the heel pad toward the area of tenderness. About 0.5 cc of corticosteroid with 0.5 to 1 cc of lidocaine can then be injected. Repeated injections in this area should be avoided due to the risk of plantar fascia rupture.[79,80]

Metatarsal-Phalangeal Joints

The small joints of the toes are aspirated and injected using techniques similar to those of the small joints of the hands. The metarsal = phalangeal (MTP) joint of the great toe is an area of particular interest because this joint is involved so often in gout. This joint may be aspirated in patients with a history suggestive of gout, even between attacks, and may sometimes yield enough fluid to allow a diagnosis of gout to be confirmed by microscopic analysis. A small mark can be made at the joint line over the medial aspect of this joint, a 22- to 25-gauge needle inserted, and the area aspirated. Care should be taken to express the tiny amount of fluid often found in the needle hub onto a microscope slide. These joints can be injected for therapeutic benefit, usually with 0.1 to 0.25 cc of steroid.

Interdigital Neuroma

This syndrome causes pain between the metatarsal heads in the foot, usually between the second and third or third and fourth toes (Fig. 47–15). Injection into this space may reduce inflammation and relieve symptoms of nerve compression between the metatarsal heads. The area is most easily injected from the dorsal aspect. The area of tenderness should be marked, a 22- to 27-gauge needle inserted ½ to 1 inch, and 0.25 to 0.5 cc of steroid with equal volume of anesthetic injected.

Current and Future Trends in Arthrocentesis and Joint Injection

In recent years, ultrasound guidance has been the subject of a number of studies as a means to increase accuracy for needle placement for arthrocentesis and therapeutic steroid injection in joints and tendon sheaths, particularly in Europe.[110,111] One recent comparative study showed that ultrasound guidance increased the ability to obtain synovial fluid from joints to 97 percent of patients, compared to 32 percent when using conventional techniques without ultrasound.[112] Ultrasound can be utilized by having the area to be aspirated marked by the ultrasonographer or by having concurrent ultrasound monitoring while the needle is inserted into the joint or tendon sheath area. The latter approach has potential to be particularly helpful in areas difficult to assess, but it is more cumbersome and requires the use of sterile components for the ultrasound machine and sterile ultrasound gel. Cost and time constraints will probably limit the widespread use of ultrasonography in routine clinical rheumatology practice, but increased use of this procedure has the potential to improve outcomes in individual patients with pain associated with difficult-to-access periarticular structures.

The irrigation of joints in osteoarthritis with large volumes of saline, known as tidal irrigation, had been a subject of controversy during the period from 1992 = 2002. Based on observations that some patients undergoing arthroscopy seemed to improve from the process of lavage that accompanies the procedure, subsequent

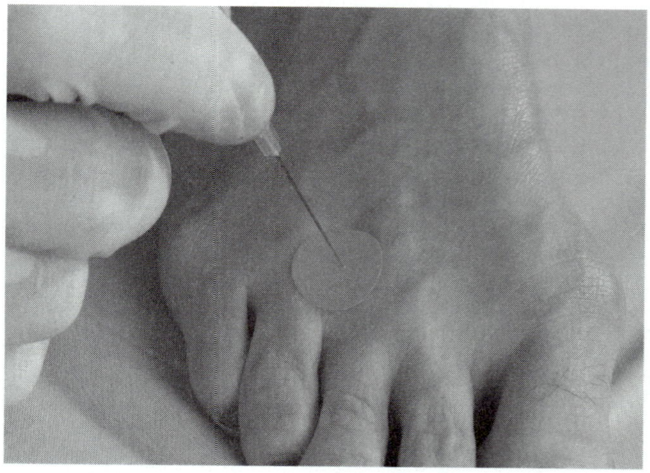

FIGURE 47–15 · Injection for Interdigital (Morton's) Neuroma. The area is most easily injected from the dorsal aspect, usually between the metarsal heads of the third and fourth toes. The area of tenderness is marked, the needle is inserted 0.5 to 1 inch, and steroid with anesthetic is injected. (See color plate 29.)

studies suggested that irrigation of the joint was superior to medical management and comparable to local steroid injection.[35,113,114] However, a recent study using a "sham" irrigation as control showed no benefit in patients receiving tidal irrigation, suggesting that most of the previously noted response was related to placebo effect.[115]

Advances in understanding of the underlying biologic processes in rheumatoid arthritis and osteoarthritis in recent years have raised hopes that intrasynovial therapy with biologic agents might have a role in the treatment of various forms of arthritis. Potential intrasynovial therapies might include agents that suppress inflammation and bone destruction (e.g., interleukin-1 receptor antagonist, interleukin-4, tumor necrosis factor inhibitors, bisphosophonates) or those that promote cartilage growth (e.g., insulin-like growth factor, transforming growth factor-β).[116] The ability to transfer genes to synoviocytes in vivo and ex vivo has led to speculation that the delivery of genes directly to the joints might lead to reduced inflammation and cartilage degradation in both rheumatoid arthritis and osteoarthritis.[117,118] In the past decade, further investigations have attempted to identify viral vectors with potential to deliver genes directly to synovial cells.[119,120] A number of strategies have been outlined to further investigate the possibility of intrasynovial gene therapy for rheumatoid arthritis, osteoarthritis, and other diseases of the joints.[121-124] The role of such therapies in the future will most likely depend on the ability to find safe and effective vectors that can deliver genetic material that will persist in synovial tissues for long periods of time at a reasonable cost.

REFERENCES

1. Committee on Rheumatology Care: Benchmarks in Rheumatology Practice. Data from the 1999 American College of Rheumatology Economic Survey. Atlanta, American College of Rheumatology, 1999.
2. Nelson RL, McCaffrey LA, Nobrega FT, et al: Altering residency curriculum in response to a changing practice environment: use of the Mayo internal medicine residency alumni survey. Mayo Clin Proc 65:809-817, 1990.
3. Pemberton R: Arthritis and Rheumatoid Conditions: Their Nature and Treatment. Philadelphia, Lea and Febiger, 1935.
4. Ropes MW, Bauer W: Synovial Fluid Changes in Joint Disease. Cambridge, Mass., Harvard University Press, 1953.
5. Woolf AEM: A surgical method of relief for intractable pain in osteoarthritis of the knee. Br J Rheumatol 1:97-108, 1938.
6. Waugh WG: Mono-articular osteo-arthritis of the hip: treatment by acid injection. Brit Med J 1:873-874, 1945.
7. Comroe BI: Arthritis and Allied Conditions. Philadelphia, Lea and Febiger, 1949.
8. Hollander JL: Hydrocortisone and cortisone injected into arthritic joints: comparative effects of and use of hydrocortisone as a local antiarthritic agent. JAMA 147:1629, 1951.
9. Hollander JL: Local anti-rheumatic effectiveness of higher esters and analogues of hydrocortisone. Ann Rheum Dis 13:297, 1954.
10. Hollander JL: Intrasynovial corticosteroid therapy: a decade of use. Bull Rheum Dis 11:239-240, 1961.
11. Hollander JL: Intrasynovial corticosteroid therapy in arthritis. Md State Med J 19:62-66, 1970.
12. McCarty DJ: Treatment of rheumatoid joint inflammation with triamcinolone hexacetonide. Arthritis Rheum 15:157-173, 1972.
13. McCarty DJ, Harman JG, Grassanovich JL, Qian C: Treatment of rheumatoid joint inflammation with intrasynovial triamcinolone hexacetonide. J Rheumatol 22:1631-1635, 1995.
14. Weitoft T, Uddenfeldt P: Importance of synovial fluid aspiration when injecting intra-articular corticosteroids. Ann Rheum Dis 59:233-235, 2000.
15. Fernandez C, Noguera R, Gonzalez JA, Pascual E: Treatment of acute attacks of gout with a small dose of intraarticular triamcinolone acetonide. J Rheumatol 26:2285-2286, 1999.
16. Green M, Marzo-Ortega H, Wakefield RJ, et al: Predictors of outcome in patients with oligoarthritis: results of a protocol of intraarticular corticosteroids to all clinically active joints. Arthritis Rheum 44:1177-83, 2001.
17. Braun J, Bollow M, Seyrekbasan F, et al: Computed tomography guided corticosteroid injection of the sacroiliac joint in patients with spondyloarthropathy with sacroiliitis: clinical outcome and followup by dynamic magnetic resonance imaging. J Rheumatol 23:659-664, 1996.
18. Maugars Y, Mathis C, Berthelot JM, et al: Assessment of the efficacy of sacroiliac corticosteroid injections in spondylarthropathies: a double-blind study. Br J Rheumatol 35:767-770, 1996.
19. Gunaydin I, Pereira PL, Daikeler T, et al: Magnetic resonance imaging guided corticosteroid injection of the sacroiliac joints in patients with therapy resistant spondyloarthropathy: a pilot study. J Rheumatol 27:424-428, 2000.
20. Hanly JG, Mitchell M, MacMillan L, et al: Efficacy of sacroiliac corticosteroid injections in patients with inflammatory spondyloarthropathy: results of a 6 month controlled study. J Rheumatol 27:719-722, 2000.
21. Allen RC, Gross KR, Laxer RM, et al: Intraarticular triamcinolone hexacetonide in the management of chronic arthritis in children. Arthritis Rheum 29:997-1001, 1986.
22. Sparling M, Malleson P, Wood B, Petty R: Radiographic followup of joints injected with triamcinolone hexacetonide for the management of childhood arthritis. Arthritis Rheum 33:821-826, 1990.
23. Ravelli A, Manzoni SM, Viola S, et al: Factors affecting the efficacy of intraarticular corticosteroid injection of knees in juvenile idiopathic arthritis. J Rheumatol 28:2100-2102, 2001.
24. Padeh S, Passwell JH: Intraarticular corticosteroid injection in the management of children with chronic arthritis. Arthritis Rheum 41:1210-1214, 1998.
25. Breit W, Frosch M, Meyer U, et al: A subgroup-specific evaluation of the efficacy of intraarticular triamcinolone hexacetonide in juvenile chronic arthritis. J Rheumatol 27:2696-2702, 2000.
26. Sherry DD, Stein LD, Reed AM, et al: Prevention of leg length discrepancy in young children with pauciarticular juvenile rheumatoid arthritis by treatment with intraarticular steroids. Arthritis Rheum 42:2330-2334, 1999.
27. Neidel J, Boehnke M, Kuster RM: The efficacy and safety of intraarticular corticosteroid therapy for coxitis in juvenile rheumatoid arthritis. Arthritis Rheum 46:1620-1628, 2002.
28. Creamer P: Intra-articular corticosteroid treatment in osteoarthritis. Curr Opin Rheumatol 11:417-421, 1999.
29. Towheed TE, Hochberg MC: A systematic review of randomized controlled trials of pharmacological therapy in osteoarthritis of the knee, with an emphasis on trial methodology. Semin Arthritis Rheum 26:755-770, 1997.
30. Miller JH, White J, Nortan TH: The value of intra-articular corticosteroids for osteoarthritis of the knee. J Bone Joint Surg Br 40:636, 1958.
31. Dieppe PA, Sathapatayavongs B, Jones HE, et al: Intra-articular steroids in osteoarthritis. Rheumatol Rehabil 19:212-217, 1980.
32. Friedman DM, Moore ME: The efficacy of intraarticular steroids in osteoarthritis: a double-blind study. J Rheumatol 7:850-856, 1980.
33. Jones A, Doherty M: Intra-articular corticosteroids are effective in osteoarthritis but there are no clinical predictors of response. Ann Rheum Dis 55:829-832, 1996.
34. Gaffney K, Ledingham J, Perry JD: Intra-articular triamcinolone hexacetonide in knee osteoarthritis: factors influencing the clinical response. Ann Rheum Dis 54:379-381, 1995.
35. Ravaud P, Moulinier L, Giraudeau B, et al: Effects of joint lavage and steroid injection in patients with osteoarthritis of the knee: results of a multicenter, randomized, controlled trial. Arthritis Rheum 42:475-482, 1999.

36. Raynauld JP: Clinical trials: impact of intraarticular steroid injections on the progression of knee osteoarthritis. Osteoarthritis Cartilage 7:348-349, 1999.
37. Plant MJ, Borg AA, Dziedzic K, et al: Radiographic patterns and response to corticosteroid hip injection. Ann Rheum Dis 56:476-480, 1997.
38. Margules KR: Fluoroscopically directed steroid instillation in the treatment of hip osteoarthritis: safety and efficacy in 510 cases. Arthritis Rheum 44:2449-2450, 2455-2456, 2001.
39. Shupak R, Teitel J, Garvey MB, Freedman J: Intraarticular methylprednisolone therapy in hemophilic arthropathy. Am J Hematol 27:26-29, 1988.
40. Felson DT, Anderson JJ: Hyaluronate sodium injections for osteoarthritis: hope, hype, and hard truths. Arch Intern Med 162:245-247, 2002.
41. Kim PS: Role of injection therapy: review of indications for trigger point injections, regional blocks, facet joint injections, and intra-articular injections. Curr Opin Rheumatol 14:52-57, 2002.
42. Cummings TM, White AR: Needling therapies in the management of myofascial trigger point pain: a systematic review. Arch Phys Med Rehabil 82:986-992, 2001.
43. Green S, Buchbinder R, Glazier R, Forbes A: Systematic review of randomised controlled trials of interventions for painful shoulder: selection criteria, outcome assessment, and efficacy. BMJ 316:354-360, 1998.
44. van der Windt DA, Koes BW, Deville W, et al: Effectiveness of corticosteroid injections versus physiotherapy for treatment of painful stiff shoulder in primary care: randomised trial. Br Med J 317:1292-1296, 1998.
45. Hay EM, Paterson SM, Lewis M, et al: Pragmatic randomised controlled trial of local corticosteroid injection and naproxen for treatment of lateral epicondylitis of elbow in primary care. Br Med J 319:964-968, 1999.
46. Smidt N, van der Windt DA, Assendelft WJ, et al: Corticosteroid injections, physiotherapy, or a wait-and-see policy for lateral epicondylitis: a randomised controlled trial. Lancet 359:657-662, 2002.
47. Shbeeb MI, O'Duffy JD, Michet CJ Jr, et al: Evaluation of glucocorticosteroid injection for the treatment of trochanteric bursitis. J Rheumatol 23:2104-2106, 1996.
48. Larsson LG, Baum J: The syndrome of anserina bursitis: an overlooked diagnosis. Arthritis Rheum 28:1062-1065, 1985.
49. Green DP: Diagnostic and therapeutic value of carpal tunnel injection. J Hand Surg [Am] 9:850-854, 1984.
50. Dammers JW, Veering MM, Vermeulen M: Injection of methylprednisolone proximal to the carpal tunnel: randomised double blind trial. Br Med J 319:884-886, 1999.
51. Neustadt DH: Local corticosteroid injection therapy in soft tissue rheumatic conditions of the hand and wrist. Arthritis Rheum 34:923-926, 1991.
52. Anderson BC, Manthey R, Brouns MC: Treatment of De Quervain's tenosynovitis with corticosteroids: a prospective study of the response to local injection. Arthritis Rheum 34:793-798, 1991.
53. Harvey FJ, Harvey PM, Horsley MW: De Quervain's disease: surgical or nonsurgical treatment. J Hand Surg [Am] 15:83-87, 1990.
54. Lane LB, Boretz RS, Stuchin SA: Treatment of de Quervain's disease: role of conservative management. J Hand Surg [Br] 26:258-260, 2001.
55. Avci S, Yilmaz C, Sayli U: Comparison of nonsurgical treatment measures for de Quervain's disease of pregnancy and lactation. J Hand Surg [Am] 27:322-324, 2002.
56. Marks MR, Gunther SF: Efficacy of cortisone injection in treatment of trigger fingers and thumbs. J Hand Surg [Am] 14:722-727, 1989.
57. Fauno P, Andersen HJ, Simonsen O: A long-term follow-up of the effect of repeated corticosteroid injections for stenosing tenovaginitis. J Hand Surg [Br] 14:242-243, 1989.
58. Lapidus PW, Guidotti FP: Report on the treatment of one hundred and two ganglions. Bull Hosp Joint Dis 28:50-57, 1967.
59. Kaplan PE, Kernahan WT Jr: Tarsal tunnel syndrome: an electrodiagnostic and surgical correlation. J Bone Joint Surg Am 63:96-99, 1981.
60. Strong G, Thomas PS: Conservative treatment of Morton's neuroma. Orthop Rev 16:343-345, 1987.
61. Crawford F, Atkins D, Young P, Edwards J: Steroid injection for heel pain: evidence of short-term effectiveness—a randomized controlled trial. Rheumatology (Oxford) 38:974-977, 1999.
62. Marks RC, Houston T, Thulbourne T: Facet joint injection and facet nerve block: a randomised comparison in 86 patients with chronic low back pain. Pain 49:325-328, 1992.
63. Lilius G, Harilainen A, Laasonen EM, Myllynen P: Chronic unilateral low-back pain: predictors of outcome of facet joint injections. Spine 15:780-782, 1990.
64. Nelemans PJ, deBie RA, deVet HC, Sturmans F: Injection therapy for subacute and chronic benign low back pain. Spine 26:501-515, 2001.
65. Carette S, Marcoux S, Truchon R, et al: A controlled trial of corticosteroid injections into facet joints for chronic low back pain. N Engl J Med 325:1002-1007, 1991.
66. Barnsley L, Lord SM, Wallis BJ, Bogduk N: Lack of effect of intraarticular corticosteroids for chronic pain in the cervical zygapophyseal joints. N Engl J Med 330:1047-1050, 1994.
67. Luukkainen RK, Wennerstrand PV, Kautiainen HH, et al: Efficacy of periarticular corticosteroid treatment of the sacroiliac joint in non-spondylarthropathic patients with chronic low back pain in the region of the sacroiliac joint. Clin Exp Rheumatol 20:52-54, 2002.
68. Blyth T, Hunter JA, Stirling A: Pain relief in the rheumatoid knee after steroid injection: a single-blind comparison of hydrocortisone succinate, and triamcinolone acetonide or hexacetonide. Br J Rheumatol 33:461-463, 1994.
69. Brandt K, Smith G, Simon L: Review: intraarticular injection of hyaluronan as treatment for knee osteoarthritis: what is the evidence? Arthritis Rheum 43:1192-1203, 2000.
70. Petrella RJ, DiSilvestro MD, Hildebrand C: Effects of hyaluronate sodium on pain and physical functioning in osteoarthritis of the knee: a randomized, double-blind, placebo-controlled clinical trial. Arch Intern Med 162:292-298, 2002.
71. Thumboo J, O'Duffy JD: A prospective study of the safety of joint and soft tissue aspirations and injections in patients taking warfarin sodium. Arthritis Rheum 41:736-739, 1998.
72. Gray RG, Tenenbaum J, Gottlieb NL: Local corticosteroid injection treatment in rheumatic disorders. Semin Arthritis Rheum 10:231-254, 1981.
73. Ostensson A, Geborek P: Septic arthritis as a non-surgical complication in rheumatoid arthritis: relation to disease severity and therapy. Br J Rheumatol 30:35-38, 1991.
74. Glaser DL, Schildhorn JC, Bartolozzi AR, et al: Do you really know what is on the tip of your needle? The inadvertent introduction of skin into the joint (Abstract). Arthritis Rheum 43:S149, 2000.
75. McCarty DJ, Hogan JM: Inflammatory reaction after intrasynovial injection of microcrystalline adrenocorticosteroid esters. Arthritis Rheum 7:359, 1964.
76. Sweetnam R: Corticosteroid arthropathy and tendon rupture. J Bone Joint Surg Br 51:397-398, 1969.
77. Gottlieb NL, Riskin WG: Complications of local corticosteroid injections. JAMA 243:1547-1548, 1980.
78. Gray RG, Kiem IM, Gottlieb NL: Intratendon sheath corticosteroid treatment of rheumatoid arthritis-associated and idiopathic hand flexor tenosynovitis. Arthritis Rheum 21:92-96, 1978.
79. Sellman JR: Plantar fascia rupture associated with corticosteroid injection. Foot Ankle Int 15:376-381, 1994.
80. Acevedo JI, Beskin JL: Complications of plantar fascia rupture associated with corticosteroid injection. Foot Ankle Int 19:91-97, 1998.
81. Koehler BE, Urowitz MB, Killinger DW: The systemic effects of intra-articular corticosteroid. J Rheumatol 1:117-125, 1974.
82. Lazarevic MB, Skosey JL, Djordjevic-Denic G, et al: Reduction of cortisol levels after single intra-articular and intramuscular steroid injection. Am J Med 99:370-373, 1995.
83. Emkey RD, Lindsay R, Lyssy J, et al: The systemic effect of intraarticular administration of corticosteroid on markers of bone formation and bone resorption in patients with rheumatoid arthritis. Arthritis Rheum 39:277-282, 1996.
84. Chandler G, Wright V: Deleterious effect of intra-articular hydrocortisone. Lancet 2:661, 1958.
85. Alarcon-Segovia D, Ward LE: Marked destructive changes occurring in osteoarthritic finger joints after intra-articular injection of corticosteroids. Arthritis Rheum 9:443-463, 1966.
86. Bentley G, Goodfellow JW: Disorganisation of the knees following intra-articular hydrocortisone injections. J Bone Joint Surg Br 51:498-502, 1969.

87. Mankin HJ, Conger KA: The acute effects of intra-articular hydrocortisone on articular cartilage in rabbits. J Bone Joint Surg Am 48:1383-1388, 1966.
88. Behrens F, Shepard N, Mitchell N: Alterations of rabbit articular cartilage by intra-articular injections of glucocorticoids. J Bone Joint Surg Am 57:70-76, 1975.
89. Moskowitz RW, Davis W, Sammarco J, et al: Experimentally induced corticosteroid arthropathy. Arthritis Rheum 13:236-243, 1970.
90. Gibson T, Burry HC, Poswillo D, Glass J: Effect of intra-articular corticosteroid injections on primate cartilage. Ann Rheum Dis 36:74-79, 1977.
91. Williams JM, Brandt KD: Triamcinolone hexacetonide protects against fibrillation and osteophyte formation following chemically induced articular cartilage damage. Arthritis Rheum 28:1267-1274, 1985.
92. Pelletier JP, Martel-Pelletier J: Protective effects of corticosteroids on cartilage lesions and osteophyte formation in the Pond-Nuki dog model of osteoarthritis. Arthritis Rheum 32:181-193, 1989.
93. Pelletier JP, Mineau F, Raynauld JP, et al: Intraarticular injections with methylprednisolone acetate reduce osteoarthritic lesions in parallel with chondrocyte stromelysin synthesis in experimental osteoarthritis. Arthritis Rheum 37:414-423, 1994.
94. Hills BA, Ethell MT, Hodgson DR: Release of lubricating synovial surfactant by intra-articular steroid. Br J Rheumatol 37:649-652, 1998.
95. Young L, Katrib A, Cuello C, et al: Effects of intraarticular glucocorticoids on macrophage infiltration and mediators of joint damage in osteoarthritis synovial membranes: findings in a double-blind, placebo-controlled study. Arthritis Rheum 44:343-350, 2001.
96. Roberts WN, Babcock EA, Breitbach SA, et al: Corticosteroid injection in rheumatoid arthritis does not increase rate of total joint arthroplasty. J Rheumatol 23:1001-1004, 1996.
97. Cawley PJ, Morris IM: A study to compare the efficacy of two methods of skin preparation prior to joint injection. Br J Rheumatol 31:847-848, 1992.
98. Abeles M, Garjian P: Do spray coolant anesthetics contaminate an aseptic field? Arthritis Rheum 29:576, 1986.
99. Cleary AG, Ramanan AV, Baildam E,et al: Nitrous oxide analgesia during intra-articular injection for juvenile idiopathic arthritis. Arch Dis Child 86:416-418, 2002.
100. Neustadt DH: Intra-articular therapy for rheumatoid synovitis of the knee: effects of the postinjection rest regimen. Clin Rheumatol Pract 3:65-68, 1985.
101. Chatham W, Williams G, Moreland L, et al: Intraarticular corticosteroid injections: should we rest the joints? Arthritis Care Res 2:70-74, 1989.
102. Chakravarty K, Pharoah PD, Scott DG: A randomized controlled study of post-injection rest following intra-articular steroid therapy for knee synovitis. Br J Rheumatol 33:464-468, 1994.
103. Alarcon GS: Treatment of rheumatoid joint inflammation with intrasynovial triamcinolone. J Rheumatol 24:1849-1850, 1997.
104. Nitzan DW, Price A: The use of arthrocentesis for the treatment of osteoarthritic temporomandibular joints. J Oral Maxillofac Surg 59:1154-1159, 1160, 2001.
105. Minamikawa Y, Peimer CA, Kambe K, et al: Tenosynovial injection for carpal tunnel syndrome. J Hand Surg [Am] 17:178-181, 1992.
106. Leopold SS, Battista V, Oliverio JA: Safety and efficacy of intraarticular hip injection using anatomic landmarks. Clin Orthop 1(391):192-197, 2001.
107. Roberts WN, Hayes CW, Breitbach SA, Owen DS Jr: Dry taps and what to do about them: a pictorial essay on failed arthrocentesis of the knee. Am J Med 100:461-464, 1996.
108. Jackson DW, Evans NA, Thomas BM: Accuracy of needle placement into the intra-articular space of the knee. J Bone Joint Surg Am 84A:1522-1527, 2002.
109. Handy JR: Popliteal cysts in adults: a review. Semin Arthritis Rheum 31:108-118, 2001.
110. Grassi W, Farina A, Filippucci E, Cervini C: Sonographically guided procedures in rheumatology. Semin Arthritis Rheum 30:347-353, 2001.
111. Koski JM: Ultrasound guided injections in rheumatology. J Rheumatol 27:2131-2138, 2000.
112. Balint PV, Kane D, Hunter J, et al: Ultrasound guided versus conventional joint and soft tissue fluid aspiration in rheumatology practice: a pilot study. J Rheumatol 29:2209-2213, 2002.
113. Ike RW, Arnold WJ, Rothschild EW, Shaw HL: Tidal irrigation versus conservative medical management in patients with osteoarthritis of the knee: a prospective randomized study. Tidal Irrigation Cooperating Group. J Rheumatol 19:772-779, 1992.
114. Chang RW, Falconer J, Stulberg SD, et al: A randomized, controlled trial of arthroscopic surgery versus closed-needle joint lavage for patients with osteoarthritis of the knee. Arthritis Rheum 36:289-296, 1993.
115. Bradley JD, Heilman DK, Katz BP, et al: Tidal irrigation as treatment for knee osteoarthritis: a sham-controlled, randomized, double-blinded evaluation. Arthritis Rheum 46:100-108, 2002.
116. Cocco R, Tofi C, Fioravanti A, et al: Effects of clodronate on synovial fluid levels of some inflammatory mediators, after intra-articular administration to patients with synovitis secondary to knee osteoarthritis. Boll Soc Ital Biol Sper 75:71-76, 1999.
117. Tomita T, Takeuchi E, Tomita N, et al: Suppressed severity of collagen-induced arthritis by in vivo transfection of nuclear factor kappaB decoy oligodeoxynucleotides as a gene therapy. Arthritis Rheum 42:2532-2542, 1999.
118. Bandara G, Robbins PD, Georgescu HI, et al: Gene transfer to synoviocytes: prospects for gene treatment of arthritis. DNA Cell Biol 11:227-231, 1992.
119. Bakker AC, van de Loo FA, Joosten LA, et al: C3-Tat/HIV-regulated intraarticular human interleukin-1 receptor antagonist gene therapy results in efficient inhibition of collagen-induced arthritis superior to cytomegalovirus-regulated expression of the same transgene. Arthritis Rheum 46:1661-1670, 2002.
120. Ijima K, Murakami M, Okamoto H, et al: Successful gene therapy via intraarticular injection of adenovirus vector containing CTLA4IgG in a murine model of type II collagen-induced arthritis. Hum Gene Ther 12:1063-1077, 2001.
121. Evans CH, Ghivizzani SC, Kang R, et al: Gene therapy for rheumatic diseases. Arthritis Rheum 42:1-16, 1999.
122. Evans CH, Robbins PD: Potential treatment of osteoarthritis by gene therapy. Rheum Dis Clin North Am 25:333-344, 1999.
123. Gouze E, Ghivizzani SC, Robbins PD, Evans CH: Gene therapy for rheumatoid arthritis. Curr Rheumatol Rep 3:79-85, 2001.
124. van de Loo FA, van den Berg WB: Gene therapy for rheumatoid arthritis: lessons from animal models, including studies on interleukin-4, interleukin-10, and interleukin-1 receptor antagonist as potential disease modulators. Rheum Dis Clin North Am 28:127-149, 2002.

48 Arthroscopy

WILLIAM J. ARNOLD • ERIN L. ARNOLD

Arthroscopy was introduced as a diagnostic tool to allow the orthopedic surgeon to directly visualize the interior of a painful knee joint in a minimally invasive fashion.[1] It is now possible for rheumatologists to perform arthroscopy and obtain biopsies from an involved joint in an outpatient setting with few complications. The performance of arthroscopy by rheumatologists has been stimulated both by the recognition that the synovium is the primary site of disease pathogenesis in patients with inflammatory arthritis and that the direct inspection of the joint surface is a valuable way to assess the progress of the disease process and the response to treatment.[2-5] Although it has been suggested that the performance of these procedures by rheumatologists be called "rheumatologic arthroscopy," the best terminology, regardless of who performs the procedure, remains simply *arthroscopy,* appended with a description of the procedure(s) performed (i.e., arthroscopy with synovial biopsy).[6]

Arthroscopic surgical procedures are performed for patients with all forms of arthritis. The primary clinical indications are for the treatment of pain and limited function. Arthroscopic surgical procedures, such as meniscectomy and débridement, are typically performed by orthopedic surgeons, are more invasive, and are associated with a greater risk of serious complications.[7] More than 650,000 of these arthroscopic surgical procedures were performed for patients with OA of the knee in 1998.[8] However, a recent study has called into question the efficacy of arthroscopic surgical procedures for this group of patients.[9] The appeal of the minimally invasive nature and reduced complication rate of arthroscopic treatments, coupled with the reduced cost and more rapid rehabilitation compared to open procedures such as total joint replacement, ensures that further studies will be performed to better define the appropriate clinical indications for arthroscopic procedures in patients with arthritis.

Arthroscopy by Rheumatologists

The history of the subspecialty of rheumatology in the United States centers on the discoveries of rheumatoid factor, the lupus erythematosus (LE) cell, and cortisone in the late 1940s.[10] When compared to other medical subspecialists, rheumatologists have not acquired many technical skills to use in the day-to-day care of patients. Only the Polley-Bickell needle, introduced at the Mayo Clinic in 1951 for use in closed synovial biopsies, and a later modification by Parker and Pearson are exceptions.[11,12]

From 1991 to 1993, the American College of Rheumatology sponsored six introductory courses for rheumatologists interested in arthroscopy. A survey of 22 attendees at the first course indicated that 30 percent of those responding had begun to do arthroscopy within 6 months after taking the course.[13] In a survey of National Institutes of Health (NIH)-funded multipurpose arthritis and musculoskeletal disease centers in 1992, of the 13 centers responding to the survey, six had active programs in arthroscopy, two had faculty members who were actively training, three indicated that arthroscopy would begin in 12 months, and the remaining two centers thought it would take between 1 and 5 years to begin arthroscopy in their programs.[14]

In 2002, the results of a survey indicated that 72 rheumatologists in 36 centers worldwide were performing arthroscopy. Twenty-five of the 36 centers had begun doing the procedure since 1990,[15] for a total of 16,532 arthroscopies.

The European Synovitis Study Group[2] has subsequently widened its membership to include North America and Australia and serves as a forum for studies of synovial tissue analysis and disease progression using biopsies obtained by arthroscopy.

The International League Against Rheumatism has convened a task force to create arthroscopy training guidelines for rheumatologists and rheumatology training programs. These guidelines were approved in 2000 and have been submitted for publication.[16] They outline the minimum faculty, facility, and curriculum requirements necessary for a rheumatology training program to offer trainees an opportunity to acquire expertise in arthroscopy.

Arthroscopic Equipment

The #22 arthroscope, which most closely resembles those now available, was used by Dr. Masaki Watanabe in Japan to produce the first edition of his *Atlas of Arthroscopy* in 1957.[17,18] In 1934, Dr. Michael Burman at the Hospital for Joint Diseases in New York published his work on using arthroscopy for patients with OA of the knee.[19] Current arthroscopes use fiber optics to transmit the light and glass rod bundles to transmit the image. These arthroscopes have angled tips that permit a wider field of vision than nonangulated, forward-viewing arthroscopes. The most common angulation in use is the 30-degree foreoblique.[20] Arthroscopes based on fiber-optic technology to transmit both the image and the light are also available. These "needle arthroscopes" have the advantage of being only 1.7 mm in diameter (Optical Catheter System, Medical Dynamics, Englewood, CO). It was thought that the smaller portal incision necessary to insert the 1.7-mm fiber-optic arthroscope compared to the larger, standard 2.9-mm glass rod arthroscope conferred the advantage of fewer potential complications. However, glass rod arthroscopes, which require only slightly larger portals, were not found to produce more complications and to give superior images.[6,21,22] The glass rod arthroscope is the instrument of choice for arthroscopy for research or clinical applications.[6,21]

Instrumentation has also improved. Motorized suction shavers have greatly enhanced the performance of arthroscopic synovectomy. Basket forceps of various angulations have been designed to permit meniscal resection in the back, middle, and front portions of the meniscus. Biopsy forceps and graspers facilitate synovial biopsy and removal of loose bodies. Specialized cartilage biopsy instruments can be used to obtain reproducible cartilage biopsies for research purposes.[23]

Arthroscopic Technique Used by Rheumatologists

Arthroscopic visualization and biopsy of synovium and cartilage under local anesthesia on an outpatient basis has been utilized by rheumatologists in patients with rheumatoid arthritis (RA) and osteoarthritis (OA)[4,22,24-28] The most frequently examined joint is the knee; small joints including the wrists, ankles, and metacarpophalangeal joints are also accessible.

Although techniques for outpatient arthroscopy vary, the necessary steps for a successful procedure are universal. The patient is usually premedicated with a mild anxiolytic drug and then is positioned supine on a standard examination table. Usually two portals are used, the inferomedial and the inferolateral. The inferolateral portal is located at the lateral margin of the patellar ligament at the level of the inferior pole of the patella. The inferomedial portal is located one thumbbreadth above the medial tibial plateau on a line dropped perpendicularly from the medial border of the patella. A superolateral portal can be used instead of, or in addition to, the inferomedial portal. A superomedial portal location has been associated with a delayed recovery due to inadvertent violation of the vastus medialis obliquus muscle.[29]

Following antiseptic skin preparation, marcaine with adrenaline is used to anesthetize the skin, subcutaneous, and capsular tissues (Fig. 48-1*A*). Then, the joint space is entered and 20 cc of the same anesthetic is injected to achieve intra-articular anesthesia.

After applying sterile drapes, arthroscopy is begun in the anterolateral portal by using a #10 blade to make an incision of 5 to 7 mm long in the skin, subcutaneous, and capsular tissues (see Fig 48–1*B*). The sharp edge of the blade should always be directed upward to avoid unintentionally cutting the upper margin of the meniscus upon entering the joint. The medial portal is established next, under direct visualization from the interior of the joint to ensure proper placement. The medial portal can be used to insert biopsy instruments, or the arthroscope may be switched to the medial portal to allow visualization of additional intra-articular structures. With two portals, inflow and outflow can be separated. This is better for continuous visualization and actually shortens the procedure time because the arthroscopist does not have to stop to irrigate and evacuate the joint.

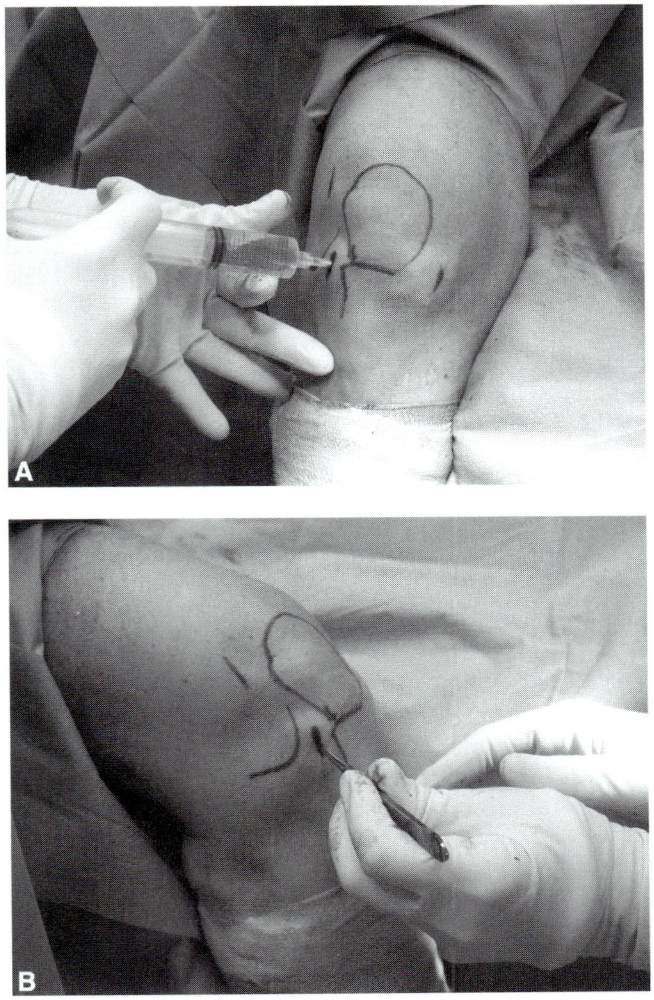

FIGURE 48–1 · A, Injection of anesthetic into the skin, subcutaneous and capsular tissues of the inferolateral portal. Intra-articular anesthesia can be achieved by injection of anesthetic solution through the same portal into the joint space. B, A#10 blade (sharp edge up) is used to make a 5 to 7 mm long incision in the skin and the capsule, which permit entry of the arthroscope into the joint.

Most arthroscopic procedures that involve biopsies will be performed with the two-portal technique. Biopsies of synovium can be obtained with specialized biopsy forceps.[26,27] In this instance, individual pieces can be obtained from directly visualized areas of the joint. Recording equipment can be used to provide a permanent record of the site and size of the biopsy. A motorized suction shaver[30] permits removal of a large amount of tissue from multiple areas. A thigh tourniquet is not necessary and cannot be employed when only local anesthesia is used. If bleeding obscures visualization, adrenaline (1 mg/1000 ml irrigation fluid) can be used or pressure on the inflow fluid increased to help tamponade bleeding vessels.

Single-portal arthroscopy in the inferolateral portal with irrigation in and out through the arthroscope can be sufficient for a simple diagnostic arthroscopy. Most areas of the joint can be inspected with a 30-degree foreoblique arthroscope inserted through the inferolateral portal. The entire cartilage surface of the femoral condyle and tibial plateau, the medial and lateral menisci, the intercondylar notch and anterior cruciate ligament, the lateral aspect of the lateral femoral condyle, and the joint capsule (the lateral gutter), as well as the lateral and inferior facet of the patella, can be well seen from this portal. The medial patellar facet, the posterior aspect of the medial gutter, and the anterior margin of the lateral meniscus are difficult to see through this portal. However, for diagnostic arthroscopy, the inferolateral portal is the single portal of choice.

No sutures are required to close the arthroscopy portals. Usually tape closures or no closures are used.[31] Gauze dressings and a loosely wrapped elastic bandage are applied. The patient may be fully weight-bearing immediately after the procedure. However, when synovial or cartilage biopsies are taken, restricted activity for 24 to 72 hours is indicated. Drainage usually stops within 24 hours. Patients may shower after 72 hours and be back at full activity as tolerated, usually within a week.

Complications

Complication rates of outpatient arthroscopy performed by rheumatologists as described previously have been reported.[15,22,26,32] An overall 1.5-percent complication rate has been reported in 16,532 arthroscopies performed by 72 rheumatologists.[15] Major complications, such as septic arthritis, are rare when the arthroscopic procedures are confined to irrigation and synovial biopsy.[15,26,32] Minor complications including portal irritation and postarthroscopy effusion occur in up to 13 percent of patients, but these conditions often go unreported.[22]

The overall complication rates of 0.8 to 1.7 percent reported in the orthopedic literature compare favorably to the rates reported by rheumatologists.[7] Major complications such as septic arthritis have been found to be more frequent in arthroscopic procedures that last more than an hour and in patients over the age of 50.[33]

These data indicate that office-based diagnostic arthroscopy with joint lavage and synovial biopsy as performed by rheumatologists can be a safe procedure.

Diagnostic Arthroscopy

There are very few clinical indications for the use of arthroscopy as a purely diagnostic tool in patients with arthritis.[35] Although the majority of patients with painful OA of the knee will have intra-articular abnormalities such as torn menisci, the diagnosis can usually be made by noninvasive means using clinical examination or magnetic resonance imaging (MRI).[36] Also, most rheumatologists should not perform meniscal débridement if a meniscal tear is found during a diagnostic arthroscopy (Figs. 48–2). The rare case of culture-negative infectious monoarthritis can be diagnosed using a blind synovial biopsy or during a therapeutic arthroscopic débridement and lavage.[37,38]

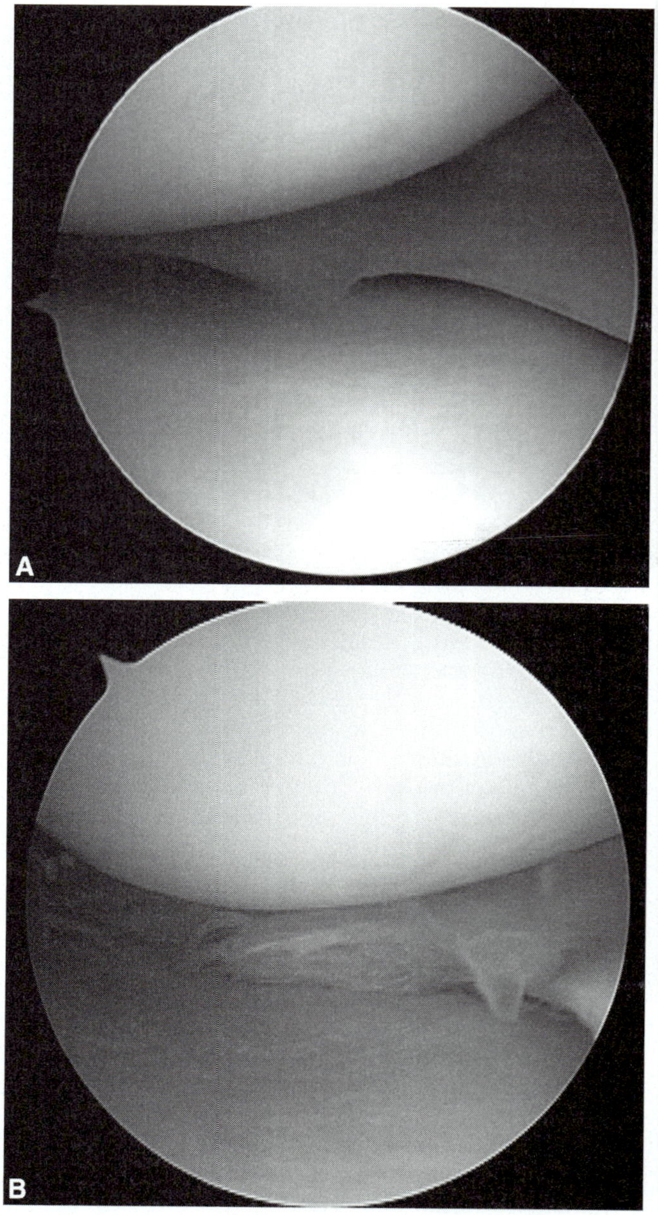

FIGURE 48–2 · Arthroscopic View of the Medical Compartment of the Knee. *A*, With the arthroscope in the inferolateral portal, the smooth margin and the body of the middle one third of the medial meniscas are seen between the cartilage of the medial femoral condyle (above) and the medial tibial plateau (below). *B*, Using the same portal, but in a different patient, the inner margin and body of the middle one third of the medial meniscus are torn and frayed.

Abnormalities of the cartilage surface in patients with OA can be directly inspected and graded[39,40] (Figs. 48–3). This technique, called chondroscopy, has been used as an outcome measure for studies of patients with OA of the knee.[4,5,41,42] Grading systems to describe cartilage abnormalities seen during arthroscopy have been devised and interobserver reliability determined.[39,40, 43,44] The SFA grading system, which assigns five categories of severity of chondropathy to each of the tibiofemoral compartments, and a 100-mm visual analogue system (VAS) scoring system were found to have the highest interobserver reliability.[43]

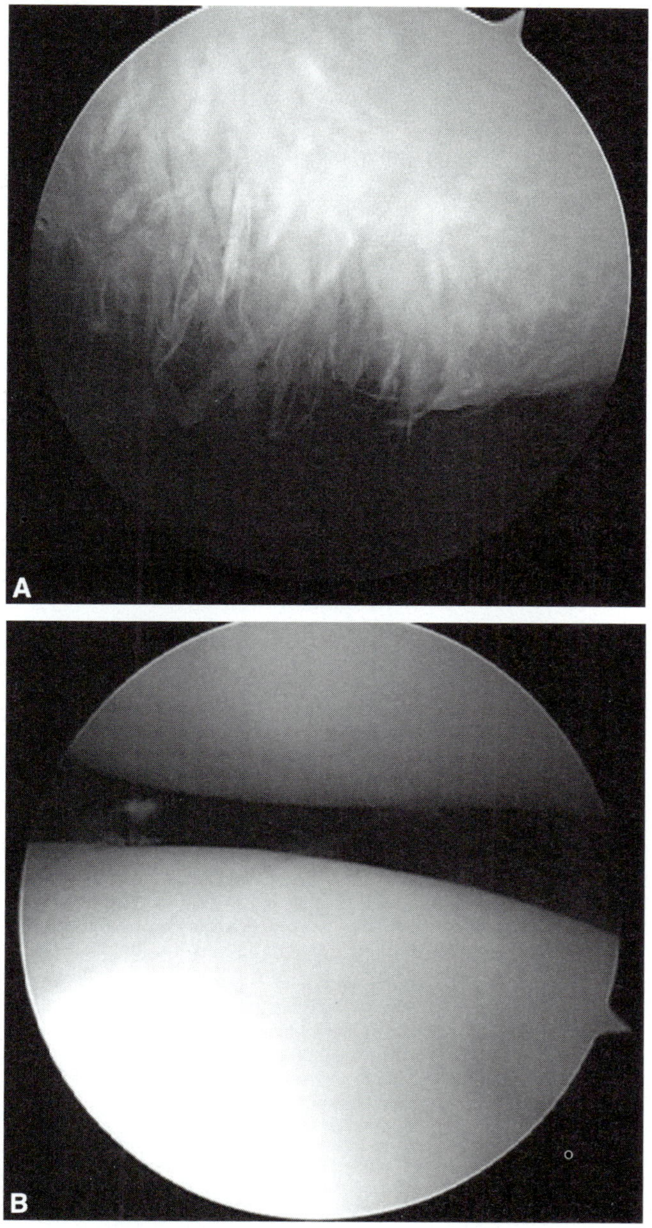

FIGURE 48–3 · Arthroscopic View of the Cartilage Surface of the Patella. *A*, With the arthroscope in the inferolateral portal, the roughened and fibrillated surface of the patella is seen. *B*, By comparison, this is a view of the smooth, normal cartilage surface of the patella above the normal cartilage on the femoral condyle.

Biopsies of cartilage obtained under direct arthroscopic visualization can add valuable biochemical and histologic information to the visual evaluation of the cartilage surface.[23]

Noninvasive imaging techniques have been compared to arthroscopic evaluation of cartilage surfaces.[45-47] Joint-space narrowing in the medial compartment on the standard anteroposterior weight-bearing radiograph of the knees has been found to be insensitive to cartilage abnormalities detected at arthroscopy. The sensitivity and specificity of medial joint-space narrowing found on radiographs was only 61 percent when followed by arthroscopic examination,[45] and false-positive rates were high on radiographs.

In contrast to plain radiographs, the specificity and sensitivity of MRI to detect cartilage abnormalities is improving.[47,48] In one study, cartilage damage determined by arthroscopy and MRI were highly correlated ($r = .83$).[47]

T_2-weighted fast spin-echo MRI in the axial and coronal planes for the detection of cartilage lesions has been found to have a sensitivity of 94 percent and a specificity of 99 percent compared to arthroscopy.[48] Fifty-five lesions (64%) were graded identically on MRI and arthroscopy. Seventy-eight lesions (90%) were within one grade, and 84 lesions were within two grades (97%) of severity using MRI and arthroscopy. These studies indicate that MRI of cartilage lesions correlates significantly with arthroscopic grading systems.

Future clinical trials of interventions designed to prevent the progression of cartilage deterioration in patients with OA are likely to involve both direct observation of cartilage integrity as determined by arthroscopy and quantification of cartilage volume and cartilage damage as determined by MRI.[49,50]

Miniarthroscopy (MA) and MRI have been used to evaluate the metacarpophalangeal (MCP) joints in patients with RA.[28,51] MA of the second MCP can be performed as an outpatient procedure and is well tolerated. Both MA and MRI were shown to be sensitive techniques for the detection of synovitis and early abnormalities of cartilage and subchondral bone. MRI revealed synovial proliferation in 21 of 22 patients, whereas MA revealed macroscopic signs of synovitis in all 22 patients. MRI found bony abnormalities in 20 of the 22 patients and MA in 19 of the 22 patients in the study.

Arthroscopy with Synovial Biopsy

Prior to arthroscopy, samples of synovial tissue were often obtained by blind synovial biopsy or at the time of arthroplasty.[52] The availability of arthroscopy and synovial biopsy has allowed synovial tissue to be obtained from many sites within large and small joints at even the earliest phases of the disease. Analysis of synovial biopsies has shown the following.

- Microscopic synovitis is present in joints that are not yet inflamed clinically.[53]

- Immunologic features of serial biopsy specimens change as the clinical manifestations change in response to treatment.[54,55]
- Early findings of synovial proliferation can identify patients at increased risk of developing joint erosions.[56]

An important question is whether synovial samples selected under direct arthroscopic visualization are better than those obtained by blind synovial biopsy techniques(Fig. 48–4), because the histologic features may differ according to the site of synovial biopsy in a joint.[57] When synovial biopsies obtained blindly with a Parker-Pearson needle from the suprapatellar pouch (SPP) were compared to arthroscopically guided biopsies from the SPP and the cartilage-pannus junction (CPJ) from the same patients, synovial tissue from the SPP showed fewer macrophages than did biopsies obtained from synovium closer to cartilage surfaces at the CPJ.[58] However, other investigators have reported that arthroscopic biopsies taken from the SPP, medial gutter, and CPJ did not vary significantly in measures of synovial histology, immunohistology, or cytokine mRNA expression.[59,60] Therefore, arthroscopic biopsies are most useful when tissue from specific sites is required or when a larger size sample of synovium is desired.[2]

Synovial biopsies obtained from the knee, wrist, and second MCP in the same patient have been compared and found to be equivalent.[61] Therefore, it may be possible to follow treatment effects by obtaining synovial biopsies from either small or large joints.

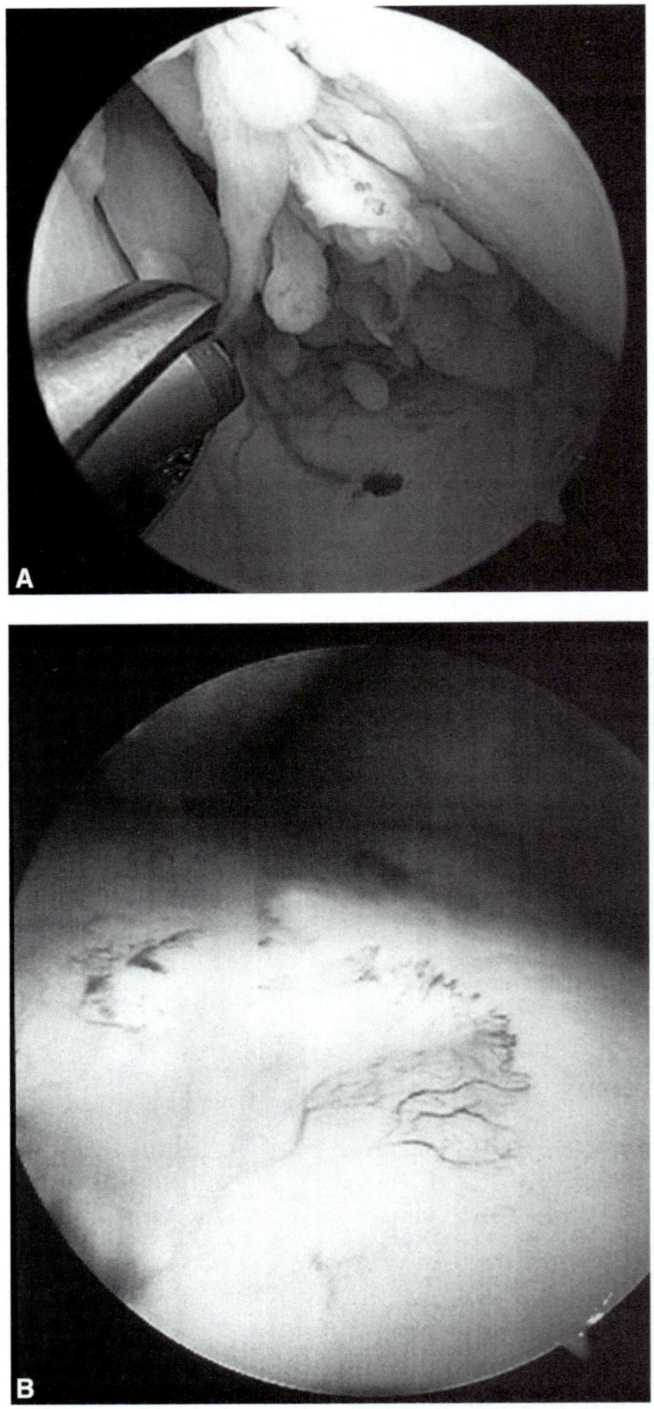

FIGURE 48–4 · Arthroscopic Synovial Biopsy. *A,* With the arthroscope in the inferolateral portal, a motorized shaver in the inferomadial portal can be used to obtain samples of proliferative, inflamed synovial tissue on the medial capsular wall. *B,* Highly vascular rheumatoid synovial pannus adherent to the cartilage surface of the medial femoral condyle. Biopsy samples of this tissue only could be obtained with direct visualization through the arthroscope.

Arthroscopic Irrigation

Arthroscopy includes irrigation of the joint as an integral part of the procedure. Irrigation improves visualization by clearing debris from the joint and distending the joint capsule to move soft tissues out of view. It is hypothesized that irrigation also removes phlogistic material and debris that causes pain, such as cartilage fragments or other “wear particles,” crystals, cytokines, eicosanoids, or enzymes.[62] Numerous reports of the beneficial effects of joint irrigation associated with arthroscopy have appeared in the literature.[1,19,63-67] These are retrospective and uncontrolled observations of reduction of pain in patients who received a joint irrigation as part of an arthroscopic procedure that also included surgical treatments.

In one controlled study, tidal irrigation (TI) of the knee with 1000 ml of normal saline was compared to continued conservative medical management in a multicenter, single-blind, randomized study of 77 patients with grade 1 through 3 OA of the knee.[68] All the patients entering the trial had failed a conservative management program consisting of physical therapy, intra-articular steroid injection, and analgesic and anti-inflammatory drug therapy. Statistically significant differences ($p < 0.05$) in joint pain, pain after 50-foot walk, and physician assessment all favored TI over medical management. Similarly, two studies that compared TI to either arthroscopic débridement or steroid injection found that TI produced significant improvement at up to 1 year.[69,70]

An American College of Rheumatology (ACR) sponsored, multicenter study comparing arthroscopic irrigation with either a large volume (3000 ml) or a small volume (250 ml) of fluid in patients with OA of the knee revealed a significant decrease in WOMAC aggregated scores at 1 year in both groups.[71] Appro-ximately 60 percent of the patients had evidence of positively birefringent crystals (consistent with calcium pyrophosphate dihydrate) adherent to synovium at the time of arthroscopy. Patients with crystals had a 40-percent greater improvement in their WOMAC scores compared to the group that did not have crystals. The authors noted that the crystals seen at the time of arthroscopy were not always found in synovial fluid analyses or observed on radiographs. In a prior study, the importance of crystals seen at the time of arthroscopy as a predictor of a positive response to arthrosocpic irrigation was also noted.[62]

TI has been compared to sham irrigation (SI) in a randomized, double-blind, controlled trial in 180 patients with OA of the knee.[72] The patients were blinded from the procedure by a curtain placed between themselves and the operator. At 1 year, both the TI and SI patients had improved over baseline to a similar degree in pain relief, stiffness, and physical function as measured by WOMAC scales, global assessments, 50-foot walk time, and knee swelling and tenderness. Blinding of patients was successfully achieved, with 91 percent of those receiving SI believing they had received TI.

This study casts strong doubt on the intrinsic validity of widespread, routine utilization of joint irrigation to provide pain relief for patients with OA of the knee. For patients who have failed comprehensive medical management and who cannot tolerate or are at high risk from oral nonsteroidal anti-inflammatory drug (NSAID) therapy, joint irrigation may still be a viable therapeutic option. This may be particularly true if the patients demonstrate chondrocalcinosis on radiograph or are found to have crystalline material in synovium at the time of arthroscopy.

Arthroscopic Débridement

In 1941, Magnuson coined the term *joint débridement* to describe open operative procedures performed on the knees of patients with OA.[73] Open débridement included drilling of exposed subchondral bone, as well as removal of osteophytes, inflamed synovium, softened or fibrillated cartilage, torn or degenerated menisci, and loose bodies.[74-76] Not surprisingly, the open débridement resulted in considerable morbidity, including required hospitalization, prolonged time for postoperative healing, loss of joint motion despite intensive physical therapy, and frequent complications, including hemarthrosis.[76] The availability of total joint replacement and high tibial osteotomy in the early 1970s caused open joint débridement for the treatment of OA of the knee to fall into disfavor.

In direct contrast, in uncontrolled case reports, arthroscopic débridement has been accompanied by relatively few complications and more than 80 percent good to excellent results in patients with OA of the knee followed for up to 2 years.[77-79] Patients with angular deformity of the knee, either varus or valgus, have been noted to do less well.[78] Casscells[80] editorialized that "the enthusiasm for arthroscopic procedures appears to know no limits at the present time." He noted the similarity of the arthroscopic procedures performed to those used by Magnusson in 1941 and suggested that the lower incidence and risk of complications from arthroscopy was primarily responsible for the enthusiasm, rather than the effectiveness of arthroscopic débridement.

Numerous reports of uncontrolled series of arthroscopic procedures for patients with OA of the knee have subsequently appeared.[81-85] Characteristically, patients who have the best outcomes from arthroscopic débridement have early disease with minimal radiographic changes, normal alignment of joint surfaces, a relatively short duration of symptoms (which are primarily mechanical), and a comprehensive medical management program employed before and after the arthroscopic procedure.[86,87]

The efficacy of arthroscopic débridement in OA of the knee has been called into question by the results of a recent randomized, double-blind, sham-controlled trial.[9] One hundred and eighty patients with OA of the knee were randomized to three groups: arthroscopic débridement, arthroscopic irrigation only, or sham arthroscopy. The sham, or placebo, group received only skin incisions and no intra-articular treatments. The irrigation group received only a washout unless there was a large, mechanically significant meniscal lesion, which was then débrided. The arthroscopic débridement group was treated with an aggressive débridement performed by an experienced arthroscopist who also performed all the procedures for the other two groups of patients. Follow-up was carried out to 2 years. The results clearly showed that there was no difference in the primary outcome measures between the three groups at any of the assessment points over the 2-year follow-up. In fact, patients who received the sham procedure experienced more pain relief sooner than the two other groups who received treatments.

The results and conclusions of this study have been widely debated, including the ethics of placebo surgery.[88-96] This study courageously attempted to answer some of the vexing questions about efficacy that have gone unanswered despite the performance of millions of arthroscopic débridement procedures for patients with OA of the knee.[88] Uncontrolled observational studies continue to be published and suggest that arthroscopic débridement for OA of the knee can have a favorable outcome, depending on patient selection.[84,85] Until further randomized, controlled studies appear, arthroscopic débridement should be reserved for those patients with OA of the knee who have failed a comprehensive medical management program and who have mechanical symptoms with minimal or moderate radiographic changes and little or no angular deformity. There is no place for the utilization of arthroscopic débridement as first-line therapy for pain in patients with OA of the knee.

Arthroscopic Synovectomy

The effect of open surgical synovectomy for the treatment of RA has been examined in a multicenter trial.[97] Open synovectomy resulted in reduced knee pain for 3 years, which then returned to baseline value despite continued decreased joint swelling. There was no difference in the progression of the disease as measured by new joint erosions between operated and control knees. Because the open synovectomy procedures were performed through peripatellar arthrotomies, a major complication of the procedure was scar development anteriorly with significant knee contracture and loss of joint motion.[98,99] The overall conclusion of the multicenter trial, published in 1977, was that open surgical synovectomy added no value to the general treatment of patients with RA.

Arthroscopic synovectomy has since supplanted the open approach for patients with inflammatory arthritis[100-102] (Figs. 48–5 and 48–6). Arthroscopic synovec-

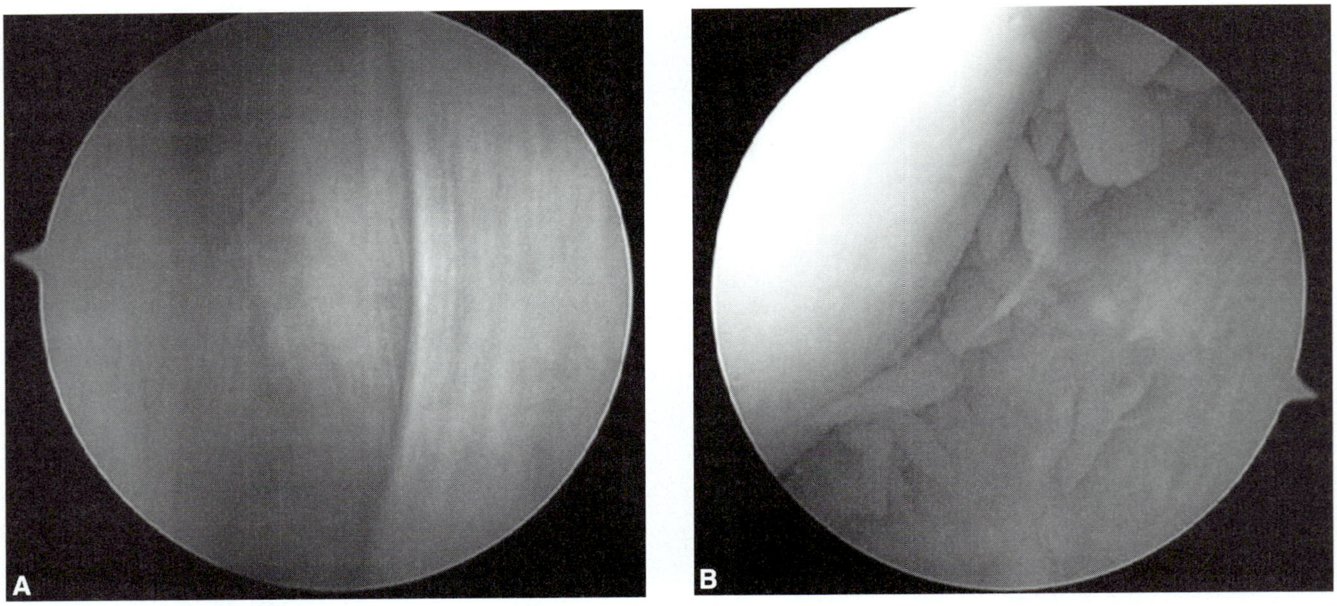

FIGURE 48–5 · Arthroscopic View of the Medial Capsular Wall. *A*, With the arthroscope in the inferolateral portal, the normal medial capsular wall can be seen through the thin covering of the normal synovial membrane. *B*, In this patient with rheumatoid arthritis, proliferative, inflamed synovial tissue covers the medial capsular wall. The cartilage of the medial femoral condyle is to the left.

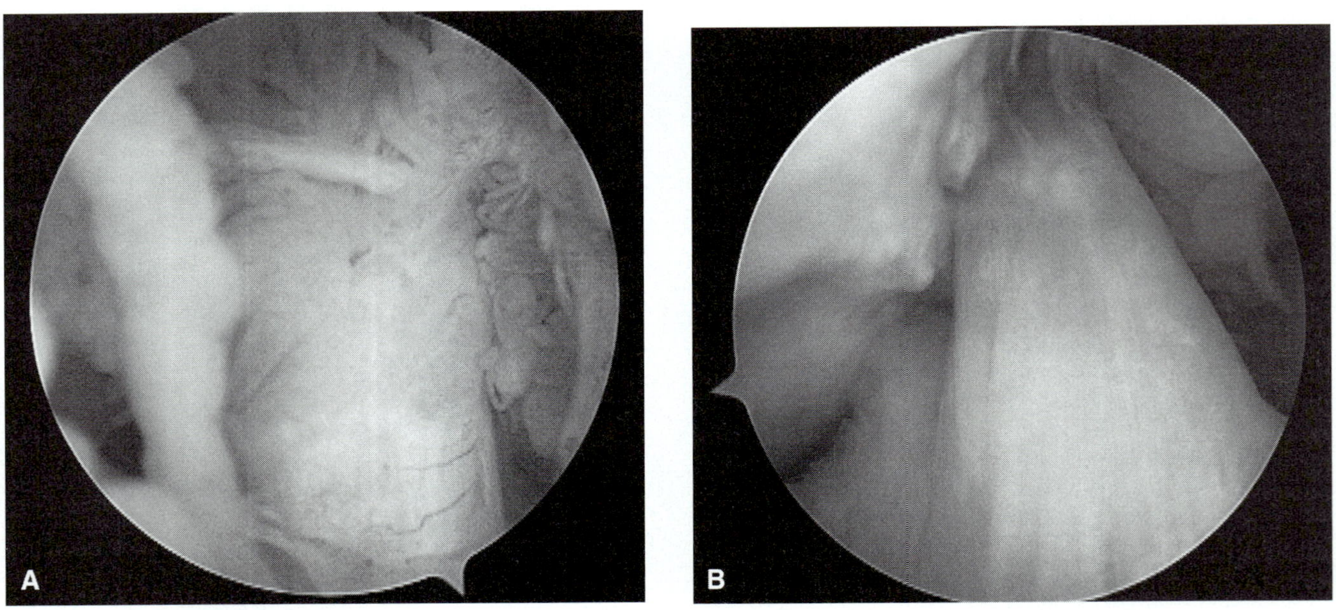

FIGURE 48–6 · Arthroscopic View of the Anterior Cruciate Ligament. *A*, With the arthroscope in the inferolateral portal, the anterior cruciate is covered with and surrounded by proliferative and inflamed synovial tissue. *B*, The normal anterior-cruciate ligament is visualized in the intercondylar notch.

tomy produces significant reduction in pain and swelling with improved function and few complications. A series of 211 arthroscopic synovectomies with at least 2 years of follow-up have been reported.[102] Of 112 patients with RA, the results were classified as good or excellent in 80 percent. Of 32 patients with seronegative arthritis, only 60 percent had similar results. Seventeen of 19 patients with pigmented villonodular synovitis achieved good to excellent results with only two recurrences. All 17 patients with synovial chondromatosis had excellent results with no recurrences.

Two other studies of arthroscopic synovectomy in patients with RA combined arthroscopic synovectomy with a chemical or radiation synovectomy.[103,104] The use of osmic acid or yttrium-90 injected locally as treatment for recalcitrant knee synovitis has been studied extensively in Europe.[100] Arthroscopic synovectomy was seen to be effective, but more difficult to carry out than osmic acid or yttrium-90 injection.

Because of the nature of inflammatory arthritis, the response to the arthroscopic synovectomy over the long term is likely to be better with improved medical management of the arthritis. Usually no comments are made on the preoperative and postoperative medical management programs for patients with inflammatory arthritis who undergo arthroscopic synovectomy. The need for arthroscopic synovectomy and the results of the procedure are likely to change with the introduction of the new biologic medications for the treatment of inflammatory arthritis, which include etanercept, infliximab, and adalimumab.[105-107] These medications offer the opportunity for better control of the inflammatory and destructive process, which could obviate the need for synovectomy.

REFERENCES

1. Jackson RW, Abe I: The role of arthroscopy in the management of disorders of the knee. J Bone Joint Surg Br 54-B:310-322, 1972.
2. Bresnihan B, Tak PP, Emery P, et al: Synovial biopsy in arthritis research: five years of concerted European collaboration. Ann Rheum Dis 59:506-510, 2000.
3. Tak PP, Bresnihan B: The pathogenesis and prevention of joint damage in rheumatoid arthritis. Arthritis Rheum 43: 2619-2633, 2000.
4. Ayral X, Dougados M, Listrat V, et al: Arthroscopic evaluation of chondropathy in osteoarthritis of the knee. J Rheum 23:698-706, 1996.
5. Listrat V, Ayral X, Patarnello F, et al: Arthroscopic evaluation of potential structure modifying activity of hyaluronan (Hyalgan) in osteoarthritis of the knee. Osteo Cart 5:153-160, 1997.
6. Ayral X, Dougados M: Rheumatological arthroscopy or research arthroscopy in rheumatology? Br J Rheum 37: 1039-1041, 1998.
7. Alum R: Complications of arthroscopy of the knee (review). J Bone Joint Surg Br 84-B:937-945, 2002.
8. Owings MF, Kozak LJ: Ambulatory and inpatient procedures in the United States, 1996. Vital and Health Stastistics. Series 13. No.139. Hyattsville, Md, National Center for Health Statistics, November 1998. (Department of Health and Human Services PHS 99-1710.)
9. Moseley JB, O'Malley K, Petersen NJ, et al: A controlled trial of arthroscopic surgery for osteoarthritis of the knee. N Engl J Med 347:81-88, 2002.
10. Benedek TG: A century of American rheumatology. Ann Int Med 106:304-312, 1987.
11. Polley HF, Bickel WH: Punch biopsy of synovial membrane. Ann Int Med 10:277-287, 1951.
12. Parker HR, Pearson CM: A simplified synovial biopsy needle. Arthritis Rheum 6:172-176, 1963.
13. Arnold WJ: Training for office-based arthroscopy: Evaluation of a pilot course sponsored by the ACR. Arthritis Rheum 35(Suppl):S220, 1992.
14. Ike RW, Fox DA: Arthroscopy in rheumatology training programs associated with NIH multipurpose arthritis centers: results from a survey of program directors. Arthritis Rheum 36:1329-1331, 1993.
15. Kane D, Veale DHJ, Fitzgerald O, Reece R: Survey of arthroscopy performed by rheumatologists. Rheum 41:210-215, 2002.
16. Reece R, Ayral X, Breedveld F, et al: Training in rheumatologic arthroscopy: ILAR minimum standards. Ann Rheum Dis, in press.
17. Jackson RW: The introduction of arthroscopy to North America. Clin Orthop 372:183-186, 2000.
18. Watanabe M, Takeda S, Ikeuchi H: Atlas of Arthroscopy. Tokyo, Igaku-Shoin, Ltd, 1957.
19. Burman MS, Finkelstein H, Mayer L: Arthroscopy of the knee joint. J Bone Joint Surg 16:255-268, 1934.
20. Goble EM, Kane SM, Wilcox TR, Olsen RE: Advanced arthroscopic instrumentation. *In* McGinty JB, Caspari RB, Jackson RW, Poehling GG (eds): Operative Arthroscopy, 2nd ed. New York, Raven Press, 1996, pp 7-12.
21. Ike RW, O'Rourke KS: Detection of intraarticular abnormalities in osteoarthritis of the knee: A pilot study comparing needle arthroscopy with standard arthroscopy. Arthritis Rheum 36:1353-1363, 1993.
22. Szachnowski P, Wei N, Arnold WJ, Cohen LM: Complications of office based arthroscopy of the knee. J Rheum 22:1722-1725, 1995.
23. Nebelung W, Pap G, Machner A, et al: Evaluation of arthroscopic articular cartilage biopsy for osteoarthritis of the knee. Arthroscopy 17:286-289, 2001.
24. Veale DJ: The role of arthroscopy in early arthritis. Clin Exp Rheum 17:37-38, 1999.
25. Rozmaryn LM, Wei N: Metacarpophalangeal arthroscopy. Arthroscopy 15:333-337, 1999.
26. Baeten D, Van den Bosch F, Elewaut D, et al: Needle arthroscopy of the knee with synovial biopsy sampling: Technical experience in 150 patients. Clin Rheum 18:434-444, 1999.
27. Wei N, Delauter SK, Erlichman MS, et al: Arthroscopic synovectomy of the metacarpophalangeal joint in refractory rheumatoid arthritis: a technique. Arthroscopy 15:265-268, 1999.
28. Ostendorf B, Peters R, Dann P, et al: Magnetic resonance imaging and miniarthroscopy of metacarpophalangeal joints. Arthritis Rheum 44:2492-2502, 2001.
29. Stetson WB, Templin K: Two-versus three-portal technique for routine knee arthroscopy. 30:108-114, 2002.
30. Moreland LW, Calvo-Alen J, Koopman WJ: Synovial biopsy of the knee joint under direct visualization by needle arthroscopy. J Clin Rheum 1:1-6, 1995.
31. Hussein R, Southgate GW: Management of knee arthroscopy portals. Knee 8:329-331, 2001.
32. Wollaston S, Brion P, Kumar A, et al: Complications of knee arthroscopy performed by rheumatologists. J Rheumatol 28: 1871-1873, 2001.
33. Babcock HM, Matava MJ, Fraser V: Postarthroscopy surgical site infections: review of the literature. Clin Infect Dis 43:6571-6580, 2002.
34. Delis KT, Hunt N, Strachan RK, Nicolaides AN: Incidence, natural history and risk factors of deep vein thrombosis in elective knee arthroscopy. Thromb Haemost 86:817-821, 2001.
35. O'Rourke KS, Ike RW: Diagnostic arthroscopy in the arthritis patient. Rheum Dis Clin North Am 20:321-342, 1994.
36. Buckland-Wright C: Current status of imaging procedures in the diagnosis, prognosis and monitoring of osteoarthritis. Baill Clin Rheum 11:727-748, 1997.
37. Vispo Seara JL, Barthel T, Schmitz H, Eulert J: Arthroscopic treatment of septic joints: prognostic factors. Arch Othop Trauma Surg 122:204-211, 2002.

38. Broy SB, Schmid FR: A comparison of medical drainage (needle aspiration) and surgical drainage (arthrotomy or arthroscopy) in the initial treatment of infected joints. Clin Rheum Dis 12:501-522,1986.
39. Klashman D, Ike R, Moreland L, et al: Validation of an osteoarthritis data report form for knee arthroscopy. Arthritis Rheum 38(Suppl):S178, 1995.
40. Dougados M, Ayral X, Listrat V, et al: The SFA system for assessing articular cartilage lesions at arthroscopy of the knee. Arthroscopy 10:69-77, 1994.
41. Ayral X, Dougados M, Listrat V, et al: Chondroscopy: A new method for scoring chondropathy. Sem Arthritis Rheum 22: 289-297, 1993.
42. Ayral X: Diagnostic and quantitative arthroscopy. Baillieres Clin Rheumatol 10:477-494, 1996.
43. Ayral X, Gueguen A, Ike RW, et al: Inter-observer reliability of the arthroscopic quantification of chondropathy of the knee. Osteo Cart 6:160-166, 1998.
44. Noyes FR, Stabler CL: A system for grading articular cartilage lesions of arthroscopy. Am J Sports Med 17:505-513, 1989.
45. Fife RS, Brandt KD, Braunstein EM, et al: Relationship between arthroscopic evidence of cartilage damage and radiographic evidence of joint space narrowing in early osteoarthritis of the knee. Arthritis Rheum 34:377-382, 1991.
46. Brandt KD, Fife RS, Braunstein EM, Katz B: Radiographic grading of the severity of knee osteoarthritis: relation of the Kellgren and Lawrence grade to a grade based on joint space narrowing, and correlation with arthroscopic evidence of articular cartilage degeneration. Arthritis Rheum 34:1381-1386, 1991.
47. Drape J-L, Pessis E, Auleley GR, et al: Quantitative MR imaging evaluation of chondropathy in osteoarthritic knees. Radiology 208:49-55, 1998.
48. Bredella MA, Tirman PF, Peterfy CG, et al: Accuracy of T2-weighted fast spin-echo MR imaging with fat saturation in detecting cartilage defects in the knee: Comparison with arthroscopy in 130 patients. Am J Roentgenol 172:1073-1080, 1999.
49. Burgkart R, Glaser C, Hyhlik-Durr A, et al: Magnetic resonance imaging-based assessment of cartilage loss in severe osteoarthritis. Arthritis Rheum 44: 2072-2077, 2001.
50. Biswal S, Hastie T, Andriacchi TP, et al: Risk factors for progressive cartilage loss in the knee: A longitudinal MRI imaging study in forty-three patients. Arthritis Rheum 46:2884-2892, 2002.
51. Ostendorf B, Dann P, Wedekind F, et al: Miniarthroscopy of metacarpophalangeal joints in rheumatoid arthritis: Rating of diagnostic value in synovitis staging and efficiency of synovial biopsy. J Rheum 26:1901-1908, 1999.
52. Allard SA, Muirden KD, Maini RN: Correlation of histopathologic features of pannus with patterns of damage in different joints in rheumatoid arthritis. Ann Rheum Dis 50:278-283, 1991.
53. Kraan MC, Versendaal H, Jonker M, et al: Asymptomatic synovitis precedes clinically manifest arthritis. Arthritis Rheum 41:1481-1488, 1998.
54. Wong P, Cuello C, Bertouch JV, et al: The effects of pulse methylprednisolone on matrix metalloproteinase and tissue inhibitor of metalloproteinase-1 expression in rheumatoid arthritis. Rheumatology 39:1067-1073, 2000.
55. Young L, Katrib A, Cuello C, et al: Effects of intraarticular glucocorticoids on macrophage infiltration and mediators of joint damage in osteoarthritis synovial membranes: Findings in a double-blind, placebo-controlled study. Arthritis Rheum 44:343-350, 2001.
56. Cunnane G, Fitzgerald O, Hummel KM, et al: Synovial tissue protease gene expression and joint erosions in early rheumatoid arthritis. Arthritis Rheum 44:1774-1753, 2001.
57. Lindblad S, Hedfors E: Arthroscopic and immunohistologic characterization of knee joint synovitis in osteoarthritis. Arthritis Rheum 30:1081-1088, 1987.
58. Youssef PP, Kraan M, Brredveld F, et al: Quantitative microscopic analysis of inflammation in rheumatoid arthritis synovial membrane samples selected at arthroscopy compared with samples obtained blindly by needle biopsy. Arthritis Rheum 41:663-669, 1998.
59. Kirkham B, Portek I, Lee CS, et al: Intraarticular variability of synovial membrane histology, immunohistology, and cytokine mRNA expression in patients with rheumatoid arthritis. J Rheum 26:777-784, 1999.
60. Smeets TJM, Kraan MC, Galjaard S, et al: Analysis of the cell infiltrate and expression of matrix metalloproteinases and granzyme B in paired synovial biopsy specimens from the cartilage-pannus junction in patients with RA. Ann Rheum Dis 60:561-565, 2001.
61. Kraan MC, Reece RJ, Smeets TJM, et al: Comparison of synovial tissues from the knee joints and the small joints of rheumatoid arthritis patients. Arthritis Rheum 46:2034-2038, 2002.
62. Evans CH, Mears DC, Stanitski CL: Ferrographic analysis of wear in human joints. J Bone Joint Surg Br 64-B:572-578, 1982.
63. O'Connor RL: The arthroscope in the management of crystal-induced synovitis of the knee. J Bone Joint Surg 55-A:1443-1449, 1973.
64. Watanabe M, Takeda S, Ikeuchi H: Atlas of Arthroscopy, 3rd ed. Tokyo, Igaku-Shoiu, Ltd., 1979.
65. Jackson RW, Silver R, Marans H: Arthroscopic treatment of degenerative joint disease. Arthroscopy 2:114-120, 1986.
66. Edelson R, Burks RT, Bloebaum RD: Short-term effects of knee washout for osteoarthritis. Am J Sports Med 23:345-349, 1995.
67. Shannon FJ, Devitt AT, Poynton AR, et al: Short-term benefit of arthroscopic washout in degenerative arthritis of the knee. Int Orthop (SICOT) 25:242-245, 2001.
68. Ike RW, Arnold WJ, Rothschild EW, et al: Tidal irrigation versus conservative medical management in patients with osteoarthritis of the knee: A prospective randomized study. J Rheum 19: 772-779, 1992.
69. Chang RW, Falconer J, Stulberg SD, et al: A randomized, controlled trial of arthroscopic surgery versus closed-needle joint lavage for patients with osteoarthritis of the knee. Arthritis Rheum 36:289-296, 1993.
70. Ravaud P, Moulinier L, Giraudeau B, et al: Effects of joint lavage and steroid injection in patients with osteoarthritis of the knee. Arthritis Rheum 42:475-482, 1999.
71. Kalunian KC, Moreland LW, Klashman DJ, et al: Visually-guided irrigation in patients with early knee osteoarthritis: A multicenter randomized, controlled trial. Osteo Cartilage 8:412-418, 2000.
72. Bradley JD, Heilman DK, Katz BP, et al: Tidal irrigation as treatment for knee osteoarthritis-a sham-controlled, randomized, double-blinded evaluation. Arthritis Rheum 46:100-108, 2002.
73. Magnuson PB: Joint débridement: Surgical treatment of degenerative arthritis. Surg Gyne Obst 73:1-9, 1941.
74. Haggart GE: The surgical treatment of degenerative arthritis of the knee joint. J Bone Joint Surg 22:717-729, 1941.
75. Isserlin B: Joint débridement for osteoarthritis of the knee. J Bone Joint Surg Br 32B:302-306, 1950.
76. Insall JN: Intra-articular surgery for degenerative arthritis of the knee. J Bone Joint Surg Br 49B: 211-228, 1967.
77. Sprague NF: Arthroscopic débridement for degenerative knee joint disease. Clin Orthop 160:118-123, 1981.
78. Salisbury RB, Nottage WM, Gardner V: The effect of alignment on results in arthroscopic débridement of the degenerative knee. Clin Orthop 198:268-272, 1985.
79. Burks RT: Arthroscopy and degenerative arthritis of the knee: A review of the literature. Arthroscopy 6:43-47, 1990.
80. Casscells SW: What, if any, are the indications for arthroscopic débridement of the osteoarthritic knee? [Editorial] Arthroscopy 6:169-170, 1990.
81. McGinley BJ, Cushner FD, Scott WN: Débridement arthroscopy: 10 year follow-up. Clin Orthop 367:190-194, 1999.
82. Crevoisier X, Munzinger U, Drobny T: Arthroscopic partial meniscectomy in patients over 70 years of age. Arthroscopy 17:732-736, 2001.
83. Andersson-Molina H, Karlsson H, Rockborn P: Arthroscopic partial and total meniscectomy: A long-term follow-up study with matched controls. Arthroscopy 10:183-189, 2002.
84. Fond J, Rodin D, Ahmad S, Nirschl RP: Arthroscopic débridement for the treatment of osteoarthritis of the knee: 2- and 5-year results. Arthroscopy 18: 829-834, 2002.
85. Hunt SA, Jazrawi LM, Sherman OH: Arthroscopic management of osteoarthritis of the knee. J Am Acad Orthop Surg 10: 356-363, 2002.
86. Jackson RW: Arthroscopic surgery and a new classification system. Am J Knee Surg 11:51-54, 1998.

87. Harwin SF: Arthroscopic débridement for osteoarthritis of the knee: Predictors of patient satisfaction. Arthroscopy 15:142-146, 1999.
88. Felson DT, Buckwalter J: Débridement and lavage for osteoarthritis of the knee [Editorial]. N Engl J Med 347:132-133, 2002.
89. Horng S, Miller FG: Is placebo surgery unethical? N Engl J Med 347:137-139, 2002.
90. Johnson LL: Degenerative arthritis arthroscopy and research [Letter]. Arthroscopy 18:683-685, 2002.
91. Chambers K, Schulzer M, Sobolev B: Degenerative arthritis arthroscopy and research [Letter]. Arthroscopy 18:685-687, 2002.
92. Jackson RW: Arthroscopic surgery for osteoarthritis of the knee [Letter]. N Engl J Med 347:1717, 2002.
93. Ewing W, Ewing JW: Arthroscopic surgery for osteoarthritis of the knee [Letter]. N Engl J Med 347:1717, 2002.
94. Chambers KG, Schulzer M: Arthroscopic surgery for osteoarthritis of the knee [Letter]. N Engl J Med 347:1718, 2002.
95. Morse LJ: Arthroscopic surgery for osteoarthritis of the knee [Letter]. N Engl J Med 347:1719, 2002.
96. Wray NP, Moseley JB, O'Malley K: Arthroscopic surgery for osteoarthritis of the knee [Response]. N Engl J Med 347:1719, 2002.
97. Arthritis Foundation Committee on Evaluation of Synovectomy: Multicenter evaluation of synovectomy in the treatment of rheumatoid arthritis. Arthritis Rheum 20:765-771, 1977.
98. Marmor L: Surgery of the rheumatoid knee: Synovectomy and débridement. J Bone Joint Surg Am 55:535-538, 1973.
99. Marmor L: Synovectomy of the knee joint. Orthop Clin North Am 10:211-218, 1979.
100. Combe B, Krause E, Sany J: Treatment of chronic knee synovitis with arthroscopic synovectomy after failure of intraarticular injection of radionuclide. Arthritis Rheum 32:10-14, 1989.
101. Arnold WJ, Kalunian K: Arthroscopic synovectomy by rheumatologists: Time for a new look. Arthritis Rheum 32:108-111, 1989.
102. Ogilvie-Harris DJ, Weisleder L: Arthroscopic synovectomy of the knee: Is it helpful? Arthroscopy 11:91-95, 1995.
103. Ayral X, Bonvarlet JP, Simmonet J, et al: Arthroscopy-assisted synovectomy in the treatment of chronic synovitis of the knee. Rev Rhum [Engl] 64:215-226, 1997.
104. Klug S, Wittmann G, Weseloh G: Arthroscopic synovectomy of the knee joint in early cases of rheumatoid arthritis: Follow-up results of a multi-center study. Arthroscopy 16:262-267, 2000.
105. Weinblatt ME, Kremer JM, Bankhurst AD, et al: A trial of etanercept, a recombinant tumor necrosis factor receptor: Fc fusion protein, in patients with rheumatoid arthritis receiving methotrexate. N Engl J Med 340:253-259, 1999.
106. Lipsky PE, van der Heijde DM, St Clair EW, et al: Anti-tumor necrosis factor trial in rheumatoid arthritis with concomitant therapy study group: Infliximab and methotrexate in the treatment of rheumatoid arthritis. N Engl J Med 343:1594-1602, 2000.
107. Weinblatt ME, Keystone EC, Furst DE, et al: Adalimumab, a fully human anti-tumor necrosis factor-a monoclonal antibody for the treatment of rheumatoid arthritis in patients taking methotrexate. Arthritis Rheum 48:35-45, 2003.

49 Laboratory Evaluation of Inflammation

STANLEY P. BALLOU • IRVING KUSHNER

The Concept of Inflammation

A major problem in using laboratory tests to quantify severity and extent of inflammation stems from ambiguity associated with the very concept of *inflammation* itself.[1] A precise definition of inflammation is difficult to express. (The definition of inflammation given on the first page of the definitive text on inflammation differs in the three consecutive editions published in 1988, 1992, and 1999.[2]) For centuries, inflammation was defined primarily in clinical terms: redness, swelling, heat, and pain on use. The introduction of light microscopy led to a histologic definition: infiltration by inflammatory cells. In the modern era, inflammation has been described in terms of the changes observed at biochemical, ultrastructural, and molecular levels. Amid the complexity of inflammatory processes,[3] the usual definition of inflammation has been relatively imprecise: the local response to tissue injury. Such a vague definition highlights the difficulty of evaluating inflammation with a laboratory test.

Two points are inadequately appreciated: (1) Inflammation is not a single process; it may be acute or chronic, and different stimuli (e.g., staphylococci, schistosomes, allergens, urate crystals, myocardial infarction, tubercle bacilli) induce different types of inflammatory responses; and (2) each type of inflammatory response represents a complex, highly orchestrated set of interactions between cells, soluble mediators, and tissue matrix. It is not reasonable to expect a single laboratory test to accurately reflect all these diverse processes. We should be aware that a single systemic marker (e.g., any constituent of blood) may not accurately reflect local inflammatory processes. In addition, the varied stimuli capable of inducing different clinical types of inflammation (e.g., acute or chronic) can be associated with distinct patterns of laboratory abnormalities. Thus, acute gout and active rheumatoid arthritis each entail inflammation and are associated with elevation of the erythrocyte sedimentation rate (ESR), but leukocytosis is more frequently associated with gout, whereas anemia of chronic disease is more characteristic of rheumatoid arthritis.

Despite these problems, physicians have exploited the acute-phase response to obtain objective but imperfect information about the extent or degree of inflammation. During the past 75 years, this role has been filled by measurement of the ESR and, more recently, the serum C-reactive protein (CRP) concentration. Several new inflammatory markers have been recognized in the last few years, but none has yet proved substantially more helpful in the clinical setting.

Acute-phase Response

A large number of systemic and metabolic changes, collectively referred to as the acute-phase response (APR), begin to occur within hours after an inflammatory stimulus.[4,5] Many elements of the APR represent early defensive mechanisms or adaptations to the stress of an inflammatory stimulus and can be regarded as participants in the innate immune response.[6]

A major component of the APR is alteration of synthesis of plasma proteins by hepatocytes. These "acute-phase proteins" display variable changes in plasma concentration and kinetics after tissue injury (Fig. 49–1). Concentrations of some, such as ceruloplasmin and complement components, rise about 50 percent above normal; others, such as α_1-acid glycoprotein, α_1-proteinase inhibitor, haptoglobin, and fibrinogen, can increase several-fold. The two major acute-phase proteins in humans, CRP and serum amyloid A (SAA), often increase to levels several hundred times above those normally present in health and may increase more than 1000-fold in severe inflammatory states, usually infections. In contrast, concentrations of several negative acute-phase proteins, such as albumin, may fall.

Acute-phase protein synthesis by hepatocytes is induced largely by the cytokines that participate in the local inflammatory process and are secreted by activated monocytes, macrophages, endothelial cells, and certain other cells. Interleukin-6 (IL-6) is the major inducer of acute-phase changes. Other cytokines, such as IL-1 and tumor necrosis factor (TNF)-α, play more limited roles. These effects are also influenced by modulators of cytokine function, such as IL-1 receptor antagonist and soluble cytokine receptors, and by other humoral molecules.[4] Acute-phase protein levels do not always change coordinately, which suggests independently regulated mechanisms for regulation of synthesis, probably involving different combinations and interactions of cytokines and their modulators in varying circumstances. Teleo-logic considerations suggest that changes in concentration of the acute-phase proteins lead to improved functional capacity to cope with the consequences of tissue injury or infection. Functional activities that have been attributed to acute-phase proteins include direct involvement in host defense (e.g., by activation of the complement pathway), proteinase inhibition, and antioxidant activity.[5,7] Some in vitro effects of acute-phase proteins, however, may not be relevant to in vivo phenomena, and in some cases the APR may be injurious rather than beneficial.

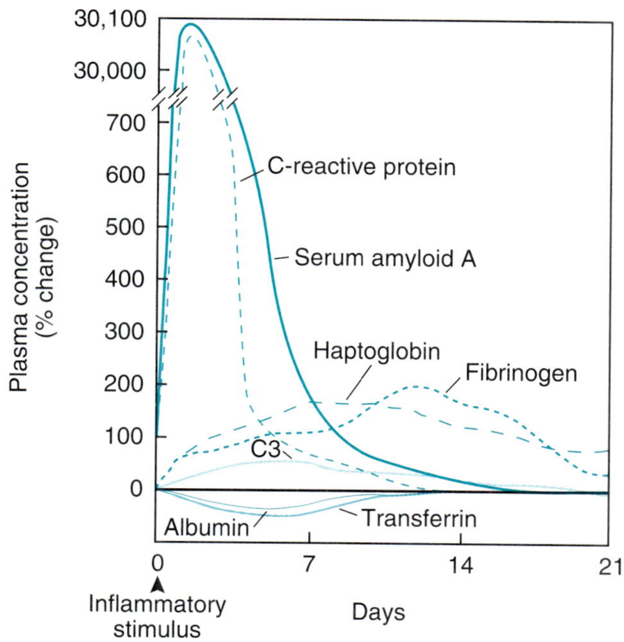

FIGURE 49–1 · Typical plasma acute-phase protein (APP) changes after a moderate inflammatory stimulus. Several patterns of response are seen: Major APP increase up to 100-fold (e.g., C-reactive protein and serum amyloid A); moderate APP increase twofold to fourfold (e.g., fibrinogen, haptoglobin); minor APP increase 50 to 100 percent (e.g., complement C3); and negative APP decrease (e.g., albumin, transferrin). (Adapted from Gitlin JD, Colten HR: Molecular biology of the acute phase plasma proteins. *In* Pick E, Landy M [eds]: Lymphokines. Vol. 14. San Diego, Academic Press, 1987, pp 123-153.)

C-REACTIVE PROTEIN

CRP is present in trace concentrations in the plasma of all humans. It is a pentamer consisting of five identical noncovalently linked 23-kD subunits and has been highly conserved over hundreds of millions of years of evolution; a homologous protein is found in the ancient organism *Limulus polyphemus,* the horseshoe crab. Although the precise function of CRP is unknown, it exhibits important recognition and activation capabilities. Among the major biologic ligands recognized by CRP are phosphocholine, other phospholipids, and histone proteins. These constituents of cell membranes and nuclei may be exposed at sites of tissue damage. Major activation functions of CRP are activation of the classic complement pathway after interaction with many of its biologic ligands and interaction with cells of the immune system by binding to Fc gamma receptors.[8] Thus, CRP bridges the gap between innate and adaptive immunity and can provide an early, effective inflammatory response. Other CRP functions appear to be anti-inflammatory, suggesting that CRP may play many pathophysiologic roles during the course of the inflammatory process.[9,10]

Following acute inflammatory stimuli, the concentration of CRP may rapidly rise for 2 or 3 days to peaks that generally reflect the extent of tissue injury. In the absence of continuing stimulus, serum CRP levels then fall relatively rapidly, with a half-life of about 18 hours.[11] However, persistently elevated serum-CRP concentrations are often seen in chronic inflammatory states, such as active rheumatoid arthritis or pulmonary tuberculosis, or in the presence of extensive malignant disease.

Serum levels of CRP can be accurately quantified by immunoassay or laser nephelometry at a modest cost. Most apparently healthy adults have serum CRP levels of less than 0.2 mg/dl, although concentrations up to 1 mg/dl are not unusual. The significance of such minor CRP elevation is discussed in a following section. It is generally accepted that concentrations over 1 mg/dl reflect significant inflammatory disease.[12,13] Concentrations between 1 and 10 mg/dl can be considered moderate increases and concentrations greater than 10 mg/dl as marked increases. Most patients with very high levels (e.g., greater than 15 to 20 mg/dl) have bacterial infections. Examples of clinical conditions associated with CRP elevations of varying degrees are shown in Table 49–1, and the range of CRP concentrations generally seen in a number of rheumatologic diseases is shown in Figure 49–2.

There are several additional caveats regarding clinical interpretation of CRP levels. Clinicians must be aware that there is no uniformity in reporting CRP concentrations; some laboratories report CRP as mg/L or µg/ml and some as mg/dl. Also, population studies of CRP reveal a skewed, rather than normal, distribution, rendering parametric statistical tests inappropriate for interpretation of CRP data. Finally, a minimal but significant elevation of CRP level that has been observed with normal aging[14,15] may reflect age-related disorders, whose pathogenesis may involve low-grade inflammatory processes, as discussed in a following section.

SERUM AMYLOID A

SAA consists of a family of proteins, some of which are constitutively expressed, whereas others display marked acute-phase behavior.[16] SAA is associated with high-density lipoproteins, but its function is not clear. Studies indicate that SAA may function as a chemoattractant,[17] induce IL-8 secretion,[18] and promote export of macrophage cholesterol.[19] As with CRP, levels of acute-phase SAA rise within hours after stimulus, and the magnitude of increase may be greater than that of CRP. Relatively trivial inflammatory stimuli can lead to

TABLE 49–1 · SOME CONDITIONS ASSOCIATED WITH VARIOUS C-REACTIVE PROTEIN LEVELS

Normal or Minor Elevation (<1 mg/dl)	Moderate Elevation (1–10 mg/dl)	Marked Elevation (>10 mg/dl)
Vigorous exercise	Myocardial infarction	Acute bacterial infection (80–85%)
Common cold	Malignancies	Major trauma
Pregnancy	Pancreatitis	Systemic vasculitis
Gingivitis	Mucosal infection (bronchitis, cystitis)	
Seizures	Most connective tissue diseases	
Depression	Rheumatoid arthritis	
Insulin resistance and diabetes		
Several genetic polymorphisms		
Obesity		

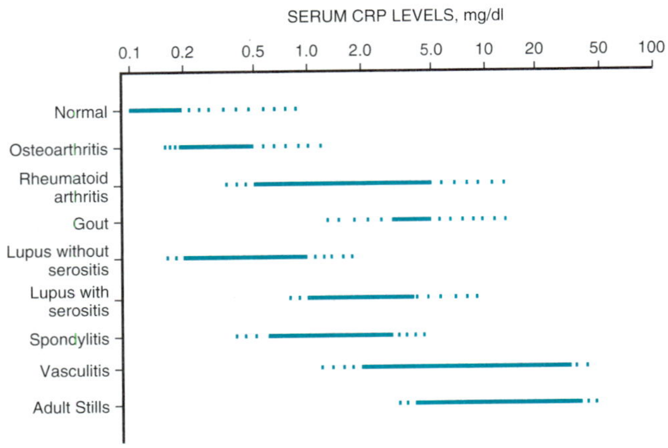

FIGURE 49–2 • Approximate serum levels of C-reactive protein (CRP) in some rheumatic diseases.

SAA responses.[16] Clinical studies have demonstrated correlation of SAA levels with disease activity in a variety of inflammatory disorders and in myocardial infarction.[20] It has recently been suggested that SAA levels correlate better with disease activity in early inflammatory joint disease than do ESR and CRP.[21] The normal level of SAA in healthy adults is probably less than 1 mg/dl. Reliable testing for acute-phase SAA is not yet widely available, and data about levels expected in health and disease are limited. The recent introduction of an enzyme immunoassay for quantifying acute-phase SAA levels may lead to greater use of SAA measurement in clinical situations.

OTHER ACUTE-PHASE PROTEINS

Measurement of other acute-phase proteins has limited value for assessment of inflammation because their responses to inflammatory stimuli are relatively slower, and the magnitudes of change in concentrations are relatively smaller than those of CRP and SAA. Serum levels of ferritin, a moderate acute-phase reactant, may be extremely high in adult-onset Still's disease (see following) and may reflect disease activity in lupus erythematosus,[22] but they are also influenced by total-body iron stores.

CYTOKINES

Plasma concentrations of cytokines and cytokine receptors are potentially useful clinically, but their quantification presents several problems related to their short plasma half-lives, the presence of blocking factors and natural inhibitors, and other technical considerations.[23] IL-6 may respond dramatically to inflammatory stimuli, with changes that are even more rapid in onset and greater in magnitude than those of CRP and SAA. Both acute and chronic inflammation and trauma have been associated with increases in IL-6, and serum levels of this cytokine have been correlated with the severity and course of disease in rheumatoid arthritis, juvenile arthritis, ankylosing spondylitis, and polymyalgia rheumatica.[24,25] Increased levels of several other cytokines and circulating cytokine receptors, some of which are listed in Table 49–2, have also been associated with inflammation or disease activity in such conditions.[26,27] Different patterns of cytokine responses have been reported in different diseases, suggesting that cytokine determinations may ultimately have diagnostic value,[28,29] as does a report that IL-6 is more sensitive than ESR for detecting disease activity in giant cell arteritis.[30] At present, the high cost, limited availability, and absence of standardization discourage measurement of plasma cytokines and their receptors in clinical practice.

Erythrocyte Sedimentation Rate

Over many years, the ESR has been the most widely used marker of the APR. Indeed, elevation of the ESR was recognized as a correlate of illness by the ancient Greeks. In this test, anticoagulated blood is placed in a vertical tube and the rate of fall of erythrocytes is measured. The ESR is an indirect way of screening for elevated concentrations of the acute-phase plasma proteins, particularly fibrinogen, that result in increased aggregation of erythrocytes (rouleaux formation), causing them to fall more rapidly.

We continue to be ignorant of many of the complex physicochemical factors that affect the ESR.[31] The ESR is known to be influenced by changes in concentrations of plasma proteins and the number and morphology of red blood cells. Two types of changes in plasma proteins commonly lead to elevation of the ESR. First, an increase in concentration of asymmetric, charged proteins decreases the natural tendency of erythrocytes to repel each other, leading to red blood cell aggregation and rouleaux formation. Fibrinogen, a moderate acute-phase reactant, is the most prevalent of the asymmetric acute-phase proteins in plasma and has the greatest effect on the ESR. Second, a major increase in concentration of a single molecular species, such as the immunoglobulin elevations that occur in multiple myeloma, may also lead to ESR elevation, although such changes do not reflect inflammatory states. In addition, anemia and polycythemia may affect the ESR, and alterations in size and shape of erythrocytes may physically interfere with rouleaux formation. It is not possible to accurately correct for alterations in size,

TABLE 49–2 • MARKERS OF INFLAMMATION THAT ARE NOT ACUTE-PHASE PROTEINS

Cytokines and Related Molecules	Products of Inflammatory and Endothelial Cells
Cytokines: IL-1	Calprotectin
IL-6	von Willebrand factor
IL-12	Adhesion molecules (e.g., vascular cell adhesion molecule-1)
Interferon-γ	Hyaluronic acid
TNF-α	Collagen and aggrecan degradation products
Granulocyte-macrophage colony-stimulating factor	Osteocalcin

Abbreviations: IL, interleukin; TNF, tumor necrosis factor.

shape, or concentration of erythrocytes. The ESR is elevated in obesity, as is CRP, presumably as a result of IL-6 secretion by adipocytes.[32]

The International Committee for Standardization in Hematology has recommended that the Westergren technique be designated as the preferred method of ESR determination.[33] The generally accepted upper limits of normal levels are 15 mm/hour for males and 20 mm/hr for females, but, in fact, the ESR progressively increases with aging, resulting in great uncertainty about "normal" levels, particularly in the elderly. Values up to 40 mm/hr are not uncommon in healthy elderly people. A simple formula for calculating maximum normal ESR at any age has been proposed.[34] A racial difference in ESR has also been reported.[35] As with CRP levels, the population distribution of ESR determinations is nongaussian. Other problems with the ESR are indicated in Table 49–3. The ESR has retained an important place in medical practice, probably because the test is both easy to perform and inexpensive, and because a wealth of information about its clinical significance has accumulated over many years. Many older physicians believe, rightly or wrongly, that they know how to compensate for its flaws, but the relative virtues of CRP determination are propelling it to a more important role in clinical practice.

TABLE 49–3 • ADVANTAGES AND DISADVANTAGES OF ERYTHROCYTE SEDIMENTATION RATE AND C-REACTIVE PROTEIN DETERMINATION

	Erythrocyte Sedimentation Rate	C-Reactive Protein
Advantages	Much clinical information in the literature	Rapid response to inflammatory stimuli
	May reflect overall health status	Wide range of clinically relevant values are detectable
		Unaffected by age and gender
		Reflects value of a single acute-phase protein
		Can be measured on stored sera
		Quantification is precise and reproducible
Disadvantages	Affected by age and gender	None
	Affected by red blood cell morphology	
	Affected by anemia and polycythemia	
	Reflects levels of many plasma proteins, not all of which are acute-phase proteins	
	Responds relatively slowly to inflammatory stimuli	
	Requires fresh sample	
	May be affected by drugs	

Laboratory Evaluation of Inflammation in Management of Rheumatic Diseases

Measurement of ESR and CRP can be clinically helpful in three ways: evaluating the extent or severity of inflammation, monitoring changes in disease activity over time, and assessing prognosis. Because neither test possesses diagnostic specificity, results cannot be used to definitely confirm or exclude any particular disease—even polymyalgia rheumatica or giant-cell arteritis (see following).

RHEUMATOID ARTHRITIS

The ESR and CRP have little place in the differential diagnosis of rheumatoid arthritis (see chapter 66), osteoarthritis, or systemic lupus erythematosus (SLE). A more appropriate application of these tests in rheumatoid arthritis is as prognostic indicators or for monitoring disease activity. Although the ESR has been more widely used for these purposes, many studies have suggested that CRP levels correlate better with disease activity.[36] CRP levels average 2 to 3 mg/dl in adult rheumatoid arthritis patients with moderate disease activity.[37] There is considerable variation: Five to 10 percent of patients have values in the normal range, whereas a few patients with severe disease activity show levels greater than 10 mg/dl. ESR values have been found to remain relatively stable over extended periods.[38] Elevated acute-phase reactant levels are associated with early synovitis and erosions as detected by magnetic resonance imaging (MRI),[39] with inflammatory cellular infiltrates in synovium,[40] and with osteoclastic activation and reduced bone mineral density.[41] Both CRP and ESR predict radiographic progression,[42,43] as do the matrix metalloproteinases MMP-3 and MMP-1.[44] Long-term studies have identified time-integrated values of ESR and CRP[45-47] as significant correlates of disease progression over periods of up to 20 years. Finally, and perhaps most importantly, acute-phase reactants correlate with work disability on long-term follow-up.[45]

Serum or synovial fluid levels of a number of other tissue products (see Table 49–2) have been correlated with clinical measures of disease activity, severity, and radiographic damage. Recent interest has focused on matrix metalloproteinase-3, pro-matrix metalloproteinase-3, and E-selectin. In general, serum levels of these markers correlate with CRP levels.[44,48-51]

ESR and CRP have long been employed to follow the response to therapy; in general, disease modifying antirheumatic drugs decrease CRP levels by about 40 percent. Even more striking improvement has been seen with the recently introduced biologic agents, providing objective laboratory support for the encouraging clinical responses observed. Thus, in a 1999 study of anti–TNF-α therapy, CRP and SAA levels fell by 75 percent and 85 percent, respectively, in about a week.[52] However, progression of joint damage can occur despite decreases in ESR and CRP.[53]

SYSTEMIC LUPUS ERYTHEMATOSUS

Although serum CRP and ESR levels are elevated in many patients with active SLE (see Chapter 75), a number do not show even mild elevation of CRP. Lupus patients with acute serositis[54] or chronic synovitis[55] are most likely to have substantially elevated levels of CRP, whereas those with other manifestations of lupus, such as nephritis, may have only modest or no elevation. It is not clear whether antibodies to CRP that have been detected in some SLE patients explain their lower CRP levels.[56] Data are insufficient to evaluate the potential use of some of the other newer markers described previously, but many SLE patients with normal CRP levels show elevated IL-6 concentrations.[57]

CRP elevation in most SLE patients is more likely to result from superimposed infection than activation of lupus. Accordingly, CRP levels in excess of 6 mg/dl in these patients should serve as an impetus to exclude the possibility of infection, just as they should in other diseases.[12] However, such levels should not be regarded as proof of infection; as indicated earlier, marked CRP elevation related to active SLE can be seen in the absence of infection.

POLYMYALGIA RHEUMATICA AND GIANT CELL ARTERITIS

The diagnosis of polymyalgia rheumatica (PMR) or giant-cell arteritis (GCA) is supported by an elevated ESR, often higher than 100 mm/hr (see Chapter 82). Such an elevation is no longer regarded as a sine qua non of these disorders; continuing reports suggest that up to 20 percent of patients with PMR can have "normal" ESRs, depending on which value (30, 40, or 45 mm/hr) is taken as the limit of normal. Such patients tend to have fewer systemic symptoms and less anemia, but the same frequency of positive temporal artery biopsies as those with high ESR.[58,59] In contrast, ESR under 40 is found in only about 5 percent of patients with GCA; these patients have fewer visual and systemic symptoms than those with higher ESR values.[60] Extreme elevation of the ESR in the absence of symptoms of PMR or GCA is more likely to be due to infection, malignancy, or renal disease.

In these diseases, CRP and ESR have in the past been regarded as equally valuable in assessing disease activity. However, recent reports indicate that CRP is more sensitive for both conditions and should be included in the diagnostic workup.[59,61,62] In addition, the uncertainty as to what ESR values are "normal" in the elderly suggests that CRP may be more valuable in this population. The report that IL-6 is more sensitive than ESR for indicating disease activity in GCA is of particular interest.[30] Finally, a number of markers of endothelial perturbation, not acute-phase reactants in the strict sense, are elevated in plasma in various inflammatory disorders of vessels, particularly PMR, GCA, and other vasculitides.[63] These molecules include von Willebrand factor, thrombomodulin, some vasoactive prostanoids, and a variety of adhesion molecules, such as vascular cell adhesion molecule-1 (VCAM-1). Of course, clinical manifestations of disease, even in the presence of a normal ESR or CRP level, should not be ignored.

ADULT-ONSET STILL'S DISEASE

Markedly elevated concentrations of ferritin, disproportionately high compared to other acute-phase reactants, have long been noted in adult-onset Still's disease (see Chapter 96).[64] It has recently been observed that only a low percentage—commonly less than 20 percent—of ferritin is glycosylated in adult-onset Still's disease,[65] a criterion included in a recently proposed set of classification criteria for this condition.[66] Swiss investigators reported extremely elevated ferritin levels in the reactive macrophage-activation syndrome as well.[67] They noted that 40 percent of individuals with this condition meet the criteria for adult-onset Still's disease and questioned whether these are indeed two distinct entities.[68] Concentrations of serum IL-18 were extremely elevated in patients with active adult-onset Still's disease, compared to those with other connective tissue diseases or healthy individuals, and correlated with serum ferritin values and disease severity.[69] It has been suggested that interferon-α may be responsible for the hyperferritinemia of adult-onset Still's disease.[64] CRP levels are usually markedly elevated in this disease as well.

ANKYLOSING SPONDYLITIS

Ankylosing spondylitis (AS) ordinarily does not lead to substantial increase in CRP or ESR. Median CRP levels are 1.6 mg/dl in patients with spinal involvement only and 2.5 mg/dl with peripheral involvement or associated inflammatory bowel disease as well. Median ESR is 13 and 21, respectively, in these groups.[70] Infliximab treatment of AS patients led to an average decrease in CRP concentration of 75 percent after 12 weeks. However, patients with basal CRP levels of 1.0 mg/dl or less showed little improvement, raising the possibility that patients with higher CRP values should be preferentially considered for infliximab treatment.[71] It has recently been reported that IL-8 levels may reflect clinical activity in spondyloarthropathies.[72]

OSTEOARTHRITIS

Minor CRP elevations, between 0.2 and 1.0 mg/dl, have been reported in patients with knee osteoarthritis, particularly those with progressive joint damage. However, one recent study has failed to confirm this finding,[73] whereas others cast doubt on the clinical usefulness of this association because of the association between CRP levels and obesity, a common accompaniment of osteoarthritis of the knee.[74]

Practical Use of Laboratory Reflectors of Inflammation

When recently surveyed, rheumatologists were found to employ ESR more than twice as frequently as they did CRP.[75] However, we know that ESR reflects many complex, poorly understood changes in blood not necessarily associated with inflammation. Moreover, it is a mistake to take the reference "normal" values for ESR seriously. It is well established that mean ESR values increase substantially with age; normal at age 20 is different from normal at 70, and normal is different in men than in women. Many rheumatologists are familiar with the clinical experience of being called upon to interpret an elevated ESR in an individual who, by history and examination, appears healthy and on further testing displays a low CRP. The "baggage" associated with interpretation of the ESR, its uncertain "normal" value, and increasing positive clinical experience with CRP all suggest that it is time to move on and that we should rely more on CRP than ESR testing.[76,77]

Discrepancies between ESR and CRP may result from the effects of blood constituents that are not related to inflammation but can influence the ESR, as discussed previously. In addition, however, patterns of acute-phase protein changes differ for different conditions.[4] For example, as indicated previously, the ESR may be markedly elevated in many patients with active SLE, while CRP is normal. Undoubtedly a number of other clinical situations exist in which similar discrepancies occur. Although many noninflammatory physicochemical causes for falsely high ESR exist (some known and many undoubtedly unknown), CRP values greater than 1 mg/dl invariably reflect an inflammatory process. In light of these considerations, many feel that several tests, rather than a single test, should be performed and interpreted in clinical context. For example, it has been suggested that ESR, which is sensitive to anemia and immunoglobulin levels, may reflect "general severity" in rheumatoid arthritis, whereas CRP is a better test of inflammation per se.[78,79]

Significance of Minor C-reactive Protein Elevation

Although most ostensibly healthy individuals have CRP concentrations of 0.2 mg/dl or less, some have concentrations as high as 1.0 mg/dl. The latter finding has long been attributed to trivial injury or to minimal inflammatory processes such as gingivitis. However, recent data indicate that CRP concentrations between 0.2 and 1.0 mg/dl may have clinical relevance. Employing a "high-sensitivity CRP" assay (HS-CRP), minimally elevated CRP levels have been found to predict the risk of a first myocardial infarction in apparently healthy individuals,[80,81] as well as "failure to thrive" and even increased mortality in the elderly.[82] This phenomenon may indeed reflect an ongoing inflammatory process in coronary arteries (or elsewhere). However, CRP values in this range are also associated with many states not ordinarily regarded as inflammatory, including insulin resistance, obesity, poor physical conditioning, high-protein diet, depression, and notably, high or low alcohol intake.[83-87] It may be that minimally elevated CRP levels identify individuals who bear an increased burden of tissue damage resulting from cumulative oxidative stress, a process strongly implicated in the pathogenesis of aging.[83] Such individuals are biologically (not necessarily chronologically) older and would be expected to have a greater likelihood of disease or death. Aging itself is associated with a minimal but statistically significant rise in CRP levels.[14,15] In addition, baseline CRP levels are heritable and a number of genetic polymorphisms, including the IL-6 gene (−174G/C), are associated with high CRP levels.[88] At present, it is not clear that HS-CRP screening to identify individuals at risk for atherosclerosis, as has been recommended,[89] will be an effective tool.[90-92] Certainly, because of the high prevalence of underlying inflammation in rheumatologic patients, it is unlikely that this screening strategy will be of much value in such patients.

REFERENCES

1. Kushner I: Semantics, inflammation, cytokines and common sense. Cytokine Growth Factor Rev 9:191-196, 1998.
2. Gallin JI, Snyderman R: Inflammation: Basic Principles and Clinical Correlates. Philadelphia, Lippincott Williams & Wilkins, 1999.
3. Nathan C: Points of control in inflammation. Nature 420:846-852, 2002.
4. Gabay C, Kushner I: Acute-phase proteins and other systemic responses to inflammation. N Engl J Med 340:448-454, 1999.
5. Samols D, Agrawal A, Kushner I: Acute phase proteins. In Oppenheim JJ, Feldman M (eds): Cytokine Reference On-Line: www.academicpress.com/cytokinereference. London, Academic Press, Harcourt, 2002.
6. Yoo JY, Desiderio S: Innate and acquired immunity intersect in a global view of the acute-phase response. Proc Natl Acad Sci U S A 100:1157-1162, 2003.
7. Volanakis JE: Acute phase proteins in rheumatic disease. In Koopman WJ (ed): Arthritis and Allied Conditions: A Textbook of Rheumatology. Vol. 13. Baltimore, Williams & Wilkins, 1997, pp 505-514.
8. Du Clos TW, Mold C: The role of C-reactive protein in the resolution of bacterial infection. Curr Opin Infect Dis 14:289-293, 2001.
9. Volanakis JE: Human C-reactive protein: Expression, structure, and function. Mol Immunol 38:189-197, 2001.
10. Mortensen RF: C-reactive protein, inflammation, and innate immunity. Immunol Res 24:163-176, 2001.
11. Vigushin DM, Pepys MB, Hawkins PN: Metabolic and scintigraphic studies of radioiodinated human C-reactive protein in health and disease. J Clin Invest 91:1351-1357, 1993.
12. Morley JJ, Kushner I: Serum C-reactive protein levels in disease. Ann N Y Acad Sci 389:406-418, 1982.
13. Macy EM, Hayes TE, Tracy RP: Variability in the measurement of C-reactive protein in healthy subjects: implications for reference intervals and epidemiological applications. Clin Chem 43:52-58, 1997.
14. Ballou SP, Lozanski FB, Hodder S, et al: Quantitative and qualitative alterations of acute-phase proteins in healthy elderly persons. Age Ageing 25:224-230, 1996.
15. Wener MH, Daum PR, McQuillan GM: The influence of age, sex, and race on the upper reference limit of serum C-reactive protein concentration. J Rheumatol 27:2351-2359, 2000.
16. Chambers RE, Hutton CW, Dieppe PA, Whicher JT: Comparative study of C reactive protein and serum amyloid A protein in experimental inflammation. Ann Rheum Dis 50:677-679, 1991.
17. Su SB, Gong W, Gao JL, et al: A seven-transmembrane, G protein-coupled receptor, FPRL1, mediates the chemotactic activity of serum amyloid A for human phagocytic cells. J Exp Med 189:395-402, 1999.
18. He R, Sang H, Ye RD: Serum amyloid A induces IL-8 secretion through a G protein-coupled receptor, FPRL1/LXA4R. Blood 26:26, 2002.
19. Tam SP, Flexman A, Hulme J, Kisilevsky R: Promoting export of macrophage cholesterol: The physiological role of a major acute-phase protein, serum amyloid A 2.1. J Lipid Res 43:1410-1420, 2002.
20. Liuzzo G, Biasucci LM, Gallimore JR, et al: The prognostic value of C-reactive protein and serum amyloid a protein in severe unstable angina. N Engl J Med 331:417-424, 1994.

21. Cunnane G, Grehan S, Geoghegan S, et al: Serum amyloid A in the assessment of early inflammatory arthritis. J Rheumatol 27:58-63, 2000.
22. Nishiya K, Hashimoto K: Elevation of serum ferritin levels as a marker for active systemic lupus erythematosus. Clin Exp Rheumatol 15:39-44, 1997.
23. Barnes A: Measurement of serum cytokines [Letter]. Lancet 352:324-325, 1998.
24. Tutuncu ZN, Bilgie A, Kennedy LG, Calin A: Interleukin-6, acute phase reactants and clinical status in ankylosing spondylitis. Ann Rheum Dis 53:425-426, 1994.
25. Uddhammar A, Sundqvist KG, Ellis B, Rantapaa-Dahlqvist S: Cytokines and adhesion molecules in patients with polymyalgia rheumatica. Br J Rheumatol 37:766-769, 1998.
26. Luqmani R, Sheeran T, Robinson M, et al: Systemic cytokine measurements: Their role in monitoring the response to therapy in patients with rheumatoid arthritis. Clin Exp Rheumatol 12:503-508, 1994.
27. Pountain G, Hazleman B, Cawston TE: Circulating levels of IL-1beta, IL-6 and soluble IL-2 receptor in polymyalgia rheumatica and giant cell arteritis and rheumatoid arthritis [Letter]. Br J Rheumatol 37:797-798, 1998.
28. Gabay C, Cakir N, Moral F, et al: Circulating levels of tumor necrosis factor soluble receptors in systemic lupus erythematosus are significantly higher than in other rheumatic diseases and correlate with disease activity. J Rheumatol 24:303-308, 1997.
29. Gabay C, Gay-Croisier F, Roux-Lombard P, et al: Elevated serum levels of interleukin-1 receptor antagonist in polymyositis/dermatomyositis: A biologic marker of disease activity with a possible role in the lack of acute-phase protein response. Arthritis Rheum 37:1744-1751, 1994.
30. Weyand CM, Fulbright JW, Hunder GG, et al: Treatment of giant cell arteritis: interleukin-6 as a biologic marker of disease activity. Arthritis Rheum 43:1041-1048, 2000.
31. Bedell SE, Bush BT: Erythrocyte sedimentation rate: From folklore to facts. Am J Med 78:1001-1009, 1985.
32. Bastard JP, Maachi M, Van Nhieu JT, et al: Adipose tissue IL-6 content correlates with resistance to insulin activation of glucose uptake both in vivo and in vitro. J Clin Endocrinol Metab 87:2084-2089, 2002.
33. International Council for Standardization in Haematology (Expert Panel on Blood Rheology): ICSH recommendations for measurement of erythrocyte sedimentation rate. J Clin Pathol 46:198-203, 1993.
34. Miller A, Green M, Roberson D: Simple rule for calculating normal erythrocyte sedimentation rate. Br Med J 286:266, 1983.
35. Gillum RF: A racial difference in erythrocyte sedimentation. J Natl Med Assoc 85:47-50, 1993.
36. Cohick CB, Furst DE, Quagliata S, et al: Analysis of elevated serum interleukin-6 levels in rheumatoid arthritis: Correlation with erythrocyte sedimentation rate or C-reactive protein. J Lab Clin Med 123:721-727, 1994.
37. Aletaha D, Smolen JS: The rheumatoid arthritis patient in the clinic: Comparing more than 1300 consecutive DMARD courses. Rheumatology 41:1367-1374, 2002.
38. Wolfe F, Pincus T: The level of inflammation in rheumatoid arthritis is determined early and remains stable over the longterm course of the illness. J Rheumatol 28:1817-1824, 2001.
39. Graudal N, Tarp U, Jurik AG, et al: Inflammatory patterns in rheumatoid arthritis estimated by the number of swollen and tender joints, the erythrocyte sedimentation rate, and hemoglobin: Longterm course and association to radiographic progression. J Rheumatol 27:47-57, 2000.
40. Fujinami M, Sato K, Kashiwazaki S, Aotsuka S: Comparable histological appearance of synovitis in seropositive and seronegative rheumatoid arthritis. Clin Exp Rheumatol 15:11-17, 1997.
41. Gough A, Sambrook P, Devlin J, et al: Osteoclastic activation is the principal mechanism leading to secondary osteoporosis in rheumatoid arthritis. J Rheumatol 25:1282-1289, 1998.
42. Jansen LM, van der Horst-Bruinsma IE, van Schaardenburg D, et al: Predictors of radiographic joint damage in patients with early rheumatoid arthritis. Ann Rheum Dis 60:924-927, 2001.
43. Combe B, Dougados M, Goupille P, et al: Prognostic factors for radiographic damage in early rheumatoid arthritis: A multiparameter prospective study. Arthritis Rheum 44:1736-1743, 2001.
44. Green MJ, Gough AK, Devlin J, et al: Serum MMP-3 and MMP-1 and progression of joint damage in early rheumatoid arthritis. Rheumatology 42:83-88, 2003.
45. Wolfe F, Sharp JT: Radiographic outcome of recent-onset rheumatoid arthritis: A 19-year study of radiographic progression. Arthritis Rheum 41:1571-1582, 1998.
46. Plant MJ, Jones PW, Saklatvala J, et al: Patterns of radiological progression in early rheumatoid arthritis: Results of an 8 year prospective study. J Rheumatol 25:417-426, 1998.
47. van Leeuwen MA, van der Heijde DM, van Rijswijk MH, et al: Interrelationship of outcome measures and process variables in early rheumatoid arthritis: A comparison of radiologic damage, physical disability, joint counts, and acute phase reactants. J Rheumatol 21:425-429, 1994.
48. Cheung NT, Dawes PT, Poulton KV, et al: High serum levels of pro-matrix metalloproteinase-3 are associated with greater radiographic damage and the presence of the shared epitope in patients with rheumatoid arthritis. J Rheumatol 27:882-887, 2000.
49. Ribbens C, Andre B, Jaspar JM, et al: Matrix metalloproteinase-3 serum levels are correlated with disease activity and predict clinical response in rheumatoid arthritis. J Rheumatol 27:888-893, 2000.
50. Roux-Lombard P, Eberhardt K, Saxne T, et al: Cytokines, metalloproteinases, their inhibitors and cartilage oligomeric matrix protein: Relationship to radiological progression and inflammation in early rheumatoid arthritis—A prospective 5-year study. Rheumatology 40:544-551, 2001.
51. Kuuliala A, Eberhardt K, Takala A, et al: Circulating soluble E-selectin in early rheumatoid arthritis: A prospective five year study. Ann Rheum Dis 61:242-246, 2002.
52. Charles P, Elliott MJ, Davis D, et al: Regulation of cytokines, cytokine inhibitors, and acute-phase proteins following anti-TNF-alpha therapy in rheumatoid arthritis. J Immunol 163:1521-1528, 1999.
53. McQueen FM, Stewart N, Crabbe J, et al: Magnetic resonance imaging of the wrist in early rheumatoid arthritis reveals progression of erosions despite clinical improvement. Ann Rheum Dis 58:156-163, 1999.
54. ter Borg EJ, Horst G, et al: C-reactive protein levels during disease exacerbations and infections in systemic lupus erythematosus: A prospective longitudinal study. J Rheumatol 17:1642-1648, 1990.
55. Moutsopoulos HM, Mavridis AK, Acritidis NC, Avgerinos PC: High C-reactive protein response in lupus polyarthritis. Clin Exp Rheumatol 1:53-55, 1983.
56. Sjowall C, Eriksson P, Almer S, Skogh T: Autoantibodies to C-reactive protein is a common finding in SLE, but not in primary Sjögren's syndrome, rheumatoid arthritis or inflammatory bowel disease. J Autoimmun 19:155-160, 2002.
57. Gabay C, Roux-Lombard P, de Moerloose P, et al: Absence of correlation between interleukin 6 and C-reactive protein blood levels in systemic lupus erythematosus compared with rheumatoid arthritis. J Rheumatol 20:815-821, 1993.
58. Proven A, Gabriel SE, O'Fallon WM, Hunder GG: Polymyalgia rheumatica with low erythrocyte sedimentation rate at diagnosis. J Rheumatol 26:1333-1337, 1999.
59. Cantini F, Salvarani C, Olivieri I, et al: Erythrocyte sedimentation rate and C-reactive protein in the evaluation of disease activity and severity in polymyalgia rheumatica: A prospective follow-up study. Semin Arthritis Rheum 30:17-24, 2000.
60. Salvarani C, Hunder GG: Giant cell arteritis with low erythrocyte sedimentation rate: Frequency of occurence in a population-based study. Arthritis Rheum 45:140-145, 2001.
61. Larrosa M, Gratacos J, Sala M: Polymyalgia rheumatica with low erythrocyte sedimentation rate at diagnosis. J Rheumatol 27: 1815-1816, 2000.
62. Liozon E, Jauberteau-Marchan MO, LyK, et al: Giant cell arteritis with a low erythrocyte sedimentation rate: Comments on the article by Salvarani and Hunder. Arthritis Care Res 47:692-694, 2002.
63. Pearson JD: Markers of endothelial perturbation and damage. Br J Rheumatol 32:651-652, 1993.
64. Stam TC, Swaak AJ, Kruit WH, Eggermont AM: Regulation of ferritin: a specific role for interferon-alpha (IFN-alpha)? The acute

phase response in patients treated with IFN-alpha-2b. Eur J Clin Invest 32(Suppl 1):79-83, 2002.

65. Fautrel B, Le Moel G, Saint-Marcoux B, et al: Diagnostic value of ferritin and glycosylated ferritin in adult onset Still's disease. J Rheumatol 28:322-329, 2001.
66. Fautrel B, Zing E, Golmard JL, et al: Proposal for a new set of classification criteria for adult-onset Still disease. Medicine 81:194-200, 2002.
67. Emmenegger U, Frey U, Reimers A, et al: Hyperferritinemia as indicator for intravenous immunoglobulin treatment in reactive macrophage activation syndromes. Am J Hematol 68:4-10, 2001.
68. Emmenegger U, Reimers A, Frey U, et al: Reactive macrophage activation syndrome: A simple screening strategy and its potential in early treatment initiation. Swiss Med Wkly 132:230-236, 2002.
69. Kawashima M, Yamamura M, Taniai M, et al: Levels of interleukin-18 and its binding inhibitors in the blood circulation of patients with adult-onset Still's disease. Arthritis Rheum 44:550-560, 2001.
70. Spoorenberg A, van der Heijde D, de Klerk E, et al: Relative value of erythrocyte sedimentation rate and C-reactive protein in assessment of disease activity in ankylosing spondylitis. J Rheumatol 26:980-984, 1999.
71. Braun J, Brandt J, Listing J, et al: Treatment of active ankylosing spondylitis with infliximab: a randomised controlled multicentre trial. Lancet 359:1187-1193, 2002.
72. Sonel B, Tutkak H, Duzgun N: Serum levels of IL-1 beta, TNF-alpha, IL-8, and acute phase proteins in seronegative spondyloarthropathies. Joint Bone Spine 69:463-467, 2002.
73. Nevitt M, Felson D, Peterfy C, et al: Inflammation markers (CRP, TNF-a, IL-6) are not associated with radiographic or MRI findings of knee OA in the elderly: The health ABC study. Arthritis Rheum 46:S372, 2002.
74. Sowers M, Jannausch M, Stein E, et al: C-reactive protein as a biomarker of emergent osteoarthritis. Osteoarthritis Cartilage 10:595-601, 2002.
75. Donald F, Ward MM: Evaluative laboratory testing practices of United States rheumatologists. Arthritis Rheum 41:725-729, 1998.
76. Weinstein A, Del Giudice J: The erythrocyte sedimentation rate—time honored and tradition bound. J Rheumatol 21:1177-1178, 1994.
77. Giacomello A, Quaratino CP, Zoppini A: Erythrocyte sedimentation rate within rheumatic disease clinics [Letter; comment]. J Rheumatol 24:2263-2265, 1997.
78. Bull BS, Westengard JC, Farr M, et al: Efficacy of tests used to monitor rheumatoid arthritis. Lancet 2:965-967, 1989.
79. Wolfe F: Comparative usefulness of C-reactive protein and erythrocyte sedimentation rate in patients with rheumatoid arthritis. J Rheumatol 24:1477-1485, 1997.
80. Ridker PM, Cushman M, Stampfer MJ, et al: Inflammation, aspirin, and the risk of cardiovascular disease in apparently healthy men. N Engl J Med 336:973-979, 1997.
81. Haverkate F, Thompson SG, Pyke SD, et al: Production of C-reactive protein and risk of coronary events in stable and unstable angina: European Concerted Action on Thrombosis and Disabilities Angina Pectoris Study Group. Lancet 349:462-466, 1997.
82. Harris TB, Ferrucci L, Tracy RP, et al: Associations of elevated interleukin-6 and C-reactive protein levels with mortality in the elderly. Am J Med 106:506-512, 1999.
83. Kushner I: C-reactive protein (CRP) elevation can be caused by conditions other than inflammation and may reflect biologic aging. Cleveland Clin J Med 68:535-537, 2001.
84. Geffken DF, Cushman M, Burke GL, et al: Association between physical activity and markers of inflammation in a healthy elderly population. Am J Epidemiol 153:242-250, 2001.
85. Fleming RM: The effect of high-protein diets on coronary blood flow. Angiology 51:817-826, 2000.
86. Imhof A, Froehlich M, Brenner H, et al: Effect of alcohol consumption on systemic markers of inflammation. Lancet 357: 763-767, 2001.
87. Temelkova-Kurktschiev T, Siegert G, Bergmann S, et al: Subclinical inflammation is strongly related to insulin resistance but not to impaired insulin secretion in a high risk population for diabetes. Metabolism 51:743-749, 2002.
88. Vickers MA, Green FR, Terry C, et al: Genotype at a promoter polymorphism of the interleukin-6 gene is associated with baseline levels of plasma C-reactive protein. Cardiovasc Res 53: 1029-1034, 2002.
89. Pearson TA, Mensah GA, Alexander RW, et al: Markers of inflammation and cardiovascular disease: application to clinical and public health practice—statement for healthcare professionals from the Centers for Disease Control and Prevention and the American Heart Association. Circulation 107:499-511, 2003.
90. Mosca L: C-reactive protein: To screen or not to screen? N Engl J Med 347:1615-1617, 2002.
91. Kushner I, Sehgal AR: Is high-sensitivity C-reactive protein an effective screening test for cardiovascular risk? Arch Intern Med 162:867-869, 2002.
92. Campbell B, Badrick T, Flatman R, Kanowski D: Limited clinical utility of high-sensitivity plasma C-reactive protein assays. Ann Clin Biochem 39:85-88, 2002.

50 Biological Markers

JEROEN DEGROOT • JOHAN M. TEKOPPELE • EDWARD D. HARRIS, JR.
• PAUL-PETER TAK

Biomarkers in the broad sense are anatomic, physiologic, biochemical, or molecular parameters associated with the presence and severity of specific diseases and are detectable by a variety of methods including physical examination, laboratory assays, and imaging. This chapter concentrates on biomarkers in senso stricto: markers that can be measured in patient samples such as blood, urine, synovial fluid, and synovial tissue and that provide information for diagnosis, prognosis, monitoring of disease progression, or the assessment of the efficacy of treatment. Such markers often first appear in studies on the pathobiology of a disease, with their application as biomarker being secondary. Due to the importance and potential of biological markers, the identification and validation of novel biomarkers is now often a primary objective in many studies.

For both osteoarthritis (OA) and rheumatoid arthritis (RA), the most important common feature is progressive destruction of articular tissues, resulting in impaired joint function and pain. Diagnosis is based on clinical symptoms and laboratory tests, in combination with radiography to visualize often irreversible degenerative and destructive changes in the joint. Radiologic evaluation of joints mainly images bone and is relatively insensitive: A follow-up period of at least 1 and more likely 2 years is needed to assess disease progression and the effect of therapy. Magnetic resonance imaging (MRI) has the ability to simultaneously visualize all joint tissues; it is currently being optimized but has as yet not reached its full potential.[1] Moreover, all imaging techniques provide a cumulative, historic view of damage that has already occurred, rather than assessing the current rate of disease progression (Fig. 50–1).

Alternative methods that detect changes in the joints in an early stage of the disease in a quantitative, reliable, and sensitive manner are, therefore, needed. Molecular markers (i.e., markers that are used to monitor molecular events taking place during disease) are well suited for this purpose. A good marker is disease-specific, reflects actual disease activity, is sensitive to change after therapy, and can predict disease outcome. Most likely, all these requirements are not met by one single marker; different (combinations of) markers will have to be applied for different purposes. The molecular markers described for joint diseases can be classified in the following categories.

1. Immunological and inflammatory markers
2. Markers that reflect extracellular matrix remodeling (Table 50–1)
3. Markers present in synovial tissue biopsies
4. Genetic markers, which have been shown to provide important information on risk factors for development and progression of OA and RA are reviewed elsewhere[2,3] and are not included in this chapter

Extensively studied markers in inflammatory arthritis that are routinely used in clinical practice include C-reactive protein (CRP) levels and the erythrocyte sedimentation rate (ESR), both of which provide information about the systemic inflammatory process. Although such markers of inflammation are neither disease nor tissue specific, they may reflect disease activity,[4] the effects of immunosuppressive and immunomodulatory therapies,[5] and to a certain extent predict disease progression in RA.[6] Although synovial inflammation is regarded as a secondary process in OA, cytokines and other signal molecules have also been proposed as markers in this disease. Serum nitrate and nitrite (reflecting nitric oxide levels) are, for instance, increased in OA compared to healthy controls, but not as much as in inflammatory conditions such as RA.[7] In addition, using a genomics approach, chondrocytes from OA cartilage have been shown to upregulate the transcription of a variety of inflammatory genes.[8] Synovial tissue from OA patients also shows signs of hyperplasty and inflammation.[9] Therefore, although OA is traditionally viewed as a non-inflammatory arthropathy, the osteoarthritic joint could be considered a mildly inflamed organ.

The focus of this chapter is on markers that mirror disease-related changes in the joints, especially markers for remodeling (i.e., degradation as well as synthesis) of the extracellular matrix.[10] Concomitant changes occur in all joint tissues (cartilage, bone, and synovium) and for a comprehensive assessment of these changes, molecular markers are needed for each of these tissues.[11,12] It should be noted that, for the markers derived from these different tissues, there can be a substantial difference in which biological fluid biomarker levels are determined. The concentration of markers in body fluids not only reflects the dynamics of the disease, but also the rate of clearance and the amount of remaining tissue. Cartilage-derived markers diffuse out of the tissue and enter the synovial fluid, which may vary in volume depending on the severity of ongoing inflammation.

Of interest, recent data suggest that synovial fluid urea levels may be used to correct for this "dilution,"[13] Clearance from the synovial fluid predominantly occurs via lymphatic drainage, and partial degradation

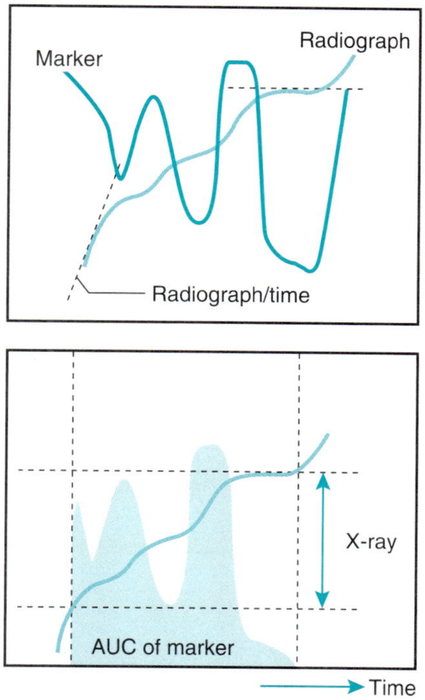

FIGURE 50–1 · Relation between radiology and biomarkers. Radiology and magnetic resonance imaging (MRI) provide a cumulative, historic view of joint destruction, whereas biomarkers provide dynamic information on the current rate of joint destruction or disease activity. At any given time, the slope of the radiograph versus time plot should, therefore, be compared to biomarker levels (upper panel). Consequently, the progression of radiographic damage (Δ radiograph) must be related to the time-integrated marker levels (area under the curve, lower panel).

may occur in the lymph nodes, depending on the marker studied. Again, synovial clearance may be dependent on the severity of the ongoing synovitis and may be determined by the permeability of the synovial membrane microvasculature.[14] Once the marker enters the systemic circulation, dilution occurs (5 ml synovial fluid versus approximately 5 l blood), and marker levels are confounded by molecules from other (non-) affected joints or even from nonarticular cartilage.

Bone- and synovium-derived markers may also enter the circulation directly. Once the marker enters the systemic circulation it will be diluted, mixed with markers derived from other joints or tissues, and potentially metabolized in the liver and kidneys. Excretion in the urine depends on the marker and the previously mentioned metabolic processes. In the discussion that follows, examples are given from studies of both OA and RA to illustrate their use in assessing disease-related tissue remodeling.

Collagen Markers

The main constituent of the extracellular matrix of connective tissues is collagen, which plays an essential role in the maintenance of tissue shape, strength, and integrity. The fibrillar collagen types I, II, and III are synthesized as propeptide-containing α-chains that are post-translationally modified by hydroxylation of lysyl and prolyl residues and by glycosylation of hydroxylysyl residues (see Chapter 2). Triple-helical collagen molecules are secreted from the cell, the propeptides are cleaved off, and fibrils are formed that are stabilized by intermolecular cross-links. This unique sequence of events provides a variety of tools used to study collagen synthesis (especially propeptides) and degradation (especially cross-links) in rheumatic diseases (Fig. 50–2).

In bone, type I collagen comprises 90 percent of the organic matrix, and markers of bone collagen turnover have proven valuable in monitoring diseases, such as osteoporosis.[15] For the bone metabolites it should be kept in mind that there is a significant menopausal effect that requires properly matched control groups and careful interpretation of the data.

Several assays have been used to assess collagen type I degradation in RA and OA. The cross-linked carboxyterminal telopeptide (ICTP) is released by matrix metalloproteinase (MMP) cleavage of type I collagen, and its levels reflect MMP-mediated soft tissue degradation.[16] Of note, cathepsin K–mediated osteoclastic bone resorption destroys ICTP antigenicity.[16] In contrast, both the carboxyterminal (CTx) and the aminoterminal (NTx) telopeptide of type I collagen are generated by cathepsin K–mediated bone collagen degradation. Previous work has shown slightly elevated serum ICTP levels in RA compared to controls in association with disease activity measured by ESR, CRP levels, and swollen joint counts.[17] In OA patients, serum and urinary CTx levels are decreased compared to controls, which suggests decreased bone remodeling in OA.[12,18] Urinary CTx levels strongly correlate with serum levels.[19] In RA, urinary NTx levels and CTx levels are increased compared to healthy controls and are sensitive to change after treatment.[20-22]

Although at first sight CTx and ICTP appear to provide identical information, closer inspection reveals that these two markers, although based on the same principle of detecting type I collagen telopeptides, may provide valuable complementary information. For instance, both CTx and NTx levels are very low in patients suffering from pycnodysostosis, which is caused by a deficient activity of cathepsin K, whereas ICTP levels are high. It has also been shown that in postmenopausal women, anti–bone resorption therapy by hormone replacement reduced serum CTx levels, whereas ICTP levels did not change.[19]

In cartilage, type II collagen comprises 80 percent of the dry weight of the tissue. Damage to the collagen network (collagen degradation and subsequent denaturation) is one of the first features of OA and contributes significantly to the decreased mechanical properties of osteoarthritic cartilage.[23] Using monoclonal antibodies, release of type II collagen telopeptides (C-telopeptide, CTx-II) was shown to reflect cartilage degradation with high tissue specificity.[24] Urinary CTx-II levels were significantly increased in RA and OA patients compared to healthy controls, although the ranges overlapped considerably.[24-26] In

TABLE 50–1 • MOLECULAR MARKERS OF EXTRACELLULAR MATRIX REMODELING

Marker	Joint Tissue	References
Synthesis		
Collagen type I		
N-propeptide (PINP)	bone, soft tissues	11
C-propeptide (PICP)	bone, soft tissues	11
Collagen type II		
N-propeptide (PIINP; PIIANP)	cartilage	30
C-propeptide (PIICP; chondrocalcin)	cartilage	27-29
Collagen type III		
N-propeptide (PIIINP)	soft tissues	12, 36-37
Proteoglycans and GAGs		
Chondroitin sulfate (epitopes 846, 3-B-3, 7-D-4)	cartilage	35-39, 48-51
Miscellaneous		
Bone specific alkaline phosphatase	bone	11
Osteocalcin	bone	12
YKL-40 (CYLK-40, gp-39, chondrex)	cartilage	11-12
Hyaluronan	cartilage, synovium	57-61
Degradation		
Collagen type I degradation		
cross-linked N-telopeptide (NTx)	bone	11-21
cross-linked C-telopeptide (CTx)	bone	12, 18-20, 22
cross-linked C-telopeptide (ICTP)	soft tissue	16-17
Collagen type II degradation		
crosslinked C telopeptide (CTx-II; 2B4 epitope)	cartilage	24-27, 30-31
Collagenase cleavage neoepitope (9A4 epitope, Col2-3/4C)	cartilage	32-35
Pyridinolines		
hydroxylysylpyridinoline (HP, PYR)	bone, cartilage	29, 38-39
lysylpyridinoline (LP, DPD)	bone	29, 39
glucosylgalactosyl-hydroxypyridinoline (GGHP)	synovium	26, 40
Proteoglycans and GAGs		
Aggrecan core protein (fragments)	cartilage	11
Keratan sulfate (epitopes 5-D-4, AN9P1)	cartilage	29, 35, 39, 43-47
Chondroitin sulfate	cartilage	11
Miscellaneous		
Matrix metalloproteinases	cartilage, synovium	26, 71, 73-77
Aggrecanases	cartilage	52-56
Cartilage oligomeric matrix protein (COMP)	cartilage, synovium	12, 62-72
Bone sialoprotein (BSP)	bone	10, 39

OA patients, CTx-II levels correlated with radiologic joint space narrowing and joint surface area, but did not correlate with WOMAC indices of clinical status in these OA patients.[12] In RA patients, increased baseline CTx-II levels were associated with progression of joint damage, which was independent of baseline damage, treatment, and disease activity.[26]

In an attempt to repair tissue damage, collagen synthesis is increased in OA cartilage, leading to increased tissue levels of the C-terminal propeptide of type II collagen (PIICP, chondrocalcin).[27] The rate of PIICP release is proportional to the rate of collagen synthesis; the propeptide has a half-life of approximately 18 hours.[27] Synovial fluid levels are also increased and correlate with OA severity and body mass index.[28] Surprisingly, PIICP levels were lower in serum of OA patients than in that of healthy controls.[29] Similarly, the serum N-propeptide of collagen type IIA (PIIANP), an alternative splice variant that is expressed in embryonic and osteoarthritic cartilage, is lowered in OA serum versus controls. Preliminary studies indicate that the balance between cartilage synthesis (indicated by PIIANP) and cartilage degradation (indicated by urinary CTX-II) could be used to discriminate between patients with rapid compared to slow progression.[30] In addition CTX-II can be used to monitor therapy effects: In osteoporosis patients CTX-II levels suggested that bisphosphonates attenuate not only bone degradation but also cartilage degradation.[31] These initial results hold promise that type II collagen–specific markers may actually reflect ongoing cartilage destruction, and that such markers may eventually be used in clinical practice.

Apart from telopeptide fragments, neoepitopes resulting from the cleavage of type II collagen by collagenases (MMP-1, MMP-8, and MMP-13) have been used to monitor cartilage collagen damage.[32,33] Urinary excretion of collagen fragments containing the carboxyterminal neoepitope (using antibody 9A4) was increased in OA patients compared to age-matched healthy controls.[34] In synovial fluid, levels of a similar carboxyterminal neoepitope (Col2-3/$4C_{long\ mono}$) using a different antibody were significantly higher in OA

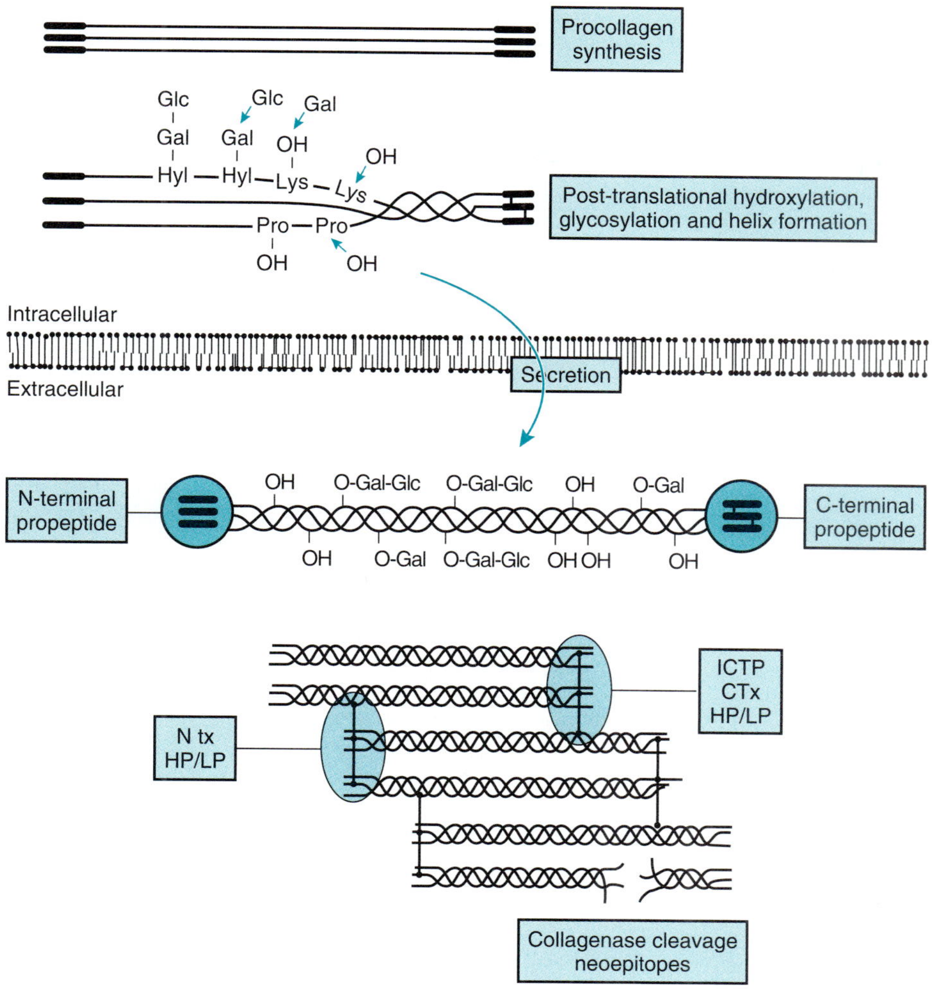

FIGURE 50–2 · Collagen-based markers for joint destruction. Collagen is synthesized as propeptide-containing α-chains that are post-translationally modified by hydroxylation of lysyl and prolyl residues and by glycosylation of hydroxylysyl residues. These modifications cease when three α-chains entwine to form a collagen triple helix. Triple-helical collagen molecules are secreted from the cell, and the propeptides are cleaved off extracellularly. Subsequently, collagen molecules spontaneously assemble into fibrils with quarter-staggered overlap of the individual triple helices. Finally, the fibrils are stabilized by formation of intermolecular pyridinoline cross-links.

than in RA.[35] These collagen-derived markers are also promising candidates to serve as biomarkers for cartilage degradation and disease progression.

In inflamed synovial tissue, the synthesis of type III collagen is upregulated, resulting in the production of its aminoterminal propeptide. In both OA and RA patients with knee involvement, serum PIIINP levels are increased compared to age-matched controls.[12,36] In RA patients, prednisolone treatment that resulted in clinical improvement also reduced serum PIIINP levels by 25 percent, and levels remained suppressed until treatment was withdrawn.[37] Thus far, collagen type III–specific degradation markers have not been described, and because type III collagen has a broad distribution in soft tissues and blood vessels, its potential as specific biomarker seems less likely.

Collagen Cross-Links

Degradation of fibrillar collagen types I, II, and III results in the quantitative excretion of the cross-links hydroxylysylpyridinoline (HP), which is derived from bone and soft tissue, including cartilage, and lysylpyridinoline (LP), derived from bone, in the urine. In RA patients who received combination therapy (sulphasalazine, methotrexate, and prednisolone in the COBRA trial), time-integrated urinary HP levels correlated with the progression of radiographic joint damage (Sharpe/van der Heide score) and bone mineral density.[38] In OA patients, both urinary HP and LP levels were increased compared to age-matched controls.[29] In the same patient population followed for 1 year, of the 14 molecular markers measured, only the cluster of baseline bone metabolism markers (HP, LP, and serum bone sialoprotein) was significantly correlated with baseline clinical scores for pain, stiffness, and disease activity.[39] None of the baseline cartilage or bone metabolism markers correlated with disease progression after 1 year of follow-up.[39] In these patients, HP that is not derived from bone (extraosseous HP) showed a highly significant correlation with the acute-phase response, suggesting that in OA, cartilage degradation is related to the degree of inflammation.[29]

The glycosylated analogue of HP, glucosyl-galactosyl-pyridinoline (GGHP), is present in human synovial tissue and is released during its degradation in vitro. GGHP is virtually absent in bone, whereas low levels have been detected in muscle and liver and intermediate levels in cartilage. Methodologic problems, such as the stability of HP during the alkaline hydrolysis needed to liberate glycosylated molecules from tissues, have so far prevented gathering of solid data on tissue distribution.[40] Urinary GGHP levels were increased in early RA patients versus controls, and baseline levels correlated with disease progression, albeit weakly.[26] Pending definite information on its tissue distribution, urinary GGHP might prove to be a marker for synovial tissue degradation.

Overall, collagen cross-links appear useful in measuring bone and cartilage catabolism and contribute to our understanding of the pathophysiology of OA and RA. In this respect it should be kept in mind that age-related changes in articular cartilage may significantly affect its susceptibility to proteinase-mediated degradation.[41,42] This underscores the use of proper age-matched control groups. Moreover, results obtained in studies with young animals cannot necessarily be extrapolated to the adult human situation.

Proteoglycan Markers

The main noncollagenous constituent of articular cartilage is aggrecan, a large proteoglycan composed of a core protein to which glycosaminoglycan chains (e.g., keratan sulfate [KS] and chondroitin sulfate) are attached. A variety of assays to measure aggrecan metabolism have been described, but the available information is not always consistent. Depending on the antibodies used, serum KS levels were reported to be either increased (antibody 5D4[43-45]) or decreased (antibody AN9P1[46]) in OA patients compared to controls. Additionally, previous work has suggested that serum 5D4-reactive KS levels are either similar[45] or higher in OA than in RA.[35] In a recent study the serum KS levels (antibody AN9P1) were 30-percent lower in OA patients than in age-matched controls.[29,39] For RA patients, a negative correlation between serum KS levels and inflammation has been found.[47]

The aggrecan epitope 846, which reflects the synthesis of proteoglycans in an attempt to repair, was increased in cartilage of OA patients,[48] and synovial fluid levels correlated with other markers such as artilage oligomeric matrix protein (COMP), CPII, tissue inhibitor of metalloproteinases-1 (TIMP-1), MMP-1, and MMP-3, as well as with the degree of radiologic damage.[49] However, the epitope 846 levels in serum were lower in OA patients than in healthy controls[39,50] and RA patients.[35] In the RA patients, elevated levels of epitope 846 could predict a benign course.[51] Taken together, none of the aggrecan-derived markers has shown sufficient power to discriminate between patients and controls, nor to provide consistent information that can be used in clinical studies.

The recent identification of two members of the ADAM-TS family of proteases (ADAM-TS4 and ADAM-TS5) as aggrecanases[52] supplied new tools to develop aggrecan-based markers for cartilage destruction. Antibodies directed at aggrecanase and MMP-generated neoepitopes in aggrecan core protein have been produced and applied in a variety of in vitro studies aimed at unraveling mechanisms of cartilage destruction in OA. In synovial fluid from patients suffering from a variety of joint diseases, both MMP and aggrecanase-released aggrecan fragments have been detected.[53-55] These studies have also shown that these two groups of proteases may have distinct roles in articular cartilage catabolism.[56]

Hyaluronan

The glucuronic acid chain hyaluronan (hyaluronic acid) is a constituent of both cartilage and synovium and is synthesized by many cell types. It functions as anchor for proteoglycans such as aggrecan, allowing the formation of the large aggregates responsible for the resilience of cartilage. In the synovial membrane, hyaluronan is synthesized by synovial fibroblasts and secreted into the synovial fluid to provide lubrication of the joint and, therefore, to facilitate joint movement. Synovial fluid hyaluronan levels are decreased in OA patients,[57] and may explain, in part, impaired joint function and pain. This provides the rationale for viscosupplementation therapy in OA patients, consisting of intra-articular injections with hyaluronan derivatives.

Surprisingly, elevated blood hyaluronan levels have been reported for both OA and RA patients. In RA, some studies failed to show a relationship between plasma hyaluronan levels and measures of disease activity,[58] whereas others demonstrated significant correlations between serum hyaluronan levels and a variety of measures of inflammation and destruction (e.g., CRP, ESR, Ritchie index, radiologic damage).[59] In OA patients, elevated serum hyaluronan levels correlated weakly with the degree of cartilage degeneration.[58] In addition, baseline hyaluronan levels could predict 5-year progression of OA,[60] and serum levels were shown to increase with disease severity.[61] These results suggest that an increase in circulating systemic hyaluronan levels could reflect synovial inflammation rather than cartilage destruction, thereby prompting the need for care in use of hyaluronan as joint-destruction marker.

Cartilage Oligomeric Matrix Protein

Since its discovery in the early 1990s, COMP has received much attention as a putative cartilage-destruction marker. Although its exact function is as yet unclear, COMP has been implicated in collagen fibrillogenesis. Increased COMP levels have been detected in the synovial fluid of OA patients.[62] In addition, COMP levels are increased in the serum of OA patients compared to healthy controls,[12,63] and they are associated with progression of radiographic signs of OA.[64] Interestingly, in OA, the serum COMP levels were even higher than in RA patients.[65] In early-RA patients, increased serum COMP levels were identified as a strong predictor of early large-joint destruction.[66-68] These data raised interest in the use of measurement of COMP levels as selective cartilage-destruction marker.

The expression of COMP in joint tissues other than cartilage, including synovium, tendons, ligaments, and menisci, raised concerns about its tissue specificity. Moreover, upregulation of COMP mRNA expression has been shown in murine OA, indicating that synovial fluid COMP levels may not only reflect tissue degradation, but also the rate of new synthesis.[69] The concerns about the use of COMP measurement as a specific cartilage-degradation marker are further fuelled by a recent study, which showed that the extent of synovial inflammation is one of the factors determining serum COMP levels.[70] On the other hand, other investigators did not observe a relationship between markers of inflammation and serum COMP levels (using a polyclonal antiserum that recognizes all COMP forms) in RA patients.[71] It should be noted that in this same study, COMP levels did not have any prognostic value with respect to progression of joint damage.[71] Similar to the CTx and ICTP assays for collagen degradation, the use of antibodies or antiserum recognizing different epitopes within (fragments of) the COMP molecule might explain the apparent inconsistent results in the literature.[72]

Matrix Metalloproteinases

In addition to cartilage breakdown products, metalloproteinases (MMPs and aggrecanases) and their endogenous inhibitors (TIMPs), which are involved in the pathologic degradation of joint tissues, could serve as useful markers. Data on MMP levels as predictor for the progression of joint erosion in early RA are rapidly accumulating. Serum and synovial fluid MMP-3 (stromelysin) levels are increased in RA patients compared to controls.[26,73] MMP-3 levels correlate with inflammation markers and disease activity in patients with untreated active RA,[74] as well as in early-RA patients who received nonsteroidal anti-inflammatory drugs (NSAIDs) only.[71,73] In these studies, serum MMP-3 levels were not related to radiographic progression.[71,73] Of interest, another study revealed an association between serum proMMP-3 concentrations at disease onset and progression of joint destruction, which was independent of known risk factors such as the presence of the shared epitope and serum levels of rheumatoid factor and CRP.[75] In line with these observations, MMP-1 (collagenase) levels have also been shown to indicate joint erosion independent of inflammation. In early-RA patients, there was a positive correlation between the area under the curve measurements of MMP-1 serum levels (but not the area under the curve of CRP levels) and the number of new joint erosions after 18 months of follow-up.[73] These data suggest that MMP levels, although they may be correlated with parameters of inflammation, do not reflect exactly the same pathways as do acute-phase reactants and, therefore, could provide valuable additional information on joint destruction in RA.

Extrapolated to OA, in which secondary inflammation is usually mild, this suggests that MMP levels may provide valuable predictive markers. In a cross-sectional study in OA patients, MMP-3 serum levels were, however, similar to those in healthy controls.[76] In addition, on average, the serum levels of TIMP-1 did not differ significantly between unilateral or bilateral hip OA patients and healthy controls.[77] On the other hand, within the OA group, patients with rapid disease progression (joint-space narrowing >0.6 mm/year at 1-year follow-up) had significantly lower serum TIMP-1 levels than patients with slow progression (joint-space narrowing <0.6 mm/year).[77] Apart from these, comprehensive studies for predictive MMP markers in OA are as yet not available and information about the use of MMP levels in OA is still incomplete.

Biological Markers in Synovial Tissue

Because many inflammatory arthropathies, including RA, primarily involve the synovial tissue, there has been increased interest in investigations of the pathologic changes in samples of synovial biopsies. This development has further been stimulated by technical advances, such as the advent of new methods to obtain synovial tissue specimens from both actively inflamed joints and clinically quiescent joints under local anesthesia, as well as because of the development of immunohistologic methods, in situ hybridization, quantitative polymerase chain reaction, and microarray technology. Previous work has clearly shown the relationship between the features of rheumatoid synovial tissue, on the one hand, and arthritis activity[78] and joint destruction[79] on the other (see also Chapter 65).

The importance of evaluation of synovial tissue samples has been underscored by the observation that the activity of clinical arthritis is accompanied by histologic signs of synovitis after treatment of RA patients with the monoclonal antibody Campath-1H, despite profound depletion of circulating lymphocytes.[80] Serial biopsy samples from RA patients who received either placebo or unsuccessful treatment did not reveal any synovial changes.[81,82] Thus, changes in serial biopsy samples cannot be explained by placebo effects, regression to the mean, expectation bias, or by the arthroscopy procedure itself. Rather, they reflect biological effects of the treatment.

The observation that synovial inflammation can occasionally be reduced in the absence of clinical improvement[83,84] suggests that examination of serial synovial biopsies is more sensitive to change than, for example, the ACR 20-percent criterion for clinical improvement. Consistent with this notion, another study revealed synovial changes in subjects with only a modest decrease in serum levels of acute-phase reactants.[85] Taken together, these studies suggest that analyses of serial biopsies can be used as a screening method to test new drug candidates requiring relatively small numbers of subjects. The absence of changes after treatment would suggest that the therapy is probably not effective. However, the demonstration of biological changes at the site of inflammation could provide the rationale for larger, placebo-controlled trials.

Several methodologic questions needed to be answered before this approach could be used to screen for potentially relevant effects in synovial tissue. It has been shown that biopsy samples can be acquired by both blind-needle technique and by miniarthroscopy.[86] However, miniarthroscopy has the potential of specifically selecting regions of interest, such as the cartilage-pannus junction, which reduces sampling error in serial sampling. Comparison of the features of synovial inflammation in biopsy samples from inflamed knee joints and paired inflamed small joints of RA patients revealed that inflammation in one inflamed joint is generally representative of that in other inflamed joints.[87] Therefore, it is possible to use serial samples from the same joint, selecting either large or small joints, for the evaluation of antirheumatic therapy. Sampling error can be reduced by selecting at least six biopsies from multiple regions, resulting in variance of less than 10 percent.[88] Obviously, an extensive quality-control system is required to allow reliable analysis by immunohistochemistry or real-time PCR. Finally, recent sophisticated computer systems allow reliable and efficient evaluation of the cell infiltrate and the expression of adhesion molecules, cytokines, and MMPs in the synovium.[89-91] Using this approach, successful treatment with disease-modifying antirheumatic drugs, such as gold,[92] methotrexate,[93-95] and leflunomide,[95] was shown to be associated with decreased mononuclear cell infiltration. Similarly, successful treatment of RA patients with infliximab,[96-98] etanercept,[99] and anakinra[82] results in reduced synovial inflammation. Of interest, the number of macrophages in the synovium was already significantly decreased 48 hours after initiation of infliximab treatment (Fig. 50–3). Similarly, high-dose intravenous methylprednisolone reduced expression of TNF-α in synovial biopsy samples 24 hours after treatment, a result that correlated with a clinical response to, and subsequent relapse after, methylprednisolone therapy.[100] Most of the biopsy studies have been performed in RA patients, but recent work suggests that the same approach can be used for the evaluation of novel therapies in patients with other rheumatologic diseases, such as spondylarthropathies.[101,102]

Synovial biopsy is now widely used by a limited number of centers with standardized methodology.[103] Because it can be anticipated that studies of serial synovial tissue samples will increasingly be used in multicenter studies, further standardization and validation of the methodology will be essential.

Combinations of Markers

None of the markers for OA that are currently used can successfully distinguish between patients and controls on an individual basis, although average marker levels differ between groups. Principal component analysis of 14 biochemical markers revealed that the markers segregate into five clusters: inflammation (IL-6, CRP, TNF-receptor (R)I, TNF-RII, and eosinophil cationic protein), bone (HP, LP, and BSP), cartilage synthesis (CPII, epitope 846, and hyaluronan), cartilage degradation (COMP and KS), and transforming growth factor (TGF)-a1, which is independent of all other markers.[29] The combination of

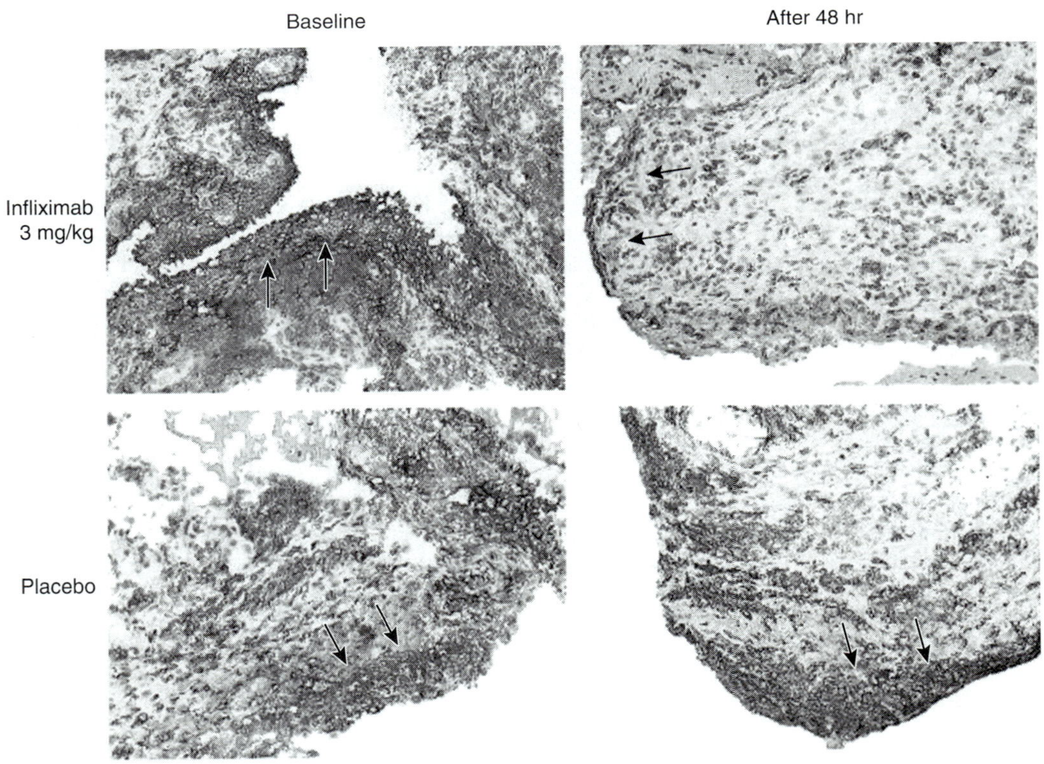

FIGURE 50–3 · Paired synovial tissue samples obtained from patients with rheumatoid arthritis before and 48 hours after initiation of infliximab or placebo treatment. Notice the marked decrease in the number of CD68+ macrophages (red-brown cells) after anti–tumor necrosis factor (TNF)-α therapy, especially in the intimal lining layer (*arrows*).

three of the markers (TNF-RII, COMP, and epitope 846) from the independent clusters inflammation, cartilage degradation, and cartilage synthesis, respectively, could correctly discriminate between OA patients and controls in approximately 90 percent of the cases.[29] Similarly, in RA, a combination of seven clinical scores and molecular markers provided a clinical prediction model that could discriminate, at the first visit, between three forms of arthritis, namely self-limiting arthritis, persistent nonerosive arthritis, and persistent erosive arthritis.[104]

The current technical progress in genomics, proteomics, and metabonomics, in combination with advanced bioinformatics[105] makes it possible to analyze a large number of markers in one sample, which could be serum, synovial fluid, or synovial tissue. The resulting profile combines the levels of a variety of markers to create a "disease fingerprint" that can serve as a powerful marker by itself. In addition to specific markers for early diagnosis, markers are needed that specifically reflect cartilage degradation. The progressive destruction of the articular cartilage is considered a major determinant of disability in patients with joint disease. A recent report showed that the balance between cartilage synthesis and degradation discriminates between OA patients with rapid versus slow progression, as assessed by the change in joint-space width and arthroscopically scored chondropathy.[106] This study using two markers supports the idea that the "-omics" approaches to combining multiple markers may not only be successful in the identification of disease-specific fingerprints, but may also provide tools to monitor tissue-specific degradation.

Conclusion

Over the years, many reports have been published that employ molecular markers in body fluids to assess inflammation and tissue destruction in joint diseases. Starting from single markers with limited tissue or disease specificity, panels of biomarkers are increasingly used, and these become more and more tissue specific. The novel markers include collagen-based markers (telopeptides, neoepitopes, and cross-links), COMP, and MMPs which are often included in clinical trials. However, apart from well-known markers such as CRP, ESR, rheumatoid factor, anticyclic citrullinated antibodies, and a few other autoantibodies, none of the markers has made it to the clinic for routine evaluation of patient disease status. The requirements for such a clinically useful marker are high, because it should be superior to existing markers in predicting disease progression or monitoring therapy efficacy in individual patients. In this respect, biomarkers for OA provide the greatest challenge, as joint destruction often proceeds without signs of inflammation. In early-RA patients, suppression of inflammation often, although not always, coincides with decreased joint destruction, and monitoring inflammation may fulfill a role as surrogate destruction marker. In later stages of the disease, when inflammation and destruction appear more uncoupled,[107] specific destruction markers are also needed for RA patients. In general, the combination of multiple markers bears most promise to meet these needs to increase disease specificity, tissue specificity, or both and to reduce the extensive overlap in marker levels that exists between patients and controls.

Moreover, analysis of molecular markers in synovial tissue is increasingly used, especially in clinical trials on targeted therapies. Obviously, tissue specificity is not a problem and examination of serial biopsy samples may be used to monitor the response in individual patients and to screen for interesting biological effects at the site of inflammation. This approach is, however, more invasive and requires a demanding setup. It can be anticipated that future development will include the use of more extensive markers of joint degradation—in addition to the available markers of inflammation—as well as the use of panels of biomarkers in synovial tissue samples.

REFERENCES

1. Biswal S, Hastie T, Andriacchi TP, et al: Risk factors for progressive cartilage loss in the knee. Arthritis Rheum 46:2884-2892, 2002.
2. Brandi ML, Gennari L, Cerinic MM, et al: Genetic markers of osteoarticular disorders: Facts and hopes. Arthritis Res 3: 270-280, 2001,
3. Williamson AA, McColl GJ: Early rheumatoid arthritis: Can we predict its outcome? Intern Med J 31:168-180, 2001.
4. Otterness IG: The value of C-reactive protein measurement in rheumatoid arthritis. Semin Arthritis Rheum 24:91-104, 1994.
5. Maini R, St Clair EW, Breedveld F, et al: Infliximab (chimeric anti-tumour necrosis factor alpha monoclonal antibody) versus placebo in rheumatoid arthritis patients receiving concomitant methotrexate: A randomised phase III trial. ATTRACT Study Group. Lancet 354:1932-1939, 1999.
6. Scott DL: Prognostic factors in early rheumatoid arthritis. Rheumatology (Oxford) 39(Suppl 1):24-29, 2000.
7. Ersoy Y, Ozerol E, Baysal O, et al: Serum nitrate and nitrite levels in patients with rheumatoid arthritis, ankylosing spondylitis, and osteoarthritis. Ann Rheum Dis 61:76-78, 2002.
8. Attur MG, Dave M, Akamatsu M, et al: Osteoarthritis or osteoarthrosis: The definition of inflammation becomes a semantic issue in the genomic era of molecular medicine. Osteoarthritis Cartilage 10:1-4, 2002.
9. Oehler S, Neureiter D, Meyer-Scholten C, et al.: Subtyping of osteoarthritic synoviopathy. Clin Exp Rheumatol 20:633-640, 2002.
10. Saxne T, Heinegard D: Matrix proteins: potentials as body fluid markers of changes in the metabolism of cartilage and bone in arthritis. J Rheumatol 43(Suppl):71-74, 1995.
11. Garnero P, Rousseau JC, Delmas PD: Molecular basis and clinical use of biochemical markers of bone, cartilage, and synovium in joint diseases. Arthritis Rheum 43:953-968, 2000.
12. Garnero P, Piperno M, Gineyts E, et al: Cross sectional evaluation of biochemical markers of bone, cartilage, and synovial tissue metabolism in patients with knee osteoarthritis: Relations with disease activity and joint damage. Ann Rheum Dis 60:619-626, 2001.
13. Kraus VB, Huebner JL, Fink C, et al: Urea as a passive transport marker for arthritis biomarker studies. Arthritis Rheum 46:420-427, 2002.
14. Myers SL, Brandt KD, Eilam O: Even low-grade synovitis significantly accelerates the clearance of protein from the canine knee: Implications for measurement of synovial fluid "markers" of osteoarthritis. Arthritis Rheum 38:1085-1091, 1995.
15. Szulc P, Delmas PD: Biochemical markers of bone turnover in men. Calcif Tissue Int 69:229-234, 2001.
16. Sassi ML, Eriksen H, Risteli L, et al: Immunochemical characterization of assay for carboxyterminal telopeptide of human type I collagen: loss of antigenicity by treatment with cathepsin K. Bone 26:367-373, 2000.

17. Jensen T, Hansen M, Madsen JC, Kollerup G, Stoltenberg M, Florescu A, Schwarz P: Serum levels of parathyroid hormone and markers of bone metabolism in patients with rheumatoid arthritis: Relationship to disease activity and glucocorticoid treatment. Scand J Clin Lab Invest 2001; 61:491-501.
18. Takahashi M, Suzuki M, Naitou K, et al: Comparison of free and peptide-bound pyridinoline cross-links excretion in rheumatoid arthritis and osteoarthritis. Rheumatology (Oxford) 38:133-138, 1999.
19. Rosenquist C, Fledelius C, Christgau S, et al: Serum CrossLaps One Step ELISA: First application of monoclonal antibodies for measurement in serum of bone-related degradation products from C-terminal telopeptides of type I collagen. Clin Chem 44:2281-2289, 1998.
20. St Clair EW, Moak SA, Wilkinson WE, et al: A cross sectional analysis of 5 different markers of collagen degradation in rheumatoid arthritis. J Rheumatol 25:1472-1479, 1998.
21. al-Awadhi AM, Olusi SO, al-Zaid NS, et al: Urine levels of type 1 collagen cross-linked N-telopeptides and deoxypyridinoline correlate with disease activity in rheumatoid arthritis. Clin Exp Rheumatol 16:569-572, 1998.
22. Seriolo B, Ferretti V, Sulli A, et al: Serum osteocalcin levels in premenopausal rheumatoid arthritis patients. Ann N Y Acad Sci 966:502-507, 2002.
23. Bank RA, Soudry M, Maroudas A, et al: The increased swelling and instantaneous deformation of osteoarthritic cartilage is highly correlated with collagen degradation. Arthritis Rheum 43:2202-2210, 2000.
24. Christgau S, Garnero P, Fledelius C, et al: Collagen type II C-telopeptide fragments as an index of cartilage degradation. Bone 29:209-215, 2001.
25. Garnero P, Christgau S, Delmas PD: The bisphosphonate zoledronate decreases type II collagen breakdown in patients with Paget's disease of bone. Bone 28:461-464, 2001.
26. Garnero P, Gineyts E, Christgau S, et al: Association of baseline levels of urinary glucosyl-galactosyl-pyridinoline and type II collagen C-telopeptide with progression of joint destruction in patients with early rheumatoid arthritis. Arthritis Rheum 46:21-30, 2002.
27. Nelson F, Dahlberg L, Laverty S, et al: Evidence for altered synthesis of type II collagen in patients with osteoarthritis. J Clin Invest 102:2115-2125, 1998.
28. Kobayashi T, Yoshihara Y, Samura A, et al: Synovial fluid concentrations of the C-propeptide of type II collagen correlate with body mass index in primary knee osteoarthritis. Ann Rheum Dis 56:500-503, 1997.
29. Otterness IG, Swindell AC, Zimmerer RO, et al: An analysis of 14 molecular markers for monitoring osteoarthritis: segregation of the markers into clusters and distinguishing osteoarthritis at baseline [In Process Citation]. Osteoarthritis Cartilage 8:180-185, 2000.
30. Garnero P, Zhu Y, Rousseau JC, et al: Prediction of osteoarthritis progression using molecular markers of cartilage metabolism [Abstract]. Trans Orthop Res Soc 27:153, 2002.
31. Lehmann HJ, Mouritzen U, Christgau S, et al: Effect of bisphosphonates on cartilage turnover assessed with a newly developed assay for collagen type II degradation products. Ann Rheum Dis 61:530-533, 2002.
32. Otterness IG, Downs JT, Lane C, et al: Detection of collagenase-induced damage of collagen by 9A4, a monoclonal C-terminal neoepitope antibody. Matrix Biol 18:331-341, 1999.
33. Billinghurst RC, Wu W, Ionescu M, et al: Comparison of the degradation of type II collagen and proteoglycan in nasal and articular cartilages induced by interleukin-1 and the selective inhibition of type II collagen cleavage by collagenase. Arthritis Rheum 43:664-672, 2000.
34. Downs JT, Lane CL, Nestor NB, et al: Analysis of collagenase-cleavage of type II collagen using a neoepitope ELISA. J Immunol Methods 247:25-34, 2001.
35. Ishiguro N, Ito T, Oguchi T, et al: Relationships of matrix metalloproteinases and their inhibitors to cartilage proteoglycan and collagen turnover and inflammation as revealed by analyses of synovial fluids from patients with rheumatoid arthritis. Arthritis Rheum 44:2503-2511, 2001.
36. Hakala M, Aman S, Luukkainen R, et al: Application of markers of collagen metabolism in serum and synovial fluid for assessment of disease process in patients with rheumatoid arthritis. Ann Rheum Dis 54:886-890, 1995.
37. Sharif M, Salisbury C, Taylor DJ, Kirwan JR: Changes in biochemical markers of joint tissue metabolism in a randomized controlled trial of glucocorticoid in early rheumatoid arthritis. Arthritis Rheum 41:1203-1209, 1998.
38. Verhoeven AC, Boers M, J.M., et al: Bone turnover, joint damage and bone mineral density in early rheumatoid arthritis treated with combination therapy including high-dose prednisolone. Rheumatology (Oxford) 40:1231-1237, 2001.
39. Otterness IG, Weiner E, Swindell AC, et al: An analysis of 14 molecular markers for monitoring osteoarthritis: Relationship of the markers to clinical end-points. Osteoarthritis Cartilage 9:224-231, 2001.
40. Gineyts E, Garnero P, Delmas PD: Urinary excretion of glucosyl-galactosyl pyridinoline: a specific biochemical marker of synovium degradation. Rheumatology (Oxford) 40:315-323, 2001.
41. DeGroot J, Verzijl N, Jacobs KM, et al: Accumulation of advanced glycation endproducts reduces chondrocyte-mediated extracellular matrix turnover in human articular cartilage. Osteoarthritis Cartilage 9:720-726, 2001.
42. DeGroot J, Verzijl N, Wenting-van Wijk MJG, et al: Age-related decrease in susceptibility of human articular cartilage to matrix metalloproteinase-mediated degradation: the role of advanced glycation end products. Arthritis Rheum 44:2562-2571, 2001.
43. Sweet MB, Coelho A, Schnitzler CM, et al: Serum keratan sulfate levels in osteoarthritis patients. Arthritis Rheum 31:648-652, 1988.
44. Campion GV, McCrae F, Schnitzer TJ, et al: Levels of keratan sulfate in the serum and synovial fluid of patients with osteoarthritis of the knee. Arthritis Rheum 34:1254-1259, 1991.
45. Mehraban F, Finegan CK, Moskowitz RW: Serum keratan sulfate: Quantitative and qualitative comparisons in inflammatory versus noninflammatory arthritides. Arthritis Rheum 34:383-392, 1991.
46. Poole AR, Ionescu M, Swan A, et al: Changes in cartilage metabolism in arthritis are reflected by altered serum and synovial fluid levels of the cartilage proteoglycan aggrecan: Implications for pathogenesis. J Clin Invest 94:25-33, 1994.
47. Poole AR, Witter J, Roberts N, et al: Inflammation and cartilage metabolism in rheumatoid arthritis: Studies of the blood markers hyaluronic acid, orosomucoid, and keratan sulfate. Arthritis Rheum 33:790-799, 1990.
48. Rizkalla G, Reiner A, Bogoch E, et al: Studies of the articular cartilage proteoglycan aggrecan in health and osteoarthritis. Evidence for molecular heterogeneity and extensive molecular changes in disease. J Clin Invest 90:2268-2277, 1992.
49. Lohmander LS, Ionescu M, Jugessur H, et al.: Changes in joint cartilage aggrecan after knee injury and in osteoarthritis. Arthritis Rheum 42:534-544, 1999.
50. Otterness IG, Saltarelli MJ: Using molecular markers to monitor osteoarthritis. (in press).
51. Mansson B, Carey D, Alini M, et al: Cartilage and bone metabolism in rheumatoid arthritis: Differences between rapid and slow progression of disease identified by serum markers of cartilage metabolism. J Clin Invest 95:1071-1077, 1995.
52. Tortorella MD, Burn TC, Pratta MA, et al: Purification and cloning of aggrecanase-1: A Member of the ADAMTS family of proteins. Science 284:1664-1666, 1999.
53. Fosang AJ, Last K, Maciewicz RA: Aggrecan is degraded by matrix metalloproteinases in human arthritis: Evidence that matrix metalloproteinase and aggrecanase activities can be independent. J Clin Invest 98:2292-2299, 1996.
54. Little CB, Hughes CE, Curtis CL, et al: Matrix metalloproteinases are involved in C-terminal and interglobular domain processing of cartilage aggrecan in late stage cartilage degradation. Matrix Biol 21:271-288, 2002.
55. Sandy JD, Flannery CR, Neame PJ, et al: The structure of aggrecan fragments in human synovial fluid. Evidence for the involvement in osteoarthritis of a novel proteinase which cleaves the Glu 373-Ala 374 bond of the interglobular domain. J Clin Invest 89:1512-1516, 1992.
56. Sandy JD, Verscharen C: Analysis of aggrecan in human knee cartilage and synovial fluid indicates that aggrecanase (ADAMTS) activity is responsible for the catabolic turnover and loss of whole aggrecan whereas other protease activity is

required for C-terminal processing in vivo. Biochem J 358:615-626, 2001.

57. Brandt KD, Smith GNJ, Simon LS: Intraarticular injection of hyaluronan as treatment for knee osteoarthritis: what is the evidence? Arthritis Rheum 43:1192-1203, 2000.
58. Goldberg RL, Huff JP, Lenz ME, et al: Elevated plasma levels of hyaluronate in patients with osteoarthritis and rheumatoid arthritis. Arthritis Rheum 34:799-807, 1991.
59. Paimela L, Heiskanen A, Kurki P, et al: Serum hyaluronate level as a predictor of radiologic progression in early rheumatoid arthritis. Arthritis Rheum 34:815-821, 1991.
60. Georges C, Vigneron H, Ayral X, et al: Serum biologic markers as predictors of disease progression in osteoarthritis of the knee [letter; comment]. Arthritis Rheum 40:590-591, 1997.
61. Sharif M, Osborne DJ, Meadows K, et al: The relevance of chondroitin and keratan sulphate markers in normal and arthritic synovial fluid. Br J Rheumatol 35:951-957, 1996.
62. Neidhart M, Hauser N, Paulsson M, et al: Small fragments of cartilage oligomeric matrix protein in synovial fluid and serum as markers for cartilage degradation. Br J Rheumatol 36:1151-1160, 1997.
63. Clark AG, Jordan JM, Vilim V, et al: Serum cartilage oligomeric matrix protein reflects osteoarthritis presence and severity. The Johnston County Osteoarthritis Project. Arthritis Rheum 42:2356-2364, 1999.
64. Vilim V, Olejarova M, Machacek S, et al: Serum levels of cartilage oligomeric matrix protein (COMP) correlate with radiographic progression of knee osteoarthritis. Osteoarthritis Cartilage 10:707-713, 2002.
65. Volck B, Johansen JS, Stoltenberg M, et al: Studies on YKL-40 in knee joints of patients with rheumatoid arthritis and osteoarthritis: Involvement of YKL-40 in the joint pathology. Osteoarthritis Cartilage 9:203-214, 2001.
66. Kuhne SA, Neidhart M, Everson MP, et al: Persistent high serum levels of cartilage oligomeric matrix protein in a subgroup of patients with traumatic knee injury. Rheumatol Int 18:21-25, 1998.
67. Mansson B, Geborek P, Saxne T: Cartilage and bone macromolecules in knee joint synovial fluid in rheumatoid arthritis: relation to development of knee or hip joint destruction. Ann Rheum Dis 56:91-96, 1997.
68. Wollheim FA, Eberhardt KB, Johnson U, Saxne T: HLA DRB1* typing and cartilage oligomeric matrix protein (COMP) as predictors of joint destruction in recent-onset rheumatoid arthritis. Br J Rheumatol 36:847-849, 1997.
69. Salminen H, Perala M, Lorenzo P, et al: Up-regulation of cartilage oligomeric matrix protein at the onset of articular cartilage degeneration in a transgenic mouse model of osteoarthritis. Arthritis Rheum 43:1742-1748, 2000.
70. Vilim V, Vytasek R, Olejarova M, et al: Serum cartilage oligomeric matrix protein reflects the presence of clinically diagnosed synovitis in patients with knee osteoarthritis. Osteoarthritis Cartilage 9:612-618, 2001.
71. Roux-Lombard P, Eberhardt K, Saxne T, et al: Cytokines, metalloproteinases, their inhibitors and cartilage oligomeric matrix protein: Relationship to radiological progression and inflammation in early rheumatoid arthritis: A prospective 5-year study. Rheumatology (Oxford) 40:544-551, 2001.
72. Vilim V, Lenz ME, Vytasek R, et al: Characterization of monoclonal antibodies recognizing different fragments of cartilage oligomeric matrix protein in human body fluids. Arch Biochem Biophys 341:8-16, 1997.
73. Cunnane G, Fitzgerald O, Beeton C, et al: Early joint erosions and serum levels of matrix metalloproteinase 1, matrix metalloproteinase 3, and tissue inhibitor of metalloproteinases 1 in rheumatoid arthritis. Arthritis Rheum 44:2263-2274, 2001.
74. Ribbens C, Andre B, Jaspar JM, et al: Matrix metalloproteinase-3 serum levels are correlated with disease activity and predict clinical response in rheumatoid arthritis. J Rheumatol 27:888-893, 2000.
75. Tchetverikov I, Lard LR, Verzijl N, et al: metalloproteinase-3, -8, -9 as markers of disease activity and joint damage progression in early rheumatoid arthritis [Abstract]. Trans Orthop Res Soc 28:15, 2003.
76. Ribbens C, Porras M, Franchimont N, et al: Increased matrix metalloproteinase-3 serum levels in rheumatic diseases: relationship with synovitis and steroid treatment. Ann Rheum Dis 61:161-166, 2002.
77. Chevalier X, Conrozier T, Gehrmann M, et al: Tissue inhibitor of metalloprotease-1 (TIMP-1) serum level may predict progression of hip osteoarthritis. Osteoarthritis Cartilage 9:300-307, 2001.
78. Tak PP, Smeets TJ, Daha MR, et al: Analysis of the synovial cell infiltrate in early rheumatoid synovial tissue in relation to local disease activity. Arthritis Rheum 40:217-225, 1997.
79. Cunnane G, Fitzgerald O, Hummel KM, et al: Synovial tissue protease gene expression and joint erosions in early rheumatoid arthritis. Arthritis Rheum 44:1744-1753, 2001.
80. Ruderman EM, Weinblatt ME, Thurmond LM, et al: Synovial tissue response to treatment with Campath-1H. Arthritis Rheum 38:254-258, 1995.
81. Smeets TJ, Kraan MC, Versendaal J, et al: Analysis of serial synovial biopsies in patients with rheumatoid arthritis: Description of a control group without clinical improvement after treatment with interleukin 10 or placebo. J Rheumatol 26:2089-2093, 1999.
82. Cunnane G, Madigan A, Murphy E, et al: The effects of treatment with interleukin-1 receptor antagonist on the inflamed synovial membrane in rheumatoid arthritis. Rheumatology (Oxford) 40:62-69, 2001.
83. Tak PP, van der Lubbe PA, Cauli A, et al: Reduction of synovial inflammation after anti-CD4 monoclonal antibody treatment in early rheumatoid arthritis. Arthritis Rheum 38:1457-1465, 1995.
84. Smeets TJ, Dayer JM, Kraan MC, et al: The effects of interferon-beta treatment of synovial inflammation and expression of metalloproteinases in patients with rheumatoid arthritis. Arthritis Rheum 43:270-274, 2000.
85. Youssef PP, Smeets TJ, Bresnihan B, et al: Microscopic measurement of cellular infiltration in the rheumatoid arthritis synovial membrane: A comparison of semiquantitative and quantitative analysis. Br J Rheumatol 37:1003-1007, 1998.
86. Youssef PP, Kraan M, Breedveld F, et al: Quantitative microscopic analysis of inflammation in rheumatoid arthritis synovial membrane samples selected at arthroscopy compared with samples obtained blindly by needle biopsy. Arthritis Rheum 41: 663-669, 1998.
87. Kraan MC, Reece RJ, Smeets TJ, et al: Comparison of synovial tissues from the knee joints and the small joints of rheumatoid arthritis patients: Implications for pathogenesis and evaluation of treatment. Arthritis Rheum 46:2034-2038, 2002.
88. Dolhain RJ, Ter Haar NT, De Kuiper R, et al Distribution of T cells and signs of T-cell activation in the rheumatoid joint: Implications for semiquantitative comparative histology. Br J Rheumatol 37:324-330, 1998.
89. Kraan MC, Smith MD, Weedon H, et al: Measurement of cytokine and adhesion molecule expression in synovial tissue by digital image analysis. Ann Rheum Dis 60:296-298, 2001.
90. Kraan MC, Haringman JJ, Ahern MJ, et al: Quantification of the cell infiltrate in synovial tissue by digital image analysis. Rheumatology (Oxford) 39:43-49, 2000.
91. Youssef PP, Triantafillou S, Parker A, et al: Variability in cytokine and cell adhesion molecule staining in arthroscopic synovial biopsies: quantification using color video image analysis. J Rheumatol 24:2291-2298, 1997.
92. Rooney M, Whelan A, Feighery C, Bresnihan B: Changes in lymphocyte infiltration of the synovial membrane and the clinical course of rheumatoid arthritis. Arthritis Rheum 32:361-369, 1989.
93. Firestein GS, Paine MM, Boyle DL: Mechanisms of methotrexate action in rheumatoid arthritis: Selective decrease in synovial collagenase gene expression. Arthritis Rheum 37:193-200, 1994.
94. Dolhain RJ, Tak PP, Dijkmans BA, et al: Methotrexate reduces inflammatory cell numbers, expression of monokines and of adhesion molecules in synovial tissue of patients with rheumatoid arthritis. Br J Rheumatol 137:502-508, 1998.
95. Kraan MC, Reece RJ, Barg EC, et al: Modulation of inflammation and metalloproteinase expression in synovial tissue by leflunomide and methotrexate in patients with active rheumatoid arthritis: Findings in a prospective, randomized, double-blind, parallel-design clinical trial in thirty-nine patients at two centers. Arthritis Rheum 43:1820-1830, 2000.
96. Tak PP, Taylor PC, Breedveld FC, et al: Decrease in cellularity and expression of adhesion molecules by anti-tumor necrosis factor alpha monoclonal antibody treatment in patients with rheumatoid arthritis. Arthritis Rheum 39:1077-1081, 1996.

97. Taylor PC, Peters AM, Paleolog E, et al: Reduction of chemokine levels and leukocyte traffic to joints by tumor necrosis factor alpha blockade in patients with rheumatoid arthritis. Arthritis Rheum 43:38-47, 2000.
98. Ulfgren AK, Andersson U, Engstrom M, et al: Systemic anti-tumor necrosis factor alpha therapy in rheumatoid arthritis down-regulates synovial tumor necrosis factor alpha synthesis. Arthritis Rheum 43:2391-2396, 2000.
99. Verschueren PC, Markusse HM, Smeets TJ, et al: Reduced cellularity and expression of adhesion molecules and cytokines after treatment with soluble human recombinant TNF receptor (P75) in rheumatoid arthritis patients [Abstract]. Arthritis Rheum 42:Σ197, 1999.
100. Youssef PP, Haynes DR, Triantafillou S, et al: Effects of pulse methylprednisolone on inflammatory mediators in peripheral blood, synovial fluid, and synovial membrane in rheumatoid arthritis. Arthritis Rheum 40:1400-1408, 1997.
101. Baeten D, Kruithof E, Van den BF, et al: Immunomodulatory effects of anti-tumor necrosis factor alpha therapy on synovium in spondylarthropathy: Histologic findings in eight patients from an open-label pilot study. Arthritis Rheum 44:186-195, 2001.
102. Kraan MC, Van Kuijk AW, Dinant HJ, et al: Alefacept treatment in psoriatic arthritis: Reduction of the effector T cell population in peripheral blood and synovial tissue is associated with improvement of clinical signs of arthritis. Arthritis Rheum 46:2776-2784, 2002.
103. Bresnihan B, Tak PP, Emery P, et al: Synovial biopsy in arthritis research: five years of concerted European collaboration. Ann Rheum Dis 59:506-511, 2000.
104. Visser H, le Cessie S, Vos K, et al: How to diagnose rheumatoid arthritis early: a prediction model for persistent (erosive) arthritis. Arthritis Rheum 46:357-365, 2002.
105. McDonald WH, Yates JR III: Shotgun proteomics and biomarker discovery. Dis Markers 18:99-105, 2002.
106. Garnero P, Ayral X, Rousseau JC, et al: Uncoupling of type II collagen synthesis and degradation predicts progression of joint damage in patients with knee osteoarthritis. Arthritis Rheum 46:2613-2624, 2002.
107. Vandenberg WB: Joint inflammation and cartilage destruction may occur uncoupled. Springer Semin Immunopathol 20:149-164, 1998.

51 Imaging

LEYLA ALPARSLAN • JOSEPH S. YU • BARBARA N. WEISSMAN

In recent years, imaging techniques available for use in evaluation of rheumatologic diseases have greatly expanded beyond the conventional radiographic studies. In this chapter an introduction to the general principles of various imaging modalities is provided to emphasize the strengths and weaknesses of each of these techniques and their musculoskeletal applications. Characteristic imaging findings of several arthritic diseases and related conditions are then discussed by integrating the findings of conventional radiography with those of more advanced imaging techniques such as magnetic resonance imaging (MRI), computed tomography (CT), ultrasound, and scintigraphy.

Overview of Imaging Modalities

CONVENTIONAL RADIOGRAPHY

Conventional radiographic examination is traditionally the first step in the radiologic evaluation of patients with suspected arthritis. Apart from its role in diagnosing and confirming the presence of arthritis, conventional radiography has also been used for monitoring the progression of the disease and the efficacy of treatment. Assessment of radiographic changes in rheumatoid arthritis (RA), using several scoring methods, is one of the pivotal measures in clinical trials. However, conventional radiography has major deficiencies in imaging arthritis. Its poor sensitivity to soft tissue contrast does not allow direct visualization of inflamed synovial tissues, articular cartilage, bone marrow edema, menisci, ligaments, and periarticular tendons. Conventional radiography can only detect the osseous erosions and joint-space narrowing that are the late irreversible sequela of preceding synovitis. It provides limited information about disease activity. Despite its limitations, conventional radiography is inexpensive and universally available, and remains the mainstay in the basic imaging of arthritis.

ARTHROGRAPHY

In arthrography, radiopaque contrast material is injected into the joint, occasionally with air (double-contrast arthrography), to delineate the intra-articular structures and joint capsule. In the past, arthrography has been frequently used to evaluate injuries of the articular cartilage, menisci, ligaments, and rotator cuff, and to investigate monoarticular arthritis (Fig. 51–1). However, recently these procedures have been replaced by other imaging modalities, particularly MRI.

The primary indication for an aspiration arthrogram is the diagnosis of a septic joint. Aspiration arthrography is also helpful in the evaluation of patients with painful joint arthroplasty to differentiate between infection and aseptic loosening of the prosthesis.

Among other uses of arthrography is diagnosis and treatment of adhesive capsulitis. Joint distention during arthrography, the "brisement procedure" may aid in the treatment of this condition.[1] Corticosteroid or long-acting anesthetic may be injected into the joints to provide pain relief.

Arthrography combined with MRI can provide better visualization of loose bodies, fibrocartilaginous and labrocapsular abnormalities, and osteochondral lesions.

COMPUTED TOMOGRAPHY

Technical Considerations

Since its development in the early 1970s, CT has had wide applications in almost all the subspecialties of radiology and has effectively replaced conventional tomography.

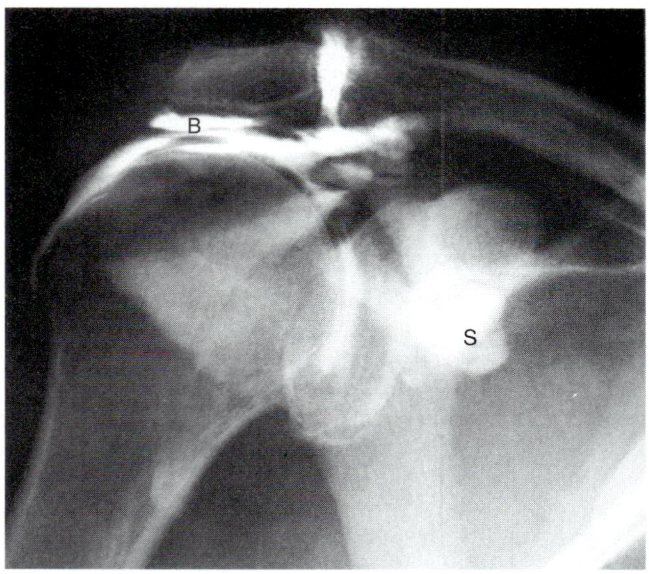

FIGURE 51–1 · Rotator Cuff Tear Demonstrated on Single-Contrast Arthrography. Anteroposterior radiographs after injection of iodinated contrast material into the joint shows filling of the normal shoulder joint and subscapularis recess (S). The contrast has filled the subacromial-subdeltoid bursa (B) indicating a full-thickness rotator cuff tear and has also extended into the acromioclavicular (AC) joint. The AC joint distention may be palpable.

In CT, a collimated x-ray beam is passed through the body from multiple directions, and the exiting attenuated x-ray is measured by detectors.

The data obtained from the detectors with each set of exposures are transferred to the computer for image reconstruction.[2] With few exceptions, CT is generally performed in the axial plane. It is possible, however, to reformat images in other planes.

The CT images are formed in arrays of individual picture elements (pixels), each of which is assigned a CT number known as a Hounsfield unit (HU). These attenuation values are expressed on an arbitrary scale with water density being 0 HU, bone density being +1000 HU, and air density being −1000 HU. To optimally visualize a specific tissue, the range and level of densities to be displayed can be adjusted on monitors. Accordingly, for musculoskeletal scans, the images are reviewed in bone and soft tissue settings.

There are two methods of CT scanning: conventional (nonspiral) and volumetric (spiral or helical) acquisition. In conventional CT systems, the images are acquired sequentially with a delay of a few seconds between each exposure. In spiral (helical) CT scans, the data are collected continuously. Thus, once a volume of data is acquired with spiral CT, images can be reconstructed at any desired increments from this volumetric dataset. The advantages of spiral CT are significant reduction of scan time, contiguous slices eliminating gaps from respiratory misregistration, and superior multiplanar reformation.[3] More recently, the introduction of multidetector (multislice) spiral CT technology has led to even faster and better-quality images with high spatial resolution (Fig. 51–2). In these new scanners, the data are collected with two or more parallel arcs of detectors that enable the coverage of long anatomic segments within seconds. Multidetector CT scanning also improves the imaging of obese patients and patients with metal hardware.[4,5]

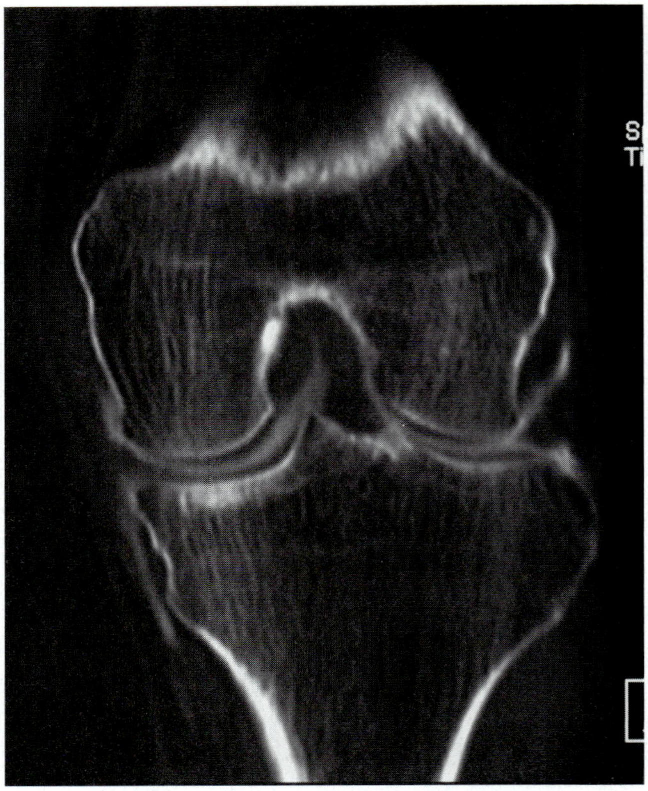

FIGURE 51–2 · Coronal reformatted image of the knee acquired by multidetector CT following intraarticular injection of iodinated contrast. Excellent spatial resolution can be achieved with multidetector CT for reformatted images by using submillimeter reconstruction increments.

Clinical Application

The main advantages of CT scanning over conventional radiography are greater contrast resolution, cross-sectional display of the acquired images, and the capability of reformatting images in different planes.

The tomographic nature of CT allows better visualization of the joints that have complex anatomy and those obscured by overlying structures such as sacroiliac, subtalar, and sternoclavicular joints.

The role of CT in evaluation of sacroiliac joint disorders has been investigated in several studies. CT images of sacroiliac joints are generally considered to be more consistently interpretable and sensitive for early pathologic changes than conventional radiography.[6-9] CT can also provide guidance for aspiration of the sacroiliac joints and intra-articular injection of corticosteroids.

Although CT offers high contrast between bone and adjacent soft tissues and is excellent for evaluation of osseous structures and calcification, its sensitivity for soft tissue contrast is relatively poor and insufficient to visualize intra-articular structures. The limited contrast resolution of CT for evaluation of articular cartilage, synovial tissue, and ligaments can be overcome to some extent by injection of iodine-containing contrast, air, or both into the joint (CT arthrography). In recent studies, it has been reported that dual-detector spiral CT arthrography of the knee enables accurate detection of meniscal tears and open cartilage lesions.[10,11]

Another application of CT in rheumatologic imaging is preoperative evaluation of arthritic patients who are candidates for various surgical procedures.[12] In surgical planning of total shoulder and hip arthroplasties, CT can be used in assessment of the glenoid body angle, bone stock, and acetabular protrusio. CT is also helpful in evaluation of many congenital diseases including tarsal coalition, patellar tracking abnormalities, femoral anteversion, and tibial torsion.

MAGNETIC RESONANCE IMAGING

MRI produces high-quality tomographic images of the body in any plane by portraying the distribution of hydrogen nuclei within the tissue imaged. MRI does not involve ionizing radiation; it uses radiofrequency (RF) pulses and a strong magnetic field to create images. When the patient is placed in a strong magnetic field, the hydrogen nuclei (protons) in the body align with the axis of the external magnetic field. RF pulses are then applied to change the orientation of aligned protons. After the cessation of the RF pulses, the excited protons relax and return to their initial state by emitting electromagnetic energy. It is the emitted electromagnetic energy that is detected, localized by, and ultimately converted into the MRI image.[13,14]

The MRI signal intensity (brightness) of a particular tissue is dependent on the number of the mobile hydrogen nuclei and also on two relaxation times: T1 and T2.

Tissues or materials with low proton density such as calcium, air, cortical bone, tendons, menisci, and ligaments exhibit low or no signal intensity in all pulse sequences. Fat, fluid, and edematous tissues containing high proton density show a variable appearance, depending on the pulse sequence.[13]

Relaxation time refers to the time required for tissue magnetization to return to equilibrium conditions after the RF pulse is turned off. T1 relaxation time represents the time the hydrogen protons take to return to the axis of the external magnetic field; T2 relaxation time depends on the time the protons take to dephase. T1 and T2 values, expressed in milliseconds, are constant for a particular type of tissue.

An MRI is said to be "T1-weighted" if image contrast is based on T1 differences between tissues. Similarly, image contrast on a T2-weighted image is based on different T2 relaxation times of tissues.[15]

The type of MRI is determined by altering 1) the repetition time (TR), the time that elapses between applying sequential RF pulses to the patient; or 2) the echo time (TE), the time interval between the incident RF pulse and when the signal is recorded. A T1-weighted imaging sequence uses short TR and TE, and T2-weighted images are produced with long TR and TE. A third type of image is a proton density (PD) or intermediate-weighted image with long TR and short TE.

A typical MRI examination includes series of different types of imaging sequences; T1- and PD-weighted images provide anatomic information, and T2-weighted and inversion-recovery images are sensitive to fluid, and therefore to pathologic processes.

Although MRI provides great inherent soft tissue contrast, intravenous contrast agents may be used to further enhance the contrast difference between normal and pathologic or vascular tissues. The most widely used agents are gadolinium compounds, which have a T1-shortening effect on nearby water protons. This results in increased signal intensity on T1-weighted images.[16] Its uptake depends on tissue vascularity and capillary permeability. Gadolinium is also used in dilute solution as an MRI arthrographic contrast agent, although it has not been approved by the Food and Drug Administration (FDA) for this use.

Clinical Application

MRI is the only available imaging modality that can directly display the osseous, cartilaginous, and soft tissue components of the joint simultaneously. This uniqueness of MRI derives from its excellent soft tissue contrast. In the past decade, application of MRI in the assessment of arthritis has rapidly increased both in clinical practice and research. A number of factors have contributed to this, including better access to scanners, improved resolution of scanners and development of new MRI sequences for evaluating different tissues.[17]

MRI offers several distinct advantages over both conventional radiography and clinical examination in evaluating early RA. MRI is capable of demonstrating inflammatory synovitis with or without contrast enhancement (Fig. 51–3). MRI detects bone erosions in early RA before they appear on plain radiographs. Bone marrow edema is another important MRI finding associated with inflammatory arthritis and is thought to be a forerunner of erosion. This valuable information provided by MRI may be used to improve diagnostic accuracy, predict prognosis, and monitor the effectiveness of therapies in clinical practice.[18-20]

In the near future, MRI is likely to play a major role as a prognostic marker and also as an outcome measure in the management of RA. However to achieve these goals, further development is required in terms of longitudinal studies and standardization of MRI scanning protocols, nomenclature, and scoring systems to make them reproducible and reliable.[21]

In addition to the potential applications of MRI mentioned previously, the most widely accepted, practical application of MRI in inflammatory arthritis is in evaluation of some of the complications that may arise because of the disease or its treatment, such as tendon tears, insufficiency fractures, osteonecrosis, and brain stem and spinal cord compression (Fig. 51–4).

At present, the main drawbacks of MRI are its high cost and limited availability.

MRI requires a longer scan time, as compared to most of the other imaging modalities. The patients have to stay still during the scanning procedure, because motion often degrades the image. MRI is contraindicated in patients with cardiac pacemakers, certain types of aneurysm clips, cochlear implants, and intraocular metallic foreign bodies among others.

ULTRASOUND (US)

Technical Considerations

Ultrasound imaging is based on detection and display of sound waves reflected from various interfaces within the body. Sound waves are produced and transmitted by transducers, which convert electric energy to sound energy. The transducers are also receivers. Returning ultrasound signals are displayed in grayscale; images are produced in a black-and-white format, and each gray dot represents a reflected sound wave of a particular intensity.

Transducers are described in megahertz (MHz) indicating their sound wave frequencies. High-resolution linear transducers are best applied to musculoskeletal examination. Superficial structures are imaged with 7.5- to 15-MHz transducers, whereas deeper structures, such as the hip joint, require low-frequency transducers.[22]

Doppler ultrasound is a technique developed for evaluation of blood flow. Doppler information can be displayed as color maps simultaneously with standard ultrasound image. Power Doppler ultrasound is a recent development in Doppler imaging that offers greater sensitivity for detection of low-velocity blood

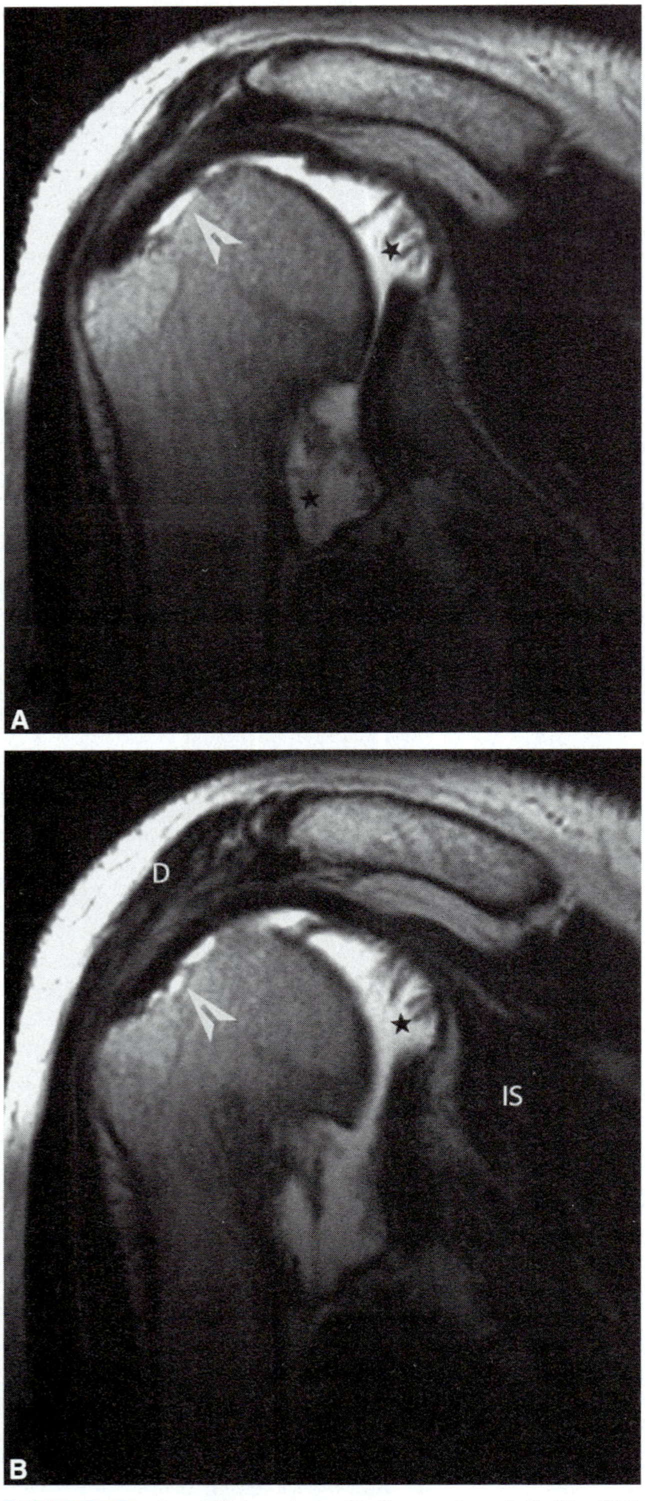

FIGURE 51–3 · MR Imaging of Inflammatory Arthritis. Oblique coronal FSE proton density images *(A,B)* from an MR-shoulder arthrogram of a patient with ankylosing spondylitis shows frond-like synovitis (stars). Erosions (arrow heads) at the superior aspect of the humeral head give the appearance of hatchet deformity. There is thinning/partial tear of the rotator cuff without evidence of full thickness tear. The infraspinatus (IS) and deltoid (D) muscles are atrophic.

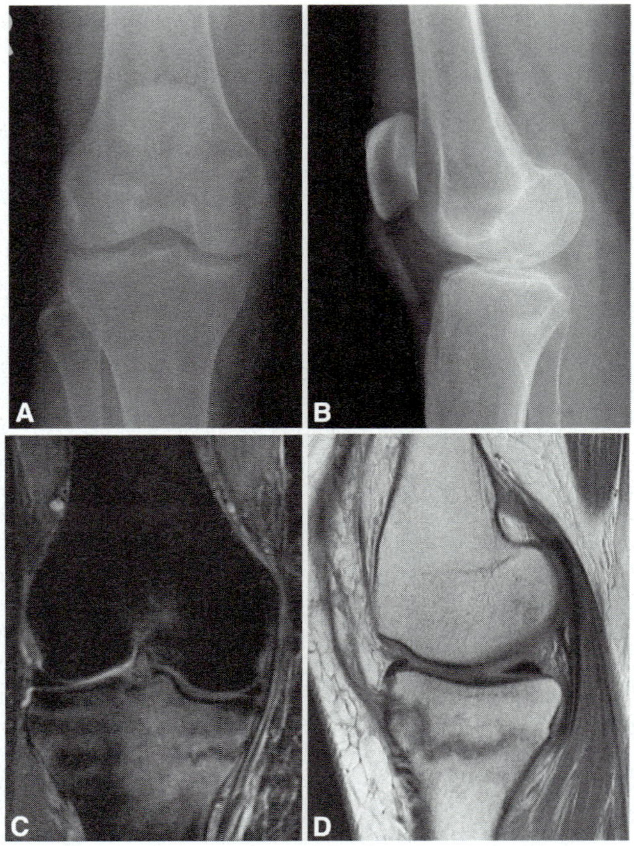

FIGURE 51–4 · Imaging Occult Insufficiency Fractures with MRI. AP *(A)* and Lateral *(B)* radiographs of a patient with rheumatoid arthritis show no visible fracture. Coronal STIR (short tay inversion recovery) *(C)* and sagittal proton density FSE MR images show a linear area of low signal in the medial tibial condyle, indicating a fracture. The surrounding bone marrow edema is evident as diffuse increased signal on the STIR image (c).

flow and small vessels than conventional color Doppler ultrasound.[23,24] The addition of microbubble-based US contrast agents increases Doppler signal intensity and improves the detection of low-volume and low-velocity blood flow, as well as deeply located vessels.[25]

Clinical Application

Recent developments in ultrasound technology have expanded the application of ultrasound in the musculoskeletal system. Introduction of high-resolution linear transducers has allowed excellent panoramic imaging of tendons, muscles, and vessels. Three-dimensional imaging permits multiplanar reformatting, enabling visualization of the optimal image plane, which may or may not be directly accessible.[26,27]

Advantages of ultrasound include its noninvasiveness, portability, relative low cost, and lack of ionizing radiation. The major weakness of ultrasound is that the ultrasound waves cannot penetrate bones; for this reason, the bones and structures deep to bones are obscured. Likewise, evaluation of intra-articular structures is limited, depending on their accessibility by the sonographic beam; only portions of articular cartilage, synovial tissue, and intra-articular ligaments can be examined.

One of the more widely accepted applications of musculoskeletal ultrasound is evaluation of rotator cuff tears. Any tendon that is located in a site accessible by the ultrasound beam can be examined for tear, tenosynovitis, and subluxation or dislocation. The real-time capability of ultrasound permits dynamic evaluation of tendons.

Because fluid is a good conductor of sound, fluid collections such as Baker's cysts, bursitis, and ganglions can be readily identified by ultrasound. Ultrasound can also provide easy guidance for aspiration, biopsy, and intra-articular anesthetic or steroid injections.

Potential applications of ultrasound in the evaluation of RA are under investigation. Preliminary data have suggested that Doppler ultrasound with or without contrast agent is a potential method for assessing the activity of synovitis in RA by measuring alterations in the vascularity of the synovial membrane.[28-31] Also, in recent studies, the diagnostic efficacy of high-resolution ultrasound for detecting osseous erosions of small joints in early RA has been reported.[32,33]

RADIONUCLIDE SCINTIGRAPHY

Unlike other imaging modalities, nuclear medicine imaging provides physiologic and metabolic information about the tissues using gamma ray–emitting radioisotopes. Scintigraphic images are obtained by mapping the spatial distribution and concentration of radioisotopes administered into the body. Scintigraphy tends to produce images with less detail and more noise than other modalities. This is due to the relatively few photons used to generate scintigraphic images. Conven-tional scintigraphic images are projectional and subject to superimposition. Single photon–emission computed tomography (SPECT), a tomographic technique analogous to that of CT and performed with a rotating camera, provides better lesion localization because of its ability to separate normal overlying activity from target activity.

The most commonly used compounds in imaging of bone disorders and articular disease are 99mTc-methylene diphosphonate (99mTc-MDP) and hydroxymethylene diphosphonate (HDP). Although the exact mechanism of uptake of the radiolabeled diphosphonates is not well understood, it has been suggested that these compounds label bone by adsorption to the hydroxyapatite crystal. The amount of tracer uptake depends on both local osteoblastic activity and blood flow. 99mTc-MDP scintigraphy is highly sensitive for changes in physiology, but the information provided is relatively nonspecific. A large variety of bone disorders, such as infection, arthritis, neoplasms, and trauma, lead to increased bone metabolism and elevated blood flow with resultant increased uptake. Therefore, a positive bone scan finding requires close correlation with other imaging modalities and clinical information to establish a correct diagnosis.

The other radiotracers used as markers of inflammatory processes are gallium 67 citrate and 111 indium chloride. These radiotracers are iron analogues and attach to iron-carrying proteins, particularly transferrin. The tracer deposition at sites of inflammation may occur by several mechanisms, including passage of the tracer through leaky capillaries and binding to transferrin receptors of dendritic and T cells in inflammatory arthritis. The suboptimal physical characteristics and high radiation dose are major drawbacks of these radiotracers.[13,34]

Clinical Application

The role of scintigraphy in the evaluation of arthritides has been limited. Scintigraphy with 99mTc-diphosphonates appears to be a more sensitive method for detecting inflammatory joint disease than conventional radiographs. A negative bone scintigraphy accurately excludes active arthritis in patients with persistent polyarthralgia. In addition, scintigraphy is a convenient way of surveying the entire skeleton for the extent and distribution of the arthritic involvement. Its major disadvantages are that 99mTc-MDP bone scan remains positive for a long time after synovitis subsides, and the information it provides is nonspecific.[35]

Several new scintigraphic techniques such as radiolabeled cell determinant 4 (CD4), E-selectin antibodies, cytokines, and somatostatin receptor imaging, and 99mTc–immunoglobulin G (IgG) scintigraphy are under investigation for assessment of disease activity in arthritis. It has been reported that compared to conventional bone scan, 99mTc-IgG scintigraphy is a more specific method of detecting synovitis activity and differentiating between the various degrees of activity in RA.[36,37]

Bone scan has been widely used for assessment of insufficiency fractures and avascular necrosis associated with arthritides; however, MRI has been shown to be a more sensitive and specific modality in detecting these complications.[38]

Conditions Primarily Affecting Peripheral Joints

INFLAMMATORY CONDITIONS

Rheumatoid Arthritis

General Imaging Features

Symmetry

The hallmark of RA is the symmetric involvement of synovial joints.

Osteoporosis

Osteoporosis is a characteristic feature of RA. Early in the course of the disease, it tends to be localized to the juxtaarticular region of the small peripheral joints. Later, generalized osteoporosis may be present in the axial and appendicular skeleton, often exacerbated by medications (e.g., steroids) and disuse.

Soft Tissue Changes

One of the earliest radiographic changes seen in the hands and feet is symmetrical soft tissue swelling around the joints involved. Soft tissue swelling is caused by a summation of joint effusion, synovial proliferation, and periarticular soft tissue edema. Occasionally, joint effusion and edema may produce transient subtle joint-space widening in the small joints of the hand early in the course of the disease.[39] Displacement of the fat pads in the elbow, knee, and ankle is an indirect sign of the presence of joint distension on radiographs. Swelling the around the joints may also occur as a result of bursitis or tenosynovitis and is usually eccentric.

Rheumatoid nodules appear as noncalcified, eccentric, lobular subcutaneous masses on radiographs (Fig. 51–5). Typical locations include olecranon, heel, Achilles tendon region, and areas about the femoral trochanters and ischial tuberosities—sites that are subjected to pressure. On MRI, they exhibit low signal on T1-weighted and heterogenous low and high signal intensity on T2-weighted images.[40]

Bony Erosions

Erosive changes indicate the aggressiveness of the arthritis. Erosions appear first in the "bare areas" of the joints where the articular cartilage is absent or thinnest. These marginal erosions may be very subtle and first appear as disruption of the white cortical line, especially at the radial aspect of the metacarpal heads under the collateral ligaments. In addition to marginal erosions, two other types of erosions have been described in RA.

Compressive erosions describes remodeling of osteoporotic bone with gradual invagination of one bone into another or the effect of muscular forces acting on osteoporotic bone. The most characteristic site of compressive erosion is the hip, where protrusio acetabuli may be identified. Other sites are at the metacarpophalangeal joints, where chronic subluxation leads to remodeling of the base of a proximal phalanx by the adjacent metacarpal head.

The third type of erosion seen in RA is surface resorption, usually due to inflammation of an adjacent tendon sheath. The typical location of this kind of erosion is at the outer margin of the ulnar styloid process due to extensor carpi ulnaris tenosynovitis.[41]

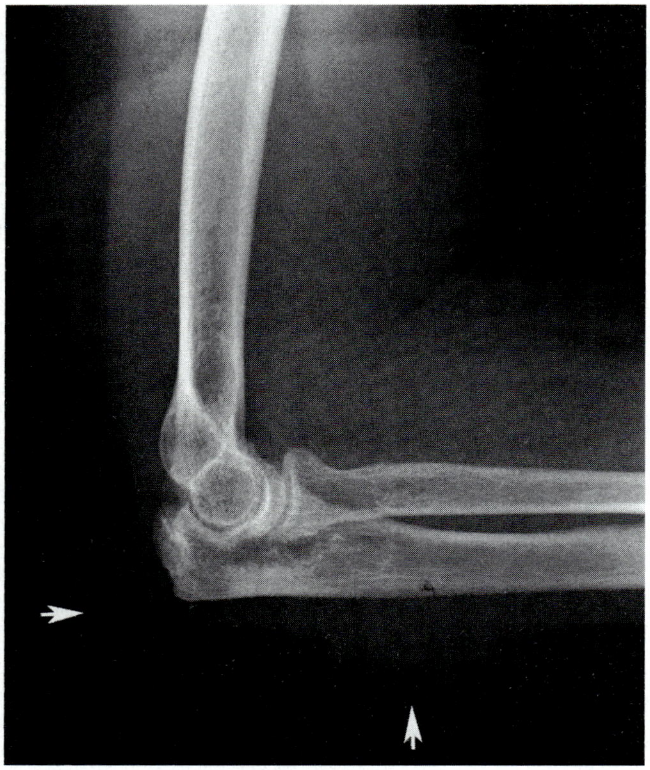

FIGURE 51–5 · Rheumatoid nodules appearing as lobulated subcutaneous soft tissue swellings *(arrows)* at the extensor surface of the elbow and forearm.

Joint-Space Narrowing

Progressive destruction of articular cartilage leads to joint-space narrowing. Joint-space narrowing in RA tends to be diffuse, and this feature may allow differentiation from the focal or asymmetric type of joint-space loss that occurs in osteoarthritis (OA). With continuing cartilage damage, the joint space may become partially or completely obliterated by fibrous ankylosis. In end-stage disease bony ankylosis may eventually develop, characteristically in the wrist and midfoot.

Bone Cysts

Subchondral cysts are almost invariably described as radiographic features of RA. These subchondral radiolucent areas are referred to as cysts, geodes, or pseudocysts. They may develop as a result of intraosseous extension of pannus, nutritional, and metabolic injury to the bone or true intraosseous rheumatoid nodules. Mechanical factors may also accentuate the development of cystic lesions. A cystic pattern of RA has been described in the hands and wrists of patients who maintain high physical activity and is termed RA of robust reaction type.[42]

Occasionally, very large cystic lesions may be encountered in the elbow (olecranon process of ulna, distal humerus), femoral neck, or knee (distal femur, proximal tibia, patella) and have been described as pseudocystic RA. These large cysts may lead to pathologic fractures.

Deformities and Instabilities

Joint malalignment and deformities are due to capsular, ligamentous, and tendinous laxity and disruption, and associated muscular contraction. The deformities are most characteristic in the wrist, the metacarpophalangeal, metatarsophalangeal, interphalangeal joints of the hand and foot, and the atlantoaxial region. The cartilage and bone loss may also lead to deformity such as is seen in protrusio acetabuli. Malalignments may be reduced when positioning for the radiographs.

Abnormalities in Specific Sites

Hand and Wrist

The usual sites of involvement in the hands are the metacarpophalangeal and proximal interphalangeal joints. The early changes consist of fusiform soft tissue swelling, juxta-articular osteoporosis, diffuse joint-space loss, and marginal erosions. These changes tend to be bilaterally symmetric in involved joints. Cartilage loss may occur without bone erosions. With progression of the disease, large erosions and complete obliteration of joint spaces appear. Finger deformities such as swan neck and boutonnière deformities and ulnar deviation at the metacarpophalangeal joints are common findings (Fig. 51–6). In the end stage of the disease, fibrous ankylosis may occur in the affected joints of the hand, and eventually arthritis mutilans may develop.

RA involves all the compartments of the wrist, with relative sparing of first carpometacarpal compartment. The distal ulna is a characteristic target area with surface erosions along the outer surface of the ulnar styloid secondary to tenosynovitis of the extensor carpi ulnaris. Inflammatory changes in the prestyloid recess and inferior radioulnar compartment may produce erosions at the tip and base of the ulnar styloid, respectively. Early erosions may be encountered in any carpal bone, typically at the radial styloid, the waist of the scaphoid, triquetrum, and pisiform (Fig. 51–7). As the disease progresses, greater amounts of cartilage and bone are destroyed, leading to bony ankylosis and carpal collapse. Drift of the entire carpus in an ulnar direction, volar direction, or both and scapholunate dissociation are frequently encountered deformities.

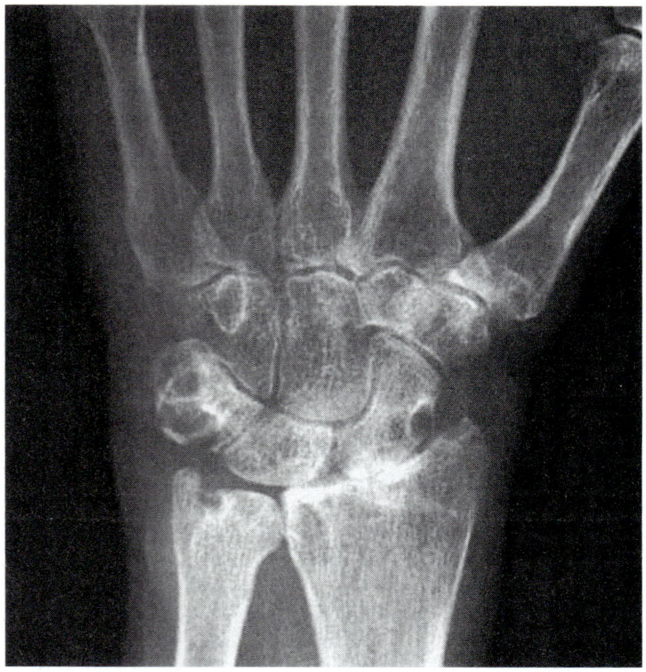

FIGURE 51–7 · Rheumatoid Arthritis. Typical sites of osseous erosion of a rheumatoid wrist shown here include triquetrum, pisiform, scaphoid and radius. There are also erosions at the ulnar aspect of the distal radius and the distal ulnar styloid process secondary to involvement of inferior radioulnar compartment. Diffuse cartilage loss is also evident in the radiocarpal compartment.

Elbow

Elbow involvement occurs in at least half of patients with RA. Earliest changes are soft tissue abnormalities including joint effusion identified by elevation of anterior and posterior fad pads, olecranon bursitis, and rheumatoid nodules along the extensor surface of the elbow. Diffuse cartilage loss and erosive changes occur in all compartments. Eventually, extensive osteolysis of the bones can simulate a neuropathic osteoarthropathy. Large intramedullary cystic erosions of the distal humerus and olecranon may predispose to pathologic fracture.[43]

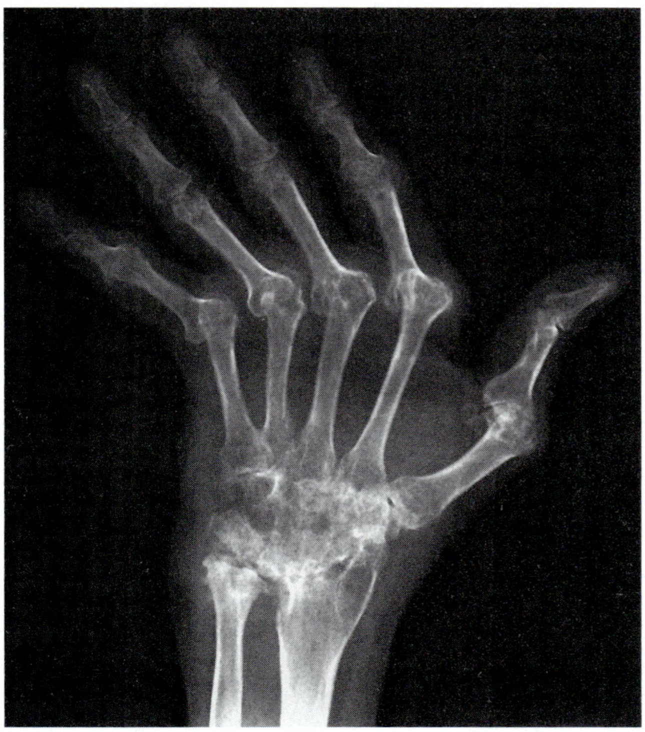

FIGURE 51–6 · Ulnar Deviation in Rheumatoid Arthritis. Severe ulnar deviation is present at the metacarpophalangeal joints with extensive erosions. Pancompartmental bony ankylosis and erosion are also seen in the wrist.

Shoulder

At the shoulder, both glenohumeral and acromioclavicular joints are involved. Cartilage loss in the glenohumeral joint is an early finding. Erosions are typically seen at the superolateral aspect of the humeral head, resembling the Hill-Sachs fracture associated with anterior shoulder dislocation. The subacromial-subdeltoid bursa may be distended due to bursitis. Involvement of the acromioclavicular joint may lead to resorption of the distal clavicle and joint widening. Rotator cuff tear or atrophy is a common complication with resultant superior migration of the humeral head and pressure erosion of the under surface of the acromion (Fig. 51–8).

Foot

RA of the foot is about as common as involvement of the hand. In the forefoot, early erosions occur at the lateral aspect of the fifth and medial aspect of the first metatarsal heads. With progression, diffuse cartilage loss and larger erosions may be seen in all

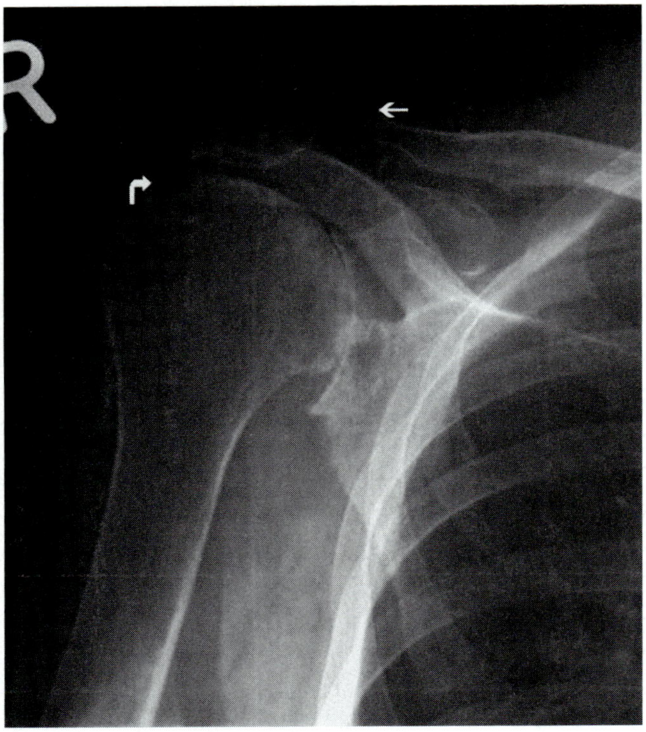

FIGURE 51–8 · Abnormalities of the Shoulder in Rheumatoid Arthritis. The Grashey posterior oblique view of a shoulder shows severe glenohumeral joint space narrowing with a marginal erosion and cystic change of the humeral head adjacent to the greater tuberosity *(curved arrow)*. Elevation of the humeral head with respect to the in the glenoid indicates chronic rotator cuff tear. There is also tapering of the distal end of the clavicle and widening of the acromioclavicular joint *(arrow)*.

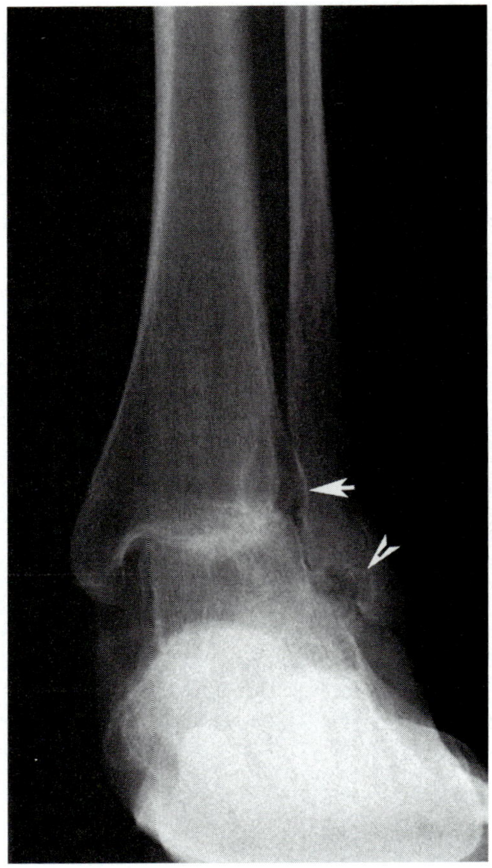

FIGURE 51–9 · Rheumatoid Arthritis of the Ankle. There is diffuse loss of cartilage space with erosions of the fibula *(arrow and arrow head)*. The scalloping along the medial border of the distal fibula *(arrow)* is designated the fibular notch sign and is a characteristic finding in rheumatoid arthritis. The hindfoot is in valgus alignment.

metatarsophalangeal joints leading to forefoot deformities. These include hallux valgus, hammer toes, and "cock up" deformity of the metatarsophalangeal joints, as well as fibular deviation of the toes and plantar subluxation of the metatarsal heads.

In long-standing RA, bony ankylosis of the midfoot is relatively common. Subluxation at the talonavicular joint may indicate posterior tibialis tendon rupture. In the heel, soft tissue findings are commonly encountered including retrocalcaneal bursitis, Achilles tendinosis, peritendinitis, plantar fasciitis, and rheumatoid nodules. Erosive changes may develop at the posterior and plantar surface of the calcaneus as a result of synovitis of the adjacent bursae.

Ankle

Approximately 60 percent of patients with long-standing RA have significant ankle involvement. The radiographic changes in the tibiotalar joint include joint effusion, diffuse cartilage loss, and erosions. A scalloped erosion along the medial border of the distal fibula is a characteristic finding and is called the fibular notch sign[44] (Fig. 51–9). Progressive osteoporosis may be complicated by an insufficiency fracture in the distal tibial metaphysis or calcaneus.

Knee

The knee is frequently affected in RA. Distension of the suprapatellar pouch of the knee joint by effusion, synovial hypertrophy, or both is identifiable on the lateral projection. Cartilage loss is uniform involving patellofemoral and femorotibial articulations. Erosions develop usually at the periphery of the articular margins. Subchondral cysts may be seen in the femoral condyles or proximal tibia and may lead to bony collapse. Varus or valgus deformity of the knee joint may be present. Rupture of the quadriceps or patellar tendon may occur with corresponding soft tissue abnormalities. Baker's cysts are well-known manifestation of RA. They can extend far down the calf and cause compartment syndrome. They can also rupture with resultant inflammation, mimicking deep-vein thrombosis clinically.

Hip

Hip involvement in RA is less common than knee involvement. Radiographic abnormalities of the hip are generally bilateral and symmetric in distribution. The hip joints show concentric loss of articular space with axial migration of the femoral head, which may lead to acetabular protrusio (Fig. 51–10). Insufficiency frac-

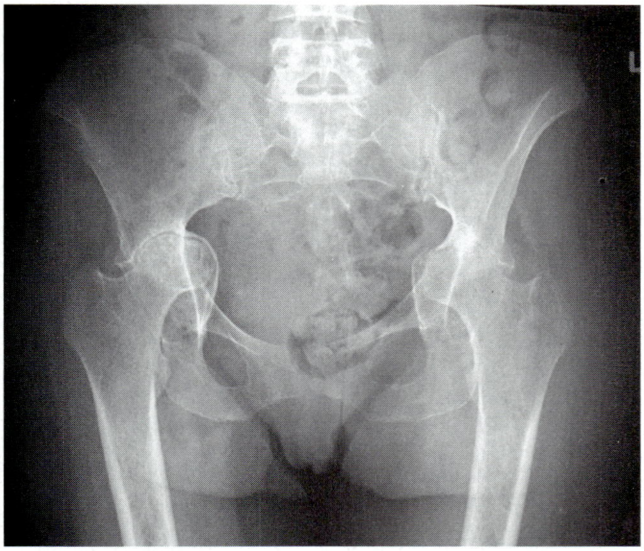

FIGURE 51–10 · **Bilateral Acetabular Protrusio in Rheumatoid Arthritis.** The medial acetabular margins protrude into the pelvis. There is severe accompanying cartilage loss.

tures of the femoral neck and avascular necrosis of the head may be encountered, usually associated with steroid therapy. Occasionally, large cystic changes of the femoral neck occur and predispose to pathologic fracture.

Other Sites

Asymptomatic erosive changes are reported to be common in sacroiliac joints. Other synovial joints that may be involved include the temporomandibular and sternoclavicular joints. Cartilaginous articulations, such as the sternomanubrial joint and symphysis pubis, may show erosive changes.

Magnetic Resonance Imaging in Rheumatoid Arthritis

The superior soft tissue contrast of MRI offers greater sensitivity for detection of early changes of RA than conventional radiography. MRI has proven to be useful in determining the extent of the inflammatory and structural changes in early stages of the disease. MRI has also the potential to monitor patients' response to therapy.

Perhaps the most frequent application of MRI in RA is in diagnosis of various complications encountered during the course of the disease and its treatment.

Inflammatory changes characterized by joint effusion, acute synovitis, pannus, and synovial sheath effusions can be recognized on MRI images. The conspicuity of inflammatory synovial tissue in contrast to joint effusion appears to vary depending on the nature of the tissue and the MRI sequence. Differentiation of inflamed sy-novium and joint effusion on non–contrast-enhanced standard spin echo T1-weighted and T2-weighted (TE less than 80 msec) sequences may not be always possible. Fast spin echo (FSE) with heavily T2-weighted sequences (80 to 180 msec) allow excellent contrast between the hyperintense fluid and relatively hypointense pannus (Fig. 51–11). The newer MRI sequences such as fat-suppressed, T1-weighted, three-dimensional spoiled-gradient echo imaging or magnetization transfer contrast sequences may also allow differentiation of inflamed synovium and joint fluid.[45-47]

Contrast-enhanced MRI has been proposed by several authors for evaluation of inflammatory synovial tissue.[48-50] After the intravenous administration of contrast agent, correct timing of aquisition of MRI images is necessary to differentiate inflamed synovial tissue from joint fluid.[51,52] Because the synovial intima has no tight junction or basement membrane, gadolinium compounds can diffuse into the synovial fluid on delayed images. Thus, the images must be obtained immediately after the injection of contrast to display only the synovial enhancement.

The enhancement of inflamed synovial tissue may vary. An active proliferative pannus is hypervascular and shows rapid enhancement after intravenous injection of gadolinium containing agents.[53] In long-standing "burned out" cases of RA, the hypervascular pannus changes into more fibrotic tissue, which is accompanied by a gradual loss of vascularization.

Quantitative MRI has been suggested to estimate the volume of enhancing pannus before and after treatment to monitor treatment efficacy. Ostergaard and colleagues[55] have also proposed that MRI-determined synovial membrane volume may prove to be useful as a marker of joint disease activity and a predictor of

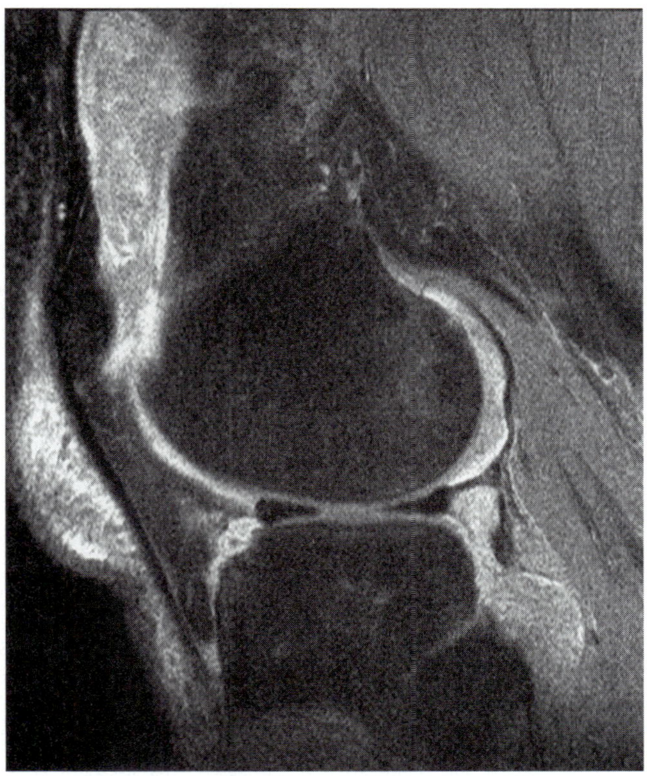

FIGURE 51–11 · **MR Imaging in Rheumatoid Arthritis.** Sagittal FSE T2 weighted (TR 3625/TE133) fat suppressed image allows excellent contrast between intermediate (gray) signal intensity, annus and (white) joint fluid.

progressive joint destruction. Synovial membrane volume can be estimated using manual or semiautomated volume measures with MRI.[54-60]

MRI is convincingly more sensitive than conventional radiography in detection of early structural changes of RA, including cartilage damage, meniscal degeneration, subchondral cysts, and erosions.[18,61-64] Erosions appear as subcortical areas of dark signal on T1-weighted images in the marrow adjacent to the bony margin or beneath the chondral surface. The content of the erosions or bone cysts may exhibit fluid-like bright signal on T2-weighted images, synovium-like intermediate signal, or both. In recent studies, the bone marrow edema detected on MRI is found to be a strong predictor of erosions in the wrist.[18]

MRI is the preferred method of imaging of the musculoskeletal complications of RA such as tendon ruptures, ischemic necrosis, insufficiency fractures, and cord compression in cervical spine.

Rheumatoid synovitis may invade ligaments and tendons directly and may eventually lead to their disruption (Fig. 51–12). Tendon injury and rupture most frequently affect the wrist, shoulder, foot, and knee in patients with RA, specifically the posterior tibialis tendon, rotator cuff tendons, quadriceps tendon, and the extensor tendons of the wrist, in particular the extensor carpi ulnaris. MRI is sensitive for diagnosis of tenosynovitis and subclinical tendon ruptures.[64] Normal tendons have smooth margins and show homogeneously low signal intensity in all MRI sequences. Increased sig-

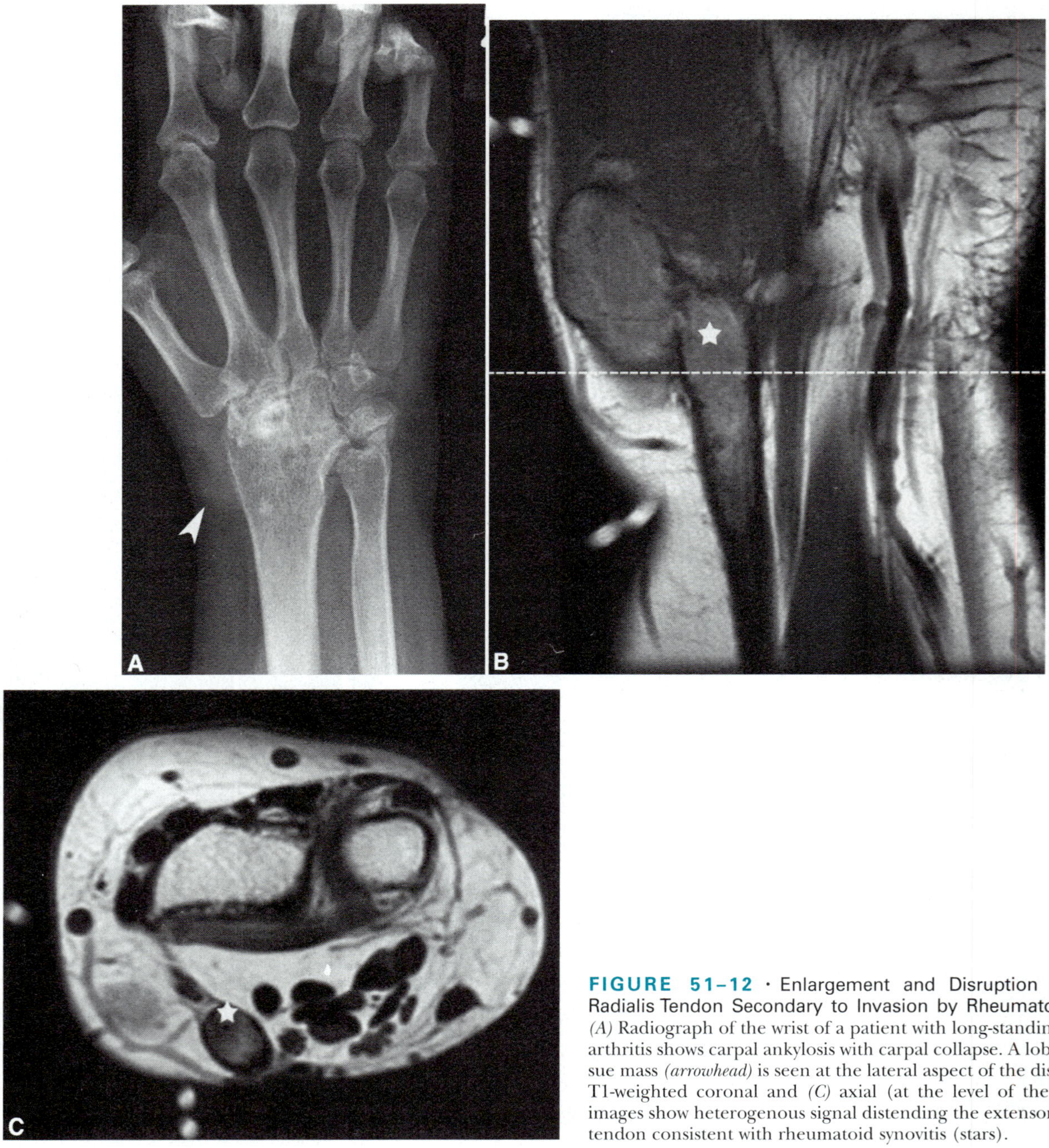

FIGURE 51–12 · Enlargement and Disruption Flexor Carpi Radialis Tendon Secondary to Invasion by Rheumatoid Synovitis. *(A)* Radiograph of the wrist of a patient with long-standing rheumatoid arthritis shows carpal ankylosis with carpal collapse. A lobulated soft tissue mass *(arrowhead)* is seen at the lateral aspect of the distal radius. *(B)* T1-weighted coronal and *(C)* axial (at the level of the dashed line) images show heterogenous signal distending the extensor carpi radialis tendon consistent with rheumatoid synovitis (stars).

nal intensity on PD and T2-weighted spin echo images indicates tendon injury, which may be due to erosion from invasion by pannus or partial tear. Partial tear may also result in thickening or thinning of the tendon. Tendon discontinuity indicates complete tear. Tenosynovitis appears as fluid and hyperplastic synovium distending the tendon sheath.[46]

Juvenile Chronic Arthritis

The term *juvenile chronic arthritis* describes a heterogeneous group of chronic inflammatory arthritides that begin in childhood. Juvenile chronic arthritis (JCA) is used synonymously with juvenile rheumatoid arthritis (JRA) and juvenile idiopathic arthritis (JIA).[65,66] A new classification of JCA is summarized in Table 51–1.[66]

The radiologic changes in JCA are largely determined by the age of onset and type of the arthritis. The types of arthritis according to the onset of the disease have been recognized as follows:

1. Systemic illness that is not usually associated with radiologic changes
2. Oligoarticular disease where growth anomalies are frequent
3. Generalized polyarthritis in which osteoporosis and periostitis occur early with subsequent development of cartilage loss and bone erosion[67]

Although the radiographic appearance of each specific type of JCA have some distinctive features, most of them share common radiographic changes.

Osteopenia

Regional or diffuse osteopenia is characteristically present. Regional osteopenia may be juxta-articular or may appear as bandlike metaphyseal lucent zones, particularly in the distal end of the femur, proximal portion of the tibia, and the distal ends of the radius, tibia, and the fibula. These lucent bands are similar to those seen in childhood leukemia. In these regions, subsequent development of transverse radiodense "growth recovery" lines has been noted.[68] Osteoporosis may lead to compression fractures of epiphysis, fractures of the tubular bones, and compression fractures of the vertebral bodies.

TABLE 51–1 • INTERNATIONAL LEAGUE OF ASSOCIATIONS FOR RHEUMATOLOGY (ILAR) CLASSIFICATION OF JUVENILE CHRONIC ARTHRITIS (JUVENILE IDIOPATHIC ARTHRITIS)

1. Systemic arthritis
2. Oligoarthritis
   Persistent: no more than 4 joints throughout the disease course
   Extended: affects cumulative total of 5 joints or more after the first 6 months of disease
3. Polyarthritis (rheumatoid factor negative)
4. Polyarthritis (rheumatoid factor positive)
5. Psoriatic arthritis
6. Enthesitis-related arthritis
7. Other arthritis

Joint-Space Abnormalities

Joint-space narrowing is usually a late finding in JCA, as opposed to adult-onset RA. In the later stages of the disease, intraarticular bony ankylosis can ultimately develop, especially affecting small joints of the hands, wrists, and feet and apophyseal joints of the cervical spine.

Bone Erosion

The development of bone erosions is also a relatively late finding in JCA. The erosions may occur at the margins of the joint or along the entire articular surface of the bone.

Periostitis

One of the most common findings of all types of JCA on presentation is periostitis along with soft tissue swelling and osteoporosis. It is most frequent in the phalanges, metacarpals, and metatarsals and occasionally is seen along the metaphyses and diaphyses of long tubular bones. In some cases, the extensive periosteal proliferation may produce an enlarged, rectangular appearance of the tubular bones of the hands and feet.

Growth Disturbance

Growth disturbance is a striking feature of JCA. Overgrowth of epiphysial centers as a result of hyperemia may result in deformity and premature fusion of epiphysis. Commonly affected locations include metacarpals, metatarsals, carpal and tarsal bones, proximal and distal femur, proximal tibia, and radial head. Asymmetric growth of paired bones may cause discrepancy of the lengths of fibula and radius.

Epiphyseal Compression Fractures

Deformity and flattening of the epiphyseal centers secondary to epiphyseal compression fractures are frequently encountered in JCA. These changes develop as a result of abnormal stress on weakened osteoporotic bone. In a similar way, cupping of the ossification centers of the proximal phalanges in response to compression by metacarpal and metatarsal heads may be encountered.[69]

Abnormalities in Specific Sites

Hand and Wrist

In the early cases of generalized polyarthritis, radiologic abnormalities are demonstrated most frequently in the wrist and consist of squaring of carpal ossification centers, followed by loss of joint space. Ultimately, bony ankylosis can develop (Fig. 51–13).

Any joint of the hand can be affected, typically in an asymmetric fashion. Early radiographic changes of the

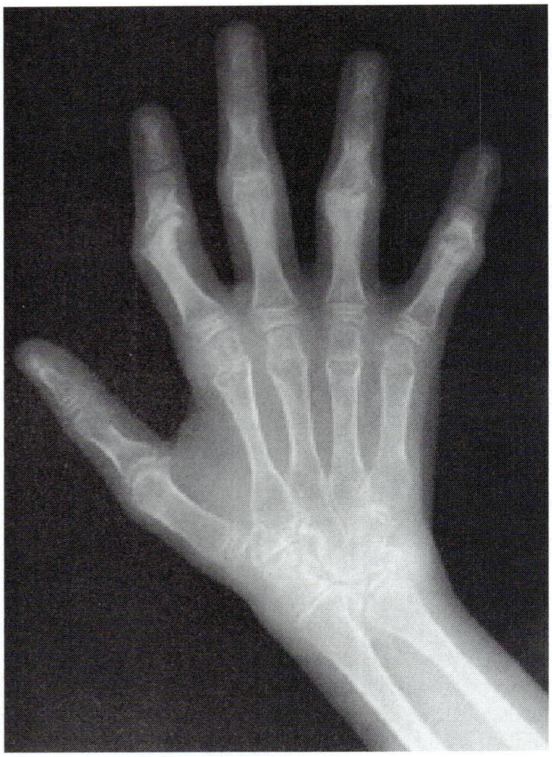

FIGURE 51–13 • **Juvenile Chronic Arthritis.** Severe abnormalities of the hand and wrist include ankylosis of carpal bones, growth disturbance of the distal radius and ulna, erosion, compression and flexion deformities of the proximal interphalangeal joints and periosteal bone formation along the proximal phalanges.

hands are soft tissue swelling and periarticular osteoporosis and periostitis of the metacarpal and phalangeal shafts. Joint-space narrowing and bone erosions tend to occur late. Epiphyseal deformity, growth disturbance, and a variety of finger deformities are characteristic changes appearing during the course of the disease.

Foot and Ankle

The radiologic changes in the tarsus are similar to those observed in the carpus, with initial enlargement and irregularity of the tarsal bones, which may fuse and show premature osteoarthritic changes. Deformities due to growth disturbance around the metatarsophalangeal joints are relatively common. Late deformities include clawing of the toes, hammer toes, hindfoot and valgus, pes cavus, and hallux valgus (Fig. 51–14).

Knee

Characteristic radiographic abnormalities of the knee related to disturbance of growth usually become obvious within a year of involvement and consist of "ballooning" of the distal femoral and proximal tibial epiphyses, flattening of femoral condyles, widening of intercondylar notch and squaring of the patella (Fig. 51–15). Other radiographic findings are diffuse narrowing of joint space and marginal and central osseous erosions.

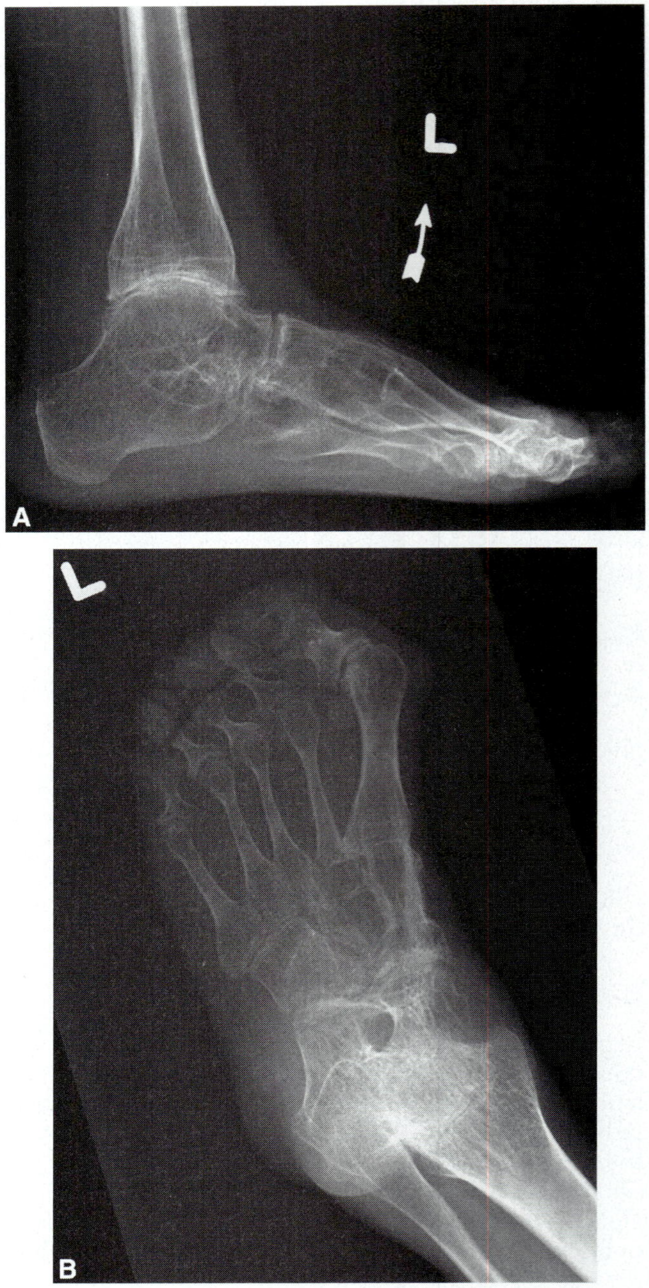

FIGURE 51–14 • **Foot Abnormalities of Juvenile Chronic Arthritis.** Lateral *(A)* and oblique *(B)* views of the foot show diffuse osteopenia, bony ankylosis of intertarsal and tarsometatarsal joints with relative preservation of the talonavicular and calcaneocuboid joints, secondary osteoarthritis of the ankle and growth disturbance of the metatarsals with erosive changes in the metatarsophalangeal joints. There is a hallux valgus deformity.

Hip

Involvement of the hip is common and can be recognized radiologically in 40 percent of patients 10 years after disease onset. Overgrowth of the femoral capital epiphysis is a characteristic initial radiologic finding, followed by premature fusion and failure of growth of the femoral neck. Coxa valga and protrusio acetabuli deformities are common. Intra-articular bony ankylosis

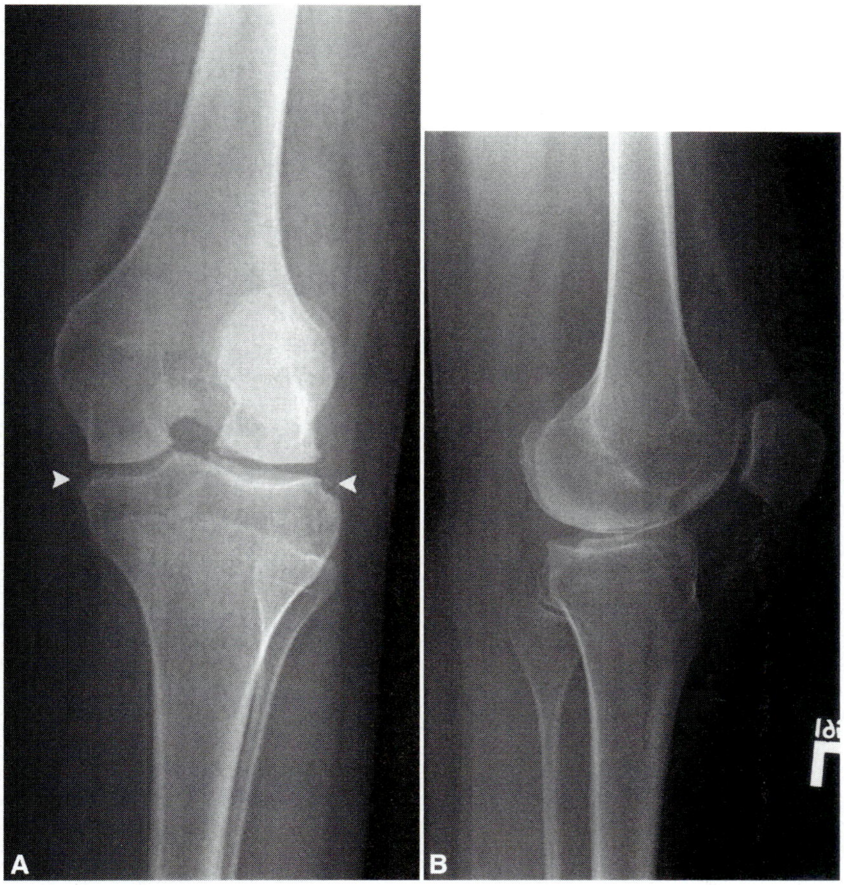

FIGURE 51–15 · Juvenile Chronic Arthritis. *(A)* Anteroposterior view of the knee shows overgrowth of the femoral epiphysis, constriction of epiphysis at the joint and widening of the intercondylar notch *(arrow)*. Old corticated, marginal erosions *(arrowhead)* are present. *(B)* The square shape of the patella is visible on the lateral view.

of the hip can be occasionally encountered. Development of iliac bones is also impaired, especially in younger children. Rarely, improvement in hip cartilage space is seen.

Sacroiliac Joints

Radiographic findings of sacroiliitis in juvenile-onset ankylosing spondylitis can become evident usually several years after onset. Early sacroiliac joint changes may be overlooked due to difficulty in radiographic analysis of the sacroiliac joints in children. Conventional radiographs of the sacroiliac joints are of limited value in patients between 8 and 16 years of age because widened articular joint-spaces and indistinct subchondral bone are normal findings in this age group.[70] Sacroiliac joint changes in juvenile-onset ankylosing spondylitis may initially be unilateral or asymmetric in distribution; however, they soon become bilateral and symmetric. Joint-space widening, indistinct joint margins, erosions, sclerosis, and eventually bony ankylosis can be detected.

Bollow and coworkers reported that contrast-enhanced MRI is superior to conventional radiography for detection of sacroiliitis in children. In their study, unenhanced MRI alone was also more sensitive in identifying sacroiliitis than conventional radiography.[71]

Cervical Spine

As in adult disease, JCA affects, in particular, the cervical spine, sparing the thoracic and lumbar regions. Ankylosis may result in growth disturbance with underdeveloped vertebral bodies. Ankylosis affects both intervertebral and apophyseal joints. Growth disturbances of the vertebral bodies occur at the levels of apophyseal joint ankylosis and consist of decreased vertical and anteroposterior diameters (Fig. 51–16). Atlantoaxial subluxation occurs most frequently in juvenile-onset adult-type RA.

Underdevelopment of the mandible with antegonial notching and articular involvement of the temporomandibular joints are additional radiographic findings in JCA.

Adult-Onset Still's Disease

Rarely, an adult patient may be encountered with a febrile illness identical to classic Still's disease. The radiographic changes involve the hands, wrists, knees, and hips. Bony erosions are unusual. Predilection for narrowing and ankylosis of carpometacarpal joints, especially the second and third metacarpal bones and the intercarpal joints in a pericapitate distribution, are characteristic.[72]

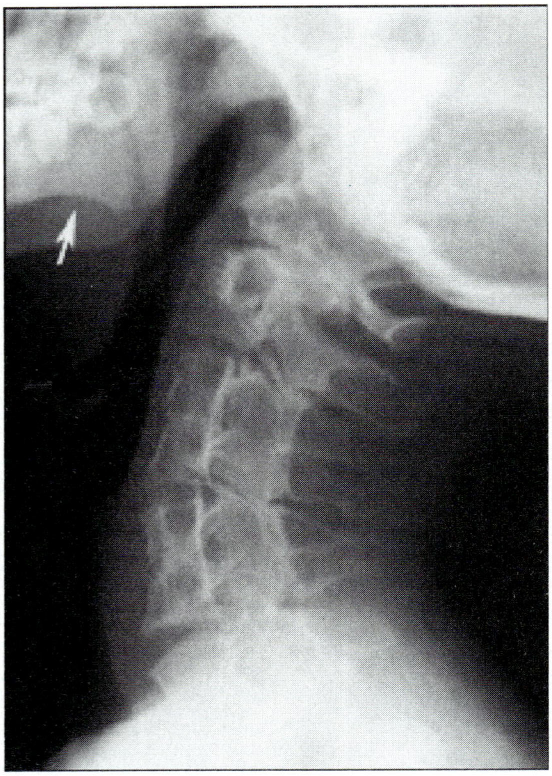

FIGURE 51–16 · Cervical Spine Abnormalities in Juvenile Chronic Arthritis. There is segmental fusion at various levels including vertebral bodies and posterior elements. The involved vertebral bodies are hypoplastic. Antegonial notching *(arrow)* of the mandible, a manifestation of JCA, is secondary to growth disturbance of the mandible and altered muscle pull.

Psoriatic Arthritis

The radiologic manifestations of psoriatic arthritis can be seen in the synovial and cartilaginous joints and at the osseous attachment sites of tendons and ligaments, involving both the axial and the appendicular skeleton. At least five patterns of clinical presentation have been described in psoriatic arthritis:

1. Polyarthritis with distal interphalangeal joint involvement
2. Symmetric seronegative polyarthritis simulating RA
3. Arthritis mutilans
4. Monoarthritis or asymmetric oligoarthritis
5. Spondyloarthropathy

Of these, asymmetric or unilateral polyarthritis seems to be the most common presentation.[73]

Psoriatic arthritis affects mainly the interphalangeal joints of the hands and feet, the metacarpophalangeal and metatarsophalangeal joints. The knees, ankles, elbows, and wrists, as well as manubriosternal and sternoclavicular joints are other sites of involvement. In the axial skeleton, sacroiliac joint and spinal abnormalities predominate. Involvement of the hip and shoulder is uncommon in psoriatic arthritis.

General radiographic abnormalities typically seen in the affected peripheral joints of the upper and lower extremities are soft tissue swelling, joint-space widening or narrowing, erosions, bone proliferation, malalignment, and ankylosis. The findings in large joints are less distinctive and are similar to those of RA. Bone proliferation is a characteristic feature of psoriatic arthritis, accompanying the bone erosions as a healing response. Bone proliferation also occurs at sites of tendon and ligament insertion. Absence of osteoporosis is a useful sign in differentiating psoriatic arthritis from RA.

Hand and Foot

The radiographic changes in the hands and feet are highly distinctive. At these sites, bilateral symmetric, asymmetric, or unilateral involvement of interphalangeal joints, as well as metacarpophalangeal and metatarsophalangeal joints, is observed. Sometimes involvement occurs along a digit (the "ray distribution").

An early soft tissue finding of psoriatic arthritis is periarticular soft tissue swelling or diffuse fusiform swelling of an entire digit, the so called "sausage digit." Fingernail thickening and irregularity may sometimes be discernable.

Initial erosions occur at the joint margins and proceed centrally. Fluffy new bone formation associated with marginal erosions produces a "whiskered" appearance (Fig. 51–17). Further destruction of the articular surfaces may lead to apparent widening of the joint space, a "pencil-and-cup" appearance, and opera glass ("main en lorgnette") deformities. The pencil-and-cup appearance describes the deformity created by protrusion of one

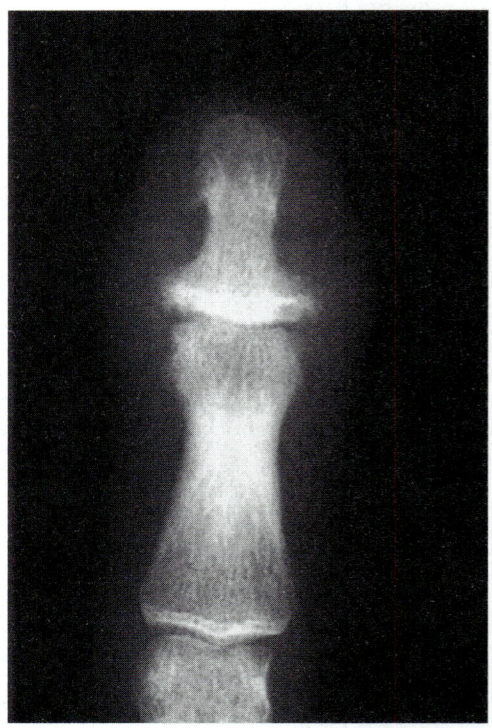

FIGURE 51–17 · Psoriatic Arthritis. Classic radiographic findings about the distal interphalangeal joints include soft tissue swelling, erosions with accompanying bone proliferation and lack of osteoporosis.

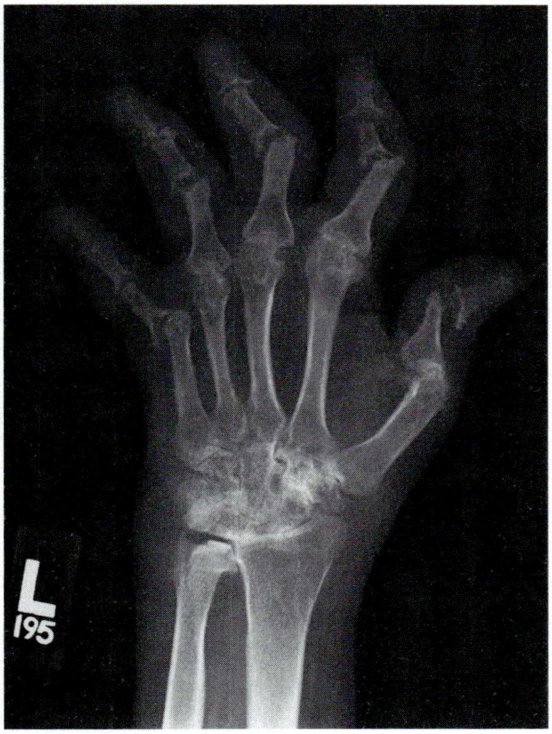

FIGURE 51–18 · Arthritis mutilans due to psoriatic arthritis with destructive changes and joint deformity of the hand and pancompartmental ankylosis of the wrist.

articular surface into its opposing articular counterpart (Fig. 51–18).

Proliferative bone changes may result in sclerosis of an entire phalanx, which is termed an *ivory phalanx*. This is most frequently seen in the terminal phalanx of the great toe. Intra-articular osseous fusion is another manifestation of bone proliferation, and it particularly affects the interphalangeal joints. Resorption of the tufts (acroosteolysis) and of the distal phalanges of hands and feet is also a characteristic finding of psoriatic arthritis.[74,75]

Bony proliferation with erosions at the posterior and plantar aspects of the calcaneus is a common finding in psoriatic arthritis as in the other seronegative spondyloarthropathies. Retrocalcaneal bursitis, thickening of the adjacent Achilles tendon, and poorly defined enthesophytes at the attachment sites of the plantar aponeurosis and the Achilles tendon are associated abnormalities.[76] New bone production along the malleoli may indicate adjacent tenosynovitis.

Sacroiliac Joints

Radiographic changes of the sacroiliac joints are observed in approximately 30 to 50 percent of patients with psoriatic arthritis. Bilateral abnormalities are much more frequent than unilateral changes. The changes in the sacroiliac joints may or may not be symmetric. Radiographic changes include erosions and sclerosis, predominantly on the iliac side, and widening and subsequent narrowing of the articular space.

Unlike ankylosing spondylitis, the disease rarely progresses to complete joint fusion. Sacroiliitis can appear without spondylitis.

Reactive Arthritis (Reiter's Syndrome)

The radiographic features of articular involvement of Reiter's syndrome are similar to those of the other seronegative spondyloarthropathies. Reiter's syndrome produces asymmetric arthritis with predilection for the lower extremity. The most characteristic sites of abnormality are the small joints of the feet, calcaneus, ankles, and knees. The upper extremity joints are less frequently affected, in contrast to psoriatic arthritis. In the axial skeleton, the sacroiliac joints, spine, symphysis pubis, and manubriosternal joints are frequently involved.

The general radiologic findings are soft tissue swelling, erosions, joint-space narrowing, and bone proliferation. Osteopenia is not a prominent finding, although periarticular osteopenia may accompany acute episodes of the arthritis.

Foot and Ankle

The most frequently affected joints in the foot are the metatarsophalangeal and interphalangeal joints. Radiographic changes include joint-space loss, marginal erosions with adjacent bony proliferation, and periostitis of the shafts of affected metatarsals and phalanges. Joint ankylosis is less common than in psoriatic arthritis. Occasionally, severe destruction and dorsolateral subluxation of the metatarsophalangeal joints are observed. Such deformity associated with Reiter's syndrome has been called Launios' deformity.[77,78]

The most characteristic radiographic feature of Reiter's syndrome is exuberant, fluffy bone proliferation. The calcaneus is a target site for such proliferative new bone formation. Bone proliferation and poorly defined erosions usually develop on the plantar and posterior aspects of the calcaneus. Retrocalcaneal bursitis can be observed as can thickening of the Achilles tendon (Fig. 51–19). Heel changes may be the sole or predominant radiographic finding of Reiter's syndrome.[76]

Radiographic changes in the ankles include soft tissue swelling, joint-space narrowing, and periostitis along the malleoli. Erosions are infrequently encountered.

Knee

Radiographic abnormalities of the knee are apparent in 25 to 40 percent of patients. The most common abnormality is joint effusion, although osteoporosis, joint-space narrowing, and periostitis of the distal femur or proximal tibia and shallow erosions can be detected.

Sacroiliac Joints

Sacroiliac joint changes are usually bilateral, but often can be persistently asymmetric.

Sacroiliitis has radiographic features similar to ankylosing spondylitis and psoriatic arthropathy, although bony ankylosis is less frequent in Reiter's syndrome (Fig. 51–20).

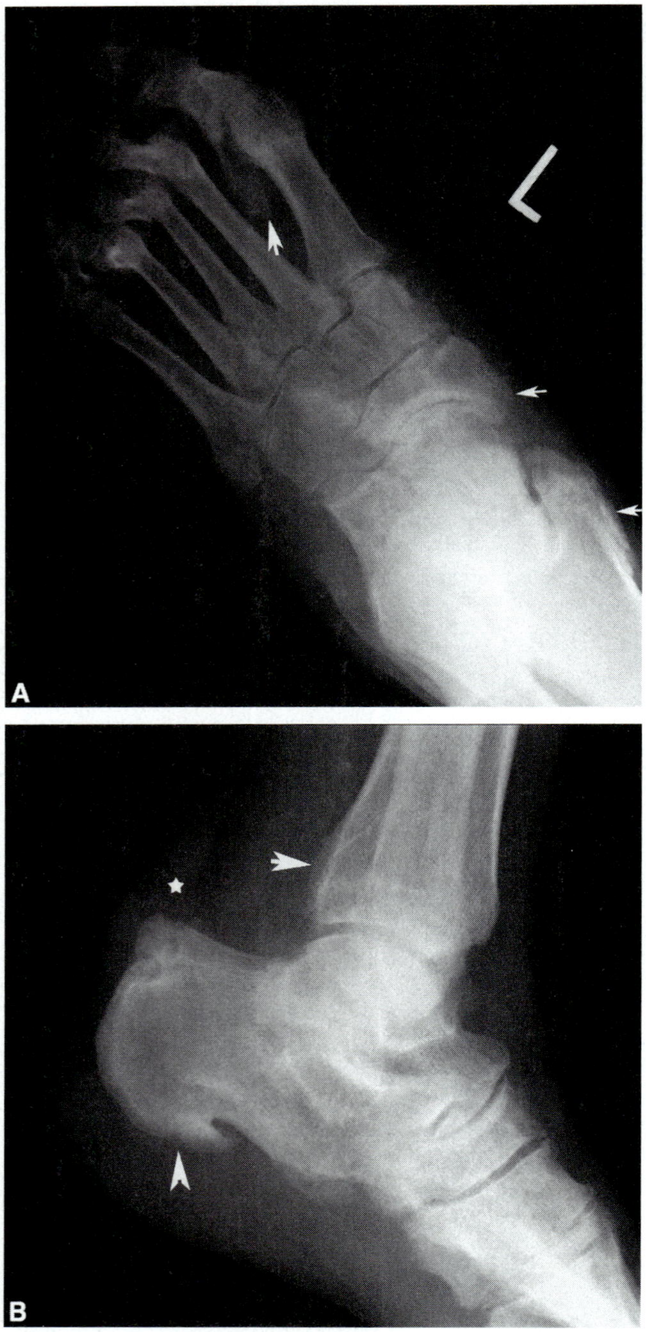

FIGURE 51–19 · Radiographic Findings of the Foot in Reactive Arthritis *(A)* AP view of the foot reveals erosions and bony proliferation of the first through fourth metatarsophalangeal joints with subluxation. Fluffy bony proliferation is noted along the medial malleolus, midfoot and sesamoid bones of the first metatarsal head *(arrows)*. *(B)* Lateral view of the hindfoot demonstrates ill-defined plantar calcaneal enthesophytes *(arrowhead)*, periosteal new bone formation along the posterior aspect of the distal tibia *(arrow)*, retrocalcaneal bursitis and thickening of the Achilles tendon (star) and erosions at the subjacent calcaneus.

Enteropathic Arthropathies

The rheumatologic manifestations of inflammatory bowel disease are sacroiliitis, spondylitis, and nondestructive, asymmetric, and usually transient arthritis of peripheral joints.

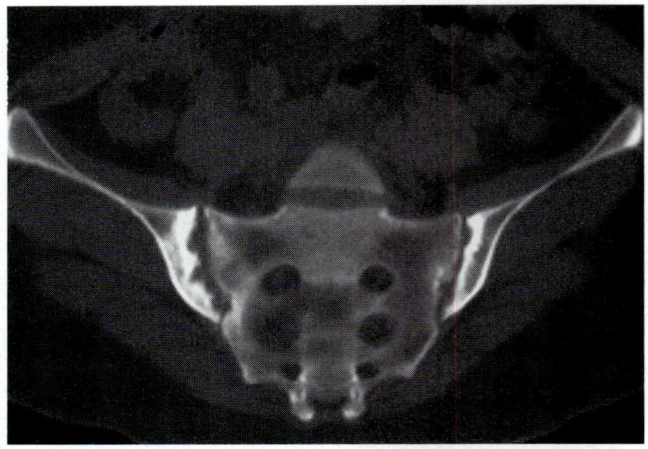

FIGURE 51–20 · CT Scanning in Reactive Arthritis. An oblique axial image through the sacroiliac joints shows erosions with associated new bone formation predominating in the iliac bones.

The radiographic features of the sacroiliac joint and spinal abnormalities are virtually indistinguishable from those in ankylosing spondylitis. Sacroiliac joint changes are usually bilateral and symmetric.

Peripheral joint involvement is usually monoarticular or pauciarticular in distribution, although it can be polyarticular. The knees are involved most commonly, followed by the ankles, elbows, wrists, shoulders, and small joints of hands and feet. The radiographic findings at these sites are nonspecific. Soft tissue swelling and regional osteoporosis may be observed, whereas cartilage loss and bone erosions are rare.

Septic Arthritis

In all varieties of septic arthritis, the earliest radiographic change is symmetric soft tissue swelling about the joint secondary to soft tissue edema, hypertrophied synovium, and joint effusion. The synovial hyperemia and early disuse atrophy may result in periarticular osteopenia. Joint effusions may be identified in elbow, wrist, hip, knee, or ankle by displacement of the capsular fat planes. Initially, edema and joint effusion may produce widening of the joint space, a finding seen fairly commonly in the pediatric septic hip.

These erosions occur at the synovium-bone interface where the cartilage is lacking and are indistinguishable from the erosion of inflammatory arthritides. As the infection progresses, the pannus extends between cartilage and bone, leading to destruction of central cartilage and subchondral cortex. Radiographically, these pathologic changes are identified as central erosion with disruption of the white line of the articular cortex (a finding strongly suggesting septic arthritis) (Fig. 51–21). Further destruction of cartilage results in narrowing of the joint space. In late stages, ankylosis of the joint may be seen.[79]

In chronic septic arthritis, the adjacent bones may show signs of osteomyelitis with periostitis and bone destruction.

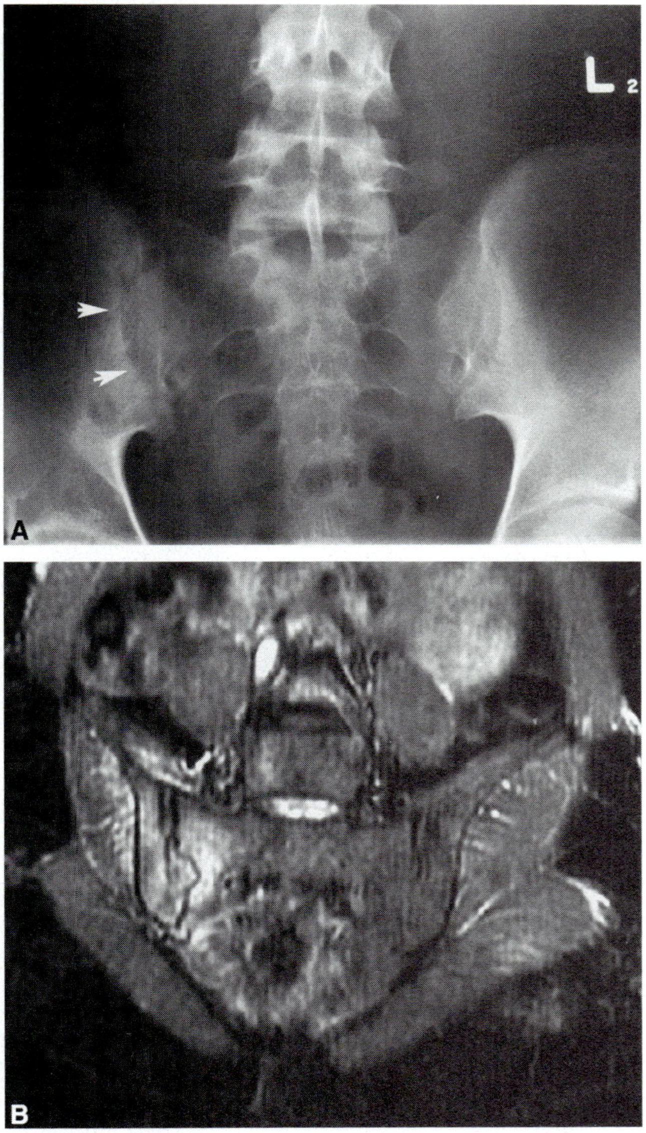

FIGURE 51–21 · Septic Arthritis of the Right Sacroiliac Joint. *(A)* Anteroposterior view of the sacroiliac joints shows destruction of the right sacroiliac joint. *(B)* In a different patient a STIR (short tau inversion recovery) coronal MR image through sacroiliac joints shows erosive changes in the right sacroiliac joint with extensive bone marrow edema.

Early diagnosis is the most important prognostic factor in septic arthritis. When there is clinical suspicion of septic arthritis, a joint aspiration should be performed without delay to avoid irreversible articular damage. Instillation of a radiographic contrast during arthrocentesis helps to confirm the site of fluid sampling, demonstrate the extent of articular and periarticular destruction, and define any cavities or fistulae.[80]

Although the radiologic abnormalities in septic arthritis are not specific for the offending organism, certain generalizations apply. Bacterial arthritis is characterized by rapid destruction of bone and articular cartilage. The bone mineralization is relatively preserved.

In tuberculous arthritis, a triad of radiographic findings (Phemister's triad) is characteristic and consists of juxta-articular osteoporosis, marginal erosions, and absent or mild joint-space narrowing. Sequestra at articular margins may be identified. Periostitis and bone production are not as prominent as in bacterial arthritis. The eventual outcome of tuberculous arthritis is a fibrous ankylosis of the affected joint. Bony ankylosis is seen occasionally but is more frequently observed with bacterial arthritis. The radiographic manifestations of fungal arthritis are similar to those of tuberculosis.[81]

The MRI appearance of septic arthritis is nonspecific, and similar findings can be observed in inflammatory arthropathies and evolving neuropathic joints. MRI may be helpful in the diagnosis of complications of septic arthritis such as abscesses and osteomyelitis. Differentiation of osteomyelitis from nonspecific reactive bone marrow edema may not be always possible in the early stages of the disease and may lead to a false-positive MRI diagnosis of osteomyelitis.[82-84]

In septic arthritis, the three-phase bone scan shows increased periarticular uptake in the distribution of the synovium, soft tissues, or both during blood flow and blood pooling phases. The delayed phase reveals minimal increased uptake in the underlying bone. Bone scintigraphy, although very sensitive, is not specific in differentiating septic from inflammatory arthritis. Generally, bone scintigraphy is used to rule out concomitant osteomyelitis.[85]

DEGENERATIVE JOINT DISEASE

Osteoarthritis

The most characteristic sites of OA include the proximal and distal interphalangeal joints of the hand, first carpometacarpal and trapezioscaphoid joints of the wrist, acromioclavicular and sacroiliac joints, hip, knee, and first metatarsophalangeal joint of the foot. Degenerative joint disease may also affect cartilaginous joints (such as the manubriosternal joint and symphysis pubis) and tendinous and ligamentous attachments to bone (such as in the pelvis, patella, and calcaneus). Degenerative disease of the spine will be discussed separately.

In spite of diversity of etiologies of OA, certain common radiographic characteristics allow a confident diagnosis in most instances. Joint-space narrowing is a key diagnostic feature of the disease (Fig. 51–22). In contrast to the inflammatory arthropathies, in which diffuse joint-space narrowing of an involved articulation is expected, the joint-space loss in OA tends to involve the portion of the joint exposed to the greatest stress (i.e., the lateral aspect of the hip, the medial compartment of the knee). Subchondral bone abnormalities are also characteristic of OA and include sclerosis and cyst formation, both of which predominate in the most stressed area of the articulation. Subchondral eburnation results from cartilage denudation and subsequent bone-to-bone contact. The origin of subchondral cysts remains in debate; joint fluid may intrude into the subchondral bone through a cartiligenous defect, or necrosis of subchondral bone may become cystic.

Osteophytes are the single most characteristic abnormality in OA.[86] They tend to arise from enchondral

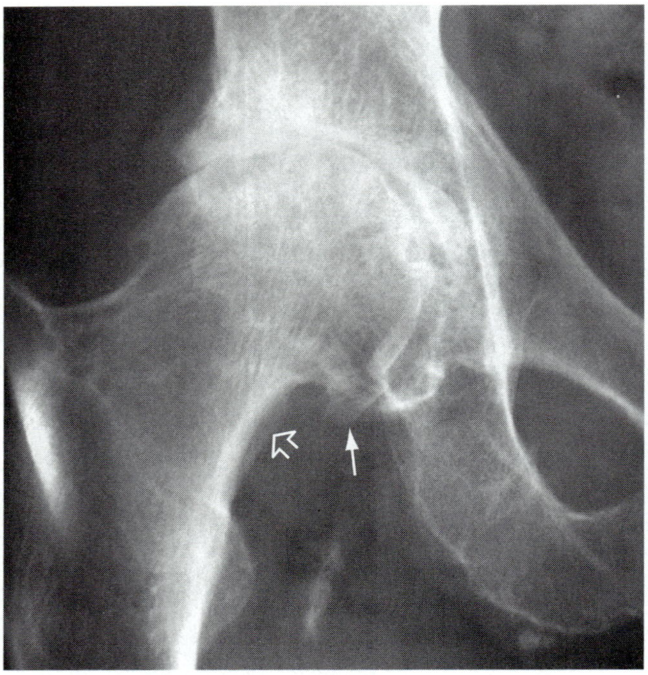

FIGURE 51–22 · **Osteoarthritis of the Hip.** The anteroposterior view of the hip shows complete cartilage space loss superiorly. There is osteophytic lipping from the femoral head, especially medially *(arrow)*, and buttressing bone *(open arrow)* is present along the femoral neck.

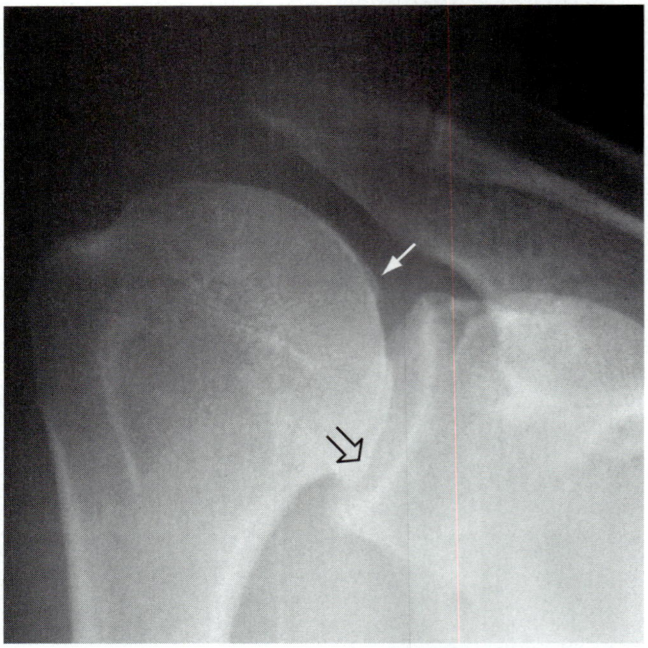

FIGURE 51–23 · **Ostearthritis of the Shoulder.** There is osteophytic lipping *(open arrow)* from the humeral head including new bone formation deep to the cartilage *(arrow)*.

ossification in areas of low stress where islands of cartilage are preserved, most commonly in joint margins (Fig. 51–23, see Fig 51–22). The presence of tibial spine or intercondylar osteophytes alone, however, may not indicate OA as cartilage-space narrowing or pain do not necessarily follow osteophyte formation in these locations.[87]

Articular Cartilage

MRI allows direct assessment of the thickness, surface contour, and internal architecture of articular cartilage and the changes in these areas that may accompany OA or other conditions.[88-91]

Direct imaging of articular cartilage would be extremely helpful in staging and following OA. Detailed cartilage imaging protocols are still being developed and are not yet widely applied clinically. Cartilage imaging requires very high spatial resolution, while at the same time, examination times must remain reasonable to avoid motion artifact. The signal intensities of the articular structures must be manipulated to allow articular cartilage to be differentiated both from subjacent bone and from adjacent joint fluid. Although a large number of techniques have been investigated, the Brigham & Women's Hospital fat-suppressed, fast-spin, echo PD images are normally used to evaluate articular cartilage. Imaging after intravenous contrast (indirect arthrographs) is used in specific circumstances, such as after cartilage repair surgery.[89]

Waldschmidt and coworkers have found normal articular cartilage to consist of three laminae: a superficial hypointense lamina, a deeper hyperintense lamina, and a heterogeneous deep zone.[92] These laminae appear to correspond to the histologic structure of articular cartilage. Eckstein found MRI to provide accurate assessment of articular cartilage volume and thickness in cadaver knees.[91]

Patients otherwise thought to have bicompartmental OA have been found on MRI to demonstrate tricompartmental disease.[93] Unfortunately, MRI generally allows detection of only intermediate-to-advanced osteoarthritic change in clinical cases.[94]

Ultrasound has also been utilized for evaluation of articular cartilage, which is seen as a hypoechoic band with sharp margins.[95] Unfortunately, evaluation of articular cartilage by ultrasonography is of limited use because the weight-bearing knee articular cartilage and patellar cartilage cannot be assessed.

Hand and Wrist

The interphalangeal joints of the hand are frequent target areas of OA (Fig. 51–24). The appearance of articular-space narrowing with closely apposed interdigitating bony surfaces and marginal osteophytes is characteristic. Metacarpophalangeal joint involvement may occur but not as an isolated event; rather, such involvement is associated with alterations at interphalangeal articulations and consists of cartilage-space narrowing as the predominant abnormality. Osseous erosions are not a feature of osteoarthrits. The first carpometacarpal (trapeziometacarpal) joint is the characteristic site of degenerative abnormalities in the wrist. Joint-space narrowing with bony eburnation, subchondral cysts, and osteophyte formation is typical. Radial subluxation of the

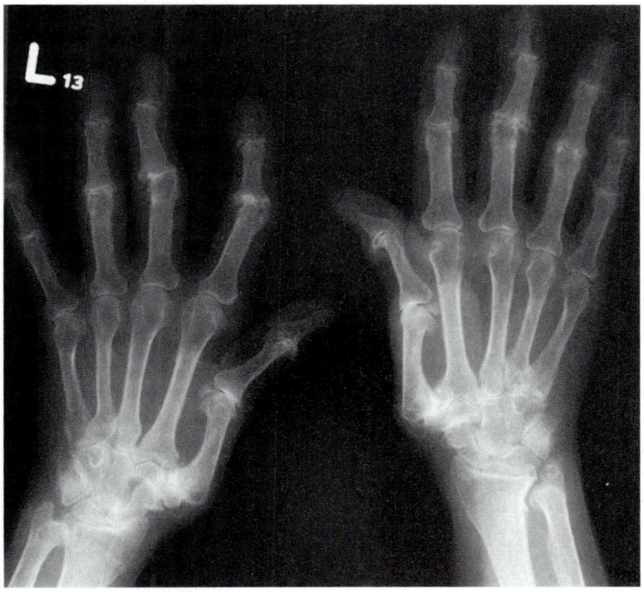

FIGURE 51–24 · Osteoarthritis of the Hands. There is asymmetric cartilage space narrowing at the proximal and distal interphalangeal joints, thumb carpometacarpal joints, and the scaphoid trapezium trapezoid articulations. Subluxation at the thumb carpometacarpal joints and secondary hyperextension at the metacarpophalangeal joints (MCP's) are characteristic deformities of osteoarthritis. Some secondary signs of osteoarthritic changes are noted at the thumb MCP's, but the other MCP's show only minimal cartilage narrowing. The osteoarthritic changes of the right radioulnar joint are likely posttraumatic.

first metacarpal base is common. The trapezioscaphoid cartilage space is the only other common site of OA in the wrist; involvement at this site is generally combined with that at the first carpometacarpal joint. Trapezioscaphoid joint disease in the absence of first carpometacarpal joint involvement should suggest another diagnosis, especially calcium pyrophosphate dihydrate (CPPD) crystal deposition disease. Similarly, a degenerative arthropathy elsewhere in the wrist, especially at the radiocarpal joint, in the absence of significant occupational or accidental trauma, is generally related to a disease other than primary OA.

Sacroiliac Joint

OA of the sacroiliac joint is extremely common in the older age-group. Joint-space narrowing with a thin, well-defined band of subchondral sclerosis, especially in the ilium, is typically present. Osteophyte formation is most common at the superior and inferior margins of the synovial portion of the joint. At the former location, these osteophytes may appear as localized radiodensities projected over the joint in the anteroposterior radiographic projection. Bony erosion and intra-articular osseous fusion are not features of sacroiliac joint OA.

Hip

OA of the hip is exceedingly common and may lead to significant patient disability. In the typical case, cartilage loss is focal, involves the superolateral aspect of the joint, and leads to upward migration of the femoral head[96] (see Fig. 51–22). Osteophyte formation is most prominent at the lateral acetabular and medial femoral margins, often in combination with thickening (buttressing) of the cortex along the medial aspect of femoral neck. Subchondral sclerosis and cyst formation on both sides of the joint space may be marked. Focal loss of cartilage on the medial aspect of the articulation occurs in approximately 20 percent of patients with OA. Diffuse loss of cartilage with axial migration of the femoral head (along the axis of the femoral neck) is uncommon in primary OA. This latter feature is important in the differentiation of OA from inflammatory arthropathies such as RA and in identifying secondary OA such as may be due to underlying calcium pyrophosphate lihydrate arthropathy, (COPD) arthrography. Abnormal juxta-articular bone, as seen in Paget's disease, increases the incidence of OA.

Knee

The knee is a common site of OA. The most characteristic pattern of disease is involvement of the medial femorotibial compartment with joint-space narrowing, osseous eburnation, subchondral cysts, and marginal osteophytes[97] (Fig. 51–25). Women often have lateral femorotibial disease. A true assessment of cartilage thinning may not be possible on standard supine anteroposterior radiographs but is better provided on radiographs obtained either in the "tunnel" projection (Fig. 51–26) or with the patient standing in a weight-bearing position.[98] Boegard and Jonsson and others suggest obtaining weight-bearing radiographs with the knee flexed, although the correct degree of flexion for a specific individual depends on the location of cartilage loss, which is not known a priori.[87] Cartilage-space narrowing is present in standing, not flexed, views if the joint space width is less than 3 mm, is narrower than half the width of the other articulation in same knee or the same articulation in the other knee or decreases on weight-bearing as compared with non–weight-bearing radiographs.[87] Varus angulation of the knee is the most common deformity in OA, reflecting the more severe involvement of the medial femorotibial compartment compared to the lateral one. Standing views of the lower extremities from hips to ankles show knee alignment in relation to the mechanical axis of the leg. Symmetric medial and lateral femorotibial compartment disease is unusual. OA changes in the patellofemoral compartment are common, either in isolation or accompanying medial femorotibial compartment disease.

Osseous or cartilaginous debris may be present as intra-articular bodies, either free within the joint cavity ("joint mice") or attached to the synovial membrane. Degeneration of the fibrocartilaginous menisci is a typical feature of advanced OA. Degenerative tears are most common in the posterior horn of the medial meniscus. On an MRI examination, grade 3 signal (linear signal reaching the articular surface of the meniscus) or diffusely abnormal meniscal signal is found in 60 percent of persons in the sixth decade of life and usually indicates degeneration

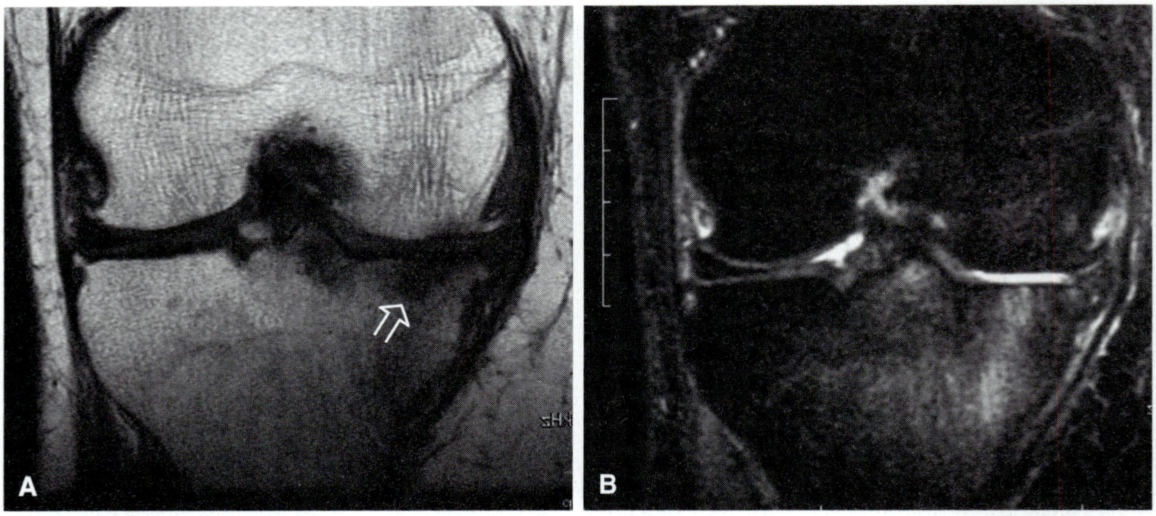

FIGURE 51–25 · Osteoarthritis of the Knee on MRI. *(A)* T1-weighted coronal image of the knee. There are osteophytes at the joint margins. There are discrete areas of low signal replacing the subchondral fat *(open arrow)* and more diffuse low signal extending into the tibial metaphysis. *(B)* Inversion recovery image of the knee shows that most of the low signal area has become bright and is poorly marginated, consistent with edema. Bright joint fluid is adjacent to the bone medially, documenting complete absence of cartilage.

and likely a tear. Also, if OA is present, it, rather than the meniscal tear, may be the cause of symptoms.

Foot

OA in the foot typically affects the first metatarsophalangeal joint. Articular space narrowing, bony eburnation, osteophyte formation, and subchondral cysts are

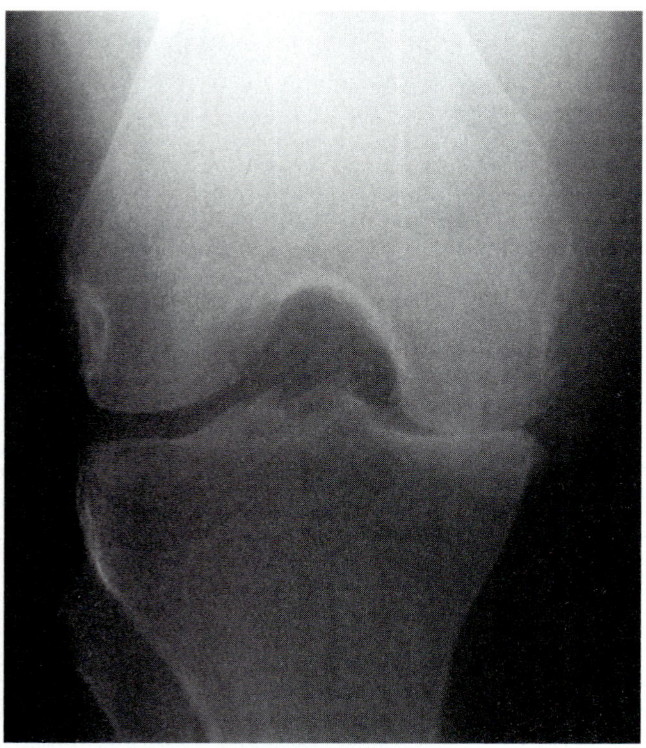

FIGURE 51–26 · Osteoarthritis with medial compartment cartilage narrowing shown to advantage on tunnel view.

common. Hallux rigidus is a specific pattern of OA characterized by painful restriction of dorsiflexion at the first metatarsophalangeal joint. Dorsal osteophytes are characteristic; sclerosis, cyst formation, and osteophytes on the medial aspect of the metatarsal head are also seen.

Other Locations

Typical OA changes in the elbows, acromioclavicular and glenohumeral joints, and ankles may be encountered, usually in patients with a history of trauma or preexisting disease. In general, without such a history, a radiographic pattern consistent with OA[87] at an unusual site should suggest another process, such as acromegaly, CPPD, hydroxyapatite deposition disease (HADD), ochronosis, or epiphyseal dysplasia.

Inflammatory Osteoarthritis

Inflammatory OA is a disorder most common in middle-aged women. It is characterized by acute episodic inflammation of interphalangeal joints of the hand. On radiographs, typical marginal osteophytes with or without bony erosions are seen. The erosions are first evident in the central portion of the subchondral bone, appearing as sharply marginated defects and producing a "gull wing" deformity[87] (Fig. 51–27). Intra-articular bony ankylosis may result. It must be emphasized that the clinical syndrome of inflammatory OA can occur in the absence of radiographically demonstrated bony erosions; therefore, the term *erosive OA* is not an ideal one for this disorder.

Magnetic Resonance Imaging in Osteoarthritis

MRI in patients with OA reflects the underlying pathologic changes. Osteophytes are well seen on MRI both at the

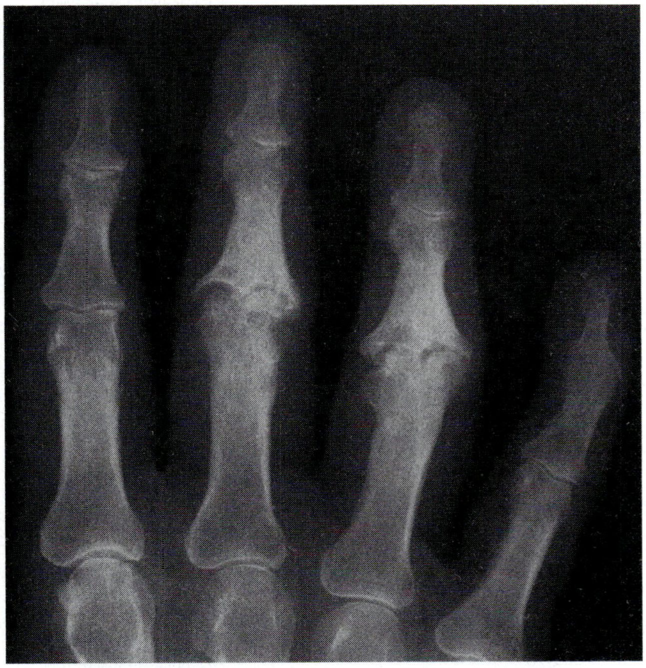

FIGURE 51–27 · Gull Wing Deformities in Erosive Arthritis. There is cartilage loss and bone remodeling at the middle and ring finger proximal interphalangeal joints, producing a "gull wing" appearance.

joint margins and beneath the articular cartilage. Often the osteophytes are better seen on MRI than on radiographs owing to the tomographic nature of MRI.[94] As in radiographs, the cortex of the osteophyte and the marrow are continuous from the host bone to the osteophyte.

Subchondral changes consist of edema, sclerosis, and cyst formation. Edema results from venous congestion and microfracture[94] (Fig. 51–25). These areas exhibit inhomogeneous, intermediate to low signal on T1-weighted or intermediate-weighted images and bright signal on fluid-sensitive sequences. Subchondral fibrosis and trabecular thickening replacing normal marrow result in hemispherical subchondral areas that are intermediate in signal on T1-weighted images and intermediate to low in signal on T2-weighted images.[99] Cystic changes may occur within the areas of subchondral sclerosis and produce well-defined lesions, usually with internal fluid signal.[95]

Synovial hypertrophy occurs in OA to a lesser degree than in RA but may be visible on MRI.[100] Investigation of the knees of patients with idiopathic OA by Fernandez-Madrid and colleagues showed synovial thickening in nearly three quarters of the patients.[101] The synovial change was unusual in that it appeared as nodules or grapelike clusters in the intercondylar region, around the cruciate ligaments, involved the infrapatellar fat pad with extension to the anterior horn of the lateral meniscus, or appeared as extensive involvement.[102] Synovial volume can be quantified.[103]

Crystal-Related Arthropathies

A variety of microcrystals can deposit in and about the joints and induce an inflammatory response. The crystals most frequently associated with arthropathy are monosodium urate (MSU), CPPD, and calcium hydroxyapatite (HA). The other entities that may be included in this group are hemochromatosis, ochronosis, and Wilson's disease.

Gout

The radiologic findings in acute gouty arthritis are nonspecific. These include soft tissue swelling, joint effusion, and periarticular osteopenia. Once the acute arthritic attack subsides, the bone remineralizes and more chronic, slowly progressive bony changes may develop.

Chronic tophaceous gout presents as an asymmetric, erosive, polyarticular disease, especially involving the feet, hands, wrists, elbows, and knees. The most common site of involvement is the first metatarsophalangeal joint. The shoulders, ankles, hips, sacroiliac joints, and spine are uncommon sites of involvement.

The radiologic changes in long-standing gout are related to tophi and their effect on soft tissue and bone. Tophi appear as eccentric, nodular soft tissue masses about the joints. They may have an amorphous increased density or patchy calcification.[104]

Intraosseous tophi may form, and these are usually recognized as small, well-marginated subchondral cystic lucencies. Calcification of urate deposits may produce intraosseous calcifications, similar to those of enchondromas and bone infarcts.[105]

The enlarging tophi can erode the adjacent bone or destroy bone from within, finally breaking out to produce erosions. The erosions may be intra-articular, para-articular, or remote from the joint. These erosions are usually well defined and round or oval, with sclerotic borders. The overhanging margin of bone is a characteristic feature of gout[106] (Fig. 51–28). This new bone develops at the margin of the erosion and forms as a result of stimulated periosteal bone apposition partially covering a tophus.

The preservation of joint space and bone density are characteristic of gouty arthritis until the destructive erosive changes lead to secondary OA and disuse osteopenia. Extensive destructive changes occasionally produce a mutilating arthritis. Bony ankylosis has also been described.[107]

Bursal inflammation commonly produces soft tissue swelling about the olecranon and in a prepatellar location. Adjacent tophi are frequently present as are adjacent bony erosions.

Chondrocalcinosis is occasionally detected in patients with gout, usually localized in knees, symphysis pubis and wrists, predominantly involving fibrocartilage.

MRI and CT imaging characteristics of gouty tophi have been described in several reports.[108-111] CT attenuation of tophi has been shown to measure about 160 HU, corresponding to the attenuation of monosodium crystal deposits measured in vitro.

On MRI, the tophi present as masses of low-to-intermediate signal on both T1- and T2-weighted images and show variable enhancement, including peripheral enhancement, after the intravenous administration of

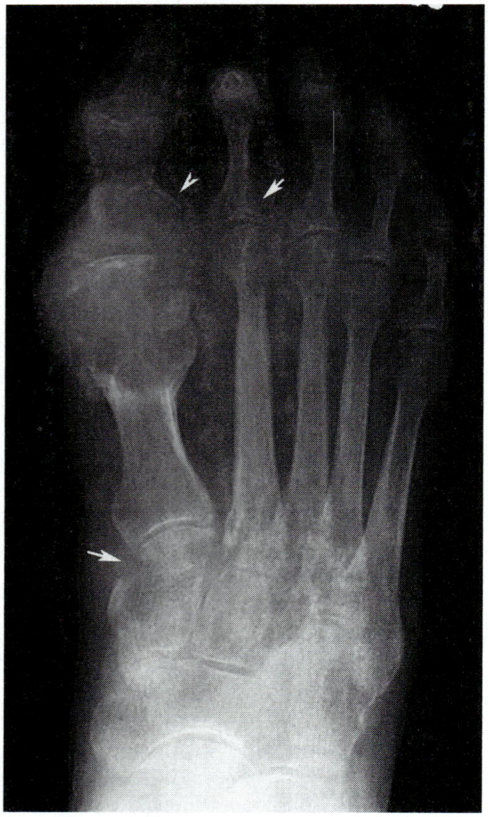

FIGURE 51–28 · **Radiographic Forefoot Abnormalities in Tophaceous Gout.** Extensive bone destruction is seen at the great toe metatarsophalangeal joint with overhanging edges *(arrowhead)* and soft tissue swelling. Smaller erosions are present involving the first tarsometatarsal and second metatarsophalangeal joints *(arrows)*.

gadolinium (Fig. 51–29). MRI may prove to be useful in the evaluation of various complications of gout, such as avascular necrosis, dissecting popliteal cysts, carpal tunnel syndrome, tendon ruptures, and spinal cord and nerve root compression.[111]

Calcium Pyrophosphate Dihydrate Crystal Deposition Disease

CPPD crystal deposition disease is the general term that includes asymptomatic CPPD crystal deposition, pseudogout, pyrophosphate arthropathy, and other less-frequent presentations such as pseudo–rheumatoid arthritis and pseudoneuropathic joints. Chondrocalcinosis refers to calcification of cartilage within one or more joints, regardless of its etiology. These calcium compounds may consist of CPPD, dicalcium phosphate dihydrate, or HA crystals.[112]

During acute attacks of pseudogout, the usual radiographic findings are soft tissue swelling and joint effusion. Chondrocalcinosis may or may not be present.

The radiologic changes in pyrophosphate arthropathy are joint-space narrowing, sclerosis, and subchondral cysts, similar to OA, with or without radiographically detectable intra- or periarticular calcifications. Intra-articular calcifications can occur in both fibrocartilage

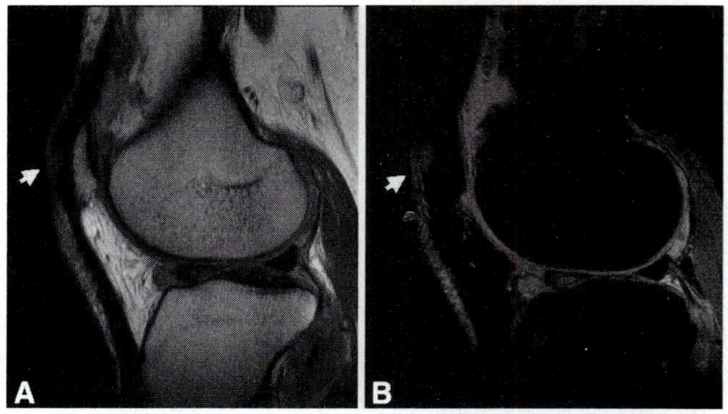

FIGURE 51–29 · **MR Imaging in Gout.** Sagittal FSE (fast spin echo) proton density *(A)* and fat suppressed FSE T2-weighted *(B)* images of the knee show a small tophus *(small arrows)* of low to intermediate signal intensity eroding the lateral aspect of the patella. The joint fluid also contains low to intermediate signal tophaceous material or synovitis.

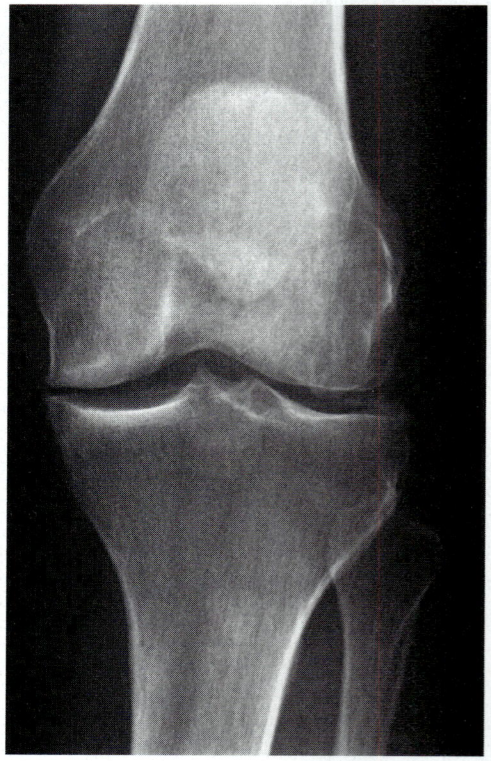

FIGURE 51–30 · **Calcium Pyrophosphate Dihydrate Crystal Deposition Disease Producing Chondrocalcinosis.** There is linear calcification within the hyaline cartilage and lateral meniscus.

and hyaline cartilage (Fig. 51–30). Fibrocartilaginous calcifications are most frequently observed in the menisci of the knee, triangular fibrocartilage of the wrist, acetabular labra, symphysis pubis, and annulus fibrosus of the intervertebral disk. Calcifications may also be deposited in bursae, synovium, ligaments, and tendons (Fig. 51–31). MRI detects calcification of hyaline cartilage as an area of low signal intensity, especially on gradient echo images, whereas the meniscal chondrocalcinosis exhibits increased signal on T1-weighted and PD images and may simulate meniscal degeneration or tear.[113,114]

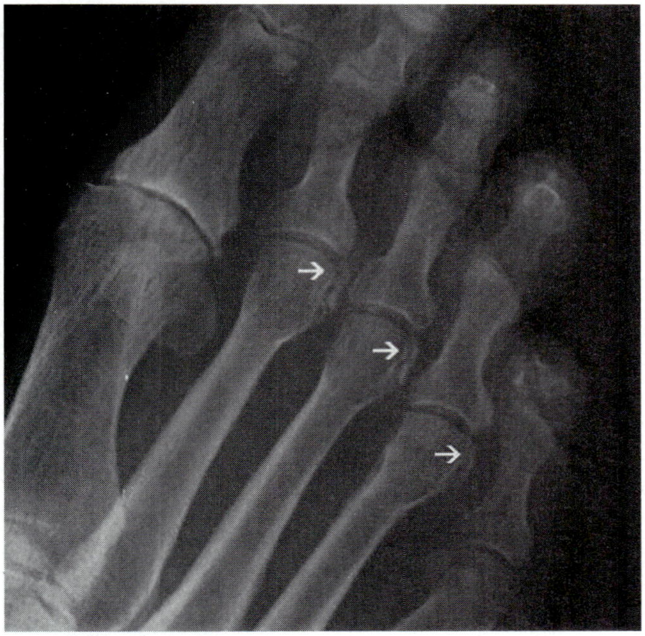

FIGURE 51–31 · Calcium Pyrophosphate Dihydrate Crystal Deposition Disease. Cartilaginous and capsular calcifications *(arrows)* are seen within 2nd through 4th metatarsophalangeal joints. A nondisplaced fracture of 4th metatarsal neck is noted.

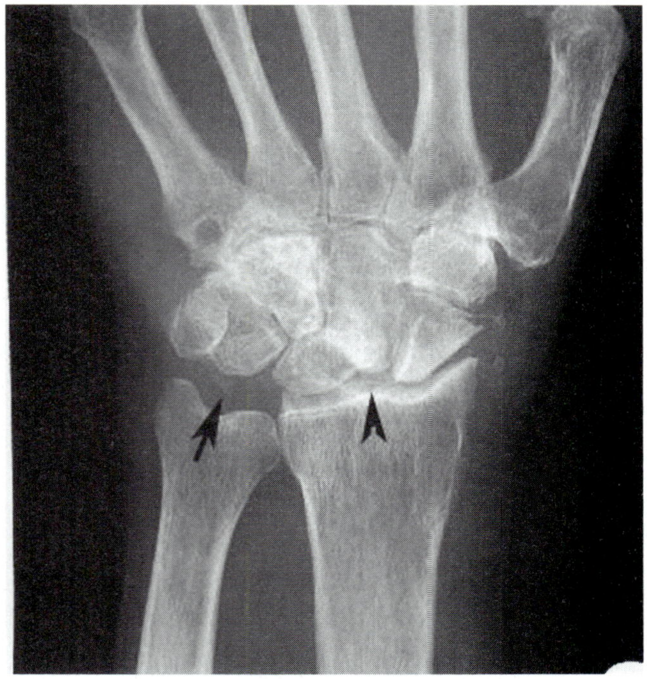

FIGURE 51–32 · Scapholunate Advanced Collapse (SLAC wrist) Secondary to CPPD Arthropathy. A posteroanterior view of the wrist shows widening of the scapholunate distance *(arrow)* with proximal migration of capitate and calcification of hyaline cartilage, triangular fibrocartilage *(arrow)* and interosseous lunoattriquetral ligament. Subchondral cysts are also seen in the carpal bones and at the base of the 5th metacarpal.

The subchondral cystic changes are one of the hallmarks of this arthropathy. They may have a distinctive radiologic appearance not usually observed in ordinary OA. These cysts appear as clusters of coalescent lucencies, varying in size and shape, with slightly sclerotic, smudged, and indistinct margins.[115]

The patellofemoral, radiocarpal, and metacarpophalangeal joints (especially the second and third metacarpophalangeal joints) are typical sites of involvement in pyrophosphate arthropathy. The distribution is usually bilateral and often symmetric. In addition to the usual target sites, arthritic changes may be observed in the hip, elbow, shoulder, and sacroiliac joints.[116]

In the wrist, the radiocarpal compartment is the most common site of involvement. CPPD crystal deposition within the scapholunate ligament may predispose to its disruption with consequent scapholunate dissociation and carpal instability. Characteristic findings of scapholunate advanced collapse (SLAC) wrist may be observed with narrowing of radioscaphoid joint and proximal migration of the capitate[117] (Fig. 51–32). Narrowing of the capitolunate joint space is also common, as is involvement of the trape-zioscaphoid joint with or without involvement of the first carpometacarpal joint. Calcification of the triangular cartilage, intercarpal ligaments, or articular cartilage also may be encountered.

Although the structural joint changes superficially resemble OA, the distribution of joints or components of joints in pyrophosphate arthropathy is different from that of OA. Non–weight-bearing joints such as the wrist, elbow, and shoulder are commonly affected in pyrophosphate arthropathy as opposed to OA. The preferential involvement of the radiocarpal joint of the wrist and patellofemoral compartment of the knee are distinctive features of pyrophosphate arthropathy. The anterior talocalcaneonavicular joint is selectively affected when CPPD crystal deposition disease involves the foot.[116]

Pyrophosphate arthropathy may be associated with extensive and rapid subchondral bone collapse and fragmentation with intra-articular loose bodies, resembling neuropathic osteoarthropathy. Tumorous CPPD crystal deposits that resemble gouty tophi are occasionally observed, most frequently in digits, and are referred to as "tophaceous pseudogout."[118]

The most common spine abnormalities of CPPD crystal deposition disease are intervertebral disk and ligamentous calcifications. In the cervical spine, CPPD crystals may deposit around the odontoid process in the region of transverse ligament and produce cord compression and bone erosion, which may result in spontaneous fracture of odontoid process.[119]

Calcium Hydroxyapatite Crystal Deposition Disease

HADD is associated with a spectrum of abnormalities from monoarticular periarthritis to a destructive arthropathy, depending in large part on the peri- or intra-articular location of crystal deposition.

Periarticular calcium hydroxyapatite deposits generally appear as amorphous and fluffy calcifications without internal trabeculation. These deposits develop within tendons, ligaments, joint capsule, bursae, and periarticular soft tissues. Calcification may change in size over time, becoming larger, smaller, or disappearing

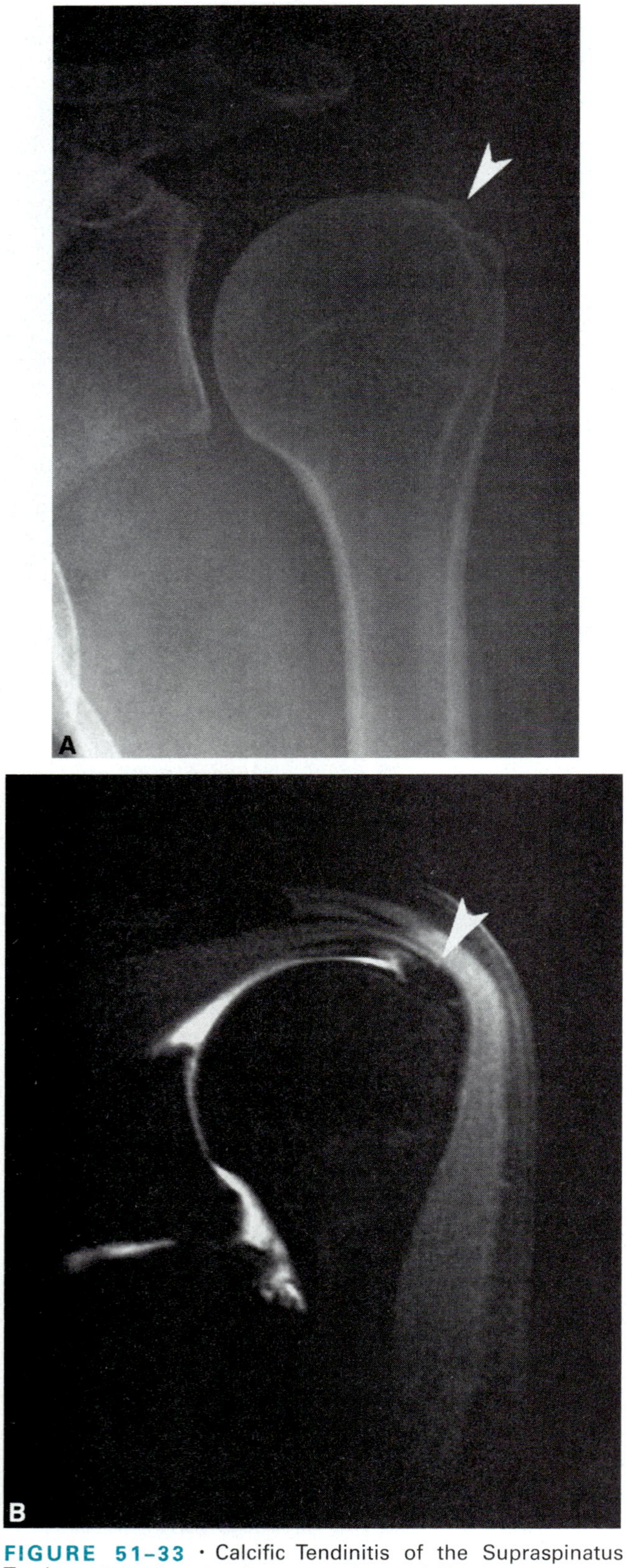

FIGURE 51–33 · Calcific Tendinitis of the Supraspinatus Tendon. *(A)* Grashey view shows amorphous calcifications *(arrowhead)* at the site of insertion of supraspinatus tendon on the greater tuberosity, *(B)* On corresponding MR arthrography; calcification appears as an area of low signal intensity *(arrowhead)* within the supraspinatus tendon and is less conspicuous.

completely. HADD is most commonly identified in the supraspinatus tendon of the rotator cuff (Fig. 51–33). Other sites include the longus colli muscle in the neck, gluteal insertion about the proximal femur, and the flexor carpi ulnaris tendon in the wrist.[120] Osseous erosion may develop adjacent to the involved tendon or ligament insertion site.

On MRI, the calcification itself is difficult to appreciate with most sequences unless it is large. The calcific deposits are of low signal intensity on all sequences. The surrounding inflamed and edematous soft tissues and muscles show high signal on T2-weighted images. Calcifications and the bone erosions beneath the calcified tendons are best shown on CT scan.[121,122]

Intra-articular HADD may be seen in association with OA or destructive arthropathy. When the accumulation of HA crystal is sufficient, amorphous or cloud-like radiodense areas within the joint can be detected; this may be accompanied by calcification in the synovial membrane and joint capsule. Structural joint changes include bone destruction, loss of cartilage, and joint deformity. The small joints of the hand are most frequently affected.[123]

HA-associated destructive arthritis of the shoulder has been described under the title "Milwaukee shoulder syndrome." The radiographic findings include bone destruction, intra-articular osseous debris, joint disorganization, and massive joint and bursal effusion. Osteophyte and subchondral cyst formation are infrequent. Associated massive rotator cuff tear results in superior displacement of humeral head so that it articulates with the undersurface of the acromion. Although shoulder involvement predominates, knees and hips may also be affected.[124]

Hemochromatosis

The radiologic features of the arthropathy of hemochrotic include signs of degenerative joint disease, chondrocalcinosis, and diffuse osteoporosis. Radiologic evidence of OA is present in approximately 50 percent of patients with hemochromatosis, and chondrocalcinosis is present in approximately 30 percent of the patients.[125,126]

The metacarpophalangeal joints, particularly the second and third, are the most frequently affected. The proximal interphalangeal and carpal joints, and the large joints such as those of the hip, knee, shoulder, ankle, and elbow are other sites of involvement. The spine may also be affected.[127]

The typical radiologic findings of the metacarpophalangeal joints in hemochromatosis are uniform joint-space narrowing, osteophytes, sharply marginated subchondral cysts, and subchondral sclerosis. Beak-like osteophytes arising from the radial aspect of the metacarpal heads are characteristic this disorder (Fig. 51–34). Wrist abnormalities consisting of joint-space narrowing, sclerosis, and cystic changes are seen in 30 to 50 percent of patients. The arthropathy of hemochromatosis has similar radiographic findings to CPPD crystal deposition disease. The presence of distinctive beak-like osteophytes of the metacarpal heads and osteoporosis may facilitate the differential diagnosis. The radiocarpal joint involve-

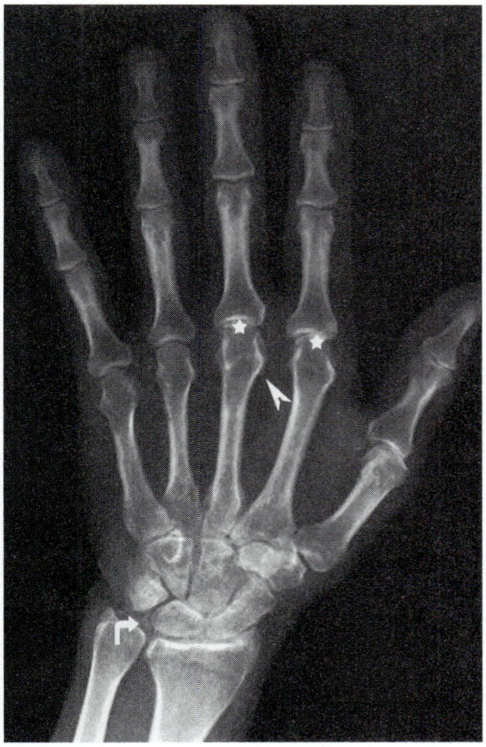

FIGURE 51–34 · Hemochromatosis. Hook-like osteophyte *(arrowhead)* at the third metacarpal head with cartilage loss at metacarpophalangeal joints (stars) and chondrocalcinosis of triangular fibrocartilage *(arrow)* are typical features of hemochromatosis.

ment and scapholunate dissociation are less frequent in hemochromatosis than in CPPD arthritis. The arthropathy of the hemochromatosis is usually slowly progressive, in contrast to idiopathic pyrophosphate arthropathy, in which a rapidly progressive arthropathy may be seen.[128]

MRI in hemochromatosis demonstrates the presence of hepatic iron overload as decreased signal intensity on both T1- and T2-weighted images due to the paramagnetic effect of iron. However, to date, MRI has not proven to be reliable in the detection of intraarticular iron.[129]

Wilson's Disease

The radiographic features of Wilson's disease include osteopenia, arthropathy, and chondrocalcinosis. Osteopenia is most apparent in the hands, feet, and spine. Osteoma-lacia and rickets have been reported in patients with Wilson's disease. In these patients, radiologic signs of rickets, retardation of skeletal maturation, and pseudofractures may be observed. Articular abnormalities described in Wilson's disease are subchondral bone fragmentation, cyst formation, and cortical irregularities, most commonly identified in the wrist, hand, foot, hip, shoulder, elbow, and knee. Irregularity and indistinctness of the subchondral bone may form a characteristic "paintbrush" appearance (Fig. 51–35). Additional characteristic radiographic findings are small, distinctly corticated ossicles about the affected joint and periosteal bone formation at the attachment sites of tendons and ligaments. Chondrocalcinosis is a rare finding, usually limited to the knees.[130,131]

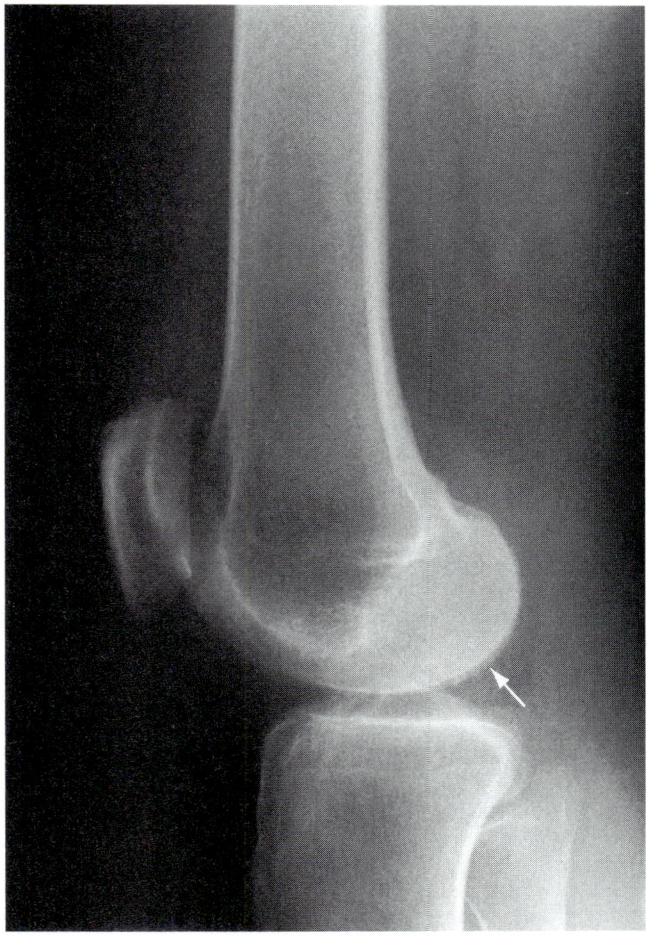

FIGURE 51–35 · Wilson's Disease. The lateral radiograph of the knee shows brush like calcifications *(arrow)* along the articular surface.

Ochronosis (Alkaptonuria)

The radiologic manifestations of skeletal involvement in alkaptonuria can be divided into spinal and extraspinal abnormalities. Spinal abnormalities include calcification and ossification of intervertebral disks, disk-space narrowing with vacuum phenomena, and osteoporosis (Fig. 51–36). Disk calcifications are usually distributed diffusely throughout the spine in a wafer-like configuration. The lumbar spine is affected first, followed by the dorsal and cervical spine. Calcifications are found predominantly in the inner fibers of the annulus fibrosis. Progressive ossification of disks and peripheral bony bridges may produce variable degrees of fusion of the vertebral bodies, simulating the "bamboo spine" appearance of ankylosing spondylitis. Osteoporosis may be associated with vertebral collapse.[132]

Extraspinal sites of calcification and ossification include the symphysis pubis, costal cartilage, helix of the ear, and peripheral tendons and ligaments. In the peripheral skeleton, the knees, hips, and shoulders are most commonly involved; more peripheral joint changes are rare. In these locations, radiologic changes resemble those of OA; however, osteophytes and subchondral cysts are not prominent in ochronosis. Occasionally, a rapidly progressing destructive peripheral arthropathy characterized by fragmentation of articular surfaces may be observed.[133]

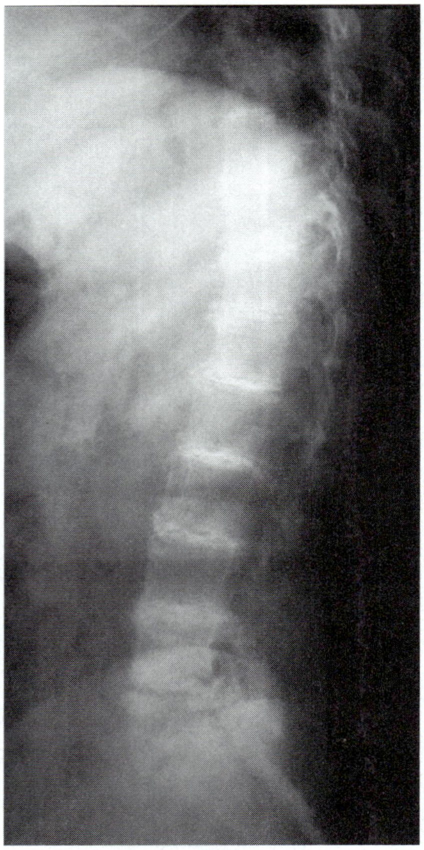

FIGURE 51–36 • Alkaptonuria. Spinal abnormalities; widespread disc space narrowing, disc calcification and osteoporosis are typical features of this disorder.

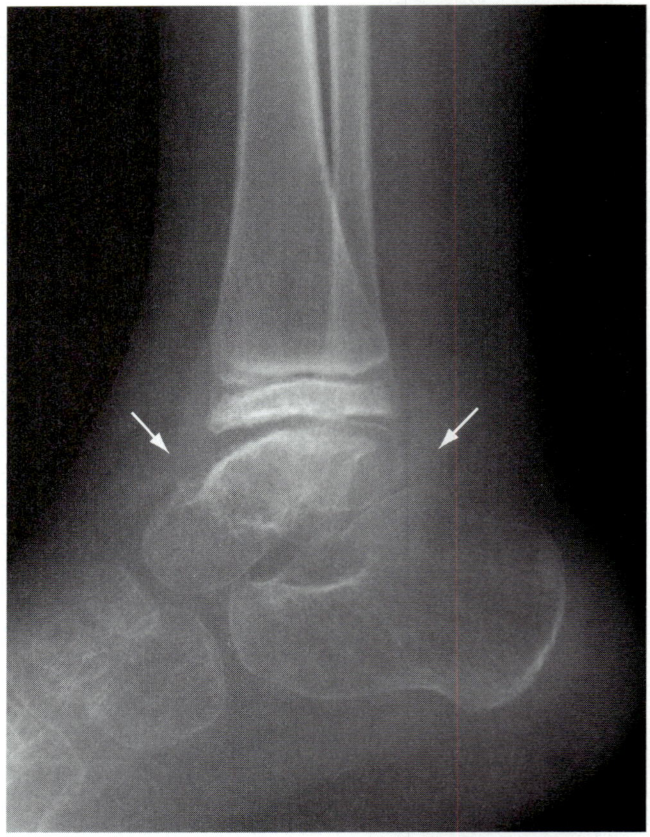

FIGURE 51–37 • Hemophilia. A lateral view of the ankle shows ankle joint distention *(arrows)*. The effusion appears more dense than the other soft tissues, consistent with hemosiderin deposition.

HEMATOLOGIC AND VASCULAR DISORDERS

Hemophilia

The arthropathy of hemophilia is related to destructive changes associated with repeated episodes of intra-articular hemorrhage (hemarthrosis) and the subsequent inflammatory reaction.[134] Any joint may be involved, but changes in the knee, ankle, and elbow are most frequently identified. The joint lining becomes thickened and brown, with hemosiderin present as fine particles within phagocytic cells.[135] The earliest radiographic findings are due to the large intra-articular effusions. Chronic effusions may appear dense because of the presence of hemosiderin (Fig. 51–37). This development is followed by osteoporosis and, in the immature skeleton, by epiphyseal overgrowth (Fig. 51–38). Subchondral cysts and bony erosions appear with subsequent cartilage destruction and joint-space narrowing. Late abnormalities include complete joint destruction with obliteration of the articular space, large bony erosions, and joint instability. In the knee, radiographic features of hemophilia include widening of the intercondylar notch of the distal femur and squaring of the inferior pole of the patella. The radiographic features of hemophilia may be difficult to differentiate from those of JCA.

MRI in patients with hemophilia may be helpful to assess the degree of damage present. The hemarthrosis, however, is not distinguishable from other types of joint effusion on MRI examination. Cyst formation and synovitis are more apparent on MRI than on radiographs. The synovitis in patients with hemophilia typically shows fronds of tissue with low-to-intermediate signal on all pulse sequences owing to its hemosiderin content (Fig. 51–39). MRI signal within the cysts varies depending on the content (e.g., low signal contents on T1-weighted and bright signal intensity on T2-weighted images suggest blood- or fluid-filled cysts).[136]

Osteonecrosis (Avascular Necrosis)

Osteonecrosis of the femoral head is the end result of a number of conditions that interrupt the blood supply to the femoral head. These conditions include traumatic disruption (e.g., femoral neck fractures, hip dislocations), vascular occlusion (e.g., sickle cell anemia, Caisson workers disease), vessel wall abnormalities (vasculitis), joint distention (e.g., sepsis) and other conditions including corticosteroid treatment and pancreatitis.

Radiographs are insensitive indicators of osteonecrosis (Fig. 51–40). Radiographic staging, usually a modification of the Ficat and Arlet classification,[137] is summarized in Table 51–2.

MRI is more sensitive than radiographs, CT scan, or bone scanning for the identification of osteonecrosis,

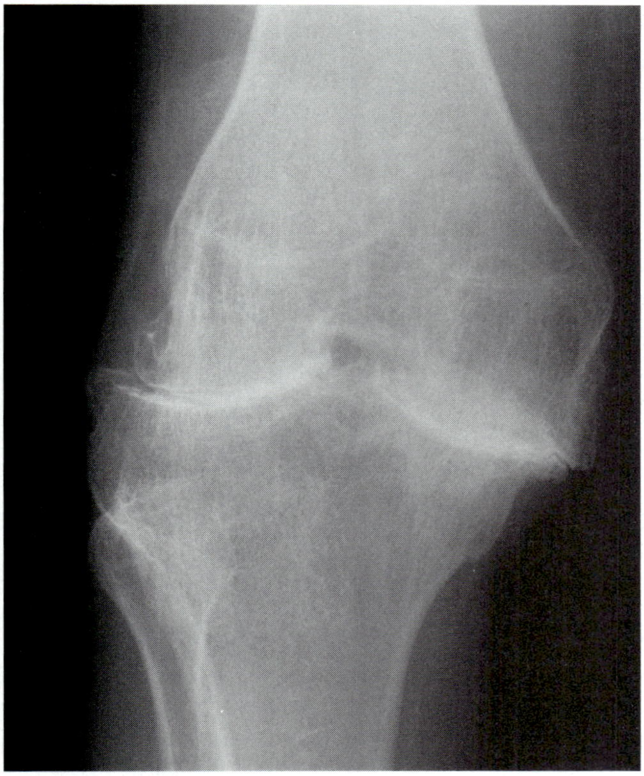

FIGURE 51–38 · **Hemophilia.** An anteroposterior radiograph of the knee shows severe cartilage space loss and secondary osteoarthritis with marginal osteophytes. There is widening of the intercondylar notch of the femur.

although occasional cases of osteonecrosis that are normal on MRI but abnormal on bone scintigraphy have been documented. Sensitivity of 97 percent and specificity of 98 percent have been reported for the MRI diagnosis of osteonecrosis.[138]

MRI findings depend on the replacement of normal bone marrow signal by abnormal signal resulting from cell death and the ensuing repair process. In adults, the femoral epiphyses are filled with yellow (fatty) marrow. Following vascular occlusion, cell death occurs, with hematopoietic cells dying within 6 to 12 hours, osteocytes dying at 12 to 48 hours, and fat cells dying 2 to 5 days after the insult.[138] After the fat cells die, the normal fat signal of the femoral head is altered.[137] Thus, theoretically, MRI findings could be abnormal within the first week after infarction. Healing proceeds from the periphery of the affected area centrally, with a hyperemic zone and granulation tissue developing around the infarcted area.

The signal abnormalities present on MRI in the center of femoral head lesions vary and have been characterized by Mitchell and coworkers as follows[139]:

Class A (fatlike lesions): The center of the lesion demonstrates the signal characteristics of fat
Class B (bloodlike lesions): The center of the lesion exhibits high signal on both T1- and T2-weighted images
Class C (fluid-like lesions): The center of the lesion has fluid-type signal; low on T1-weighted images and high signal on T2-weighted images
Class D (fibrous lesions): The center of the lesion demonstrates low signal on both T1- and T2-weighted images

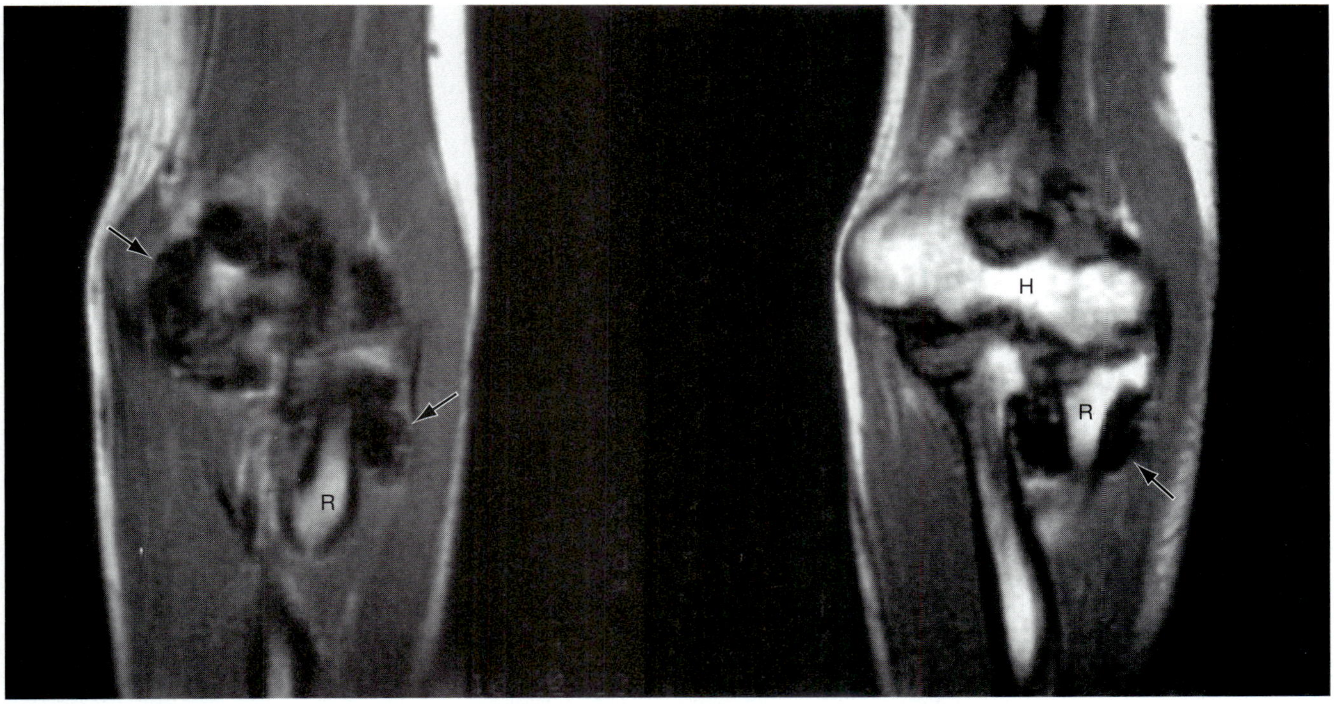

FIGURE 51–39 · **Hemophilia of the Elbow with Low Signal Synovial Tissue on MRI.** Two coronal T1-weighted images of the elbow the left more anterior, shows the low signal tissue *(arrows)*. R indicates radius, H humerus.

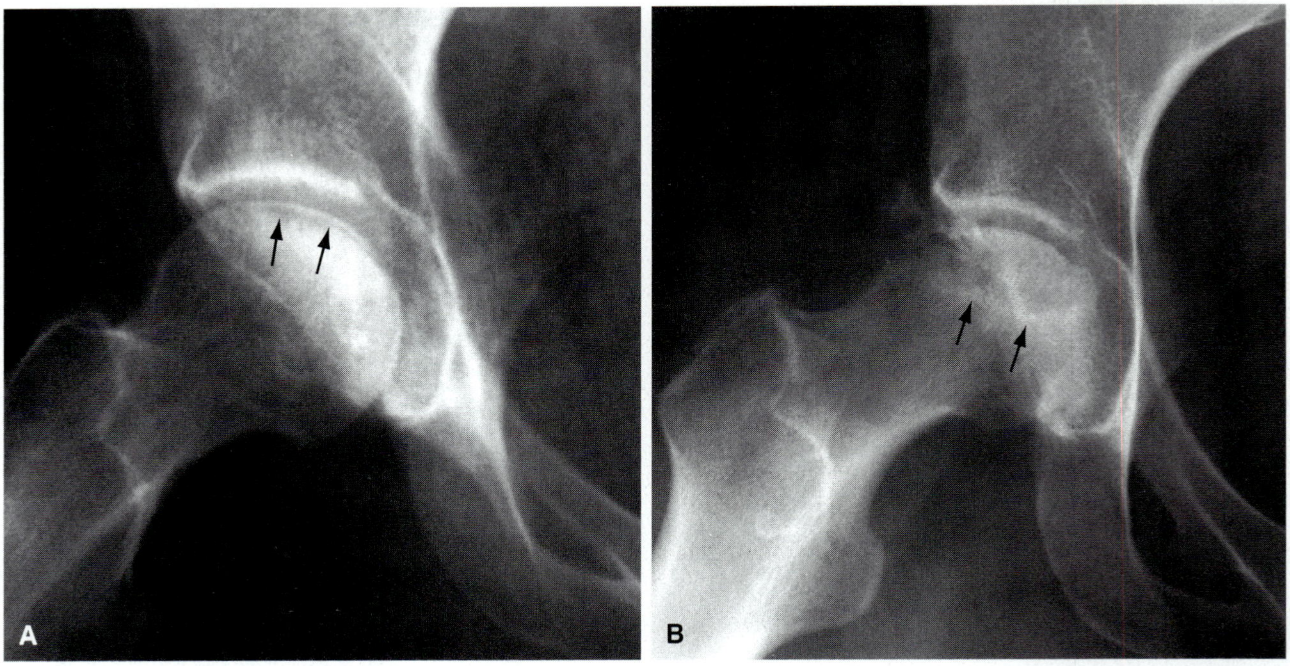

FIGURE 51–40 · Avascular Necrosis. *A*, The frog leg lateral view of the hip shows a lucency *(the cresent sign, arrows)* between the living subchondral bone and the dead bone of the femoral head. *B*, Late avascular necrosis is present with flattening of the articular surface. The area of infarcted bone appears largely lucent in this case with a rim of sclerosis *(arrows)* at the junction with the living bone.

Generally, class A lesions are early and class D lesions are the most chronic. Many lesions actually exhibit mixed signal.

As healing occurs, the periphery of the infarcted area becomes delimited by a low signal rim on T1-weighted images. On T2-weighted images, the inner portion of this rim exhibits bright signal, producing an appearance termed *the double line sign*[138] (Fig. 51–41). The inner bright zone most likely corresponds to granulation tissue, and the outer rim corresponds to sclerosis. Chemical shift artifact may accentuate the low signal rim. This double-line sign is diagnostic of osteonecrosis and is seen in up to 80 percent of cases.[138]

Other findings present in patients with osteonecrosis include premature conversion of intertrochanteric femoral hematopoietic marrow to fatty marrow, joint effusion, and a complete ("sealed off") epiphyseal scar.[140]

MRI may help determine the prognosis of avascular necrosis. In one series, involvement of less than 25 percent of the femoral head was unlikely to be associated with collapse of the femoral head, whereas when involvement of more than half of the head was seen, collapse was common.[141] As emphasized by Conway and Totty, MRI abnormalities occurring in the absence of clinical findings do not predict subsequent clinical avascular necrosis (AVN).[137]

In the knee, a particular form of "spontaneous" osteonecrosis is seen, most commonly involving the medial femoral condyle. The condition affects elderly persons, and the onset is abrupt. Radiographic changes

TABLE 51–2 · STAGING OSTEONECROSIS

Stage	Symptoms	Radiographic Findings	Bone Scintigraphic Findings	Magnetic Resonance Imaging Findings
0	None	Normal	+/– decreased flow	+/– low signal in head and focal marrow edema
I	Pain	Normal, +/– osteopenia	Decreased flow, increased uptake in reactive zone at edge of infarct	
II	Pain	Osteopenia and sclerosis	Larger area, increased uptake	Larger nonhomogeneous decreased signal on T1- and T2-weighted images
III	Pain	Crescent sign (fracture)	Focal cold area with surrounding increased activity	Heterogenous marrow abnormalities
IV	Pain	Flattening	Same as III	Femoral head flattening
V	Pain	Osteoarthritis	Same as III	Osteoarthritis

Adapted from Conway WF, Totty WG: Hip. *In* Stark DD, Bradley JR (eds): MR imaging. St. Louis, Mosby, 1999, 795-810.

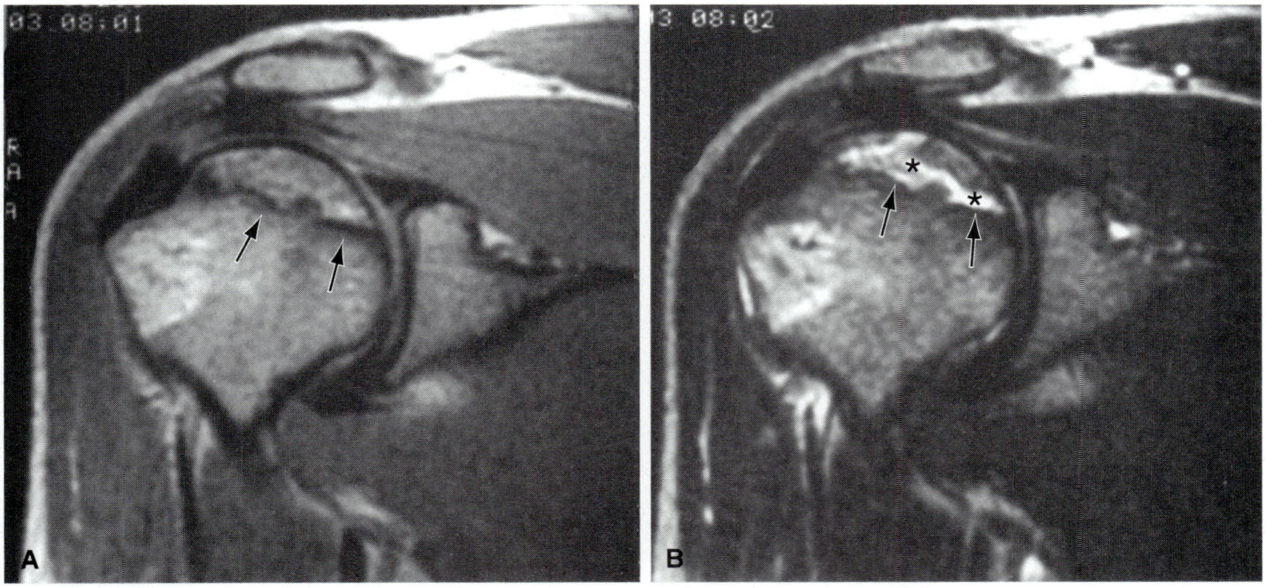

FIGURE 51–41 · Avascular Necrosis of the Humeral Head. *A*, T1-weighted SE image shows a black demarcation zone *(arrows)* between the avascular portion of the humeral head and the viable bone distally. *B*, The T1-weighted image shows the "double line" sign with an area of bright signal intensity (asterisks). The brighter signal region corresponds to granulation tissue.

are delayed, but eventually sclerosis, flattening, and irregularity of the femoral surface occur (Fig. 51–42). MRI is able to show marrow changes prior to radiographic abnormalities.

Bone Marrow Edema

Bone marrow edema may be an early feature of osteonecrosis or a finding accompanying a variety of disorders including stress fracture, osteomyelitis, tumor, transient osteoporosis, or transient marrow edema syndrome.[142] The MRI features of the edema pattern consist of poorly defined, diffusely abnormal signal intensity in the femoral head that extends to some degree into the femoral neck and intertrochanteric regions. The normal marrow signal is replaced by fluid signal, which is low on T1-weighted images and bright on T_2-weighted images (Fig. 51–43). Distinguishing patients with early osteonecrosis from those with transient osteoporosis and from those with transient bone marrow edema syndrome may be problematic. In transient osteoporosis, marked osteopenia is noted on radiographs, sometimes with the loss of the subchondral bone but with preservation of cartilage space. Infection must be excluded in these cases. Transient osteoporosis resolves spontaneously. The distinction between bone marrow edema and osteonecrosis is also difficult. Radiographs are normal in the transient marrow edema syndrome and in early osteonecrosis. Conway and Totty suggest that if no osteopenia is present on radiographic follow-up at 4 to 6 weeks, patients should be evaluated clinically and with MRI; those with high risk factors for osteonecrosis should be considered for early surgical intervention, and those without risk factors should be carefully followed clinically and with radiographs and MRI.[137] Vande Berg and coworkers found that analysis of subchondral signal was helpful.[143] The absence of any signal abnormality in the subchondral region (besides the edema) on T2-weighted or contrast-enhanced T1-weighted images was evidence of a transient lesion rather than osteonecrosis in all cases.

Neuropathic Osteoarthropathy

Neuropathic osteoarthropathy (Charcot joint) is a progressive destructive arthropathy associated with a number of diseases that produce loss of pain sensation and proprioception. The majority of the cases of neuropathic osteoarthropathy occur in patients with diabetes; less-frequent causes are syringomyelia, syphilis, congenital insensitivity to pain, myelomeningocele, and alcohol abuse.

There are two different hypotheses proposed for the pathogenesis of neuroarthropathy: The "neurotraumatic" theory postulates that the loss of joint sensation, unperceived repetitive trauma, ligamentous laxity, and continued joint use all lead to permanent damage to the bone and articular structures. The second mechanism, known as the "neurovascular" theory, postulates a neurovascular reflex with regional hyperemia causing osteoclastic stimulation and active bone resorption. It seems likely that both mechanisms play a role, and the resultant hypertrophic and resorptive appearance of the joint reflects the final balance of the two.[144]

The radiographic abnormalities of neuropathic osteoarthropathy have been subdivided into hypertrophic and atrophic types. The earliest radiographic findings are joint effusion and soft tissue swelling. At this stage the bony contours may remain well defined. Abnormal joint alignment from subluxation may be found before any bony changes are visible. Subsequently, fragmentation of the articular surfaces occurs leading to disorganization of the joint with large amounts of intra- and extra-articular osseous and calcified debris. Osseous

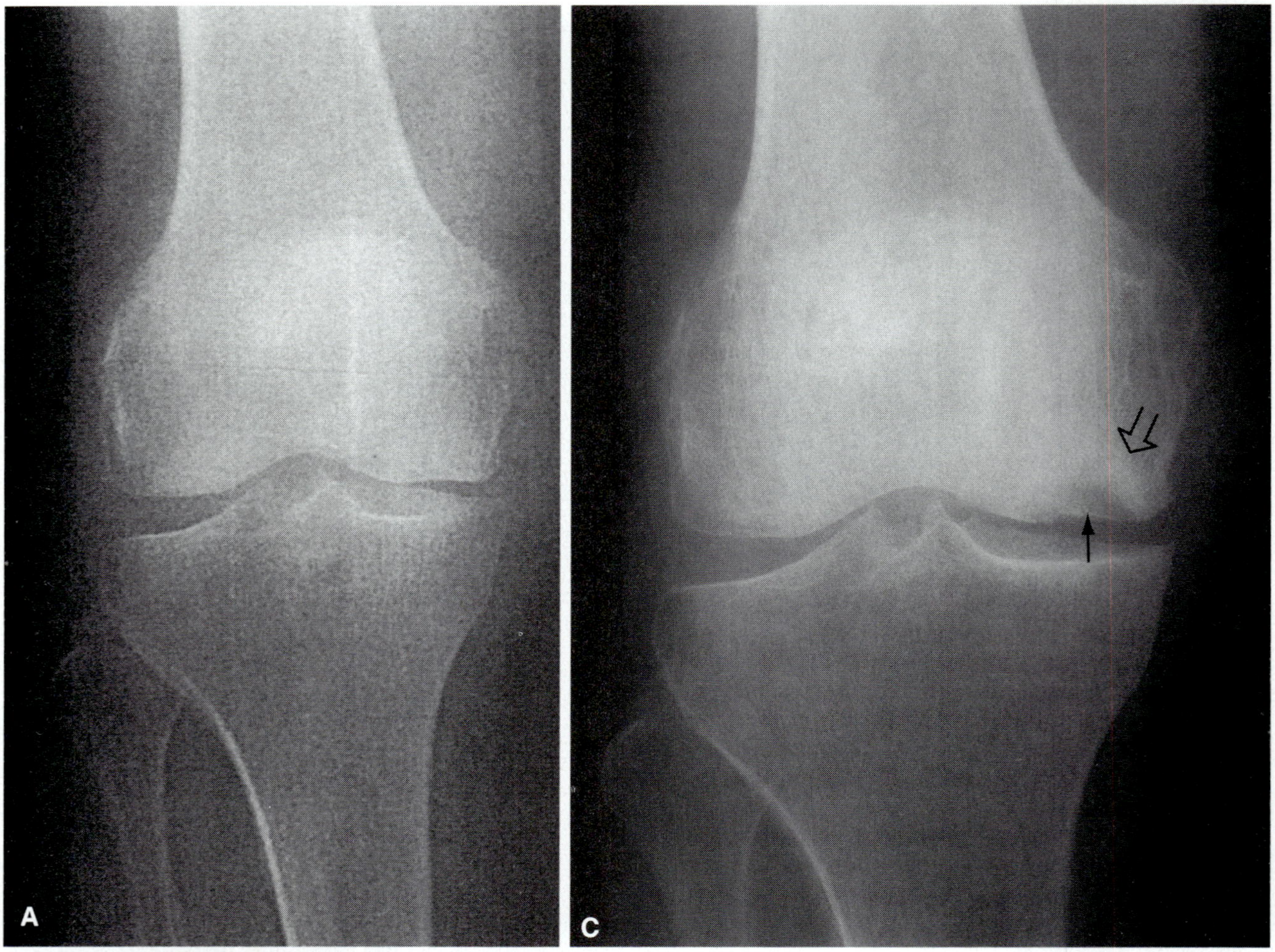

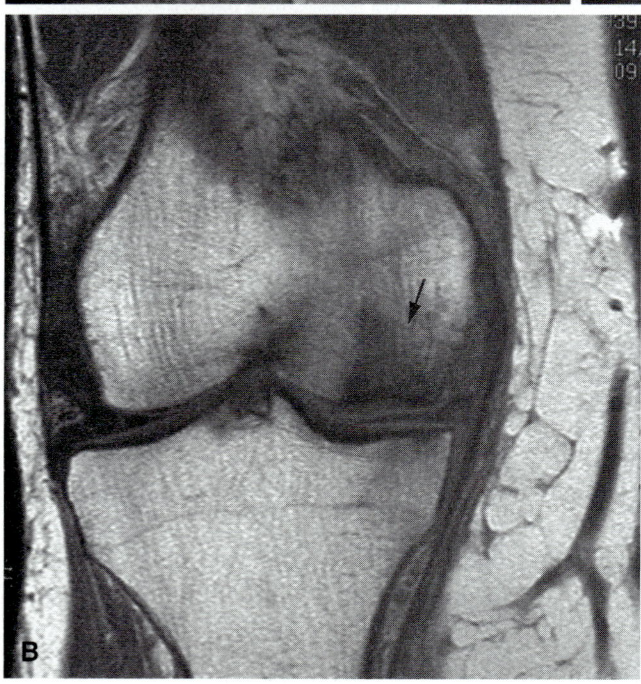

FIGURE 51–42 · Spontaneous Osteonecrosis. *A*, Initial radiograph shows mild medial cartilage space narrowing. Questionable subchondral lucency of the medial femoral condyle is noted. *B*, The T1-weighted shows coronal image a prominent focal area of low in the medial femoral condyle. *C*, Radiograph obtained months later shows diagnostic features of osteonecrosis with a subchondral area of lucency surrounded by sclerosis *(open arrow)* and a depressed cortical bone fragment *(arrow)*. The medial cartilage space is slightly narrow, and there are tiny osteophytes.

proliferation in the form of periosteal new bone formation, sclerosis, and osteophytes is also a characteristic finding. These findings are referred to as the "Ds" of neuropathic arthropathy: debris, destruction, dislocation, and no demineralization (Fig. 51–44).

Fractures of the neighboring bones are often demonstrated in neuropathic arthropathy. These fractures may occur spontaneously or with minor trauma and tend to be transverse, unlike the fractures associated with trauma, which are often spiral or oblique. In the atrophic form,

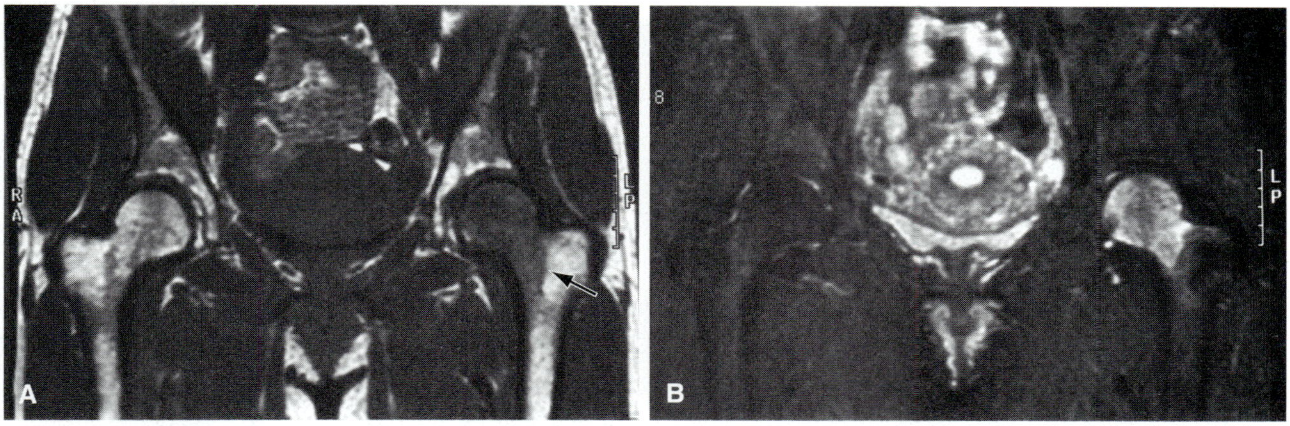

FIGURE 51–43 · Bone Marrow Edema. *A*, The T1-weighted image shows replacement of normal left proximal femoral marrow fat by intermediate signal *(arrow)*. *B*, The STIR (short tau inversion recovery) image shows the poorly defined increased signal in the proximal femur consistent with edema.

the affected joint has sharp edges, resembling surgical amputation with little or absent bone repair (Fig. 51–45).

Diabetes Mellitus

Diabetes mellitus is the most common cause of neuropathic osteoarthropathy. The joints involved are almost always in the lower extremity, especially the feet. The tarsal, tarsometatarsal, and metatarsophalangeal joints are most commonly affected. Arthropathy of the ankle and knee is also seen. Spinal, elbow, and wrist involvement have also been reported.[145-147]

The most common radiographic finding is a longstanding Lisfranc fracture-dislocation with eburnation and fragmentation of the tarsometatarsal joints. Calcaneal fractures, talocalcaneal joint dissolution, collapse of the talus, talar angulation within the ankle mortise, and distal fibular fractures are also encountered. In the forefoot, osseous resorption may result in tapering or sharpening of metatarsal and phalangeal shafts.[148]

Neuropathic joint changes and infection may coexist in the affected foot in diabetes.

The radiologic changes of neuropathic joint make the diagnosis of superimposed infection a diagnostic challenge. The presense of fuzzy bone margins and osteoporosis may suggest infection. Scintigraphy is sensitive, but not specific; 99mTc-MDP, gallium, and indium-111–labeled WBC scans cannot reliably distinguish between osteomyelitis and neuropathic arthropathy because of extensive bone remodeling and inflammation, which are present in both conditions.[149]

MRI may play a role in the evaluation of the neuropathic joint.[82,150-152] On MRI, marrow and soft tissue edema, joint effusion, articular destruction with fragmentation, and malalignment characterize neuropathic osteoarthropathy (Fig. 51–46). If the bone marrow changes around the affected joint exhibit decreased signal intensity on both T1- and T2-weighted images, superimposed infection can be virtually excluded. If bone marrow has decreased signal intensity on T1-weighted and increased signal intensity on T2-weighted images and similar changes of signal intensity in the adjacent soft tissues, it may represent acutely evolving neuropathic arthropathy with or without concomitant infection. Evaluation of adjacent soft tissue for ulceration and underlying cortical destruction are helpful in suggesting osteomyelitis.

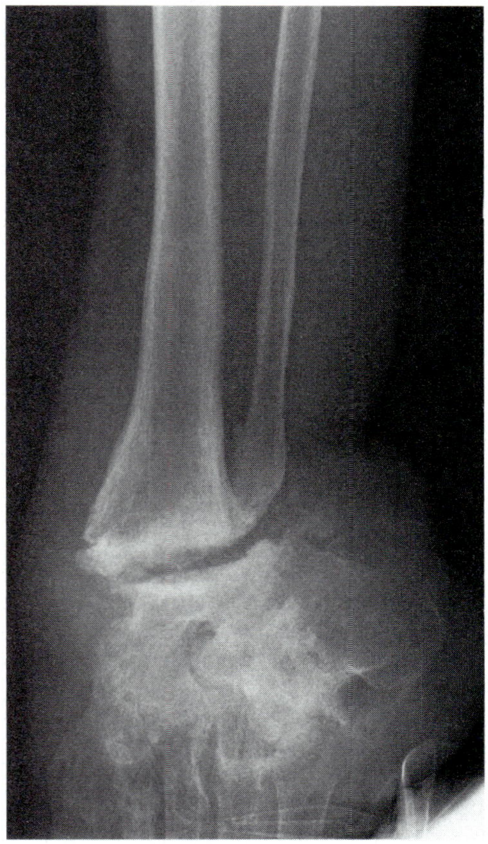

FIGURE 51–44 · Severe Neuropathic Changes in the Ankle of a Diabetic Patient. Complete destruction of the joint with sclerosis and fragmentation of the joint margins is noted.

Syringomyelia

Approximately 20 to 25 percent of the patients with syringomyelia develop neuroarthropathy. There is a distinct predilection for the joints of the upper extremity,

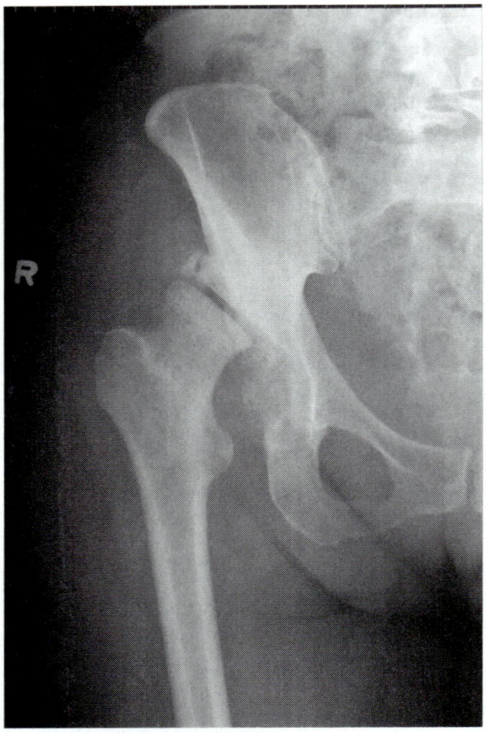

FIGURE 51–45 · Atrophic neuropathic osteoarthropathy of right hip, secondary to spinal dysraphism

especially the glenohumeral joint, elbow, and wrist. Lower extremity or spinal alterations may also occur.

Tabes Dorsalis

Five to 10 percent of patients with tabes dorsalis demonstrate neuroarthropathy. The joints of the lower extremity are most affected, with knee and hip being the most frequent target sites. Involvement of the axial skeleton is not uncommon in tabes. The thoracolumbar junction and lumbar spine are most frequently affected, and one or more vertebral segments may be involved.

The radiologic appearance of spinal neuroarthropathy may be similar to that of severe degenerative disease, spinal infection, or metastatic disease. The CT and MRI findings, such as presence of vacuum disk, facet involvement, spondylolisthesis, joint disorganization, and debris and gadolinium enhancement in the periphery of the disk, help to differentiate spinal neuropathic arthropathy from infection, favoring the former.[153,154]

Connective Tissue Disorders

PROGRESSIVE SYSTEMIC SCLEROSIS (SCLERODERMA)

Soft tissue or bony involvement in progressive systemic sclerosis (PSS) is common. The radiographic abnormalities can be divided into four main categories[155]: 1) soft tissue resorption, 2) soft tissue calcification, 3) osteolysis, and 4) erosive articular disease.

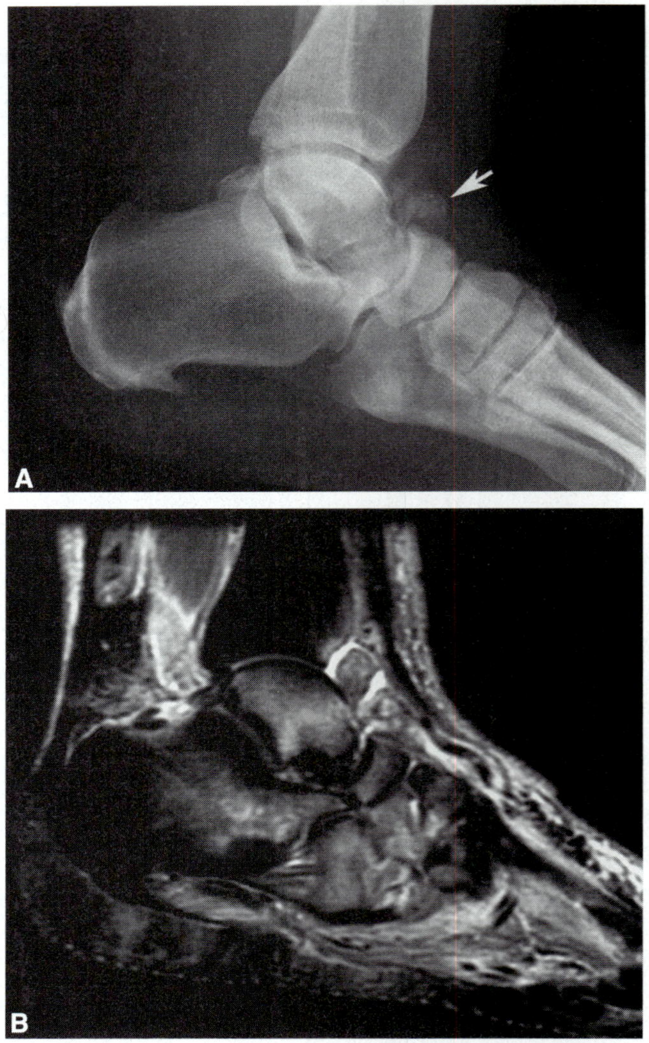

FIGURE 51–46 · Early Changes of Neuropathic Osteoarthropathy involving the Talonavicular joint in a Diabetic patient. *A*, Lateral view reveals calcific debris at the dorsal aspect of the talonavicular joint which shows subtle incongruity. *B*, Sagittal STIR (short-term inversion recovery) MR image shows extensive bone marrow edema in tarsal bones and soft tissue edema. Subluxation of the talonavicular joint appears more conspicuous. The calcific debris detected on plain film appears as material of inhomogeneous signal outlined by bright joint fluid about the talonavicular joint.

Soft tissue resorption is most commonly noted in the fingertips in association with Raynaud's phenomenon (Fig. 51–47). Early changes can be identified by noting a reduction in the normal distance between the phalangeal tips and the skin (the normal distance is approximately 20 percent of the transverse diameter of the base of the same phalanx).[156] In time, the fingertip assumes a conical shape, and soft tissue calcification is often present.

Soft tissue calcification is most common in the hand but may occur at virtually any site.[157,158] Calcification may be present in subcutaneous tissue, joint capsule, tendons, or ligaments. The calcification typically is composed of hydroxyapatite crystals and has a cloudlike radiographic appearance. Occasionally, large tumoral collections may be present adjacent to a joint. Intra-articular or intraosseous calcification may also be noted.

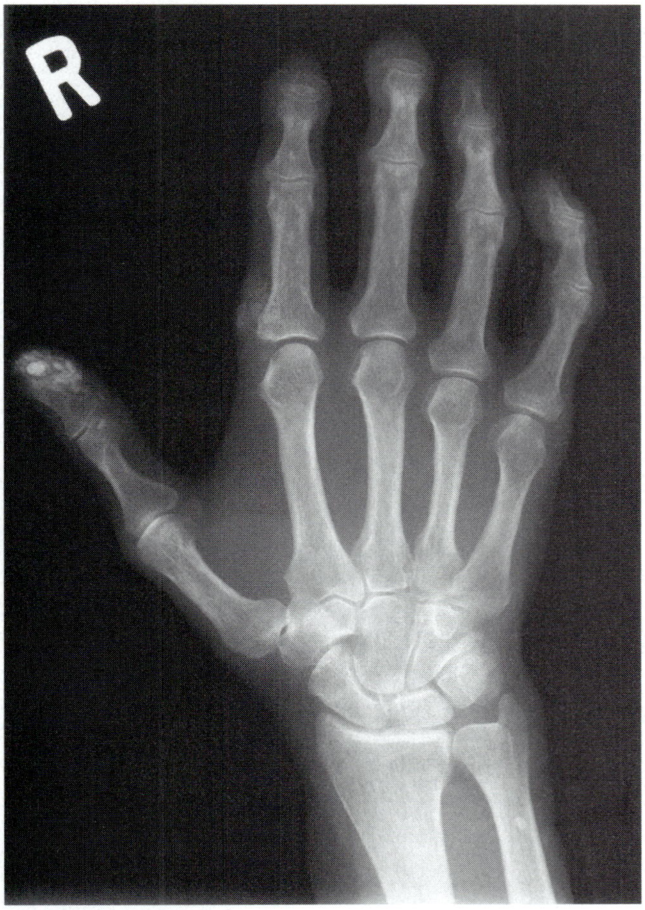

FIGURE 51–47 · Scleroderma. This posterioranterior radiograph demonstrates flexion of the fingers, loss of the tufts of the index finger and middle finger distal phalanges and calcification including finger tip calcification.

Extra-articular osteolysis is frequently a manifestation of PSS. The most common sites are the tufts of the distal phalanges of the hand, or occasionally of the foot, usually in association with Raynaud's phenomenon and soft tissue calcification. The earliest change is in the volar aspect of the tuft with continuing resorption, leading to a "sharpened" appearance of the phalanx. Elsewhere, thickening of the periodontal membrane about the roots of the teeth[159] or localized mandibular osteolysis may be seen, the latter predisposing to pathologic fracture. Localized osteolysis involving the ribs, acromion, clavicle, radius, ulna, and cervical spine has also been reported.[160-163]

A severe articular disease consisting of joint-space narrowing, marginal and central osseous erosions, and deformity may occur.[164] There is a tendency toward involvement of the first carpometacarpal joint.[165] Indeed, bilateral destructive changes of the first carpometacarpal articulation with joint subluxation should arouse suspicion of PSS. Other relatively common sites of joint involvement in PSS include the distal interphalangeal, proximal interphalangeal, distal radioulnar, and metatarsophalangeal joints.

Patients with scleroderma may exhibit a spectrum of muscle disease ranging from fatigue, most likely without objective findings, to an inflammatory myositis resembling dermatomyositis.[166] MRI is useful for evaluating the presence and extent of inflammatory muscle disease.

SYSTEMIC LUPUS ERYTHEMATOSUS

The roentgenographic changes of systemic lupus erythematosus (SLE) include symmetric polyarthritis, deforming nonerosive arthropathy, spontaneous tendon rupture (Fig. 51–48), osteonecrosis, soft tissue calcification, acral sclerosis, and tuft resorption.[167-175] The radiographic changes of polyarthritis in SLE are nonspecific and consist of soft tissue swelling and periarticular osteoporosis.[167,168] Joint-space narrowing and bony erosions are unusual. Deforming nonerosive arthropathy is seen in 5 to 40 percent of patients with SLE. Symmetric involvement of the hands is typical. The specific type of deformity is variable.[167-169] Swan neck or boutonnière deformity can be evident. Other deformities include hyperextension of the interphalangeal joint of the thumb, ulnar drift at the metacarpophalangeal joints, and subluxation of the first carpometacarpal joint. The prominent thumb deformity is especially characteristic of lupus arthropathy (see Fig. 51–48).

Although bony and cartilaginous abnormalities are generally not present, joint-space narrowing, "hook-like" erosions of the radial and volar aspects of the metacarpal heads, and subchondral cyst formation are occasionally encountered.

Linear and nodular calcific deposits in the subcutaneous tissues, particularly in the lower extremities, may occasionally be seen in SLE.[173] Sclerosis (acrosclerosis) or resorption of the tufts of the terminal phalanges is also occasionally evident in SLE.[175]

The prevalence and severity of avascular necrosis (AVN) in SLE patients on glucocorticoid treatment are reported to be higher than in patients without SLE.[176]

Osteonecrosis in patients may affect small bones. MRI prognostication of AVN in SLE patients with normal radiographs was performed by Sugano and coworkers,[177] who concluded that the location and size of AVN were major elements of prognosis. This study also showed that if the MRI findings were normal 1 year after treatment, progression to femoral head collapse was unlikely.

DERMATOMYOSITIS AND POLYMYOSITIS

Articular abnormalities in dermatomyositis and polymyositis are usually without radiographic manifestations, although periarticular soft tissue swelling and osteoporosis are noted occasionally.[178] More dramatic radiographic changes occur in the skeletal musculature, especially the large proximal muscle groups of the thorax, arm, forearm, thigh, and calf. Initial inflammation produces increased bulk and radiodensity of muscles with loss of the normal intermuscular fat planes.[179] In later stages, muscle atrophy or contractures may be prominent. The most characteristic soft tissue abnormality is calcification in subcutaneous tissue, intermuscular fascia, tendons, or fat (Fig. 51–49). Subcutaneous calcific deposits simulate those of progressive systemic sclerosis,

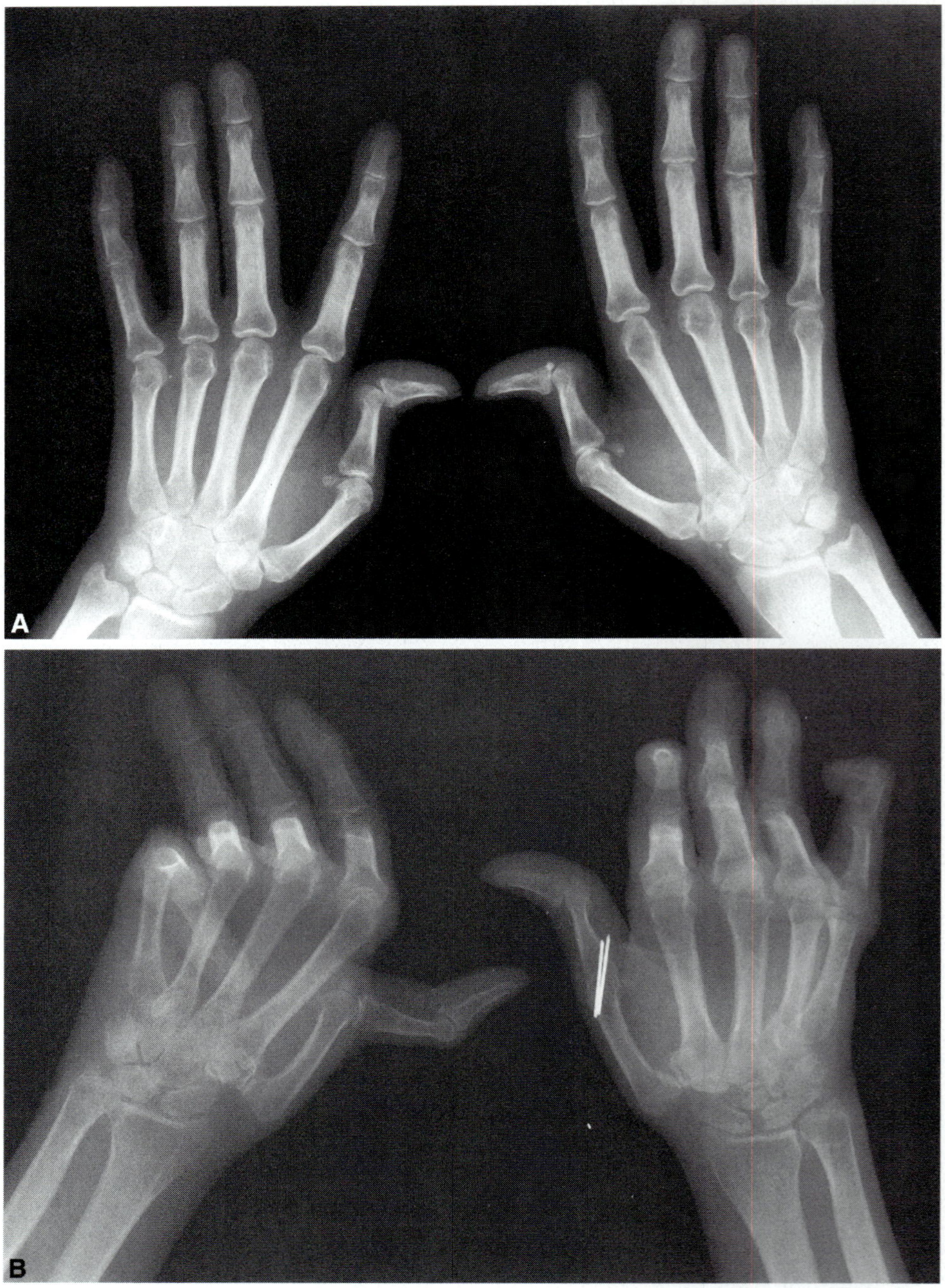

FIGURE 51–48 · Systemic lupus Erythematosus. *A*, A posteroanterior (PA) view of the hands and wrists shows hyperextension of the thumb interphalangeal joints. There are small calcifications at the radial aspect of the right wrist. *B*, PA view of the hands and wrists show multiple finger deformities. No erosions are present. (From Weissman BN, Rappoport AS, Sosman JL, Schur PH: Radiographic findings in patients with systemic lupus erythematosus. Radiology 126:313, 1978, Fig 1A.)

but the presence of marked linear calcification favors the diagnosis of polymyositis or dermatomyositis.

MRI of patients with polymyositis or dermatomyositis lesions has shown abnormal muscle signal consisting of either isointense signal on T1-weighted images with hyperintense signal on T2-weighted images (suggesting inflammation or edema) or fatty atrophy (Fig. 51–50). Inflammatory changes usually involve the entire muscle, whereas fatty atrophy often begins at the distal myotendinous junction. Muscle involvement may be asymmetric, and distal leg muscles as well as proximal are often involved. Inflammatory changes on MRI mirror the clinical findings.[180] MRI may be used to select a biopsy site and to follow the inflammatory response after treatment.[181]

Conditions Primarily Affecting the Spine

INFLAMMATORY DISORDERS

Rheumatoid Arthritis

Cervical spine involvement occurs in approximately two thirds of patients with RA.[182] In contrast to the frequency of cervical spine involvement, changes in thoracic and lumbar spine are uncommon in this disease.

The radiographic findings include osteoporosis, atlantoaxial and subaxial subluxations, erosions involving the vertebral endplates, apophyseal joints and spinous

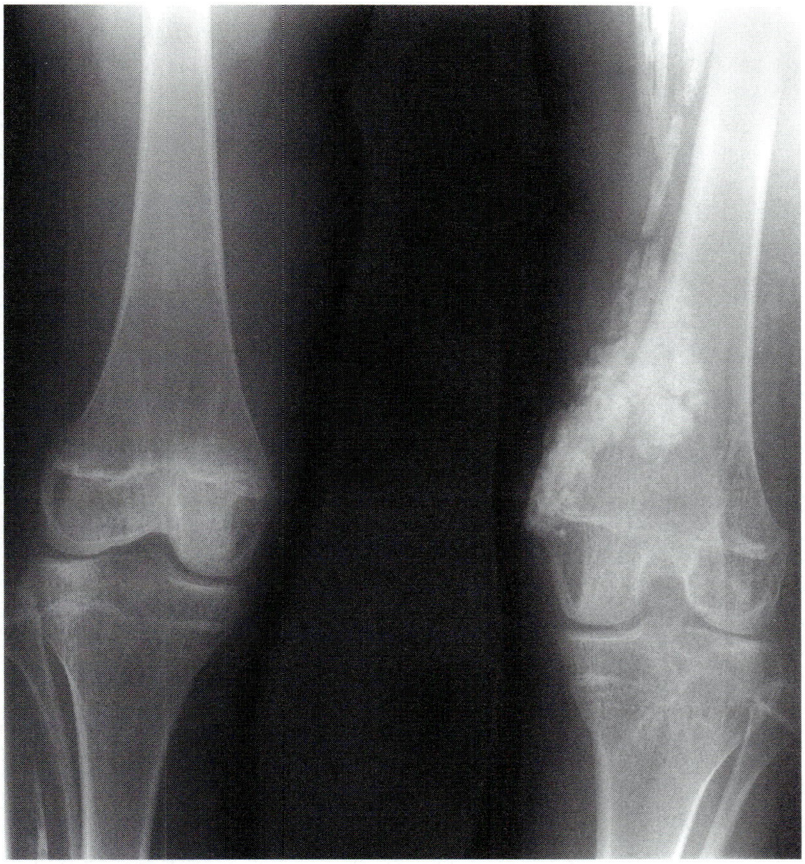

FIGURE 51–49 · Dermatomyositis. There is extensive soft tissue calcification.

processes, intervertebral disk-space narrowing, and, rarely, bony ankylosis of the apophyseal joints.

Although any segment of the cervical spine may be affected, the destructive changes at the occipitoatlantoaxial junction predominate. Erosive synovitis involving the atlantoaxial, atlantoodontoid, and atlantooccipital joints causes atlantoaxial subluxation. Atlantoaxial subluxation can be anterior, posterior, vertical, lateral, rotational, or a combination of these.

Anterior atlantoaxial subluxation (AAS) is the most common type of subluxation and is due to weakening and destruction of the transverse, alar, and apical liga-

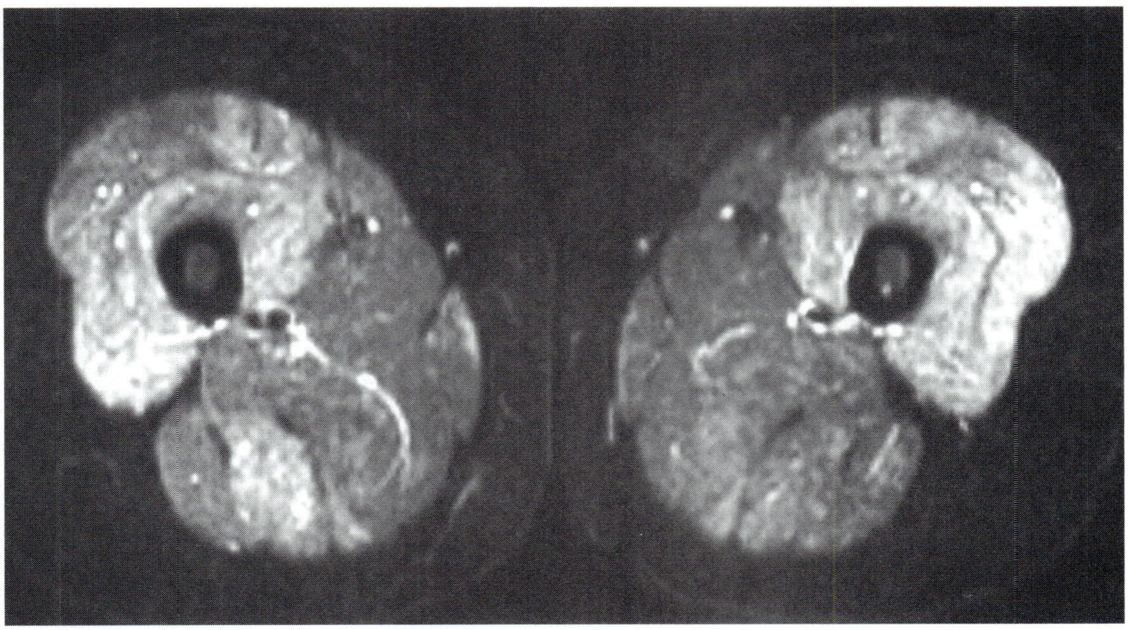

FIGURE 51–50 · Dermatomyositis. An axial STTR image through the thighs shows scattered muscle involvement demonstrated as increased signal in the involved muscles.

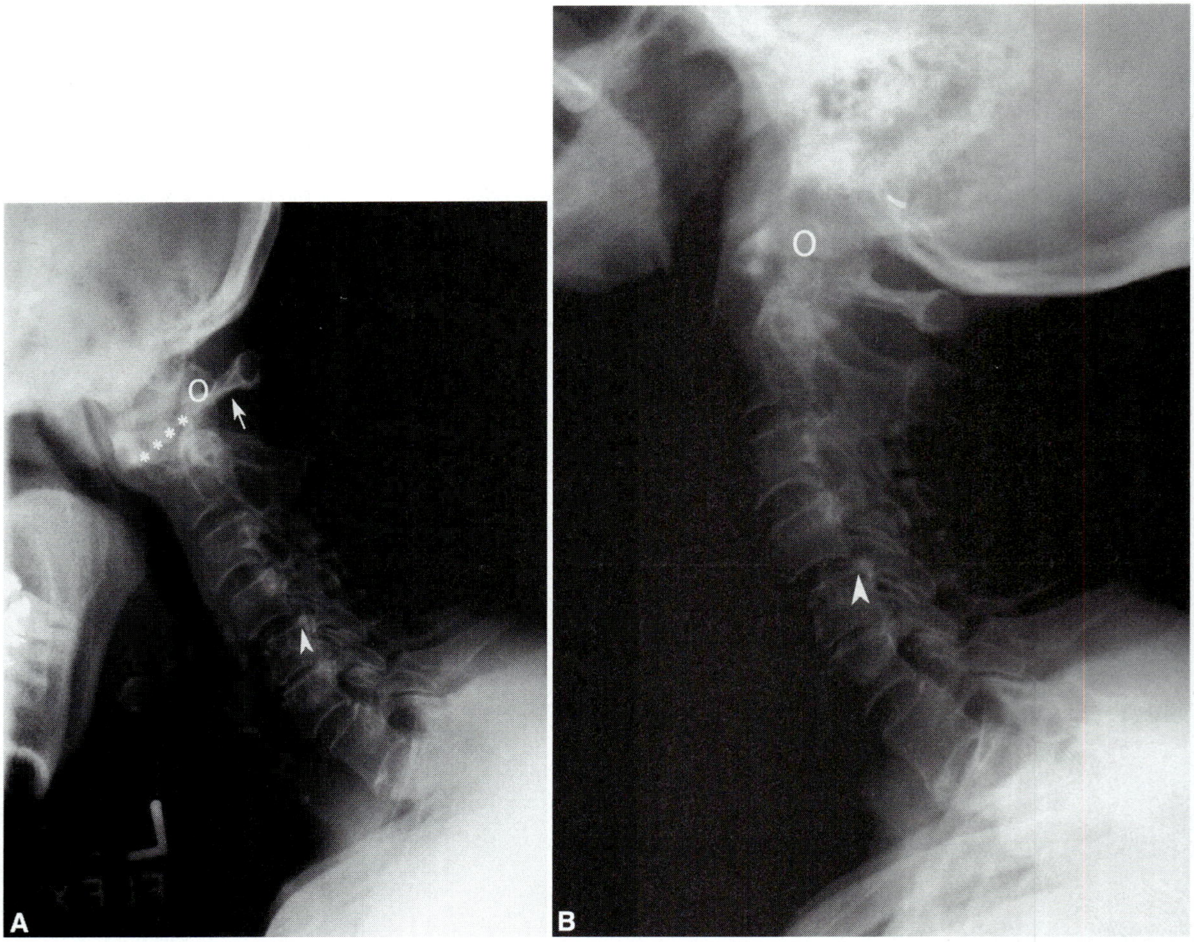

FIGURE 51–51 · **Rheumatoid Arthritis of Cervical Spine.** Lateral radiograph in flexion *(A)* demonstrates severe anterior atlanto-axial subluxation with a wide anterior atlantodental interval (AADI) (asterisks) and decreased posterior atlantodental interval (PADI) *(arrow)*. Almost complete reduction of subluxation is noted on the lateral view in extension *(B)*. There is also subaxial subluxation at the level of C4-C5 *(arrow heads)* with erosive changes in various facet joints. O indicates odontoid.

ments. Resultant anterior displacement of the atlas narrows the spinal canal and eventually causes spinal cord compression (Fig. 51–51). On lateral radiographs of the cervical spine, an anterior atlantodental interval (AADI) greater than 2.5 mm is considered abnormal in adults. The measurement is made from the posteroinferior arch of the atlas to the anterior surface of the odontoid. Radiographs should be obtained in both the flexion and extension positions, because radiographs taken in the neutral position may miss 48 percent of cases of anterior atlantoaxial subluxation, and subluxation may reduce extension.[183]

Vertical subluxation, also as known atlantoaxial impaction and cranial settling, is the least common, but clinically most dangerous, form of instability. Destruction of atlantoaxial and atlantooccipital joints leads to superior migration of the odontoid and surrounding pannus through the foreman magnum, impinging on the brain stem and spinal cord (Fig. 51–52).

Posterior atlantoaxial subluxation may occur in the setting of pathologic fracture or severe erosion of the odontoid. Asymmetric bony erosion and collapse of the lateral masses of C1 and C2 may lead to lateral atlantoaxial subluxation. Lateral subluxation is defined as more than 2 mm offset of the lateral masses of C1 and C2. Rotational deformity usually accompanies it. Clinically, these patients reveal fixed head tilt toward the side of osseous collapse and rotation of the face toward the opposite site.

In the lower cervical spine, involvement of apophyseal and uncovertebral joints, intervertebral disks, and interspinous ligaments results in subaxial subluxations and diskovertebral joint abnormalities (see Fig.51–51). Subaxial subluxations tend to occur at multiple levels giving the "stepladder" appearance of the cervical vertebral bodies.

The radiologic examination plays a key role in identifying patients who are at increased risk of developing neurologic sequelae. On the basis of plain radiographs, anterior atlantoaxial subluxation greater than 9 mm and the presence of atlantoaxial impaction have been defined as risk factors for cord compression.[184] Recent literature suggests that the posterior atlantodental interval (PADI), the distance measured between the posterior surface of the odontoid and the anterior margin of the posterior ring of atlas, is a better method

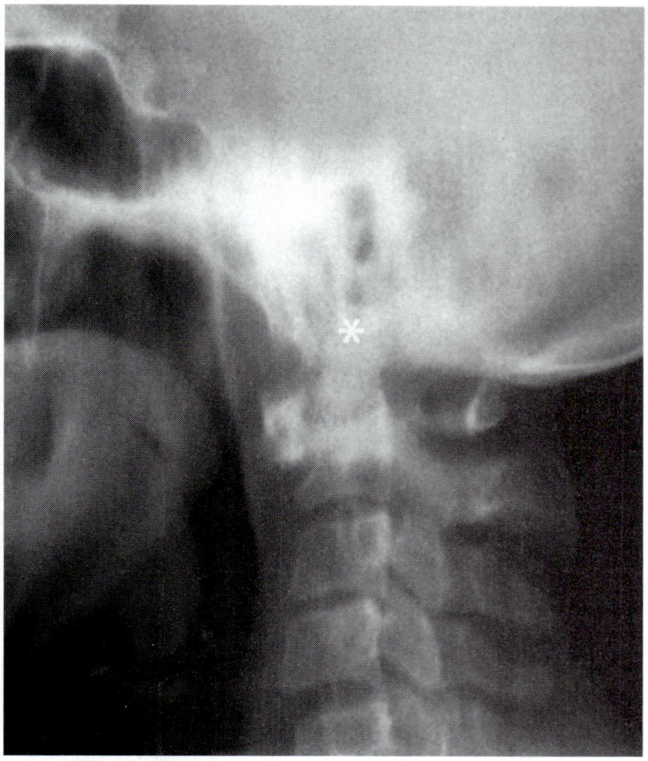

FIGURE 51–52 · Vertical Subluxation of C1 on C2. Lateral tomogram shows protrusion of odontoid (asterisk) through the foramen magnum.

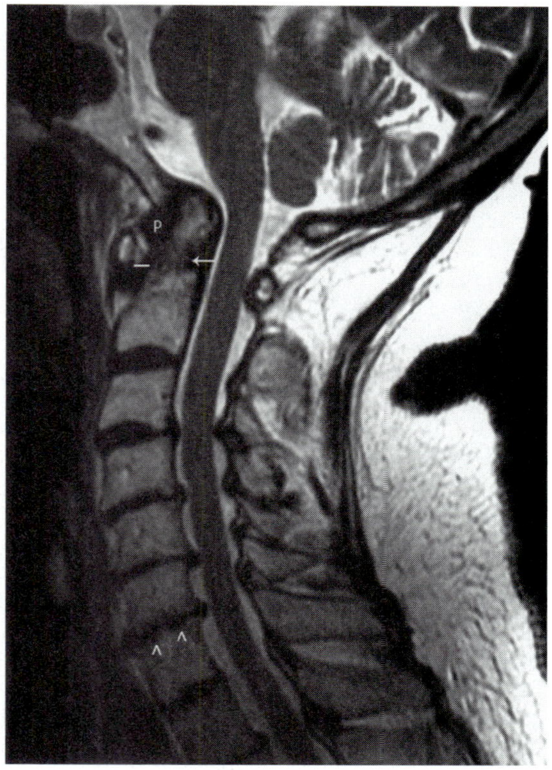

FIGURE 51–53 · Rheumatoid Arthritis of Cervical Spine. T2-weighted sagittal image shows low signal periodontoid pannus (P). Odontoid process appears irregular secondary to erosions *(arrow)*. The atlantodental distance shows mild widening (solid line). There is also vertical subluxation without signs of cord compression. Anterior subarachnoid space is compromised by disc protrusions at multiple levels. Erosions *(arrow heads)* are seen at the vertebral endplates at the C6-C7 level.

of assessing anterior atlantoaxial subluxation than the AADI. A minimum distance of 14 mm for PADI is required to avoid cord compression.[185]

MRI is the preferred method for evaluation of spinal cord and brain stem compression. MRI has been recommended for the patients who have progressive and severe subluxations, intractable cervical or suboccipital pain, patients who have symptoms or signs of spinal cord or brain stem compression, and those who have signs of vertebral artery compromise.[186] MRI allows direct visualization of periodontoid pannus, subarachnoid space, spinal cord, and brain stem (Fig. 51–53). Distortion of the spinal cord (cervicomedullary angle less than 135 degrees) correlates with clinical evidence of cervical myelopathy.[187] Internal spinal cord damage due to cord compression is best shown on T2-weighted images as an area of increased signal. This increased signal may represent myelomalacia or cord gliosis, with or without associated edema, and correlates with a poor response to medical and surgical treatment.[188]

MRI obtained in neck flexion may better demonstrate the degree of spinal cord compromise, but the necessity and safety of this maneuver are debated.

SERONEGATIVE SPONDYLOARTHROPATHIES

Ankylosing Spondylitis

Synovial and cartilaginous joints, as well as sites of tendon and ligament insertion (entheses), may be involved in ankylosing spondylitis and other seronegative spondyloarthropathies.[189,190] Axial skeletal involvement is characteristic, with predilection for the sacroiliac, apophyseal, diskovertebral, and costovertebral articulations. The initial sites of involvement are the sacroiliac joints and the lumbosacral and thoracolumbar vertebral junctions. Subsequently, ascending and descending spinal disease may be encountered.[191,192] Peripheral joint involvement, although common (50%), is usually mild.[193] The hips and glenohumeral joints are the most common extraspinal locations of disease.

Sacroiliac Joints

Involvement of the sacroiliac (SI) joints is the hallmark of ankylosing spondylitis, and it is difficult to verify the diagnosis of this disease in the absence of such involvement. Sacroiliitis occurs early in the course of ankylosing spondylitis and is characteristically bilateral and symmetric in its distribution.[192,194-196] Occasionally, initial unilateral or asymmetric SI joint changes are observed, and rarely, spinal disease occurs in the absence of significant SI joint abnormality. Changes occur in both the synovial and the ligamentous portions of the joint, with the abnormalities being more prominent on the iliac side of the articulation. Osteoporosis, subchondral bony resorption with loss of definition of the articular margins and superficial osseous erosions, are interspersed with focal areas of bony sclerosis. Radiographically, in this stage, the articulation may appear widened. With progression of the disease, a wide, ill-defined band of sclerosis is seen on the iliac side of the joint with larger subchondral erosions (Fig. 51–54). In the late proliferative stage, bony bridges traverse the joint space, initially isolating islands of intact cartilage. Such segmental ankylosis may be followed by complete intra-articular bony fusion and disappearance of the periarticular sclerosis. The ligamentous (syndesmotic) portions of the SI joint may also be affected, leading to bony erosions and proliferation.

CT and MRI better delineate the complex anatomy of the SI joints than do conventional radiographs. Good indicators of sacroiliitis on CT include increased subchondral sclerosis in patients younger than 40 years of age, unilateral or bilateral diffuse joint space loss (less than 2 mm), erosions, and intra-articular ankylosis. The superiority of CT over plain films in the study of sacroiliitis is controversial. In most patients with clinical signs of sacroiliitis, high-quality radiographs of the SI joints are diagnostic. When CT is used, however, it may reveal that the disease is more advanced than had been suspected. In cases of ankylosing spondylitis not responding to conventional therapy, intra-articular corticosteroid injection can be guided by CT (or fluoroscopy).

MRI allows detection of sacroiliitis before conventional radiography or CT. This sensitivity is due to the ability of MRI to detect bone marrow edema on fluid-sensitive sequences. Contrast-enhanced MRI studies further increase the sensitivity for detecting early sacroiliitis.[197] Cartilage abnormalities may be visible on MRI with the normal thin band of intermediate signal intensity representing cartilage on T1-weighted images replaced by areas of inhomogeneous, mixed signal intensity.

Spine

The initial sites of spinal involvement, especially in men, are the lumbosacral and thoracolumbar junctions. In women, the cervical spine may be affected at an early stage of disease. Osteitis is an initial finding, related to inflammation of the anterior portion of the diskovertebral junction. Erosions at the anterosuperior and anteroinferior vertebral margins lead to loss of the normal concavity of the anterior aspect of the vertebral body, resulting in a "squared" vertebral configuration on the lateral radiographic projection. This appearance is more easily identified in the lumbar spine, as the thoracic vertebral bodies may normally have a straight, squared appearance. In ankylosing spondylitis, bony sclerosis adjacent to the sites of erosion produces a "shining corner" sign on radiographs (Fig. 51–55).

Syndesmophytes are vertically oriented bony excrescences that represent ossification of the outer fibers of the annulus fibrosus of the intervertebral disk.[198] They predominate on the anterior and lateral aspects of the spine and eventually bridge the intervertebral disk (Fig 51–56). In the late stages of the disease, extensive syndesmophyte formation produces a smooth, undulating spinal contour termed the *bamboo spine.*

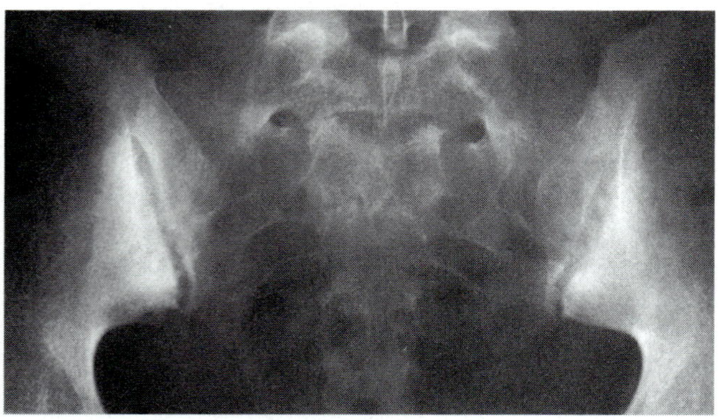

FIGURE 51–54 · Sacroiliitis in Ankylosing Spondylitis. There is sclerosis along the iliac sides of the sacroiliac joints and loss of portions of the iliac subchondral bone indicating erosion. Small linear bony bridges or residual bone are noted overlying the cartilage space.

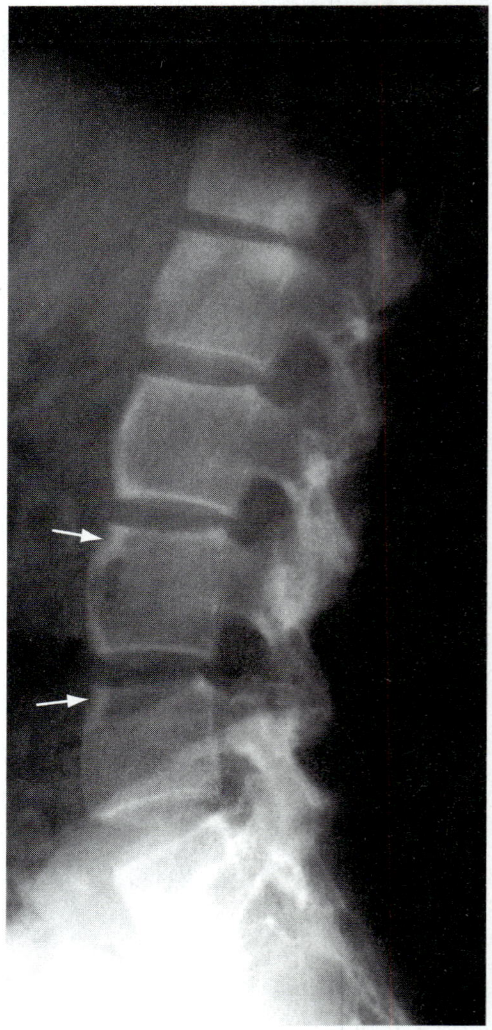

FIGURE 51–55 · Ankylosing Spondylitis with Shining Corners and Vertebral Squaring. There has been marked erosion at the vertebral margins producing straight or slightly convex anterior vertebral surfaces. New bone formation has resulted in shining corners *(arrows)*. The facet joints are fused.

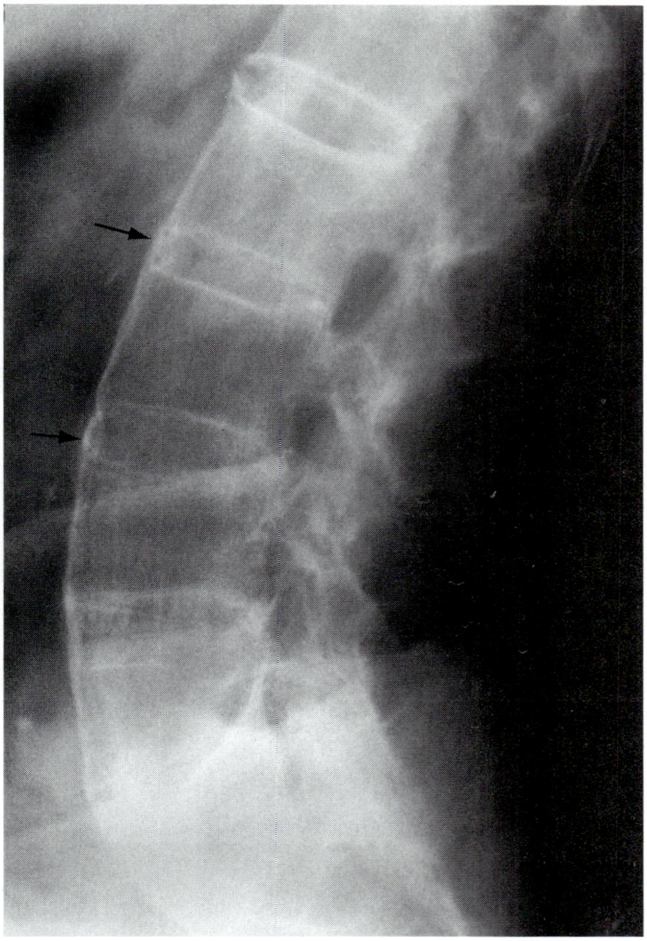

FIGURE 51–56 · **The Syndesmophytes of Ankylosing Spondylitis.** Extensive bony bridging *(arrows)* extends from the edge of one vertebral body to the next.

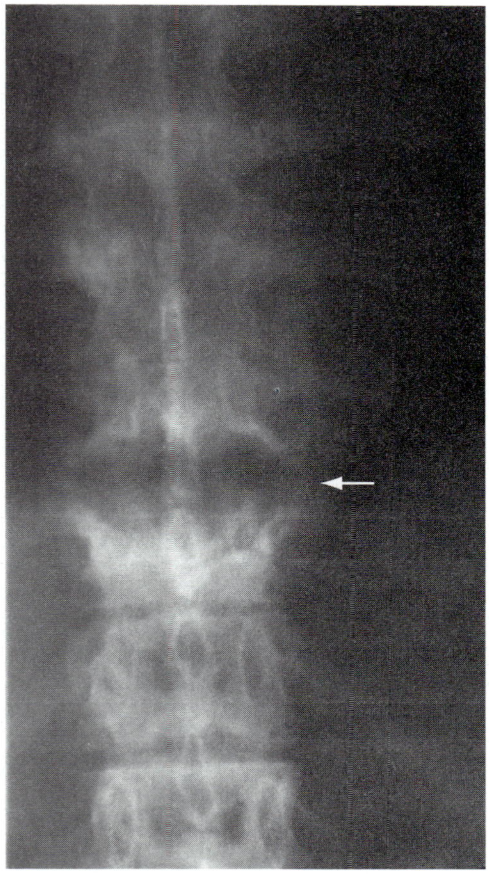

FIGURE 51–57 · **Ankylosing Sponcylitis with Pseudoarthrosis.** There is marked bone resorption from vertebral bodies and posterior elements at the site of pseudoarthrosis *(arrow)*. In this patient, syndesmophytes were not prominent.

It is important to differentiate the syndesmophytes that characterize ankylosing spondylitis (and enteropathic spondyloarthritis) from other spinal and paraspinal bony excrescences. Vertebral excrescences in spondylosis deformans arise several millimeters from the diskovertebral junction, are triangular in shape, and demonstrate a horizontally oriented segment of variable length at their point of origin. In diffuse idiopathic skeletal hyperostosis (DISH), bone formation in the anterior longitudinal ligament results in a flowing pattern of ossification, thicker than that seen in ankylosing spondylitis. Such ossification is best demonstrated on lateral spine radiographs. Furthermore, in DISH there is absence of erosion and widespread bony ankylosis of the SI joints. The paravertebral ossifications that characterize psoriatic arthritis and Reiter's syndrome arise, asymmetrically, in the soft tissues adjacent to the outer layer of annulus fibrosus. Initially, they are unattached to the vertebral bodies, but with time, they fuse with the margins of the vertebral body at a point several millimeters from the diskovertebral junction. Bridging identical to that observed in ankylosing spondylitis may occur, however, in psoriatic arthritis or Reiter's syndrome. Disk calcification may occur at levels of ankylosis in all these conditions.

Erosions at one or more diskovertebral junctions can be prominent radiographic findings in ankylosing spondylitis. These erosions may be classified as focal or diffuse.[199] Focal lesions may relate to intraosseous protrusion of disk material (cartilaginous or Schmorl's node) or enthesis. Diffuse destruction of the diskovertebral junction may be related to a pseudoarthrosis that follows a fracture in a previously ankylosed spine (Fig. 51–57).

Early alterations in the apophyseal joints in the lumbar, thoracic, and cervical segments consist of ill-defined erosions accompanied by reactive sclerosis. Capsular ossification or intra-articular bony ankylosis may occur subsequently. On frontal radiographs of the spine, such ossifications produce vertically oriented, parallel radiodense bands, which when combined with a central radiodense band related to ossification of the interspinous and supraspinous ligaments, lead to the "trolley-track" sign (Fig. 51–58).

Erosions of the odontoid process and sclerosis of the odontoid process and atlantoaxial subluxation may be observed in ankylosing spondylitis, although with less frequency than in RA.[194,200] Ankylosis of the atlantoaxial articulation, either in its normal position or in a position of subluxation, may occasionally be noted. At other lev-

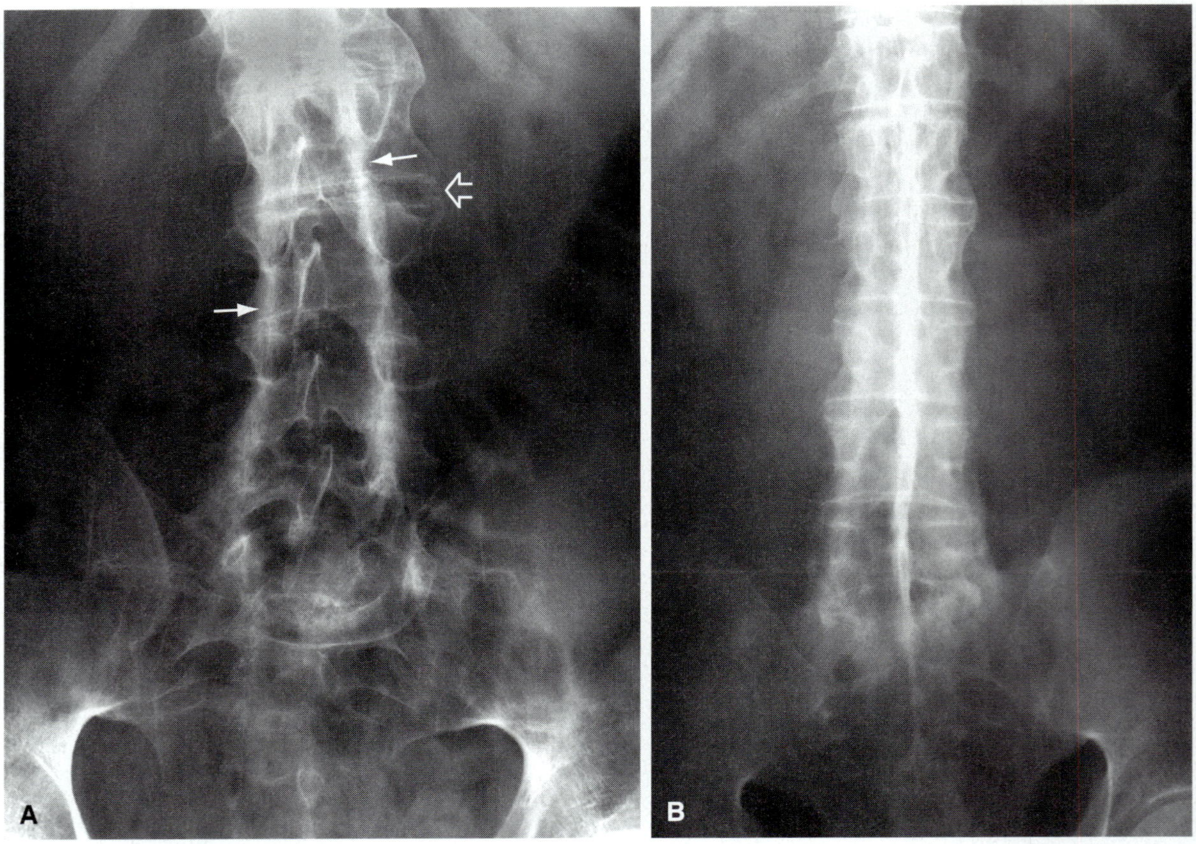

FIGURE 51–58 · Ankylosing Spondylitis. *A*, Fusion of the facet joints and ossification of the adjacent soft tissue has produced a "trolley track" appearance *(arrows)*. The sacroiliac joints are fused. Syndesmophytes *(open arrow)* are present. *B*, In another patient, there is a prominent fusion of the interspinous ligaments producing a saber sheath appearance.

els in the cervical spine, the changes, when present, are identical to those in the thoracolumbar spine.

MRI can be utilized to detect spinal involvement, even before the onset of clinical symptoms related to the spine or before changes detectable by other imaging modalities such as radiographs or bone scans. On MRI, the low signal at the affected enthesis enhances after intravenous gadolinium on T1-weighted images with fat saturation, and there is a high signal on T2-weighted images. These findings correspond to hypervascularity and inflammation of the subchondral bone at the involved enthesis.

Spinal complications include functional limitation from severe kyphosis, acute fracture of the ankylosed spine, pseudoarthrosis after spinal fracture (usually from minor trauma), and cauda equina syndrome. Detection of pseudoarthrosis or of acute spinal fracture may be difficult (Fig. 51–59). CT with reformatted images may detect spinal fracture that is not apparent on radiographs or on axial CT images. In patients who develop pseudarthrosis, MRI helps differentiate this condition from other causes of diskovertebral destruction, such as infection or tumor. Spinal cord compression can also be delineated with MRI, enabling early intervention to prevent catastrophic consequences. CT examination of the lumbar region in patients with ankylosing spondylitis who have cauda equina syndrome may reveal enlargement of the spinal canal with multiple scalloped erosions involving the adjacent bone (Fig. 51–60).

Extraspinal Locations

The hip is the most commonly involved peripheral articulation in ankylosing spondylitis, and the changes are most frequently bilateral and symmetric in distribution.[201] Concentric joint-space narrowing with axial migration of the femoral head and marginal osteophyte formation is characteristic (Fig. 51–61). Osteophytes are first observed at the lateral margin of the femoral head-neck junction and, with progression, proliferate circumferentially to produce a "ring osteophyte."[201,202] Subchondral cysts and erosions as well as intra-articular bony ankylosis may be seen. Surgical intervention may be required, but patients with ankylosing spondylitis who undergo total hip replacement are prone to develop exuberant heterotopic bone, which may restrict postoperative motion.

The shoulder is the second most common site of peripheral involvement in ankylosing spondylitis.[193] Bilateral involvement is common; changes are osteoporosis, joint-space narrowing, bony erosions, and rotator

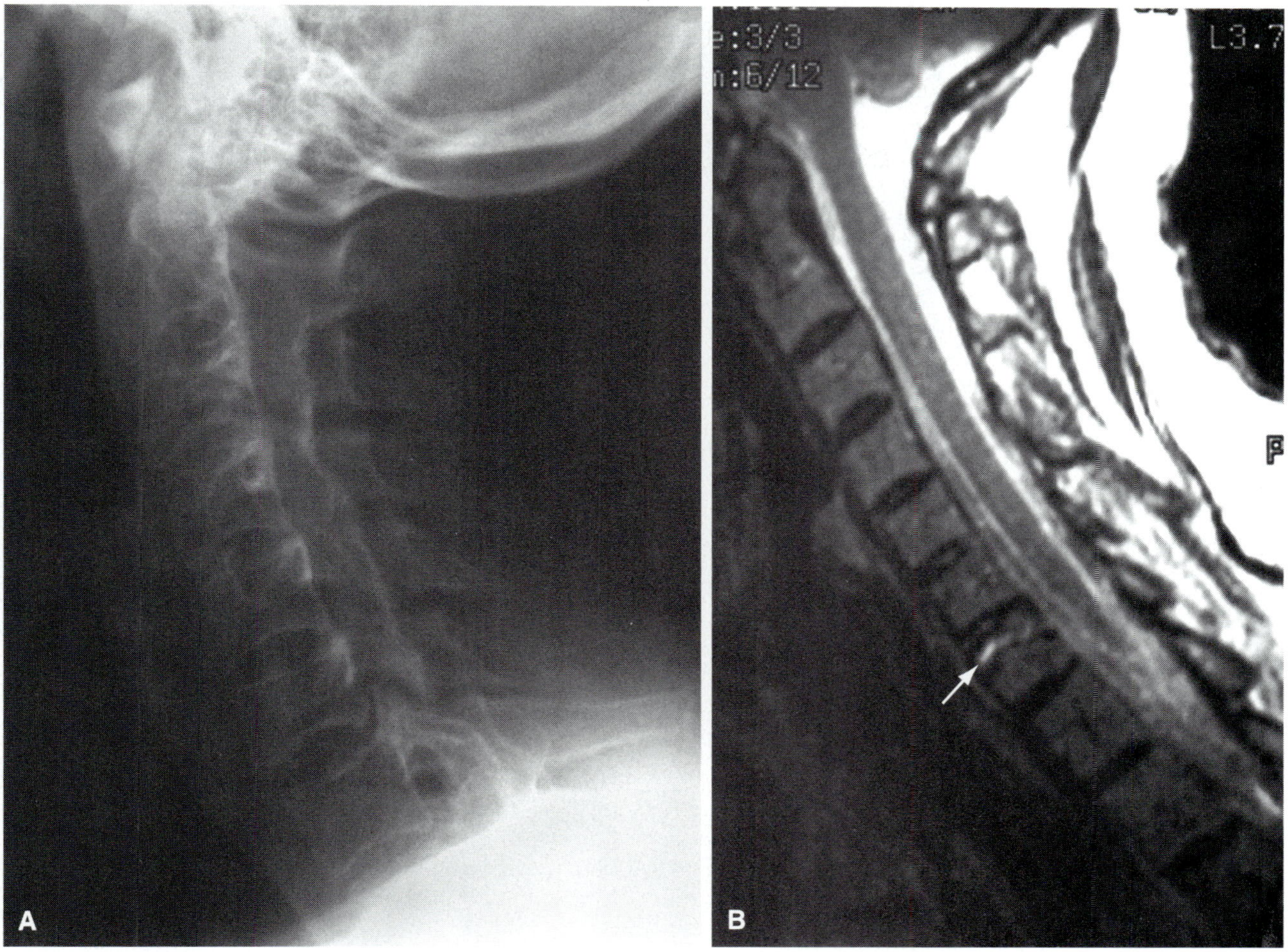

FIGURE 51–59 · Fracture in Ankylosing Spondylitis. *A*, The radiograph demonstrates disruption of the previously fused C6-C7 facet joints and slight anterior subluxation. *B*, A sagittal T2-weighted image confirms a high signal fracture line *(arrow)* through the superior aspect of C7.

cuff disruption. A characteristic large destructive abnormality involving the superolateral aspect of the humeral head in this disease has been termed the *hatchet sign*.[203]

Changes in other peripheral joints occur with variable frequency. In general, these changes, which are similar to but less extensive than those in the other seronegative spondyloarthropathies, include soft tissue swelling, mild osteoporosis, joint-space narrowing, bony erosions, and osseous proliferation.[190] The erosions tend to be less prominent than in RA. The presence of bone proliferation (whiskering) and periostitis in ankylosing spondylitis (and the other seronegative spondyloarthropathies) is another helpful diagnostic feature.

Inflammation with bony proliferation at sites of tendon and ligament insertion (enthesitis) is prominent in ankylosing spondylitis (as well as in the other seronegative spondyloarthropathies). Plantar and posterior calcaneal enthesophytes are common and may be either well defined or indistinct with feathery margins, representing the combination of erosive and proliferative change. Erosions of the posterior calcaneal margin due to inflammation in the retrocalcaneal bursa and

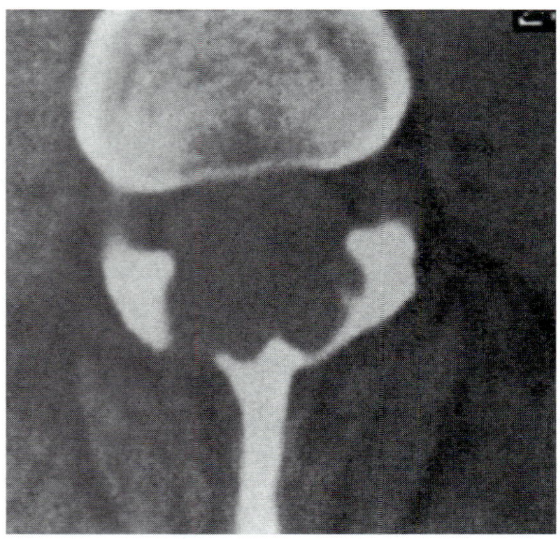

FIGURE 51–60 · Cauda Equine Syndrome in Ankylosing Spondylitis. Ankylosing Spondylitis and thecal diverticula. A CT image of a lumbar vertebra demonstrates scalloped erosions of the posterior elements. (From Resnick D, Niwayama G: Diagnosis of Bone and Joint Disorders. Philadelphia, WB Saunders, 1988; Fig. 42-6)

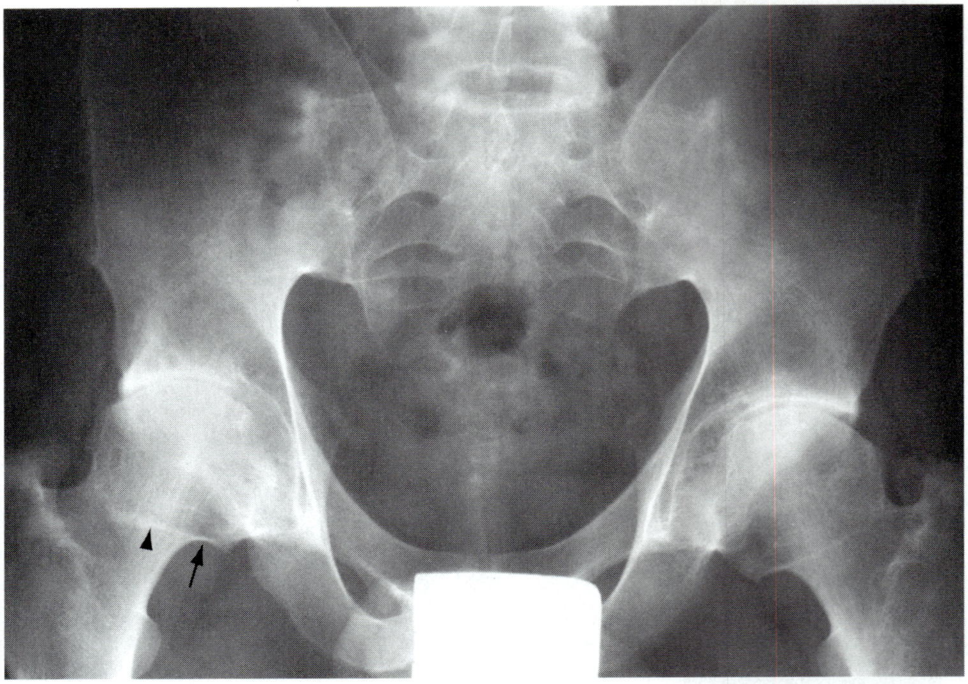

FIGURE 51–61 · Ankylosing Spondylitis Involving the Hips. There is bilateral cartilage space narrowing. A ring of osteophytes is noted at the capsular insertion *(arrows)* on each femoral head. The sacroiliac joints are fused.

thickening of the Achilles tendon may be present.[204] The inflammatory enthesopathy of the seronegative spondyloarthropathies[205] differs from the degenerative enthesopathy seen in DISH. In DISH, bony outgrowth (enthesophytes) are sharply marginated and well defined. Other sites of involvement in ankylosing spondylitis include the symphysis pubis, manubriosternal, temporomandibular, and sternoclavicular joints.

Psoriatic Arthritis and Reactive Arthritis

The characteristic spinal lesion of psoriatic arthritis (as well as reactive arthritis) is paravertebral ossification.[206] These ossifications initially appear as either thick and irregular or thin and curvilinear densities, asymmetrically distributed parallel to the lateral surface of the intervertebral disk and vertebral body (Fig. 51–62). At this stage, the outgrowths are unattached to the vertebral body, although in later stages, the ossific densities merge with the lateral margins of the vertebral body several millimeters from the diskovertebral junction. Occasionally, syndesmophytes identical to those in ankylosing spondylitis occur in psoriatic arthritis and reactive arthritis; however, in the great majority of cases, they are interspersed with the more characteristic paravertebral ossifications. "Corner osteitis," vertebral body "squaring," and apophyseal joint ankylosis are less common than in ankylosing spondylitis.

Cervical spine changes in psoriatic arthritis may be dramatic, even in patients with minimal thoracolumbar spinal involvement.[207,208] Diskovertebral joint irregularity with extensive bony proliferation about the anterior aspect of the vertebra and extensive apophyseal joint erosion and narrowing may be seen. Atlantoaxial subluxation may occur.

Spinal involvement is less frequent in reactive arthritis than in ankylosing spondylitis and psoriatic arthritis. Although in some instances the changes may be identical to those of ankylosing spondylitis, a more characteristic finding consists of asymmetrically distributed paravertebral ossifications involving the thoracolumbar spine.[209] Cervical spine involvement is unusual, and atlantoaxial subluxation is rare.

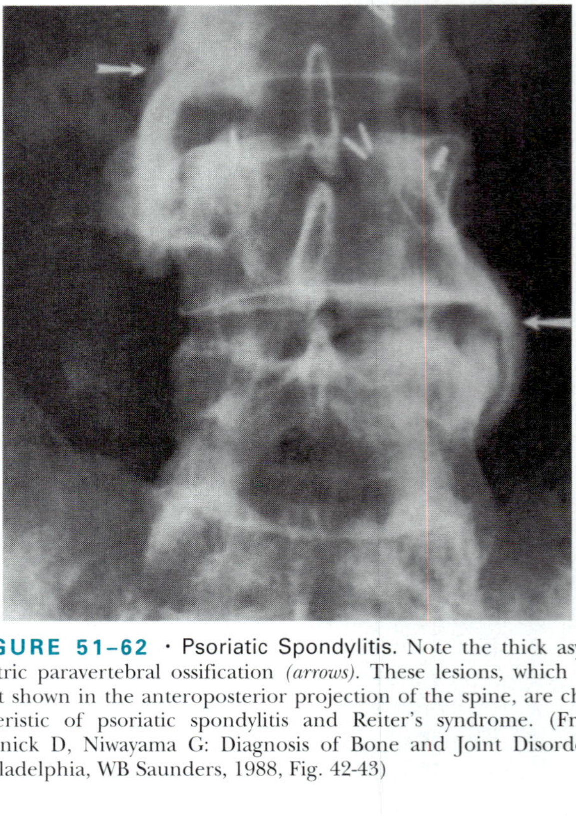

FIGURE 51–62 · Psoriatic Spondylitis. Note the thick asymmetric paravertebral ossification *(arrows)*. These lesions, which are best shown in the anteroposterior projection of the spine, are characteristic of psoriatic spondylitis and Reiter's syndrome. (From Resnick D, Niwayama G: Diagnosis of Bone and Joint Disorders. Philadelphia, WB Saunders, 1988, Fig. 42-43)

Infectious Spondylitis

Infectious spondylitis represents 2 to 7 percent of all cases of osteomyelitis.[210] Pathogenic organisms reach the spine by hematogenous or contiguous spread or direct inoculation from penetrating wounds or diagnostic or surgical procedures. The most common offending organism is *Staphylococcus aureus*. Other organisms include *Streptococcus*, gram-negative organisms, and *Mycobacterium*. In adults, the infection almost always starts at the vertebral body and involvement of disk is secondary.

The initial radiographs are often normal in early infection. There is usually 2 to 3 weeks' delay between the onset of clinical symptoms and detection of radiographic changes. The earliest radiographic findings include blurring of end plates of the involved vertebral bodies followed by narrowing of intervertebral disk height and gradual development of destruction of the vertebral end plates. Depending on host resistance and the virulence of the organism, the destruction may progress to vertebral collapse. Reparative sclerosis with new bone formation ensues at about 10 to 12 weeks. Bony bridging between the involved vertebral bodies or complete bony ankylosis can be the late sequela of infectious spondylitis.[211]

In tuberculous spondylitis, the lower thoracic and upper lumbar vertebrae are most frequently affected. The infection typically starts at the anterior part of the vertebral body near the end plate and spreads by subligamentous extension with multilevel involvement and skip levels. Initially, the cortical end plates are often focally destroyed with little or no reactive sclerosis (Fig. 51–63). With progression of destruction, collapse and anterior wedging of vertebral bodies can occur, leading to characteristic sharp angulation and gibbus deformity. Large calcified paravertebral abscesses are characteristic findings in tuberculous spondylitis. On MRI, intraosseous abscesses with ringlike, peripheral enhancement, and meningeal involvement can be demonstrated on postcontrast images.

Although there is an overlap in the radiologic appearances of tuberculous and pyogenic spondylitis, involvement of multiple levels, a delay in destruction of the intervertebral disks, and the presence of large calcified paravertebral abscesses favor tuberculous spondylitis.[212,213]

Bone scintigraphy will be positive in spinal infection well before bone destruction becomes obvious on radiographs. The combined accuracy of technetium and gallium scans has been reported to be as high as 94 percent. For follow-up studies, gallium scan alone is recommended. During the healing phase, the technetium scan remains abnormal despite the resolution of infection due to its sensitivity for bone remodeling and

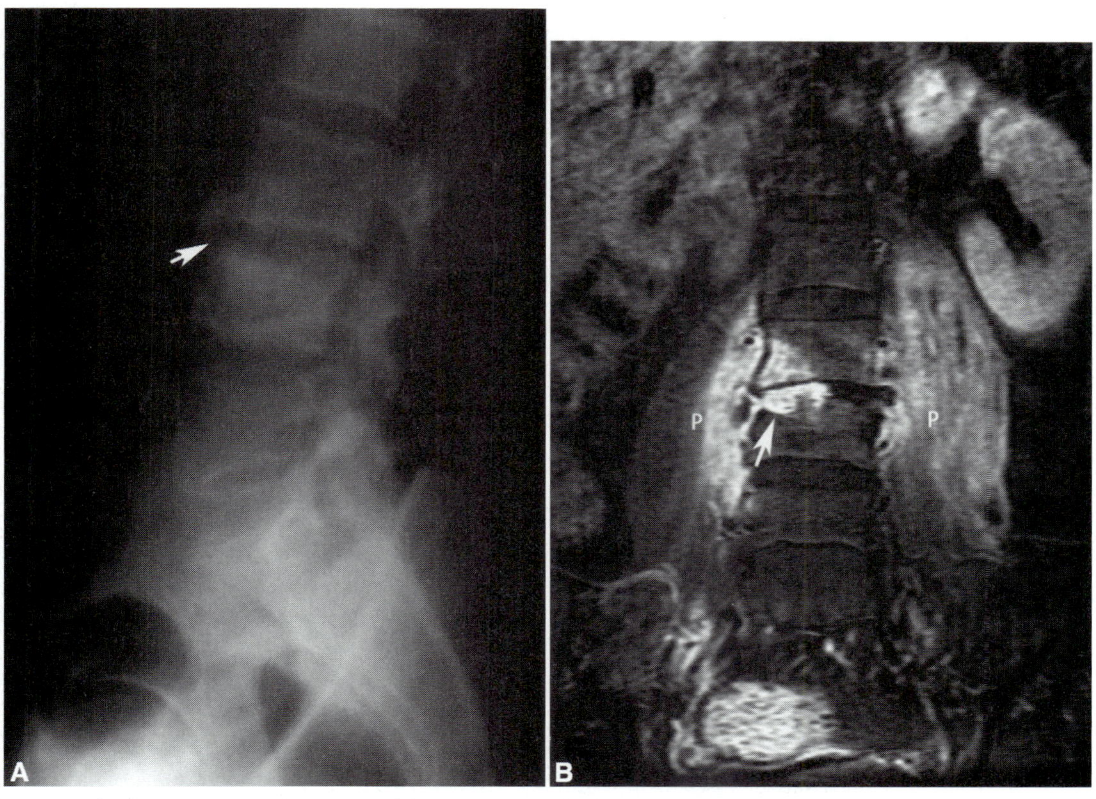

FIGURE 51–63 · Tuberculous Spondylitis. *(A)* A lateral view of the lumbar spine shows disc space narrowing at L3-L4 level with destructive changes involving the superior endplate of the L4 vertebral body (arrow). *(B)* Coronal STIR (short tau inversion recovery) MR image of the lumbar spine of the same patient confirms the focal destruction of the L4 vertebral body *(arrow)*. Enlargement of both psoas muscles (P) with increased signal is noted due to paraspinal extension of the infection.

repair; the gallium scan, however, returns to normal when the infection is eradicated.[214,215]

CT with reformatted images in the sagittal and coronal planes may play a role in the assessment of spinal infection. CT scans allow better definition of the extent of bone destruction and spinal canal compromise than radiographs. Paravertebral and epidural abscesses are easily identified after contrast administration. CT also facilitates guidance for percutaneous biopsy.

MRI has become the imaging modality of choice for the diagnosis and evaluation of the extent and complications of infectious spondylitis. The reported sensitivity, specificity, and accuracy of MRI in the diagnosis of infectious spondylitis are 96, 92, and 94 percent, respectively.[216] The appearance of pyogenic spondylitis on MRI has been characterized as 1) decreased signal intensity on T1-weighted images with corresponding increased signal on T2-weighted and short tau inversion (STIR) images in the involved vertebral body, 2) abnormal increased signal of the intervertebral disk with obliteration of the normal low-signal central cleft on T2-weighted images, and 3) increased signal of the vertebral end plates at the abnormal disk level on T2-weighted images.[216] Gadolinium-enhanced images are helpful in precise characterization and delineation of any paravertebral and epidural extension of the infection. On postcontrast images, a phlegmon shows fairly uniform enhancement, whereas an abscess demonstrates rim enhancement.[217,218]

MRI is also helpful in monitoring the efficacy of conservative treatment. Resolution of soft tissue inflammation, reduced enhancement of tissues, and quiescence of signal changes within the intervertebral disk and adjacent bone marrow reflect a favorable response to treatment.[219,220]

DEGENERATIVE DISORDERS

Intervertebral (Osteo)chondrosis

The vertebral column is composed of a complex series of synovial, cartilaginous, and fibrous articulations. Degenerative diseases of the spine can involve any of these articulations as well as ligamentous insertions (entheses).[221] Many distinct degenerative processes can be identified.

Primary degenerative disease of the nucleus pulposus of the intervertebral disk, termed *intervertebral (osteo)chondrosis,* is a common disorder, especially in the elderly. It may occur at any level but is more commonly identified in the lumbar and cervical regions. The earliest radiographic change consists of a linear or circular collection of gas ("vacuum phenomenon") within the disk substance[222] (Fig. 51–64). These gas collections are more prominent on radiographs obtained with the spine in extension and may disappear in flexion. The presence of a vacuum phenomenon is a useful observation, because it virtually excludes the possibility of infection. Progressive narrowing of the intervertebral disk and sclerosis beneath the subchondral bone plate are additional manifestations of intervertebral (osteo)chondrosis. Displacement of portions of the intervertebral

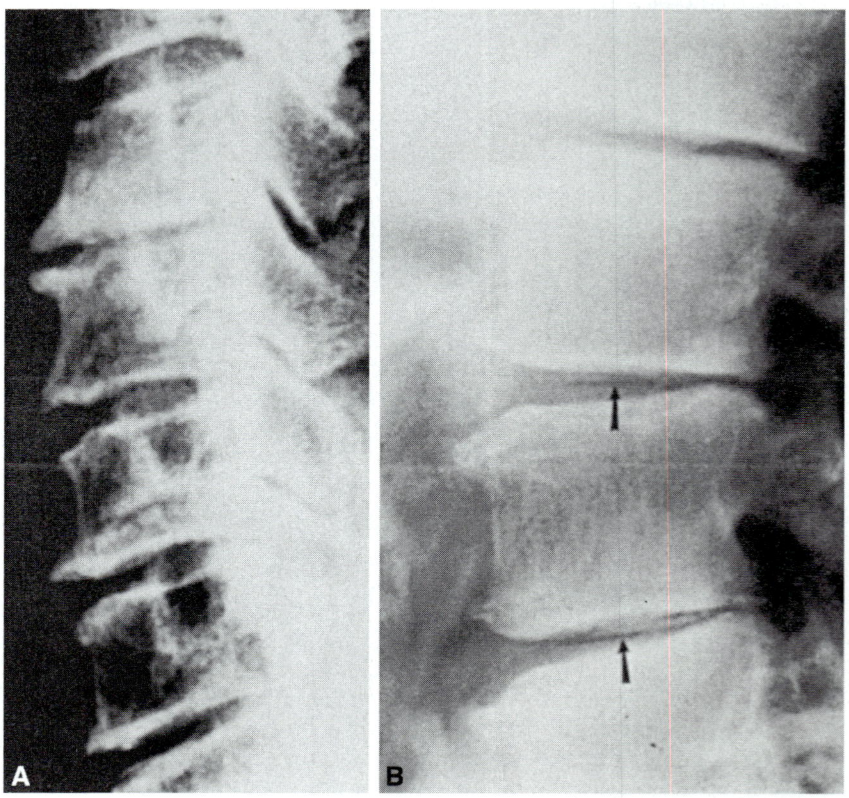

FIGURE 51–64 · Intervertebral (osteo) Chondrosis. Lateral Projections of the Cervical Spine *(A)* and the lumbar spine *(B)* reveal typical abnormalities of intervertebral (osteo)chondrosis. Intervertebral disk space narrowing with sclerosis of the vertebral end plates and the formation of small triangular osteophytes from the anterior vertebral margins are evident. Prominent vacuum phenomena *(arrows in B)* are present in the lumbar spine. (From Resnick D, Niwayama G: Diagnosis of Bone and Joint Disorders. Philadelphia, WB Saunders, 1988, Fig 42-57.)

disk into the adjacent vertebral body (Schmorl's node, cartilaginous node) is a further, although not specific, radiographic sign. Small, triangular osteophytes at the diskovertebral junction are also seen.

Spondylosis Deformans

Spondylosis deformans refers to the formation of multiple large osteophytes predominantly along the anterior and lateral aspects of the vertebral bodies[223] (Fig. 51–65). These osteophytes may occur at any level; in the thoracic spine, they predominate on the right side, presumably because their formation is inhibited on the left side by the constant pulsation of the descending thoracic aorta.[224] Narrowing of the intervertebral disk space, vacuum phenomena, and endplate bony sclerosis are not features of spondylosis deformans.

Apophyseal Joint Osteoarthritis

The synovium-lined apophyseal joint is a frequent site of degenerative disease.[225] Changes are most common in the mid- and lower cervical spine, the midthoracic spine, and the lower thoracic spine. The radiographic changes are identical to those of OA in peripheral articulations, with joint-space narrowing, osseous eburnation, and marginal osteophyte formation. Capsular laxity may result in apophyseal joint malalignment. In this setting or with large osteophytes arising from the joint margins, impingement of a spinal nerve root within the neural foramen may occur.

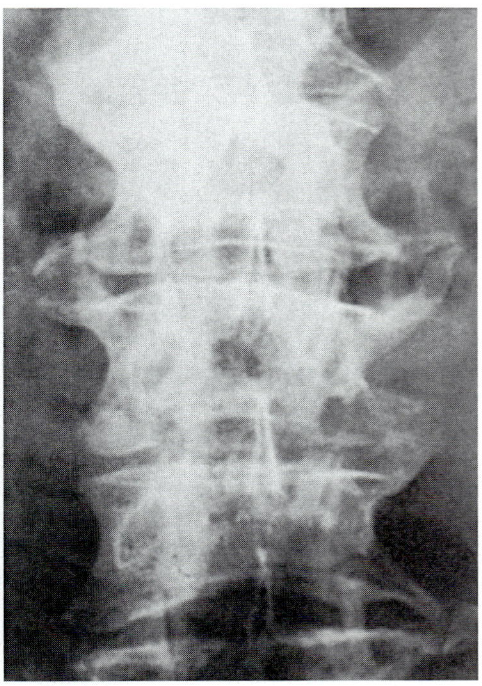

FIGURE 51–65 · Spondylosis Deformans. The frontal projection of the spine reveals multiple, large interdigitating osteophytes arising from the lateral margins of the vertebral bodies. Note that the initial portion of the osteophytes has a horizontal orientation. (From Resnick D, Niwayama G: Diagnosis of Bone and Joint Disorders. Philadelphia, WB Saunders, 1988, Fig 42-58.)

Uncovertebral Arthrosis

Degenerative changes in the cervical uncovertebral (Luschka) articulations are often identified on the frontal radiograph of the cervical spine. The nature of this process is debated, because these articulations have been shown to represent intervertebral disk extensions in early life and to contain synovial-like tissue in later life. Radiographic changes consist of osseous sclerosis, joint space loss, and osteophyte formation.

Diffuse Idiopathic Skeletal Hyperostosis

DISH is a common degenerative enthesopathy and has been described with a variety of terms,[226-229] including *Forestier's disease, spondylitis ossificans ligamentosa, spondylosis hyperostotica,* and *ankylosing hyperostosis of the spine.* Although radiographic changes are evident in both the axial and the appendicular skeleton, the diagnosis of DISH is based on the presence of characteristic spinal alterations. Resnick and colleagues have advocated that three criteria must be present before a diagnosis of DISH can be made: 1) the presence of flowing calcification or ossification along the anterolateral aspect of at least four contiguous vertebral levels; 2) relative preservation of intervertebral disk heights in the involved vertebral segments without the extensive changes of primary degenerative disk disease; and 3) the absence of apophyseal joint ankylosis or sacroiliac joint erosions, sclerosis, or widespread intra-articular bony ankylosis.[228]

The most characteristic radiographic abnormality of DISH is calcification and ossification of the anterior longitudinal ligament of the spine.[228] This finding is most commonly identified in the midthoracic spine but is also evident in the cervical and lumbar levels. Early in the disease, an undulating radiodense band forms along the anterolateral aspect of the spine and is separated from the anterior aspect of the vertebral body by a thin radiolucent line (Fig. 51–66); with progression of the disease, the lucency may disappear. These changes, which are best demonstrated in the lateral radiographic projection of the thoracic spine, may resemble the "bamboo spine" of ankylosing spondylitis, but several important differentiating features exist. Syndesmophytes arise from anterosuperior and anteroinferior margins of the vertebral body, whereas the ossification in DISH attaches to the vertebral body several millimeters from these margins. In addition, syndesmophytes may be best seen in the frontal projection, in contrast to DISH, in which changes are most prominent on the lateral radiographic projection. The presence of sacroiliac joint erosions and extensive intra-articular bony ankylosis of the sacroiliac and apophyseal joints in ankylosing spondylitis constitute another important differential point.

In the cervical spine, bony outgrowths characteristically appear at the anteroinferior margin of the vertebral body and extend inferiorly around the disk space. With progression, a thick, armor-like mass bridges the intervertebral disk, leading to markedly diminished cervical motion and, in some cases, dysphagia. Linear or Y-shaped radiolucencies in the bony mass may be noted at the

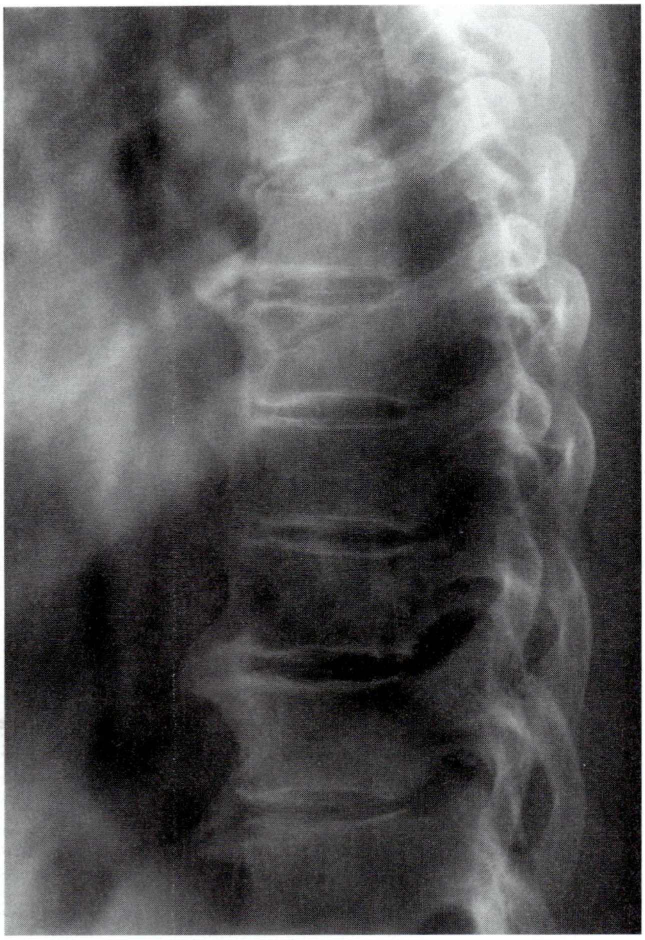

FIGURE 51–66 · Diffuse Idiopathic Skeletal Hyperostosis (DISH). There is bone formation along the anterior aspects of more than four vertebral bodies. The disk spaces are maintained and the sacroiliac joints were normal.

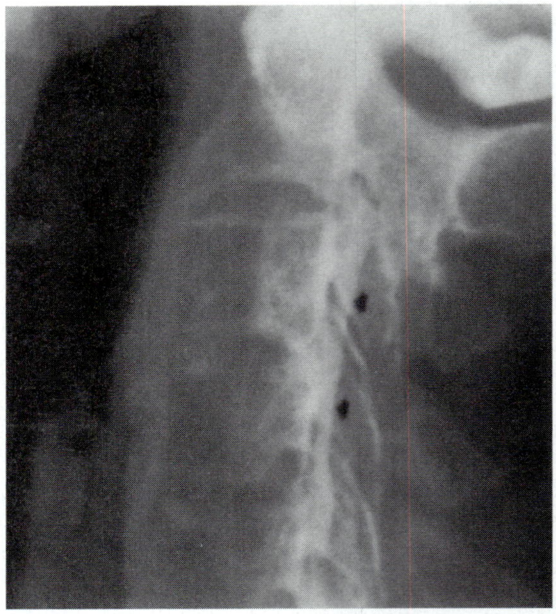

FIGURE 51–67 · Ossification of the Posterior Longitudinal Ligament (OPLL). In a patient with diffuse idiopathic skeletal hyperostosis (DISH) there is flowing ossification along the anterior margins of the vertebral bodies. Ossification of the posterior longitudinal ligament (PLL) is also present *(arrowheads)* just behind the C2 to C5 vertebral bodies.

level of the intervertebral disk space, owing to displacement of disk material into the ossific mass. Ossification adjacent to the posterior margin of the posterior longitudinal ligament may be seen as a distinct entity but occurs with increased frequency in patients with DISH[230] (Fig. 51–67). DISH-like changes also occur in a rare syndrome, sternoclavicular hyperostosis, in which extensive ossification of the soft tissues is evident between the anterior ribs, medial clavicle, and sternum.

Extraspinal manifestations of DISH[231] are especially common in the pelvis. Bony proliferation at sites of ligamentous and tendinous attachment (enthesopathy) results in the formation of coarse, well-marginated bony excrescences, in contrast to the finely spiculated, ill-defined bony proliferative changes of the seronegative spondyloarthropathies (Fig. 51–68). Calcification of the iliolumbar and sacrotuberous ligaments is an additional characteristic feature. Para-articular osteophytes are commonly noted about the hip and along the inferior aspect of the SI joints.

Other extraspinal sites of prominent bony proliferation include the patellar poles, calcaneus, and olecranon process of the ulna. The "spurs" that form at these sites

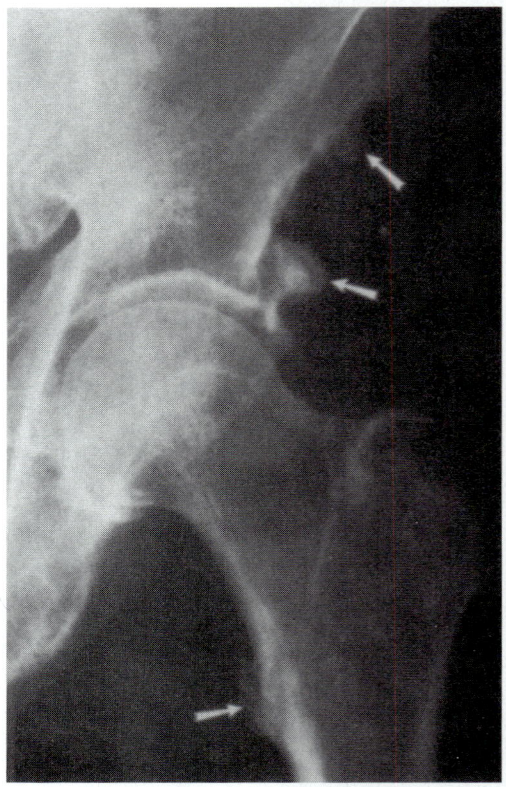

FIGURE 51–68 · Extraspinal Manifestation of Diffuse Idiopathic Skeletal Hyperostosis (DISH). The degenerative enthesopathy of DISH is well demonstrated with coarse bony excrescences arising from sites of ligament and tendon insertion along the lateral aspect of the ilium, superior acetabular margin, and lesser trochanter *(arrows)*. This appearance differs from that of the finely spiculated inflammatory enthesopathy of the seronegative spondyloarthropathies. (From Resnick D, Niwayama G: Diagnosis of Bone and Joint Disorders. Philadelphia, WB Saunders, Fig 42-61.)

may be identical in appearance to localized degenerative changes in otherwise normal persons, but they demonstrate a tendency toward increased size and multiplicity. In the hand, hyperostotic changes of the metacarpal and phalangeal heads, with proliferation in the terminal tufts, may be noted. Irregular excrescences may also be seen at the femoral trochanters, deltoid tuberosity of the humerus, anterior tibial tuberosity, and at the interosseous membranes of the forearm and leg.

Spinal Stenosis

Spinal stenosis is either congenital or acquired, or a combination of the two. The congenital form is related to developmental aberrations such as short pedicles, whereas the acquired form results from a reduction in diameter of the spinal canal caused by any combination of disk bulging, ligamentum flavum hypertrophy, postoperative changes, and facet hypertrophy. The most common form of spinal stenosis that is studied by MRI is the acquired form.[232] The thecal sac may be compressed or even obliterated by bulging disks, osteophytes, or a hypertrophied ligamentum flavum. The resulting appearance of the thecal sac is an hourglass deformity. Multilevel disk degeneration illustrated by abnormal low-signal-intensity disks and disk-space narrowing also may be present. On transaxial images, the stenotic spinal canal has a triangular shape owing to encroachment by hypertrophied facets. If questions about the osseous anatomy remain after MRI examination, CT or CT myelography may be done.

Sacral Insufficiency Fractures

Insufficiency fractures occur when normal stress is applied to a bone with deficient elastic resistance, typically in elderly osteoporotic patients. The most common presenting symptom is low back pain, accompanied by hip and buttock pain. The fractures may go unrecognized on plain radiographs, until visible areas of linear sclerosis are seen in the sacral alae. Radionuclide bone scan shows intense uptake along one or both sacral ala, and, occasionally, if the fracture crosses from one side to the other, it will produce characteristic H-shaped uptake (Honda sign).[233] CT may be used to confirm the diagnosis. It has been reported that the presence of vacuum phenomena at the fracture site on CT scan can be a clue for the diagnosis of insufficiency fracture.[234] MRI is the most sensitive and specific tool in detection of occult fractures. MRI demonstrates fractures as linear low signal intensity paralleling the SI joints on both T1- and T2-weighted images with surrounding bone marrow edema[38,235] (Fig. 51–69).

Miscellaneous Disorders

PIGMENTED VILLONODULAR SYNOVITIS

Pigmented villonodular synovitis (PVNS) is a proliferative synovitis of unknown cause. It may be intra-articular or extra-articular in location and diffuse or localized in distribution. The extra-articular form, sometimes termed *giant-cell tumor of tendon sheath,* is most often seen in the fingers and is usually localized, and the articular form is usually present in the knee, hip, or ankle and is usually diffuse.[135]

Pathologic examination reveals nodular or villous enlargement of the synovial lining, which appears red, brown, or yellow. Histiocytic cells and lipid-laden foam cells are present in fibrous stroma. Intra- and extracellular hemosiderin is present. The joint fluid is typically brown or red-brown.

Radiographic examination may suggest the diagnosis. Only one joint is involved in nearly all cases. Erosions and cysts on both sides of the joint are seen with normal bone density and cartilage space[236-238] (Fig. 51–70). During arthrography, nodular soft tissue masses may be demonstrated, and aspiration of joint fluid will yield the characteristic "rusty" fluid.

MRI signal characteristics can be highly suggestive of nodular or diffuse PVNS but are not always specific enough to differentiate it from other forms of synovitis associated with hemosiderin deposition or caused by amyloid (Table 51–3). The MRI signal characteristics reflect the fat, fibrous tissue, and iron present in the tissues; iron appears dark on all pulse sequences, and the size of the lesion may appear slightly larger on T2-weighted images (the blooming effect). PVNS deposits usually display intermediate signal intensity on T1-weighted or intermediate-weighted images with some low signal regions, and show very dark signal intensity on T2-weighted sequences.[135] These deposits are enhanced with intravenous gadolinium administration. Bright regions on T2-weighted sequences are noted and may represent trapped fluid within the synovial membrane.[239] MRI must include the entire joint to evaluate the extent and location of intra-articular and periarticular masses for surgical removal. Post-treatment recurrence can also be assessed on MRI.

PRIMARY SYNOVIAL (OSTEO) CHONDROMATOSIS

This disorder is due to metaplasia of the synovial lining with the formation of hyaline cartilage nodules that may protrude into the joint and eventually detach to form loose bodies. Calcification or ossification of these nodules may occur. *"Primary" synovial (osteo)chondromatosis* is the term used when no underlying cause of loose body formation, such as OA, can be identified. Joints, tendon sheaths, or bursae may be affected. The disorder is monarticular.

The typical radiographic picture of synovial (osteo) chondromatosis is that of numerous calcific (or ossific) densities confined to the joint cavity (Fig. 51–71). The calcified bodies are fairly uniform in size. Pressure erosions of adjacent bony surfaces may be seen and may predispose to fracture. Osteoporosis and joint-space narrowing are generally not prominent. In cases in which the bodies are not calcified, MRI may confirm the diagnosis.

MRI appearances may be diagnostic, even when no calcification is present, because uncalcified cartilage nodules exhibit a characteristic lobulated appearance and are isointense or slightly brighter in signal intensity

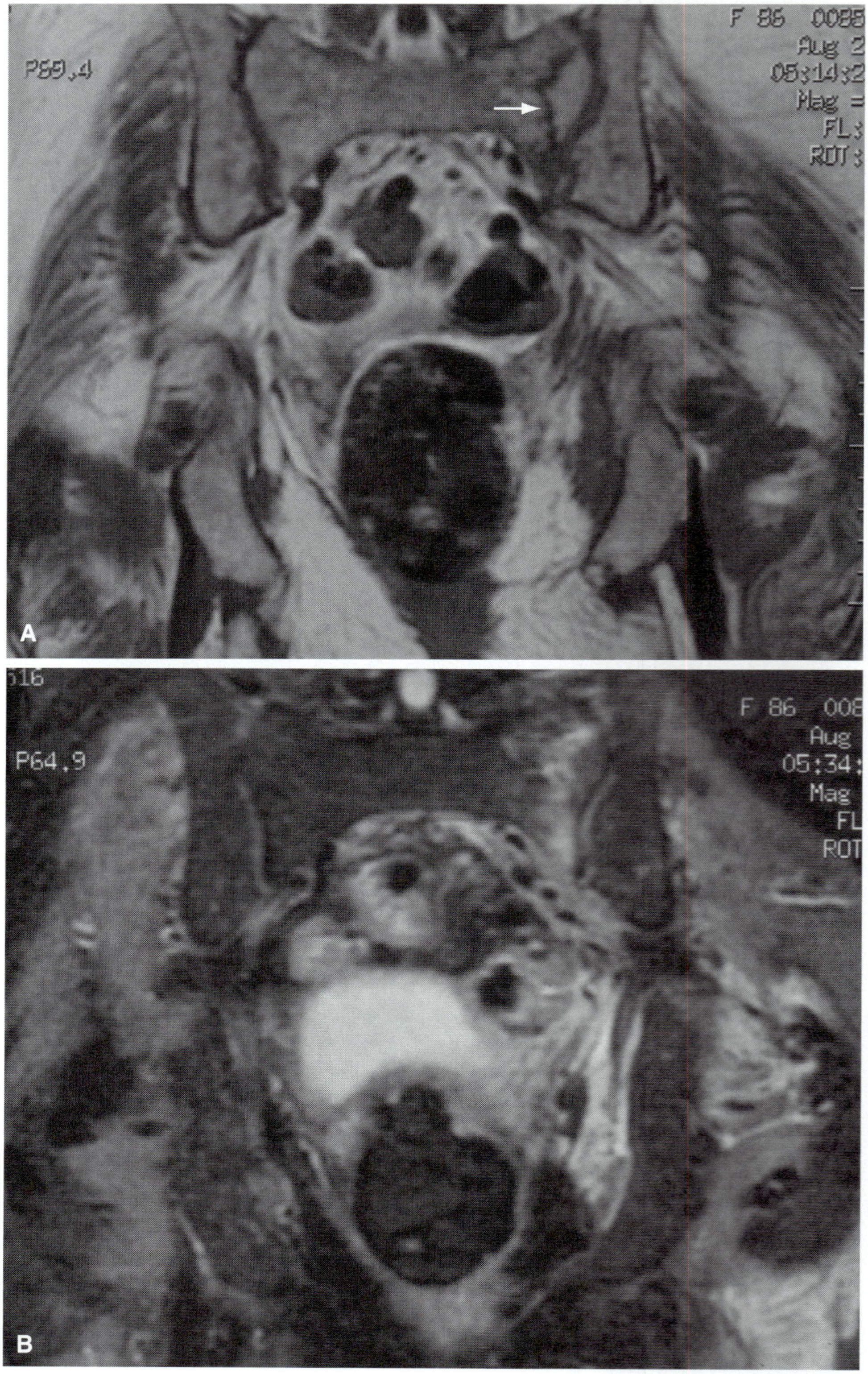

FIGURE 51–69 · Sacral Insufficiency Fracture shown on MRI. *A*, A T1-weighted image of the posterior portion of the pelvis in an elderly woman with pain shows a band of low signal in the left side of the sacrum *(arrow)*. *B*, STIR image shows a linear area of very bright signal intensity with adjacent high signal in the left sacral ala.

than muscle on T1- and T2-weighted images.[135] Low-signal fibrous septae separate the cartilage nodules and aid in the differentiation of the nodules from joint effusion, which has similar signal characteristics on these sequences. Arc-like enhancement around the nodules may be seen within the cartilage. Ossification is identified by its peripheral low-signal calcified rim and central fat signal marrow (Fig. 51–72).

BETA2-MICROGLOBULIN AMYLOIDOSIS

β_2-microglobulin amyloid arthropathy is a sequela of long-term hemodialysis but may also occur in patients on peritoneal dialysis or with uremia without dialysis treatment.[135,240,241] β_2-microglobulin amyloidosis is found in synovial tissue, joint capsules, periarticular tissues, articular cartilage, and bone—the last likely by

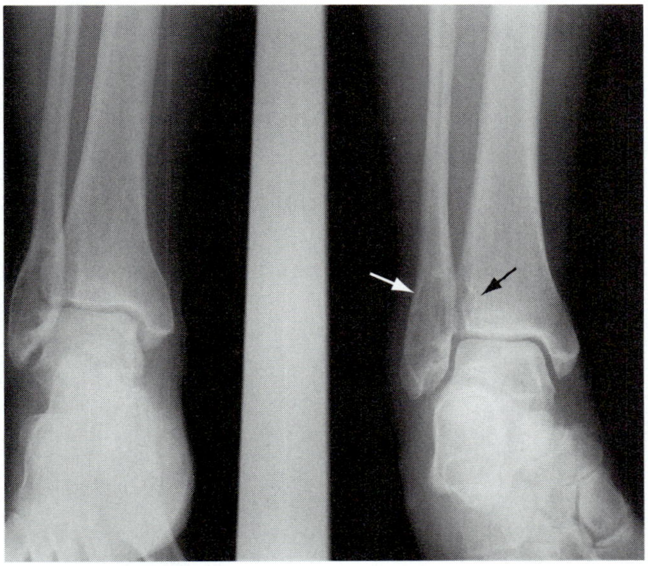

FIGURE 51–70 · Pigmented Villonodular Synovitis. The anteroposterior and mortise radiographs of the ankle show the classical but not entirely specific features of pigmented villonodular synovitis: erosion on both sides of the joint *(arrows)*, preservation of the cartilage space, and normal bone density. The location at the tibiofibular joint recess is unusual.

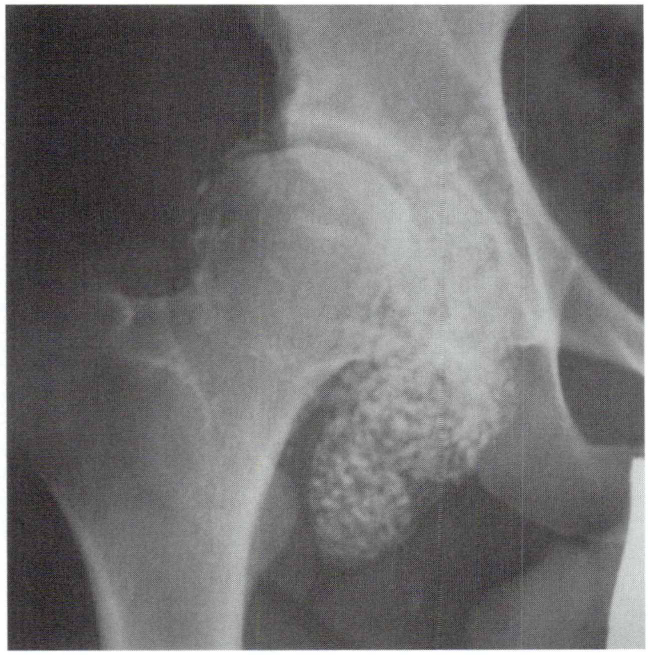

FIGURE 51–71 · Synovial Osteochondromatosis. Multiple calcified bodies that are uniform in size are noted within a distended ilio psoas bursa and the hip joint. The cartilage space is not narrowed, and bone density is normal; these features are typical of the condition.

extension from the adjacent soft tissue deposits.[242-245] The wrists, shoulders, hips, and knees are most often involved. Carpal tunnel syndrome and large joint arthralgias are the most common clinical complaints.[246] Pathologic fracture of the femur may follow cystic bone changes.[242,244] A peripheral arthro-pathy is seen in hemodialyzed patients, but its relation to amyloid is uncertain.[246] A destructive spondylo-arthropathy may occur that usually involves the cervical spine, often the atlantoaxial region.[241,247]

Radiographically, juxta-articular cysts or erosions are present with relatively preserved articular cartilage spaces. Unlike PVNS, multiple joints may be involved and osteopenia is usually present. Nodular soft tissue swelling may be seen. The wrists, hips, and shoulders are often involved. Hip erosion seems to favor the anterosuperior aspect of the femoral necks.[248] The spondyloarthropathy may be rapidly progressive with vertebral collapse, end plate erosion, disk narrowing, and subluxation.[241] Ultrasonography has been particularly helpful about the shoulder in identifying the echogenic nature of the amyloid deposits.[249]

MRI of β_2-microglobulin amyloidosis typically shows masses of tissue in joints and bursae that are intermediate to low in signal intensity on T1-weighted images and usually low in signal intensity on T2-weighted images (Fig 51–73). MRI, therefore, can distinguish amyloid deposition from inflammatory conditions or tumors, which usually demonstrate high signal on T2-weighted images.[135,250,251] Tendon and capsular thickening is noted particularly in the supraspinatus tendon and the iliofemoral portion of the hip capsule. The masses of amyloid extend into the bone defects, although the signal of bone lesions seems more variable, possibly because of the presence of fluid in some of the erosions.[243] As in other erosive processes, MRI is able to demonstrate erosions that are not visible on radiographs.[243] Amyloid deposition may be documented on MRI even in asymptomatic subjects but is more marked when symptoms are present.[243]

TABLE 51–3 · SOME INTRA-ARTICULAR AND PERIARTICULAR CONDITIONS PRODUCING LOW SIGNAL INTENSITY MASSES ON T2-WEIGHTED MAGNETIC RESONANCE IMAGING (MRI)

Chronic rheumatoid arthritis
Pigmented villonodular synovitis
Chronic hemarthrosis
Amyloidosis
Calcified loose bodies
Benign fibroblastic tumors
Gouty tophus

LIPOMA ARBORESCENS

Lipoma arborescens is a rare disorder in which collections of fat develop beneath the synovial lining.[252] Their large size and frondlike configuration distinguish them from other intrasynovial collections of fat. The condition is usually unilateral but may be bilateral or may involve multiple joints,[252] with the knee most often affected. Painless swelling of the joint over many years occurs with periodic effusions.[253]

Occasionally the fatty deposits will be visible on standard radiographs. However, CT and MRI are better

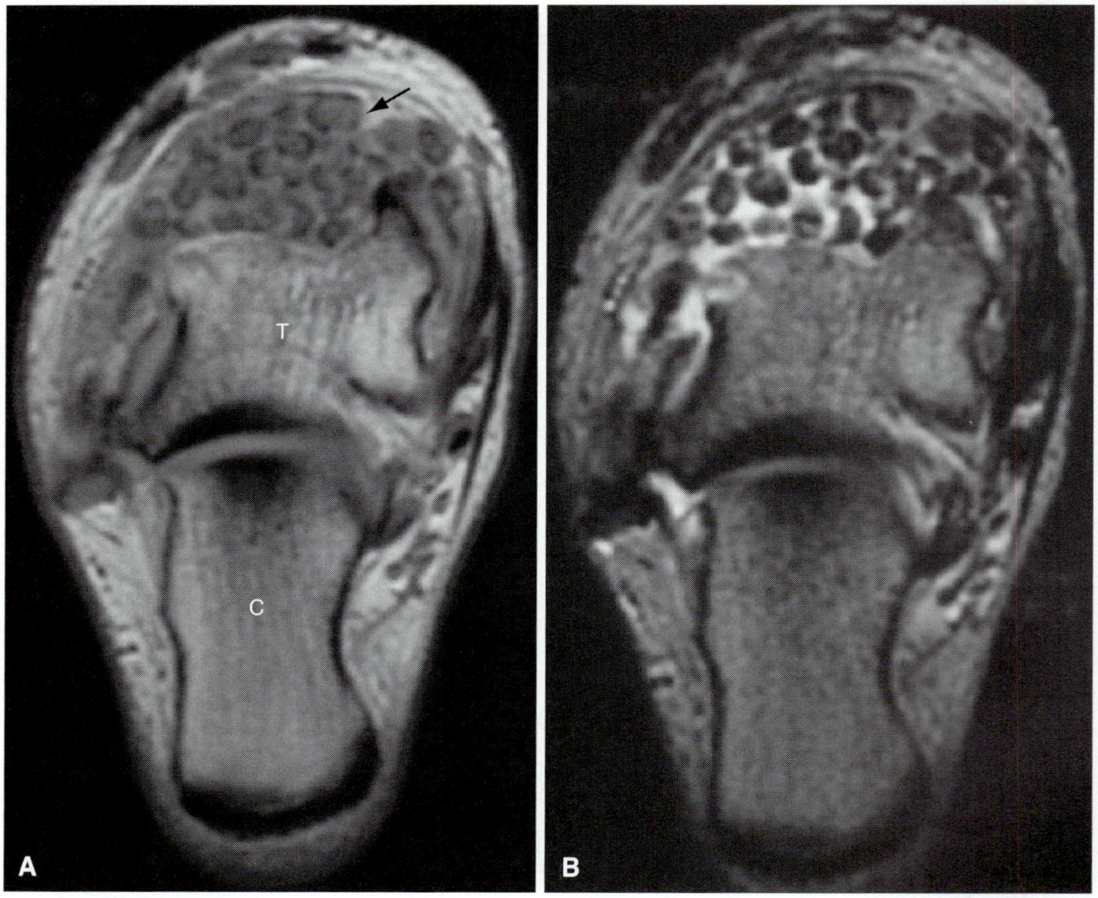

FIGURE 51–72 · Synovial Osteochondromatosis shown on MRI. *A* Oblique axial proton density image of the ankle shows multiple fairly uniformly sized bodies *(arrow)* with low signal rims and intermediate signal centers. *B*, The corresponding T2-weighted image shows the periphery of the nodules to remain dark, consistent with calcification or bone, and the centers of the nodules to remain intermediate in signal intensity. The joint fluid is very bright on the T2-weighted image. C, calcaneus; T, talus.

able to establish the specific diagnosis because the villous fatty nature of the lesion and the accompanying effusions are well seen with these modalities.[252,254,255]

The lesion does not enhance after intravenous gadolinium injection[255] (Fig. 51–74).

SILICONE SYNOVITIS

Silicone synovitis or prosthetic synovitis is a form of chronic foreign-body synovitis caused in response to shedding of silicone particles from damaged silicone polymer prostheses. Silicone synovitis has been most frequently reported in cases with carpal implants. The interval between surgical implantation and the complication of synovitis varies between 1 to 9 years with a mean of 5.5 years. The most common clinical features are local pain, limitation of motion, and swelling.[256,257]

Radiologic changes in silicone synovitis, when present, include nodular soft tissue swelling and well-defined subchondral lytic lesions (Fig. 51–75). These lytic lesions vary in size and may or may not have a sclerotic rim.[258] The cartilage space is relatively preserved. The prosthesis is often fragmented, deformed, or subluxed. On MRI, the lytic lesions show intermediate to mildly increased signal on PD and T2-weighted images, which are not typical of fluid-filled cysts. The internal signal characteristic of these lytic lesions is consistent with the presence of inflammatory and fibrous tissue. Disintegrated silicone fragments appear as hypointense regions on all sequences, as does the prosthesis itself[259] (Fig. 51–76).

IMPINGEMENT SYNDROME AND ROTATOR CUFF TEARS

The impingement syndrome is a well-recognized clinical entity, defined as painful compression of the supraspinatus tendon, subacromial bursa, and long head of the biceps tendon between the humeral head and the coracoacromial arch. The coracoacromial ligament, anterior third of acromion, and acromioclavicular joint comprise the coracoacromial arch.[260]

Impingement syndrome produces a spectrum of rotator cuff tendon abnormalities, beginning with degenerative tendinopathy and eventually progressing to a full-thickness tear. Many causes have been proposed for impingement of subacromial soft tissues.[260,261] These factors can be classified as extrinsic and intrinsic. The extrinsic causes include abnormal shape and slope of the

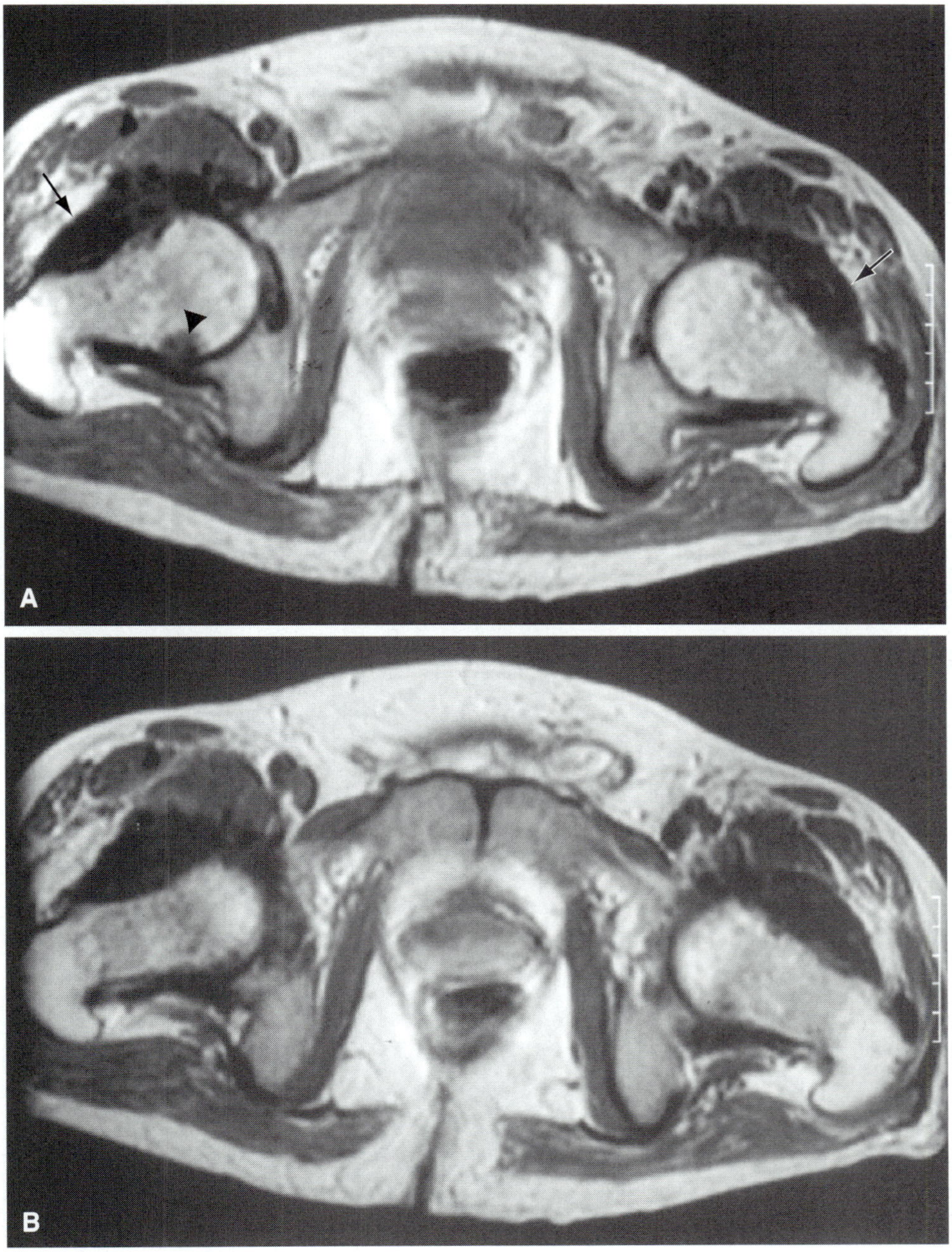

FIGURE 51–73 · **Beta 2-Microglobulin Amyloid in a Renal Transplant Recipient.** *A* Proton density image shows low signal material filling the hip joints bilaterally *(arrows)*. There is erosion of the right femoral head-neck junction *(arrowhead)*. *B*, The T2-weighted image shows the material around the femoral head and within the erosions of the right hip to remain low in signal, typical of amyloidosis.

acromion, subacromial spur formation, thickened coracoacromial ligament, and degenerative changes of the acromioclavicular joint. Rotator cuff disease may also occur as a result of repetitive microtrauma (overuse syndrome) without morphologic abnormalities of the coracoacromial arch. Intrinsic causes such as aging and decreased vascularity of the tendons are other contributing factors.

Radiographic findings suggesting subacromial impingement include osteophytes about the acromioclavicular joint and spur formation of the anterior acromion (Fig. 51–77) with corresponding areas of sclerosis and subchondral cysts of the greater tuberosity. An unfused acromial apophysis at the anterior aspect of the acromion (os acromiale), best seen on axillary view, may also predispose to subacromial impingement.[263] An outlet view is helpful for evaluating the shape of acromion. Rotator cuff tears are not generally apparent on radiographs, but chronic rotator cuff tear may be suggested on radiographs when there is superior migration of humeral head with relation to glenoid and an acromioclavicular distance less than 7 mm.

MRI findings used in diagnosing rotator cuff impingement and tear have been described in several reports.[264-269] The normal rotator cuff tendons appear uniformly low in signal intensity on all sequences. In early stages of impingement, the supraspinatus tendon shows thickening and inhomogeneous increased signal, representing

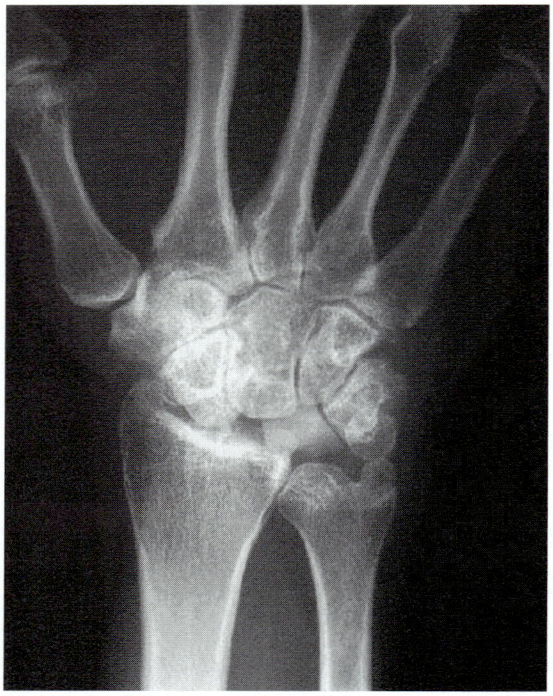

FIGURE 51–74 · Silicon Synovitis. A PA view of the wrist shows a silicone implant of the lunate for the treatment of Kienbock's disease. Multiple periarticular subchondral lytic lesions involving the carpal bones and distal ulna and radius are typical features of silicone synovitis. The prosthesis shows medial migration with a deformed and eroded proximal surface. There is also rotary subluxation of the scaphoid.

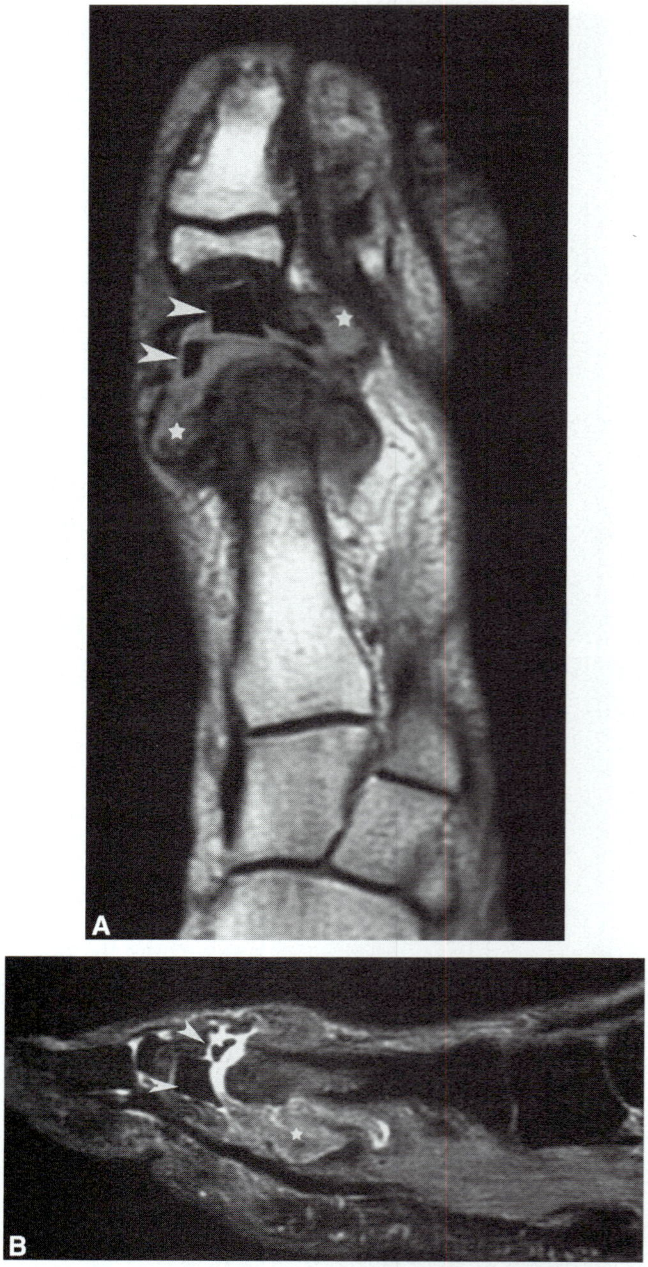

FIGURE 51–75 · Silicon Synovitis. *(A)* Coronol FSE proton density and *(B)* Sagittal STIR images of the great toe show fragments of a metatarsophalangeal silicone rubber prosthesis *(arrowheads)* with extensive surrounding synovitis (stars).

degenerative tendinopathy or tendinosis. There may be associated subacromial-subdeltoid bursitis. Further damage to the tendon results in partial tear as manifested on MRI by the presence of focal fluid signal intensity through a portion of the tendon on T2-weighted images. Partial rotator cuff tears can be seen inferiorly at the articular surface, superiorly at the bursal surface or within the tendon substance. Partial tears can be mistaken for full-thickness tears or tendinopathy with MRI. MR arthrography has been shown to be more accurate than conventional MRI for evaluation of partial tears, especially for articular surface tears.[270]

Full thickness rotator cuff tear is characterized on MRI by a fluid-filled gap in the tendon, with or without tendon retraction (Fig. 51–78). However, up to 10 percent of the tears may not show high signal intensity on T2-weighted images.[267] This may be due to replacement of the chronic tears with fibrous or granulation tissue that is low on T2-weighted images. Indirect signs of rotator cuff tears include a high-riding humeral head, fluid in subacromial-subdeltoid bursa, obliteration of the peribursal fat stripe, and joint effusion in the glenohumeral joint.[271]

Overall reported sensitivity of MRI for identification of rotator cuff tears ranges from 90 to 100 percent and specificity from 80 to 95 percent.[264-266,272,273]

Ultrasound is also an effective tool for the evaluation of rotator cuff tears, when performed by experienced sonographers. The tendons of a normal rotator cuff appear as hyperechoic, fibrillar structures on ultrasound. The diagnosis of a large retracted tear is made when there is nonvisualization of the supraspinatus tendon, and the deltoid muscle is directly apposed to the humeral cortex. A focal full-thickness tear is visualized as a hypoechoic or anechoic area extending through the rotator cuff with subacromial bursal fluid supporting the diagnosis. Ultrasound is less sensitive in diagnosing partial-thickness tears that may appear hypoechoic or of mixed echogenicity if the hyperechoic free edges of the torn tendon are surrounded by hypoechoic fluid or granulation tissue.[260,274]

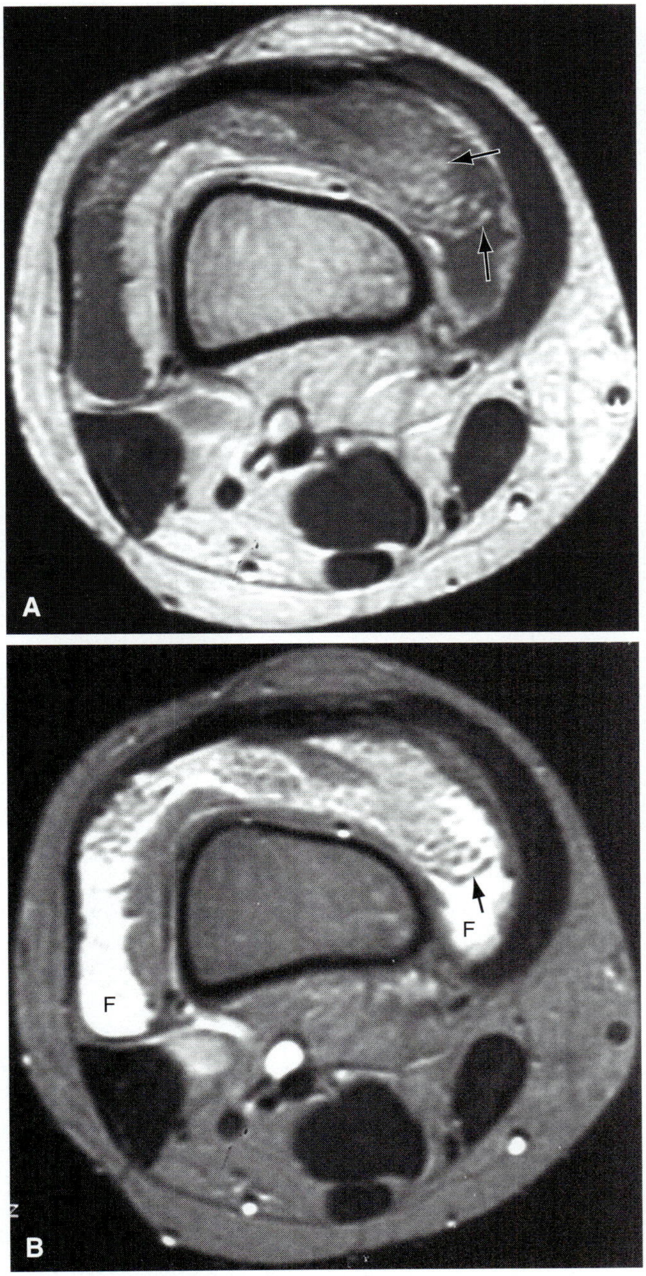

FIGURE 51–76 · Lipoma Arborescens. Proton density *(A)* and T2-weighted *(B)* images show frondlike collections of fat *(arrows)* within the joint separated by synovial fluid (F).

CARPAL TUNNEL SYNDROME

Carpal tunnel syndrome is the most common peripheral entrapment neuropathy, caused by pressure on the median nerve as it passes through the carpal tunnel. The nerve compression may result from a decrease in the volume of the canal (e.g., malalignment, fractures of the distal radius or carpal bones) or from an increase in the size of the soft tissues within the canal (e.g., tenosynovitis, soft tissue masses, persistent median artery, anomalous lumbrical muscles, amyloid deposition, excessive fat, hemorrhage).

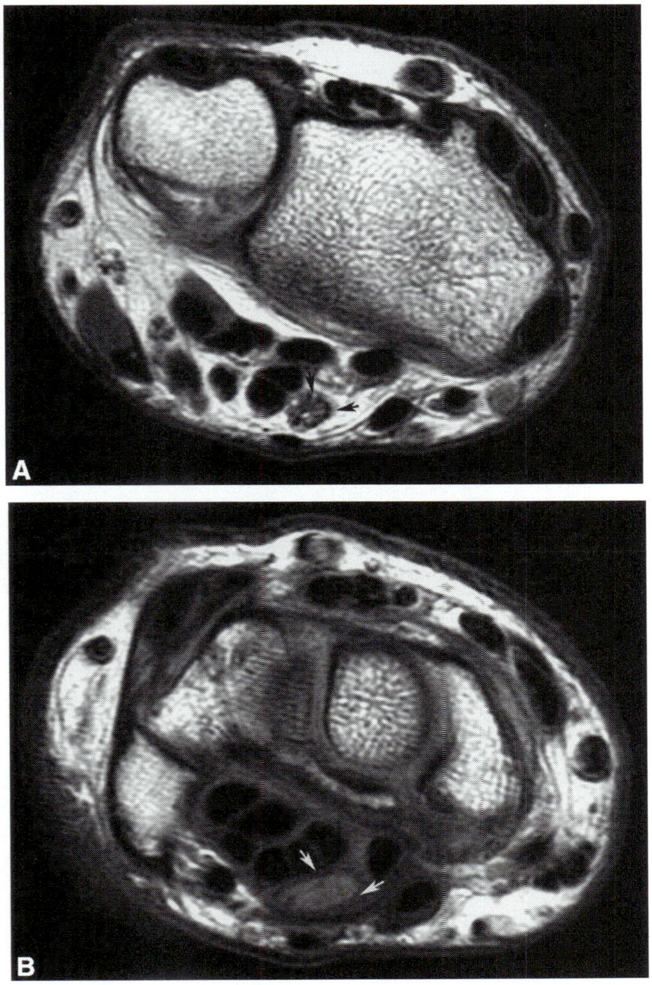

FIGURE 51–77 · Carpal Tunnel Syndrome. *A*, FSE Proton density axial image at the level of the distal radius. The median nerve *(black arrows)* has normal size prior to entering the carpal tunnel. *B*. FSE Proton density axial image at the level of pisiform. The median nerve *(arrows)* shows enlargement and high signal.

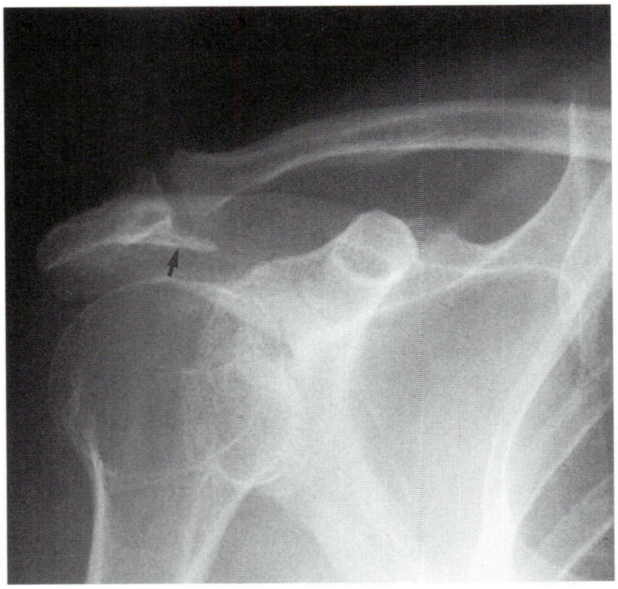

FIGURE 51–78 · The frontal radiograph of the shoulder of the shows a large spur *(arrow)* projecting from the inferior, anterior acromion process. Subsequent MR imaging examination showed full thickness tears of both the supraspinatus and infraspinatus tendons.

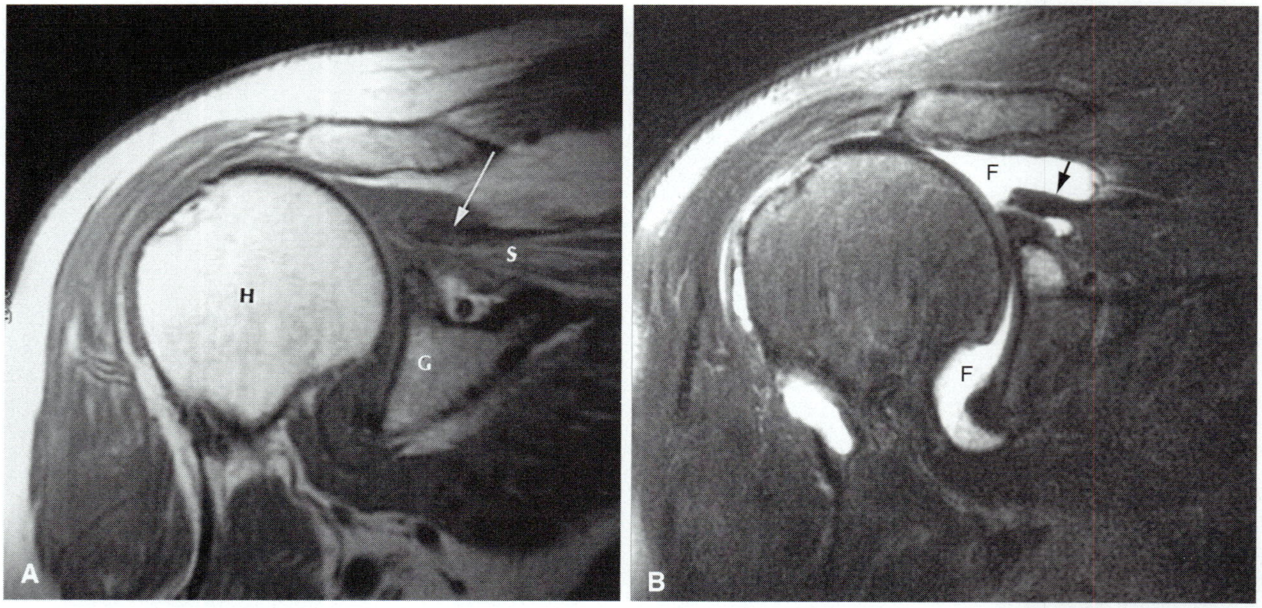

FIGURE 51–79 · Rotator Cuff Tear with Retraction. *A*, The T1-weighted oblique coronal MRI of the shoulder shows elevation of the humeral head (H) with relation of the glenoid (G). There is narrowing of the distance between the humeral head and the acromion. The supraspinatus is atrophic and infiltrated with fat. The dark tendon *(arrow)* is seen retracted proximally. *B*, The oblique coronal T2-weighted image better shows the torn, retracted edge of the supraspinatus tendon *(arrow)*. The joint fluid (F) is bright on this sequence and communicates through the rotator cuff defect with the subacromial subdeltoid bursal fluid.

In most cases, the diagnosis of carpal tunnel syndrome can be made with clinical examination and confirmed by nerve conduction studies[275]; generally, imaging is not necessary. MRI is reserved for the patients with atypical clinical presentation and inconclusive electrophysiologic tests. MRI findings of carpal tunnel syndrome, irrespective of the underlying etiology, are diffuse or segmental enlargement of the median nerve, increased signal intensity of the median nerve on T2-weighted images, bowing of the flexor retinaculum, and flattening of the nerve[276,277] (Fig. 51–79). MRI may also be helpful in the evaluation of patients with recurrent or persistent symptoms after surgical division of the flexor retinaculum by demonstrating incomplete release of the flexor retinaculum, postsurgical fibrosis around the median nerve, or a mass lesion within the carpal tunnel.[278]

Morphologic changes of the median nerve in carpal tunnel syndrome have been also described with ultrasound.[279,280] When the cross-sectional area of median nerve exceeds 10 to 15 mm^2, it is considered abnormal. Tenosynovitis and a ganglion are among the causes of carpal tunnel syndrome that can be evaluated with sonography.

REFERENCES

1. Andren L, Lundberg BJ: Treatment of rigid shoulders by joint distention during arthrography. Acta Orthop Scan 36:45, 1965.
2. Bushong S: Computed tomography. *In* (eds): Radiologic Science for Technologists, 3rd ed. St. Louis, Mosby, 1984, pp 363-886.
3. Padhani AR, Adrian KD: Whole body computed tomography. *In* Grainger RG, Allison D, Adam A, Dixon AK (eds): Grainger & Allison's Diagnostic Radiology: A Textbook of Medical Imaging, 4th ed., Churchill Livingstone, 2001, pp 81-99.
4. Cinnoman J: Multislice volumetric spiral CT. Picker Multislice Volumetric Spiral CT Principles & Applications. Picker International, 1999, pp 27-35.
5. Buckwalter KA, Rydberg J, Crow K, et al: Musculoskeletal imaging with multislice CT. AJR 176:979-986, 2001.
6. Winalski CS, Shapiro AW: Computed tomography in the evaluation of arthritis: Imaging of Rheumatic diseases. Rheum Dis Clin North Am 17:543-557, 1991.
7. Carrera GF, Foley WD, Kozin F, et al: CT of sacroiliitis. AJR 136:41-46, 1981.
8. Borzala GS, Seigel R, Huhns LR, et al: Computed tomography in the evaluation of sacroiliac arthritis. Radiology 139:437-440, 1981.
9. Morgan GJ, Schlegelmilch JG, Spiegel PK: Early diagnosis of septic arthritis of the sacroiliac joint by use of computed tomography. J Rheumatol 8:979-982, 1981.
10. Vande Berg BC, Lecouvet FE, Poilvache P, et al: Dual detector spiral CT arthrography of the knee: Accuracy for detection of meniscal abnormalities and unstable meniscal tear. Radiology 216: 851-857, 2000.
11. Vande Berg BC, Lecouvet FE, Poilvache P, et al: Assessment of knee cartilage in cadavers with dual-detector spiral CT arthrography and MR imaging. Radiology 222:430-436, 2002.
12. Kaye JJ: Arthritis: Roles of radiography and other imaging techniques in evaluation. Radiology 177:601-608, 1990.
13. Peterfy CG: Imaging techniques. *In* Maddison PJ, Isenberg DA, Woo P, et al (eds): Oxford Textbook of Rheumatology, 2nd ed. Oxford, Oxford Medical Publications, 1998.
14. Wood ML, Werhli FW: Principles of magnetic resonance imaging. *In* Stark DD, Bradley WG (eds): Magnetic Resonance Imaging, 3rd ed. St. Louis, Mosby,1999, pp 1-14.
15. Tung GA, Brody JM: Contemporary imaging of athletic injuries. Clin Sports Med 16:393-417, 1997.
16. Paley MNJ, Wilkinson ID, van Beek E, et al: Magnetic resonance imaging: basic principles. *In* Grainger RG, Allison D, Adam A, Dixon

AK (eds): Grainger & Allison's Diagnostic Radiology: A Textbook of Medical Imaging, 4th ed. Churchill Livingstone, 2001, pp 101-135.
17. McGonagle D, Conaghan PG, Wakefield R, et al: Imaging of the joint in early rheumatoid arthritis. Best Prac Res Clin Rheum 15:91-104, 2001.
18. Savnik A, Malmskov H, Thomsen HS, et al: MRI of the wrist and finger joints in inflammatory joint diseases at 1-year interval: MRI features to predict bone erosions. Eur Radiol 12:1203-1210, 2002.
19. Weissman BN: Imaging techniques in rheumatoid arthritis. J Rheumatology 21(Suppl 42):14-19, 1994.
20. McQueen FM: Magnetic resonance imaging in early inflammatory arthritis: what is its role? Rheumatology 39:700-706, 2000.
21. Taouli B, Guermazi A, Sack K, Genant HK: Imaging of the hand and wrist in RA. Ann Rheum Dis 61:867-869, 2002.
22. Backhaus M, Burmester GR, Gerber T, et al: Guidelines for musculoskeletal ultrasound in rheumatology. Ann Rheum 60:641-649, 2001.
23. Rubin JM, Bude RO, Carson PL, et al: Power Doppler: a potentially useful alternative to mean-frequency based color Doppler sonography. Radiology 190:853-856, 1994.
24. Newman JS, Adler RS, Bude RO, et al: Detection of soft tissue hyperemia: Value of power Doppler sonography. AJR 163:385-389, 1994.
25. Correas JM, Bridal L, Lesavre A, et al: Ultrasound contrast agents: properties, principles of action, tolerance, and artifacts. Eur Radiol 11:1316-1328, 2001.
26. Barberia JE, Wong AD, Cooprg PL, et al: Extended field-of-view sonography in musculoskeletal disorders. AJR 171:751-757, 1998.
27. Adler RS: Future and new developments in musculoskeletal ultrasound. Radiol Clin North Am 37:623-631, 1999.
28. Qvistgaard E, Rogind H, Torp-Pederson S, et al: Quantitative ultrasound in arthritis: rheumatoid evaluation of inflammation in Doppler technique. Ann Rheum Dis 60:690-693, 2001.
29. Klauser A, Frauscher F, Schirmer M, et al: The value of contrast-enhanced color Doppler ultrasound in the detection of vascularization of finger joints in patients with Rheumatoid arthritis. Arthritis Rheum 46:647-653, 2002.
30. Stone M, Bergin D, Whelan B, et al: Power Doppler ultrasound assessment of rheumatoid hand synovitis. J Rheumatol 28: 1979-1982, 2001.
31. Szkudlarek M, Court-Payen M, Strandberg C, et al: Power Doppler ultrasonography for assessment of synovitis in the metacarpophalangeal joints of patients with rheumatoid arthritis: A comporison with dynamic magnetic resonance imaging. Arthritis Rheum 9:2018-2023, 2001.
32. Wakefield RJ, Gibbon WW, Conaghan PG, et al: The value of sonography in the detection of bone erosions in patients with rheumatoid arthritis: a comparison with conventional radiography. Arthritis Rheum 43:2762-2770, 2000.
33. Grassi W, Filipucci E, Farina A, et al: Ultrasonography in the evaluation of bone erosions. Ann Rheum Dis 60:98-103, 2001.
34. Rosenthall L: Nuclear medicine techniques in arthritis. Imaging of rheumatic diseases. Rheum Dis Clin North Am 17:585-597, 1991.
35. Vos K, Van der Linden E, Pauwels EK: The clinical role of nuclear medicine in rheumatoid arthritis patients; A comparison with other imaging modalities. Q J Nucl Med 43:38-45, 1999.
36. Bois de MHW, Pauwels EKJ, Breedveld FC: New agents for scintigraphy in rheumatoid arthritis. Eur J Nuc Med 22:1339-1346, 1995.
37. Bois de MHW, Arndt J-W, van der Velde EA, et al: 99m Tc human immuno-globulin scintigraphy: a reliable method to detect joint activity in rheumatoid arthritis. J Rheumatol 19:1371-1376, 1992.
38. Miller IL, Savory CG, Polly DW Jr., et al: Femoral head osteonecrosis: Detection with magnetic resonance imaging versus single-photon emission compute tomography. Clin Orthop Rel Res 247:152-162, 1989.
39. Renner WR, Weinstein AS: Early changes of rheumatoid arthritis in the hand and wrist. Radiol Clin North Am 26:1185-1193, 1988.
40. Sanders TG, Linares R, Su A: Rheumatoid nodule of the foot: MRI appearances mimicking an intermediate soft tissue mass. Skeletal Radiol 27:457-460, 1998.
41. Resnick D: Rheumatoid arthritis. *In* Resnick D (ed): Diagnosis of Bone and Joint Disorders, 4th ed. Philadelphia, WB Saunders, 2002, pp 891-987.
42. Barker JA, Sebes JI: Rheumatoid arthritis of the robust-reaction type. Arthritis Rheum 41:1131-1132, 1998.
43. Maher MM, Kennedy J, Hynes D, et al: Giant distal humeral geode. Skeletal Radiol 29:165, 2000.
44. Karasick D, Schweitzer ME, O'Hara BJ: Distal fibular notch: a frequent manifestation of the rheumatoid ankle. 26:529-532, 1997.
45. Beltran J, Caudill JL, Herman LA, et al: Rheumatoid arthritis: MR imaging manifestations. Radiology 165:153-157, 1987.
46. Winalski CS, Palmer WE, Rosenthal DI, Weissman BN: Magnetic resonance imaging of rheumatoid arthritis. Radiol Clin North Am 34:243-258, 1996.
47. Peterfy CG, Majumdar S, Lang P, et al: MR imaginag of arthritic knee: improved discrimination of cartilage, synovium, and effusion with pulsed saturation transfer and fat-suppressed T1-weighted sequences. Radiology 191:413-419,1994.
48. Kursunoglu-Brahme S, Riccio T, Weisman MH, et al: Rheumatoid knee: Role of gadopentetate-enhanced MR imaging. Radiology 176:831-835, 1990.
49. Bjorkengren AG, Gebcrek P, Rydholm U, et al: MR imaging of the knee in acute rheumatoid arthritis: synovial uptake of gadolinium-DOTA. AJR 155:329-332, 1990.
50. Reiser MF, Bongartz GP, Erleman R, et al: Gadolinium-DTPA in rheumatoid arthritis and related diseases: first results with dynamic magnetic resonance imaging. Skeletal Radiol 18:591-597, 1989.
51. Winalski CS, Aliabadi P, Wright JR, et al: Enhancement of joint fluid with intravenously administered gadopentetate dimenglumine: Technique, rationale and implications. Radiology 187:179-185, 1993.
52. Drape J-L, Thelen P, Gay-Depassier, et al: Intraarticular diffusion of Gd-DOTA after intravenous injection in the knee: MR imaging evaluation. Radiology 188:227-234, 1993.
53. Konig H, Sieper J, Wolf KJ: Rheumatoid arthritis: Evaluation of hypervascular and fibrous pannus with dynamic MR imaging enhanced with Gd-DTPA. Radiology 176:473-477, 1990.
54. Kalden-Nemeth D, Grebmeier J, Antoni C, et al: NMR monitoring of rheumatoid arthritis patients receiving anti-TNF monoclonal antibody therapy. Rheumatol Int 16 249-255, 1997.
55. Ostergaard M, Stoltenberg M, Henricksen O, Lorenzen I: Quantitative assessment of synovial inflammation by dynamic gadolinium-enhanced magnetic resonance imaging. A study of the effect of intra-articular methylprednisolone on the rate of early synovial enhancement. Br J Rheumatol 35:50-59, 1996.
56. Sugimoto H, Takeda A, Kano S: Assessment of disease activity in rheumatoid arthritis using magnetic resonance imaging: quantification of pannus volume in the hands. Br J Rheumatol 37: 854-861, 1998.
57. Ostergaard M, Hansen M, Stoltenberg M, et al: Magnetic resonance imaging-determined synovial membrane volume as a marker of disease activity and predictor of progressive joint destruction in wrists of patients with rheumatoid arthritis. Arthritis Rheum 42:918-928, 1999.
58. Ostergaard M, Gideon P, Lorenzen I: Synovial volume-A marker of disease severity in rheumatoid arthritis? Quantification by MRI. Scand J Rheumatol 23:197-202, 1994.
59. Ostergaard M: Different approaches to synovial membrane volume determination by magnetic resonance imaging: manual vs automated segmentation. Br J Rheumatol 36:1166-1177, 1997.
60. Sugitomo H, Takeda A, Hyodoh K: Early-stage rheumatoid arthritis: Prospective study of the effectiveness of MR imaging for diagnosis. Radiology 216:569-575, 2000.
61. Sugitomo H, Takeda AT, Masuyama J, Furuse M: Early stage rheumatoid-arthritis: diagnostic accuracy of MR imaging. Radiology 198:185-192, 1996.
62. Rominger MB, Bernreuter WK, Kenney PJ, et al: MR imaging of the hands in early rheumatoid arthritis: preliminary results. RadioGraphics 13:37-36, 1993.
63. McQueen FM, Stewart N, Crabbe J, et al: Magnetic resonance imaging of the wrist in early rheumatoid arthritis reveals high prevalence of erosions at 4 months after symptoms onset. Ann Rheum Dis 57:350-356, 1998.
64. Rubens DJ, Bleba JS, Totterman SMS, et al: Rheumatoid arthritis: evaluation of wrist tendons with clinical examination versus MR imaging. Radiology 187:831-838, 1993.
65. Cohen PA, Job-Deslandre CH, Lalande G, et al: Overview of the radiology of juvenile idiopathic arthritis. Eur J Radiol 33:94-101, 2000.

66. Petty RE, Southwood TR, Baum J, et al: Revision of the proposed classification criteria for juvenile idiopathic arthritis: Durban 1997. J Rheum 25:1991-1994, 1998.
67. Ansell BM, Kent PA: Radiological changes in juvenile chronic polyarthritis. Skeletal Radiol 1:129-144, 1977.
68. Martel W, Holt JF, Cassidy JT: Roentgenologic manifestations of juvenile rheumatoid arthritis. AJR 88:400, 1962.
69. Resnick D: Juvenile chronic arthritis. *In* Resnick D (ed): Diagnosis of Bone and Joint Disorders, 4th ed. Philadelphia,WB Saunders, 2002, pp 988-1022.
70. Bollow M, Braun J, Biederman T, et al: Use of contrast-enhanced MR imaging to detect sacroiliitis in children. Skeletal Radiol 27:606-616, 1998.
71. Bollow M, Braun J, Kannenberg J, et al: Normal morphology of sacroiliac joints in children: magnetic resonance studies related to age and sex. Skeletal Radiol 26:697-704,1997.
72. Medsger TA Jr., Christy WC: Carpal arthritis with ankylosis in late-onset Still's disease. Arthritis Rheum 19:232, 1976.
73. Moll JHM, Wright V: Psoriatic arthritis. Semin Arthritis Rheum 3:55-78, 1973.
74. Porter GG: Psoriatic arthritis; Plain radiology and other imaging techniques. Bailliere's Clin Rheumatol 8(2):465-482, 1994.
75. Resnick D: Psoriatic arthritis. *In* Resnick D (ed): Diagnosis of Bone and Joint Disorders, 4th ed. Philadelphia, WB Saunders, 2002, pp 1082-1109.
76. Resnick D, Feingold ML, Curd J, et al: Calcaneal abnormalities in articular disorders: Rheumatoid arthritis, ankylosing spondylitis, psoriatic arthritis and Reiter's syndrome. Radiology 125:355-366, 1977.
77. Sholkoff SD, Glickman MG, Steinbach HL: Roentgenology of Reiter's syndrome. Radiology 97:497-503, 1970.
78. Resnick D: Reiter's syndrome. *In* Resnick D (ed): Diagnosis of Bone and Joint Disorders, 4th ed. Philadelphia, WB Saunders, 2002, pp 1010-1126.
79. Mitchell M, Howard B, Haller J, et al: Septic arthritis. Radiol Clin North Am 26:1295-1313, 1988.
80. Goldman AB: Arthrography for rheumatic disease; when, why and for whom: Imaging of rheumatic diseases. Rheum Dis Clin North Am 17:505-542, 1991.
81. Resnick D: Osteomyelitis, septic arthritis and soft tissue infection: organisms. *In* Resnick D (ed): Diagnosis of Bone and Joint Disorders, 4th ed. Philadelphia, WB Saunders, 2002, pp 2510-2624.
82. Brower A: Septic arthritis. Radiol Clin North Am 34:293-309, 1996.
83. Graif M, Schweitzer ME, Deely D, et al: The septic versus nonseptic inflamed joint: MRI characteristics. Skeletal Radiol 28:616-620, 1999.
84. Learch TJ, Farooki S: Magnetic resonance imaging of septic arthritis. J Clin Imaging 24:236-342, 2000.
85. Tumeh SS, Tohmeh A: Nuclear medicine techniques in septic arthritis and osteomyelitis. Rheum Clin Rheumatol 17:559-583, 1991.
86. Resnick D, Niwayama G: Degenerative disease of extraspinal locations. *In* Resnick D, Niwayama G (eds): Diagnosis of Bone and Joint Disorders. Philadelphia, WB Saunders, 1981, p 1270.
87. Boegard T, Jonsson K: Radiography in osteoarthritis of the knee. Skeletal Radiol 28(11):605, 1999.
88. Marshall KW, Mikulis DJ, Gunthrie BM: Quantitation of articular cartilage using magnetic resonance imaging and three-dimensional reconstruction. J Orthop Res 13:184, 1995.
89. Drape JL, Pessis E, Auleley GR, et al: Quantitative MR imaging evaluation of chondropathy in osteoarthritis knees. Radiology 208:49, 1998.
90. Reddy R, Insko EK, Noyszeski EA, et al: Sodium MRI of human cartilage in vivo. Magn Reson Med 39:697, 1998.
91. Eckstein F, Schnier M, Haubner M, et al: Accuracy of cartilage volume and thickness measurements with magnetic resonance imaging. Clin Orthop Rel Res 352:137, 1998.
92. Waldschmidt JG, Rilling RJ, Kajdacsy-Balla AA, et al: In vitro and in vivo MR imaging of hyaline cartilage: Zonal anatomy, imaging pitfalls, and pathologic conditions. Radiographics 17:1387, 1997.
93. Chan WP, Lang P, Stevens MP, et al: Osteoarthritis of the knee: Comparison radiography, CT and MR imaging to assess extent and severity. AJR 157:799, 1991.
94. Waldschmidt JG, Braunstein EM, Buckwalter KA: Magnetic resonance imaging of osteoarthritis. Rheum Dis Clin North Am 25:451, 1999.
95. Ostegaard M, Court-Payan M, Gideon P, et al: Ultrasonography in arthritis of the knee: A comparison with MR imaging. Acta Radiol 36:19, 1995.
96. Resnick D: Patterns of migration of the femoral head in osteoarthritis of the hip: Roentgenographic-pathologic correlation and comparison with rheumatoid arthritis.AJR 124:62, 1975.
97. Thomas RH, Resnick D, Alazraki NP, et al: Compartmental evaluation of osteoarthritis of the knee: A comparative study of available diagnostic modalities. Radiology 116:585, 1975.
98. Leach RE, Grett T, Ferris JS: Weight-bearing radiography in osteoarthritis of the knee. Radiology 97:265, 1970.
99. Bergman AG, Willen HK, Lindstran AL, et al: Osteoarthritis of the knee: Correlation of subchondral MR signal abnormalities with histopathologic and radiographic features. Skeletal Radiol 23:445, 1994.
100. Ostegaard M, Soltenberg M, Lovgreen-Nielson P, et al: Magnetic resonance imaging: determined synovial membrane and joint effusion volumes in rheumatoid arthritis and osteoarthritis: Comparison of the macroscopic and microscopic appearance of the synovium. Arthritis Rheum 40:1856, 1997.
101. Fernandez-Madrid F, Karvonen RL, Teitge RA, et al: MR features of osteoarthritis of the knee. Magn Reson Imaging 12:703, 1994.
102. Fernandez-Madrid F, Karvonen RL, Teitge RA, et al: Synovial thickening detected by MR imaging in osteoarthritis of the knee confirmed by biopsy as synovitis. Magn Reson Imaging 13:177, 1995.
103. Ostegaard M: Different approaches to synovial membrane volume determination by magnetic resonance imaging: Manual versus automated segmentation. Br J Rheum36:1166, 1997.
104. Cornelius R, Schneider HJ: Gouty arthritis in the adult. Radiol Clin North Am 26:1267-1276, 1988.
105. Resnick D, Broderick TW: Intraosseous calcifications in tophaceous gout. AJR 137:1157-1161,1981.
106. Martel W: The overhanging margin of bone: A roentgenologic manifestation of gout. Radiology 91:755-756, 1968.
107. Good AE, Rapp R: Bony ankylosis: a rare manifestation of gout. J Rheumatol 5:335-337, 1978.
108. Chen KHC, Yeh LR, Pan HB, et al: Intraarticular gouty tophi of the knee: CT and MR imaging in 12 patients. Skeletal Radiol 28:75-80, 1999.
109. Gerster JC, Landry M, Dufresne L, et al: Imaging of tophaceous gout: computed tomography provides images compared with magnetic resonance imaging and ultrasonography. Ann Rheum Dis 61:52-54, 2002.
110. Yu JS, Chung C, Recht M, et al: MR imaging of tophaceous gout. AJR 168:523-527, 1997.
111. King JG, Nicholas CN: Gouty arthropathy of the lumbar spine. Spine 22:2309-2312, 1997.
112. Jensen PS: Chondrocalcinosis and other calcifications. Radiol Clin North Am 26(6):1315-1325, 1988.
113. Beltran J, Marthy-Delfault E, Bencardino J, et al: Chondrocalcinosis of the hyaline cartilage of the knee: MRI manifestation. Skeletal Radiol 27:369-374, 1998.
114. Kaushik S, Erickson JK, Palmer WE, et al: Effect of chondrocalcinosis on the MR imaging of knee menisci. AJR 177:905-909, 2001.
115. Martel W, McCarter DK, Solsky MA, et al: Further observations on the arthropathy of calcium pyrophosphate deposition disease. Radiology 141:1-15, 1981.
116. Steinbach LS, Resnick D: Calcium pyrophosphate dihydrate crystal deposition disease revisited. Radiology 200:1-9, 1996.
117. Helfgott SM, Skoff H: Scapholunate dissociation associated with crystal induced synovitis. J Rheumatol 19:485-487, 1992.
118. Ishida T, Dorfman HD, Bullough PG: Tophaceous pseudogout tumoral calcium pyrophosphate dihydrate crystal deposition. Hum Pathol 26:587-593, 1995.
119. Kakisubata Y, Boutin RD, Theodorou DJ, et al: Calcium pyrophosphate crystal deposition in and around atlantoaxial joint: association with type 2 fractures in nine patients. Radiology 216:213-219, 2000.
120. Holt PD, Keats TE: Calcific tendinitis: a review of the usual and unusual. Skeletal Radiol 22:1-9, 1993.
121. Resnick D: Calcium hydroxyapatite crystal deposition disease. *In* Resnick D (ed): Diagnosis of Bone and Joint Disorders, 4th ed. Philadelphia, WB Saunders, 2002, pp 1619-1657.

122. Kraemer EJ, El-Khoury GY: Atypical calcific tendinitis with cortical erosions. Skeletal Radiol 29:690-696, 2000.
123. Uri DS, Dalinka MK: Crystal disease. Radiol Clin North Am 34:359-374, 1996.
124. Nguyen VD: Rapid destructive arthritis of the shoulder. Skeletal Radiol 25:107-112, 1996.
125. Jensen PS: Hemachromatosis: a disease often silent but not visible. AJR 126:343-351, 1976.
126. Dymock IW, Hamilton EBD, Laws JW, Williams R: Arthropathy of hemochromatosis: clinical and radiological analysis of 63 patients with iron overload.Ann Rheum Dis 29:469-476, 1970.
127. Hirsch JH, Killien FC, Troupin RH: The arthropathy of hemochromatosis. Radiology 118:591-596, 1976.
128. Adamson TC, Resnik CS, Guerra J, et al: Hand and wrist arthropathies of hemochromatosis and calcium pyrophosphate deposition disease: distinct radiologic features. Radiology 147: 377-381, 1983.
129. Eustace S, Buff B, McCarthy C, et al: Magnetic resonance imaging of hemochromatosis arthropathy. Skeletal Radiol 23: 547-549, 1994.
130. Mindelzun R, Elkin M, Scheinberg IH, et al: Skeletal changes in Wilson's disease. Radiology 94:127-132,1970.
131. Resnick D: Hemochromatosis and Wilson's disease. *In* Resnick D (ed): Diagnosis of Bone and Joint Disorders, 4th ed. Philadelphia, WB Saunders, 2002, pp 1658-1677.
132. Cervenansky J, Sitaj S, Urbanek T: Alkaptonuria and ochronosis. J Bone Joint Surg 41-A:1169-1182,1959.
133. Resnick D: Alkaptopnuria. *In* Resnick D (ed): Diagnosis of Bone and Joint Disorders, 4th ed. Philadelphia, WB Saunders, 2002, pp 1678-1691.
134. Pettersson H, Ahlberg A, Nilsson IM: A radiologic classification of hemophilic arthropathy. Clin Orthop Rel Res 149:153, 1980.
135. Winalski CS, Foldes K, Gravallese EM, et al: Synovial membrane disorders. Magn Reson Imaging 2:1079-1096, 1999.
136. Idy-Peretti I: MR imaging of hemophilic arthropathy of the knee: Classification and evolution of the subchondral cysts. Magn Reson Imaging 10:67, 1992.
137. Conway WE, Totty WG: Hip in Magnetic Resonance Imaging, 3rd ed. St. Louis, Mosby, 1999.
138. Zurla JV: The double line sign. Radiology 212:541, 1999.
139. Mitchell DG, Rao JM, Dalinka MK, et al: Femoral head avascular necrosis: Correlation of MR imaging, radiographic staging, radionuclide imaging, and clinical findings. Radiology 162:709, 1987.
140. Jiang CC, Shih TTF: Epiphyseal scar of the femoral head: Risk factor of osteonecrosis. Radiology 191:409, 1994.
141. Beltran J, Herman IJ, Burk JM, et al. Femoral head avascular necrosis: MRI with clinical-pathologic correlation. Radiology 166:215, 1988.
142. Hayes CW, Conway WF, Daniel CW: MR imaging of bone marrow edema pattern: Transient osteoporosis, transient bone marrow edema syndrome, or osteonecrosis. Radiographics 13:1001, 1993.
143. Vande Berg BC, Malghem JJ, Lecouvert FE, et al: Idiopathic bone marrow lesions of the femoral head: Predictive value of MR imaging findings. Radiology 212:527, 535.
144. Brower AC, Almann RM: Pathogenesis of the neurotrophic joint: Neurotraumatic versus neurovascular. Radiology 139: 349-354, 1981.
145. Phillips S, Williams AL, Peters JR: Neuropathic arthropathy of the spine in diabetes. Diabetes Care 18:867-869, 1995.
146. Feldman MJ, Becker KL, Reefe WE, Longo A: Multiple neuropathic joints, including wrist, in a patient with diabetes mellitus. JAMA 209:1690-1692, 1969.
147. Deirmengian CA, Lee SG, Jupiter JB: Neuropathic arthropathy of the elbow: A report of five cases. J Bone Joint Surg 83-A: 839-844, 2001.
148. Reinhardt K: The radiological residue of healed diabetic arthropathies. Skeletal Radiol 7:167-172, 1981.
149. Seabold JE, Flicker FW, Kao SC, et al: Indium-111-leukocyte/technetium-99m-MDP bone and magnetic resonance imaging: difficulty of diagnosing osteomyelitis with neuropathic osteoarthropathy. J Nuclear Med 31:549-556, 1990.
150. Beltran J, Campanini DS, Knight C, et al: The diabetic foot: magnetic resonance imaging evaluation. Skeletal Radiol 19:37-41, 1990.
151. Yu J: Diabetic foot and neuroarthropathy: magnetic resonance imaging evaluation. Topics Magn Res Imag 9:295-310, 1998.
152. Greenstein AS, Marzo-Ortega H, Emery F, et al: Magnetic resonance imaging as a predictor of progressive joint destruction in neuropathic disease. Arthritis Rheum 46:2814-2815, 2002.
153. Park YH, Taylor JAM Szollar SM, et al: Imaging findings in spinal neuropathy. Spine 13:1499-1504, 1994.
154. Wagner SC, Schweitzer ME, Morrison WB, et al: Can imaging findings help differentiate spinal neuropathic arthropathy from disk space infection? Initial experience. Radiology 214:693-699, 2000.
155. Resnick D: Scleroderma (progressive systemic sclerosis). *In* Resnick D, Niwayama G (eds): Diagnosis of Bone and Joint Disorders. Philadelphia, WB Saunders, 1981, p 1204.
156. Poznanski AK: The Hand in Radiologic Diagnosis. Philadelphia, WB Saunders, 1974.
157. Thibierge G, Weissenbach RJ: Concretions calcare souscutanees et sclerodermie. Ann Dermatol Syph 2:129, 1911.
158. Muller SA, Brunsting LA, Winkelmann RK: Calcinosis cutis: Its relationship to scleroderma. Arch Dermatol Venereal 80:15, 1959.
159. Rowell NR, Hopper FE: The periodontal membrane in systemic lupus erythematosus. Br J Dermatol 93(suppl):23, 1975.
160. Mezarsos WT: The regional manifestations of scleroderma. Radiology 70:313, 1958.
161. Kemp Harper RA, Jackson DC: Progressive systemic sclerosis. Br J Radiol 38:825, 1965.
162. Keats TE: Rib erosions in scleroderma. AJR 100:530, 1967.
163. Seifert MH, Steigerwald JC, Cliff MM: Bone resorption of the mandible in progressive systemic sclerosis. Arthritis Rheum 18:507, 1977.
164. Haverbush TJ, Wilde AH, Hawk WA Jr, et al: Osteolysis of the ribs and cervical spine in progressive systemic sclerosis (scleroderma): A case report. J Bone Joint Surg 56 Am :637, 1974.
165. Lovell CR, Jayson MIV: Joint involvement in systemic sclerosis. Scand J Rheumatol 8:154, 1979.
166. Olsen NJ, King LE, Park JH: Muscle abnormalities in scleroderma. Scleroderma 22:783, 1996.
167. Labowitz R, Schumacher H: Articular manifestations of systemic lupus erythematosus. Ann Intern Med 74:911, 1971.
168. Weissman BN, Rappoport AS, Sosman JL, et al: Radiographic findings in the hands in patients with systemic lupus erythematosus. Radiology 126:313, 1978.
169. Bleifield CJ, Inglis AE: The hand in systemic lupus erythematosus. J Bone Joint Surg 56(A):1207, 1974.
170. Bywaters EGL: Jaccoud's syndrome: A sequel to the joint involvement in systemic lupus erythematosus. Clin Rheum Dis 1:125, 1975.
171. Twinning RH, Marcus WY, Carey JL: Tendon rupture in systemic lupus erythematosus. JAMA 189:377, 1964.
172. Klippel JH, Gerber LH, Pollack L, et al: Avascular necroses in systemic lupus erythematosus: Silent symmetric osteonecrosis. Am J Med 67:83, 1979.
173. Budin JA, Feldman F: Soft tissue calcifications in systemic lupus erythematosus. AJR 124:358, 1975.
174. Staples PJ, Gerding DN, Decker JL, et al: Incidence of infection in systemic lupus erythematosis. Arthritis Rheum 17:1, 1971.
175. Goodman N: The significance of terminal phalangeal osteosclerosis. Radiology 89:709, 1967.
176. Houssiau FA, N'Zeusseu Toukap A, Depresseux G, et al: Magnetic resonance imaging-detected avascular osteonecrosis in systemic lupus erythematosus: Lack of correlation with antiphospholipid antibodies. Br J Rheumatol 37:448, 1998.
177. Sugano N, Ohzono K, Masuhara K, et al: Prognostication of osteonecrosis of the femoral head in patients with systemic lupus erythematosus by magnetic resonance imaging. Clin Orthop Rel Res 305:190, 1994.
178. Schumacher HR, Schimmer B, Gordon GV, et al: Articular manifestations of polymyositis and dermatomyositis. Arthritis Rheum 23:491, 1980.
179. Ozonoff MB, Flynn FJ Jr.: Roentgenologic features of dermatomyositis of childhood. AJR 118:206, 1973.
180. Fujitake J, Ishikawa Y, Fujii H, et al: Magnetic resonance imaging of skeletal muscles in polymyositis. Muscle Nerve 20:1463, 1997.
181. Fleckenstein JL, Reimers CD: Inflammatory myopathies. Radiol Clin North Am 34(2):427, 1996.

182. Park WM, O'Neil M, McCall IW: The radiology of rheumatoid involvement of the cervical spine. Skeletal Radiol 4:1-7, 1979.
183. Kauppi M, Neva MH: Sensivity of lateral view taken in the neutral view position in atlantoaxial subluxation in rheumatic disease. Clin Rheumatol 17:511-514, 1998.
184. Weissman BN, Aliabadi P, Weinfeld MS, et al: Prognostic features of atlantoaxial subluxation in rheumatoid arthritis patients. Radiology 144:745-751, 1982.
185. Boden S, Dodge L, Bohlmann H, et al: Rheumatoid arthritis of cervical spine: A long-term analysis with predictors of paralysis and recovery. J Bone Joint Surg Am:1282-1297, 1993.
186. Kramer J, Jolesz F, Kleefield J: Rheumatoid arthritis of the cervical spine. Rheum Dis Clin North Am 17:757-772, 1991.
187. Bundschuh C, Modic MT, Kearney F, et al: Rheumatoid arthritis of the cervical spine: surface coil MR imaging AJNR 9:565-571, 1988.
188. Takahashi M, Yamashita Y, Sakamoto Kojima R, et al: Chronic cervical cord compression: Clinical significance of increased signal intensity on MR images. Radiology 173:219-224, 1989.
189. Bluestone R: Histocompatibility antigens and rheumatic disease. Current Concepts. Kalamazoo, Mich., Upjohn, 1978, p 17.
190. Resnick D, Niwayama G: Ankylosing spondylitis. *In* Resnick D, Niwayama G (eds): Diagnosis of Bone and Joint Disorders, Philadelphia, WB Saunders, 1981, p 1040.
191. Kleinman P, Rivelas M, Schneider R, et al: Juvenile ankylosing spondylitis. Radiology 125:775, 1977.
192. Rosen PS, Graham DC: Ankylosing (Strumpell-Marie) spondylitis: A clinical review of 128 cases. AJR 5:158, 1962.
193. Resnick D: Patterns of peripheral joint disease in ankylosing spondylitis. Radiology 110:523, 1977.
194. Wilkinson M, Bywaters EGL: Clinical features and course of ankylosing spondylitis as seen in a follow-up referred cases. Ann Rheum Dis 17:209, 1958.
195. Berens DL: Roentgen features of ankylosing spondylitis. Clin Orthop Rel Res 74:20, 1971.
196. Resnick D, Niwayama G, Goergen TG: Comparison of radiographic abnormalities of the sacro-iliac joint in degenerative joint disease and ankylosing spondylitis. AJR 128:189,1977.
197. Bollow M, Braun J, Biederman T, et al: Use of contrast-enhanced MR imaging to detect sacroiliitis in children. Skeletal Radiol 27:606, 1998.
198. Forestier J, Jacqueline F, Rotes-Querol J: Ankylosing Spondylitis. Springfield, Ill, Charles C. Thomas, 1956.
199. Cawley MID, Chalmers TM, Kellgren JH, et al: Destructive lesions of vertebral bodies in ankylosing spondylitis. Ann Rheum Dis 13:345, 1972.
200. Martel W: The occipito-atlanto-axial joints in rheumatoid arthritis and ankylosing spondylitis. AJR 86:223, 1961.
201. Dwosh IL, Resnick D, Becker MP: Hip involvement in ankylosing spondylitis. Arthritis Rheum 19:683, 1976.
202. Glick EN: A radiological comparison of the hip in rheumatoid arthritis and ankylosing spondylitis. Proc R Soc Med 59:1229, 1976.
203. Rosen PS: A unique shoulder lesion in ankylosing spondylitis: Clinical comment. J Rheumatol 7:109, 1980.
204. Bywaters EGL: Heel lesions in rheumatoid arthritis. Ann Rheum Dis 13:42, 1954.
205. Ball J: Enthesopathy of rheumatoid and ankylosing spondylitis. Ann Rheum Dis 30:213, 1971.
206. Sundaram M, Patton JT: Paravertebral ossification in psoriasis and Reiter's disease. Br J Radiol 48:628, 1975.
207. Killebrew K, Gold RH, Sholkoff SD: Psoriatic spondylitis. Radiology 108:9, 1973.
208. Kaplan D, Plotz CM, Nathanson L, et al: Cervical spine in psoriasis and psoriatic arthritis. Ann Rheum Dis 23:50, 1964.
209. Cliff JM: Spinal bony bridging and carditis in Reiter's disease. Ann Rheum Dis 30:171, 1971.
210. Currier BL, Eismont FJ: Infection of spine. *In* Rothman RH, Simone FA (eds): The Spine, 3rd ed. Philadelphia, WB Saunders, 1992, pp ***.
211. Stabler A, Reiser MF: Imaging of spinal infection. Radiol Clin North Am 39:115-135, 2001.
212. Yao DC, Sartoris D: Musculoskeletal tuberculosis. Radiol Clin North Am 33:679-688, 1995.
213. Moore SL, Rafii M: Imaging of musculoskeletal and spinal tuberculosis. Radiol Clin North Am 39:329-342, 2001.
214. Varma R, Lander P, Assat A: Imaging of pyogenic infectious spondylodiskites. Radiol Clin Radiol 39:203-213, 2001.
215. Hadjipavlou AG, Cesani-Vazquez F, Villaneuva-Meyer, et al: The effectiveness of gallium citrate 67 radionuclide imaging in vertebral osteomyelitis revisited. Am J Orthop 27:179-183, 1998.
216. Modic MT, Feiglin DH, Piraino DW, et al: Vertebral osteomyelitis: Assessment using MR. Radiology 157:157-166, 1985.
217. Thrush A, Enzmann D: MR imaging of infectious spondylitis. AJNR 11:1171-1180, 1990.
218. Dagirmanjian A, Schils J, McHenry MC: MR imaging of spinal infections. Magn Res Clin North Am 7:525-538, 1999.
219. Gilliams AR, Chadda B, Carter AP: ME appearance of the temporal evaluation and resolution of infectious spondylitis. AJR 166:903-907, 1996.
220. Tyrrell PNM, Cassar-Pullicino VN, McCall IW: Europ Radiol 9:1066-1077, 1999.
221. Resnick D, Niwayama G: Degenerative disease of the spine. *In* Resnick D, Niwayama G (eds): Diagnosis of Bone and Joint Disorders. Philadelphia, WB Saunders, 1981, p 1368.
222. Knutson F: The vacuum phenomenon in the intervertebral discs. Acta Radiol 23:173, 1942.
223. Bick EM: Vertebral osteophytosis: pathologic basis of its roentgenology. AJR 73:979, 1955.
224. Goldberg RP, Carter BL: Absence of thoracic osteophytosis in the area adjacent to the aorta: Computed tomography demonstration. J Comput Assist Tomogr 2:173, 1978.
225. Schmorl G, Junghanns H: The Human Spine in Health and Disease. New York, Grune & Stratton, 1971.
226. Oppenheimer A: Calcification and ossification of vertebral ligaments. Radiology 38:160, 1940.
227. Forestier J, Rotes-Querol J: Senile ankylosing hyperostosis of the spine. Ann Rheum Dis 9:321, 1950.
228. Resnick D, Niwayama G: Radiographic and pathologic features of spinal involvement in diffuse idiopathic skeletal hyperostosis (DISH). Radiology 119:559, 1976.
229. Resnick D, Niwayama G: Diffuse idiopathic skeletal hyperostosis (DISH): Ankylosing hyperostosis of Forestier and Rotes-Querol. *In* Resnick D, Niwayama G (eds): Diagnosis of Bone and Joint Disorders. Philadelphia, WB Saunders, 1981, p 1416.
230. Resnick D, Guerra J Jr., Robinson CA, et al: Association of diffuse idiopathic skeletal hyperostosis (DISH) and calcification and ossification of posterior longitudinal ligament. AJR 131:1049, 1978.
231. Resnick D, Shaul SR, Robins JM: Diffuse idiopathic skeletal hyperostosis (DISH): Forestier's disease with extraspinal manifestations. Radiology 115:513, 1975.
232. Heithhoff KB, Ray CD, Schellhas KP, et al: CT and MRI of lateral entrapment syndromes. *In* Genant HK (ed): Spine Update 1987. San Francisco, Radiology Research and Education Foundation, 1987, pp 203-234.
233. Tumeh SS: Scintigraphy in the evaluation of arthropathy. Radiol Clin North Am 34:215-231.
234. Stabler A, Beck R, Bartl R, et al: Vacuum phenomena in insufficiency fractures of the sacrum. Skeletal Radiol 24:31-35, 1995.
235. Kursunoglu Brahme S, Cervillo V, Vint V, et al: Magnetic resonance appearance of sacral insufficiency fractures. Skeletal Radiology 19:489-493, 1990.
236. Resnick D: Tumors and tumor-like lesions in or about joints. *In* Resnick D, Niwayama G (eds): Diagnosis of Bone and Joint Disorders. Philadelphia, WB Saunders, 1981, pp 2638.
237. Prager RJ, Mall JC: Arthrographic diagnosis of synovial chondromatosis. AJR 127:344, 1976.
238. Breimer CW, Freiberger RH: Bone lesions associated with villonodular synovitis. AJR 79:618, 1958.
239. Weissman BN: Imaging of arthritis. Syllabus: A categorical course in musculoskeletal radiology. Advanced imaging of joints: Theory and Practice. Presented at the 79th Scientific Assembly of Annual Meeting of the Radiological Society of North America:37-50, 1993.
240. Cornelis F, Bardin T, Faller B, et al: Rheumatic syndromes and beta2-microglobulin amyloidosis in patients receiving long-term peritoneal dialysis. Arthritis Rheum 32(6):785, 1989.
241. Goldman AB, Bansal M: Amyloidosis and silicone synovitis updated classification, updated pathophysiology, and synovial articular abnormalities. Imaging Arthropathies 34(2):375, 1996.
242. Campistol JM, Sole M, Munoz-Gomez J, et al: Pathological fractures in patients who have amyloidosis associated with dialysis. Bone Joint Surg 72A:568, 1990.
243. Escobedo EM: Magnetic resonance imaging of dialysis-related amyloidosis of the shoulder and hip. Skeletal Radiol 25:41, 1996.

244. Kokubo T: MR demonstration of intraosseous beta 2-microglobulin amyloidosis. J Comput Assist Tomogr 14:1030, 1990.
245. Claudon M: MR patterns of dialysis arthropathy. J Comput Assist Tomogr 14:968, 1990.
246. Friman C, Pettersson T: Amyloidosis. Curr Opin Rheumatol 8:62, 1996.
247. Orzincolo C, Bedani PL, Scutellari PN, et al: Destructive spondyloarthropathy and radiographic follow-up in hemodialysis patients. Skeletal Radiol 19:483, 1990.
248. Naito M, Ogata K, Shiota E, et al: Amyloid bone cysts of the femoral neck. Bone Joint Surg 76:922, 1994.
249. Kaye J, Benson CB, Lester S, et al: Utility of high-resolution ultrasound for the diagnosis of dialysis-related amyloidosis. Arthritis Rheum 35:926, 1992.
250. Bernageau J, Bardin T, Goutallier D, et al: Magnetic resonance imaging findings in shoulders of hemodialyzed patients. Clin Orthop Rel Res 304:91, 1994.
251. Cobby MJ, Adler RS, Swartz R, et al: Dialysis-related amyloid arthropathy: MR findings in four patients. AJR 157:1023, 1991.
252. Armstrong SJ, Watt I: Lipoma arborescens of the knee. Br J Radiol 62:178, 1989.
253. Hallel TSL, Bansal M: Villous lipomatous proliferation of the synovial membrane (lipoma arborescens). J Bone Joint Surg 70:264, 1988.
254. Laorr A, Peterfy CG, Tirman PFJ, et al: Lipoma arborescens of the shoulder: Magnetic resonance imaging findings. Can Assoc Radiol J 46:311, 1995.
255. Chaljub G, Johnson PR: In vivo MRI characteristics of lipoma arborescens utilizing fat suppression and contrast administration. J Comput Assist Tomogr 20:85, 1996.
256. Shergy WJ, Urbaniak JR, Polisson RP, et al: Silicone synovitis: Clinical, radiologic and histologic features. South Med J 82: 1156-1158, 1989.
257. Goldman AB, Bansal M: Amyloidosis and silicone synovitis. Radiol Clin North Am 34:375-394, 1996.
258. Rosenthal DI, Rosenberg AE, Schiller AL, et al: Destructive arthritis due to silicone: A foreign body reaction. Radiology 149:69-72, 1983.
259. Man-Kwong C, Prathana C, Workman T, et al: Silicone synovitis: MR imaging in five patients. Skeletal Radiol 27:13-17, 1999.
260. Bigliani LU, Levine WN: Subacromial impingement syndrome. J Bone Joint Surg. 79-A:1854-1868, 1997.
261. Neer CS II: Anterior acromioplasty for chronic impingement syndrome in shoulder. A preliminary report. J Bone Joint Surg 54-A:41-50, 1972.
262. Neer CS II: Impingement lesions. Clin Orthop 173:70-77, 1983.
263. Neer CS: Rotator cuff tears associated with os acromiale. J Bone Joint Surg 66-A:1320-1321, 1984.
264. Kneeland BJ, Middleton WD, Carrera GF, et al: MR imaging of shoulder: Diagnosis of rotator cuff tears. AJR 149:333-337, 1987.
265. Reeder JD, Andelman S: The rotator cuff tear: MR evaluation. Magn Res Imag 5:331-338, 1987.
266. Seeger LL, Gold RH, Bassett LW, et al: Shoulder impingement syndrome: MR findings in 53 shoulders. AJR 150:343-347, 1988.
267. Rafii M, Firooznia H, Sherman O: Rotator cuff lesions: signal patterns at MR imaging. Radiology 177:817-823, 1990.
268. Buirski G: Magnetic resonance imaging in acute and chronic rotator cuff tears. Skeletal Radiol 19:109-111, 1990.
269. Farley TE, Neumann CH, Steinbach LS, et al: Full-thickness tears of the rotator cuff of the shoulder: Diagnosis with MR imaging. AJR 158:347-351, 1992.
270. Flannigan B, Kursunoglu-Brahme S, Snyder S, et al: MR arthropathy of the shoulder: Comparison with conventional MR imaging. AJR 155:829-832, 1990.
271. Liou JTS, Wilson AJ, Totty WG, et al: The normal shoulder: Common variations that simulate pathologic conditions at MR imaging. Radiology 186:435-441, 1993.
272. Zlatkin MB, Iannotti JP, Roberts MC, et al: Rotator cuff tears: diagnostic performance of MR imaging. Radiology 172:223-229, 1989.
273. Burk DL Jr., Karasick D, Kurtz AB, et al: Rotator cuff tears: prospective comparison of MR imaging with arthroscopy, sonography, and surgery. AJR 153:87-92, 1989.
274. Jacobsen JA, van Holsbeeck MT: Musculoskeletal ultrasonography. Orthop Clin North Am 29:135-167, 1998.
275. Omer GE Jr: Median nerve compression at the wrist. Hand Clin 8:317-324, 1992.
276. Middleton WD, Kneeland JB, Kellman GM, et al: MR imaging of the carpal tunnel: Normal anatomy and preliminary findings in the carpal tunnel syndrome. AJR 148:307-316, 1987.
277. Mesgarahzade M, Schneck CD, Bonakdarpour A: Carpal tunnel MR imaging part II: Carpal tunnel syndrome. Radiology 171:749-754, 1989.
278. Murphy RX Jr., Chernofsky MA, Osborne MA, et al: Magnetic resonance imaging in the evaluation of persistent carpal tunnel syndrome. J Hand Surg 18:113-120, 1993.
279. Lee D, van Holsbeeck MT, Janevski PK, et al: Diagnosis of carpal tunnel syndrome: Ultrasound versus electromyography. Radiol Clin North Am 37:859-872, 1999.
280. Chen P, Maklad N, Redwine M, et al: Dynamic high-resolution sonography of carpal tunnel. AJR 168(2) 533-537, 1997.

SECTION

VII

Modalities of Therapy in Rheumatic Diseases: Non-pharmacologic Interventions

52

Education of Patients

KATE R. LORIG

Most arthritis treatment guidelines place patient education or patient self-management at a pivotal point in the treatment plan. For the first time, the Healthy People 2010 objectives for the nation include a developmental objective to: "Increase the proportion of persons with arthritis who have had effective, evidence-based arthritis education as an integral part of the management of their condition."[1]

Despite the almost universal recognition among rheumatology professionals of the importance of patient education, it is estimated that fewer than 5 percent of all arthritis patients receive any formal or standardized education. This chapter will discuss the evidence for patient education, make some suggestions about how patient education can be included in clinical practice, and will end with some suggested key messages for patients.

The suggestions in this chapter are supported by evidence that while there are many different types of arthritis, the problems faced by patients are more similar across conditions than they are different. These concerns include the medical management of the disease, such as adherence to medication taking and exercise.[2]

Evidence: What Should be Taught

The key symptoms of arthritis—pain, fatigue, disability, and depression—are all linked and feed into each other in complex patterns that are difficult to distinguish. One key to patient education is to break these patterns and, thus, lessen these symptoms by the use of self-management behaviors such as exercise, fatigue management, use of assisting aids, and cognitive coping. The following is a short examination of each of these behaviors.

Probably the strongest evidence is for the effectiveness of conditioning exercise, both endurance and strengthening, in people with osteoarthritis (OA) and rheumatoid arthritis (RA).[3,4] Walking, cycling, water aerobics, strength training, and low-impact exercise programs report decreased pain and improved range of motion, cardiovascular fitness, strength, endurance, function, and gait in people with arthritis.[5] Well-controlled studies of aerobic exercise consistently report that people with arthritis can safely exercise regularly and vigorously enough to improve fitness and health without exacerbation of disease or increased joint symptoms.[6] The training regimens in most aerobic exercise studies progressively increase the intensity and duration of the exercise sessions to achieve the guidelines for cardiovascular fitness set by the American College of Sports Medicine (30 to 45 minutes of moderate intensity whole body exercise such as walking, cycling, or swimming on 3 to 5 days a week).

Controlled trials of exercise interventions designed specifically for people with knee OA include strengthening, aerobic, and functional exercises. These studies use a short period of initial instruction followed by several months of self-directed home exercise and report improved strength, proprioception, and function, as well as decreased pain.[7,8]

Low-intensity, active range-of-motion exercise, the traditional home exercise program for people with arthritis, can provide benefits in addition to flexibility and joint motion. Gentle exercise performed using some Thai Chi motions can significantly reduce morning stiffness for persons with RA. An exercise program of active exercise and relaxation (the Range of Motion Dance) has shown significant improvements in self-reported function and pain.[5]

In addition to the previously mentioned benefits, exercise also appears to improve depression. Although the exact mechanism is not understood, it may be that depression and other negative mood states are mediated by self-efficacy, or the belief (confidence) that one can effect disease symptoms.

Keefe, Parker, and others have published studies indicating that patients who cope with pain in an overly negative fashion (catastrophizing) have much more severe pain and disability; and patients who avoid catastrophizing and who report they can use more adaptive strategies (e.g., distraction, calming self-statements) to control and decrease pain have much lower levels of pain and disability.[9-11] Furthermore, it has been shown that systematic training in pain-coping skills can lessen pain and disability in both RA and OA patients.[12-16]

Assistive devices are frequently recommended for people with arthritis to improve their functional capabilities by compensating for limitations in dexterity, joint range of motion, muscle strength, and endurance. The devices most frequently used by patients with RA are wrist splints, followed by silver ring splints, raised toilet seats, bath or shower benches, and dressing sticks.[17] It has been ascertained that a majority of assistive-device users with RA and OA had positive impressions of assistive devices, including their ability to make task performance more independent, easier, and safer.[18-20] In another study, it was found that the use of devices or altered methods reduced perceived task difficulty for 42 percent of the task items.[21]

Evidence: The Effectiveness of Structured Programs

Several modes of patient education have demonstrated effectiveness in terms of improved health status and or decreased health care use. These include small-group education led by both peers (patients) and health professionals, telephone interventions, mail-delivered interventions, computer-delivered interventions, and group medical visits. Let us examine each of these more closely.

Although there is substandard evidence for the effectiveness of arthritis patient education there are also many studies demonstrating little to no effect. In fact, one of the problems with any patient education meta-analysis (such as those done by the Cochrane collaboration) is that such analyses tend to suffer from the syndrome of "mixing apples and oranges"; early studies are compared with later studies, many different delivery modes are used, and interventions have variable duration and content.[22]

Probably the most studied interventions are those offered in small, face-to-face groups. In a professionally led 6-week group series emphasizing behavioral change, Lindroth and colleagues found that participants, when compared to randomized controls, demonstrated improvements in knowledge, appropriate behaviors, and their disability.[23] Five years later, treatment subjects continued to demonstrate an increased ability to cope with their disease.[24] In a subsequent study for people with OA of the knee, which combined walking and educational sessions based on self-efficacy theory, it was demonstrated that the program improved functional status without worsening pain or other symptoms.[25]

Finally, a series of studies on the peer-led Arthritis Self-Management Program (also known as the Arthritis Self Help Program and Challenging Arthritis) found increases in self-management behaviors, exercise, and cognitive-symptom management, as well as a decrease in pain. Decreases in pain and outpatient visits to physicians persisted for up to 4 years.[26-28]

Weinberger has concluded a series of telephone-based interventions that consisted of regular phone calls to patients by trained students. Results from several randomized trials demonstrated that patients contacted by phone, compared to those receiving the same information in the clinic, demonstrated improved physical health and reduced pain.[29-30] The telephone intervention was also less costly.[31] In one survey of users of an "arthritis hotline," it was found that hotline users asked their doctors more questions and reported improved compliance with treatment,[32] and in a study that was not limited to people with arthritis, it was shown that for older patients with a variety of chronic and morbid conditions, proactive phone calls by their health care provider between regularly scheduled visits reduced both outpatient visits and hospitalizations.[33]

Goeppinger used both telephone and mailed intervention for patients in rural areas. This intervention demonstrated increases in self-management knowledge and behaviors and reductions in pain,[34] and the effectiveness of a mailed intervention meditated by computer-generated personalized letters over a period of 1 year has been proved.[35,36]

Computer-meditated interventions are only beginning to be utilized with arthritis patients. An early intervention in the 1980s with poor seniors demonstrated increases in knowledge, improved outlook, and an increase in self-management behaviors.[37] More recently a year-long e-mail discussion group for patients with back pain demonstrated that participants, compared to randomized nonparticipants, experienced less disability and pain with a trend toward fewer back pain–related visits.[38]

Although the previous interventions at first appear to have little in common, we are beginning to understand some of the component parts of successful interventions. Most, if not all, have been based on patient-perceived problems or symptoms rather than professionally modeled activities, such as specific exercise programs. Second, all of the successful interventions allow patients to interact in a planned, structured manner, usually with both health professionals and other patients. We often have been told by patients that they need two types of information: that offered by health professionals and that offered by other patients living with similar conditions. The best interventions offer both opportunities.

Studies have shown that self-efficacy or confidence in ability to self-manage arthritis is a key mediating variable for health outcomes. Studies of self-management intervention have demonstrated that patients can improve self-efficacy and that changes in self-efficacy mediate improvements in health status.[39] Self-efficacy, confidence, or empowerment can be accomplished by systematically using four strategies: skills mastery, modeling, reinterpretation of symptoms, and social persuasion.[41] Skills mastery involves getting patients to master self-management skills. This is typically accomplished by having them set a specific short-term goal or action plan. A typical plan would be: "This week I will walk 15 minutes before lunch on Monday, Wednesday, and Friday;" or, "this week I will not eat after 7 P.M. four days out of seven." In a meta-analysis of asthma studies, a Cochrane Review[42] found that goal setting or action planning was a key variable that separated successful from unsuccessful interventions. It is important that an action plan be something that the patient wants to do, rather than an activity demanded by the physician. One way of establishing an action plan is by asking the patient at the end of a consultation: "Given what we have discussed today, what are you going to do in the next two weeks or month?" An answer such as "exercise" is not specific enough. You may need a follow-up question asking the patient to specify what exercise, when, how long, and how many times a week.

The second self-efficacy strategy, modeling, involves having patients learn from other patients or patient models. The patient input can be accomplished through modeling. This is one of the reasons patient intervention is so important. This can be accomplished by having patients starting a new drug talk with patients successfully using this drug. The same can be done for patients contemplating joint replacement surgery. The best patient-education materials include patient vignettes as well as drawings or photos of persons like those for whom the materials are intended. When patients meet in groups, the leader should use structure that allows patients to share experiences and help each other with problems. Internet e-mail listservs, chat rooms, and discussion boards also provide for patient modeling. In a series of experiments with nonarthritic patients, Brennan[43] has found that the most-used portions of Internet education programs are those that allow patients to communicate with each other.

Patients do, or do not, take part in self-management activities based on their beliefs about the meaning of symptoms. Thus, reinterpretation of symptoms is the third efficacy-enhancing strategy. If one believes that exercise will damage joints and make arthritis worse, he or she will not exercise. If on the other hand, if a patient perceives that exercise will strengthen muscles, lessen arthritis pain, and will slow disability, exercise is more likely to be accepted as a modality. Thus, in practice it is important to always explain symptoms as having many causes, thereby opening the way for patients to try new self-management activities. At the same time, it is important not to perpetuate myths, such as that exercise makes arthritis worse or that it is important to not overuse joints. Figure 52–1 demonstrates how patient self-management activities may be enhanced by changing beliefs about pain.

The fourth means of enhancing self-efficacy is social persuasion. This involves making a new or desired behavior the social norm. If everyone around you is doing one thing, it is hard not to follow suit. This is why an individual trying to maintain a low-fat diet is encouraged to order first from a menu so as not to be influenced by others' choices. Another good example is that having a walking partner encourages exercise. On a community level, social persuasion may come about through laws such as those mandating no smoking or the provision of sidewalks, bike lanes, and curb cuts to make a community exercise friendly.

Along with social interaction and self-efficacy, there are at least two other strategies that mediate the effectiveness of patient education: tailoring or self-tailoring and the amount of exposure to the intervention.

It is accepted that patient-education efforts that are either tailored to patient's needs or allow patients to self-tailor their "curriculum" are more effective than those that do not meet these criteria. Tailoring is accomplished by learning something about a patient's motivation, beliefs, and lifestyle and subsequently offering education and other suggestions designed in the context of this knowledge. With self-tailoring, the assumption is that once the patient is given guidance and options, he or she will construct a self-management plan that fits his or her needs. Here the role of the health professional is to supply key messages (see more about this in the next section) and a scaffold structure to begin building a program. The actual changes to be made are determined by the patient.

A final mediator of effective patient education is exposure. In a meta-analysis of diabetes programs, Norris[44] found an association between the amount of exposure and effectiveness; the programs offering more exposure were more effective.

Tips for Busy Clinicians

1. Base one-to-one teaching on patients' main concerns. These can be determined by asking: "When you think about arthritis, what do you think of?" or "What are you afraid might happen?" Use the

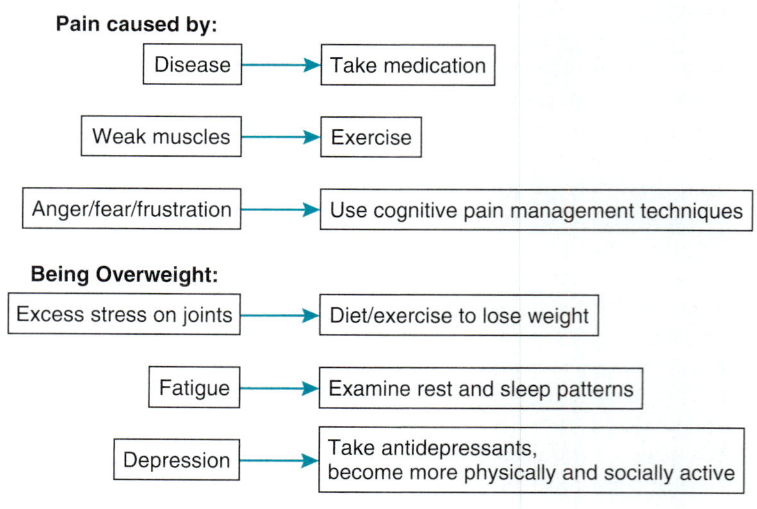

Figure 52–1 · Management Strategies Based on Beliefs About the Causes of Symptoms.

answers to tailor your education. For example, if the response to the first question is "pain," the physician can answer that pain can be caused by several different things and that there are many ways of dealing with it (see Fig. 52–1).

2. Screen frequently for depression. A good single-question screen is: "What do you do for fun?" If the patient cannot give a positive answer, further screening and possible treatment are needed. Patient education is probably not the first treatment for major depression.
3. Have a set of consistent key messages. A key message is one detailed enough to allow patients to self-tailor, while not overwhelming them with details. Examples of key messages are as follows.
   - "You should not have more pain when you finish exercising than before you start, but exercise may not be pain free."
   - "Weight loss is a function of eating less and moving more."
   - "Start an exercise program by doing what you can do now. Do this four to five times a week and add to it by 10 percent every week or two."
   - "Take your pills with some activity you do every day, such as brushing your teeth."
   - "I cannot cure your arthritis, but by working together, we can do lots of things so that you can continue living a normal life."
   - "It is easier to control pain when it is not severe. Thus, take your medicine when you have only mild pain. Do not wait to see if it will get worse."
4. Have patients set specific behavioral goals or action plans for one or two months ahead. Be sure to ask about these during the next visit.
5. Keep a list of good books and Web sites to give your patients. Update these at least yearly.
6. Know about community resources such as exercise classes, arthritis patient–education classes, meditation classes, and support groups. If at all possible, visit some of these so you really know about them. Then, refer patients with a specific name and telephone number.
7. Keep a small patient-education library in your waiting room.
8. Always tell patients when to expect new medications to start working. Many patients expect new medications to have effects in hours or at least in days. When this does not happen, they often stop taking the medications or reduce the dose before full effectiveness is reached.
9. When asking patients about their medications, assume that there may have been problems. Ask, "What problems have you had taking this medication?" This makes it much easier for the patients to say they forgot, the medicine was too expensive, or that they did not like the side effects.
10. Finally, make yourself available to your patients by phone or e-mail. This is difficult given a busy schedule, legal considerations, and the present lack of reimbursement for these services. Nevertheless, most patients do not abuse this privilege and this is an excellent way to catch problems before they grow, encourage patients, or relieve them of needless worry. Those few patients who abuse this added contact could be handled by limiting them to a set number of contacts per month.

Conclusion

In conclusion, we have growing evidence that properly administered patient education can reduce symptoms and possibly avoid health care use above and beyond usual care. Good rheumatology care requires the systematic application of this evidence.

ACKNOWLEDGEMENTS

I would like to acknowledge Marion Minor, PhD, PT; Francis Keepe, PhD; Joan Rogers, PhD, OT; and Basha Belza, PhD, RN for their assistance with this chapter.

REFERENCES

1. U.S. Department of Health and Human Services: Healthy People 2010, 2nd ed. With Understanding and Improving Health and Objectives for Improving Health. 2 vols. Washington, DC: U.S. Government Printing Office, November 2000.
2. Corbin J, Strauss A: Unending Work and Care: Managing Chronic Illness at Home. San Francisco, Jossey-Bass, 1988.
3. Van den Ende CHM, Vilet Vlieland TPM, Munneke M, Hazes JMW: Dynamic exercise therapy in rheumatoid arthritis (Cochrane Review). In The Cochrane Library, Issue 4, 2003. Chichester, UK: John Wiley & Sons, Ltd.
4. Van Baar ME, Assendelft WJJ, Dekker J, et al: Effectiveness of exercise therapy in patients with osteoarthritis of the hip or knee: A systematic review of randomized clinical trials. Arthritis Rheum 42(7):1361-1369, 1999
5. Minor MA, Westby MD: Rest and exercise. *In* Robbins L, Burckhardt CS, Hannan MT (eds): Clinical Care in the Rheumatic Diseases, 2nd ed. Atlanta, Association of Rheumatology Health Professionals, 2001.
6. Westby MD: A health professional's guide to exercise prescription for people with arthritis: a review of aerobic fitness activities. Arthritis Care Res 45(6):501-511, 2001.
7. O'Reilly S, Muir K, Doherty M: Effectiveness of a home exercise on pain and disability from osteoarthritis of the knee: A randomized controlled trial. Ann Rheum Dis 58:15-19, 1999.
8. Petrella RJ, Bartha C: Home based exercise therapy for older persons with knee osteoarthritis: A randomized clinical trial. J Rheumatol 27:2215-2221, 2000.
9. Keefe FJ, Caldwell DS, Queen KT, et al: Osteoarthritic knee pain: A behavioral analysis. Pain 28:309-321, 1987.
10. Keefe FJ, Caldwell DS, Queen KT, et al: Pain coping strategies in osteoarthritis patients. J Consult Clin Psychol 55:208-212, 1987.
11. Parker JC, Smarr KL, Buescher KL, et al: Pain control and rational thinking: Implications for rheumatoid arthritis. Arthritis Rheum 32:984-990, 1989.
12. Bradley LA, Young LD, Anderson JO, et al: Effects of psychological therapy on pain behavior of rheumatoid arthritis patients: Treatment outcome and six-month follow-up. Arthritis Rheum 30:1105-1114, 1987.
13. Bradley L, Young L, Anderson K, et al: Effects of cognitive-behavior therapy on rheumatoid arthritis pain behavior: One year follow-up. *In* Dubner R, Gebhart G, Bond M: Pain Research and Clinical Management, No.3 (Proceedings of the 5th World Congress on Pain). Amsterdam, Elsevier, 1988, pp 310-314.
14. Keefe FJ, Caldwell DS, Williams DA, et al: Pain coping skills training in the management of osteoarthritic knee pain. I. A comparative study. Behavior Therapy 21:49-62, 1990.

15. Parker J, Frank R, Beck N, et al: Pain management in rheumatoid arthritis: A cognitive-behavioral approach. Arthritis Rheum 31:593-601, 1988.
16. Parker JC, Smarr KL, Buckelew SP, et al: Effects of stress management on clinical outcomes in rheumatoid arthritis. Arthritis Rheum 38:1807-1818, 1995.
17. Kulp CS: The Use of Adaptive Equipment by Rheumatoid Arthritis Patients. Unpublished master's thesis. Richmond, Virginia Commonwealth University, 1988.
18. Rogers JC, Holm MB: Assistive technology device use in patients with rheumatic disease: A review of literature. Am J Occupational Therapy 46:120-127, 1992.
19. Rogers JC, Holm MB, Perkins L: Trajectory of assistive device usage and user and non-user characteristics: Long-handled bath sponge. Arthritis Care Res (in press).
20. Rogers JC, Poole JL, Holm MB, et al: Assistive devices: Prescription, patient education, patient perceptions. Arthritis Rheum 32:S195, 1989.
21. Nordenskiöld U, Grimby G, Dahlin-Ivanoff S: Questionnaire to evaluate the effects of assistive devices and altered working methods in women with rheumatoid arthritis. Clin Rheumatol 17:6-16, 1998.
22. Riemsma RP, Kirwan JR, Taal E, Rasker JJ: Patient education for adults with rheumatoid arthritis (Cochrane Review). In the Cochrane Library, Issue 4, 2003. Chichester, UK: John Wiley & Sons, Ltd.
23. Lindroth Y, Bauman A, Barnes C, et al: A controlled evaluation of arthritis education. Br J Rheumatol 28(1):7-12, 1989.
24. Lindroth Y, Bauman A, Brooks PM, Priestley D: A 5-year follow-up of a controlled trail of an arthritis education programme. Br J Rheumatol 34(7):647-652, 1995.
25. Kovar PA, Allegrante JP, MacKenzie CR, et al: Supervised fitness walking in patients with osteoarthritis of the knee: A randomized, controlled trial. Annals Intern Med 116(7):529-534, 1992.
26. Lorig K, Lubeck D, Kraines R, et al: Outcomes of self-help education for patients with arthritis. Arthritis Rheum 28(6):680-685, 1985.
27. Lorig K, Mazonson P, Holman H: Evidence suggesting that health education for self-management in patients with chronic arthritis has sustained health benefits while reducing health care costs. Arthritis Rheum 36(4):439-446, 1993.
28. Lorig K, González V, Laurent D: The Chronic Disease Self-Management Leader's Manual (revised). Palo Alto, Calif., Stanford University, Stanford Patient Education Research Center, 1999.
29. Weinberger M, Tierney WM, Boher P, Katz BP: Can the provision of information to patients with osteoarthritis improve functional status? A randomized, controlled trial. Arthritis Rheum 32(12):1577-1583, 1989.
30. Rene J, Weinberger M, Mazzuca SA, et al: Reduction of joint pain in patients with knee osteoarthritis who have received monthly telephone calls from lay personnel and whose medical treatment regimens have remained stable. Arthritis Rheum 35(5):511-515, 1992.
31. Weinberger M, Tierney WM, Cowper PA, et al: Cost-effectiveness of increased telephone contact for patients with osteoarthritis: A randomized, controlled trial. Arthritis Rheum 36(2):243-246, 1993.
32. Maisiak R, Koplon S, Heck LW: Subsequent behavior of users of an arthritis information telephone service. Arthritis Rheum 33(2):212-218, 1990.
33. Wasson J, Gaudette C, Whaley F, et al: Telephone care as a substitute for routine clinic follow up. JAMA 267(13):1788-1793, 1992.
34. Goeppinger J, Arthur MW, Baglioni AJ Jr, et al: A reexamination of the effectiveness of self-care education for persons with arthritis. Arthritis Rheum 32(6):706-716, 1989.
35. Gale F, Kirk J, Davis R: Patient education and self-management: randomized study of effects on health status of a mail-delivered program. Arthritis Rheum 37(9):S197, 1994.
36. Fries J, Carey C, McShane D: Patient education in arthritis: Randomized controlled trial of a mail-delivered program. J Rheumatol 24(7):1378-1383, 1997.
37. Wetstone SL, Sheehan TJ, Votaw RG, et al: Evaluation of a computer based education lesson for patients with rheumatoid arthritis. J Rheumatol 12(5):907-912, 1985.
38. Lorig K, Laurent D, Deyo R, et al: Can a back pain e-mail discussion group improve health status and lower health care costs? Arch Intern Med 162:792-796, 2002.
39. Lorig K, Lubeck D, Holman H: Nonassociations of new behaviors with favorable outcome in effective arthritis health education. Arthritis Rheum 25(25):S148, 1982.
41. Bandura A: Self-efficacy: The Exercise of Control. New York, WH Freeman and Co., 1997.
42. Gibson PG, Coughlan J, Wilson AJ, et al: Self-management education and regular practitioner review for adults with asthma (Cochrane Review). In the Cochrane Library, Issue 4, 2003. Chichester, UK: John Wiley & Sons, Ltd.
43. Brennan P, Moore S, Smyth K: Alzheimer's disease caregivers' uses of a computer network. J Nurs Res 14:662-673, 1992.
44. Norris SL, Lau J, Smith SJ, et al: Self-management education for adults with type 2 diabetes: A meta-analysis of the effect on glycemic control. Diabetes Care 25(7):1159-1171, 2002.

53 Psychosocial Management of the Rheumatic Diseases

W. NEAL ROBERTS, JR.

The Illness Experience in Rheumatic Disease

What the illness means to the patient is difficult to grasp. Reading what patients have written about arthritis is not having arthritis; listening and talking and teaching are not the same as the experience. Physicians who have become patients note in retrospect that the "illness experience" was much more complex than anticipated. The thing that seems to make the experience of rheumatic diseases different from that of other medical and surgical conditions is the combination of pain with chronicity.

> *"Since the pain never goes away, the emotions never go away. So it's a matter of finding out how to escape from the emotions. That's what gets to you; it's like a bloodhound pursuing you. The doctors say, 'Most patients feel somewhat better in 6 to 8 weeks.' Six to 8 weeks feels like an eternity, and there's nothing left to do, nowhere to go."*

These words were spoken by a 50-year-old woman after 10 years of rheumatoid arthritis (RA) and five different disease-modifying antirheumatic drugs (DMARD's).

The average course of RA is about 27 years. The usual psychologic defenses wear out. The illness becomes an unwelcome but integrated part of the person, perhaps.

> *"I used to believe that 'my arthritis' was separate from myself. I have come to understand, after 30 years of living with JRA (juvenile rheumatoid arthritis), that this is no less a part of me than my fingers, my voice. My appreciation for pain, especially that which goes unseen, for recognizing the reality of potential (not everyone can be whatever they want), and for the ability to work at accepting one's limitations has guided and still guides my perspective. Everything about who I am is wrapped in and around this illness."*

These are the words of a woman who has had polyarticular JRA since age 6.

Equal to pain for many is loss of control and self confidence.

> *"But when my symptoms are present, my self image changes....I am aging, tentative, dependent, tinged with self-pity and regret. I am more willing to accept, rather than strive. In short, my confidence in my life and myself is reduced by how I feel physically. Despite this, a part of me rebels against this lowered self-esteem. It effectively refuses to accept the disease, it will not admit to not being able to the things I once did with ease or even skill. These two conflicting personae—the hesitant, reflective sick person and the unaccepting person who does what he wants despite how he feels—arise from each other in uninterrupted, shifting patterns. The self-pity, which is the last stage of my sick person, awakens my healthy person. When he is eventually confronted with a task, however mundane, that symptoms prevent him from doing, the sick person reemerges, and the cycle begins anew."*

These reflections are from a man who has had 20 years of ankylosing spondylitis.

Initial events of chronic pain and loss of control and confidence give rise to reactions and adaptations analogous to the stages of reaction to acute losses in general: anger, denial, anxiety, resignation. Management of these reactions and adaptations in the chronic setting may present new problems of their own from the patient's point of view, and these are dependent upon the responses of the patient's social support system (family, friends, coworkers). During this series of emotional events, there is always the possibility of depression developing.

> *"Any patient with RA who tells you they haven't ever been depressed is lying. When I see those questionnaires about depression, I just mark something in the middle of the scale. It's embarrassing to admit how bad you feel."*

Remarks from a 50-year-old registered nurse with 10 years of RA.

Landmarks of Psychosocial Adaptation in Rheumatic Disease

There are four landmark events that virtually every rheumatology patient faces and that routinely require some active management. These are: not getting a diagnosis; getting a diagnosis; repeatedly struggling to understanding risks and benefits; and dealing with the impact of the disease on relationships with others. Everyone either receives a diagnosis or does not. If there is no immediate diagnosis, it may help to realize that that ambiguity is a good prognostic factor. If it is clinically and serologically obvious what you have, things may turn out worse. Second, a clear diagnosis entails facing the fact of having a chronic illness. The risk-benefit decisions about therapies are ongoing. The disease changes. Decisions have to be made again.

The Influence of Reading and Educational Levels

In general, people with the lowest literacy have the worst health. Whether reading level per se is an independent cofactor or is dependent on other sociodemographic features such as poverty is uncertain. A mechanism by which impaired literacy might have direct effects is clear enough, however. Patient information pamphlets, medication sheets, and other materials are written at reading levels too difficult for most American adults, putting a premium on non–literacy-dependent patient education. This persistent fact may be among the reasons why face-to-face programs that involve therapists interacting with groups of patients have a beneficial effect (Table 53–1) (see Chapter 52). The Internet promises to multiply the effects of reading and education and research,[1] but to the extent it does, it may contribute to a digital divide effect in care of rheumatic diseases. On a theoretic basis, sociologic intervention touching on fundamental factors such as reading and education levels of the population as a whole might be expected to be the most effective psychosocial interventions for arthritis and other rheumatic diseases. It is, therefore, logical that most proven psychosocial interventions are individual or small-group provider-patient communication or patient education interventions that have a potential to overcome educational deficits and compensate for uncoordinated care (see Table 53–1).

Many variables other than the level of education and reading comprehension make real contributions to outcome of rheumatic diseases. As an example, there is a moderately strong relationship between physical workload and the incidence of hip OA. Farming and heavy lifting mediate this association with an odds ratio of 3:1.[2] In that context, educational attainment is inversely related to exposure to heavy labor. Likewise, if high-salaried people with gratifying jobs and bonuses in their salary structures avoid disability applications for rheumatoid arthritis, whereas hourly workers do not, that tendency may generate an understandable indirect effect of education on continued employment. These complex sorts of relationships of education to clinical outcome should not obscure more direct effects. Education and reading level can also operate directly on visit and medication compliance, having particularly noticeable effects on the outcome of complex diseases with threatening outcomes such as RA and systemic lupus erythematosus (SLE).

Epidemiology of Psychiatric Disorders in Rheumatology

In general, diagnosable psychiatric disorders occur no more frequently in patients with rheumatic diseases than in those with other chronic diseases. Two exceptions stand out. People with SLE often suffer from cognitive deficits, particularly as related to learning new concepts. People with widespread, nonarticular, axial aching have more diagnosable psychiatric illnesses and are more likely to somatasize their symptoms. A comparison of patients across the spectrum of those usually seen in an office practice for rheumatology was made in an attempt to map out the relationship between pain, disability, and abnormal psychology across the diagnostic groups.[3] Those with serious peripheral joint disease from RA had the most disability, but the least pain, and the most normal psychologic test scores. The highest pain scores and most psychologic distress was reported by people with the axial disorders, including fibromyalgia, back pain, and neck pain.

CHRONIC WIDESPREAD PAIN, FIBROMYALGIA, AND LOW BACK PAIN

Arguably, fibromyalgia and chronic widespread pain are physiologically distinct. Nonetheless, they form part of the same differential diagnostic group of nonarticular axial aching and may overlap in surveys or population-

TABLE 53–1 • EVIDENCE-BASED PSYCHOSOCIAL INTERVENTIONS

Intervention	Target	Method	Results
Arthritis self-help courses*, self-management programs	All arthritis diagnoses; fund of knowledge	4 to 12 hrs of didactic sessions with a trained leader; includes flip charts; overheads; handouts; discussion aimed at problem solving; pain, stress and depression management; and information on medications and communicating with providers	43% decrease in office visits over 4-year follow-up; decreased pain satisfying criteria for clinical significance (15-20% on visual analogue scale), increased exercise, increased fund of knowledge and self-efficacy, 9% decrease in disability[38] Most annual cost savings by patients with RA ($162); sustained effect 4 years after the intervention
Aquatics exercise at the YMCA*	All arthritis diagnoses; range of motion, strength	12 to 30 hrs over 6 to 10 weeks in a heated pool with a lifeguard, trained instructor, and physical therapist	13-17% improvement in range of motion, strength in the lower extremities, and also self-efficacy; exercise compliance drops off over time
Land-based exercise programs such as Arthritis Foundation PACE or walking programs	All arthritis diagnoses; range of motion, strength	Varied	Decreased depression and increased self-efficacy with respect to activities of daily living; decreasing adherence to exercise regimen over time[39]
Phone follow-up of osteoarthritis patients	Symptomatic, radiographic knee OA	Symptom-monitoring phone call on a scheduled basis	Pain improvement similar in magnitude to treatment with nonsteroidal anti-inflammatory drugs[35]

*Organized, current effort of Arthritis Foundation local chapters with certified instructor.

based studies applicable to office practice. Chronic widespread pain in unselected general populations is associated with a 17-percent incidence of psychiatric diagnosis in Australia;[4] one quarter of a community sample of similar patients in Manchester, England had a psychiatric diagnosis.[5] Mood and anxiety disorders predominate in these patients. In the Manchester group, the odds ratio for having a psychiatric illness if accompanied by self-reported chronic widespread pain was 4.9 CI (2.6, 9.5). In the Australian phone survey (n = 17,545), 18 percent of the population had widespread chronic pain sufficient to interfere with daily activity two thirds of this cohort. Psychosocial markers statistically associated with widespread chronic pain were less education, less income, lack of health insurance, and pending unemployment or disability payments. Finally, in prospective studies, people initially without generalized axial aching, but who somatasize their physical symptoms, have increased risk of developing chronic widespread pain later.

RHEUMATOID ARTHRITIS

Most patients with moderately severe RA have been depressed. However, patients are resilient and they adapt. Even the distress accompanying chronic joint pain in RA, described previously as the "illness experience," does not uniformly lead to sustained, treatable clinical depression. In RA, depression is no more common than among other rheumatology office patients.[6] Their pain causes psychological distress rather than the other way around.[7]

KNEE OSTEOARTHRITIS

Self-reported knee pain in the United States has its highest prevalence among elderly people and non-Hispanic black women.[8] Younger and less-educated patients presenting with knee OA are more likely to be depressed, however.[9] Multiple regression analysis of a study of a mixed Asian population in Singapore revealed a number of independent variables associated with better outcome; some were biologic, some fixed psychosocial, and some potentially modifiable. The best functioning patients with knee OA were not only those with less pain and less radiographic severity, but those with better education and fewer feelings of helplessness ("learned helplessness") and who were of Chinese ethnicity.

SYSTEMIC LUPUS ERYTHEMATOSUS

Psychological complaints, especially mild cognitive deficits and emotional responses to them, are a prominent aspect of SLE, perhaps caused by subtle brain disease, and are as common as more easily recognized features such as arthritis and skin lesions. Reported increased frequency of mild cognitive deficits in African Americans with SLE has been attributed, by hierarchical regression analysis, to the additive effects of psychosocial variables, not race.

Overall, generalizable population-based studies show chronic, nonarticular, axial aching groups of rheumatic syndromes to be those most likely to have an underlying psychiatric diagnosis, usually a mood disorder or anxiety. Somatazation is an important causal factor, at least for chronic widespread pain ascertained at the community level. Patients with SLE are particularly subject to mild cognitive deficits, such as difficulty in finding words to speak. Patients with RA psychologically adapt over time and are usually as well adjusted and productive as their damaged joints permit.

Psychosocial Factors' Effects on the Course of Rheumatic Diseases

Psychologic and social factor effects on the presentation of a number of important diseases have been studied. These illnesses include the most statistically and economically important of the rheumatic diseases: OA, RA, and low back pain, as well as SLE and fibromyalgia. A number of important critical clinical situations requiring management during the course of these illnesses have also been delineated in the same way. These range from joint replacement in OA to fatigue in RA and SLE.

LARGE-JOINT OSTEOARTHRITIS, EARLY COURSE

Depression appeared to influence the younger patients and the less-educated patients to seek attention for OA of the hip or knee among a community interview sample of 108 patients older than 50 years of age. In this study, {9} about half of the variance in the incidence of depression was explained by the effects or interactions of age, education, and self-assessment of the impact of OA. Biologic and sociologic variables were analyzed together in a second community-based, much larger (n = 1272) study. Pain and three other factors, none of which were modifiable psychosocial features, were independent influences upon disability. Of several psychosocial variables affecting disability and utilization, only the psychologic one, depression in a younger patient, is amenable to direct intervention.

LARGE-JOINT OSTEOARTHRITIS, LATE COURSE, TOTAL JOINT ARTHROPLASTY

In contrast, later in the course of OA, patient education, rather than detection and treatment of depression, plays the strongest role. When total joint replacement is proposed for OA, the subsets of both African Americans and elderly patients tend to accept fewer arthroplasties. In a study of 596 older Cleveland veterans with symptomatic hip or knee OA, African-American men were only about half as likely (odds ratio 0.50, 95% confidence interval 0.30-0.84) to accept a recommendation for total joint arthroplasty (TJA). The underlying reasons for this racial disparity seemed to be predominantly fear and expectations on the part of the African-American subset of a more prolonged and troublesome postoperative period. These people were also less familiar overall with details about TJA than were non-blacks. Socioeconomic status per se has not been found to determine acceptance of TJA. A Canadian survey of 48,218 people older than

55 found 3307 with hip and knee problems verified as OA by clinical examination and radiographs. The individuals with the lowest levels of schooling were equally willing to undergo treatment, and they actually needed it more than others, as might be expected due to their lower educational attainment.

In-depth interviews of elderly patients have revealed three common misconceptions influencing decisions about TJA. Specifically, older patients expect that if their doctor fails to make an explicit recommendation for TJA, this means they are not appropriate candidates. These patients felt their provider was actively screening for the procedure and they had already been screened out. Elderly patients also tend to believe that more pain and daily impairment is needed to make a favorable risk-benefit tradeoff than do their orthopedic surgeons.[10] It has been suggested that this perspective is in part due to the fact that elderly patients are much more sensitive than their doctors to risk of mild postanesthesia cognitive deficits. The third misconception is a philosophic difference; the elderly patients revealed in the interview study that they viewed OA as a normal aging process to be tolerated rather than as a disease to be operated upon.[10] These data may also reflect an unproved but suspected desire on the part of orthopedic surgeons to replace as many joints in as many patients as possible.

FATIGUE IN RHEUMATOID ARTHRITIS AND SYSTEMIC LUPUS ERYTHEMATOSUS

Fatigue is the most common chief complaint of patients with SLE.[11] For patients with RA, fatigue is prevalent,[12] correlates well with depression when that occurs,[13] and becomes the focus of elaborate coping strategies.[14] The rapid, dramatic response of fatigue in RA to tumor necrosis factor (TNF) blockade in some patients implies that fatigue must be due in part to circulating cytokines rather than to deconditioning and psychologic factors. In contrast to RA, in SLE there is no association between fatigue and disease activity or markers of inflammation. Unless cytokines are acting locally within the central nervous system (CNS) with no concentration in serum, psychosocial factors may the dominant cause of SLE fatigue.[15] The other key reason for fatigue is clearly treatable deconditioning. When 93 patients with SLE were compared to 44 sedentary controls, the patients were about 20-percent more deficient with regard to muscular strength, FEV, and VO2 max. A smaller interventional study of exercise physiology found the same baseline.[16] The patients were selected or pretreated to suppress SLE disease activity and underwent 8 weeks of aerobic conditioning, which was successful in reducing their fatigue by about half. A stepwise regression model explaining 37 percent of variation in SLE fatigue featured abnormal illness-related behaviors, greater age, greater degree of helplessness, and lack of health insurance as potentially responsible psychosocial variables.[11]

FAMILY RELATIONSHIPS

Among the landmark situations that almost every rheumatology patient encounters while facing the diagnosis of a chronic disease are understanding repetitive cost-benefit decisions and the threats to family relationships. There are particular challenges when the patient is a child. In the latter case the reestablishment of a peer group—through school, camp, or any other setting—is a primary goal (see Chapter 96). In other sectors of consideration, despite the loss of self confidence and the effects of pain, fatigue, and deformity, patients with RA have the same divorce rate as the general population. However, they have fivefold less remarriages once divorced. Rates of progression of disability in married people are substantially the same as for those who are married.[17] Healthy husbands of women with RA are affected by realization of the vulnerability of their own health. Marriage, in summary, increases social support and is a favorable psychosocial variable. Childhood and adolescence are particularly unfortunate times to encounter rheumatic disease.[18]

EMPLOYMENT AND DISABILITY

In understanding disability and communicating that understanding to patients, four different funds of knowledge are of special value. These are a detailed knowledge of the mechanics and criteria of Social Security Disability Insurance (SSDI);[19] cross-cultural disease comparisons, which include an appreciation of the major criticism raised in critique of the logical assumptions underlying the current system;[20] and finally, knowledge of research results showing what determines disability in specific diseases. Achieving reasonable expectations on the part of the patient and less frustration for the provider and the patients are two attainable goals of disability management.

The mechanics of the SSDI system vary from state to state but are simple and easily caricatured. The patient submits a two-page form along with medical records for the past18 months. The result depends on the clerk matching the medical record with an index of diseases and criteria, known as the "blue book." The book is thin, the criteria strict. Typical criteria for disability caused by SLE are stroke and renal failure with dialysis. For back pain, it is leg paresis and bowel or bladder dysfunction. Due to backlogs, each reapplication typically takes 6 months, and the clerk has no recourse with the administrative law judge until the third application. At that stage attorneys' and doctors' opinions have an effect, but not before. At this stage the court is empowered to ask and answer the question, for example, of whether a lupus patient's skin lesions, joint symptoms, and cognitive deficits are equivalent in severity to a stroke or renal failure.

Cross-cultural comparisons offer little help to individual patients suffering economic losses that constitute the indirect costs of rheumatic diseases. It is interesting that between 1983 and 1996, a number of countries passed a milestone at which the absolute numbers of persons drawing disability payments surpassed the official number of unemployed for the first time. The United States and the United Kingdom both passed this marker in about 1993. Economists think that both political incentives to record low unemployment numbers and the personal incentive of more payments for disability than for unemployment favor continuation of this trend for as long as it is fiscally sustainable. In the long term, it may be that disability insurance will become more like unemployment insurance. Such a change would have to involve acknowledgement that disability and unemployment are related aspects of a single work problem.

The major philosophic underpinning of the current SSDI system is the assumption that the amount of disease determines the amount of work disability.[20] A necessary corollary is that the amount of disease is objectively quantifiable. From the rheumatologic standpoint, two things are wrong. First, pain is self-reported and, by definition, not objectively quantifiable. Second, and more critically, psychosocial factors are stronger determinants of disability than are disease factors in many cases. Examples of this have been studied in a range of illnesses as outlined in the following paragraphs.

In one multivariate analysis of knee OA, only age, female sex, obesity, and severity of knee pain maintained independent effects ($p < 0.0009$). All of these factors, individually and together, had more influence on HAQ-determined disability than did radiographic severity.[21] For 180 English patients with low back pain,[22] the best predictor of some pain persisting at 1-year follow-up was concomitant widespread pain (odds ratio 6.4). Other factors, from the most clinical (radicular pain) to the most psychologic (job dissatisfaction), all showed equal odds ratios of about 3. The lack of influence over work environment and poor social relations with coworkers[23] are specific job-related factors influencing work disability from back pain. Whiplash injury was definitively studied[24] in an "experiment of nature" when Saskatchewan switched from tort to no-fault auto insurance in 1995, which abruptly disallowed claims for pain and suffering. Analysis of 7462 claims showed that both the number of claims and the prognosis of the neck injuries improved by about 30 percent. Depression was found to influence duration of the neck pain. The relative parity of psychosocial factors with clinical disease factors seen in the spine seems to be maintained in analyses of more peripheral musculoskeletal problems, such as forearm pain.[25] Patients with RA and those with fibromyalgia report equal disability on self-report scales, but people with RA report less pain. Labeling a patient with widespread pain or nonarticular axial aching as having fibromyalgia probably will not increase work impairment.[26] Disablility awards are heavily influence by objective radiographic data, such as the presence of erosions and narrowing. However, it is the age, pain score, and a depressed mood secondary to physical disability that determine overall disability in RA from the patient's point of view.[27] Odds are 2 to 3 to 1 against returning to work for a patient with RA who stops working. SSDI, older age, and less education decrease the odds.[28] In SLE multivariate models for patients at university centers, predictors of early disability in the first 3 years were low educational level ($p = 0.0004$), a physical job ($p = 0.0028$), plus disease activity at diagnosis ($p = 0.0078$). Cumulative organ damage and disease duration, race, and gender did not predict stopping work.[29]

Psychosocial Factors as Determinants of Outcome and Targets of Interventions

To be a target for intervention, a psychosocial factor should be shown to be a potential cause of a clinical outcome and should be somewhat modifiable. Psychosocial factors such as education and mood fit these criteria and bear directly upon psychosocial outcomes such as patient satisfaction and job preservation. In addition, however, socioeconomic and psychosocial factors help determine biologic outcome. Effects of psychosocial factors on biologic outcome are mediated primarily by visit compliance, medication adherence, and availability, plus funds of knowledge about disease and the health care system. Psychosocial interventions effective in randomized clinical trials tend to revolve around the most modifiable factors, such as funds of knowledge.

There is an obvious logic to studying psychologic and social factors together. Distinct features separate psychologic factors and socioeconomic factors as they apply to practice, however. First, psychologic characteristics of both doctors and patients are made up of some fairly fixed personality traits combined with some states, such as mood, and other modifiable factors such as fund of knowledge about a disease or medication. In contrast to psychologic states, sociologic features are almost certainly fixed. As Virchow wrote of the turbulent 1840s in Germany, "Politics is medicine written large." His observation remains applicable.[30] In addition, because sociologic variables cannot be easily changed in a hypothesis-testing experiment, inference of causality is problematic, though analysis of variance can help. Even when the biology of the disease is complex, the genetics heterogeneous, and access barriers likely—such as in US urban or rural populations with SLE—detailed analysis suggests that education and counseling, coordinated with medical care, would improve outcome.[19] These studies found SLE disease activity and overall health status to be most strongly associated with potentially modifiable psychosocial factors, such as self-efficacy for disease management. SLE organ damage, in contrast, was best predicted by conventional biologic factors such as duration of disease. Notably, outcomes were not associated with race. In patients with SLE, then, even when the sociologic factors seem overwhelming and the biology of the disease and its therapies complex, targeted psychosocial interventions[20] concentrating on patient education seem to have potential to change outcome (see Chapter 52).

Psychosocial Interventions

Psychosocial interventions fall into three main categories: efforts to improve doctor-patient communication in usual care, organized programs aimed at teaching or influencing groups of patients, and psychopharmacology or psychotherapy.

DOCTOR-PATIENT COMMUNICATION

What do patients want? Canadian patients (n = 197) with established diagnoses representative of office practice, except for the omission of widespread pain and fibromyalgia, answered this question fundamental to improving doctor-patient communication.[31] Factor analysis condensed questionnaires covering 32 possible concerns down to eight points. Patients asked for help in five areas and extra information in two. The five areas mentioned for help were psychologic, coping, getting medication, social, and financial. The information deficits were in disease-specific areas of natural history and therapy, both conventional and unproven remedies. Physician sources and written material were preferred. The scleroderma patients were particularly interested in support groups. The most-common worry for patients across the diagnostic groups, progression of the disease, was probably the same as their physicians'. However, from other studies, it seems that patients with SLE and their physicians have particularly divergent worries.[32] Patients and physicians rate disease activity in SLE differently because physicians place more emphasis on laboratory features, whereas patients place more emphasis on function,[33] particularly the detrimental effect of fatigue.

Data-based recommendations for improving doctor-patient communications have been derived in part from taped usual care visits and post hoc interviews with the participants[34] (Box 53–1).

TIME CONSTRAINTS

Time constraints in the context of usual-care office visits argue for maximum use of organized programs, as well as self-completed questionnaires and forms, such as the ACR new patient form. Patients sometimes see forms as an imposition if they are not referred to in the subsequent interview. If the form is part of the conversation, even marked with a few highlights or marginal notes, it is interpreted as an element of thoroughness. Scheduled telephone contact is poorly reimbursed but was effective enough to reduce knee pain from OA in a randomized study.[35] Legal and institutional restrictions not withstanding, a reasonable rule of thumb for clinical e-mail is to use it for nothing more sensitive than what would be said over the telephone.[1]

ORGANIZED PROGRAMS

A variety of interventional programs improve outcome, measured in their own terms, when other psychosocial variables or a health status scale are the primary outcomes. These programs include support groups, which improve coping more than half the time,[36] and stress management.[37] A smaller number (see Table 53–1) also save the patient money, improve pain, protect anatomy, and have a durable affect. Exercise programs are very effective, but patients have difficulty sustaining the effort they require over time.

PSYCHOTHERAPY AND PSYCHOPHARMACOLOGIC INTERVENTIONS

Depression goes unrecognized a good part of the time. With psychiatric telephone interviews in a survey study taken as the gold standard, only about 19 percent of depressed people are diagnosed and treated in the course of 1 year of usual care.[40] Treatment was less likely for men, African Americans, and those with lower educational level. People aged 30 to 60 were more likely to get treatment. Depression in rheumatology appears more frequently in particular settings, including patients reporting widespread chronic pain, patients coming to grips with work disability, and patients presenting at a young age for knee OA. Recent findings in relevant psychopharmacology include SSRI equivalence for efficacy across the class.[41] There is also more recognition of large relative increases in the risk of sudden cardiac deaths on moderate doses of antipsychotics.[42]

Summary: Effect Size, the Measurable, and the Important

The results of patient education and psychosocial intervention seem modest compared to very effective, biologically based interventions such as TNF blockade.

Techniques to Improve Communication in Usual Care Office Visits*

1. Encourage patients to write down their concerns before each visit.
2. Addressing each concern specifically, even if just briefly.
3. Ask patients what they think has caused their problems.
4. Tailor treatments to patients' goals and preferences, as much as possible.
5. Explain the purpose, dosage, common side effects, and inconveniences of each treatment, and tell patients how to judge the efficacy, including length of trial.
6. Checking patients' understanding of information they have received.
7. Anticipate problems in compliance with treatment plans and discuss methods for coping with common problems.
8. Write down the diagnosis and treatment plan to help patients remember.
9. Give patients written materials, which are now widely available;.
10. Reinforce patients' confidence in their ability to manage their regimen.
11. Use ancillary personnel in patient education.
12. Refer patients to organized programs in their community.

*Taken from Daltroy LH: Doctor-patient communication in rheumatological disorders. Baillieres Clin Rheumatol 7(2):221-239, 1993.

The latter costs about $15,000 per year and promises to make inroads into the lifetime loss of 16 QUALYs per average 27-year course of RA, including 6.6 years of lost survival. In contrast, the best organized and delivered psychosocial intervention administered on a group basis, the Arthritis Foundation Self Help Course, has minimal costs and cuts outpatient visits 40 percent, saving each OA patient $47and each RA patient $162 per year. Specific psychosocial management techniques, therefore, stand as modest adjuncts to powerful specific therapy, but they must be understood as the middle part of a range of promising opportunities. It is likely that increasing literacy and improvement of the individual doctor-patient communication are the two most effective psychosocial interventions. Interpreted broadly over their whole range, then, psychosocial management techniques are potentially as powerful as a biologic therapy. However, only techniques and experiments confined to the middle of the range of psychosocial intervention (i.e., organized programs applied to defined patient subgroups) are easily measured and discussed in a scientific sense. This confinement of thought illustrates French anthropologist-philosopher Rene Dubois' dictum that "the measurable drives out the important." However, that still leaves individual patients and their physicians a fascinating set of possibilities to study, apply, and from which to benefit.

REFERENCES

1. Edworthy SM: World wide web: opportunities, challenges, and threats. Lupus 8(8):596-605, 1999.
2. Lievense A, Bierma-Zeinstra S, Verhagen A, et al: Influence of work on the development of osteoarthritis on the hip: a systematic review. J Rheumatol 28:2520-2528, 2001.
3. Hawley DJ, Wolfe F: Pain, disability, and pain/disability relationships in seven rheumatic disorders: a study of 1,522 patients. J Rheumatol 18(10):1552-1557, 1991.
4. Blyth FM, March LM, Brnabic AJ, et al: Chronic pain in Australia: a prevalence study. Pain 89(2-3):127-134, 2001.
5. Macfarlane GJ, Morris S, Hunt IM, et al: Chronic widespread pain in the community: the influence of psychological symptoms and mental disorder on healthcare seeking behavior. J Rheumatol 26(2):413-419, 1999.
6. Hawley DJ, Wolfe F: Depression is not more common in rheumatoid arthritis: a 10-year longitudinal study of 6,153 patients with rheumatic disease. J Rheumatol 20(12):2025-2031, 1993.
7. Smedstad LM, Vaglum P, Kvien TK, Moum T: The relationship between self-reported pain and sociodemographic variables, anxiety, and depressive symptoms in rheumatoid arthritis. J Rheumatol 22(3):514-520, 1995.
8. Andersen RE, Crespo CJ, Ling SM, et al: Prevalence of significant knee pain among older Americans: results from the Third National Health and Nutrition Examination Survey. J Am Geriatr Soc 47(12):1435-1438, 1999.
9. Dexter P, Brandt K: Distribution and predictors of depressive symptoms in osteoarthritis. J Rheumatol 21(2):279-286, 1994.
10. Hudak PL, Clark JP, Hawker GA, et al: "You're perfect for the procedure! Why don't you want it?" Elderly arthritis patients' unwillingness to consider total joint arthroplasty surgery: a qualitative study. Med Decis Making 22(3):272-278, 2002.
11. Zonana-Nacach A, Roseman JM, McGwin G Jr, et al: Systemic lupus erythematosus in three ethnic groups. VI: Factors associated with fatigue within 5 years of criteria diagnosis. LUMINA Study Group. Lupus in Minority populations: Nature vs Nurture. Lupus 9(2):101-109, 2000.
12. Tack BB: Fatigue in rheumatoid arthritis. Conditions, strategies, and consequences. Arthritis Care Res 3(2):65-70, 1990.
13. Tack BB: Self-reported fatigue in rheumatoid arthritis. A pilot study. Arthritis Care Res 3(3):154-157, 1990.
14. Tan G, Jensen MP, Robinson-Whelen S, et al: Coping with chronic pain: a comparison of two measures. Pain 90(1-2):127-133, 2001.
15. Omdal R, Mellgren SI, Koldingsnes W, et al: Fatigue in patients with systemic lupus erythematosus: lack of associations to serum cytokines, antiphospholipid antibodies, or other disease characteristics. J Rheumatol 29(3):482-486, 2002.
16. Robb-Nicholson LC, Daltroy L, Eaton H, et al: Effects of aerobic conditioning in lupus fatigue: a pilot study. Br J Rheumatol 28(6):500-505, 1989.
17. Ward MM, Leigh JP: Marital status and the progression of functional disability in patients with rheumatoid arthritis. Arthritis Rheum 36(5):581-588, 1993.
18. Ehrlich GE: Social, economic, psychologic, and sexual outcomes in rheumatoid arthritis. Am J Med 75(6A):27-34, 1983.
19. Karlson EW, Daltroy LH, Lew RA, et al: The independence and stability of socioeconomic predictors of morbidity in systemic lupus erythematosus. Arthritis Rheum 38(2):267-273, 1995.
20. Karlson EW, Daltroy LH, Lew RA, et al: The relationship of socioeconomic status, race, and modifiable risk factors to outcomes in patients with systemic lupus erythematosus. Arthritis Rheum 40(1):47-56, 1997.
21. Jordan JM, Luta G, Renner JB, et al: Self-reported functional status in osteoarthritis of the knee in a rural southern community: the role of sociodemographic factors, obesity, and knee pain. Arthritis Care Res 9(4):273-278, 1996.
22. Thomas E, Silman AJ, Croft PR, et al: Predicting who develops chronic low back pain in primary care: a prospective study. BMJ 318(7199):1662-1667, 1999.
23. Thorbjornsson CB, Alfredsson L, Fredriksson K, et al: Physical and psychosocial factors related to low back pain during a 24-year period. A nested case-control analysis. Spine 25(3):369-374, 2000.
24. Cassidy JD, Carroll LJ, Cote P, et al: Effect of eliminating compensation for pain and suffering on the outcome of insurance claims for whiplash injury. N Engl J Med 342(16):1179-1186, 2000.
25. Macfarlane GJ, Hunt IM, Silman AJ: Role of mechanical and psychosocial factors in the onset of forearm pain: prospective population based study. BMJ 321(7262):676-679, 2000.
26. White KP, Nielson WR, Harth M, et al: Does the label "fibromyalgia" alter health status, function, and health service utilization? A prospective, within-group comparison in a community cohort of adults with chronic widespread pain. Arthritis Rheum 47(3):260-265, 2002.
27. Salaffi F, Ferraccioli GF, Carotti M, et al: [Disability in rheumatoid arthritis: the predictive value of age and depression]. Recenti Prog Med 83(12):675-679, 1992.
28. Straaton KV, Maisiak R, Wrigley JM, et al: Barriers to return to work among persons unemployed due to arthritis and musculoskeletal disorders. Arthritis Rheum 39(1):101-109, 1996.
29. Partridge AJ, Karlson EW, Daltroy LH, et al: Risk factors for early work disability in systemic lupus erythematosus: results from a multicenter study. Arthritis Rheum 40(12):2199-2206, 1997.
30. Jackson RH, Davis TC Explaining the connection between privilege and health. N Engl J Med 330(2):139, 1994.
31. Neville C, Fortin PR, Fitzcharles MA, et al: The needs of patients with arthritis: the patient's perspective. Arthritis Care Res 12(2):85-95, 1999.
32. Yen JC, Neville C, Fortin PR: Discordance between patients and their physicians in the assessment of lupus disease activity: relevance for clinical trials. Lupus 8(8):660-670, 1999.
33. Alarcon GS, McGwin G Jr, Brooks K, et al: Systemic lupus erythematosus in three ethnic groups. XI. Sources of discrepancy in perception of disease activity: a comparison of physician and patient visual analog scale scores. Arthritis Rheum 47(4):408-413, 2002.
34. Daltroy LH: Doctor-patient communication in rheumatological disorders. Baillieres Clin Rheumatol 7(2) 221-239, 1993.
35. Maisiak R, Austin J, Heck L: Health outcomes of two telephone interventions for patients with rheumatoid arthritis or osteoarthritis. Arthritis Rheum 39(8):1391-1399, 1996.
36. Baker PR, Groh JD, Kraag GR, et al: Impact of patient with patient interaction on perceived rheumatoid arthritis overall disease status. Scand J Rheumatol 25(4):207-212, 1996.

37. Parker JC, Smarr KL, Buckelew SP, et al: Effects of stress management on clinical outcomes in rheumatoid arthritis. Arthritis Rheum 38(12):1807-1818, 1995.
38. Lorig KR, Mazonson PD, Holman HR: Evidence suggesting that health education for self-management in patients with chronic arthritis has sustained health benefits while reducing health care costs. Arthritis Rheum 36(4):439-446, 1993.
39. Sullivan T, Allegrante JP, Peterson MG, et al: One-year followup of patients with osteoarthritis of the knee who participated in a program of supervised fitness walking and supportive patient education. Arthritis Care Res 11(4):228-233, 1998.
40. Young AS, Klap R, Sherbourne CD, Wells KB: The quality of care for depressive and anxiety disorders in the United States. Arch Gen Psychiatry 58(1):55-61, 2001.
41. Kroenke K, West SL, Swindle R, et al: Similar effectiveness of paroxetine, fluoxetine, and sertraline in primary care: a randomized trial. JAMA 286(23):2947-2955, 2001.
42. Ray WA, Meredith S, Thapa PB, et al: Antipsychotics and the risk of sudden cardiac death. Arch Gen Psychiatry 58(12):1161-1167, 2001.

54 Nutrition and Rheumatic Diseases

JOEL M. KREMER

Although it has been appreciated for some time that disease processes can interfere with adequate nutrition, we are only now beginning to understand how altered nutritional status contributes to the pathogenesis of disease. As a corollary, it is now known that certain dietary manipulations can result in improvements in the inflammatory disease process. These principles represent an evolution of thinking from the relatively recent past when contributors to the field believed it extremely unlikely that dietary manipulation could affect patients with inflammatory disease. Appreciation of the possible role of nutritional manipulation in inflammatory disease has increased, however, along with the understanding of immunity, eicosanoid metabolism, and cellular biology. Epidemiologic studies have confirmed the role of diet in other disease processes, such as vascular and gastrointestinal disease.[1,2] Surprisingly, improvements in mortality rates from cardiovascular disease in some large population studies are not linked solely to favorable changes in cholesterol, hypertension, or smoking profiles but also to alteration of other biologic processes through the intake of dietary fatty acids.[3] Paralleling the emergence of data on the role of diet in disease states is the realization that our current dietary habits are altered from those our species adapted to during almost the entire span of human history[4,5] (Table 54–1). Circumstantial evidence has linked an increased incidence of cancer and cardiovascular and gastrointestinal disease to high-fat, low-fiber diets.

Role of Protein-Energy Malnutrition and Metabolic Response to Inflammation

The catabolic effect of inflammatory disease is multifactorial and may lead to weight loss through a variety of mechanisms. Fever is associated with increased energy expenditure and, thus, increased caloric requirements to maintain body weight. Catecholamine-mediated increases in lipolysis and hepatic and muscular glycogenolysis occur, along with hyperglycemia and hypoinsulinemia, to increase energy substrates in the acute-phase response to injury.[6] After a few days, hyperinsulinemia and increased protein catabolism occur in what Blackburn and Bistrian called the "adaptive phase" of metabolic response to stress or injury.[6] The increased amino acids may then serve as precursors for hepatic production of acute-phase reactants and gluconeogenesis. Increased production of eicosanoids and cytokines associated with the inflammatory state lead to an enhanced catabolic effect and increased protein breakdown.

Weight loss of 5 to 10 percent is associated with little functional impairment,[7] although it should be considered of potential clinical significance if it occurs over a period of 1 to 6 months. Protein-calorie malnutrition is subdivided into marasmus and kwashiorkor. Marasmus is defined as a weight below 80 percent of ideal weight, as calculated from standardized tables of height and weight, with preservation of serum protein levels and immune function. Kwashiorkor may be associated with a similar degree of weight loss, but it has the additional factor of lowered serum protein levels and compromised immune function. Patients with the hypoalbuminemic malnutrition of kwashiorkor have a significantly higher mortality rate as a result of infections and other metabolic stress.

Role of Nutrition

RHEUMATOID ARTHRITIS

Interest in the possible role of nutrition in the pathogenesis of the rheumatic diseases is not new. An early study analyzed dietary intake in the period preceding the onset of rheumatoid arthritis (RA) in an attempt to determine whether altered nutrition could be linked to the development of disease.[8] Information obtained from patient recall indicated that there were no significant dietary differences between patients with RA and the population at large. A later investigation compared the nutritional status of patients with RA to those with osteoarthritis (OA).[9] Patients with OA were found to be 15 lbs overweight on average, whereas patients with RA were an average of 10.3 lbs underweight. The groups did not differ in intake of protein, fat, carbohydrate, vitamins, or minerals, although both groups had a high prevalence of deficient vitamin intake.

More recent investigations have assessed nutrition in patients with RA using a 3-day food record, which is a reliable method of diet assessment. Deficient dietary intake of folic acid, zinc, magnesium, and pyridoxine have been reported by three independent groups of investigators.[10-14] Intake of other nutrients, including fat, protein, and carbohydrate, was reported to be similar to age-matched subjects in one investigation.[10]

A nutritional assessment of 50 patients with RA involved anthropometric measurements, including triceps skin-fold thickness and body mass index calculated from height, weight, and upper-arm muscle circumference, as well as biochemical measurements of nutrition.[12]

TABLE 54–1 • COMPARISON OF THE LATE PALEOLITHIC DIET, CURRENT AMERICAN DIET, AND U.S. DIETARY RECOMMENDATIONS

	Late Paleolithic Diet	Current American Diet	U.S. Senate Select Committee Recommendations*
Total dietary energy (%)			
Protein	34	12	12
Carbohydrate	45	46	58
Fat	21	42	30
P:S ratio	1.41	0.44	1
Cholesterol (mg)	591	600	300
Fiber (g)	45.7	19.7	30-60
Sodium (mg)	690	2300-6900	1100-3300
Calcium (mg)	1580	740	800-1200
Ascorbic acid (mg)	392.3	87.7	45

*Select committee on Nutrition and Human Needs, United States Senate: Dietary Goals for the United States. Washington, DC, Government Printing Office, 1977.

Abbreviation: P:S, polyunsaturated:saturated fats.

From Eaton SB, Konner M: Paleolithic nutrition: a consideration of its nature and current implications. N Engl J Med 312:283, 1985. Reprinted with permission from *The New England Journal of Medicine*.

Patients were judged to be malnourished if they had a reduction in one anthropometric measurement in conjunction with a reduction in two or more biochemical indices. By these criteria, 13 patients (26%) were malnourished. When the dietary history was assessed, no differences in dietary intake could be found between these individuals and those with normal nutritional status. Malnourished patients were more likely to have severe RA than those without malnutrition. In addition, significantly lower values were obtained for all anthropometric measurements in the patients with RA compared to a control population. Decreased weight and triceps skin-fold thickness occurred twice as frequently as a significant reduction in upper arm-muscle circumference. Because dietary intake was judged to be adequate in these patients, it was suggested that the increased demand of the inflammatory state placed a greater burden on the metabolism of certain essential nutrients. The etiology of the catabolic state is related to increased cytokine production, primarily tumor necrosis factor-α (TNF-α).[15] Of interest is the observation that the increased protein breakdown seen in patients with RA is normalized with either methotrexate (MTX) treatment or strength training.[16]

JUVENILE RHEUMATOID ARTHRITIS

Dietary assessments of children with juvenile rheumatoid arthritis (JRA) were reported in two Swedish studies.[17,18] Biochemical measures and anthropometric measurements were examined in 26 11- to 16-year-old girls with JRA and matched healthy control subjects. Arm-muscle circumference and serum creatinine levels were lower in the children with arthritis. Significant inverse correlations were observed between disease activity and concentrations of albumin, prealbumin, and retinol-binding protein. Using the same definition of malnutrition as in the previously discussed study of adult patients with RA,[14] the researchers found that five girls with chronic arthritis (19%) fit the definition of malnutrition. Their intake of calories and protein did not differ from that of the control population. An analysis of nutrient intake, by means of a 4-day dietary history, in the same population failed to reveal any significant differences from controls. Children with arthritis were, however, observed to derive a greater percentage of their energy requirements from fat and a lower percentage from carbohydrates than controls. Another study observed increased spinal bone mass in children with arthritis given supplemental calcium and vitamin D.[19]

Independent investigations have, thus, reached similar conclusions about the nutritional status of patients with RA and JRA: Patients with active disease require increased dietary energy and protein and frequently exhibit deficiencies in micronutrients, including selenium, zinc, magnesium, vitamin C, and vitamin A. They have a high intake of fat, particularly saturated fatty acids, which could have significant effects on immune function. These nutritional alterations are at times associated with frank malnutrition. The appreciation of the less than optimal dietary and nutritional status of patients with rheumatic disease is poor among most practitioners who treat these conditions. It is, therefore, apparent that considerable potentials exist for improving general well-being if greater attention is given to the overall nutritional status of patients with rheumatic problems.

Gout

The potential contribution of various foods to the onset and frequency of gouty attacks has been well described.[20] Many patients with gout may also be obese, hypertensive, and diabetic and may fulfill criteria for an insulin-resistance syndrome.[20]

Free Radicals and Nutrition

A compound with unpaired free electrons is termed a *free radical*, and some of the most reactive of these compounds contain oxygen. Free radicals extract electrons from stable compounds in an attempt to stabilize themselves, and in the process they create new free radicals.[21] The rapidly proliferating cells of the immune system are uniquely prone to oxidative damage from free radicals, which can also affect the activity of thromboxane, prostaglandin, and leukotriene species.[22]

The phospholipid bilayer of cell membranes contains polyunsaturated fatty acids, which can be common sites for free-radical reactions (Fig. 54–1). Membrane damage from lipid peroxidation results in the formation of unstable lipid peroxyl radicals, which can further damage the membrane in a "snowball effect".[21] Potentially toxic products of lipid membrane peroxidation include malondialdehyde, volatile substances such

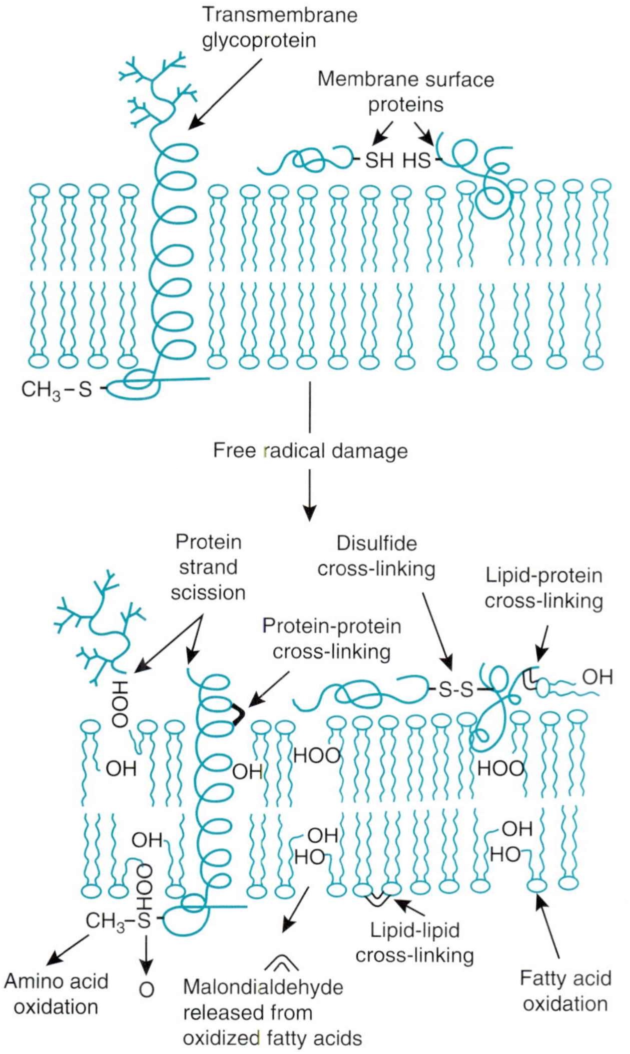

FIGURE 54–1 · **Free Radical Damage to Lipid Membranes and Proteins Associated with Cell Membranes.** (From Bendich A: Antioxidant micronutrients and immune functions. Ann N Y Acad Sci 587:168-180, 1990.)

$$O_2^{\bullet-} + O_2^{\bullet-} + 2H^+ \xrightarrow[\text{Superoxide dismutase}]{\text{Cu/Zn, Mn}} H_2O_2 + O_2$$
Superoxide radical anion → Hydrogen peroxide

$$H_2O_2 + H_2O_2 \xrightarrow{\text{Fe-catalase}} 2H_2O + O_2$$

$$H_2O_2 + 2GSH \xrightarrow[\text{peroxidase}]{\text{Se-glutathione}} 2H_2O + GSSG$$
glutathione → Oxidized glutathione

$$LOOH + 2GSH \xrightarrow[\text{peroxidase}]{\text{Se-glutathione}} LOH + GSSG + H_2O$$
Lipid hydroperoxide → Lipid aldehyde

FIGURE 54–2 · **Antioxidant Metalloenzyme Reactions.** Nutritionally essential elements are not antioxidants until they are incorporated into their metalloenzyme ligand. Cu, copper; Zn, zinc; Mn, manganese; Fe, iron; Se, selenium. (From Bendich A: Antioxidant micronutrients and immune functions. Ann N Y Acad Sci 587:168-180, 1990.)

as ethane and pentane, cross-linked membrane lipids, conjugated dienes, and protein-lipid adducts.[23-24]

Free radicals are also essential to normal immune competence.[25,26] Intracellular free-radical production is part of the host response necessary for the killing of invading microorganisms. Free-radical reactions are associated with the release of arachidonic acid and the conversion of arachidonate to eicosanoids and subsequent eicosanoid metabolism.[27] These substances are, in turn, essential in the functioning of a normal immune system.[28] When considering the production and modulation of free radicals, therefore, the critical issue is the balance between potentially destructive reactions and naturally occurring free-radical generation that is essential for normal immune competence.

Several naturally occurring enzymes inactivate reactive oxygen molecules. Antioxidant metalloenzymes interfere with the production of free radicals by inactivating precursor molecules. Superoxide dismutase exists in two forms, either of which can inactivate the superoxide anion. There is a manganese-containing superoxide dismutase in mitochondria and a copper-zinc–containing superoxide dismutase in the cytoplasm (Fig. 54–2). Both of these reactions produce hydrogen peroxide (H_2O_2). An iron-containing catalase found in cytoplasmic peroxisomes catalyzes the decomposition of H_2O_2 to oxygen and water. Selenium is an essential component of two glutathione peroxidases that inactivate H_2O_2, lipid peroxides, and phospholipid peroxides.

The nutritionally essential mineral elements copper, zinc, iron, manganese, and selenium are not antioxidants until they are incorporated into the antioxidant enzymes.[21] Further addition of these elements to the system by dietary intake does not enhance the activity of the antioxidative enzymes once the system is saturated. Circulating levels of these enzymes are lower than intracellular concentrations. The balance between extracellular free-radical formation and release and antioxidant enzyme protection may be important in the inflammation and tissue destruction of several immune-mediated inflammatory diseases. Observations in an animal model of OA have suggested that oxidized low density lipoprotein LDL receptors may be associated with leukocyte infiltration and cartilage destruction.[23]

Antioxidant Vitamins

BETA CAROTENE

The carotenoids are red-yellow pigments found in all photosynthesizing plants. There are more than 500 carotenoids, but only a small number of these compounds can be metabolized to vitamin A. Cleavage of beta carotene, however, results in two molecules of vitamin A, which makes it unique among the carotenoids. In contrast to vitamin A, beta carotene is a potent antioxidant and can also function as an immunostimulant. Enhancement of activation markers of human peripheral blood mononuclear cells was observed in vitro after exposure to carotenoids.[29] In models of animal tumorigenesis, both cytotoxic T lymphocyte functions and macrophage secretion of TNF were increased following carotenoid administration.[30] A recent study, however, presents data showing all cause mortality is increased in patients taking B-carotene, but not Vitamin E.[30a]

VITAMIN E

Vitamin E (α-tocopherol) is the major lipid-soluble antioxidant found in cells. Vitamin E protects the unsaturated double bonds of the fatty acids in the phospholipid bilayer from oxidation. It accomplishes this by donating electrons to lipid peroxide and other radicals and in this way can interrupt the chain reaction of free-radical damage to the cell membrane. The antioxidant activity of vitamin E is regenerated by electron donation from vitamin C, glutathione, and other antioxidants.

Vitamin E is critical to maintaining the normal function of the immune system. T cells are more susceptible to membrane peroxidative damage than B cells, and peroxidative damage has been associated with the loss of certain T cell receptor (TCR) activities.[31] T cells are, therefore, more sensitive to vitamin E status, even though the vitamin E content of both T and B lymphocytes is more than 10 times that found in red blood cells.[32] The macrophage membrane expresses decreased Ia antigen in the vitamin E–deficient state. Phagocytic function is diminished in the presence of vitamin E deficiency in both animal and human studies.[33]

VITAMIN C

Vitamin C (ascorbic acid) is water soluble and is important in decreasing free-radical reactions in both intracellular and extracellular fluids. It is also required for the hydroxylation of proline and lysine in the production of collagen and is involved in several enzymatic reactions in the formation of neuropeptides. Neutrophils and mononuclear cells maintain concentrations of vitamin C that are approximately 150 times that found in serum.[34] Vitamin C has been shown to increase neutrophil and monocyte chemotaxis in vitro in experimental models.[35]

Plasma and platelet ascorbic acid levels have been demonstrated to be low in patients with RA who take high doses of aspirin.[36] The decrease was thought to be from either impaired tissue uptake or increased urinary excretion. Lowered ascorbate levels may be caused by superoxide-associated oxidation at inflammatory sites. Scorbutic guinea pigs develop lesions resembling rheumatoid arthropathy, prompting a suggestion that synovial vitamin C deficiency could contribute to rheumatoid synovitis.[36] An early study of vitamin C supplementation in patients with RA failed to show any effect.[37]

Free radicals derived from phagocytes are autotoxic to cells in their immediate environment, causing inhibition of chemotaxis, phagocytosis, and antimicrobial activity.[38] Reactive oxygen species also inhibit proliferation of T and B lymphocytes, as well as the cytotoxic activity of natural killer (NK) cells.[39] Neutrophil-derived production of hydrogen peroxide and hypochlorous acid (HOC1) are the most potent mediators of immunosuppression.[40] At physiologically relevant concentrations, ascorbate protects neutrophil metabolic activity and function from HOCl- but not H_2O_2-mediated inhibition.[41] Ascorbate is the first-line plasma antioxidant in the defense against phagocyte-derived reactive oxidants; only when it is depleted does lipid peroxidation occur.[42] By neutralizing granulocyte-derived HOCl, ascorbate maintains host defenses by sustaining the function of phagocytes and bystander lymphocytes by protecting them from oxidative damage. Vitamin C may also enhance immune responses indirectly by maintaining optimal levels of vitamin E. It does this by donating an electron to the α-tocopherol molecule to reestablish the latter's antioxidant activity.

VITAMIN D

Dietary deficiency of vitamin D may contribute to osteopenia in patients with RA and has been linked to cortical thinning and spontaneous fractures of long bones in this condition.[43] Vitamin D supplementation may have some beneficial effect in the treatment of psoriasis.[44] 1,25-Dihydroxyvitamin D_3 has inhibitory effects in vitro on psoriatic fibroblast proliferation[45] and has been shown to inhibit the effects of interleukin (IL)-1β on prostaglandin production from human fibroblasts. It has significant effects on the T lymphocyte proliferative response to mitogen stimulation[46] and has demonstrated effects on cytokine production.[47] 1,24-dihydroxyvitamin D_3 can potentiate the inhibitory effects of cyclosporine on helper T cells from patients with RA.[48] An open, uncontrolled study using increasing dosages of 1,25 $(OH)_2D_3$ over 6 months showed significant improvement in several clinical parameters of psoriatic arthritis disease activity in a small number of patients who completed the study.[49]

Folic Acid

Treatment with MTX may be associated with decreases in plasma levels of folic acid, which are associated with hyperhomocysteinemia.[50,51] This is because MTX interferes with the conversion of dihydrofolic acid to tetrahydrofolic acid. As the latter is a critical cofactor for the conversion of homocysteine to methionine, it is easy to understand why the addition of supplemental folic acid will lower levels of circulating homocysteine, which has been found to be associated with an increased risk for atherosclerosis.

Trace Elements

Before considering the effects of certain trace elements on the immune response and inflammatory disease, it is appropriate to examine certain related areas of their metabolism and processing. Copper, zinc, and iron are, in many cases, integral components of metalloproteinases found within the intestinal mucosa.[52] Because these different metals compete for binding with the same proteins, there may be a reciprocal relation between high dietary levels of certain elements and a deficiency in others.[53]

Increased circulating levels of the cytokines IL-1, IL-6, and TNF-α may affect the availability of trace elements by inducing the increased production of metalloproteinases within the liver and intestine. This increased metalloproteinase production results in sequestration of these elements, so they are less readily available to peripheral tissues.[53] Thus, the diets of patients with inflammatory disease may have adequate iron and zinc but inadequate levels at metabolically important sites, with iron bound to cytokine-induced ferritin within the macrophages and liver and zinc bound to the excess metalloproteinases in liver and gut.[54] Teleologically, the cytokine-induced decreased concentrations of iron and zinc may have enhanced host defenses against infection or parasitism, because iron is required for bacterial replication and zinc has a natural anti-inflammatory role.[55]

ZINC

Zinc has been known to be an essential element for growth for more than 100 years. It is essential for a large and diverse collection of enzymes involved in multiple areas of normal metabolic functioning. Only iron exceeds zinc in total body-tissue concentrations. It is considerably less reactive and less toxic than copper. Dietary sources include protein derived from meat, fish, or dairy products, and total body storage reserves are thought to be somewhat limited. Absorption of zinc is diminished by ingestion of copper or iron. As is the case with iron and copper, increased cytokine production in inflammatory disease can result in increased binding of zinc to metallothioneins and decreased serum and leukocyte zinc concentrations.[55] This situation may be compounded in patients who regularly consume iron supplements, because this interferes with zinc absorption. In addition, dietary surveys have documented that zinc intake is low in patients with RA.[10–13]

The unexpected incidence of autoimmune disease after treatment with D-penicillamine has been linked to the ability of D-penicillamine to chelate zinc, as well as magnesium and pyridoxine.[56] Zinc can function as a lymphocyte mitogen when added in vitro to experimental systems.[57] The process of activation is thought to be initiated through monocyte processing of a zinc-transferring complex. Zinc has been demonstrated to enhance NK cell activity in vitro in the presence of interferon-α (IFN-α) or IFN-γ.

The rationale for trials using zinc in inflammatory diseases has been summarized by Whitehouse.[58] It is derived from a collection of evidence showing the following:

- A tendency for decreased zinc concentrations at critical tissue stores in inflammatory disease
- Decreased absorption associated with iron therapy
- The importance of zinc to normal immune functioning
- The tendency of certain drugs such as D-penicillamine and corticosteroids to suppress zinc concentrations
- Depressed oral intake of zinc in dietary surveys[10,11] and serum measurements of patients with RA
- The anti-inflammatory effect of zinc complexes in chronic models of inflammation[59]

The clinical studies of zinc supplementation, however, have yielded unconvincing mixed results.[60] Nevertheless, researchers in the field retain a good deal of interest in the potential role of zinc therapy in the rheumatic diseases.

SELENIUM

Selenium was recognized to be an essential nutrient in 1957. It exerts myriad effects on the immune system and functions through several different pathways that have been extensively reviewed.[61] Spallholz and colleagues[62] have summarized its three major functions: 1) reduction of organic and inorganic peroxides; 2) metabolism of hydroperoxides, which are intermediate steps in the metabolism of prostaglandins and leukotrienes derived from arachidonic acid; and 3) modulation of the respiratory burst through the control of superoxide (O_2^-) and hydrogen peroxide generation.

The effect of selenium on immune function is derived from the selenium-dependent enzymes glutathione peroxidase and phospholipidhydroperoxide. The former is responsible for antioxidant activities in reactions described earlier in this chapter (see Fig. 54–2). Both enzymes participate in the reduction of prostaglandin (PG) G_2 in the arachidonic acid cascade, leading to the production of thromboxane A_2, prostacyclin, and prostaglandins.[62] They also participate in the production of leukotrienes and lipoxins through the reduction of the hydroperoxy intermediates.[63] Eicosanoid synthesis is significantly diminished in the absence of selenium.[64] It is likely that both the anti-inflammatory and immune-modulating effects of selenium are mediated by means of the effect of its ligand enzymes on the production of eicosanoids and the reduction of hydroperoxides. Dietary supplementation of selenium is associated with increased production of superoxide in an animal model.[65] It may, therefore, exert cytotoxic, protective, or modulatory effects in different biologic systems.

Because selenium's ligand enzyme, glutathione peroxidase, catalyzes the reduction of peroxides and increased levels of these reactive elements are found in serum and synovial fluid of some patients with RA, there has been some interest in the selenium status of these patients, as well as those with other arthritic conditions. There are conflicting reports of selenium-glutathione peroxidase status in patients with RA.[66,67] Selenium has been administered to patients with RA[68] and OA[69] without apparent effect. A *reduction* in serum selenium has been found inpatients with systemic sclerosis.[70] Patients with RA but not OA showed an improved pain score in one study of selenium supplementation.[71]

COPPER

Copper is an essential nutrient for biologic systems, including the immune system. Copper is the third largest trace element found in human tissues, after iron and zinc. Free copper ion is rapidly complexed to specific ligands, through which it expresses its biologic activity. Most serum copper is bound to ceruloplasmin, which increases as part of the acute-phase response.

The mechanisms of the effects of copper on the immune system are unknown, although several hypotheses are plausible. As mentioned, along with zinc and manganese, copper is a cofactor in the enzyme superoxide dismutase, which has an essential role in inhibiting free-radical damage in tissues and the immune system (see Fig. 54–2). Altered glutathione levels have also been reported in copper-deficient rats.[72] The circulating cuproenzyme ceruloplasmin also has antioxidant properties. Increased levels of ceruloplasmin produced as a result of the acute-phase response to inflammation may directly scavenge superoxide, although this is thought to be inefficient.[35] Of more importance, ceruloplasmin can oxidize Fe(II) to Fe(III), thus inhibiting the Fe(II)-catalyzed reactions of lipid peroxidation and the scavenging of reactive hydroxyl radicals. It also transports copper for synthesis of intracellular copper-zinc superoxide dismutase, which is critical in the reduction of highly reactive oxygen free radical species.

Two copper-dependent enzymes present within lymphocytes are important in immune function: cytochrome C oxidase and sulfhydryl oxidase. The former acts in intracellular energy metabolism, and the latter is located in lymphocyte plasma membranes and is a cofactor in pentamer immunoglobulin M (IgM) formation and B cell differentiation.[73]

IRON

Asymptomatic tissue iron deficiency is the most common nutritional deficiency in the world. It occurs along with the more severe iron deficiency, anemia, and is particularly common in infants, children, and pregnant and menstruating females. Iron-deficient populations have a high rate of infectious diseases, which may paradoxically be worsened with iron supplementation. This is thought to be due to the improved replication of many microorganisms that also require iron for optimal growth.[76]

Iron has many well-documented effects on immune function. The iron-containing enzyme catalase is found in cytoplasmic peroxisomes and catalyzes the decomposition of hydrogen peroxide to water and O_2, protecting the cellular environment from free radical–induced damage (see Fig. 54–2). Like zinc, serum levels of iron decrease in inflammation and infection, probably by a mechanism of cytokine-stimulated withdrawal from the circulation and enhanced synthesis of ferritin.[74] The immune effects of iron may be at least partially mediated through alterations in prostaglandin synthesis. Prostaglandin endoperoxide synthase is an iron-dependent enzyme critical in the synthesis of prostaglandin species.[74] Because PGE_2 can, in turn, regulate the production of IL-1, impaired prostaglandin production secondary to iron deficiency could affect the production of this important cytokine. The precise mechanism responsible for the effects of iron on the immune response has not been established and may have to do with a general role in cellular growth and protein synthesis, as well as more specific effects on the immune system.

Fatty Acids

BACKGROUND

Certain long-chain fatty acids are deemed essential in our diet because their deficiency can result in severe growth retardation and death. Early experiments showed that rats fed a fat-free diet failed to grow or reproduce and eventually died. Linoleic acid has been found to be the primary essential fatty acid, together with its derivative n-6 fatty acid compounds. The n-3 fatty acids have also been found to be essential. They represent the largest species of fatty acids in the cerebral cortex and retina and can be derived only from the diet. Animals lack two important desaturase enzymes that are present in plants and phytoplankton and that convert the monounsaturate oleic acid to linoleic acid and linoleic acid to α-linolenic acid. Once animals and humans consume linoleic acid or α-linolenic acid, the basic n-6 and n-3 fatty acids, they can then be metabolized to the longer-chain fatty acids, including arachidonic, eicosapentaenoic acid (EPA), and docosahexaenoic acid (DHA).

Because of the mammalian inability to interconvert n-3 and n-6 fatty acids, the composition of phospholipids in cellular membranes is determined by nutritional intake.[75] The fatty acids found in the membrane bilayer are substrates for the production of prostaglandin and leukotriene species essential for many biologic activities, including modulation of the inflammatory and immune response. It is becoming widely recognized that reproducible metabolic alterations in these pathways can be engineered by consistent modifications in dietary fatty acid content. These fatty acid–induced changes have been documented in trials in animals[76] and normal humans,[77] as well as in large epidemiologic studies of populations that consume relatively homogeneous diets.[78]

Fatty acids are designated with a number followed by a colon, another lesser number, a lowercase *n* and yet another number; for example, 18:2 n-6. The first number designates the number of carbon atoms in the molecule. The number appearing after the colon represents the number of double bonds. The number after the *n* indicates the position of the first double bond starting from the methyl or *omega* end of the fatty-acid chain. Linoleic acid, 18:2 n-6, thus, has 18 carbons and two double bonds, and the first double bond is found six carbon atoms from the terminal methyl group. It is, therefore, an n-6 fatty acid. In discussing fatty acid dietary studies in inflammatory disease, we will consider n-6 and n-3 intervention separately.

N-6 FATTY ACIDS

By far the most common fatty acid constituents in the Western diet are the n-6 fatty acids. They are derived predominantly from terrestrial sources and are ubiquitous in plant seeds. Linoleic acid (18:6 n-6) is essential to life, as it is the precursor of arachidonic acid (20:4 n-6) (Fig. 54–3). Arachidonate is present in cellular membranes, where it is esterified to phospholipids in the 2 position. It is released by phospholipase A_2 to form the eicosanoid derivatives of the prostaglandin and leukotriene families through the enzymes cyclooxygenase (COX) and 5-lipoxygenase, respectively, which catalyze the insertion of molecular oxygen into arachidonic acid. Gamma-linolenic acid (GLA), 18:3 n-6, is found in seeds from the evening primrose and borage plants. It may be converted by an elongase enzyme to dihomogammalinolenic acid (DGLA), 20: 3 n-6. DGLA is oxidized by COX to PGE_1 (Fig. 54–4), a monoenoic prostaglandin that has altered biologic activities from the dienoic PGE_2. For example, PGE_1 can inhibit platelet aggregation in humans and rats in vivo and in vitro, whereas PGE_2 cannot.[79] PGE_1 dietary supplementation can suppress inflammation and joint-tissue injury in several animal models of inflammation[80] and can inhibit neutrophil function. GLA dietary supplementation can suppress acute and chronic inflammation in several experimental animal models.

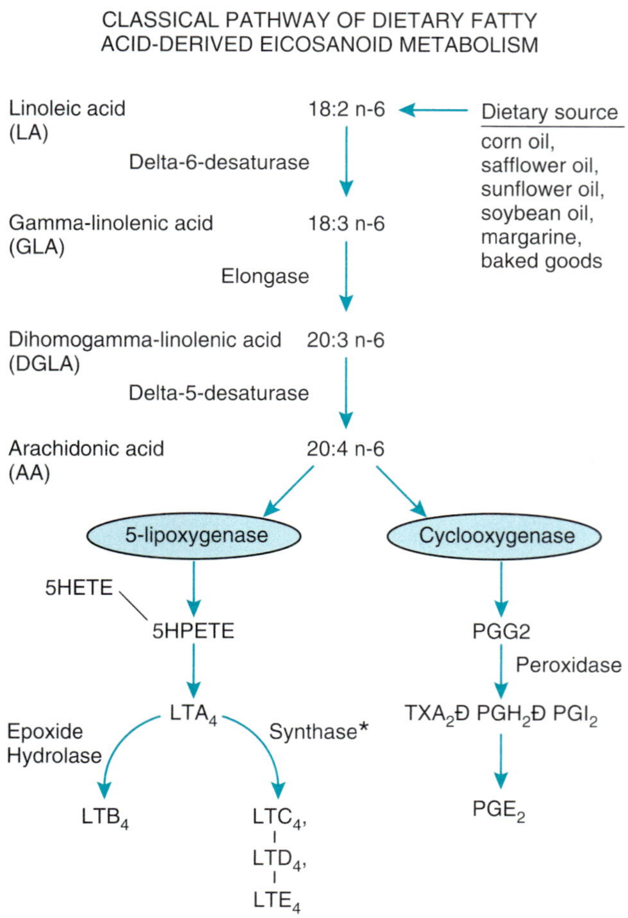

FIGURE 54–3 · Metabolism of Linoleic Acid to Eicosanoids. Synthase is also known as glutathione S transferase. 5-HPETE, 5S-hydroperoxyeicosatetraenoic acid; 5-HETE 5S-hydroperoxyeicosatetraenoic acid; LT, leukotriene; PG, prostaglandin; TXA_2, thromboxane A_2; PGI_2, prostacylin I_2.

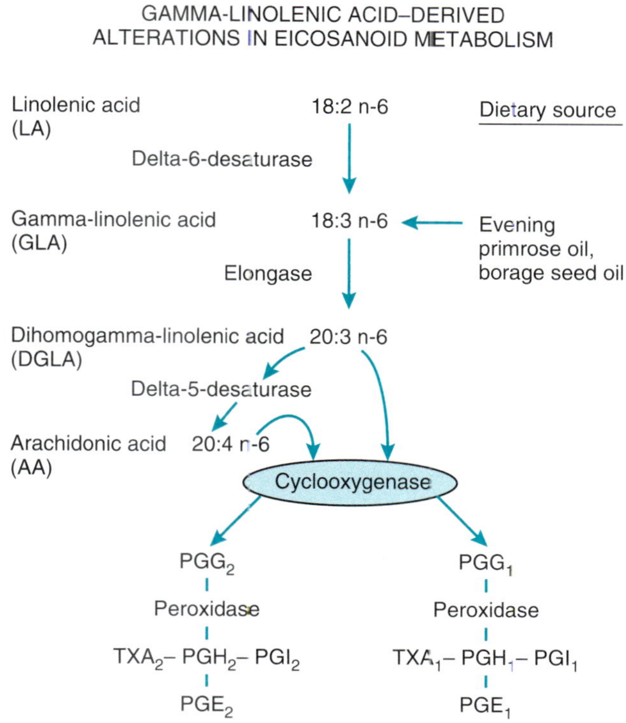

FIGURE 54–4 · Metabolism of Gamma-Linolenic Acid (GLA) to Prostaglandin Species with One Double Bond. Dihomogammalinolenic acid (DGLA) cannot be converted to a leukotriene compound. Instead, it is converted by 15-lipoxygenase to 15-hydroxy DGLA (reaction not shown), which can inhibit 5-lipoxygenase activities.

Animal Studies

The "subcutaneous air pouch" model of inflammation was used to assess response to monosodium urate crystals, or Freund's adjuvant, in Sprague-Dawley rats that consumed diets enriched with either safflower oil, as a source of linoleic acid, or borage seed oil, as a source of GLA.[81] Animals that consumed GLA had a marked reduction of neutrophil exudate and lysosomal enzyme activity compared to those fed sunflower oil. PGE_2 and leukotriene B_4 (LTB_4) concentrations were significantly diminished in pouch exudates in the GLA-fed rats. The fatty acid profiles in the serum and inflammatory cells from animals that consumed primrose oil exhibited significant increases in GLA and dihomogammalinolenic acid.

When DGLA is added to human synovial cells grown in tissue culture, IL-1β–stimulated growth is suppressed five-fold compared to cells grown in medium supplemented with arachidonic acid.[82] Cells incubated with DGLA exhibited a 14-fold increase in PGE_1 and a 70-percent decrease in PGE_2 compared to cells in control medium. The increase in PGE_1 concentrations was associated with significantly enhanced levels of cyclic adenosine monophosphate (cAMP), which the researchers suggested was responsible for the antiproliferative effects. The inhibiting effect could be blocked by indomethacin, lending further support to PGE_1 as the mediator of growth suppression.

Human Studies

Studies of dietary supplementation with GLA in humans have shown somewhat mixed results. An open study of only 20 patients with RA treated with GLA in combination with various vitamins showed no significant changes of any clinical or laboratory parameters over 12 weeks.[83] An investigation that compared evening primrose oil to olive oil as a source of GLA in 20 patients with RA over 13 weeks failed to show any significant difference between groups.[84]

In a well-designed study, investigators treated patients with RA with 1.4 g of GLA daily over 24 weeks.[85] They observed a clinically important reduction in both the tender and swollen joint counts of 36 and 28 percent, respectively; the placebo group showed no improvement in these parameters. It had previously been demonstrated that GLA can inhibit IL-2 production by peripheral blood mononuclear cells in vitro[86] and may reduce the expansion of activation markers on T lymphocytes.[87] The precise mechanism of the improvements observed was not studied.[85] Studies of GLA in patients with RA have recently been reviewed.[88]

N-3 FATTY ACIDS

n-3 fatty acids have their first double bond at the third carbon atom from the methyl end of the molecule. The primary dietary source of this class of fatty acids in human diets is fish and other marine sources, which derive the n-3 fatty acids from phytoplankton and zooplankton at the base of the food chain. EPA (20:5 n-3) (Fig. 54–5) and DHA (22:6 n-3) are the n-3 fatty acids derived from marine sources. n-3 fatty acids may also occur naturally in terrestrial sources in the form of α-linolenic acid (18:3 n-3), which is commonly found in chloroplasts of green leaves and in some plant oils, including flax, canola, and soybean oils. The ability to synthesize the longer-chain n-3 fatty acids EPA and DHA from α-linolenic acid is slow in humans and may diminish even further with aging or certain disease states[89] as a result of a loss of n-6 and n-5 desaturase enzyme activity. The shorter-chain n-3 fatty acids must also compete for these enzymes with the much larger amounts of n-6 fatty acids found in the typical Western diet. The n-6 fatty acids can competitively inhibit the formation of EPA and DHA from α-linolenic acid.[3] The primary source of n-3 fatty acids in the Western diet is, therefore, nonterrestrial—a reversal of the pattern of most of human prehistory, in which large sources of n-3 fatty acids were obtained in hunter-gatherer societies through consumption of wild game.[4] Fat of wild animals contains about 9 percent EPA and five times more polyunsaturated fat per gram than is found in domestic livestock,[90] which contains almost undetectable amounts of EPA. Throughout most of human history, hunter-gatherer societies consumed a higher percentage of polyunsaturated fat, more n-3 fatty acids, more fiber, and less total fat than are found in the present Western diet (see Table 54–1). Our current dietary fatty acid intake must be properly viewed as a relatively recent alteration of long-standing dietary patterns humans had adapted to over tens of thousands of years. Speculation has, thus, arisen about the possible influence of our changing dietary patterns on the development of some major chronic diseases of industrialized society.[4]

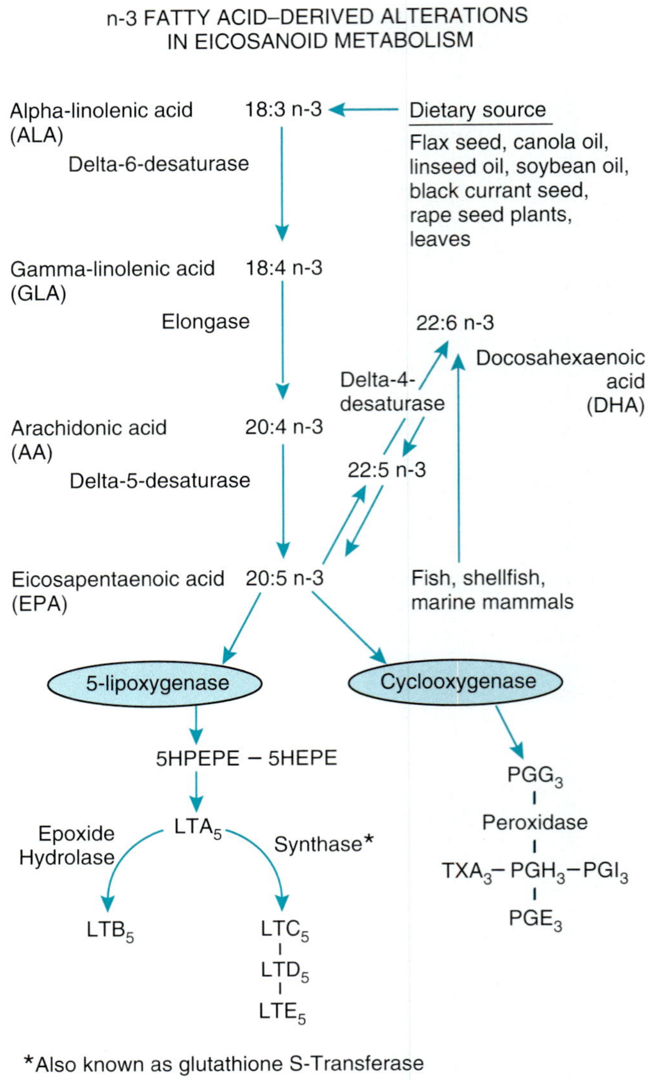

FIGURE 54–5 · Metabolism of n-3 fatty Acids to Eicosanoids. "Linolenic acid (ALA) is derived from terrestrial sources, and eicosapentaenoic acid (EPA) and docosahexaenoic acids (DHA) are derived from marine sources. n-3 fatty acids are converted to prostaglandin species with three double bonds and leukotriene species with five double bonds. They also compete with arachidonic acid as the substrate for cyclooxygenase and may selectively inhibit the epoxide hydrolase enzyme converting LTA_4 to LTB_4. 5-HPEPE, 5S-hydroperoxyeicosapentaenoic acid; 5-HEPE, 5S-hydroxyeicosapentaenoic acid; LT, leukotriene; PG, prostaglandin; TXA_3, thromboxane A_3; PGI_3, prostacyclin I_3.

EPA can be metabolized through both the COX and 5-lipoxygenase metabolic pathways to form end products with altered biologic activity. EPA is acted upon by COX to form thromboxane A_3 (TXA_3) and prostacyclin I_3 (PGI_3)[91] (see Fig. 54–5). PGI_3 retains its antiaggregatory platelet activity, but TXA_3 is not nearly as potent as TXA_2 in inducing platelet aggregation. This may partially account for the diminished risk of cardiovascular morbidity and mortality that is associated with fish consumption.[2,3] EPA is also metabolized to PGE_3, a compound with less inflammatory activity than PGE_2.[92] PGE_2 stimulates osteoclast activity, resulting in bone resorption, a process of significance in RA. The dienoic prostaglandins also increase vascular permeability in a synergistic effect with serotonin and bradykinin.[92] PGE-series prostaglandins

Other investigators have found evidence of a selective inhibition of the epoxide hydrolase enzyme (see Fig. 54–5) in neutrophils from normal persons[96] and patients with RA[98] who consume fish oil because of unaltered quantities of 5-hydroxyeicosatetraenoic acid and 5-hydroxyeicosapentaenoic acid relative to the corresponding arachidonic-acid product generated before dietary supplementation.

Chemotactic activity of neutrophils from patients with RA who had ingested fish oil was found to be enhanced compared to the pretreatment state.[98] This seems paradoxical in view of the suppression of neutrophil chemotaxis after fish oil ingestion in normal persons.[97] The improved chemotaxis in patients with RA represents a partial correction of a reduced chemotactic activity of peripheral blood neutrophils of persons with this disease. Platelet activating factor (PAF)-acether generation of stimulated monocytes is significantly diminished[97] after fish oil ingestion, suggesting an n-3 fatty acid–induced inhibitory effect of phospholipase A_2 activity on substrate alkyl phospholipids, which affects PAF generation. This is of considerable interest in the context of inflammation, in that PAF can stimulate TNF as well as other cytokines in endothelial tissue[99] and is 1000 times more potent than histamine in inducing changes in vascular permeability.[100] Evidence suggests that PAF can also modulate T cell and monocyte function.[101] n-3 fatty acids are associated with a variety of effects on mononuclear cell function, including the production of eicosanoids, nitric oxide, reactive oxygen species, adhesion-molecule expression, chemotaxis, and cytokine production.[102-105] n-3 intake has also been shown to increase apoptosis and T helper type 1 (TH1) or type 2 (Th2)–derived cytokine synthesis.[106,107]

n-3 fatty acid ingestion is associated with significant changes in the fatty acid profiles of cellular lipids. Neutrophil arachidonic acid content is reduced by 33 percent and EPA content is enhanced 20-fold compared to presupplement values obtained in patients with RA who ingested fish oil.[98] n-3 fatty acid ingestion is, thus, associated with reproducible changes in the biochemical composition of cell membranes of neutrophils and monocytes, as well as striking alterations in the production of the metabolic end products of myriad inflammatory and immunologically active compounds that may influence the course of rheumatic disease.

The lipid bilayer of cellular membranes is composed primarily of phospholipids and cholesterol (Fig. 54–6). Because cellular receptors, enzymes, and transport proteins are embedded in the phospholipid bilayer, a change in its structure could have significant implications for cellular function that extend beyond the alterations in eicosanoid and PAF-acether biosynthesis described herein. One investigation demonstrated a significant reduction of IL-1 from monocytes of normal volunteers ingesting fish oil for 6 weeks.[101] The precise mechanism of this effect is speculative, but it may be

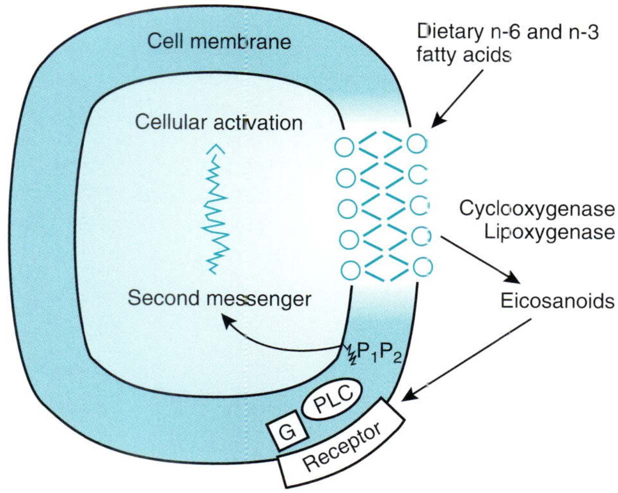

FIGURE 54–6 · **Potential Role of Dietary Fatty Acids in the Function of the Membrane Phospholipid Bilayer of Cells.** Dietary fatty acids will be incorporated into the phospholipid bilayer of cells, where they can be metabolized to eicosanoids. Biologically modified eicosanoids derived from ingesting omega-3 or omega-6 fatty acids may have a role in modulating receptor-ligand activity and cellular activation to various stimuli. Fatty-acid changes in the lipid bilayer may also result in changes in membrane fluidity that could have potential effects on the function of other receptor-related membrane activities. The stimulated receptor transmits a signal via a G-protein to phospholipase C (PLC), which splits phosphatidylinositol-4, 5-biphosphate (PIP_2) to products that eventually lead to second-messenger generation and cellular activation (biochemical steps not shown). (Modified from Weber PC: Membrane phospholipid modification by dietary ω-3 fatty acids: Effects on eicosanoid formation and cell function. *In* Karnovsky ML [ed]: Biological Membranes: Aberrations in Membrane Structure and Function. New York, Liss, 1988, pp 263-274. (Copyright 1988 Wiley-Liss. Reprinted by permission of Wiley-Liss, A Division of John Wiley & Sons, Inc.)

associated with membrane changes in phospholipid fatty acid content, leading to diminished amounts of eicosanoid products, such as LTB_4.

Before considering the effects of fish oil fatty acid supplementation in animal models of inflammation and humans with RA, it should be emphasized that controlled studies of actual increased fish consumption in patients with inflammatory disease have not been reported. Although most experts continue to recommend increased fish consumption as a healthy dietary strategy, increased mercury levels have been reported in some species of fish, such as swordfish and tuna, which may actually cancel out the beneficial biologic effects of fish.[108]

Animal Studies

Dietary modifications containing n-3 fatty acids reduce the severity of diffuse proliferative glomerulonephritis in several autoimmune strains of mice, including NZBxNZWF1, BxSB/Mpj, and MRL/1pr.[76,109] Dietary n-3 fatty acids reduce the severity of glomerulonephritis even when they are withheld until after the renal disease has begun to evolve.[109] Not all observed effects of fish oil have been beneficial in the laboratory; an increased incidence of arthritis was observed in rats immunized with type II collagen who consumed a fish oil–enriched diet compared to animals ingesting beef tallow, although the severity of the arthritis was the same in each group.[110] An increased incidence of necrotizing vasculitis was noted in renal arteries of MRL/1pr mice with systemic lupus erythematosus (SLE)-like disease, even while their glomerulonephritis was alleviated on a fish oil diet.[109] Studies indicate that a mixture of n-3 fatty acids containing both EPA and DHA may be more effective than either of these n-3 fatty acids by themselves.[111]

Human Studies

A pilot study published in 1985 suggested a possible beneficial effect of dietary supplementation with n-3 fatty acids in patients with RA.[112] In a subsequent investigation, patients received 2.8 g of EPA and 1.8 g of DHA in a blinded cross-over format in which subjects received fish oil–derived n-3 fatty acids or olive oil for a period of 14 weeks before crossing over to receive the opposite dietary supplement.[113] Patients were observed to have a highly statistically significant decrease in the number of tender joints after they took fish oil in contrast to when they consumed olive oil. Fatigue, which was quantitated as the time interval from awakening to the first feeling of tiredness, also lessened significantly in patients who consumed fish oil. All of 12 clinical parameters measured favored fish oil, although only two achieved statistical significance. LTB_4 from stimulated neutrophils decreased by 57.8 percent in patients who consumed the fish oil n-3 supplement compared to those who consumed olive oil. A significant correlation was observed between the decrease in the number of tender joints and the decrease in neutrophil LTB_4 production in individual patients.

LTB_4 production from stimulated neutrophils was significantly reduced at week 4 in patients taking fish oil, even though significant clinical improvement did not occur until week 12.[114] There is, thus, an asynchrony between n-3–induced decreases in neutrophil LTB_4 production that occur after only 4 to 6 weeks[97,98,114] and the clinical benefits, which are delayed until at least week 12.[112-114] This might be due, in part, to the delayed suppressive effects of fish oil ingestion on the production of IL-1.[101]

The effects of different doses of fish oil versus olive oil were studied in a 6-month randomized, double-blind, parallel investigation of 49 patients with active RA.[115] Fish oil supplements were supplied according to body weight, not as a uniform dose as in previous studies. A "low-dose" group consumed 27 mg/kg/day of EPA and 18 mg/kg/day of DHA. A "high-dose" group ingested exactly twice that amount. Patients maintained their background medications and diets without change, as in the previously described studies on patients with RA. Multiple clinical parameters improved from baseline in the groups consuming fish oil, with statistically significant improvements in joint swelling and tenderness scores; morning stiffness and physician evaluation of global disease activity occurred with significantly greater frequency in the high-dose group. Significant decreases were also observed in stimulated neutrophil production of LTB_4 and monocyte IL-1, and the greatest decreases in IL-1 were observed in the patients consuming the higher dose of fish oil. The clinical effects of long-term dietary supplementation with n-3 fatty acids have recently been summarized.[116]

It, thus, appears that the beneficial effects of n-3 fatty acid ingestion in humans with inflammatory disease may be dose dependent, as in the autoimmune animal model[111] and studies of the antihypertensive effects of fish oil ingestion in humans.[117] Significant clinical benefits were observed more commonly after 18 and 24 weeks of fish oil ingestion. Fish oil dietary supplementation has not been effective in patients with stable lupus nephritis[118] or OA,[119] but it does appear to offer a protective effect in the prevention of renal transplant rejection[120] and treatment of IgA nephropathy.[121]

VASCULAR DISEASES

The role of n-3 fatty acids in cardiovascular disease is well established and has been recently reviewed.[3] Effects of n-3 fatty acids that may improve the status of individuals with impaired circulation include the following:

- Improved rheologic status secondary to increased erythrocyte deformability
- Decreased plasma viscosity
- A more favorable vascular response to ischemia
- A reduced vasospastic response to catecholamines and angiotensin
- Increased levels of tissue plasminogen activator
- Increased endothelial-dependent relaxation of arteries in response to bradykinin, serotonin, adenine diphosphate, and thrombin

Fish oil dietary intervention, thus, differs from present interventions for vascular disease because of the potential for beneficial benefits at multiple physiologic loci.

In an investigation of the effect of fish oil ingestion in patients with Raynaud's phenomenon, 32 patients with primary or secondary disease consumed daily dietary supplements of 3.96 g of EPA and 2.64 g of DHA or olive oil for 12 weeks.[122] Digital systolic blood pressure and blood flow were evaluated by a strain gauge plethysmograph in room air and in water baths of different temperatures. Results showed significant improvements in the time to onset of symptoms and in digital systolic pressure in the cold water baths in patients with primary, but not secondary, Raynaud's phenomenon. The mechanism of these benefits was not studied.

Recent attention has been directed to the inflammatory component of atherosclerosis. Elevations in C-reactive protein (CRP) have been associated with an increased risk of myocardial infarction.[123,124] It is apparent that inflammation and oxidized LDL particles may contribute to the rupture of an atheromatous plaque, with resultant vascular occlusion.[124] As vascular disease accounts for much of the increased mortality seen in patients with RA, the potential contribution of a possible inflammatory vascular process to the generalized poor outcomes seen in many patients with this diagnosis has become a subject of much emerging interest.

Allergic Arthritis

The idea that rheumatologic disease might be etiologically linked to ingestion of food is not a new one.[125,126] The idea has gained some support from sporadic but convincing case reports of the reproducible onset of joint symptoms shortly after the ingestion of certain foodstuffs. Patients with Behçet's syndrome had striking exacerbations of disease within 48 hours of ingestion of English walnuts.[127] Lymphocytes from these patients also had significantly decreased reactivity to a walnut extract ex vivo within 2 days of ingestion of English walnuts, and leukocyte incorporation of tritiated thymidine after mitogen stimulation was increased.[127] A hypersensitivity to certain foods has been speculated to be the cause of at least some cases of palindromic rheumatism[126] and was documented to occur in a report of an individual with a hypersensitivity to sodium nitrate in food preservatives.[128] L-Canavanine, a nonprotein amino acid found in alfalfa, has been linked to exacerbations of SLE in both monkeys[129] and humans.[130] For a response to food to be plausibly linked to a hypersensitivity reaction resulting in articular symptoms, it is necessary to implicate an altered intestinal permeability that would allow passage of intact food antigens into the circulation. Circumstantial evidence exists to link arthritis to damaged intestinal function in ulcerative colitis,[131] Crohn's disease,[132] and the polyarthritis that follows jejunal bypass surgery for obesity.[133] Moreover, immune complexes that contain intact food antigens complexed to IgE or IgG have been documented in normal and atopic subjects[134] and have been observed to cause bronchospasm and pruritus in allergic individuals. A study of intestinal permeability that used oral ^{51}Cr-EDTA (edetic acid) showed that patients with RA who took nonsteroidal anti-inflammatory drugs (NSAIDs) exhibited abnormalities, whereas patients not taking NSAIDs did not have abnormal permeability.[135] Indium-III–labeled leukocyte scans showed ileocecal inflammation in six of nine patients taking NSAIDs.

A food antigen can be convincingly linked to arthritis if a flare of clinical symptoms occurs within 48 hours of a blinded challenge with the putative offending antigen. An elimination diet, in which a patient totally discontinues ingestion of the food in question, with total clearing of articular symptoms would also provide implicative evidence, albeit weaker than that of a flare after a blinded challenge. Two cases have been reported involving significant flares in articular symptoms after ingestion of milk or dairy products.[136,137] The challenges were open[136] and blinded,[137] and symptoms peaked within 24 to 48 hours. IgE antibodies to milk were demonstrated using the radioallergosorbent test in one patient,[136] and large amounts of IgG_4 antimilk antibodies directed to α-lactalbumin were detected in the other.[137] A flare in articular disease manifestations has also been documented after blinded challenges with shrimp and nitrates.[138]

Interest in the possible role of food intolerance in the etiology of arthritic symptoms has been renewed[139,140] as a result of these case reports. It is difficult to assess the incidence of this syndrome, in that patients may not necessarily be aware of possible sensitivities to commonly ingested foods in their diet. Because of the small number of documented cases of food intolerance in the literature, however, the syndrome is probably rare.

Complementary and Alternative Medicine

Complementary and alternative medicine (CAM) encompasses an expanding array of approaches to disease. These include, but are not limited to, traditional Chinese medicine, dietary macro- and micronutrients, as well as dietary non-nutrient factors. Other natural agents, as well as physical, psychologic, and spiritual approaches, are also included in CAM.[141,142] Drugstore shelves display CAM products prominently, and the consumer may purchase these products without either the knowledge or approval of a physician. Asterisks in both the lay press and medical journals have described inconsistent formulations, may even contain pharmacologically relevant doses of adulterants and other potentially toxic substances.[143-148] Because of these well-publicized problems and the medical community's understandable reluctance to empower patients to shop for their own remedies without medical supervision, most practitioners are skeptical of, if not hostile to, CAM.

At the same time, use of these treatments is expanding. Patients are intrigued by the possible benefits offered by CAM, and a growing number are trying these approaches. It is increasingly clear that clinicians need to have some working knowledge of CAM to adequately advise patients and follow developments in the scientific literature. The National Institutes of Health (NIH) has established a branch to study CAM.

Macronutrients such as dietary fats may inhibit inflammation through a variety of mechanisms discussed elsewhere in this chapter. Other macronutrients, such as sugar, fiber, vegetarian foods, and amino acids, have also been shown to affect inflammatory disease. Micronutrients, including vitamins, are also discussed elsewhere in this chapter. Substances such as coenzyme Q10 (ubiquinone) are purported to have a variety of potentially beneficial effects—both as antioxidants and as facilitators of mitochondrial energy metabolism.[192]

Dietary non-nutrient factors include phytoestrogens, which are estrogen-like compounds produced by bacterial action on precursors such as soy and a variety of meats in human intestines. By competing with natural estrogens for receptor sites, they may lower the bioavailability of circulating estrogens. It has been suggestted that phytoestrogens may protect against breast cancer and perhaps SLE.

Flavonoids are a large group of phenolic compounds occurring naturally in most fruits and vegetables, as well as beer, wine, tea, and coffee. These compounds may exhibit a variety of effects on the immune and inflammatory system, including inhibition of eicosanoid-mediated inflammation. The flavonoids quercetin and those found in extracts of ginkgo biloba are potent free-radical scavengers that decrease rat lymphocyte proliferation, perhaps by inhibiting the respiratory burst.[145] In different doses, flavonoids derived from green tea have been observed to stimulate lymphocyte proliferation and NK activity in mice. They may also be associated with a variety of antitumor and antiplatelet activities. Usifkav-ibes are flavanoid compounds found in a variety of plants including soy. Genistein is an isoflavone that induces apoptosis and inhibits platelet assresation, DNA topoisomerase II, leukotriene production, and angiogenesis, whereas it reduces the bioavailability of sex hormones.[142]

Much attention has been directed to the hormonal effects of stress on immune function. Through relief of stress, increased spirituality, and the correcting of emotional imbalances, traditional Chinese and Ayurvedic medicine seek to harness the body's own natural healing powers. Although few studies have been conducted on the possible benefits of mediation of inflammatory disease, there is a growing interest in the potential of mind-body interactions to favorably effect a variety of disease states.

Space does not allow for a full discussion of all the interventions included in the category of CAM. Even as we recognize the possible placebo effect of these interventions, it will be important to cultivate an open mind and remain aware of the malpractice responsibility that could be associated with the recommendation of their use.[146] Recently, proposals for actual credentialing of alternative-medicine providers have been suggested.[147]

REFERENCES

1. Hirai A, Terano T, Saito H, et al: Eicosapentaenoic acid and platelet function in Japanese. *In* Lovenburg W, Yamori Y (eds): Nutritional Prevention of Cardiovascular Disease. New York, Academic Press, 1984, pp 231-239.
2. Kromhout D, Bosschieter EB, de Lezenne Coulander C: The inverse relation between fish consumption and 20-year mortality from coronary heart disease. N Engl J Med 312:1205-1209, 1985.
3. Leaf A, Weber PC: Cardiovascular effects of n-3 fatty acids. N Engl J Med 318:549, 1988.
4. Eaton SB, Konner M: Paleolithic nutrition: a consideration of its nature and current implications. N Engl J Med 312:283, 1985.
5. Hecht A: Hocus-pocus as applied to arthritis. FDA Consumer 14:24, 1980.
6. Blackburn GL, Bistrian BR: Nutritional care of the injured and/or septic patient. Surg Clin North Am 56:1195, 1976.
7. Silberman H, Eisenberg D: Consequences of malnutrition. *In* Parenteral and Enteral Nutrition for the Hospitalized Patient. East Norwalk, Conn, Appleton-Century-Crofts, 1982, pp 1–18.
8. Bayles TB, Richardson H, Hall FC: The nutritional background of patients with rheumatoid arthritis. N Engl J Med 229:319, 1943.
9. Eising L: Dietary intake in patients with arthritis and other chronic diseases. J Bone Joint Surg Ann 45:69, 1963.
10. Kowsari B, Finnie SK, Carter RL, et al: Assessment of the diet of patients with rheumatoid arthritis and osteoarthritis. J Am Diet Assoc 82:657, 1983.
11. Bigaouette J, Timchalk MA, Kremer J: Nutritional adequacy of diet and supplements in patients with rheumatoid arthritis who take medications. J Am Diet Assoc 87:1687, 1987.
12. Kremer JM, Bigaouette J: Nutrient intake of patients with rheumatoid arthritis is deficient in peridoxine, zinc, copper and magnesium. J Rheumatol 23:6, 1996.
13. Stone J, Drube A, Dadson D, Wallace J: Inadequate calcium, folic acid, vitamin E, zinc, and selenium intake in rheumatoid arthritis patients: results of a dictary survey. Semi Arthritis Rheum 27:180, 1997.
14. Helliwell M, Coombes EJ, Moody BJ, et al: Nutritional status in patients with rheumatoid arthritis. Ann Rheum Dis 43:386, 1984.
15. Roabenoff R, Roubonoff RA, Cannon JG, et al: Rheumatoid cachexia: cytokine-driven hypermetabolism and loss of lean body mass in chronic inflammation. J Clin Invest 93:2379, 1994.
16. Rall LC, Rosen CJ, Daluikowski G, et al: Protein metabolism in rheumatoid arthritis and aging: effects of muscle strengthening and tumor necrosis factor-α. Arthritis Rheum 39:1115, 1996.
17. Johansson U, Portinsson S, Akesson A, et al: Nutritional status in girls with juvenile chronic arthritis. Hum Nutr Clin Nutr 40C:57, 1986.
18. Portinsson S, Akesson A, Svantesson H, et al: Dietary assessment in children with juvenile chronic arthritis. J Hum Nutr Diet 1:133, 1988.
19. Warady B, Lindsley R, Robinson R, Lukert B: Effects of nutritional supplementation on bone mineral status of children with rheumatic diseases receiving corticosteroid therapy. J Rheumatol 21(3): 530-535, 1994.
20. Fam FG: Gout, diet and the insulin resistance syndrome. J Rheumatol 29(7):1350-1355, 2002.
21. Bendich A: Antioxidant nutrients and immune functions. Adv Exp Med Biol 262:1-12, 1990.
22. Tengerdy RP, Mathias MM, Nockels CF: Effect of vitamin E on immunity and disease resistance. *In* Prasad KN (ed): Vitamins, Nutrition and Cancer. Basel, Karger, 1984, pp 118-122.
23. Nagakawa T, Akagi M, Hoshikawa H, et al: Lectin-like oxidized low-density lipoprotein receptor 1 mediates leukocyte infiltration and articular cartilage destruction in rat zymaosan-induced arthritis. Arthritis Rheum 46:2486-2494, 2002.
24. Halliwell B, Gutteridge JMC: Lipid peroxidation: a radical chain reaction. *In* Free Radicals in Biology and Medicine. Oxford, Clarendon Press, 1985, pp 139-189.
25. Fidelius RK: The generation of oxygen radicals: a positive signal for lymphocyte activation. Cell Immunol 113:175, 1988.
26. Dornand J, Gerber M: Inhibition of murine T-cell responses by antioxidants: the targets of lipoxygenase pathway inhibitors. Immunology 68:384, 1989.
27. Austen KF, Soberman RJ: Perspectives on additional areas for research in leukotrienes. N Y Ann Acad Sci 524:xi, 1988.
28. Goodwin JS, Behrens T: Role of lipoxygenase metabolites of arachidonic acid in T cell activation. Ann N Y Acad Sci 524:201, 1988.
29. Bendich A: A role for carotenoids in immune function. Clin Nutr 7:113, 1988.
30. Boxer LA: Functional effects of leukocyte antioxidants on polymorphonuclear leukocyte behavior. Adv Exp Med 262:19-34, 1990.
31. Grever MR, Thompson VN, Balcerzak SP, et al: The effect of oxidant stress on human lymphocyte cytotoxicity. Blood 56:284, 1980.
32. Hatam CJ, Cayden HJ: A high performance lipid chromatographic method for the determination of tocopherol in plasma and cellular elements of the blood. J Lipid Res 20:639, 1979.
33. Boxer LS, Oliver JM, Spielberg SP, et al: Protection of granulocytes by vitamin E in glutathione synthetase deficiency. N Engl J Med 301:901, 1979.
34. Moser J, Weber F: Uptake of ascorbic acid by human granulocytes. Int J Vitam Nutr Res 54:47, 1983.
35. Goetzl EJ, Wasserman SI, Gigli I, Austen KF: Enhancement of random migration and chemotactic response of human leukocytes by ascorbic acid. J Clin Invest 53:813, 1974.
36. Sahud MA, Cohen R: Effect of aspirin ingestion on ascorbic acid levels in rheumatoid arthritis. Lancet 1:937, 1971.
37. Hall MG, Darling RC, Taylor FH: The vitamin C requirement in rheumatoid arthritis. Ann Intern Med 13:415, 1939.
38. Baehner RL, Boxer A, Allen JM, et al: Autooxidation as a basis for altered function by polymorphonuclear leukocytes. Blood 50:327, 1977.
39. El-Hag A, Lipsky PE, Bennett M, et al: Immunomodulation by neutrophil myeloperoxidase and hydrogen peroxide: differential susceptibility of human lymphocyte functions. J Immunol 136:3420, 1986.
40. El-Hag A, Clark RA: Immunosuppression by activated human neutrophils: dependence on the myeloperoxidase system. J Immunol 139:2406, 1987.
41. Anderson R, Smit M, Joone GK, VanStaden AM: Vitamin C and cellular immune functions. Ann N Y Acad Sci 587:34-48, 1990.
42. Frei BR, Stocker R, Ames BN: Antioxident defenses and lipid peroxidation in human blood plasma. Proc Natl Acad Sci 85:9748, 1988.
43. Maddison PJ, Bacon PA: Vitamin D deficiency, spontaneous fractures and osteopenia in rheumatoid arthritis. Br Med J 4:433, 1974.

44. Smith EL, Pincus SH, Donovan L, et al: A novel approach for the evaluation and treatment of psoriasis. J Am Acad Dermatol 19:516, 1988.
45. MacLaughlin JA, Gange W, Taylor D, et al: Cultured psoriatic fibroblasts from involved and uninvolved sites have a partial but not absolute resistance to the proliferation-inhibition activity of 1,25-dihydroxyvitamin D3. Proc Natl Acad Sci U S A 82:5409, 1985.
46. Rigby WFC, Stacy T, Ganger MW: Inhibition of T lymphocyte mitogenesis by 1,25-dihydroxyvitamin D3 (calcitriol). J Clin Invest 74:1451, 1984.
47. Ghalla AK, Amento EP, Krane SM: Differential effects of 1,25-dihydroxyvitamin D_3 on human lymphocytes and monocyte/macrophages: inhibition of interleukin-2 and augmentation of interleukin-1 production. Cell Immunol 98:311, 1986.
48. Gepner P, Amor B, Fournier C: 1,25-dihydroxyvitamin D_3 potentiates the in vitro inhibitory effects of cyclosporin A on T cells from rheumatoid arthritis patients. Arthritis Rheum 32:31, 1989.
49. Huckins D, Felson DT, Holick M: Treatment of psoriatic arthritis with oral 1,25-dihydroxyvitamin D_3: a pilot study. Arthritis Rheum 33:1732, 1990.
50. Morgan SI, Baggott JE, Lee JY, Alarcon GS: Folic acid supplementation prevents deficient blood folate levels and hpyerhomocysteinemia during longterm, low dose methotrexate therapy for rheumatoid arthritis: implications for cardiovascular disease prevention. J Rheumatol 25:441-446, 1998.
51. Haagsma CJ, Blom HJ, van Riel PLCM, et al: Influence of sulphasalazine, methotrexate, and the combination of both on the plasma homocysteine concentrations in patients with rheumatoid arthritis. Ann Rheum Dis 58:79-84, 1999.
52. Fukushima T, Iijima Y, Kosaka F: Endotoxin-induced zinc accumulation by liver cells is mediated by metallothionein synthesis. Biochem Biophys Res Commun 152:874-878, 1988.
53. Cousins RJ: Absorption, transport and hepatic metabolism of copper and zinc: special reference to metallothionein and ceruloplasmin. Physiol Rev 65:238-309, 1985.
54. Kluger MJ, Rothenburg BA: Fever and reduced iron: their interaction as a host defense response to bacterial infection. Science 203:374, 1979.
55. Svenson KLG, Hallgren R, Johansson E: Reduced zinc in peripheral blood cells from patients with inflammatory connective tissue diseases. Inflammation 9:189, 1985.
56. Seelig MS: Auto-immune complications of *D*-penicillamine: a possible result of zinc and magnesium depletion and of pyridoxine inactivation. J Am Coll Nutr 1:207, 1982.
57. Ruhl J, Kirshner H: Monocyte-dependent stimulation of human T cells by zinc. Clin Exp Immunol 32:484, 1978.
58. Whitehouse MW: Trace element supplements for inflammatory disease. *In* Dixon J, Furst D (eds): Second Line Agents in the Rheumatic Diseases. New York, Marcel Dekker, 1991, pp 184-189.
59. Whitehouse MW, Rainsford KD, Taylor RM, Vernon-Roberts B: Zinc monoglycerolate: a slow-release source of zinc with antiarthritic activity in rats. Agents Actions 31:47, 1990.
60. Cimmino MA, Mazzucotelli A, Rovetta G, Cutolo M: The controversy over zinc sulfate efficacy in rheumatoid and psoriatic arthritis. Scand J Rheumatol 13:191, 1984.
61. Spallholz JE: Anti-inflammatory immunologic and carcinostatic attributes of selenium in experimental animals. Adv Exp Med Biol 135:43, 1981.
62. Spallholz JE, Boyland LM, Larsen HS: Advances in understanding selenium's role in the immune system. Ann N Y Acad Sci 587: 123-139, 1990.
63. Ursini F, Maiorino M, Gregolin C: The selenoenzyme phospholipid hydroperoxide glutathione peroxidase. Biochem Biophys Acta 839:62, 1985.
64. Bryant RW, Bailey JM, King JC, Levander OA: Altered platelet glutathione peroxidase activity and arachidonic acid metabolism during selenium repletion in a controlled human study. *In* Spallholz JE, Martin JL, Ganther HE (eds): Selenium in Biology and Medicine. Westport, Conn, AVI, 1981, pp 395-399.
65. Spallholz JE, Boylan LM: Effect of dietary selenium on peritoneal macrophage chemiluminescence. Fed J 3:A778, 1989.
66. Sonne M, Helleberg L, Jenson PT: Selenium status in patients with rheumatoid arthritis. Scand J Rheumatol 14:318, 1985.
67. Borgland M, Akesson A, Adesson B: Distribution of selenium and glutathione peroxidase in plasma compared in healthy subjects and rheumatoid arthritis patients. Scand J Clin Lab Invest 48:27, 1988.
68. Tarp U, Overvad K, Thorling EB, et al: Selenium treatment in rheumatoid arthritis. Acta Pharmacol Toxicol 59(Suppl 7):382, 1986.
69. Hill J, Bird HA: Failure of selenium-ACE to improve osteoarthritis. Br J Rheumatol 29:211, 1990.
70. Herrick A, Rieley F, Schofield D, et al: Micronutrient antioxidant status in patients with primary Raynaud's phenomenon and systemic sclerosis. J Rheumatol 21:8:1477-1483, 1994.
71. Wagner E, Gruber FO: The trace element selenium in rheumatic diseases (abstract P-682). Rio de Janeiro, XVII ILAR Congress of Rheumatology, 1989.
72. Allen KGD, Arthur JR, Morrice PC, et al: Copper deficiency and tissue glutathione concentration in the rat. Proc Soc Exp Biol Med 187:38, 1988.
73. Roth RA, Koshland ME: Identification of a lymphocyte enzyme that catalyzes pentamer immunoglobulin M assembly. J Biol Chem 256:4633, 1981.
74. Sherman AR: Influence of iron on immunity and disease resistance. N Y Acad Sci 587:140-146, 1990.
75. Weber PC: Membrane phospholipid modification by dietary n-3 fatty acids: Effects on eicosanoid formation and cell function. *In* Karnovsky ML (ed): Biological Membranes: Aberrations in Membrane Structure and Function. New York, Liss, 1988, pp 263-274.
76. Prickett JD, Robinson DR, Steinberg AD: Dietary enrichment with the polyunsaturated fatty acid eicosapentaenoic acid prevents proteinuria and prolongs survival in (NZB × NZW) F1 mice. J Clin Invest 68:556, 1981.
77. Lee TH, Hoover RL, Williams JD, et al: Effect of dietary enrichment with eicosapentaenoic and docosahexaenoic acids on in vitro neutrophil and monocyte leukotriene generation and neutrophil function. N Engl J Med 312:1217, 1985.
78. Shekelle RB, Missell LV, Paul O, et al: Fish consumption and mortality from coronary heart disease. N Engl J Med 313:820, 1985.
79. Willis AL, Comai K, Kuhn DC, et al: Dihomogammalinolenate suppresses platelet aggregation when administered in vitro or in vivo. Prostaglandins 7:509, 1974.
80. Zurier RB: Prostaglandins, immune responses, and murine lupus. Arthritis Rheum 25:804-809, 1982.
81. Tate GA, Mandell BF, Karmali RA, et al: Suppression of monosodium urate crystal-induced acute inflammation by diets enriched with gammalinolenic acid and eicosapentaenoic acid. Arthritis Rheum 31:1543, 1988.
82. Baker DG, Krakauer KA, Tate G, et al: Suppression of human synovial cell proliferation by dihomogammalinolenic acid. Arthritis Rheum 32:1273, 1989.
83. Hansen TM, Lerche A, Kassis V, et al: Treatment of rheumatoid arthritis with prostaglandin E1 precursors cis-linoleic acid and gamma-linolenic acid. Scand J Rheumatol 12:85, 1983.
84. Jantti J, Nikkari T, Solakivi T, et al: Evening primrose oil in rheumatoid arthritis: changes in serum lipids and fatty acids. Ann Rheum Dis 48:124, 1989.
85. Leventhal LJ, Boyce EG, Zurier RB: Treatment of rheumatoid arthritis with gammalinolenic acid. Ann Intern Med 119(9): 867-873, 1993.
86. Santoli D, Zurier RB: Prostaglandin E precursor fatty acids inhibit human IL-2 production by a prostaglandin E-independent mechanisms. J Immunol 143:1303-1309, 1989.
87. Santoli D, Philips PD, Zurier RB: Suppression of interleukin 2-dependent human T cell growth by prostaglandin E (PGE) and their precursor fatty acids: Evidence for a PGE-independent mechanism of inhibition by the fatty acids. J Clin Invest 85: 424-432, 1990.
88. Zurier RB: Gammalinolenic acid treatment of rheumatoid arthritis. *In* Kremer JM (ed): Medicinal Fatty Acids in Inflammation. Basel, Birkhauser, 1998, p 29-43.
89. Lands WEM: Fish and Human Health. Orlando, Fla, USA, Academic Press, 1986, p 103.
90. Crawford MA: Fatty-acid ratios in free-living and domestic animals. Lancet 1:1329, 1968.

91. Fischer S, Weber PC: Prostaglandin I3 is formed in vivo in man after dietary eicosapentaenoic acid. Nature 307:165, 1984.
92. Robinson DR, Tateno S, Balkrishna P, Hirai A: Lipid mediators of inflammatory and immune reactions. *In* Karnovsky ML (ed): Biological Membranes: Aberrations in Membrane Structure and Function. New York, Liss, 1988, pp 295-303.
93. Ferretti A, Flanagan VP: Modification of prostaglandin metabolism in vivo by longchain omega-3 polyunsaturates. Biochem Biophys Acta 1045:299, 1990.
94. Holman RT: Nutritional and metabolic interrelationships between fatty acids. Fed Proc 23:1062, 1964.
95. Simopoulos AP, Kifer RR, Martin RE (eds): Health Effects of Polyunsaturated Fatty Acids in Seafoods. New York, Academic Press, 1986.
96. Lee TH, Mencia-Huerta JM, Shih C, et al: Characterization and biologic properties of 5,12-dihydroxy derivatives of eicosapentaenoic acid, including leukotriene B5 and the double lipoxygenase product. J Biol Chem 259:2383, 1984.
97. Lee TH, Hoover RL, Williams JD, et al: Effect of dietary enrichment with eicosapentaenoic and docosahexaenoic acids on in vitro neutrophil function. N Engl J Med 312:1217, 1985.
98. Sperling RI, Weinblatt M, Robin JL, et al: Effects of dietary supplementation with marine fish oil on leukocyte lipid mediator generation and function in rheumatoid arthritis. Arthritis Rheum 30:988, 1987.
99. Dulioust A, Salem P, Vivier E, et al: Immunoregulatory functions of PAF-acether (platelet-activating factor). *In* Karnovsky ML (ed): Biological Membranes: Aberrations in Membrane Structure and Function. New York, Liss, 1988, pp 87-96.
100. Humphrey DM, McManase L, Satouchi K, et al: Vasoactive properties of acetyl glyceryl ether phosphorylcholine and analogs. Lab Invest 46:422, 1982.
101. Endres S, Chorbani R, Kalley VE, et al: The effects of dietary supplementation with n-3 polyunsaturated fatty acids on the synthesis of interleukin-1 and tumor necrosis factor by mononuclear cells. N Engl J Med 320:265, 1989.
102. Calder PC: Effects of fatty acids and dietary lipids on cells of the immune system. Proc Nutr Soc 55:127, 1996.
103. Meydani SN: Effect of n-3 polyunsaturated fatty acids on cytokine production and their biologic function. Nutrition 12:58, 1996.
104. Endres S, von Schacky C: n-3 polyunsaturated fatty acids and human cytokine synthesis. Curr Opin Lipidol 7:48, 1996.
105. Calder PC: n-3 Polyunsaturated fatty acids and mononuclear phagocyte function. *In* Kremer JM (ed): Medicinal Fatty Acids in Inflammation. Basel, Birkhauser, 1998, pp 1–27.
106. Fernandes G, Jolly CA: Nutrition and autoimmune disease. Nutr Rev 56:S161, 1998.
107. Fernandes G: n-3 Fatty acids on autoimmune disease. *In* Kremer JM (ed): Medicinal Fatty Acids in Inflammation. Basel, Switzerland, Birkhauser, 1998, pp 73-89.
108. Guallar E, Sanz-Gallardo I, van't Veer P, et al: Mercury, fish oils, and the risk of myocardial infarction. New Engl J Med 347: 1747-1754, 2002.
109. Robinson DR, Prickett JD, Makoul GT, et al: Dietary fish oil reduces progression of established renal disease in (NZB × NZW) F1 mice and delays renal disease in BXSB and MRL/1 strains. Arthritis Rheum 29:539-546, 1986.
110. Prickett JD, Trentham DE, Robinson DR: Dietary fish oil augments the induction of arthritis in rats immunized with type II collagen. J Immunol 132:725-729, 1984.
111. Robinson DR, Tateno S, Knoell C, et al: Dietary marine lipids suppress murine autoimmune disease. J Intern Med 225(Suppl 1):211, 1989.
112. Kremer JM, Bigauoette J, Michalek AU, et al: Effects of manipulating dietary fatty acids on clinical manifestations of rheumatoid arthritis. Lancet 1:184, 1985.
113. Kremer JM, Jubiz W, Michalek A, et al: Fish-oil fatty acid supplementation in active rheumatoid arthritis: a double blinded, controlled crossover study. Ann Intern Med 106:498, 1987.
114. Cleland LG, French JK, Betts WH, et al: Clinical and biochemical effects of dietary fish-oil supplements in rheumatoid arthritis. J Rheumatol 15:1471-1475, 1988.
115. Kremer JM, Lawrence DA, Jubiz W, et al: Dietary fish oil and olive oil supplementation in patients with rheumatoid arthritis: clinical and immunologic effects. Arthritis Rheum 33:810, 1990.
116. Geusens PP: n-3 Fatty acids in the treatment of rheumatoid arthritis. *In* Kremer JM (ed): Medicinal Fatty Acids in Inflammation. Basel, Switzerland, Birkhauser, pp 111-123, 1998.
117. Knapp HR, FitzGerald GA: The antihypertensive effects of fish oil: a controlled study of polyunsaturated fatty acid supplements in essential hypertension. N Engl J Med 320:1037, 1989.
118. Clark WF, Parbtani A, Naylor CD, et al: Fish oil in lupus nephritis: clinical findings and methodological implications. Kidney Int 44:75-85, 1993.
119. Stammers T, Sibbald B, Freeling P: Efficacy of cod liver oil as an adjunct to non-steroidal anti-inflammatory drug treatment in the management of osteoarthritis in general practice. Ann Rheum Dis 51:128-129, 1992.
120. Homan van der Heide JJ, Bilo HJG, Donker JM, et al: Effect of dietary fish oil on renal function and rejection in cyclosporine-treated recipients of renal transplants. N Engl J Med 329(11): 769-773, 1993.
121. Donadio JV Jr, Bergstralh EJ, Offord KP, et al: A controlled trial of fish oil in IgA nephropathy. N Engl J Med 331(18):1194-1199, 1994.
122. DiGiacomo RA, Kremer JM, Shah DM: Fish oil supplementation in patients with Raynaud's phenomenon: a double-blind controlled prospective study. Am J Med 86:158, 1989.
123. Koenig W, Sund M, Froelich M, et al: C-reactive protein, a sensitive marder of inflammation, predicts future risk of coronary heart disease in initially healthy middle-aged men: results from the MONICA (Monitoring Trends and Determinants in Cardiovascular Disease) Augsburg Cohort Sudy, 1984 to 1992. Circulation 99:237-242, 1999.
124. Kost NS, Solf PA, Dase CS, et al: Plasma concentration of C-reactive protein and risk of ischemic stroke and transient ischemic attack: The Framingham Study. Stroke 32:2575-2579, 2002.
125. Lewis P, Taub SJ: Allergic synovitis due to ingestion of English walnuts. JAMA 106:214-244, 1936.
126. Zeller M: Rheumatoid arthritis food allergy as a factor. Ann Allergy 7:200, 1947.
127. Marquardt JC, Synderman R, Oppenheim JJ: Depression of lymphocyte transformation and exacerbation of Behçet's syndrome by ingestion of English walnuts. Cell Immunol 9:263, 1973.
128. Epstein S: Hypersensitivity to sodium nitrate: a major causative factor in case of palindromic rheumatism. Ann Allergy 27:343, 1969.
129. Malinow MR, Bardana EJ, Pirofsky B, et al: Systemic lupus erythematosus-like syndrome in monkeys fed alfalfa sprouts: role of a non protein amino acid. Science 216:415, 1982.
130. Roberts JL, Hayashi JA: Exacerbation of SLE associated with alfalfa ingestion [Letter]. N Engl J Med 308:1361, 1983.
131. Wright V, Watkinson G: The arthritis of ulcerative colitis. Br Med J 2:670, 1965.
132. von Potter WN: Regional enteritis. Gastroenterology 26:347, 1954.
133. Wands JR, LaMont JT, Mann E, Isselbacher K: Arthritis associated with intestinal by-pass procedure for morbid obesity: complement activation and character of circulating cryoproteins. N Engl J Med 294:121, 1976.
134. Paganelli R, Levinsky RJ, Brostoff J, et al: Immune complexes containing food proteins in normal and atopic subjects after oral challenge and effect of sodium cromoglycate on antigen absorption. Lancet 1:1270, 1979.
135. Bjarnason I, So A, Levi AJ, et al: Intestinal permeability and inflammation in rheumatoid arthritis: effects of non-steroidal anti-inflammatory drugs. Lancet 2:1171, 1984.
136. Parke EL, Hughes GRV: Rheumatoid arthritis and food: a case study. BMJ 282:2027, 1981.
137. Panush RS, Stroud RM, Webster EM: Food-induced (allergic) arthritis. Arthritis Rheum 29:220, 1986.
138. Panush RS: Food induced ("allergic") arthritis: clinical and serologic studies. J Rheumatol 17:291, 1990.
139. Darlington LG: Does food intolerance have any role in the aetiology and management of rheumatoid disease? Ann Rheum Dis 44:801, 1985.
140. Panush RS: Possible role of food sensitivity in arthritis. Ann Allergy 19(Suppl):31, 1988.
141. Spencer JW, Jacobs JJ (eds): Complementary Alternative Medicine: An Evidence-Based Approach. St. Louis, Mosby, 1999.

142. Boik J (ed): Cancer and Natural Medicine. Princeton, Minn., Oregon Medical Press, 1996.
143. Eisenberg DM, Kessler RC, Foster C, et al: Unconventional medicine in the United States: prevalance, costs and patterns of use. N Engl J Med 328:246, 1993.
144. Ko RJ: Adulterants in Asian patent medicines. N Engl J Med 339:847, 1998.
145. Ernst E: The risk-benefit profile of commonly used herbal therapies: Ginkgo, St. John's wort, ginseng, echinacea, saw palmetto, and kava. Ann Intern Med 136:42-53, 2002.
146. Cohen MH, Eisenberg DM: Potential physician malpractice liability associated with complementary and integrative medical therapies. Ann Intern Med 136:596-603, 2002.
147. Eisenberg DM, Cohen MG, Hrbek A, et al: Credentialing complementary and alternative medical providers. Ann Intern Med 137:965-973, 2002.
148. Angell M, Kassirer JP: Alternative medicine: the risks of untested and unregulated remedies. N Engl J Med 339:839, 1998.

55 Rehabilitation of Patients with Rheumatic Diseases

JOSEPH J. BIUNDO, JR • PERRY J. RUSH

The aim of rehabilitation is to maximize function and minimize the disability and handicap resulting from the underlying impairment or disease. Rehabilitation of inflammatory rheumatic diseases should begin early and continue throughout the disease course. The impairment and resulting disability caused by rheumatic diseases can be ameliorated by a rehabilitation program even when the disease remains active. Even short-term, 6-week programs, consisting of exercise, education, and pain-relief modalities, have been shown to benefit rheumatoid arthritis (RA) patients.[1] A home physical therapy program including education, exercise, and removal of environmental hazards can reduce disability, even in the elderly.[2]

In the rehabilitation of patients with rheumatic diseases, a wide variety of allied health professionals may be involved, usually under the direction of a physiatrist or a rheumatologist. These health professionals may include nurses, physical therapists, occupational therapists, speech therapists, recreational therapists, psychologists, social workers, orthotists, and prosthetists. The comprehensive rehabilitation of arthritis employs medical, surgical, psychologic, and physical methods of treatment. Above all, patients must be enlisted as willing participants in their treatment. Rehabilitation can only succeed when the patient is motivated, cooperative, and capable of learning new information.

International Classification of Functioning, Disability, and Health

The International Classification of Functioning, Disability and Health (ICF) of the World Health Organization (WHO) provides an international classification to code a wide variety of information about health (e.g., diagnosis, functioning, and disability).[3] This WHO classification scheme is an international statistical, research, clinical, social policy, and educational tool. *Impairments* are defined as problems in body function or structure, such as significant deviation or loss. *Body functions* are the physiologic functions of body systems (including psychologic functions). *Body structures* are anatomic parts of the body, such as organs, limbs, and their components. Typical impairments in rheumatology patients include loss of joint range of motion and muscular weakness. Such impairments may lead to activity limitations or participation restrictions or both (*disability*). An *activity* is the execution of a task by an individual. *Activity limitations* are difficulties an individual may have in executing activities. *Participation* is involvement in a life situation. *Participation restrictions* are problems an individual may experience in involvement in life situations. Environmental factors interact with the components of body functions, body structures, activities, and participation. Disability is characterized as the outcome of a complex relationship between an individual's health condition and personal factors with which the individual lives. Society may hinder an individual's performance because it either creates barriers (e.g., inaccessible buildings) or it does not provide facilitators (e.g., lack of available assistive devices).

In the United States, arthritis and other rheumatic conditions are said to be the leading cause of disability. Three percent of all adults have disability due to arthritis and other rheumatic conditions. Among all adults with disability, about 16 percent attribute their disability to arthritis and other rheumatic conditions.[4,5] Based on self-reported data, the estimated prevalence of arthritis, chronic joint symptoms, or both among U.S. adults in 2001 was 33 percent.[4] The prevalence of self-reported arthritis increases with age. By age 65, there is an estimated 45-percent prevalence of self-reported arthritis, and about 22 percent of these have activity limitations.[6] In Canada, it is estimated that the prevalence of self-reported arthritis will increase from about 17 percent in 1991 to about 24 percent in 2031 and that the arthritis disability in the general population will increase from 2.3 percent in 1991 to 3.3 percent in 2031.[7]

Work disability occurs commonly during the course of rheumatic diseases. In a Canadian survey, about 18 percent of men and 36 percent of women with arthritis were not in the labor force because of arthritis disability.[8] About 40 percent of RA patients stopped working within 5 years after the onset of their disease,[9] and about 40 percent of systemic lupus erythematosus (SLE) patients stopped working within 3.4 years after their diagnosis.[10]

Assessment of Function

EVALUATION AND CLASSIFICATION

Each patient's the level of function should be determined so a specific rehabilitation program can be planned and the outcome can be measured. Functional disability is frequently unrecognized in outpatients and inpatients in acute and chronic care.[11] The level of function is determined by the ability to perform activities of daily living (ADL), home activities, and activities outside the home. Activities of daily living are self-care activities and consist of grooming, dressing, feeding, bathing, toileting, ambulating, transfers, continence, and communication. Instrumental activities of daily living (IADL) require a combination of cognitive and physical ability and consist of functions in the home (e.g., cleaning, cooking, doing laundry, using the telephone, climbing stairs, managing medication) and functions external to the home (e.g., working, using public transportation, shopping, money management, social interaction).

Although most physicians managing patients with RA are appropriately concerned about the degree of inflammation, they may not ascertain which functional activities the patient is capable of performing or not performing. It is important to know how the patient spends a typical day and what his or her difficulties may be in carrying out tasks and recreational activities.

The original American Rheumatism Association classification of functional impairment was a general four-point scale and was not very specific or useful for measuring improvement in functional activities.[12] Subsequently, other scales have been devised. Some scales are limited to functional assessment for a specific disease, such as RA, multiple sclerosis, or juvenile rheumatoid arthritis, or even to a specific joint, such as the shoulder.[13,14] The functional independence measure (FIM), commonly used in rehabilitation units[15] is designed for general use and classifies each ADL into categories: independent, independent with aids, requires supervision, requires assistance, and dependent. Other scales include IADL such as the sickness impact profile (SIP). Each scale has advantages and disadvantages. These tools provide semiquantitative measures of patient function, which can be described and communicated to other health professionals and to the family. Functional assessment measurements can help determine the patient's length of stay in hospital programs, monitor ongoing treatment, predict prognoses, help plan the placement of patients, estimate patient-care requirements, and provide an estimate of future care requirements for medical and legal purposes.[16] But perhaps the most important reason for measuring functional outcome today is to justify program funding to third-party payors, federal government officials, Congress, and even to local hospital administrators.[17]

The most widely used scales for rheumatic diseases are the Arthritis Impact Measurement Scale (AIMS), the Health Assessment Questionnaire (HAQ), and the McMaster Toronto Arthritis Patient Preference Disability Questionnaire (MACTAR).[18-21] The MACTAR is unique in that it allows the patients to choose which activities are important to them.[22] The HAQ is also a self-administered questionnaire and includes activities of daily living inside and outside the home.[23] The AIMS and HAQ scales correlate with one another.[24] The AIMS has also been adapted for use in the elderly,[25] and the HAQ has been adapted for children.[26] The HAQ appears to be useful in monitoring disease severity and response to a drug therapy over time.[27] However, the validity of the HAQ for measuring disability of an individual patient has been questioned.[18,28] The HAQ also has been modified by reducing the number of items (MHAQ) and by having a disease-specific version (RA-HAQ). However, the shorter HAQ versions may not be as sensitive to change as the full version.[29]

BIOMECHANICAL AND COMPUTERIZED DEVICES

Various biomechanical and computerized devices such as the Baltimore Therapeutic Equipment work simulator (Baltimore Therapeutic Equipment, Hanover, Md.), the LIDO WorkSet, and the ERGOS system have been used to measure impairment and disability. Testing relies on full patient participation, motivation, and cooperation to give accurate and valid results. The motivation of a patient desiring to keep his or her job is different from that of a patient who is applying for disability.

A complete functional-abilities evaluation with these machines should include tests to evaluate level and consistency of effort. These measurements may include coefficient of variation of repeated testing of the same activity, bell curve analysis of grip strength, rapid exchange of grip strength, measurement of heart rate during activities, and nonorganic physical signs.[30]

INDEPENDENT MEDICAL EVALUATIONS

Physicians are commonly requested to perform independent medical evaluations by third parties. The Social Security Administration publishes a detailed guide of impairments that lead to disability.[31]

The American Medical Association (AMA) guide to the evaluation of permanent impairment describes a specific joint examination that emphasizes range of motion to determine impairment.[32] However, the degree of medical impairment measured using the AMA guide may not be predictive of the degree of associated disability, and the guide itself states "impairment ratings are not intended for use as direct determinants of work disability."[32]

The results of such assessments have enormous financial and social implications for the patient and for society. These assessments and the resulting diagnoses should be based on objective evidence of an impairment or disease.

The determination of physical disability is difficult because nonmedical factors have a significant influence, such as level of education, occupation, income, job satisfaction, motivation, and the presence or absence of psychiatric illness. Objective findings, such as joint swelling, may not correlate with disability. Even when objective evidence of a disease exists, the associated level of function in rheumatic diseases may fluctuate during the day and from day to day so that one assessment may not be representative of a patient's true abilities.[33,34] Reported symptoms or disability in osteoarthritis (OA) of the hip and knee may not correlate with radiographic changes.[35] Objective test results may not correlate with perceived disability, as in cases of fibromyalgia.[36,37]

Components of Rheumatic Disease Rehabilitation

REST

Active inflammatory joint disease may disappear from limbs that have become paralyzed, from all joints after prolonged systemic rest (bed rest), or from joints given local rest (with splints and braces).[38] However, complete bed rest has no place in the long-term management of rheumatic diseases because of the deleterious effects on the musculoskeletal, cardiovascular, nervous, and integumentary systems. In healthy subjects, cast immobilization causes a loss of muscle mass as determined by computed tomography and biopsy within 4 weeks.[39] If a few days of bed rest are required to treat an acute flare of RA, passive and active exercises in bed should be advised to prevent loss of muscle mass. A program of rest for a limited period each day, or rest of particular joints, is preferable to complete bed rest. For ambulatory patients, 1 hour of bed rest during the day may help decrease the fatigue caused by systemic inflammation. Rest of specific joints can be provided by orthoses, most commonly by resting and working wrist splints (see following).

EXERCISE

The importance of therapeutic exercise in the management of rheumatic diseases is often inadequately appreciated. There is no scientific evidence that shows exercise to be deleterious for arthritis patients.[40] Exercise is safe and helpful for SLE and polymyositis.[41,42] Inflammatory muscle, joint, and connective tissue diseases and adverse effects of medications may result in loss of joint range of motion, muscle strength, and bone density. The immediate reaction to a painful stimulus, such as in a joint, is to stop using that joint. For example, knee and hip pain are strongly associated with quadriceps weakness.[43,44] Accumulation of fluid within a joint also inhibits movement. A knee effusion inhibits quadriceps contractions, and quadriceps training is less effective when a persistent effusion is present.[45] Inflamed joints are usually more comfortable in a slightly flexed position because of a reduction in intra-articular pressure. As a result of immobilization, the joint capsule tightens, and a permanent joint contracture may occur that is resistant to any treatment. A shortening of the surrounding muscles and tendons may also occur, further contributing to contracture. Inflammation can directly injure muscles and joints. Widespread muscle or polyarticular inflammation may also cause fatigue and reduce endurance.

Exercise therapy can increase aerobic capacity, joint range of motion, endurance, muscle strength, and coordination and can improve joint stability and physical function.[46] Exercises may be prescribed for specific joints or muscles or for part of a program to maintain or improve overall cardiovascular fitness and endurance. Task-specific exercise training can improve the ability to perform specific functions such as rising from a bed or chair.[47] A hand exercise program can increase grip strength in OA of the hand.[48] In OA of the knee, aerobic and resistive exercise can decrease disability by improving function and decreasing pain.[49,50] Even the elderly, following falls or hip surgery, can benefit from progressive resistance exercise programs.[51] Loss of muscle cells normally occurs with aging.[52]

Therapeutic exercise may be broadly classified into three groups:

1. Range of motion or stretching
2. Strengthening (resistive)
3. Aerobic (endurance)

Exercises are divided into those that are active and those that are passive. The types of strengthening exercises are isometric, isotonic, and isokinetic (Fig. 55–1).

Generally, an exercise program progresses from passive to active assisted to active and then to resistive exercises. With passive exercises, a therapist or assistive device moves the joint without any muscle contraction exerted by the patient. With active-assisted exercises, the patient exerts some muscle contraction in attempting joint movement but is assisted in achieving the desired range. In active exercises, the individual exerts his or her own muscle activity to achieve the desired range of motion.

In resistive exercises, which are strengthening exercises, a force from a therapist, free weights, or a machine applies resistance in opposition to the attempted movement of a specific muscle group by the subject. In progressive resistive exercises, an increase in resistance is applied over time as muscle strength improves.

Inflamed joints should be exercised daily, preferably passively, through the usual range of motion, including flexion and extension and, when appropriate, abduction, adduction, and rotation. At least 10 repetitions should be performed twice each day for each joint. Stretching may be carried out more effectively after the use of heat for superficial analgesia or medication for systemic analgesia.

Active exercise includes free exercises, which may be assisted, if necessary, and resistive exercises, which are manually resisted or defined by weighing devices such as pulley systems and sandbags. Isometric (or static) exercise is performed without a change in joint range or muscle length. These exercises are particularly recommended in RA because they are easy to perform and require no special equipment. Isometric exercise causes the least strain on joints and places less stress on the cardiovascular system than dynamic exercise.[53] Dynamic exercises involve a change in joint motion. A program of dynamic and isometric exercises may be more effective than isometric and range-of-motion exercises in improving muscle strength without increasing disease activity.[54] Dynamic exercises are divided into isotonic and isokinetic. Isotonic exercise consists of muscle shortening *(concentric)* and muscle lengthening *(eccentric)* contractions. This form of strengthening, however, is not usually recommended for patients with inflamed joints. Isokinetic exercise involves movement through a fixed range of motion at a fixed rate of motion (velocity) against variable resistance that matches exactly the force generated by the patient at any point in the

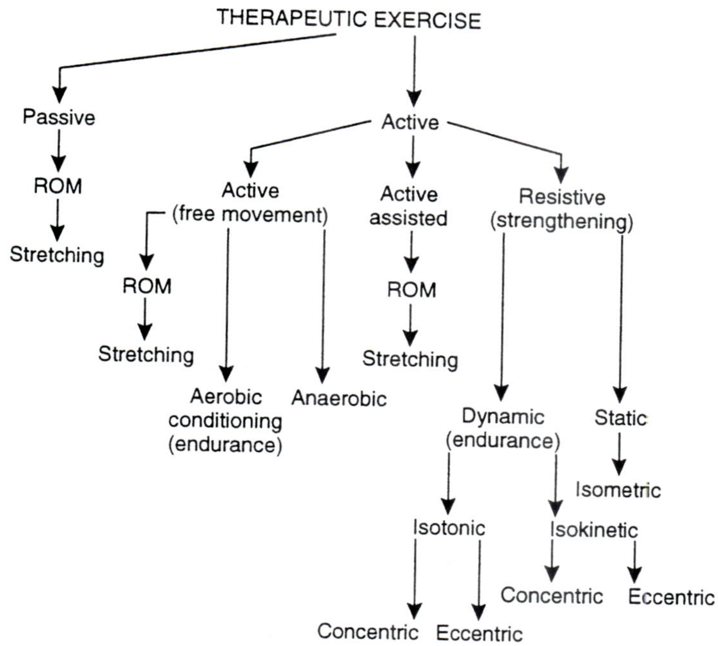

FIGURE 55–1 · Summary of Exercises. ROM, Range of Motion.

range. The stronger the force applied by the user, the greater is the resistance supplied. Equipment providing the latter type of accommodating resistance (e.g., Cybex system) is highly sophisticated and expensive. This equipment can also provide a printout of the torque developed during the exercise activity.

Quadriceps muscle strength can be maintained by isometric exercises.[55,56] An isometric contraction held for 6 seconds against two thirds of a maximal contracture strengthens the muscle if performed daily for 4 to 6 weeks.[57] A usual program consists of 10 to 20 repetitions with about one half of the maximal power performed two to three times daily. Quadriceps strengthening also results from straight leg raising performed from the sitting position.[58] The patient should sit in a chair and extend the leg, placing the heel on a second chair or stool of nearly the same height. The leg is held straight, raised about 8 inches, and then returned to the chair. Twenty repetitions should be performed at least three times per day.

The gluteal muscles are also important for gait and mobility and work in tandem with the quadriceps muscles. Tightening the buttocks and holding the contraction for several seconds 10 to 20 times twice per day is advisable. To avoid shoulder weakness, the patient can strengthen rotator cuff muscles by using a 1- to 3-pound weight while performing 10 to 20 repetitions of internal and external rotations; the elbow is flexed at 90 degrees, and the arm is held adjacent to the thorax. Elastic band devices, such as the Theraband, may be used to strengthen various muscles, including the shoulder.[59]

Because patients with ankylosing spondylitis find it difficult to maintain cardiorespiratory fitness and spinal mobility, general exercises, such as swimming and cycling, are appropriate. The goals of an exercise program in ankylosing spondylitis are to relieve pain and stiffness and maintain posture and should include specific joint and back passive stretching and active exercises. Consistent home exercise programs help increase and maintain spinal mobility and reduce pain and stiffness.[60-62] Group exercises may also encourage patient compliance, support patients psychologically, and are cost effective.[63,64] Patients with ankylosing spondylitis who exercise two to four hours per week may have less disability and less disease activity than those who exercise more or not at all.[65]

Compliance in exercise programs is improved by having an individual join a group with a structured program and keep an exercise diary, which should be reviewed on each clinic visit. Pool therapy provides buoyancy and support through reduction of the effects of gravity by the water. Pool therapy may permit exercising and independent walking even when walking aids or assistance are required on dry land. The water temperature should be 33°C to 34°C (92°F to 94°F) for pool exercises.[66]

Swimming, bicycling, and other non–weight-bearing conditioning exercises are especially suitable for patients with arthritis. Exercises such as tennis and racquetball are best avoided because of the sudden stresses and strains placed on ligaments and joints from rapid acceleration and deceleration movements that occur during these activities.

PHYSICAL MODALITIES

Physical modalities, such as hot packs, paraffin wax baths, ultrasound, and ice packs, are commonly used to treat the inflammation and pain of rheumatic diseases. However, clinical trials proving their effectiveness in improving objective measures of disease activity, such as joint range of motion and swelling, are often lacking.[67,68] Their usage is variable among rheumatologists.[69] Modalities are probably more effective when used along with exercise in a physical therapy program, occupational therapy program, or both.[70] In essence, modalities should be considered as a prelude to exercise therapy.

The physical treatment with modalities of nonspecific pain syndromes remains problematic. A systematic review of randomized control trials found little evidence to support the use of common interventions for managing shoulder pain, including mobilizations, ultrasound, and exercise.[67] A trial with a 6-month follow-up showed no efficacy of traction for the treatment of nonspecific low back pain.[71]

The use of physical modalities should be goal oriented and time limited. Close cooperation between the physician and therapist is needed regarding the goals and duration of treatment to achieve maximal patient benefit without excessive cost.

HEAT AND COLD

For centuries, heat has been used to alleviate the pain of joint and other diseases. Heat therapy probably began with mud baths, mineral waters, hot springs, and spas. Although the application of heat is known to produce analgesia and sedation, the mechanism by which the heating of tissues results in a subjective decrease in symptoms is unclear. It is possible that heating affects sensory and muscle nerve endings. However, placebo effects may play an important role in the effectiveness in any pain treatment, including surgery.[72] Superficial ice has been shown to reduce intra-articular temperature by about six or seven degrees C, and superficial heating may increase intra-articular temperature by about 2 degrees.[73-75] By a secondary effect on the viscoelastic properties (i.e., extensibility) of collagen, heat has also been shown to enhance stretching.[76]

Cold applications raise the pain threshold, producing local analgesia. Cold may also temporarily decrease spasticity and muscle spasms by direct action on the muscle spindle.[77] Topical ice therapy has been found to reduce pain in gouty arthritis.[78]

Some evidence suggests that, in arthritic joints, intra-articular temperature may be indirectly increased by superficial heat and decreased by superficial cold.[79] It has been further suggested that increasing intra-articular temperature may increase collagenase activity.[80] Experimentally, superficial cold reduced intra-articular temperature in dog knees.[81] The clinical implications of these findings are unclear,[79] and they may be insignificant because the long-term use of heat or cold treatments has not been shown to have deleterious effects on joint pathology in controlled trials.[82]

Common methods of superficial heating include hot packs, heating pads, Hydrocollator packs, paraffin wax (Fig. 55–2), hot water bottles, heated pools and whirlpools, and infrared lamps. Heating pads should be set with a timer to avoid burns, which can occur if the patient falls asleep.

A Hydrocollator pack contains silica gel covered by cloth; it is warmed in a hot water bath. The silica allows prolonged retention of heat. Because the temperature of these packs can be high, they are usually wrapped in a towel before application to prevent burns.

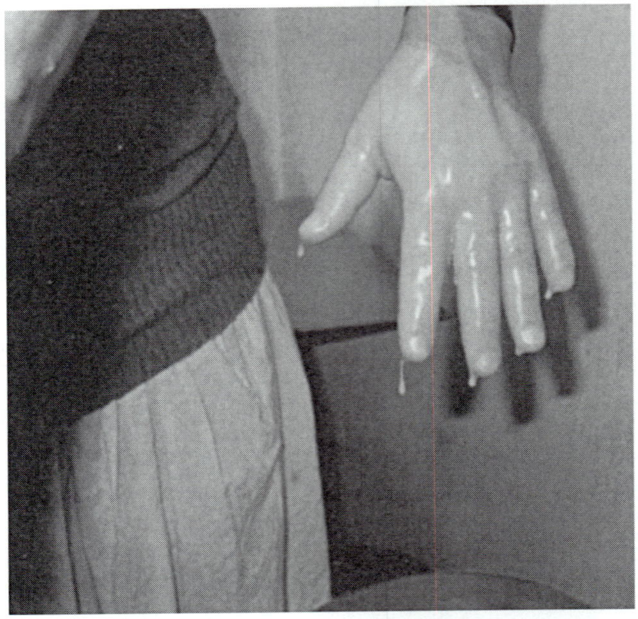

FIGURE 55–2 • Paraffin wax molds to any surface to provide superficial heating of tissues.

Paraffin wax treatment, a principal method to heat the hands, can be set up at home. A wax mixture is first heated to a liquid form. The patient then dips a hand in and out of the wax until several layers have adhered. The hand can be wrapped with a towel to maintain the heat. The partially solidified glove of wax retains warmth for about 20 minutes. Although a somewhat messy application, wax is particularly useful for patients with hand arthritis and deformities because the wax can mold to any surface. In one study, when this treatment was combined with an exercise program, patients reported decreased stiffness and increased range of motion in the hand.[83]

Hydrotherapy in a Hubbard tank can provide superficial heat to multiple joints and may help reduce morning stiffness. However, Hubbard tanks are now infrequently used. At home, hot baths and showers, especially in the morning, can be used for relief. Fertility problems have been reported in men after prolonged immersion in hot baths.[84] Spa therapy, which includes bathing in thermal or mineral waters (balneotherapy), is common in Europe and has been shown to be helpful for patients with ankylosing spondylitis and possibly other rheumatic diseases.[85,86] Objective benefits of hydrotherapy over land exercises have not been shown.[87]

More expensive modalities that theoretically can heat deeper structures include short waves, microwaves, and ultrasound. However, the available frequencies permitted for the medical application of short waves and microwaves allow for only superficial heating. Only ultrasound may heat deeper structures. No study has unequivocally demonstrated the advantage of presumed deep heating methods over less expensive hot packs, and it has been difficult to demonstrate a benefit of ultrasound over placebo.[88] However, ultrasound treatment was shown to improve grip strength in rheumatoid arthritis.[89]

Cooling of tissues can be obtained with ice packs or frozen food packages. The patient's skin should be protected from ice with a towel or other barrier to prevent tissue damage. Only superficial tissues can be cooled, because no deep cooling devices are available. Cooling causes vasoconstriction, with a reduction of blood flow and a decrease in metabolic activity in the region treated.

Heat and cold modalities should be avoided in patients who cannot communicate feelings of discomfort, such as very young, comatose, or demented patients. Tumors; eyes; fresh hematomas; open wounds; ischemic areas; areas with metal implants, pacemakers, or other electric-mechanical devices; and uteruses of pregnant women generally should not be heated. Ultrasound should not be used near metal implants. Patients with cold-related diseases, such as cold agglutinin disease, Raynaud's phenomenon, cold hypersensitivity, cryoglobulinemia, and paroxysmal cold hemoglobinuria, should not be treated with tissue cooling.

The decision whether to use superficial heat or cold is subjective. Because neither modality appears to affect inflammation adversely, the primary considerations for use are cost, availability, experience of the physician, and patient preference.[90] Based on the observation that heat increases intra-articular temperature, it is suggested that cooling be used for joints that are acutely inflamed. Cooling is also used in the first 24 hours after acute musculoskeletal trauma because of bleeding and swelling of the tissues. The pain of subacute and chronic inflammation is more responsive to superficial moist heat and is often preferred by patients (Table 55–1).

ELECTROTHERAPY

Transcutaneous electrical nerve stimulation (TENS) is another physical modality commonly used for the treatment of pain. An intermittent low-voltage current is applied to the skin. TENS is noninvasive and has few side effects but should probably not be used in patients with pacemakers. The mechanism of action remains unknown, but the most popular concept embraces the gate theory of pain of Melzack and Wall. Presumably, the current produced by the device closes the gate and prevents transmission of pain impulses.

TENS units are battery powered and self-contained. They can be worn by the patient and used when and where desired. Location of electrodes, duration of treatment, and electrical parameters are arbitrary. The effectiveness of electrotherapy for pain treatment over placebo, however, has been difficult to demonstrate in controlled trials.[91]

Electrotherapy can also be used to stimulate muscles by causing muscle contractions in the hope of improving muscle strength in a patient unable to exercise on his or her own because of pain or active inflammatory disease. However, this passive method of exercising has not been proven to be effective for improving the strength of atrophied muscles or function.[92]

TABLE 55–1 • SUMMARY OF HEAT AND COLD MODALITIES

Superficial Heat	Deep Heat	Cold
Conductive		
Hot packs	Ultrasound	ColPac†
Thermaphore*	Short wave	Ice massage
Electric heating pad	Microwave	Ice pack
Paraffin wax		Fluorotherapy
Convection		
Jacuzzi		
Whirlpool		
Hubbard tank		
Radiation		
Infrared		

*Battle Creek Equipment Co., 307 W. Jackson St., Battle Creek, MI 49016.
†Chattanooga Pharmacal Co., 2413 Lyndon Ave., Chattanooga, TN 37415.

ORTHOTICS

Orthotic devices include braces, splints, corsets, collars, and shoe modifications. A properly prescribed orthosis restores lost function or helps to maintain optimal function by altering biomechanics and reducing pain.[93] Orthoses decrease forces passing through painful weight-bearing joints, stabilize subluxating joints, improve motion patterns, and maximize functional positioning. Unless the underlying inflammation is treated, orthotic devices cannot prevent deformity. An orthosis may also allow a highly inflamed joint to fuse in the best functional position.

Advances in thermodynamic plastics have removed the need for heavy metal and plaster in orthotic construction. Lighter orthoses require less energy and oxygen consumption in their use.[94] Two types of plastics are commonly used: thermoplastic and thermoset.

Thermoplastic (e.g., Sansplint) is a plastic that can be reheated multiple times to change its shape. This is advantageous because, as joint swelling decreases, the old splint can simply be reheated and remolded, saving the expense of a new one. Thermoplastic is lightweight and ideally suited for non–weight-bearing splints. After heating, thermoplastic can be applied to the patient directly over a cloth and then molded as it cools.

Thermoset plastic, in contrast, requires a higher temperature for molding. It cannot be reheated or remolded, but it is stronger and more durable. Thermoset is suited for use in such applications as an ankle-foot orthosis. Because of the higher temperatures required for molding, the plastic cannot be applied to the patient directly. A plastic cast must first be molded on the patient, increasing the time and expense required for construction.

Perforations may be incorporated into both materials to allow air to circulate. Fastening tape (e.g., Velcro) straps are attached, which assist patients with hand or wrist deformities in fastening the orthosis more easily. Although a wrist splint can reduce pain while worn, the splint may also impede the speed of functional performance.[95]

SPLINTS

Splints may be static or dynamic and resting or working. Static rest splints are worn during periods when joint movement is not needed, usually at night, and provide pain relief.[96] Static work splints are worn during the day and must accommodate some movement (e.g., a wrist splint that allows a child with juvenile rheumatoid arthritis to write at school).

Dynamic splints have movable parts that may include metal, gas, electrical, and elastic components. Such devices may replace lost muscle power or may be used to strengthen weak muscles or reduce or prevent contractures. For example, loss of finger extension from rupture of the extensor tendons in RA may be replaced by elastic bands on a splint, which hold the fingers in extension.

Ready-made wrist splints can be as effective as custom-made splints.[97] However, prefabricated splints ("off the shelf") should be used with caution, as an improperly fitted device may lead to skin breakdown and may even aggravate the joint pain.

BRACES

Braces are used on the lower limbs to decrease weight-bearing or to provide stability. In the past, they were composed of heavy metal and required a large energy expenditure for their use. Today, braces can be fabricated from lightweight metal, such as aluminum, with plastic components, increasing their usefulness and compliance by the patient. Compliance is a major problem with splints and braces.

Specific Types of Orthoses

Ring splints, composed of metal, may be used for a swan neck deformity to improve hand function by reducing hyperextension of the proximal interphalangeal (PIP) joint. When this splint is placed upside down on the PIP joint, it can be used to reduce excessive flexion seen in the boutonniere deformity.

Wrist splints are the most commonly prescribed splints in RA. Resting or night wrist splints have 10 to 40 degrees of extension at the wrist, 20 to 70 degrees flexion of the metacarpophalangeal (MCP) joints, and 10 to 20 degrees of flexion at the PIP joints and distal interphalangeal joints. Resting splints for the wrist may have finger dividers added to each finger to prevent ulnar deviation, or a single ulnar lip may be attached to the ulnar side of the fifth finger. Working splints that allow greater joint movement and function are used during the day. The thumb is separated with a C-bar to prevent adduction deformity.

In juvenile rheumatoid arthritis, wrist splints are of paramount importance, because gravity and the other forces across the joint result in volar subluxation (i.e., dropped wrist). Working wrist splints for patients with juvenile rheumatoid arthritis are cut short at the MCP level, and the thumb remains free so the child is able to use the fingers to grasp and write at school (Fig. 55–3).

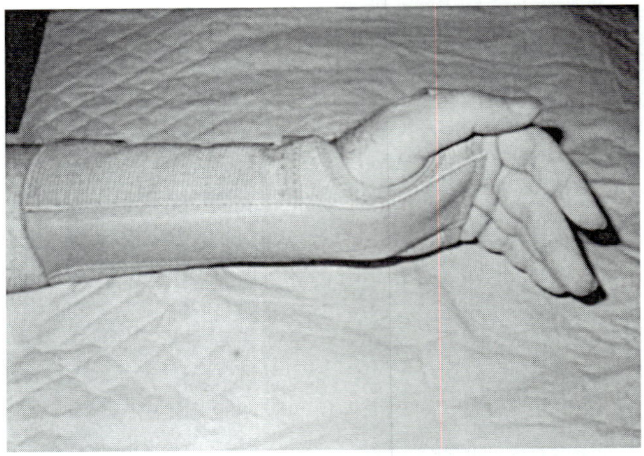

FIGURE 55–3 · Daytime resting splints for wrist involvement should permit normal function at school.

Wrist splints are also useful in the initial treatment of carpal tunnel syndrome. Dynamic wrist splints are used to replace finger extension in patients with extensor tendon rupture. In osteoarthritis, pain and instability at the first carpometacarpal joint can be treated with an opponens splint, which stabilizes the joint in opposition (Fig. 55–4).

Subluxation of the atlantoaxial joint can occur in RA, and when surgery is not indicated, cervical collars may be prescribed. Cervical collars include soft collars, the Philadelphia collar, and the sterno-occipital–mandibular immobilizer. None of these collars is effective in severely restricting neck motion, and their effectiveness varies among patients.[98] Soft collars can also be used at night by any patient with a cervical neck syndrome and may provide some comfort. Corsets and abdominal binders may assist weak abdominal muscles and provide support to the lumbar spine. These devices do not replace abdominal muscle exercises but are useful in cases of acute pain, such as compression fractures of the spine, or for an older, noncompliant patient.

In OA and RA, long and short leg braces are sometimes used to try to reduce instability and control knee movements. A brace to support the knee usually consists

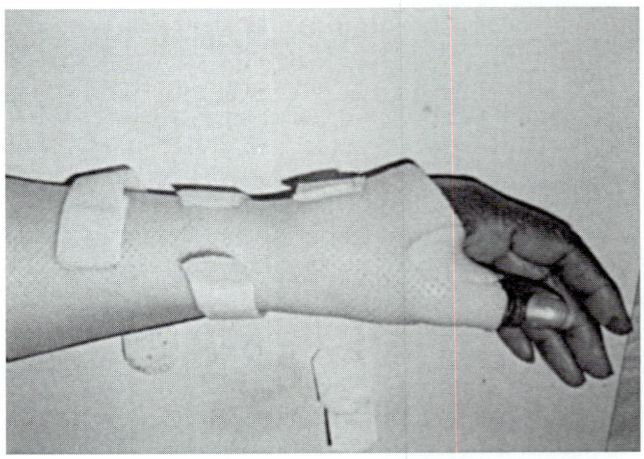

FIGURE 55–4 · A static wrist-hand orthotic (long opponens), which stabilizes the wrist and the first carpometacarpal joint.

of thigh and calf enclosures, two uprights, and a hinge at the level of the knee that permits flexion and extension. The long leg (knee) brace may begin just below the hip and extend to just above the ankle. A short knee brace has hinges and a leather elastic enclosure but provides much less support because it is restricted to the region of the knee itself. Although they provide better support, the long leg braces, which are heavier than short braces and cosmetically less appealing, are less acceptable to patients. Arthritis of the hand with deformities may make it difficult for patients to don the knee brace. When ankle stability is lacking, a high shoe boot or a plastic ankle-foot orthosis is recommended. An ankle-foot orthosis provides medial and lateral stability in place of lax ligaments and controls ankle plantar and dorsiflexion in a patient with foot drop. In patients with anesthetic feet, an external ankle-foot orthosis composed of double metal uprights, a fixed or movable ankle, and metal stirrups directly fixed to the shoe is preferred. Inversion and eversion straps can be added to further control ankle stability.

Destructive changes of the ankle or subtalar joint from RA or other inflammatory arthritis can be painful and cause a major limitation in ambulation. A patellar tendon-bearing orthosis (PTB) is helpful for this problem. This brace, which provides weight-bearing on the patellar tendon and tibial condyles through a molded upper calf band, has a fixed ankle and a rocker-bottom sole; the weight of the upper body can be transmitted directly from the knee region and calf to the floor (Fig. 55–5). In addition to inflammatory arthritis, this brace is used to decrease stress on the ankle or subtalar joints in other conditions such as severe osteoarthritis, Charcot's joint, and nonunion fractures of the lower limb.

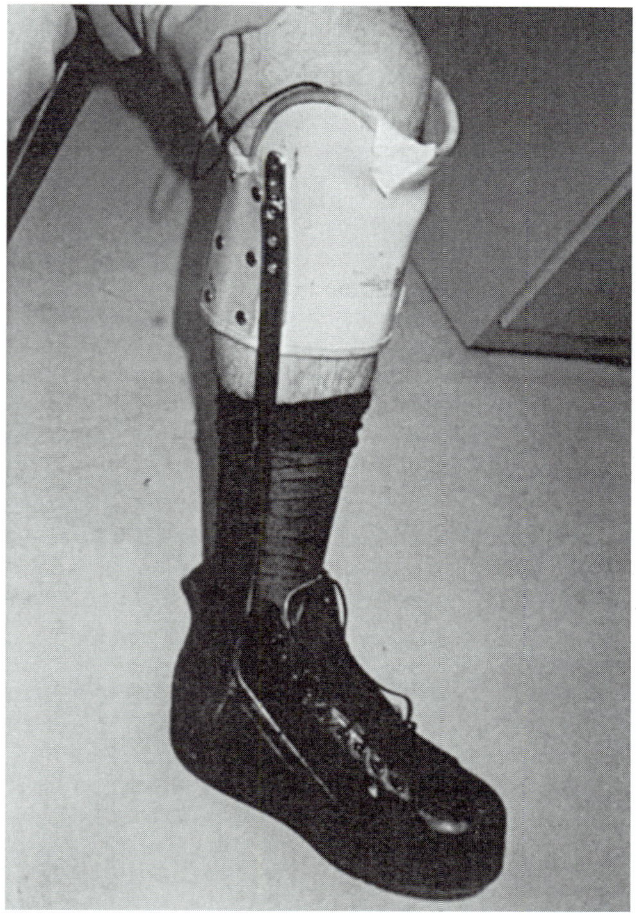

FIGURE 55–5 · A patellar tendon-bearing ankle-foot orthotic allows transfer of body weight from the knee to the floor, bypassing the ankle.

Ligament laxity is common in inflammatory rheumatic diseases, often resulting in subluxation of joints. Metatarsophalangeal (MTP) joint subluxation results in broadening of the forefoot, clawing of toes, and painful weight bearing on MTP heads (Fig. 55–6). Callus forms on the bottom of the foot. An internal or external metatarsal bar can be placed on each shoe to redistribute the weight away from the MTP heads. Alternatively, a metatarsal pad attached directly to a toe inside the sock (metatarsal corset) may be used in any shoe.

Joint subluxation also results in loss of foot arches, uneven weight distribution, and pain. Arch supports placed in shoes can help reform these arches.

Heel pain due to plantar fasciitis may be treated with a heel cup or spur pad in the shoe or with a medial longitudinal arch support. Extra-depth shoes must be used to provide room for these orthoses, clawed toes, and bunions. Otherwise, corns may develop where the PIP or first MTP joints rub on the superior part or side of the shoe.

Asymmetric joint involvement in adult RA or OA may also lead to differences in leg lengths if bone or articular cartilage is destroyed on one side. A lift may be added to the shoe of the short leg. The amount of the shoe rise should be one half to three quarters of the leg length discrepancy. If the leg length discrepancy is not a recent event and is asymptomatic, it is probably better not to treat it.

ASSISTIVE DEVICES

When needed, a wide variety of assistive devices are available to reduce disability[99] (Fig. 55–7). An experienced occupational therapist can recommend which devices are appropriate for each patient, including those that aid the patient in dressing, such as button hooks, long-handled reachers, and sock aids. A rocker knife allows the patient to cut food with one hand. High toilet seats, bathroom-wall grab bars, and bath seats aid in hygiene (Figs. 55–8 and 55–9). It is important to determine patient compliance with and the usefulness of the aids provided and whether modifications are needed.[100]

MOBILITY DEVICES

Mobility devices, such as walkers, crutches, canes, and wheelchairs, are easily accessible and provide immediate assistance. These devices are used when lower extremity joint instability, pain, weakness, fatigue, paralysis, or balance problems limit independent ambulation. Weight-bearing is reduced through the diseased limb or limbs.

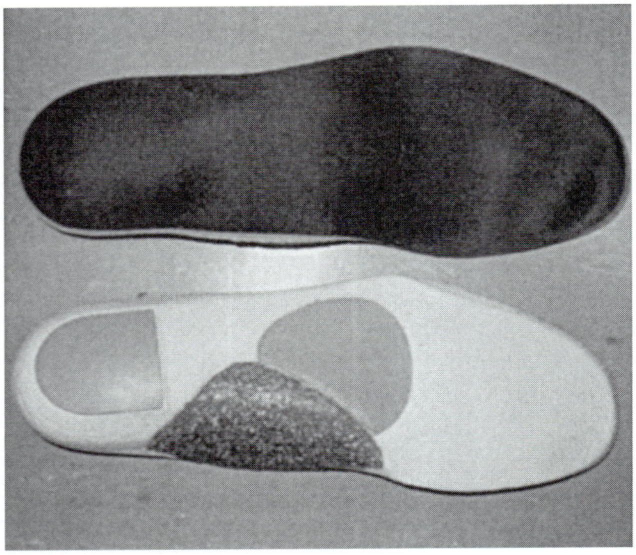

FIGURE 55–6 • Shoe orthosis with a cushioned insole to which a metatarsal pad, heel pad, and cork arch support have been added.

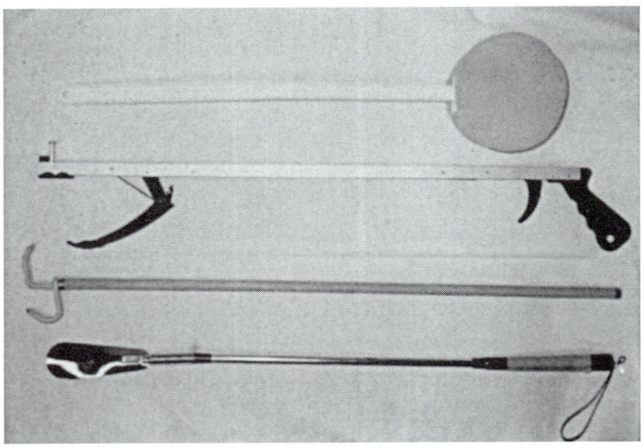

FIGURE 55–7 • A long-handled reacher, bath sponge, hook, and shoehorn substitute for lost joint range of motion caused by rheumatic diseases.

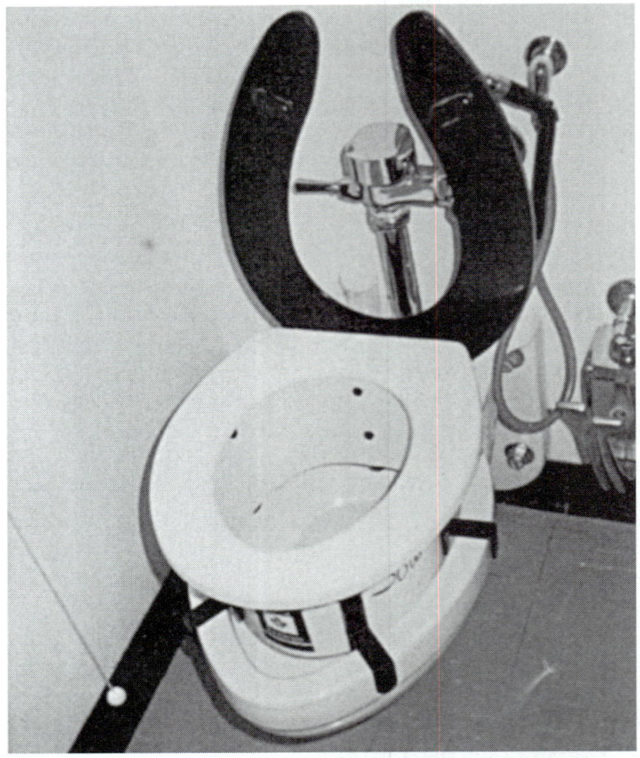

FIGURE 55–8 • Raising the height of the toilet seat assists in transfers from a wheelchair to the toilet and can compensate for proximal lower extremity weakness.

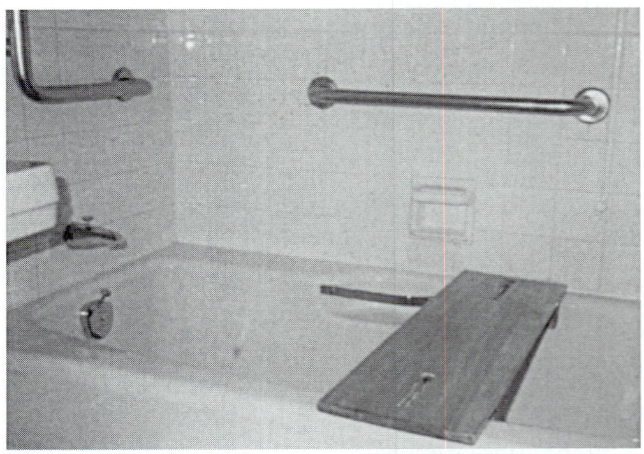

FIGURE 55–9 • A bathboard and grab bars improve safety and ease access to the bathtub.

Balance is improved by widening the base of support so that the patient's center of gravity can be shifted, safely enhancing proprioceptive input. However, any type of assisted mobility requires more physical effort than normal walking.[101]

The choice of an assistive device is based on the impairment and the resulting disability. Such devices add to safety in ambulation and can prevent falls in the elderly, which can result in devastating hip fractures. The use of hip protectors can also decrease the risk of fractures in the elderly. Unfortunately, compliance with this device is poor.[102]

Canes

A properly used cane can reduce more than 25 percent of the body weight supported by the contralateral limb during gait.[103] To determine cane length, a measurement should be taken from the level of the greater trochanter or distal wrist crease to the heel of the shoe.[104] With cane use, the shoulders should be level and the elbow flexed at about 30 degrees. Canes can be constructed of metal or wood. Metal is more durable and can be adjusted, whereas wood is cheaper.

C and T Handles

The common cane handle is in the shape of a C. However, a C cane is difficult to grasp and may increase falls in the unstable patient, because the line of gravity falls behind the cane shaft. An alternate choice is a T-shaped handle. This type fits the contour of the hands better, and the line of gravity falls through the cane shaft, providing greater stability. The cane base can have a rubber or metal tip, depending on the ground surface. A reversible metal spike is available for use on ice.

Single-Point, Tripod, and Quadripod Bases

Although a single-point cane (i.e., straight cane) is most common, tripod and quadripod bases are also available. These canes provide a broader base of support with three or four points of floor contact. The cane legs that are closest to the lower limb of the patient are usually shorter to allow clearance of the foot. Tripod and quadripod canes, however, are not practical on stairs and usually result in a slower gait pattern, because all three or four legs must contact the floor to maintain patient stability.

Crutches

Crutches are prescribed when more stability is required than is provided by a cane or when one leg must be kept off the ground. Types of crutches include axillary, forearm, and platform (i.e., trough) crutches (Fig. 55–10).

Axillary Crutches

Axillary crutches are held under the arm against the chest wall. For effective crutch use, the patient must have good upper extremity strength and range of motion. The crutch prescription must include accurate patient measurements to ensure effective use and prevent adverse effects on the upper extremities, including axillary tissue trauma and brachial plexus and radial nerve injuries. Proper instruction in crutch use is most important to avoid weight-bearing through the axilla. The height of the crutch handle should be measured from 6 inches lateral to the fifth toe to the distal wrist crease with the elbow extended. The top of the crutch should be 1 inch, or two to three finger breadths, below the axillary fold.

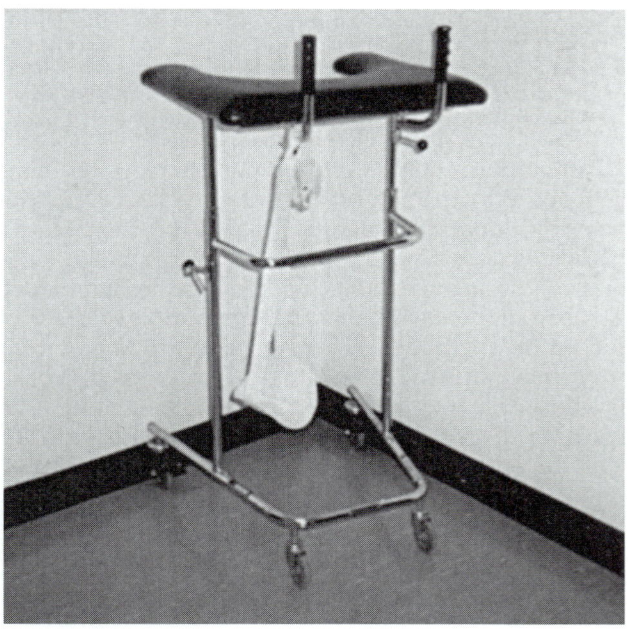

FIGURE 55–10 · A high-wheeled platform walker allows weight-bearing through the forearms.

Forearm and Platform Crutches

For more chronic conditions, including RA, in which hand function may be problematic, forearm and platform (i.e., trough) crutches are suggested. Joint stability, strength, and coordination are needed to use them.

Forearm crutches are more expensive than axillary crutches but are more functional for patients requiring long-term ambulation aids. A forearm crutch usually consists of a single metal shaft attached to two uprights that extend to below the elbow. It is lightweight and easily adjustable. Freedom is allowed for hand movements such as opening doors.

Platform crutches are top heavy and unstable. However, no weight-bearing occurs through the hand or wrist. These devices are useful when these joints are impaired from arthritis.

Several types of gait are possible with canes, crutches, and walkers, and proper training is required for each type.[105] Normal ambulation is a two-point gait with alternate upper and lower extremities advancing forward during the swing phase.

Walkers

Walkers are prescribed for patients who require considerable external support. Good bilateral grasp and upper extremity strength are required for their use. Walkers are cumbersome and can be difficult to maneuver, especially on deep carpeting. They cannot be used on stairs.

Walkers are available in different heights. Safety is improved by increasing the height of the walker, but efficiency is decreased. High walkers may be indicated in very weak patients, such as those with limited upper extremity function or chronic cardiopulmonary conditions. They also provide space for oxygen tanks to be attached. Standard-height walkers can have two or four wheels or no wheels. Wheels permit the walker to be pushed along the floor, but if there are no brakes, patients may have difficulty stopping. Traditional walkers must be lifted before stepping and place greater demands on the cardiovascular system than walkers with wheels.[106] Some walkers may also have baskets and a seat (see Fig. 55–10).

Wheelchairs

Wheelchairs are underused, possibly because of their cost and the failure to recognize their benefit for the disabled.[107] For patients unable to propel a wheelchair manually, an electric wheelchair, although expensive, is a consideration because it can improve the quality of life by maintaining independent mobility. Electric scooters are an alternative to wheelchairs. The safe use of wheelchairs requires proper training and practice. Wheelchair accidents are not uncommon, especially in the elderly, and typically occur at home.[108] Most accidents involve falls or tips and occur while a person is traversing ramps or transferring in and out of the chair.[109] Modifications of homes for wheelchair users may prevent falls.

ENVIRONMENTAL MODIFICATIONS

A home visit by a qualified occupational therapist can result in suggestions to modify the home to improve accessibility and patient safety. Most problems occur in bathrooms, kitchens, bedrooms, and doorways.[110] A ramp may be installed to bypass steps. Doorways may be widened to accommodate a wheelchair. Bars and railings can be installed in strategic areas. Area rugs can be removed. Counters can be raised or lowered. Assistive devices can be added to the kitchen. Chair features such as height and armrests can be altered.[111] A home visit by the therapists also gives an indication of the functional level that must be achieved by the patient in order to return home.

Patient Education

Patient education increases compliance with exercise, energy conservation, joint protection, and in taking medication.[112] Education and exercise provided by a physical therapist in the community can be beneficial and improve disease management knowledge and reduce morning stiffness.[113] Joint protection programs may slow the progression of RA and increase function.[114] Appropriate sexual, psychosocial, and vocational counseling should be available. Educational materials and information on specific self-help groups can be obtained from local arthritis societies. Patient education should be part of a comprehensive program. Simply providing a booklet alone does not seem to be sufficient as the success of the educational process can be measured with a questionnaire.[114] Considerable patient and professional education information can be obtained from the Internet.

REFERENCES

1. Lineker SC, Bell MJ, Wilkins AL, Badley EM: Improvements following short term home based physical therapy are maintained at one year in people with moderate to severe rheumatoid arthritis. J Rheumatol 28:165, 2001.
2. Hammond A, Freeman K: One-year outcomes of a randomized controlled trial of an educational-behavioural joint protection programme for people with rheumatoid arthritis. Rheumatology 40:1044, 2001.
3. International Classification of Functioning, Disability and Health, World Health Organization, 2001. Accessed December 14, 2003. www.who.int.
4. Prevalence of self-reported arthritis or chronic joint symptoms among adults: United States, 2001. MMWR Morb Mortal Wkly Rep 51:948, 2002.
5. Verbrugge L, Juarez L: Epidemiology and determinants profile of arthritis disability. Public Health Rep 116(Suppl):157, 2001.
6. Lawrence RC, Helmick CG, Arnett FC, et al: Estimates of the prevalence of arthritis and selected musculoskeletal disorders in the United States. Arthritis Rheum 41:778, 1998.
7. Badley EM: Arthritis and the aging population: projections of arthritis prevalence in Canada 1991 to 2031. J Rheumatol 25:138, 1998.
8. Badley EM, Wang PP: The contribution of arthritis and arthritis disability to nonparticipation in the labor force: a Canadian example. J Rheumatol28:1077, 2001.
9. Young A, Dixey J, Kulinskaya E, et al: Which patients stop working because of rheumatoid arthritis? Results of five years' follow up in 732 patients from the early RA study (ERAS). Ann Rheum Dis 61:335, 2002.
10. Partridge AJ, Karlson EW, Daltroy LH, et al: Risk factors for early work disability in systemic lupus erythematosus. Arthritis Rheum 40:2199, 1997.
11. Gill TM, Hardy SE, Williams CS: Underestimation of disability in community living older persons. J Am Geriatr Soc 50:1492, 2002.
12. Steinbrocker O, Traeger CH, Batterman RC: Therapeutic criteria in rheumatoid arthritis. JAMA 140:659-662, 1949.
13. Oen K, Malleson PN, Cabral DA, et al: Disease course and outcome of juvenile rheumatoid arthritis in a multicenter cohort. J Rheumatol 29:1989, 2002.
14. van der Heijden GJMG, Leffers P, Bouter LM: Shoulder disability questionnaire design and responsiveness of a functional status measure. J Clin Epidemiol 53:29, 2000.
15. Valach L, Steck GC, Roschli C, Selz B: Rehabilitation of cognitive and motor functions in younger and older patients with vascular brain damage, rheumatological illness and in post-surgery patients. Int J Rehab Res 25:133, 2002.
16. Ward MM: Functional disability predicts total costs in patients with ankylosing spondylitis. Arthritis Rheum 46:223, 2002.
17. Maravic M, Bozonnat MC, Sevezan A, et al: Preliminary evaluation of medical outcomes (including quality of life) and costs in incident RA cases receiving hospital-based multidisciplinary management. Joint Bone Spine 67:425, 2000.
18. Greewood MC, Doyle DV, Ensor M: Does the Stanford Health Assessment Questionnaire have potential as a monitoring tool for subjects with rheumatoid arthritis? Ann Rheum Dis 60:344, 2001.
19. Soderlin MK, Nieminen P, Hakala M: Arthritis impact measurement scales in a community-based rheumatoid arthritis population. Clin Rheumatol 19:30, 2000.
20. Verhoeven AC, Boers M, van der Linden S: Validity of the MACTAR Questionnaire as a functional index in a rheumatoid arthritis clinical trial. J Rheumatol 27:2801, 2000.
21. Soderlin MK, Mieminen P, Hakala M: Arthritis impact measurement scales in a community-based rheumatoid arthritis population. Clin Rheumatol 19:30, 2000.
22. Tugwell P, Bombardier C, Buchanan W, et al: The MACTAR patient preference disability questionnaire: an individualized functional priority approach for assessing improvement in physical disability in clinical trials in rheumatoid arthritis. J Rheum 14:446-451, 1987.
23. Fries JF, Spitz P, Kraines RG, et al: Measurement of patient outcome in arthritis. Arthritis Rheum 23:137-145, 1980.
24. Hakala M, Nieminen P, Manelius J: Joint impairment is strongly correlated with disability measured by self-report questionnaires: functional status assessment of individuals with rheumatoid arthritis in a population based series. J Rheum 21:64-69, 1994.
25. Hughes SL, Edelman P, Chang RW, et al: The GERIAIMS: Reliability and validity of the arthritis impact measurement scales adapted for elderly respondents. Arthritis Rheum 34:856, 1991.
26. Tennant A, Kearns S, Turner F, et al: Measuring the function of children with juvenile arthritis. Rheumatology 40:1274, 2001.
27. Scott DL, Strand V: The effects of disease-modifying anti-rheumatic drugs on the Health Assessment Questionnaire score: lessons from the leflunomide clinical trials database. Rheumatology 41:899, 2002.
28. Wolfe F: A reappraisal of HAQ disability in rheumatoid arthritis. Arthritis Rheum 43:2751, 2000.
29. Wolfe F: Which HAQ is best? A Comparison of the HAQ, MHAW and RA-HAQ, a difficult 8 Item HAQ (DHAQ), and a record for 20 items HAQ (HAQ20): analysis in 2491 rheumatoid arthritis ratients following leflunomide initiation. J Rheumatol 28:982, 2001.
30. Lechner DE, Bradbury SF, Bradley LA: Detecting sincerity of effort: a summary of methods and approaches. Physical Therapy 78:867, 1998.
31. U.S. Department of Health and Human Services, Social Security Administration: Disability Evaluation Under Social Security. SSA Publication No. 64-039. Washington, DC, Department of Health and Human Services, January 2003.
32. Cocchiarella L, Andersson GBJ: Guides to the Evaluation of Permanent Impairment, 5th ed. Chicago, American Medical Association, 2002.

33. Dekkers JC, Geenen R, Godaert GLR, et al: Diurnal courses of cortisol, pain, fatigue, negative mood, and stiffness in patients with recently diagnosed rheumatoid arthritis. Int J Behav Med 7:353, 2000.
34. Godaert GLR, Hartkamp A, Geenen R, et al: Fatigue in daily life in patients with primary Sjögren's syndrome and systemic lupus erythematosus: neuroendocrine immune basis of the rheumatic disease II. Ann Acad 966:320, 2002.
35. van Barr ME, Dekker J, Lemmens AL, et al: Pain and disability in patients with osteoporosis of hip or knee: the relationship with articular, kinesiological, and psychological characteristics. J Rheumatol 25:125, 1998.
36. Wolfe F: The fibromyalgia problem. J Rheumatol 24:1247, 1997.
37. Gervais RO, Russell AS, Green P,et al: Effort testing in patients with fibromyalgia and disability incentives. J Rheumatol 28:1892, 2001.
38. Ouguchi Y, Yoshida H: Sparing effect of hemiparesis on palindromic rheumatism. Clin Rheumatol 16:204, 1997.
39. Veldhuizen JW, Verstappen FT, Vroemen JP, et al: Functional and morphological adaptations following four weeks of knee immobilization. Int J Sports Med 14:283, 1993.
40. Van den Ende CHM, Vliet Vlietland TPM, Munneke M, Hazes JMW: Dynamic exercise for treating rheumatoid arthritis (Cochrane Review). Cochrane Library Issue 4, 2003.
41. Alexanderson H, Stenstrom CH, Jenner G, Lundberg I: The safety of a resistive home exercise program in patients with recent onset active polymyositis or dermatomyositis. Scand J Rheum 29:295, 2000.
42. Ramsey-Goldman R, Schilling EM, Dunlop D, et al: A pilot study on the effects of exercise in patients with systemic lupus erythematosus. Arthritis Care Res 13:262, 2000.
43. O'Reilly SC, Jones A, Muir KR, Doherty M: Quadriceps weakness in knee osteoarthritis: the effect on pain and disability. Ann Rheum Dis 57:588, 1998.
44. Robben SGF, Lequin MH, Meradji M, et al: Atrophy of the quadriceps muscle in children with a painful hip. Clin Physiol 19:385, 1999.
45. Bolgla LAA, Keskula DR: A review of the relationship among knee effusion, quadriceps inhibition and knee function. J Sport Rehab 9:160, 2000.
46. Hakkinen A, Sokka T, Kotaniemi A, Hannonen P: A randomized two-year study of the effects of dynamic strength training on muscle strength, disease activity, functional capacity, and bone mineral density in early rheumatoid arthritis. Arthritis Rheum 44:515, 2001.
47. Alexander NB, Galecki AT, Grenier ML, et al: Task-specific resistance training to improve the ability of activities of daily living: impaired older adults to rise from a ced and from a chair. J Am Geriatr Soc 49:1418, 2001.
48. Stamm TA, Machold KP, Smolen JS, et al: Joint protection and home hand exercises improve hand function in patients with hand osteoarthritis: a randomized controlled trial. Arthritis Care Res 47:44, 2002.
49. Fransen M, McConnell S, Bell M: Therapeutic exercise for people with osteoarthritis of the hip or knee. J Rheumatol 29:1737, 2002.
50. Thomas KS, Muir KR, Doherty M, et al: Home based exercise programme for knee pain and knee osteoarthritis: randomized controlled trial. BMJ 325:1, 2002.
51. Hauer K, Specht N, Schuler M, et al: Intensive physical training in geriatric patients after severe falls and hip surgery. Age Ageing 31:49, 2002.
52. Vandervoort AA: Aging of the human neuromuscular system. Muscle Nerve 25:17, 2002.
53. Iellamo F, Legramante JM, Raimondi G, et al: Effects of isokinetic, isotonic submaximal exercise on heart rate and blood pressure. Euro J Applied Physiol Occupat Physiol 75:89, 1997.
54. van den Ende CHM, Breedveld FC, le Cessie S, et al: Effect of intensive exercise on patients with active rheumatoid arthritis: a randomised clinical trial. Ann Rheum Dis 59:615, 2000.
55. DeLateur B, Lehman JF, Warren CG, et al: Comparison of effectiveness of isokinetic and isotonic exercise in quadriceps strengthening. Arch Phys Med Rehabil 53:60-64, 1972.
56. DeLateur B, Lehman J, Stonebridge J, et al: Isotonic versus isometric exercise: a double-shift transfer-of-training study. Arch Phys Med Rehabil 53:212-226, 1972.
57. Lieberson WT: Brief isometric exercises. *In* Basmajian J (ed): Therapeutic Exercise, ed 4. Baltimore, Williams and Wilkins, 1984, pp 236-256.
58. Biundo JJ, Hughes GM: Rheumatoid arthritis rehabilitation: practical guidelines. I. J Musculoskel Med 8(6):85-96, 1991.
59. Brox JI, Gjengedal E, Uppheim G, et al: Arthroscopic surgery versus supervised exercises in patients with rotator cuff disease (stage II impingement syndrome): a prospective, randomized, controlled study in 125 patients with a 2 ½ year follow-up. J Shoulder Elbow Surg 8:102, 1999.
60. Kraag G, Stokes B, Groh J, et al: The effects of comprehensive home physiotherapy and supervision on patients with ankylosing spondylitis: an 8 month follow up. J Rheum 21:261-3, 1994.
61. Sweeney S, Taylor G, Calin A: The effect of a home based exercise intervention package on outcome in ankylosing spondylitis: a randomized controlled trial. J Rheumatol 29(4): 763-766, 2002.
62. Uhrin Z, Kuzis S, Ward MM: Exercise and changes in health status in patients with ankylosing spondylitis. Arch Intern Med 160:2969, 2000.
63. Baaker C, Hidding A, van der Linden S, et al: Cost effectiveness of group physical therapy compared to individualized therapy for ankylosing spondylitis: a randomized controlled trial. J Rheum 21:264-8, 1994.
64. Rasmussen JO, Hansen TM: Physical training for patients with ankylosing spondylitis. Arthritis Care Res 2:25-27, 1989.
65. Santos H, Brophy S, Calin A: Exercise in ankylosing spondylitis: How much is optimum? J Rheumatol 25:2156, 1998.
66. Basmajian JV: Exercises in water. *In* Basmajian JV(ed): Therapeutic Exercise, 4th ed. Williams & Wilkins, 1984, pp 303-308.
67. Philadelphia panel evidence-based clinical practice guidelines on selected rehabilitation interventions for shoulder pain. Phys Ther 81:1719, 2001.
68. Robinson V, Brosseau L, Casimiro L, et al: Thermotherapy for treating rheumatoid arthritis (Cochrane Review). Cochrane Library Issue 4, 2003.
69. Zink A, Listing J, Ziemer S, Zeidler H Practice variation in the treatment of rheumatoid arthritis among German rheumatologists. J Rheum 28:2201, 2001.
70. Buljina AI, Taljanovic MS, Avdic DM, Hunter TB: Physical and exercise therapy for treatment of the rheumatoid hand. Arthritis Care Res 45:392, 2001.
71. Beurskens AJ, De Vet HC, Koke AJ, et al: Efficacy of traction for nonspecific low back pain. Spine 23:2756, 1997.
72. Turner JA, Deyo RA, Loeser JD, et al: The importance of placebo effects in pain treatment and research. JAMA 271:1609-1614, 1994.
73. Martin SS, Spindler KP, Tarter JW, et al: Cryotherapy: an effective modality for decreasing intraarticular temperature after knee arthroscopy. Am J Sports Med 29:288, 2001.
74. Ohkoshi Y, Ohkoshi M, Nagasaki S, et al: The effect of cryotherapy on intraarticular temperature and postoperative care after anterior cruciate ligament reconstruction. Am J Sports Med 27(3): 357-362, 1999.
75. Martin SS, Spindler KP, Tarter JW, Detwiler KB: Does cryotherapy affect intraarticular temperature after knee arthroscopy? Clin Orthop Rel Res 400:184, 2002.
76. Warren CG, Lehmann JF, Koblanski JN: Heat and stretch procedures: evaluation using rat tail tendon. Arch Phys Med Rehabil 57:122-126, 1976.
77. Price R, Lehmann JF, Boswell-Bessette S, et al: Influence of cryotherapy on spasticity at the human ankle. Arch Phys Med Rehabil 74:300, 1993.
78. Schlesinger N, Detry MA, Holland BK, et al: Local ice therapy during bouts of acute gouty arthritis. J Rheumatol 29, 331, 2002.
79. Oosterveld FGJ, Rasker JJ: Effects of local heat and cold treatment on surface and articular temperature of arthritic knees. Arthritis Rheum 37:1578-1582, 1994.
80. Oosterveld FGJ, Rasker JJ, Jacobs WG, et al: The effect of local heat and cold therapy on the intraarticular and skin surface temperature of the knee. Arthritis Rheum 35:146-151, 1992.
81. Bocobo C, Fast A, Kingery W, et al: The effect of ice on intra-articular temperature of the dog. Am J Phys Med Rehabil 70:181-185, 1991.
82. Mainardi CL, Walter JM, Spiegel PK, et al: Rheumatoid arthritis: failure of daily heat therapy to affect its progression. Arch Phys Med Rehab 60:390-393, 1979.

83. Dellhag B, Wollersjo I, Bjelle A: Effect of active hand exercise and wax bath treatment in rheumatoid arthritis patients. Arthritis Care Res. 5:87-92, 1992.
84. Peter RU, Meurer M: Back pain as a risk factor for azoospermia: it's not the pain, it's hot baths. Arch Androl 28:71, 1992.
85. Van Tubergen A, Landewe R, Van der Heijde D, et al: Combined spa-exercise therapy is effective in patients with ankylosing spondylitis: a randomized controlled trial. Arthritis Care & Research 45:430, 2001.
86. van Tubergen A, van der Linden: A brief history of spa therapy. Ann Rheum Dis 61:273, 2002.
87. Lineker SC, Badley EM, Hawker G, Wilkins A: Determining sensitivity to change in outcome measures used to evaluate hydrotherapy exercise programs for people with rheumatic diseases. Arthritis Care Res 13:62, 2000.
88. Green S, Buchbinder R, Glazier R, Forbes A: Systemic review of randomized controlled trials of interventions for painful shoulder: selection criteria, outcome assessment, and efficacy. BMJ 316:354, 1998.
89. Casimiro L, Brosseau L, Robinson V, et al: Therapeutic ultrasound for the treatment of rheumatoid arthritis (Cochrane Review). Cochrane Library Issue 4, 2003.
90. Biundo JJ, Hughes GM: Rheumatoid arthritis rehabilitation: practical guidelines.II. J Musculoskel Med 8(7):37-46, 1991.
91. Milne S, Welch V, Brosseau L, et al: Transcutaneous electrical nerve stimulation (TENS) for chronic low back pain. Cochrane Library Issue 4, 2003.
92. Pelland L, Brosseau L, Casimiro L, et al: Electrical stimulation for the treatment of rheumatoid arthritis (Cochrane Review). Cochrane Library Issue 4, 2003.
93. Woodburn J, Barker S, Helliwell PS: A randomized controlled trial of foot orthoses in rheumatoid arthritis. J Rheumatol 29:1377, 2002.
94. Barnett SL, Bagley AM, Skinner HB: Ankle weight effect on gait: orthotic implications. Orthopedics 16:1127-31, 1993.
95. Pagnotta, A, Baron M, Korner-Bitensky N: The effect of a static wrist orthosis on hand function in individuals with rheumatoid arthritis. J Rheumatol 25:879, 1998.
96. Callinan NJ, Mathiowetz V: Soft versus hard resting hand splints in rheumatoid arthritis: pain relief, preference, and compliance. Am J Occupat Ther 50:347, 1996.
97. Tijhuid GJ, Vlieland TPMV, Zwinderman AH, Hazes JMW: A comparison of the future wrist orthosis with a synthetic ThermoLyn orthosis: utility and clinical effectiveness. Arthritis Care Res 11:217, 1998.
98. Sandler AJ, Dvrak J, Humke T, et al: The effectiveness of various cervical orthoses: an in vivo comparison of the mechanical stability provided by several widely used models. Spine 21:1624, 1996.
99. Nordenskiold U, Grimby G, Dahlin-Ivanoff S: Questionnaire to evaluate the effects of assistive devices and altered working methods in women with rheumatoid arthritis. Clin Rheumatol 17:6, 1998.
100. Nordenskiold U, Grimby G, Hedberg M, et al: The structure of an instrument for assessing the effects of assistive devices and altered working methods in women with rheumatoid arthritis. Arthritis Care Res 9:358, 1996.
101. Waters RL, Mulroy S: The energy expenditure of normal and pathologic gait. Gait Posture 9:207, 1999.
102. Kannus P, Parkkari J, Niemi S, et al: Prevention of hip fracture in elderly people with the use of a hip protector. New Engl J Med 343:1506, 2000.
103. McGibbon CA, Krebs DE, Mann RW: In vivo hip pressures during cane and load carrying. Arthritis Care Res 10:300, 1997.
104. Kumar R, Roe MC, Scremin OU: Methods for estimating the proper length of a cane. Arch Phys Med Rehab 76:1173, 1995.
105. Hoberman M, Basmajian JV: Crutch and cane exercises and use. *In* Basmajian JV (ed): Therapeutic Exercise, ed. 4. Baltimore, Williams & Wilkins, 1984, pp 267-284.
106. Foley MP, Prax B, Browell R, Boone T: Effects of assistive devices on cardiorespiratory demands in older adults. Phys Ther 76:1313, 1996.
107. Brooks LL, Wertsch JJ, Duthie EH Jr: Use of devices for mobility by the elderly. Wisconsin Med J 93:16-20, 1994.
108. Berg K, Hines M, Allen S: Wheelchair users at home: few home modifications and many injurious falls. Am J Public Health 92:48, 2002.
109. Ummat S, Kirby RL: Nonfatal wheelchair-related accidents reported to the National Electronic Injury Surveillance System. Am J Phys Med Rehab 73:163-167, 1994.
110. Gitlin LN, Mann W, Tomit M, Marcus SM: Factors associated with home environment problems among community-living older people 23:777, 2001.
111. Alexander NB, Koester DJ, Grunawalt JA: Chair design affects how older adults rise from a chair. J Am Geriatr Soc 44:356, 1996.
112. Hill J, Bird H, Johnson S: Effect of patient education on adherence to drug treatment for rheumatoid arthritis: a randomised controlled trial. Ann Rheum Dis 60:869, 2001.
113. Bell MJ, Lineker SC, Wilkins AL, et al: A randomized controlled trial to evaluate the efficacy of community based physical therapy in the treatment of people with rheumatoid arthritis. J Rheumatol 25:231, 1998.
114. Lubrano E, Helliwell P, Parsons W, et al: Patient education in psoriatic arthritis: a cross sectional study on knowledge by a validated self-administered questionnaire. J Rheumatol 25:1560, 1998.

56 Nonsteroidal Anti-Inflammatory Drugs

LESLIE J. CROFFORD

The use of nonsteroidal anti-inflammatory drugs (NSAIDs) is ubiquitous in the practice of medicine because of their effectiveness as anti-inflammatory, analgesic, and antipyretic agents. NSAIDs differ widely in their chemical class, but they share the property of blocking production of prostaglandins. This is accomplished by inhibiting the activity of the enzyme prostaglandin H synthase (PGHS), also called cyclooxygenase (COX).

In recent years, important progress has been made toward understanding the clinical effects of NSAIDs by clarifying prostaglandin biosynthetic pathways. This advance came with the discovery of COX-2, the isoform whose expression is increased during inflammation. Specific inhibition of COX-2 blocks prostaglandin production at sites of inflammation while preserving production via COX-1 in certain other tissues, most importantly platelets and the gastroduodenal mucosa. The therapeutic and adverse actions of nonspecific NSAIDs compared to COX-2–specific NSAIDs can be understood in terms of the biology of prostaglandin production and action.

In addition to their use in rheumatoid arthritis (RA) and osteoarthritis (OA), NSAIDs are widely used in the symptomatic management of other rheumatic diseases characterized by chronic musculoskeletal pain and diverse forms of acute pain (e.g., headache, dysmenorrhea, postoperative pain). Aspirin is used by millions more for primary and secondary prevention of cardiovascular thrombosis. Therapeutic application of NSAIDs as chemopreventive agents for cancer is under investigation. In light of the widespread use of these drugs for common diseases, which is likely to increase in prevalence with the aging of the population, it is critically important to appreciate the potential adverse events and drug interactions associated with NSAIDs.

This chapter reviews the class characteristics of the COX-2–specific and nonspecific NSAIDs. acetaminophen (paracetamol), an antipyretic and analgesic drug without anti-inflammatory activity, inhibits COX enzymes by a different mechanism than NSAIDs and will also be discussed. Colchicine possesses anti-inflammatory characteristics similar to those of NSAIDs in some situations and will be discussed in this chapter, although it differs in its mechanism of action and profile of adverse effects.

History

Botanicals containing salicylates have been used since antiquity to treat pain, inflammation, and fever. About 3500 years ago, the Egyptian Ebers papyrus recommended use of a decoction of dried myrtle leaves applied to the abdomen and back for relief of rheumatic pains. About 1000 years later, Hippocrates recommended poplar tree juices for eye disease treatment and willow bark to alleviate fever and the pain of childbirth. Throughout Roman times, the use of botanical treatments, including willow bark, for pain and inflammation was recommended. The medicinal use of salicylate-containing plants also occurred in China and other parts of Asia. In addition, the curative effects of other botanicals were known to the indigenous populations of North America. Colchicine-containing extracts of the autumn crocus plant were used for treatment of acute gout as early as the sixth century A.D.[1,2]

The first modern report of the therapeutic application salicylate-containing plants was reported to the Royal Society of London by the Reverend Edward Stone, who provided an account of the success of the dried bark of the willow for fever.[1] Salicylate was identified as the active ingredient of willow bark by Leroux in 1929 and synthesized in its pure form in Germany in 1860.[1,3] The bitter taste of salicylic acid prompted the chemist Felix Hoffman in 1860 to synthesize the more palatable acetylsalicylic acid. After demonstration of its anti-inflammatory effects, Dr. Heinrich Dreser of Bayer introduced this compound into medicine in 1899 as aspirin, and it remains the most widely used drug in the world.[1]

Phenylbutazone came into clinical practice in 1949 and was followed by indomethacin, fenamates, naproxen, and others. Despite the diversity of their chemical structures, these drugs share therapeutic properties with aspirin. Furthermore, adverse events, including gastric upset, gastrointestinal (GI) ulceration and bleeding, hypertension, edema, and renal damage are also shared by all these drugs. As stated by Sir John Vane, "When a chemically diverse group of drugs all share the same therapeutic qualities and the same side effects, it is fairly certain that the actions of those drugs are based on a single biochemical intervention."[1] The discovery in 1971 that each of the chemically diverse members of this large group of drugs all act by inhibiting prostaglandin biosynthesis provided a unifying explanation of their therapeutic actions.[1]

The enzyme inhibited by these drugs, PGHS or COX, was isolated in 1976 from the endoplasmic reticulum of prostaglandin-forming cells.[4] An inducible COX activity was predicted in 1990 based on the observation of a cellular COX induced by endotoxin and suppressed by dexamethasone in mice.[5] In 1991, the second isoform of COX was cloned and characterized as a gene product induced by inflammatory or mitogenic stimuli.[6]

Because of the prediction that inhibiting COX-2 would block prostaglandin biosynthesis participating in the inflammatory response, but not prostanoids required for homeostasis, there was a tremendous push to develop drugs that specifically inhibit COX-2. This was accomplished with astonishing speed as existing NSAIDs were tested for differential inhibition of the two COX isoforms, and crystal structures revealed differences in the protein structures on which new drug development could be based.[7] By 1999, 100 years after aspirin was introduced, two drugs that specifically inhibit COX-2, celecoxib and rofecoxib, were approved for treatment of arthritis and pain.

Cyclooxygenase Biology

Therapeutic and adverse effects of NSAIDs are best understood in the context of COX biology. The COX enzymes are the first committed step in the synthesis of prostaglandins from arachidonic acid (Fig. 56–1). Arachidonate is a 20-carbon–containing polyunsaturated fatty acid cleaved from the *sn*-2 position of cell membrane glycerophospholipids by one of several different phospholipase A_2 enzymes.[8] Although the synthesis of prostaglandins is regulated acutely by activation of phospholipases and release of arachidonate, the net level of individual prostanoids is determined by expression of COX and terminal synthase enzymes.

PROSTAGLANDIN PRODUCTION AND ACTION

Prostaglandins act as autocrine and paracrine mediators with effects limited to the immediate vicinity of their synthetic sites. For this reason, all of the enzymes required for production of a specific prostanoid must be localized at its site of action, and the receptor mediating the action of this prostanoid be locally available.[9] The diversity of prostaglandin actions is due to the wide range of stable prostaglandins generated from arachidonic acid, but most cell types produce only one or a few of the possible prostanoids depending on the terminal prostaglandin synthases expressed.[6] Prostaglandin E_2 (PGE_2), the most abundant prostaglandin at sites of inflammation such as arthritis, can be produced by many different cell types via at least three different PGE synthases.[10-12] Expression of the inducible form of PGE synthase, microsomal PGE synthase-1 (mPGES-1), is similar to expression of COX-2, and mPGES-1 may act in concert with COX-2 to produce high levels of PGE_2 during inflammation.[13-15] Prostaglandins are released from cells predominantly by facilitated transport through a prostaglandin transporter of the organic anion transporter polypeptide family, and possibly by other transporters.[16]

The actions of prostaglandins are local due to their evanescent nature and are mediated by cell surface G protein–coupled receptors (GPCR). There are at least nine known prostaglandin receptors, with additional splice variants.[17] The prostaglandin receptors

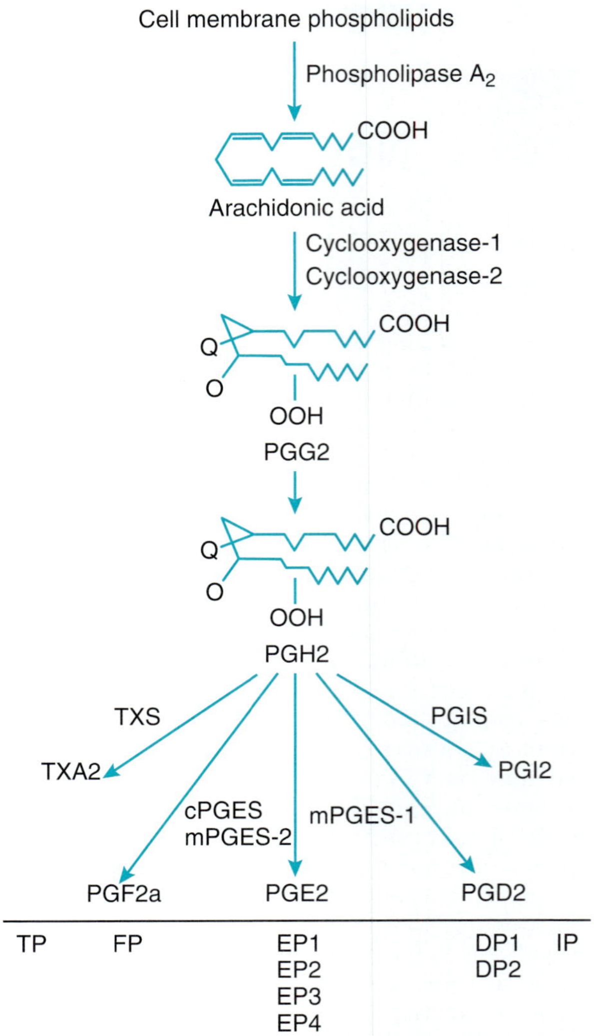

FIGURE 56–1 • Prostaglandin Biosynthetic Pathway. Arachidonic acid is released from cell membrane phospholipids, usually nuclear membrane or perinuclear endoplasmic reticulum, by phospholipase A_2. Cyclooxygenase(COX)-1 or COX-2 catalyzes formation of cyclic endoperoxides. Prostaglandin (PG) H_2, an unstable intermediate, is further metabolized to stable prostaglandins by synthase enzymes. These bioactive prostaglandins interact with G protein–coupled receptors. cPGES, cytosolic prostaglandin E synthase; DP, prosta-glandin D receptor; EP, prostaglandin E receptor; FP, prostaglandin $F_{2\alpha}$ receptor; IP, prostacyclin receptor; mPGES, microsomal prostaglandin E synthase; PGDS, prostaglandin D synthase, both hematopoietic and neuronal forms exist; PGIS, prostacyclin synthase; TP, thromboxane receptor; TXS, thromboxane synthase.

belong to three clusters within a distinct subfamily of the GPCR superfamily, with the lone exception of one of the PGD_2 receptors (DP_2), which belongs to the chemokine receptor subfamily. The relaxant receptors for prostacyclin (IP), PGD_2 (DP_1), and PGE_2 (EP_2 and EP_4) signal through G_s-mediated increases in intracellular cyclic adenosine monophosphate (cAMP). The contractile receptors for thromboxane A_2 (TP), $PGF_{2\alpha}$ (FP), and PGE_2 (EP_1) signal through a G_q-mediated increase in intracellular calcium. An inhibitory receptor for PGE_2 (EP_3) couples to G_i and decreases cAMP formation. Note that PGE_2 has at least four different receptors with a broad range of potential actions.

BIOCHEMISTRY AND STRUCTURAL BIOLOGY

COX-1 and COX-2 are bifunctional enzymes that mediate a COX reaction whereby arachidonate plus two molecules of O_2 are converted to the cyclic endoperoxide PGG_2, followed by a hydroperoxidase reaction in which PGG_2 undergoes a two-electron reduction to PGH_2.[8] COX enzymes are integral membrane proteins that sit within the inner leaflet of the lipid bilayer of intracellular phospholipid membranes of the nuclear envelope and the endoplasmic reticulum. COX-1 and COX-2 are 70- to 72-kD proteins with multiple N-glycosylation sites.[6] The crystal structures of COX-1 and COX-2 have been solved, and they have essentially identical domain structures (Fig. 56–2).[7] The COX enzymes are homodimers, with each monomer consisting of three structural domains. The epidermal growth factor–like domain located at the N-terminus is likely to be involved in dimerization. The membrane-binding domain consists of four amphipathic α-helices that are inserted into one half of the lipid bilayer. These α-helices are arranged to form an entrance to a hydrophobic channel in the center of the large, globular catalytic domain.

COX and hydroperoxidase reactions occur at distinct but structurally and functionally interconnected sites. The peroxidase activity occurs at a heme-containing site located near the protein surface, whereas the COX reaction occurs in the hydrophobic core of the enzyme. The COX reaction is peroxide-dependent and requires that the heme group at the peroxidase site undergo a two-electron oxidation. A tyrosine residue located at the cyclooxygenase active site is involved as a reaction intermediate.[8] The physiological heme oxidant in vivo is not known, but it has been shown that the COX activity of COX-2 can be activated at tenfold lower concentrations of hydroperoxide than that of COX-1.[8] NSAIDs function by blocking access of arachidonic acid to the COX active site within the hydrophobic channel.

Most of the amino acids that form the hydrophobic channel of the COX-1 and COX-2 molecules are identical, with the exception of the substitution of the small amino acid valine in COX-2 for the isoleucine with a bulky side chain in COX-1 at position 523 (Fig. 56–3). This substitution opens a side pocket to the hydrophobic channel in COX-2 and was found to be critical for the development of drugs that specifically inhibit COX-2.[7] The interaction of arachidonic acid with COX-1 and COX-2 may also be different, as demonstrated by experiments in which different amino acid substitutions are made for the arginine at position 120, located at the mouth of the hydrophobic channel.[8] It is likely that an ionic bond with arachidonate is formed in COX-1 and a hydrogen bond is formed in COX-2 Overall, COX-2 has a wider and somewhat more flexible interior channel that has been exploited for the development of specific inhibitors.

MOLECULAR BIOLOGY

The most striking difference between the COX isoforms is in their expression and regulation (Table 56–1).[18] COX-1 is constitutively expressed in most cells, and its expression is not altered by inflammatory stimuli. The promoter region of COX-1 has the characteristics of a gene that is continuously transcribed and stably expressed. COX-1 is available to increase prostaglandin production acutely when an abrupt increase in arachidonic acid substrate occurs. COX-1 is the only isoform expressed in mature platelets and is the dominant isoform in normal gastroduodenal mucosa.[18]

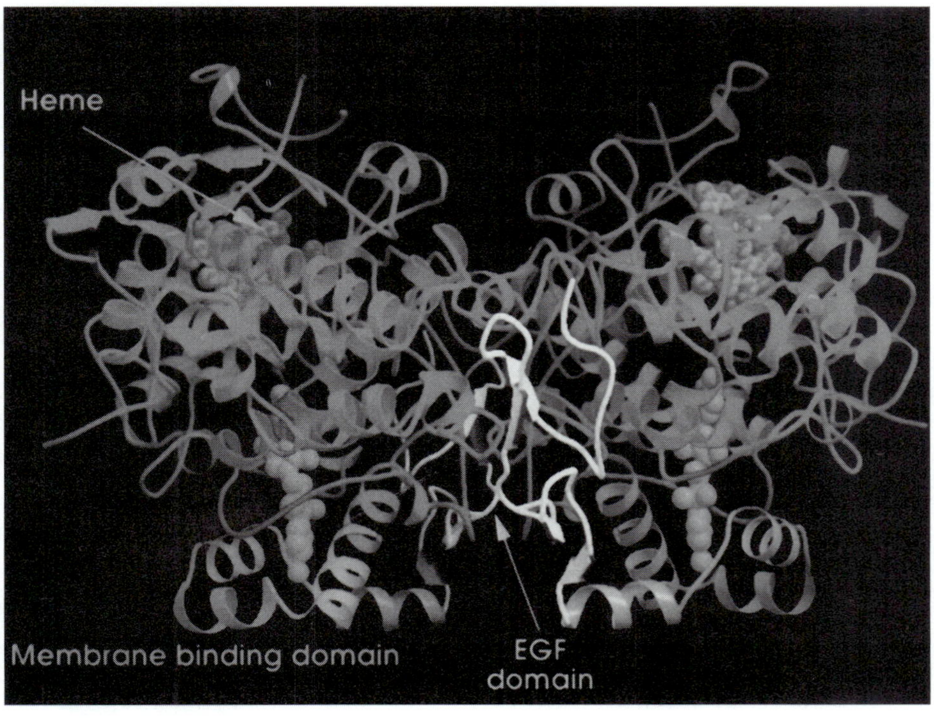

FIGURE 56–2 · Crystal Structure of the Cyclooxygenase (COX)-2 Dimer. The axis of dimerization is in the middle of this representation. The COX site is in the center of the globular domain, marked by the location of a COX-2 inhibitor shown as a space-filling model. The peroxidase site is adjacent to the heme. Reprinted with permission from Browner MF: X-ray crystal structure of human cyclooxygenase-2. *In* Bazan N, Botting J, and Vane J (eds): New Targets in Inflammation. Kluwer Academic Publishers and William Harvey Press, London, 1996.

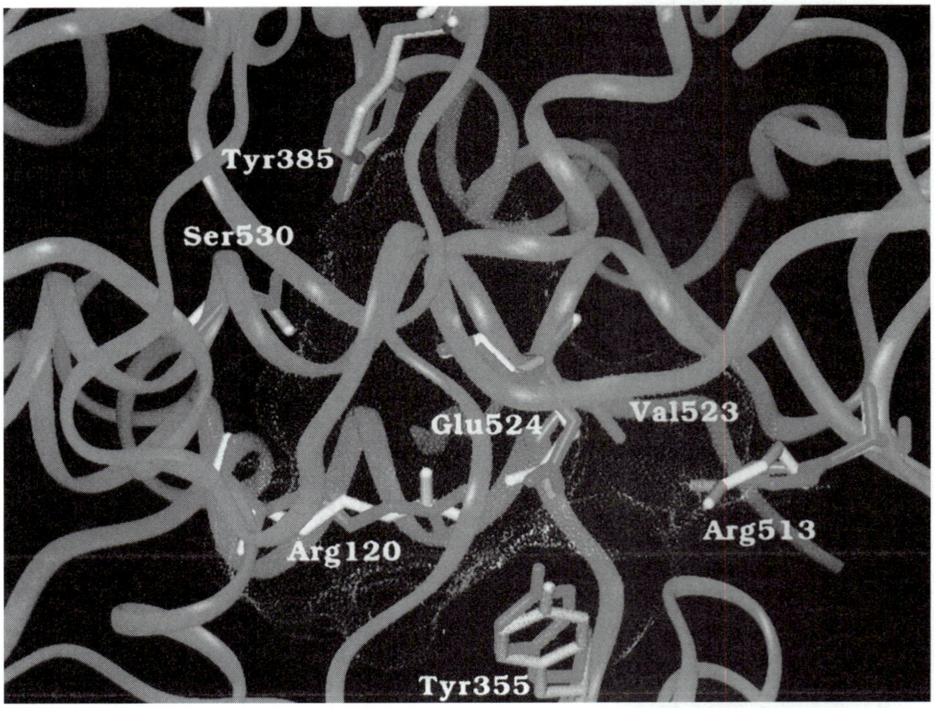

FIGURE 56–3 • Hydrophobic Channel of Cyclooxygenase (COX)-2. Close up view of the nonsteroidal anti-inflammatory drug (NSAID) binding site of COX-2. The ribbon diagram for COX-2 is shown, with side chains of the specified amino acids and their positions in COX-2. The dotted white surface indicates the size and shape of the NSAID binding site of COX-2. Reprinted with permission from Browner MF: X-ray crystal structure of human cyclooxygenase-2. *In* Bazan N, Botting J, and Vane J (eds): New Targets in Inflammation. Kluwer Acade-mic Publishers and William Harvey Press, London, 1996.

COX-2 has the structure of a highly regulated gene product with binding sites for transcription factors, such as nuclear factor-κB (NF-κB) and activating protein-1 (AP-1), that rapidly increase transcription in response to inflammatory signals.[18] As anticipated from analysis of the COX-2 promoter, COX-2 expression is highly induced by proinflammatory cytokines (e.g., tumor necrosis factor-α and interleukin-1β), microbial products (e.g., lipopolysaccharide), and mitogens (e.g., phorbol ester and growth factors).[8,18] Increased levels of COX-2 mRNA are seen as early as 15 to 30 min after a stimulus, and protein levels increase in 1 to 2 hours. Similar to other proteins involved in inflammation, COX-2 expression is inhibited by glucocorticoids.[18] Another feature of the COX-2 gene important in its regulation is the presence of multiple AUUUA instability sequences in the 3′ region that promote rapid degradation of the mRNA. One mechanism by which interleukin-1β increases COX-2 expression is by interfering with post-transcriptional regulation.[19]

Although the role of COX-2 in inflammation is now clear, there is a growing awareness that COX-2 is expressed

TABLE 56–1 • EXPRESSION AND REGULATION OF CYCLOOXYGENASE (COX) ISOFORMS

	COX-1	COX-2
Inflammation, Tissue Damage and Repair	**Constitutive.** Acutely increased prostaglandin (PG) production. No change during inflammation or damage.	**Induced.** Mediates inflammatory symptoms, role in resolution and repair in normal physiology.
Gastrointestinal Tract	**Constitutive.** Cytoprotection of normal gastroduodenal mucosa.	**Induced.** Increased by inflammation and injury, important for mucosal defense in the colon. Increased in colonic adenomas and adenocarcinoma.
Kidney	**Constitutive.** Expressed in vasculature, glomerulus, medullary collecting ducts. Role in glomerular filtration rate (GFR) and solute homeostasis.	**Constitutive.** Expressed in vasculature, macula densa, medullary interstitium. Role in GFR, renin secretion, and solute homeostasis. **Induced.** In glomerulus during inflammation, and in macula densa with salt/water deprivation.
Cardiovascular	**Constitutive.** Platelet thromboxane production, activation, hemostasis/thrombosis, vasoconstriction.	**Constitutive.** Prostacyclin production in normal arteries, inhibits platelet activation, vasodilation. **Induced.** In atherosclerosis, vasculitis.
Reproductive	**Constitutive.** Null mice are fertile.	**Induced.** Acute increase during ovulation, implantation, parturition.
Bone	**Constitutive.** Role unclear.	**Induced.** Osteoclastogenesis, endochondrol bone formation.
Pulmonary	**Constitutive.** Counterbalances leukotriene synthesis in aspirin-enhanced respiratory disease.	**Constitutive/Induced.** May provide protective PGs during lung remodeling.

constitutively in several organ systems and regulated by physiologic as well as pathologic stimuli. The most important sites of basal COX-2 expression are the brain and kidney.[20,21] COX-2 plays an important role in normal reproductive, renal, cardiovascular, and skeletal physiology.[18,22-24]

Mechanism of Action

The cardinal manifestations of inflammation include rubor (redness), calor (warmth), tumor (swelling), and dolor (pain). These signs result predominantly from the local effects of inflammatory mediators, including prostaglandins. However, pain is generated as a consequence of both peripheral and central mechanisms, and there is increasing evidence that prostaglandin production in the spinal cord and brain may be important mediators of pain. Fever is generated by hypothalamic centers as a consequence of increased circulating endogenous pyrogens. NSAIDs and acetaminophen function as antipyretic and analgesic agents by virtue of actions in the central nervous system (CNS).

CYCLOOXYGENASE INHIBITION

The most important mechanism of NSAID action is to inhibit production of prostaglandins by competing with arachidonic acid for binding in the COX catalytic site[8,25] (see Fig. 56–3). NSAIDs exhibit different kinetic modes of inhibition: 1) rapid, reversible binding; 2) time-dependent, slowly reversible binding; and 3) covalent modification as exhibited by aspirin.[8] Time-dependent inhibition of COX enzymes appears to depend on the arginine at position 120 near the entrance to the hydrophobic channel, which serves as the counter ion for the carboxylate group of many nonspecific NSAIDs. Time-dependent inhibition of COX-2 by specific inhibitors appears to depend on the arginine at position 513 located in the side pocket of the hydrophobic channel. Many NSAIDs are optical isomers or enantiomers in which the S-, but not the R-, enantiomers are active COX inhibitors. The tyrosine at position 355 near the closed end of the hydrophobic channel governs the stereospecificity of NSAIDs.[8] Aspirin covalently acetylates the serine at position 530 in the hydrophobic channel. Serine 530 is important in positioning arachidonic acid with respect to the tyrosine 385 radical of the COX active site. Aspirin acetylated COX-1 forms no eicosanoid product.[8] However, due to the wider hydrophobic channel of COX-2, aspirin acetylation results in formation of alternate eicosanoid products including anti-inflammatory lipoxins.[26]

CYCLOOXYGENASE-2 SPECIFICITY

All currently available COX-2–specific NSAIDs exhibit time-dependent inhibition of COX-2. The specificity for COX-2 is based on the structural difference between the hydrophobic channels of COX-1 and COX-2, with the NSAID binding site being about 20 percent larger than COX-1 and also including the side pocket. The specific COX-2 inhibitors contain a bulky sulfa-containing side chain that fits into the side pocket. Mutagenesis of COX-1 to create access to the side pocket completely abrogates differential sensitivity of specific inhibitors.[7]

Most NSAIDs inhibit COX-1 and COX-2 to a similar extent. COX-2 specificity can be determined in a number of ways. The ability of a drug to inhibit a COX enzyme is expressed as the IC_{50}, the concentration that inhibits 50 percent of prostanoid synthesis in the assay system. Calculation of a COX-2 to COX-1 ratio (i.e., the ratio of the IC_{50} value for COX-2 divided by the IC_{50} value for COX-1) can provide a standard for comparing the selectivity of an NSAID for one or the other of the isoforms.[27] However, caution must be used when interpreting in vitro assays because comparisons are limited by the variability in the assay conditions (e.g., purified enzymes, intact cell systems, cells transfected with recombinant enzymes, animal models, whole blood assay systems).[27-29] Some of these differences reflect characteristics of the study agents, such as protein binding and lipophilicity, which differentially affect the free drug concentration or the drug's ability to access the COX enzyme in each assay system. Others reflect the assay conditions themselves, such as the duration and temperature of incubation. Some of the differences may be related to the animal species from which the cells or COX enzymes for the assay were taken, because COX enzymes are not completely conserved among mammals.

The most widely accepted definition of a specific COX-2 inhibitor is based on the in vitro whole blood assay[30] (Table 56–2). The magnitude of COX-1 inhibition is measured by determining the degree of inhibition of thromboxane produced by platelets after the sample is allowed to clot. In a heparinized blood sample, inhibition of COX-2 is determined by the degree of inhibition of PGE_2 after stimulation by lipopolysaccharide.[30] Specific COX-2 inhibitors lack inhibitory effect on platelet COX-1 at doses at or above those that maximally inhibit COX-2.[28,30]

TABLE 56–2 • IN VITRO* WHOLE BLOOD ASSAY FOR CYCLOOXYGENASE (COX) SPECIFICITY[30]

COX-1 Inhibition
Whole blood sample collected Drug added over a range of concentrations Blood allowed to clot × 60 min Serum thromboxane B_2 measured
COX-2 Inhibition
Whole blood sample collected and heparinized Drug added over a range of concentrations Blood treated with lipopolysaccharide (LPS) for 24 hr to induce COX-2 Plasma PGE_2 measured

*Ex vivo whole blood assays are performed by having human subjects ingest either a single dose or multiple doses of drug to achieve steady state, usually 7 days. Whole blood samples are collected, stimulated, and assayed as above. Ex vivo methodology takes pharmacologic variability into account but is rarely performed systematically.[30]

CYCLOOXYGENASE-INDEPENDENT MECHANISMS OF ACTION

COX-independent actions typically are seen only at very high doses, and their relevance to in vivo activity of most NSAIDs remains unclear. Various investigators have demonstrated, under carefully controlled in vitro conditions, that NSAIDs inhibit phosphodiesterase; this leads to potentiation of PGE_1-mediated increased intracellular cAMP levels and subsequent inhibition of proinflammatory cellular functions, peripheral blood lymphocyte responses to mitogen stimulation, neutrophil and monocyte migration, and various neutrophil functions.[3] NSAIDs inhibit the aggregation of human neutrophils in vitro and in vivo, as well as in cells of the marine sponge that do not contain COX and are unresponsive to stable prostaglandins.[31] NSAIDs may also scavenge radicals, inhibit superoxide generation by polymorphonuclear neutrophils (PMNs), inhibit mononuclear cell phospholipase C activity, and inhibit inducible nitric oxide synthase.[32] Salicylate may stimulate endogenous anti-inflammatory mechanisms. It has been shown that the anti-inflammatory effect of salicylate can be inhibited by an adenosine A_2 receptor antagonist in a murine model of inflammation, suggesting that salicylate may stimulate adenosine release.[33]

Sodium salicylate and aspirin also inhibit activation of the transcription factor NF-κB, suggesting another potentially important anti-inflammatory mechanism.[34] However, in mice genetically deficient for the p105 subunit of NF-κB, salicylates retain their anti-inflammatory activity.[33] Other NSAIDs, including inactive enantiomers of flurbiprofen, were also found to inhibit NF-κB.[35] There are reports that other cell-signaling molecules, such as mitogen-activated protein kinases and the transcription factor AP-1, may also be modulated by NSAIDs.[35] Some NSAIDs bind to and activate members of the peroxisome proliferator-activated receptor (PPAR) family and other intracellular receptors.[35] PPAR activation is thought to mediate anti-inflammatory activities.[36] Specific COX-2 inhibitors may have unique structural features that promote COX-independent apoptosis and angiogenesis.[37]

MECHANISM OF ACETAMINOPHEN ACTION

The mechanism of action of acetaminophen is not completely clear, but most believe that the antipyretic and analgesic actions of acetaminophen are due to inhibition of COX in the central nervous system. At therapeutic doses, acetaminophen does not inhibit COX in peripheral tissues, which could explain its very weak anti-inflammatory activity.[38] It has been shown that inhibition of recombinant COX by acetaminophen is dependent on hydroperoxide concentrations, which suggests a mechanism by which acetaminophen acts to reduce the active oxidized form of COX to the inactive form.[38,39] Peroxide levels are high in inflammatory sites but low in the CNS, possibly accounting for the site of acetaminophen activity in vivo. Other authors have speculated that alternatively spliced forms of COX-1 or COX-2 may be more sensitive to inhibition by acetaminophen.[40,41] These COX variants are present at higher levels in the CNS than in the periphery, which may account for the observed central site of activity for acetaminophen.

MECHANISM OF COLCHICINE ACTION

Colchicine appears to interfere predominantly with steps of the inflammatory response in which neutrophils play a central role.[3] Colchicine appears to act predominantly by interfering with the organization of the fibrillar microtubules involved in cell morphology and movement. This leads to disaggregation of microtubules and decreased neutrophil motility and chemotaxis. Furthermore, colchicine inhibits release of chemotactic factors (e.g., leukotriene B_4), formation of digestive vacuoles, and lysosomal degranulation.[42] This results in an inhibition of neutrophil migration into an area of inflammation and a reduction of the metabolic and phagocytic activity of the neutrophils already present. Clinically, this results in an interruption in the inflammatory process of gout and other neutrophil-dominated acute inflammatory diseases.

Pharmacology

NONSTEROIDAL ANTI-INFLAMMATORY DRUG CLASSIFICATION

The NSAIDs can be classified in several different ways: chemical class, plasma half-life, and COX-1/COX-2 inhibition. By chemical class, most are organic acids with relatively low pKa values, which may allow higher concentrations of active drug in inflamed tissue where the pH is lower[3] (Fig. 56–4). Generally, the lower the pKa, the shorter the half-life of an NSAID. However, nonacidic compounds such as nabumetone have well-documented anti-inflammatory effects. Plasma half-life has been commonly used for classifying NSAIDs, but the concentration of NSAIDs in the synovial fluid undergoes much less variation over the dosing interval and is sustained over a longer period than the plasma concentration. This means that many NSAIDs with a short half-life (Table 56–3) can be given less frequently than would be suggested by their plasma half-lives, and they can provide pain relief over a significant period.

NSAIDs with a longer half-life take a longer time to reach steady-state concentrations (Table 56–4). Drugs with a half-life of 12 hours or more can be administered once or twice daily. Because five half-lives are required to approach steady state, plasma concentrations of these drugs continue to rise for 3 days to several weeks, depending on the half-life, but thereafter tend to be fairly stable between doses. The long half-life allows ample time for equilibration of drug between plasma and synovial fluid, and synovial fluid concentrations of unbound drug usually are equal to those in plasma. The sum of the bound and unbound drug concentrations is lower in synovial fluid, reflecting the lower quantity of albumin in the fluid.

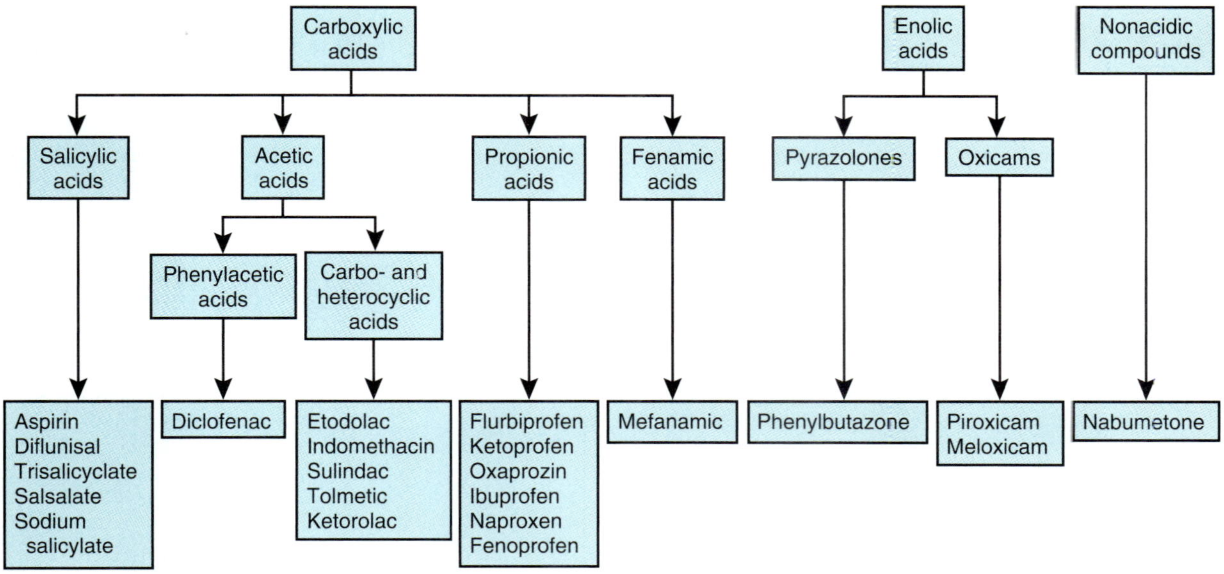

FIGURE 56–4 • Classification of nonspecific nonsteroidal anti-inflammatory drugs (NSAIDs) based on chemical class.

TABLE 56–3 • NONSTEROIDAL ANTI-INFLAMMATORY DRUGS (NSAIDS) WITH SHORT HALF-LIVES

Drug	Brand Name	Available Formulations (mg)	Maximal Daily Dose (mg)	T_{max} (hr)	T½ (hr)	Dose Adjustment or Special Precautions
Diclofenac	Voltaren, Voltaren XR, Cataflam	Tabs: 25, 50, 75 Extended release: 100	225	1-2	2	Incidence of increased transaminase levels higher than other NSAIDs.
Diclofenac + misoprostol	Arthrotec	Tabs: 50 or 75 Plus misoprostel 200 mcg	200	1-2	2	Incidence of increased transaminase levels higher than other NSAIDs.
Etodolac	Lodine, Lodine XL	Caps: 200,300 Tabs: 400 Extended release: 400, 500, 600	1200	1-2	6-7	
Fenoprofen	Nalfon	Caps: 200, 300, 600	3200	1-2	2-3	Idiosyncratic nephropathy more frequent than other NSAIDs.
Flurbiprofen	Ansaid	Tabs: 50, 100	300	1.5-2	3-4	
Ibuprofen	Motrin, Advil, Nupren, Rufen	Tabs: 200 (OTC), 300, 400, 600, 800	3200	1-2	2	Avoid in severe hepatic disease.
Indomethacin	Indocin, Indocin SR,	Caps: 25, 50 Sustained release: 75 Oral suspension: 25 mg/5 ml Suppositories: 50	200	1-4	2-13	Approved for treatment of patent ductus arteriosus.
Ketoprofen	Orudis, Oruvail,	Tabs: 12.5 (OTC), Caps: 25, 50, 75 Sustained release: 100, 150, 200	300	0.5-2	2-4	Decrease dose with severe renal disease, hepatic disease, elderly.
Ketorolac	Toradol	IM/IV: 15 or 30 mg/ml Tabs: 10	120 IV/IM 40 mg PO	0.3-1	4-6	Decrease dose by 50% in renal failure and in elderly patients. Do not use longer than 5 days.
Meclofenamate	Meclomen	Caps: 50, 100	400	0.5	2-3	
Tolmetin	Tolectin	Tabs: 200, 600 Caps: 400	1800	0.5-1	1-1.5	

Abbreviations: IM/IV, intramusscular-intravenous; PO, per Oral. Data taken from MICROMEDEX(R) Healthcare Series Vol. 119: Micromedex, Greenwood Village, CO. (Edition expires 3/2004.)

TABLE 56–4 • NONSTEROIDAL ANTI-INFLAMMATORY DRUGS (NSAIDS) WITH LONG HALF-LIVES

Drug	Brand Name	Available Formulations (mg)	Maximal Daily Dose (mg)	T_{max} (hr)	T½ (hr)	Dose Adjustment or Special Precautions
Celecoxib	Celebrex	Caps: 100, 200, 400	400 (800 mg in FAP)	3	11	Contraindicated with sulfonamide allergy.
Diflunisal	Dolobid	Tabs: 250, 500	1500	2-3	7-15	Decrease dose by 50% in renal failure.
Etoricoxib*	Arcoxia	Tabs: 30, 60	120	1-1.5	22	
Meloxicam	Mobic	Tab: 7.5	15	5-6	20	
Nabumetone	Relafen	Tabs: 500, 750	2000	3-6	24	Food increases peak concentration. Reduce dose in renal disease. Avoid in severe liver disease. Limit dose to 1 g/day in elderly.
Naproxen	Naprosyn, Aleve, Anaprox, EC-Naprosyn, Naprelan	Tabs: 125 (OTC), 250, 375, 500 Sustained release: 375, 500 Suspension: 125 mg/5 ml	1500	2-4	12-15	Decrease dose in renal disease, liver disease, and the elderly.
Oxaprozin	Daypro	Tabs: 600	1800 or 26 mg/kg/d	3-6	49-60	Decrease dose in renal failure and weight <50 kg.
Parecoxib*		IM/IV		<1-2.5	8	Prodrug metabolized to valdecoxib in <1 hr. Contraindicated with sulfonamide allergy.
Piroxicam	Feldene	Caps: 10, 20	20	2-5	3-86	Decrease dose in hepatic disease and elderly.
Rofecoxib	Vioxx	Tabs: 12.5, 25, 50 Suspension: 12.5 or 25 mg/5 ml	50	2-9	17	Dose of 50 mg/day for acute pain limited to 5 days. Caution in severe renal or liver diseases.
Sulindac	Clinoril	Tabs: 150, 200	400	2-4	16	Prodrug metabolized to active compound. Decrease dose in renal disease, liver disease, and the elderly.
Valdecoxib	Bextra	Tabs: 10, 20	20	1-3	8-11	Contraindicated with sulfonamide allergy. Caution in severe renal and liver disease.

Data taken from MICROMEDEX(R) Healthcare Series Vol. 119: Micromedex, Greenwood Village, CO (Edition expires 3/2004).
*Not yet FDA approved.

Classification of NSAIDs as nonspecific versus COX-2–specific yields important information regarding adverse event profile, particularly with respect to the risk for GI ulceration and bleeding (Table 56–5).

NONSTEROIDAL ANTI-INFLAMMATORY DRUG METABOLISM

NSAIDs are produced in a variety of dosage forms, including slow-release preparations, sustained-release preparations, and suppositories. Most NSAIDs are completely absorbed from the GI tract. After absorption, almost all NSAIDs are more than 90-percent bound to plasma proteins. If total drug concentrations are increased beyond the point at which the binding sites on albumin are saturated, biologically active free drug concentrations increase disproportionately to the increasing total drug concentration. The clearance of NSAIDs is usually by hepatic metabolism with production of inactive metabolites that are excreted in the bile and urine. Most NSAIDs are metabolized through the microsomal cytochrome P450–containing mixed-function oxidase system. NSAIDs are most often metabolized by CYP3A, CYP2C9, or both. However, some are metabolized by other cytosolic hepatic enzymes.

SALICYLATE METABOLISM

Salicylates are acetylated (e.g., aspirin) or nonacetylated (e.g., sodium salicylate, choline salicylate, choline magnesium trisalicylate, salicylsalicylic acid).[43] Although the nonacetylated salicylates are only weak inhibitors of COX in vitro, they are able to reduce inflammation in vivo. Aspirin is rapidly deacetylated to salicylate, both spontaneously and enzymatically. Formulation of these agents affects the absorption properties, but not bioavailability.

TABLE 56–5 • RELATIVE INHIBITION OF CYCLOOXYGENASE (COX)-1 AND COX-2 BY SELECTED NONSPECIFIC AND COX-2–SPECIFIC NONSTEROIDAL ANTI-INFLAMMATORY DRUGS (NSAIDS) BY IN VITRO WHOLE BLOOD ASSAY (IC_{50} COX-1:COX-2)[29]

Highly COX-2 Specific	Somewhat COX-2 Selective§	Nonselective
Etoricoxib (106.0)	Nimesulide (7.3)	Indomethacin (0.4)
Rofecoxib (35.0)	Diclofenac (3.0)	Ibuprofen (0.2)
Valdecoxib (30.0)	Etodolac (2.4)	6-MNA‡ (0.2)
Parecoxib* (30.0)	Meloxicam (2.0)	Naproxen (0.7)
Celecoxib† (7.6)		

*Parenteral formulation of valdecoxib.
†There is disagreement among authors as to whether celecoxib should be considered highly or somewhat selective, but it behaves clinically as a highly specific drug.
§Clinical significance of this degree of selectivity has not been demonstrated.
‡Active metabolite of nabumetone.

Buffered aspirin tablets contain antacids that increase the pH of the microenvironment, whereas enteric coating slows absorption. The bioavailability of rectal aspirin suppositories increases with retention time.

Albumin is the dominant protein to which salicylates bind, and these drugs diffuse into most body fluids fairly rapidly. Salicylate is metabolized principally by the liver and excreted primarily by the kidney. In the kidney, salicylate and its metabolites are freely filtered by the glomerulus, then reabsorbed and secreted by the tubules.

The serum levels of salicylate bear only a modest relationship to the dose, and small increments in dose may lead to a profound increase in serum level. The rate of disappearance varies with serum level. The major determinant of serum salicylate levels are urinary pH and the activity of the metabolic enzyme.

PHARMACOLOGIC VARIABILITY

Variability in response to NSAIDs exists among patients, although the exact cause is not fully understood. Several pharmacologic factors related to NSAIDs may influence this variability, such as dose response, plasma half-life, enantiomeric conversion, urinary excretion, and pharmacodynamic variation.[44] Such drug factors include protein binding, the metabolic profile of the drug, and the percentage of the drug that is available as the active (S) enantiomer. Some NSAIDs exist as two enantiomers; these include the propionic acid derivatives ibuprofen, ketoprofen, and flurbiprofen, which exist as mixtures of inactive (R) and active (S) enantiomers. Naproxen is composed of the active (S) enantiomer. Conversion of the propionic acid NSAIDs from the inactive (R) enantiomer to the active (S) enantiomer occurs in vivo to various degrees, providing some basis for the variability in patient response.[3] There is also genetic variability in the cytochrome P450 metabolic enzymes such that some individuals or ethnic groups metabolize drugs more slowly. For example, Asians are frequently slow metabolizers through the CYP2C9 pathway. Finally, the pharmacokinetics of some NSAIDs are affected by hepatic disease, renal disease, or old age.

Therapeutic Effects

ANTI-INFLAMMATORY EFFECTS

NSAIDs are frequently used as first-line agents for the symptomatic relief of inflammatory conditions. In double-blind, randomized clinical trials of inflammatory arthritis, NSAIDs have been compared with placebo, aspirin, and each other. Clinical trials of NSAID efficacy in RA (and OA) most often employ a design whereby the current NSAID is discontinued and the patient must have an increase in symptoms, or flare, to enter the study. Although there is some variation in primary outcome measures, most include parameters that make up the American College of Rheumatology (ACR)-20. Efficacy superior to that of placebo is easily demonstrated for nonspecific and COX-2–specific NSAIDs within 1 to 2 weeks in patients with active RA who are not receiving corticosteroids or other anti-inflammatory medications.[45] Comparisons of adequate doses of nonspecific NSAIDs or COX-2–specific NSAIDs with one another almost always show comparable efficacy. Despite improvement in pain and stiffness with NSAIDs, these agents do not usually reduce erythrocyte sedimentation rate or C-reactive protein levels. Furthermore, there are no data to suggest that NSAIDs modify disease as measured by radiographs. The anti-inflammatory effects of NSAIDs have also been demonstrated in rheumatic fever, juvenile rheumatoid arthritis, ankylosing spondylitis, gout, OA, and systemic lupus erythematosus (SLE).[3] Although not as rigorously proven, their efficacy is also widely accepted in the treatment of Reiter's syndrome, psoriatic arthritis, acute and chronic bursitis, and tendinitis.

Colchicine exhibits excellent anti-inflammatory activity in acute gouty arthritis. Treatment of acute attacks can be accomplished by oral or intravenous dosing (intravenous rarely used) Colchicine dose is usually limited by GI toxicity, including nausea, vomiting, diarrhea, cramping, and pain. Dosing should be stopped if these symptoms occur. In patients with normal renal and hepatic function, the maximum cumulative dose is 6.0 mg orally. Dose should be reduced in the elderly (even if they have apparently normal renal function) and those with hepatic or renal disease. Patients who receive a full dose of colchicine should not receive additional drug by any route for at least 7 days afterward.[46,47]

Colchicine is also used to prevent acute gouty attacks. Prophylactic treatment appears to reduce the frequency of attacks by 75 to 85 percent and mitigates the severity of attacks that occur.[48] However, there is concern that prophylactic therapy should be initiated only if hyperuricemia is controlled, because tophi may develop without the usual warning signs of acute gouty attacks. Albeit with less efficacy, colchicine treatment may also benefit patients with acute episodes of pseudogout and arthritis due to other crystals.

Daily colchicine (1.2 to 1.8 mg) is the mainstay of treatment for familial Mediterranean fever (FMF).[49] It is effective in preventing acute attacks and amyloidosis. Daily colchicine sometimes ameliorates attacks in patients with tumor necrosis factor (TNF) receptor–associated periodic syndromes (TRAPS), but is not as effective as in FMF. Colchicine has been used for treatment of other periodic fevers such as hyperimmunoglobulinemia D and Muckle-Wells syndrome, but again is not as effective as in FMF.[49] Colchicine has been used empirically in other rheumatologic disorders, such as Behçet's disease, sarcoidosis, calcific tendinitis, amyloidosis, cutaneous necrotizing vasculitis, and Sweet's syndrome.[3]

ANALGESIC EFFECTS

Virtually all the NSAIDs relieve pain when used in doses substantially lower than those required to demonstrate suppression of inflammation. The analgesic action of NSAIDs is likely to be due to inhibition of prostaglandin production both peripherally and centrally. Prostaglandins sensitize peripheral nociceptors to other chemical mediators of pain, such as bradykinin, histamine, nitric oxide, and others.[50] However, prostaglandins also play a role in central sensitization at the spinal level. In the dorsal horn of the spinal cord, COX-2 is constitutively expressed and is upregulated during inflammation.[51] The analgesic activity of COX-2–specific NSAIDs is correlated with decreased cerebrospinal fluid prostaglandin levels. The analgesic effect of acetaminophen occurs in the absence of significant anti-inflammatory activity, suggesting a central mechanism of action.

ANTIPYRETIC EFFECTS

The NSAIDs and acetaminophen effectively suppress fever in humans and experimental animals. It has been postulated that PGE_2 generates neuronal signals that activate the thermoregulatory center in the preoptic area of the anterior hypothalamus.[3] PGE_2 synthesis is stimulated by endogenous (e.g., interleukin-1) or exogenous (e.g., lipopolyshaccharide) pyrogens. This likely occurs by induced expression of COX-2 and microsomal PGES-1 in blood vessel endothelial cells of the CNS.[52] Mice with a targeted deletion of the COX-2 gene fail to develop fever in response to inflammatory stimuli.[53] There is little evidence that suggests that any nonspecific or COX-2–specific NSAID has superior efficacy as an antipyretic. However, in fever associated with viral illnesses, aspirin should be avoided due to the association with hepatocellular failure (Reye's syndrome).[54]

OTHER THERAPEUTIC EFFECTS

Antiplatelet Effects

Aspirin and nonspecific NSAIDs inhibit platelet COX-1. Except for aspirin, inhibition of platelet aggregation is reversible and depends on the concentration of drug in the platelet. Aspirin acetylates platelet COX-1, which cannot be resynthesized. The antiaggregation effect of as little as 80 mg of aspirin can last for up to 4 to 6 days, until the bone marrow can resupply new platelets. Aspirin is indicated for secondary prevention of cardiovascular disease.[55] The role of aspirin in preventing cardiovascular events in patients without a prior history of cardiovascular disease is less clear. However, recent recommendations from the U.S. Preventive Services Task Force suggest that those patients with an increased risk for coronary heart disease events may receive greater benefit than harm from low-dose aspirin.[56] There is no consensus that any NSAID other than aspirin is effective for prophylaxis of cardiovascular thrombotic events. However, recent data suggest that some NSAIDs (e.g., ibuprofen) may interfere with the protective effect of aspirin.[57]

Cancer Chemoprevention

Epidemiologic studies suggest that NSAIDs prevent carcinogenesis or progression of some cancers, particularly colon cancer.[20] The first prospective data were in those patients at very high risk of developing colon cancer due to a genetic defect. Clinical trials demonstrated that NSAIDs could cause regression of polyps in patients with familial adenomatous polyposis (FAP).[58] COX-2 is implicated in this effect of NSAIDs because human colorectal cancers overexpress COX-2, and COX-2–specific NSAIDs or genetic deficiency of COX-2 are associated with a marked reduction in tumor burden in animal models of FAP.[20] Celecoxib was subsequently approved by the U.S. Food and Drug Administration (FDA) for reduction of polyps in patients with FAP on the basis of prospective clinical trials.[59]

In support of epidemiologic studies of sporadic colorectal cancer, two prospective randomized placebo-controlled trials suggest a chemopreventive effect of aspirin.[60,61] Patients with a history of either previous colorectal cancer or colorectal adenomas were randomized to take either aspirin or placebo. Those patients taking low-dose aspirin had a reduced risk of developing new adenomas. It should be noted that in these prospective studies, adenomas did develop in aspirin-treated patients. Therefore, chemoprevention with aspirin or other NSAIDs does not replace screening colonoscopy.

Studies are ongoing in many different forms of cancer to determine whether NSAIDs, generally COX-2–specific NSAIDs, will be useful as chemopreventive agents either as single agents or in combination.[62] Chemopreventive activity of COX-2–specific NSAIDs, particularly celecoxib, may be COX dependent and independent.

Alzheimer's Disease

Epidemiologic studies have suggested that use of NSAIDs, particularly long-term use, may reduce the risk of developing Alzheimer's disease (AD).[63-65] The mechanism underlying this putative protective effect is not known. Anti-inflammatory mechanisms have been proposed, but not proved. Certain NSAIDs may also preferentially decrease secretion of the highly amyloidogenic Aβ42 peptide (the 42-residue isoform of the amyloid-β peptide) in cultured cells and in transgenic mice.[66] Prospective therapeutic trials of NSAIDs in AD have, however, been disappointing. The apparent inconsistency may be due to the fact that the epidemiologic evidence is based on studies examining AD before clinical manifestations are apparent, whereas therapeutic studies have been carried out on people with illnesses severe enough to exceed the clinical detection threshold. Therefore, it is conceivable that therapeutic strategies administered during early AD dementia or moderate dementia may not be optimally effective.[67]

TABLE 56–6 • SHARED TOXICITIES OF NONSTEROIDAL ANTI-INFLAMMATORY DRUGS (NSAIDS)

Organ System	Toxicity
Gastrointestinal (GI)	Dyspepsia
	Gastroduodenal ulcers*
	Ulcer complications (bleeding, perforation, obstruction)*
	GI bleeding (upper and lower)*
	Exacerbates colitis
Renal	Sodium retention
	Weight gain and edema
	Hypertension
	Type IV renal tubular acidosis and hyperkalemia
	Acute renal failure
	Papillary necrosis
	Acute interstitial nephritis
	Accelerated chronic renal failure§
Hepatic	Elevated transaminases
	Reye's syndrome§
Asthma/Allergic	Exacerbates aspirin-exacerbated respiratory disease*
	Cutaneous hypersensitivity
Hematologic	Cytopenias
Nervous	Dizziness, confusion, drowsiness
	Seizures
	Aseptic meningitis
Cardiovascular	Hypertension
	Thrombosis†‡
Skeletal	Reduced fracture healing‡
Reproductive	Infertility‡

*Reduced with COX-2–specific NSAIDs.
§Aspirin.
†Seen only with rofecoxib at doses >25 mg/day in patients at risk for cardiovascular thrombosis.
‡Somewhat speculative.

Adverse Effects

The NSAIDs share a common spectrum of clinical toxicities, although the frequency of particular side effects varies with the compound. Important toxicities occur in the GI tract, kidney, and other organ systems (Table 56–6). Hypersensitivity reactions occur with all of the NSAIDs. COX-2–specific NSAIDs are associated with a reduced risk of GI ulceration and ulcer complications.

GASTROINTESTINAL TRACT EFFECTS

Dyspepsia

Nonulcer dyspepsia is the most common adverse event associated with use of nonspecific and COX-2–specific NSAIDs. At least 10 to 20 percent of patients taking NSAIDs report dyspepsia.[68] Poor correlation has always been observed for the subjective symptoms of dyspepsia, fecal blood loss, and endoscopic findings. Furthermore, only a minority of patients with serious GI events report antecedent dyspepsia.[69]

Epidemiology of Nonsteroidal Anti-inflammatory Drug–Induced Ulcers

Injury to the upper GI tract in the form of ulcers and their complications is the most important toxicity associated with the use of nonspecific NSAIDs. This risk is reduced, but not eliminated, by opting for COX-2–specific NSAIDs. Epidemiologic studies have shown that the use of nonspecific NSAIDs increases the risk of ulcer complications by a factor of four compared with nonuse, and low-dose aspirin (325 mg/d or less) doubles the risk of bleeding ulcers.[70-72] The absolute risk of serious ulcer complications (bleeding, perforation, or obstruction) in a patient with no other risk factors is about 0.5 percent per year, and the risk in RA patients is about 2 to 4 percent per year.[69] By life-table analysis of prospectively collected data from multiple NSAID submissions, the U.S. FDA estimates that GI ulcers, bleeding, and perforation occur in approximately 1 to 2 percent of patients who use NSAIDs for 3 months and approximately 2 to 5 percent of patients who use them for 1 year. Based on Arthritis, Rheumatism and Aging Medical Information System (ARAMIS) data, Fries[73] estimates that NSAID-induced gastropathy is responsible for 76,000 hospitalizations and 7600 deaths each year in the United States.[73] The mortality rate among patients hospitalized for NSAID-induced upper GI bleeding is 5 to 10 percent.[68]

Mechanism of Gastroduodenal Injury

Mucosal damage associated with inhibiting prostaglandin synthesis is associated with a decrease in epithelial mucus production, a reduction of bicarbonate secretion, decreased mucosal blood flow, reduced epithelial proliferation, and decreased mucosal resistance to injury.[68] Impaired mucosal resistance permits injury, thereby amplifying risk due to new mucosal lesions. Topical mucosal injury is initiated by the acidic properties of aspirin and many other NSAIDs. In addition, topical injury may occur indirectly via biliary excretion and subsequent duodenogastric reflux of active NSAID metabolites. Indomethacin, sulindac, and meclofenamate sodium have extensive enterohepatic recirculation, which probably increases GI exposure to these drugs and enhances their GI toxicity. Regardless of topical injury, systemic inhibition of prostaglandin production is the principal mechanism underlying development of gastroduodenal ulceration, illustrated by the fact that enteric-coating and parenteral or rectal administration fails to reduce ulcer risk.[68] Lastly, inhibition of platelet aggregation mediated by aspirin and nonspecific NSAIDs may increase the risk of bleeding from gastroduodenal ulcers.[74]

In the normal gastroduodenal mucosa, COX-1 is the isoform responsible for prostaglandin production. However, inhibition of COX-2 may contribute to ulcer risk in situations in which damage is already present. During injury of the GI tract, as in other tissues, COX-2 is induced. Prostaglandins derived from COX-2 would normally exert suppressive effects on inflammatory cells, notably neutrophils, which contribute to mucosal damage.[75]

Risk of Nonsteroidal Anti-inflammatory Drug–induced Gastroduodenal Ulcers and Ulcer Complications

Patients differ in their risk for NSAID-related GI ulceration and bleeding. Factors consistently associated with increased risk for developing NSAID-associated ulcers are shown in Table 56–7.[68] These risk factors can be identified in prospective clinical trials of gastroprotective strategies, and risk reduction is higher in those at greatest risk.[76] Concomitant corticosteroid use increases the risk of a GI event over that with the use of one NSAID alone (odds ratio = 1.83).

Risk Reduction for Ulcers and Ulcer Complications

In those patients at risk for developing ulcers and ulcer complications, it is important to employ gastroprotective strategies (Table 56–8). Using the lowest effective dose of an NSAID can reduce risk compared to using higher doses.[72] Although high doses of acetaminophen may also cause ulcers and bleeding, doses lower than 2 grams daily are not associated with upper GI toxicity.[72] Other available strategies include the use of COX-2–specific NSAIDs, replacement of gastric prostanoids with misoprostol, a stable analogue of PGE_1, or coadministration of a proton pump inhibitor. Unfortunately, despite a number of strategies available for risk reduction, there is a high level of failure to adequately protect patients using NSAIDs.[77]

TABLE 56–7 • RISK FACTORS FOR NONSTEROIDAL ANTI-INFLAMMATORY DRUG (NSAID)-INDUCED ULCER COMPLICATIONS

Definite
Advanced age (substantial risk after age 65)
Prior ulcer disease or ulcer complications
High-dose, multiple NSAIDs (including low-dose aspirin)
Concomitant use of anticoagulants
Concomitant use of corticosteroid therapy
Serious systemic disorder
Possible
Cigarette smoking
Alcohol consumption
Infection with *Helicobacter pylori*

Modified from Wolfe MM, Lichtenstein DR, Singh G: Gastrointestinal toxicity of nonsteroidal antiinflammatory drugs. New Engl J Med 340:1888, 1999.

TABLE 56–8 • STRATEGIES TO PROTECT PATIENTS FROM NONSTEROIDAL ANTI-INFLAMMATORY DRUG (NSAID)-INDUCED UPPER GASTROINTESTINAL ULCERATION AND ULCER COMPLICATIONS

Use the lowest possible dose[70,72]
Avoid using more than one NSAID (including low-dose aspirin)[72]
Use a COX-2–specific NSAID[78,79]
Add misoprostol (200 mcg four times daily)[82]
Add a proton pump inhibitor[86]

Two large randomized, controlled clinical trials were performed to evaluate the occurrence of clinically significant ulcers and ulcer complications in patients treated with COX-2–specific NSAIDs compared to nonspecific NSAIDs.[78-80] The Vioxx GI Outcome Research (VIGOR) study enrolled 8076 patients with RA and randomized subjects to receive rofecoxib (50 mg daily) or naproxen (500 mg twice daily). There was a highly significant reduction of clinical GI events defined as symptomatic ulcers and ulcer complications (2.1 per 100 patient-years compared with 4.5 per 100 patient-years) in rofecoxib-treated patients.[78] This difference translates into a relative risk of 0.46 percent (95% CI, 0.33-0.64) for rofecoxib. It was calculated that 41 patients would need to be treated to prevent one clinical GI event. Furthermore, the higher the risk, the greater the absolute risk reduction associated with the use of rofecoxib.[76]

The Celecoxib Long-Term Safety Study (CLASS) enrolled 7968 patients with OA or RA to receive treatment with celecoxib (400 mg twice daily), ibuprofen (800 mg three times daily), or diclofenac (75 mg twice daily); randomization was performed as two parallel trials comparing celecoxib to one or the other nonspecific NSAID.[79] Patients were allowed to use low-dose (≤325 mg daily) aspirin, which occurred in 22 percent of enrolled patients. The primary outcome measure was complicated ulcer, with a secondary outcome that included symptomatic ulcers and ulcer complications. After 6 months, the annualized incidence of ulcer complications was 0.76 percent in the celecoxib-treated patients and 1.45 percent in the ibuprofen or diclofenac groups, a nonsignificant difference ($p = 0.09$). There was a significant reduction in clinical GI events, particularly notable in patients not receiving aspirin. In aspirin-treated patients, there was no reduction in the incidence of complicated ulcers. Celecoxib was associated with a significant reduction of upper GI bleeding compared with patients taking nonspecific NSAIDs in an observational study of elderly Canadian patients.[81]

The Misoprostol Ulcer Complications Outcome Safety Assessment (MUCOSA) trial was a double-blind, randomized, placebo-controlled, 6-month study of serious clinical upper GI events 8843 patients with RA (at least 52 years old; mean age, 68 years) in a protocol designed to reflect normal clinic practice.[82] The misoprostol group (200 μg four times daily) showed a 40-percent reduction in the rate of serious GI complications compared to the placebo group. Misoprostol is often poorly tolerated at high doses, with diarrhea as the most important side effect. A combination agent consisting of diclofenac plus misoprostol (200 μg) used twice daily is available. In observational studies, this combination agent is less effective than COX-2–specific NSAIDs in preventing upper GI bleeding.[81]

There are endoscopic studies that suggest proton pump inhibitors are more effective than ranitidine or misoprostol in healing of gastroduodenal ulcers and reducing recurrence of gastroduoenal ulcers in patients taking NSAIDs.[83,84] In patients with a history of upper GI bleeding who continued taking either low-dose aspirin or nonspecific NSAIDs and were also infected with *Helicobacter pylori*, omeprazole was superior to eradication of *H. pylori* in preventing recurrent bleeding in those taking nonspecific NSAIDs.[85] In patients taking NSAIDs and with a recent history of ulcer bleeding, the risk of recurrent ulcer bleeding was similar in patients receiving celecoxib (4.9%; 95% CI, 3.1-6.7) and in patients receiving diclofenac plus omeprazole (6.4%; 95% CI, 4.3-8.4).[86]

Other Sites of Gastrointestinal Injury

NSAIDs are potentially toxic to the entire GI tract. The use of NSAIDs is associated with buccal ulceration, reflux esophagitis, and esophageal strictures. Ulcers may develop in the stomach, duodenum, jejunum, ileum, and colon, where they can cause perforation or malabsorption.[87,88] Rarely, obstructive valve-like lesions form in the terminal ileum; these lesions are associated with increased mortality. NSAIDs may also contribute to the frequent anemia and small bowel protein loss observed in RA patients taking these drugs. A number of NSAIDs have intrinsic secretory properties, which lead to diarrhea.

RENAL EFFECTS

Cyclooxygenase Expression in the Kidney

Prostaglandins play a vital role in solute and renovascular homeostasis.[89] It is becoming quite clear that prostaglandins are produced by both COX-1 and COX-2, generally in different locations within, the kidney and that these prostaglandins may play opposing physiologic roles in renal function.[22,90] COX-1 is highly expressed in the renal vasculature, glomerular mesangial cells, and collecting duct.[91] COX-2 expression is restricted to the vasculature, cortical thick ascending limb (specifically in cells associated with the macula densa), and medullary interstitial cells. COX-2 expression in the macula densa increases in high-renin states (e.g., salt restriction, angiotensin-converting enzyme inhibition, renovascular hypertension), and selective COX-2 inhibitors significantly decrease plasma renin levels and renal renin activity. COX-2 expression in the macula densa is reduced by angiotensin II and mineralocorticoids. Dehydration or hypertonicity appears to regulate COX-2 expression in the medullary interstitium. COX-2 is also necessary for normal renal development.[91]

Prostaglandin and Nonsteroidal Anti-Inflammatory Drug Effects on Renal Physiology

At the current time, there is no indication of differences between COX-2–specific and nonspecific NSAIDs with regard to renal effects.[89] Prostaglandins are known to regulate renal sodium resorption by their ability to inhibit active transport of sodium in both the thick ascending limb and the collecting duct and to increase renal water excretion by blunting the actions of vasopressin.[21] The cellular source of COX-2–derived prostanoids that promote natriuresis remains uncertain, but it is possible that they may in large part be derived from the medullary interstitial cells. Sodium retention has been reported to occur in up to 25 percent of NSAID-treated patients and may be particularly apparent in patients who have an existing avidity for sodium, such as those with mild heart failure or liver disease[21] (Table 56–9). Decreased sodium excretion in NSAID-treated patients can lead to weight gain and peripheral edema. This effect may be sufficiently important to cause clinically important exacerbations of congestive heart failure.

In addition to sodium retention, NSAIDs may cause altered blood pressure, with average increases of mean arterial pressure of between 5 and 10 mm Hg. It has also been reported that using NSAIDs may increase the risk of initiating antihypertensive therapy in older patients, with the magnitude of increased risk being proportional to the NSAID dose.[92] Furthermore, in a large (n = 51,630) prospective cohort of women age 44

TABLE 56–9 • CONDITIONS ASSOCIATED WITH INCREASED RISK OF NONSPECIFIC AND CYCLOOXYGENASE (COX)-2–SPECIFIC NONSTEROIDAL ANTI-INFLAMMATORY DRUG (NSAID)-INDUCED RENAL ADVERSE EVENTS

Condition	Risk
Congestive heart failure	ARF, edema, ↑CHF
Cirrhosis (with or without ascites)	ARF, edema
Nephrotic syndrome	ARF, edema
Chronic renal insufficiency	ARF, ↑CRF, edema, hyperkalemia
Volume depletion	ARF
Diabetes mellitus	Hyperkalemia
Hypertension*†	Exacerbated HTN
Advanced age§	ARF, induced HTN

*NSAIDs interfere with effectiveness of diuretics, angiotensin-converting enzyme inhibitors, and beta-blockers.

†Patients on angiotensin-converting enzyme inhibitors are at risk for hyperkalemia.

§ARF most likely in the elderly with other risk factors.

Abbreviations: ARF, acute renal failure; CRF, chronic renal failure; HTN, hypertension; CHF, congestive heart failure.

Modified from Brater DC: Effects of nonsteroidal anti-inflammatory drugs on renal function: Focus on cyclooxygenase-2-selective inhibition. Am J Med 107:65S, 1999.

to 69 without hypertension in 1990, incident hypertension over the following 8 years was significantly more likely in frequent users of aspirin, acetaminophen, and NSAIDs.[93] NSAIDs can attenuate the effects of antihypertensive agents, including diuretics, angiotensin-converting enzyme inhibitors, and beta blockers, thereby interfering with blood pressure control.

Prostaglandins stimulate renin release that, in turn, increases secretion of aldosterone and, subsequently, potassium secretion by the distal nephron. For this reason, NSAID-treated patients may develop hyporeninemic hypoaldosteronism that manifests as type IV renal tubular acidosis and hyperkalemia.[94] The degree of hyperkalemia is generally mild; however, patients with renal insufficiency or those that may otherwise be prone to hyperkalemia (e.g., patients with diabetes mellitus and those on angiotensin-converting enzyme inhibitors or potassium-sparing diuretics) may be at greater risk.[94]

Acute renal failure is an uncommon consequence of NSAID treatment. This is due to the vasoconstrictive effects of NSAIDs and is reversible. In most cases, renal failure occurs in patients who have a depleted actual or effective intravascular volume (e.g., congestive heart failure, cirrhosis, or renal insufficiency).[21]

Marked reduction in medullary blood flow may result in papillary necrosis. This is speculated to be the result of apoptosis of medullary interstitial cells. Inhibition of COX-2 may be a predisposing factor.[91] Specific COX-2 inhibitors, like nonspecific NSAIDs, have been reported to cause papillary necrosis.[95]

Another adverse renal effect resulting from NSAIDs involves an idiosyncratic reaction accompanied by massive proteinuria and acute interstitial nephritis. Hypersensitivity phenomena, such as fever, rash, and eosinophilia, may occur. This syndrome has been observed with most NSAIDs.

Aspirin, Acetaminophen, and Chronic Renal Failure

Use of analgesics, particularly acetaminophen and aspirin, has been associated with nephropathy leading to chronic renal failure. In one large case-control study, the regular use of aspirin or acetaminophen was associated with a risk of chronic renal failure 2.5 times as high as that for nonuse, and the risk increased significantly with an increasing cumulative lifetime dose.[96] In subjects regularly using both acetaminophen and aspirin, the risk was also significantly increased compared to users of either agent alone. No association between the use of nonaspirin NSAIDs and chronic renal failure could be detected after adjusting for acetaminophen and aspirin use. Preexisting renal or systemic disease was a necessary precursor to analgesic-associated renal failure, and those without preexisting renal disease had only a small risk of end-stage renal disease.[96,97]

HEPATIC EFFECTS

Small elevations of one or more liver tests may occur in up to 15 percent of patients taking NSAIDs, and notable elevations of alanine amino transferase (ALT) or aspartate amino transferase (AST) (approximately three or more times the upper limit of normal) have reported in approximately 1 percent of patients in clinical trials of NSAIDs. Patients usually have no symptoms, and discontinuation or dose reduction generally results in normalization of the transaminase values, although rare, fatal outcomes have been reported with almost all NSAIDs.[3] Those NSAIDs that appear most likely to be associated with hepatic adverse events are diclofenac and sulindac.

In clinical trial reports to the U.S. FDA, 5.4 percent of patients with RA who were treated with aspirin experienced persistent elevations of results in more than one liver function test. In children with viral illnesses, hepatocellular failure and fatty degeneration (Reye's syndrome) is associated with aspirin ingestion.[54]

At therapeutic doses, acetaminophen is unlikely to cause hepatic abnormalties. In large doses, the detoxification system is overwhelmed leading to fulminant hepatic injury.[98]

ASTHMA AND ALLERGIC REACTIONS

Asthma

Up to 10 to 20 percent of the general asthmatic population, especially those with the triad of vasomotor rhinitis, nasal polyposis, and asthma, are hypersensitive to aspirin. In these patients, ingestion of aspirin and nonspecific NSAIDs leads to severe exacerbations of asthma with naso-ocular reactions. Formerly termed *aspirin-sensitive asthma*, these patients are now characterized as having aspirin-exacerbated respiratory disease (AERD) because they have chronic upper and lower respiratory mucosal inflammation, sinusitis, nasal polyposis, and asthma independent of their hypersensitivity reactions. It is now thought that production of protective prostaglandins in the setting of AERD is derived from COX-1. A number of studies have been reported demonstrating that the COX-2–specific NSAIDs, rofecoxib and celecoxib, fail to trigger asthma exacerbation or naso-ocular symptoms in patients with AERD.[99,100] Nevertheless, these studies were performed as challenge tests rather than long-term placebo-controlled trials, and caution is advised. The fact that specific COX-2 inhibitors appear safe in AERD does not imply that other hypersensitivity reactions do not occur.

Allergic Reactions

A wide variety of cutaneous reactions have been associated with NSAIDs. Almost all the NSAIDs have been associated with cutaneous vasculitis, erythema multiforme, Stevens-Johnson syndrome, or toxic epidermal necrolysis. NSAIDs are also associated with urticaria/angioedema, anaphylactoid, or anaphylactic reactions. Special note should be made that celecoxib and valdecoxib contain a sulfonamide group and should not be given to patients who report allergy to sulfa-containing drugs.

HEMATOLOGIC EFFECTS

Aplastic anemia, agranulocytosis, and thrombocytopenia rarely are associated with NSAIDs, but they are prominent among the causes of deaths attributed to these drugs. Because of the risk of hematologic effects, phenylbutazone is no longer recommended for use in any condition in the United States and has been taken off the market.[3]

CENTRAL NERVOUS SYSTEM EFFECTS

Severe headaches occur in patients taking indomethacin, and dizziness, confusion, depression, drowsiness, hallucinations, and seizures have been reported. Elderly patients may be particularly susceptible to developing cognitive dysfunction and other CNS effects. Acute aseptic meningitis, perhaps an unusual type of hypersensitivity reaction, has been reported in patients with SLE or mixed connective tissue disease treated with ibuprofen, sulindac, tolmetin, or naproxen. Aseptic meningitis has been reported with rofecoxib.[101]

CARDIOVASCULAR EFFECTS

Consideration of the cardiovascular effects of COX inhibition has accompanied the development of COX-2–specific NSAIDs. The hypothesis that specific inhibition of COX-2 may increase risk of thrombosis is due to the fact that platelet-derived thromboxane A_2 is synthesized via a COX-1 pathway, whereas endothelial prostacyclin production is largely synthesized via COX-2.[30] Prostacyclin is functionally antagonistic to thromboxane in the vasculature, inhibiting platelet activation and acting as an important mediator of vasodilation. Nevertheless, it is now clear that COX-2–specific NSAIDs are not likely to be associated with adverse vascular events in otherwise healthy, low-risk patients.[102] In patients at high risk for thrombosis, specific inhibition of COX-2–derived prostacyclin represents a theoretic hazard. In the VIGOR trial, patients with RA taking twice the recommended dose of rofecoxib were five times more likely to have a myocardial infarction than those taking naproxen.[78] Furthermore, a retrospective case-control study reported an increased risk for serious coronary heart disease in patients using rofecoxib at doses higher than recommended.[103] At usual doses of rofecoxib (25 mg/d or less), no increase in cardiovascular events has been reported.[103] There is no data suggesting an increased cardiovascular risk with celecoxib in clinical trials or retrospective case-control studies.[102,103]

EFFECTS ON BONE

The complex effects of prostanoids on bone formation and remodeling have been appreciated for many years. It is now clear that COX-2 is required for many functions of both osteoblasts and osteoclasts. COX-2 is rapidly inducible and highly expressed and regulated in osteoblasts, the cells responsible for bone formation. The production of prostaglandins by osteoblasts is an important mechanism for the regulation of bone turnover. Furthermore, PGE_2 is a potent stimulator of bone resorption and osteoclastogenesis. Genetic deletion of the COX-2 gene or COX-2–specific NSAIDs partially block the PTH- or 1,25-OH vitamin D-induced formation of osteoclasts in organ cultures. The mechanism underlying this effect may be related to a reduction of receptor activator of NF-κB (RANK) ligand on marrow stromal cells when COX-2 is inhibited. Despite the observations that prostaglandins are important in many aspects of bone physiology, the skeletal development of mice null for either COX-1 or COX-2 is normal.[23]

It has long been appreciated that NSAIDs can inhibit experimental fracture healing and reduce formation of heterotopic bone in patients.[104] This effect of NSAIDs is due to inhibition of COX-2 and is demonstrated in experiments that show induction of COX-2 is crucial for lamellar bone formation elicited by mechanical strain.[105] Furthermore, fracture healing is impaired in rats treated with specific COX-2 inhibitors and in mice with genetic deletion of the COX-2 gene.[24] Based on these findings, it is prudent to avoid use of both nonspecific and COX-2–specific NSAIDs during a period of bone healing.[104]

EFFECTS ON OVARIAN AND UTERINE FUNCTION

Prostaglandins derived from COX-2 have been implicated as mediators in multiple stages of the female reproductive cycle. Induction of COX-2 immediately after the luteinizing hormone surge was the first observation involving the isoenzyme during a normal physiologic event. It has been suggested that COX-2–derived prostaglandins may be an important signal that sets the time of ovulation in mammals.[106,107] Studies using COX-2–null mice show reproductive failure at ovulation, fertilization, implantation, and decidualization.[108] COX-2–dependent prostanoid production probably leads to the generation of proteolytic enzymes that rupture the follicles. After fertilization, COX-2 also plays a role in embryo implantation in the myometrium.[108] Prostaglandins are important for inducing uterine contractions during labor. Murine studies have shown that the mechanism of uterine contraction involves fetal release of PGF_{2}, a compound that induces luteolysis. This pathway leads to reduced maternal progesterone levels, induction of oxytocin receptors in the myometrium, and parturition.

Based on these observations in animals, one could hypothesize that NSAIDs may have an influence on fertility. In fact, studies to suggest that luteinized unruptured follicle syndrome as a cause of reversible infertility can be related to ingestion of NSAIDs.[109] For this reason, women should be cautioned that chronic NSAID use may impair fertility.

SALICYLATE INTOXICATION AND NONSTEROIDAL ANTI-INFLAMMATORY DRUG OVERDOSE

The new appearance of tachypnea, confusion, ataxia, oliguria or a rising blood urea nitrogen (BUN)/creatinine in a patient—particularly an elderly patient—taking aspirin or salicylates should suggest the possibility of salicylate intoxication. In adults, metabolic acidosis is masked by hyperventilation due to stimulation of respiratory centers, which is a direct effect of salicylates. Sudden increases in salicylate levels can occur even if there is no change in dose. This is particularly common in patients who develop acidosis from any cause, dehydration, or the ingestion of other drugs that displace salicylate from protein binding sites. Therapy consists of removing residual drug from the GI tract, forced diuresis while maintaining the urinary pH in the alkaline range and with potassium replacement, or hemodialysis if diuresis is unsatisfactory. Vitamin K is recommended because large doses of salicylate may interfere with the synthesis of the vitamin K–dependent clotting factors.

Acute overdoses of NSAIDs are much less toxic than are overdoses of aspirin or salicylates. This subject has been most carefully evaluated for ibuprofen, prompted by its approval for over-the-counter sale to the general public. Symptoms with overdoses ranging up to 40 grams include CNS depression, seizures, apnea, nystagmus, blurred vision, diplopia, headache, tinnitus, bradycardia, hypotension, abdominal pain, nausea, vomiting, hematuria, abnormal renal function, coma, and cardiac arrest. Treatment includes prompt evacuation of the stomach contents, observation, and administration of fluids.

ADVERSE EFFECTS OF ACETAMINOPHEN

Acetaminophen is used widely as the first-line treatment of pain, chiefly because it is viewed as effective and safer than NSAIDs. Used in doses below 2 grams daily, there is little evidence of toxicity.[98] In higher doses, gastrointestinal ulcers and bleeding have been reported.[72,110] Furthermore, regular use of acetaminophen has been associated with an increased risk for chronic renal failure.[96] Intentional self-poisoning with acetaminophen remains an important problem due to fulminant hepatic failure. Treatment of acetaminophen overdose includes aspiration of the stomach, intensive support measures, and early treatment with *N*-acetylcysteine.

ADVERSE EFFECTS OF COLCHICINE

The mechanism of colchicine actions is different from NSAIDs, so the adverse event profile is also different. More than 80 percent of patients who take a traditional full, oral, therapeutic dose of colchicine for an acute gouty attack experience cramping, abdominal pain, diarrhea, nausea, or vomiting, and these symptoms usually limit the dose.[47]

Bone marrow depression, hair loss, amenorrhea, dysmenorrhea, oligospermia, and azoospermia have been reported with chronic colchicine treatment.[3] There may be an increase in trisomy 21 in the offspring of FMF patients taking colchicine at the time of conception.[49] Colchicine can cause subacute onset muscle and peripheral nerve toxicity, particularly in patients with chronic renal failure. For this reason, colchicine should be used cautiously in patients with chronic renal failure, and dose adjustment should be considered. Patients with colchicine-induced neuromyopathy present with proximal muscle weakness, elevated serum creatine kinase (CK) levels, and neuropathy or myopathy on electromyography (EMG).[111]

Death has occurred after ingestion of as little as 8 mg of colchicine, but it is inevitable after the ingestion of more than 40 mg. Treatment includes aspiration of the 0stomach, intensive support measures, and hemodialysis, although there is no specific evidence that colchicine can be removed by dialysis.[3]

Effects of Concomitant Drugs, Diseases, Aging, and Patient Characteristics

Because of the widespread use of prescription and nonprescription NSAIDs, there are ample opportunities for interaction with other drugs and for interactions with patient-specific factors.[112] Specific drug interactions are listed on the package inserts of individual agents.

DRUG-DRUG INTERACTIONS

Table 56–10 provides a partial list of potential interactions involving NSAIDs. Although the degree to which individual patients exhibit these interactions varies considerably, the risks should be considered when prescribing drug combinations that include NSAIDs.

Because most NSAIDs are extensively bound to plasma proteins, they may displace other drugs from binding sites or may themselves be displaced by other agents. Aspirin and other NSAIDs may increase the activity or toxicity of sulfonylurea, hypoglycemic agents, oral anticoagulants, phenytoin, sulfonamides, and methotrexate by displacing these drugs from their protein binding sites and increasing the free fraction of the drug in plasma.[112] NSAIDs may blunt the antihypertensive effects of β-blockers, angiotensin-converting enzyme inhibitors, and thiazides. Ethanol increases the gastrointestinal toxicity of NSAIDs.[3]

DRUG-DISEASE INTERACTIONS

RA and other diseases (e.g., hepatic and renal disease) that decrease serum albumin concentrations are associated with increased concentrations of free drug. Hepatic and renal diseases may also impair drug metabolism or excretion, and thereby increase the toxicity of a given dose of NSAID to an individual patient. Renal insufficiency may also be accompanied by accumulated endogenous organic acids that may displace NSAIDs from protein binding sites. Unbound drug concentrations of naproxen and oxaprozin are doubled in patients with moderate to severe renal insufficiency, and for these drugs, doses should be reduced by one half.[3]

DRUG REACTIONS IN THE ELDERLY

Aging is accompanied by changes in physiology resulting in altered pharmacokinetics and pharmacodynamics. Decreased drug clearance may be the consequence of reductions in hepatic mass, enzymatic activity, blood flow, renal plasma flow, glomerular filtration rate, and tubular function associated with aging. The elderly are more likely to experience adverse GI and renal effects related to NSAIDs.[68,89] The elderly have more illnesses than younger patients and, therefore, take more medications, increasing the possibility of drug–drug interactions. Older patients may also be more likely to self-medicate or make errors in drug dosing. For these reasons, frequent

TABLE 56–10 • DRUG INTERACTIONS

Drug	Mechanism	Comments
Anticoagulants • Warfarin	• Protein binding displacement, altered metabolism	• Beware all NSAIDs and aspirin. • Check PT INR whenever initiating treatment
Anticonvulsants • Phenytoin	• Altered metabolism	• Monitor phenytoin plasma levels.
Anti-inflammatory • Aspirin • Other NSAIDs • Glucocorticoids	• Aspirin and NSAIDs compete for protein binding sites; altered metabolism • Glucocorticoids increase salicylate metabolism • Glucocorticoids increase GI toxicity of NSAIDs	• Avoid combining multiple NSAIDs. • Ibuprofen interferes with cardioprotective effect of aspirin. • Use lowest dose of NSAID possible when combined with glucocorticoids.
Antihypertensives • β-Blockers • ACE inhibitors • Peripheral vasodilators • Diuretics	• Loss of antihypertensive effect • Loss of natriuretic and diuretic effects of furoxemide • Loss of hypotensive, but not natriuretic or diuretic, effect of thiazides	• Adjust antihypertensives or choose alternate drug. • Thiazides may be preferred diuretic.
Cardiac • Digoxin	• Altered metabolism	• Monitor digoxin levels.
Hypoglycemic agents • Sulfonylurea	• Altered metabolism	• Beware hypoglycemia and adjust dose.
Immunosuppressives • Methotrexate	• Altered metabolism; decreased clearance	• Monitor CBC and LFT. • No interaction reported for celecoxib and rofecoxib.
Gastrointestinal • Antacids • H_2-blockers (cimetidine)	• Increased urine pH results in reduced salicylate levels • Reduced absorption of some NSAIDs • Cimetidine can increase concentraion of some NSAIDs (piroxicam)	• Review interference with absorption between individual NSAID and antacids. • Do not use cimetidine with piroxicam.
Uricosuric • Probenecid	• Reduced NSAID excretion • Salicylates, including aspirin, reduce uricosuric effect of probenecid	• Adjust NSAID dose when used with probenecid. • Avoid combining probenecid with salicylates.
Psychoactive • Lithium	• Altered metabolism	• Elderly and patients with renal insufficiency most susceptible. • Monitor lithium levels. • Use lowest dose of NSAID.

Abbreviations: PT INR, protime international normalized ratio; ACE, angiotensin converting enzyme; GI, gastrointestinal; CBC, complete blood count; LFT, liver function test.

monitoring for compliance should be a part of the use of NSAIDs in this population.[3]

Distinctive Characteristics of Individual Drugs

A valuable source for information about individual drugs is the package insert for that drug or its reproduction in the *Physician's Desk Reference.* The package inserts for individual NSAIDs represent the most current, reliable, and conservative summaries of information about each drug. They contain published information, unpublished information from the manufacturer's files, and additional information about adverse effects from the FDA. The quantitative estimates of the frequency of adverse effects associated with each NSAID are given. Furthermore, advice about dosage for each approved conditions can be found. Information about drug-drug interactions and the need for dose reduction for renal and hepatic insufficiency are located in the package inserts.

Choosing Anti-inflammatory Analgesic Therapy

In choosing an NSAID for a particular patient, the clinician must consider efficacy, potential toxicity related to concomitant drugs and patient factors, and cost. Furthermore, patient preference for factors such as dosing regimen may be taken into account. In addition to choices from the perspective of the individual patient and physician, it may be important to take a broader view. Choice of anti-inflammatory analgesic therapy can also be considered from the perspective of health care institutions and payors. The symptoms (e.g., pain) and conditions (e.g., arthritis) for which NSAIDs are used are extraordinarily common. Consequently, the cost of NSAIDs as a proportion of total drug costs can be high when drugs are expensive. The increased cost of COX-2–specific and other branded NSAIDs has an important pharmacoeconomic impact. On the other hand, adverse events can have important economic consequences, and improved safety may be cost effective. It seems reasonable at this time to limit use of COX-2–specific NSAIDS to those individuals at risk for adverse GI events. The use of COX-2–specific NSAIDs in low-risk populations may be more difficult to justify since their cost is substantially higher than generic forms of nonspecific NSAIDs.

NONSTEROIDAL ANTI-INFLAMMATORY DRUGS VERSUS ACETAMINOPHEN

Absence of anti-inflammatory activity reduces the effectiveness of acetaminophen for diseases accompanied by a significant component of inflammation (e.g., RA, gout). However, acetaminophen is a safe and effective alternative for milder pain conditions, including OA. With respect to patient preference, a survey study demonstrated that only 14 percent of a large group of rheumatic disease patients (n = 1799) with RA, osteoarthritis, or fibromyalgia preferred acetaminophen to NSAIDs, whereas 60 percent preferred NSAIDs.[113] In a head-to-head clinical trial of acetaminophen versus diclofenac plus misoprostol, there was significantly greater improvement in pain scores in patients in the diclofenac group. This finding was magnified in those patients with more severe disease at baseline.[114] The COX-2–specific inhibitor rofecoxib (25 mg daily) was shown to provide significantly greater relief of pain and stiffness at 6 weeks than acetaminophen in a randomized, controlled, clinical trial of patients with osteoarthritis.[115]

Acetaminophen should be tried as the initial therapy in patients with mild to moderate pain for reasons of safety and cost. However, if patients have moderate to severe symptoms or if evidence of inflammation is present, moving to treatment with NSAIDs may provide more rapid and effective relief.[116]

CYCLOOXYGENASE-2–SPECIFIC VERSUS NONSPECIFIC NONSTEROIDAL ANTI-INFLAMMATORY DRUGS

If cost were not a consideration, an argument could be made that there is no situation in which nonspecific NSAIDs, other than aspirin for cardiovascular prophylaxis, have an advantage over COX-2–specific NSAIDs. Nonspecific NSAIDs have an inferior GI safety profile, there is no difference with respect to renal or other toxicities, and there are no measurable efficacy advantages, though some patients may have a preference for older agents. However, in patients at low risk for gastroduodenal toxicities, the extra cost of COX-2–specific NSAIDs may not be justified. Furthermore, patients at high risk for ulcers and ulcer complications that require aspirin for cardioprophylaxis require ulcer prophylaxis with misoprostel or proton pump inhibitors regardless of NSAIDs. Studies to examine incremental benefits of two strategies for ulcer prophylaxis have not yet been reported, and use of COX-2–specific NSAIDs with other gastroprotective agents may provide little added safety benefit for the increased cost. Unless new safety concerns arise or it becomes clear that there is an increased risk of thrombosis associated with COX-2–specific NSAIDs, these agents are likely to replace nonspecific NSAIDs for most patients as their costs decline.

Future Prospects

Advances in the understanding of prostaglandin biology and the development of COX-2–specific inhibitors resulted in important changes in the treatment of pain and inflammation. However, even with the reduced GI toxicity of COX-2–specific NSAIDs, important adverse effects on renal and other organ systems remain. New insights into prostaglandin biosynthesis and action have suggested several other novel approaches for development of drugs. These potential targets include phospholipase A_2, prostaglandin synthases (e.g., microsomal prostaglandin E synthase-1), and specific prostanoid receptors (e.g., EP_4 receptors). In other approaches, nonspecific NSAIDs, including aspirin, have been complexed with nitric oxide in an effort to reduce GI toxicity, renal toxicity, and the potential for cardiovascular toxicity. With a rapidly aging population, the prevalence of diseases in which NSAIDs are useful will continue to increase. Continuing to develop safer drugs and developing strategies to use existing drugs wisely are important goals.

REFERENCES

1. Vane JR, Botting RM: The history of anti-inflammatory drugs and their mechanism of action. *In* Bazan N, Botting J, Vane J (eds): New Targets in Inflammation: Inhibitors of COX-2 or Adhesion Molecules. London, Kluwar Academic Publishers and William Harvey Press, 1996, p 1.
2. Rodnan GP, Benedek TG: The early history of antirheumatic drugs. Arthritis Rheum 13:145, 1970.
3. Santana-Sahagun E, Weisman MH: Nonsteroidal anti-inflammatory drugs. *In* Harris ED (ed): Kelley's Textbook of Rheumatology. Philadelphia, Elsevier Science, 2000.
4. Hemler M, Lands WEM, Smith WL: Purification of the cyclooxygenase that forms prostaglandins: demonstration of the two forms of iron in the holoenzyme. J Biol Chem 251:5575, 1976.
5. Masferrer JL, Zweifel BS, Seibert K, et al: Selective regulation of cellular cyclooxygenase by dexamethasone and endotoxin in mice. J Clin Invest 86:1375, 1990.
6. Crofford LJ: Prostaglandin biology. Gastroenterol Clin North Am 30:863, 2001.
7. Kurumbail RA, Stevens AM, Gierse JK, et al: Structural basis for selective inhibition of cyclooxygenase-2 by anti-inflammatory agents. Nature 384:644, 1996.
8. Smith WL, DeWitt DL, Garavito RM: Cyclooxygenases: structural, cellular, and molecular biology. Ann Rev Biochem 69:145, 2000.
9. Breyer MD: Beyond cyclooxygenase. Kidney Int 62:1898, 2002.
10. Jakobsson P-J, Thorén S, Morgenstern R, et al: Identification of human prostaglandin E synthase: a microsomal, glutathione-dependent, inducible enzyme, constituting a potential novel drug target. Proc Natl Acad Sci U S A 96:7220, 1999.
11. Tanioko T, Nakatani Y, Semmyo N, et al: Molecular identification of cytosolic prostaglandin E2 synthase that is functionally coupled with cyclooxygenase-1 in immediate prostaglandin E2 biosynthesis. J Biol Chem 42:32775, 2000.
12. Tanikawa N, Ohmiya Y, Ohkubo H, et al: Identification and characterization of a novel type of membrane-associated prostaglandin E synthase. Biochem Biophys Res Commun 291:884, 2002.
13. Murakami M, Naraba H, Tanioka T, et al: Regulation of prostaglandin E_2 biosynthesis by inducible membrane-associated prostaglandin E_2 synthase that acts in concert with cyclooxygenase-2. J Biol Chem 42:32783, 2000.
14. Stichtenoth DO, Thoren S, Bian H, et al: Microsomal prostaglandin E synthase is regulated by pro-inflammatory cytokines and glucocorticoids in primary rheumatoid synovial cells. J Immunol 167:469, 2001.
15. Uematsu S, Matsumoto M, Takeda K, et al: Lipopolysaccharide-dependent prostaglandin E2 production is regulated by the glu-

tathione-dependent prostaglandin E2 synthase gene induced by the toll-like receptor 4/MyD88/NF-IL6 pathway. J Immunol 168:5811, 2002.
16. Funk CD: Prostaglandins and leukotrienes: advances in eicosanoid biology. Science 249:1871, 2001.
17. Narumiya S, FitzGerald GA: Genetic and pharmacological analysis of prostanoid receptor function. J Clin Invest 108:25, 2001.
18. Crofford LJ, Lipsky PE, Brooks P, et al: Basic biology and clinical application of specific COX-2 inhibitors. Arthritis Rheum 43:4, 2000.
19. Dixon DA, Kaplan CD, McIntyre TM, et al: Post-transcriptional control of cyclooxygenase-2 gene expression: the role of the 3′-untranslated region. J Biol Chem 275:11750, 2000.
20. DuBois RN, Abramson SB, Crofford L, et al: Cyclooxygenase in biology and disease. FASEB J 12:1063, 1998.
21. Brater DC, Harris C, Redfern JS, et al: Renal effects of COX-2 selective inhibitors. Am J Nephrol 21:1, 2001.
22. FitzGerald GA: The choreography of cyclooxygenases in the kidney. J Clin Invest 110:33, 2002.
23. Okada Y, Lorenzo JA, Freeman AM, et al: Prostaglandin G/H synthase-2 is required for maximal formation of osteoclast-like cells in culture. J Clin Invest 105:823, 2000.
24. Simon AM, Manigrasso MB, O'Connor JP: Cyclo-oxygenase 2 function is essential for bone fracture healing. J Bone Min Res 17:963, 2002.
25. Browner MF: X-ray crystal structure of cyclooxygenase-2. *In* Bazan N, Botting J, Vane JR (eds): New Targets in Inflammation Inhibitors of COX-2 or Adhesion Molecules. London, Kluwer Academic Press, 1996, p 71.
26. Serhan CN: Lipoxins and novel aspirin-triggered 15-epi-lipoxins (ATL): a jungle of cell-cell interactions or a therapeutic opportunity? Prostaglandins 53:107, 1997.
27. Brooks P, Emery P, Evans JF, et al: Interpreting the clinical significance of the differential inhibition of cyclooxygenase-1 and cyclooxygenase-2. Rheumatology 38:779, 1999.
28. Lipsky PE, Abramson SB, Crofford L, et al: The classification of cyclooxygenase inhibitors (Editorial). J Rheumatol 25:2298, 1998.
29. Riendeau D, Percival MD, Brideau C, et al: Etoricoxib (MK-0663): preclinical profile and comparison with other agents that selectively inhibit cyclooxygenase-2. J Pharmacol Exp Ther 296:558, 2000.
30. FitzGerald GA, Patrono C: The coxibs, selective inhibitors of cyclooxygenase-2. N Engl J Med 345:433, 2001.
31. Abramson SB, Weissman G: The mechansisms of action of nonsteroidal antiinflammatory drugs. Arthritis Rheum 32:1, 1989.
32. Amin AR, Vyas P, Attur M, et al: The mode of action of aspirin-like drugs: effect on inducible nitric oxide synthase. Proc Natl Acad Sci U S A 92:7926, 1995.
33. Cronstein BN, Montesinos MC, Weissmann G: Salicylates and sulfasalazine, but not glucocorticoids, inhibit leukocyte accumulation by an adenosine-dependent mechanisms that is independent of inhibition of prostaglandin synthesis and p105 of NFkappaB. Proc Natl Acad Sci U S A 96:6377, 1999.
34. Kopp E, Gosh S: Inhibition of NF-kappa B by sodium salicylate and aspirin. Science 265:956, 1994.
35. Tegeder I, Pfeilschifter J, Geisslinger G: Cyclooxygenase-independent actions of cyclooxygenase inhibitors. FASEB J 15:2057, 2001.
36. Harris SG, Padilla J, Koumas L, et al: Prostaglandins as modulators of immunity. TRENDS Immunol 23:144, 2002.
37. Zhu J, Song X, Lin HP, et al: Using cyclooxygenase-2 inhibitors as molecular platforms to develop a new class of apoptosis-inducing agents. J Natl Cancer Inst 94:1745, 2002.
38. Ouellet M, Percival MD: Mechanism of acetaminophen inhibition of cyclooxygenase isoforms. Arch Biochem Biophys 387:273, 2001.
39. Boutaud O, Aronoff DM, Richardson JH, et al: Determinants of the cellular specificity of acetaminophen as an inhibitor of prostaglandin H2 synthases. Proc Natl Acad Sci U S A 99:7130, 2002.
40. Botting R: Paracetamol-inhibitable COX-2. J Physiol Pharmacol 51:609, 2000.
41. Chandrasekharan NV, Dai H, Roos KLT, et al: COX-3, a cyclooxygenase-1 variant inhibited by acetaminophen and other analgesic/antipyretic drugs: cloning, structure, and expression. Proc Natl Acad Sci U S A 99: 13926, 2002.
42. Chang Y-H, Silverman SL, Paulus HE: Colchicine. *In* Paulus HE, Furst DE, S D (eds): Drugs for Rheumatic Diseases. New York, Churchill Livingstone, 1987, p 431.
43. Kimberly RP, Plotz PH: Salicylates including aspirin and sulfasalazine. *In* Kelley WN, Harris ED, Ruddy S, Sledge CB (eds): Textbook of Rheumatology, 3rd ed. Philadelphia, WB Saunders, 1989, p 739.
44. Vane JR, Botting RM: Anti-inflammatory drugs and their mechanism of action. Inflam Res 47(Suppl 2):S78, 1997.
45. Hochberg MC: New directions in symptomatic therapy for patients with osteoarthritis and rheumatoid arthritis. Semin Arthritis Rheum 32:4, 2002.
46. Emmerson BT: The management of gout. N Engl J Med 334:445, 1996.
47. Bridges SL: Gout treatment. *In* Klippel JH (ed): Primer on the Rheumatic Diseases. Atlanta, Arthritis Foundation, 2001, p 320.
48. Paulus HE, Schlosstein LH, Godfrey RG, et al: Prophylactic colchicine therapy of intercritical gout: a placebo-controlled study of probenecid-treated patients. Arthritis Rheum 17:609, 1974.
49. Kastner DL: Periodic syndromes. *In* Klippel JH (ed): Primer on the Rheumatic Diseases. Atlanta, Arthritis Foundation, 2001, p 194.
50. Ito S, Okuda-Ashitaka E, Minami T: Central and peripheral roles of prostaglandins in pain and their interactions with novel neuropeptides nociceptin and nocistatin. Neuroscience Res 41:299, 2001.
51. Yaksh TL, Dirig DM, Conway CM, et al: The acute antihyperalgesic action of nonsteroidal, anti-inflammatory drugs and release of spinal prostglandin E2 is mediated by inhibition of constitutive spinal cyclooxygenase-2 (COX-2) but not COX-1. J Neurosci 21:5847, 2001.
52. Ek M, Engblom D, Saha S, et al: Inflammatory response: pathway across the blood-brain barrier. Nature 410:430, 2001.
53. Li S, Wang Y, Matsumura K, et al: The febrile response to lipopolysaccharide is blocked in cyclooxygenase-2(−/−), but not in cyclooxygenase-1(−/−) mice. Brain Res 825:86, 1999.
54. Belay ED, S BJ, Holman RC, et al: Reye's syndrome in the United States from 1981 through 1997. N Engl J Med 340:1377, 1999.
55. Antithrombotic Trialists' Collaboration: Collaborative meta-analysis of randomised trials of antiplatelet therapy for prevention of death, myocardial infarction, and stroke in high risk patients. British Med J 324:71, 2002.
56. Hayden M, Pignone M, Phillips C, et al: Aspirin for the primary prevention of cardiovascular events: a summary of the evidence for the U.S. Preventive Services Task Force. Ann Intern Med 136:161, 2002.
57. Catella-Lawson F, Reilly M, Kapoor SC, et al: Cyclooxygenase inhibitors and the antiplatelet effects of aspirin. New Engl J Med 345:1809, 2001.
58. Giardeillo FM, Offerhaus GJA, DuBios RN: The role of nonsteroidal antiinflammatory drugs in colorectal cancer prevention. Eur J Cancer 31A:1071, 1995.
59. Phillips RK, Wallace MH, Lynch PM, et al: A randomised, double blind, placebo controlled study of celecoxib, a selective cyclooxygenase 2 inhibitor, on duodenal polyposis in familial adenomatous polyposis. Gut 50:857, 2002.
60. Baron JA, Cole BF, Sandler RS, et al: A randomized trial of aspirin to prevent colorectal adenomas. N Engl J Med 348:891, 2003.
61. Sandler RS, Halabi S, Baron JA, et al: A randomized trial of aspirin to prevent colorectal adenomas in patients with previous colorectal cancer. N Engl J Med 348:883, 2003.
62. Hawk ET, Viner JL, Dannenberg A, et al: COX-2 in cancer: a player that's defining the rules. J Natl Cancer Inst 94:545, 2002.
63. in t' Veld BA, Ruitenberg A, Hofman A, et al: Nonsteroidal anti-inflammatory drugs and the risk of Alzheimer's disease. N Engl J Med 345:1515, 2001.
64. Zandi PP, Anthony JC, Hayden KM, et al: Reduced incidence of AD with NSAID but not H2 receptor antagonists: the Cache County Study. Neurology 59:880, 2002.
65. Lindsay J, Laurin D, Verreault R, et al: Risk factors for Alzheimer's disease: a prospective analysis from the Canadian Study of Health and Aging. Am J Epidemiol 156:445, 2002.
66. Weggen S, Eriksen JL, Das P, et al: A subset of NSAIDs lower amyloidogenic Abeta42 independently of cyclooxygenase activity. Nature 414:212, 2001.
67. Pasinetti GM: From epidemiology to therapeutic trials with anti-inflammatory drugs in Alzheimer's disease: the role of NSAIDs

and cyclooxygenase in beta-amyloidosis and clinical dementia. J Alzheimers Dis 4:435, 2002.
68. Wolfe MM, Lichtenstein DR, Singh G: Gastrointestinal toxicity of nonsteroidal antiinflammatory drugs. New Engl J Med 340:1888, 1999.
69. Singh G, Ramey DR, Morfeld D, et al: Gatrointestinal tract complications of nonsteroidal anti-inflammatory drug treatment in rheumatoid arthritis: a prospective observational cohort study. Arch Intern Med 156:1530, 1996.
70. Garcia Rodriguez LA, Jick H: Risk of upper gastrointestinal bleeding and perforation associated with individual non-steroidal anti-inflammatory drugs. Lancet 343:769, 1994.
71. Lanas A, Bajador E, Serrano P, et al: Nitrovasodilators, low-dose aspirin, other nonsteroidal antiinflammatory drugs, and the risk of upper gastrointestinal bleeding. N Engl J Med 343:834, 2000.
72. Garcia Rodriguez LA, Hernandez-Diaz S: Relative risk of upper gastrointestinal complications among users of acetaminophen and nonsteroidal anti-inflammatory drugs. Epidemiology 12:570, 2001.
73. Fries JF: The epidemiology of NSAID gastropathy: the ARAMIS experience. J Clin Rheumatol 4:S11, 1998.
74. Patrono C, Patrignani P, Garcia-Rodrigues LA: Cyclooxygenase-selective inhibition of prostanoid formation: transducing biochemical selectivity into clinical read-outs. J Clin Invest 108:7, 2002.
75. Wallace JL: Nonsteroidal anti-inflammatory drugs and gastroenteropathy: the second hundred years. Gastroenterology 112:1000, 1997.
76. Laine L, Bombardier C, Hawkey CJ, et al: Stratifying the risk of NSAID-related upper gastrointestinal clinical events: results of a double-blind outcomes study in patients with rheumatoid arthritis. Gastroenterol 123:1006, 2002.
77. Bakowsky VS, Hanly JG: Complications of nonsteroidal antiinflammatory drug gastropathy and use of gastric cytoprotection: experience at a tertiary care health center. J Rheumatol 26:1557, 1999.
78. Bombardier C, Laine L, Reicin A, et al: Comparison of upper gastrointestinal toxicity of rofecoxib and naproxen in patients with rheumatoid arthritis. N Engl J Med 343:1520, 2000.
79. Silverstein FE, Faich G, Goldstein JL, et al: Gastrointestinal toxicity with celecoxib vs nonsteroidal anti-inflammatory drugs for osteoarthritis and rheumatoid arthritis: the CLASS study—randomized controlled trial. JAMA 284:1247, 2000.
80. Simon LS, Smolen JS, Abramson SB, et al: Controversies in COX-2 selective inhibtion. J Rheumatol 29:1501, 2002.
81. Mamdani M, Rochon PA, Juurlink DN, et al: Observational study of upper gastrointestinal haemorrhage in elderly patients given selective cyclo-oxygenase-2 inhibitors or conventional non-steroidal anti-inflammatory drugs. BMJ 325:624, 2002.
82. Silverstein FE, Graham DY, Senior JR, et al: Misoprostol reduces serious gastrointestinal complications in patients with rheumatoid arthritis receiving nonsteroidal anti-inflammatory drugs. Ann Intern Med 123:241, 1995.
83. Hawkey CJ, Karrasch JA, Szczepanski L, et al: Omeprazole compared with misoprostol for ulcers associated with nonsteroidal antiinflammatory drugs. N Engl J Med 338:727, 1998.
84. Yeomans ND, Tulassay Z, Juhasz L, et al: A comparison of omeprazole with ranitidine for ulcers associated with nonsteroidal antiinflammatory drugs. N Engl J Med 338:719, 1998.
85. Chan FKL, Chung SCS, Suen BY, et al: Preventing recurrent upper gastrointestinal bleeding in patients with Helicobacter pylori infection who are taking low-dose aspirin or naproxen. N Engl J Med 344:967, 2001.
86. Chan FKL, Hung LCT, Suen BY, et al: Celecoxib versus diclofenac and omeprazole in reducing the risk of recurrent ulcer bleeding in patients with arthritis. N Engl J Med 347:2104, 2002.
87. Houchen CW: Clinical implications of prostaglandin inhibition in the small bowel. Gastroenterol Clin North Am 30:953, 2001.
88. Wallace JL: Prostaglandin biology in inflammatory bowel disease. Gastroenterol Clin North Am 30:971, 2001.
89. Brater DC: Anti-inflammatory agents and renal function. Semin Arthritis Rheum 32:33, 2002.
90. Qi Z, Hao C-M, Langenbach RI, et al: Opposite effects of cyclooxygenase-1 and -2 activity on the pressor response to angiotensin II. J Clin Invest 110:61, 2002.
91. Harris RC, Breyer MD: Physiological regulation of cyclooxygenase-2 in the kidney. Am J Physiol Renal Physiol 281:F1, 2001.
92. Gurwitz JH, Avorn J, Bonh RL, et al: Initiation of antihypertensive treatment during nonsteroidal anti-inflammatory drug therapy. JAMA 272:781, 1994.
93. Dedier J, Stampfer MJ, Hankinson SE, et al: Nonnarcotic analgesic use and the risk of hypertension in US women. Hypertension 40:604, 2002.
94. Brater DC: Effects of nonsteroidal anti-inflammatory drugs on renal function: focus on cyclooxygenase-2-selective inhibition. Am J Med 107:65S, 1999.
95. Akhund L, Quinet RJ, Ishaq S: Celecoxib-related renal papillary necrosis. Arch Intern Med 163:114, 2003.
96. Fored CM, Ejerblad E, Lindblad P, et al: Acetaminophen, aspirin, and chronic renal failure: a nationwide case-control study in Sweden. N Engl J Med 2001.
97. Rexrode KM, Buring JE, Glynn RJ, et al: Analgesic use and renal function in men. JAMA 286:315, 2001.
98. Prescott LF: Paracetamol: Past, present, and future. Am J Therapeutics 7:143, 2000.
99. Woessner KM, Simon RA, Stevenson DD: The safety of celecoxib in patients with aspirin-sensitive asthma. Arthritis Rheum 46:2201, 2002.
100. Stevenson DD, Simon RA: Lack of cross-reactivity between rofecoxib and aspirin in aspirin-sensitive patients with asthma. J Allergy Clin Immunol 108:47, 2001.
101. Bonnel RA, Villalba ML, Karwoski CB, et al: Aseptic meningitis associated with rofecoxib. Arch Intern Med 162:713, 2002.
102. Strand V, Hochberg MC: The risk of cardiovascular thrombotic events with selective cyclooxygenase-2 inhibitors. Arthritis Care Res 47:349, 2002.
103. Ray WA, Stein CM, Daugherty JR, et al: COX-2 selective nonsteroidal anti-inflammatory drugs and risk of serious coronary heart disease. Lancet 360:1071, 2002.
104. Einhorn TA: Do inhibitors of cyclooxygenase-2 impair bone healing? J Bone Miner Res 17:977, 2002.
105. Forwood MR: Inducible cyclo-oxygenase (COX-2) mediates the induction of bone formation by mechanical loading in vivo. J Bone Miner Res 11:1688, 1996.
106. Sirois J, Dore M: The late induction of prostaglandin G/H synthase in equine preovulatory follicles supports its role as a determinant of the ovulatory process. Endocrinology 138:4427, 1997.
107. Richards JS: Sounding the alarm: does induction of the prostaglandin endoperoxide synthase-2 control the mammalian ovulatory clock? [Editorial]. Endocrinology 138:4047, 1997.
108. Lim H, Paria BC, Das SK, et al: Multiple female reproductive failures in cyclooxygenase 2-deficient mice. Cell 91:197, 1997.
109. Stone S, Khamashta MA, Nelson-Piercy C: Nonsteroidal anti-inflammatory drugs and reversible female infertility: is there a link? Drug Saf 25:545, 2002.
110. Rahme E, Pettitt D, LeLorier J: Determinants and sequelae associated with utilization of acetaminophen versus traditional nonsteroidal antiinflammatory drugs in an elderly population. Arthritis Rheum 46:3046, 2002.
111. Altiparmak MR, Pamuk ON, Pamuk GE, et al: Colchicine neuromyopathy: a report of six cases. Clin Exp Rheumatol 20:S13, 2002.
112. Brater DC: Drug-drug and drug-disease interactions with nonsteroidal anti-inflammatory drugs. Am J Med 80:62, 1986.
113. Wolfe F, Zhao S, Lane N: Preference for nonsteroidal antiinflammatory drugs over acetaminophen by rheumatic disease patients: a survey of 1,799 patients with osteoarthritis, rheumatoid arthritis, and fibromyalgia. Arthritis Rheum 43:378, 2000.
114. Pincus T, Koch GG, Sokka T, et al: A randomized, double-blind, crossover clinical trial of diclofenac plus misoprostol versus acetaminophen in patients with osteoarthritis of the hip or knee. Arthritis Rheum 44:1587, 2001.
115. Geba GP, Weaver AL, Polis AB, et al: Efficacy of refecoxib, celecoxib, and acetaminophen in osteoarthritis of the knee. JAMA 287:64, 2002.
116. American College of Rheumatology Subcommittee on Osteoarthritis Guidelines: Recommendations for the medical management of osteoarthritis of the hip and knee: 2000 update. Arthritis Rheum 43:1905, 2000.

57 Glucocorticoid Therapy

JOHANNES W.G. JACOBS • JOHANNES W.J. BIJLSMA

Glucocorticoids are widely used for the treatment of patients with rheumatic diseases. The first to be isolated, in 1935, was the naturally occurring corticosteroid hormone cortisone. It was synthesized in 1944 and subsequently became available for clinical use. In 1948, for the first time cortisone (then called *compound E*) was administered by American rheumatologist Philip Hench (1896-1965) to a 29-year-old woman with active rheumatoid arthritis (RA) of more than 4 years' duration. Her joints were so painful she could "hardly get out of bed." After 2 days of treatment with 100 mg of intramuscular compound E daily, "she rolled over in bed with ease, and noted much less muscular soreness." The next day, she was able to walk with "only a slight limp." Hench published this case of dramatic improvement in 1949,[1] and won for his research the 1950 Nobel Prize in Physiology or Medicine, which he shared with colleagues at the Mayo Clinic Foundation. Later on, by chemical modification of natural steroids, different synthetic glucocorticoids were produced, some of which have proved to be very effective antiphlogistic and immune-suppressive substances with instant effect.

Initially, there was considerable enthusiasm about glucocorticoids, because of the striking relief of symptoms seen in patients treated with supraphysiologic dosages. However, when the wide array of potentially serious adverse side effects became apparent, the use of glucocorticoids decreased. Nevertheless, because glucocorticoids can be considered the most effective antiphlogistic and immune-suppressive substances currently known,[2] they have become the cornerstone in the treatment of many rheumatic disorders, such as systemic lupus erythematosus (SLE), vasculitis, polymyalgia rheumatica, and myositis.[3] Careful administration of glucocorticoids to patients with RA has also become accepted.

During the past decades, our knowledge about glucocorticoids has increased, but there is still much to learn about the modes of actions of these drugs in rheumatic autoimmune disorders. Hopefully, the unraveling of these mechanisms may eventually lead to new classes of therapy.[4]

Characteristics of Glucocorticoids

STRUCTURE AND CLASSIFICATION

The main precursor molecule of all steroid hormones is cholesterol. Steroid hormones and cholesterol are characterized by a sterol-skeleton, formed by three six-carbon hexane rings and one five-carbon pentane ring. The carbon atoms of this sterol-nucleus are numbered in a specific sequence; the term *steroid* refers to this basic sterol nucleus (Fig. 57–1).

Steroid hormones can be classed on the basis of their main function into (male and female) sex hormones, mineralocorticoids, and glucocorticoids. Sex hormones are synthesized mainly in the gonads, but also in the adrenal cortex. Mineralocorticoids and glucocorticoids are only synthesized in the adrenal cortex; the terms *corticosteroid* and *corticoid* for these hormones refer to the adrenal cortex. Some glucocorticoids have also a mineralocorticoid effect and vice versa. The main natural mineralocorticoid is aldosterone, and the main natural glucocorticoid is cortisol (hydrocortisone). Although the separation of corticoids into the classes mineralocorticoids and glucocorticoids is not absolute, it is better (more precise) to use the term *glucocorticoid* than the term *corticosteroid* when referring to one of these compounds.[5] The importance of standardized nomenclature is illustrated by the knowledge that an electronic literature search can be complicated by multiple synonyms.

In the 1950s, chemical modification of natural steroids revealed a number of structural features essential for specific biologic activities. Synthetic steroid hormones more potent than natural steroid hormones and steroid hormones with altered biologic activity were developed.

These studies proved that the 17-hydroxy, 21-carbon steroid configuration (see Fig. 57–1) is required for glucocorticoid activity through binding to the glucocorticoid receptor. Glucocorticoids with an 11-keto, instead of an 11-hydroxy, group such as cortisone and prednisone are prohormones that must be reduced in the liver to their 11-hydroxy configurations. Cortisone is converted to cortisol and prednisone to prednisolone to become biologically active.[6] Practically speaking, in patients with severe liver disease, it is rational to prescribe prednisolone instead of prednisone.

There are no qualitative differences between the glucocorticoid effect of endogenous cortisol and exogenously applied synthetic glucocorticoids, because these effects are, except for higher doses, predominantly genomic (i.e., mediated through the glucocorticoid receptor).[5,7] There are quantitative differences, however. The potency and other biologic characteristics of the glucocorticoids depend on structural differences in the steroid configuration. For example, the introduction of a double bond between the 1 and 2 positions of cortisol yields prednisolone, which has about four times more glucocorticoid activity than cortisol[6] (Table 57–1).

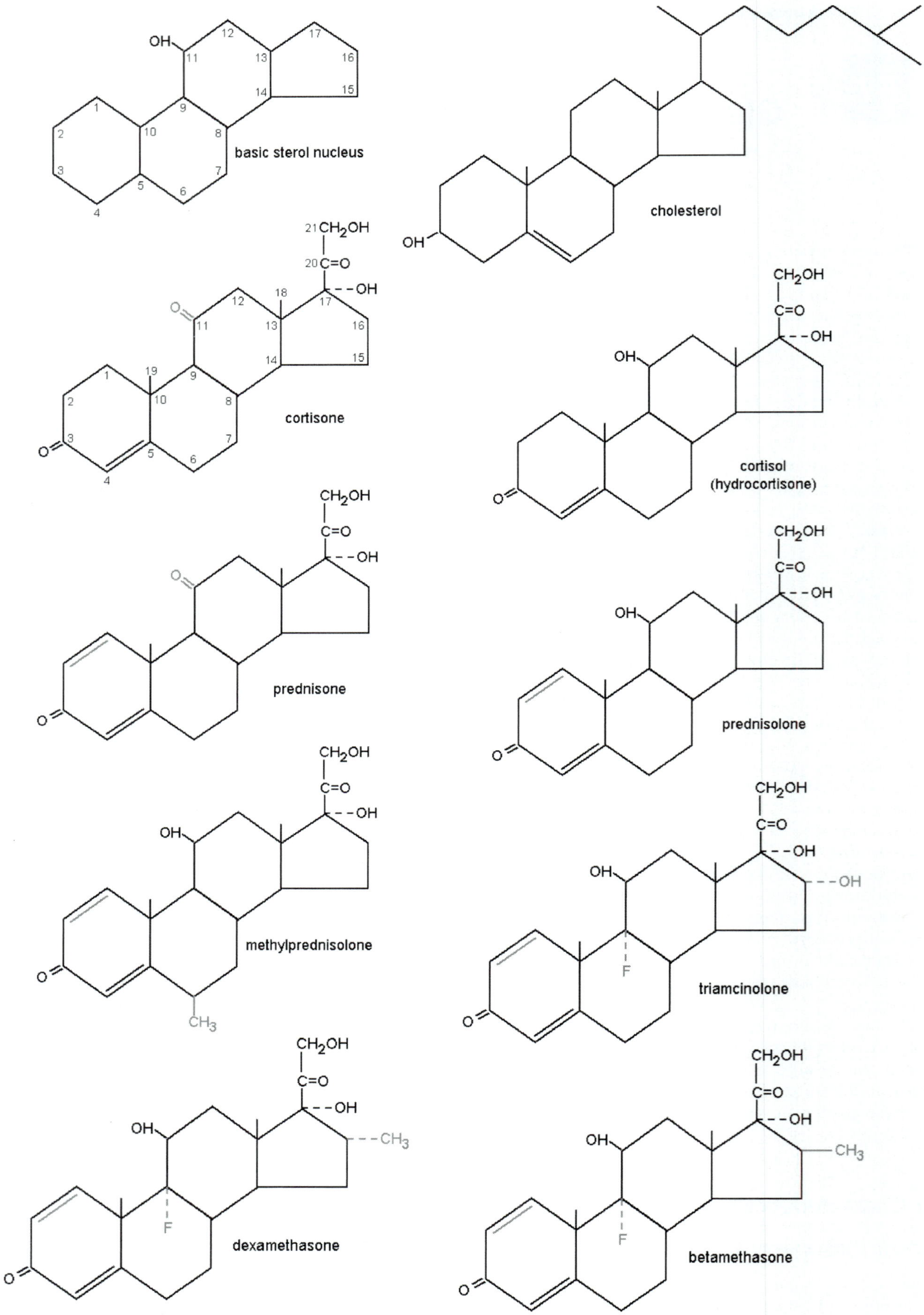

FIGURE 57–1 · Basic steroid configuration and structure of cholesterol and of natural and some synthetic glucocorticoid.

TABLE 57–1 • PHARMACODYNAMICS OF GLUCOCORTICOIDS USED IN RHEUMATOLOGY

	Equivalent Glucocorticoid Dose (mg)	Relative Glucocorticoid Activity	Relative Mineralocorticoid Activity*	Protein Binding†	Half-life in Plasma (hr)	Biologic Half-life (hr)
Short Acting						
Cortisone	25	0.8	0.8	–	0.5	8-12
Cortisol	20	1	1	++++	1.5-2	8-12
Intermediate Acting						
Methylprednisolone	4	5	0.5	–	>3.5	18-36
Prednisolone	5	4	0.6	++	2.1-3.5	18-36
Prednisone	5	4	0.6	+++	3.4-3.8	18-36
Triamcinolone	4	5	0	++	2->5	18-36
Long Acting						
Dexamethasone	0.75	20-30	0	++	3-4.5	36-54
Betamethasone	0.6	20-30	0	++	3-5	36-54

*Clinically: sodium and water retention, potassium depletion.
†*Symbols:* –, none; ++, high; +++, high to very high; ++++, very high.

Addition of a six-methyl group to prednisolone yields methylprednisolone, which is about five times more potent than cortisol. All the aforementioned glucocorticoids also have a mineralocorticoid effect. The synthetic glucocorticoids triamcinolone and dexamethasone, however, have negligible mineralocorticoid activity.

BIOLOGIC CHARACTERISTICS AND THERAPEUTIC CONSEQUENCES

Apart from the steroid configuration, biologic characteristics of glucocorticoids also depend on whether they are in free form (as an alcohol) or chemically bound (as an ester or salt). In their free form, glucocorticoids are virtually insoluble in water, so they can be used in tablets, but not in parenteral preparations. For that reason, synthetic glucocorticoids are formulated as either organic esters or as salts. Esters, such as (di)acetate and (hex)acetonide, are lipid soluble but have limited water solubility and are suitable for oral use and intramuscular, intralesional, and intra-articular injection. Salts, such as sodium phosphate and sodium succinate, are, in general, more water soluble and, therefore, also suitable for intravenous use. So, dexamethasone sodium phosphate can be used intravenously, whereas dexamethasone acetate cannot. When given intramuscularly, dexamethasone sodium phosphate will be absorbed much faster from the injection site than dexamethasone acetate. If an immediate effect is required, dexamethasone sodium phosphate given intravenously is more effective than the same preparation given intramuscularly, and the least adequate in this case is intramuscular dexamethasone acetate. For local use, less solubility means longer duration of the local effect, which, in general, is beneficial.

PHARMACOKINETICS AND PHARMACOLOGY

Water insolubility does not impair absorption in the digestive tract. Most orally administered glucocorticoids, whether in free form or as an ester or salt, are absorbed readily, probably within about 30 minutes.[6] Bioavailability of prednisone and prednisolone is high; commercially available oral and rectal prednisone and prednisolone preparations are considered approximately bioequivalent.[8]

The affinity of the different glucocorticoids for various plasma proteins varies (see Table 57–1). Of cortisol in plasma, 90 to 95 percent is bound to plasma proteins, primarily transcortin (also called corticosteroid-binding globulin) and, to a lesser degree, albumin. Protein-bound cortisol is not biologically active, but the remaining 5 to 10 percent of free cortisol is. Prednisolone has—in contrast to methylprednisolone, dexamethasone and triamcinolone—a high affinity for transcortin and competes with cortisol for this binding protein. The synthetic glucocorticoids, other than prednisolone, with little or no affinity for transcortin are two-thirds bound (weakly) to albumin, and about one third circulates as free glucocorticoid.[6]

Because only unbound glucocorticoids are pharmacologically active, patients with low levels of plasma protein such as albumin (e.g., because of liver diseases or chronic active inflammatory diseases) are more susceptible to effects and side effects of glucocorticoids; adjusting doses should be considered in these patients. In liver disease, an additional argument for dose adjustment is reduced clearance of glucocorticoids (see following).

Glucocorticoids have biologic half-lives two to 36 times longer than their plasma half-lives (see Table 57–1). That is why prednisolone, with a plasma half-life of about 3 hours, can be dosed once daily for most diseases. Maximal effect of glucocorticoids lags behind peak serum concentrations. Transcortin binds these compounds more strongly than does albumin. The plasma elimination of glucocorticoids bound to transcortin is slower than that of glucocorticoids that do not bind. However, transcortin binding is not a major determinant of the glucocorticoids' biologic half-lives, in contrast to distribution to different compartments of the body and binding to cytosolic glucocorticoid receptor. Synthetic glucocorticoids have lower affinity for transcortin but higher affinity for the cytosolic glucocorticoid receptor than cortisol (see following). The affinity of prednisolone and triamcinolone for the glucocorticoid receptor is approximately two times higher and of dexamethasone is seven times higher. Prednisone and cortisone have negligible glucocorticoid bioactivity before they have been chemically reduced because of their very low affinity for the glucocorticoid receptor.

Another important factor determining biologic half-lives of glucocorticoids is the rate of metabolism. Synthetic glucocorticoids are subject to the same reduction, oxidation, hydroxylation, and conjugation reactions as cortisol. Pharmacologically active glucocorticoids are metabolized primarily in the liver into inactive metabolites and are excreted by the kidneys; only small amounts of unmetabolized drug are also excreted in the urine.[6] There is an inverse correlation between prednisolone clearance and age, which means that a given dose may have a greater effect in older persons.[9] In addition, prednisolone clearance is also slower in African Americans compared to Caucasians.[10] Serum half-life of prednisolone ranges from 2.5 to 5 hours, but it is increased in renal disease and liver cirrhosis, and the elderly, presumably. Prednisolone can be removed by hemodialysis, but overall, the amount removed does not require dose adjustment in patients on hemodialysis. In patients with liver cirrhosis, however, the clearance of unbound steroid is about two thirds of normal, a difference that should be taken into account with dosing.

DRUG INTERACTIONS

It is important to realize that certain drugs (e.g., barbiturates, phenytoin, rifampin)[11] (Fig. 57–2)) increase the metabolism of synthetic and natural glucocorticoids, particularly by increasing hepatic hydroxylase activity by inducing cytochrome P-450 (CYP) isoenzyme 3A4 and, thus, reducing glucocorticoid concentrations.[6] Rifampin-induced nonresponsiveness to prednisone in inflammatory diseases has been described,[11-13] as has rifampin-induced adrenal crisis in patients on glucocorticoid replacement therapy.[14] Clinicians should consider increasing the dosage of glucocorticoids in patients who are cotreated with these medications.

Conversely, drugs that inhibit CYP3A4, such as ketoconazole, decrease glucocorticoid clearance and lead to higher concentrations of glucocorticoids and increased risk of side effects. Concomitant administration of prednisolone and cyclosporin may result in increased plasma concentrations of the former drug; and concomitant administration of methylprednisolone and cyclosporin may result in increased plasma concentrations of the latter drug. The mechanism of this probably is competitive inhibition of microsomal liver enzymes.[6] Antibiotics such as erythromycin may raise plasma concentrations of glucocorticoids. Synthetic estrogens in oral contraceptives increase the level of transcortin and, thus, total (sum of bound and unbound) glucocorticoid levels. Thus, in women taking oral contraceptives, care is required in the interpretation of cortisol measurements: Adrenal insufficiency might be present even if total cortisol levels are within the normal range.[15]

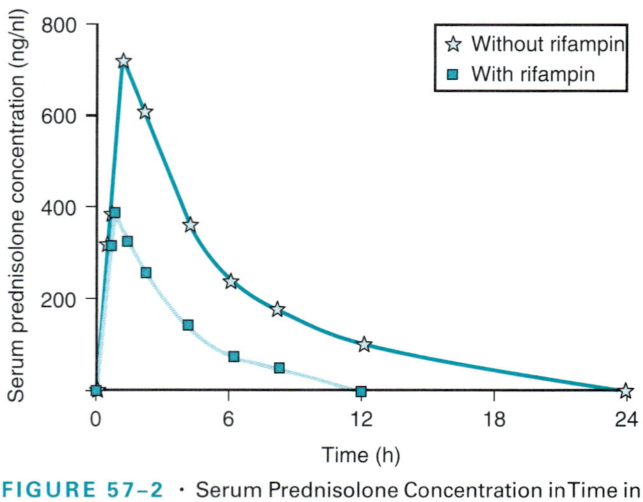

FIGURE 57–2 • Serum Prednisolone Concentration in Time in One Patient, Following 0.9 mg/kg Prednisone Orally Daily, in Presence and Absence of Therapy with Rifampin. Curve with rifampin: during a priod of continuous administration of both drugs; curve without rifampin: after a washout of rifampin of 4 weeks. With rifampin reduced area under the curve, indicating reduced biovailability.

PREGNANCY AND LACTATION

In pregnancy, glucocorticoids seem to be well tolerated by mother and child. The maternal-to-child prednisolone blood concentration ratio is about 10:1, due to transformation of biologically active prednisolone into inactive prednisone by the placenta. In contrast, dexamethasone is not metabolized by the placenta; the maternal-to-child dexamethasone blood concentration ratio is about 1:1. So when the pregnant mother has to be treated with glucocorticoids, prednisolone would be a good choice; but if the unborn child has to be treated, dexamethasone would be indicated. Prednisolone and prednisone are excreted in only small quantities in breast milk; breast feeding is considered safe for a child whose mother is taking these drugs.

CONCLUSIONS

It is, thus, important in daily clinical use to carefully choose which preparation of a particular glucocorticoid to use in various settings.

Basic Mechanisms of Glucocorticoids

GENOMIC AND NONGENOMIC EFFECTS

Glucocorticoids at any therapeutically relevant dosage exhibit pharmacologic effects via classic *genomic* mechanisms. The lipophilic glucocorticoid passes across the cell membrane, attaches to the cytosolic glucocorticoid receptor and heat-shock protein, then binds to glucocorticoid-responsive elements on genomic DNA, and interacts with nuclear transcription factors. This takes time; when acting through genomic mechanisms, it takes at least 30 minutes before the clinical effect of a glucocorticoid begins to show.[16] Only when high dosages are given, such as in pulse therapy, can glucocorticoids act within minutes by *nongenomic* mechanisms. This occurs either via specific receptor-mediated activity or via nonspecific membrane-associated physicochemical activity.[7] The response to high-dose pulse methylprednisolone therapy, for instance, may therefore be biphasic, with an early, rapid, nongenomic effect and a delayed and more sustained classic genomic effect.[17] Clinically, genomic and nongenomic effects cannot be separated.

GENOMIC MECHANISMS

Most of the effects of glucocorticoids are exerted via genomic mechanisms, by binding to the glucocorticoid receptor located in the cytoplasm of the target cells. Only one type of glucocorticoid receptor, which is common to all target tissues, binds all types of glucocorticoids, as has been described previously. The activated glucocorticoid receptor-glucocorticoid complex is rapidly translocated into the nucleus, where it binds to specific consensus sites in the DNA (glucocorticoid-response elements), directly or indirectly regulating the transcription of a large variety of target genes. This process is called transactivation. Binding to glucocorticoid-response elements results in either stimulation or suppression of transcription of these target genes.[18] Suppression of genes may also be mediated by indirect mechanisms involving the interaction of the glucocorticoid receptor with other transcriptional factors, such as activator protein-1 and nuclear factor-κB. This process is called transrepression. The nature and availability of these transcriptional factors may be pivotal in determining the differential sensitivity of different tissues to glucocorticoids,[19] because they play a critical role in regulating the expression of a wide variety of proinflammatory genes induced by cytokines. The binding of transcriptional factors to DNA is inhibited by glucocorticoids, resulting in depressed expression of these genes and inhibition of their amplifying role in inflammation. Activated glucocorticoid receptors may also inhibit protein synthesis by decreasing the stability of mRNA through the induction of ribonucleases. This mechanism has been proposed to mediate glucocorticoid-induced inhibition of the synthesis of interleukin (IL)-1, IL-6, granulocyte-macrophage colony-stimulating factor (GMC-SF), and inducible cyclooxygenase (COX)-2.[20]

There is increasing acceptance of the hypothesis that side effects of glucocorticoids may be due to transactivation of genes following binding of glucocorticoid receptor dimers to DNA, whereas the therapeutic, anti-inflammatory effects may be due to the binding of a single glucocorticoid receptor to transcription factors or coactivators, resulting in gene repression (transrepression).[21] Further unraveling of molecular mechanisms of these processes may hopefully lead to development of novel glucocorticoids with a more favorable balance of transactivation and transrepression and, clinically, thus to a more favorable balance of side effects and therapeutic effects.[22]

GLUCOCORTICOID EFFECTS ON THE IMMUNE SYSTEM

Glucocorticoids reduce activation, proliferation, differentiation, and survival of a variety of inflammatory cells, including macrophages and T lymphocytes, and promote apoptosis, especially in immature and activated T cells. This is mainly mediated by changes in cytokine production and secretion. In contrast, B lymphocytes and neutrophils are less sensitive to glucocorticoids, and their survival may actually be increased by glucocorticoid treatment. The main effect of glucocorticoids on neutrophils seems to be inhibition of adhesion to endothelial cells. Glucocorticoids inhibit not only the expression of adhesion molecules, but also the secretion of complement pathway proteins and prostaglandins. At supraphysiologic concentrations, glucocorticoids suppress fibroblast proliferation, and IL-1 and tumor necrosis factor-α (TNF-α)–induced metalloproteinase synthesis. By these effects, glucocorticoids may retard bone and cartilage destruction.[23]

Leukocytes

Administration of glucocorticoids leads to a rise in the total leukocyte blood count due to an increase in neutrophils in the blood, though the number of other leukocytes in blood decreases. Table 57–2 summarizes the effects of glucocorticoids on specific leukocytes. The redistribution of lymphocytes, which is maximal 4 to 6 hours after administration of a single high dose of prednisone and returns to normal within 24 hours, has no clinical consequences; B cell function and immunoglobulin production are hardly affected. The effects of glucocorticoids on monocytes and macrophages might increase susceptibility to infection, however.[24]

Cytokines

The influence of glucocorticoids on cytokine production and action represents one of the major mechanisms for glucocorticoid action in chronic inflammatory diseases such as RA. Glucocorticoids exert potent inhibitory

TABLE 57–2 • ANTI-INFLAMMATORY EFFECTS OF GLUCOCORTICOIDS ON IMMUNOMODULATORY CELLS

Cell Type	Effects
Neutrophils	Increased blood count, decreased trafficking, relatively unaltered functioning
Macrophages and Monocytes	Decreased blood count, decreased trafficking, decreased phagocytosis and bactericidal effects, inhibited antigen presentation, decreased cytokine and eicosanoid release
Lymphocytes	Decreased blood count, decreased trafficking, decreased cytokine production, decreased proliferation and impaired activation, little effect on immunoglobulin synthesis
Eosinophils	Decreased blood count, increased apoptosis
Basophils	Decreased blood count, decreased release of their mediators of inflammation

effects on the transcription and action of a large variety of cytokines with pivotal importance in the pathogenesis of RA. Most proinflammatory, T helper type 1 (Th1) cytokines are inhibited by glucocorticoids, including IL-1β, IL-2, IL-3, IL-6, TNF-α, interferon-γ, and GMC-SF. These cytokines are, in RA, considered responsible for synovitis, cartilage degradation, and bone erosion. Conversely, the production of Th2 cytokines, such as IL-4, IL-10, and IL-13, is either stimulated or not affected by glucocorticoids.[25] These cytokines have been related to the extra-articular features of erosive RA associated with B cell overactivity, such as immune complex formation and vasculitis. Activation of Th2 cells can inhibit rheumatoid synovitis and joint destruction through the release of IL-4 and IL-10, which inhibit Th1 activity and downregulate a number of monocyte and macrophage functions.[26]

Inflammatory Enzymes

An important part of the inflammatory cascade is arachidonic acid metabolism, leading to the production of prostaglandins and leukotrienes, most of which are strongly proinflammatory. Through the induction of lipocortin (an inhibitor of phospholiphase A2), glucocorticoids inhibit the formation of arachidonic acid metabolites. Glucocorticoids have also been shown to inhibit the production of COX-2 and phospholipase A2 induced by cytokines in monocytes and other inflammatory cells. In addition, glucocorticoids are potent inhibitors of the production of metalloproteinases in vitro and in vivo, especially collagenase and stromelysin, which are the main effectors of cartilage degradation induced by IL-1 and TNF-α.[27]

Adhesion Molecules and Permeability Factors

Pharmacologic doses of glucocorticoids dramatically inhibit exudation of plasma and migration of leukocytes into inflammatory sites. Adhesion molecules play a central role in chronic inflammatory diseases by controlling the trafficking of inflammatory cells into sites of inflammation. Glucocorticoids reduce the expression of adhesion molecules through the inhibition of proinflammatory cytokines and by direct inhibitory effects on the expression of adhesion molecules, such as intercellular adhesion molecule-1 and E-selectin.[28] Chemotactic cytokines attracting immune cells to the inflammatory site, such as IL-8 and the macrophage chemoattractant proteins, are also inhibited by glucocorticoids. Nitric oxide production in inflammatory sites is increased by proinflammatory cytokines and results in an increased blood flow, exudation, and probably amplification of the inflammatory response. The inducible form of nitric oxide synthase by cytokines is potently inhibited by glucocorticoids.[29]

THE HYPOTHALAMIC-PITUITARY-ADRENAL AXIS

Pathophysiology

Proinflammatory cytokines, such as IL-1 and IL-6, as well as eicosanoids, such as prostaglandin E2, and endotoxines, all activate corticotropin-releasing hormone (CRH) at the hypothalamic level. This, in turn, stimulates the secretion of adrenocorticotropic hormone (ACTH) by the pituitary gland and, thus, of glucocorticoids by the adrenal glands. In otherwise healthy individuals in situations with severe infections or other major physical stress, cortisol production may increase to six times the normal amount.[15] However, in patients with active RA (and other chronic inflammatory diseases) the increase of cortisol driven by elevated cytokines might be inappropriately low,[4] meaning that cortisol levels—although normal or elevated in the absolute sense—are insufficient to control the inflammatory response. This is the concept of relative adrenal insufficiency.[15,30,31] Both endogenous and exogenous glucocorticoids exert negative feedback control on the hypothalamic-pituitary-adrenal axis, directly by suppressing secretion of pituitary ACTH and indirectly on the level of CRH, via suppression of release from inflammatory tissues of proinflammatory cytokines (Fig. 57–3). This latter counterregulation mechanism is possibly also less effective in RA.[32]

ACTH is secreted in brief, episodic bursts, resulting in sharp rises in plasma concentrations of ACTH and cortisol, followed by slower declines in cortisol levels: the normal diurnal rhythm in cortisol secretion. The secretory ACTH episodic bursts increase in amplitude but not in frequency after 3 to 5 hours of sleep, reach a maximum in the hours before and the hour after awakening, decline throughout the morning, and are minimal in the evening. So cortisol levels are highest at about the time of awakening in the morning, are low in the late afternoon and evening, and reach their lowest level an hour or so after falling asleep (see Fig. 57–3). Glucocorticoids are not stored in the adrenal glands in significant amounts; therefore, continuing synthesis and release are required to maintain basal secretion or to increase blood levels during stress. The total daily basal secretion of cortisol in humans has been estimated at 5.7 mg/m^2/day.[33] This rather low daily cortisol production rate may explain the cushingoid symptoms, which are sometimes observed in patients with adrenal insufficiency using glucocorticoids at a dose previously regarded to be a normal replacement dose.

Effects of Glucocorticoids on the Hypothalamic-Pituitary-Adrenal Axis

Chronic suppression of the hypothalamic-pituitary-adrenal axis by pathologically increased endogenous glucocorticoid secretion or administration of exogenous glucocorticoids leads to adrenal atrophy and loss of cortisol secretory capability. The patients have both a failure of pituitary ACTH–release and adrenal responsiveness to ACTH; serum cortisol and ACTH levels are low. Glucocorticoid-induced secondary adrenal insufficiency is characterized by a selective ACTH deficit; other hypopituitary axes are normal. The time required to achieve suppression depends on the dosage and the serum half-life of the glucocorticoid used, but it also varies among patients, probably because of individual differences in rates of glucocorticoid metabolism and in

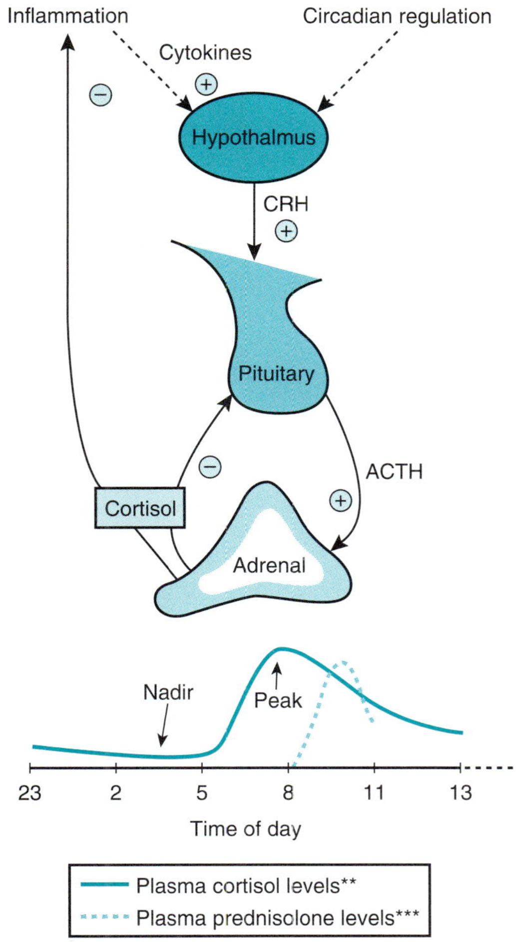

FIGURE 57–3 • Simplified scheme showing the hypothalamic-hypopituitary-adrenal axis, plasma cortisol levels in rheumatoid arthritis, and plasma prednisolone levels after an oral dose at 8 o'clock*
*negative feedback loops of cortisol and exogenous glucocorticoids via pituitary (fast, major determinant serum half life) and via inflammation (slow, major determinant biological half life)
**scheme for control persons. Probably, induced by cytokines, circadian rhythms are changed in RA, with a shift to an earlier cortisol peak (about 1.5 h earlier)
***oral administration of prednisolone at 8 o'clock, peak plasma concentration in 1-3 h, plasma half life 2-3.5 h, biological half life 6 h

glucocorticoid sensitivity. This means that prediction with certainty of chronic suppression of the hypothalamic-pituitary-adrenal axis and adrenal insufficiency is not possible. The duration of anti-inflammatory effect of one dose of a glucocorticoid approximates the duration of hypothalamic-pituitary-adrenal suppression. After a single oral dose of 250 mg hydrocortisone or cortisone, 50 mg prednisone or prednisolone, and 40 mg methylprednisolone, suppression for 1.25 to 1.5 days has been described. Duration of suppression after 40 mg triamcinolone and 5 mg dexamethasone was 2.25 and 2.75 days, respectively.[6] Following intramuscular administration of a single dose of 40 to 80 mg triamcinolone acetonide, duration of hypothalamic-pituitary-adrenal suppression is 2 to 4 weeks, and after 40 to 80 mg methylprednisolone, suppression lasts 4 to 8 days.[6]

In the case of chronic therapy, for patients who have had less than 10 mg of prednisone or its equivalent per day in one dose in the morning, the risk of clinical (symptomatic) adrenal insufficiency is not very high, but is also not nil. A recent review on adrenal insufficiency states that if the daily dose is 7.5 mg prednisolone or equivalent or more for at least 3 weeks, adrenal hypofunctioning should be anticipated and acute cessation of glucocorticoid in this situation could lead to problems.[15] Patients who have received glucocorticoids for less than 3 weeks or have been treated with alternate-day prednisolone therapy do not have an absent risk of suppression of the hypothalamic-pituitary-adrenal axis,[34,35] but the risk depends on the dose. After 5 to 30 days of at least 25 mg prednisone or equivalent daily, suppression of adrenal response (measured by a low-dose corticotropin test) was present in 34 of 75 patients studied (45%).[36] In these patients, a basal plasma cortisol concentration below 100 nmol/liter was highly suggestive of adrenal suppression, whereas levels of basal cortisol above 220 nmol/liter predicted a normal adrenal response in most, but not all, patients. It seems prudent to treat these patients as having secondary adrenal insufficiency.

Treatment with Glucocorticoids

Glucocorticoids are widely used for several rheumatic diseases in various dosages. Often it is not clear what is meant with the semiquantitative terms used for dosages, such as "low" or "high." Based on pathophysiologic and pharmacokinetic data, standardization has been recently proposed to minimize problems in interpretation of these generally used terms[5] (Table 57–3).

INDICATIONS

For each disease, indications for glucocorticoid therapy will be discussed in the specific chapters. Here, an overview is given (Table 57–4), which only summarizes the general use and dosages of glucocorticoids. Without detailed description, some of the indications could be considered questionable at first glance. For instance, in systemic sclerosis, glucocorticoids, especially in high doses, are contraindicated because of the risk of scleroderma renal crisis,[37] but they may be useful for myositis or interstitial lung disease. As can be seen, glucocorticoids are basic part of the therapeutic strategy in myositis, polymyalgia rheumatica, and systemic vasculitis; for other diseases, glucocorticoids are adjunctive therapy or are not used at all. In osteoarthritis, for example, glucocorticoids

TABLE 57–3 • TERMINOLOGY OF DOSAGES OF GLUCOCORTICOIDS FOR USE IN RHEUMATOLOGY

Low dose	≤7.5 mg prednisone or equivalent per day
Medium dose	>7.5 mg, but ≤ 30 mg prednisone or equivalent per day
High dose	>30 mg, but ≤ 100 mg prednisone or equivalent per day
Very high dose	>100 mg prednisone or equivalent per day
Pulse therapy	≥250 mg prednisone or equivalent per day for one day or a few days

TABLE 57–4 • USE OF GLUCOCORTICOIDS IN RHEUMATOLOGY IN THE GENERAL PATIENT, EXCLUDING EXCEPTIONAL CLINICAL SITUATIONS

	Initial* Oral Dose			Intravenous, Very High Dose† or Pulse	Intra-articular Injection
	Low†	*Medium*†	*High*†		
Arthritides					
Gouty arthritis, acute	-	-	-	-	2
Juvenile idiopathic arthritis	-	1	1	-	1
Osteoarthritis	-	-	-	-	1
Pseudogout	-	-	-	-	2
Psoriatic arthritis	-	1	-	-	2
Reactive arthritis, Reiter's syndrome	-	-	-	-	1
Rheumatic fever	-	1	1	-	-
Rheumatoid arthritis	2	2	1	1	2
Collagen Disorders					
Dermatomyositis, polymyositis	-	-	3	1	-
Mixed connective tissue disease	-	1	-	1	1
Polymyalgia rheumatica	-	3	-	1	-
Sjögren's syndrome, primary	-	-	1	-	-
Systemic lupus erythematosus	-	2	1	1	-
Systemic sclerosis	-	1	-	-	-
Systemic Vasculitides					
In general	-	-	3	1	-

*Initial dose is the dose at the start of therapy and will often be decreased in time depending on disease activity.
† Dose in prednisone equivalents a day: low: ≤7.5 mg; medium: >7.5 but ≤30 mg; high: >30 but ≤100 mg; very high: >100 mg.
Symbols: –, rare use; 1, infrequent use or use for therapy-resistant disease, complications, severe flare, and major exacerbation; 2, frequently added to the basic therapeutic strategy; 3, basic part of the therapeutic strategy.

are not given, except for intra-articular injection when there are signs of synovitis of the osteoarthritic joint.[38] For generalized soft tissue disorders, glucocorticoids are not indicated, and for localized soft tissue disorders, they should only be used for intralesional injection.

GLUCOCORTICOID THERAPY IN RA

Signs and Symptoms

As can be seen in Table 57–4, RA is the only disease in which glucocorticoid therapy is often started and maintained at a low dose as additional therapy.[39] The rationale for this therapy is a probable relative insufficiency of the adrenal gland in patients with RA.[30,31] Glucocorticoids are highly effective for relieving symptoms in patients with active RA in doses of less than 10 mg/d; many patients become functionally dependent on this therapy and continue it long term.[40] A review of seven studies (253 patients) concluded that glucocorticoids, when administered for a period of approximately 6 months, are effective for the treatment of RA.[41] After 6 months of therapy, the beneficial effects of glucocorticoids seem to diminish.[42-44] However, if this therapy then is tapered off and stopped, patients often—during some months—experience aggravation of symptoms.

More patients are given glucocorticoids in the United States than in Europe. In the European leflunomide study for instance, 27 percent of the patients used concomitant glucocorticoids,[45] whereas in the U.S. leflunomide study, 54 percent did.[46]

Radiologic Joint Damage

Awareness of disease-modifying properties of glucocorticoids in RA is particularly interesting. In 1995, joint-preserving effects of 7.5 mg of prednisolone daily for 2 years in patients with RA of short and intermediate duration who also were treated with disease-modifying antirheumatic drugs (DMARDs) were described. The group of RA patients participating in this randomized, placebo-controlled trial was heterogeneous, not only in respect to disease duration but also to stages of the disease and the kind and dosages of DMARDs.[44] In another trial published in 1997, patients with early RA were randomized to either step-down therapy with two DMARDs (sulphasalazine and methotrexate) and prednisolone (start 60 mg/day, tapered in six weekly steps to 7.5 mg/day and stopped at 28 weeks), or sulfasalazine alone. In the combined-drug-strategy group, a statistically significant and clinically relevant effect in retarding joint damage was shown, compared to the effect of sulfasalazine alone.[47] In an extension of this study, long-term (4 to 5 year) beneficial benefits were also shown regarding radiologic damage following the combination strategy.[48] It has been hypothesized that the superior effect of the combination therapy in this trial can be ascribed to the prednisolone, because in two double-blind, randomized trials, the effect of the combination of methotrexate and sulfasalazine was not superior to that of either drug alone.[49,50] Published as an abstract is a study in which 200 patients with early RA were treated with methotrexate or intramuscular gold and, in addition, were randomized for additional treatment with 5 mg of prednisolone or placebo. After 2 years, progression of radiologic damage proved to be less in the prednisolone-treated patients than in those patients treated with placebo prednisolone.[51] In 2002, the results of a placebo-controlled trial on the effects of prednisolone in DMARD-naïve patients with early RA was published. Ten mg of prednisolone daily in these patients (who only got DMARD therapy as rescue) clearly inhibited the progression of radiologic joint damage[43] (Fig. 57–4). In this study, a 40-percent decreased need for intra-articular glucocorticoid injections, 49-percent decreased need for acetaminophen use, and 55-percent decreased need for NSAID use was found in the prednisolone group, compared to the placebo group. This explains the study finding that the effect of glucocorticoids on parameters of inflammation waned after some months.[43] In clinical trials evaluating the clinical effect of DMARDs or glucocorticoids, additional therapies should, thus, be taken into account.

There are also negative studies on the effect of glucocorticoids on radiologic damage,[42,52] but in early RA, evidence of joint-sparing properties of glucocorticoids seems convincing. The jury is still out, however, on whether or not glucocorticoids can also inhibit progression of erosions in RA of longer duration. It could well be that there is a so-called "window of opportunity" in the treatment of RA.[53] If this window exists, effective treatment of early RA with glucocorticoids, as well as DMARDs, may result in an effect that lasts for a long period of time, whereas if effective treatment starts later, this opportunity may be lost and erosive progression may continue.

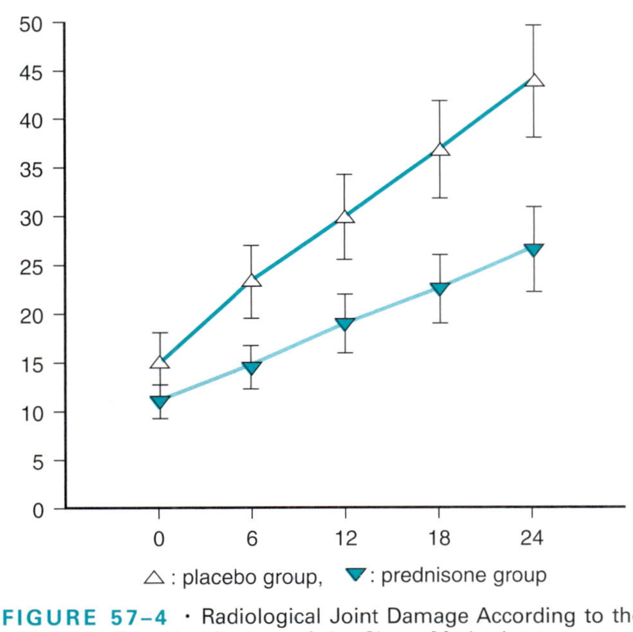

FIGURE 57–4 · Radiological Joint Damage According to the van der Heijde Modification of the Sharp Method. Means (standard errors) of total scores for erosions and joint space narrowing in hands and feet. On the y-axis is displayed the total Sharp score, on the x-axis the time, in months. From 12 months on, joint damage is significantly less among patients treated with prednisone compared to patients taking placebo; p=0.04 at 12 months and 0.02 at 24 months.

Also, because glucocorticoid-induced osteoporosis and peptic complications (if glucocorticoids are combined with NSAIDs) can be prevented much more effectively now than a decade ago, the joint-protective effect of prednisolone in early RA is a very interesting finding. A toxicity index score for DMARDs has been published (based on symptoms, laboratory abnormalities, and hospitalization data), evaluating 3000 patients with more than 7300 patient-years from the Arthritis, Rheumatism, and Aging Medical Information System (ARAMIS) database. Though this score is not yet validated and is clearly influenced by confounding by indication, it gives an impression of the relative toxicity of glucocorticoids.[54] It is comparable with that of other immune-suppressive medications used in RA, such as methotrexate and azathioprine. However, as many questions yet remain to be answered, such as how the effect of glucocorticoids compares with that of high dosages of methotrexate or that of TNF-α–blockers and for how long glucocorticoids should be prescribed and in what dosages, the final place of chronic glucocorticoid therapy in RA still has to be determined[3] (see Chapter 67).

CHRONOBIOLOGY

The diurnal rhythm in the rheumatoid inflammatory process and symptoms is known. Early in the morning, patients experience the most extensive joint stiffness and other symptoms and signs. This is due to the long rest period during the night and the circadian rhythm of cortisol[55] (see Fig. 57–3). In patients with RA with low or medium disease activity, serum cortisol maximum and minimum shift to earlier times of the day and night, whereas in patients with high disease activity, the circadian rhythm is markedly reduced or even lost. So the timing of glucocorticoid administration may be of importance for both efficacy and side effects. However, data in literature are not unequivocal in their findings. In one study, administration of low doses of prednisolone at 2:00 A.M. had favorable effects on more of the clinical variables than administration at 7:30 A.M. However, the difference in the time period from the last dose of prednisolone to assessment could have been a bias.[56] In another study, 12 patients with RA took low-dosage prednisolone (mean 5.6 mg daily) at either 0800 h, 1300 h, or 2300 h in a double-blind within-patient controlled fashion. Subjective and objective assessments showed no differences in effectiveness among the three times of administration of prednisolone. Urinary excretion patterns of 11-hydroxycorticosteroids provided no evidence of adrenal cortical suppression at the dose levels studied, even when this dose was taken in the evening. Therefore, it was concluded in this study that it is reasonable to administer therapy in the morning to diminish as much adrenopituitary suppression as possible.[57]

ALTERNATE-DAY REGIMENS

For oral, long-term use of glucocorticoid therapy, alternate-day regimens were devised in an attempt to alleviate the undesirable side effects such as hypothalamic-pituitary-adrenal axis suppression. Alternate-day therapy uses a single dose administered every other morning, which is usually equivalent to, or somewhat higher than, twice the usual or preestablished daily dose. The rationale of this regimen is that the body, including the hypothalamic-pituitary-adrenal axis is exposed to exogenous glucocorticoid only on alternate days. This only makes sense in cases of usage of a class and dosage of a glucocorticoid that suppresses the hypothalamic-pituitary-adrenal axis activity for less than 36 hours following a single dose.[58] And, of course, the patient should have a responsive hypothalamic-pituitary-adrenal axis; the alternate-day schedule does not work in patients on a chronic, intermediate, or high dose of glucocorticoids.

Unfortunately, alternate-day therapy is unsuccessful in most patients who require glucocorticoids; patients with RA often experience exacerbation of symptoms on the second day. This is in line with the clinical impression that a single dose of glucocorticoids daily is less effective in RA than half that dose, given twice daily. In giant-cell arteritis, alternate-day glucocorticoid therapy is also less effective than daily administration.[59,60] In general, alternate-day regimens are used rarely in rheumatology today, except in patients with juvenile idiopathic arthritis, in whom alternate-day glucocorticoid usage results in less inhibition of body growth than does daily usage. If treatment has been initiated with daily administration, the change to alternate-day therapy should preferably be made after the disease has stabilized.

GLUCOCORTICOID SENSITIVITY AND RESISTANCE

A small proportion of patients does not react favorably to glucocorticoids or even fails to respond to high doses. Also, the susceptibility to adverse effects of glucocorticoids varies widely. Several different factors are involved in the variability of glucocorticoid sensitivity in patients with rheumatic diseases, and understanding of the mechanisms involved might eventually allow their modulation.

Hereditary glucocorticoid resistance (rare) and increased susceptibility to glucocorticoids have been related to specific polymorphisms of the glucocorticoid-receptor gene.[61] The glucocorticoid receptor exists as an alpha and beta isoform, but only the alpha isoform binds glucocorticoids. The beta isoform functions as an endogenous inhibitor of glucocorticoids and is expressed in several tissues. Glucocorticoid resistance has been associated with an enhanced expression of this β receptor.[62]

The protein lipocortin-1 (or annexin-1) inhibits eicosanoid synthesis. Glucocorticoids are thought to stimulate lipocortin-1. In patients with RA, autoantibodies to lipocortin-1 have been described; the titers in these patients correlate with the height of maintenance doses of glucocorticoids, suggesting that these antibodies may also lead to glucocorticoid resistance.[63]

Although glucocorticoids exert most of their immunosuppressive actions through inhibition of cytokine production, high concentrations of cytokines, especially IL-2, antagonize the suppressive effect of glucocorticoids in a dose-dependent manner.[64] The balance is usually in favor of glucocorticoids, but high local concentrations of cytokines may result in a localized glucocorticoid resistance that cannot be overridden by exogenous glucocorticoids. Also, macrophage migration inhibitory factor (MIF) may play a role in steroid resistance in RA. MIF is a proinflammatory cytokine whose involvement in TNF-α synthesis and T cell activation suggests a role in the pathogenesis of RA. MIF is suppressed by higher concentrations of glucocorticoids, but it is induced by low concentrations, leading to stimulation of inflammation.[65]

GLUCOCORTICOID WITHDRAWAL REGIMENS

Because of potential side effects, glucocorticoids generally are tapered off as soon as the disease being treated is under control. Tapering must be done carefully to avoid both recurrent activity of the disease and, infrequently, cortisol deficiency resulting from chronic hypothalamic-pituitary-adrenal axis suppression; gradual tapering permits recovery of the adrenal function. There is no best scheme based on controlled, comparative studies for tapering glucocorticoids; furthermore, tapering depends on the individual's disease, the disease activity, doses and duration of therapy, and clinical response, which is also dependent on each individual's glucocorticoid sensitivity. Therefore, only generic guidelines can be offered. To taper the dose of prednisone, decrements of 5 to 10 mg every 1 to 2 weeks can be used when the prednisone dose is more than 40 mg/day, followed by 5-mg decrements every 1 to 2 weeks at a dose between 40 and 20 mg/day, and finally 1- to 2.5-mg/day decrements every 2 to 3 weeks at a prednisone dose of less than 20 mg/day. Another scheme is to taper 5 to 10 mg every 1 to 2 weeks down to 30 mg/day of prednisone, and when the dose is less than 20 mg/day, taper 2.5 to 5 mg every 2 to 4 weeks down to 10 mg/day; thereafter, dose is tapered 1 mg each month or 2.5 mg (half a 5-mg tablet of prednisolone) each 7 weeks. For tapering every 7 weeks or longer periods, a printed schedule can be given to the patient, such as the one shown in Table 57–5.

ADAPTATIONS OF GLUCOCORTICOID DOSES, STRESS REGIMENS, AND PREOPERATIVE CARE

Patients on chronic low-dose glucocorticoid medication who, therefore, have suppressed adrenal activity should be advised to double their daily glucocorticoid dose, or increase the dose to 15 mg prednisolone or equivalent, if they develop fever attributed to infection and to seek medical help. In case of major surgery, given the unreliable prediction of adrenal suppression on the basis of duration and dose of glucocorticoid therapy (see the section "Effects of glucocorticoids on the hypothalamic-pituitary-adrenal axis"), many physicians recommend "stress doses" of glucocorticoids for patients with a low risk of adrenal suppression. The scheme of 100 mg hydrocortisone intravenously just before the operation, followed by an additional 100 mg

TABLE 57–5 • GLUCOCORTICOID TAPERING SCHEME TO HAND OUT TO PATIENTS*

	Monday	Tuesday	Wednesday	Thursday	Friday	Saturday	Sunday
period 1	high	high	high	high	low	high	high
period 2	high	low	high	high	high	low	high
period 3	high	low	high	low	high	low	high
period 4	low	high	low	high	low	high	low
period 5	low	high	low	low	low	high	low
period 6	low	low	low	high	low	low	low
period 7	low	low	low	low	low	low	low

*At each consecutive period (e.g., one week or some weeks), the number of days during which a low dose should be taken increases by one. After completion of period 7, the next step in tapering can be taken; the dose called "low" during the previous 7 periods now is "high", and so on. In case of aggravation of symptoms, patient should not diminish the dose, but contact the specialist instead.

every 6 hours for 3 days is not always necessary. A scheme with a lower dose, possibly reducing the risk of postoperative bacterial infectious complications, is to continuously infuse 100 mg of hydrocortisone intravenously the first day of surgery, followed by 25 to 50 mg of hydrocortisone every 8 hours for 2 or 3 days. Another option is to administer the usual dose of oral glucocorticoid orally or (the equivalent) parenterally on the day of surgery, followed by 25 to 50 mg of hydrocortisone every 8 hours for 2 or 3 days. In cases of minor surgery, it is probably sufficient to double the oral dose or to increase the dose to 15 mg prednisolone or equivalent for 1 to 3 days. However, no comparative randomized studies on different perioperative glucocorticoid stress schemes have been published. Because in glucocorticoid-induced loss of adrenal responsiveness aldosterone secretion is preserved, mineralocorticoid therapy is not necessary.

GLUCOCORTICOID-SPARING AGENTS

For most inflammatory rheumatic diseases, including SLE, vasculitis, RA, and myositis, other immunomodulatory drugs are often added to therapy with glucocorticoids, such as azathioprine and methotrexate, and, especially in case of systemic vasculitis, cyclophosphamide. Exception is polymyalgia rheumatica, which is managed with glucocorticoids alone. Combination therapy is applied early in the disease when the disease is one for which it is known that the effect of the combination is better than that of glucocorticoids alone (e.g., in case of systemic vasculitis) or if the disease (e.g., inflammatory myositis) seems relatively resistant to the high initial doses of glucocorticoids.

If in a later stage of the disease immunomodulatory drugs are added to therapy with glucocorticoids to enable further reduction of the dose to decrease the risk of side effects, these immunomodulatory drugs are often called glucocorticoid-sparing agents. For this purpose, azathioprine and methotrexate are often used.

GLUCOCORTICOID PULSE THERAPY

Glucocorticoid pulse therapy (GPT) is used in rheumatology, especially for disease induction or treatment of flares of collagen disorders and vasculitides (see Table 57–4). In RA, pulse therapy is applied to treat some of the serious complications of the disease and to induce remission in active disease, often in the initiation phase of second-line antirheumatic treatment. In the latter patients, pulse therapy with schemes of 1000 mg methylprednisolone intravenously or equivalents has been proven to be effective in most studies; the beneficial effect generally lasts for about 6 weeks, with a large variation in the duration of the effect.[66] Therefore, it does not seem sensible to apply pulse therapy in active RA unless there is also a change in the therapeutic strategy (e.g., with second-line antirheumatic treatment aimed to stabilize in the long term the remission induced by the pulse therapy). The short-term effects of pulse therapy in patients with established, active RA on various dimensions of health status closely resemble the long-term effects of effective conventional DMARD therapy, such as methotrexate, in patients with early RA.

The risk of some of the adverse effects of pulse therapy is not the same for all rheumatic disorders. In SLE, osteonecrosis and psychosis seem to be more frequent side effects of pulse therapy compared to patients with RA.[67] However, osteonecrosis and psychosis can also be complications of SLE itself.

INTRALESIONAL AND INTRA-ARTICULAR GLUCOCORTICOID INJECTIONS

Injections with glucocorticoids are widely used for arthritis (see Table 57–4), tenosynovitis, bursitis, enthesitis, and compression neuropathies such as carpal tunnel syndrome (see also Chapter 47). In general, the effect occurs within days, but if the underlying disease is active, the effect is temporary. Administration of a local anesthetic concurrently with intra-articular or soft tissue injection of a glucocorticoid may provide immediate relief of pain.

Soluble glucocorticoids (e.g., phosphate salts) have a more-rapid onset of action with probably less risk of subcutaneous tissue atrophy and depigmentation of the skin when given intralesionally. Insoluble glucocorticoids are longer acting and might decrease the soft tissue fibrous matrix more, so they should be used with caution in places with thin skin, especially in elderly and patients with peripheral vascular disease. Insoluble glucocorticoids are more safely given into deep sites. Short-acting soluble glucocorticoids can be mixed with long-acting insoluble glucocorticoids to combine rapid onset with long-acting effect.

The effect of intra-articular glucocorticoid injection probably depends on several factors. These are the underlying disease (e.g., RA or osteoarthritis), the treated joint (size, weight-bearing or non–weight-bearing), the activity of arthritis, volume of synovial fluid of the treated joint,[38] application of arthrocentesis (synovial fluid aspiration) before injection, the choice and dose of the glucocorticoid preparation, application of rest to the injected joint, and the injection technique. The effect of injections seems to be less favorable in osteoarthritis compared to RA. In a retrospective study, especially knee joints in OA often required at least one additional injection.[68] Arthrocentesis before injecting the glucocorticoid preparation reduces the risk for relapse of arthritis.[69] Triamcinolone hexacetonide, which among the injectable glucocorticoids is the least-soluble preparation, shows the longest effect.[68,70,71]

Theoretically, rest of the injected joint minimizes leakage of the injected glucocorticoid preparation to the systemic circulation (via the hyperemic, inflamed synovium by enhanced pressure in the joint during activity), minimizes the risk of cartilage damage, and provides rest for repair of inflammatory tissue damage. Advices and procedures for the postinjection period in terms of activity vary from no restrictions, to minimal activity of the injected joint for a couple of days, to bed rest for 24 hours following injection of a knee joint or splinting of injected joints.[68,72,73] Based on the literature, no definite evidence-based recommendation can be made, but it seems prudent to rest and certainly not to overuse the injected joint, even if pain is relieved.

It is recommended that intra-articular glucocorticoid injections be repeated no more often than once every 3 weeks and be given no more frequently than 3 times a year in a weight-bearing joint (e.g., the knee) to minimize glucocorticoid-induced joint damage. This recommendation also seems sensible, but there is no definite clinical evidence to support it. As one would expect, accuracy of steroid placement influences the clinical outcome of glucocorticoid injections into the shoulder and probably also into other joints as well.[74] This is important, as it is estimated that a little more than half of shoulder injections are inaccurately placed.[74,75]

The reported infection rate of joints following local injections with glucocorticoids is low, ranging from one case in 13,900 to 77,300 injections.[76-78] Introduction of disposable needles and syringes has helped to reduce the risk. A prospective study during 3 years in an urban area of 1,000,000 people in the Netherlands has been performed. In 214 joints (including 58 joints with a prosthesis or osteosynthetic material) of 186 patients, bacterial infections were detected; only three of these joint infections were attributed to an intra-articular injection.[79]

Other adverse effects of local glucocorticoid injections are systemic adverse effects of the glucocorticoid, such as disturbance of the menstrual pattern,[80] hot flush–like symptoms the day of or the day after injection,[81] and hyperglycemia in diabetes mellitus.[82] Local complications include subcutaneous fat tissue atrophy (especially after improper local injection),[83] local depigmentation of the skin,[84] tendon slip and rupture,[68,85] and lesions to local nerves.[86]

Adverse Effects and Monitoring

Given the diversity of their mechanisms and sites of action, it is not surprising that glucocorticoids can cause a wide array of adverse effects (Table 57–6). Most of these side effects cannot be avoided. The risk of most complications is dosage- and time-dependent; minimizing the amount of glucocorticoids minimizes the risk of complications. It is a striking clinical observation that some patients develop severe adverse effects after relatively small doses of glucocorticoids, although other patients receive rather high dosages without serious adverse effects. The apparent individual susceptibility to adverse effects does not seem to parallel the individual susceptibility to beneficial effects.

SKELETAL ADVERSE EFFECTS

Osteoporosis

Osteoporosis is a well-known adverse effect of glucocorticoids, which can be prevented to a large degree. Internationally accepted guidelines have been developed to minimize the occurrence of glucocorticoid-induced osteoporosis.[87] Preventive and therapeutic management of glucocorticoid-induced osteoporosis is discussed in detail in Chapter 90.

Osteonecrosis

High-dose (more than 30 mg prednisone or equivalent) glucocorticoids are implicated as a cause for osteonecro-

TABLE 57–6 • COMMON ADVERSE EFFECTS OF GLUCOCORTICOIDS

System	Adverse Effect
Skeletal	Osteoporosis, osteonecrosis, myopathy
Gastrointestinal	Peptic ulcer disease (in combination with NSAIDs), pancreatitis, fatty liver
Immunologic	Predisposition to infections, suppressed delayed hypersensitivity
Cardiovascular	Fluid retention, hypertension, accelerated arteriosclerosis, arrhythmias
Ocular	Glaucoma, cataract
Cutaneous	Skin atrophy, striae, ecchymoses, impaired wound healing, acne, buffalo hump, hirsutism
Endocrine	Cushinoid appearance, diabetes mellitus, changes in lipid metabolism, enhanced appetite and weight gain, electrolyte abnormalities, HPA-axis suppression, suppression of gonadal hormones
Behavioral	Insomnia, psychosis, emotional instability, cognitive effects

Abbreviations: HPA, hypothalamic-pituitary-adrenal; NSAIDs, nonsteroidal anti-inflammatory drugs.

sis, especially in children and patients with SLE. Vascular mechanisms seem to be involved; possibly ischemia is caused by microscopic fat emboli or impingement of the sinusoidal vascular bed by increased intraosseous pressure due to fat accumulation.[88] An early symptom is diffuse pain, which becomes persistent and increases with activity. Most frequently hip or knee joints are involved, less frequently ankle and shoulder joints. For early assessment, bone scan imaging and especially magnetic resonance imaging (MRI) are the most sensitive investigations; bone scans give less specific information. Plain radiographs are only adequate for follow-up. Treatment in the early stage includes immobilization and decreased weight-bearing. Surgical decompression, joint replacement, or both follow this if needed. Prevention is not possible; awareness is the most important factor in early detection.

Myopathy

Weakness in proximal muscles, especially of the lower extremities, occurring within weeks to months after the onset of treatment with glucocorticoids, or after an increase in the dosage, may indicate steroid myopathy. It is often suspected, but infrequently found and, when it is found, occurs almost exclusively in patients treated with high dosages (more than 30 mg prednisone or equivalent). Diagnosis can be made by muscle biopsy that reveals atrophy of type II fibers with a lack of inflammation. In the blood there is no elevation of muscle enzymes.[89] Treatment is withdrawal of the steroids. If this is possible, quite often there is a prompt improvement of symptoms.

A rare syndrome of rapid-onset, acute steroid myopathy, occurring within days of the start of high-dosage glucocorticoids or pulse therapy has been described; muscle biopsies show necrosis with atrophy of all muscle fibers.

GASTROINTESTINAL ADVERSE EFFECTS

Peptic Ulcer Disease

Data from literature on peptic upper gastrointestinal (GI) safety of oral glucocorticoids are nonconclusive. The fact that glucocorticoids inhibit the production of COX-2 without hampering that of COX-1 supports the studies that found no increased risk. In other studies, a relative risk of serious upper GI peptic complications of about 2 was found.[90] When glucocorticoids are used in combination with nonsteroidal anti-inflammatory drugs (NSAIDs) the relative risk of peptic ulcer and associated complications is about 4.[91] In patients treated with glucocorticoids without concomitant use of NSAIDs, there is no indication for gastroprotective agents if there are no (other) risk factors for peptic complications.

Other Gastrointestinal Adverse Effects

Although glucocorticoids are usually listed as one of the many potential causes of pancreatitis, evidence for such an association is weak and difficult to separate from the underlying disease such as SLE or vasculitis.[92] Asymptomatic and symptomatic colonization of the upper GI tract with *Candida albicans* is increased in patients treated with glucocorticoids, especially when other risk factors are present, such as advanced age, diabetes mellitus, and concomitant use of other immunosuppressive agents. Glucocorticoids may mask symptoms and signs usually associated with the occurrence of intra-abdominal complications, such as perforation of the intestine and peritonitis, and, thus, can lead to a delay in diagnosis with increased morbidity and mortality.

IMMUNOLOGIC ADVERSE EFFECTS

Predisposition to Infections

At high dosage, glucocorticoids diminish neutrophil phagocytosis and bacterial killing in vitro, whereas in vivo, normal bactericidal and phagocytic activities are found. Monocytes are more susceptible; during treatment with medium to high dosages of glucocorticoids, bactericidal and fungicidal activity in vivo as well as in vitro are reduced. These factors may influence the risk of infection. However, from epidemiologic studies it seems that treatment with a daily dosage of less than 10 mg prednisone or equivalent leads to no or only a slightly increased risk of infection, whereas if dosages between 20 and 40 mg daily are used, an increased risk of infection is found (relative risk [RR] 1.3 to 3.6).[93] This risk increases with increase of dosage and duration of treatment.

In a meta-analysis of 71 trials involving more than 2000 patients with different diseases and different dosages of glucocorticoids, an increased RR of infection was found of 2.0. The risk varied according to the type of disease being treated. Five of these trials involved patients with rheumatic diseases and showed no increased risk (RR = 1.0).[93]

The same was found in a recent double-blind, placebo-controlled, 2-year trial in patients with early RA; the study compared the effect of 10 mg prednisone daily with that of placebo.[43] However, in patients treated with glucocorticoids, especially at high dosages, clinicians should anticipate infections with both usual and unusual organisms, realizing that glucocorticoids may blunt classic clinical features and delay diagnosis.

CARDIOVASCULAR ADVERSE EFFECTS

Mineralocorticoid Effects

Some glucocorticoids have clear mineralocorticoid actions (see Table 57–1), including reduced excretion of sodium and chloride and increased excretion of potassium, calcium, and phosphate. This may lead to edema, weight gain, increased blood pressure, and heart failure (due to reduced excretion of sodium and chloride), cardiac arrhythmia (due to increased excretion of potassium), or tetany and electrocardiographic changes (due to hypocalcemia). There are no direct effects of glucocorticoids on the kidneys or on renal function.

Doses of less than 10 mg prednisolone or equivalent per day have only minor effects on blood pressure and are not a relevant cause of hypertension.[94] No formal studies addressing the effects of glucocorticoids in previously hypertensive patients have been reported. Detrimental effects of glucocorticoids on cardiac function in patients with congestive heart failure are to be expected, but have not been documented. Two randomized, controlled studies in patients with myocarditis and idiopathic cardiomyopathy showed no differences between placebo- or glucocorticoid-treated groups after 1 year, nor in survival at 2 and 4 years.[95,96]

Atherosclerosis

Accelerated atherosclerosis has been reported in patients with SLE and, more recently, also in RA.[97] In the pathogenesis of this complication, the use of glucocorticoids has been directly and indirectly implicated through alterations in serum lipoproteins, blood pressure, and vascular effects.[98] On the other hand, atherosclerosis itself has now been recognized as an inflammatory disease, for which glucocorticoids may be theoretically effective.[99] Though the use of glucocorticoids has been found to be an independent risk factor for coronary artery disease in SLE, it is difficult to eliminate the confounding factor of the underlying inflammatory disease.[100]

OCULAR ADVERSE EFFECTS

Cataract

Glucocorticoids tend to stimulate the formation of posterior subcapsular cataract especially,[101] but the risk of cortical cataract also seems increased, with an odds ratio of 2.6.[102] To some extent, the likelihood or severity of this cataract's formation is dependent on dose and duration of treatment.[103] In patients treated long term with glucocorticoids at a dosage of 15 mg prednisone or more daily during 1 year, cataract is observed frequently; in patients receiving long-term therapy with less than 10 mg prednisone daily, the percentage of cataract is less, approximately 10 percent. Posterior subcapsular cataract may develop in as few as 2 years on as little as 5 mg/day of prednisone. These cataracts are usually bilateral but progress relatively slowly. They may cause glare disturbance, but usually cause little visual impairment, except for end stages.

Glaucoma

By increasing intraocular pressure glucocorticoids may cause or aggravate glaucoma. Patients with a familial propensity to develop open-angle glaucoma are prone to develop this adverse effect; they need to be treated with pressure-lowering medications, often for a prolonged period of time after stopping the glucocorticoids.[104] Topical application of glucocorticoids in the eye has much more effect on the intraocular pressure than do systemic glucocorticoids.[105] A family history of glaucoma or high dosages of glucocorticoids demand occasional pressure checks for patients on chronic systemic glucocorticoids.

DERMATOLOGIC ADVERSE EFFECTS

Clinically relevant adverse effects of glucocorticoids on skin include cushingoid appearance, easy bruising, ecchymoses, skin atrophy, striae, disturbed wound healing, acne, perioral dermatitis, hyperpigmentation, rubeosis faciei, and increased hair growth—excluding scalp hair.[106] The physician often considers these changes as of relatively minor clinical importance, but they may be disturbing to the patient. No reliable data on the occurrence of these adverse effects are available, but many physicians recognize immediately the skin of a patient who has chronically used glucocorticoids.

ENDOCRINE ADVERSE EFFECTS

Glucose Intolerance and Diabetes Mellitus

Glucocorticoids increase hepatic glucose production and induce insulin resistance by inhibiting insulin-stimulated glucose uptake and metabolism by peripheral tissues.[107] There probably is also a direct effect of glucocorticoids on the beta cells of the pancreas, resulting in enhanced insulin secretion during glucocorticoid therapy.[108] It may take only a few weeks before glucocorticoid-induced hyperglycemia occurs. One case-control, population-based study suggested, in previously nondiabetic subjects, an odds ratio of 1.8 for the need to initiate antihyperglycemic drugs during glucocorticoid therapy in dosages of up to 10 mg prednisone or equivalent per day.[109] This risk increased with higher daily dosages of glucocorticoids: The odds ratio was 3.0 for 10 to 20 mg, 5.8 for 20 to 30 mg, and 10.3 for 30 mg or more prednisone or equivalent per day. It is likely that this risk is further increased in patients with other risk factors for diabetes mellitus, such as a family history of the disease, increasing age, obesity, and previous gestational diabetes. Postprandial hyperglycemia and only mildly elevated fasting glucose concentrations are characteristic of glucocorticoid-induced diabetes mellitus.[110] Worsening of glycemic control in patients with established glucose intolerance or diabetes mellitus can be expected. Usually, glucocorticoid-induced diabetes is reversible when the drug is discontinued.

Fat Redistribution and Body Weight

One of the most notable effects of chronic endogenous or exogenous glucocorticoid excess is the redistribution of body fat. A centripetal fat accumulation with sparing of the extremities is a characteristic feature of patients exposed to long-term high-dose glucocorticoids. Potential mechanisms include increased conversion of cortisone to cortisol in visceral adipocytes, hyperinsulinemia, and a change in expression and activity of adipocyte-derived hormones and cytokines, such as leptin and TNF-α.[111] Protein loss resulting in muscle atrophy also contributes to the change in body appearance. Increased appetite and energy intake influence body weight during glucocorticoid therapy. Recent trials in patients with RA given low-dose glucocorticoids for a prolonged period of time showed only minor effects in fat redistribution and body weight.[43,47]

Dyslipidemia

Long-term treatment with glucocorticoids increases plasma levels of low-density lipoprotein (LDL) cholesterol, very low-density lipoprotein (VLDL) cholesterol, total cholesterol, and triglycerides—the so-called dyslipidemia of glucocorticoid therapy. These changes are very likely mediated by increased plasma insulin levels, impaired lipid catabolism, and increased lipid production in the liver. The ensuing increased plasma level of LDL represents one of the most important risk factors for the development of atherosclerosis, next to glucocorticoid-induced hypertension. On the other hand, the association of RA with a higher risk of cardiovascular disease may be due to the direct deleterious impact of prolonged inflammation on vessel walls. Glucocorticoids have been found to inhibit macrophage accumulation in injured arterial wall in vitro, possibly resulting in attenuation of the local inflammatory response.[112] Because dyslipidemia and increased cardiovascular risk are mainly found during long-term and high-dose glucocorticoid therapy, it is possible that the use of low-dosage glucocorticoids, especially when initiation of this therapy prompts the physician to check for the presence of (preexisting) dyslipidemia, could even decrease the incidence of atherosclerosis in patients with RA.

Suppression of the Hypothalamic-Pituitary-Adrenal Axis

In the section on 'effects of glucocorticoids on the hypothalamic-pituitary-adrenal axis,' mechanisms of chronic suppression of the hypothalamic-pituitary-adrenal axis by administration of exogenous glucocorticoids are described. In such a situation, acute discontinuation of glucocorticoid therapy may lead to acute adrenal insufficiency with possible circulatory collapse and death.[113] About 10 years after glucocorticoid therapy became available, the first well-documented case of adrenal insufficiency after withdrawal of exogenous glucocorticoid was reported.[114] Acute cessation of glucocorticoid therapy without tapering is indicated for corneal ulceration by herpes virus, which can rapidly lead to perforation of the cornea, and glucocorticoid-induced acute psychosis. In these patients, assessment of the adrenal responsiveness on a corticotropin test seems prudent. Not all patients with a blunted cortisol response have signs or symptoms of adrenal insufficiency, however.

Clinical signs and symptoms of chronic adrenal hypofunctioning are not very specific. They include fatigue and weakness, lethargy, orthostatic hypotension, nausea, loss of appetite, vomiting, diarrhea, arthralgia, and myalgia. These symptoms partly overlap glucocorticoid withdrawal symptoms such as fatigue, arthralgia, and myalgia. When in doubt, measurements of serum cortisol levels and the corticotropin stimulation test are indicated. The glucocorticoid withdrawal symptoms are sometimes also difficult to discriminate from those of the primary disease, such as polymyalgia rheumatica. Because mineralocorticoid secretion remains intact via the renin-angiotensin-aldosterone axis, hypokalemia is uncommon.[15]

ADVERSE BEHAVIORAL EFFECTS

Glucocorticoid treatment is associated with a variety of behavioral symptoms. Although most attention has been dedicated to specific, rather dramatic, disturbances collectively described under the term *glucocorticoid psychosis*, less florid effects also occur that may cause distress to a patient and deserve medical attention. Similar manifestations may occur upon withdrawal of glucocorticoids.

Steroid Psychosis

Overt psychosis is rare and is usually associated with high-dose glucocorticoids or GPT, especially in patients with SLE, but psychosis is also a complication of this disease itself. This makes it difficult to distinguish in the individual SLE patient whether the psychosis is a complication of the disease, the therapy, or both.

Isolated psychosis represents about 10 percemt of glucocorticoid-related cases, but in most patients, affective disorders are present as well. Around 40 percent of cases of glucocorticoid-induced psychosis present as depression, whereas mania, often dominated by irritability, is predominant in 30 percent of cases.[115] Psychotic symptoms usually start just after initiation of treatment (60% within the first 2 weeks, 90% within the first 6 weeks), and remission after drug lowering or withdrawal follows the same pattern. Occasionally, remission occurs without dose reduction.

Minor Mood Disturbances

Glucocorticoids have been associated with a wide variety of low-grade disturbances such as depressed or elated mood (euphoria), irritability or emotional instability, anxiety and insomnia, memory failure, and cognition impairments. Although the symptoms may not reach severity for a specific diagnosis, they warrant attention—not only because they cause distress to the patient, but also because they may interfere with evaluation and treatment of the underlying disease. Most physicians recognize the occurrence of such symptoms in a considerable number of their glucocorticoid treated patients; these symptoms can occur in varying degrees in up to 50 percent of treated patients within the first week. The exact incidence in rheumatic patients exposed to the usual dosages of glucocorticoids is not known; most studies dedicated to mood disturbances studied high dosages.[116] It is important to inform patients about these minor mood disturbances before starting glucocorticoid therapy.

MONITORING

Monitoring of adverse effects should include assessments even before therapy is started. Indications for what and how to monitor are given in Table 57–7.

TABLE 57–7 • RISK AND MONITORING OF ADVERSE EFFECTS OF GLUCOCORTICOID THERAPY*

Before treatment is started, screen:
Blood pressure, check for peripheral edema and cardiac insufficiency
Risk factors for osteoporosis
Comedication, especially nonsteroidal anti-inflammatory drugs (NSAIDs)
History of peptic ulcer
Family history of glaucoma
Serum lipids
Urine glucose
During treatment, screen (frequency depends on individual patient's risk and glucocorticoid dose):
Blood pressure, check for peripheral edema and cardiac insufficiency
Serum lipids
Urine glucose
Ocular pressure (in patients with a family history of glaucoma or on a high dose of glucocorticoids)
Preventive measures:
Always provide calcium and vitamin D supplementation and biphosphonates on indication (see international guidelines).
In case of comedication with NSAIDs, consider comedication with proton pump inhibitors or prescribe a cyclooxygenase (COX)-1–sparing NSAID.

*International guidelines do not yet exist for monitoring.

The discovery of glucocorticoids as a therapeutic tool still stands as one of the most significant advances in clinical medicine of the last century; we cannot do without glucocorticoids in many rheumatic diseases. However, because of the many adverse effects, prudent application of glucocorticoids is needed, based on knowledge of these drugs.

REFERENCES

1. Hench PS, Kendall EC, Slocumb CH, Polley HF: The effect of a hormone of the adrenal cortex (17-hydroxy-11-dehydrocorticosterone: compound E) and of pituitary adrenocorticotropic hormone on rheumatoid arthritis: preliminary report. Proceedings Staff Meetings Mayo Clinic 24:181-197, 1949.
2. Bijlsma JW, Straub RH, Masi AT, et al: Neuroendocrine immune mechanisms in rheumatic diseases. Trends Immunol 23:59-61, 2002.
3. Moreland LW, O'Dell JR: Glucocorticoids and rheumatoid arthritis: back to the future? Arthritis Rheum 46:2553-2563, 2002.
4. Neeck G: Fifty years of experience with cortisone therapy in the study and treatment of rheumatoid arthritis. Ann N Y Acad Sci 966:28-38, 2002.
5 Buttgereit F, da Silva JA, Boers M, et al: Standardised nomenclature for glucocorticoid dosages and glucocorticoid treatment regimens: current questions and tentative answers in rheumatology. Ann Rheum Dis 61:718-722, 2002.
6. American Society of Health-System Pharmacists, Inc. AHFS Drug Information. Bethesda, MD, 2001.
7. Buttgereit F, Wehling M, Burmester GR: A new hypothesis of modular glucocorticoid actions: steroid treatment of rheumatic diseases revisited. Arthritis Rheum 41:761-767, 1998.
8. Garg DC, Wagner JG, Sakmar E, et al: Rectal and oral absorption of methylprednisolone acetate. Clin Pharmacol Ther 26:232-239, 1979.
9. Tornatore KM, Logue G, Venuto RC, Davis PJ: Pharmacokinetics of methylprednisolone in elderly and young healthy males. J Am Geriatr Soc 42:1118-1122, 1994.
10. Tornatore KM, Biocevich DM, Reed K, et al: Methylprednisolone pharmacokinetics, cortisol response, and adverse effects in black and white renal transplant recipients. Transplantation 59: 729-736, 1995.
11. Carrie F, Roblot P, Bouquet S,et al: Rifampin-induced nonresponsiveness of giant cell arteritis to prednisone treatment. Arch Intern Med 154:1521-1524, 1994.
12. Kawai S, Ichikawa Y, Homma M: [Rifampicin-induced resistance to prednisolone treatment in collagen disease: a pharmacokinetic study]. Ryumachi 24:32-37, 1984.
13. McAllister WA, Thompson PJ, Al Habet SM, Rogers HJ: Rifampicin reduces effectiveness and bioavailability of prednisolone. Br Med J (Clin Res Ed) 286:923-925, 1983.
14. Kyriazopoulou V, Parparousi O, Vagenakis AG: Rifampicin-induced adrenal crisis in addisonian patients receiving corticosteroid replacement therapy. J Clin Endocrinol Metab 59: 1204-1206, 1984.
15. Cooper MS, Stewart PM: Corticosteroid insufficiency in acutely ill patients. N Engl J Med 348:727-734, 2003.
16. Barnes PJ: Anti-inflammatory actions of glucocorticoids: molecular mechanisms. Clin Sci (Lond) 94:557-572, 1998.
17. Lipworth BJ: Therapeutic implications of non-genomic glucocorticoid activity. Lancet 356:87-89, 2000;
18. Truss M, Beato M: Steroid hormone receptors: interaction with deoxyribonucleic acid and transcription factors. Endocr Rev 14:459-479, 1993.
19. da Silva JA, Bijlsma JW: Optimizing glucocorticoid therapy in rheumatoid arthritis. Rheum Dis Clin North Am 26:859-880, 2000.
20. Ristimaki A, Narko K, Hla T: Down-regulation of cytokine-induced cyclo-oxygenase-2 transcript isoforms by dexamethasone: evidence for post-transcriptional regulation. Biochem J 318(Pt 1):325-331, 1996.
21. Belvisi MG, Brown TJ, Wicks S, Foster ML: New glucocorticosteroids with an improved therapeutic ratio? Pulm Pharmacol Ther 14:221-227, 2001.
22. Resche-Rigon M, Gronemeyer H: Therapeutic potential of selective modulators of nuclear receptor action. Curr Opin Chem Biol 2:501-507, 1998.
23. Boumpas DT, Chrousos GP, Wilder RL, et al: Glucocorticoid therapy for immune-mediated diseases: basic and clinical correlates. Ann Intern Med 119:1198-1208, 1993.
24. Leonard JP, Silverstein RL: Corticosteroids and the haematopoietic system. *In* Lin AN, Paget SA (eds): Principles of Corticosteroid Therapy. New York, Arnold, 2002, pp 144-149.
25. Verhoef CM, van Roon JA, Vianen ME, et al: The immune suppressive effect of dexamethasone in rheumatoid arthritis is accompanied by upregulation of interleukin 10 and by differential changes in interferon gamma and interleukin 4 production. Ann Rheum Dis 58:49-54, 1999.
26. Morand EF, Jefferiss CM, Dixey J, et al: Impaired glucocorticoid induction of mononuclear leukocyte lipocortin-1 in rheumatoid arthritis. Arthritis Rheum 37:207-211, 1994.
27. DiBattista JA, Martel-Pelletier J, Wosu LO, et al: Glucocorticoid receptor mediated inhibition of interleukin-1 stimulated neutral metalloprotease synthesis in normal human chondrocytes. J Clin Endocrinol Metab 72:316-326, 1991.
28. Cronstein BN, Kimmel SC, Levin RI, et al: A mechanism for the antiinflammatory effects of corticosteroids: the glucocorticoid receptor regulates leukocyte adhesion to endothelial cells and expression of endothelial-leukocyte adhesion molecule 1 and intercellular adhesion molecule 1. Proc Natl Acad Sci U S A 89: 9991-9995, 1992.
29. Di Rosa M, Radomski M, Carnuccio R, Moncada S: Glucocorticoids inhibit the induction of nitric oxide synthase in macrophages. Biochem Biophys Res Commun 172:1246-52, 1990.
30. Gudbjornsson B, Skogseid B, Oberg K, et al: Intact adrenocorticotropic hormone secretion but impaired cortisol response in patients with active rheumatoid arthritis: effect of glucocorticoids. J Rheumatol 23:596-602, 1996.
31. Chikanza IC, Petrou P, Kingsley G, et al: Defective hypothalamic response to immune and inflammatory stimuli in patients with rheumatoid arthritis. Arthritis Rheum 35:1281-1288, 1992.

32. Bijlsma JW, Cutolo M, Masi AT, Chikanza IC: The neuroendocrine immune basis of rheumatic diseases. Immunol Today 20:298-301, 1999.
33. Esteban NV, Loughlin T, Yergey AL, et al: Daily cortisol production rate in man determined by stable isotope dilution/mass spectrometry. J Clin Endocrinol Metab 72:39-45, 1991.
34. Ackerman GL, Nolsn CM: Adrenocortical responsiveness after alternate-day corticosteroid therapy. N Engl J Med 278:405-409, 1968.
35. Schlaghecke R, Kornely E, Santen RT, Ridderskamp P: The effect of long-term glucocorticoid therapy on pituitary-adrenal responses to exogenous corticotropin-releasing hormone. N Engl J Med 326:226-30, 1992.
36. Henzen C, Suter A, Lerch E, et al: Suppression and recovery of adrenal response after short-term, high-dose glucocorticoid treatment. Lancet 355:542-545, 2000.
37. DeMarco PJ, Weisman MH, Seibold JR, et al: Predictors and outcomes of scleroderma renal crisis: the high-dose versus low-dose D-penicillamine in early diffuse systemic sclerosis trial. Arthritis Rheum 46:2983-2989, 2002.
38. Gaffney K, Ledingham J, Perry JD: Intra-articular triamcinolone hexacetonide in knee osteoarthritis: factors influencing the clinical response. Ann Rheum Dis 54:379-381, 1995.
39. Buchanan WW, Stephen LJ, Buchanan HM: Are 'homeopathic' doses of oral corticosteroids effective in rheumatoid arthritis? Clin Exp Rheumatol 6:281-284, 1988.
40. ACR Subcommittee on Rheumatoid Arthritis Guidelines. Guidelines for the management of rheumatoid arthritis: 2002 Update. Arthritis Rheum 46:328-346, 2002.
41. Criswell LA, Saag KG, Sems KM, et al: Moderate-term, low-dose corticosteroids for rheumatoid arthritis. Cochrane Database Syst Rev CD001158, 2000.
42. Hansen M, Podenphant J, Florescu A, et al: A randomised trial of differentiated prednisolone treatment in active rheumatoid arthritis: clinical benefits and skeletal side effects. Ann Rheum Dis 58:713-718, 1999.
43. Van Everdingen AA, Jacobs JW, Siewertsz Van Reesema DR, Bijlsma JW: Low-dose prednisone therapy for patients with early active rheumatoid arthritis: clinical efficacy, disease-modifying properties, and side effects: a randomized, double-blind, placebo-controlled clinical trial. Ann Intern Med 136:1-12, 2002.
44. Kirwan JR: The effect of glucocorticoids on joint destruction in rheumatoid arthritis: the Arthritis and Rheumatism Council Low-Dose Glucocorticoid Study Group. N Engl J Med 333:142-146, 1995.
45. Smolen JS, Kalden JR, Scott DL, et al: Efficacy and safety of leflunomide compared with placebo and sulphasalazine in active rheumatoid arthritis: a double-blind, randomised, multicentre trial. European Leflunomide Study Group. Lancet 353:259-266, 1999.
46. Weinblatt ME, Kremer JM, Coblyn JS, et al: Pharmacokinetics, safety, and efficacy of combination treatment with methotrexate and leflunomide in patients with active rheumatoid arthritis. Arthritis Rheum 42:1322-1328, 1999.
47. Boers M, Verhoeven AC, Markusse HM, et al: Randomised comparison of combined step-down prednisolone, methotrexate and sulphasalazine with sulphasalazine alone in early rheumatoid arthritis. Lancet 350:309-318, 1997.
48. Landewe RB, Boers M, Verhoeven AC, et al: COBRA combination therapy in patients with early rheumatoid arthritis: long-term structural benefits of a brief intervention. Arthritis Rheum 46:347-356, 2002.
49. Haagsma CJ, van Riel PL, de Jong AJ, van de Putte LB: Combination of sulphasalazine and methotrexate versus the single components in early rheumatoid arthritis: a randomized, controlled, double-blind, 52 week clinical trial. Br J Rheumatol 36:1082-1088, 1997.
50. Dougados M, Combe B, Cantagrel A, et al: Combination therapy in early rheumatoid arthritis: a randomised, controlled, double blind 52 week clinical trial of sulphasalazine and methotrexate compared with the single components. Ann Rheum Dis 58: 220-225, 1999.
51. Wassenberg S, Rau R, Zeidler H: Low dose prednisolone therapy (LDPT) retards radiographically detectable destruction in early rheumatoid arthritis. Arthritis Rheum 42(suppl):S243, 2002.
52. Paulus HE, Di Primeo D, Sanda M, et al: Progression of radiographic joint erosion during low dose corticosteroid treatment of rheumatoid arthritis. J Rheumatol 27:1632-1637, 2000.
53. O'Dell JR: Treating rheumatoid arthritis early: a window of opportunity? Arthritis Rheum 46:283-285, 2002.
54. Fries JF, Williams CA, Ramey D, Bloch DA: The relative toxicity of disease-modifying antirheumatic drugs. Arthritis Rheum 36: 297-306, 1993.
55. Neeck G, Federlin K, Graef V, et al: Adrenal secretion of cortisol in patients with rheumatoid arthritis. J Rheumatol 17:24-29, 1990.
56. Arvidson NG, Gudbjornsson B, Larsson A, Hallgren R: The timing of glucocorticoid administration in rheumatoid arthritis. Ann Rheum Dis 56:27-31, 1997.
57. Kowanko IC, Pownall R, Knapp MS, et al: Time of day of prednisolone administration in rheumatoid arthritis. Ann Rheum Dis 41:447-452, 1982.
58. Fauci AS: Alternate-day corticosteroid therapy. Am J Med 64: 729-731, 1978.
59. Bengtsson BA, Malmvall BE: An alternate-day corticosteroid regimen in maintenance therapy of giant cell arteritis. Acta Med Scand 209:347-350, 1981.
60. Hunder GG, Sheps SG, Allen GL, Joyce JW: Daily and alternate-day corticosteroid regimens in treatment of giant cell arteritis: comparison in a prospective study. Ann Intern Med 82:613-618, 1975.
61. Huizenga NA, Koper JW, De Lange P, et al: A polymorphism in the glucocorticoid receptor gene may be associated with and increased sensitivity to glucocorticoids in vivo. J Clin Endocrinol Metab 83:144-151, 1998
62. Chikanza IC: Mechanisms of corticosteroid resistance in rheumatoid arthritis: a putative role for the corticosteroid receptor beta isoform. Ann N Y Acad Sci 966:39-48, 2002.
63. Podgorski MR, Goulding NJ, Hall ND, et al: Autoantibodies to lipocortin-1 are associated with impaired glucocorticoid responsiveness in rheumatoid arthritis. J Rheumatol 19:1668-1671, 1992.
64. Molijn GJ, Spek JJ, van Uffelen JC, et al: Differential adaptation of glucocorticoid sensitivity of peripheral blood mononuclear leukocytes in patients with sepsis or septic shock. J Clin Endocrinol Metab 80:1799-1803, 1995.
65. Leech M, Metz C, Hall P, et al: Macrophage migration inhibitory factor in rheumatoid arthritis: evidence of proinflammatory function and regulation by glucocorticoids. Arthritis Rheum 42: 1601-1608, 1999.
66. Weusten BL, Jacobs JW, Bijlsma JW: Corticosteroid pulse therapy in active rheumatoid arthritis. Semin Arthritis Rheum 23:183-192, 1993.
67. Jacobs JW, Geenen R, Evers AW, et al: Short term effects of corticosteroid pulse treatment on disease activity and the wellbeing of patients with active rheumatoid arthritis. Ann Rheum Dis 60: 61-64, 2001.
68. McCarty DJ, Harman JG, Grassanovich JL, Qian C: Treatment of rheumatoid joint inflammation with intrasynovial triamcinolone hexacetonide. J Rheumatol 22:1631-1635, 1995.
69. Weitoft T, Uddenfeldt P: Importance of synovial fluid aspiration when injecting intra-articular corticosteroids. Ann Rheum Dis 59:233-235, 2000.
70. Blyth T, Hunter JA, Stirling A: Pain relief in the rheumatoid knee after steroid injection: a single-blind comparison of hydrocortisone succinate, and triamcinolone acetonide or hexacetonide. Br J Rheumatol 33:461-463, 1994.
71. Gray RG, Gottlieb NL: Intra-articular corticosteroids: an updated assessment. Clin Orthop 177:235-263, 1983.
72. Chatham W, Williams G, Moreland L, et al: Intraarticular corticosteroid injections: should we rest the joints? Arthritis Care Res 2:70-74, 1989.
73. Chakravarty K, Pharoah PD, Scott DG: A randomized controlled study of post-injection rest following intra-articular steroid therapy for knee synovitis. Br J Rheumatol 33:464-468, 1994.
74. Eustace JA, Brophy DP, Gibney RP, et al: Comparison of the accuracy of steroid placement with clinical outcome in patients with shoulder symptoms. Ann Rheum Dis 56:59-63, 1997.
75. Jones A, Regan M, Ledingham J, et al: Importance of placement of intra-articular steroid injections. BMJ 307:1329-1330, 1993.
76. Hollander JL: Intrasynovial corticosteroid therapy in arthritis. Md State Med J 19:62-66, 1970.

77. Gray RG, Tenenbaum J, Gottlieb NL: Local corticosteroid injection treatment in rheumatic disorders. Semin Arthritis Rheum 10:231-254, 1981.
78. Seror P, Pluvinage P, d'Andre FL, et al: Frequency of sepsis after local corticosteroid injection (an inquiry on 1160000 injections in rheumatological private practice in France). Rheumatology (Oxford) 38:1272-1274, 1999.
79. Kaandorp CJ, Krijnen P, Moens HJ, et al: The outcome of bacterial arthritis: a prospective community-based study. Arthritis Rheum 40:884-92, 1997.
80. Mens JM, Nico DW, Berkhout BJ, Stam HJ: Disturbance of the menstrual pattern after local injection with triamcinolone acetonide. Ann Rheum Dis 57:700, 1998.
81. DeSio JM, Kahn CH, Warfield CA: Facial flushing and/or generalized erythema after epidural steroid injection. Anesth Analg 80:617-619, 1995.
82. Black DM, Filak AT: Hyperglycemia with non–insulin-dependent diabetes following intraarticular steroid injection. J Fam Pract 28:462-463, 1989.
83. Di Stefano, V, Nixon JE: Skin and fat atrophy complications of local steroid injection. Pa Med 77:38, 1974.
84. Stapczynski JS: Localized depigmentation after steroid injection of a ganglion cyst on the hand. Ann Emerg Med 20:807-809, 1991.
85. Kleinman M, Gross AE: Achilles tendon rupture following steroid injection. Report of three cases. J Bone Joint Surg Am 65:1345-1347, 1983.
86. Linskey ME, Segal R: Median nerve injury from local steroid injection in carpal tunnel syndrome. Neurosurgery 26:512-515, 1990.
87. American College of Rheumatology Ad Hoc Committee on Glucocorticoid-Induced Osteoporosis: Recommendations for the prevention and treatment of glucocorticoid-induced osteoporosis: 2001 update. Arthritis Rheum 44:1496-503, 2001.
88. Lukert BP: Glucocorticoid-induced osteoporosis. *In* The American Society for Bone and Mineral Research (eds): Primer on the Metabolic Bone Diseases and Disorders of Mineral Metabolism. Philadelphia, Lippincott Williams & Wilkins, 1999, pp 292-296.
89. Dekhuijzen PN, Decramer M: Steroid-induced myopathy and its significance to respiratory disease: a known disease rediscovered. Eur Respir J 5:997-1003, 1992.
90. Garcia Rodriguez LA, Hernandez-Diaz S: The risk of upper gastrointestinal complications associated with nonsteroidal anti-inflammatory drugs, glucocorticoids, acetaminophen, and combinations of these agents. Arthritis Res 3:98-101, 2001.
91. Piper JM, Ray WA, Daugherty JR, Griffin MR: Corticosteroid use and peptic ulcer disease: role of nonsteroidal anti-inflammatory drugs. Ann Intern Med 114:735-740, 1991.
92. Saab S, Corr MP, Weisman MH: Corticosteroids and systemic lupus erythematosus pancreatitis: a case series. J Rheumatol 25:801-806, 1998.
93. Stuck AE, Minder CE, Frey FJ: Risk of infectious complications in patients taking glucocorticosteroids. Rev Infect Dis 11: 954-963, 1989.
94. Jackson SH, Beevers DG, Myers K: Does long-term low-dose corticosteroid therapy cause hypertension? Clin Sci (Lond) 61(Suppl 7):381S-383S, 1981.
95. Mason JW, O'Connell JB, Herskowitz A, et al: A clinical trial of immunosuppressive therapy for myocarditis: The Myocarditis Treatment Trial Investigators. N Engl J Med 333:269-275, 1995.
96. Latham RD, Mulrow JP, Virmani R, et al: Recently diagnosed idiopathic dilated cardiomyopathy: incidence of myocarditis and efficacy of prednisone therapy. Am Heart J 117:876-882, 1989.
97. Van Doornum S, McColl G, Wicks IP: Accelerated atherosclerosis: an extraarticular feature of rheumatoid arthritis? Arthritis Rheum 46:862-873, 2002.
98. Maxwell SR, Moots RJ, Kendall MJ: Corticosteroids: do they damage the cardiovascular system? Postgrad Med J 70:863-870, 1994.
99. Ross R: Atherosclerosis is an inflammatory disease. Am Heart J 138:S419-S420, 1999.
100. Petri M, Perez-Gutthann S, Spence D, Hochberg MC: Risk factors for coronary artery disease in patients with systemic lupus erythematosus. Am J Med 93:513-519, 1992.
101. Carnahan MC, Goldstein DA: Ocular complications of topical, peri-ocular, and systemic corticosteroids. Curr Opin Ophthalmology 11:478-483, 2000.
102. Klein BE, Klein R, Lee KE, Danforth LG: Drug use and five-year incidence of age-related cataracts: The Beaver Dam Eye Study. Ophthalmology 108:1670-1674, 2001.
103. Urban RC Jr., Cotlier E: Corticosteroid-induced cataracts. Surv Ophthalmol 31:102-110, 1986.
104. Garbe E, LeLorier J, Boivin JF, Suissa S: Risk of ocular hypertension or open-angle glaucoma in elderly patients on oral glucocorticoids. Lancet 350:979-982, 1997.
105. Tripathi RC, Parapuram SK, Tripathi BJ, et al: Corticosteroids and glaucoma risk. Drugs Aging 15:439-450, 1999.
106. Cooper C, Kirwan JR: The risks of local and systemic corticosteroid administration. Baillieres Clin Rheumatol 4:305-332, 1991.
107. Tayek JA, Katz J: Glucose production, recycling, Cori cycle, and gluconeogenesis in humans: relationship to serum cortisol. Am J Physiol 272:E476-E484, 1997.
108. Delaunay F, Khan A, Cintra A, et al: Pancreatic beta cells are important targets for the diabetogenic effects of glucocorticoids. J Clin Invest 100:2094-2098, 1997.
109. Gurwitz JH, Bohn RL, Glynn RJ, et al: Glucocorticoids and the risk for initiation of hypoglycemic therapy. Arch Intern Med 154:97-101, 1994.
110. Hirsch IB, Paauw DS: Diabetes management in special situations. Endocrinol Metab Clin North Am 26:631-645, 1997.
111. Stewart PM, Tomlinson JW: Cortisol, 11 beta-hydroxysteroid dehydrogenase type 1 and central obesity. Trends Endocrinol Metab 13:94-96, 2002.
112. Poon M, Gertz SD, Fallon JT, et al: Dexamethasone inhibits macrophage accumulation after balloon arterial injury in cholesterol fed rabbits. Atherosclerosis 155:371-380, 2001.
113. Oelkers W: Adrenal insufficiency. N Engl J Med 335:1206-1212, 1996.
114. Sampson PA, Brooke BN, Winstone NE: Biochemical conformation of collase due to adrenal failure. Lancet i:1377, 1961.
115. Patten SB, Neutel CI: Corticosteroid-induced adverse psychiatric effects: incidence, diagnosis and management. Drug Saf 22:111-122, 2000.
116. Naber D, Sand P, Heigl B: Psychopathological and neuropsychological effects of 8-days' corticosteroid treatment: A prospective study. Psychoneuroendocrinology 21:25-31, 1996.

58 Second Line Agents

DUNCAN A. GORDON • ALICE V. KLINKHOFF

Sulfasalazine

Professor Nanna Svartz of Stockholm, believing that infection was the cause of rheumatoid arthritis (RA), collaborated in 1938 with the Swedish pharmaceutical company Pharmacia to synthesize salicylazosulfapyridin, now known as sulfasalazine (SSZ), consisting of salicylic acid (antiarthritic) and sulfapyridine (antibacterial) joined by an azo bond (Fig. 58–1). She reported a 60-percent improvement in her patients with chronic polyarthritis and also observed good responses in ankylosing spondylitis (AS).[1,2]

PHARMACOLOGY OF SULFASALAZINE

Absorption of SSZ is only 10 to 20 percent. Most of the drug reaches the colon, where the azo bond is reduced by colonic bacteria. Sulfapyridine, possibly the active component in rheumatic diseases,[3] and 5-aminosalicylic acid (ASA), active in ulcerative colitis, are liberated[4,5] (Fig. 58–2).

Sulfapyridine appears in plasma 4 to 6 hours after a dose of SSZ and is extensively metabolized in the liver by N4-acetylation and ring hydroxylation with subsequent glucuronidations.[6] Wide intersubject variation in metabolic rates of sulfapyridine, and thus in blood concentrations, is observed, in part owing to genetically determined variation in acetylation and oxidative capacities, respectively.[6] However, no relationship between plasma concentrations of sulfapyridine and efficacy has been demonstrated.[7] The pharmacokinetics, efficacy, and adverse effect rate of SSZ are unaffected by age.[8,9]

In ulcerative colitis, the active moiety is believed to be 5-ASA with the sulfapyridine acting as a carrier to the site of action in the colon. In RA, the mechanism of action remains unclear. Immunomodulatory activity of SSZ is suggested by the reduction of circulating activated lymphocytes after 12 weeks of therapy, the inhibition of B cell activation, significant falls in immunoglobulin M (IgM) and rheumatoid factor titers, an incidence of hypogammaglobulinemia of up to 10 percent, and the hyperreactivity or restoration of normal responses of lymphocytes to various stimuli ex vivo after SSZ treatment.[10] SSZ treatment for 16 weeks altered the distribution of lymphocyte subtypes in the intestinal mucosa without corresponding changes in peripheral blood in patients with RA.[11]

SSZ significantly reduced interleukin-1α (IL-1α), IL-1β, and tumor necrosis factor-α (TNF-α) in patients with RA of less than a year's duration in association with clinical and laboratory evidence of response to the drug, but whether the cytokine effects were primary or secondary to disease improvement was uncertain.[12] Another study has shown that SSZ reduces basal IL-6 production.[13]

Carlin and associates[14] demonstrated that SSZ and sulfapyridine inhibit the flux of second messengers, such as cytosolic calcium, diacylglycerol, and inositol triphosphate, induced by stimulation of human leukocytes

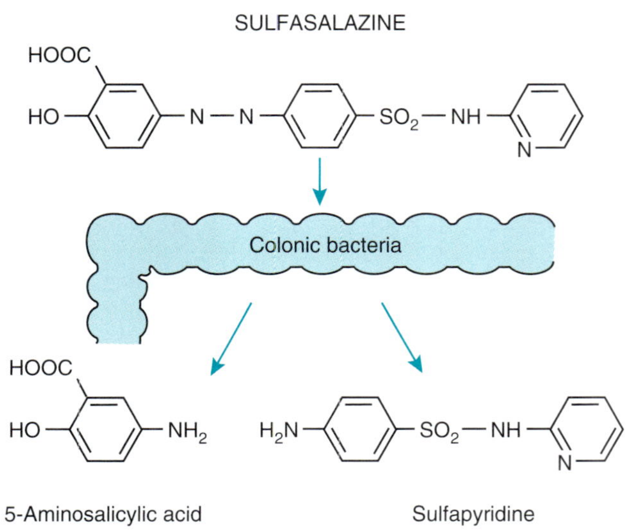

FIGURE 58–1 • Sulfasalazine and its Major Metabolites.

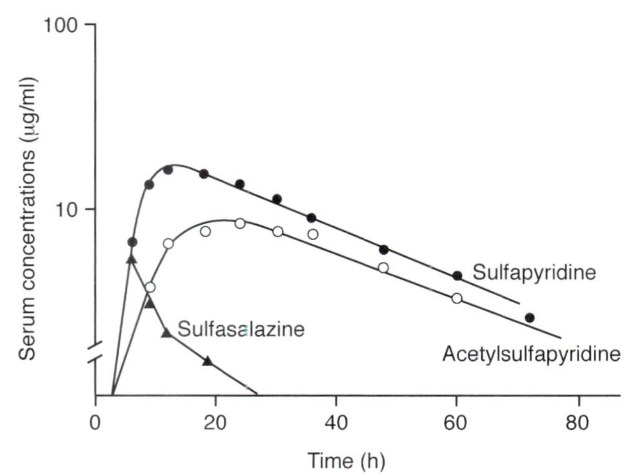

FIGURE 58–2 • Serum concentrations of sulfasalazine, sulfapyridine, and acetylsulfapyridine after dose of 2 g orally in a 40-year-old woman. (From Taggart A, McDermott B, Delargy M, et al: The pharmacokinetics of sulphasalazine in young and elderly patients with rheumatoid arthritis. Scand J Rheumatol 64:32, 1987.)

in vitro. These effects may depend on drug action at the level of phospholipase C or its regulatory guanosine triphosphate (GTP)-binding protein and could explain some of the other effects of SSZ on mediators of inflammation and lymphocyte function.

CLINICAL APPLICATIONS

Selection of Patients

SSZ has been a popular disease-modifying antirheumatic drug (DMARD) in Europe for more than 30 years. It is approved by the Food and Drug Administration (FDA) and recommended by the American College of Rheumatology (ACR) for use in RA[15] and is effective in psoriatic arthritis (PsA) and other spondyloarthropathies, as well as pauciarticular and polyarticular juvenile rheumatoid arthritis (JRA). In systemic-onset JRA and in adult-onset Still's disease (AOSD) there are reports of frequent and serious side effects and no evidence for benefit.

EFFICACY

Rheumatoid Arthritis

Between 1983 and 1995 eight double-blind, placebo-controlled trials were published. A meta-analysis published in 1999 of these studies involving 552 RA patients treated with SSZ and 351 with placebo showed superior effectiveness of SSZ in all measures evaluated except physician global assessment (measured in only three of eight trials).[16] The articular index improved by 46 percent for SSZ versus 20 percent for placebo ($p < .0001$). The number of swollen joints was reduced by 54 percent, versus 38 percent for placebo ($p = .004$). The erythrocyte sedimentation rate, (ESR) fell by 37 percent, compared to 14 percent for placebo $p < .0001$), and pain improved by 42 percent compared to 14 percent for placebo ($p < .0001$). In this meta-analysis, 27 percent withdrew due to adverse events and 11 percent due to lack of effect compared to 7 percent and 28 percent for placebo, respectively. In six of eight trials the dose of SSZ was 2 g daily and in remaining two the dose was 3 g. No study compared these two doses. Compared to gold sodium aurothioglucose (GSTG) in trials and with D-penicillamine (DP) in three trials results showed similar efficacy and greater withdrawals due to side effects in patients randomized to GSTG compared with hydroxychloroquine (HCQ). Two studies suggest superior efficacy of SSZ and similar incidence of side effects resulting in withdrawal. In a 48-week study comparing SSZ to HCQ in early RA, SSZ had a faster onset of action and was associated with less radiographic progression at 24 and 48 weeks[17] and at 3-year follow up.[18] A controlled trial comparing SSZ to leflunomide and with placebo showed similar clinical effectiveness of the active agents and superiority compared to placebo for both clinical outcomes and radiographic progression after 6 months.[19] However, a follow-up of this group at 24 months showed more improvement in patients taking lefluminide than SSZ.[20]

In recent years methotrexate (MTX), SSZ, and HCQ have each been used more commonly than GSTG and DP.[21] As with other traditional DMARDS, long-term adherence to therapy is disappointing. About 50 percent discontinue treatment within 2 years due to either lack of effect or side effects. There are no clinical or laboratory predictors of response.[22] Moreover, although MTX, SSZ, and HCQ are each effective, it has been reported that patients with RA continue taking MTX longer than SSZ or HCQ alone.[23]

Combination Therapy of Rheumatoid Arthritis

Combination of SSZ with HCQ and MTX was more effective than MTX and SSZ alone and barely better than MTX and HCQ in a 2-year randomized control trial, (RCT).[24] In contrast two European trials in patients with early active RA failed to show any advantage of combining MTX with SSZ or MTX, cyclosporine A (CSA) and intra-articular corticosteroids versus SSZ alone.[25,26] The combination of SSZ with MTX and prednisone using an intensive 6-month step-down strategy was superior to SSZ monotherapy for up to 1 year after prednisone was discontinued in the Dutch COBRA trials[27] and in terms of radiographic progression measured after 4 to 5 years.[28]

A delay as short as 4 months in starting single-dose second-line therapy also reduced remission compared to a DMARD combination of SSZ, MTX, HCQ, and prednisone.[29] Earlier, this same group had reported prevention of cervical spine involvement after combination treatment.[30]

Seronegative Spondyloarthropathies

A placebo-controlled trial has shown SSZ to be effective in PsA for the peripheral joints.[31] Similar findings were reported in a series of 619 patients with seronegative spondyloarthopathies in terms of improvement in peripheral arthritis but not in terms of axial disease.[32] A randomized, double-blind trial of SSZ versus placebo in 76 patients with reactive arthritis showed earlier remission in SSZ-treated patients ($p + .013$) but no difference when compared to placebo at 6 months.[33] In AS patients without peripheral arthritis, a placebo-controlled trial by Dougados showed benefit of SSZ after 3 months measured in terms of patient global assessment, functional index[25], use of nonsteroidal anti-inflammatory drugs (NSAIDs), and serum IgG. A meta-analysis by Ferraz of five randomized, controlled trials indicated clinical benefit in AS favoring SSZ over placebo in duration of morning stiffness, severity of morning stiffness, pain, patient global assessment, ESR and serum IgA.[34]

SSZ has been found effective in the treatment of PsA without worsening rash. A case of nail-loss recovery[35] was reported, but its use was poorly tolerated in a series of cases with PsA.[36]

Comparing cyclosporin A, (CSA) to SSZ and placebo, CSA resulted in greater improvement in most clinical measures, as well as the psoriatic arthritis skin index, (PASI) score; spondylitis functional index and ESR were statistically significantly improved in the SSZ-treated patients when compared to placebo-treated patients.[37] In seronegative spondyloarthropathies, flares of acute anterior uveitis may also be reduced by treatment with SSZ.[38]

Juvenile Rheumatoid Arthritis

SSZ has been widely and safely used in the treatment of childhood inflammatory bowel disease, (IBD), but it is poorly tolerated in juveniles with arthritis.

A randomized, double-blind, 24-week trial in 69 JRA patients in the Netherlands demonstrated effectiveness in terms of all global assessments, number of swollen joints total active joints physician global assessment, ESR, and C-reactive protein, (CRP).[39] In an intent-to-treat analysis, 69 percent of treated patients versus 45 percent of placebo patients met predetermined response criteria; there was statistically significant ($p < .001$) benefit using the Pavia core set of criteria for improvement in JRA. Gastrointestinal (GI) side effects occurred in 24 of 35 SSZ patients and 18 of 34 placebo patients. Eighteen percent of placebo and 31 percent of SSZ patients withdrew prior to 24 weeks. It has also been reported that systemic-onset disease responds poorly to SSZ and may be associated with a serum-sickness reaction.[40] Patients with AOSD taking SSZ also show frequent severe side effects.[41]

Dosing Schedules

The common dosage for adults with rheumatic disease is in the 2-g range (1.5 to 3 g) of the enteric-coated formulation taken as 1 g twice a day with meals. Starting doses of 500 mg to 1 g per day are usually employed to minimize the risk of side effects. If tolerated, dosage increase in increments of 500 mg/day at intervals of a week or longer are prescribed. However, increased doses from 2 to 3 g/day do not always improve response. In some patients, GI side effects can be controlled by dose reduction.

DRUG INTERACTIONS

Broad-spectrum antibiotics that alter gut flora may reduce the bioavailability of sulfapyridine, and 5-ASA as the azo link between these two metabolites of SSZ is cleaved by bacterial metabolism. Concomitant cholestyramine is likely to reduce the systemic availability of sulfapyridine because the resin binds SSZ, rendering it unavailable for bacterial digestion. SSZ absorption is reduced if it is coadministered with oral iron preparations, but sulfapyridine concentrations are unaffected.

Toxicity of Sulfasalazine

The majority of adverse effects are seen within 3 months. In a large series with long-term follow-up, 205 of 774 RA patients discontinued therapy due to adverse effects.[38] Sixty percent of withdrawals were due to GI side effects. There were no deaths and no permanent sequellae. The most frequent side effects of SSZ are listed in Table 58–1. Serious ones are rare.

TABLE 58–1 • MOST FREQUENT ADVERSE EFFECTS OF SULFASALAZINE

Adverse effect	Frequency
Nausea, malaise, or dyspepsia	30%
Rash	5%
Neutropenia	2-4%
Megaloblastic anemia	0.3%
Neurologic effects: headache, fever, lightheadedness, dizziness	4%
Elevated liver function tests	2.5%

Gastrointestinal

Nausea and upper abdominal discomfort, often in association with headache and dizziness, are the most common adverse effects, and their incidence is reduced by starting at a low dose and increasing dosage gradually. These effects are often less of a problem after 2 to 3 months. Hepatitic reactions, sometimes accompanied by fever, rash, and lymphadenopathy, are a well-known adverse effect of SSZ.[42]

Blood

The incidence of leukopenia and neutropenia varies from 1 to 5 percent and is most common in the first 3 months of therapy. The drug has to be stopped in about one third to one half of patients who become leukopenic. However, leukopenia and neutropenia can occur at any time, necessitating some continued surveillance[43] (Fig. 58–3). Timely recognition is usually associated with recovery, although some cases of fatal agranulocytosis have been described.[44] There are conflicting data concerning the effect of SSZ on serum or red cell folate concentrations; some studies show lowered folate. Although some degree of macrocytosis and hemolysis has been common in patients taking higher doses of SSZ for ulcerative colitis, frank hemolytic anemia is unusual; it is typically associated with methemoglobinemia, Heinz bodies, and reticulocytosis. Glucose-6-phosphate dehydrogenase deficiency is a risk factor for hemolysis, and assessment of baseline enzyme levels is recommended.

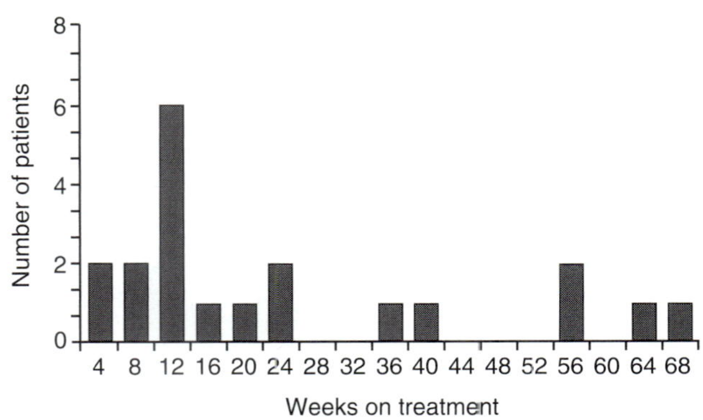

FIGURE 58–3 · Patients develop leukopenia during sulfasalazine treatment, indicating that most cases occur in the first few months of therapy. (From Marabani M, Madhok R, Capell H, et al: Leucopenia during sulphasalazine treatment for rheumatoid arthritis. Ann Rheum Dis 48:506, 1989.)

Skin

Rashes occur in 1 to 5 percent of patients. Pruritic, maculopapular, and generalized rashes are most common, but occasional patients have urticarial reactions, and reversible and dose-dependent cases of lichen planus have been reported.[45] Desensitization to SSZ has been successfully accomplished.[46] Some cases of alopecia have been noted. Classic serum sickness has been described, and toxic epidermal necrolysis and Stevens-Johnson syndrome have been reported rarely.

Pulmonary

A number of cases manifesting reversible pulmonary infiltrates accompanied by eosinophilia, dyspnea, fever, and weight loss have been described. Fibrosing alveolitis has been reported; the condition slowly resolves with prednisone therapy and cessation of SSZ.

Reproduction

SSZ is safe in pregnancy and does not interfere with conception in women with RA.[47] In men, a reversible reduction in sperm count and sperm motility has been seen in some patients.[48] Little drug is excreted in breast milk.

Other Adverse Effects

Changes in mood including irritability and depression are not unusual in the early months of therapy. A range of central nervous system adverse effects has been documented, including aseptic meningitis.[49] Hypogammaglobulinemia has been described,[7] as have multiple cases of drug-induced lupus and induction of DNA antibodies.[7,50] Nevertheless, positive antinuclear antibody, (ANA) titers are common in patients with RA, but its presence does not imply reaction to SSZ or the likelihood of drug-induced lupus.[51] In another series, however, an increased frequency of speckled ANA may be a risk factor for lupus-like disease in association with SLE-HLA haplotypes and increased levels of serum IL-10 levels.[52]

Treatment Monitoring

Rheumatologists with experience using SSZ recommend baseline hematology and liver function tests monitoring and hematology tests every 2 to 4 weeks for 3 months. Beyond 3 months it is debatable whether formal monitoring is required,[42] but some authorities recommend monitoring every 3 months. It should be used with caution in patients with hepatic or renal disease. SSZ is contraindicated in patients with an ileostomy.[53]

Antimalarial Drugs

Antimalarial medications were first derived from the bark of the Peruvian cinchona tree. The active agents, quinine and cinchonine, were isolated by Pelletier and Caventau in 1820. In 1894, J. P. Payne, physician to St. Thomas' Hospital in London, in a postgraduate lecture on lupus, first described the successful use of quinine for a rheumatic disease.[54] Page's landmark publication in 1951[55] provided impetus for the widespread use of antimalarials to treat connective tissue diseases. He used quinacrine for patients with systemic lupus erythematosus (SLE) and reported that skin lesions improved in 17 of 18 patients. Associated "rheumatoid arthritis" also remitted in two of these patients, and systemic symptoms, including arthritis, cleared in a third.

Chloroquine (CQ) and hydroxychloroquine (HCQ) were developed in an effort to minimize antimalarial toxicity.[56] In 1959, however, Hobbs and associates[57] recognized that treatment might result in serious retinal toxicity, and this led to a diminished antimalarial use. Retinal toxicity is primarily related to high daily doses[58] but may still occur.[59] Many rheumatic diseases have been shown to respond to antimalarials.[60-66] In the 1990s, the early use of second-line treatment for active RA has gained acceptance and with it the widespread use of antimalarials alone or in combination.[67]

PHARMACOLOGY OF ANTIMALARIALS

Only three antimalarial compounds are now used to treat rheumatic diseases (Fig. 58–4). Of these, two

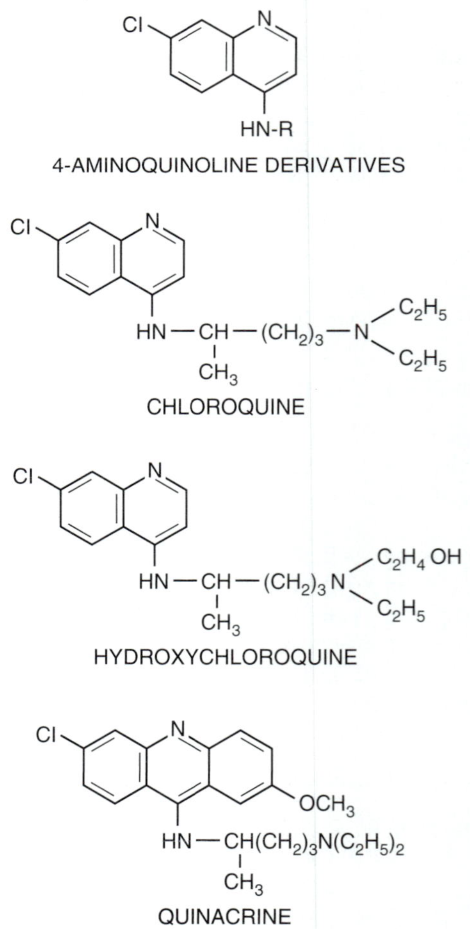

FIGURE 58–4 · Chemical structures of antimalarial drugs used to treat rheumatic disease and the basic structure of 4-aminoquinolines. R represents the side chain.

4-aminoquinoline derivatives, CQ and HCQ, are virtually the only drugs prescribed. They differ only by the substitution of a hydroxyethyl group for an ethyl group on the tertiary amino nitrogen of the side chain of CQ. HCQ is more commonly prescribed in the United States.

Quinacrine, although not a 4-aminoquinoline, does include the CQ structure (see Fig. 58–4). It is occasionally used in patients with discoid lupus but may cause yellowish skin discoloration. In the United States, this drug is currently formulated only by pharmacists.

Distribution

Both HCQ and CQ are rapidly are rapidly absorbed after oral administration, cleared from plasma, and distributed extensively in tissues including liver, spleen, kidney, and red and white blood cells. Mononuclear cells have a higher concentration than do neutrophils. There are high concentrations in intracellular lysomes and in pigmented eye tissue. Steady-state concentrations are achieved after 3 to 4 months.[68] The large volume of distribution accounts for the extended half-life of 40 to 50 days.[69]

Most of the absorbed medication is excreted in urine up to 50 percent unchanged, but about one third is metabolized to a desethyl derivative formed by alkyl degradation of a terminal amino ethyl group in the side chain.[70] About 9 percent can be found in feces, some of which is a result of excretion.[70] Small amounts of CQ can be found in plasma, red blood cells, and urine for as long as 5 years after the last dose[71], and more in mononuclears than neutrophils.

Pharmacokinetics

Various drug actions that can affect rheumatic diseases are listed in Table 58–2. Some of the references are documented in previous editions.[73]

The mechanism of action of antimalarial drugs in rheumatic diseases is controversial. It is likely that the major effect is due to inhibition of antigen-processing ability by macrophages and monocytes, including inhibition of lymphocyte transformation, chemotaxis, and monocyte secretion of IL-1. Because antimalarial drugs are weak bases, they may interfere with enzymatic activities that require an acid milieu, including action of acid hydrolases and processing of antigenic peptides. Some cell surface receptors and ligands are transported by endosomes to lysosomes, where receptors are separated from ligands and returned to the cell surface. Antimalarial drugs interfere with this receptor recycling.[74]

CQ may inhibit protein secretion and the intracellular processing of proteins by blocking the proteolytic conversion of secretory protein precursors, such as the complement component precursor pro-C3.[75] These biochemical changes are associated with morphologic changes.

Antimalarials affect multiple aspects of the immunologic cascade. Animal studies document that they do not inhibit antibody production to exogenous antigens.[76] Fox and Kang,[77] however, suggested that higher pH in the endoplasmic reticulum stabilizes major histocompatibility protein with invariant chains, preventing their displacement by low-affinity autoantigens that may result in a block of autoantibody production. In fact, rheumatoid factor disappears in some patients with RA who are responding to antimalarials.[5]

Interference with immunologic cell function has been documented. CQ inhibits the proliferative response of stimulated cultured human lymphocytes.[56,73] Decreased responsiveness to phytohemagglutinin has been demonstrated by lymphocytes of treated patients.[78] Natural killer cell action is inhibited both in vitro[56] and in vivo.[79] Changes in immune function are further documented by studies of cytokines and receptors on lymphocyte membranes that are crucial in the development of RA. Antimalarials block the in vitro production of IL-1, IL-6, TNF-α, and interferon-γ (IFN-γ) through reduced cytokine messenger RNA expression,[80-82] limiting their release into plasma and whole blood.[81] There appears to be a greater effect on release from monocytes than from lymphocytes,[82] and not all studies are in agreement.[80,82]

TABLE 58–2 • ANTIMALARIAL ACTIONS

Primary Actions
Interferes with intracellular function dependent on an acidic microenvironment*
Inhibits enzyme activity, including phospholipase A_2
Anti-inflammatory Activity
Stabilizes lysosomal membranes
Inhibits polymorphonuclear cell chemotaxis and phagocytosis
Affects superoxide generation
Inhibits connective tissue encapsulation
Decreases fibronectin production
Decreases histamine production
Decreases intravascular erythrocyte aggregation
Decreases platelet aggregation
Is photoprotective†
Inhibits interleukin-1–induced cartilage degradation
Effects on Immune Function
Inhibits cytokine production[31-33]
Inhibits lymphocyte membrane receptor formation
May decrease autoantibody production
Inhibits proliferative response of stimulated lymphocytes[35]
Inhibits natural killer cell activity
Inhibits immune complex formation
Increases apoptosis[36]
Effects on Infectious Agents
Inhibits bacterial replication
Protects tissue culture from virus infection
Prevents virus replication
Induces expression of Epstein-Barr virus early antigen
Miscellaneous Actions
Forms complexes with DNA
May interfere with sulfhydryl-disulfide interchange reactions

*References not listed are cited in previous editions: Kelley WN, et al (eds): Textbook of rheumatology, 2nd, 4th, and 5th eds. Philadelphia, WB Saunders, 1985, 1993, 1996, 2001.

†May in part be related to increased activation of the gene coding for *c-jun*.[38]

Reductions in IL-2R expression[83] and IL-6, soluble CD8, and soluble IL-2R levels in lupus patients treated with HCQ[83] have also been shown. CQ inhibits T cell proliferation by decreasing both IL-2 production and T cell responsiveness to IL-2.[84]

Other immune actions include increased in vitro apoptosis in lymphocytes from normal subjects and patients with SLE.[85] This increased apoptosis was not confined to a particular T cell subset.

Antimalarials reduce the activity of many enzymes,[57] including phospholipase A_2.[80] Total prostaglandin production decreases, and in an experimental test system, leukotriene release from lung was diminished.[86] In addition to causing direct enzyme inhibition, these drugs stabilize lysosomal membranes, thereby inhibiting the release of lysosomal enzymes.[73]

Among miscellaneous actions, antimalarials protect against ultraviolet light damage. Besides causing damage, ultraviolet light leads to activation of the gene *c-jun*, which is protective. 4-Aminoquinolines increase this activation,[87] perhaps through membrane-associated Src tyrosine kinase.

Antimalarials also form complexes with DNA by binding of the quinoline ring to the phosphate groups and nucleotide bases and thereby interfere with nuclear events.[73] Reactions between DNA and anti-DNA antibodies may be blocked.[73] This may explain the inhibition of the lupus erythematosus cell phenomenon observed by Dubois.[88] Furthermore, they decrease proliferation of some viruses.[89] Finally, HCQ leads to an increase in pain thresholds,[90] which could help patients with a variety of diseases.

CLINICAL APPLICATIONS

Selection of Patients

Antimalarials have been widely used in adults and children for the treatment of RA, lupus, and their variants, as well for the treatment of peripheral arthritis in the seronegative arthropathies of AS and psoriasis. Recently there have been publications suggesting possible effectiveness in erosive osteoarthritis and calcium pyrophosphate crystal-deposition disease, (CPPD).

Efficacy

Rheumatoid Arthritis

The effectiveness of antimalarial drugs in improving clinical outcomes has been repeatedly demonstrated in placebo-controlled trials lasting from 15 weeks to 1 year.[56] Studies have not been done to demonstrate benefit in terms of prevention of damage measured radiographically. A meta-analysis comparing effectiveness of HCQ to that of CQ showed the latter was more effective.[91] Choice and dosing of antimalarial drugs depends largely on the minimizing risks of retinal toxicity. Hence, HCQ is the preferred agent in North America, and the dose of 6.5 mg/kg/day for ideal body weight or lean body weight, whichever is the lesser, is recommended to maximize safety and effectiveness. Exceeding this recommended daily dose sharply increases the risk of retinal toxicity.[67]

When using antimalarial drugs, the value of instituting therapy early in the course of RA was supported by the results of a 3-year follow-up of the HERA study.[92] A delay of 9 months in initiating therapy with HCQ resulted in worse outcomes measured 3 years later.

Onset of action is from several weeks to 6 months. Using a loading dose of 800 mg/day results in earlier onset of benefit but no difference in 6-month outcomes compared to 400 mg/day.[93]

Comparisons with Other Disease-Modifying Antirheumatic Drugs

Antimalarial drugs are relatively weak disease-modifying drugs. Nevertheless, their role in early RA has been clearly established in the HERA trial, and they continue to be popular, particularly in North America, both as monotherapy and in combination with other disease-modifying agents.[94]

An evaluation by Hurst and colleagues using the Health Assessment Questionaire, (HAQ) disability index, treatment data collected on 1160 RA patients, and area-under-the-curve analysis measured extent and duration of benefit in HAQ disability units.[95] DMARD naïve patients treated with HCQ improved at a rate of −.18 annualized HAQ area units compared to −.33 and −.38 for MTX and gold, respectively. Effectiveness was better for all drugs with earlier treatment, including HCQ −.74 versus −.47 when comparing RA patients treated before 1 year to those treated after 1 year from disease onset.[95]

A controlled trial comparing HCQ to SSZ demonstrated similar clinical response at 48 weeks and less radiographic damage with SSZ both at 48 weeks and at 3-year follow-up.[96,97] In early RA, a 24-week, double-blind trial found similar efficacy comparing HCQ and CSA and greater renal side effects and paresthesias with CSA. A 2-year, double-blind RCT comparing minocycline to HCQ showed superior benefit from minocycline in terms of ACR-50, prednisone dose, and adherence to therapy.[98] Moreover, in a metanalysis of DMARD-continuation rates, Maetzel showed discontinuation of antimalarial drugs by more than 40 percent of patients by 2 years, primarily due to lack of efficacy.[76]

Combination Therapy

The safety of antimalarial drugs makes them attractive agents for use in combination. In a placebo-controlled trial involving 88 patients a combination of MTX (7.5 mg) and CQ was more effective than MTX (7.5 mg) and placebo.[99] Another pharmacokinetic study showed changes in bioavailability of MTX when administered with HCQ. In 10 subjects, the time to onset of maximum MTX concentration and the area under the curve of serum MTX levels were increased with combination MTX/HCQ, and there were no changes in the pharmacokinetics of HCQ.[100]

A triple combination of HCQ, SSZ, and MTX has been shown to be significantly more effective than MTX alone or HCQ and SSZ in a 2-year study involving 100 patients.[101] Efficacy failures were only 15 percent in the triple combination compared to 60 percent in each of the other groups. Therapy had failed in all patients with at least one slow-acting antirheumatic drug. Toxicity was not increased in the combination group. Furthermore, patients who had failed to respond to MTX or HCQ/SSZ showed significant clinical improvement with triple therapy.[102]

HCQ may decrease corticosteroid toxicity by lessening the hyperlipidemic effect of the steroids.[103,104] One analysis showed lowered cholesterol and low-density lipoproteins,[104] and another showed improved high-density lipoprotein cholesterol and triglycerides compared to gold.[105] Another showed no effect on cholesterol but a lowering of triglycerides and its associated apolipoprotein C.[103] Antimalarials may decrease MTX-induced nodulosis,[106] but amelioration of liver-enzyme elevations has not been established.[100,107]

Palindromic Rheumatism

CQ and HCQ have been reported to be beneficial in treating palindromic rheumatism in uncontrolled studies.[61,64] The largest series reviewed 71 patients with an average follow-up of 3.6 years.[61] Forty-seven were treated with CQ and four with HCQ. Forty-one patients responded, with a 77-percent reduction in frequency and a 63-percent reduction in duration of attacks.

Juvenile Rheumatoid Arthritis

Several groups have found antimalarials to be efficacious in treatment of JRA.[56] In an open, parallel study, hydroxychloroquine was equal in efficacy to and better tolerated than gold sodium thiomalate (GSTM) or DP. A collaborative placebo-controlled study found neither HCQ nor DP to be more effective than placebo.[108]

Sjögren's Syndrome

In a study of 50 consecutive patients treated with HCQ, local eye and mouth symptoms, arthralgias, and myalgias improved.[109] Laboratory abnormalities were improved in this and another study.[73,109]

Virus-Associated Arthritis

Anecdotal reports suggest that antimalarials may be beneficial for hepatitis C–associated arthritis[65] and acquired immunodeficiency syndrome (AIDS)-associated arthritis.[64]

Systemic Lupus Erythematosus

The variability of the natural course of SLE and of the response of different manifestations of disease to various medications makes treatment evaluation difficult, but antimalarials are beneficial.

Patients in uncontrolled studies have shown improvement in arthralgias, fever, and constitutional symptoms with antimalarial use. A placebo-controlled study found that joint pain and tenderness but not joint swelling decreased with HCQ therapy.[110] Antimalarials may have a corticosteroid-sparing effect, improve lipid abnormalities, and have a protective effect in preventing bone loss,[111] but they are not appropriate for the more severe lupus manifestations (e.g., renal lesions).

The strongest evidence supporting the efficacy of antimalarials in treating SLE comes from studies in which medication was discontinued in successfully treated patients.[73] A 6-month double-blind, placebo-controlled drug-discontinuation study provided substantial evidence that HCQ prevents lupus flare-ups.[112] Forty-seven patients, all of whom were being treated with HCQ, were studied. Sixteen of the 22 patients in whom placebo was substituted for HCQ experienced flare-ups, whereas only nine of 25 who continued HCQ therapy suffered a disease exacerbation ($p = .02$). Most manifestations were minor. Flares often involved abnormalities that had been present before treatment. Only one severe exacerbation occurred in the group that continued treatment, compared to five in patients receiving placebo ($p = .06$). Overall, the risk of disease flare-up was increased by a factor of 2.5 for the placebo group.

In one series, reasons for discontinuation of HCQ in SLE included noncompliance in 15 percent, disease remission in 42 percent, lack of efficacy in 8 percent, and miscellaneous in 6 percent.[113] The benefit of antimalarial drugs in pediatric-onset lupus appears to be similar to that seen in adult-onset disease.

Discoid Lupus

Antimalarials are also effective against discoid lesions. Compared with the spontaneous remissions in 15 percent of untreated patients, remissions or major improvements have been reported in 60 to 90 percent of treated patients.[56]

The effectiveness of antimalarials in discoid lupus and cutaneus may be seen within the first week. Remission of skin disease has been reported in 60 to 90 percent of treated patients,[56] compared to 15 percent of untreated patients.

Quinacrine alone or in combination is occasionally helpful when discoid lesions fail to respond adequately to HCQ or CQ,[59,114] but its long-term use is limited by the potential development of yellowish skin pigmentation.

The effectiveness of antimalarials in the treatment of skin lesions is often apparent within the first week, when erythematous changes start to regress. Most patients who respond to antimalarial medication experience relapse after the drug is discontinued.[73] Antimalarials are particularly effective in treating subacute cutaneous lupus erythematosus.

Childhood Systemic Lupus Erythematosus

Antimalarials have been used in 25 to 100 percent of childhood SLE by 15 rheumatologists observing 400 patients. These drugs are considered moderately effective, and toxicity paralleled that reported in adults.[115]

Antiphospholipid Syndrome

Although anticoagulants and antiaggregant therapy remain the cornerstone of treatment for this condition, HCQ has been used in uncontrolled fashion as adjunct immunomodulation for it.[116,117]

Childhood Dermatomyositis

HCQ has been effective against childhood dermatomyositis in patients who had been unresponsive or partially responsive to corticosteroids.[118] All seven patients in one report had improvement of rash, with complete clearing in three.[116] Myositis did not appear to improve, but corticosteroid dosage was tapered in two patients. A retrospective review of nine patients showed significant improvement in rash and in abdominal and proximal muscle strength.[116,118] After 6 months of treatment with HCQ, prednisone dosage had been significantly reduced.

Seronegative Arthropathies

The reports of response of PsA arthritis and of the peripheral arthritis of AS to antimalarials are anecdotal. Several investigators have reported responses similar to those seen for RA.[56] Kammer and coworkers[119] reported 68-percent benefit in 50 courses of HCQ treatment of patients with PsA. Exacerbation of psoriatic skin lesions may occur with antimalarial treatment.[73]

Eosinophilic Fasciitis

Eosinophilic fasciitis has been successfully treated with antimalarials in uncontrolled studies.[56,62] In one series of 52 patients with this disease, two of eight patients who failed to respond to prednisone and two of eight who had not received prednisone had complete resolution with HCQ treatment, whereas six had a partial response, one had no response, and five of the 16 patients treated with HCQ were lost to follow-up.[62] Responses occurred in 3 to 6 months with a daily dose of 200 or 400 mg.

Erosive Osteoarthritis

A retrospective review of eight patients with erosive osteoarthritis treated with HCQ after failure to respond to NSAIDs revealed improvement in morning stiffness, synovitis, and patient global assessment in six, with a partial response in one.[63] One patient experienced a flare-up after drug discontinuation and went into remission again after reinstitution of HCQ therapy.

Calcium Pyrophosphate Crystal–Deposition Disease

One controlled study of CPPD lasting more than 3 months revealed a greater response rate and decreased numbers of active joints in the 17 patients treated with HCQ compared to the placebo group.[66]

Dosage

To prevent ocular toxicity, the dosage of HCQ should be maintained at or below 6.5 mg/kg for ideal body weight or body weight, whichever is less, and the dose of CQ should be 3.5 mg/kg for body weight or ideal body weight. Exceeding this recommended daily dose sharply increases the risk of retinopathy. It is important to review antimalarial drug doses intermittently during follow-up and particularly if the patient's weight declines below ideal body weight for any reason.[67]

An Australian study compared HCQ (200 mg/day) in RA with 400 mg/day and showed no statistically significant difference in outcomes of RA patients.[120] Furst and coworkers evaluated the effect of a loading dose of 800 mg of HCQ for 6 months; there was a more rapid onset of action in RA patients, more GI side effects, and ultimately no difference compared to the standard 400-mg dosage at 24 weeks.[93]

Drug Interactions

HCQ is reported to reduce the requirement for hypoglycemic agents in diabetic patients taking oral hypoglycemic agents. These patients should have their blood glucose levels monitored more closely when antimalarial drug therapy is initiated. In one study, coadministration of CQ reduced MTX levels. In another, combination of HCQ with MTX resulted in a reduction in the maximum serum MTX level, but a greater exposure to MTX based on area-under-the-curve analysis. In one report, adding CQ to CSA appeared to increase renal toxicity of CSA. HCQ in patients taking digoxin may result in an increase in serum digoxin levels.

TABLE 58–3 • TOXIC EFFECTS OF CHLOROQUINE AND HYDROXYCHLOROQUINE[73]

Gastrointestinal
Anorexia Abdominal bloating Abdominal cramps Diarrhea Heartburn Nausea Vomiting Weight loss
Skin and Hair

Alopecia
Bleaching of hair
Dryness of skin
Exacerbation of psoriasis
Increased pigmentation of skin and hair
Pruritus
Rashes
  Exfoliative
  Lichenoid
  Maculopapular
  Morbilliform
  Urticarial

TABLE 58–3 • TOXIC EFFECTS OF CHLOROQUINE AND HYDROXYCHLOROQUINE[73]—cont'd

Neuromuscular
Convulsive seizures Difficulty in visual accommodation Headache Insomnia Involuntary movements Lassitude Myasthenic reaction Mental confusion Nervousness or irritability Neuromyopathy Ototoxicity Nerve deafness Tinnitus Polyneuropathy Toxic psychosis Vestibular dysfunction Weakness
Ocular
Corneal deposits: halos around lights Diplopia Defects in accommodation and convergence: various mild visual difficulties Loss of corneal reflex Retinopathy Loss of vision Pigment abnormalities Scotomas Visual field abnormalities
Cardiac[70,71]
Conduction disturbances Electrocardiographic changes Congestive heart failure Restrictive cardiomyopathy
Miscellaneous
Birth defects Blood dyscrasias Leukopenia Agranulocytosis Aplastic anemia Leukemia Death from overdosage: peripheral circulatory collapse Precipitation of porphyria cutanea tarda Renal: decreased creatinine clearance

Toxicity of Antimalarials

Although HCQ and CQ are relatively safe, the list of reported side effects is extensive (Table 58–3). The incidence of adverse effects varies according to daily dosage. Up to 55 percent of patients may have some side effects, but two thirds of these remit spontaneously, and another quarter respond to dosage reduction.[73] HCQ is half as toxic as CQ on a weight basis.[73]

In a cohort of 224 patients with lupus, 20 of 156 taking HCQ had it withdrawn because of side effects.[113] GI side effects were most frequent in 11 patients; headaches, dizziness, rash, or hearing loss in six; myopathy in two; and retinopathy after 6 years of HCQ in one patient was another reason for stopping HCQ.

Mucocutaneous

Rash is the most common side effect leading to cessation of treatment. Patients taking HCQ may show increased photosensitivity. The lesions produced are variable in type. Patients with PsA arthritis may experience an exacerbation of psoriatic skin lesions,[73] including exfoliative dermatitis.[73] Pigmentary changes of skin or hair include either grayish hypopigmentation or blue-black hyperpigmentation.[73] Alopecia may develop[73] and must be differentiated from the alopecia that is a manifestation of lupus erythematosus.

Heart

Cervera reviewed 12 cases of conduction disorders.[121] Cardiomyopathy occurs rarely.

Metabolic

When HCQ is initiated for treatment of RA in patients with type II diabetes mellitus requiring insulin or sulfonylurea treatment, blood glucose concentration should be monitored closely because insulin may have to be reduced to prevent hypoglycemic reactions.[122]

Gastrointestinal

GI side effects of antimalarial drugs can mimic those of NSAIDs and include epigastric burning, nausea, and vomiting. Abdominal cramps, bloating, and diarrhea are unique to antimalarial agents. Antimalarials do not cause peptic ulcer disease or GI bleeding.

Reproduction

Because of the long half-life and extensive tissue deposition of antimalarial drugs, discontinuation of therapy at the time of conception or pregnancy does not prevent fetal exposure. Although transplacental passage of HCQ has been demonstrated, there is no evidence to support harm to the fetus.[123] Eye examinations showed no abnormalities in 21 children whose mothers had taking antimalarial drugs in pregnancy.[124] Because discontinuation of antimalarial drugs may precipitate lupus flares, it is generally considered appropriate to continue antimalarial drugs in pregnant lupus patients.[113] In the RA patient, the decision to continue or discontinue antimalarial drugs in pregnancy should be individualized, taking into account the likelihood of natural disease remission in pregnancy and postpartum disease exacerbation.

Neuromuscular

The more frequently seen neurologic manifestations are often of little significance because of their mildness and reversibility when the daily dosages are lowered. These include headaches, giddiness, insomnia, and nervousness.[56] HCQ may be associated with nightmares.

Neuromyopathy is a rare syndrome characterized by proximal muscle weakness with normal creatine phosphokinase, (CPK) levels.

More important, but uncommon, is a neuromuscular syndrome[4,69] that includes proximal lower-extremity muscle weakness (which may start months after treatment is begun), normal CPK, and abnormal muscle and nerve biopsy results. Neuromyopathy may be confused with glucocorticoid-induced muscle weakness and may be attributed to the disease being treated.[125]

Eye

Early symptoms may include defects in accommodation or conversion and blurred vision. These are not serious and resolve with dose reduction or temporary medication discontinuation. Corneal deposits, which may be associated with halos around lights, are both benign and reversible. Retinopathy has been extensively reviewed in previous editions of this book. HCQ is associated with reduced risk of retinopathy compared to CQ. The earliest phase of retinopathy is characterized by lack of visual symptoms, shallow scotomata on Amsler and automated visual-field testing, and normal central vision, color vision, and fundi. Patients with these ophthalmologic findings should discontinue therapy; normally these visual changes do not progress if antimalarial drugs are promptly discontinued. True retinopathy is characterized by loss of central or clear vision and absolute scotomata with or without visual symptoms. In these patients, vision may deteriorate even if the drug is discontinued. Corneal deposition is suggestive of drug overdosage. To prevent retinal toxicity, careful adherence to dosing guidelines is recommended, and dose should be reevaluated on a regular basis, particularly in the face of weight loss or the presence or development of renal or hepatic impairment, which might affect drug metabolism and excretion. Reports of retinal toxicity have declined due to improved understanding of factors that contribute to risk of retinopathy. With careful ophthalmology evaluation on an annual basis, it is possible to detect the distinctive central visual field changes of antimalarial retinopathy well before patients become symptomatic.

Gold

Gold has been advocated for the treatment of many human diseases for centuries. After Koch, in 1890, reported the in vitro inhibition of tubercle bacilli by gold cyanide, gold compounds were used for treating tuberculous disorders.[126,127] In 1929, Forestier pioneered the use of gold for the treatment of RA on the basis of the mistaken notion that the disease might be caused by a tuberculous infection.[127]

The beneficial effects of parenteral gold therapy were conclusively documented later in placebo-controlled trials in Europe and in the United States.[126-131]

Gold treatment is also used in PsA, juvenile RA, and AOSD. Since 1990, the use of gold has declined in North America. This has paralleled the emergence of MTX as a second-line agent that is more convenient by virtue of its oral administration and its superior long-term cumulative tolerability.[95]

PHARMACOLOGY OF GOLD

Gold Preparations

Two products, each containing 50-percent gold in solution, are currently available for parenteral administration. Their structural formulas are shown in Figure 58–5.

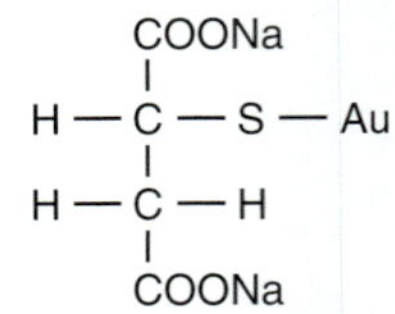

GOLD SODIUM THIOMALATE
(MYOCHRYSINE)

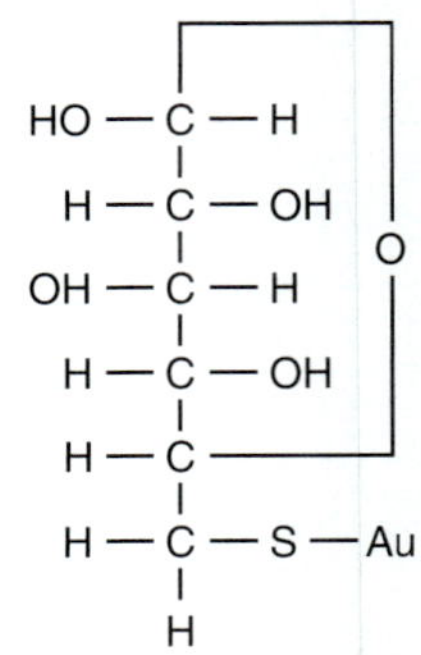

AUROTHIOGLUCOSE
(SOLGANAL)

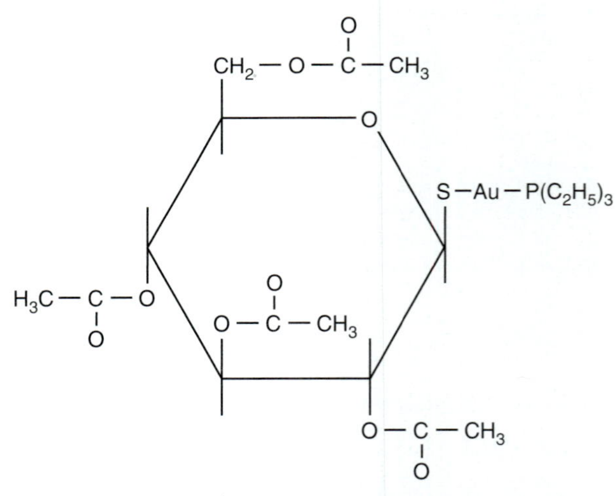

(2, 3, 4, 6-TETRA-*O*-ACETYL-1-THIO-β-D-GLUCOPYRANOSATO-*S*)
(TRIETHYLPHOSPINE) GOLD

AURANOFIN

FIGURE 58–5 · Gold sodium thiomalate and aurothioglucose, the two intramuscular gold preparations most widely used in the United States, are aurous salts, contain 50 percent gold by weight, and are attached to a sulfur moiety. Auranofin, a conjugated gold compound with two ligands, contains sulfur and is 29 percent gold by weight.

GSTM is water soluble and rapidly absorbed after intramuscular injection. GSTG, a suspension in sesame seed oil, reaches peak levels about 24 hours after administration and rises to 30-percent lower peak serum levels compared to GSTG; this may account for observed lower incidence of adverse effects.

Auranofin is a triethylphosphine gold compound absorbed orally. First studied in the 1970s, it was found to have different clinical and pharmacologic properties compared to parenteral gold.[132]

In plasma, approximately 95 percent of gold is bound to albumin; 70 percent is eliminated in urine and 30 percent in feces[133,134] (Fig. 58-56).

Following the standard weekly-injection schedule, 40 percent of the dose is excreted each week, and the remainder is retained and eliminated more slowly. The biologic half-life of gold, following a 50-mg dose, has been reported to range from 3 to 27 days early in treatment and up to 168 days after 10 weekly injections, with considerable individual variation.[133-134]

After several months, serum levels are stabilized with weekly injections; a steady decline in serum levels occurs when intervals between injections are increased. With prolonged administration, gold is stored in bone marrow, liver, spleen, lymph nodes, skin, and kidneys.

About 25 percent of auranofin is absorbed orally. With the standard dose of 3 mg bid, serum gold levels rise gradually over 8 to 12 weeks to a median of 500 ng/ml. This compares to serum gold levels of 3000 ng/ml with weekly intramuscular GSTM.[133]

Numerous immunologic, cellular, and enzymatic effects are ascribed to gold compounds, but there is uncertainty as to which mechanisms are responsible for the therapeutic benefits of gold. In vivo experiments, including serial synovectomy studies, have demonstrated selective accumulation of gold in macrophages of many tissues and abundance, during gold treatment, in lysomes of synovial macrophages of inflamed synovium. It is probable that the beneficial effects of gold result from its action to influence multiple arthritis-perpetuating effects of the monocytes and macrophages.[135]

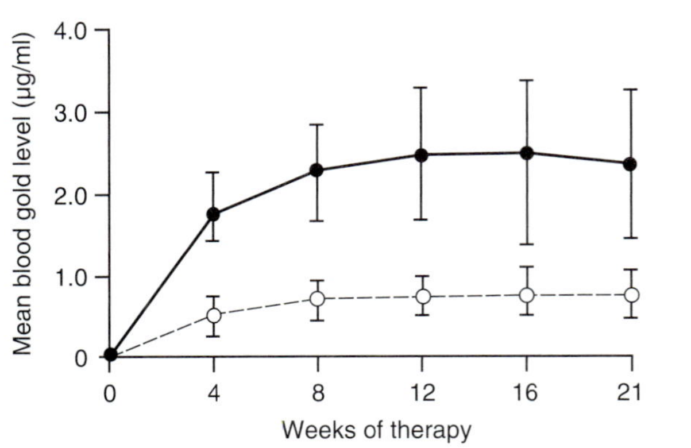

FIGURE 58–6 · Mean whole blood gold concentrations in 59 auranofin-treated patients (o) and 51 gold sodium thiomalate–treated patients (•) after 21 weeks of therapy. Higher blood gold concentrations are achieved with conventional doses of gold sodium thiomalate than with auranofin (triethylphosphine gold). Gold levels reach a plateau after 6 to 8 weeks of injectable treatment and after 12 weeks of auranofin, reflecting the longer half-life of the oral compound. Bars show standard deviations. (Adapted from Dahl SL, Coleman ML, Williams HJ, et al: Lack of correlation between blood gold concentrations and clinical response in patients with definite or classic rheumatoid arthritis receiving auranofin or gold sodium thiomalate. Arthritis Rheum 28:1211, 1985. Reprinted with permission of the American College of Rheumatology.)

Monocytes and macrophages are key players in RA pathogenesis; they act as antigen-presenting cells, produce complement, release proteolytic enzymes, and produce and release cytokines. With chronic use, gold reduces IL-1 production of synovial macrophages. This has been measured in synovial fluid samples and has been demonstrated by reduction of IL-1 staining in the synovium of gold-treated patients.[136]

In the synovium, there is a decrease in macrophage numbers, and IL-6 and IL-8 production. In vitro experiments show a reduction of angiogenic properties of macrophages.[133] In monocytes, gold compounds inhibit fragment crystallizable (Fc) and C3 receptor expression and oxygen radicals. Gold compounds inhibit lymphocyte-proliferative responses by their action on the monocyte and macrophage.[134] GSTG inhibits spontaneous and IFN-γ–induced production of the second component of complement by monocytes and macrophages, as well as IFN-γ–induced expression of DR antigens.[137]

Clinical Applications

Selection of Patients

Gold is used primarily for RA. Response to treatment appears unaffected by age, sex, race, extra-articular features, and rheumatoid factors. We have also found it effective in controlling monoarticular or pauciarticular RA. It has been demonstrated to be effective and safe for use in Felty's syndrome; anemia, neutropenia, and splenomegaly improve without undue toxicity.

Preexisting proteinuria or renal failure is a relative contraindication to the use of gold because it confuses monitoring for nephrotoxicity. Patients with blood dyscrasias or lupus and persons taking angiotensin coventing enzyme, (ACE) inhibitors should not take gold. Care should also be taken when injecting patients on anticoagulants. Parenteral therapy does not appear to affect babies born to mothers treated with gold, but any newborn exposed to maternal gold during pregnancy or lactation should be monitored closely.

Efficacy

Between 1960 and 1983, there were four prospective placebo-controlled trials; these are summarized in Table 58–4. Each trial demonstrated statistically significant improvement in gold-treated RA patients compared to those treated with placebo in terms of active joint counts and laboratory measures of inflammation (Fig. 58–7). Three of the four trials evaluated radiographic outcomes and two of three showed reduction in erosions in gold-treated patients compared to those assigned to placebo.[128-130,138]

Lukainen and colleagues compared radiographic progression according to the Larson scale in patients

TABLE 58–4 • SUMMARY OF PUBLISHED TRIALS COMPARING PARENTERAL GOLD WITH PLACEBO

Trial	No. of Patients Enrolled	Months of RX/Months of Follow-up	Improvement Versus Placebo	Withdrawals LOE G/P	Withdrawals SE G/P
Empire Rheumatism Council, ERC[128]	200	20/210	Newly affected and quiescent joints Grip strength, ESR Hgb, analgesic use. Radiographic progression (p =.06)	3/3	14/4
Sigler[129] 1974	32	104/104	Active joints, ring size, grip strength ESR, radiographic progression	1/8	2/1
American Rheumatism Association (ARA)[130] 1973	68	27/27	ESR Physician Global Assessment	2/12	8/1
Ward[131] 1983	193 46 placebo 72 Auranofin 75 GST	21/21	Both GST and auranofin for tender joints, ESR, and platelets. GST and not auranofin for swelling scores, Hgb, and physician global assessment	P/A/G =5/2/0	P/A/G=1/5/22

Abbreviations: P, placebo; A, Auranolin; LOE, lack of effect; SE, side effect.

who had received more than 500 mg of gold to those who had received less.[139] The mean cumulative dose of gold in the high-dose gold group was 1858 mg and in the low-dose gold group was 254 mg. Radiographs were evaluated prior to the start of gold treatment and 5 years later. The reduction in damage after 5 years in the high-gold group was statistically significant ($p < .001$) Buckland-Wright and coworkers compared radiographs of patients who received gold early in their disease to RA patients whose treatment was delayed by 6 months using quantitative microfocal radiography; there was a decrease in erosion area after 6 months of gold treatment in the group treated early.[140]

In a 12-month, prospective, blind, parallel study comparing 15 mg of parenteral MTX to 50 mg of GSTM in 174 patients with early erosive RA, clinical and laboratory results were similar (Fig. 58–8). In addition, the slope of radiographic progression was reduced in the second 6 months of therapy for both DMARDs, with no difference between the two regimens at baseline, or after 6 and 12 months (Fig. 58–9). A 3-year follow-up in this group, however, showed an overall reduction in radiographic progression somewhat better in the gold group.[141] Interestingly, in the same study, patients with early RA who stopped gold because of side effects had sustained improvement over 3 years similar to those who continued taking gold and MTX.[142]

In a retrospective analysis of RA deaths in Finland, where gold use is high, the mortality rate during 25 years was highest (69.8%) in patients without intramuscular gold treatment and lowest (25.2%) in patients with the longest duration of intramuscular gold treatment.[143]

The advantage of combining study results was shown in two meta-analyses that examined comparable controlled studies.[144,145] Both analyses confirmed a favorable magnitude of efficacy for parenteral gold. Although some have questioned the long-term effectiveness of gold as a second-line agent, the weight of evidence, including these meta-analyses, radiographic outcomes, and mortality data, does not support these concerns.[146-148] Moreover, good evidence of efficacy during a 1-year period in a group of 98 RA patients was reported, despite a dropout rate of 36 percent.[146,147] In addition, patients starting gold with disease duration of less than 2 years show longer-lasting functional improvement than those starting later.[148]

There is an association between treatment response and rash. Patients with RA possessing HLA-DR3 may be more responsive to gold treatment than patients without HLA-DR3, and they may be more likely to develop mucocutaneous reactions and proteinuria.[149] Treatment efficacy for PsA has traditionally been regarded as the same as for RA. However, a retrospective comparison of patients with PsA taking gold or MTX showed that both were safe and effective.[150]

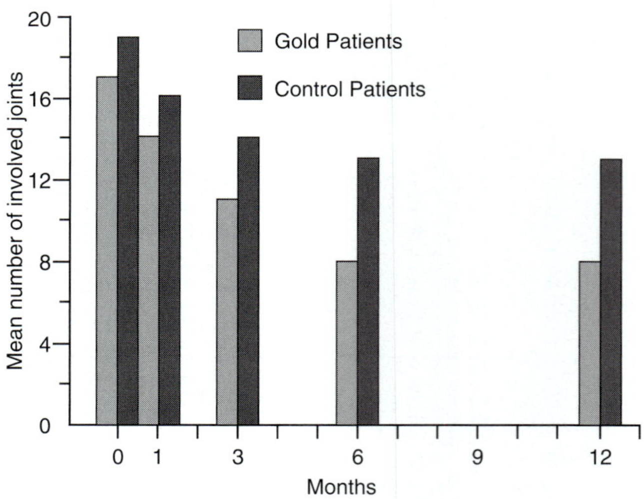

FIGURE 58–7 • Mean number of involved joints declined significantly in gold-treated rheumatoid arthritis patients during 6 months. Improvement compared with control patients was maintained up to 12 months in spite of no further administration of gold. This study is important for many reasons. It includes 18 months of follow-up with control subjects. It shows effectiveness of gold lasting for 6 months after gold was stopped. (Adapted from the Empire Rheumatism Council Study: Gold therapy in rheumatoid arthritis. Ann Rheum Dis 19:1995, 1960 and 20:315, 1961.)

Disease-Modifying Antirheumatic Drug Combinations with Gold

Combinations of second-line agents are increasingly employed when single agents provide insufficient benefit. A formal overview of the topic has compared the benefits and risks of combinations of agents with the single drugs.[151]

Adding CSA, mean dose 2.5 mg/kg, to baseline gold therapy has showed benefit without unexpected toxicity or drug interaction after 6 months.[152] Adding HCQ to gold showed no measurable benefit in one study.[153] A 48-week, double-blind, placebo-controlled trial showed benefit in terms of ACR-20 response and no important drug interactions when weekly 50-mg ATG doses were given to partial responders on MTX (mean MTX dose 18.5 mg).[154]

Dosage Schedules

The gold treatment protocol in common use was derived from the dosing schedule used by the Empire Rheumatism Council after its first blinded trial (Table 58–5). The test dose of 10 mg occasionally elicits a skin or allergic reaction. As long as the test dose induces no side effects, the second injection is 25 mg, and subsequent weekly injections, in the absence of side effects, are 50 mg. As with other older DMARDS, no dose-finding studies have been done to determine optimal dosing. Nevertheless, both high and lower weekly doses of gold have been studied.[155]

All doses studied have been shown to be effective; higher doses are associated with an increase in toxicity, but there is substantial individual variation with regard to efficacy and tolerability. The typical patient is improved by 3 months of treatment and achieves further improvement during the course of 6 to 18 months of therapy. Although the traditional gold regimen includes weekly injections until a cumulative dose of 1 g has been given, the maintenance regimen of injections every 2 to 4 weeks has not been evaluated well for effectiveness in the long term; loss of effect with increase of dosing interval is such a common scenario that unless there is limiting toxicity, weekly or every-other-week injections may be administered indefinitely. Clinical trials and long-term follow-up studies have demonstrated that the major cause of early discontinuation of gold is toxicity, most commonly mucocutaneous reactions. When the patient develops symptoms of toxicity that are not potentially serious, the gold should be held temporarily and reintroduced at a 50-percent lower dose once side effects have subsided.[156]

Low-dose gold in the range of 2 to 20 mg weekly may produce acceptable improvement or remission when toxicity prohibits use of standard dose.[157] Intermittent intramuscular injections of corticosteroids may improve tolerability of chrytsotherapy. In patients who have discontinued gold due to side effects, effectiveness may be maintained for months or longer. In patients who discontinue gold due to remission, eventually RA will recur. In these individuals, a second course of gold is commonly effective.[158,159]

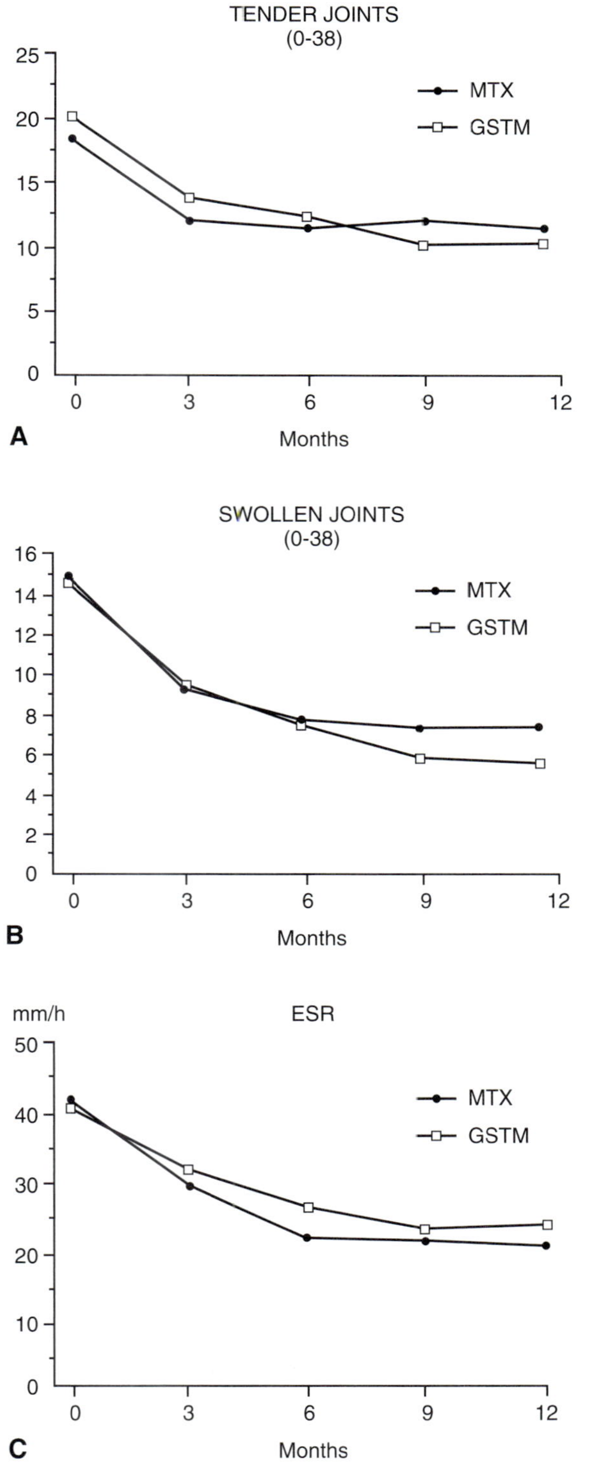

FIGURE 58–8 · Mean values of the number of tender (A) and swollen (B) joints for both treatment groups at baseline and after months 3, 6, 9, and 12. Thirty-eight peripheral joints were counted. Significant improvement from baseline in both groups without significant intergroup differences. *C*, Mean values of the erythrocyte sedimentation rate (ESR) (mm/h, Westergren method) for both treatment groups at baseline and after months 3, 6, 9, and 12. Significant improvement from baseline in both groups without significant intergroup differences. (After Rau R, Herborn N, Menninger H, Blechschmidt J: Comparison of intramuscular methotrexate and gold sodium thiomalate in the treatment of early erosive rheumatoid arthritis. Br J Rheumatol 36:345, 1997. Reprinted with permission.)

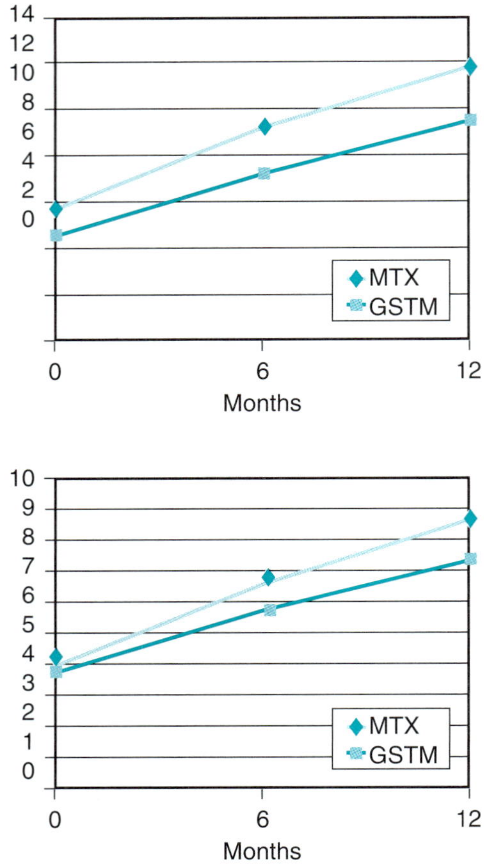

FIGURE 58–9 • The distribution of radiographic scores for patients treated with methotrexate (MTX) and GSTM shows no statistical difference between the two treatment groups at baseline and or after 6 and 12 months (top). Similarly, there were no differences in the main number of eroded joints between the two treatment groups (bottom). (From Rau R, Herborn G, Menninger H, Sangha O: Progression in early erosive RA: 12 month results from a randomized controlled trial comparing MTX and GSTM. Br J Rheumatol 37:1220, 1998.)

TABLE 58–5 • GOLD TREATMENT PROTOCOL: DOSE AND SIDE-EFFECT MONITORING

Dose	
• Week 1	10 mg
• Week 2	25 mg
• Weekly	50 mg—until rheumatoid arthritis (RA) is optimally controlled or side effects develop
• q 2 weeks*	When optimal control is achieved
Side Effects Monitoring	
CBC PLTs and Urinalysis	
• Weekly	For 4 weeks
• q2 weeks	Until 20 weeks
• q3 weeks	Until 52 weeks
• q4-8 injections	After 52 weeks
Prior to Injection Ask About the Following	
• Rash, pruritus	
• Postinjection reaction	
• Any unusual complaints	
Management of Common Side Effects	
• Rash, pruritus, stomatitis, proteinuria	Hold gold until side effects subside and reintroduce at 50% lower dosage
• Postinjection reactions	Reduce dose by 50% until reactions no longer occur, or switch from GST to ATG
• Thrombocytopenia	Discontinue gold; treat with prednisone (30-60 mg)

*Intervals between injections may be increased to 3 to 4 weeks in the event of remission. When RA flares, resume weekly regimen.

Discontinue gold in the event of potentially serious side effects such as cholestatic hepatitis, colitis, gold-induced interstitial pneumonitis, encephalitis, or peripheral neuritis.

Cost of Gold Treatment

Gold treatment includes medication and administration costs, laboratory monitoring costs, and costs attributable to management of toxicity. Strategies to reduce cost include less frequent laboratory testing and administration of gold at home by the patient or a family member.[160]

Toxicity of Gold

When a patient with RA does poorly despite treatment, symptoms may be related to the disease itself or to side effects from the antirheumatic medications. Adverse reactions occur in up to 40 percent of treated patients and frequently result in discontinuation of therapy (Table 58–6). Most toxicity develops during the first 6 months of therapy. Side effects that are not serious can be managed by interruption of therapy and careful dose adjustment. Eosinophilia may precede or accompany side effects. Mucocutaneous reactions, proteinuria, and thrombocytopenia are associated with HLA-DR3.[149] Anti-Ro (SSA) antibodies have been associated with mucocutaneous side effects.[161]

Postinjection Reactions

Vasomotor nitritoid reactions have been reported with all therapeutic gold compounds, most commonly with GSTM (about 4% incidence).[162] Reactions are due to vasodilatation and hypotension and can occur at any stage of gold therapy. Symptoms, which include facial flushing, lightheadedness, sweating, weakness, nausea, syncope, and occasionally vomiting, occur within seconds to 30 minutes after injection. Patients with underlying cerebrovascular or coronary artery disease and patients receiving ACE inhibitors appear to be at greater risk for this reaction, generally described as benign and self limiting, and for rarely reported cerebral or coronary ischemia that follows hypotension.[163] Management should include early recognition, injection of gold in the recumbent position, observation for 20 minutes after injection in individual patients, temporary reduction of dose, and switching to GSTG.[163] Anaphylactoid reactions occur rarely.

Nonvasomotor postinjection reactions, with transient arthralgia, joint swelling, fatigability, and malaise, have developed in 15 percent of patients treated with

TABLE 58–6 • TOXICITY PROFILE WITH GOLD COMPOUNDS

Adverse Effects	Aurothiomalate	Aurothioglucose	Auranofin
Postinjection Reactions			
Vasomotor (nitritoid)	Uncommon* (5%)	Rare	Rare*
Anaphylaxis or syncope	Rare	Unknown	Unknown
Myalgias or arthralgias	Common	Rare	Unknown
Mucocutaneous Effects			
Dermatitis or stomatitis	Common† (10%)	Less common	Common
Pruritus	Common (30-40%)	Less common	Common
Alopecia	Rare	Rare	Rare
Urticaria	Rare	Rare	Uncommon
Trophic nails	Rare	Rare	Unknown
Chrysiasis or pigmentation	Rare (unless dose >89)	Rare	Unknown
Photosensitivity	Rare	Rare	Unknown
Kidney			
Proteinuria	Common‡ (2-7%)	Less common	Rare
Hematuria	Uncommon	Less common	Rare
Nephrotic syndrome	Rare	Rare	Rare
Renal insufficiency	Rare	Rare	Unknown
Blood			
Eosinophilia	Common (10-20%)	Common	Rare
Thrombocytopenia	Rare‡ (1%)	Rare	Rare
Granulocytopenia	Rare (<1%)	Rare	Rare
Lymphocytopenia	Uncommon	Rare	Rare
Hypogammaglobulinemia	Rare	Rare	Unknown
Aplastic anemia	Rare (<1/1000)	Rare	Unknown
Pulmonary Complications			
Diffuse infiltrates	Rare (<1/1000)	Rare	Rare
Intestinal Effects			
Upper gastrointestinal symptoms	Rare	Rare	Uncommon
Mild enterocolitis	Rare	Rare	Common
Severe enterocolitis	Rare	Rare	Rare
Liver			
Cholestatic jaundice	Rare (<1/1000)	Rare	Unknown
Hepatocellular effects	Rare	Rare	Uncommon
Pancreas			
Pancreatitis	Rare	Rare	Rare
Nervous System			
Peripheral or cranial neuropathies	Rare	Rare	Rare
Encephalopathy	Rare	Rare	Rare
Eye			
Corneal or lens chrysiasis	Common-dose related	Common	Unknown
Conjunctivitis	Rare	Rare	Uncommon
Iritis or corneal ulcer	Rare	Rare	Unknown
Miscellaneous			
Metallic taste	Common	Common	Common
Headaches	Rare	Rare	Rare

* Reported in hypertensive patients receiving angiotensin-converting enzyme inhibitors.

†HLA-DR3: possible relationship.

‡HLA-DR3: relationship proved.

Data from Wooley PH, Griffin J, Panayi GS, et al: HLA-DR antigens and toxic reaction to sodium thiomalate and D-penicillamine in patients with rheumatoid arthritis. N Engl J Med 303:300, 1980.

GSTM.[164] The reaction comes about 6 to 24 hours after injection but can appear within an hour and last as long as a few days. Postinjection reactions are not a reason to abandon gold treatment because a temporary dose reduction or a switch to GSTG can obviate them.[165]

Mucocutaneous Effects

Dermatitis and stomatitis account for 60 percent of adverse reactions. Virtually all gold dermatitis is pruritic. Any part of the body may be affected; vaginal irritation and vaginal pruritus are reactions the patient may not disclose. The histologic appearance of gold dermatitis is variable but may distinguish it from other conditions.

When pruritus, rash, or both appear, chrysotherapy should be discontinued until the eruption resolves. Treatment may then be reinstituted, using a reduced dosage schedule of 5 to 10 mg of gold weekly, with 5- to 10 mg increment increases every 1 to 4 weeks if toxicity does not recur. When doses greater than 10 mg are not tolerated, individualized reductions should be tried because doses as low as 5 to 10 mg monthly may be effective.[157]

Careful dose titration avoids serious exfoliative dermatitis. Symptomatic management includes antihistamines and topical corticosteroids. Steroid gel or pellets sucked three or four times daily may improve healing of stomatitis.

Chrysiasis, a grey-blue discoloration of the sun-exposed skin, may develop after a cumulative dosage of 10 g. Caucasians with fair skin are particularly susceptible. Except for cosmetic effects, chrysiasis is asymptomatic. Localized chrysiasis a disfiguring hyperpigmentation and has been described after laser cosmetic surgery using Q switched dermatologic laser in a patient receiving gold[166]; as the deposition of gold in skin is long lasting, patients who are currently receiving gold or who have received gold in the past must avoid Q-switched laser dermatologic treatment.

Metallic taste is rare with gold. It occurs early in treatment and resolves with ongoing therapy.

Kidney

Proteinuria due to membranous glomerulonephritis develops in 1 to 3 percent of gold-treated patients, typically within the first year of therapy. Studies that include long-term follow-up show complete resolution of proteinuria in 88 percent of patients within 4 to 18 months of discontinuation of therapy.[167] With appropriate monitoring, nephrotic syndrome occurs rarely. To avoid nephrotic syndrome, proteinuria of greater than 500 mg in 24 hours should lead to cessation of gold until proteinuria subsides, but treatment may be safely restarted at 50-percent lower dosage.

Blood

The most serious side effect of gold is aplastic anemia. No incidence figures are available; however, based on large series of treated patients without an incidence, an estimate of less than 1 in 1000 is reasonable. Most reported cases describe this side effect early in the treatment course. Bone marrow aplasia due to gold is treated similarly to other drug-induced aplasias with discontinuation of the offending agent, supportive care, immunosuppression, and, when necessary, transplantation.[168] Excellent supportive care has improved the outcome of this condition. Immune thrombocytopenia develops in 1 percent of patients, typically within the first 6 months of treatment. Cases of delayed gold-induced thrombocytopenia have been reported as long as 18 months after drug discontinuation. An association with HLA-DR3 has been reported.[169] Appropriate management includes early detection, permanent discontinuation of gold, and administration of prednisone (30 to 60 mg/d) until thrombocytopenia resolves. Isolated neutropenia is an uncommon manifestation of myelotoxicity.[170] Other causes of neutropenia in gold-treated patients must be considered, including Felty's syndrome, viral illness, and other drugs. Neutropenia due to Felty's syndrome is not a contraindication to gold treatment because it normally responds well to chrysotherapy with improvement in neutrophil counts over time.[171] A benign and nonprogressive leukopenia may develop in patients on long-term therapy and need not lead to drug discontinuation.[170] A red cell aplasia has been described.[172] Eosinophilia may be an early sign of gold sensitivity and warrants increased vigilance for common gold side effects. In itself, it is not a reason to alter treatment. Hypogammaglobulinemia is a rare side effect of gold.

Other Toxicity of Gold

Acute respiratory distress associated with diffuse pulmonary infiltration characteristically causes cough productive of small amounts of sputum, shortness of breath, pleuritic chest pain, and pulmonary crackles.[173] The clinical picture develops after parenteral administration of about 500 mg of gold. Radiographs show patchy pulmonary consolidation, and pulmonary function test results are consistent with restrictive lung disease. Dramatic improvement follows withdrawal of chrysotherapy and systemic administration of glucocorticoids.

Enterocolitis, a rare but serious complication of parenteral gold therapy, occurs primarily in middle-aged women after small total doses of gold. Symptoms may include abdominal pain, bloody or nonbloody diarrhea, nausea, vomiting, and fever. Despite supportive treatment, the mortality rate is high. Successful treatment of gold-induced enteritis with octreotide has been reported.[174]

Patients with RA taking auranofin have twice the frequency of diarrhea as do patients taking parenteral gold.

Cholestatic jaundice, with hyperbilirubinemia, elevated transaminases, and high alkalinephosphatase levels, is a rare complication of gold. Liver biopsy may show bile stasis and thrombi in the biliary tree or ballooning hepatocytes with sinusoidal compression and minimal cholestasis. Hepatic necrosis and pancreatitis are rare complications of oral or injectable gold.

Neurologic complications of chrysotherapy are rare but reversible and include peripheral neuropathy, a Guillain-Barré–type syndrome, cranial nerve palsies including ophthalmoplegia, and encephalopathy.[175] They usually arise after 3 months of weekly injections, and myokymia is a characteristic clinical sign. Sural nerve biopsy shows both axonal degeneration and segmental demyelination, and computed tomographic brain scan may show evidence of cerebral demyelination.

Corneal and lens chrysiasis is benign and directly related to cumulative dose. It occurs in 75 percent of patients receiving more than 1500 mg of gold intramuscularly.

Treatment Monitoring

Efforts to reduce untoward gold reactions have been fairly successful. The mortality rate has fallen from an estimated 4 percent in the early years of chrysotherapy to less than 0.05 percent at present. Precautionary measures do not prevent gold complications; they merely permit their recognition.

The patient must be instructed to report unexpected symptoms and carefully questioned before each injection about pruritus, rash, or mucous membrane reaction. Mucocutaneous side effects occurring early in therapy are best managed conservatively by interruption of therapy and careful dose adjustment aimed at preventing serious reactions. Laboratory monitoring during the first year includes complete blood indices, platelet count, and urinalysis every one to three injections. Because most hematologic and renal toxicity occurs within the first year, laboratory monitoring may be done less frequently with successful long-term therapy. Proteinuria and cytopenia should result in prompt discontinuation of therapy followed by appropriate investigation and management.

D-Penicillamine

DP is a component of the penicillin molecule obtained by acid hydrolysis. In rheumatology, it is approved for the treatment of RA.[176]

Enthusiasm for use of DP in RA was greatest in the mid-1970s to mid-1980s. Thereafter, there has been a gradual and consistent decrease in its use as a DMARD due to slow onset of action, autoimmune side effects, and safer, more effective therapies. Use in diffuse scleroderma continued until recent multicenter, controlled trials were published showing lack of benefit.

PHARMACOLOGY OF D-Penicillamine

Chemistry

The structural formula of DP is shown in Figure 58–10. It is a sulfhydryl amino acid that differs from the naturally occurring cysteine because of the two methyl groups that replace hydrogen in the β-carbon position. It may be made from penicillin by a semisynthetic process, or it may be made entirely synthetically. All of the DP in clinical use is the D-isomer.

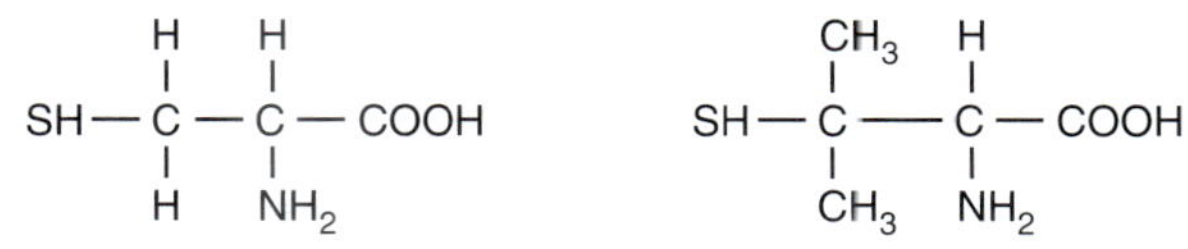

CYSTEINE PENICILLAMINE

FIGURE 58–10 · The Chemical Structure of Penicillamine. The drug is an analogue of the naturally occurring amino acid cysteine, with CH_3 groups replacing H^+ at the β-carbon position.

Biochemistry

The biochemical and pharmacologic properties of DP in humans form the basis for certain of its clinical applications. Chelation of divalent cations such as copper and trace metals accounts for its usefulness in the treatment of Wilson's disease and heavy-metal poisoning. It forms a thiazolidine with pyridoxal phosphate, which may result in antagonism to vitamin B_6, although it is much weaker in this regard than L-penicillamine. A thiazolidine bond may also be formed between DP and the aldehyde groups of collagen, thereby inhibiting collagen cross-linking. This is the biochemical basis for its application to the treatment of systemic sclerosis. Which, if any, of these actions is responsible for the efficacy of DP in RA is unknown.

Pharmacokinetics and Mechanisms of Action

DP is well absorbed from the upper GI tract when it is given in the postabsorptive state. About half of an orally administered dose can be accounted for in urine and feces. When DP administration is discontinued, free DP rapidly disappears from the urine, but oxidized forms can be recovered for more than 3 months.[177] Plasma binding is greatest to albumin, α-globulin, and ceruloplasmin. In tissues, radioactive DP is found in the greatest amount in collagen-containing structures, skin, and tendons.

The mechanism of action of DP in RA is unknown. The DP molecule is so highly reactive that the demonstration of an effect in an in vitro test system cannot be extrapolated to explain its mode of action in RA. In test systems, DP is neither anti-inflammatory nor immunosuppressive, and it has no effect on animal models of arthritis. DP effects a consistent reduction of rheumatoid factor titer and immune complexes with treatment.

Clinical Applications

Selection of Patients

DP is indicated for the treatment of active RA and selected patients with JRA. The efficacy of DP for RA was first established by the United Kingdom Multi-Centre Trial.[178] Use of DP was greatest between 1975 and 1985 and subsequently has declined in North America. DP is currently used in RA when the disease cannot be controlled with antimalarial drugs, MTX, SSZ, gold, CSA, and combinations of these agents. It has been particularly useful in some patients with RA with extra-articular manifestations, such as vasculitis, Felty's syndrome, amyloidosis, and rheumatoid lung disease. Successful treatment of MTX-induced nodulosis after the addition of DP has been reported.[179] DP is not of value in the seronegative spondyloarthropathies, PsA, and other types of inflammatory connective tissue disease.

Efficacy

The pattern of improvement in a DP-responsive patient is similar to that of chrysotherapy. Objective signs of a decrease in synovitis may be found by 6 months. In responsive patients, there is a gradual improvement in the ESR and the C-reactive protein level and a rise in hemoglobin. A reduction in the titer of serum rheumatoid factor is consistent and usually correlates with clinical improvement.

Because of the latent period of 8 to 12 weeks before improvement is evident, analgesic and anti-inflammatory drugs must be maintained. Exacerbations in disease activity may be observed and may require an increase in maintenance dose to regain control. Antibodies to DP may develop during treatment, and this may explain the loss of efficacy in some patients.[180]

After 5 years, only about 25 percent of patients given DP continue with a satisfactory result. Withdrawals are largely due to adverse reactions and less to loss of efficacy.[181]

Dosing Schedule

DP is available as a 250- or 125-mg capsule or as a 250-mg scored tablet. Various dosage regimens have been studied in RA, and it is recommended that treatment be initiated with 125 or 250 mg/day for 4 to 8 weeks. The dosage may then be raised by a similar increment every 1 to 3 months until improvement commences or a daily maximum of 1000 mg/day is reached. Intermittent thrice-weekly dosage has been reported to be as effective as daily doses with fewer side effects.[182] The average patient requires a dose of 500 to 750 mg/day for at least 3 months before a satisfactory response is achieved.

Absorption of DP is hindered by food, antacids, and oral iron; hence, it is optimally given in the postabsorptive state. It may be given in a single daily dose, 1 to 2 hours apart from food or other medicines.

Contraindications and Precautions

DP is contraindicated in pregnancy. If a patient with RA becomes pregnant while receiving DP, the drug should be stopped, but termination of the pregnancy is not indicated. A history of previous allergic or hypersensitivity reaction to penicillin is not a contraindication to the use of DP, and no additional precautions are required.

Toxicity of D-Penicillamine

The adverse effects of DP administration have been the major factor limiting its usefulness. Some of these effects can be favorably influenced by the "go low, go slow" dosage regimens, but others can occur regardless of the maximal maintenance dose or the duration of treatment.[48] Most of the side effects are encountered during the first 18 months of therapy (Fig. 58–11). There is an association between HLA-B8 and HLA-DR3 and toxic reactions to both gold salts and DP, particularly with respect to nephropathy. RA patients with Sjögren's syndrome appear more prone to DP toxicity. Antibodies to DP are also associated with a higher incidence of adverse reactions.[180]

Blood

Hematologic conditions are certainly the most serious of the adverse reactions. Leukopenia, immune thrombocytopenia, and aplastic anemia may occur. Complete blood counts with platelets should be done every 2 weeks for the first 6 months of therapy and monthly thereafter.

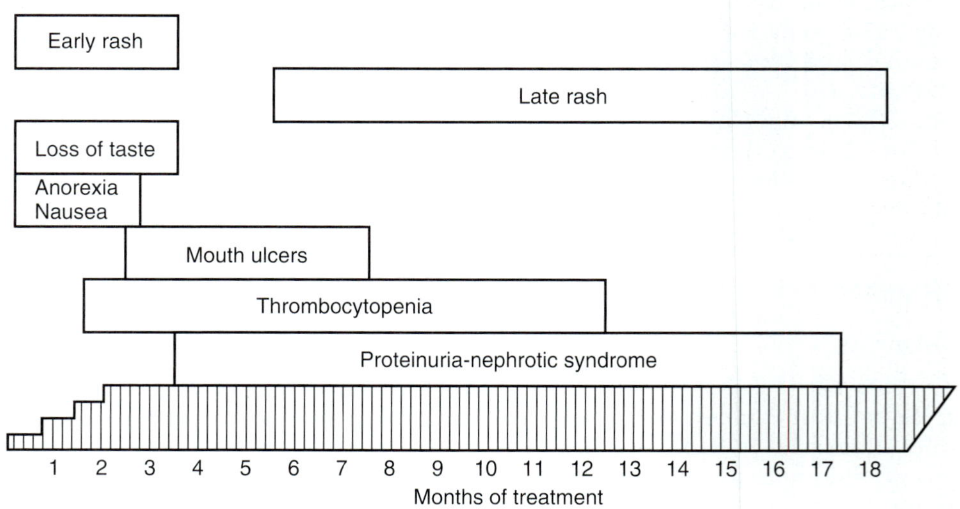

FIGURE 58–11 • The Chronopharmacology of Penicillamine. This diagram depicts the peak incidence of some of the more common side effects of penicillamine during a course of therapy with a maintenance dose of 1 g/day. Most of the serious reactions will have developed during the first 18 months of treatment. Aplastic anemia was not included in this illustration, but it may occur at any time, particularly after an increase in dosage. (After Balme HW, Huskisson EC: Chronopharmacology of penicillamine and gold. Scand J Rheumatol 4[Suppl 8]:21, 1975.)

Kidney

The most common renal side effect is a membranous glomerulonephritis, presenting with proteinuria alone. Goodpasture's syndrome occurs rarely. Biweekly monitoring for the first 6 months should include a urinalysis.

Mucocutaneous Effects

Pruritus and a variety of early and late rashes are the most common side effects of the drug. Simple pruritus can often be managed by a temporary interruption of DP therapy and the addition of an antihistamine. Aphthous ulcers and stomatitis may occur, but these often resolve with a modest reduction in dosage. The appearance of bullous dermatitis might herald the development of DP-induced pemphigus. Administration of the drug must be stopped, and immunosuppressive therapy may be required.

Other Toxicity

GI symptoms due to DP are usually not serious but are commonly dose limiting. Anorexia, nausea, hypogeusia, dysgeusia, and metallic taste may disappear with continued use or temporary dose reduction. There have been reports of cholestatic jaundice, but serious hepatotoxicity is extremely rare.[183]

Pulmonary complications are also rare. A Goodpasture-like syndrome has been described.[184] There have been reports of DP-associated bronchiolitis obliterans. The appearance of dyspnea associated with midinspiratory rhonchi should alert the physician to this serious event.[185]

Neuromuscular disorders may infrequently be caused by DP. Myasthenia gravis is the most common in this category, and it is identical to the spontaneously occurring disease.[186] There are antibodies to the acetylcholine receptor, and the patients respond to anticholinesterase drugs. Myasthenia, often with ocular symptoms, is reversible after DP withdrawal, but months may be required before dependence on anticholinesterase drugs ends. Whereas spontaneous myasthenia is associated with HLA-DR3 and HLA-B1, DP-induced myasthenia is almost always associated with HLA-DR1 and HLA-Bw35.[3] Polymyositis and dermatomyositis can also be produced by DP, sometimes with cardiac involvement.[54]

Autoimmune syndromes have been described in the other diseases for which DP is given, such as Wilson's disease and cystinuria, indicating that they are a feature of the drug rather than an altered immune responsiveness in rheumatoid patients. Autoantibodies to insulin and the insulin receptor have been described.[180] DP-induced lupus has been well recognized, and these patients differ from those with drug-induced lupus because they have antibody to native, double-stranded DNA.[187]

Drug fever, often with a morbilliform rash, usually develops shortly after treatment is begun and recurs on rechallenge.

Other Sulfhydryl Compounds

Numerous attempts have been made to find a sulfhydryl compound with a DP-like beneficial effect in RA but with greater safety. Bucillamine, developed in Japan, has a molecular structure similar to that of DP. Clinical effects in patients suggest that bucillamine might suppress RA as effectively as and with fewer side effects than DP.[188] T cells, 5-thiopyridoxine, pyrithioxin (pyritinol), tiopronin (α-mercaptopropionylglycine), and captopril have been studied. All were effective; captopril was the weakest. Unfortunately, they all displayed a similar and characteristic spectrum of adverse effects, including induction of autoimmune disease.

REFERENCES

1. Svartz N: Salazopyrin, a new sulfanilamide preparation. Acta Med Scand 110:577, 1942.
2. Day RO: Sulfasalazine. *In* Ruddy S, Harris ED Jr., Sledge CB (eds): Kelley's Textbook of Rheumatology, 6th ed. Philadelphia, WB Saunders, 2001, pp 869-878.
3. Pullar T, Hunter J, Capell H: Which component of sulphasalazine is active in rheumatoid arthritis? BMJ 290:1535, 1985.
4. Peppercorn M, Goldman P: The role of Intestinal bacteria in the metabolism of salicylazosulapyridine. J Pharm Exp Ther 181:555, 1972.
5. Azad Khan A, Truelove S, Aronson J: The disposition and metabolism of sulphasalazine (salicylazosulphapyrdine) in man. Br J Clin Pharmacol 13:523, 1982.
6. Schroder H, Campbell D: Absorption, metabolism and excretion of salicylazo-sulfapyridine in man. Clin Pharmacol Ther 13:539, 1972.
7. Chalmers I, Sitar D, Hunter T: A one-year, open, prospective study of sulfasalazine in the treatment of rheumatoid arthritis: Adverse reactions and clinical response in relating to laboratory variables, drug and metabolite serum levels and acetylator status. J Rheumatol 17:764, 1990.
8. Taggart A, McDermott B, Delargy M, et al: The pharmacokinetics of sulphasalazine in young and elderly patients with rheumatoid arthritis. Scand J Rheumatol 64:29, 1987.
9. Wilieson CA, Madhok R, Hunter JA, et al: Toleration, side-effects and efficacy of sulfasalazine in rheumatoid arthritis patients of different ages. Q J Med 86:501, 1993.
10. Imai F, Suzuki R, Ishigashi T, et al: Effect of sulfasalazine on B cell hyperactivity in patients with rheumatoid arthritis. J Rheumatol 21:612, 1994.
11. Kanerud L, Scheynius A, Hafstorm I: Evidence of a local intestinal immunomodulatory effect of sulfasalazine in rheumatoid arthritis. Arthritis Rheum 37:1138, 1994.
12. Danis VA, Franic GM, Rathjen DA, et al: Circulating cytokine levels in patients with rheumatoid arthritis: Results of a double blind trial with sulphasalazine. Ann Rheum Dis 51:945, 1992.
13. Crilly A, Madhok R, Watson J, et al: Production of interleukin-6 by monocytes isolated from rheumatoid arthritis patients receiving second-line drug therapy. Br J Rheumatol 33:821, 1994.
14. Carlin G, Djursater R, Smedegard G: Sulphasalazine inhibition of human granulocyte activation by inhibition of second messenger compounds. Ann Rheum Dis 51:1230, 1992.
15. American College of Rheumatology Ad Hoc Committee on Clinical Guidelines: Guidelines for monitoring drug therapy in rheumatoid arthritis. Arthritis Rheum 39:723, 1996.
16. Weinblatt ME, Reda D, Henderson W, et al: Sulfasalazine treatment for RA: A meta-analysis of 15 randomized Trials. J Rheumatol 26:2123, 1999.
17. Van der Heijde D, van Riel P, Nuver-Zwart E, et al: Effect of hydroxychloroquine and sulphasalazine on progression of joint damage in rheumatoid arthritis. Lancet 13:1036, 1989.

18. Van der Heijde D, van Riel P, Nuver-Zwart E, et al: Sulphasalazine versus hydroxychloroquine in rheumatoid arthritis: 3-year follow-up Lancet 335:539, 1990.
19. Smolen JS, European Leflunomide Study Group: Efficacy and safety of leflunomide compared with placebo and sulphasalazine in active rheumatoid arthritis: a double-blind, randomized, multicenter trial. Lancet 353:259, 1999.
20. Kalden JR, Scott DL, Smolen JS, et al: Improved functional ability in patients with rheumatoid arthritis: long-term treatment with leflunomide versus sulfasalazine. J Rheumatol 28:1983, 2001.
21. Aletaha D, Smolen JS: Effectiveness profiles and dose dependent retention of traditional disease modifying antirheumatic drugs for rheumatoid arthritis: An observational study. J Rheumatol 29:1631, 2002.
22. Bax DE, Amas RS: Sulphasalazine: a safe, effective agent for prolonged control of rheumatoid arthritis—a comparison with sodium aurothiomalate. Ann Rheum Dis 44:194, 1985.
23. Maetzel A, Wong A, Strand V, et al: Meta-analysis of treatment termination rates among rheumatoid arthritis patients receiving disease-modifying anti-rheumatic drugs. Rheumatology 39:975, 2000.
24. O'Dell, Leff R, Paulsen G, et al: Treatment of rheumatoid arthritis with methotrexate and hydroxychloroquine, methotrexate and sulfasalazine, or a combination of the three medications: results of a two-year, randomized, double-blind, placebo-controlled trial. Arthritis Rheum 46:1164, 2002.
25. Dougados M, Combe B, Cantagrel A, et al: Combination therapy in early rheumatoid arthritis—a randomized, controlled, double blind 52 week clinical trial of sulphasalazine and methotrexate compared with the single components. Ann Rheum Dis 58:220, 1999.
26. Proudman SM, Conaghan PG, Richardson C, et al: Treatment of poor-prognosis early rheumatoid arthritis: a randomized study of treatment with methotrexate, cyclosporine A, and intraarticular corticosteroids compared with sulfasalazine alone. Arthritis Rheum 43:1809, 2000.
27. Boers M, Verhoeven AC, Markusse HM, et al: Randomized comparison of combined step-down prednisolone, methotrexate and sulphasalazine with sulphasalazine alone in early rheumatoid arthritis. Lancet 350:309, 1997.
28. Landewe RBM, Boers M, Verhoeven AC, et al: COBRA combination therapy in patients with early rheumatoid arthritis: Long-term structural benefits of a brief intervention. Arthritis Rheum 46:347, 2002.
29. Mottonen T, Hannonen P, Korpela M, et al: Delay to institution of therapy and induction of remission using single-drug or combination-disease-modifying antirheumatic drug therapy in early rheumatoid arthritis. Arthritis Rheum 46:894, 2002.
30. Neva MH, for the FIN-RA Co Trial Group: Combination drug therapy retards the development of rheumatoid atlantoaxial subluxations. Arthritis Rheum 43:2397, 2000.
31. Clegg DO, Reda DJ, Mejias E, et al: Comparison of sulfasalazine and placebo in the treatment of psoriatic arthritis. Arthritis Rheum 39:2013, 1996.
32. Clegg DO, Reda DJ, Abdellatif M: Comparison of sulfasalazine and placebo for the treatment of axial and peripheral articular manifestations of the seronegative spondylarthropathies: A Department of Veterans Affairs cooperative study. Arthritis Rheum 42:2325, 1999.
33. Egsmose C, Hansen TM, Andersen LS, et al: Limited effect of sulphasalazine treatment in reactive arthritis: A randomized double blind placebo controlled trial. Ann Rheum Dis 56:32, 1997.
34. Ferraz MB, Tugwell P, Goldsmith CH, et al: Meta-analysis of sulfasalazine in ankylosing spondylitis. J Rheumatol 17:1482, 1990.
35. Gerster JC: Nail lesions in psoriatic arthritis: recovery with sulfasalazine treatment [letter]. Ann Rheum Dis 61:277, 2002.
36. Rahman P, Gladman DD, Cook RJ, et al: The use of sulfasalazine in psoriatic arthritis: a clinical experience. J Rheumatol 25:1957, 1998.
37. Salvarani C, Macchioni, P. Olivieri I, et al: A comparison of cyclosporine, sulfasalazine, and symptomatic therapy in the treatment of psoriatic arthritis. J Rheumatol 28(28):2274, 2000.
38. Munoz-Fernandez S, Hidlago V, Fernandez-Melon J, et al: Sulfasalzine improves the numbers of flares of acute anterior uveitis over a one-year period. J Rheumatol 30:1277, 2003.
39. van Rossum MAJ, Fiselier, TJW, Franssen MJAM, et al: Sulfasalazine in the treatment of juvenile chronic arthritis: a randomized, double-blind, placebo-controlled, multicenter study. Arthritis Rheum 41:808, 1998.
40. Brooks CD: Sulfasalazine for the management of juvenile rheumatoid arthritis. J Rheumatol 28:845, 2001.
41. Jung, JH, Jun JB, Yoo DH, et al: High toxicity of sulfasalazine in adult-onset Still's disease. Clin Exp Rheumatol 18:245, 2000.
42. Amos R, Pullar T, Capell H: Sulphasalzine for rheumatoid arthritis: Toxicity in 774 patients monitored for one to 11 years. BMJ 293:420, 1986.
43. Marabani M, Madhok R, Capell H, et al: Leucopenia during sulphasalazine treatment for rheumatoid arthritis. Ann Rheum Dis 48:505, 1989.
44. Canvin JMG, El-Gaalawy HS, Chalmers IM: Fatal agranulocytosis with sulfasalazine therapy in rheumatoid arthritis. J Rheumatol 20:909, 1993.
45. Kaplan S, McDonald E, Marino C: Lichen planus in patient with rheumatoid arthritis treated with sulfasalazine. J Rheumatol 20:909, 1993.
46. Farr M, Scott D, Bacon P: Sulphasalazine desensitization in rheumatoid arthritis. BMJ 284:118, 1982.
47. Mogadam M, Dobbins W, Korelitz B, et al: Pregnancy in inflammatory bowel disease: Effect of sulphasalazine and corticosteroids on fetal outcome. Gastroentrology 80:72, 1981.
48. Toovey S, Hudson E, Hendry W, et al: Sulphasalazine and male infertility: Reversibility and possible mechanism. Gut 22:445, 1981.
49. Alloway JA, Mitchell SR: Sulfasalazine neurotoxicity: A report of aseptic meningitis and a review of the literature. J Rheumatol 20:409, 1993.
50. Caulier M, Dromer C. Andrieu V, et al: Sulfasalzine induced lupus in rheumatoid arthritis. J Rheumatol 21:750, 1994.
51. Gordon M-M, Porter DR, Capell HA: Does sulphasalazine cause drug induced systemic lupus erythematosis? No effect evident in a prospective randomized trial of 200 rheumatoid patients treated with sulphasalazine or auranofin over five years. Ann Rheum Dis 58:288, 1999.
52. Gunnarson I, Normark B, Bakri AH, et al: Development of lupus-related side-effects in patients with early RA during sulphasalazine treatment: The role of IL-10 and *HLA*. Rheumatology 39:886, 2000.
53. Dougados M: *In* van de Putte LB (ed): Sulfasalazine in Therapy of Systemic Rheumatic Disorders. New York, Marcel Dekker, 1988, pp 165-183.
54. Payne JP: A post-graduate lecture on lupus erythematosus. Clin J 4:223, 1894.
55. Page F: Treatment of lupus erythematosus with mapacrine. Lancet 2:755, 1951.
56. Rynes RI: Antimalarial drugs. *In* Kelley WN, Harris ED Jr, Ruddy S, Sledge CB (eds): Textbook of Rheumatology, 4th ed. Philadelphia, WB Saunders, 1993, pp 731-742.
57. Hobbs HE, Sorsby A, Freedman A: Retinopathy following chloroquine therapy. Lancet 2:478, 1959.
58. Rynes RI, Bernstein HN: Ophthalmologic safety profile of antimalarial drugs. Lupus 2(Suppl 1):S17, 1993.
59. Maurikakis M, Papazoglou S, Sfolalos PP, et al: Retinal toxicity in long-term hydroxychloroquine treatment. Ann Rheum Dis 55:187, 1996.
60. Woo TY, Callen JP, Voorhees JJ, et al: Cutaneous lesions of dermatoloyositis are improved by hydroxychloroquine. J Am Acad Dermatol 10:592, 1984.
61. Youssef W, Yan A, Russell A: Palindromic rheumatism: A response to chloroquine. J Rheumatol 18:1, 1991.
62. Lakhanpal S, Ginsberg WW, Michet CJ, et al: Eosinophilic fasciitis: Clinical spectrum and therapeutic response in 52 cases. Semin Arthritis Rheum 17:221, 1988.
63. Bryant LR, DesRosier KF, Carpenter MT: Hydroxychloroquine in the treatment of erosive osteoarthritis. J Rheumatol 22:1527, 1995.
64. Hannonen P, Mottonen T, Oka M: Treatment of palindromic rheumatism with chloroqine. BMJ 294:1289, 1987.
65. Lovy MR, Starkebaum G, Uberoi S: Hepatitis C infection presenting with rheumatic manifestations: A mimic of rheumatoid arthritis J Rheumatol 23:97, 1996.
66. Rothschild BM: Prospective six-month double-blind trial of Plaquenil treatment of calcium pyrophosphate deposition disease (CPPD). Arthritis Rheum 37(Suppl 9):S414, 1994.
67. Esdaile JM: Canadian Rheumatology Association consensus conference on hydroxychloroquin. J Rheumatol 2919, 2000.

68. Tett SE, Cutler DJ, Day R: Antimalarials in rheumatic diseases. Baillieres Clin Rheumatol 4:467, 1990.
69. Furst DE: Pharmacokinetics of hydroxychloroquine and chloroquine during treatment of rheumatic diseases. Lupus 5(Suppl):S11, 1996.
70. McChesney EW, Conway WD, Banks WF Jr, et al: Studies on the metabolism of some compounds of the 1-amino-7-chloroquinoline series. J Pharmacol Exp Ther 151:482, 1966.
71. Rubin M, Bernstein HN, Zvaifler NJ: Studies on the pharmacology of chloroquine. Arch Ophthalmol 70:474, 1962.
72. French JK, Hurst NP, O'Donnell ML, Betts WH: Uptake of hydroxychloroquine by human blood leukocytes in vitro: Relation to cellular concentrations during antirheumatic therapy. Ann Rheum Dis 46:42, 1987.
73. Rynes RI: Antimalarial drugs. *In* Ruddy S, Harris ED Jr., Sledge CB (eds): Kelley's Textbook of Rheumatology, 6th ed. Philadelphia, WB Saunders, 2001, pp 859-867.
74. Gonzalez-Noriega A, Grubb JH, Talkad V, Sly WS: Chloroquine inhibits lysosomal enzyme pinocytosis and enhances lysosomal enzyme secretion by impairing receptor recycling. J Cell Biol 85:839, 1980.
75. Oda K, Koriyama Y, Yamada E, Ikehara Y: Effects of weakly basic amines on proteolytic processing and terminal glycosylation of secretory proteins in cultured rat hepatocytes. Biochem J 240:739, 1986.
76. Thompson GR, Bartholomew LE: The effect of chloroquine on antibody formation. Univ Mich Med Cent J 30:227, 1964.
77. Fox RI, Kang HI: Mechanism of action of antimalarial drugs: Inhibition of antigen processing and presentation. Lupus 2(Suppl 1):S9, 1993.
78. Panayi GS, Neill WA, Duthie J Jr, et al: Action of chloroquine phosphate in rheumatoid arthritis. I: Immunosuppressive effect. Ann Rheum Dis 32:316, 1973.
79. Ausiello CM, Barbiere P, Spagnoli GC, et al: In vivo effects of chloroquine treatment on spontaneous and interferon-induced natural killer activities in rheumatoid arthritis patients. Clin Exp Rheumatol 1:225, 1986.
80. Bondeson J, Sundler R: Antimalarial drugs inhibit phospholipase A_2 activation and induction of interleukin 1beta and tumor necrosis factor alpha in macrophages: Implications for their mode of action in rheumatoid arthritis. Gen Pharmacol 30:357, 1998.
81. Karres I, Kremer JP, Dietl I, et al: Chloroquine inhibits proinflammatory cytokine release into human blood. Am J Physiol 274:R1058, 1998.
82. van den Borne BE, Dijkmans BA, de Rooij HH, et al: Chloroquine and hydroxychloroquine equally affect tumor necrosis factor-alpha, interleukin 6 and interferon-gamma production by peripheral blood mononuclear cells. J Rheumatol 24:55, 1997.
83. Wallace DJ, Linker-Israeli M, Metzger AL, Stecher VJ: The relevance of antimalarial therapy with regard to thrombosis, hypercholesterolemia and cytokines in SLE. Lupus 2(Suppl 1):S13, 1993.
84. Landewe RBM, Miltenburg AMM, Verdonk MJA, et al: Chloroquine inhibits T cell proliferation by interfering with IL-2 production and responsiveness. Clin Exp Immunol 14:144, 1995.
85. Pittman, SM, Ireland CM: Induction of apoptosis in peripheral blood lymphocytes following treatment in vitro with hydroxychloroquine. Arthritis Rheum 40:927, 1997.
86. Kench, JG, Seale JP, Temple DM, Tennant C: The effects of nonsteroidal inhibitors of phospholipase A_2 on leukotriene and histamine release from human and guinea-pig lung. Prostaglandins 20:199, 1985.
87. Nguyen TQ, Capra JD, Sontheimer RD: 4-Aminoquinoline antimalarials enhance UV-B induced c-jun transcriptional activation. Lupus 7:148, 1998.
88. Dubois EL: Effect of quinacrine (Atabrine) upon lupus erythematosus phenomenon. Arch Dermatol 71:570, 1955.
89. Mayer L: Inhibition of human immunodeficiency virus type 1 replication by hydroxychloroquine in T cells and monocytes. AIDS Res Hum Retrovirus 9:91, 1993.
90. Middleton GD, McFarlin JE, Lipsky PE: Hydroxychloroquine and pain thresholds. Arthritis Rheum 38:445, 1995.
91. Felson DT, Anderson JJ, Meenan RF: The comparative efficacy and toxicity of second-line drugs in rheumatoid arthritis. Arthritis Rheum 33:1449, 1990.
92. Tsakonas E, Fitzgerald A, Fitzcharles M-A, et al: Consequences of delayed therapy with second-line agents in rheumatoid arthritis: A 3 year followup on the hydroxychloroquine in early rheumatoid arthritis (HERA study). J Rheumatol 27:623-629, 2000.
93. Furst DE, Lindsley H. Baethge B, et al: Dose-loading with hydroxychloroquine improves the rate of response in early, active rheumatoid arthritis. Arthritis Rheum 42:357-363, 1999.
94. HERA Study Group: A randomized trial of hydroxychloroquine in early rheumatoid arthritis. Arthritis Rheum 27:267, 1984.
95. Hurst S, Kallan MJ, Wolfe FJ, et al: Methotrexate, hydroxychloroquine, and intramuscular gold in rheumatoid arthritis: relative area under the curve effectiveness and sequence effects. J Rheumatol 29:1639, 2002.
96. Van der Heijde DMFM, Van Riel PL, Zuver-Zwart IH, et al: Effects of hydroxychloroquine and sulfasalazine on progression of joint damage in rheumatoid arthritis. Lancet 1:1036, 1989.
97. Van Der Heijde DMFM, Van Riel PLCM, Nuver-Zwart IH, et al: Alternative methods for analysis of radiographic damage in a randomized, double blind, parallel group clinical trial comparing hydroxychloroquine and sulfasalazine. J Rheumatol 27:535-539, 2000.
98. O'Dell JR, Blakely KW, Mallek JA, et al: Treatment of early seropositive rheumatoid arthritis: A two-year, double-blind comparison of minocycline and hydroxychloroquine. Arthritis Rheum 44:2235, 2001.
99. Ferraz MB, Pinheiro GRC, Helfenstein M, et al: Combination therapy with methotrexate and chloroquine in rheumatoid arthritis. Scand J Rheumatol 23:231, 1994.
100. Carmichael SJ, Beal J, Day RO, et al: Combination treatment with methotrexate and hydrochloroquine and rheumatoid arthritis increases exposure to methotrexate. J Rheumatol 29:2077, 2002.
101. O'Dell JR, Haire CE, Erikson N, et al: Treatment of rheumatoid arthritis with methotrexate alone, sulfasalazine and hydroxychloroquine or a combination of all three medications. N Engl J Med 334:1287, 1996.
102. O'Dell JR, Haire C, Erickson N, et al: Efficacy of triple DMARD therapy in patients with suboptimal response to methotrexate. J Rheumatol 23(Suppl 44):72, 1996.
103. Hodis HN, Quismorio FP Jr., Wickham E, Blankenthorn DH: The lipid, lipoprotein and apolipoprotein effects of hydroxychloroquine in patients with SLE. J Rheumatol 20:661, 1993.
104. Wallace JD, Metzger AL, Stecher VJ, et al: Cholesterol-lowering effect of hydroxychloroquine (Plaquenil) in rheumatoid disease patients: Reversal of deleterious effects of steroids on lipids. Am J Med 89:322, 1990.
105. Munro R, Morrison E, McDonald AG, et al: Effects of disease modifying agents on the lipid profiles of patients with rheumatoid arthritis. Ann Rheum Dis 56:374, 1997.
106. Combe B, Guitierrezz M, Anaya JN, Sany J: Possible efficacy of hydroxychloroquine on accelerated noculosis during methotrexate therapy for rheumatoid arthritis. J Rheumatol 20:755, 1993.
107. Fries JR, Gurkipal S, Lenert L, Furst DE: Aspirin, hydroxychloroquine and hepatic enzyme abnormalities with methotrexate in rheumatoid arthritis. Arthritis Rheum 33:1161, 1990.
108. Brewer EJ, Giannini EH, Kuzima N, Alekseev L: Penicillamine and hydroxychloroquine in the treatment of severe juvenile rheumatoid arthritis. N Engl J Med 315:1269, 1986.
109. Fox RI, Dixon R, Guarrasi V, Krubel S: Treatment of primary Sjögren's syndrome with hydroxychloroquine: A retrospective open-label study. Lupus 5(Suppl 1):S31, 1996.
110. Williams HJ, Egger MJ, Singer JZ, et al: Comparison of hydroxychloroquine and placebo in the treatment of the arthropathy of mild systemic lupus erythematosus. J Rheumatol 21:1457, 1994.
111. Lakshminarayana S, Walsh S, Mohanraj M, et al: Factors associated with low bone mineral density in female patients with systemic lupus erythematosus. J Rheumatol 28:102, 2001.
112. Canadian Hydroxychloroquine Study Group: A randomized study of the effects of withdrawing hydroxychloroquine sulfate in systemic lupus erythematosus. N Engl J Med 324:150, 1991.
113. Wang C, Fortin PR, Li Yin, et al: Discontinuation of antimalarial drugs in systemic lupus erythematosus. J Rheumatol, 26:808-815, 1999.

114. Toubi E, Rosner I, Rozenbaum M, et al. The benefit of combining hydroxychloroquine with quinacrine in the treatment of SLE patients. Lupus 9:92, 2000.
115. Workshop Report: Aspects of use of antimalarials in systemic lupus erythematosus. J Rheumatol 25:983, 1998.
116. Yoon KH: Sufficient evidence to consider hydrochloroquine as an adjunct therapy in antiphospholipid antibodies (Hughes Syndrome) [letter]. J Rheumatol 29:1574, 2002.
117. McCarty GA: Hydrochloroquine HCQ treatment in antiphospholipid syndrome (APS): Time course of clinical improvement in antiphospholipid antibodies (aPL)—time changes over 4 years [abstract]. Arthritis Rheum 43(Suppl 9):S1061, 2000.
118. Olson NY, Lindsley CB: Adjunctive use of hydroxychloroquine in childhood dermatomyositis. J Rheumatol 16:12, 1989.
119. Kammer GM, Soter NA, Gibson DJ, Schur PH: Psoriatic arthritis: A clinical, immunologic and HLA study of 100 patients. Semin Arthritis Rheum 9:75, 1979.
120. Tett SE, Cutler DJ, Beck C, et al: Concentration-effect relationship of hydroxychloroquine with rheumatoid arthritis: A prospective, dose ranging study. J Rheumatol 27:1656, 2000.
121. Cervera A, Espinosa G, Cervera R, et al: Cardiac toxicity secondary to long term treatment with chloroquine [letter]. Ann Rheum Dis 60:301-304, 2001.
122. Shojania K, Koehler BE, Elliott T: Hypoglycemia induced by hydroxychloroquine in a type II diabetic treated for polyarthritis. J Rheumatol 26:195, 1999.
123. Costeoat-Chalumeau Z, Amoura G, Aymard M, et al: Evidence of transplacental passage of hydroxychloroquine in humans [letter]. Arthritis Rheum 46:1123, 2002.
124. Klinger G, Mora Y, Westall CA, et al: Ocular toxicity and antenatal exposure to chloroquine or hydroxychloroquine for rheumatic disease [letter]. Lancet 358:812, 2001.
125. Stein M, Bell MJ, Ang L-C: Hydroxychloroquine neuromyotoxicity. J Rheumatol 27:2927, 2000.
126. Gordon DA, Klinkhoff AV: Gold and penicillamine. *In* Ruddy S, Harris ED Jr., Sledge CB (eds): Kelley's Textbook of Rheumatology, 6th ed. Philadelphia, WB Saunders, 2001, pp 869-878.
127. Forestier J: Rheumatoid arthritis and its treatment by gold salts. J Lab Clin Med 20:827, 1935.
128. Empire Rheumatism Council Research Sub-committee: Gold therapy in rheumatoid arthritis: Final report of a multicentre controlled trial. Ann Rheum Dis 20:315, 1961.
129. Sigler JW, Bluhm GB, Duncan H, et al: Gold salts in the treatment of rheumatoid arthritis: A double-blind study. Ann Intern Med 80:21, 1974.
130. Cooperating Clinics Committee: A controlled trial of gold salt therapy in rheumatoid arthritis. Arthritis Rheum 16:353, 1973.
131. Ward J, Williams HJ, Egger MJ, et al: Comparison of auranofin, gold sodium thiomalate, and placebo in the treatment of rheumatoid arthritis: A controlled clinical trial. Arthritis Rheum 26:1303, 1983.
132. Prete PE, Zane J, Krailo M, Bulanowski M: Randomized trial of switching rheumatoid arthritis patients in remission with injectable gold to auranofin. Clin Rheumatol 13:60, 1994.
133. Riesta RA, Noriega JL, Harth M: Pharmacology of gold compounds in rheumatoid arthritis: A review. Can J Clin Pharmacol 4:127, 1997.
134. Repchinsky C, Welbanks L, Bisson R (eds): Compendium of Pharmaceuticals and Specialties. Correction Pharmacits Association. Ottawa, Canadian Pharmacists Association, 2002, p 1569.
135. Kinne RW, Stuhlmuller B, Palombo-Kinne E, et al: The role of macrophages in rheumatoid arthritis. *In* Firestein GS, Panay GS, Wollheim FA (eds): Rheumatoid Arthritis New Fronters in Pathogenesis and Treatment. Oxford, Oxford University Press, 2000, p 80.
136. Kirkham BW, Navarro FJ, Corkill MM, et al: In vivo analysis of disease-modifying drug therapy activity in RA by sequential immunohistological analysis of synovial membrane IL1b. J Rheumatol 21:1615, 1994.
137. Kawakami A, Eguchi K, Migiti K, et al: Inhibitory effects of gold sodium thiomalate on the proliferation and interferon gamma induced HLA DR expression in human endothelial cells J Rheumatol;17, 430, 1990.
138. The Research Subcommittee of the Empire Rheumatism Council: Gold therapy in rheumatoid arthritis: Report of a multi-centre controlled trial. Ann Rheum Dis;19:95, 1960.
139. Luukkainen R, Kajander A, Isomaki H: Effect of gold on progression of erosions in rheumatoid arthritis: Better results with early treatment. Scand J Rheumatol 6:189, 1977.
140. Buckland-Wright JC, Clarke GS, Chikanza IC, et al: Quantitative microfocal radiography detects changes in erosion area in patients with early rheumatoid arthritis treated with Myochrisine. J Rheumatol 20:243, 1993.
141. Rau R, Herborn G, Menninger H, et al: Radiographic outcome after three years of patients with early erosive rheumatoid arthritis treated with intramuscular methotrexate or parenteral gold. Extension of a one-year double blind study in 174 patients. Rheumatology (Oxford) 41:196, 2002.
142. Sander O, Herborn G, Bock E, et al: Prospective six year follow up of patients withdrawn from a randomized study comparing parenteral gold salt and methotrexate. Ann Rheum Dis 58:281, 1999.
143. Lehtinen K, Isomaki H: Intramuscular gold therapy is associated with long survival in patients with rheumatoid arthritis. J Rheumatol 18:524, 1991.
144. Clark P, Tugwell P, Bennett K, Bombardier C: Meta-analysis of injectable gold in rheumatoid arthritis. J Rheumatol 16:442, 1989.
145. Felson DT, Anderson JJ, Meenan RF: The comparative efficacy and toxicity of second-line drugs in rheumatoid arthritis. Arthritis Rheum 33:1449, 1990.
146. Wolfe F, Hawley DJ, Cathey MA: Measurement of gold treatment effect in clinical practice: Evidence for effectiveness of intramuscular gold therapy. J Rheumatol 20:797, 1993.
147. Wolfe F: The curious case of intramuscular gold (review). Rheum Dis Clin North Am 19:173, 1993.
148. Munro R, Hampson R, McEntengart A, et al: Improved functional outcome in patients with early rheumatoid arthritis treated with intramuscular gold: Results of a 5 year prospective study. Ann Rheum Dis 57:88, 1998.
149. Speerstra F, Van Riel PLCM, Reekers P, et al: The influence of HLA phenotypes on the response to parenteral gold in rheumatoid arthritis. Tissue Antigens 28:1, 1986.
150. Lacaille D, Stein HB, Raboud J, et al: Longterm therapy of psoriatic arthritis: intramuscular gold or methotrexate? J Rheumatol 27:1922, 2000.
151. Boers M, Ramsden M: Long-acting drug combinations in rheumatoid arthritis: A formal overview. J Rheumatol 18:316, 1991.
152. Bensen W, Tugwell P, Roberts RM, et al: Combination therapy of cyclosporine with methotrexate and gold in rheumatoid arthritis (2 pilot studies). J Rheumatol 21:2034, 1994.
153. Porter DR, Capell HA, Hunter J: Combination therapy in rheumatoid arthritis: No benefit of addition of hydroxychloroquine to patients with a suboptimal response to intramuscular gold therapy. J Rheumatol 20:654, 1993.
154. Lehman AF, Esdaile JM, Klinkhoff A, et al: A 48 week double blind double observer placebo controlled multicentre trial of intramuscular gold in combination with methotrexate in rheumatoid arthritis [Abstract]. Arthritis Rheum 46:5240, 2002.
155. Furst DE, Levine S. Srinivasan R, et al: A double blind trial of high versus conventional dosage of gold salts for rheumatoid arthritis. Arthritis Rheum 20:1473, 1977.
156. Arthur AB, Klinkhoff A, Teufel A: Nitritoid reactions: case report, review, and recommendations for management. J Rheumatol 28:2209, 2001.
157. Klinkhoff AV, Teufel A: How low can you go? Use of very low dosage of gold in patients with mucocutaneous reactions. J Rheumatol 22:1657, 1995.
158. Ten Wolde S, Hermans J, Breedveld FC, Dijkmans RA: Effect of resumption of second line drugs in patients with rheumatoid arthritis that flared up after treatment discontinuation. Ann Rheum Dis 56:235, 1997.
159. Klinkhoff AV, Teufel A: The second course of gold. J Rheumatol 22:1625, 1995.
160. Arthur AB, Klinkhoff AV, Teufel A: Safety of self-injection of gold and methotrexate. J Rheumatol 26:302, 1999.
161. Tishler M, Goldbrut B, Shoenfeld Y, Yaron M: Anti-Ro (SSA) antibodies in patients with rheumatoid arthritis: A possible marker for gold induced side effects. J Rheumatol 21:1040, 1994.

162. Ho M, Pullar T: Vasomotor reactions with gold [editorial]. Br J Rheumatol 36:154, 1997.
163. Healey LA, Backes MB: Nitritoid reactions and angiotensin-converting-enzyme inhibitor [letter]. N Engl J Med 321:763, 1989.
164. Arthur AB, Klinkhoff A, Teufel A: Nitritoid reactions: case report, review, and recommendations for management. J Rheumatol 28:2209-2212, 2001.
165. Halla JT, Hardin JG, Linn JE: Postinjection nonvasomotor reactions during chrysotherapy. Arthritis Rheum 20:1188, 1977.
166. Trotter MJ, Tron VA, Hollingdale J, Rivers JK: Localized Chrysiasis induced by laser therapy Arch Dermatol 131:1411, 1995.
167. Hall CC: The natural course of gold and penicillamine nephropathy: Long term study of 54 patients. Adv Exp Med Biol 252:247, 1989.
168. Yan A, Davis P: Gold induced marrow suppression: a review of 10 cases. J Rheumatol 17:47, 1990.
169. Coblyn JS, Weinblatt M, Holdsworth D, et al: Gold induced thrombocytopenia: A clinical and immunogenetic study of twenty-three patients. Ann Intern Med 95:178, 1981.
170. Aaron S, Davis P, Percy J: Neutropenia occurring during the course of crysotherapy: Review of 25 cases. J Rheumatol 12:897, 1985.
171. Dillon AM, Luthra HS, Conn D, et al: Parenteral gold therapy in the Felty syndrome. Medicine, 65:107, 1986.
172. Reid C, Patterson AC: Pure red cell aplasia after gold treatment. BMJ ii 1457, 1977.
173. Tomioka R, King TE Jr: Gold-induced pulmonary disease: Clinical features, outcome, and differentiation from rheumatoid lung disease. Am J Respir Crit Care Med 155:1011, 1997.
174. Dorta G, Schnegg G, Schmied P: Treatment of gold-induced enteritis with octreotide. Lancet 342:179, 1993.
175. Fam AG, Gordon DA, Sarkozi J, et al: Neurologic complications associated with gold therapy for rheumatoid arthritis. J Rheumatol 11:700, 1984.
176. Clements PJ, Wong WK, Hurwitz, et al: The disability index of the Health Assessment Questionnaire is a predictor and correlate of outcome in the high-dose versus low-dose penicillamine in systemic sclerosis trial. Arthritis Rheum 44:653, 2001.
177. Joyce DA: D-Penicillamine pharmacokinetics and pharmacodynamics in man. Pharmacol Ther 42:405, 1989.
178. Multi-Centre Trial Group: Controlled trials of D-penicillamine in severe rheumatoid arthritis. Lancet 1:275, 1973.
179. Dash S, Seibold JR, Tiku ML: Successful treatment of methotrexate-induced nodulosis with D-penicillamine. J Rheumatol 26:1396, 1999.
180. Vardi P, Brik R, Barzilai D, et al: Frequent induction of insulin autoantibodies by D-penicillamine in patients with rheumatoid arthritis. J Rheumatol 19:1527, 1992.
181. Proceedings of the 7th French Conference of Rheumatology, Paris, 1985. Rev Rhum 53:1, 1986.
182. Hakoda M, Taniguchi A, Kamatani N, et al: Intermittent treatment with D-penicillamine is effective in lower doses and with fewer adverse effects in patients with rheumatoid arthritis. J Rheumatol 21:1637, 1994.
183. Langan MN, Thomas P: Penicillamine-induced liver disease. Am J Gastroenterol 82:1318, 1987.
184. Gaskin G, Thompson EM, Pusey CD: Goodpasture-like syndrome associated with anti-myeloperoxidase antibodies following penicillamine treatment. Nephrol Dial Transplant 10:1925, 1995.
185. Pegg SJ, Lang BA, Mikhail EL, Hughes DM: Fatal bronchiolitis obliterans in a patient with juvenile rheumatoid arthritis receiving chrysotherapy. J Rheumatol 21:549, 1994.
186. Andonopoulos AP, Terzis E, Tsibri E, et al: D-Penicillamine induced myasthenia gravis in rheumatoid arthritis: An unpredictable common occurrence? Clin Rheumatol 13:586, 1994.
187. Chin GL, Kong NCT, Lee BC, Rose IM: Penicillamine-induced lupus syndrome in a patients with classical rheumatoid arthritis. J Rheumatol 18:947, 1991.
188. Kim HA, Song YW: A comparison between bucillamine and D-penicillamine in the treatment of rheumatoid arthritis. Rheumatol Int 17:5, 1997.

59 Methotrexate, Leflunomide, and Combination Therapies

JAMES R. O'DELL

Methotrexate

It would be difficult to overstate the importance of methotrexate (MTX) in the contemporary management of rheumatic disease and, in particular, rheumatoid arthritis (RA). Because of its antiproliferative effects, MTX was introduced over 50 years ago to treat cancer. Over the last 20 years, it has become the disease-modifying antirheumatic drug (DMARD) of choice in the treatment of RA and is used in many other rheumatic diseases as well.

CHEMICAL STRUCTURE

MTX is a structural analogue of folic acid and has substitutions in the pteridine group and *para*-aminobenzoic acid structure (Fig. 59–1). The structure of folic acid (pteroylglutamic acid) consists of three elements: a multiring pteridine group, linked to a *para*-aminobenzoic acid, which is connected to a terminal glutamic acid residue (see Fig. 59–1).

PHARMACOLOGY

After ingestion, folic acid is reduced by the enzyme dihydrofolate reductase (DHFR) to the metabolically active folates dihydrofolate and tetrahydrofolate. These reduced folates are essential in the conversion of homocysteine to methionine, in the metabolism of histidine, and in the synthesis of purines and thymidylate. As a folate acid analogue, MTX acts as an antimetabolite, binding and inactivating the enzyme DHFR. Inhibition of DHFR results in the cessation of the synthesis of thymidylate, inosinic acid, and other purine metabolites. MTX also inhibits protein synthesis by preventing the conversion of glycine to serine and homocysteine to methionine.

MTX is metabolized from a monoglutamate to a polyglutamated derivative. MTX polyglutamates remain within the cell in the absence of extracellular drugs and are more potent than the monoglutamate.[1] The synthesis of MTX polyglutamates increases with the duration of therapy. MTX polyglutamates inhibit other folate-dependent enzymes, including thymidylate synthetase and 5-aminoimidazole-4-carboxamide ribonucleotide (AICAR) transformylase.

Folinic acid, also known as leucovorin (see Fig. 59–1), is a fully reduced and, therefore, metabolically active folate coenzyme and does not require reduction by the enzyme DHFR. Folinic acid restores thymidylate, purine, and methionine biosynthesis, even in the presence of MTX. Folinic acid is used to "rescue" normal cells from the toxicity induced by MTX and is used with high-dose MTX in cancer chemotherapy and as a treatment for acute MTX overdose and hematologic toxicity.

ACTIONS OF METHOTREXATE

The mechanisms of action whereby MTX exerts its therapeutic effects in rheumatic disease are incompletely understood. Therapeutic effects may result from MTX's antifolate activity by inhibition of DHFR; inhibition of other folate-dependent enzymes, including AICAR transformylase; immunosuppressive properties; or anti-inflammatory effects. It appears most plausible that a combination of these factors account for the drug's therapeutic profile in RA.

Inhibition of the enzyme AICAR transformylase by MTX interferes with de novo purine biosynthesis.[2] Inhibition of AICAR transformylase increases the intracellular concentration of its substrate, AICAR, which stimulates the release of adenosine (Fig. 59–2). Adenosine is a potent inhibitor of stimulated neutrophil function and has potent anti-inflammatory properties. In the murine air sac model of inflammation, MTX increased intracellular accumulation of AICAR, which led to increased adenosine concentrations in the exudates that inhibited leukocyte accumulation.[3] This reduction of leukocyte accumulation was partially reversed by adenosine deaminase and completely reversed by an adenosine A_2 receptor antagonist. Adenosine also inhibits the production of several proinflammatory cytokines, including tumor necrosis factor-α (TNF-α), interleukin-6 (IL-6), and IL-8.

The high doses of MTX used as chemotherapy for cancer result in severe immunosuppression. In RA, profound immunosuppressive effects have not been demonstrated with low-dose MTX. Global suppression of T cell function or phenotypes has not been reported with MTX in RA.[4-6] MTX in vitro induces apoptosis of activated T cells and clonal deletion of activated T cells.[7] Adenosine release accounts for only a small portion of this effect. This process can be blocked by the addition of folinic acid.

MTX's effects on humoral immunity include a decrease in serum levels of immunoglobulin G (IgG), IgM, and IgA,[5] suppression of IgM rheumatoid factor synthesis in vitro,[8] and a reduction in IgA and IgM rheumatoid factor levels in vivo.[9]

In a rabbit corneal model,[10] MTX inhibits neovascularization, suggesting an antiangiogenic effect. MTX also inhibits the formation of *S*-adenosyl methionine, the methyl donor required for protein and lipid methylation.[11]

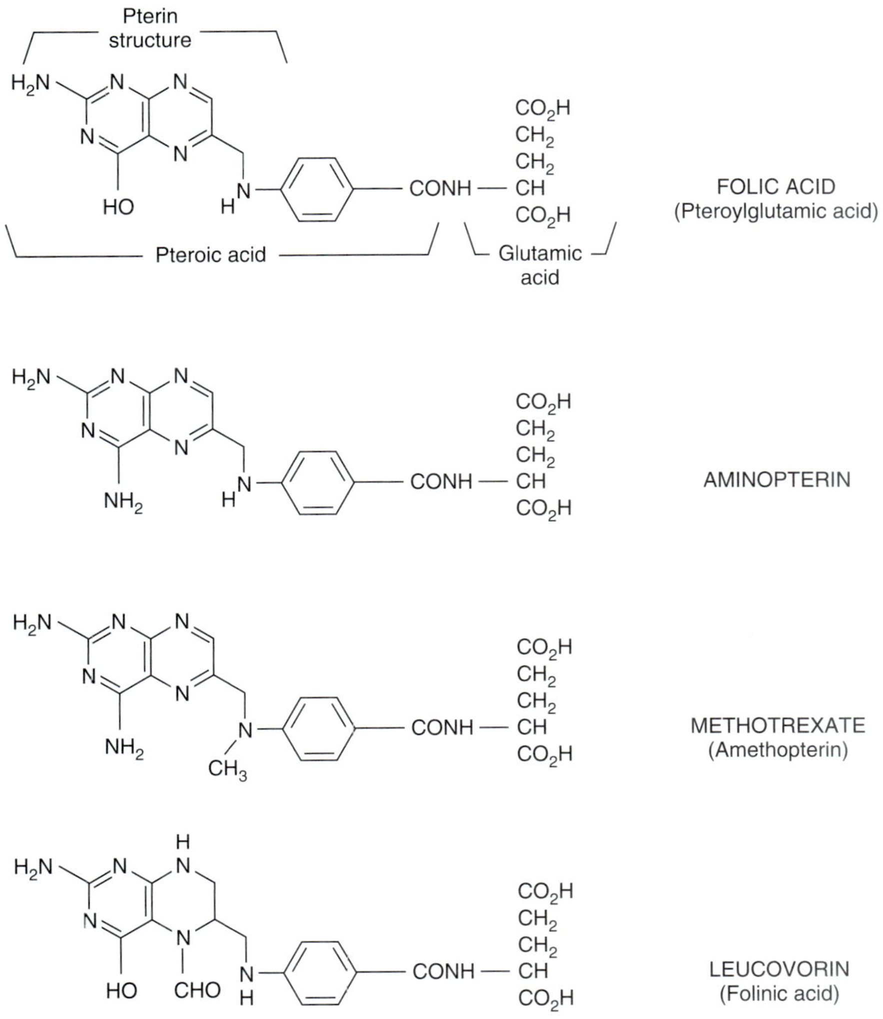

FIGURE 59–1 · Structure of folic acid, aminopterin, methotrexate, and leucovorin.

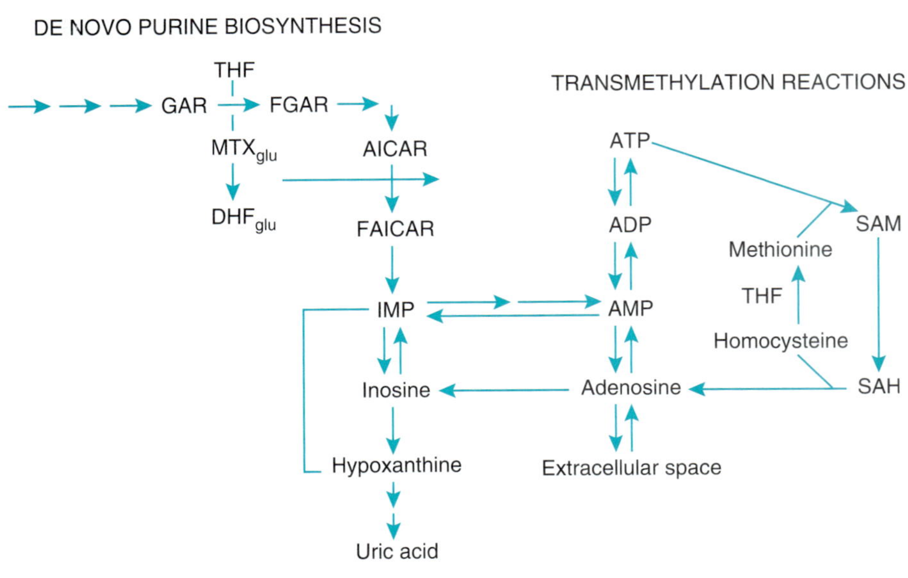

FIGURE 59–2 · Proposed Mechanism of Action of Methotrexate. (From Cronstein BN, Naime D, Ostad E: The anti-inflammatory mechanism of methotrexate: increased adenosine release at inflamed sites diminishes leukocyte accumulation in one in vivo model of inflammation. J Clin Invest 92:2675, 1993.)

MTX has multiple effects on cytokine levels, production, and activity. In vitro, MTX inhibits IL-1 activity, but not IL-1 production or secretion.[12] Inhibition of IL-1 activity can be blocked by folinic acid, but not folic acid.[13] No consistent effects on IL-1 levels or stimulated IL-1 production from peripheral blood mononuclear cells were observed in RA patients receiving MTX.[14] A reduction in IL-6, IL-8, soluble TNF receptor, and soluble IL-2 receptor levels has been observed with MTX.[15] In vitro MTX has been shown to increase T helper type 2 (Th2) cytokines, IL-10, and IL-4 gene expression with a corresponding decrease in T helper type 1 (Th1) cytokines, IL-2, and interferon gamma (IFN-γ).[16]

An anti-inflammatory effect has been suggested by MTX's rapid onset of action and the flare after drug discontinuation. The C-reactive protein level and erythrocyte sedimentation rate decrease several days after a single injection of MTX.[17] In vivo chemotaxis, after stimulation with leukotriene B_4, was blocked in psoriasis patients with MTX.[18] In RA patients, low-dose MTX decreased the generation of leukotriene B_4 from stimulated neutrophils ex vivo.[19] MTX also reduces in vitro prostaglandin E_2 release[20] and superoxide production.[21] Recently, MTX and leflunomide have both been shown to substantially inhibit neutrophil chemotaxis in RA, both ex vivo[22] and in vivo.[23]

Synovial tissue metalloproteinase levels decrease after MTX therapy,[24] including a significant decrease in collagenase gene expression, but not stromelysin mRNA levels or levels of tissue inhibitor of metalloproteinase-1 (TIMP-1).[25]

PHARMACOKINETICS

At low doses, MTX can be administered either orally or parenterally. The bioavailability of low-dose oral MTX (less than 20 mg/week) is relatively high, but there is significant individual-patient variability. Absorption is not reduced by concomitant food intake.[26] Forty-one RA patients who received 10 mg/m^2 of oral MTX had a mean bioavailability of 70 percent with a range of 40 to 100 percent.[27] The mean absorption time was 1.2 hours with a terminal half-life of 6 hours. Four hours after MTX administration, synovial fluid concentrations equal serum levels.[27] The pharmacokinetics of subcutaneous MTX are equivalent to intramuscular MTX; maximum serum concentration is attained within 2 hours of injection by either route.[28] Patients responding incompletely to oral MTX should be given a trial of parenteral MTX to ensure the bioavailability of the drug. There is also equivalent bioavailability between tablets and orally administered parenteral solution[29]; the parenteral solution is much less expensive.

MTX undergoes some hepatic metabolism by the enzyme aldehyde oxidase to the 7-hydroxymethotrexate metabolite; this metabolite has unknown significance in RA. MTX and metabolites are excreted by the kidney by glomerular filtration and proximal tubular secretion. Organic acids such as sulfonamides, salicylates, and probenecid competitively inhibit tubular secretion, which delays MTX clearance. Accumulation of MTX in malignant effusions has been reported.

MTX is 50 to 60 percent bound to plasma proteins. An increase in free MTX because of displacement from albumin by more highly protein-bound drugs such as aspirin, nonsteroidal anti-inflammatory drugs (NSAIDs), and sulfonamides can occur. This is generally of limited clinical significance with low MTX doses, because the increase in free MTX is usually only modest. A significant pharmacokinetic or clinical interaction has not been reported between low-dose MTX and a variety of NSAIDs.[30] There is a wide variation in the kinetics of MTX with NSAIDs in juvenile RA.[31] Although not a common problem in rheumatic diseases, administration of NSAIDs or aspirin with high-dose MTX (as used in cancer chemotherapy) may be toxic and is contraindicated.

Drugs that affect renal function should be used with caution because of the renal clearance of MTX and, therefore, the increased risk of MTX toxicity that could occur because of decreased clearance. Probenecid should be avoided because it inhibits tubular secretion of MTX. Trimethoprim-sulfamethoxazole should also be avoided, or used with extreme caution, because of possible hematologic toxicity with MTX.[32] Mechanisms for this toxicity include an additive antifolate effect from trimethoprim, decreased MTX clearance due to inhibition of tubular secretion by sulfamethoxazole, and altered MTX plasma protein binding.

METHOTREXATE USE IN RHEUMATOID ARTHRITIS

Because of its effects on proliferation, aminopterin (a closely related compound) was first used by Gubner and colleagues[33] to treat eight patients with arthritis; they reported these results in 1951. Six of their eight patients appear to have had RA, and five of these patients improved, in some cases quite dramatically. All patients, however, flared when the aminopterin was stopped. These early findings of significant benefit did not receive much attention, in part because there was a great deal of excitement about corticosteroids, which were introduced at approximately this same time. MTX has been utilized extensively to treat malignancies and psoriasis (including psoriatic arthritis) since the early 1950s. In 1972, Hoffmeister[34] reported his extensive experience with MTX in RA and followed this up with a more detailed report in 1983.[35] These observations led to a flurry of activity and to the double-blind, controlled studies of the mid-1980s (detailed later in chapter) that have established MTX as the preferred treatment for RA.

The efficacy of MTX in RA has been clearly established by three different, but critically important, paths. Initially, as is usually the case, the process was set in motion by clinicians reporting their uncontrolled observations of the efficacy of MTX in their clinical practice. Next, it was necessary to rigorously prove the short-term benefits of MTX in carefully controlled, randomized, double-blind studies in which MTX was first compared to placebo and later to other accepted DMARDs. More recently, open, prospective, longitudinal studies have played a critical role in establishing the long-term benefit and tolerability of MTX. These later studies have been particularly significant because RA is a lifelong disease;

and although other DMARDs have been successful in the short-term treatment of RA (6 months to 1 year),[36] none compare to the durable response seen with MTX.[37-42]

After the initial reports by Gubner and colleagues and Hoffmeister, other investigators also reported favorable clinical experiences at about the same time (e.g., Willkens[43] and Wilke[44]). These reports provided the impetus and enthusiasm for the controlled studies that followed. Four well-designed, blinded, placebo-controlled trials[4,5,45,46] published in 1984 and 1985 had a tremendous impact on the treatment of RA (Table 59–1). These trials varied in design and duration: Two of these trials used oral MTX and two used intramuscular (IM) MTX; two trials had a crossover and two were parallel; and the duration of treatment varied from 6 to 28 weeks. Although the design and duration of therapy in these trials varied, the conclusions did not; all showed MTX to be superior to placebo in the short-term treatment of RA. A meta-analysis of these trials by Tugwell and coworkers[47] showed that MTX-treated patients received a 37-percent greater improvement in swollen joint and tender joint scores, a 39-percent greater improvement in joint pain, and a 46-percent greater improvement in morning stiffness. MTX was generally well tolerated in these trials; withdrawal rates ranged from 0 to 32 percent and were mostly for minor toxicities (i.e., stomatitis, nausea). Taken together, the results of these trials firmly established MTX as an effective therapy for the treatment of RA, at least in the short term.

MTX has been shown to be both more effective and better tolerated than oral gold,[48] but it has appeared to have similar short-term efficacy to IM gold in four trials.[49-52] MTX appeared to offer more clinical benefit than azathioprine in three trials,[53-56] although no difference was found in a fourth trial.[57] The meta-analysis done by Felson and coworkers[36] showed MTX superior to placebo, auranofen, and probably hydroxychloroquine, and comparable to penicillamine, sulfasalazine, and IM gold. This meta-analysis probably underestimates the difference between MTX and the other DMARDs, because the patients enrolled in the MTX trials were, in general, felt to be more refractory patients. Notably, no trial has ever suggested that any other synthetic DMARD is superior to MTX.

RA is a lifelong disease process, and part of the paradox of treatment has been that, as the previously discussed meta-analysis suggests, some DMARDs have shown short-term effectiveness but have not had a significant impact on the long-term outcome of patients with RA. This paradox is apparently explained by the accumulating evidence that the short-term benefit of most DMARDs is not sustained; few patients continue to take these drugs after 3years.[40,42] Wolfe[42] found that median time to discontinuation of MTX was 4.61 years, more than three times longer than auranofen, IM gold, or D-penicillamine. Pincus and colleagues[40] have shown that 60 percent of patients continued MTX at 5 years, compared to less than 25 percent for penicillamine, gold, hydroxychloroquine, and azathioprine. As important as the short-term, blinded studies (see Table 59–1) have been in establishing MTX as a viable treatment option for RA patients, the prospective, long-term, observational studies[40,42] have really separated MTX from the other DMARDs as the long-term treatment of choice for RA. Of all the DMARDs, MTX appears to have the best efficacy-to-toxicity ratio.[58]

Despite all the favorable efficacy reports mentioned previously, MTX rarely induces remissions of RA.[59-61] In fact, even if we lower the standards considerably and accept 50-percent improvement by Paulus criteria, only approximately one third of RA patients treated with MTX achieve this modest goal at 2[62] or 4 years.[63] The gold standard of efficacy for a DMARD has been its ability to halt, or at least retard, the progression of erosions. MTX does not halt erosive disease,[56,64-72] but studies have shown that it does slow the progression of erosions when compared to auranofen,[64-66] IM gold,[64,67] azathioprine,[56,64,68] leflunomide,[69] and NSAIDs.[64] Other studies, however, have failed to show an advantage of MTX; similar rates of progression of erosions have been reported before and during MTX therapy,[70] with MTX compared to IM gold,[71] leflunomide[72] or azathioprine.

OTHER RHEUMATIC DISEASES

MTX has been used for several decades for psoriatic arthritis, despite the paucity of clinical trials. There is a clinical impression that higher doses of MTX are required to treat psoriatic arthritis than are needed to treat RA. There has been a small open experience with Reiter's syndrome[73] using MTX doses of 15 to 30 mg/week.

MTX has been used successfully in treating Felty's syndrome[74] and the large granulocytic lymphocyte syndrome when it is found in patients with RA.[75] Improvement in neutrophil count occurs within 4 to 8 weeks of MTX initiation in both cases. Doses of MTX from 7.5 to 20.0 mg/week are required to improve the neutrophil count.

TABLE 59–1 • METHOTREXATE PLACEBO-CONTROLLED, RANDOMIZED TRIALS

Trial Feature	Weinblatt[4]	Williams[45]	Thompson[46]	Anderson[5]
Number of subjects	35	189	48	15
Design crossover	Parallel	Parallel	Crossover	Crossover
Duration	24 weeks	18 weeks	6 weeks	26 weeks
Methotrexate dose (mg/wk)	7.5-15.0	7.5-15.0	10.0-25.0	5.0-25.0
Administration	Oral	Oral	Intramuscular	Intramuscular
Clinical response	Improvement	Improvement	Improvement	Improvement
Withdrawal due to adverse events	1	30	2	1

Open studies of cutaneous vasculitis of RA,[76] adult-onset Still's disease,[77] multicentric reticulohistiocytosis,[78] systemic lupus erythematosus,[79,80] non–life-threatening Wegener's granulomatosus,[81] and Takayasu's arteritis[82] all report improvement with MTX. A small, randomized trial reported a response in treating scleroderma.[83] Adjuvant MTX in polymyalgia rheumatica has not been shown to be helpful.[84]

MTX has also been successfully used in juvenile RA. A definitive, randomized, placebo-controlled trial with 127 children demonstrated that MTX at a dose of 10.0 mg/m^2 was superior to 5.0 mg/m^2 or placebo.[85] Sixty-three percent of the children who received the higher dose (10.0 mg/m^2) of MTX improved, compared to 32 percent in the lower-dose group (5.0 mg/m^2), and 36 percent in the placebo group. Only three children discontinued MTX because of mild to moderate side effects; none had severe toxicity. MTX is an effective treatment for children with resistant juvenile RA, but higher mean doses based on body weight are used than for adults.

DOSE AND DRUG ADMINISTRATION

MTX is given only on a weekly basis. More frequent administration is associated with a significantly increased risk of liver toxicity.[86] MTX can be administered orally or by parenteral injection. The starting dose is usually 5 to 10 mg given as a single weekly dose; occasionally, to improve tolerability, the MTX dose may be divided and each half given 12 hours apart. The dosage of MTX can be escalated, usually every 4 to 8 weeks to 20 to 30 mg/week, to achieve the desired clinical response. The bioavailability of orally administered MTX is variable, averaging approximately 70 percent at low doses, but decreasing at higher doses.[27] Because the bioavailability is variable (some patients may absorb only 40%) and appears to decrease at higher doses, a trial of parenteral MTX is generally recommended if patients have active disease despite approximately 20 mg/week orally. The bioavailability of subcutaneous MTX is similar to IM[28] and is generally recommended. Injectable MTX is well absorbed if given orally[29] and, although somewhat cumbersome, may result in substantial cost savings.

Concomitantly, administration of folic acid (1 to 3 mg/day) decreases the frequency of toxicities, including mucositis, nausea, hematologic abnormalities, and liver enzyme elevations without seemingly interfering with the clinical efficacy.[87-89] There are no data to address the question of whether folic acid can decrease the pulmonary toxicity of MTX. Folic acid administration will also decrease the hyperhomocystinemia that patients on MTX may get, and this may be important to help decrease the already high cardiovascular risk of patients with RA.

High-dose folinic acid (leucovorin) rescue is a common practice when high-dose MTX is used in the treatment of malignancies. Low-dose folinic acid has been used and can also markedly reduce MTX toxicity in rheumatic disease therapy without interfering with efficacy if given in doses of 2.5 to 5 mg/week and not administered until 24 hours after the MTX dose. Because folic acid is widely available and less expensive, it is preferred by most.

TOXICITY

The initial enthusiasm for the efficacy of MTX in RA was tempered by a fear of its potential toxicity. In particular, great concern about its effects, especially on the liver, grew out of the experience of using MTX on a daily basis to treat psoriasis. With accumulating clinical experience, these concerns have been alleviated.

Some of the toxicities of MTX (stomatitis, nausea, bone marrow depression) are dose dependent, appear to be related to folate deficiencies, and respond to folate replacement; other toxicities appear to be idiosyncratic or allergic and in most cases require discontinuation of MTX (e.g., pneumonitis). Still other toxicities, such as liver fibrosis and cirrhosis, appear to be multifactorial and may depend on the presence of concomitant risk factors, total dose, and frequency of administration.

Hepatic

The risk of clinically significant liver toxicity and the belief that this toxicity could be evaluated only by frequent liver biopsies were major factors that slowed the acceptance of MTX as a first-line therapeutic option for RA. This risk of MTX, when given once weekly to patients who abstain from alcohol consumption and are monitored carefully, appears to be low—on the order of 1 case per 1000 after 5 years of use.[90] The accumulated clinical experience that led to the American College of Rheumatology (ACR) subcommittee's guidelines on monitoring liver toxicity of MTX[86] has greatly aided the clinical use of this drug in RA and have stood the test of time.[91]

These guidelines recommend that liver blood tests (asparate aminotransferase [AST], alanine aminotransferase [ALT]) be done every 4 to 8 weeks, and that MTX be stopped if more than half of these tests are abnormal in a 1-year period. Additionally, they recommend following the serum albumin and making modifications if a previously normal albumin level falls below 3.5 g/dl. Practically, modification in the dose or administration should be made so that patients do not have multiple liver blood test elevations. Biopsies are recommended only in those patients who continue to have enzyme abnormalities and for whom continuation of MTX therapy is contemplated.

The pathophysiology of MTX liver injury is still poorly understood and appears to be multifactorial. The experience in patients with psoriasis clearly shows that toxicity is significantly decreased if the interval between doses is increased. Of interest in this regard is a report by Kremer and colleagues[92] that some patients can successfully take MTX every other week rather than on the usual weekly schedule. Additionally, psoriasis itself may be a risk factor for MTX liver toxicity. Alcohol consumption, alpha-1-antitrypsin deficiency, morbid obesity, diabetes, and chronic hepatitis B or C have all been implicated as possible risk factors for MTX toxicity.[93]

Hematologic

Bone marrow toxicity, in most cases, is dose dependent and responds to folate acid administration. To prevent toxicity, MTX is usually started at a low dose (10 mg/wk) and increased every month to 2 months (up to a dose of 20 to 30 mg/wk) as needed to achieve the desired clinical efficacy. Complete blood count (CBCs) with platelet counts every 4 to 8 weeks are recommended, as are serum creatinines.[90,94] Rising mean corpuscular volume (MCVs) may be a harbinger of toxicity, but this response may be unreliable in patients who are also receiving folate.[95,96] Folic acid is often given prophylactically and may be increased if bone marrow suppression is present. Severe, life-threatening bone marrow toxicity can be treated with folinic acid (leucovorin), and, in some cases, success has been reported with granulocyte-stimulating factor (GSF).[97]

Because the elimination of MTX is dependent on the kidney function, decreases in renal function may precipitate bone marrow and other toxicities in MTX-treated patients who have been previously stable.

Pulmonary

MTX lung toxicity continues to be an enigma. Recent studies have helped shed some light on this problem.[98,99] Patients generally present with shortness of breath, tachypnea, dry cough, and fevers. Chest radiographs most typically show a bilateral interstitial infiltrate (although this varies). Infectious causes, including opportunistic organisms, must always be ruled out. A bronchoscopy with transbronchial biopsy and bronchoalveolar lavage is recommended, especially to help exclude infections. The absence of infectious causes and the presence of eosinophilia, desquamative lesions, and pneumocyte proliferation favor MTX as the cause. After discontinuation of the MTX, treatment should be supportive, with the use of steroids in the more severe cases. Some patients with this toxicity have been successfully restarted on MTX,[100] but some clinicians have reported mortality in up to 50 percent of retreated patients.[98]

Factors that appear to predispose to MTX lung toxicity include age, blue-collar occupation, smoking (in women), diabetes, pleuropulmonary rheumatoid disease, and skin rashes from MTX.[99,101] Most experts recommend a baseline chest radiograph before starting MTX.[94]

Mucocutaneous

The mucocutaneous toxicities of MTX, which have been reported to occur in up to one third of patients, are dose dependent and respond to folate replacement. Patients generally complain of fairly minor oral ulcerations; but severe ulceration of the mouth, esophagus, bowel, and vagina can occur, especially at higher doses. The use of folic acid replacement in these patients has minimized this toxicity,[87-89] which previously precluded the use of MTX in many patients.

Malignancies

The induction of malignancies by MTX is a concern, and several studies have examined this question with conflicting conclusions. Recently, some reports of lymphoma in MTX-treated RA patients have appeared. Because the incidence of lymphoma is increased in RA patients anyway,[102] these reports are hard to interpret. The case for a causative role of MTX has been strengthened, however, because a number of these cases have been B cell lymphomas[103-105] of the type commonly seen in association with immunosuppression and that regress after the discontinuation of MTX.[103,104] This question has been reviewed by Moder and colleagues.[106] The potential benefits of MTX for most RA patients, however, far outweigh these statistically small risks.[107]

Miscellaneous

Nausea is a common problem with MTX and usually occurs within 24 to 48 hours after ingestion. Patients taking MTX may also describe flu-like symptoms shortly after taking their weekly dose. Nausea, low-grade fevers, myalgias, and chills are the most common signs of the so-called "methotrexate flu." These side effects usually respond to supplementation with folic acid, decreasing the dose, switching from oral to parenteral administration, or changing the time of the dose (so the patient takes MTX right before going to bed).

The development of, or increase in, the number or size of rheumatoid nodules (nodulosis) has been reported to occur in RA patients treated with MTX,[108,109] even when the synovitis is under excellent control. The mechanism of this nodule formation has been suggested to be due to an increase in adenosine, which appears to promote nodule formation.[110] This reaction can be quite problematic and no treatment is known; although some have suggested treatment with sulfasalazine, hydroxychloroquine, or colchicine. Conversely, nodules have also been reported to decrease during MTX therapy. Leukocytoclastic vasculitis has also been attributed to MTX therapy.[111]

PATIENT SELECTION AND MONITORING

Not all patients with RA will be candidates for MTX therapy. Patients with very mild disease, those with renal insufficiency, those with liver or lung disease, or those who desire to continue to drink alcohol should, in most cases, not be treated with MTX.

Two sets of guidelines published by the ACR provide excellent recommendations for starting and monitoring MTX therapy.[84,94] The ACR guidelines for monitoring liver toxicity recommend AST, ALT, albumin, and hepatitis serology in all patients prior to starting MTX. Additionally, a serum creatinine, a CBC with platelet count, and a chest radiograph are recommended by the ACR guidelines for monitoring MTX. With an eye toward cost effectiveness, most clinicians routinely do the hepatitis B and C screening only in patients with abnormal AST, albumin, or both or a history of high-risk behaviors. This recommendation should be adjusted based on practice environment. Liver biopsies prior to initiating MTX are not routinely recommended. The rare patients whom one wants to treat with MTX despite abnormalities in screening lab or other significant risk factors may require liver biopsy before starting MTX. Liver biopsy before treatment may also be considered in patients with remote or questionable histories of significant alcohol intake.

Leflunomide

Leflunomide, a novel isoxazole derivative, is the newest synthetic DMARD to be approved for the treatment of RA. It emerged from a specific anti-inflammatory drug development program and has potent immunomodulatory effects first demonstrated in mouse models of inflammatory arthritis.

CHEMICAL STRUCTURE

Leflunomide is a low molecular weight isoxazole compound (Fig. 59–3). It is chemically unrelated to any previous immunosuppressant. Leflunomide is a prodrug and is rapidly and completely converted to its active metabolite, the malononitriloamide A77 1726 (see Fig. 59–3).

PHARMACOLOGY

The gastrointestinal tract and liver rapidly and completely convert ingested leflunomide into the active metabolite, A77 1726. Circulating A77 1726 is highly bound (more than 99%) to plasma proteins, predominantly albumin. The plasma concentration of A77 1726 is linearly correlated with ingested dose over a range of 5 to 25 mg after single oral doses.[112]

ACTIONS OF LEFLUNOMIDE

Like MTX, the precise mechanism of action responsible for the effects of leflunomide in rheumatic disease is not completely understood.[113] Leflunomide is immunomodulatory with the net effect being a reduction in the activated T lymphocytes. Its effects vary depending on concentration: At the concentration of the active metabolite (A77 1726) achieved in patients, its major effect appears to be a reversible inhibition of the enzyme dihydroorotate dehydrogenase (DHODH), which results in inhibition of pyrimidine ribonucleotide synthesis. At higher concentrations, A77 1726 also inhibits tyrosine kinases.

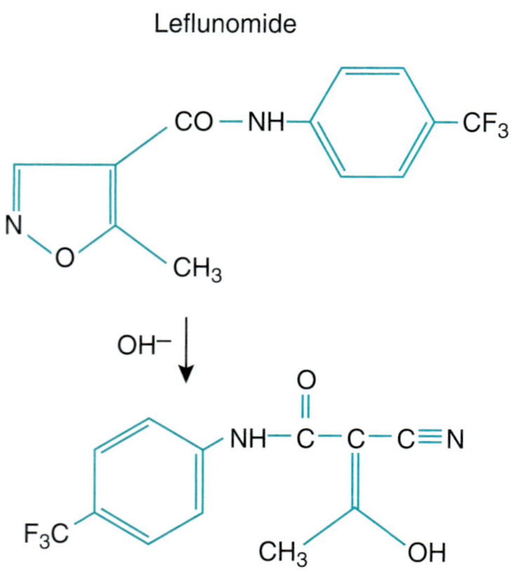

FIGURE 59–3 • Leflunomide is rapidly and completely metabolized to its active metabolite, A77 1726.

Activation of T cells requires significant increases in pyrimidine biosynthesis. In vitro, mitogen-stimulated activation of T cells is blocked by A77 1726. Experiments that demonstrated that the addition of uridine to these cultures could reverse A77 1726 inhibition[114] suggested that this active metabolite of leflunomide was working via an inhibition of pyrimidine ribonucleotide biosynthesis.[115-119] Other experiments confirmed that leflunomide acts at a site within the pathway for de novo pyrimidine ribonucleotide synthesis.[114,116-121] Further, the only enzyme inhibited by A77 1726 in this pathway, at concentration obtained in vivo, is DHODH.[118] Resting lymphocytes are essentially unaffected by leflunomide because this pathway is inactive in resting lymphocytes, which maintain ribonucleotide requirements largely through salvage pathways.[122,123] A critical step in this pathway that occurs in the mitochondria (Fig. 59–4) is the conversion of dihydroorotate to orotate; this step is catalyzed by DHODH and results in the production of uridine monophosphate (rUMP).

Further evidence to support this effect of leflunomide are experiments that confirm that inhibition of DHODH results in accumulations of dihydroorotate and decreased amounts of rUMP[117] (see Fig. 59–4) and that inhibition of DHODH produces an arrest of lymphocytes in the G1 phase of the cell cycle.[115,124] In cultures of human T cells, A77 1726 depletes pyrimidine ribonucleotide rUMP pools and results in an accumulation of nuclear p53. Induction of the proto-oncogene p53 correlates with cell-cycle arrest.[125] Cell-cycle arrest also results in accumulation of p53 in the nucleus, where it initiates the activation of p21,[125-127] a potent inhibitor of cyclin-dependent kinase (CDK). CDK activates cyclin D and E; therefore, the accumulation of nuclear p53 results in cell-cycle arrest in the G1 phase.[128]

At higher concentrations, A77 1726 inhibits phosphorylation of tyrosine kinases[129-134] that are critical for cell growth and differentiation of activated cells.[135] This inhibition has been proposed to partially or completely explain leflunomide's antiproliferative effects; however, it is unclear whether concentrations sufficient to achieve this effect are obtained in vivo.

Leflunomide also appears to have the ability to block the activation of nuclear factor κB (NFκB).[136,137] NF-κB regulates the expression of genes important in inflammatory processes, including those seen in inflammatory arthritis.[138-140] In vitro studies have also shown that leflunomide blocks TNF-induced NFκB activation, I-κBα phosphoralation, I-κBα kinase (IKK) activation, activation of activator protein-1 (AP-1) and the c-Jun N-terminal protein kinase, and suppresses TNF-induced apoptosis.[137] Finally, ex vivo and in vitro studies in humans have shown that leflunomide and MTX both significantly inhibit neutrophil chemotaxis, which may significantly decrease the recruitment of inflammatory cells into the joints.[22,23]

Leflunomide has been shown to be effective in a number of animal models of RA. In the commonly used

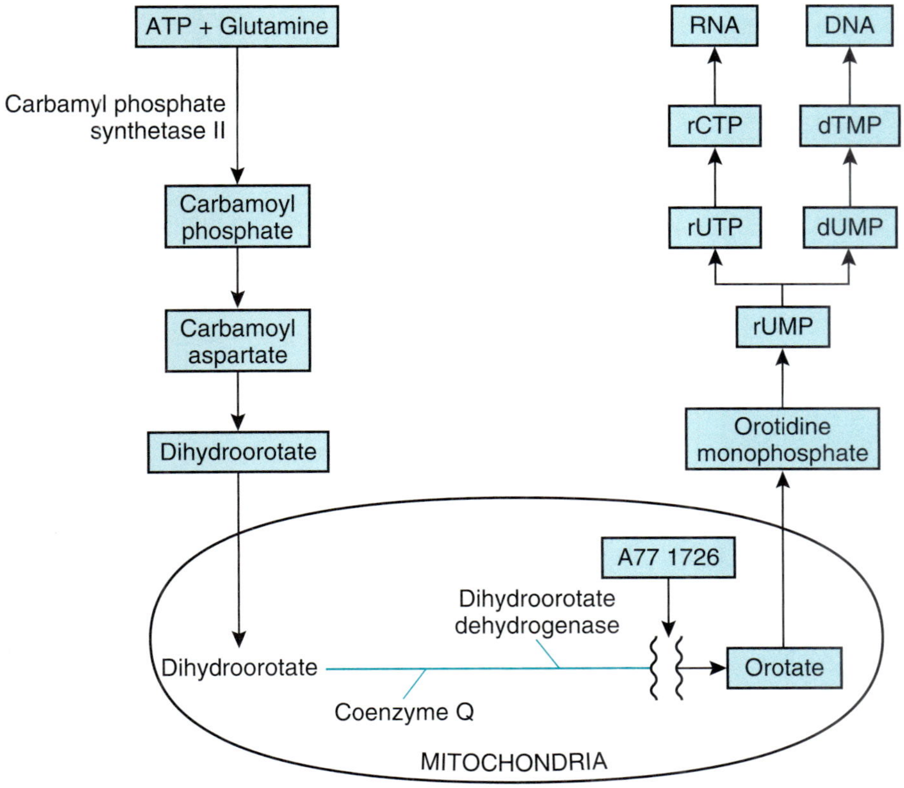

FIGURE 59–4 · Leflunomide's active meta-bolite, A77 1726, blocks the conversion of dihydroorotate to orotate within the mitochondria.

rat model, adjuvant-induced arthritis (AIA), orally administered leflunomide given during the induction of arthritis appears to almost completely abrogate the development of the disease.[141-143] In another rat model of RA, bovine serum albumin (BSA)-induced arthritis, leflunomide reduces both the clinical manifestations of arthritis and the production of antibodies to collagen and proteoglycans, which, in general, correlate with arthritis severity.[144] Leflunomide has also been shown to reduce arthritis in mouse models of RA.[145,146]

PHARMACOKINETICS

Leflunomide's active metabolite (A77 1726) has a half-life of approximately 2 weeks (mean 15.5 days).[112] A77 1726 undergoes enterohepatic recirculation. In healthy subjects, 90 percent of leflunomide is excreted by 28 days,[112] but some may be present for much longer periods. In healthy subjects, the proportion excreted by the kidney and gut are nearly equal. Because enterohepatic recirculation occurs and may be responsible for detectable A77 1726 being present in the body months or years later, the ability to rapidly and effectively eliminate A77 1726 with cholestyramine is important. Because of the very long half-life of A77 1726, initial recommendations advocate giving a loading dose of leflunomide (100 mg/day for 3 days) to achieve more rapid steady-state, therapeutic levels.

LEFLUNOMIDE IN RHEUMATOID ARTHRITIS

Leflunomide was first shown to be safe and effective in treating RA in a European placebo-controlled, dose-ranging, 6-month trial.[112] In this 402-patient trial, leflunomide at doses of 5, 10, and 25 mg/day were compared to placebo. Efficacy and toxicity were dose dependent with patients in both the 10 and 25 mg/day groups; these groups showed significant improvement (ACR-20) compared to the placebo-treated patients, but with a higher rate of withdrawals for adverse events. A subsequent population-based analysis suggested that a dose of 20 mg/day was the optimal dose of leflunomide to best balance efficacy and toxicity.[147]

This initial trial was followed by two pivotal trials, one in Europe and one in the United States. The European trial had three arms: leflunomide (20 mg/day after a loading dose), sulfasalazine (escalated to 2 g/day), and placebo[148] (Fig. 59–5). In this trial, both leflunomide and sulfasalazine were superior to placebo in terms of swollen and tender joint counts, as well as physicians' and patients' overall assessments (ACR-20 responses were not reported). Importantly, both the leflunomide and sulfasalazine groups reported statistically significant effects on slowing radiographic progression of disease compared to placebos. The initial U.S. trial, also three-armed, compared patients treated with leflunomide (20 mg/day after a loading dose), MTX (7.5 to 15 mg/week) or placebo[72] (Fig. 59–6). Again, both active drugs, leflunomide and MTX, were found to be superior to placebo but not different than each other. Both leflunomide and MTX also slowed radiographic progression of disease compared to the placebo group.

A second trial compared leflunomide (20 mg/day with loading) to MTX (10 to 15 mg/wk) in a 1-year trial with a 1-year extension and was completed in Europe[69] (Table 59–2). In this trial, MTX was shown to be statisti-

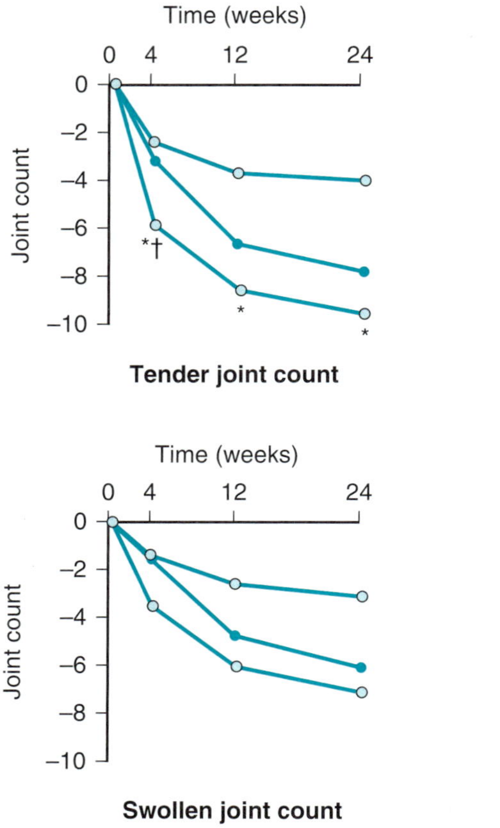

FIGURE 59–5 · Changes from baseline and outcome measures at weeks 4, 12, and 24.
*p ≤ 0.001 versus placebo.
†p ≤ 0.03 versus sulfasalazine.
(From: Smolen JS, Kalden JR, Scott LD, et al: Efficacy and safety of leflunomide compared with placebo and sulfasalazine in active rheumatoid arthritis: a double-blind, randomized, multicenter trial. Lancet 353:259, 1999.)

cally superior to leflunomide for the clinical outcomes measured (tender and swollen joint counts, and patient and physician global assessments), as well as the rate of radiographic progression after 2 years. Reconciliation of the disparate results of the U.S. and European trials with regard to the efficacy of leflunomide relative to MTX is difficult. Several possibilities exist; the European trial was longer, had more power (included more patients), had slightly higher mean MTX doses, and did not mandate folic acid supplementation. This latter point has again raised speculation that folic acid may interfere with some of the actions of MTX.

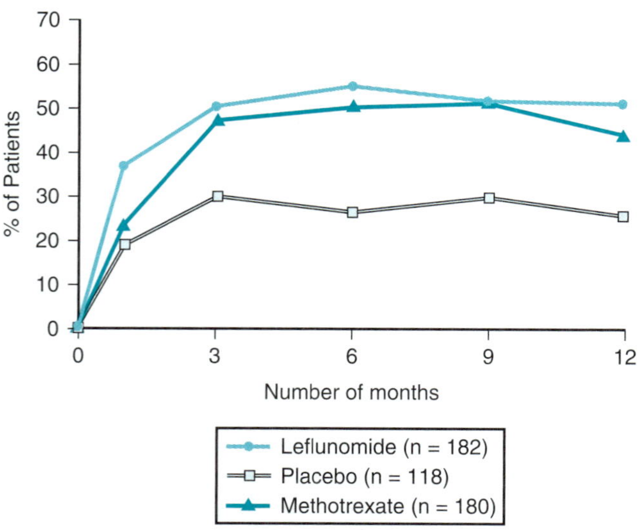

FIGURE 59–6 · Percent of patients receiving an ACR 20 response by month. (From Strand V, Cohen S, Schiff M, et al: Treatment of active rheumatoid arthritis with leflunomide compared with placebo and methotrexate. Arch Intern Med 159:2542, 1999.)

The leflunomide trials (see Figs. 59–5 and 59–6 and Table 59–2), in addition to proving the efficacy of leflunomide, have taught us a lot about sulfasalazine and MTX. These trials, particularly the first two with their placebo controls, have clearly demonstrated the clinical and radiographic benefits of sulfasalazine and MTX, as well as leflunomide, in patients with RA.

LEFLUNOMIDE IN OTHER RHEUMATIC DISEASES

Leflunomide is used to treat various aspects of systemic lupus and has been reported to be effective and well tolerated in an uncontrolled trial.[149] It has also been used successfully in both psoriasis and psoriatic arthritis.[150] Leflunomide or its active metabolite (A77 1726) have been effective in preventing rejection of transplanted organs in a number of animal models.[151-154]

DOSE AND ADMINISTRATION

Oral leflunomide is rapidly metabolized to A77 1726, which has a very long half-life (approximately 2 weeks). Therefore, the standard recommendation is to start therapy with a loading dose of 100 mg daily for 3 days, then switch to the standard maintenance dose of 20 mg daily. Despite this recommendation, many clinicians no longer prescribe a loading dose because it is felt that loading increases the drug's gastrointestinal toxicity.[155] Also, it is common practice to decrease the dose to 10 mg daily if toxicity occurs or if complete control of the disease can be maintained. Further, again because of its long half-life, some clinicians give leflunomide less often (three to five times per week).

Leflunomide should be used with caution in patients with renal insufficiency and is not recommended in patients with hepatic disease.[156] In renal insufficiency, the levels of circulating A77 1726 do not appear to be increased, but the component of free A77 1726 is. Liver failure is a concern; the liver is necessary to convert leflunomide to its active metabolite and is involved in the enterohepatic recirculation. Animal studies have demonstrated substantial teratogenic effects with leflunomide. Therefore, women with childbearing potential should be strongly counseled about this and should be practicing reliable methods of birth control; pregnancy tests before starting leflunomide should be considered. Leflunomide excretion in milk has not been studied; therefore, nursing mothers should not receive leflunomide.

It is critically important to note that leflunomide's active metabolite (A77 1726), largely because of its enterohepatic circulation, may remain in the body for years. Therefore, if toxicity occurs or a woman who has previously received leflunomide desires to become preg-

TABLE 59–2 • CHANGES IN PRIMARY CLINICAL EFFICACY ENDPOINTS (MEAN ± S.D.) AFTER 1 YEAR OF TREATMENT WITH LEFLUNOMIDE (LEF) OR METHOTREXATE (MTX)

	LEF (n = 495)	MTX (n = 489)	p
Tender joint count			
Baseline	17.2 ± 6.8	17.7 ± 6.7	
Δ	−8.3 ± 7.9	− 9.7 ± 7.9	0.006
Swollen joint count			
Baseline	15.8 ± 6.0	16.5 ± 5.9	
Δ	− 6.8 ± 7.3	− 9.0 ± 7.3	0.0001
Physician global assessment			
Baseline	3.5 ± 0.6	3.6 ± 0.6	
Δ	− 0.9 ± 1.0	− 1.2 ± 1.0	< 0.001
Patient global assessment			
Baseline	3.6 ± 0.6	3.6 ± 0.7	
Δ	− 0.9 ± 1.1	− 1.2 ± 1.0	< 0.001

From Emery P, Breedvell FC, Lemmel EM et al: A comparison of the efficacy and safety of leflunomide and methotrexate for the treatment of rheumatoid arthritis. Rheumatology 39:655, 2000.

nant, active elimination of leflunomide from the body should be considered. This can be achieved by the oral administration of cholestyramine for 11 days (8 g three times daily).[156] The success of this program, or the need for it, can be ascertained by plasma levels of A77 1726. If levels are greater than 0.02 g/ml, cholestyramine administration may be helpful.[156]

TOXICITY

For the three major controlled trials that have used leflunomide at the dose of 20 mg/day, the incidence of adverse events that resulted in trial withdrawal are shown in Table 59–3. Leflunomide-associated withdrawals (19%) were more frequent than those associated with MTX (14%), were similar in frequency to those associated with sulfasalazine (19%), but more frequent than those associated with placebo treatment (8%).

The most common adverse advents leading to trial withdrawal during the U.S. trial are shown in Table 59–4. Elevated transaminase levels and gastrointestinal events were the major differences between leflunomide and placebo. In this trial, withdrawal was mandated if transaminase levels were greater than three times normal or levels were repeatedly greater than two times normal despite dosage adjustments of study medications.

Hepatic

Early recommendations for monitoring patients on leflunomide did not include hepatic monitoring, but it is now apparent that liver toxicity may occur. Elevations of liver blood tests, ALT, AST, or both, was the most common reason for withdrawal for leflunomide-treated patients in the U.S. trial (7.7% of patients versus 4.4% of MTX-treated patients). In the European trial that compared leflunomide and MTX, withdrawals for elevated transaminases occurred more commonly in the MTX-treated patients (withdrawal of 3.2% of patients versus 1.6% of leflunomide-treated patients). This difference may reflect the more liberal use of folic acid in the U.S. trial and the different criteria for trial withdrawal in the European trial. The incidence of elevations of transaminase levels out of the normal range in clinical trials is not published; some studies report information on levels that are two or three times the upper limits of normal. There is paucity of data from clinical trials on liver biopsies in leflunomide-treated patients (one patient biopsied). It is apparent from recent reports that liver toxicity, although rare, does occur in association with leflunomide administration. The European Agency for Evaluation of Medicinal Products (EMEA) reported 296 cases of hepatic abnormalities and 15 patients with liver failure and death while taking leflunomide,[157] and additional cases of liver toxicity in patients taking leflunomide have been reported in Australia.[158] Conversely, data from a large RA database failed to show any difference in liver abnormalities in patients receiving leflunomide compared to those treated with MTX.[159] Until further information is available, it seems prudent to follow transaminase levels and adjust the dose of leflunomide for any elevations, as is done for MTX.

TABLE 59–3 • TRIAL WITHDRAWALS FOR ADVERSE EVENTS[69,72,148]

	No. of Patients	Withdrawals
Leflunomide	816	154 (19%)
Methotrexate	680	94 (14%)
Sulfasalazine	133	25 (19%)
Placebo	210	16 (8%)

Gastrointestinal

The most common side effect that limits the use of leflunomide is diarrhea. In clinical trials, this is reported in 13 to 34 percent of patients and is significantly increased over placebo (Table 59–5). In clinical practice, diarrhea responds to dose reduction and may be less common if the loading dose is not used.[155] Importantly, no long-term adverse effects have been reported from

TABLE 59–4 • ADVERSE EVENTS LEADING TO TREATMENT WITHDRAWAL

	Patients Withdrawn, (%)		
Adverse Event	*Leflunomide* (n = *182)*	*Placebo* (n = *118)*	*Methotrexate* (n = *182)*
Total	22.0	8.5	10.4
Elevated transaminase level	7.1	1.7	4.4
Gastrointestinal	5.5	1.7	1.7
Rash	2.2	2.5	0.0
Hypertension	1.1	0.8	0.0
Hyperlipidemia	1.6	0.0	0.0
Myocardial infarction	0.5	0.0	0.5
Pneumonia	0.5	0.0	0.5
Interstitial pneumonitis	0.0	0.0	0.5
Alopecia	0.5	0.8	1.1
Other	3.0	1.0	1.7

From Strand V, Cohen S, Schiff M, et al: Treatment of active rheumatoid arthritis with leflunomide compared with placebo and methotrexate. Arch Intern Med 159: 2542, 1999.

the diarrhea in leflunomide-treated patients. Abdominal pain, dyspepsia, and nausea from leflunomide appear to be slightly increased over placebo rates.

Cardiovascular

Hypertension has consistently been reported to occur more frequently in leflunomide-treated compared to placebo-treated patients.[72,148] In the U.S. trial, 11 percent of leflunomide-treated patients, compared to 5.1 percent of placebo-treated patients, had hypertension.[72] Additionally, elevation of cholesterol levels has also been reported in association with leflunomide use.[160] Both of these effects should be monitored because the major cause of excess mortality in patients with RA is cardiovascular.

Miscellaneous

An increased incidence of alopecia (see Table 59–5) has been reported in clinical trials in association with leflunomide. Weight loss has also been reported to occur with leflunomide.[161]

PATIENT SELECTION AND MONITORING

Most patients with RA are potential candidates for leflunomide therapy, which has been shown to have similar efficacy to sulfasalazine or moderate-dose MTX. Because pregnancy is contraindicated for patients taking leflunomide and for patients who have previously taken leflunomide (until plasma levels confirm it has been cleared from the body), women with childbearing potential must be practicing reliable forms of birth control to receive leflunomide. In patients with early RA, most clinicians opt for MTX before leflunomide because MTX is less costly and has a longer proven track record. Leflunomide is most commonly used as monotherapy in patients who do not tolerate MTX or in combination with MTX in those patients who have active disease despite MTX therapy.

TABLE 59–5 • SIDE EFFECTS INCIDENCE: THREE MAJOR TRIALS[69,72,148]

Trial	Lef-Ssz-Placebo	Lef-Mtx-Placebo	Lef-Mtx
No. patients	133 (92)*	182 (118)*	501
Diarrhea %	13% (5%)*	34% (17%)*	18%
Hypertension	5% (3%)*	11% (5%)*	7%
Alopecia	6% (2%)*	10% (1%)*	17%
Rash/allergic Rxn	8% (4%)*	24% (14%)*	7%
Abd pain	4% (8%)*	14% (7%)*	6%

*Incidence of side effects for placebo-treated patients is in parentheses.
Ssz, sulfasalazine.

Combination Disease-Modifying Antirheumatic Drug Therapy in Rheumatoid Arthritis

In the early 1990s, the use of combinations of DMARDs to treat RA was rare; now this strategy is employed by essentially all rheumatologists to treat more than one quarter of their patients.[162] Currently, the timing and make-up of combinations selected to treat RA is one of the most important decisions clinicians face as they care for patients with RA.

Monotherapy with MTX is considered by most as the initial treatment of choice for early RA. Four major studies[62,163-165] have demonstrated the superiority of combinations of DMARDs over monotherapy in head-to-head comparisons; the latter three studies have done so in early RA. Trials with multiple conventional DMARDs[166-168] and biologicals[169-173] have shown them to be more effective than placebo when added to the baseline MTX in patients who have active disease despite MTX therapy. With very few exceptions, successful combination trials have included MTX as part of the combination. Thus, MTX remains the cornerstone of combination therapy.[174]

THE HISTORY OF COMBINATION DISEASE-MODIFYING ANTIRHEUMATIC DRUG THERAPY

Early combination DMARD studies were initiated in the late 1970s; the combination of cyclophosphamide, azathioprine, and hydroxychloroquine produced substantial responses in an open-label trial of 17 patients with severe refractory RA.[175] Remission was reported in five patients, and an additional two patients achieved "near remissions," with "excellent responses" reported in all but three patients. Four years later, results were expanded to a total of 31 patients.[176] Remissions were reported in 52 percent, near remissions in 23 percent, and only one patient failed to have at least a good response. Unfortunately, five malignancies developed in four patients with three related deaths. These early reports revealed both the promise and perils of combination therapy.

Inadequate dosing, the use of DMARDs with marginal efficacy, and problematic trial design contributed to the less-than-exciting results reported with combination therapy in the 1980s. Suboptimal dosing of MTX and azathioprine in the combination arms of studies reported by Willkens and colleagues[56] was the likely explanation for the inability of these trials to show a significant benefit of combination therapy. In this trial, the dose of MTX and azathioprine in the combination group was half of what it was in the monotherapy groups. Trials that combined oral gold with other DMARDs were an example of the use of DMARDs with marginal efficacy.[177] In the European combination trials of MTX and sulfasalazine, only a marginal benefit of this combination over monotherapy was seen,[178,179] presumably because of trial design issues, such as the fact that doses of the medications were escalated without clear guidelines or end points. The result was lower doses of the medications in the combination arms, but efficacy that was only marginally better.

In 1994, the first trial to convincingly show the superiority of combination DMARD therapy in a head-to-head comparison with state-of-the-art mono-DMARD therapy was reported.[180] In this 2-year, randomized, double-blind, parallel study of 102 patients (mean disease duration 8.6 years), triple-drug therapy with MTX, sulfasalazine, and hydroxychloroquine (Fig. 59–7) was superior to the combination therapy of hydroxychloroquine and sulfasalazine and monotherapy with MTX.[62] Seventy-seven percent of patients receiving the triple-drug therapy achieved a modified Paulus 50-percent response,[181] compared to 40 percent of the sulfasalazine-and-hydroxychloroquine patients and 33 percent of the MTX-alone patients ($p = 0.003$). This combination was well tolerated, with numerically fewer withdrawals in the combination group compared to the other two groups. This therapy has also been shown to be durable; follow-up of the patients who continued on triple-drug therapy over a 5-year period revealed that 62 percent (36 of 58) continued to maintain a 50-percent efficacy response while tolerating therapy well.[182] A similar long-term response rate (67%) occurred in 15 patients who switched to triple-drug therapy after suboptimal response to monotherapy with MTX (17.5 mg/week).[183]

EARLY RHEUMATOID ARTHRITIS

Studies have clearly shown that delays in disease-modifying therapy for as little as 4 to 9 months may result in less-optimal outcomes for patients.[184-186] More than a decade ago, Wilske and Healey[187] proposed a step-down bridge approach for the treatment of early RA. The central tenet of this approach was to completely control disease as early as possible and later to taper the patient off a number of these drugs, leaving him or her on the simplest possible long-term maintenance regimen.

Researchers in the Netherlands recently reported on such an approach: the COBRA (Combinatietherapie

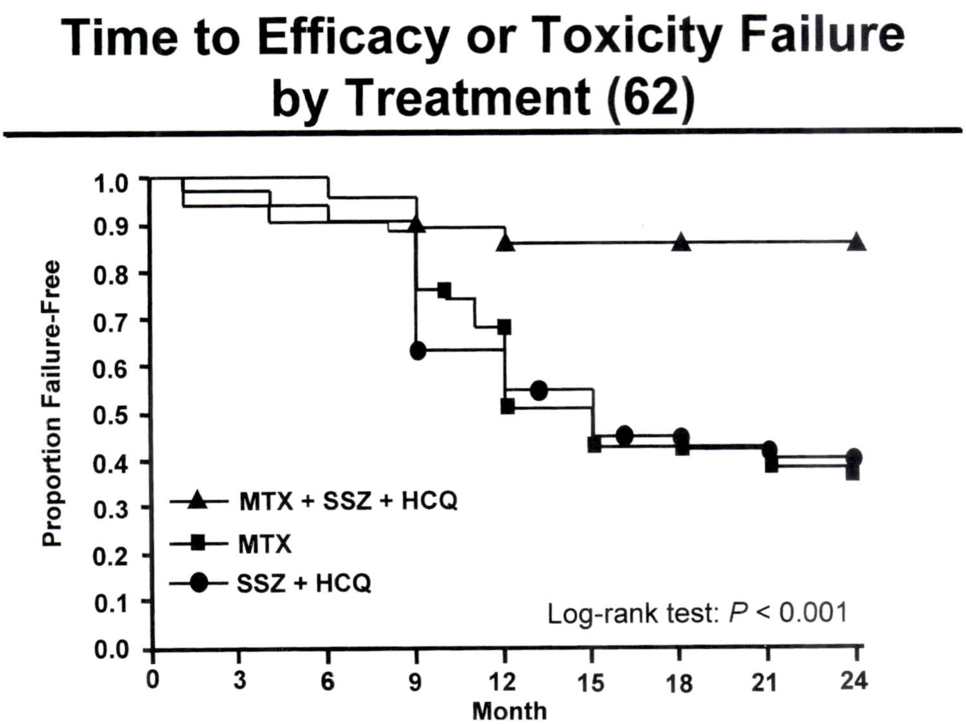

FIGURE 59–7 · Kaplan-Meyer plot of patients who achieve and maintain a modified Paulus 50% response as a function of time. (Adapted from O'Dell J, Haire C, Erikson N, et al: Treatment of rheumatoid arthritis with methotrexate alone, sulfasalazine and hydroxychloroquine, or a combination of all three. N Engl J Med 334:1287, 1996.)

Bij Reumatoide Artritis) trial.[163] In this trial, 155 patients with early disease (< 2 years) were randomly assigned to two groups. A combination of prednisolone, MTX, and sulfasalazine was compared to sulfasalazine alone. Prednisolone was started at 60 mg/day and rapidly tapered to 7.5 mg/day over the course of several weeks; it was discontinued by week 28. MTX (7.5 mg/wk) was given until week 40. The dose of sulfasalazine was the same in both groups and was rapidly accelerated to 2 g per day. At 28 weeks, the combination group was significantly better than the sulfasalazine-alone group, with ACR-20 score of 72 percent versus 49 percent (p = 0.006), and ACR-50 of 49 percent versus 27 percent (p = 0.007). As the prednisolone and MTX were tapered, the clinical responses became similar in the two groups. However, in terms of a number of important parameters, significant benefits existed in patients in the combination-treated group, at 54 and 80 weeks and also at 4 to 5 years.[188] Importantly, the withdrawal rate was much higher in the sulfasalazine-alone group (39% versus 8%), demonstrating that combination therapy was not more toxic. Recent data confirm that the radiographic benefits (radiographs read in a blinded fashion) conferred by COBRA in the initial trial extend at least 5 years[188] (Fig. 59–8). COBRA therapy was effective in rapidly suppressing acute-phase reactants; erythrocyte sedimentation rates were suppressed by 75 percent by 2 weeks, as compared to the 20 weeks necessary for the monotherapy group to achieve this degree of suppression (Boers, personal communication, 2002).

In another important early RA study (disease duration of less than two years), the Finland Rheumatoid Arthritis (Fin-RA) trial, 195 patients were randomized to receive combination DMARD therapy (MTX, sulfasalazine, hydroxychloroquine, and low-dose prednisolone) or monotherapy with sulfasalazine. Patients in the sulfasalazine-alone group had the option of receiving prednisolone as well, and also of switching to MTX if they had suboptimal responses to sulfasalazine alone. The major endpoint of this prospective, randomized, but open, trial was remission at 2 years. Patients who received combination therapy achieved remission more frequently, (37% versus 18%; odds ratio 2.7, p = 0.003). A follow-up of this trial at 5 years demonstrated that patients treated initially with the combination were less likely to have evidence of C1-C2 subluxation on cervical spine radiographs.[189] In a trial from Turkey,[165] 180 patients with early RA (mean duration 2.3 years) were randomized equally to single DMARD therapy (20 patients each to MTX, sulfasalazine, and hydroxychloroquine), two-drug therapy (30 patients each to MTX and sulfasalazine or MTX and hydroxychloroquine), or three-drug therapy (60 patients to all three drugs). This trial was a randomized, open, 2-year trial with end points of Paulus 50 response, ACR remission, and no radiographic progression (radiographs read blinded). For all end points measured, two drugs were shown to be statistically superior to monotherapy (p = 0.007 or better), and three were statistically superior to the two-drug regimens for Paulus 50 and ACR remission endpoints (p = 0.007 or better) and showed a trend for no radiographic progression (Table 59–6).

With the data provided from the COBRA trial,[163,188] the Fin-RA trial,[164,189] and the Turkish trial,[165] a convincing case can be made to treat patients initially with combination therapy. However, trials to define whether an approach that uses initial combinations is superior to a rapid step-up program, for only those patients who need it, have not been done.

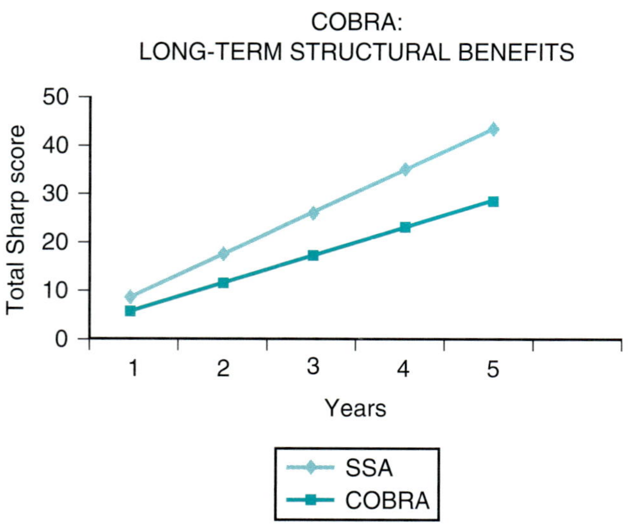

FIGURE 59–8 • Change in radiographic scores during longterm follow-up based on original randomization. (From: Landewe RBM, Boars M, ver Hoeven AC, et al: COBRA combination therapy in patients with early rheumatoid arthritis. Arthritis Rheum 46:347, 2002).

PATIENTS WITH ACTIVE DISEASE DESPITE METHOTREXATE

Many patients fail to have a complete response to MTX and are labeled "incomplete responders," "suboptimal responders," or "active disease despite MTX." Usually, these patients are further characterized by the weekly dose of MTX they have received, and currently, patients who have received somewhere between 15 and 25 mg/week of MTX have been so labeled. As a practical matter, most patients should switch to subcutaneous or IM MTX, and the dose should be escalated to 25 mg/week before they are considered suboptimal MTX-responders. Most of the studies reviewed in the coming paragraphs used dif-

TABLE 59–6 • COMBINATION VERSUS MONOTHERAPY IN EARLY RHEUMATOID ARTHRITIS

				p Values		
	Mono (%)	*Double (%)*	*Triple (%)*	*I vs II*	*I vs III*	*II vs III*
Paulus 50	49.1	73.2	87.9	<0.001	<0.001	<0.001
Remission	31.5	44.6	60.3	0.007	0.007	0.007
No X-ray Progression	24.5	64.2	68.9	0.001	0.001	0.210

Calguneri M, Pay S, Caliskaner Z, et al: Combination therapy versus monotherapy for the treatment of patients with rheumatoid arthritis. Clin Exp Rheumatol. 17(6):699-704, 1999.

ferent and less-rigorous definitions of MTX suboptimal responders. A host of trials have been directed at this group of patients.[166-173] Other studies have been designed to compare combination therapy head-to-head with MTX therapy.[62] All the trials that compare an active drug to placebo in MTX suboptimal responders (Fig. 59–9) suffer from an obvious flaw: Clinicians sorely need head-to-head comparisons of active products to make critical clinical judgments for their patients. The first study to show the advantage of combination therapy with MTX and another DMARD compared to continued therapy with MTX alone in this group of patients was the cyclosporine-MTX trial[166] (see Fig, 59–9). In this trial, 148 patients with active disease (despite MTX in doses up to 15 mg/week; mean dose of MTX 10.2 mg/week) were randomized to receive either cyclosporine in low-to-moderate doses or placebo, in addition to their baseline MTX. Forty-eight percent of the patients in the cyclosporine treatment group had achieved an ACR-20 response by 6 months, compared to 16 percent of the patients in the placebo group ($p = 0.001$). Creatinine elevations did occur and dosage adjustments were necessary; creatinines at the end of the trial were greater in the cyclosporine-treated group than in those treated with placebo ($p = 0.02$). More importantly, long-term use of cyclosporine in RA is associated with a high rate of withdrawal, most commonly because of elevated creatinine levels, hypertension, lack of efficacy, or some combination of these. Of the 335 patients enrolled in an open-label extension study, only 22 percent continued cyclosporine for 3 years.[190]

The newest synthetic DMARD, leflunomide, is comparable in efficacy to other conventional therapies, such as MTX[72] and sulfasalazine.[148] A double-blind, placebo-controlled trial[168] (see Fig. 59–9) has compared the addition of leflunomide or placebo to baseline MTX in 266 patients selected for suboptimal responses to MTX (mean 16.4 mg/week). Leflunomide (10 mg/day with an option to increase to 20 mg/day) or placebo was added to MTX. The ACR-20 criteria for clinical response were met at 24 weeks by 46 percent of the group randomized to receive leflunomide, compared to 20 percent of the placebo-treated patients ($p < 0.0001$). The combination was reasonably well-tolerated clinically, but side effects were increased in the combination arm, with 22 percent of patients reporting diarrhea, 12 percent reporting nausea, and 5 percent reporting dizziness. Elevated alanine aminotransferase levels (more than 1.2 times normal) occurred more frequently in patients on combination therapy than those on MTX alone (32% compared to 7%), with increases leading to withdrawal in 2.3 percent of patients who received the combination. In a previous, small, open-labeled trial of 30 patients who received this combination, 60 percent of patients had liver enzyme elevations at some time during the trial, but only two patients were withdrawn.[191] Recently, reports of liver toxicity with leflunomide have surfaced in Europe (EMEA) and Australia.[159] Whether these liver blood test abnormalities will prove to be problematic for the clinical use of this combination remains to be seen.

Therapy with the combination of MTX, sulfasalazine, and hydroxychloroquine, so called "triple therapy," has been shown by three different groups (four trials) to not only be well tolerated,[62,164,165,167] but also to be more effective than MTX monotherapy,[62,165] sulfasalazine monotherapy,[164] and, in an open trial of patients with early disease, more effective than the double combinations of MTX and sulfasalazine or MTX and hydroxychloroquine.[165]

In a 2-year, double-blind trial on patients with moderately advanced disease, the triple combination was compared to the two double combinations (MTX and

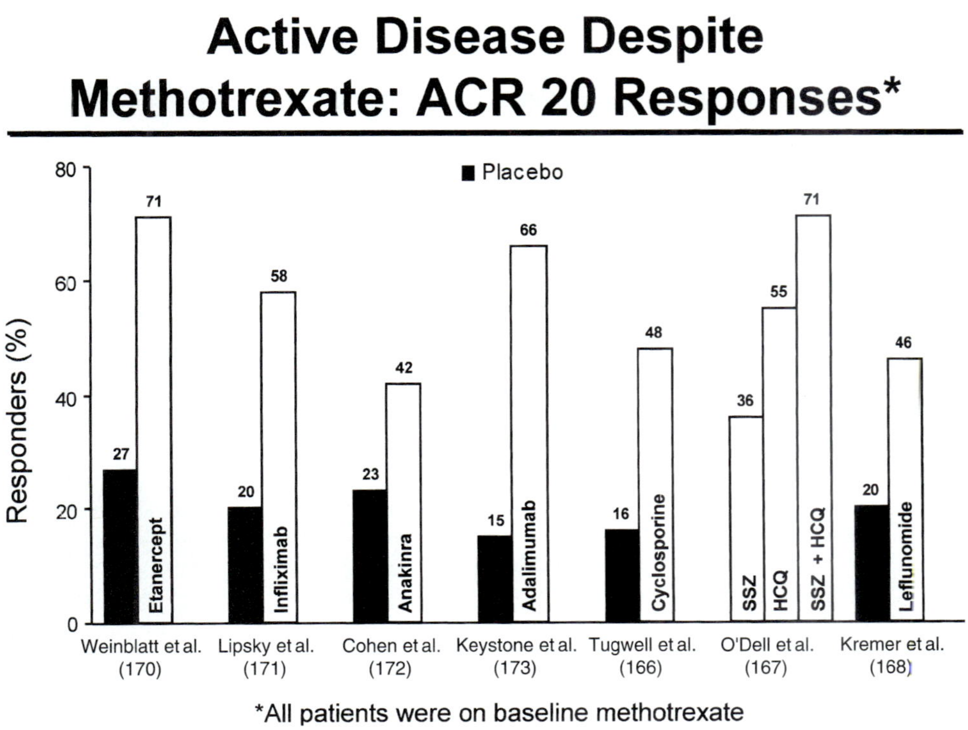

FIGURE 59–9 · Summary of data taken from seven different clinical trials of therapies in patients with active disease despite methotrexate therapy.

sulfasalazine, and MTX and hydroxychloroquine) in a head-to-head comparison.[167] Patients were stratified for previous MTX use, and the previous users had to have active disease despite receiving 17.5 mg/week. Triple therapy and both double therapy groups tolerated their treatments well, with only 8 percent withdrawing for toxicities, which were mostly minor. Triple therapy was shown to be superior to either of the double combinations. The primary outcome variable for this trial was ACR-20 response at 2 years; this was achieved by 78 percent of the triple-therapy patients, 60 percent of those on MTX and hydroxychloroquine ($p = 0.05$ for triple comparison), and 49 percent of those on MTX and sulfasalazine ($p = 0.002$ compared to triple[see Fig. 59–9]). A subanalysis of the MTX naïve and MTX suboptimal responders demonstrated that, in the MTX-naïve group of patients, MTX-and-sulfasalazine-treated patients did better than MTX-and-hydroxychloroquine-treated patients (ACR-20 of 71 and 56%, respectively). However, in the patients who entered the study as MTX suboptimal responders, the MTX and hydroxychloroquine combination was superior to the MTX andsulfasalazine combination (ACR-20 of 55 and 36%, respectively). For years, despite the paucity of data, the MTX and hydroxychloroquine combination has been by far the most popular combination used by clinicians; these data would lend support to this long-standing clinical preference.

CORTICOSTEROIDS IN DISEASE-MODIFYING ANTIRHEUMATIC DRUG COMBINATIONS

Corticosteroids have not traditionally been considered DMARDs. However, they clearly fulfill all the criteria for DMARDs, including retarding radiographic progression.[192-195] Few clinicians that care for patients with RA dispute their efficacy. Indeed, they have been used as baseline therapy for well over half of the patients included in the combination trials discussed previously.

Prednisolone undoubtedly was a critical component for the success of the COBRA protocol[163] and may have played a role in the success of the combination group in the Fin-RA trial.[164] Kirwan and colleagues' report of the ability of prednisolone to significantly retard radiographic progression of RA compared to placebo[194,195] is testament to the efficacy of steroids when used in combination with other DMARDs; all patients in this trial were receiving routine background DMARD therapy. In this 2-year, double-blind trial, 128 patients with early RA were randomized to receive prednisolone (7.5 mg/day) or placebo in addition to background DMARD therapy.[194] At the end of the 2 years, Larsen scores had increased by 0.72 units for the prednisolone group and by 5.37 units in the placebo group ($p = 0.004$). In a follow-up study, prednisolone was tapered, and the rate of radiographic progression increased and matched that of the placebo-treated group,[195] further supporting the efficacy of prednisolone in this cohort.

Steroids clearly deserve further formal investigation as a component of combination therapy. The COBRA trial (particularly the follow-up report of this group of patients),[188] as well as the Kirwan data, have raised another interesting question: Should/could short courses of high-dose steroids be used as a form of induction therapy?[196]

OTHER COMBINATIONS WITH METHOTREXATE

After their combination therapy protocols of the early 1980s, which showed considerable efficacy, but unfortunately also considerable toxicity, McCarty and colleagues[197] have reported on a cohort of patients treated with combinations that did not include cyclophosphamide. In an observational study of 169 patients followed in their clinic, McCarty and coworkers reported a complete remission rate of 43 percent when MTX, hydroxychloroquine, and azathioprine were added in a sequential, as-needed fashion. In general, patients were started on either hydroxychloroquine or MTX alone, or a combination of these two medications; azathioprine was added for patients who were not optimally controlled. Overall, satisfactory control of inflammatory disease was reported in 167 of 169 patients. The triple combination of MTX, hydroxychloroquine, and azathioprine was well tolerated and was needed in 69 patients (41% of cohort). The remission rate in the group that needed three-drug therapy was 45 percent, similar to the overall rate of 43 percent.

THE BIOLOGICALS IN DISEASE-MODIFYING ANTIRHEUMATIC DRUG COMBINATIONS

Biologicals have been combined with conventional DMARDs (particularly in the much-studied "MTX suboptimal responder" group) and have significantly improved patient responses over background therapy (see Fig. 59–9). Strategies that combine biologicals, particularly inhibition of TNF-α and IL-1, have been effective in animal models of inflammatory arthritis, but early trials in humans have resulted in an apparent increased risk of infections.

SELECTING THE RIGHT PATIENTS FOR COMBINATION THERAPY

Factors that predict a poor prognosis for patients with RA are well accepted and include rheumatoid factor, elevated erythrocyte sedimentation rate or C-reactive protein (CRP), the number of joints involved, erosions, and the presence of certain genetic markers. However, unless these factors can be shown to predict response to certain therapies in a differential fashion, they are of limited therapeutic use. Although patient characteristics recommending one therapeutic regimen over another remain to be fully elucidated, genetic differences have been suggested to influence outcomes in a differential fashion. In an attempt to predict response to specific RA treatment regimens, patients with late disease (described previously)[62] were tested for the presence of shared HLA-DRB1 epitope alleles.[198] Patients who were shared-epitope positive were much more likely to achieve a 50-percent response if treated with triple therapy (MTX, sulfasalazine, and hydroxychloroquine) compared to MTX alone (94 vs. 32% responders, $p < 0.0001$). In contrast, shared-epitope negative patients did equally well regardless of the treatment provided (88% responders for triple-drug therapy vs. 83% for MTX monotherapy). Until this observation can be corroborated and factors that predict response to other therapies elucidated, choices will remain largely empirical.

Treatment of RA using MTX combinations should be the gold standard against which future therapies are compared; available data demonstrate that a variety of combinations are more effective than MTX alone. Many questions remain to be answered regarding the appropriate timing of combination therapy and the optimal combinations for specific patients and for specific clinical situations (e.g., induction, maintenance therapy, and suboptimal response to MTX). Future research is needed to clarify the role of corticosteroids and, particularly, biological response modifiers (specifically anti-TNF therapies), both as components of and alternatives to MTX combination regimens.

REFERENCES

1. Jolivet J, Cowan KH, Curt GA, et al: The pharmacology and clinical use of methotrexate. N Engl J Med 309:1094, 1983.
2. Cronstein BN, Eberle MA, Gruber HE, et al: Methotrexate inhibits neutrophil function by stimulating adenosine release from connective tissue cells. Proc Natl Acad Sci U S A 88:2441, 1991.
3. Cronstein BN, Naime D, Ostad E: The antiinflammatory mechanism of methotrexate: increased adenosine release at inflamed sites diminishes leukocyte accumulation in an in vivo model of inflammation. J Clin Invest 92:2675, 1993.
4. Weinblatt ME, Coblyn JS, Fox DA, et al: Efficacy of low-dose methotrexate in rheumatoid arthritis. N Engl J Med 312:818, 1985.
5. Andersen PA, West SG, O'Dell JR, et al: Weekly pulse methotrexate in rheumatoid arthritis: clinical and immunologic effects in a randomized, double-blind study. Ann Intern Med 103:489, 1985.
6. Weinblatt ME, Trentham DE, Fraser PA, et al: Long-term prospective trial of low-dose methotrexate in rheumatoid arthritis. Arthritis Rheum 31:167, 1988.
7. Genestier L, Paillot R, Fournel S, et al: Immunosuppressive properties of methotrexate: apoptosis and clonal deletion of activated peripheral T cells. J Clin Invest 102:322, 1988.
8. Olsen NJ, Callahan LF, Pincus T: Immunologic studies of rheumatoid arthritis patients treated with methotrexate. Arthritis Rheum 30:481, 1987.
9. Alarcón GS, Schrohenloher RE, Bartolucci AA, et al: Suppression of rheumatoid factor production by methotrexate in patients with rheumatoid arthritis: evidence for differential influences of therapy and clinical status on IgM and IgA rheumatoid factor expression. Arthritis Rheum 33:1156, 1990.
10. Hirata S, Matsubara T, Saura R, et al: Inhibition of in vitro vascular endothelial cell proliferation and in vivo neovascularization by low-dose methotrexate. Arthritis Rheum 32:1065, 1989.
11. Nesher G, Moore TL: The in vitro effects of methotrexate on peripheral blood mononuclear cells: modulation by methyl donors and spermidine. Arthritis Rheum 33:954, 1990.
12. Segal R, Mozes E, Yaron M, et al: The effects of methotrexate on the production and activity of interleukin-1. Arthritis Rheum 32:370, 1989.
13. Segal R, Yaron M, Tartakovsky B: Rescue of interleukin-1 activity by leucovorin following inhibition by methotrexate in a murine in vitro system. Arthritis Rheum 33:1745, 1990.
14. Chang D-M, Weinblatt ME, Schur PH: The effects of methotrexate on interleukin 1 in patients with rheumatoid arthritis. J Rheumatol 19:1678, 1992.
15. Barrera P, Boerbooms AMT, Janssen EM, et al: Circulating soluble tumor necrosis factor receptors, interleukin-2 receptors, tumor necrosis factor-α, and interleukin-6 levels in rheumatoid arthritis: longitudinal evaluation during methotrexate and azathioprine therapy. Arthritis Rheum 36:1070, 1993.
16. Constantin A, Loubet-Lescoulié P, Lambert N, et al: Antiinflammatory and immunoregulatory action of methotrexate in the treatment of rheumatoid arthritis: evidence of increased interleukin-4 and interleukin-10 gene expression demonstrated in vitro by competitive reverse transcriptase polymerase chain reaction. Arthritis Rheum 41:48, 1998.
17. Segal R, Caspi D, Tishler M, et al: Short term effects of low dose methotrexate on the acute phase reaction in patients with rheumatoid arthritis. J Rheumatol 16:914, 1989.
18. van de Kerkhof PC, Bauer FW, Maassen-de Grood RM: Methotrexate inhibits the leukotriene B4 induced intraepidermal accumulation of polymorphonuclear leukocytes. Br J Dermatol 113:251a, 1985.
19. Sperling RI, Benincaso AI, Anderson RJ, et al: Acute and chronic suppression of leukotriene B_4 synthesis ex vivo in neutrophils from patients with rheumatoid arthritis beginning treatment with methotrexate. Arthritis Rheum 35:376, 1992.
20. Vergne P, Liagre B, Bertin P, et al: Methotrexate and cyclooxygenase metabolism in cultured human rheumatoid synoviocytes. J Rheumatol 25:433, 1998.
21. Laurindo IMM, Mello SBV, Cossermelli W: Influence of low doses of methotrexate on superoxide anion production by polymorphonuclear leukocytes from patients with rheumatoid arthritis. J Rheumatol 22:633, 1995
22. Kraan MC, de Koster BM, Elferink JG, et al: Inhibition of neutrophil migration soon after initiation of treatment with leflunomide or methotrexate in patients with rheumatoid arthritis: findings in a prospective, randomized, double-blind clinical trial in fifteen patients. Arthritis Rheum 43: 1488, 2000.
23. Kraan MC, Reece RJ, Barg EC, et al: Modulation of inflammation and metalloproteinase expression in synovial tissue by leflunomide and methotrexate in patients with active rheumatoid arthritis: findings in a prospective, randomized, double-blind, parallel-design clinical trial in thirty-nine patients at two centers. Arthritis Rheum 43: 1820, 2000.
24. Martel-Pelletier J, Cloutier J-M, Pelletier J-P: In vivo effects of antirheumatic drugs on neutral collagenolytic proteases in human rheumatoid arthritis cartilage and synovium. J Rheumatol 15:1198, 1988.
25. Firestein GS, Paine MM, Boyle DL: Mechanisms of methotrexate action in rheumatoid arthritis: selective decrease in synovial collagenase gene expression. Arthritis Rheum 37:193, 1994.
26. Kozloski GD, De Vito JM, Kisicki JC, et al The effect of food on the absorption of methotrexate sodium tablets in healthy volunteers. Arthritis Rheum 35:761, 1992.
27. Herman RA, Veng-Pedersen P, Hoffman J, et al: Pharmacokinetics of low-dose methotrexate in rheumatoid arthritis patients. J Pharm Sci 78:165, 1989.
28. Brooks PJ, Spruill WJ, Parish RC, et al: Pharmacokinetics of methotrexate administered by intramuscular and subcutaneous injections in patients with rheumatoid arthritis. Arthritis Rheum 33:91, 1990.
29. Marshall PS, Gertner E: Oral administration of an easily prepared solution of injectable methotrexate diluted in water: a comparison of serum concentrations vs methotrexate tablets and clinical utility. J Rheumatol 23:455, 1996.
30. Skeith KJ, Russell AS, Jamali F, et al: Lack of significant interaction between low dose methotrexate and ibuprofen or flurbiprofen in patients with arthritis. J Rheumatol 17:1008, 1990.
31. Dupuis LL, Koren G, Shore A, et al: Methotrexate-nonsteroidal antiinflammatory drug interaction in children with arthritis. J Rheumatol 17:1469, 1990.
32. Thomas MH, Gutterman LA: Methotrexate toxicity in a patient receiving trimethoprim-sulfamethoxazole. J Rheumatol 13:440, 1986.
33. Gubner R, August S, Ginsberg V: Therapeutic suppression of tissue reactivity. II. Effect of aminopterin in rheumatoid arthritis and psoriasis. Am J Med Sci 22:176, 1951.
34. Hoffmeister RT: Methotrexate in rheumatoid arthritis [Abstract]. Arthritis Rheum 15:114, 1972.
35. Hoffmeister RT: Methotrexate therapy in rheumatoid arthritis: 15 years' experience. Am J Med 75:69, 1983.
36. Felson DT, Anderson JJ, Meenan RF: The comparative efficacy and toxicity of second-line drugs in rheumatoid arthritis. Arthritis Rheum 33: 1449, 1990.

37. Kremer JM, Phelps CT: Long-term prospective study of the use of methotrexate in rheumatoid arthritis: update after a mean of 90 months. Arthritis Rheum 35:138, 1992.
38. Kremer JM: Safety, efficacy, and mortality in a long-term cohort of patients with rheumatoid arthritis taking methotrexate: follow-up after a mean of 13.3 years. Arthritis Rheum 40:984, 1997.
39. Weinblatt ME, Kaplan H, Germain BF, et al: Methotrexate in rheumatoid arthritis: a five year prospective multicenter trial. Arthritis Rheum 37:1492, 1994.
40. Pincus T, Marcum SB, Callahan LF: Long-term drug therapy for rheumatoid arthritis in seven rheumatology private practices. II. Second line drugs and prednisone. J Rheumatol 19:1885, 1992.
41. Weinblatt ME, Maier AL, Fraser PA, et al: Longterm prospective study of methotrexate in rheumatoid arthritis: conclusion after 132 months of therapy. J Rheumatol 25:238, 1998.
42. Wolfe F: The epidemiology of drug treatment failure in rheumatoid arthritis. Baillieres Clin Rheumatol 9(4):619, 1995.
43. Willkens RF, Watson MA, Paxson CS: Low dose pulse methotrexate therapy in rheumatoid arthritis. J Rheumatol 7:501, 1980.
44. Wilke WS, Calabrese LH, Scherbel AL: Methotrexate in the treatment of rheumatoid arthritis. Cleve Clin Q 47:305, 1980.
45. Williams HJ, Willkens RF, Samuelson CO Jr., et al: Comparison of low-dose oral pulse methotrexate and placebo in the treatment of rheumatoid arthritis: a controlled clinical trial. Arthritis Rheum 28:721, 1985.
46. Thompson RN, Watts C, Edelman J, et al: A controlled two-centre trial of parenteral methotrexate therapy for refractory rheumatoid arthritis. J Rheumatol 11:760, 1984.
47. Tugwell P, Bennett K, Gent M: Methotrexate in rheumatoid arthritis. Ann Int Med 107:358, 1987.
48. Weinblatt ME, Kaplan H, Germain BF, et al: Low-dose methotrexate compared with auranofin in adult rheumatoid arthritis: a thirty-six-week, double-blind trial. Arthritis Rheum 33:330, 1990.
49. Morassut P, Goldstein R, Cyr M, et al: Gold sodium thiomalate compared to low dose methotrexate in the treatment of rheumatoid arthritis: a randomized double-blind, 26-week trial. J Rheumatol 16:302, 1984.
50. Rau R, Herborn G, Menninger H, et al: Comparison of intramuscular methotrexate and gold sodium thiomalate in the treatment of early erosive rheumatoid arthritis: 12 month data of a double-blind parallel study of 174 patients. Br J Rheumatol 36:345, 1997.
51. Suarez-Almozaor M, Fitzgerald A, Grace M, Russell AS: A randomized controlled trial of parenteral methotrexate compared with sodium aurothiomalate (Myochrysine) in the treatment of rheumatoid arthritis. J Rheumatol 15:753, 1998.
52. Rau R, Schleusser B, Herborn G, et al: Long-term combination therapy of refractory and destructive rheumatoid arthritis with methotrexate (MTX) and intramuscular gold or other disease modifying antirheumatic drugs compared to MTX monotherapy. J Rheumatol 25:1485, 1998.
53. Hamdy H, McKendry RJR, Mierins E, Liver JA: Low-dose methotrexate compared with azathioprine in the treatment of rheumatoid arthritis. Arthritis Rheum 30:361, 1987.
54. Jeurissen MEC, Boerbooms AMT, van de Putte LBA, et al: Methotrexate versus azathioprine in the treatment of rheumatoid arthritis: a forty-eight-week randomized, double-blind trial. Arthritis Rheum 34:961, 1991.
55. Jeurissen MEC, Boerbooms AMT, van de Putte LBA, et al: Influence of methotrexate and azathioprine on radiologic progression in rheumatoid arthritis: a randomized, double-blind study. Ann Intern Med 114:999, 1991.
56. Willkens RF, Sharp JT, Stablein D, et al: Comparison of azathioprine, methotrexate, and the combination of the two in the treatment of rheumatoid arthritis. Arthritis Rheum 38:1799, 1995.
57. Arnold MH, O'Callaghan J, McCredie M, et al: Comparative controlled trial of low-dose weekly methotrexate versus azathioprine in rheumatoid arthritis: 3 year prospective study. Br J Rheumatol 29:120, 1990.
58. Felson DT, Anderson JJ, Meenan RF: Use of short-term efficacy/toxicity tradeoffs to select second-line drugs in rheumatoid arthritis: a metaanalysis of published clinical trials. Arthritis Rheum 35:1117, 1992.
59. Kremer JM, Joong KL: A long-term prospective study of the use of methotrexate in rheumatoid arthritis: update after a mean of fifty-three months. Arthritis Rheum 31:577, 1988.
60. Tugwell P, Bennett K, Gent M: Methotrexate in rheumatoid arthritis. Ann Intern Med 107:358, 1987.
61. Weinblatt ME, Weissman BN, Holdsworth DE, et al: Long-term prospective study of methotrexate in the treatment of rheumatoid arthritis: 84-month update. Arthritis Rheum 35:129, 1992.
62. O'Dell J, Haire C, Erickson N, et al: Treatment of rheumatoid arthritis with methotrexate alone, sulfasalazine and hydroxychloroquine, or a combination of all three medications. N Engl J Med 334:1287, 1996.
63. Weinblatt ME: Methotrexate (MTX) in rheumatoid arthritis (RA): a 5-year multicenter prospective trial. Arthritis Rheum 36:S79, 1993.
64. Alacron GS, Lopez-Mendez A, Walter J, et al: Radiographic evidence of disease progression in methotrexate treated and non-methotrexate disease modifying antirheumatic drug treated rheumatoid arthritis patients: a meta-analysis. J Rheumatol 19:1868, 1992.
65. Lopez-Mendez A, Daniel WW, Reading JC, et al: Radiographic assessment of disease progression in rheumatoid arthritis patients enrolled in the Cooperative Systemic Studies of the Rheumatic Diseases Program randomized clinical trial of methotrexate, auranofin, or a combination of the two. Arthritis Rheum 36:1364, 1993.
66. Weinblatt ME, Polisson R, Blotner SD, et al: The effects of drug therapy on radiographic progression of rheumatoid arthritis: results of a 36-week randomized trial comparing methotrexate and auranofin. Arthritis Rheum 36:613, 1993.
67. Rau R, Herborn G, Karger T, Werdier D: Retardation of radiologic progression in rheumatoid arthritis with methotrexate therapy: a controlled study. Arthritis Rheum 34:1236, 1991.
68. Jeurissen MEC, Boerbooms MT, van de Putte LBA, et al: Influence of methotrexate and azathioprine on radiologic progression in rheumatoid arthritis: a randomized, double-blind study. Ann Intern Med 114:999, 1991.
69. Emery P, Breedveld FC, Lemmel EM, et al: A comparison of the efficacy and safety of leflunomide and methotrexate for the treatment of rheumatoid arthritis. Br Soc Rheum 39:655, 2000.
70. Nordstrom DM, West SG, Andersen PA: Pulse methotrexate therapy in rheumatoid arthritis: a controlled prospective roentgenographic study. Ann Intern Med 107:797, 1987.
71. Rau R, Herborn G, Karger T, et al: A double-blind randomized parallel trial of intramuscular methotrexate and gold sodium thiomalate in early erosive rheumatoid arthritis. J Rheumatol 18:328, 1991.
72. Strand V, Cohen S, Schiff M, et al, for the Leflunomide Rheumatoid Arthritis Investigators Group: Treatment of active rheumatoid arthritis with leflunomide compared with placebo and methotrexate. Arch Intern Med 159:2542, 1999.
73. Lally EV, Ho G Jr: A review of methotrexate therapy in Reiter syndrome. Semin Arthritis Rheum 15:139, 1985.
74. Fiechtner JJ, Miller DR, Starkebaum G: Reversal of neutropenia with methotrexate treatment in patients with Felty's syndrome: correlation of response with neutrophil-reactive IgG. Arthritis Rheum 32:194, 1989.
75. Loughran TP, Kidd PG, Starkebaum G: Treatment of large granular lymphocyte leukemia with oral low-dose methotrexate. Blood 84(7):2164, 1994.
76. Espinoza LR, Espinoza CG, Vasey FB, et al: Oral methotrexate therapy for chronic rheumatoid arthritis ulcerations. J Am Acad Dermatol 15:508, 1986.
77. Aydintug AO, D'Cruz D, Cervera R, et al: Low dose methotrexate treatment in adult Still's disease. J Rheumatol 19:431, 1992.
78. Gourmelen O, Le Loët X, Fortier-Beaulieu M, et al: Methotrexate treatment of multicentric reticulohistiocytosis. J Rheumatol 18:627, 1991.
79. Rahman P, Humphrey-Murto S, Gladman DD, et al: Efficacy and tolerability of methotrexate in antimalarial resistant lupus arthritis. J Rheumatol 25:243, 1998.
80. Carneiro JR, Sato EI: Double blind, randomized, placebo controlled clinical trial of methotrexate in systemic lupus erythematosus. J Rheumatol 26(6):1275, 1999.

81. Langford CA, Talar-Williams C, Sneller MC: Use of methotrexate and glucocorticoids in the treatment of Wegener's granulomatosus: long-term renal outcome in patients with glomerulonephritis. Arthritis Rheum 43(8):1836, 2000.
82. Hoffman GS, Leavitt RY, Kerr GS, et al: Treatment of glucocorticoid-resistant or relapsing Takayasu arteritis with methotrexate. Arthritis Rheum 37:578, 1994.
83. Van den Hoogen FHJ, Boerbooms AMT, Swaak AJG, et al: Comparison of methotrexate with placebo in the treatment of systemic sclerosis: a 24 week randomized double-blind trial, followed by a 24 week observational trial. Br J Rheumatol 35:364, 1997.
84. Hoffman GS, Cid MC, Hellmann DB, et al: A multicenter, randomized, double-blind, placebo-controlled trial of adjuvant methotrexate treatment for giant cell arteritis. Arthritis Rheum 46(5):1309, 2002.
85. Giannini EH, Brewer EJ, Kuzmina N, et al: Methotrexate in resistant juvenile rheumatoid arthritis: results of the U.S.A.-U.S.S.R. double-blind, placebo-controlled trial. N Engl J Med 326:1043, 1992.
86. Kremer JM, Alarcón GS, Lightfoot RW Jr, et al: Methotrexate for rheumatoid arthritis: suggested guidelines for monitoring liver toxicity. Arthritis Rheum 37:316, 1994.
87. Morgan SL, Baggott JE, Vaughn WH, et al: The effect of folic acid supplementation on the toxicity of low-dose methotrexate in patients with rheumatoid arthritis. Arthritis Rheum 33:9, 1990.
88. Morgan SL, Baggott JE, Vaughn WH, et al: Supplementation with folic acid during methotrexate therapy for rheumatoid arthritis: a double-blind, placebo-controlled trial. Ann Intern Med 121:833, 1994.
89. van Ede AE, Laan RF, Rood MJ, et al: Effect of folic acid supplementation on the toxicity and efficacy of methotrexate in rheumatoid arthritis: a forty-eight week, multicenter, randomized, double-blind, placebo-controlled study. Arthritis Rheum 44(7): 1515, 2001.
90. Kremer JM, Lee RG, Tolman KG, et al: Liver histology in rheumatoid arthritis patients receiving long-term methotrexate therapy: a prospective study with baseline and sequential biopsy samples. Arthritis Rheum 32:121, 1989.
91. Kremer JM: Not yet time to change the guidelines for monitoring methotrexate liver toxicity: they have served us well. J Rheumatol 29(8): 1590, 2002.
92. Kremer JM, Davies JMS, Rynes RI, et al: Every-other-week methotrexate in patients with rheumatoid arthritis. Arthritis Rheum 38:601, 1995.
93. Erickson AR, Reddy V, Vogelgesang SA, West SG: Usefulness of the American College of Rheumatology recommendations for liver biopsy in methotrexate-treated rheumatoid arthritis patients. Arthritis Rheum 38:1115, 1995.
94. Simms RW, Kwoh K, Anderson LG, et al: Guidelines for monitoring drug therapy in rheumatoid arthritis. Arthritis Rheum 39:723, 1996.
95. Stewart KA, Mackenzie AH, Wilke WS: Folate supplementation in methotrexate-treated rheumatoid arthritis patients. Semin Arthritis Rheum 20:332, 1991.
96. Weinblatt ME, Fraser P: Elevated mean corpuscular volume as a predictor of hematologic toxicity due to methotrexate therapy. Arthritis Rheum 32:1592, 1989.
97. Mathers D, Russell AS: Methotrexate. In Dixon JS, DE, Furst (eds): Second-Line agents in the Treatment of Rheumatic Diseases. New York, Marcel Dekker, 1992, pp 287-310.
98. Kremer JM, Alarcón GS, Weinblatt ME, et al: Clinical, laboratory, radiographic, and histopathologic features of methotrexate-associated lung injury in patients with rheumatoid arthritis: a multicenter study with literature review. Arthritis Rheum 40:1829, 1997.
99. Alarcón GS, Kremer JM, Macaluso M, et al: Risk factors for methotrexate-induced lung injury in patients with rheumatoid arthritis: a multicenter, case-control study. Ann Intern Med 127:356, 1997.
100. Cook NJ, Carroll GJ: Successful reintroduction of methotrexate after pneumonitis in two patients with rheumatoid arthritis. Ann Rheum Dis 51:272, 1992.
101. Searles G, McKendry RJ: Methotrexate pneumonitis in rheumatoid arthritis: potential risk factors. Four case reports and a review of the literature. J Rheumatol 14:1164, 1987.
102. Isomaki HA, Hakulinen T, Joutsenlahti U: Excess risk of lymphomas, leukemia and myeloma in patients with rheumatoid arthritis. J Chronic Dis 31:691, 1978.
103. Kamel OW, Van de Rijn M, Weiss LM, et al: Reversible lymphomas associated with Epstein-Barr virus occurring during methotrexate therapy for rheumatoid arthritis and dermatomyositis. N Engl J Med 328:1317, 1993.
104. Salloum E, Cooper DL, Howe G, et al: Spontaneous regression of lymphoproliferative disorders in patients treated with methotrexate for rheumatoid arthritis and other rheumatic diseases. J Clin Oncol 14:1943, 1996.
105. Ferraccioli GF, Casatta L, Bartoli E, et al: Epstein-Barr virus–associated Hodgkin's lymphoma in a rheumatoid arthritis patient treated with methotrexate and cyclosporin A. Arthritis Rheum 38:867, 1995.
106. Moder KG, Tefferi A, Cohen MD, et al: Hematologic malignancies and the use of methotrexate in rheumatoid arthritis: a retrospective study. Am J Med 99:276, 1995.
107. Thoburn R, Katz P: Lymphoproliferative disease in patients with autoimmune disease on low-dose methotrexate. American College of Rheumatology Hotline June 1, 1995.
108. Kerstens PJSM, Boerbooms AMT, Jeurissen MEC, et al: Accelerated nodulosis during low dose methotrexate therapy for rheumatoid arthritis: an analysis of ten cases. J Rheumatol 19:867, 1992.
109. Karam NE, Roger L, Hankins LL, Reveille JD: Rheumatoid nodulosis of the meninges. J Rheumatol 21:1960, 1994.
110. Merrill JT, Shen C, Schreibman D, et al: Adenosine A_1 receptor promotion of multinucleated giant cell formation by human monocytes: a mechanism for methotrexate-induced nodulosis in rheumatoid arthritis. Arthritis Rheum 40:1308, 1997.
111. Marks CR, Willkens RF, Wilske KR, Brown PB: Small-vessel vasculitis and methotrexate. Ann Intern Med 100:916, 1984.
112. Mladenovic V, Domljan Z, Rozman B, et al: Safety and effectiveness of leflunomide in the treatment of patients with active rheumatoid arthritis: results of a randomized, placebo-controlled, phase II study. Arthritis Rheum 38:1595, 1995.
113. Fox RI, Herrmann MH, Frangou CG, et al: Mechanism of action of leflunomide in rheumatoid arthritis. Clin Immunol 93:198, 1999.
114. Silva HT, Cao W, Shorthouse R, et al: Mechanism of action of leflunomide: in vivo uridine administration reverses its inhibition of lymphocyte proliferation. Transplant Proc 28:3082-3084, 1996.
115. Cherwinski HM, McCarley D, Schatzman R, et al: The immunosuppressant leflunomide inhibits lymphocyte progression through cell cycle by a novel mechanism J Pharmacol Exp Ther 272:460, 1995.
116. Cherwinski HM, Byars N, Ballaron SJ, et al: Leflunomide interferes with pyrimidine nucleotide biosynthesis. Inflamm Res 44:317, 1995.
117. Cherwinski HM, Cohn RG, Cheung P, et al: The immunosuppressant leflunomide inhibits lymphocyte proliferation by inhibiting pyrimidine biosynthesis. J Pharmacol Exp Ther 275:1043, 1995.
118. Greene S, Watanabe K, Braatz-Trulson J, et al: Inhibition of dihydroorotate dehydrogenase by the immunosuppressive agent leflunomide. Biochem Pharmacol 50:861, 1995.
119. Cao WW, Kao PN, Chao AC, et al: Mechanism of the antiproliferative action of leflunomide. J Heart Lung Transplant 14:1016, 1995.
120. Williamson RA, Yea CM, Robson AP, et al: Dihydroorotate dehydrogenase is a target for the biological effects of leflunomide. Transplant Proc 28:3088, 1996.
121. Nair RV, Cao W, Morris RE: The antiproliferative effect of leflunomide on vascular smooth muscle cells in vitro is mediated by selective inhibition of pyrimidine biosynthesis. Transplant Proc 28:3081, 1996.
122. Fairbanks LD, Bofill M, Rickemann K, et al: Importance of ribonucleotide availability to proliferating T-lymphocytes from healthy humans. J Biol Chem 50:29682, 1995.
123. Marijnen YM, de Korte D, Haverkort WA, et al: Studies on the incorporation of precursors into purine and pyrimidine nucleotides via "de novo" and "salvage" pathways in normal lymphocytes and lymphoblastic cell-line cells. Biochim Biophys Acta 1012:148, 1989.

124. Ruckemann K, Fairbanks LD, Carrey EA, et al: Leflunomide inhibits pyrimidine de novo synthesis in mitogen-stimulated T-lymphocytes from healthy humans. J Biol Chem 273:21682, 1998.
125. Linke SP, Clarkin KC, De Leonardo A, et al: A reversible, p53-dependent G_0/G_1 cell cycle arrest induced by ribonucleotide depletion in the absence of detectable DNA damage. Genes Dev 10:934, 1996.
126. Herrmann M, Frangou CG, Kirschbaum B. Cell cycle control of the de novo pyrimidine synthesis inhibitor leflunomide through the p53 and p21WAF-1 pathways [Abstract]. Arthritis Rheum 40:S177, 1997.
127. Levine AJ: p53: The cellular gatekeeper for growth and division. Cell 88:323, 1997.
128. Wahl GM, Linke SP, Paulson TG, et al: Maintaining genetic stability through TP53 mediated checkpoint control. Cancer Surv 29:183, 1997.
129. Bartlett RR, Dimitrijevic M, Mattar T, et al: Leflunomide (HWA 486): a novel immunomodulating compound for the treatment of autoimmune disorders and reactions leading to transplantation rejection. Agents Actions 32:10, 1991.
130. Mattar T, Kochhar K, Bartlett RR, et al: Inhibition of the epidermal growth factor receptor tyrosine kinase activity by leflunomide. FEBS Lett 334:161, 1993.
131. Xu X, Williams JW, Bremer EG, et al: Inhibition of protein tyrosine phosphorylation in T cells by a novel immunosuppressive agent, leflunomide. J Biol Chem 270:12398, 1995.
132. Gong H, Finnegan A, Chong AS-F: Two activities of the immunosuppressive metabolite of leflunomide, A77 1726. Biochem Pharmacol 52:527, 1996.
133. Xu X, Blinder L, Shen J, et al: In vivo mechanism by which leflunomide controls lymphoproliferative and autoimmune disease in MRL/MpJ-lpr/lpr mice. J Immunol 159:167, 1997.
134. Elder RT, Xu X, Williams JW, et al: The immunosuppressive metabolite of leflunomide, A77 1726, affects murine T cells through two biochemical mechanisms. J Immunol 159:22, 1997.
135. Manna SK, Aggarwal BB: Immunosuppressive leflunomide metabolite (A77 1726) blocks TNF-dependent nuclear factor-κB activation and gene expression. J Immunol 162:2095, 1999.
136. Hunter T: Protein kinases and phosphatases: the yin and yang of protein phosphorylation and signaling. Cell 80:225, 1995.
137. Manna SK, Mukhopadhyay A, Aggarwal BB: Leflunomide suppresses TNF-induced cellular responses: effect on NF-kappaB, Activator protein-1, c-Jun N-terminal protein kinase, and apoptosis. J Immunol 165:5962, 2000.
138. Miagkov AV, Kovalenko DV, Brown CE, et al: NF-kappaB activation provides the potential link between inflammation and hyperplasia in the arthritic joint. Proc Natl Acad Sci U S A 95:13859, 1998.
139. Foxwell B, Browne K, Bondeson J, et al: Efficient adenoviral infection with IkappaB alpha reveals that macrophage tumor necrosis factor alpha production in rheumatoid arthritis is NF-kappaB dependent. Proc Natl Acad Sci U S A 95:8211, 1998.
140. Bondeson J, Foxwell B, Brennan F, et al: Defining therapeutic targets by using adenovirus: blocking NF-kappaB inhibits both inflammatory and destructive mechanisms in rheumatoid synovium but spares antiinflammatory mediators. Proc Natl Acad Sci U S A 95:5668, 1999.
141. Bartlett RR, Schleyerbach R: Immunopharmacological profile of a novel isoxazol derivative, HWA 486, with potential antirheumatic activity. I. Disease modifying action on adjuvant arthritis of the rat. Int J Immunopharmacol 7:7, 1985.
142. Hambleton P, McMahon S: Drug actions on delayed-type hypersensitivity in rats with developing and established adjuvant arthritis. Agents Actions 29:328, 1990.
143. Pasternak RD, Wadopian NS, Wright RN, et al: Disease modifying activity of HWA 486 in rat adjuvant-induced arthritis. Agents Actions 21:241, 1987.
144. Thoss K, Henzgen S, Petrow PK, et al: Immunomodulation of rat antigen-induced arthritis by leflunomide alone and in combination with cyclosporin A. Inflamm Res 45:103, 1996.
145. Glant TT, Mikecz K, Bartlett RR, et al: Immunomodulation of proteoglycan-induced progressive polyarthritis by leflunomide. Immunopharmacology 23:105, 1992.
146. Glant TT, Mikecz K, Brennan F, et al: Suppression of autoimmune responses and inflammatory events by leflunomide in an animal model for rheumatoid arthritis. Agents Actions 41:C267, 1994.
147. Weber W, Harnisch L: Use of a population approach to the development of leflunomide: a new disease-modifying drug in the treatment of rheumatoid arthritis. In Aarons L, Balant LP, Danhof M, et al (eds): European Cooperation in the Field of Scientific and Technical Research. Brussels, European Commission, 1997, p 239.
148. Smolen JS, Kalden JR, Scott DL, et al: Efficacy and safety of leflunomide compared with placebo and sulphasalazine in active rheumatoid arthritis: a double-blind, randomized, multicentre trial. Lancet 353:259, 1999.
149. Remer CF, Weisman MH, Wallace DJ: Benefits of leflunomide in systemic lupus erythematosus: a pilot observational study. Lupus 10(7):480, 2001.
150. Salvarani C, Cantini F, Olivieri I: Disease-modifying antirheumatic drug therapy for psoriatic arthritis. Clin Exp Rheumatol 20(Suppl 28):S71, 2002.
151. Kuchle CC, Thoenes GH, Langer KH, et al: Prevention of kidney and skin graft rejection in rats by leflunomide: a new immunomodulating agent. Transplant Proc 23:1083, 1991.
152. Yuh DD, Gandy KL, Morris RE, et al: Leflunomide prolongs pulmonary allograft and xenograft survival. J Heart Lung Transplant 14:1136, 1995.
153. Krook H, Wennberg L, Hagberg A, et al: Immunosuppressive drugs in islet xenotransplantation: a tool for gaining further insights. Transplantation 74(8):1084, 2002.
154. Jin MB, Nakayama M, Ogata T, et al: A novel leflunomide derivative, FK778, for immunosuppression after kidney transplantation. Surgery 132(1):72, 2002.
155. Chokkalingam S, Shepherd R, Cunningham F, Eisen S: Leflunomide use in the first 33 months after FDA approval: experience in a national cohort of 3325 patients. Arthritis Rheum 46(9):S538, 2002.
156. ARAVA, US prescribing information. September 1998.
157. Leflunomide hepatotoxicity: European Agency for the Evaluation of Medicinal Products (EMEA). February, 2001.
158. Leflunomide: serious hepatic, blood, skin and respiratory reactions. Australian Adverse Drug Reactions Bulletin 20(2), 2001.
159. Low rates of serious liver toxicity to leflunomide (LEF) and methotrexate (MTX): a longitudinal surveillance study of 14,997 LEF and MTX exposures in RA. Arthritis Rheum 46(9):S375, 2002.
160. Prokopowitsch AS, Diogenes AHM, Borges CT, et al: Leflunomide induces progressive increase in rheumatoid arthritis lipid profile. Arthritis Rheum 46(9):S164, 2002.
161. Coblyn JS, Shadick N, Helfgott S: Leflunomide-associated weight loss in rheumatoid arthritis. Arthritis Rheum 44(5):1048, 2001.
162. Mikuls T, O'Dell J: The changing face of rheumatoid arthritis therapy: results of a survey. Arthritis Rheum 43:464, 2000.
163. Boers M, Verhoeven AC, Markusse HM, et al: Randomized comparison of combined step-down prednisolone, methotrexate and sulphasalazine with sulphasalazine alone in early rheumatoid arthritis. Lancet 350:309, 1997.
164. Mottonen T, Hannonsen P, Leirasalo-Repo M, et al: Comparison of combination therapy with single-drug therapy in early rheumatoid arthritis: a randomised trial. Lancet 353:1568, 1999.
165. Calguneri M, Pay S, Caliskaner Z, et al: Combination therapy versus monotherapy for the treatment of patients with rheumatoid arthritis. Clin Exp Rheumatol, 17:699, 1999.
166. Tugwell P, Pincus T, Yocum D, et al: Combination therapy with cyclosporine and methotrexate in severe rheumatoid arthritis. N Engl J Med 333:137, 1995.
167. O'Dell J, Leff R, Paulsen G, et al: Treatment of rheumatoid arthritis with methotrexate and hydroxychloroquine, methotrexate and sulfasalazine, or a combination of the three medications. Arthritis Rheum 46(5):1164, 2002.
168. Kremer JM, Genovese MC, Cannon GW, et al: Concomitant leflunomide therapy in patients with active rheumatoid arthritis despite stable doses of methotrexate. a randomized, double-blind, placebo-controlled trial. Ann Intern Med 137(9):726, 2002.

169. Maini RN, Breedveld FC, Kalden JR, et al: Therapeutic efficacy of multiple intravenous infusions of anti-tumor necrosis factor alpha monoclonal antibody combined with low-dose weekly methotrexate in rheumatoid arthritis. Arthritis Rheum 41:1552, 1998.
170. Weinblatt ME, Kremer JM, Bankhurst AD, et al: A trial of etanercept, a recombinant tumor necrosis factor receptor:Fc fusion protein, in patients with rheumatoid arthritis receiving methotrexate. N Engl J Med 340:253, 1999.
171. Lipsky P, Van der Heijde D, St. Clair EW, et al: Infliximab and methotrexate in the treatment of rheumatoid arthritis. N Engl J Med 343(22):1594, 2000.
172. Cohen S, Hurd E, Cush J, et al: Treatment of rheumatoid arthritis with anakinra, a recombinant human interleukin-1 receptor antagonist, in combination with methotrexate. Arthritis Rheum 46(3):614, 2002.
173. Keystone E, Weinblatt M, Furst D, et al: The ARMADA trial: a double-blind placebo controlled trial of the fully human anti-TNF monoclonal antibody, adalimumab (D2E7), in patients with active RA on methotrexate (MTX). Arthritis Rheum 44(9):S213, 2001.
174. Kremer JM: Combination therapy with biologic agents in rheumatoid arthritis: perils and promise. Arthritis Rheum 41:1548, 1998.
175. McCarty DJ, Carrera GF: Treatment of intractable rheumatoid arthritis with combined cyclophosphamide, azathioprine, and hydroxychloroquine. JAMA 248:1718, 1982.
176. Csuka ME, Carrero GF, McCarty DJ: Treatment of intractable rheumatoid arthritis with combined cyclophosphamide, azathioprine, and hydroxychloroquine: a follow-up study. JAMA 255:2315, 1986.
177. Williams HJ, Ward JR, Reding JC, et al: Comparison of auranofin, methotrexate, and the combination of both in the treatment of rheumatoid arthritis: a controlled clinical trial. Arthritis Rheum 35:259, 1992.
178. Haagsma CJ, van Riel PL, de Rooj DJ, et al: Combination of methotrexate and sulphasalazine vs methotrexate alone: a randomized open clinical trial in rheumatoid arthritis patients resistant to sulphasalazine therapy. Br J Rheumatol 33:1049, 1994.
179. Dougados M, Combe B, Cantagrel A, et al: Combination therapy in early rheumatoid arthritis: a randomised, controlled, double blind 52 week clinical trial of sulphasalazine and methotrexate compared with the single components. Ann Rheum Dis 58:220, 1999.
180. O'Dell J, Haire C, Erickson N, et al: Triple DMARD therapy for rheumatoid arthritis: efficacy. Arthritis Rheum 37:S295, 1994.
181. Paulus HE, Egger MJ, Ward JR, William JH: Analysis of improvement in individual rheumatoid arthritis patients treated with disease-modifying antirheumatic drugs, based on the findings in patients treated with placebo. Arthritis Rheum 33:477, 1990.
182. O'Dell J, Paulsen G, Haire C, et al: Combination DMARD therapy with methotrexate (M) - Sulfasalazine (S) - Hydroxychloroquine (H) in rheumatoid arthritis (RA): continued efficacy with minimal toxicity at 5 years. Arthritis Rheum 41(9 Suppl):S132, 1998.
183. O'Dell JR, Haire C, Erikson N, et al: Efficacy of triple DMARD therapy in patients with RA with suboptimal response to methotrexate. J Rheumatol 23(Suppl 44):72, 1996.
184. Egsmose C, Lung B, Borg G, et al: Patients with rheumatoid arthritis benefit from early second-line therapy: 5-year follow-up of a prospective double-blind placebo-controlled study. J Rheumatol 22:2208, 1995.
185. Tsakonas E, Fitzgerald AA, Fitazcharles MA, et al: Consequences of delayed therapy with second-line agents in rheumatoid arthritis: a 3 year followup on the hydroxychloroquine in early rheumatoid arthritis (HERA) study. J Rheumatol 27(3):623, 2000.
186. Lard LR: Early versus delayed treatment in patients with recent-onset rheumatoid arthritis: comparison of two cohorts who received different treatment strategies. Am J Med 111(6):446, 2001.
187. Wilske KR, Healey LA: Remodeling the pyramid: a concept whose time has come. J Rheumatol 16:565, 1989.
188. Landewe RBM, Boers M, Verhoeven AC, et al: COBRA combination therapy in patients with early rheumatoid arthritis. Arthritis Rheum 46(2):347, 2002.
189. Neva MH: FIN-RACo Trail Group. Combination drug therapy retards the development of rheumatoid atlantoaxial subluxations. Arthritis Rheum 43(11):2397, 2000.
190. Yocum DE, Stein M, Pincus T: Long-term safety of cyclosporin/Sandimmune(tm) (CsA/SIM) alone and in combination with methotrexate (MTX) in the treatment of active rheumatoid arthritis (RA): analysis of open-label extension studies [Abstract]. Arthritis Rheum 41(Suppl):S364, 1998.
191. Weinblatt ME, Kremer JM, Coblyn JS, et al: Pharmacokinetics, safety, and efficacy of combination treatment with methotrexate and leflunomide in patients with active rheumatoid arthritis. Arthritis Rheum 48(7):1322, 1999.
192. The Joint Committee of the Medical Research Council and Nuffield Foundation on Clinical Trials of Cortisone, ACTH, and Other Therapeutic Measures in Chronic Rheumatic Diseases: A comparison of prednisolone with aspirin or other analgesics in the treatment of rheumatoid arthritis. Ann Rheum Dis 18:173, 1959.
193. The Joint Committee of the Medical Research Council and Nuffield Foundation on Clinical Trials of Cortisone, ACTH, and Other Therapeutic Measures in Chronic Rheumatic Diseases: A comparison of prednisolone with aspirin or other analgesics in the treatment of rheumatoid arthritis. Ann Rheum Dis 19:331, 1960.
194. Kirwan JR, Arthritis and Rheumatism Council Low-Dose Glucocorticoid Study Group: The effect of glucocorticoids on joint destruction in rheumatoid arthritis. N Engl J Med 333:142, 1995.
195. Hickling P, Jacoby RK, Kirwan JR: Joint destruction after glucocorticoids are withdrawn in early rheumatoid arthritis. Br J Rheumatol 37:930, 1998.
196. O'Dell JR: Treating rheumatoid arthritis early: a window of opportunity. Arthritis Rheum 46:283, 2002.
197. McCarty DJ, Harman JG, Grassanovich JL, et al: Combination drug therapy of seropositive rheumatoid arthritis. J Rheumatol 22(9):1636, 1995.
198. O'Dell JR, Nepom BS, Haire C, et al: HLA-DRB1 typing in rheumatoid arthritis: predicting response to specific treatments. Ann Rheum Dis 57:209, 1998.

60 Immunoregulatory Drugs

C. MICHAEL STEIN

Our understanding of the complex cellular and subcellular mechanisms that regulate immune function is sophisticated, but our understanding of the specific immunologic factors that trigger and sustain most inflammatory rheumatic diseases remains rudimentary. The immunologic triggers of rheumatic disease and the specific functionally important mechanisms of antirheumatic drugs are both poorly characterized; thus, therapy has until recently evolved empirically rather than in an hypothesis-based, targeted fashion. This trial and error approach has led to the relatively slow evolution of immunoregulating treatment regimens, which are often based on clinical practice rather than controlled trials. Current regimens (Table 60–1) are not ideal, as they have suboptimal efficacy and often substantial toxicity, but they continue to evolve.

This chapter outlines the clinical pharmacology of both the older cytotoxic agents, where our major advance has been an improved understanding of how to use the drugs, and newer immunoregulating drugs, where optimal clinical use remains to be defined. Methotrexate, leflunomide, and biologic agents are discussed elsewhere.

Alkylating Agents

Alkylating agents, widely used as anticancer drugs, substitute alkyl radicals into DNA, resulting in cross-linking of DNA, impaired DNA synthesis, and cell death. Nitrogen mustard (mechlorethamine) was the alkylating agent first used in rheumatic diseases in the 1950s, but the requirement for intravenous (IV) administration and toxicity led to it being replaced by cyclophosphamide and chlorambucil.

CYCLOPHOSPHAMIDE

Cyclophosphamide is an analogue of nitrogen mustard that was developed to be a less-reactive drug more selectively cytotoxic to neoplastic cells than to healthy cells.[1] The original concept that tumor cells would selectively activate cyclophosphamide, an inactive prodrug, thus resulting in selective cytotoxicity to neoplastic cells, was incorrect. Nevertheless, cyclophosphamide does have a better therapeutic index than nitrogen mustard and is the alkylating agent of choice for most rheumatic disease requiring such therapy.

Mechanisms of Action

Cyclophosphamide is inactive. Its effects are mediated predominantly through phosphoramide mustard and, to a lesser extent, other active metabolites (Fig. 60–1). The primary mechanism of action is through the alkylation of DNA by active metabolites, such as phosphoramide mustard. These positively charged, reactive intermediates alkylate nucleophilic bases resulting in the cross-linking of DNA, breaks in DNA, decreased DNA synthesis, and apoptosis.[1-3] The cytotoxicity of alkylating agents correlates with the amount of DNA cross-linking,[4] but the relationship between cytotoxicity and immunoregulatory effects is unclear.

The effects of cyclophosphamide are not limited to any particular cell type; however, sensitivity varies among cell populations. Several mechanisms of cellular resistance to alkylating agents have been proposed. These include increased intracellular concentrations of glutathione and other thiols, increased activity of enzymes, such as aldehyde dehydrogenase, that produce inactive metabolites of cyclophosphamide, and increased DNA repair mechanisms.[2,5] Cyclophosphamide has a marked effect not only on rapidly dividing cells, but also throughout the cell cycle, resulting in alterations of most humoral and cellular immune responses.[6,7] The effects of cyclophosphamide include decreased numbers of both T and B lymphocytes, decreased lymphocyte proliferation, decreased antibody production, and suppression of delayed hypersensitivity to new antigens with relative preservation of established delayed hypersensitivity.[6,7] A marked effect on B lymphocyte function, in both resting and stimulated cells, is thought to be an important component of the clinical mechanism of action of cyclophosphamide.[3,7]

Clinical Pharmacology

Absorption and Distribution

Oral and IV administration of cyclophosphamide result in similar plasma concentrations.[8] Peak plasma concentrations of cyclophosphamide occur 1 hour after oral administration, and formation of the active phosphoramide mustard is rapid.[1,8] Protein binding of cyclophosphamide is low (20 percent), and it is widely distributed, with concentrations of cyclophosphamide in most body fluids approaching 50 to 80 percent of plasma concentrations.[1,9]

TABLE 60–1 • MECHANISM OF ACTION OF IMMUNOREGULATORY DRUGS

Drugs	Class	Mechanism of Action
Cyclophosphamide, chlorambucil	Alkylating cytotoxics	Active metabolites alkylate DNA
Azathioprine 6-Mercaptopurine	Purine analog cytotoxics	Inhibit purine synthesis
Cyclosporine Tacrolimus (FK506)	Calcineurin inhibitors	Inhibit calcium-dependent T cell activation and interleukin-2 (IL-2) production
Sirolimus (rapamycin)	Non–calcineurin-binding macrolide immunoregulator	Blocks IL-2– and growth factor–mediated signal transduction
Mycophenolate mofetil	Purine synthesis inhibitor	Mycophenolic acid inhibits inosine monophosphate dehydrogenase
Thalidomide	Glutamic acid derivative	Inhibition of tumor necrosis factor-α (TNF-α) production and angiogenesis
Dapsone	Sulfone antimicrobial	Inhibition of neutrophil function

Metabolism and Elimination

Cyclophosphamide, itself inactive, is rapidly metabolized, largely by the liver, to active and inactive metabolites (see Fig. 60–1). The initial formation of 4-hydroxycyclophosphamide is mediated by cytochrome P450 (CYP) enzymes. However, the relative contribution of specific isoforms is unclear with CYP2B6, CYP2C9, CYP2C19, and CYP3A4 reported to play a role.[10-12] The formation of 4-hydroxycyclophosphamide, which is cytotoxic, but not at physiologic pH, allows entry of the drug into cells and subsequent formation of the active phosphoramide mustard.

The elimination half-life of cyclophosphamide is 2 to 8 hours, and alkylating activity is not detectable in the plasma of most patients 24 hours after a dose of 12 mg/kg.[13] Plasma concentrations of cyclophosphamide are not clinically useful predictors of either efficacy or toxicity. Cyclophosphamide is eliminated predominantly in the urine, mostly as inactive metabolites; however, 10 to 20 percent is eliminated as unaltered cyclophosphamide, and some active metabolites, such as phosphoramide mustard and acrolein, are present in urine.[1,2,9,13]

Pharmacokinetic Considerations in Special Circumstances

Liver Disease

The half-life of cyclophosphamide is increased to 12 hours in patients with liver failure as compared to 8 hours in controls.[14] However, toxicity is not increased, suggesting that exposure to cytotoxic metabolites is not increased and dose modification in liver disease is generally not required.[1,2]

Renal Impairment

Some studies have shown little alteration in drug disposition with no increased toxicity in patients with impaired renal function.[1,9] However, small amounts of unchanged cyclophosphamide and its active metabolites are excreted by the kidneys. Thus, some accumulation of these would be expected. In two groups of patients with autoimmune disease and a creatinine clearance of 25 to 50 ml/min and 10 to 25 ml/min, exposure to cyclophophamide increased 44 and 77 percent, respectively.[15] In clinical practice, initial cyclophosphamide doses are decreased by

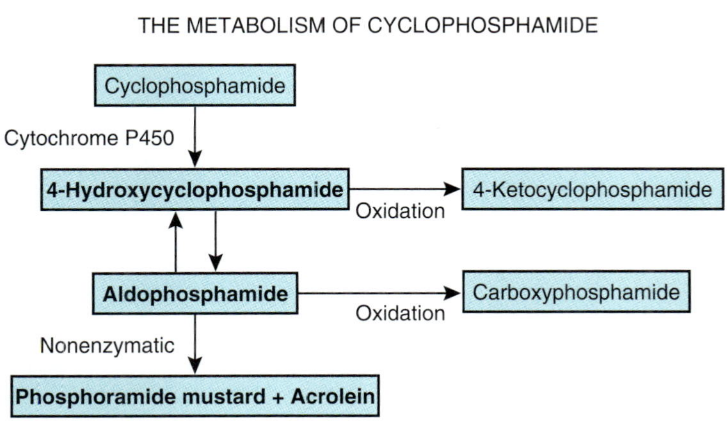

FIGURE 60–1 • Cyclophosphamide is converted to 4-hydroxycyclophosphamide, in equilibrium with its tautomer aldophosphamide, by cytochrome P450 enzymes. Subsequent nonenzymatic processes lead to the formation of phosphoramide mustard and acrolein. Oxidation of 4-hydroxycyclophosphamide and aldophosphamide through enzymes, including aldehyde dehydrogenase, result in inactive metabolites. Cytotoxic metabolites are shown in bold type.

approximately 25 percent in patients with mild to moderate renal impairment (creatinine 2.0 to 2.5 mg/dl or creatinine clearance 25 to 50 ml/min) and decreased 30 to 50 percent in patients with more severe renal impairment. Subsequent doses are titrated according to clinical response and effects on the leukocyte (WBC) count.[16] Cyclophosphamide is removed by dialysis and is, therefore, administered after dialysis,[1] or, alternatively, dialysis can be initiated the day after cyclophosphamide administration.[15]

Drug Interactions

Cimetidine

Cimetidine inhibits the activity of several hepatic enzymes. Coadministration with cyclophosphamide results in increased exposure to alkylating metabolites and increased bone marrow toxicity in an a mouse model.[17] Ranitidine,[18] and presumably other H_2-receptor antagonists that have little effect on hepatic drug metabolism, are not associated with increased cyclophosphamide toxicity.

Allopurinol

Allopurinol increases the half-life of cyclophosphamide[19] and the frequency of leukopenia.[20]

Succinylcholine

Cyclophosphamide decreases plasma pseudocholinesterase activity and can potentiate the effect of succinylcholine.[21]

Adverse Effects

Hematologic

Reversible myelosuppression is common. The degree of leukopenia and neutropenia, and the consequent increased risk of infection, is related to the dose of cyclophosphamide administered. Platelet counts are generally not affected with pulse doses of less than 50 mg/kg, but with chronic oral use a mild decrease in platelet count is common. After a single dose of cyclophosphamide, the approximate times to nadir and recovery of leukocyte counts are 8 to 14 days, and 21 days, respectively.[22] The WBC nadir is about 3000 cells/mm^3 after a dose of 1 g/m^2 (approximately 25 mg/kg) and 1500 cells/mm^3 after 1.5 g/m^2.[9] With chronic use there is increased sensitivity to the myelosuppressive effects of cyclophosphamide, and doses usually need to be decreased over time.

Infection

Infection with a range of common and opportunistic pathogens is a frequent complication (Table 60–2). In 100 patients with systemic lupus erythematosus (SLE), infection occurred in 45 during treatment with a cyclophosphamide-based regimen and was the primary cause of death in seven patients.[23] In this study, infection was equally common in patients receiving oral or IV cyclophosphamide and was associated with a WBC nadir at some point in treatment of less than 3000/mm^3 (55 percent infection rate versus 36 percent). However, at the time of infection, the average WBC count was within the normal range.[23] A higher maximum corticosteroid dose was also associated with increased risk of infection.

TABLE 60–2 • INFECTIONS THAT OCCURRED IN 45 OF 100 PATIENTS WITH SYSTEMIC LUPUS ERYTHEMATOSUS DURING TREATMENT WITH CYCLOPHOSPHAMIDE AND GLUCOCOCORTICOIDS

Type of Infection	Total Infections	Organisms (Number of infections)	Sites
Bacterial	33 (five patients had multiple, simultaneous infections)	*Escherichia coli* (5)	Urine, blood
		Pseudomonas (4)	Urine, blood, lung
		Klebsiella (4)	Urine, pancreas, skin
		Staphylococcus aureus (3)	Blood, skin, urine
		Citrobacter (2)	Urine, pancreas
		Proteus (2)	Skin, urine
		Enterobacter (2)	Urine
		Streptococcus pneumoniae (2)	Lung, blood
		Others (9)	Lung, blood, central nervous system (CNS), sinus
Opportunistic	20	*Candida albicans* (4)	Lung, urine, blood, esophagus
		Pneumocystis carinii (3)	Lung
		Cryptococcus neoformans (2)	CNS, urine, lung
		Torulopsis glabrata (2)	Blood, lung, urine
		Unidentified viral (2)	Esophagus, lung
		Aspergillus fumigatus (1)	Lung
		Cytomegalovirus (1)	Adrenal
		Others (5)	lung, skin, CNS
Other	10	*Herpes zoster* (10)	Skin

From Pryor BD, Bologna SG, Kahl LE: Risk factors for serious infection during treatment with cyclophosphamide and high-dose corticosteroids for systemic lupus erythematosus. Arthritis Rheum 39:1475-1482, 1996.

Half the infections occurred at prednisone doses of less than 40 mg/day, and a quarter of the infections occurred at doses less than 25 mg/day. Lower rates of infection (25 to 30 percent) have been reported in patients with SLE receiving cyclophosphamide in National Institutes of Health (NIH) protocols.[24]

Oral cyclophosphamide regimens generally pose a greater risk of infection than IV pulse regimens. For example, the treatment of vasculitis with cyclophosphamide and corticosteroids was associated with serious infections in 41 percent and 70 percent of patients with Wegener's granulomatosis treated with pulse IV or daily oral cyclophosphamide, respectively.[25] These rates of infection are higher than those reported in long-term NIH protocols in which 48 percent of 158 patients experienced 140 infections requiring hospitalization.[26] The reported frequency of cyclophosphamide-associated infection varies, probably as a function of the stage and severity of the underlying disease, the degree of cyclophosphamide-induced immunosuppression, and variations in concomitant glucocorticoid regimens.[25,27] Despite differences in clinical experience, infections are a common and potentially serious complication of all cyclophosphamide-based regimens.

Pneumocystis carinii pneumonia (PCP) has been recognized as a preventable, serious opportunistic infection that complicates treatment of systemic vasculitis with cyclophosphamide and methotrexate-based regimens. The risk is highest during the initial "induction" phase and is greater with oral than IV cyclophosphamide regimens.[25,28]

Urologic

The bladder toxicities of cyclophosphamide, hemorrhagic cystitis, and bladder cancer are related to route of administration, duration of therapy, and cumulative cyclophosphamide dose. Pulse IV cyclophosphamide regimens in rheumatology, in contrast to the high-dose oncology regimens, do not generally result in bladder toxicity. Bladder toxicity, a particular problem with long-term oral cyclophosphamide, is largely due to acrolein, a metabolite of cyclophosphamide.[29] Bladder toxicity can be prevented in patients receiving pulse doses of IV cyclophosphamide by administering mesna, a sulphydryl compound that binds acrolein in the urine and inactivates it.[30] The short half-life of mesna renders it suboptimal for the prevention of bladder toxicity in the patients at greatest risk—those receiving daily oral cyclophosphamide—but oral mesna administered three times a day with daily oral cyclophosphamide decreased the incidence of bladder toxicity to 12 percent and may decrease the risk of bladder cancer.[31] Nonglomerular hematuria, which may range from minor, microscopic blood loss to severe, macroscopic bleeding, is the most common manifestation of cyclophosphamide-induced cystitis.[32,33] Nonglomerular hematuria occurred at some time in 50 percent of 145 patients treated with oral cyclophosphamide and was related to the duration of therapy and cumulative cyclophosphamide dose.[33] The absolute risk of bladder cancer is difficult to quantify. In a large study, the risk of bladder cancer was increased 31-fold (95 percent confidence interval 13- to 65-fold) and seven of 145 patients (5 percent) have developed bladder cancer to date.[33] Bladder cancer developed 7 months to 15 years after initiating therapy and was preceded by nonglomerular hematuria in all patients. In six of the seven patients, bladder cancer was associated with a cumulative dose of more than 100 g cyclophosphamide and a cumulative duration of therapy of more than 2.7 years.[33] Smokers are at increased risk of both hemorrhagic cystitis and bladder cancer.[33]

Malignancy

In addition to the increased risk of bladder cancer cyclophosphamide increases the risk of other malignancies two- to fourfold[34,35]; however, the absolute risk is difficult to quantify because long-term studies have been performed on relatively few patients. In the largest study, 119 patients with rheumatoid arthritis (RA) who had been treated with oral cyclophosphamide were followed for 20 years. There were 50 cancers in 37 patients in the cyclophosphamide group compared to 26 cancers in 25 of 119 control RA patients.[34] Bladder, skin, myeloproliferative, and oropharangeal malignancies occurred more commonly in the cyclophosphamide group.[34] The risk of bladder and other malignancies increased with the cumulative dose of cyclophosphamide, and 53 percent of patients who received more than 80 g of cyclophosphamide developed malignancy.[34] Few malignancies have been reported in patients treated with pulse IV cyclophosphamide regimens.[34] Current data do not allow quantification of the long-term risk of malignancy associated with pulse IV cyclophosphamide treatment, but it is likely to be substantially smaller than that associated with oral regimens.

Reproductive

The adverse effects of alkylating agents on subsequent fertility in both men and women who have undergone cancer chemotherapy are well recognized[36]; however, it is reassuring that there was no increase in genetic disease in the offspring of adults who underwent cancer chemotherapy in childhood.[37] Cyclophosphamide, as used in autoimmune disease, results in significant gonadal toxicity. The risk of sustained amenorrhea after cyclophosphamide therapy has ranged from 11 to 59 percent.[38] The risk of ovarian failure may be lower with IV pulse cyclophosphamide regimens than oral regimens, but the difference is not substantial. For example, ovarian failure occurred in 5 of 11 patients (45 percent) receiving IV pulse cyclophosphamide as compared with 13 of 22 (59 percent) receiving oral cyclophosphamide for lupus nephritis.[39] Irrespective of the route of cyclophosphamide administration, the risk of ovarian failure increases with the age of the patient and the cumulative dose of cyclophosphamide.[38,40,41] For example, patients younger than 25 years of age receiving six pulses of IV cyclophosphamide had a very low frequency of ovarian failure (none of four patients), whereas patients older than 31 years of age receiving 15 to 24 pulses all had ovarian failure (four of four patients).[40] In men undergoing chemotherapy with regimens that include an alkylating agent, the frequency of azoospermia has ranged from 50 to 90 percent.[36,42] Less information is available in autoimmune disease but azoospermia or severe oligospermia were found in 11 of 17 men receiving cyclophosphamide for Behçet's syndrome.[43]

If the clinical situation allows, sperm or ova can be banked before starting treatment with cyclophosphamide to preserve future fertility in selected patients. Various strategies, usually involving suppression of luteinizing hormone (LH) and follicle-stimulating hormone (FSH), have been used to protect against cyclophosphamide-induced gonadal toxicity. Data are, however, limited.[44] A small study suggested that an oral contraceptive with a high dose of estrogen was protective, but in a retrospective cohort study, low-dose oral contraceptives were not.[41] Preliminary findings in women treated with a gonadotropin-releasing hormone analog while undergoing chemotherapy for lymphoma[44] and SLE[45] suggested a protective effect. None of eight women with SLE treated with an alkylating agent and a monthly injection of a gonadotropin-releasing hormone agonist developed ovarian failure, whereas five of nine treated only with an akylating agent did.[45] In men, an LH-releasing analog was not protective,[46] but testosterone (100 mg intramuscularly every 15 days) was protective in five patients.[42]

Pulmonary

Cyclophosphamide-induced pulmonary toxicity occurs in less than 1 percent of patients.[22] Early-onset pneumonitis 1 to 6 months after exposure to cyclophosphamide may respond to withdrawal of the drug and treatment with corticosteroids. A more insidious, irreversible, late-onset pneumonitis and fibrosis with radiographic findings of diffuse reticular or reticulonodular infiltrates may occur after treatment with oral cyclophosphamide for 1 to13 years.[47]

Miscellaneous

A varying degree of reversible alopecia occurs with both daily oral and monthly pulse cyclophosphamide. There are considerable differences in sensitivity among patients. Cardiotoxicity, a dose-limiting adverse effect in oncology, and water intoxication due to inappropriate antidiuretic hormone secretion, are rare.[48] Unusual hypersensitivity reactions include urticaria and anaphylaxis[22,49]; however, allergic reactions to the bladder protectant mesna are a more likely cause of allergic responses in patients who receive both mesna and cyclophosphamide.[30,50] Cyclophosphamide is teratogenic, particularly in the first trimester, and should be avoided in pregnancy.[51]

Clinical Considerations

Efficacy in Rheumatic Diseases

In long-term studies in patients with SLE, monthly IV cyclophosphamide regimens preserve renal function better than oral cyclophosphamide or azathioprine-based regimens.[52] IV cyclophosphamide pulses can also be effective in patients with other serious complications of SLE, including central nervous system involvement and thrombocytopenia,[53] as well as interstitial lung disease associated with scleroderma and other autoimmune diseases.[54,55] The use of cyclophosphamide for the treatment of Wegener's granulomatosis and other forms of systemic vasculitis has evolved through careful observational studies. Oral daily cyclophosphamide regimens (Table 60–3) remain the standard against which other treatments are compared. IV cyclophosphamide is less effective than oral cyclophosphamide for the treatment of Wegener's granulomatosis, particularly in terms of inducing a sustained response to therapy,[16,25] although this opinion is not universal.[56] In RA, oral cyclophosphamide is effective but the benefit seldom justifies the risks.[57] In rheumatoid vasculitis, IV cyclophosphamide improves the vasculitis but, interestingly, does not improve the arthritis.[57] The bioavailability of oral cyclophosphamide is excellent, and monthly oral pulse therapy with cyclophosphamide (0.5 to 1 g/m^2) has been successful.[58] Low-dose (500 mg) IV cyclophosphamide infusions weekly have been used to initiate therapy to induce remission more rapidly in patients who would otherwise be treated with daily oral cyclophosphamide.[59]

Strategies to Minimize Toxicity

Strategies to minimize toxicity include adjusting the dose of cyclophosphamide to avoid a significant degree of leukopenia (WBC less than 3000/mm^3 for daily oral therapy or a nadir of less than 2000/mm^3 for pulse IV therapy) and granulocytopenia.[27,60] The blood count is monitored initially at 1- to 2-week intervals and monthly thereafter in patients on stable oral doses. To decrease the risk of infection added by concomitant high-dose corticosteroids, the dose of corticosteroids should be reduced after a clinical response has been obtained, and alternate-day glucocorticoids should be considered in the maintenance phase. Oral cyclophosphamide is best administered as a single dose in the morning with the patient drinking plenty of fluids and emptying the bladder frequently to dilute the urinary concentration of acrolein and to minimize the time the bladder is exposed to it. Prophylaxis against PCP is often prescribed, particularly during the "induction" phase when doses of cyclophosphamide and corticosteroids are higher.[27] Many clinicians administer mesna with IV cyclophosphamide (see Table 60–3) to decrease bladder toxicity, and limited data suggest it may also be beneficial with oral therapy.[31] Urinalysis should be performed monthly and nonglomerular hematuria evaluated by a urologist. Patients who receive cyclophosphamide, particularly those who develop cyclophosphamide-induced cystitis, are at greater risk of developing bladder cancer, and life-long surveillance is required with urinalysis, urine cytology and, if indicated, cystoscopy.[33] Lastly, drugs that are less toxic than cyclophosphamide, such as methotrexate, are an option for inducing remission in patients with less severe Wegener's granulomatosis[61]

TABLE 60–3 • TYPICAL NATIONAL INSTITUTES OF HEALTH–DERIVED PROTOCOLS FOR THE MANAGEMENT OF SYSTEMIC VASCULITIS WITH ORAL CYCLOPHOSPHAMIDE AND THE MANAGEMENT OF LUPUS NEPHRITIS WITH INTRAVENOUS (IV) PULSE CYCLOPHOSPHAMIDE

	Wegener's Granulomatosis Oral Cyclophosphamide Regimen	Lupus Nephritis Intravenous Cyclophosphamide Regimen
Glucocorticoid	Prednisone 1mg/kg/day for 4 weeks decreasing, if possible, to achieve a prednisone dose of approximately 60 mg alternate days at 3 months	Prednisone 0.5-1 mg/kg/day for 4 weeks decreasing the every other day dose each week, if possible, by 5 mg to reach a goal of 0.25 mg/kg on alternate days
Cyclophosphamide (initial dose)	2 mg/kg/day by mouth; very ill patients receive 3-5 mg/kg/day for 2-3 days then 2 mg/kg/day; decrease dose 25-50% for renal impairment	0.5-0.75 g/m² infused IV in saline over 30-60 minutes; decrease dose by approximately 30% if the glomerular filtration rate is less than one-third normal
Cyclophosphamide (subsequent dose)	Increase daily dose in 25-mg increments at 1-2 week intervals if disease active; adjust dose to avoid leukopenia (WBC <3000/mm³) and granulocytopenia	If WBC nadir 10-14 days after the previous dose is >4000/mm³ increase the dose 25% to a maximum of 1 g/m²; adjust dose to avoid WBC nadir < 2000/mm³; if WBC nadir <1500/mm³ decrease dose by at least 25%
Adjunct Treatment	Pneumocystis prophylaxis, particularly during "induction" phase	Optional mesna every 3 hours for 4 doses orally or IV; each mesna dose approximately 20% of cyclophosphamide dose; antiemetics: ondansetron 4-8 mg po every 4 hours for 3-4 doses and one dose of dexamethasone 10 mg po
Treatment Plan	Taper cyclophosphamide after 1 year of remission; alternatively, after remission induced, consider alternative maintenance therapy such as methotrexate	Monthly cyclophosphamide for 6 months then a maintenance dose every 3 months; continue maintenance cyclophosphamide for 1 year after remission

Data from McCune WJ, Golbus J, Zeldes W, et al: Clinical and immunologic effects of monthly administration of intravenous cyclophosphamide in severe systemic lupus erythematosus. New Engl J Med 318:1423, 1988. Gourley MF, Austin HA, Scott D, et al: Methylprednisolone and cyclophosphamide, alone or in combination, in patients with lupus nephritis: a randomized, controlled trial. Ann Intern Med 125:549, 1996. Hoffman GS: Treatment of Wegener's granulomatosis: time to change the standard of care? Arthritis Rheum 40:2099, 1997. Hoffman GS, Kerr GS, Leavitt RY, et al: Wegener granulomatosis: an analysis of 158 patients. Ann Intern Med 116:488, 1992. Balow JE, Boumpas DT, Fessler BJ, Austin HA: Management of lupus nephritis. Kidney Int 53(Suppl):S88, 1996.

or for maintenance therapy in some patients after remission has been induced with cyclophosphamide and prednisone.[62]

Clinical Role

Cyclophosphamide remains the drug of choice for most patients with systemic necrotizing vasculitis or Goodpasture's syndrome, for many patients with SLE, and for some patients with autoimmune disease–associated interstitial lung disease and inflammatory eye disease. In other diseases, such as RA, unless complicated by vasculitis, less toxic and more effective drugs have replaced cyclophosphamide. High doses of cyclophosphamide, with or without stem-cell rescue, are being studied as therapies for RA and SLE. Cyclophosphamide may be a lifesaving drug, but it can also induce life-threatening adverse effects. Meticulous monitoring and good clinical judgment are required to use it effectively.

CHLORAMBUCIL

Chlorambucil is an alkylating agent widely used to treat lymphomas and other malignancies. It has also been used, usually as an alternative to cyclophosphamide, in rheumatologic diseases. The mechanism of action of chlorambucil is similar to that of cyclophosphamide; however, the onset of action is slower.

Clinical Pharmacology

Chlorambucil is well absorbed (>70 percent) after oral administration with peak concentrations occurring within 2 hours.[63] Chlorambucil is extensively metabolized by β-oxidation to a metabolite, phenylacetic acid mustard, which is also cytotoxic.[63,64] Less than 1 percent of the oral dose of chlorambucil appears in the urine as unchanged drug.[63] The plasma half-life of chlorambucil and the phenylacetic acid mustard metabolite is 30 to 180 minutes.[63,64]

Adverse Effects

Hematologic

Myelosuppression is common and may be abrupt in onset. The degree of leukopenia and neutropenia is dose related, but there are considerable interindividual differences in sensitivity. The frequency of leukopenia in patients receiving chlorambucil for RA has ranged from 14 to 50 percent.[65] Myelosuppression is usually reversible; however, it may take several months for the WBC count to return to the normal range, and some patients remain relatively leukopenic. Irreversible, fatal bone marrow suppression has been reported in patients receiving chlorambucil for rheumatic disease.[65]

Infection

The average frequency of herpes zoster infection is 13 percent and, as is the case with cyclophosphamide, infections due to a wide range of bacterial and nonbacterial pathogens occur.[65]

Malignancy

Treatment with chlorambucil increases the risk of leukemia, particularly myeloid leukemia, and has been associated with a range of lymphomas.[65-67] Various solid organ tumors have occurred in association with chlorambucil, but no causal relationship has been established.[65]

Miscellaneous

Other adverse effects of chlorambucil include azoospermia and amenorrhea, which are usually reversible; pulmonary fibrosis; oral ulceration; hepatotoxicity; nausea; fever; and rashes. Chlorambucil is teratogenic.

Clinical Considerations

Chlorambucil is moderately effective in RA, with approximately 70 percent of patients showing benefit in uncontrolled studies.[65] Alternative, safer drugs are preferred for the treatment of RA. Chlorambucil is effective for some patients with inflammatory eye disease, including Behçet's syndrome,[68] and occasionally for refractory dermatomyositis.[69] Chlorambucil is used as an alternative alkylating agent for patients unable to tolerate cyclophosphamide because of bladder toxicity or gastrointestinal intolerance. However, chlorambucil does not appear to be as effective as cyclophosphamide in the treatment of vasculitis or glomerulonephritis.[70] Chlorambucil is often started in a dose of 0.1 mg/kg/day and the dose increased or decreased according to clinical response and toxicity. Doses of 0.2 mg/kg/day or higher are associated with more frequent myelosuppression. Alternatively, a "start low, go slow" approach, with chlorambucil started at a dose of 4 mg/day and increased in 1-mg increments at 1- to 2-month intervals, if required, may be better tolerated. However, even with this approach, 75 percent of patients discontinued therapy because of chlorambucil-related toxicity.[65] Regular monitoring, particularly of the WBC, at approximately 2-week intervals initially, and then monthly once stable, is required.

Purine Analogs

AZATHIOPRINE AND 6-MERCAPTOPURINE

Azathioprine, a prodrug of 6-mercaptopurine (6-MP), is a purine analog, cycle-specific antimetabolite that is widely used as an immunosuppressant for organ transplantation, the treatment of malignancy, and autoimmune diseases such as RA, SLE, and Behçet's syndrome. Azathioprine has a better therapeutic index than 6-MP and has largely replaced it in the treatment of autoimmune disease. Azathioprine is rapidly converted to 6-MP in vivo by the removal of an imidazole group.[71] Thus, the clinical pharmacology of azathioprine and 6-MP are similar and will be discussed together.

Mechanisms of Action

Azathioprine is converted to 6-MP and then to active intracellular thiopurine metabolites as discussed later. The exact mechanism of action of the active thiopurine metabolites of azathioprine and 6-MP in autoimmune disease is not known. Thiopurine metabolites, such as thioguanine nucleotides, decrease the de novo synthesis of purine nucleotides by inhibiting amidotransferase enzymes and purine ribonucleotide interconversion and are incorporated into DNA and RNA.[71] The incorporation of thioguanine nucleotides into the nucleic acids of cells is thought to mediate the cytotoxicity of azathioprine, whereas inhibition of purine synthesis may be more important in decreasing cellular proliferation.[71] Leukopenia is not necessary for immunosuppression. Azathioprine and 6-MP decrease the circulating lymphocyte count, suppress lymphocyte proliferation, inhibit antibody production, inhibit monocyte production, suppress natural killer (NK) cell activity,[72] and inhibit cell-mediated and humoral immunity.

Clinical Pharmacology

Absorption and Distribution

After absorption, azathioprine is rapidly converted to 6-MP enzymatically by glutathione-*S*-transferase and nonenzymatically by sulfhydryl groups[71] (Fig. 60–2). The bioavailability of azathioprine, measured as the concentrations of 6-MP achieved after oral administration, is variable. In healthy volunteers, bioavailability ranged from 27 to 83 percent with an average of 47 percent.[73] 6-MP is widely distributed with a volume of distribution of 4 to 8 L/kg.[73]

Metabolism and Elimination

The metabolism of 6-MP is complex[71,74] and has been simplified in Figure 60–2. Two enzymes, xanthine oxidase and thiopurine methyltransferase (TPMT), shunt 6-MP metabolites to relatively inactive compounds, whereas other enzymes such as hypoxanthine-guanine-phosphoribosyl-transferase (HGPRT) lead to the formation of cytotoxic thiopurine nucleotides. Low TPMT activity or inhibition of xanthine oxidase by drugs such as allopurinol will, therefore, lead to decreased detoxification and increased formation of cytotoxic metabolites after the administration of azathioprine or 6-MP. Maximum concentrations of 6-MP occur 1 to 3 hours after administration of azathioprine, and the half-life of 6-MP is 1 to 2 hours.[73] However, the half-life of the intracellular, active 6-thioguanine nucleotides is estimated to be 1 to 2 weeks, and concentrations do not change over the 24-hour dose period in patients receiving daily azathioprine.[75,76] Measurement of plasma

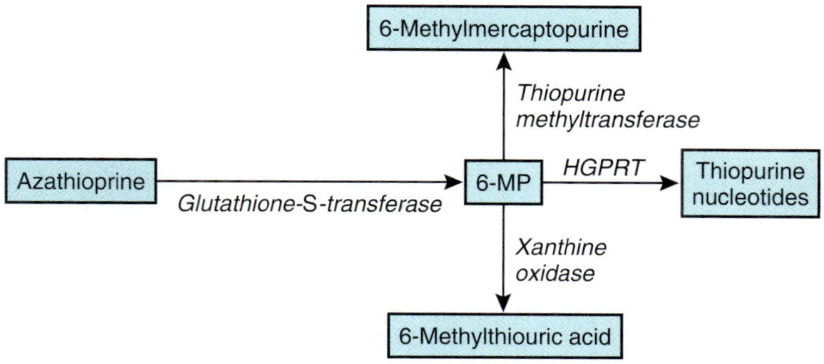

FIGURE 60–2 · Azathioprine is converted to 6-Mercaptopurine (6-MP) enzymatically by glutathione-S-transferase and nonenzymatic mechanisms. Xanthine oxidase and thiopurine methyltransferase metabolize 6-MP to the inactive metabolites methylthiouric acid and 6-methylmercaptopurine, respectively. Hypoxanthine-guanine-phosphoribosyl-transferase (HGPRT) metabolizes 6-MP to active, cytotoxic thiopurine nucleotides.

concentrations of azathioprine or 6-MP are not useful predictors of efficacy or toxicity. Therapeutic monitoring using the active 6-thioguanine nucleotides has been attempted in rheumatic diseases but has not been established to be useful.[77] At conventional rheumatologic doses, approximately 1 percent of 6-MP is excreted unchanged in the urine[75]; however, increased toxicity can occur with renal impairment, and a modest dose reduction is usually needed. The substantial interindividual variability in azathioprine disposition and TPMT activity are more important determinants of sensitivity to azathioprine than renal function.[78] Azathioprine and 6-MP cross the placenta, but fetal concentrations are low, suggesting placental metabolism.[51] Studies in renal allograft recipients who have received azathioprine during pregnancy have generally not found an increased frequency of birth defects.[51] There are limited data in rheumatologic diseases and, if possible, azathioprine is avoided in pregnancy.

Drug Interactions

Allopurinol

One of the most important, and potentially fatal, drug interactions in rheumatology is the ability of allopurinol, through inhibition of xanthine oxidase–mediated inactivation of 6-MP, to dramatically increase the cytotoxic effects of azathioprine and 6-MP.[79] Various strategies have been employed to treat hyperuricemia and gout in patients receiving azathioprine, a common clinical problem after transplantation. Reduction of the dose of azathioprine by at least two thirds in patients who are also receiving allopurinol is advocated. However, because myelosuppression can still occur after a 75-percent reduction in dose, careful monitoring is required.[79] Alternatively, uricosurics such as benzbromarone, have been effective and safe,[79] and mycophenolate mofetil has been substituted for azathioprine as an alternative immunosuppressant.[80]

Sulfasalazine

Sulfasalazine is commonly used in combination with azathioprine or 6-MP for the management of refractory inflammatory bowel disease. This combination may increase the frequency of myelosuppression, perhaps because sulfasalazine inhibits TPMT activity.[81,82]

Warfarin

Azathioprine has been associated with resistance to warfarin in four case reports.[83]

Adverse Effects

Azathioprine is not as well tolerated as weekly methotrexate.[84] Approximately 15 to 30 percent of patients discontinue azathioprine within 6 months, most often because of gastrointestinal adverse effects.[74,85]

Hematologic

Reversible myelosuppression is common, dose related, and varies substantially among individuals. Low-dose azathioprine (1 to 2 mg/kg/day) resulted in leukopenia in 4.5 percent and thrombocytopenia in 2 percent of subjects.[85] Pure red-cell aplasia is rare. Severe myelosuppression in uncommon and has until recently been thought to be an idiosyncratic response to azathioprine. It is now evident that the majority of patients with severe azathioprine-induced myelosuppression have low or absent TPMT activity. Decreased TPMT activity leads to a decreased ability to detoxify 6-MP and results in increased formation of cytotoxic thioguanine metabolites and clinical toxicity. TPMT activity is affected by genetic polymorphism, and several point mutations are associated with impaired enzyme activity.[86] TPMT activity in white and black Americans is similarly polymorphic with a trimodal distribution. Approximately 90 percent of subjects show high activity, 10 percent intermediate activity, and 0.3 percent (the subjects homozygous for the poorly functional polymorphisms) very low activity.[86,87] The median TPMT activity in black Americans is approximately 17 percent lower than in white Americans.[87] The 1 in 300 subjects with low or absent TPMT activity is at great risk of severe azathioprine-induced myelosuppression, which has a delayed but sudden onset, most commonly between 4 and 10 weeks after azathioprine has been started.[88] Subjects with intermediate TPMT activity may have more frequent adverse effects, including gastrointestinal effects.[74]

Gastrointestinal

Nausea, vomiting, and diarrhea are among the most common adverse effects of azathioprine. A mild increase in liver enzymes occurs in 5 to 10 percent of patients, but serious liver toxicity, severe cholestasis, hepatic veno-occlusive disease, and nodular regenerative hyperplasia are rare.

Malignancy

Data regarding the risk of malignancy in patients treated with azathioprine for rheumatologic disease are conflicting. Some studies found an increased risk, particularly of lymphoproliferative malignancies, whereas others did not.[57]

Azathioprine Hypersensitivity

Acute hypersensitivity syndromes, usually occurring within 2 weeks of starting therapy, with a range of manifestations including shock, fever, rash, pancreatitis, renal failure, and hepatitis, are rare.[89]

Others

Infection is less common with azathioprine than with alkylating agents; however, infections with a range of bacterial and nonbacterial pathogens, including herpes zoster and cytomegalovirus, may occur. The rate of infection when azathioprine is administered alone or with low doses of glucocorticoids is approximately 2.5 per 100 person-years of exposure.[85] Maculopapular or urticarial rashes can occur. Eosinophilia and drug fever are rare.

Clinical Considerations

Efficacy in Rheumatic Diseases

Azathioprine is often started at a dose of 50 mg daily and, if this is tolerated, the dose is increased to 2 to 2.5 mg/kg after 1 to 2 weeks. A more gradual increase in dose of 25 mg every 1 to 2 weeks is better tolerated. The onset of immunomodulatory effects is relatively slow, over several weeks, presumably because the active thioguanine metabolites slowly accumulate intracellularly. Azathioprine is effective in the treatment of RA with a slow clinical response over several months,[57] but it is not as effective as methotrexate. The combination of azathioprine and methotrexate is no more effective than methotrexate alone in RA.[84] Azathioprine is used to treat some patients with lupus nephritis and, although more effective than corticosteroids alone, is not as effective as IV pulse cyclophosphamide.[52] For other manifestations of SLE, including cutaneous disease, azathioprine is widely used as a corticosteroid-sparing agent.[90] Azathioprine in combination with corticosteroids is useful in the treatment of a range of other autoimmune diseases including inflammatory muscle disease. For refractory myositis the combination of azathioprine, methotrexate, and corticosteroids has been effective.[91] Efficacy is reported in inflammatory eye disease including Behçet's syndrome,[92] psoriatic arthritis,[93] Reiter's syndrome, and various forms of vasculitis.[94] In systemic vasculitis, azathioprine is most often used as a steroid-sparing agent, and because it is less effective than cyclophosphamide, it is not used to induce remission.

Strategies to Minimize Toxicity

The tests to identify the one out of 300 individuals with low or absent TPMT activity are now available from commercial and research laboratories. TPMT activity can be measured directly in red blood cell (RBC) membranes or, alternatively, the known polymorphisms can be identified by polymerase chain reaction (PCR). In the absence of genetic testing, a low initial dose and careful monitoring of the WBC in patients starting azathioprine is required; some suggest monitoring as often as weekly during the first 15 weeks of azathioprine treatment.[88] Once patients are on a stable dose of azathioprine, blood counts are monitored monthly and liver function tests are given every 3 to 4 months.

Clinical Role

Azathioprine is seldom used to treat RA except in patients who are unable to tolerate or do not respond to other therapies. The most common clinical use of azathioprine is as a steroid-sparing agent in the management of SLE and other autoimmune diseases.

Cyclosporine, Tacrolimus (FK506), and Sirolimus (rapamycin)

CYCLOSPORINE A

Cyclosporine A, a lipophilic endecapeptide derived from a fungus, has revolutionized organ transplantation and has more recently become an established therapeutic option for a range of autoimmune diseases from RA to autoimmune eye disease.

Mechanism of Action

Cyclosporine is a prototype drug that impairs production of interleukin-2 (IL-2) and other cytokines and, thus, decreases lymphocyte proliferation. Cyclosporine complexes with cyclophilin, one of a group of a cytosolic-binding proteins known as immunophilins. This complex binds to and inhibits calcineurin, a serine/threonine phosphatase. Inhibition of calcineurin phosphatase activity prevents the translocation of cytosolic nuclear factor of activated T cells (NF-AT) to the nucleus, a translocation that is required for the transcription of genes for cytokines such as IL-2 and for T cell activation[95-97] (Fig. 60–3).

Clinical Pharmacology

There are two formulations of cyclosporine for oral use: the older, oil-based Sandimmune formulation and the newer, microemulsion Neoral formulation. The active drug, cyclosporine, is identical in both formulations, but the microemulsion formulation results in better bioavailability and less inter- and intrasubject variability. Neoral or equivalent generic formulations will replace the Sandimmune formulation of cyclosporine, which is no longer universally available.

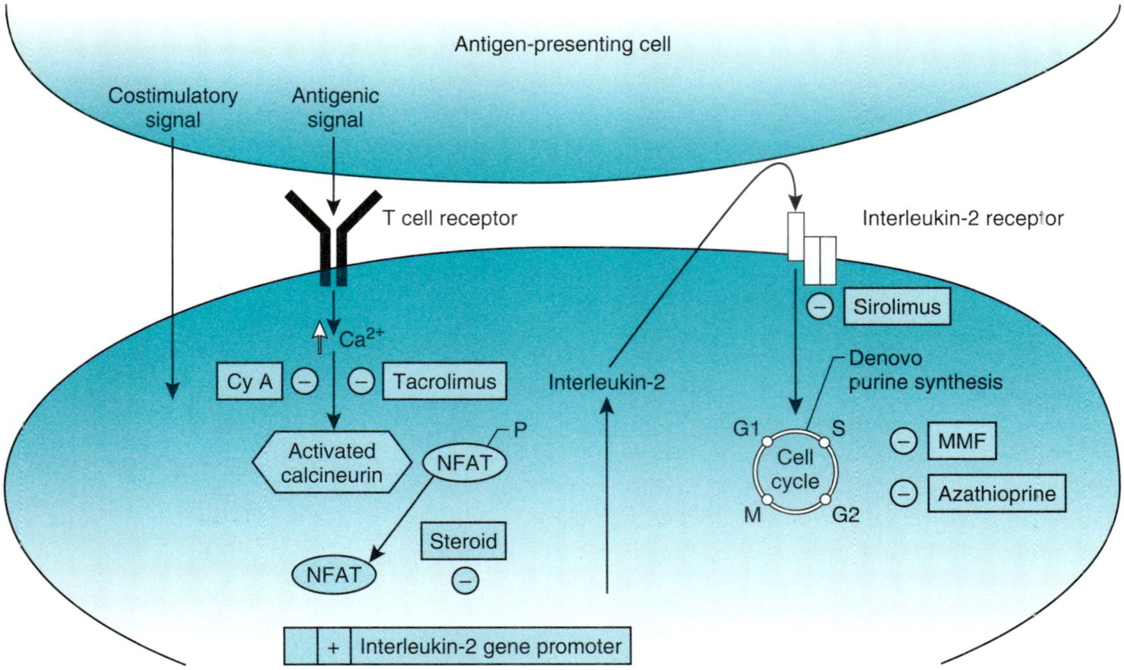

FIGURE 60–3 · Stages of T Cell Activation. Multiple targets for immunosuppressive agents. Stimulation of T cell receptor (TCR) results in calcineurin activation, a process inhibited by cyclosporin (CyA) and tacrolimus. Calcineurin dephosphorylates nuclear factor of activated T cells (NF-AT) enabling it to enter nucleus and bind to interleukin-2 (IL-2) promoter. Corticosteroids inhibit cytokine gene transcription in lymphocytes and antigen-presenting cells by several mechanisms. Costimulatory signals are necessary to optimize T cell IL-2 gene transcription, prevent T cell anergy, and inhibit T cell apoptosis. Experimental agents, but not current immunosuppressive agents, interrupt these intracellular signals. IL-2 receptor stimulation induces cell to enter cell cycle and proliferate. Signal 3 may be blocked by IL-2 receptor antibodies or by sirolimus, which inhibits second messenger signals induced by IL-2 receptor ligation. Following progression into cell cycle, azathioprine and mycophenolate mofetil interrupt DNA replication by inhibiting purine synthesis. (Reproduced with permission from Denton MD, Magee CC, Sayegh MH: Immunosuppressive strategies in transplantation. Lancet 353: 1083-1091, 1999.)

Absorption and Distribution

Cyclosporine is poorly and variably absorbed from the gut with a bioavailability of approximately 30 percent. A high-fat meal increases absorption. There is substantial interindividual (three-fold) and intraindividual (two-fold) variability in cyclosporine disposition.[98] The time to peak concentration is highly variable (1 to 8 hours) as is the elimination half-life (3 to 20 hours). Cyclosporine is lipophilic and widely distributed in body tissues, particularly in the lean body mass.[98] Higher concentrations of cyclosporine are found in RBCs than in plasma; thus, for monitoring of cyclosporine concentrations, which is seldom required in autoimmune diseases, whole blood cyclosporine concentrations are measured. With the microemulsion formulation, as compared to the Sandimmune formulation, the time to maximum concentration is approximately 25 percent shorter, and the maximum cyclosporine concentration and area under the concentration curve (AUC) are increased by approximately 50 percent.[99,100] More importantly, inter- and intraindividual variability in cyclosporine disposition is decreased by approximately 50 percent with the microemulsion formulation.[99,100]

Metabolism and Elimination

There are two major determinants of cyclosporine disposition. First, P-glycoprotein (P-GP), a drug efflux pump, pumps substrates such as cyclosporine out of cells. P-GP, the product of the multidrug resistance (MDR) gene, is expressed on intestinal epithelial cells and in the liver. Second, cyclosporine is extensively metabolized by the cytochrome P4503A (CYP3A) enzyme system, which is active not only in the liver but also in intestinal epithelium. Thus, P-GP, by limiting drug uptake, and CYP3A4, by facilitating drug metabolism in the gut and liver, both act to limit the bioavailability of cyclosporine and to determine its disposition.[101] Cyclosporine is extensively metabolized to more than 20 metabolites. The rate-limiting step in the elimination of cyclosporine is the formation of metabolites, not their clearance. Cyclosporine elimination is not altered in renal failure; however, because of its nephrotoxicity, cyclosporine is avoided in patients with impaired renal function. Liver disease impairs the excretion of cyclosporine metabolites.

Drug Interactions

Cyclosporine and tacrolimus, because of the influence of P-GP and CYP3A4 enzyme activity on their disposition, have many clinically important drug interactions. Selected clinically important interactions are listed in Table 60–4 and have been reviewed by others.[102] Many drugs such as erythromycin, azole antifungal drugs, and some of the calcium channel antagonists that

TABLE 60–4 • CLINICALLY IMPORTANT DRUG INTERACTIONS WITH CYCLOSPORINE*

Increased Cyclosporine Concentrations
• Erythromycin, clarithromycin • Azole antifungals: ketoconazole, fluconazole, itraconazole • Calcium channel antagonists: diltiazem, verapamil, amlodipine† • Grapefruit juice • Others: amiodarone, danazol, allopurinol, colchicine
Decreased Cyclosporine Concentrations
• Inducers of hepatic enzymes (rifampicin, phenytoin, phenobarbitone, nafcillin, St. John's wort)
Increased Cyclosporine Toxicity
• Increased renal toxicity with aminoglycosides, quinolone antibiotics, amphotericin B, (?) nonsteroidal anti-inflammatory drugs (NSAIDs), (?) angiotensin converting enzyme (ACE) inhibitors
Cyclosporine Increasing the Toxicity of Another Drug
• Increased risk of myopathy and rhabdomyolysis with lovastatin and other statins • Increased risk of colchicine neuromyopathy and toxicity • Increased digoxin concentrations • Increased risk of hyperkalemia with K^+ sparing diuretics and K^+ supplements

*Most of the interactions with cyclosporine are also likely to apply to tacrolimus.
†There are conflicting data that amlodipine does and does not increase cyclosporine concentrations.

inhibit CYP3A4 (thus inhibiting the metabolism of cyclosporine) also inhibit P-GP. Drug interactions mediated by these dual mechanisms may result in a two-to five-fold increase in cyclosporine concentrations.

Azithromycin, in contrast to erythromycin, appears unlikely to alter cyclosporine levels. The plasma concentrations and clinical toxicity of several statin lipid-lowering agents are increased substantially by cyclosporine, but the disposition of fluvastatin and pravastatin, because they are not metabolized primarily by CYP3A4, are less likely to be altered by cyclosporine.[103] Nevertheless, the pravastatin AUC, a measure of drug exposure was five times higher in patients also receiving cyclosporine.[104] Of the calcium channel antagonists, nifedipine and isradipine have little effect on cyclosporine concentrations, compared to diltiazem, which does affect cyclosporine concentrations. It is controversial whether nonsteroidal anti-inflammatory drugs (NSAIDs) increase cyclosporine nephrotoxicity. In many clinical studies, cyclosporine and NSAIDs have been safely coadministered[105–107]; however, increased cyclosporine-associated nephrotoxicity with NSAIDs has been reported. Currently, many patients starting cyclosporine also take an NSAID. If their creatinine increases, then in addition to decreasing the dose of cyclosporine, discontinuing the NSAID may be tried.

Adverse Effects

In many clinical trials performed over 6 to 12 months, cyclosporine has generally been well tolerated with little serious toxicity. Gastrointestinal upset is common but usually mild and transient. A few patients, however, discontinue cyclosporine therapy for this reason. Other adverse effects that are relatively common but usually of minor significance include hypertrichosis, gingival hyperplasia, tremor, paresthesia, breast tenderness, hyperkalemia, hypomagnesemia, and an increase in serum uric acid.[108] Cyclosporine may result in a clinically insignificant increase in alkaline phosphatase concentrations but does not increase the frequency of abnormal transaminase concentrations in patient also receiving methotrexate.[109]

Hypertension

Hypertension occurs in approximately 20 percent of patients with autoimmune disease receiving cyclosporine. The hypertension is usually relatively mild and can be controlled by either reducing the dose of cyclosporine or by antihypertensive drug therapy.[108]

Nephrotoxicity

Virtually all patients who take cyclosporine have a small but measurable decrease in renal function that is reversible after cyclosporine is discontinued. Serum creatinine concentrations have increased approximately 20 percent in 6- to12-month clinical trials, but few patients have had to withdraw because of this.[105,106,110] Long-term data regarding renal function in RA patients treated with cyclosporine are limited. In one 12-month study, a rise in serum creatinine of more than 30 percent occurred in 50 percent of patients; half these patients responded to cyclosporine dose reduction and half did not, requiring discontinuation of the drug.[108] The small rise in serum creatinine observed in most studies occurs mainly during the first 2 to 3 months of treatment and then remains relatively stable over 12 months.[106,108] Other data, however, suggest that over periods of treatment longer than 1 year, many patients, who over the first year had a stable, acceptable increase in creatinine concentration, subsequently have a rise in creatinine to more than 30 percent of baseline that is not controlled by cyclosporine dose reduction and have to discontinue treatment.[111]

Irreversible cyclosporine-induced nephrotoxicity is a potentially more serious problem which, although most often described in transplant patients, may occur even with low-dose cyclosporine regimens in autoimmune disease. The mechanisms underlying cyclosporine-induced nephrotoxicity are unknown but may include increased production of the vasoconstrictors thromboxane and endothelin, decreased production of vasodilator prostaglandins, and altered vascular sensitivity.[112] Chronic cyclosporine nephrotoxicity is characterized by irreversible histopathologic changes such as focal interstitial (striped) fibrosis, tubular atrophy, and arteriolar abnormalities.[113] Preventable risk factors are a high dose of cyclosporine (more than 5 mg/kg/day) and an increase in serum creatinine concentration of more than 50 percent of the baseline value.[114] The risk of cyclosporine nephropathy is low in patients treated according to the clinical guidelines discussed later (Table 60–5).[114] Renal biopsies in 11 patients with RA who received cyclosporine (average dose 3.3 mg/kg/day) for 26 months and had an average increase in serum creatinine of 31 percent showed no significant cyclosporine-induced renal changes.[115]

Malignancy

In transplant recipients, cyclosporine use has been associated with an increased risk of skin cancer and lymphoma. The number of patients with RA treated with cyclosporine is too small, and the duration of treatment too short, to provide definitive data about the risks of malignancy. In 208 patients with RA treated with cyclosporine for an average of 1.6 years, the incidence of malignancy and mortality was similar to that of RA controls.[116] Epstein-Barr virus–induced B cell lymphoma, which may be reversible when cyclosporine is discontinued, has been reported in a small number of patients receiving cyclosporine for a variety of indications.

Clinical Considerations

Efficacy in Rheumatic Diseases

Several large and well-performed studies have shown that cyclosporine is effective in the treatment of RA, both as a single agent[110] and in combination with methotrexate[105] or hydroxychloroquine. Cyclosporine slows the rate of radiologic progression.[117] As monotherapy, the mean stabilization dose of cyclosporine (old formulation) was 3.8 mg/kg/day and resulted in an approximately 25-percent improvement in clinical outcome measures.[110] Clinical trials comparing the efficacy of cyclosporine to that of other second-line treatments for RA suggest comparable efficacy; however, comparative data over long periods of time and in a large number of patients are limited.

Cyclosporine is effective for both the skin and joint manifestations of psoriasis.[118,119] Less data are available regarding the use of cyclosporine in other rheumatic diseases. In uncontrolled, small studies in SLE,[120] cyclosporine has been reported improve disease activity; have a steroid-sparing effect; and to improve proteinuria, thrombocytopenia, and leukopenia. Cyclosporine has also been reported to be effective in many other autoimmune conditions including pyoderma gangrenosum, Behçet's disease, maintenance therapy of antineutrophil cytoplasmic antibody (ANCA) associated vasculitis,[121] and the macrophage-activation syndrome in juvenile rheumatoid arthritis.[122]

Clinical Use

Effective use of cyclosporine requires that appropriate patients be selected for treatment and carefully monitored. Guidelines are shown in Table 60–5. The starting dose of cyclosporine is 2.5 mg/kg/day, usually administered in divided doses. In obese patients, the dose is based on the approximate ideal body weight. Clinical response is relatively slow, occurring over 4 to 8 weeks, and may only be maximal after 12 weeks or more of treatment. To improve efficacy, the dose can be increased by 0.5 mg/kg/day at 4- to 8-week intervals to a maximum dose of 4.0 mg/kg/day of the microemulsion formulation. If there is no clinical response in 4 to 6 months, cyclosporine should be discontinued. In patients who are well controlled, the dose of cyclosporine can be decreased by 0.5 mg/kg/day at 4- to 8-week intervals to determine the minimum effective dose for the individual patient. In patients receiving the older Sandimmune formulation of cyclosporine who convert to the microemulsion formulation, a 1:1 dose conversion is generally used. However, because of the greater and more predictable bioavailability of the microemulsion formulation, a greater exposure to cyclosporine is likely and blood pressure and creatinine should initially be monitored at 2-week intervals after the conversion and the dose of cyclosporine decreased if required.

TABLE 60–5 • CLINICAL USE OF CYCLOSPORINE IN RHEUMATIC DISEASE

- Select appropriate patients
  Contraindications: Current or past malignancy other than basal call carcinoma, renal impairment, uncontrolled hypertension, hepatic dysfunction
  Cautions: Elderly, obesity, controlled hypertension, premalignant lesions, drugs that interact with cyclosporine, pregnancy
- Obtain two or more creatinine concentrations before starting cyclosporine and average these to provide a baseline creatinine value
- Start low: cyclosporine 2.5 mg/kg/day in divided doses
- Stay low: maximum 4.0 mg/kg/day (microemuslion formulation)
- Monitor blood pressure and creatinine initially every 2 weeks for 3 months, then monthly if stable
- If serum creatinine rises more than 30 percent above the patient's baseline, reduce dose of cyclosporine by 1.0 mg/kg/day; recheck serum creatinine in 1 to 2 weeks and temporarily discontinue cyclosporine if the creatinine remains more than 30 percent above baseline
- When creatinine level returns to within 15 percent of baseline, cyclosporine can be restarted at a lower dose

For Consensus Guidelines see Panayi GS, Tugwell P: The use of cyclosporin A microemulsion in rheumatoid arthritis: conclusions of an international review. Br J Rheumatol 36:808, 1997 for international; and Cush JJ, Tugwell P, Weinblatt M, Yocum D: US consensus guidelines for the use of cyclosporin A in rheumatoid arthritis. J Rheumatol 26:1176-1186, 1999.

The outcome of pregnancy in transplant recipients receiving cyclosporine-based and non–cyclosporine-based regimens are similar, but cyclosporine use in pregnancy is not recommended unless the potential benefit exceeds the potential risk to the fetus. Breast feeding should be avoided.

Strategies to Minimize Toxicity

Because cyclosporine may increase liver enzymes, potassium, uric acid, and lipid concentrations and decrease magnesium concentrations, it is prudent to measure these before, and occasionally after, initiating therapy. At least two, and preferably more, recent normal blood pressure and serum creatinine determinations should be obtained before starting treatment. Many patients with RA have low serum creatinine concentrations, and it is important not to overlook significant cyclosporine-induced elevations in serum creatinine, which may remain within the normal laboratory reference range. For example, if a patient has a baseline creatinine level of 0.6 mg/dl that after cyclosporine increases to 0.9 mg/dl (still in the normal range), this represents a 50-percent increase above baseline and requires dose reduction. Monitoring and cyclosporine dose reduction should be performed as shown in Table 60–5.

Cyclosporine concentrations are not useful predictors of efficacy or toxicity in rheumatic diseases and are not routinely performed. Cyclosporine trough concentrations, measured approximately 12 hours after the last dose, can be useful if there are concerns about compliance or unusual drug disposition in individual patients.

Clinical Role

The role of cyclosporine in the treatment of rheumatic diseases continues to evolve. Cyclosporine as monotherapy for RA currently offers few advantages over more established disease-modifying antirheumatic drugs (DMARDs) that are often cheaper and require less intensive monitoring. The combination of cyclosporine and methotrexate is more effective than methotrexate alone[105] and has an acceptable safety profile over 1 year.[106] In a population-based study, approximately 50 percent of patients with RA starting cyclosporine were still taking it 5 years later, suggesting reasonable efficacy and tolerability.[123] Thus, cyclosporine offers a useful therapeutic alternative for patients with RA who have not responded to, or are intolerant of, other DMARDs, and in combination therapy, it is a useful option for patients with an incomplete response to methotrexate. In patients with psoriatic arthritis and Behçet's syndrome, cyclosporine offers an alternative to current drugs. Clinical use in a range of other rheumatic diseases, including SLE, remains experimental and is based on limited information. More data regarding the long-term tolerability of cyclosporine, particularly as combination therapy in RA, are awaited.

TACROLIMUS (FK506)

Tacrolimus, previously known as FK506, is a macrolide derived from an actinomycete and is widely used in organ transplantation as an alternative to cyclosporine. Studies in autoimmune disease are less advanced.

Mechanisms of Action

Tacrolimus is more potent than cyclosporine, and although structurally different, it has a similar mechanism of action. Tacrolimus binds to an intracellular binding protein (FK binding protein) and this drug-immunophilin complex, in association with calcineurin, suppresses transcription of cytokines, such as IL-2, that mediate lymphocyte activation[97] (see Fig. 60–3).

Clinical Pharmacology

Absorption of tacrolimus after oral administration is poor and highly variable (range 4 percent to 93 percent, average 25 percent).[124] Tacrolimus is lipophilic, widely distributed in tissues, and is almost completely metabolized with an elimination half-life ranging from 5 to 16 hours.[125] As with cyclosporine, P-GP and CYP3A4 in liver and gut are important determinants of the metabolism and disposition of tacrolimus. Drugs that inhibit CYP3A4 or P-GP can increase tacrolimus concentrations[124] (see Table 60–4). Impaired hepatic function, but not impaired renal function, increases tacrolimus concentrations.[125] The adverse effects of tacrolimus are dose related and include nephrotoxicity, hypertension, hyperkalemia, hyperuricemia, tremor, hyperglycemia, and gastrointestinal intolerance.[124]

Clinical Considerations

Tacrolimus is effective in animal models of arthritis but data in humans are limited. In a phase II, randomized, double-blind, placebo-controlled monotherapy study, 268 patients with RA were randomized to receive 1, 3, or 5 mg of tacrolimus or placebo daily for 24 weeks. An American College of Rheumatology (ACR)-20 response was observed in 16 percent of patients receiving placebo and in 29, 34, and 50 percent of patients receiving tacrolimus in doses of 1, 3, and 5 mg, respectively.[126] The incidence of creatinine elevation more than 40 percent above baseline increased in a dose-dependent manner, with 3 and 11 percent of patients receiving 3 and 5 mg, respectively, discontinuing for this reason. These data suggest that further studies will be needed to define the optimal dose of tacrolimus for RA. The potential efficacy of tacrolimus in RA and other autoimmune diseases and its tolerability, particularly in comparison with current immunomodulating agents, will be of interest.

SIROLIMUS (RAPAMYCIN)

Sirolimus, isolated from an actinomycete, has been developed as an immunosuppressant for organ transplantation. Sirolimus, in contrast to cyclosporine and tacrolimus, does not act through calcineurin. It binds to FK binding protein and then targets proteins variously known as targets of rapamycin (TOR) proteins or FK-rapamycin associated proteins (FRAP), blocking progression of the cell cycle from G_1- to S-phase by inhibiting several downstream signal transduction pathways.[95] Clinical trials and experience have shown efficacy in transplantation, but there are no clinical trials in RA or autoimmune disease. The mechanism of action of sirolimus distinguishes it from cyclosporine and tacrolimus. It has a different adverse effect profile and potentially a different efficacy profile in autoimmune disease.

Mycophenolate Mofetil

Mycophenolate mofetil is widely used in organ transplantation and studies in many rheumatic diseases are in progress. Mycophenolate mofetil, a prodrug, is the inactive 2-morpholinoester of mycophenolic acid, which is hydrolyzed to the active mycophenolic acid, a drug whose immunosuppressive effects have been recognized since the 1970s and has been used to treat psoriasis.[127]

MECHANISMS OF ACTION

There are two pathways for the synthesis of guanine nucleotides: the de novo pathway and the salvage pathway. Mycophenolic acid reversibly inhibits inosine monophosphate dehydrogenase (IMPDH), an enzyme crucial for the de novo synthesis of purines.[80,128] Lymphocytes, in contrast to many other cells, are critically dependent on the de novo purine synthesis pathway and are, thus, a relatively selective target for mycophenolic acid, accounting for the ability of the drug to reversibly inhibit B and T cell proliferation without myelotoxicity.[80] Mycophenolic acid results in decreased guanine synthesis and, thus, decreased DNA synthesis, decreased lymphocyte proliferation, and decreased antibody production.[80,128,129]

CLINICAL PHARMACOLOGY

Mycophenolate mofetil is rapidly and completely absorbed and de-esterified to the active mycophenolic acid (MPA), which is highly (98 percent) protein bound. Most MPA (more than 99 percent) is found in plasma, with very little in cells; the majority is glucuronidated to the poorly active, stable phenolic glucuronide, which is eliminated in the urine.[130] Minor metabolites, some of which may be active, have also been described. Peak levels of MPA occur 1 to 2 hours after administration, and secondary peaks, thought to be due to enterohepatic circulation, can be seen. The half-life of MPA is 16 hours and interindividual variability in drug disposition is generally less than 50 percent.[130] Both renal disease and liver disease have relatively minor effects on the disposition of the active drug, MPA. Dose adjustment is not generally required,[130] but because MPA concentrations are increased in patients with severe renal impairment, they may sometimes be necessary. The major glucuronide metabolite of MPA accumulates in patients with impaired renal function and may cause increased gastrointestinal side effects. Decreased protein binding resulting in an increase in free MPA, and potentially greater effect, has been described in patients with severe renal impairment, but the clinical significance is uncertain.[131] MPA is highly protein bound and, therefore, not cleared by hemodialysis.[132] Because MPA is glucuronidated and not metabolized by cytochrome P450 oxidation, there are few clinically significant drug interactions. Antacids reduce bioavailability by approximately 15 percent[133] and cholestyramine by approximately 40 percent. Coadministration with azathioprine is not recommended.

ADVERSE EFFECTS

Mycophenolate mofetil is relatively well tolerated over 2 to 3 years in transplant recipients, but there are limited data available in rheumatic diseases. Sixteen percent of 325 patients with RA who received mycophenolate mofetil daily withdrew for adverse events, most commonly gastrointestinal side effects such as diarrhea, nausea, abdominal pain, and vomiting.[134] Occasional leukopenia, lymphocytopenia, and elevated liver enzymes occurred. Seven nonskin malignancies, four skin malignancies, and seven deaths (three from pneumonia) were reported.[134]

CLINICAL CONSIDERATIONS

Mycophenolate mofetil is currently undergoing clinical trials in several rheumatic diseases. The drug is active in animal models of arthritis and autoimmune disease[135] and shows promise in several uncontrolled reports and a more recent controlled study in patients with SLE,[136] preliminary reports from a controlled trial in RA,[137] and observational reports in vasculitis,[138] myasthenia gravis, and inflammatory muscle disease.[139]

Patients with SLE and diffuse proliferative nephritis were randomized to receive prednisolone and mycophenolate mofetil (1 g) twice daily for 12 months (n = 21) or prednisolone and daily oral cyclophosphamide for 6 months followed by prednisolone and azathioprine for 6 months, (n = 21).[136] The two treatments were equally effective in inducing remission of renal disease, but mycophenolate mofetil caused fewer adverse effects. This small study has several limitations. Oral cyclophosphamide, rather than the more usual IV pulse therapy, was used, and the study does not provide information about long-term preservation of renal function. Nevertheless, it suggests that mycophenolate mofetil has potential as a therapy for lupus nephritis.

In RA, clinical benefit was noted within 4 weeks. The percentage of patients meeting the ACR criteria for a 20-percent improvement receiving 1g twice daily (29.3 percent) and 2 g twice daily (37.1 percent) is in the range reported with other treatments for RA but indicates that the mycophenolate mofetil, as monotherapy, will not control RA in the majority of patients.[137,140] Mycophenolate mofetil may be useful as an alternative immunosuppressant to azathioprine in transplant patients with gout who require therapy with allopurinol because, in contrast to azathioprine, it does not appear to interact significantly with allopurinol.[80] Further studies regarding the comparative efficacy and long-term safety of mycophenolate mofetil in RA, SLE, and vasculitis will be of interest.

Thalidomide

Thalidomide was introduced in the 1950s as a hypnotic that was remarkably safe, even in overdose. The recognition that thalidomide was a potent teratogen resulting in characteristic congenital malformations led to its withdrawal in 1961. The rediscovery of the immunomodulating effects of thalidomide has led to the cautious and closely regulated, but highly controversial, reintroduction of thalidomide for a specific indication: the treatment of erythema nodosum leprosum. Preliminary studies have explored other potential therapeutic roles.

MECHANISMS OF ACTION

Thalidomide has immunosuppressive effects in several transplant models.[141] Multiple mechanisms have been proposed, the most plausible being the inhibition of angiogenesis and the inhibition of tumor necrosis factor-α (TNF-α) production.[142,143]

CLINICAL PHARMACOLOGY

Pharmacokinetics

Thalidomide is a derivative of glutamic acid and exists as racemic compound that, in vivo, interconverts between isomers.[141] Peak concentrations of thalidomide occur 2 to 4 hours after oral administration. The elimination half-life is approximately 5 hours, with elimination being virtually entirely through nonenzymatic hydrolysis.[141,144] The pharmacokinetics of thalidomide are relatively poorly characterized, and there is little information regarding drug interactions or use in patients with impaired renal or hepatic function. The sedative effects of other central depresants such as barbiturates are enhanced by thalidomide.

Adverse Effects

The most serious, best known, and preventable adverse effect of thalidomide is its ability to cause birth defects. In clinical studies, peripheral neuropathy has been the most common serious adverse effect. The reported incidence of peripheral neuropathy, usually manifesting as symmetrical paresthesias that may be painful, varies widely from 1 percent to more than 50 percent.[141,145] Electrophysiologic changes precede clinical neuropathy and most studies reporting higher rates of neuropathy have used this diagnostic technique. The neuropathy may only become evident after thalidomide has been discontinued and, in most patients (75 percent), may not resolve completely.[141] Other relatively common adverse effects include sedation, skin rash, limb edema, and constipation. Neutropenia is less common. Ovarian failure[146] and arterial and venous thromboses have been reported.

CLINICAL CONSIDERATIONS

Efficacy in Rheumatic Diseases

Thalidomide is Food and Drug Administration (FDA) approved only for the treatment of erythema nodosum leprosum. Prescription of thalidomide for this indication and its off-label use is, and should be, very closely regulated. Thalidomide (200 mg/day for 4 weeks) healed oral aphthous ulcers associated with human immunodeficiency virus (HIV) infection in approximately half the patients studied.[147] Thalidomide (100 mg/day and 300mg/day) for 24 weeks both improved the mucocutaneous lesions of Behçet's syndrome; however, clinical response was lost rapidly after discontinuation of the drug.[148] Small, largely uncontrolled reports suggest possible benefit in graft-versus-host disease, the skin manifestations of lupus, sarcoidosis, RA, ankylosing spondylitis, systemic-onset juvenile rheumatoid arthritis, and pyoderma gangrenosum.[141,145,149-152]

Strategies to Minimize Toxicity

Strategies to prevent fetal exposure to thalidomide are outlined in the System for Thalidomide Education and Prescribing Safety (STEPS) program developed by the drug's manufacturer, Celgene, and in guidelines developed in the United Kingdom.[153] Registration in the STEPS program is required before thalidomide is used. The program involves mandatory patient registration, education, surveys, and contraception for males and females. Electrophysiologic monitoring for thalidomide-induced neuropathy has been advocated[153] and should be considered, particularly if long-term therapy is planned. Thalidomide should be discontinued if peripheral neuropathy occurs.

Clinical Role

The frequent side effects of thalidomide limit its potential for chronic use. This, together with its teratogenic effects and the rapid relapse of autoimmune disease after discontinuation of thalidomide, severely limit its therapeutic potential. Research is being directed toward safer analogs of thalidomide.

Dapsone

Dapsone, a sulfone antimicrobial that has been used for decades to treat leprosy, is also a second-line component of regimens for the prophylaxis of PCP and malaria. The anti-inflammatory effects of dapsone have led to its use in a range of autoimmune disorders.

MECHANISMS OF ACTION

The antimicrobial action of dapsone, as with sulfonamides, occurs through the inhibition of folate synthesis. The mechanisms of the anti-inflammatory effects of dapsone are poorly understood, but effects on neutrophil function are prominent. Inhibition of chemoattractant-induced signal transduction by dapsone may decrease neutrophil recruitment and neutrophil chemotaxis, thus inhibiting neutrophil function.[154]

CLINICAL PHARMACOLOGY

Absorption and Distribution

After oral administration of dapsone, 70 to 80 percent is absorbed with peak concentrations occurring 2 to 6 hours after administration.[155] Dapsone is 70 to 90 percent protein bound, and its major circulating metabolite, monoacetyldiaminodiphenylsulfone (MADDS) is even more tightly protein bound (99 percent).[155] Dapsone is widely distributed, crosses the placenta, and appears in breast milk.[155]

Metabolism and Elimination

There are two major metabolic pathways: acetylation and hydroxylation. Dapsone is acetylated by hepatic *N*-acetyltransferases to form MADDS. There is substantial interindividual variability in acetylation activity, and in populations there is a polymorphic, bimodal distribution. However, because deacetylation of MADDS back to dapsone takes place and an equilibrium in this cycling exists, "slow acetylators" and "fast acetylators" show no differences in dapsone pharmacokinetics, therapeutic response, or toxicity.[155] Dapsone also undergoes N-hydroxylation by the cytochrome P450 (CYP) system. The resulting hydroxylamine metabolite is the cause of the methemoglobinemia associated with dapsone. The half-life of dapsone is 20 to 30 hours. The major route of elimination from the body is renal, largely as conjugated metabolites. There is little information to guide the use of dapsone in individuals with impaired renal or hepatic function. Rifampin, through enzyme induction, decreases the half-life of dapsone.[155] Probenecid reduces excretion of dapsone.[155]

Adverse Effects

Hematologic

The most frequent adverse effects of dapsone are methemoglobinemia and hemolysis. The hematologic effects dapsone are dose dependent, often detectable at doses of 75 mg/day or greater, and are observed in almost all individuals receiving 250 mg/day.[156,157] A mild degree of asymptomatic methemoglobinemia (2 to 5 percent) and hemolytic anemia, resulting in a decrease in hemoglobin concentration of 1 to 2 g/liter, is common in patients receiving 100 mg/day of dapsone.[156] The hemotoxic effects are often most marked in the first 6 weeks, then improve and stabilize, and are generally well tolerated.[157] Individuals vary in their susceptibility to dapsone-induced methemoglobinemia and hemolysis. Subjects with glucose-6-phosphate dehydrogenase (G6PD) deficiency are particularly susceptible to the oxidative stress imposed by dapsone that results in lipid peroxidation, red blood cell membrane damage, and hemolysis.[156,157]

Agranulocytosis, which is reversible if dapsone is discontinued, may develop in one of every 250 to 500 patients treated.[158,159] The median time of onset of agranulocytosis is 6 to 8 weeks and, although it may occur suddenly, a gradual decrease in granulocyte count preceding agranulocytosis is often noted.[159]

Sulfone Syndrome

A rare, potentially serious syndrome thought to be due to a hypersensitivity reaction that manifests as fever, rash that may be exfoliative, jaundice with elevated liver enzymes, lymphadenopathy, and hemolytic anemia may occur even after low doses (e.g., 50 mg/d) of dapsone.[160]

Miscellaneous

Other adverse effects are uncommon and include rash, peripheral neuropathy, psychosis, hepatitis, headache, and insomnia.

CLINICAL CONSIDERATIONS

Efficacy in Rheumatic Diseases

There are almost no adequate clinical trials guiding the use of dapsone in rheumatology. Empirical use, often when standard therapies have failed, has evolved. Thus, occasional efficacy has been reported in a small number of patients over a range of conditions including pustular dermatoses, erythema elevatum diutinum,[161] leukocytoclastic and urticarial vasculitis,[162,163] cutaneous and bullous lupus erythematosus (LE)[164] orogenital ulceration in Behçet's syndrome, and RA.[157] In relatively few small, double-blind, randomized studies, dapsone (100 mg/day) was more effective than placebo and equal in efficacy to antimalarials in the treatment of RA.[157] In cutaneous LE, an excellent response is estimated to occur in only about 25 percent of patients, and dapsone is seldom a drug of first choice.[164]

Clinical Use

In most clinical studies, the starting dose of dapsone has been 50 mg/day for a few days, increasing rapidly to a maintenance dose of 100 mg/day. However, a more gradual increase from a starting dose of 25 mg twice daily to 50 mg twice daily over several months may be better tolerated.[157] Higher doses, up to 350 mg/day, have been used in dermatologic conditions, but dose-related toxicity is limiting.

Strategies to Minimize Toxicity

Screening patients for G6PD deficiency before treatment with dapsone is prudent, particularly in population groups in which G6PD deficiency is more frequent (i.e., African, Mediterranean, East Asian). Cimetidine, because it inhibits the formation of the toxic hydroxylamine metabolite of dapsone, has been used in subjects receiving high doses of dapsone to reduce the degree of methemoglobinemia and to improve tolerability.[159] Regular monitoring of the blood count, initially weekly for a month, every 2 weeks for the next 2 months, and monthly thereafter, as well as intermittent monitoring of the liver function tests is recommended.[157] Because of increased RBC turnover, folate supplementation may be required.

Clinical Role

Dapsone, because of its dose-related toxicity and the limited efficacy data, has a very limited role in rheumatology, usually as a drug that is tried in occasional patients when more standard therapies have failed.

Conclusion

The use of immunoregulatory drugs for rheumatic diseases has evolved out of the use of glucocorticoids and the older anticancer alkylating and purine analog cytotoxic drugs to now include a generation of noncytotoxic immunomodulators. The clinical use of immunomodulating drugs provides a therapeutic challenge unique to the art of rheumatology. It often involves the selection of a drug, or combinations of drugs, based on inadequate data; a highly variable individual response to that therapy; long-term treatment with drugs that have potentially serious adverse effects; and the goal of halting or controlling a disease that can have an unpredictable clinical course.

REFERENCES

1. Moore MJ: Clinical pharmacokinetics of cyclophosphamide. Clin Pharmacokinet 20:194-208, 1991.
2. Fleming RA: An overview of cyclophosphamide and ifosfamide pharmacology. Pharmacotherapy 17:146S-154S, 1997.
3. Hemendinger RA, Bloom SE: Selective mitomycin C and cyclophosphamide induction of apoptosis in differentiating B lymphocytes compared to T lymphocytes in vivo. Immunopharmacology 35: 71-82, 1996.
4. Garcia ST, McQuillan A, Panasci L: Correlation between the cytotoxicity of melphalan and DNA crosslinks as detected by the ethidium bromide fluorescence assay in the F1 variant of B16 melanoma cells. Biochem Pharmacol 37:3189-3192, 1988.
5. Vendrik CP, Bergers JJ, De JW, Steerenberg PA: Resistance to cytostatic drugs at the cellular level. Cancer Chemother Pharmacol 29:413-429, 1992.
6. Makinodan T, Santos GW, Quinn RP: Immunosuppressive drugs. Pharmacol Rev 22:189-247, 1970.
7. Fauci AS, Wolff SM, Johnson JS: Effect of cyclophosphamide upon the immune response in Wegener's granulomatosis. New Engl J Med 285:1493-1496, 1971.
8. Struck RF, Alberts DS, Horne K, et al: Plasma pharmacokinetics of cyclophosphamide and its cytotoxic metabolites after intravenous versus oral administration in a randomized, crossover trial. Cancer Res 47:2723-2726, 1987.
9. Grochow LB, Colvin M: Clinical pharmacokinetics of cyclophosphamide. Clin Pharmacokinet 4:380-394, 1979.
10. Ren S, Yang JS, Kalhorn TF, Slattery JT: Oxidation of cyclophosphamide to 4-hydroxycyclophosphamide and deschloroethylcyclophosphamide in human liver microsomes. Cancer Res 57:4229-4235, 1997.
11. Chang TK, Yu L, Goldstein JA, Waxman DJ: Identification of the polymorphically expressed CYP2C19 and the wild-type CYP2C9-ILE359 allele as low-Km catalysts of cyclophosphamide and ifosfamide activation. Pharmacogenetics 7:211-221, 1997.
12. Huang Z, Roy P, Waxman DJ: Role of human liver microsomal CYP3A4 and CYP2B6 in catalyzing N-dechloroethylation of cyclophosphamide and ifosfamide. Biochem Pharmacol 59:961-972, 2000.
13. Bagley CMJ, Bostick FW, DeVita VT Jr: Clinical pharmacology of cyclophosphamide. Cancer Res 33:226-233, 1973.
14. Juma FD: Effect of liver failure on the pharmacokinetics of cyclophosphamide. Eur J Clin Pharmacol 26:591-593, 1984.
15. Haubitz M, Bohnenstengel F, Brunkhorst R, et al: Cyclophosphamide pharmacokinetics and dose requirements in patients with renal insufficiency. Kidney Int 61:1495-1501, 2002.
16. Hoffman GS, Leavitt RY, Fleisher TA, et al: Treatment of Wegener's granulomatosis with intermittent high-dose intravenous cyclophosphamide. Am J Med 89:403-410, 1990.
17. Anthony LB, Long QC, Struck RF, Hande KR: The effect of cimetidine on cyclophosphamide metabolism in rabbits. Cancer Chemother Pharmacol 27:125-130, 1990.
18. Alberts DS, Mason-Liddil N, Plezia PM, et al: Lack of ranitidine effects on cyclophosphamide bone marrow toxicity or metabolism: a placebo-controlled clinical trial. J Nat Cancer Instit 83:1739-1742, 1991.
19. Boston Collaborative Drug Surveillance Program: Allopurinol and cytotoxic drug: interaction in relation to bone marrow depression. JAMA 227:1036-1040, 1974.
20. Yule SM, Boddy AV, Cole M, et al: Cyclophosphamide pharmacokinetics in children. Br J Clin Pharmacol 41:13-19, 1996.
21. Koseoglu V, Chiang J, Chan KW: Acquired pseudocholinesterase deficiency after high-dose cyclophosphamide. Bone Marrow Transplant 24:1367-1368, 1999.
22. Fraiser LH, Kanekal S, Kehrer JP: Cyclophosphamide toxicity: characterising and avoiding the problem. Drugs 42:781-795, 1991.
23. Pryor BD, Bologna SG, Kahl LE: Risk factors for serious infection during treatment with cyclophosphamide and high-dose corticosteroids for systemic lupus erythematosus. Arthritis Rheum 39:1475-1482, 1996.
24. Gourley MF, Austin HA, Scott D, et al: Methylprednisolone and cyclophosphamide, alone or in combination, in patients with lupus nephritis: a randomized, controlled trial. Ann Intern Med 125:549-557, 1996.
25. Guillevin L, Cordier JF, Lhote F, et al: A prospective, multicenter, randomized trial comparing steroids and pulse cyclophosphamide versus steroids and oral cyclophosphamide in the treatment of generalized Wegener's granulomatosis. Arthritis Rheum 40:2187-2198, 1997.
26. Hoffman GS, Kerr GS, Leavitt RY, et al: Wegener granulomatosis: an analysis of 158 patients. Ann Intern Med 116:488-498, 1992.
27. Hoffman GS: Treatment of Wegener's granulomatosis: time to change the standard of care? Arthritis Rheum 40:2099-2104, 1997.
28. Godeau B, Mainardi JL, Roudot-Thoraval F, et al: Factors associated with Pneumocystis carinii pneumonia in Wegener's granulomatosis. Ann Rheum Dis 54:991-994, 1995.
29. Cox PJ: Cyclophosphamide cystitis: identification of acrolein as the causative agent. Biochem Pharmacol 28:2045-2049, 1979.
30. Goren MP: Oral mesna: a review. Semin Oncol 19:65-71, 1992.
31. Reinhold-Keller E, Beuge N, Latza U, et al: An interdisciplinary approach to the care of patients with Wegener's granulomatosis: long-term outcome in 155 patients. Arthritis Rheum 43: 1021-1032, 2000.
32. Stillwell TJ, Benson RCJ, DeRemee RA, et al: Cyclophosphamide-induced bladder toxicity in Wegener's granulomatosis. Arthritis Rheum 31:465-470, 1988.
33. Talar-Williams C, Hijazi YM, Walther MM, et al: Cyclophosphamide-induced cystitis and bladder cancer in patients with Wegener granulomatosis. Ann Intern Med 124:477-484, 1996.
34. Radis CD, Kahl LE, Baker GL, et al: Effects of cyclophosphamide on the development of malignancy and on long-term survival of patients with rheumatoid arthritis: a 20-year followup study. Arthritis Rheum 38:1120-1127, 1995.
35. Baltus JA, Boersma JW, Hartman AP, Vandenbroucke JP: The occurrence of malignancies in patients with rheumatoid arthritis treated with cyclophosphamide: a controlled retrospective follow-up. Ann Rheum Dis 42:368-373, 1983.
36. Nicholson HS, Byrne J: Fertility and pregnancy after treatment for cancer during childhood or adolescence. Cancer 71: 3392-3399, 1993.
37. Byrne J, Rasmussen SA, Steinhorn SC, et al: Genetic disease in offspring of long-term survivors of childhood and adolescent cancer. Am J Hum Genet 62:45-52, 1998.
38. Mok CC, Lau CS, Wong RW: Risk factors for ovarian failure in patients with systemic lupus erythematosus receiving cyclophosphamide therapy. Arthritis Rheum 41:831-837, 1998.

39. Austin HA, Klippel JH, Balow JE, et al: Therapy of lupus nephritis: controlled trial of prednisone and cytotoxic drugs. New Engl J Med 314:614-619, 1986.
40. Boumpas DT, Austin HA, Vaughan EM, et al: Risk for sustained amenorrhea in patients with systemic lupus erythematosus receiving intermittent pulse cyclophosphamide therapy. Ann Intern Med 119:366-369, 1993.
41. McDermott EM, Powell RJ: Incidence of ovarian failure in systemic lupus erythematosus after treatment with pulse cyclophosphamide. Ann Rheum Dis 55:224-229, 1996.
42. Masala A, Faedda R, Alagna S, et al: Use of testosterone to prevent cyclophosphamide-induced azoospermia. Ann Intern Med 126:292-295, 1997.
43. Fukutani K, Ishida H, Shinohara M, et al: Suppression of spermatogenesis in patients with Behçet's disease treated with cyclophosphamide and colchicine. Fertil Steril 36:76-80, 1981.
44. Blumenfeld Z, Haim N: Prevention of gonadal damage during cytotoxic therapy. Ann Med 29:199-206, 1997.
45. Blumenfeld Z, Shapiro D, Shteinberg M, et al: Preservation of fertility and ovarian function and minimizing gonadotoxicity in young women with systemic lupus erythematosus treated by chemotherapy. Lupus 9:401-405, 2000.
46. Johnson DH, Linde R, Hainsworth JD, et al: Effect of a luteinizing hormone releasing hormone agonist given during combination chemotherapy on posttherapy fertility in male patients with lymphoma: preliminary observations. Blood 65:832-836, 1985.
47. Malik SW, Myers JL, DeRemee RA, Specks U: Lung toxicity associated with cyclophosphamide use: two distinct patterns. Am J Respir Crit Care Med 154:1851-1856, 1996.
48. Bressler RB, Huston DP: Water intoxication following moderate-dose intravenous cyclophosphamide. Arch Intern Med 145: 548-549, 1985.
49. Knysak DJ, McLean JA, Solomon WR, et al: Immediate hypersensitivity reaction to cyclophosphamide. Arthritis Rheum 37: 1101-1104, 1994.
50. Reinhold-Keller E, Mohr J, Christophers E, et al: Mesna side effects which imitate vasculitis. Clin Invest 70:698-704, 1992.
51. Ostensen M: Optimisation of antirheumatic drug treatment in pregnancy. Clin Pharmacokinet 27:486-503, 1994.
52. Balow JE, Boumpas DT, Fessler BJ, Austin HA: Management of lupus nephritis. Kidney Int 53(Suppl):S88-S92, 1996.
53. McCune WJ, Golbus J, Zeldes W, et al: Clinical and immunologic effects of monthly administration of intravenous cyclophosphamide in severe systemic lupus erythematosus. New Engl J Med 318:1423-1431, 1988.
54. White B, Moore WC, Wigley FM, et al: Cyclophosphamide is associated with pulmonary function and survival benefit in patients with scleroderma and alveolitis. Ann Intern Med 132:947-954, 2000.
55. Schnabel A, Reuter M, Gross WL: Intravenous pulse cyclophosphamide in the treatment of interstitial lung disease due to collagen vascular diseases. Arthritis Rheum 41:1215-1220, 1998.
56. Haubitz M, Schellong S, Gobel U, et al: Intravenous pulse administration of cyclophosphamide versus daily oral treatment in patients with antineutrophil cytoplasmic antibody-associated vasculitis and renal involvement: a prospective, randomized study. Arthritis Rheum 41:1835-1844, 1998.
57. Gaffney K, Scott DG: Azathioprine and cyclophosphamide in the treatment of rheumatoid arthritis. Brit J Rheumatol 37:824-836, 1998.
58. Dawisha SM, Yarboro CH, Vaughan EM, et al: Outpatient monthly oral bolus cyclophosphamide therapy in systemic lupus erythematosus. J Rheumatol 23:273-278, 1996.
59. Haga HJ, D'Cruz D, Asherson R, Hughes GR: Short term effects of intravenous pulses of cyclophosphamide in the treatment of connective tissue disease crisis. Ann Rheum Dis 51:885-888, 1992.
60. Langford CA, Klippel JH, Balow JE, et al: Use of cytotoxic agents and cyclosporine in the treatment of autoimmune disease. Part 2: Inflammatory bowel disease, systemic vasculitis, and therapeutic toxicity. Ann Intern Med 129:49-58, 1998.
61. Hoffman GS, Leavitt RY, Kerr GS, Fauci AS: The treatment of Wegener's granulomatosis with glucocorticoids and methotrexate. Arthritis Rheum 35:1322-1329, 1992.
62. de Groot K, Reinhold-Keller E, Tatsis E, et al: Therapy for the maintenance of remission in sixty-five patients with generalized Wegener's granulomatosis: methotrexate versus trimethoprim/sulfamethoxazole. Arthritis Rheum 39:2052-2061, 1996.
63. Newell DR, Calvert AH, Harrap KR, McElwain TJ: Studies on the pharmacokinetics of chlorambucil and prednimustine in man. Brit J Clin Pharmacol 15:253-258, 1983.
64. Hartvig P, Simonsson B, Oberg G, et al: Inter-and intraindividual differences in oral chlorambucil pharmacokinetics. Eur J Clin Pharmacol 35:551-554, 1988.
65. Cannon GW, Jackson CG, Samuelson COJ, et al: Chlorambucil therapy in rheumatoid arthritis: clinical experience in 28 patients and literature review. Semin Arthritis Rheum 15:106-118, 1985.
66. Patapanian H, Graham S, Sambrook PN, et al: The oncogenicity of chlorambucil in rheumatoid arthritis. Br J Rheumatol 27: 44-47, 1988.
67. Palmer RG, Denman AM: Malignancies induced by chlorambucil. Cancer Treat Rev 11:121-129, 1984.
68. O'Duffy JD, Robertson DM, Goldstein NP: Chlorambucil in the treatment of uveitis and meningoencephalitis of Behçet's disease. Am J Med 76:75-84, 1984.
69. Sinoway PA, Callen JP: Chlorambucil. An effective corticosteroid-sparing agent for patients with recalcitrant dermatomyositis. Arthritis Rheum 36:319-324, 1993.
70. Branten AJ, Reichert LJ, Koene RA, Wetzels JF: Oral cyclophosphamide versus chlorambucil in the treatment of patients with membranous nephropathy and renal insufficiency. QJM 91: 359-366, 1998.
71. Van SK, Johnson CA, Porter WR: The pharmacology and metabolism of the thiopurine drugs 6-mercaptopurine and azathioprine. Drug Metabol Rev 16:157-174, 1985.
72. Pedersen BK, Beyer JM, Rasmussen A, et al: Azathioprine as single drug in the treatment of rheumatoid arthritis induces complete suppression of natural killer cell activity. APMIS 92:221-225, 1984.
73. Van OE, Zins BJ, Sandborn WJ, et al: Azathioprine pharmacokinetics after intravenous, oral, delayed release oral and rectal foam administration. Gut 39:63-68, 1996.
74. Stolk JN, Boerbooms AM, de AR[AU10], et al: Reduced thiopurine methyltransferase activity and development of side effects of azathioprine treatment in patients with rheumatoid arthritis. Arthritis Rheum 41:1858-1866, 1998.
75. Bergan S, Rugstad HE, Bentdal O, et al: Kinetics of mercaptopurine and thioguanine nucleotides in renal transplant recipients during azathioprine treatment. Ther Drug Monit 16:13-20, 1994.
76. Chan GL, Erdmann GR, Gruber SA, et al: Azathioprine metabolism: pharmacokinetics of 6-mercaptopurine, 6-thiouric acid and 6-thioguanine nucleotides in renal transplant patients. J Clin Pharmacol 30:358-363, 1990.
77. Schmiegelow K, Kriegbaum NJ: 6-Thioguanine nucleotide accumulation in erythrocytes during azathioprine treatment for systemic connective tissue diseases: a possible index for monitoring treatment. Ann Rheum Dis 52:152-154, 1993.
78. Chocair PR, Duley JA, Simmonds HA, Cameron JS: The importance of thiopurine methyltransferase activity for the use of azathioprine in transplant recipients. Transplantation 53:1051-1056, 1992.
79. Cummins D, Sekar M, Halil O, Banner N: Myelosuppression associated with azathioprine-allopurinol interaction after heart and lung transplantation Transplantation 61:1661-1662, 1996.
80. Suthanthiran M, Strom TB: Immunoregulatory drugs: mechanistic basis for use in organ transplantation. Pediatr Nephrol 11: 651-657, 1997.
81. Lewis LD, Benin A, Szumlanski CL, et al: Olsalazine and 6-mercaptopurine-related bone marrow suppression: a possible drug-drug interaction. Clin Pharmacol Therapeut 62:464-475, 1997.
82. Szumlanski CL, Weinshilboum RM: Sulphasalazine inhibition of thiopurine methyltransferase: possible mechanism for interaction with 6-mercaptopurine and azathioprine. Brit J Clin Pharmacol 39:456-459, 1995.
83. Walker J, Mendelson H, McClure A, Smith MD: Warfarin and azathioprine: clinically significant drug interaction. J Rheumatol 29:398-399, 2002.
84. Willkens RF, Sharp JT, Stablein D, et al: Comparison of azathioprine, methotrexate, and the combination of the two in the treatment of rheumatoid arthritis: a forty-eight-week controlled clinical trial with radiologic outcome assessment. Arthritis Rheum 38:1799-1806, 1995.

85. Singh G, Fries JF, Spitz P, Williams CA: Toxic effects of azathioprine in rheumatoid arthritis: a national post-marketing perspective. Arthritis Rheum 32:837-843, 1989.
86. Szumlanski CL, Honchel R, Scott MC, Weinshilboum RM: Human liver thiopurine methyltransferase pharmacogenetics: biochemical properties, liver-erythrocyte correlation and presence of isozymes. Pharmacogenetics 2:148-159, 1992.
87. McLeod HL, Lin JS, Scott EP, et al: Thiopurine methyltransferase activity in American white subjects and black subjects. Clin Pharmacol Therapeut 55:15-20, 1994.
88. Leipold G, Schutz E, Haas JP, Oellerich M: Azathioprine-induced severe pancytopenia due to a homozygous two-point mutation of the thiopurine methyltransferase gene in a patient with juvenile HLA-B27-associated spondylarthritis. Arthritis Rheum 40:1896-1898, 1997.
89. Fields CL, Robinson JW, Roy TM, et al: Hypersensitivity reaction to azathioprine. South Med J 91:471-474, 1998.
90. Rahman P, Humphrey-Murto S, Gladman DD, Urowitz MB: Cytotoxic therapy in systemic lupus erythematosus: experience from a single center. Medicine 76:432-437, 1997.
91. Villalba L, Hicks JE, Adams EM, et al: Treatment of refractory myositis: a randomized crossover study of two new cytotoxic regimens. Arthritis Rheum 41:392-399, 1998.
92. Hamuryudan V, Ozyazgan Y, Hizli N, et al: Azathioprine in Behçet's syndrome: effects on long-term prognosis. Arthritis Rheum 40:769-774, 1997.
93. Jones G, Crotty M, Brooks P: Psoriatic arthritis: a quantitative overview of therapeutic options: the Psoriatic Arthritis Meta-Analysis Study Group. Brit J Rheumatol 36:95-99, 1997.
94. Taylor HG, Samanta A: Treatment of vasculitis. Brit J Clin Pharmacol 35:93-104, 1993.
95. Sehgal SN: Rapamune (RAPA, rapamycin, sirolimus): mechanism of action immunosuppressive effect results from blockade of signal transduction and inhibition of cell cycle progression. Clin Biochem 31:335-340, 1998.
96. Ho S, Clipstone N, Timmermann L, et al: The mechanism of action of cyclosporin A and FK506. Clin Immunol Immunopathol 80:S40-S45, 1996.
97. Denton MD, Magee CC, Sayegh MH: Immunosuppressive strategies in transplantation. Lancet 353:1083-1091, 1999.
98. Fahr A: Cyclosporin clinical pharmacokinetics. Clin Pharmacokinet 24:472-495, 1993.
99. Choc MG: Bioavailability and pharmacokinetics of cyclosporine formulations: Neoral vs Sandimmune. Int J Dermatol 36(Suppl 1):1-6, 1997.
100. Friman S, Backman L: A new microemulsion formulation of cyclosporin: pharmacokinetic and clinical features. Clin Pharmacokinet 30:181-193, 1996.
101. Lown KS, Mayo RR, Leichtman AB, et al: Role of intestinal P-glycoprotein (mdr1) in interpatient variation in the oral bioavailability of cyclosporine. Clin Pharmacol Therapeut 62:248-260, 1997.
102. Campana C, Regazzi MB, Buggia I, Molinaro M: Clinically significant drug interactions with cyclosporin: an update. Clin Pharmacokinet 30:141-179, 1996.
103. Goldberg R, Roth D: Evaluation of fluvastatin in the treatment of hypercholesterolemia in renal transplant recipients taking cyclosporine. Transplantation 62:1559-1564, 1996.
104. Olbricht C, Wanner C, Eisenhauer T, et al: Accumulation of lovastatin, but not pravastatin, in the blood of cyclosporine-treated kidney graft patients after multiple doses. Clin Pharmacol Therapeut 62:311-321, 1997.
105. Tugwell P, Pincus T, Yocum D, et al: Combination therapy with cyclosporine and methotrexate in severe rheumatoid arthritis: The Methotrexate-Cyclosporine Combination Study Group. New Engl J Med 333:137-141, 1995.
106. Stein CM, Pincus T, Yocum D, et al: Combination treatment of severe rheumatoid arthritis with cyclosporine and methotrexate for forty-eight weeks: an open-label extension study—The Methotrexate-Cyclosporine Combination Study Group. Arthritis Rheum 40:1843-1851, 1997.
107. Tugwell P, Ludwin D, Gent M, et al: Interaction between cyclosporin A and nonsteroidal antiinflammatory drugs. J Rheumatol 24:1122-1125, 1997.
108. Landewe RB, Goei TH, van RA, et al: Cyclosporine in common clinical practice: an estimation of the benefit/risk ratio in patients with rheumatoid arthritis. J Rheumatol 21:1631-1636, 1994.
109. Stein CM, Brooks RH, Pincus T: Effect of combination therapy with cyclosporine and methotrexate on liver function test results in rheumatoid arthritis. Arthritis Rheum 40:1721-1723, 1997.
110. Tugwell P, Bombardier C, Gent M, et al: Low-dose cyclosporin versus placebo in patients with rheumatoid arthritis. Lancet 335:1051-1055, 1990.
111. Yocum DE, Stein CM, Pincus T: Longterm safety of Cyclosporin/Sandimmune alone and in combination with methotrexate in the treatment of active rheumatoid arthritis: analysis of open label extension studies. Arthritis Rheum 41:S364, 1998.
112. Stein CM, He H, Pincus T, Wood AJ: Cyclosporine impairs vasodilation without increased sympathetic activity in humans. Hypertension 26:705-710, 1995.
113. Feutren G, Mihatsch MJ: Risk factors for cyclosporine-induced nephropathy in patients with autoimmune diseases. International Kidney Biopsy Registry of Cyclosporine in Autoimmune Diseases. New Engl J Med 326:1654-1660, 1992.
114. Rodriguez F, Krayenbuhl JC, Harrison WB, et al: Renal biopsy findings and followup of renal function in rheumatoid arthritis patients treated with cyclosporin A: an update from the International Kidney Biopsy Registry. Arthritis Rheum 39:1491-1498, 1996.
115. Landewe RB, Dijkmans BA, van der Woude FJ, et al: Longterm low dose cyclosporine in patients with rheumatoid arthritis: renal function loss without structural nephropathy. J Rheumatol 23:61-64, 1996.
116. van den Borne BE, Landewe RB, Houkes I, et al: No increased risk of malignancies and mortality in cyclosporin A-treated patients with rheumatoid arthritis. Arthritis Rheum 41:1930-1937, 1998.
117. Pasero G, Priolo F, Marubini E, et al: Slow progression of joint damage in early rheumatoid arthritis treated with cyclosporin A. Arthritis Rheum 39:1006-1015, 1996.
118. Olivieri I, Salvarani C, Cantini F, et al: Therapy with cyclosporine in psoriatic arthritis. Seminars in Arthritis Rheum 27:36-43, 1997.
119. Lebwohl M, Ellis C, Gottlieb A, et al: Cyclosporine consensus conference: with emphasis on the treatment of psoriasis. J Am Acad Dermatol 39:464-475, 1998.
120. Caccavo D, Lagana B, Mitterhofer AP, et al: Long-term treatment of systemic lupus erythematosus with cyclosporin A. Arthritis Rheum 40:27-35, 1997.
121. Haubitz M, Koch KM, Brunkhorst R: Cyclosporin for the prevention of disease reactivation in relapsing ANCA-associated vasculitis. Nephrol Dial Transplant 13:2074-2076, 1998.
122. Mouy R, Stephan JL, Pillet P, et al: Efficacy of cyclosporine A in the treatment of macrophage activation syndrome in juvenile arthritis: report of five cases. J Ped 129:750-754, 1996.
123. Marra CA, Esdaile JM, Guh D, et al: The effectiveness and toxicity of cyclosporin A in rheumatoid arthritis: longitudinal analysis of a population-based registry. Arthritis Rheum 45:240-245, 2001.
124. Spencer CM, Goa KL, Gillis JC: Tacrolimus: an update of its pharmacology and clinical efficacy in the management of organ transplantation. Drugs 54:925-975, 1997.
125. Peters DH, Fitton A, Plosker GL, Faulds D: Tacrolimus: a review of its pharmacology, and therapeutic potential in hepatic and renal transplantation. Drugs 46:746-794, 1993.
126. Furst DE, Saag K, Fleischmann MR, et al: Efficacy of tacrolimus in rheumatoid arthritis patients who have been treated unsuccessfully with methotrexate: a six-month, double-blind, randomized, dose-ranging study. Arthritis Rheum 46(8):2020-2028, 2002.
127. Epinette WW, Parker CM, Jones EL, Greist MC: Mycophenolic acid for psoriasis: a review of pharmacology, long-term efficacy, and safety. J Am Acad Dermatol 17:962-971, 1987.
128. Ransom JT: Mechanism of action of mycophenolate mofetil. Therapeut Drug Monitor 17:681-684, 1995.
129. Smith KG, Isbel NM, Catton MG, et al: Suppression of the humoral immune response by mycophenolate mofetil. Nephrol Dial Transplant 13:160-164, 1998.
130. Bullingham RE, Nicholls AJ, Kamm BR: Clinical pharmacokinetics of mycophenolate mofetil. Clin Pharmacokinet 34:429-455, 1998.

131. Meier-Kriesche HU, Shaw LM, Korecka M, Kaplan B: Pharmacokinetics of mycophenolic acid in renal insufficiency. Therapeut Drug Monitor 22:27-30, 2000.
132. Johnson HJ, Swan SK, Heim-Duthoy KL, et al: The pharmacokinetics of a single oral dose of mycophenolate mofetil in patients with varying degrees of renal function. Clin Pharmacol Therapeut 63:512-518, 1998.
133. Bullingham R, Shah J, Goldblum R, Schiff M: Effects of food and antacid on the pharmacokinetics of single doses of mycophenolate mofetil in rheumatoid arthritis patients. Br J Clin Pharmacol 41:513-516, 1996.
134. Schiff MH, Leishman B: Long-term safety of CellCept (mycophenolate mofetil), a new therapy for rheumatoid arthritis. Arthritis Rheum 41(Suppl):S155, 1998.
135. Corna D, Morigi M, Facchinetti D, et al: Mycophenolate mofetil limits renal damage and prolongs life in murine lupus autoimmune disease. Kidney Int 51:1583-1589, 1997.
136. Chan TM, Li FK, Tang CS, et al: Efficacy of mycophenolate mofetil in patients with diffuse proliferative lupus nephritis: Hong Kong-Guangzhou Nephrology Study Group. New Engl J Med 343:1156-1162, 2000.
137. Schiff M, Stein G, Leishman B: CellCept (mycophenolate mofetil), a new treatment for RA: a 9-month, randomized, double-blind trial comparing 1 g bid and 2 g bid. Arthritis Rheum 40(Suppl):S194, 1997.
138. Nowack R, Gobel U, Klooker P, et al: Mycophenolate mofetil for maintenance therapy of Wegener's granulomatosis and microscopic polyangiitis: a pilot study in 11 patients with renal involvement. J Am Soc Nephrol 10:1965-1971, 1999.
139. Chaudhry V, Cornblath DR, Griffin JW, et al: Mycophenolate mofetil: a safe and promising immunosuppressant in neuromuscular diseases. Neurology 56:94-96, 2001.
140. Drossos AA: Newer immunosuppressive drugs: their potential role in rheumatoid arthritis therapy. Drugs 62:891-907, 2002.
141. Tseng S, Pak G, Washenik K, et al: Rediscovering thalidomide: a review of its mechanism of action, side effects, and potential uses. J Am Acad Dermatol 35:969-979, 1996.
142. D'Amato RJ, Loughnan MS, Flynn E, Folkman J: Thalidomide is an inhibitor of angiogenesis. Proceed Nat Acad Sci U S A 91:4082-4085, 1994.
143. Sampaio EP, Sarno EN, Galilly R, et al: Thalidomide selectively inhibits tumor necrosis factor alpha production by stimulated human monocytes. J Exper Med 173:699-703, 1991.
144. Eriksson T, Bjorkman S, Hoglund P: Clinical pharmacology of thalidomide. Euro J Clin Pharmacol 57:365-376, 2001.
145. Gunzler V: Thalidomide in human immunodeficiency virus (HIV) patients: a review of safety considerations. Drug Safety 7:116-134, 1992.
146. Ordi J, Cortes F, Martinez N, et al: Thalidomide induces amenorrhea in patients with lupus disease. Arthritis Rheum 41:2273-2275, 1998.
147. Jacobson JM, Greenspan JS, Spritzler J, et al: Thalidomide for the treatment of oral aphthous ulcers in patients with human immunodeficiency virus infection: National Institute of Allergy and Infectious Diseases AIDS Clinical Trials Group. New Engl J Med 336:1487-1493, 1997.
148. Hamuryudan V, Mat C, Saip S, et al: Thalidomide in the treatment of the mucocutaneous lesions of the Behçet syndrome: a randomized, double-blind, placebo-controlled trial. Ann Intern Med 128:443-450, 1998.
149. Stevens RJ, Andujar C, Edwards CJ, et al: Thalidomide in the treatment of the cutaneous manifestations of lupus erythematosus: experience in sixteen consecutive patients. Brit J Rheumatol 36:353-359, 1997.
150. Huizinga TW, Dijkmans BA, van der Velde EA, et al: An open study of pentoxyfylline and thalidomide as adjuvant therapy in the treatment of rheumatoid arthritis. Ann Rheum Dis 55: 833-836, 1996.
151. Lehman TJ, Striegel KH, Onel KB: Thalidomide therapy for recalcitrant systemic onset juvenile rheumatoid arthritis. J Pediatr 140:125-127, 2002.
152. Huang F, Gu J, Zhao W, et al: One-year open-label trial of thalidomide in ankylosing spondylitis. Arthritis Rheum 47: 249-254, 2002.
153. Powell RJ, Gardner-Medwin JM: Guideline for the clinical use and dispensing of thalidomide. Postgrad Med J 70:901-904, 1994.
154. Debol SM, Herron MJ, Nelson RD: Anti-inflammatory action of dapsone: inhibition of neutrophil adherence is associated with inhibition of chemoattractant-induced signal transduction. J Leukocyte Biol 62:827-836, 1997.
155. Zuidema J, Hilbers-Modderman ES, Merkus FW: Clinical pharmacokinetics of dapsone. Clin Pharmacokinet 11:299-315, 1986.
156. Jollow DJ, Bradshaw TP, McMillan DC: Dapsone-induced hemolytic anemia. Drug Metabol Rev 27 107-124, 1995.
157. Chang DJ, Lamothe M, Stevens RM, Sigal LH: Dapsone in rheumatoid arthritis. Semin Arthritis Rheum 25:390-403, 1996.
158. Hornsten P, Keisu M Wiholm BE: The incidence of agranulocytosis during treatment of dermatitis herpetiformis with dapsone as reported in Sweden, 1972 through 1988. Arch Dermatol 126:919-922, 1990.
159. Coleman MD: Dapsone toxicity: some current perspectives. Gen Pharmacol 26:1461-1467, 1995.
160. Tomecki KJ, Catalano CJ: Dapsone hypersensitivity. The sulfone syndrome revisited. Arch Dermatol 117 38-39, 1981.
161. Katz SI, Gallin JI, Hertz KC,et al: Erythema elevatum diutinum: skin and systemic manifestations, immunologic studies, and successful treatment with dapsone. Medicine 56:443-455, 1977.
162. Holtman JH, Neustadt DH, Klein J, Callen JP: Dapsone is an effective therapy for the skin lesions of subacute cutaneous lupus erythematosus and urticarial vasculitis in a patient with C2 deficiency. J Rheumatol 17:1222-1225, 1990.
163. Fredenberg MF, Malkinson FD: Sulfone therapy in the treatment of leukocytoclastic vasculitis: report of three cases. J Am Acad Dermatol 16:772-778, 1987.
164. Callen JP: Treatment of cutaneous lesions in patients with lupus erythematosus. Dermatol Clin 12:201-206, 1994.

61 Anticytokine Therapies

ZUHRE TUTUNCU • ARTHUR KAVANAUGH

In recent years, discoveries delineating the immunpathophysiologic basis of various rheumatic diseases, combined with advances in biopharmaceutical development, have allowed the introduction of biologic therapeutics. These agents target specific components of the immune response considered central to the etiology and sustenance of the disease process. In the rheumatoid synovium, for example, there is substantial evidence of an upregulation of key proinflammatory cytokines such as tumor necrosis factor-α (TNF-α) and interleukin-1 (IL-1).[1,2] Agents targeting these key mediators have proven to have considerable efficacy in patients with rheumatoid arthritis (RA), initially in research studies and subsequently in the clinic. The ability of anticytokine therapy to substantially improve signs and symptoms of disease and also inhibit disease progression has altered both physicians' and patients' expectations regarding the treatment of RA and other systemic inflammatory disorders.

Tumor Necrosis Factor-α

TNF-α is a member of a family of peptide mediators that includes lymphotoxin-α (LT-α), which was-previously known as TNF-β, Fas ligand (FasL), CD40 ligand (CD40L), and receptor activator of nuclear factor-kappa B (NF-κB) ligand (RANKL). Although initial observations of its effect were made in the 1890s, data concerning the central role of TNF-α as a mediator of inflammation, tissue destruction, and organ injury have emerged largely over the last quarter of the twentieth century.[3] TNF-α can be produced by numerous cell types; however, in inflammatory conditions it is made primarily by macrophages in response to various proinflammatory stimuli. Human TNF-α is synthesized and expressed as a 26 k-D transmembrane protein on the plasma membrane and is cleaved by a specific metalloproteinase (TNF-α converting enzyme ([TACE]). After proteolytic cleavage, TNF-α is converted to a 17-kD soluble protein, which oligomerizes to form the active homotrimer. The actions of TNF-α are mediated through two structurally distinct cell-associated receptors: TNF-RI (55 kD; CD120a) and TNF-RII (75 kD; CD120b).[3] The two receptors differ in their binding abilities and signaling properties; these differences also reflect the differences in their primary functions.[3,4] Soluble forms of CD120a and CD120b bind TNF-α with high avidity and may serve an inhibitory function. The binding of TNF-α to its receptor can initiate several signaling pathways. Signaling cascades include activation of transcription factors (e.g., NF-κB), protein kinases (intracellular enzymes that mediate cellular responses to inflammatory stimuli, e.g., c-Jun N-terminal kinase [JNK], p38 MAP kinase), and proteases (enzymes that cleave peptide bonds, e.g., caspases). Members of the TNF superfamily play important roles in programmed cell death (apoptosis). The apoptosis-inhibition pathway is NF-κB dependent, as shown by studies demonstrating that TNF-α–induced apoptosis of malignant cells was inhibited by activation of NF-κB–dependent pathways.[5]

TNF-α was first characterized as a factor that induces necrosis of tumor cells. It has subsequently been recognized to mediate numerous inflammatory and immuno regulatory activities. TNF-α facilitates lymphocyte, neutrophil, and monocyte accumulation at inflammatory sites by upregulating endothelial expression of various adhesion molecules. It also modulates growth, differentiation, and metabolism in different cell types. Of note, TNF induces the synthesis of several other key proinflammatory cytokines (including IL-1, IL-6, and granulocyte-macrophage colony-stimulating factor [GM-CSF]), chemokines (e.g., IL-8), and other inflammatory mediators (e.g., prostaglandins, leukotrienes, and platelet-activating factor [PAF]). TNF-α can stimulate macrophages and fibroblasts to produce matrix metalloproteinase (MMP) enzymes (e.g., collagenases, stromolysins) that effect damage to cartilage and bone. In addition, TNF-α can directly mediate pain, fever, and cachexia.[6,7] The pivotal role of TNF in mediating such diverse inflammatory activities provided the rationale for targeting this cytokine in systemic inflammatory diseases.[8] This was proven initially in animal studies in which inhibition of TNF with monoclonal antibodies (mAb) or soluble TNF-R constructs ameliorated the signs of inflammation and prevented joint destruction.[9]

Therapies Targeting Tumor Necrosis Factor-α

Currently there are three anti–TNF-α agents available for clinical use: infliximab, a chimeric anti–TNF-α mAb; etanercept, a soluble TNF-R construct; and adalimumab (formerly know as D2E7), a human anti–TNF-α mAb. For each agent, initial assessment in open-label studies of patients with RA was followed by double-blind, placebo-controlled, randomized clinical trials (DBPCRCT). Typically, early studies included patients with chronic refractory disease. Some studies included patients with active disease, despite concurrent methotrexate (MTX), whereas others assessed efficacy as monotherapy (Table 61–1). These agents have subsequently been studied in other RA populations (e.g., early RA) as well as in other systemic inflammatory diseases (e.g., Crohn's disease, psoriatic arthritis, psoriasis, ankylosing spondylitis).

Although all three agents are TNF inhibitors, there are differences among them. Infliximab and adalimumab are specific for TNF-α; etanercept binds both TNF-α and LT-α. Although all bind with high affinity, the avidity and, hence, duration of binding may be greater

TABLE 61–1 • CLINICAL TRIALS WITH BIOLOGIC AGENTS

	Study Design	MTX Mean Dose	Pt #	DD Mean/ Yr	SJC/ TJC at Entry	Failed DMARD Mean	Efficacy
Infliximab[14]	Single dose 0, 1, or 10 mg/kg	None	73	8	24/27 mn	3.2	Paulus 20: 79% (10 mg), 44% (1 mg), 8% (placebo)
Infliximab[12]	DB wk: 0 (0, 5, 10, 20 mg/kg) OL, wks: 12, 20, 28 (10 mg/kg)	10 mg/wk	28	6.2	21/31 mn	2.8	ACR-20 at wk 1: 86%(5 mg/kg), 71% (10 mg/kg), 86% (20 mg/kg), 14% (placebo) ACR-20 at wk 40: 28% (10 mg/kg)
Infliximab[10]	DBPCRCT 1, 3, or 10 mg/kg wks 0, 2, 6, 10, 14	7.5 mg/wk some groups	101	10	18/26 md	2.4	Paulus 20 at wk 14: 60% (3 mg or 10 mg/kg ± MTX) Paulus 20 sustained at week 26 in 3 or 10 mg/kg group + MTX
Infliximab[11]	DBPCRCT 1, 3, or 10 mg/kg every 4 or 8 wks	15 mg/kg	428	8.4	20/30 md	2.6	ACR-20 at 30 wks: 52% (infliximab), 20% (placebo) ACR-50 at 30 wks: 28% (infliximab), 5% (placebo) ACR-70 at 30 wks: 12% (infliximab), 0% (placebo)
Infliximab[15]	DBPCRCT 3 or 10 mg/kg every 4 or 8 wks	16 mg/kg	428	9	22/32	?	Radiograph at 54 wks: Arrest of progression of structural damage Sharp score median change: 0.0 (infliximab), +4.0 (placebo)
Etanercept[19]	DBPCRCT 0.25, 2, or 16 mg/m^2 twice a wk	None	180	>77% 5 yr	24/32 mn	100%	ACR-20 at 12 wks: 75% (16 mg), 46% (2 mg), 33% (0.25 mg), 14% (placebo) ACR-50 at 12 wks: 57% (16 mg), 22% (2 mg), 9% (0.25 mg), 7% (placebo)
Etanercept[20]	DBPCRCT 10 or 25 mg twice a wk	None	234	12	25/34 mn	3.2	ACR-20 at 24 wks: 59% (25 mg), 51% (10mg), 11% (placebo) ACR-50 at 24 wks: 40% (25 mg), 24% (10 mg), 5% (placebo) ACR-70 at 24 wks: 15% (25 mg), 9% (10mg), 1% (placebo)
Etanercept[21]	DBPCRCT 25 mg twice a wk	19 mg/kg	89	13	19/28 md	2.7	ACR-20 at 24 wks: 71% (etanercept), 27% (placebo) ACR-50 at 24 wks: 39% (etanercept), 3% (placebo) ACR-70 at 24 wks: 15% (etanercept), 0% (placebo)
Etanercept[22, 60]	DBPCRCT 10 or 25 mg etanercept twice a wk, or oral MTX	19 mg/wk only MTX group	632	1	24/31 mn	42%	ACR-20 at 24 months: 72% (25 mg), 61% (10 mg), 59% (MTX) ACR-50 at 24 months 49% (25 mg), 35% (10 mg), 42% (MTX) ACR-70 at 24 months: 29% (25 mg), 19% (10 mg), 24% (MTX) Radiograph at 2 years: Sharp score mean change: 1.3 (25 mg), 3.2 (MTX)
Adalimumab[29]	DBPCRCT 20 or 40 mg every or every other wk	None	544	11	20/34 md	3.7	ACR-20 at 26 wks: 53% (40 mg qwk), 46% (40 mg qowk), 39% (20 mg qwk), 36% (20 mg qowk), 19% (placebo) ACR-50 at 26 wks: 35% (40 mg qwk), 22% 40 mg qow), 21% (20 mg qwk), 19% (20 mg qow), 8% (placebo)
Adalimumab[30]	DBPCRCT 20, 40, or 80 mg. every other wk	16.8 mg/wk	271	12	17/29 mn	3.0	ACR-20 at 24 wks: 66% (80 mg), 66% (40 mg), 48% (20 mg), 15% (placebo) ACR-50 at 24 wks: 43% (80 mg), 54% (40 mg), 32% (20 mg), 8% (placebo) ACR-70 at 24 wks: 19% (80 mg), 27% (40 mg), 10% (20 mg), 5% (placebo) Radiograph at 52 wk: Sharp score mn change: 0.1 (40 mg), 0.8 (20 mg), 2.7 (placebo)

Continued

TABLE 61–1 • CLINICAL TRIALS WITH BIOLOGIC AGENTS—cont'd

	Study Design	MTX Mean Dose	Pt #	DD Mean/ Yr	SJC/ TJC at Entry	Failed DMARD Mean	Efficacy
Adalimumab[31]	DBPCRCT 40 mg every other wk, or 20 mg every wk	16.7 mg/wk	619	11	19/28 mn	2.4	ACR-20 at 24 wks: 60% (40 mg), 55% (20 mg), 24% (placebo) ACR-50 at 24 wks: 41.5% (40 mg), 38% (20 mg), 9.5% (placebo) ACR-70 at 24 wks: 23% (40 mg), 21% (20 mg), 4.5% (placebo)
Anakinra[57]	DBPCRCT 30, 75, or 150 mg	None	472	4.0	26/34 mn	75%	ACR-20 at 24 wks: 43% (150 mg), 34% (75 mg), 39% (30 mg), 27% (placebo) Radiograph at 24 wks: Genant score: 47% reduction (anakinra)
Anakinra[59]	DBPCRCT 0.04, 0.1, 0.4, 1.0, or 2.0 mg/kg/day	17 mg/wk	419	7.4	18/25 mn	1.9	ACR-20 at 24 wks: 35% (2 mg), 42% (1 mg), 23% (placebo)

Abbreviations: ACR, American College of Rheumatology; DB, double blind; DBPCRCT, double-blind, placebo-controlled clinical trial; DD, disease duration; DMARD: disease-modifying drugs; F-U, follow-up; OL, open label; md, median; mn, mean; MTX, methotrexate; pl, placebo; Pt: patient; qwk, once a week; qowk, once every other week; SJC, swollen joint count; TJC, tender joint count; wk, week; yr, year.

for the mAb. Effector functions such as induction of cell lysis and apoptosis can be demonstrated by in vitro studies with the mAb but not the soluble receptor; the in vivo relevance of this is uncertain. Given intravenously, infliximab has a high peak concentration followed by steady-state elimination, whereas etanercept and adalimumab, because they are given subcutaneously, have more "flat" pharmacokinetic profiles. Despite these potential differences, all agents are effective in controlling the signs and symptoms of RA (Table 61–2). Whether these differences in characteristics between the agents will result in differences in other outcomes in RA patients (e.g., effect on radiographic changes), efficacy in other diseases, and toxicities, remains largely to be shown.

INFLIXIMAB

Structure and Mechanism of Action

Infliximab is a chimeric mouse-human monoclonal antibody composed of constant regions of human (Hu) immunoglobulin (Ig)G1κ coupled to the variable regions of a high-affinity neutralizing murine anti-Hu TNF-α antibody. The resulting construct is approximately 70 percent human in origin (Fig. 61–1).

Infliximab neutralizes the biologic activity of TNF-α by binding with high affinity to the soluble and transmembrane forms of TNF-α, and it inhibits binding of TNF-α with its receptors.

Pharmacokinetics

Clinical pharmacology studies demonstrate that infliximab has a dose-dependent pharmacokinetic (PK) profile following infusions of 1 to 20 mg/kg. In combination therapy with MTX (7.5 mg once a week), serum infliximab concentrations tend to be slightly higher than when administered alone.[10] Infliximab behaves in a consistent manner across different demographic groups (including pediatric versus adult patients) and among patients with different diseases of varied severity. It has been estimated that the half-life of infliximab is around 8 to 9.5 days at the 3 mg/kg dose, although longer values have been reported for higher doses.[11] The volume distribution (Vd) of infliximab at steady state is independent of dose, suggesting predominantly intravascular distribution.[12,13] Median Vd ranges from 3 to 5 liters. The clearance of infliximab is approximately 0.01 liters/hr.

Drug Dose

The initial recommended dose of infliximab is 3 mg/kg given as an intravenous (IV) infusion, followed by doses at 2 and 6 weeks after the first infusion, then every 8

TABLE 61–2 • COMPARISON OF BIOLOGICAL AGENTS

	Etanercept	Infliximab	Adalimumab	Anakinra
Half-Life	3 to 4.8 days	8 to 9.5 days	10 to 13.6 days	4 to 6 hours
Binding Target	TNF-α and LT-α	TNF-α	TNF-α	IL-R1
Construct	Recombinant human soluble receptor-Fc construct	Recombinant chimeric mAb	Recombinant human mAb	Recombinant human receptor antagonist
Administration	Twice weekly, SC	Every 4 to 8 weeks, IV	Every 1 to 2 weeks, SC	Daily, SC

Abbreviations: Fc, Fragment crystallizable; IL-R1, type 1 interleukin receptor; IV, intravenous; LT-α, lymphotoxin-alpha; mAb, monoclonal antibody; SC, subcutaneous.

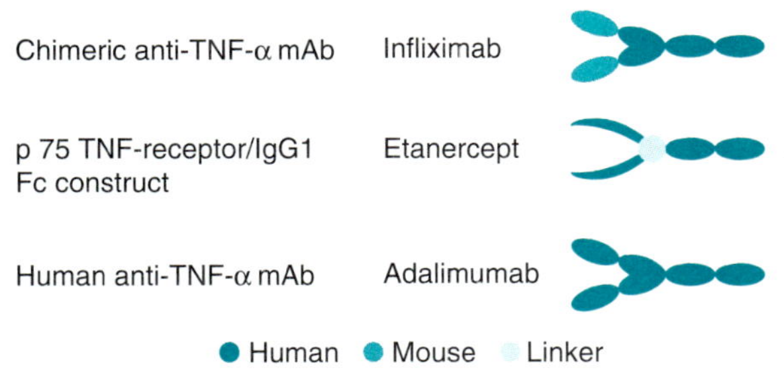

FIGURE 61–1 · Structure of TNF-α Antagonists.

weeks thereafter. Infliximab is approved for use in combination with MTX, although patients have also received infliximab with other disease-modifying antirheumatic drugs (DMARDs) or as monotherapy. At the recommended initial dose, about 25 percent of patients will have trough concentrations below 1 mg/mL; this is associated with lesser clinical response.[13] In that case, higher doses, shorter intervals, or both may be used.

Efficacy

In the earliest controlled trials, the efficacy of single doses of 1, 5, 10, and 20 mg/kg of infliximab was demonstrated; however, disease activity recurred upon discontinuation of therapy.[12,14] This, along with the growing safety experience gained with therapy, provided the rationale for studies with longer duration of therapy. In a subsequent study, concurrent therapy with MTX at a dose of 7.5 mg/week seemed to enhance the clinical response to infliximab and also decrease its immunogenicity.[10]

Further multicenter, randomized, double-blind trials have evaluated the effects of multiple doses of infliximab over longer periods of time. In the Anti-Tumor Necrosis Factor Trial in Rheumatoid Arthritis with Concomitant Therapy (ATTRACT) trial, addition of infliximab to treatment of patients with active disease, despite concurrent MTX use, was significantly superior to treatment with MTX alone. The initial promising results, based on an analysis of improvement in signs and symptoms at 6 months of treatment, have been shown to be sustained through 54 weeks of follow-up.[11,15] In addition to achieving substantial efficacy as measured by American College of Rheumatology-20 (ACR-20) clinical response criteria, the use of infliximab was associated with significant improvement in functional status and quality of life.[15] Perhaps most remarkably, patients receiving infliximab had a dramatic reduction in the progression of joint damage as assessed by radiographic change scores. The median change of the Sharp score at 1 year for infliximab treated patients was 0.0 units (mean change +0.55, baseline score 50.5), indicating no significant progression. The median change in score for patients on MTX alone was +4.0 units (mean change +7.0, baseline score 55.5); this amount of progression is roughly what would have been predicted given the severity of patient's disease.[13,15]

ETANERCEPT

Structure and Mechanism of Action

Etanercept is formed by the linkage of two p75 TNF-R extracellular domains to the fragment crystallizable (Fc) portion of human IgG_1 (see Fig. 61–1). The resultant molecule is a dimeric, soluble TNF-R that binds both TNF-α and LT-α with high affinity and specificity.[16] The TNF-R domains in etanercept bind to two of the three receptor binding sites on the TNF trimer, thus blocking the ability of TNF to interact with cell-bound TNF-R, a prerequisite for signal transduction. The dimeric structure of etanercept results in a high binding ability for TNF and thereby inhibits TNF-α–induced proinflammatory activity.[16]

Pharmacokinetics

When administered subcutaneously, etanercept is absorbed slowly, reaching a mean peak concentration approximately 50 hours after a single 25-mg dose. The Ig structure affords a half-life of 3 to 4.8 days. The volume of distribution of suggests predominantly intravascular distribution.[17] The route of clearance from the circulation is unclear, although it is presumed to be mediated through Fc binding by the reticuloendothelial system.

Drug Dose

Etanercept is given by self-administered subcutaneous injection of 25 mg twice weekly. However, recent studies have suggested comparable efficacy with a 50-mg once per week injection. Etanercept is approved for use either alone or in conjunction with MTX.

Efficacy

Initial studies have demonstrated the efficacy and tolerability of etanercept in both early and refractory disease and have also established the optimal dose as 25 mg twice weekly.[18,19]

In addition to achieving substantial efficacy as measured by ACR-20 clinical response criteria, the use of etanercept has been associated with significant improvement in functional status and quality of life. In a DBPCRCT, patients with active and long-standing RA who were refractory to DMARD therapy were treated with etanercept (10 or 25 mg twice weekly) for 6 months. Etanercept was effective in rapidly reducing disease activity.[20] In another trial, addition of etanercept to patients with active disease, despite concurrent MTX, was significantly superior to treatment with MTX alone. The addition of etanercept resulted in rapid and sustained improvement.[21] At 6 months, disease activity was significantly reduced in the combination therapy group versus those who received only MTX. In the open-label extension part of this study, the patients were able to sustain the improvement, and the majority of them were able to decrease their use of MTX, corticosteroid, or both.

The role of TNF-α inhibitors for the treatment of early disease was demonstrated in a large clinical trial in which two doses of etanercept (10 or 25 mg twice weekly) were compared to an accelerated dosing of MTX in MTX-naïve RA patients with less than 3 years of disease.[22,60] Radiographic assessments at 0, 6, 12, and 24 months showed that the rate of radiographic progression appeared to be dramatically reduced by both agents. However, the effect of 25-mg etanercept was greater than that of MTX.

In long-term, open-label follow-up studies of patients from the clinical trials, responses appear to have been sustained over the course of several years.[23,24] Based on the promising results of a clinical trial of 69 patients, etanercept has been approved for the therapy of juvenile rheumatoid arthritis (JRA) and further safety has been demonstrated.[25,26] With the growing evidence that suggests TNF-α's role in psoriatic arthritis (PsA) and ankylosing spondylitis (AS), TNF-α blockers have been studied in these conditions. The safety and efficacy of anti–TNF-α therapy have been demonstrated in DBPCRCTs with PsA and AS patients.[27,28]

ADALIMUMAB

Structure and Mechanism of Action

Adalimumab is a fully human IgG1 mAb generated through repertoire cloning. Adalimumab neutralizes the biologic activity of TNF-α by binding with high affinity to the soluble and transmembrane forms of TNF-α and inhibiting binding of TNF-α with its receptors.

Pharmacokinetics

The peak serum adalimumab concentration and the area under the curve (AUC) increases linearly with doses in the range of 0.5 to 10mg/kg. Adalimumab appears to have a low clearance and distributes mainly in the vascular compartment. Its elimination half-life is comparable to that of native IgG_1 (10 to 13.6 days).

Drug Dose

Adalimimab has been studied with different doses at different intervals. The initial recommended dose is 40 mg every other week administered subcutaneously, with the possibility of changing the dose frequency to weekly.

Efficacy

In a phase II DBPCRCT, 283 patients were treated with placebo or one of three doses of adalimumab (20, 40, or 80 mg) via weekly subcutaneous injection for 12 months (placebo patients switched to active treatment at 3 months).[29] Clinical results demonstrated the efficacy of adalimumab in comparison to placebo. Efficacy was comparable among doses. In a subsequent DBPCRCT study, adalimumab was shown to be safe and effective with concurrent MTX therapy.[30]

In a multicenter DBPCRCT, 619 patients with active RA who had inadequate response to MTX were randomized to receive 40 mg of adalimumab every other week, 20 mg of adalimumab weekly, or placebo.[31] At the end of the study, modified total Sharp scores showed significantly smaller changes in patients treated with adalimumab. In addition, significantly more patients had no new erosions compared to those taking placebo. Both adalimumab regimens were found to be significantly more effective at reducing signs and symptoms measured with ACR-20 response, and they also improved physical function compared to placebo.

TUMOR NECROSIS FACTOR-α INHIBITORS

Mechanism of Action

TNF-α inhibitors probably achieve their clinical efficacy by various mechanisms, including downregulation of local and systemic proinflammatory cytokine production, reduction of lymphocyte migration into the joint, and reduction of angiogenesis in the joints. It has been demonstrated, for example, that serum levels of IL-6 and IL-1 were significantly reduced after administration of anti–TNF-α mAb.[32,33] The reduction in TNF-α and the consequent reduction in IL-1 would be expected to reduce the synthesis of MMP and production of other degradative enzymes. Serial studies have shown that indeed there was a marked reduction in proMMP-3 and proMMP-1 after anti–TNF-α therapy.[34-36] Anti-TNF-α therapy is associated with a reduction of lymphocyte migration into the joints of patients with RA. Using radiolabeled granulocytes, it has been demonstrated that anti–TNF-α mAb significantly reduced cell movement into the affected joints.[37] In addition, post-treatment synovial biopsies showed reduced cellular infiltrates, with fewer numbers of T cells and macrophages present.[38] These effects are thought to be secondary to a reduction in the expression of endothelial adhesion molecules in the synovial tissue. Treatment with anti–TNF-α mAb resulted in a dose-dependent decrease in soluble forms of intercellular adhesion molecule-1 (ICAM-1) and E-selectin.[37] Changes in soluble E-selectin, soluble ICAM-1, and circulating lymphocytes with anti–TNF-α therapy correlated with clinical outcome. Vascular endo-thelial growth factor (VEGF) is a potent endothelial cell–specific angiogenic factor. It is produced in the synovium and is an important regulator of neovascularization in the pannus. After anti–TNF-α therapy, VEGF serum levels were reduced in patients with RA. The decrease correlated significantly with the clinical benefit observed in these patients.[39] Because angiogenesis is a prominent feature of rheumatoid synovium, the relationship between inflammation and angiogenesis has been investigated. Computerized image analysis of endothelium for multiple markers of endothelium (e.g., von Willabrand factor [VWF], CD31) and neovasculature (αvβ3) has shown reduced vascularity after anti–TNF-α therapy.

Other Considerations

Monitoring During Anti–TNF-α Therapy

No specific laboratory monitoring is currently required by regulatory agencies during therapy with TNF-α inhibitors. Nevertheless, because of the rare occurrence of myelosuppression and concern about the risk of infections, clinicians may obtain intermittent assessment of the complete blood count (CBC). Assiduous monitoring of patients for any sign and symptom of infection, demyelinating disease, and malignancy is requisite during treatment with all TNF-α inhibitors.

Pregnancy and Breast Feeding During Anti–TNF-α Therapy

Developmental toxicity studies in rats, rabbits, and mice have not revealed any maternal toxicity, embryo toxicity, or teratogenicity associated with TNF-α inhibition. However, there have been no human studies and, hence, no data to support using TNF-α blockers during pregnancy. Thus, they are not recommended for use during pregnancy. As the number of patients treated with TNF-α inhibitors increases, there are a growing number of pregnancies among treated patients. Outcome data on anecdotal observation of small numbers of pregnant mothers treated with infliximab and etanercept disease reveal that relative rates of live births, miscarriages, and therapeutic terminations observed were comparable to rates in a national cohort of healthy women. Because it is not currently known if TNF-α blockers are excreted in human milk or if they are absorbed systemically after ingestion, TNF-α blockers should not be used by nursing mothers.

Anti–TNF-α Therapy for Other Diseases

In addition to their use in RA, TNF-α inhibitors have also been assessed in patients with JRA, psoriasis, PsA, ankylosing spondylitis, and Wegener's granulomatosis, among other diseases. Other possible indications for anti–TNF-α therapy are currently being explored in preliminary studies. Open-label studies with TNF-α inhibitors in adult Still's disease, uveitis, Behçet's disease, scleroderma, Sjögren's syndrome, sarcoidosis, pyoderma gangrenosum, and polymyositis or dermatomyositis have shown promising results. However, whether anti–TNF-α therapy can be safely and efficaciously applied to these other inflammatory disorders requires further controlled studies. Of note, infliximab has proven efficacious in several studies for the treatment of Crohn's disease, whereas etanercept was ineffective.[40] The reason for this disparity is unknown, but it may relate to some of the differences between the agents noted previously.

Toxicity

In clinical trials, etanercept, infliximab, and adalimumab have generally been well tolerated.[11,15,19-21,30] Furthermore, longer-term follow-up of patients initially enrolled in clinical trials has provided additional safety data for these agents. However, TNF-α plays a key role not only in the pathogenesis of autoimmune diseases, but also in normal immune homeostasis. Therefore, there are a number of safety considerations, including the potential risk of infection and malignancy, that are germane to optimal clinical use of these agents. Additional information concerning the adverse effects associated with these agents as they are used in the clinic has come through pharmacovigilance.

Adverse events related to the use of TNF-α inhibitors can be grouped into those that are agent related versus those that are target related. Injection site and infusion reactions, and immunogenicity and its sequelae, vary depending on the particular agent. Potentially increased predisposition to infections, development of malignancy, induction of autoimmune disorders, and associations with demyelinating disorders, myelosuppression, and worse outcome with congestive heart failure might be considered target-related adverse events. Any clinically effective TNF-α inhibitor might be associated with such adverse events, although the relative risk among different agents may vary depending on characteristics such as target specificity, affinity or avidity, effector functions, and pharmacokinetic or pharmacodynamic considerations.

Infusion and Injection Site Reactions

Infliximab has been associated with infusion reactions, the most common of which are headache (20 percent) and nausea (15 percent). These are rarely severe, are usually transient, and can typically be controlled by slowing the rate of infusion or by treatment with acetaminophen or antihistamines.[11,15] The infusion reactions tend not to increase over time and seldom require discontinuation of therapy.[11] With etanercept and adalimumab, cutaneous reactions at injection sites represent the most frequent side effect, although they rarely cause discontinuation of therapy.[20,21,31] Injection site reactions, which occur in about 49 percent of patients treated with etanercept and 24 percent of those treated with adalimumab, typically consist of erythematous or urticarial lesions.[20,31] Although they can arise at sites of previous injections, these reactions seem to be limited to the skin and are not associated with other features of immediate hypersensitivity. Reactions typically occur close to initiation of treatment and abate over time, even with continued dosing.

Antigenicity

The development of antibodies to a therapeutic agent could diminish its half-life and, consequently, decrease its efficacy. They might also lead to adverse effects including immune-complex formation or hypersensitivity reactions. Any compound, for example, even a small molecule such as recombinant human insulin, has the potential to be immunogenic. Factors that affect the immunogenicity of a compound include foreign-ness (human compounds are less immunogenic than those derived from other species), size (larger molecules are more immunogenic than smaller), type (proteins are more immunogenic than carbohydrates), route of administration (oral administration tends to lead to tolerance, subcutaneous administration tends to be more immunogenic than intravenous), dose (very low doses and very high doses can lead to tolerance rather than immunogenicity), and immunmodulatory effects of the compound or concomitant therapy (compounds that suppress the immune response decrease immunogenicity). Complicating assessment of the immunogenicity of compounds such as the TNF-α inhibitors are the difficulties in interpreting results from the novel assays that must be developed for such testing. Perhaps the most extensive data currently available is with infliximab. RA trials of infliximab with or without concomitant MTX treatment revealed that immunogenicity was decreased by concomitant MTX, due perhaps in part to the increase in the half-life of infliximab associated with MTX use.[10] In studies of Crohn's patients, longer-term dosing protocols and the concurrent use of medications decreased immunogenicity. The frequency of antibody-to-infliximab formation may be inversely related to infliximab dosage. Of note, although the presence of such antibodies may increase the number of infusion reactions, it might not necessarily attenuate the clinical efficacy of the agent. Routine testing for antibodies to infliximab or other TNF-α inhibitors is not currently recommended.

Infection

Given that TNF-α is a key mediator of inflammation, a major concern surrounding the use of TNF-α inhibitors is their potential to increase the risk for infection. Although inhibition of TNF-α in animals does not appear to increase their risk for infection with most pathogens, it does interfere with the ability to mount an inflammatory response against intracellular organisms. In experimental models, TNF-α blockade impairs the resistance to infection with mycobacterium,[41,42] *Pneumocystis carinii*,[43] fungi,[44] *Listeria monocytogenes*,[45] and legionella.[46] Confounding attribution of infections to any therapeutic agent in RA is the fact that infections occur more frequently and are important contributors to the accelerated morbidity of RA patients when compared to normal population. How much of this susceptibility relates to the disease itself and how much is caused by effects of immunomodulatory drugs (e.g., steroids, cytotoxic drugs) is difficult to define. The subset of RA patients with great susceptibility to infection (i.e., those with severe, active disease[47,48]) have also been the type of patient most commonly enrolled in trials of TNF-α inhibitors; this is also the group of patients for whom these agents have perhaps the greatest utility in the clinic.

In RA trials with anti–TNF-α therapies, a number of infections have occurred among patients receiving TNF-α inhibitors. In all studies, the most frequent infection was upper respiratory both in the placebo and the drug group. Other frequent infections included sinusitis, urinary tract, bronchitis, and pharangitis. In some studies, a slightly greater propensity to develop upper respiratory infections has been seen in patients receiving TNF-α inhibitors, particularly at higher doses. However, the incidence of severe infections has typically been comparable to that seen in the placebo groups, and significant sequelae occurring as a consequence of infection also appears similar to that in placebo groups.[11,20,21] Although these results are reassuring, clinicians need to monitor the patients closely for signs and symptoms of infections. Anti–TNF-α therapy can mask the initial signs and symptoms of infection. When using TNF-α inhibitors, withholding treatment should be a consideration when there is a potential for serious infection.

Opportunistic infections, particularly disseminated *Mycobacterium tuberculosis* (TB), are a major area of concern with the use of TNF-α inhibitors.[11] To date, a greater number of cases have been seen among patients receiving infliximab than the other TNF-α inhibitors, but this may in part relate to issues such as the particular patient population exposed. Approximately three quarters of TB cases associated with infliximab were diagnosed within the first three infusions of infliximab, implying reactivation of latent infection.[49] Of note, more anti–TNF-α–treated patients have disseminated TB and other unusual illnesses compared to the overall population, highlighting the need for clinical suspicion and close follow-up. Current U.S. guidelines recommend purified protein derivative (PPD) skin testing prior to infliximab therapy. If the PPD test is positive without evidence of active infection, treatment for latent TB should commence before or concurrent with infliximab therapy. However, a screening chest radiograph and PPD test appear prudent before initiating any treatment with a TNF-α inhibitor.

Malignancy

Anti–TNF-α drugs can theoretically affect the host defense against malignancy. To date, the occurrence of malignancies in clinical trials and long-term follow-up of patients from clinical trials of the various TNF-α inhibitors in RA patients does not appear to exceed the rate that would be expected in this population.[11] As is the case for infections, the incidence of certain malignancies is higher than expected in rheumatoid patients with severe disease and who are receiving other immunosuppressant drugs. Longer-term follow-up of larger numbers of patients will provide clinicians with a better view about safety of these agents in this regard.

Autoimmune Disorders

Approximately 10 percent of the patients treated with any TNF-α inhibitor develop antibodies to double-stranded DNA (ds-DNA). However, few (0.2-0.4%) treated patients develop symptoms consistent with drug-induced lupus.[11,20,50] The mechanism and the significance of the development of antibodies are uncertain. Of note, patients did not develop life-threatening lupus involvement (e.g., nephritis, central nervous system [CNS] lupus) and rarely developed the panolopy of other autoantibodies characteristic of idiopathic SLE (e.g., anti-Sm/RNP, anti-Ro/La, anti-Scl70). A few patients have been reported to develop anticardiolipin antibodies, but they are mostly asymptomatic. Of those few patients who developed lupus-like symptoms while on TNF-α inhibition, improvement has been seen upon discontinuation of anti-TNF-α therapy. Although the rare occurrence of autoimmune disorders has not dissuaded most clinicians from using TNF-α inhibitors in RA, some remain cautious about using them in patients with a history of SLE.

Demyelinating Syndromes

Several cases of multiple sclerosis (MS) or demyelinating disease have been reported with anti–TNF-α therapy in patients with RA, PsA, and Crohn's disease.[51] In addition, two studies of TNF-α inhibitors in MS patients showed worsening of MS-related symptoms and exacerbations in the treated group.[52,53] Although there is supporting evidence that the incidence of MS may be increased in patients with RA, the association between anti–TNF-α therapy and MS remains unclear. The risk of developing a demylelinating disease is very small; however, anti–TNF-α therapy should be withheld in patients with demyelinating diseases or who are showing neurologic signs and symptoms during anti–TNF-α therapy.

Congestive Heart Failure

There is data suggesting that TNF-α may play a role in the pathogenesis of congestive heart failure (CHF). In a pilot trial designed to evaluate the effect of infliximab on clinical status in patients with stable class III or IV CHF, patients were randomized to receive either placebo or infliximab (5 mg/kg or 10 mg/kg) at 0, 2, and 6 weeks. No clinical benefit was observed; in fact, higher incidences of mortality and hospitalization for worsening of CHF were seen in patients treated with infliximab, especially those treated with higher dose. Trials of etanercept for CHF similarly failed to show clinical benefit, although no excess mortality was noted. Therefore, patients with CHF should probably not be treated with TNF-α inhibitors.

Pancytopenia

Rare reports of pancytopenia, including aplastic anemia, have been reported in patients treated with TNF-α inhibitors. The causal relationship to therapy remains unclear, but caution should be exercised in patients who have a previous history of hematologic abnormalities.

Interleukin-1

Members of the IL-1 family include IL-1α, IL-1β, and the IL-1 receptor antagonist (IL-1Ra). IL-1α and IL-1β are synthesized as leader peptides. The molecular weight of each precursor is 31 kDa. Specific cellular proteases process IL-1α and IL-1β to their 17 kDa mature forms. ProIL-1α precursor (proIL-1α) is active intracellularly. However, proIL-1β is not active before cleavage with IL-1β–converting enzyme (ICE). After cleavage it is secreted and is fully functional. IL-1Ra is a naturally occurring antagonist protein with amino acid sequence homology to IL-1α and IL-1β. Multiple forms of this protein exist. One is secreted and functions as a competitive inhibitor of IL-1α and IL-1β, binding to the same counterreceptor but transducing no signal. Other forms of IL-1Ra are intracellular; although they may serve inhibitory functions, their roles have not been fully defined. A very low level of receptor occupancy (2 to 3 percent) by IL-1 is sufficient to elicit a full response. The IL-1 polypeptides bind to two cell-surface receptors: type 1(IL-1R1) and type 2 (IL-1RII). IL-1RI is found on most cell types, whereas IL1-RII occurs mainly on the surface of neutrophils, monocytes, B cells, and bone marrow progenitor cells. When IL-1 binds to IL-1RI, the signal transduction is mediated through association of a second receptor unit, IL-R accessory protein (IL-1R-AcP). The three members of the IL-1 family bind to IL-1RI with similar affinities. Binding of IL-1 to IL1-RII does not lead to signal transduction. IL-1RII acts like a decoy receptor and competitive inhibitor. Soluble forms of IL-1RII inhibit IL-1 activity by competing with IL-1RI for IL-1 binding.

Like TNF-α, IL-1 is one of the key mediators of inflammatory response. Although IL-1 can be synthesized by many different cell types, it is produced at inflammatory sites primarily by macrophages. IL-1 exhibits both local and systemic biologic effects. Some systemic affects of IL-1 include, fever, muscle breakdown, and induction of acute-phase proteins in the liver. IL-1 induces the production of other cytokines including TNF-α, IL-6, and IL-8. IL-1 enhances the expression of adhesion molecules on endothelial cells and induces chemotaxis of neutrophils, monocytes, and lymphocytes. IL-1 has both angiogenic and angiostatic activities.[54] In addition, IL-1 is a potent inducer of collegenase and prostaglandin E_2 (PGE_2) from synovial fibroblasts and chondrocytes. It has also been shown that IL-1 blocks the repair process in the human articular cartilage by interfering with glycosaminoglycan synthesis. IL-1, together with TNF-α, plays a major role in the recruitment of osteoclasts and in the inhibition of bone formation, which causes osteopenia.[55]

Studies in animal models of arthritis have also demonstrated the therapeutic potential of IL-1 blockade. IL-1β gene knockout mice show markedly reduced levels of inflammation following immunization with type II collagen. The use of genetically modified mice has also helped to confirm the physiologic significance of IL-1Ra, as deletion of this gene in mice results in the spontaneous development of arthritis.

ANAKINRA

Structure and Mechanism of Action

Anakinra (IL-1ra) is a recombinant nonglycosylated homologue of IL-1Ra that differs from native human IL-1Ra by the addition of a single methionine residue at its amino terminus. Anakinra blocks the activity of IL-1 by competitively inhibiting IL-1 binding to the IL-1RI receptor. Levels of the naturally occurring IL-1Ra, which are elevated in the synovium and synovial fluid from RA patients, appear to be insufficient with the excess amount of locally produced IL-1.

Pharmacokinetics

In subjects with RA, maximum plasma concentrations of anakinra occurred 3 to 7 hours after subcutaneous administration clinically relevant doses (1 to 2 mg/kg). The terminal half-life ranged from 4 to 6 hours. In RA patients, no unexpected accumulation of anakinra was observed after daily subcutaneous doses for up to 24 weeks. The estimated anakinra clearance increased with increasing creatinine clearance and body weight.

Drug Dose

The recommended dose of anakinra for the treatment of patients with moderate to severely active RA is

100 mg/day administered by subcutaneous injection. Anakinra can be used alone or in combination with MTX. Because of the potential for increase in rate of infections, it is not recommended for use in conjunction with TNF inhibitors.

Efficacy

Preliminary clinical studies indicated that anakinra can be safely administered by subcutaneous injection.[56,57] The efficacy of anakinra in the treatment of active RA was confirmed in a 24-week, phase II, placebo-controlled study in which 472 patients received daily, subcutaneous injections of placebo or one of the three different doses of anakinra (30 mg, 75 mg, or 150 mg).[57] Improvements were observed in all individual clinical parameters, including swollen-tender joint counts, pain score, duration of early morning stiffness, and patient and physician assessment of disease activity. More patients on the higher dose of anakinra achieved improvement in ACR-20 criteria in comparison to placebo group. However, the overall magnitude of reductions in clinical symptoms and signs (20 to 30 percent) were relatively modest when compared to those reported in TNF-α blocking agents (60 to 70 percent).[15,19] Patients were allowed to go on to non–placebo-controlled extension study with three different doses of anakinra after completing the 24-week double-blind study. On completion of the extension study, 55 percent of the patients who had previously received placebo achieved ACR-20 response. Of the patients who continued receiving the same dose of anakinra, 49 percent maintained ACR-20 response at 48 weeks. Analysis of hand radiographs by two different methodologies after 24 weeks of treatment showed a statistically significant decrease in the rate of progressive joint damage compared to placebo.[58]

The efficacy of anakinra plus MTX was evaluated in a 24-week, randomized, double-blind, placebo-controlled study.[59] Active RA patients, despite MTX therapy, were treated with 0, 0.04, 0.1, 1.0, or 2.0 mg/kg of anakinra per day. The optimal dose of anakinra was 1.0 mg/kg. ACR-20 response at 24 weeks was seen in 42 percent of patients receiving 1.0 mg/kg of anakinra as well as methotrexate, and it was seen in 23 percent of the patients receiving placebo and MTX.

Toxicity

Anakinra is generally well tolerated. Injection site reactions (ISR) are the most frequently reported adverse event. In the randomized clinical trial, ISRs were reported in 25 percent of patients given placebo, and in 50, 73, and 81 percent of patients given anakinra in doses of 30, 75, and 150 mg/day, respectively.[57] These reactions were generally mild and transient, yet they resulted in premature withdrawal from the study in 5 percent of the patients. Infections were uncommon and occurred at a similar rate to placebo group. Infections that required antibiotic therapy occurred in 12 percent of the placebo-treated group, whereas they occured in 15 to 17 percent of the treatment group. The infections consisted primarily of bacterial events such as cellulites, pneumonia, and bone and joint infections. The incidence of pulmonary infections may be higher among patients with underlying asthma. In placebo-controlled studies, up to 8 percent of patients receiving anakinra showed reductions in their neutrophil count, compared to 2 percent of the placebo patients. Other adverse events reported were headache, nausea, diarrhea, sinusitis, influenza-like syndrome, and abdominal pain. Malignancy rate and incidences were similar to those expected for the populations studied.

Monitoring

Patients should be closely monitored for signs and symptoms of infection. Administration of anakinra needs to be discontinued if a patient develops serious infection. Neutrophil count should be assessed prior to initiating anakinra treatment, as well as while receiving anakinra therapy monthly for 3 months, and then every 4 months up to 1 year.

Pregnancy and Breast-feeding

Reproductive studies have only been performed on rats and rabbits, and they have not revealed any evidence of harm to the fetus. However, there are no well-controlled studies in pregnant women. Therefore, anakinra should only be used during pregnancy if clearly needed. It is not known if anakinra is secreted in human milk; anakinra should be discontinued in nursing mothers.

Conclusion

Treatment of RA with inhibitors of the key proinflammatory cytokines TNF-α and IL-1 is a compelling example of effective targeted biologic therapies. Not only has therapy with these agents substantially improved the signs and symptoms of disease, but for many patients, quality of life has been improved, the progression of joint damage has been inhibited, and disability has been averted. The success of this approach has "raised the bar" for the goals of treating this pernicious disease and has reinvigorated research aimed at further refining therapy.

A number of questions remain regarding the optimal use of these drugs. Longer-term safety data will allow clinicians to more fully assess the risk-to-benefit ratio for individual patients. Given the uncertainties regarding their long-term safety and the heterogeneity of clinical responses, research defining the populations of patients expected to derive the greatest benefit with the least toxicity from particular types of therapy is critical. Ongoing research, for example, correlating specific genetic polymorphisms in key immunomodulatory molecules, could optimize efficacy while minimizing toxicity. This is also relevant from a cost standpoint. Although the acquisition costs of these agents are relatively high, data supporting their cost effectiveness with gains in employment and reduced hospitalizations are emerging. These results have raised additional clinical questions. For example, the potential benefit of intervention with cytokine inhibitors early in the disease course, or of aggressive combination therapy as the initial therapeutic approach, has been suggested by several studies. Conceivably, these treatment paradigms may become the standard of care in the future.

The success of the TNF-α inhibitors has also generated substantial interest in targeting this cytokine by alternative approaches, including inhibitors of TNF-α–converting enzyme, inhibitors of phosphodiesterase IV (which regulates TNF-α production), gene transfer to overexpress the TNF-R, and inhibition of key regulatory factors—such as p38 MAP kinase and NF-kB. Advances in biopharmaceuticals could generate agents that possess desirable characteristics in terms of pharmacokinetics, immunogenicity, adverse effects, ease of administration, and cost. These developments should eventually allow clinicians to maximize their use of these novel therapies and achieve clinical benefits for their patients that were previously considered unattainable. Further developments are eagerly expected.

REFERENCES

1. Koch AE, Kunkel SL, Strieter RM: Cytokines in rheumatoid arthritis. J Investig Med 43:28-38, 1995.
2. Feldman M, Brennan FM, Maini RN: Role of cytokines in rheumatoid arthritis. Annu Rev Immunol 43:28-38, 1996.
3. Bazzoni F, Beutler B: The tumor necrosis factor ligand and receptor families. N Engl J Med 334:1717-1725, 1996.
4. Sacca R, Cuff C, Lesslauer W, et al: Differential activities of secreted lymphotoxin-alpha3 and membrane lymphotoxin-alpha1beta2 in lymphotoxin-induced inflamation: critical role of TNF receptor 1 signaling. J Immunol 160:485-491, 1998.
5. Beg A, Baltimore D: An essential role for NF-κB in preventing TNF-α-induced cell death. Science 274:782-784, 1996.
6. Cunha FQ, Poole S, Lorenzetti BB, Ferreira SH: The pivotal role of tumor necrosis alpha in the development of inflammatory hyperalgesia. Br J Pharmacol 107:660-669, 1992.
7. Dinarello C, Cannon J, Wolff S: Tumor necrosis factor is an endogeneous pyrogen and induces production of interleukin 1. J Exp Med 163:1433-1450, 1986.
8. Feldman M, Elliott MJ, Woody JN, Maini RN: Anti-tumor necrosis factor-α therapy of rheumatoid arthritis. Adv Immunol 64:283-350, 1997.
9. Seymour HE, Worsley A, Smith JM, Thomas HL: Anti-TNF agents for rheumatoid arthritis. Br J Clinic Pharmacol 51:201-208, 2001.
10. Maini RN, Breedveld FC, Kalden JR, et al: Therapeutic efficacy of multiple intraveneous infusions of anti-tumour necrosis factor-alpha monoclonal antibody combined with low-dose weekly methotrexate in rheumatoid arthritis. Arthritis Rheum 41:1552-1563, 1998.
11. Maini R, St Clair EW, Breedweld F, et al: Infliximab (chimeric anti-tumour necrosis factor α monoclonal antibody) versus placebo in rheumatoid arthritis patients receiving concomitant methotrexate: a randomized phase III trial. Lancet 354:1932-1939, 1999.
12. Kavanaugh A, St Clair EW, McCune WJ, et al: Chimeric anti-tumour necrosis factor α monoclonal antibody treatment of patients with rheumatoid arthritis receiving methotrexate therapy. J Rheumatol 27:841-850, 2000.
13. St Clair E, Wagner C, Fasanmade A, et al: Relationship of serum infliximab concentrations to clinical improvement in rheumatoid arthritis. Arthritis Rheum 46:1451-1459, 2002.
14. Elliott MJ, Maini RN, Feldman M: Randomized double-blind comparison of chimeric monoclonal antibody to tumor necrosis factor alpha (cA2) versus placebo in rheumatoid arthritis. Lancet 344:1105-1110, 1994.
15. Lipsky PE, Desiree MFM, van der Heijde, et al: Infliximab and methotrexate in the treatment of rheumatoid arthritis. N Engl J Med 343:1594-1602, 2000.
16. Mohler KM, Torrance DS, Smith CA, et al: Soluble tumor necrosis factor (TNF) receptors are effective theraupetic agents in lethal endothexemia and function simultaneously as both TNF carriers and TNF antagonists. J Immunol 151:1548-1561, 1993.
17. Korth-Bradley, Abbe SR, Roberta KH, et al: The pharmacokinetics of etanercept in healthy volunteers. Ann Pharmacothar 34:161-164, 2000.
18. Moreland LW, Margolies G, Heck LW, et al: Recombinant soluble tumor necrosis factor receptor (p80) fusion protein: toxicity and dose finding trial in refractory rheumatoid arthritis. J Rheumatol 23:1849-1855, 1996.
19. Moreland LW, Baumgartner SW, Schiff MH, et al: Treatment of rheumatoid arthritis with a recombinant human tumour necrosis factor receptor (p75)-Fc fusion protein. N Engl J Med 337: 141-147, 1997.
20. Moreland LW, Schiff MH, Baumgartner SW, et al: Etanercept therapy in rheumatoid arthritis: a randomized, controlled trial. Ann Intern Med 130:478-486, 1999.
21. Weinblatt ME, Kremer KM, Bankhurst AD, et al: A trial of etanercept, a recombinant tumor necrosis factor receptor: Fc fusion protein in patients with rheumatoid arthritis receiving methotrexate. N Engl J Med 340:253-259, 1999.
22. Genovese MC, Bathon JM, Martin R, et al: Etanercept versus methotrexate in patients with early rheumatoid arthritis: two year radiographic and clinical outcomes. Arthritis Rheum 46:1443-1450, 2002.
23. Moreland LM, Cohen SB, Baumgartner SW, et al: Long-term safety and efficacy of etanercept in patients with rheumatoid arthritis. J Rheumatol 28:1238-1244, 2001.
24. Lovell DJ, Giannini EH, Reiff A, et al: Etanercept in children with polyarticular juvenile rheumatoid arthritis. N Engl J Med 342:763-769, 2000.
25. Kietz DA, Pepmueller PH, Moore TL: Theraupetic use of etanercept in polyarticular course juvenile idiopathic arthritis over a two year period. Ann Rheum Dis 61:171-173, 2002.
26. Brandt J, Haibel H, Reddig J, et al: Successful short term treatment of severe undifferentiated spondyloarthropathy with the anti-tumour necrosis factor-alpha monoclonal antibody infliximab. J Rheumatol 29:118-122, 2002.
27. Mease PJ, Goffe BS, Metz J, et al: Etanercept in the treatment of psoriatic arthritis and psoriasis: randomized trial. Lancet 356:385-390, 2000.
28. Van den Bosch F, Kruithof E, Baeten D, et al: Randomized double-blind comparison of chimeric monoclonal antibody to tumor necrosis factor (infliximab) versus placebo in active spondyloarthropathy. Arthritis Rheum 46:755-765, 2002.
29. Van de Putte LBA, Rau R, Breedveld FC, et al: Six month efficacy of the fully human anti-TNF antibody D2E7 in rheumatoid arthritis. Ann Rheum Dis 59(Suppl 1):i47, 2000.
30. Weinblatt ME, Keystone EC, Furst DE, et al: Adalimumab, a fully human anti-tumor necrosis factor α monoclonat antibody, for the treatment for the treatment of rheumatoid arthritis in patients taking concomitant methotrexate. Arthritis Rheum 48: 35-45, 2003.
31. Keystone E, Kavanaugh A, Sharp J, et al: Adalimumab (D2E7), a fully human anti-TNFα monoclonal antibody, inhibits the progression of structural damage in patients with active rheumatoid arthritis despite concomitant methotrexate therapy. Arthritis Rheum 46(Suppl 9):S205, 2002.
32. den Broeder AA, Joosten LAB, Saxne T, et al: Long term anti-tumour necrosis factor α monotherapy in rheumatoid arthritis: effect on radiological course and prognostic value of markers of cartilage turnover and endothelial activation. Ann Rheum Dis 61:311-318, 2002.
33. Lorenz HM, Antoni C, Valerius T, et al: In vivo blockade of TNF-α by intravenous infusion of a chimeric monoclonal TNF-α antibody in patients with rheumatoid arthritis: short term cellular and molecular effects. J Immunol 156:1646-1653, 1996.
34. Charles P, Elliott MJ, Davis D, et al: Regulation of cytokines, cytokine inhibitors, and acute-phase proteins following anti-TNF alpha therapy in rheumatoid arthritis. J Immunol 153:1521-1528, 1999.
35. Brennan FM, Browne KA, Green PA, et al: Reduction of serum matrix metalloproteinase 1 and matrix metalloproteinase 3 in rheumatoid arthritis patients following anti-tumour necrosis factor-alpha (cA2) therapy. Br J Rheumatol 36:643-650, 1997.

36. Catrina AI, Lampa J, af Klint E, et al: Anti-tumour necrosis factor (TNF)-alpha therapy (etanercept) down-regulates serum matrix mettaloproteinase (MMP)-3 and MMP-1 in rheumatoid arthritis. Rheumatology 41:484-489, 2002.
37. Paleolog EM, Hunt M, Elliot MJ, et al: Deactivation of vascular endothelium by monoclonal anti-tumor necrosis factor-α antibody in rheumatoid arthritis. Arthritis Rheum 39:1082-1091, 1996.
38. Tak PP, Taylor PC, Breedveld FC, et al: Decrease in cellularity and expression of adhesion molecules by anti-tumor necrosis factorα monoclonal antibody treatment in patients with rheumatoid arthritis. Arthritis Rheum 39:1077-1081, 1996.
39. Paleolog E, Young S, McClosekey RV, et al: Angiogenesis as a therapeutic target in rheumatoid arthritis: serum vascular endothelial growth factor is decreased by anti-TNFα therapy. Clin Exp Rheumatol 16:232, 1998.
40. Sandborn WJ, Hanauer SB, Katz S, et al: Etanercept for active Crohn's disease: a randomized, double-blind, placebo-controlled trial. Gastroenterology 121:1088-1094, 2001.
41. Bean AG, Roach DR, Briscoe H, et al: Structural deficiencies in granuloma formation in TNF gene-targeted mice underlie the heightened susceptibility to aerosol Mycobacterium tuberculosis infection. J Immunol 162:3504-3511, 1999.
42. Ehlers S, Benini J, Kutsch S, et al: Fatal granuloma necrosis despite intact antibacterial functions in TNFRp55-deficient mice chronically infected with M. Avium. Infect Immun 67:3571-3579, 1999.
43. Chen W, Havell EA, Harmsen AG: Importance of endogeneous tumor necrosis factor and gamma interferon in host resistance against Pneumocystis carinii infection. Infect Immun 60:1279-1284, 1992.
44. Allendoerfer R, Deepe GS: Blockade of endogeneous TNF-α exacerbates primary and secondary pulmonary histoplasmosis by differential mechanisms. J Immunol 160:6072-6082, 1998.
45. Rothe J, Lesslauer W, Lotscher H, et al: Mice lacking the tumour necrosis factor receptor 1 are resistant to TNF-mediated toxicity but highly susceptible to infection by Listeria monocytogenes. Nature 364:798-802, 1993.
46. Skerret SJ, Bagby GJ, Schmidt RA, Nelson S: Antibody-mediated depletion of tumour necrosis factor impairs pulmonary host defenses to Legionella pneumophila. J Infect Dis 176:1019-1028, 1997.
47. Wolfe F, Mitchell D, Sibley J: The mortality of rheumatoid arthritis. Arthritis Rheum 37:481-494, 1994.
48. Doran MF, Crowson CS, Pond GR, et al: Frequency of infection in patients with rheumatoid arthritis compared with controls. Arthritis Rheum 46:2287-2293, 2002.
49. Keane J, Gerbson S, Wise RP, et al: Tuberculosis associated with infliximab, a tumor necrosis factor neutralizing agent. N Engl J Med 345:1098-1104, 2001.
50. Charles PJ, Smeenk RJT, De Jong J, et al: Assessment of antibodies to DsDNA induced in rheumatoid arthritis (RA) patients following treatment with infliximab, a monoclonal antibody to TNF alpha. Arthritis Rheum 43:2383-2390, 2000.
51. Mohan N, Edwards ET, Cupps TR, et al: Demyelination occurring during anti-tumor necrosis factor alpha therapy for inflammatory arthritides. Arthritis Rheum 44:2862-2869, 2001.
52. van Oosten BW, Barkhof F, Truyen L, et al: Increased MRI activity and immune activation in two multiple sclerosis patients treated with monoclonal anti-tumor necrosis factor antibody cA2. Neurology 47:1531-1534, 1996.
53. The Lenercept Multiple Sclerosis Study Group and the University of British Columbia MS/MRI Analysis Group: TNF neutralization in MS: results of a randomized, placebo-controlled multicenter trial. Neurology 53:457-465, 1999.
54. Arend WP, Malyak M, Smith MF Jr, et al: Binding of IL-1a, IL-1b, and IL-1 receptor antagonist by soluble IL-1 receptors and levels of soluble IL-1 receptors in synovial fluids. J Immunol 153:4766-4774, 1994.
55. Hofbauer LC, Khosla S, Dunstan CR, et al: The roles of osteoprotegerin and osteoprotegerin ligand in the paracrine regulation of the bone resorption. Bone Miner Res 15:2-12, 2000.
56. Campion GV, Lebsack ME, Lookabaugh J, et al: Dose-range and dose-frequency study of recombinant human interleukin-1 receptor antagonist in patients with rheumatoid arthritis. Arthritis Rheum 39:1092-1202, 1996.
57. Bresnihan B, Alvaro-Garcia JM, Cobby M, et al: Treatment of rheumatoid arthritis with recombinant human interleukin-1 receptor antagonist. Arthritis Rheum 41:2196-2204, 1998.
58. Jiang Y, Genant HK, Watt I, et al: A multicenter, double-blind, dose raging, randomized and placebo controlled study of recombinant human interleukin-1 receptor antagonist in patients wth rheumatoid arthritis: radiologic progression and correlation of Genant and Larsen scoring methods. Arthritis Rheum 43: 1001-1009, 2000.
59. Cohen S, Hurd E, Cush JJ, et al: Treatment of rheumatoid arthritis with anakinra, a recombinant human interleukin-1 receptor antagonist, in combination with methotrexate: results of a twenty-four-week, multicenter, randomized, double-blind, placebo-controlled trial. Arthritis Rheum 46:614-624, 2002.
60. Bathon JM, Martin RW, Fleischmann RM, et al: A comparison of entanercept and methotrexate in patients with early rheumatoid arthritis. N Engl J Med 343(22): 1586-1593, 2000.

62 Emerging Therapies in Rheumatoid Arthritis

EDWARD C. KEYSTONE • VIBEKE STRAND

The use of tumor necrosis factor-alpha (TNF-α) antagonists in the treatment of rheumatoid arthritis (RA) has demonstrated that selective targeting of pathogenic elements of disease can result in substantial improvement in disease activity and can delay or inhibit progression of joint damage.[1] Despite their impressive efficacy, only a portion of the RA population responds well to any TNF antagonist, and few patients achieve complete remission. Because of the continuing unmet clinical need in RA and other autoimmune diseases, other therapeutic agents targeting different aspects of the immune response are under development. This chapter will provide an overview of emerging therapies resulting from advances in biotechnology and a better understanding of the pathogenesis of RA.

Current dogma suggests that initiation of RA by an exogenous agent results in the induction of proinflammatory cytokines and chemokines that upregulate adhesion molecules on endothelium and recruit circulating leukocyte cells into the inflammatory synovium.[2] Subsequent interaction of antigen-presenting cells (macrophages, B cells, dendritic cells) with T cells in the Major histocompatibility complex (MHC)-antigen-T cell receptor trimolecular complex and association with adhesion and costimulatory molecules triggers release of proinflammatory cytokines.[3,4] These cytokines, in turn, stimulate synovial lining cell hyperplasia and osteoclast activation with resultant invasion of cartilage and bone, as well as proteolytic enzyme release, which causes cartilage degradation.[5] This entire pathogenic process is maintained by persistent cell trafficking to the site of inflammation and stimulation of angiogenesis[6] (Fig. 62–1).

Pathogenic elements thought critical in the perpetuation of disease have become key therapeutic targets; these include 1) adhesion molecules; 2) chemokines; 3) inflammatory cell subsets, including T cells, B cells, dendritic cells, macrophages, and synovial fibroblasts; 4) costimulatory molecules, 5) cytokines, 6) angiogenesis factors, 7) proteolytic enzymes, and 8) the intracellular signal transduction cascade that generates proinflammatory molecules.

Targeting Adhesion Molecules

Adhesion molecules have been targeted using monoclonal antibodies (mAbs) and antisense oligonucleotides. A murine immunoglobulin G2 (IgG2) mAb against intercellular adhesion molecule-1 (ICAM-1) was studied in two open-label trials in RA.[7,8] Clinical benefit was short lived, and re-treatment resulted in substantial adverse effects.[9] Parenteral administration of an antisense oligonucleotide selectively binding ICAM-1 messenger RNA inhibited cell surface ICAM expression but was not effective in early RA trials.[10] Clinical development in Crohn's disease was recently discontinued. Cyclic peptide (mAb) inhibitors of very late antigen-4 (VLA-4) were shown to be effective in collagen-induced arthritis.[11] Several other mAbs developed to target CD44[12] and platelet endothelial cell adhesion molecule-1 (PECAM-1),[13] as well as VCAM-1,[14] have been shown to ameliorate rodent models of established arthritis, but have not yet entered clinical trials in humans.

Targeting Chemokines

Chemokines selectively activate and recruit circulating leukocytes into the synovial tissue in active RA. Chemokines and their cognate receptors cause migration of neutrophils, T cells, monocytes, and basophils through the endothelium. Antagonists, including an oral inhibitor of a chemokine receptor and an mAb to interleukin-8 (IL-8), have been studied.

IL-8 is a chemotactic cytokine that affects lymphocyte and neutrophil migration through interaction with IL-8 receptors. A fully human IgG1 mAb to IL-8 (HUMAX anti–IL-8), produced using homologous recombination, has been evaluated in psoriasis and RA. Following intravenous administration in a 12-week, phase II study in RA, no benefit was observed in reducing signs and symptoms of active disease compared to placebo (unpublished observations).[15] An oral inhibitor of chemokine receptor 1 (CCR1) is under evaluation; however, no clinical data are available.

Antagonists to chemokines, including regulated on activation normal T expressed secreted (RANTES)[15] and monocyte chemoattractant protein-1 (MCP-1),[16] reduced joint swelling and bone destruction in rodent models of RA. A fully human anti–MCP-1 mAb is in early clinical development in RA. No clinical data are available.

Targeting Inflammatory Cells

T CELLS

Preclinical studies in animal models of RA have demonstrated that mAbs directed against T cells resulted in substantial reduction in T cell numbers and improved disease. These have included murine, chimeric, primatized, and humanized anti-CD4 mAbs; humanized

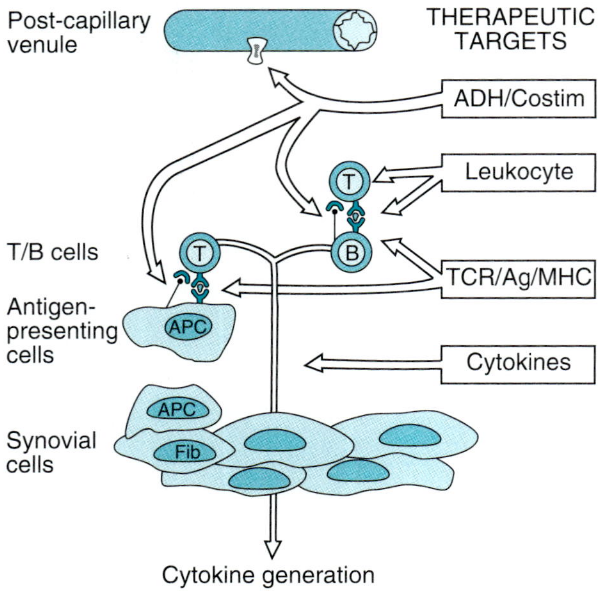

FIGURE 62–1 · Targets for Selective Immunomodulation. Adhesion and/or costimulatory (ADH/Costim) molecules to inhibit cell recruitment into the synovium and block cell-cell interaction. Immune cells to deplete or inhibit function. T cell receptor (TCR)–antigen (Ag)–major histocompatibility complex (MHC) to block antigen-specific TCR activation. Cytokines to inhibit proinflammatory effect of molecules.
Abbreviations: APC, antigen-presenting cell; Fib, fibrinogen.

anti-CD52 (CAMPATH 1-H) mAb; and two immunoconjugates: anti-CD5 and DAB–IL-2. Despite multiple positive open-label studies with murine anti-CD4 mAbs, subsequent placebo randomized controlled trials (RCTs) of chimeric, primatized, and humanized anti-CD4 mAbs[8] failed to show clinical benefit.[17] Even a fully human anti-CD4 mAb (produced by homologous recombination) has not demonstrated clinical efficacy, and development has been discontinued in RA.[18] Development of the other T cell–targeted mAbs have resulted in little or no benefit compared to placebo and have been characterized by adverse events, including prolonged T cell depletion.[19] The DAB–IL-2 mAb has been approved for treatment of cutaneous T cell lymphoma.

B CELLS

Until recently, antibody-producing B cells were thought to play a secondary role in RA by production of IgM, IgG, and IgA rheumatoid factors. Recent data support the role of B cells as antigen-presenting cells, specifically capturing antigen via cell surface immunoglobulin and presenting it to T cells.[20] A recent study indicated that B cells provide a critical function in T cell activation and may harbor the relevant antigen in RA.[21] Several therapeutics have been developed to target B cells, including anti-CD20 mAb (rituximab), anti–B cell activating factor and B-lymphocyte stimulator (BLYS). Depletion of CD20+ B cells in RA synovium– Severe combined immunodeficiency (SCID) mouse chimeras was associated with reduction of proinflammatory cytokines in the synovial tissue, suggesting a critical role for mature B cells in perpetuating the inflammatory process.[22]

Rituximab is a chimeric anti-CD20 IgG1 monoclonal antibody that is effective in treating relapsed or refractory indolent lymphomas when given in combination with chemotherapy. In non-Hodgkin's lymphoma (NHL), rituximab (RTX) is used as initial therapy and with re-treatment and maintenance regimens. It has been stated that 250,000 NHL patients have received rituximab. Interest in its use as treatment for nonmalignant autoimmune conditions has been sparked by reports of small pilot studies in idiopathic thrombocytopenia (n = 40), autoimmune hemolytic anemia (n = 20), myasthenia gravis (n = 3), polyneuropathy (n = 16), graft versus host disease (n = 16), organ transplant rejection (n = 7), and RA (n = 20).

Rituximab in Rheumatoid Arthritis

An initial open-label study in RA was conducted in five patients who received RTX, cyclophosphamide (CTX), and prednisolone.[22] At 26 weeks, three fifths of patients achieved an American College of Rheumatology (ACR) 70 response and two fifths had ACR 50 responses. These were maintained or improved to ACR 70 responses in three fifths and ACR 50 responses in two fifths of patients at 12 months, and ACR 70 responses were achieved in all at 19 months (71 weeks), with re-treatment in two patients. Peripheral B cell counts fell to undetectable levels after treatment and remained decreased for 6 to 12 months. In two patients, increases in CD19+ cells correlated with relapses. No infusion reactions were reported.

A subsequent report extended these results to a series of 22 patients.[23] A total of 29 treatments using five different regimens of RTX in combination with CTX, high dose prednisolone, or both were administered. The authors concluded that RTX should be administered in doses not less than 600 mg/m^2 and should be combined with CTX as well as prednisolone. They reported mean duration of responses to a single treatment of 14.4 months, ranging from 6 to 33.5 months. Again, peripheral B cell depletion was observed, from 5.5 to 11 months duration.

More recently, an interim analysis of a 24-week RCT of 120 patients with disease-modifying antirheumatic drug (DMARD)-refractory RA and an inadequate response to methotrexate (MTX), demonstrated substantial clinical benefit after one course of therapy with RTX in combination with MTX and corticosteroids.[24] In the RTX plus MTX group, ACR-20 responses were achieved in 80 percent of patients, ACR-50 responses in 50 percent of patients, and ACR-70 responses in 23 percent of patients. In the control MTX monotherapy group, ACR-20, -50, and -70 responses were achieved in 22, 10, and 0 percent, respectively. Despite B cell depletion, total immunoglobulin levels remained within normal range. Autoantibody levels decreased more than proportionally. IgA and IgG rheumatoid factor (RF), anticyclic citrulinated peptide Abs, and CRP levels, although IgM RF paralleled total Ig levels. Three serious adverse events were reported: Two patients had pneumonia, one case of which was fatal, and a patient had septic arthritis. One patient in the MTX group experienced a serious infection.

An open-label pilot study was conducted with RTX without immunosuppressives or corticosteroids.[25] RTX was administered in increasing doses from 100 mg week one to 375 mg/m^2 week two to 500 mg/m^2 weeks three and four. Of seven evaluable patients, three had ACR 20-percent responses at a median follow-up of 5 months. B cell depletion was evident at 8 weeks following treatment, and only infusion reactions were reported as adverse events.

The safety profile of this treatment regimen requires a larger number of patients treated over 12 months in blinded protocols and 24 months in which randomization to comparator therapies is preserved. Prolonged depletion of peripheral B cells has been observed in some patients and does not always appear to correlate with efficacy. Evaluation of tissue (i.e., synovium and lymph nodes) would be valuable because peripheral blood findings do not necessarily correlate with those in tissue. Both published reports allude to severe infections, but do not offer sufficient information to correlate their occurrence with persistent B cell depletion or other potential effects of RTX administration.

OTHER INFLAMMATORY CELL TARGETS

Fibroblast-like Synoviocytes

To date, only preclinical studies in animal models have demonstrated selective depletion of synoviocytes using a variety of techniques, which ameliorates signs of inflammation and decreases bone loss. These include mAbs to Fas antigen,[26] intra-articular gene transfer of Fas ligand,[27] as well as peroxisome proliferator-activated receptors (PPARs)[28] and intra-articular gene transfer of herpes simplex virus thymidine kinase gene, which is designed to induce apoptosis when ganciclovir is administered.[29]

Targeting the Trimolecular Complex of T Cell Receptor-Antigen-Major Histocompatibility Complex

Interference with formation of the trimolecular complex of antigen-specific T cell receptor (TcR), antigenic peptide, and MHC molecule is the principal target for antigen-specific immunotherapy that may ameliorate autoimmune disease without causing clinical immunosuppression. Therapies employing vaccination with TcR peptides[30,31] and MHC DR4/DR1 peptides[32] offered only modest benefit in RCTs in RA, and their development has been abandoned. Oral administration of bovine or chicken collagen type II, designed to result in immunologic tolerance, also demonstrated little or no efficacy compared to placebo in RCTs in RA and have also been discontinued. However, other strategies attempting to induce oral tolerance are still in various phases of investigation.

Targeting Costimulatory Molecules

T cell activation by an antigen requires two distinct signals 1) formation of the T cell receptor-antigen-MHC trimolecular complex and 2) binding of a costimulatory molecule, CD28, on the surface of T cells to CD80/CD86 on antigen-presenting cells. Following T cell activation, a protein homologous to CD28, cytotoxic lymphocyte-associated antigen-4 (CTLA-4) is upregulated on the T cell surface and downregulates T cell activation when binding to CD80/86. Several agents have been designed to inhibit interaction of costimulatory molecules on activated cells. These include a fusion protein of the fragment crystallizable (Fc) portion of IgG1 and soluble CTLA-4, an mAb to CD80, to inhibit CD28-CD80/86 interactions on activated T cells and fusion of two mAbs to CD40 ligand to interfere with interaction of CD40 with its ligand.

Based on promising preclinical studies in the New Zeland Black/New Zeland White (NZB/NZW) mouse model of systemic lupus erythematosus (SLE)[33] and the collagen II–induced rat model of arthritis,[34] CTLA-4Ig was evaluated in psoriasis. Phase I data showed a substantial improvement in approximately 50 percent of patients, without interference in assays of delayed hypersensitivity and proliferation to recall antigens.[35]

In RA, a pilot dose-finding placebo RCT compared CTLA-4Ig and LEA294 (a second-generation CTLA-4Ig product with higher binding avidity for CD80/CD86). CTLA-4Ig or LEA294 in doses of 0.5, 2, or 10 mg/kg or placebo was administered intravenously to 214 patients with active RA.[36] Patients received four infusions, at 0, 2, 4, and 8 weeks. Evaluation at day 85 revealed ACR-20, -50, and -70 responses of 23, 44, and 53 percent in CTLA-4Ig–treated patients and 34, 45, and 61 percent in LEA294-treated patients at doses of 0.5, 2.0, and 10 mg/kg, respectively, compared to 31 percent in placebo-treated patients. Both agents were well tolerated; the most common infusion-associated adverse events were nausea, vomiting, and headache, with serious adverse events reported in 4 percent of patients in the active treatment group (not considered related to study drug administration) compared with 13 percent in the placebo group.

Subsequently, a 6-month placebo RCT trial of CTLA-4Ig (2 and 10 mg/kg) in combination with MTX was completed in 339 RA patients who had active disease despite MTX treatment for at least 6 months.[37] ACR-20, -50, and -70 responses in the 10 mg/kg group were 63, 37, and 16 percent, respectively, compared to 35, 12, and 2 percent at week 24. Treatment was well tolerated; no anti-CTLA4Ig antibodies were detected. CTLA-4Ig was also evaluated in a 6-month placebo randomized control trial (PRCT) compared to placebo in combination with etanercept (25mg subcutaneously, twice per week) in patients with an inadequate response to etanercept alone.[38] Combination therapy resulted in ACR-20, -50, and -70 responses of 48, 26, and 11 percent, respectively, compared to 28, 19, and 0 percent, respectively, in patients receiving placebo and etanercept, the results of which were statistically significant for ACR-20 and ACR-70. The combination was well tolerated with a safety profile comparable to etanercept alone. These RCTs indicate that CTLA-4Ig has a therapeutic role in treatment of RA patients who are inadequately responding to MTX or etanercept.

Other strategies to inhibit costimulatory molecules are no longer in clinical development. One anti-CD40 ligand mAb was associated with thromboembolic complications in patients with SLE and ITP, and trials with an anti-CD80 mAb have been discontinued.

Targeting Cytokines

The substantial clinical benefit of TNF antagonists infliximab, etanercept, and adalimumab in RA have provided significant impetus for development of other strategies to inhibit proinflammatory cytokines in active RA. These include soluble TNF receptor type I polythyleneglycolylated (PEG) fusion protein, polyehyleneglycolylated (PEG) anti-TNF mAb Fab[1], CDP-870, TNF-α converting enzyme inhibitor (TACE) and several p38 MAP kinase inhibitors. Agents designed to inhibit interleukin-1b (IL-1b) include a soluble IL-1 receptor type II fusion protein, anti–IL-1 TRAP and anti–IL-1b mAbs, and an mAb to the soluble IL-6 receptor.

TUMOR NECROSIS FACTOR-α INHIBITORS

Soluble Tumor Necrosis Factor Receptor Type I

A construct was developed of the p55-soluble TNF receptor that was bound to polyethylene glycol (PEG) to increase its molecular weight and prolong its half-life. It was administered weekly and biweekly subcutaneously to 66 patients with active RA, and results were compared to 15 patients receiving placebo. Pharmacokinetic analysis revealed a half-life of 82 hours, plus or minus 17 hours. Most frequent adverse events were headaches, and no serious adverse events were reported. Six percent of patients developed low-titer antibodies to the soluble TNF receptor. A subsequent 3-month placebo RCT examined two doses (400 or 800 mg/kg) administered weekly in 195 RA patients.[39] At 12 weeks, a dose-response effect was evident with ACR-20 responses of 50 percent in the 800 mcg/kg group and 33 percent in the 400 mcg/kg group, compared to 26 percent in the placebo group. Mean improvements in components of the ACR criteria were statistically significant, with the exception of swollen joint counts and CRP. The most commonly reported adverse events were injection site reactions; they were encountered in 27 percent of patients with active treatment compared to 21 percent of patients receiving placebo. No treatment-related effects on laboratory variables or autoantibodies were evident. A long-term safety evaluation of this Soluble TNF-receptor-I (sTNF-RI) was initiated, comparing four dose regimens (400 or 800 mcg/kg weekly or 300 or 600 mcg/kg every 2 weeks) in 502 patients for an average of 7 months (range 3 to 11 months) of treatment.[40] The sTNF-RI was well tolerated. Additional clinical trials with this agent are proceeding.

CDP870

CDP870 is a humanized Fab anti–TNF fragment conjugated to PEG, with a half-life of 12 to 15 days. A single ascending-dose placebo RCT indicated ACR-20 responses at 8 weeks of 25, 75, and 75 percent in the 1, 5, or 20 mg/kg (n = 8) treatment groups, respectively, compared with 16.7 percent with placebo (n = 8).[41] A subsequent dose-finding placebo RCT examined CDP870 monotherapy administered in monthly subcutaneous doses of 50, 100, 200, and 400 mg in 204 patients with active RA.[42] The results demonstrated that the onset of effect was rapid, with ACR-20, -50, and -70 responses in the 400-mg treatment group of 60, 40, and 29 percent, respectively, compared to 15, 0, and 0 percent in the placebo group. The frequency of adverse events with active treatment was comparable to placebo, with few serious infections. Further clinical trials are underway.

Tumor Necrosis Factor Converting Enzymes Inhibition

TNF is synthesized in an inactive 26-kD precursor form (pro-TNF) that must be cleaved to the mature 17-kD form to be secreted into the extracellular space. Inhibition of these TACEs may provide a novel therapeutic strategy for RA. Oral administration of a TACE inhibitor was effective in the adjuvant arthritis model.[43,44] TACE inhibitors are being evaluated in early-phase studies.

Human Tumor Necrosis Factor Antisense Oligodeoxynucleotide

During DNA transcription, one of the two complementary DNA strands acts as a template on which a messenger RNA (mRNA), or sense, molecule is synthesized. The mRNA is modified and sequence elements added to control the translation process.[45,46]

Antisense oligonucleotides have nucleotide sequences complementary to the mRNA sequences encoding the targeted protein. When they bind to mRNA, translation at the ribosome is prevented, thereby blocking production of the relevant protein. Recently, a human TNF antisense oligonucleotide to ICAM-1 was developed for use in RA. Phase I studies in RA demonstrated a good safety profile, but subsequent clinical trials were disappointing, and development has been discontinued.[47] A human TNF antisense oligonucleotide is currently in clinical trials in RA.

INTERLEUKIN-1B INHIBITORS

Interleukin-1ra-Fragment Crystallizable Immunoglobulin G Fusion Protein

The interleukin-1 (IL-1) receptor antagonist (IL-1ra) has demonstrated efficacy in relieving the signs and symptoms of active RA, as well as halting radiographic progression. Its utility, however, is limited by its short half-life and requirement for daily subcutaneous administration. To prolong the half-life, a fusion protein of the recombinant Human (rHu) IL-1ra Fc portion of IgG1 has been developed and is in early-phase clinical trials.

Soluble Interleukin-1 Receptors

As with soluble TNF-α receptors, the extracellular portions of the IL-1 type I and II receptors are released from cell surfaces; these soluble IL-1 receptors (sIL-Rs) also serve as natural IL-1 antagonists. Several recombinant human (rHu) sIL-1Rs have been developed. A rHu sIL-1R type I was evaluated clinically, using subcutaneous and intra-articular administration, with very minimal clinical benefit.[47,48] A high-molecular-weight Rhu sIL-1 type II receptor has been developed and is in early, phase I clinical trials in RA.

IL-1 TRAP

Soluble receptors generally bind cytokines with low affinity, and they must be persistently present to effectively inhibit the cytokine activity. Another means to create a high-affinity cytokine antagonist is to generate cytokine "traps," fusion molecules of extracellular domains of two cytokine receptors and Fc portion of IgG1. Cytokines such as IL-1, IL-4, and IL-18 first bind a single surface receptor chain with relatively low affinity, then recruit a second protein chain. The complex of cytokine bound to both receptor chains then results in signal transduction. IL-1 first binds IL-1R type I and then recruits the cell surface IL-1R accessory protein (IL-1RAcP). IL-1 TRAP contains IL-1R type 1 and IL-1RAcP fused to the Fc portion of human IgG1. A heterodimer, IL-1 TRAP binds IL-1b with higher affinity than IL-1Ra or sIL-1R type II, and it also blocks IL-1a with high affinity.[49]

Administration of a murine version of the IL-1 TRAP was effective in the collagen II model of arthritis, and it reduced bone erosions.[49] A phase I, single-dose escalation study of IL-1 TRAP in RA revealed that IL-1 TRAP was well tolerated and has an extended serum half-life, making once-weekly dosing adequate. This small study of five patients per group (four active, one placebo) demonstrated ACR-20 and -50 responses at the 800 mcg/kg TRAP dose of 63 and 38 percent, respectively, versus placebo responses of 32 and 21 percent, respectively. There was a higher incidence of infection (mostly upper respiratory infections) in the 800 mcg/kg-dose group. Further studies are in progress.[50]

CDP484

Recently, a PEGylated humanized Fab fragment with specificity for IL-1 (CDP484) has been developed for use in RA. No clinical data is available to date.

Interleukin-1β Converting Enzyme Inhibition

IL-1β converting enzyme (ICE), also known as caspase-1, is a protease that activates both IL-1β and IL-18 in the cytoplasm by cleavage of their inactive precursors to form mature cytokines that can be secreted from the cell. Both IL-1 and IL-18 are proinflammatory cytokines that cause inflammation and promote cartilage loss and bone erosion. Preclinical data, both in vitro and in vivo, have shown that an orally active ICE inhibitor reduced inflammation and radiographic damage in animal models of arthritis.

Results of a phase II RCT were recently reported in 285 patients who had active RA despite receiving DMARDs and corticosteroids for more than 3 months. The study compared 300 and 1200 mg/day doses of ICE with placebo in a 2:2:1 randomization protocol.[51] In the intent to treat population, ACR-20 responses were 38.3, 44.0, and 32.7 percent, respectively, and failed to achieve statistical significance. When patients who had received MTX for less than 6 months were excluded from the analysis, ACR-20 responses in the 300-mg, 1200-mg, and placebo groups were 36.2, 48.9, and 28.9 percent, respectively ($p = 0.049$). This dose-response relationship correlated with similar treatment-associated changes in trologic markers of serum amyloid A protein, Matrix-metalloproteins (MMP)-1 and tissue inhibitor of matrix-metalloproteins (TIMP)-1 levels. Although a subset analysis, these data indicate further RCTs should be conducted to examine the clinical efficacy of this ICE inhibitor. When studying a promising new therapy superimposed on "failed background treatment," careful consideration must be given to ensure maximal responses to traditional DMARDs have been reached.

Interleukin-6

IL-6 plays a regulatory role in the immune system by activating T cells and inducing B cell differentiation and hepatocyte production of acute-phase reactants. IL-6 is responsible for elevated CRP level, and symptoms of malaise and fatigue in active RA. Blocking IL-6 in animal models has ameliorated arthritis. However, anti–IL-6 mAbs and soluble IL-6R fusion proteins have, in fact, acted as agonists, rather than antagonizing the inflammatory effects of IL-6. Potential therapeutic agents have, therefore, been designed to block the IL-6R.

A humanized mAb to IL-6 receptor has been evaluated in an open-label study and a placebo RCT with promising results. Preliminary data were reported in a 12-week, dose-finding placebo RCT in 45 patients (9 to 11 per group) with DMARD-refractory RA.[52] The mAb was administered monthly intravenous in doses of 0.1 to 10 mg/kg. ACR-20 (or greater) responses of 55 percent in the 5 mg/kg group compared to no responses in the placebo group (ACR-20 or greater = 0%). In a second trial, the anti–IL-6R mAb was also administered intravenously every four weeks at doses of 4 mg/kg or 8 mg/kg to 164 patients with active RA.[53] ACR-20, -50, and -70 responses were 57.4, 25.9, and 20.4 percent, respectively, in the 4 mg/kg group; 78.2, 40.0, and 16.4 percent, respectively, in the 8 mg/kg group; and 11.3, 1.9, and 0.0 percent, respectively in the placebo groups. The incidence of serious adverse events and infections were comparable in all groups. Further RCTs in active RA are in progress.

ANTI-INFLAMMATORY CYTOKINES

Several cytokines, including IL-4, IL-10, and IL-11, have been shown to possess anti-inflammatory activity by down-modulating production of proinflammatory cytokines and antagonizing their effects. Treatment with IL-4 and IL-10 has shown benefit in animal models of arthritis.

RCTs with both IL-4 and IL-10 have been conducted in RA, but disappointing results have led to discontinuation of clinical development for both cytokine products.

OTHER CYTOKINE TARGETS

IL-12, acting in concert with IL-15[54] and IL-18,[55,56] plays a key role in driving the differentiation of T cells from precursor T helper (Th0) CD4+ cells to T helper type 1 (Th1) CD4+ T cells, which is thought critical in the pathogenesis of RA. IL-15 and IL-18 also induce T cell chemotaxis and activation, as well as stimulating B cell maturation. IL-17 induces several inflammatory mediators, including TNF-α and IL-1b, and has recently been associated with cartilage destruction.[57] Inhibitors of each of these cytokines have reduced the severity of arthritis in several animal models, suggesting they represent promising targets for therapy in RA. A fully human anti–IL-15 mAb is currently in clinical trials in RA. To date no clinical data have been published.

Interferons have received much attention over the years as a therapeutic target for RA. Numerous studies of interferon-gamma (IFN-γ) in RA have yielded conflicting results, although it remains an approved treatment in Germany.[58] More recently, given its demonstrated efficacy in multiple sclerosis and preclinical studies in RA, IFN-β-1b was evaluated in RA patients. Although a small pilot study was positive, a placebo RCT failed to demonstrate benefit and clinical development in RA was discontinued.

Targeting Angiogenesis

Angiogenesis is critical to recruitment of inflammatory cells into the synovium, generation of proinflammatory molecules, and pannus formation. An important molecule inducing generation of new blood vessels, as well as osteoclast differentiation, is the integrin αVβ3. Preclinical studies using both intra-articular and systemic administration of αVβ3 inhibitors in animal models of arthritis demonstrated anti-inflammatory, as well as disease-modifying, effects.[59] A humanized anti-αVβ3 mAb is in early-phase placebo RCTs in RA. An oral αVB3 antagonist has also shown efficacy in preclinical studies. A variety of other approaches to inhibit angiogenesis have demonstrated benefit in preclinical studies, including inhibition of vascular endothelial growth factor (VEGF) with anti-VEGF mAbs,[60,61] a soluble VEGF receptor (sFlt),[62] and Trinitropheny (TNP)470. Inhibition of b-fibroblast growth factor (bFGF), which stimulates angiogenesis, has also been extensively evaluated with the small-molecule inhibitor AGM-1470.[63]

Targeting Osteoclasts

The mechanism of bone erosion in RA has been better defined through identification of factors responsible for differentiation and activation of osteoclasts.[64] A pivotal soluble factor mediating bone erosion in receptor activator of nuclear factor kappa B (NFκB) ligand (RANKL), or osteoprotegerin ligand (OPGL), acts in concert with other soluble mediators, such as TNF, IL-1, macrophage colony-stimulating factor (MCF), IL-17, and others, to induce differentiation and activation of osteoclasts. RANKL is expressed at the site of bone erosion in collagen-induced arthritis and is generated by human T cells and synovial fibroblasts. Inhibition of RANKL by its decoy receptor osteoprotegerin (OPG) inhibits bone resorption in adjuvant arthritis without affecting joint inflammation.[65] NFκB plays an essential role in signal transduction mediated by RANKL interaction with its cognate receptor on osteoclasts.[66] A number of approaches have been taken to inhibit osteoclastogenesis in preclinical studies. Several modalities are in early-phase clinical trials in RA.

Intracellular Molecules as Targets

Over the past 20 years, biotechnology has pioneered the development of genetically engineered therapies that target specific aspects of the immune response. We have learned much about the underlying pathophysiology of autoimmune disease because of their use. However, biologic agents are frequently immunogenic and often require complex and labor-intensive production processes, as well as parenteral administration, resulting in high costs that limit availability and access to treatment.

One way to avoid these issues is to develop small molecules that selectively target pathogenic elements of the immune response. The rationale leading to development of the majority of these synthetic agents stems from the concept that proinflammatory molecules, including adhesion molecules, cytokines, and proteolytic enzymes, are generated via intracellular signaling pathways using enzymes (kinases) that can be selectively inhibited by specific chemical moieties. It is expected that these small-molecule synthetic agents will gradually supplant the use of biologic agents for the treatment of RA over the next 10 to 15 years.

Once a ligand binds with its specific cell surface receptor, signal transduction pathways are initiated. Once this occurs, the signal is generated for activation of an intracytoplasmic cascade of enzymes (predominantly kinases), which act as intracellular signaling molecules or switches.[67-70] Once a series of these kinases are activated within the cytoplasm, transcription factors are generated that translocate to the cell nucleus and bind selectively to the promoter regions of DNA, resulting in gene transcription. Activation of the gene results in unwinding of the relevant segment of encoding DNA and subsequent generation of messenger RNA (mRNA) from complementary RNA sequences. Translocation of mRNA transcripts to cytoplasmic ribosomes results in translation of ribosomal RNA into protein. Protein production may, therefore, be specifically inhibited at any step in this process. Several transcription factor families have been targeted as potential treatments in RA, including mitogen-activated protein kinases (MAPK) andNFkB.[71]

MITOGEN-ACTIVATED PROTEIN KINASE INHIBITORS

There are three major MAPK signaling cascades, including extracellular signal-regulated kinase (ERK), Jun N-terminal kinase (JNK) and p38 MAPK.[71] These MAPKs are activated by upstream MAPK kinases (MAPKKs), which, in turn, have been activated by MAPK kinase kinases (MAPKKKs). ERKs are initially activated by cytokines and growth factors, whereas JNK and p38 MAPKs are activated

TABLE 62–1 • CURRENT THERAPEUTIC APPROACHES USING BIOLOGIC AGENTS

Therapeutic Agents	Agents in Clinical Trials
1. Chemokines as a Therapeutic Target	
	CCR1 inhibitor
	Anti-MCP-1 mAb
2. T and B cell Surface Antigens as Therapeutic Targets	
• CD4	Nondepleting anti-CD4 mAb
• CD20	Anti-CD20 mAb
3. Costimulation	
	CTLA4Ig
4. Cytokines as a Therapeutic Target	
Soluble receptor fusion protein	
• Cytokine receptor antagonist	IL-1ra, IgG Fc
	sIL-1R-type II
	IL-1 TRAP
• mAb to cytokines	Anti-IL-6 receptor mAb
	PEGylated Fab to IL-1
	PEGylated Fab to TNF
	Anti-IL-12, anti-IL-15, anti-IL-18
• Small molecules	Interleukin-1 converting enzyme (ICE) inhibitor
	TNF converting enzyme (TACE) inhibitor
• Antisense	TNF antisense oligodeoxynucleotide
5. Signal Transduction	
6. Intracellular Molecules as a Therapeutic Target	
• MAPK	P38 MAPK inhibitors
• NFκB	
7. Angiogenesis as a Therapeutic Target	
	Anti-αVβ3 mAb
	Taxol
8. Matrix Metalloproteinase Inhibitors as a Therapeutic Target	
9. Osteoclasts as a Therapeutic Target	
	Osteoprotegrin

Abbreviations: CCR, chemokine receptor; MCP, monocyte chemotactic protein.

in response to proinflammatory cytokines, including TNF-α and IL-1b, as well as cellular stress (e.g., heat). Activation of the MAPK cascade leads to activation of transcription factor AP-1, which binds to DNA and leads to transcription of cytokines and matrix metalloproteinases (MMPs). Recent data have demonstrated that MAPK signal transduction pathways also play a critical role in post-transcriptional regulation (control of mRNA stability and translation) of cytokines such as TNF-α.[72]

Expression of MAPK families in RA fibroblast-like cells (FLS) and AP-1 in RA synovium indicate their underlying role in the pathogenesis of this inflammatory disease.[73]

P38 MAPKs may be particularly relevant to the underlying pathogenesis of RA because they appear to play a central role in regulating production of proinflammatory cytokines TNF-α, IL-1b, IL-6, IL-8, and cyclooxygenase-2 (COX-2), as well as participating in TNF-α–induced upregulation of adhesion molecules, including VCAM-1 and E-selectin. Activation of p38 MAPKs increases synthesis of MMPs and is likely involved in angiogenesis and cell recruitment. Five isoforms of p38 MAPK have been identified; p38α is the major isoform present in most inflammatory cells.[74]

Oral administration of a selective p38a MAPK inhibitor during the established phase of collagen-induced arthritis has markedly reduced clinical manifestions and radiographic damage.[75-77] A number of oral p38 MAPK inhibitors have been developed; however, the development of several of the molecules' clinical trials has been discontinued, based on tolerability issues. Despite these setbacks a number of promising molecules continue in early-phase clinical trials in RA.

NUCLEAR FACTOR KAPPA B INHIBITORS

NFkB is one of the most important transcription factors in the inflammatory pathway.[78] It is activated by a number of different signals, including TNF-α, IL-1b, lipopolysaccharide, and oxygen free radicals. NFkB is involved in the expression of numerous proinflammatory mediators, including TNF-α; IL-1b; IL-2; IL-6; IL-8; inducer of nitric-oxide (iNOS); cyclooygenase (COX)-2; cphospholipase (cPLA2); cell adhesion molecules including intercellular adhesion molecule (ICAM)-1, vascular cell adhesion molecule (VCAM)-1, and E-selectin; chemokines including macrophage inflammatory protein 1-α (MIP-1α), monocyte chemoattractant protein-3 (MCP-3), and RANTES; and generation of MMP gene expression in articular chondrocytes.[79] Because activation of NFkB can prevent apoptosis, or programmed cell death, it is thought to play a role in synovial lining cell hyperplasia.[80]

NFκB is a dimer, the classic components of which are p50 (NFκB1) and p65 (RelA), and exists in the cytoplasm in an inactive form associated with inhibitory proteins, which are referred to as inhibitor of NFκB (IκB), that include IκBα, IκBβ, and IκBε. After an extracellular stimulus, IκB undergoes a degradation process initiated by two IκB kinases, IKK-1 (IKKα) and IKK-2 (IKKβ) that phosphorylize IκB. The phosphorylated IκB is subsequently ubiquinated and degraded by a proteosome. Degradation of the inhibitor IκB enables NFκB to be activated and translocated to the nucleus, where it binds to the DNA of the target gene to initiate gene transcription.

NFκB plays a pathogenic role in RA, which is suggested by the observation that NFκB proteins p50 and p65 are detected in abundance in the synovial lining cells, vascular endothelium, and macrophages in RA synovium.[81] IKK-1 and IKK-2 have been shown to be expressed in cultured FLS and induced by IL-1 and TNF.[82] In vitro and in vivo preclinical studies strongly support the concept of targeting NFκB in RA. Inhibition of IKK-2, and not IKK-1, has been demonstrated to prevent TNF-mediated cytokine MMP and adhesion molecule synthesis in FLS.[83] These data implicate IKK-2 as the key regulator of NFκB in RA synovium.

A number of strategies have been developed to inhibit NFκB activity, including inhibition of IκBα activation, the use of a decoy synthetic double-stranded DNA with high affinity for NFκBm and intra-articular gene transfer of IKKB.[84,85] All of these strategies have demonstrated suppression of disease activity in animal models of arthritis. Of significance, oral inhibitors of NFκB, including a proteosome inhibitor that blocks IκB degradation and a novel T cell–specific NFκB inhibitor, have significantly ameliorated established arthritis in collagen-induced and adjuvant arthritis, respectively.[86,87] In RA, a number of existing therapeutic agents inhibit NFκB as part of their activity, including nonsteroidal anti-inflammatory drugs (NSAIDs), corticosteroids, leflunomide, gold, D-penicillamine, cyclosporine, and sulfasalazine.[69] A number of selective inhibitors of NFκB have also been developed for use in RA.[88] Whether selective and pronounced inhibition of NFκB will be clinically feasible with respect to host resistance to infection remains unclear.

JUN N-TERMINAL KINASE INHIBITORS

The transcription factor AP-1 can be activated by protein kinases that phosphorylate specific amino acid residues, especially members of the MAPK family. JNK is particularly important because of its ability to phosphorylate c-JUN, a key component of AP-1. JNK has become a therapeutic target in RA because the collagenase gene, among others, is regulated by AP-1, and increased activation of JNK has been demonstrated in RA synoviocytes.[89,90] A selective JNK inhibitor decreased disease severity and radiologic damage observed in adjuvant arthritis.[91] No clinical studies have been published to date.

Metalloproteinase Inhibitors

MMPs are a group of neutral proteinases that degrade extracellular matrix of cartilage and bone. MMP activity is regulated at three levels: 1) through transcription factors (i.e., NFκB and MAPK pathways), 2) by activation (i.e., MMPs are secreted in an inactive form requiring proteolytic cleavage of the prodomain for activation), and 3) by inhibition by TIMPs, which bind activated MMPs. Any of these regulatory steps are potential targets for therapeutic intervention.

Collagen within the cartilage is at neutral pH, susceptible to degradation from collagenases MMP-1, MMP-8, MMP-13. Chondrocytes and synovial lining cells make all known collagenases. Both MMP-1 and MMP-13 are considered major collagenases involved in joint destruction and are, therefore, targets for inhibition.[92]

Early inhibitors (e.g., batimastat, or BB-94) exhibited broad-spectrum inhibition for many MMPs but had low oral availability. Marimastat, a chemically modified form of batimastat, demonstrated similar broad-spectrum MMP inhibition. With advances in crystal structure, identification of new nonpeptide inhibitors with increased specificity for individual MMPs have been made. A number of MMP inhibitors have demonstrated efficacy in menisectomy models of osteoarthritis (OA) and the guinea pig model of spontaneous OA. One inhibitor, BAY12-9566, was given to 3000 OA patients without musculoskeletal side effects and was detectable in human cartilage in patients undergoing joint replacement. Trocade, a selective collagenase inhibitor, was used in trials in RA. Unfortunately, it was found to lack efficacy in preventing radiographic progression.

With regard to safety issues, MMPs are involved in wound healing, growth, and fetal development. Because a balance exists between matrix synthesis and breakdown, MMP inhibition could cause fibrosis. Indeed, marimastat caused musculoskeletal pain and tendinitis that were time and dose dependent.

Inhibition of collagen destruction still remains an available target for preventing joint destruction. A key to success is the identification of the specific MMPs responsible for tissue destruction in the joint. Selectively targeted specific MMPs have potential to reduce side effects when used in patient treatment.

REFERENCES

1. Keystone EC: Tumor necrosis factorα blockade in the treatment of rheumatoid arthritis: Rheum Dis Clin North Am 27:427, 2001.
2. Szehanecz Z, Koch AE: Chemokines and angiogenesis. Arthritis Res 13:202, 2001.
3. Panayi GS, Corrigall VM, Pitzalis C: Pathogenesis of rheumatoid arthritis: role of T cells and other beasts. Rheum Dis Clin North Am 27:317, 2001.
4. Zhang Z, Bridges SL Jr: Pathogenesis of rheumatoid arthritis: role of B cells. Rheum Dis Clin North Am 27:335, 2001.
5. Yamanishi Y, Firestein CS: Pathogenesis of rheumatoid arthritis: the role of synoviocytes. Rheum Dis Clin North Am 27:355, 2001.
6. Koch AE: Angiogenesis implications for rheumatoid arthritis. Arthritis Rheum 41:951, 1998.
7. Kavanaugh AF, Davis LS, Nichols LA, et al: Treatment of refractory rheumatoid arthritis with a monoclonal antibody to intercellular adhesion molecule-1 (ICAM-1). Arthritis Rheum 37:992, 1994.
8. Kavanaugh AF, Jain R, McFarlin J, et al: Anti-CD54 (intercellular adhesion molecule-1; ICAM-1) monoclonal antibody therapy in early rheumatoid arthritis. Arthritis Rheum 37:S220, 1994.
9. Kavanaugh AF, Schulze-Koops N, Davis LS, et al: Repeat treatment of rheumatoid arthritis patients with a murine anti-intercellular adhesion molecular 1 monoclonal antibody. Arthritis Rheum 40:849, 1997.

10. Maksymowych WP, Blackburn WD, Tami JA, et al: A randomized placebo controlled trial of an anti-sense oligodeoxynucleotide to intercellular adhesion molecule-1 in the treatment of severe rheumatoid arthritis. J Rheumatol 29:447, 2002.
11. Dutta AS, Gormley JJ, Coath M, et al: Potent cyclic peptide inhibitors of VLA-4 (alpha 4 beta integrin) mediated cell adhesion: discovery of compounds like cyclo (MePhe-Leu-Asp-Val-D-Arg-D-Arg) (ZD7349) compatible with depot formation. J Pept Sci 6:398, 2000.
12. McKecz K, Brennan FR, Kim JH, et al: Modulation of hyaluronon receptor (CD44) function in vivo in a murine model of rheumatoid arthritis. Nat Med 1:558, 1995.
13. Ishikan J, Okada Y, Vird IN, et al: Use of anti-platelet endothelial cell adhesion molecule-1 antibody in the control of disease progression in established collagen-induced arthritis in DBA/1J mice. J Pharmacol 88:332, 2002.
14. Carter RA, Campell K, O'Donnel KL, et al: Vascular cell adhesion molecule-1 (VCAM-1) blockade in collagen-induced arthritis reduces joint involvement and alters B cell trafficking. Clin Exp Immunol 128:44, 2002.
15. Barnes DA, Tse J, Kaufhold M, et al: Polyclonal antibody directed against human RANTES ameliorates disease in the LEWIS adjuvant-induced arthritis model. J Clin Invest 101:2910, 1998.
16. Guglielmotti A, D'Onofrio E, Coletta I, et al: Amelioration of rat adjuvant arthritis by therapeutic treatment with bindarit, an inhibitor of MCP-1 and TNF-alpha production. Inflamm Res 51:252, 2002.
17. Moreland LW: Potential biologic agents for treating rheumatoid arthritis. Rheum Dis Clin North Am 27:445, 2001.
18. Fishwald DM, Strand V: Administration of an anti-CD5 immunoconjugate to patients with rheumatoid arthritis: selective decrease in synovial collagenase gene expression. Arthritis Rheum 37: 193-200, 1994.
19. Olsen NJ, Brooks RH, Cush JJ, et al: A double-blind, placebo-controlled study of anti-CD5 immunoconjugate in patients with rheumatoid arthritis: the XOMA RA Investigators Group. Arthritis Rheum 39:1102-1108, 1996.
20. De Vita S, Zaja F, Sacco S, et al: Efficacy of selective B cell blockade in the treatment of rheumatoid arthritis. Arthritis Rheum 46:2029, 2002.
21. Takemura S, Klimiuk PA, Braun A, et al: T cell activation in rheumatoid synovium is B cell dependent. J Immunol 167:4710, 2001.
22. Edwards JCW, Cambridge G: Sustained improvement in RA following a protocol designed to deplete B lymphocytes. Rheumatology. 40:205-211, 2001.
23. Leandro MD, Edwards JCW, Cambridge G: Clinical outcome in 22 patients with RA treated with B lymphocyte depletion. Ann Rheum Dis 61:883-888, 2002.
24. Edwards JCW, Szczepanski L, Szechinski J, et al: Efficacy and safety of rituximab, a B cell targeted chimeric monoclonal antibody: a placebo RCT in patients with RA. Arthritis Rheum 46(Suppl 9):S197, 2002.
25. Tuscano JM: Successful treatment of infliximab-refractor rheumatoid arthritis with rixuximab. Presented at the American College of Rheumatology. October 2002.
26. Matsuno H, Yudoh K, Nakazawa, et al: Anti-rheumatic effects of humanized anti-Fas monoclonal antibody in human rheumatoid arthritis/SCID mouse chimeric. J Rheum 29:1609, 2002.
27. Zhang H, Yang Y, Horton JL, et al: Amelioration of collagen-induced arthritis by CD95 (Apo-1/Fas) ligand gene transfer. J Clin Invest 100: 1997.
28. Kawahito Y, Kondo M, Tsubouchi Y, et al: 15-deoxy-[DELTA] 12, 14-PGJ2 induces synoviocyte apoptosis and suppresses adjuvant-induced arthritis in rats. J Clin Invest 106:189, 2000.
29. Goossens PH, Schovten GJ, Hart RA: Feasibility of adenovirus-mediated non-surgical synovectomy in collagen-induced arthritis affected rhesus monkeys. Hum Gene Ther 10:1139, 1999.
30. Moreland LW, Morgan EE, Adamson TC III, et al: T cell receptor peptide vaccination in rheumatoid arthritis: a placebo-controlled trial using a combination of V beta 3, V beta 14 and V beta 17 peptides. Arthritis Rheum 41:1919, 1998.
31. Matsumoto AK, Moreland LW, Strand V, et al: Results of phase Iib rheumatoid arthritis clinical trial using T-cell receptor peptides. Arthritis Rheum 42: S281, 1999.
32. St. Clair EW, Cohen SB, Lee ML, et al: Treatment of rheumatoid arthritis with a DR4/DR1 peptide. J Rheum 27:1855, 2000.
33. Finck BK, Kinsley PS, Wofsy D: Treatment of murine lupus with CTLA4-Ig. Science 265:1225, 1994.
34. Knoerzer DB, Karr RW, Schwartz BD, et al: Collagen-induced arthritis in the BB rat: prevention of disease by treatment with CTLA4-Ig. J Clin Invest 96: 987, 1995.
35. Abrams JR, Lebwohl MG, Guzzo CA, et al: CTLA4Ig mediated blockade of T cell costimulation in patients with psoriasis vulgaris. J Clin Invest 103:1243, 1999.
36. Moreland LW, Alten R, Van den Bosch F, et al: Co-stimulatory blockade in patients with rheumatoid arthritis: a pilot dose finding, double-blind placebo controlled clinical trial evaluating CTLA 4Ig and LEA 294 eighty-five days after the first infusion. Arthritis Rheum 46:1470, 2002.
37. Kremer J, Westhovens R, Leon M, et al: A phase IIb multi-center, randomized double-blind placebo controlled study to evaluate the safety and efficacy of two different doses of CTLA4Ig administered intravenously to subjects with active rheumatoid arthritis while receiving methotrexate. Arthritis Rheum 46(Suppl):S203, 2002.
38. Weinblatt M, Schiff M, Goldman M, et al: A pilot, multi-center, randomized, double-blind, placebo controlled trial of a co-stimulatory blocker CTLA4-Ig) (2 mg/kg) given monthly in combination with etanercept in active rheumatoid arthritis. Arthritis Rheum 46(Suppl):S204, 2002.
39. Schiff M, Furst D, Fleischmann R, et al: The efficacy and safety of PEGylated recombinant methionyl human soluble tumor necrosis factor receptor type I (PEG sTNF-RI: p55) in a randomized placebo controlled clinical study of patients with rheumatoid arthritis. Ann Rheum Dis Abstract No. FRI 0059, 2001.
40. Schiff M, Furst D, Cohen S, et al: The long term safety of PEGylated recombinant methionyl human soluble tumor necrosis factor type 1 (PEGs TNF-RI): an extension study for rheumatoid arthritis patients completing pervious PEGs TNF-RI studies. Arthritis Rheum 44:S79, 2001.
41. Hazleman B, Smith M, Moss K, et al: Efficacy of a novel PEGylated humanized anti-TNF fragment (CDP870) in patients with rheumatoid arthritis. Rheumatology 39(suppl):87, 2000.
42. Keystone EC, Choy E, Kalden J, et al: CDP-870, a novel PEGylated humanized TNFα inhibitor is effective in treating the signs and symptoms of rheumatoid arthritis. Presented at the American College of Rheumatology, San Francisco, November, 2001.
43. Conway JG, Andrews RC, Beandet B, et al: Inhibition of tumor necrosis factor alpha (TNF-alpha) production and arthritis in the rat lig GW 3333, a dual inhibitor of TNF alpha converting enzyme and matrix metalloproteinases. J Pharmacol Exp Ther 298:900, 2001.
44. Doggrell SA: TACE inhibition: a new approach to treating inflammation. Expert Opin Investig Drugs 11:1003, 2002.
45. Helene C, Toulme JJ: Specific regulation of gene expression by antisense, sense and natigene nucleic acids. Biochem Biophys Acta 99:1049, 1999.
46. Crooke ST: Progress toward oligonucleotide therapeutics: pharmacodynamicproperties. FASEBJ7:S33, 1993.
47. Drevlow B, Capezio J, Lovis R, et al: Phase I study of recombinant humaninterleukin-1 receptor (rhu IL-1R) administered intrarticularly in active rheumatoid arthritis. Arthritis Rheum 36(Suppl):S39, 1993.
48. Drevlow B, Louis R, Haag MA, et al: Recombinant human interleukin-1 receptor type I (rhu IL-1RI) in the treatment of patients with active rheumatoid arthritis. Arthritis Rheum 39:257, 1989.
49. Economides AN, Carpenter LR, Rudge JS, et al: Cytokine traps: multi-component, high-affinity blockers of cytokine action. Nature Med 9:47, 2003.
50. Guler HP, Cardwell J, Littlejohn T III, et al: A phase I, single dose escalation study of IL-1 Trap in patients with rheumatoid arthritis. Arthritis Rheum 44(Suppl 9):S371, 2001.
51. O'Hara R, Murphy EP, Whitehead AS, et al: Synovial tissue derived acute phase serum amyloid A (A-SAA) stimulates matrix metalloproteinase (MMP)-1 and MMP-3 production in inflammatory arthritis. Arthritis Rheum 46(Suppl 9):S549, 2000.
52. Choy EHS, Isenberg DA, Garrood T, et al: Therapeutic benefit of blocking interluekin-6 activity with an anti-interleukin-6 receptor monoclonal antibody in rheumatoid arthritis: a randomized,

double-blind, placebo-controlled, dose escalation trial. Arthritis Rheum 46:3143, 2002.
53. Maini RN, Paulus H, Breeveld FC, et al: rHu IL-10 in subjects with active rheumatoid arthritis (RA): a phase I cytokine response study. Arthritis Rheum 40(Suppl 9):S224, 1997.
54. McInnes IB, Lew FY: Interleukin-15: A pro-inflammatory role in rheumatoid arthritis synovitis. Immunol Today 19:75, 1998.
55. Gracie JA, Forsey RJ, Chan WL, et al: A proinflammatory role for IL-18 in rheumatoid arthritis. J Clin Invest 104:1337, 1999.
56. Bessis N, Boissier NC: Novel pro-inflammatory interleukins: potential therapeutic targets in rheumatoid arthritis. Joint Bone Spine 68:477, 2002.
57. Chabaud M, Durand JM, Buks N, et al: Human IL-17: A T-cell derived proinflammatory cytokine produced by the rheumatoid synovium. Arthritis Rheum 42:963, 1999.
58. Veys EM, Mielants H, Vergruggen G: Thymic hormones and interferons in the treatment of rheumatoid arthritis. Scan J Rheumatol 76(Suppl):297, 1988.
59. Badger AM, Blake S, Kapadia R: Disease modifying activity of SB 273005 an orally active non-peptide alphavbeta 3 (vitronecron receptor) antagonist in rat adjuvant-induced arthritis. Arthritis Rheum 44:128, 2002.
60. Sone H, Kawakami Y, Sakauchi M, et al: Neutralization of vascular endothelial growth factor prevents collagen-induced arthritis and ameliorates established disease in mice. Biochem Biophys Res Commun 28:562, 2001.
61. Lu Jing, Kasama T, Kobayashi K, et al: Vascular endothelial growth factor expression and regulation of murine collagen-induced arthritis. J Immunol 164:5922, 2000.
62. Miotla J, Maciewicz R, Kendrew J, et al: Treatment with soluble VEGF receptor reduces disease activity in murine collagen-induced arthritis. Lab Invest 80:1195, 2000.
63. Peacock DJ, Banquerigo ML, Brahn E: Angiogenesis inhibition suppresses collagen arthritis. J Exp Med 175:1135, 1992.
64. Gravellese EM, Galson DC, Golding SR, et al: The role of TNF-receptor family members and other TRAF dependent receptors in bone resorption (a review). Arthritis Rheum 43:612, 2001.
65. Kong YY, Yashida H, Sarosi I, et al: OPGL is a key regulator of osteoclastagenesis lymphocyte development and lymph node organogenessi. Nature 397:315-323, 1999.
66. Bondeson J, Foxwell B, Brennan F, et al: Defining therapeutic targets by using adenovirus: blocking NFκB inhibits both inflammatory and destructive mechanisms in rheumatoid synovium, but spares anti-inflammatory mediators. PNAS 96:S668-S673, 1999.
67. Aggarwal BB: Tumor necrosis factor receptors associated signaling molecules and their role in activation of apoptosis, JNK and NFκB. Ann Rheum 59(Suppl I):i6, 2000.
68. Piecyk M, Anderson P: Signal transduction in rheumatoid arthritis. Best practice and research. Clin Rheumatol 15:789, 2001.
69. Handel ML, Girgis L: Transcription factors. Best practice and research. Clin Rheumatol 15:657, 2001.
70. Clark A: Post-transcriptional regulation of pro-inflammatory gene expression. Arthritis Res 2:172, 2000.
71. Firestein GS, Manning AM: Signal transduction and transcription factors in rheumatic disease. Arthritis Rheum 42:609, 1999.
72. Clark A: Post-transcriptional regulation of proinflammatory gene expression. Arthritis Res 2:172-174, 2000.
73. Schett G, Tohidast-Akrad M, Smolden JS, et al: Activation, differential localization and regulation of the stress-activated protein kinases, extracellular signal regulated kinase, C-Jun N-terminal kinase and p38 mitogen activated protein kinase an synovial tissue and cells in rheumatoid arthritis. Arthritis Rheum 43:2501, 2000.
74. Adams J, Badger A, Kumar S, et al: p38 MAP Kinase: molecular target for the inhibition of pro-inflammatory cytokines. Prog Med Chem 38:1, 2001.
75. Badger AM, Bradbeer JN, Votta B, et al: Pharmacological profile of SB 203580, a selective inhibitor of cytokine suppressive binding protein/p38 kinase in animal models of arthritis, bone resorption, endotoxin shock and immune function. J Pharmacol Exp Ther 279:1453, 1996.
76. Badger AM, Griswold DE, Kapadia R, et al: Disease modifying activity of SB 242235, a selective inhibitor of p38 mitogen-activated protein kinase in rat adjuvant induced arthritis. Arthritis Rheum 43:175, 2000.
77. McLay LM, Halley F, Souness JE: The discovery of RPR200765A, a p38 MAP kinase inhibitor displaying a good oral anti-arthritic efficacy. Bioorg Med Chem 9:537, 2001.
78. Baines PJ, Karen M: Nuclear factor kappa B: A pivotal transcription factor in chronic inflammatory diseases. N Eng J Med 336:1066, 1997.
79. Liacini A, Sylvester N, Li WQ, et al: Inhibition of interleukin-1 stimulated MAP kinases activating protein-1 and nuclear factor kappa β (NF-kappa β) transcription factors down-regulates, matrix metalloproteinases gene expression in articular chondrocytes. Matrix Biol 21: 251, 2002.
80. Chen KH, Jargens J, Liu H, et al: NFkβ regulation of Flip: potential role in rheumatoid arthritis—synovial fibroblast resistance to TNFα induced apoptosis. Arthritis Rheum 44(Suppl 9):S602, 2002.
81. Handel ML, McMorrow LB, Gravallese EM, Nuclear factor kβ in rheumatoid synovium localization of p50 and p65. Arthritis Rheum 38:1762, 1995.
82. Aupperle KR, Yamanishi Y, Bennett BL: Expression and regulation of inducible I kappa β kinase (IKK-I) in human fibroblast-like synovioctyes. Cell Immunol 214:54, 2001.
83. Aupperle KR, Bennett BL, Boyle DL, et al: NFkβ regulation by I kappa β kinase primary fibroblast-like synoviocyes. J Immunol 163:427, 1999.
84. Tomita T, Takeuchi E, Tomita N, et al: Suppressed severity of collagen-induced arthritis by in vivo transfection of nuclear factor kappa β decoy oligodeoxynucleotides as a gene therapy. Arthritis Rheum 42:2532, 1999.
85. Feldmann M, Andreakos E, Smith C, et al: Is NFkβ a useful therapeutic target in rheumatoid arthritis. Ann Rheum Dis. 61:ii13, 2002.
86. Miagkov AV, Kovalenko DV, Brown CE, et al: Nfkappa β activation provides the potential link between inflammation and hyperplasia in the arthritic joint. Proc Natl Acad Sci USA 95:13859, 1998.
87. Seetharaman R, Mora AL, Nabozny G, et al: Essential role of T cell NF kappa β activation in collagen induced arthritis. J Immunol 163:1577, 1999.
88. Roshak AK, Callahan JF, Blake SM: Small molecule inhibitors of NFkB for the treatment of inflammatory joint disease. Current Opin Pharmacol 2:316-321, 2002.
89. Han Z, Boyle DL, Bennett B: et al: Activation of Jun amino-terminal kinase in rheumatoid arthritis synovitis. Arthritis Rheum 41(Suppl 9):S136, 1998.
90. Han Z, Boyle DL, Aupperle KR, et al: Jun N-terminal kinase in rheumatoid arthritis. J Pharmacol Exp Ther 291:124, 1999.
91. Han Z, Boyle D, Chang L, et al: c Jun N-terminal kinase is required for metalloproteinase expression and joint destruction in inflammatory arthritis. J Clin Invest 108:73, 2001.
92. Catterall JB, Cawston TE: Drugs in development: biosphosphonates and metalloproteinases inhibitors. Arthritis Dis Ther 5:12, 2003.

63 Pharmacology and the Elderly

STEPHANIE A. STUDENSKI • MICHAEL M. WARD

Rheumatologists are likely to encounter older adults with complex prescribing issues in daily practice. Although rheumatic conditions such as osteoarthritis (OA) and polymyalgia rheumatica are well known to occur most commonly in the older adult, less well recognized is the increasing incidence and prevalence of rheumatoid arthritis (RA) with increasing age. The median age at diagnosis is now the late fifties, and incidence increases beyond age 80.[1] Degenerative arthritis and soft tissue problems, common in the elderly, are the most frequent diagnoses in a community-based rheumatology practice.[2] Coexisting diseases and impairments such as hypertension, diabetes, ischemic heart disease, cerebrovascular disease, cognitive disorders, and vision loss are 10 to 100 times more common in persons over age 65 than in persons under age 45.[3]

Therapy for rheumatic conditions in older adults is complicated by physiologic changes with aging and by the frequent coexistence of other diseases and medications. This chapter will review the main effects of aging on clinical pharmacokinetics and pharmacodynamics, provide general principles of drug-drug and drug-disease interactions, summarize issues in treatment adherence, and recommend strategies for prescribing for the elderly. Individual interactions among specific medications and medical conditions and among different medications will then be reviewed for special issues in the older adult.

General Principles of Prescribing for the Elderly

PHARMACOKINETICS AND PHARMACODYNAMICS

The major components of pharmacokinetics are absorption, distribution, metabolism, and elimination.[4] Although degree of absorption is not altered with age, the time course may be delayed by decreased gut perfusion. Previously, gastric acidity was thought to be routinely diminished in older adults, but it has been found to be normal in otherwise healthy elders. Drug distribution is influenced by body composition, which undergoes predictable alterations with age; muscle mass and total body water decrease and fat increases. Thus, water-soluble drugs have a decreased volume of distribution and can have higher peak concentrations. In contrast, lipid-soluble drugs are more widely distributed, which can lead to slowed elimination. Metabolism by the cytochrome P450 (CYP3A) system is not systematically altered by age, but it is heavily influenced by genetic variation. Decreased liver mass and blood flow can increase the concentration of active drug in agents with large first-pass metabolism and can prolong the serum half-life of drugs metabolized by the liver. Renal elimination of many agents is decreased by both age and disease. Because muscle mass is decreased with aging, creatinine production is decreased and serum creatinine levels can often overestimate glomerular filtration rate.

Pharmacodynamic changes with age reflect a difference in drug effect at a given drug concentration. For example, narcotic analgesics often have increased pharmacodynamic effects, such as greater pain relief, at lower doses in the elderly and may require dosage reduction. Beta-blockers have reduced pharmacodynamic effects, such as less resistance to increased heart rate, perhaps due to decreased numbers or responsiveness of receptors and may require increased dosage.

INTERACTIONS BETWEEN DISEASES AND DRUGS

Common conditions in older adults that may be affected by rheumatologic therapy are listed in Table 63–1. Most interactions are associated with nonsteroidal anti-inflammatory drugs (NSAIDs) and glucocorticoids, although analgesics and antidepressant medications can also have significant effects in the elderly.[5]

Because older adults have more diseases and conditions, they take more medications and the risks of drug-drug interactions increase. Persons taking five or more drugs daily have a 50 to 60 percent risk of an adverse drug interaction.[6] Warfarin has become a commonly prescribed agent in the elderly because atrial fibrillation is highly prevalent and anticoagulation has become the standard of care. Warfarin and many oral hypoglycemic agents are highly protein bound, resulting in wide swings in drug effect when other protein-bound drugs such as NSAIDs or methotrexate (MTX) are started or stopped. Antacids can decrease absorption of many drugs.

ADHERENCE AND AGING

Aging itself has not been shown to cause increased problems with medication adherence, but many conditions and common age-associated factors have clear negative effects on adherence.[7] Complex regimens of multiple drugs and frequent schedules decrease adherence. Cognitive disorders, low vision, and poor hand function can make adherence difficult. Medication

TABLE 63–1 • COMMON CONDITIONS IN THE ELDERLY THAT ARE AFFECTED BY ANTIRHEUMATIC THERAPY

Condition	Antirheumatic Drug	Adverse Event
Cognitive deficit	Corticosteroids, narcotic analgesics, tricyclic antidepressants with high anticholinergic effects	Confusion, delirium
Congestive heart failure	NSAIDs, corticosteroids	Worsening fluid retention
Diabetes	Corticosteroids	Change in glucose tolerance and need for dosage adjustment of insulin or oral agents
Hypertension	NSAIDs, corticosteroids	Increased blood pressure, drug resistance
Anticoagulation (atrial fibrillation, pulmonary embolus)	MTX, diphenylhydantoin, NSAIDs	Competition for protein-binding sites and need for warfarin dose adjustment
Osteoporosis	Corticosteroids	Bone mineral loss, fractures
Renal insufficiency	NSAIDs	Worsening renal function, potassium retention and hyperkalemia

Abbreviations: MTX, methotrexate; NSAIDs, nonsteroidal anti-inflammatory drugs.

costs are not covered by standard Medicare and can consume a sizable portion of an older adult's income.

PRESCRIBING FOR THE OLDER ADULT

The rheumatologist can follow simple guidelines to promote safe medication prescribing and adherence (Table 63–2). Treatment goals and expectations should be defined in advance with the patient. All the medications the patient is currently taking should be brought to each appointment. These should be reviewed for changes, potential interactions, outdated bottles, and duplications, especially if both a brand name and generic form are available. An active problem list of comorbid conditions must be maintained and written instructions for all new or changing prescriptions must be provided. The physician, often the rheumatologist, should ask about affordability, difficulty with childproof bottles, and examine nonsystemic therapies for local conditions. If a planned treatment does not appear as effective as expected, the doctor should explore the possibility of a problem with adherence in a nonjudgmental manner. It is very useful in aged patients to consider tapering doses of effective drugs after a period of good control has been established.

Specific Drug-Disease Interactions

NONSTEROIDAL ANTI-INFLAMMATORY DRUGS

Gastrointestinal complications of cyclooxygenase-2 (COX-2) nonselective NSAIDs are a major cause of morbidity among elderly patients, accounting for 13 hospitalizations per 1000 patient-years of observation.[8,9] The case fatality rate among elderly patients hospitalized with an NSAID-induced gastrointestinal hemorrhage, ulcer, or perforation ranges from 5 to 17 percent.[10,11] In almost all studies, the risk of gastrointestinal complications due to NSAIDs is two to five times higher among patients who are age 70 years or older than it is in patients who are 40 to 50 years old.[12] The elderly may be more susceptible to these complications because age-associated decreases in prostaglandin-mediated gastric mucosal protection may be further compromised by NSAID treatment.[13] If NSAID therapy is required in a patient with a history of NSAID-induced gastrointestinal disease, the risk of recurrence may be reduced by using selective COX-2 inhibiting NSAIDs or by using nonacetylated salicylates. Use of misoprostol, a proton-pump inhibitor, or high-dose histamine-2 receptor blockers with nonselective NSAIDs can also

TABLE 63–2 • PRACTICAL POINTS FOR RHEUMATOLOGIC PRESCRIBING FOR OLDER ADULTS

1. Maintain and update a complete list of all active prescription and over-the-counter medications.
2. Examine actual medication bottles for outdated prescriptions, duplicates, and unreported agents.
3. Maintain and update a medical problem list of coexisting conditions.
4. Define treatment goals and expectations and provide written instructions with all new and changed prescriptions.
5. Ask about patient's ability to afford prescribed medicines.
6. Ask about problems with childproof caps.
7. Suspect drug side effects if new symptoms such as confusion, anorexia, weakness, or dizziness develop.
8. Use nonsystemic therapy such as joint injections, physical agents, and topical medications for local conditions when possible.
9. If a treatment is not working as expected, consider poor adherence prior to increasing dose.
10. Consider drug taper after a period of disease control.

decrease the risk of gastrointestinal complications and is cost effective among patients age 65 and older.[14] These strategies are underutilized, with recent findings suggesting that only 16 percent of NSAID-treated patients receive gastroprotective medications.[15] Treatment of concomitant *Helicobacter pylori* infection, which is present in more than 70 percent of the elderly,[16] can also reduce gastrointestinal complications in patients taking NSAIDs.[17]

Prostaglandins are responsible for maintaining renal blood flow and glomerular filtration in settings of decreased effective circulatory volume and hyperreninemia. Therefore, NSAIDs may precipitate acute renal failure in elderly patients with congestive heart failure, nephosis, decompensated cirrhosis, or hypovolemia. NSAID use increases the risk of hospitalization for acute renal failure from 1.5 to 4 times that of persons not using NSAIDs, but the absolute risk of acute renal failure is low.[18,19] Preexisting renal insufficiency, hypoalbuminemia, diuretic use, and use of NSAIDs with long serum half-lives all increase the risk of acute renal failure.[20,21] Dose reductions may be indicated for these patients. Renal insufficiency of any cause affects clearance of commonly used rheumatic agents, including MTX, hydroxychloroquine, colchicine, and allopurinol, requiring reduction in the doses of these medications.

NSAIDs can cause sodium and water retention, leading to peripheral edema, hypertension, and worsening of congestive heart failure. In two meta-analyses of randomized controlled trials, NSAID treatment increased mean arterial pressure by 1 mm Hg in normotensive patients and by 3 to 6 mm Hg in hypertensive patients.[22,23] Indomethacin caused the largest increases in blood pressure, whereas aspirin and sulindac influenced blood pressure the least. In observational studies, NSAID use has been reported to increase the risk of hypertension by 40 to 70 percent.[24] The renal toxicity of selective COX-2 inhibitors is similar to that of nonselective NSAIDs.[25] Use of NSAIDs has been associated with exacerbations of established congestive heart failure but not with the development of new cases.[26,27]

Specific NSAIDs have potential side effects on the central nervous system. Moderate- or high-dose salicylates may cause profound hearing loss in elderly patients, occasionally without the warning sign of tinnitus. Salicylism in the elderly may be manifested by confusion, dysarthria, agitation, hallucinations, seizures, and coma. Indomethacin and phenylbutazone can cause headache, confusion, cognitive dysfunction, depression, and paranoia in elderly patients, and they are best avoided, if possible.[28]

Not all unintended consequences of NSAID use are harmful. Regular use of NSAIDs has been consistently associated with substantially reduced risks of colon polyps and colorectal cancer.[29,30] NSAID use has also been associated with a lower risk of Alzheimer's disease, but not with other types of dementia.[31] There has been no consistent association with milder degrees of cognitive impairment.

ANALGESICS AND ANTIDEPRESSANT MEDICATIONS

Narcotic analgesics may cause excessive sedation and cognitive dysfunction in elderly patients. In particular, meperidine has been associated with postoperative delirium in the elderly.[32] The elderly may be more sensitive to the analgesic effects of narcotics and may require lower doses than younger patients. However, tolerance and dependency are no less common among the elderly than in younger individuals.[33] Severe constipation or fecal impaction may also occur, and bowel regimens should begin along with the start of any narcotic analgesic.

Tricyclic antidepressants may worsen preexisting orthostatic hypotension, as well as falling, glaucoma, dry mouth, constipation, and urinary retention through their anticholinergic effects. When a tricyclic antidepressant is indicated, nortriptyline or desipramine, which have less anticholingeric activity, should be used rather than amitriptyline. Tricyclic antidepressants can decrease cardiac conduction and cause arrhythmias and should be used cautiously in patients with preexisting heart disease. Tricyclic antidepressants may also cause confusion and excessive sedation in elderly patients. Serotonin selective reuptake inhibitors are generally safer than tricyclic antidepressants, but they can cause the syndrome of inappropriate antidiuretic hormone secretion and have been associated with an increased risk of falling in the elderly.[34]

GLUCOCORTICOIDS

Systemic steroid therapy may worsen hypertension, diabetes mellitus, osteoporosis, muscle weakness, and glaucoma. Oral glucocorticord use for more than 6 months increases the risk of new-onset diabetes mellitus in the elderly by 2.3 times that of nonusers.[35] Glucocorticoid use may worsen congestive heart failure by causing sodium retention, and may predispose to infections in elderly patients already at risk because of impaired host defenses. Risk of infection is related to the dose and duration of treatment. Elderly patients are more likely to have alterations in the hypothalamic-pituitary-adrenal axis, a condition that requires slower tapering of these drugs and closer monitoring during dose reductions.[36] Glucocorticoids also have central nervous system side effects, including depression, mania, delirium, and psychosis. The risk of depression is three times higher in patients using these drugs than in nonusers.[37] Patients with dementia may be more susceptible to these effects.[38] Glucocorticoids may also cause more subtle cognitive dysfunction in the elderly or may worsen preexisting cognitive deficits.[39]

DISEASE-MODIFYING MEDICATIONS AND BIOLOGICS

Hydroxychloroquine and chloroquine are generally avoided in patients with preexisting retinal disease, although the risk of ocular toxicity with hydroxychloroquine is low when dosed appropriately. MTX dose reductions are required in the setting of renal insufficiency to avoid drug toxicity, particularly cytopenias. Dose reductions are also indicated whenever renal blood flow is decreased, as can occur with dehydration, congestive heart failure, diuretic use, or institution of NSAID treatment. Cyclosporine can worsen hypertension and cause renal insufficiency, and it is contraindicated in patients with preexisting renal insufficiency. Infliximab has been associated with worsening congestive heart failure and death due to congestive heart failure.[40] Infliximab is contraindicated in patients with New York Heart Association class III or IV heart failure and should be discontinued if new congestive heart failure develops or if mild congestive heart failure worsens during treatment. It is not yet clear if etanercept has similar effects, but etanercept should be used with caution in patients with a history of congestive heart failure.

Specific Drug-Drug Interactions

NONSTEROIDAL ANTI-INFLAMMATORY DRUGS

NSAIDs are the antirheumatic medications most often involved in drug-drug interactions (Table 63–3). Most NSAIDs are highly protein bound, and interaction with other medications can occur if NSAIDs displace these drugs from serum protein binding sites. This mechanism accounts for the potentiation by NSAIDs of the effects of warfarin and sulfonylureas and the increase in serum levels of digoxin, sulfonamides, penicillins, phenytoin, and valproic acid.[41] NSAIDs can increase serum lithium levels by decreasing renal excretion. Concomitant use of COX-2 nonselective NSAIDs and anticoagulants, steroids, or alcohol can increase risk of bleeding. Although COX-2 selective NSAIDs have minimal effects on the prothrombin time in healthy subjects, bleeding events have occurred in elderly patients using celecoxib and rofecoxib in combination with warfarin. Use of NSAIDs with loop diuretics or angiotensin-converting enzyme inhibitors can increase the risk of acute renal failure.

NSAIDs can interfere with the effects of antihypertensive medications. This inhibition is greatest for beta-blockers but also occurs with diuretics and angiotensin-converting enzyme inhibitors.[22,42] NSAIDs may also interfere with the effects of diuretics and angiotensin-converting enzyme inhibitors in the treatment of congestive heart failure.[26,43] Comcomitant use of low-dose aspirin (325 mg per day or less) and COX-2 selective NSAIDs may decrease the gastroprotection afforded by COX-2 selective NSAIDs, limiting their therapeutic advantage.[44,45]

OTHER MEDICATIONS

Narcotic analgesics may interact with other central nervous system depressants, such as sedatives, hypnotics, major tranquilizers, tricyclic antidepressants, and alcohol, to cause excessive sedation, cognitive dysfunction, and coma. Glucocorticoids have few interactions with other drugs, but they can cause profound hypokalemia when used with potassium-wasting diuretics or amphotericin B. Barbituates, phenytoin, and rifampin can increase the metabolism of corticosteroid drugs, requiring increased dosages.

Disease-modifying medications other than cyclosporine have few drug interactions (Table 63–4).[46] The most important interactions are between azathioprine and allopurinol, and between methotrexate and trimethoprim, which can cause severe bone marrow toxicity. Although pharmacokinetic interactions occur between MTX and aspirin and other NSAIDs that result in greater bioavailability of MTX, concomitant use of these medications has not been associated with clinically important toxicity.[47] Most of the interactions between cyclosporine and other drugs are due to their common metabolism by the CYP3A enzyme.

TABLE 63–3 • COMMON DRUG INTERACTIONS INVOLVING NONSTEROIDAL ANTI-INFLAMMATORY DRUGS

Mechanism	Drug	Effect
Displacement from protein binding sites	Warfarin	Increased prothrombin time
	Sulfonylureas	Increased hypoglycemic effect
	Digoxin	Increased blood levels
	Sulfonamides	Increased blood levels
	Penicillins	Increased blood levels
	Phenytoin	Increased blood levels
	Valproic acid	Increased blood levels
Decreased renal excretion	Lithium	Increased blood levels
Worsening of adverse effects	Anticoagulants	Increased risk of gastrointestinal bleeding
	Glucocorticoids	Increased risk of gastrointestinal bleeding
	Alcohol	Increased risk of gastrointestinal bleeding
	Loop diuretics	Increased risk of acute renal failure
	ACE inhibitors	Increased risk of acute renal failure
	Quinolones	Seizures
Interference with drug action	Antihypertensives	Decreased hypotensive effect
	Diuretics	Worsening congestive heart failure
	ACE inhibitors	Worsening congestive heart failure
	Aspirin	Less gastroprotection of COX-2 selective NSAIDs
	Probenecid	Decreased hypouricemic effect

Abbreviations: ACE, angiotensin converting enzyme; COX-2, cyclooxygenase-2; NSAID, nonsteroidal anti-inflammatory drug.

TABLE 63–4 • COMMON DRUG INTERACTIONS INVOLVING DISEASE-MODIFYING MEDICATIONS

Disease-Modifying Drug	Interacting Drug	Effect
Antimalarials	Digoxin	Increased digoxin blood levels
	Cimetidine	Decreased clearance of chloroquine
Sulfasalazine	Digoxin	Decreased digoxin blood levels
	Warfarin	Increased prothrombin time
	Sulfonylureas	Increased hypoglycemic effect
	Antibiotics	Possible decreased absorption of sulfasalazine
	Vitamin C	Crystalluria
Minocycline	Digoxin	Increased digoxin blood levels
	Warfarin	Increased prothrombin time
	Iron, magnesium, aluminum	Decreased absorption of minocycline
Azathioprine	Allopurinol	Bone marrow toxicity
	ACE inhibitors	Anemia, leukopenia
Methotrexate (MTX)	Trimethoprim	Bone marrow toxicity
	Probenecid	Decreased MTX clearance
	Sulfonamides	Increased MTX toxicity
	Sulfonylureas	Increased MTX toxicity
	Phenytoin	Decreased phenytoin blood levels
Cyclosporine	Aminoglycosides	Nephrotoxicity
	Cotrimoxazole	Nephrotoxicity
	Amphotericin B	Nephrotoxicity
	NSAIDs	Nephrotoxicity
	ACE inhibitors	Nephrotoxicity
	Statins	Myopathy
	Colchicine	Myopathy, neuropathy, hepatotoxicity
	Macrolide antibiotics	Increased cyclosporine blood levels
	Azole antifungals	Increased cyclosporine blood levels
	Diltiazem, verapamil	Increased cyclosporine blood levels
	Amiodarone	Increased cyclosporine blood levels
	Metoclopramide	Increased cyclosporine blood levels
	Glipizide	Increased cyclosporine blood levels
	Danazol	Increased cyclosporine blood levels
	Allopurinol	Increased cyclosporine blood levels
	Rifampin	Decreased cyclosporine blood levels
	Phenytoin	Decreased cyclosporine blood levels
	Barbiturates	Decreased cyclosporine blood levels
	Azathioprine	Decreased cyclosporine blood levels
Cyclophosphamide	Allopurinol	Bone marrow toxicity
	Phenothiazines	Bone marrow toxicity

Abbreviations: ACEm angiotensin converting enzyme; MTX, methotrexate; NSAID, nonsteroidal anti-inflammatory drug.

REFERENCES

1. Doran MF, Pond GR, Crowson CS, et al: Trends in incidence and mortality in rheumatoid arthritis in Rochester, Minnesota, over a forty-year period. Arthritis Rheum 46:625-631, 2002.
2. Vanhoof J, Declerck K, Geusens P: Prevalence of rheumatic diseases in a rheumatological outpatient practice Ann Rheum Dis 61:453-455, 2002.
3. Blackwell DL, Collins JG, Coles R: Summary health statistics for U.S. adults: National Health Interview Survey, 1997—National Center for Health Statistics. Vital Health Stat 10:205, 2002.
4. Beyth RJ, Shorr RI: Principles of drug therapy in older patients: rational drug prescribing. Clin Geriatr Med 18:577-592, 2002.
5. Percy LA: Geropharmacology for the rheumatologist. Rheum Dis Clin North Am 26:433-454, 2000.
6. Walker J, Wynne H: The frequency and severity of adverse drug reactions in older people. Age Ageing 23:255-259, 1994.
7. Balkirshnan R: Predictors of medication adherence in the elderly. Clin Ther 20:764-771, 1998.
8. Wolfe MM, Lictenstein DR, Singh G: Gastrointestinal toxicity of nonsteroidal anti-inflammatory drugs. N Engl J Med 340:1888-1899, 1999.
9. Smalley WE, Ray WA, Daugherty JR, Griffin MR: Nonsteroidal anti-inflammatory drugs and the incidence of hospitalizations for peptic ulcer disease in elderly persons. Am J Epidemiol 141:539-545, 1995.
10. Wilcox CM, Clark WS: Association of nonsteroidal anti-inflammatory drugs with outcome in upper and lower gastrointestinal bleeding. Dig Dis Sci 42:985-989, 1997.
11. Blower AL, Brooks A, Fenn GC, et al: Emergency admissions for upper gastrointestinal disease and their relation to NSAID use. Aliment Pharmacol Ther 11:283-291, 1997.
12. Hernandez-Diaz S, Garcia Rodriquez LA: Incidence of serious upper gastrointestinal bleeding/perforation in the general population: review of epidemiologic studies. J Clin Epidemiol 55:157-163, 2002.
13. Solomon DH, Gurwitz JH: Toxicity of nonsteroidal anti-inflammatory drugs in the elderly: is advanced age a risk factor? Am J Med 102:208-215, 1997.
14. Gabriel SE, Jaakkimainen RL, Bombardier C: The cost-effectiveness of misoprostol for nonsteroidal anti-inflammatory drug-associated adverse gastrointestinal events. Arthritis Rheum 36:447-459, 1993.
15. Smalley W, Stein CM, Arbogast PG, et al: Underutilization of gastroprotective measures in patients receiving nonsteroidal anti-inflammatory drugs. Arthritis Rheum 46:2195-2200, 2002.
16. Everhart JE: Recent developments in the epidemiology of Helicobacter pylori. Gastroenterol Clin North Am 29:559-578, 2000.
17. Huang J-Q, Sridhar S, Hunt RH: Role of Helicobacter pylori infection and non-steroidal anti-inflammatory drugs in peptic-ulcer disease: a meta-analysis. Lancet 359:14-22, 2002.

18. Perez Gutthann S, Garcia Rodriguez LA, Raiford DS, et al: Nonsteroidal anti-inflammatory drugs and the risk of hospitalization for acute renal failure. Arch Intern Med 156:2433-2439, 1996.
19. Griffin MR, Yared A, Ray WA: Nonsteroidal anti-inflammatory drugs and acute renal failure in elderly persons. Am J Epidemiol 151:488-496, 2000.
20. Murray MD, Black PK, Kuzmik DD, et al: Acute and chronic effects of nonsteroidal anti-inflammatory drugs on glomerular filtration rate in elderly patients. Am J Med Sci 310:188-197, 1995.
21. Caspi D, Lubart E, Graff E, et al: The effect of mini-dose aspirin on renal function and uric acid handling in elderly patients. Arthritis Rheum 43:103-108, 2000.
22. Johnson AG, Nguyen TV, Day RO: Do nonsteroidal anti-inflammatory drugs affect blood pressure? Ann Intern Med 121:289-300, 1994.
23. Pope JE, Anderson JJ, Felson DT: A meta-analysis of the effects of nonsteroidal anti-inflammatory drugs on blood pressure. Arch Intern Med 153:477-484, 1993.
24. Johnson AG: NSAIDs and blood pressure: clinical importance for older patients. Drugs Aging 12:17-27, 1998.
25. Brater DC, Harris C, Redfern JS, et al: Renal effects of COX-2 selective inhibitors. Am J Nephrol 21:1-15, 2001.
26. Heerdink ER, Leufkens HG, Herings RM, et al: NSAIDs associated with increased risk of congestive heart failure in elderly patients taking diuretics. Arch Intern Med 158:1108-1112, 1998.
27. Feenstra J, Heerdink ER, Grobbee DE, Stricker BH: Association of nonsteroidal anti-inflammatory drugs with first occurrence of heart failure and with relapsing heart failure: the Rotterdam Study. Arch Intern Med 162:265-270, 2002.
28. Hoppmann RA, Peden JG, Ober SK: Central nervous system side effects of nonsteroidal anti-inflammatory drugs: aseptic meningitis, psychosis, and cognitive dysfunction. Arch Intern Med 151:1309-1313, 1991.
29. Garcia Rodriquez LA, Huerta-Alvarez C: Reduced incidence of colorectal adenoma among long-term users of nonsteroidal anti-inflammatory drugs: a pooled analysis of published studies and a new population-based study. Epidemiology 11:376-381, 2000.
30. Smalley W, Ray WA, Daugherty J, Griffin MR: Use of nonsteroidal anti-inflammatory drugs and incidence of colorectal cancer: a population-based study. Arch Intern Med 159:161-166, 1999.
31. in t'Veld BA, Ruitenberg A, Hofman A, et al: Nonsteroidal anti-inflammatory drugs and the risk of Alzheimer's disease. N Engl J Med 345:1515-1521, 2001.
32. Marcantonio ER, Juarez G, Goldman L, et al: The relationship of postoperative delirium with psychoactive medications. JAMA 272:1518-1522, 1994.
33. Ozdemir V, Fourie J, Busto U, Naranjo CA: Pharmacokinetic changes in the elderly: do they contribute to drug abuse and dependence? Clin Pharmacokinet 31:372-385, 1996.
34. Ensrud KE, Blackwell TL, Mangione CM, et al: Central nervous system-active medications and risk for falls in older women. J Am Geriatr Soc 50:1629-137, 2002.
35. Blackburn D, Hux J, Mamdani M: Quantification of the risk of corticosteroid-induced diabetes mellitus among the elderly. J Gen Intern Med 17:717-720, 2002.
36. Ferrari E, Cravello L, Muzzoni B, et al: Age-related changes of the hypothalamic-pituitary-adrenal axis: pathophysiological correlates. Eur J Endocrinol 144:319-329. 2001.
37. Patten SB: Exogenous corticosteroids and major depression in the general population. J Psychosom Res 49:447-449, 2000.
38. Kirby M, Lawlor BA: Biologic markers and neurochemical correlates of agitation and psychosis in dementia. J Geriatr Psychiatry Neurol 8(Suppl 1):S2-S7, 1995.
39. Belanoff JK, Gross K, Yager A, Schatzberg AF: Corticosteroids and cognition. J Psychiatr Res 35:127-145, 2001.
40. Mann DL: Inflammatory mediators and the failing heart: past, present, and the foreseeable future. Circ Res 91:988-998, 2002.
41. Seymour RM, Routledge PA: Important drug-drug interactions in the elderly. Drugs Aging 12:485-494, 1998.
42. Gurwitz JH, Everitt DE, Monane M, et al: The impact of ibuprofen on the efficacy of antihypertensive treatment with hydrochlorothiazide in elderly persons. J Gerontol A Biol Sci Med Sci 51: M74-M79, 1996.
43. Nawarskas JJ, Spinler SA: Does aspirin interfere with the therapeutic efficacy of angiotensin-converting enzyme inhibitors in hypertension or congestive heart failure? Pharmacotherapy 18:1041-1052, 1998.
44. Silverstein FE, Faich G, Goldstein JL, et al: Gastrointestinal toxicity with celecoxib vs nonsteroidal anti-inflammatory drugs for osteoarthritis and rheumatoid arthritis. The CLASS Study: a randomized controlled trial. JAMA 284:1247-1255, 2000.
45. Deeks JJ, Smith LA, Bradley MD: Efficacy, tolerability, and upper gastrointestinal safety of celecoxib for treatment of osteoarthritis and rheumatoid arthritis: systematic review of randomized controlled trials. BMJ 325:619-626, 2002.
46. Haagsma CJ: Clinically important drug interactions with disease-modifying antirheumatic drugs. Drugs Aging 13:281-289, 1998.
47. Bannwarth B, Pehoureq F, Schaeverbeke T, Dehais J: Clinical pharmacokinetics of low-dose pulse methotrexate in rheumatoid arthritis. Clin Pharmacokinet 30:194-210, 1996.

64 Chronic Musculoskeletal Pain

MAREN LAWSON MAHOWALD

List of Definitions

Hypesthesia	Partial loss of tactile sensation, not loss of sensation (anesthesia) or decrease of painful sensation (hypalgesia or analgesia)
Hyperalgesia	Normally painful stimuli cause an excess of pain (i.e., a heightened pain perception to a noxious stimulus resulting from abnormal processing of nociceptor inputs in the PNS or CNS [7])
Dysesthesia	Abnormal sensation from innocuous stimuli, (i.e., light touch produces bizarre tingling
Allodynia	Normally innocuous stimulus produces pain sensation (e.g., light touch of burned skin produces pain)
Paresthesias	Spontaneous sensation without stimulation, tingling or "pins and needles" sensation

List of Abbreviations

AMPA	Alpha-amino-3-3hydroxy-5-methyl-isoxazolepropionic acit	NE	Norepinephrine
CCK	Cholecystokinin	NK1	Neurokinin 1
CGRP	Calcitonin gene-related peptide	NMDA	*N*-methyl-*D*-aspartate
CNS	Central nervous system	P23X	Purine receptor
DRG	Dorsal root ganglia	PNS	Peripheral nervous system
DYN	Dynorphin	SNRT	Serotonin-norepinephrine reuptake inhibitors
ENK	Leukenkephalin	SOM	Somatostatin
EP	Epinephrine	SP	Substance P
FRAP	Fluoride resistant acid phosphatase	SSRI	Selective serotonin uptake inhibitor
GABA	γ aminobutyric acid	TCA	Tricyclic antidepressant
GDNF	Glial derived nerve growth factor	TrK	Nerve growth factor receptor
GRP	Gastrin releasing peptide	VIP	Vasoactive intestinal peptide
5-HT	Serotonin	VRI	Vanilloid receptor for capsaicin
		WDR	Wide dynamic range

All physicians would agree that relief of suffering is central to patient care. However, discussions about the treatment of pain, especially with opioids, reveal divergent opinions.[1,2] Suffering is the sum of all the negative affective, sensory, and cognitive components of the pain experience, and not all persons suffer to the same degree with similar pain symptoms.[3] The amount of suffering associated with pain is determined by the intensity of the nociceptive input and the individual's circumstances and cultural environment. This human variability permits the clinician to help relieve suffering even when the pain cannot be eliminated completely. Pain is a complex phenomenon that has been defined by the International Association for the Study of Pain (IASP) as "an unpleasant sensory and emotional *experience* associated with actual or potential tissue damage, or described in terms of such damage. Pain is always subjective and may appear in the absence of tissue damage."[4] Pain should be conceptualized as an experience that incorporates the sensory component nociception with important personality and environmental influences.[5] Pain can be produced by noxious stimuli, innocuous stimuli, or, in some cases, in the absence of identifiable stimuli. From the clinical standpoint, it is useful to classify pain first as acute or chronic because the differential diagnosis, diagnostic evaluation, treatments, and prognosis are likely to be different. Recent advances in knowledge of the neurobiology of pain generation, transmission, and modulation now permit more precise definitions of pathophysiology and mechanism-based treatment approaches.[6]

Acute pain is temporally associated with a noxious stimulus due to an identifiable tissue injury, disease process, or abnormal function of a muscle or viscera and is the normal physiologic survival response to potential harm. The function of acute pain is to protect tissue from actual or potential injury by a response of muscular reflexes, alerting processes, and autonomic responses in vascular, visceral, and endocrine tissues. The global response to pain is produced by a complex interaction of cognitive interpretation and emotional responses, which are influenced by one's general physical state, past experiences, psychologic state, social environment, and expectations. The source of acute pain is usually identifiable and localizable.

The pain intensity is usually proportional to the severity of tissue injury and subsides as it heals. Acute pain is associated with an autonomic nervous system response, causing tachycardia, increased blood pressure, anxiety, and stereotypic behaviors of withdrawal, splinting, rubbing, grimacing, or some combination of these. In contrast, patients with sustained or chronic pain do not have autonomic overactivity but have varying degrees of physical dysfunction, anxiety, depression, social isolation, and personality changes that result in a decrease in their quality of life. The term *chronic pain* is imprecise but refers to pain lasting longer than 3 to 6 months. In some, the pain is chronic because the underlying pathologic condition is chronic. Examples of chronic nociceptive pain include rheumatoid arthritis (RA), osteoarthritis (OA), degenerative disk and joint disease, osteoporosis fractures, chronic gout, or ankylosing spondylitis. Chronic neurogenic pain may be central pain resulting from pathology in the spinal cord, brain stem, thalamus, or cortex, and neuropathic pain may be pain arising from damage to primary afferent neurons.[7] The course of chronic pain associated with musculoskeletal disease is a combination of chronic persistent pain with intermittent acute exacerbations. The pain is usually associated with movement (incident pain), pressure (hyperalgesia or tenderness), and light touch (allodynia) if neuropathic processes are contributing. Hyperalgesia and allodynia are expressions of sensitization of peripheral nociceptors and plasticity-induced central mechanisms in the spinal cord or brain.[7]

The concept of psychogenic pain, wherein the pain is actually caused by psychiatric disease, is confusing. In some patients, psychogenic pain refers to pain that lasts beyond the time expected for healing, pain not alleviated by routine pain treatment, or pain that does not have an identified abnormal tissue source. Chronic pain that persists long after an injury has healed serves no physiologic function but may cause physical function, mental health, and personality to deteriorate. Chronic pain related to an underlying chronic disease may become complicated by emotional distress and psychiatric disorders. Pain that appears out of proportion to underlying disease or does not have an identifiable tissue pathology is termed *pain syndromes.* Such pain syndromes have standard diagnostic criteria detailed in the *Diagnostic and Statistical Manual of Mental Disorders* (DSM-IV)[8] for somatoform disorders, malingering, factitious disorder, or personality disorders, which will be reviewed. Clinically pure psychogenic cause for chronic pain is rare but must be detected to prevent unnecessary and ineffective evaluations and treatments. Similarly, most patients with chronic pain will develop anxiety and depression, which require prompt detection and directed therapies.

Epidemiology of Pain

Chronic pain is common worldwide and impacts health care utilization and health-related quality of life. Chronic-pain patients have been among the most frequent users of the Danish health care system[9] and spent 11.4 days per year in hospital, compared to 2.4 days for the general population. In Denmark, chronic musculoskeletal pain conditions are managed primarily by rheumatology services. In a study of 150 chronic pain patients referred to a specialty pain clinic in Copenhagen,[9] pathophysiologic mechanisms included 46 percent with neuropathic pain, 43 percent with somatic pain, 4 percent with psychogenic pain, and 5 percent with visceral pain, and in 2 percent the pain mechanism was unclassified (Table 64–1). The quality of sleep was poor in 42 percent, and sleep was interrupted by pain in 83.9 percent of the patients. Denmark has the highest legal opioid consumption in the world. In this study, 73 percent of patients were on opioids at the time of referral, with a mean dose of 64 mg of morphine equivalents per day. Only 25 percent of those with neuropathic pain were taking anticonvulsants. Sixty percent of the patients took aspirin, paracetamol, or other nonsteroidal anti-inflammatory drugs (NSAIDs), and 36 percent took benzodiazepines. Health-related quality of life indicators revealed 40 percent had depression and 50 percent had an anxiety disorder. Medical out comes study short form-36 MOS SF 36) subscale scores were significantly lower than the Danish general population for physical, social, and mental aspects of health-related quality of life, confirming the severe multidimensional impact of chronic pain. The SF 36 subscale scores were as low or lower than scores in patients having severe cardiopulmonary diseases or major depression. Interestingly, the SF 36 physical function scale (a disability measure) was a stronger predictor of depression than pain intensity. In 141 patients with RA, functional disability as measured by the Stanford Health Assessment Questionnaire (HAQ) had a higher correlation with pain severity ($r = .652$, $p < 0.001$) than with the Larsen score for radiographic damage ($r = .277$, $p = 0.001$).[10] In the regression analysis, the pain score was the primary explanatory variable for functional disability (the HAQ score), accounting for 41.4 percent of the variability, whereas radiologic damage accounted for only 7.3 percent and depression Beck Depression Invntory (BDI score) accounted for only 5.5 percent of the variability. Other variables of current disease activity, including age, duration of disease, serologic

TABLE 64–1 • CHRONIC PAIN IN DENMARK

Underlying Cause	Percentage Reporting
Neuropathic pain	46
Somatic pain	43
Visceral pain	4
Psychogenic pain	4
Unclassified pain	2
40% had depression and 50% had an anxiety disorder	
Treatments	
Opioids	73
Salicylates, acetaminophen, and NSAIDs	60
Benzodiazepines	36
Anticonvulsants	25 (of those with neuropathic pain)

*Location of pain: extremity 33%, low back 20%, head 14%, abdomen 12%, rectum 4%.

Abbreviations: NSAIDs, nonsteroidal anti-inflammatory drugs.

From Becker N, Bondegaard Thomsen A, Olsen AK, et al: Pain epidemiology and health related quality of life in chronic nonmalignant pain patients referred to a Danish multidisciplinary pain center. Pain 73(3):393-400, 1997.

features, and gender, did not contribute significantly to physical disability. Data on socioeconomic risk factors for chronic musculoskeletal pain are conflicting because of the differences in definitions of pain and wording of survey questions.[11] Nearly 75 percent of the Dutch population in 1998 reported having musculoskeletal pain in the preceding 12 months, and 44.4 percent reported pain lasting longer than 3 months. Sites of pain included low back pain (26.9 percent), shoulder pain (20.9 percent), and neck pain (20.6 percent). Pain complaints were more common in women than men for all age-groups. Widespread chronic pain was reported by 5 percent of men and 10 percent of women. Indicators of risk for low back pain, but not for the other anatomic sites, included vocational education and being work disabled. The course of the pain was described as continuous by 30 percent, recurrent by 55 percent, or as continuous mild pain with recurrent severe pain by 9.7 percent. Almost half those with pain had consulted a health care provider in the preceding year because of the pain, and 30 percent reported limitation in daily life due to musculoskeletal pain.[11] A Swedish survey found a prevalence of chronic musculoskeletal pain of 34.5 percent, which varied with age and gender.[12] Age-adjusted prevalences were 38.3 percent for women and 30.9 percent for men. Prevalence increased with age, and there was a peak in prevalence at ages 55 to 64 for men and 65 to 69 for women. Men had a secondary peak at 40 to 44 years of age. The highest prevalences were found in manual workers, immigrants, and those who lived in a low-income housing area. The Nuprin Pain Report of pain in the United States was commissioned by Bristol Myers Company and conducted by Louis Harris and Associates.[13] This survey of 1254 individuals found 10 percent had joint pains, 9 percent had backaches, and 5 percent had muscle pains more than 101 days in the preceding year. In contrast to the Swedish study, the frequency of pain was not higher in older individuals or those with lower household incomes.

The prevalence of pain in the elderly is variable, depending on how the survey questions are worded and the site setting for the survey (i.e., community-based or long-term-care facility–based study populations).[14] Chronic pain is reported by 25 to 50 percent of the community-dwelling elderly and 45 to 80 percent of nursing home residents.[14] A survey of residents in a nursing home with three different skill levels found 71 percent had some pain and 78 percent had an analgesic medication ordered.[15] Those in the board and care level had the highest prevalence of pain (84 percent), and only 66 percent of those in the skilled nursing facility reported pain. Pain severity was described by 52 percent as severe, horrible, or excruciating. Those who had intermittent pain related the pain to movement, weight-bearing, or overexertion. Functional impairments due to pain included impaired enjoyable activities (54 percent), impaired ambulation (53 percent), sleep disturbance (45 percent), depression (32 percent) and anxiety (26 percent). Analgesics ordered included acetaminophen in only 75 percent of the residents and codeine for 12 percent. Only 15 percent of the individuals had received any analgesic medication in the preceding 24 hours. Clearly, pain is an important problem for the elderly—especially in long-term-care facilities—and is usually undertreated. Some of the barriers to pain treatment identified included subjects not wanting to "bother the nurses," being "tired of asking," or not wanting to "give in to the pain." The consequences of chronic pain in the elderly include depression, decreased socialization, sleep disturbance, impaired ambulation, and increased health care utilization and costs.[14]

Pathophysiology of Pain Generation, Transmission, Recognition, and Modulation

Most pain syndromes can be classified into combinations of basic mechanisms: nociceptive, neuropathic, and psychogenic pain (Fig. 64–1). Somatic or nociceptive pain arises from stimulation of nociceptors in body tissues and stimulation of nerves in the peripheral and central nervous system. Pain signaling reaches the brain via multiple neuronal pathways. Cells in the higher termination regions within the forebrain and brain stem also project back to the origin of the ascending pathways.[16] Pain can also be generated from activation of central nociceptive pathways without involving peripheral nociceptors (i.e., "central pain") due to damage in the central nervous system.[17] Neurons in the ascending pathways can change phenotype during sustained peripheral injury as noxious stimulation results in new gene expression in the spinal cord and brain.[16] Therefore, chronic-pain states generate unique neurochemical signatures in the brain and spinal cord.[16] Pain generated by psychogenic mechanisms is complex and difficult to detect and analyze. It is important to distinguish conditions of persistent chronic nociceptive and neuropathic pain with reactive emotional factors from conditions of a pain disorder (i.e., chronic pain syndrome) in which psychologic factors are judged to play a significant role in the onset, severity, exacerba-tion, or maintinance of the pain.[8] Prominent psychobehavioral symptoms are disproportionate to

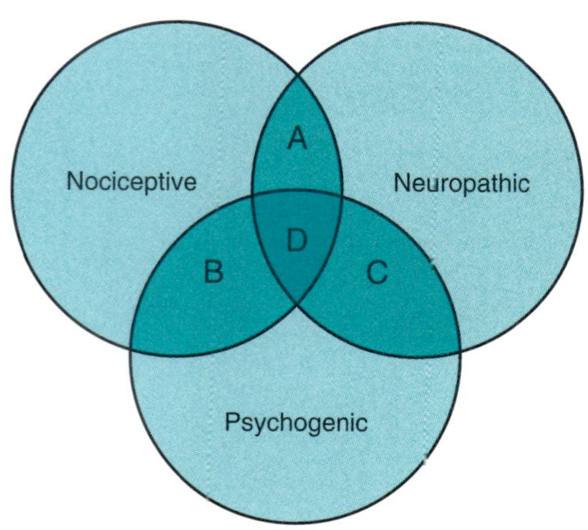

FIGURE 64–1 · Mechanisms of Chronic Pain. A, Nociceptive and neuropathic pathology such as degenerative disc disease and radiculopathy. B, Nociceptive and psychogenic pathology such as hypochondriasis and osteoporotic compression fracture (aka the "crocks revenge"). C, Psychogenic and neuropathic pathology, substance abuse disorder, and alcoholic neuropathy. D, Nociceptive, neuropathic, and psychogenic pathology such as rheumatoid arthritis with depression and herpes zoster.

objective pathologic findings in both groups of patients. The patients with a pain disorder have primary psychopathology that antedated the onset of pain (i.e., psychopathogenic pain), such as depressive disorders, anxiety disorders, somatization disorder, hypochondriasis, conversion disorder, a personality disorder, or substance-abuse disorders. They have usually seen multiple physicians, have had multiple failed treatments, and display dissatisfaction and hostility. The other group of patients had a healthy prepain personality and were functionally intact. These patients have developed significant psychologic dysfunction *because* of the effects of an organic illness. They exhibit depression, anxiety, confusion, anger, hopelessness, and feelings of isolation and loss of control. There is a tendency to "doctor shop" to "find the cure," and these patients often have a depressed, negative attitude. Pain symptoms may be intentionally feigned in malingering and factitious illness disorders. Pain symptoms are not common with psychosis (schizophrenia and psychotic depression), but a patient may present a bizarre pain symptom as a fixed delusion.[8]

PAIN GENERATION IN PERIPHERAL NOCICEPTOR

Nociception is the sensory process signaling trauma or tissue injury (Fig. 64–2). *Nociceptor* is the term used for pain-sensitive neurons or primary afferent neurons whose cell bodies are in the dorsal root ganglion adjacent to the spinal cord. Noxious stimuli threaten or produce tissue damage. The noxious stimulus is transduced by the peripheral afferent nerve endings into an action potential that is transmitted to the dorsal horn of the spinal cord. These peripheral nerve fibers can distinguish between noxious and innocuous stimuli because of their high threshold for stimulation, and they can translate the intensity of the stimulus as the frequency of impulse firing. The smallest C fibers transmit the noxious impulse at the slowest speed (second pain), and the largest A-delta fibers at the fastest (first pain). An intense thermal stimulus (a burn) may be felt as "first" pain 0.05 seconds after the injury and again as "second" pain as long as 2 seconds after the injury. Some C fibers (polymodal nociceptors) have higher thresholds and respond to intense noxious mechanical, thermal, or chemical stimuli nonselectively (Table 64–2). The conscious experience of pain has a localizing component, which enables the individual to describe the location, intensity, and nature of the noxious stimulus, and an alerting and affective component, which alerts the individual to potential body danger and alters behaviors. An unconscious component of pain is an involuntary spinal motor reflex, which produces a withdrawal response for protection.

Nociceptors have been described in skin, muscles, joints, and viscera.[17] Microneurography and microstimulation of peripheral nerves in humans have shown that the quality of pain sensation depends on the tissue innervated by the nociceptors being stimulated and the rate of stimulation (Table 64–3). Nociceptor afferents from the skin (high-threshold mechanoreceptors) are lightly myelinated A-delta fibers that conduct impulses at 2.5 to 35 m/sec or smaller unmyelinated C fibers that conduct impulses at 0.5 to 2 m/sec. Some C fibers express the P2X3 purine receptor, the IB4-lectin binding site, and receptors for glial cell–derived neurotrophic factor (GDNF), and terminate in the deeper parts of the substantia gelatinosa.[16] Other C fibers synthesize substance P (SP) and calcitonin gene-related peptide (CGRP) and express the nerve growth factor receptor TrkA.[16] All C fibers express the capsaicin vanilloid receptor 1 (VR1) receptor, which transduces noxious chemical and thermal stimuli.[16] Afferent fibers from muscle are called group III or group IV afferents and are analogous to A-delta and C fibers. Mechanoreceptors and polymodal nociceptors contain the neurotransmitter glutamate. Polymodal nociceptors also contain neuropeptides

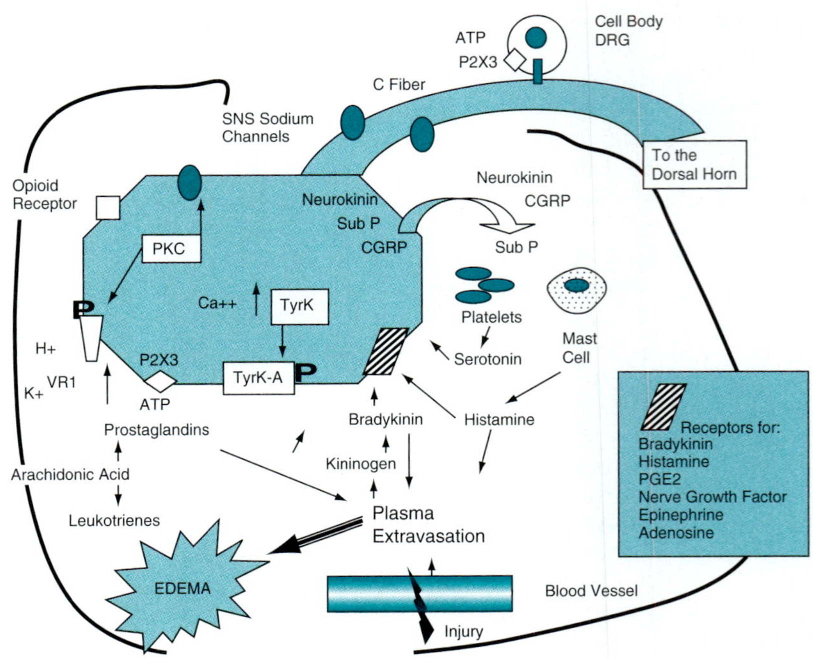

FIGURE 64–2 · Pain Generation in Peripheral Nociceptors.

TABLE 64–2 • TYPES OF AFFERENT NERVE FIBERS

Location	Nerve Fiber	Normally Activating Stimuli	Mediators Released	Quality of Pain Sensation	Process of Sensitization	Comment
Skin, tendon, joint capsule, ligament, menisci, periosteum	Group II (A-beta)	Innocuous touch, movement, pressure, temperature		Normally not painful	With neuropathy produces paresthesia, dysesthesias (buzzing, tingling)	Injured nerve expresses SP and CGRP
Skin	A-delta fiber; high-threshold mechanoreceptor; lightly myelinated	Noxious moderate-a and high-intensity mechanical stimuli and intense heat	SP and CGRP	Fast pain; pricking, sharp, aching pain	Can be sensitized by exposure to noxious stimuli	
Skin	C-polymodal; high-threshold nociceptors; unmyelinated	Mechanical, thermal, or irritant chemical stimuli	SP, CGRP, TrkA receptor for nerve growth factor; terminates in superficial dorsal horn; capsaicin; VR1 receptor	Poorly localized slow pain; burning pain	Bradykinin, histamine, acetylcholine, and KCl; prostaglandins, SP Can be sensitized by exposure to noxious stimuli and repetitive simulation	10% not pain but innocuous heat A subgroup of fibers has P2X3 purine receptor, IB4-lectin binding site and receptor for glial cell–derived neurotrophic factor; terminates in deep dorsal horn
Skin	A-delta fiber mechanothermal nociceptors	Intense noxious thermal and mechanical stimuli	Transmitter glutamate and aspartate	Well-localized fast pain; pricking, sharp, aching pain		
Muscles, fascia, tendon, vessel walls	Group III (A-delta) Group IV (C fibers)	Mechanical stimuli but not stretch, thermal		Diffuse, aching pain		
Joints, capsule plexus, ligaments, menisci, fat pads, vessel walls	Group III (A-delta) Group IV (C fiber)	Noxious mechanical and chemical stimulation		Dull aching	Inflammation increases sensitivity so fibers are activated by innocuous joint movement, pressure	
Muscle spindle	A-gamma fiber	Stretch reflex				

Abbreviations: CGRP, Calcitonin gene-related peptide; SP, substance P.

TABLE 64–3 • DESCRIPTORS OF VARIOUS SOMATOGENIC PAINS

Pain Source	Skin	Muscle	Bone	Viscera	Nerve
Descriptors	Throbbing Sharp Itchy Sore Tender Burning	Pounding Stabbing Cramping Wrenching Aching Taut Tiring	Boring Gnawing Hurting Rasping Tiring	Boring Stabbing Gnawing Cramping Squeezing Pulling Heavy Sickening	Quivering Shooting Pricking Pulling Burning Tingling Stinging Numb
Localization	Surface	Subcutaneous	Deep	Not well localized; often radiates	Follows distribution of neural structures

SP, CGRP, and neurokinin A, and are sensitized by K^+, H^+, PGE2, bradykinin, serotonin, and adenosine triphosphate (ATP). The purinergic agonist ATP can cause transient pain by increasing sodium ion permeability.[7]

Most nociceptors are normally inactive and rather unresponsive but are sensitized by inflammatiory mediators to develop spontaneous discharges and lower the threshold of activation to peripheral stimulation.[18] A consequence of this sensitization is primary hyperalgesia, an increased painfulness of a noxious stimulus and a reduced threshold for pain (i.e., tenderness to palpation and pain with movement—a mechanical stimulus that is normally not painful).

SENSITIZATION OF THE PRIMARY AFFERENT NEURON

Sensitization of peripheral nociceptors that occurs with inflammation and nerve injury[17] is the essential step to chronic nociceptive pain with hyperalgesia and allodynia. The activity of these receptors is changed by chemical actions on axon surface-membrane receptors that increase intracellular calcium and activate intracellular protein kinase C and tyrosine kinases. These kinases phosphorylate sensory neuron–specific (SNS) sodium channels and VR1 receptors[7] (see Fig. 64–2). Primary afferent nociceptors have receptors for opiates, γ aminobutyric acid (GABA), bradykinin, histamine, serotonin, and capsaicin (VR1 receptor). Changes in nerve growth factors are seen with tissue damage and inflammation. In addition, afferent joint fibers have excitatory amino acid receptors (glutamate). Nociceptors are stimulated by chemical substances released from damaged tissues (e.g., K^+) and inflammatory mediators, such as prostaglandins, serotonin, bradykinin, and histamine, as well as by sympathomimetic amines, noradrenaline, and dopamine.

Nociceptive neurons themselves release chemical stimulants of nociception, such as SP and CGRP, which amplify the local inflammatory response by interacting with the inflammatory cells and adjacent blood vessels (also known as "neurogenic" inflammation). Vasodilatation and edema resulting from neurogenic inflammation is mediated by vasoactive peptides (CGRP, SP, neurokinin A) released from perivascular C fiber afferents. Tissue injury causes local release of K^+, prostaglandins, and bradykinin, resulting in stimulation of sensory afferents. Peripheral sensory impulses cause release of SP, which causes mast cells to release histamine and platelets to release serotonin, which promotes sensitization of nearby nociceptors.[7] Recent work has demonstrated the direct sensitization of mechanical nociceptors in the rat by paw injection of tumor necrosis factor-alpha (TNF-α), interleukin-beta (IL-β) and IL-8, which could be blocked by atenolol and indomethacin, further supporting the role of eicosanoids and sympathetic amines in hyperalgesia produced by inflammation.[19] Upregulation of genes and increased expression of vanilloid receptor 1 and sensory nerve–specific sodium channels in response to injury, inflammatory mediators, and nerve growth factors decreases the threshold to noxious stimulation resulting in hyperalgesia.[7] Clustering of sodium channels in the axon membrane produces foci of irritability and ectopic discharges.[7] These sodium channels can be blocked by lidocaine, mexilitine, and anticonvulsants. Opioids bind to receptors in dorsal root ganglia, central terminals of primary afferent neurons in the spinal cord, and also the peripheral nerve fibers and terminals (nociceptors).[20] Opioids increase potassium currents and decrease calcium currents reducing neuronal firing and release of SP and other transmitters.

Damage to peripheral nerves leads to a different neurochemical signature for neuropathic pain. A-delta fibers and C fibers normally express SP and CGRP; however, expression is downregulated after nerve injury. Nonpainful sensations are normally detected by specialized corpuscle structures and free nerve endings that transduce mechanical stimuli via large myelinated A-beta afferent fibers. Injured A-beta fibers begin to express SP and CGRP; therefore, low-threshold stimuli can lead to SP release in the dorsal horn and hyperexcitability. Regenerative sprouts "rewire" the afferent sensory system, wherein non-noxious stimuli are input as noxious stimuli (allodynia).[7] Schwann cells in damaged nerves produce increased mRNA for nerve growth factors and their receptors for regenerative events. Damaged axons also express adrenoreceptors, causing discharges in response to circulating epinephrine and norepinephrine. These neurotrophins may also cause aberrant regeneration, such as the ingrowth of sympathetic postganglionic axons into dorsal root ganglia or the ingrowth of large myelinated afferents into lamina II, forming abnormal connections in the nociceptive processing circuits within the dorsal horn (which may explain allodynia).[17,21]

PAIN TRANSMISSION TO THE SPINAL CORD

The primary afferent neurons synapse onto second-order neurons in the dorsal horn of the spinal cord (Fig. 64–3) Central terminals of primary afferent neurons contain the excitatory amino acid neurotransmitters (glutamate and aspartate), neuropeptides (fluoride resistant acid phosphatase [FRAP], SP, vasoactive intestinal peptide [VIP], somatostatin [SOM], cholecystokinin [CCK], gastrin releasing peptide [GRP], angiotensin II, CGRP, leuenkephalin, and dynorphin), and receptors for cholecystokinin, opioids, and GABA-B, which modulate transmitter release. The second-order neurons express receptors for NMDA, AMPA, and metabotropic receptors that bind glutamate, neurokinin, GABA-A (a ligand-gated chloride channel), and have glycine binding sites, which decrease responses to stimulation. Noxious stimulation induces c-fos expression in dorsal horn neurons. Interneuronal networks in the dorsal horn are both excitatory and inhibitory. The neurons are either nociceptive-specific or wide dynamic range (WDR) neurons that respond to innocuous and noxious stimuli. Nociceptive neurons synapse with excitatory interneurons to stimulate flexor motor neurons for the spinal withdrawal reflex, and they stimulate nociceptive projection neurons to signal the higher centers in the brain. The interneurons that cross the anterior commisure and ascend in the contralateral spinothalamic tract transmit pain signals to the thalamus where they synapse with third-order neurons that project to the somatosensory and cingulate cortices to produce consciousness of the type and location of the tissue injury. There is another pathway for affective and motivational dimensions of pain that involves the parabrachial nucleus, amygdala, and intralaminar nucleus of the thalamus (for neurokinin 1 [NK1]-positive spinal neurons). Interneurons that inhibit the nociceptive projection neurons are activated by incoming sensory afferents and descending analgesic fibers. The balance of these excitatory and inhibitory processes in the spinal cord has been used as the gate theory of pain,[22] the theory of "diffuse noxious inhibitory controls,"[23] and as a possible explanation of the analgesic effects of acupuncture and transcutaneous nerve stimulation.

CENTRAL SENSITIZATION AT THE SPINAL CORD

Development of peripheral arthritis or damage to a peripheral nerve results in changes in levels of neurotransmitters and subsequent activation of second messenger systems (protein kinase C), which produces central sensitization with enhanced responsiveness to stimuli. Central sensitization causes allodynia to tactile stimuli in an area of secondary hyperalgesia. This "wind up phenomenon" is due to increased responsiveness of WDR neurons in the dorsal horn when sustained high-frequency impulses are delivered and the C fibers' central terminals release the excitatory transmitter glutamate (see Fig. 64–3). The WDR neurons will then respond to both noxious and innocuous stimuli. Hyperexcitability in the spinal cord depends on release of excitatory amino acids, such as glutamate and neuropeptides, from afferent nerves and interneurons. Glutamate activates multiple receptors, including NMDA receptor, non-NMDA receptors, and meta-botropic glutamate receptors. Glutamate reacts with postsynaptic AMPA receptors causing fast excitatory postsynaptic potentials (EPSPs). During intense noxious stimulation, SP and glutamate are coreleased causing sustained slow EPSPs, (depolarization), temporal summation, and removal of the magnesium blockade of the NMDA calcium channel. Increased calcium activates protein kinase C (PKC), which phosphorylates NMDA receptors, further increasing excitability of dorsal horn neurons. In contrast to sensitization from peripheral inflammation or tissue damage, nerve damage causes downregulation of SP, somatostatin, and CGRP.

Inhibitory circuits in the spinal cord release inhibitory amino acids (GABA and glycine) and the neuropeptide enkephalin. Presynaptic inhibition is mediated through opioid receptors, GABA-A, and GABA-B receptors, and postsynaptic inhibition is mediated through the glycine receptor and the two GABA receptors.[17] Peripheral afferents for position sense and vibration also have cell bodies in the dorsal root ganglia and have inhibitory feedback on nociceptive processing in the dorsal horn. These large fibers can be stimulated by transcutaneous nerve stimulators to decrease pain.

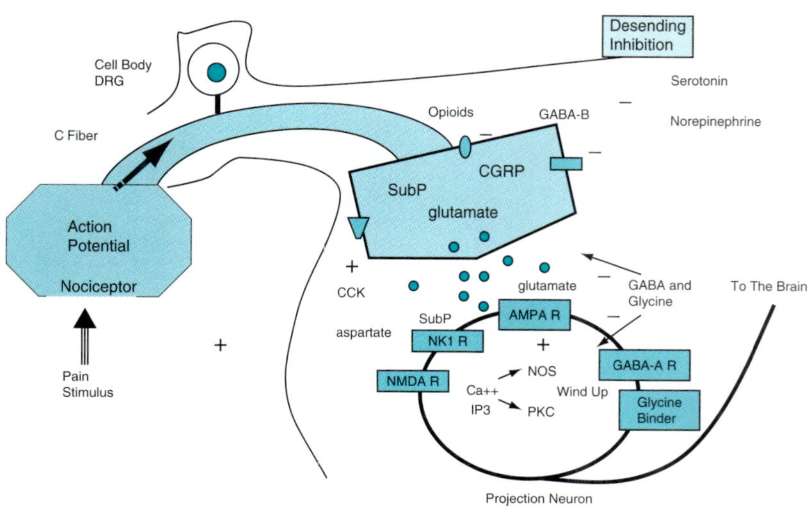

FIGURE 64–3 · Pain Transmission at the Spinal Cord.

PROJECTION OF PAIN TO THE BRAIN

Nociceptive projection neurons in the spinal cord cross the spinal cord and ascend in the spinothamic tract (STT), spinoreticular tract (SRT), and spinomesencephalic tract (SMT) (Table 64–4). Spinothalamic cells have excitatory receptive fields sensitive to noxious stimulation and inhibitory receptive fields that can be inhibited by repetitive stimulation of peripheral nerves (i.e., transcutaneous electric nerve stimulation [TENS] unit). The lateral axons of the STT synapse in the ventroposterolateral thalamus with third-order neurons that project to the somatosensory cortex in the parietal lobe (Fig. 64–4). The medial fibers of the STT ascend and send fibers to the reticular formation, periaqueductal gray (PAG) area, parabrachial nuclei, and medial thalamus to synapse with neurons that project to the limbic system (hypothalamus, amygdaloid nucleus, septal nucleus).[17] The SMT cells originate in the laminae I and IV-VI primarily and project to midbrain periaqueductal gray (PAG) nuclei and synapse in the medial thalamus. These cells often have complex receptive fields on widely separated areas of the body and serve to provoke aversive behavior and activate descending analgesia. The cells of the SRTs are in the deep laminae of the dorsal horn and ventral horn (VII and VIII), project to the caudal medulla (reticular nucleus to stimulate alertness), and send collaterals to catecholamine cell groups of the medulla and pons to signal brain stem autonomic centers, activate endogenous analgesia systems, and synapse in the medial thalamus.[17] From the medial thalamus, neurons project to the anterior cingulate gyrus and are involved in affective responses and perception of suffering with pain. Neurons from the lateral thalamus project to the somatosensory cortex to allow precise localization and characterization of the pain stimulus. Functional brain imaging studies have shown that multiple cortical areas are activated by painful stimuli including somatosensory cortices (for discrimi-native aspects of pain sensation) and cingulate cortex, insula, and prefrontal cortex (for affective motivational aspects of pain sensation).[16]

MODULATION OF PAIN TRANSMISSION IN THE CENTRAL NERVOUS SYSTEM

Transmission of a nociceptor signal to the brain initiates pain modulation via an inhibitory descending analgesia system from the cortex, limbic system, thalamus, and hypothalamus. The descending pathway projects onto the PAG area, the nucleus raphe magnus (NRM) of the pons and rostral medulla, and to the dorsal horn of the spinal cord where the nociceptive transmission is inhibited (see Fig.64–4). Analgesia produced by stimulation of PAG matter is mediated by endogenous opioids and does not affect touch, proprioception, or thermal sensation. Bind-ing of opiate receptors by endogenous enkephalin, beta-endorphin, and dynorphin, or by exogenous opiates, activates the descending analgesia tracts from the PAG to the spinal cord. Both serotonin and norepinephrine are the likely neurotransmitters in the midbrain pain-modulation system. The action of these monoamines in the descending endogenous analgesic mechanism may explain the analgesic potentiating effects of tricyclic antidepressants. Stimulation of the PAG inhibits nociceptive dorsal horn neurons and STT cells. Bilateral projections descend from the locus ceruleus to innervate laminae I, II, and V of the dorsal horn. Brain stem raphe nuclei neurons contain serotonin (5-HT) and are the major source of 5-HT in the spinal cord. Reticular-formation neurons are excited by noxious stimuli and result in aversive behavior.

The Neurobiology of Articular Pain

Articular and periarticular structures have nociceptors analgous to cutaneous nociceptors[24] (Fig. 64–5). C poly-

TABLE 64–4 • PAIN TRANSMISSION PATHWAYS

	First Synapse	Pathway	Third-Order Synapse	Destination
Ascending Nociceptive Projection Pathways				
Lateral spinothalamic tract	Dorsal horn	Contralateral	Ventral, posterior lateral thalamus	Somatosensory cortex
Medial spinothalamic tract	Dorsal horn	Contralateral	Reticular formation periaqueductal gray and hypothalamus	Limbic forebrain
Spinoreticular tract	Dorsal horn	Ipsilateral and contralateral	Midbrain reticular formation, medial thalamic nuclei	Limbic forebrain
Spinomesencephalic tract	Dorsal horn	Contralateral	Midbrain reticular formation	Limbic forebrain
Descending Pain-Modulation Pathway				
	Periaqueductal grey	Dorsolateral funiculus; serotonergic and suppresses nociception transmission	Nucleus raphe magnus, rostral ventromedial medulla (RVM), brain stem opioid receptors	Dorsal horn, opioid receptors, serotonin, norepinephrine
	Locus ceruleus	Ventrolateral funiculus, pons pathway		Dorsal horn, serotonin, norepinephrine

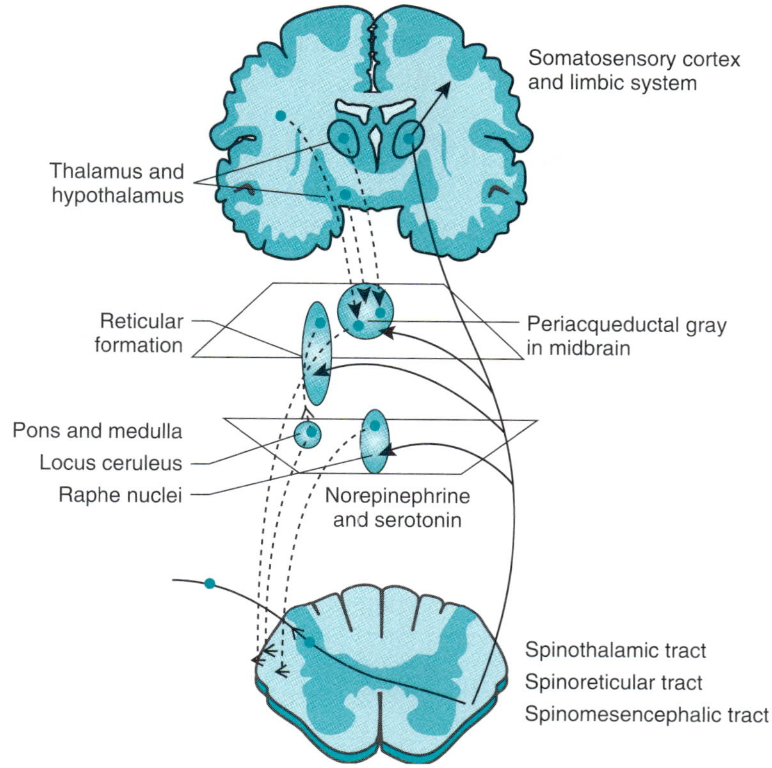

FIGURE 64–4 · Ascending and Descending Pain Tracts.

modal nociceptors form a diffuse lattice throughout the articular capsule. A-delta fiber free nerve endings are found in intra-articular and periarticular ligaments.[25] In the synovium, SP- and CGRP-positive nerve fibers are associated with blood vessels or form a network of free endings up to the intima layer. Sympathetic fibers are localized to blood vessels. Nociceptive and proprioceptive signaling is the obvious function of articular nerves; however, recent advances in the understanding of molecular mechanisms involved in afferent and efferent transmissions has led to the reciprocal concept that neurogenic inflammation might play a role in the pathogenesis of joint disorders. Antidromic (reverse) stimulation of peripheral fibers proximate to blood vessels, and tissue mast cells can cause vasodilatation and plasma extravasation.[25] Under conditions of inflammation, articular primary afferent neurons become sensitized to mechanical, thermal, and chemical stimuli, producing the characteristic inflammatory joint pain with pain on movement and palpation (i.e., allodynia and hyperalgesia).[26] Sensitization of the articular primary afferent is the essential step in the generation of inflammatory joint

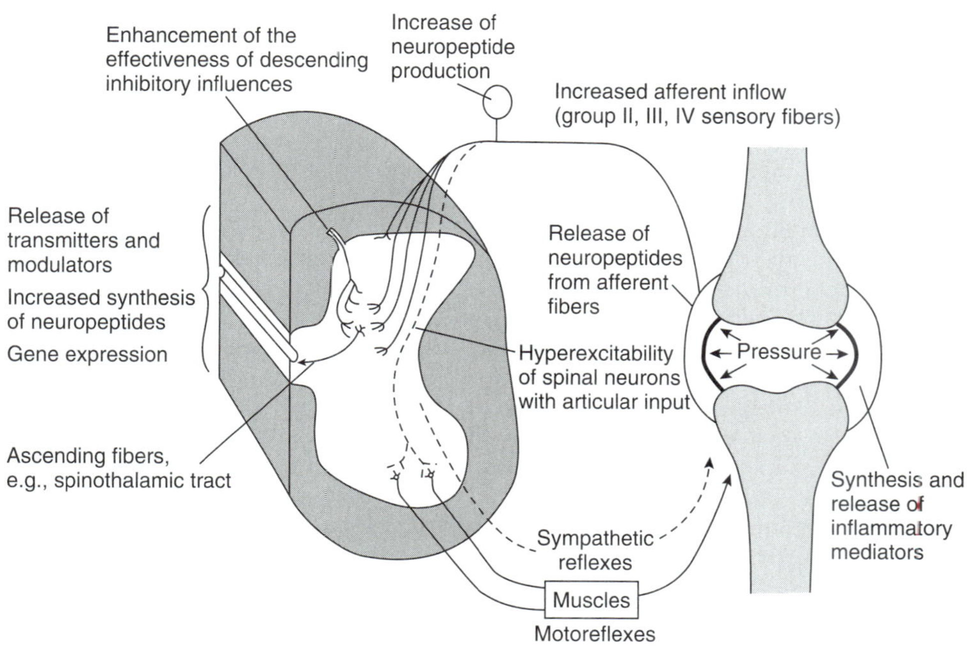

FIGURE 64–5 · Articular Innervation. Schema of nociceptive interactions that occur during joint inflammation. (From Schaible HG, Grubb BD, Afferent and spinal mechanisms of joint pain. Pain 55:6, 1993, with permission from Elsevier Science.)

pain. Spinal cord neurons also become sensitized by inflammation in the joint and have increased sensitivity to afferent inputs from the inflamed joint (i.e., central sensitization), thereby amplifying nociceptive processing. Neuropeptides synthesized in dorsal root ganglion cells of C fibers and A-delta fibers are transported centrally to the dorsal horn as neurotransmitters but also distally to interact with resident articular cells, inflammatory cells, blood vessels, and lymphatics (i.e., neurogenic inflammation). Sympathetic efferent fibers may also be involved with neurogenic inflammation. In rat adjuvant arthritis, sectioning the nerve or applying capsaicin to the limb (which depletes SP) attenuates arthritis severity.[27] Subcutaneous injection of capsaicin reduced levels of SP, CGRP, and nerve growth factor in arthritic joints and dorsal root ganglia and reduced the inflammatory response in rats.[28] Later in the course of adjuvant arthritis, SP and CGRP nerve fiber density are reduced in the synovium and periarticular bone (autodenervation), followed by a regenerative phase and altered morphology.[25] In the rheumatoid synovium there are reduced free nerve endings and sympathetic fibers on blood vessels in the superficial layer. In a mouse model of antigen-induced arthritis, immunocytochemical localization studies showed the apparent reduction in SP and CGRP nerves in arthritic synovium was likely due to failure of reinnervation by outgrowing neural fibers because they were unable to keep up with the intense proliferation of synovial tissue during the arthritic process, rather than because of the destruction of nerve tissue.[29] Sensitization of articular nociceptors by inflammation results in normally nonresponsive primary afferents becoming responsive to non-noxious movements and touch and having spontaneous activity at rest.[30] SP appears to be the principal neurotransmitter of pain in arthritis and contributes to the inflammatory response by stimulating the resident cells in the joint to produce a multitude of inflammatory mediators and cytokines.[31] SP can activate mast cells, synoviocytes, neutrophils, T cells, B cells, and macrophages, thereby amplifying the inflammatory response. Neurokinin receptors that bind SP are coupled to regulatory G proteins and activate hydrolysis of inositol-containing phospholipids for the second response in cell activation.[31] During inflammation, opioid receptors are upregulated on peripheral sensory nerves and resident immune cells express endogenous opioids; thus, intra-articular opioids reduce pain and possibly inflammation.[20] Recent studies suggested a role for nitric oxide in pain accompanying inflammation. In a rat model of polyarthritis, administration of nitric oxide synthase inhibitor N-nitro-L-arginine methyl ester (L-NAME) reversed thermal hyperalgesia but not mechanical allodynia or joint inflammation. Independent of inflammation in the joint, mechanical pain in joints may be produced by nociceptors in ligaments, joint capsule, enthises, and blood vessels that are activated by increased intra-articular pressure with effusions and abnormal forces and torque with deformities.

The spinal cord is the integrative site for afferent sensory information and reflex functions. The description of events in the spinal cord relevant in processing nociceptive information from the joint is not yet complete.[24] Following noxious stimulation of peripheral tissues, c-fos is expressed, presumably for long-term adaptations in neurons such as synthesis of neuropeptides. With acute and chronic inflammation in a peripheral joint, levels of transmitters and receptors in dorsal root ganglia and the spinal cord change. Glutamate appears to be involved with NMDA receptors in transmission of nociceptive information from an inflamed joint to the spinal cord. Transmitters involved with descending inhibition of spinal neurons include serotonin and norepinephrine, which are increased under inflammatory conditions. Neuropeptide synthesis (SP, CGRP, dynorphin, enkephalin) in dorsal ganglia, the spinal cord, or both is also increased in at least some of the stages of joint inflammation.[25] However, the functional consequences of the changes in neuropeptides, transmitters, and receptors remain to be elucidated. The role of the spinal cord in regulation of peripheral joint inflammation is just beginning to be defined.[32]

Recent work with a mouse model of bone-cancer pain, neuropathic pain, and inflammatory pain has helped to delineate neuromolecular signatures of the three different pain states. The signature for bone-cancer pain was increase in a spinal cord astrocyte marker (reflecting hypertrophy of astrocytes), increased dynorphin in deep spinal laminae, no changes in SP or CGRP, but increased internalization of SP receptor and increased c-fos expression in lamina I of the dorsal horn, demonstrating sensitization of primary afferent neurons.[21] With paw-inflammation pain there was upregulation of SP and CGRP in laminae I and II of the dorsal horn and increases protein kinase C and SP receptor. In contrast, with nerve injury there was downregulation of SP and CGRP and upregulation of galanin, neuropeptide Y, and GAP-43 in both primary afferent neurons and the spinal cord.[16] Interestingly this group of investigators has also shown that osteoprotegerin prevented cancer-induced bone destruction by osteoclasts, reduced pain, and blocked the spinal cord changes of sensitization.[33] Such advances in our understanding of the neuromolecular signatures for different pain states will provide a new framework for the mechanism-based development of new analgesics.

Pain Generation with Nervous System Disorder

Many musculoskeletal and rheumatologic conditions have an overlapping or prominent neuropathic component to the pain (intervertebral disk disease with radiculopathy, vasculitis-associated neuropathy). It is important to detect and assess the degree that neuropathic pain is contributing to the clinical picture, because the treatment approaches are different than the treatments for immune-mediated or inflammatory musculoskeletal disorders. Neuropathic pain is complex because the many signs and symptoms fluctuate in number and intensity over time.[34] Injured peripheral nerves produce intense and prolonged sensory information to the central nervous system and may cause a secondary increase in excitability of dorsal horn neurons and altered local or descending inhibition.[35] After injury, nociceptive nerves develop spontaneous ectopic discharges, become responsive to innuocuous stimuli, and develop expanded receptive fields. Spontaneous ectopic discharges in C fibers produce repetitive stimulation of spinal cord neurons and hypersensitivity mediated by glutamate interaction with NMDA, AMPA, and glutamate receptors. Glutamate can cause excitotoxic damage to the inhibitory interneurons in the dorsal horn, resulting in central disinhibition of nociceptive input. Clinically, the symptoms are those of the neurologic deficit and the abnormal sensory symptoms of dysesthesias (e.g., painful light touch), paraesthesias (e.g., tingling), expanded territory of pain (expanded receptive field gives "stocking glove distribution"), steady pain, and spontaneous paroxysms of pain. Each of these symptoms has a different underlying mechanism. Generation of pain in the peripheral neuropathies is not from nociception in the tissues of the painful area. The injured axons become the source of spontaneous activity (neuromata), which is further activated by chemicals, ischemia, inflammation, infection, or adrenergic agonists. Pain in association with polyneuropathies can be superficial or deep. Peripheral nerve sensitization results in severe allodynia and signs of autonomic dysfunction (changes in skin color, temperature, and edema). Transected nerves in amputees have ongoing spontaneous C fiber activity (burning, spontaneous pain) and contact-evoked stump pain, which results from sensitized C nociceptors, which can be blocked by lidocaine. At the site of nerve injury there is an accumulation of sodium channels, a lowered nociceptor depolarization threshold, and ectopic discharges. In regenerating nerve sprouts, novel receptors are expressed, including adrenergic receptors and N-type or L-type calcium channels. Central sensitization following peripheral nerve injury develops in the spinal cord and is called "wind up." Tachykinin release from nociceptors (SP and neurokinin A) bind to NK1 and NK2 receptors, triggering the release of intracellular calcium, which increases neuronal hyperexcitability and expression of NMDA receptors. Glutamate from the primary afferents is bound, leading to a further increase of intracellular calcium and sodium into the cells. The end result of increased intracellular calcium is activation of protein kinase C, phopholipase C, and nitric oxide synthetase and induction of early gene expression (c fos, c-jun), all processes that maintain central sensitization (see Fig. 64–4). In poststroke pain, the area of pain is within the area of abnormal sensory function, indicating that lost input causes secondary sensitization in the central neurons, which can be reduced by opioids, gabapentin, lidocaine, and lamotrigine.

PERIPHERAL NERVE DISORDERS CAUSING PAIN

Peripheral nerve disorders are classified as generalized (axonal or demyelinating) and focal (mononeuropathy simplex and segmental neuropathies). Peripheral nerves have small fibers (pain and temperature sensation and autonomic fibers) and large fibers (motor function, stretch reflex, position, vibration, touch). Focal neuropathies are simplex or multiplex and may be due to entrapment, ischemia, trauma, vasculitis, or infection (herpes virus, human immunodeficiency virus [HIV], leprosy, Lyme disease). In patients with diabetic neuropathy, acute mononeuropathies of cranial and peripheral nerves are due to ischemia or entrapment. In focal segmental neuropathy, groups of nerves are involved by neoplastic infiltration, radiation plexopathy, and postinfectious or immune-mediated cervical, brachial, or lumbosacral plexopathy. Mononeuropathies (either single or multiple), regardless of cause, produce burning pain and a neurologic deficit in the distribution of the involved nerve. Diabetic focal proximal neuropathy (previously known as amyotrophy or plexopathy) is an immune-mediated inflammatory process with vasculitis and demyelination. The clinical presentation is an elderly person with type II diabetes who develops the gradual or abrupt onset of pain in the thighs, hips, or buttocks, followed by significant weakness that may resolve in 1 to 2 years. Entrapment syndromes occur with gradual compression of the median nerve at the wrist (carpal tunnel syndrome), ulnar nerve at the cubital tunnel, and the posterior tibial nerve at the tarsal tunnel. The compression causes demyelination initially and, if chronic, axonal destruction. Pain originates from nociceptors in nervi nervorum. Patients may describe tingling with numbness in the distribution of the nerve or may have a deep aching pain in the entire extremity with atrophy and weakness. Palpation or percussion of the nerve trunk produces an electric shock-like sensation. Nerve compression produces a focal nerve injury with pain in and beyond the sensory distribution of the nerve. With carpal tunnel syndrome, numbness, tingling, and burning sensations occur in the thumb, index, and middle fingers. The pain awakens the patient at night, may radiate up the forearm to the shoulder or neck, and may include thumb muscle weakness and atrophy. With ulnar nerve entrapment in the cubital tunnel, weakness and atrophy predominate over pain. Meralgia paresthetica is entrapment of the lateral femoral cutaneous nerve under the inguinal ligament, which produces numbness and burning pain over the lateral thigh. The posterior tarsal tunnel syndrome is produced by compression of the posterior tibial nerve inferior to the medial malleolus, causing pain in the sole of the foot that has a burning, unpleasant quality. The pain typically worsens with rest and at night.

Severe injury to a major peripheral nerve due to avulsion, knife or gunshot wound, tumor invasion, or severence (as with amputation) causes post-traumatic neuralgia or causalgia. Causalgia is a devastating pain syndrome with hyperactivity of the sympathetic nervous system. There is sensory loss distal to the injury. The dysesthetic pain of a peripheral nerve injury is burning with superimposed lancinating pain thought to be due to increased firing of regenerating nerve sprouts and spontaneous firing at sites of demyelination. Nerve trunk pain is an aching pain, possibly due to firing of nociceptors in the nerve sheath (nervi nervorum) of the injured nerve. Causalgia is described as a burning, red-hot pain with vasomotor changes (mottled or red skin) edema, allodynia, hyperpathia, hyperalgesia, and later trophic changes. Palpation of the injured nerve produces electric shock-like pain, which travels down the nerve, and there may be a palpable nodule at the site of the nerve injury, which is a neuroma of axon sprouts at the site of axon regeneration. Causalgia is often relieved by wet applications and warming but is aggravated by various somatosensory, visual, auditory, emotional, or psychologic factors, movement, or touch. The pain gradually disappears in a few months to 2 years but may be helped by early sympathetic blockade. It has been theorized that damaged nociceptor fibers become sensitive to noradrenaline after injury; regenerating fibers at the injury site may synapse sympathetic fibers to afferent nociceptor fibers and give rise to a pain stimulus; or fibers in the dorsal horn may become sensitive to non-nociceptive signals by sympathetic activity. Following amputation, most patients have persistent sensations of the limb and, in some, the sensation is painful. The pain in the phantom limb is described as aching, cramping, burning, squeezing, crushing, or tearing and can persist for years or be intermittent. Phantom sensations gradually disappear; sympathetic blockade may help. Stump pain after healing is due to a neuroma at the severed nerve or other complications in the stump tissues such as ischemia, infection, osteomyelitis, or poorly fitting prosthesis.

Postherpetic neuralgia (PHN) causes spontaneous, deep, stabbing pain, allodynia (superficial burning, itching produced by touch), hyperalgesia, and altered sensation in the distribution of the involved nerve. It is a mononeuropathy caused by reactivation of herpes zoster[36] in cranial nerve V and cervical and thoracic spinal nerves. Herpes virus–induced inflammation in the dorsal root ganglion produces a sensory deficit and intractable pain in the affected dermatome. The skin is extremely tender to touch (tactile allodynia), yet firm compression relieves the pain. Cold and psychologic stress adversely affect the pain. These features suggest PHN is a deafferentation pain with activation of the sympathetic system, which renders nociceptors sensitive to tactile stimuli. The pain may persist for 2 years then disappear spontaneously. Aspirin and NSAIDs are generally ineffective. Topical preparations of aspirin, lidocaine, and capsaicin (if transient increased pain can be tolerated) may be beneficial. Tricyclic antidepressants, but not selective serotonin reuptake inhibitors (SSRIs), may help, and anticonvulsant drugs such as gabapentin[37] can reduce the pain.[38] Interestingly, the 34 percent improvement in pain was the same for doses of either 1800 mg or 2400 mg per day.[37] Transcutaneous nerve stimulation, but not acupuncture, reduced pain in some patients. Treatment of herpes zoster with corticosteroids and antiviral agents is recommended to prevent or reduce the severity of PHN.

Tic douloureux, or trigeminal neuralgia, is unilateral, recurring, sudden paroxysms of sharp, stabbing, lancinating pain in the second division, third division, or both of the fifth cranial nerve. This disorder can be caused by trauma, tumor, or demyelination, or it can be idiopathic. Mechanisms considered are an irritable focus generating nociceptive signals or an area of demyelination with spontaneous activation. The paroxysms are precipitated by touch, chewing, teeth brushing, or talking and occur in clusters lasting as long as several hours. Between episodes, patients are asymptomatic. Finding of altered cutaneous sensation between episodes should prompt a search for a structural lesion such as gasserian ganglion tumor, multiple sclerosis, or brain stem infarct. Treatment with carbamezipine, phentoin, or baclofen is usually effective.

Generalized peripheral neuropathies are categorized as demyelinating or axonal, acute, and chronic. Demyelinating neuropathies are associated with toxins, viral infections, paraproteins, and, as a paraneoplastic process, with immune-mediated and hereditary diseases. The axonal neuropathies are usually acquired and are divided into small-fiber or large-fiber involvement. This form is seen in diabetes, uremia, hereditary neuropathies, and immunologic and nutritional toxic neuropathies. The most common cause is diabetes, with a generalized distal sensory or sensorimotor neuropathy of insidious onset involving small fibers, large fibers, or both. The clinical features of large-fiber neuropathy include loss of vibration, touch, and proprioception sense with loss of deep-tendon reflexes and abnormal nerve conduction studies. Small-fiber neuropathy is associated with burning or lancinating pain, hyperalgesia, paresthesias, and loss of pain and temperature sensation but intact reflexes, touch, vibration, and position sense, and it is often complicated by foot skin ulcerations. Diabetic polyneuropathy causes gradual numbness, dull aching or burning pain with pins and needles sensation, and mild or no muscle weakness. There is decreased cutaneous and vibratory sense, decreased deep-tendon reflexes, and a gradual decrease in pain as all sensation is lost. Large-fiber neuropathies produce weakness, loss of reflexes, loss of touch sense, and various dysesthesiae.

CENTRAL NERVOUS SYSTEM DISORDERS CAUSING PAIN

Central pain has many synonyms—poststroke pain, thalamic pain, spinal cord injury pain, central deafferentation pain or "anesthesia dolorosa"—that refer to pain that originates in the central nervous system after partial, complete, or subclinical interruption of somatosensory pathways, especially the STTs. Causes of central pain are stroke, trauma, tumor, and multiple sclerosis. Deafferentation nerve injury can cause denervation in the next higher-order neuron due to excitotoxicity. Patients experience multiple pain symptoms: a spontaneous, unpleasant, burning pain; tingling or numbness; crawling, ripping, or tearing sensation; warm and cold allodynia; and hyperalgesia. Localization of the pain is diffuse and usually beyond the area of sensory loss. Weeks to months after an injury or thalamic infarct, spontaneous pain develops in the same distribution as the sensory loss, presumably from denervation hypersensitivity of sensory neurons in the midbrain reticular formation. Lesions in the spinothalamic input into the thalamus are followed by reorganization and connection of touch input to previously silent neurons with an opioid link.

The pain can be decreased with amitryptiline, lamotrigine, and IV lidocaine, all sodium channel blockers.

IV lidocaine significantly decreased spontaneous pain and evoked brush-induced allodynia and mechanic hyperalgesia but not thermal allodynia and hyperalgesia in 16 patients with central pain due to stroke or spinal cord injury.[39] Unfortunately, follow-up treatment with oral mexiletine was disappointing because of much less pain relief and more side effects. IV morphine reduced touch-evoked pain (allodynia) but not other evoked pains. Overall effects of morphine on spontaneous ongoing pain was no different than placebo; however, 46 percent of the patients responded to morphine.[40]

COMPLEX REGIONAL PAIN SYNDROMES I AND II

Reflex sympathetic dystrophy is a term for sensory, autonomic, and motor features in an extremity following an injury or operation, or it may develop spontaneously. At a consensus meeting, the term *chronic regional pain syndrome type I* for reflex sympathetic dystrophy with no definable nerve injury and *chronic regional pain syndrome type II* for causalgia with a definable nerve injury were defined.[41] Patients experience an excruciating burning pain and functional impairment with variable occurrence of evolving symptoms beyond the area of trauma. There is a cold feeling, warm feeling, or both in the affected area; edema; increased nail and hair growth; hyperhidrosis; abnormal skin color; hypoesthesia; hyperalgesia; mechanical allodynia, thermal allodynia, or both; movement disorder; and patchy demineralization of the bone (Sudek's atrophy).[42] The movement disorder with complex regional pain syndrome (CRPS) is complex and includes inability to initiate movement, tremor, spasms, weakness, and dystonia. Autonomic dysfunction is evident early as hyperemia of the limb with rapid capillary refill time, and later, the limb becomes cool, cyanotic, and mottled with diminished blood flow and prolonged capillary refill time. Recent investigations have suggested that release of SP and calcitonin gene-related peptide from sensitized C-nociceptors causes vasodilatation and increased capillary permeability to account for ongoing edema, vasodilatation, and pain (i.e., neurogenic inflammation).[43] Interestingly, bone and periosteum are densely innervated by CGRP-positive neurons, which decrease several days after a dislocated fracture, indicating nerve damage. After fracture or surgery, surviving nerve fibers undergo sprouting and regeneration, which might be the underlying pathophysiology of some patients with CRPS I and those with CRPS II.[43] Treatment with NSAIDs, gabapentin, and narcotics; physical therapy; and TENS has been only partially effective in most patients. Treatment with sympathetic block or intravenous lidocaine followed by oral mexilitine may help refractory patients. In selected patients, spinal cord stimulation decreased pain and improved quality of life.[42] Intrathecal baclofen, a GABA-receptor antagonist, reduced the dystonia in the hands and improved function with prolonged treatment.[44] CRPS is a devastating illness and underlying mechanisms are becoming known. Injury to periperal C fibers or A-delta fibers triggers neurochemical changes in the distal nociceptors, the dorsal root ganglia cells, and neurons in the dorsal horn of the spinal cord by retrograde transport of neurochemicals and nerve growth factors, with subsequent alteration in membrane channels and ectopic firing to sustain the pain and sympathetic stimulation.[16]

Psychiatric Comorbidities in the Patient with Chronic Pain

Psychiatric disorders in patients with chronic pain may be primary, secondary, or both. Psychiatric comorbidities can have a negative impact on chronic pain and functional status. Psychiatrists have expertise in elucidating a patient's life profile and special skills in analyzing psychodynamic mechanisms in these complex patients. They also have a specialized fund of knowledge and experience treating psychiatric disorders that medical specialists do not have. Axis I psychiatric disorders such as depression, anxiety, or panic disorder are common at some time in patients with chronic pain but are not thought to cause the pain. However, approximately 60 percent of patients with depression report pain at the time of diagnosis.[45] Depression is a comorbid condition that interacts with chronic pain to increase its severity and adversely affects the patient's coping strategies and function. The role of depression must be explored in detail in patients with chronic pain so that the depression, as well as the pain, can be treated. Treatment of some patients with tricyclic antidepressants (TCAs) had both a direct analgesic effect and depression-relief effect on chronic pain. In patients with chronic pain who are also depressed, the depression may be "masked" (i.e., they have only vegetative symptoms of insomnia, weight loss, reduced energy or interest, loss of libido, reduced concentration, and nonproductive activity, rather than the depressed affect). Anxiety can change pain threshold and tolerance. As many as 19 percent of chronic-pain patients have anxiety disorder, 10 percent have panic disorder, and 40 percent of patients with anxiety disorder reported chronic pain.[45] Alcohol and drug abuse affects 16 to 20 percent of general medical outpatients.[46] Substance-abuse disorders may be more prevalent in patients with chronic pain (3.2 to 18.9 percent); however, the research data are discrepant, and most individuals had the substance-abuse disorder prior to the onset of chronic pain.[47] In some patients, pain emerges without an apparent physical abnormality as the source or cause. These patients have psychiatric disorders that antedated the onset of chronic pain, and the pain has become a manifestation of psychiatric disease. These disorders have specific diagnostic criteria, stereotypic life profiles, abnormal family dynamics, and social and vocational dysfunction. The diagnosis should not be made as a diagnosis of exclusion but by positive diagnostic evidence for a somatoform disorder, depression, substance-abuse disorder, personality disorder, or psychotic disorder, such as schizophrenia or major psychotic depression. In other patients, the chronic pain state may have become complicated by the development of a comorbid psychiatric disorder such as depression, anxiety, or substance abuse. The in-depth history should be directed at "unlayering" the psychologic components of the observed pain behaviors.

In DSM-IV-TR, the diagnosis of pain disorder replaces the term *somatoform pain disorder*. Somatoform disorders, which may have pain as a symptom, include somatization disorder, hypochondriasis, conversion disorder, and pain disorder (Table 64–5). Somatization means the conversion of mental experiences or states into bodily symptoms. Somatization is a feature of a number of psychiatric disorders associated with pain and is an important cause for misdiagnosis of psychiatric disorders. More than 50 percent of patients with a psychiatric disorder present with somatic complaints to a primary care physician. Underdiagnosis of disabling psychiatric disease occurs when the diagnosis of psychiatric disease is viewed a diagnosis of exclusion. For patients who have pain as a manifestation of underlying psychiatric disorders, therapeutic attempts focused on symptomatic treatment of the pain will be unsuccessful and will delay appropriate diagnosis and treatment of the psychiatric disease. Somatization is a psychophysiologic process wherein symptom perception varies from minimalization to amplification; however, no physical illness can be found.[45] The individual attributes the symptom to some cause and decides how to react to the symptom. Over time, the list of unexplained somatic complaints accumulates and is accompanied by functional impairment, overuse of the health care system, and additional psychiatric disorders such as depression and anxiety. Somatization disorder typically begins before age 20 to 30. Symptoms are exaggerated and multifocal, involving most organ systems. The patients are preoccupied with their pain and believe they have a serious medical illness. The patients do not intentionally produce or magnify the pain and are unaware that the pain is linked to psychological factors or conflict. A neuropsychologic basis for somatization disorder has been postulated, which suggests that attentional and cognitive impairments result in

TABLE 64–5 • FEATURES OF COMORBID PSYCHIATRIC DISORDERS

Disorders	Hallmark	Additional Features	Comments
Somatoform Disorders	Symptoms but no physical abnormality	Positive evidence for link to psychologic factor or conflict	No response to antidepressants, anxiolytics, or muscle relaxants
• Somatization disorder (hysteria)	Preoccupied with the pain; dramatic or exaggerated symptoms	Polysymptomatic, often anxious, depressed; common social difficulties; onset at a young age (<20 to 30)	Complicated history with care from multiple doctors; has no insight the pain is linked to psychologic factors
• Hypochondriasis	Preoccupied with fear they have physical illness; unrealistic interpretation of sensations as abnormal	Often anxious, depressed, and frustrated with doctors	Symptoms but no loss of function. A doctor shopper, "worried well"; seeking relief from fear of illness rather than pain
• Pain disorder (psychogenic pain)	Preoccupation with pain in excess of physical abnormality	Pain nonanatomic; antecedent event in adulthood with psychologic conflict	Pain provides secondary gain of support or avoidance
• Conversion disorder	Pain as a conversion reaction with motor or sensory deficit	Indifferent to deficit	Self-limited but recurrent episodes of motor or sensory deficit and pain
Pain-Depression Syndrome	Pain as a somatic manifestation of depression, which may be masked (only vegetative signs)	Depression makes pain exaggerated and less tolerated	Tricyclic antidepressants improve both pain and depression
Personality Disorders	Pain used to carry out pathologic relationships and get attention (i.e., interpersonal exploitation, manipulation, theft)	DSM-IV Cluster B antisocial, borderline, histrionic, and narcissistic personalities	The most difficult patient to treat in an interdisciplinary setting—problems with authority and triangulate staff, impulsive and aggressive, seductive; usually oblivious to their own problems, behavior is inflexible and pervasive; they disregard and violate the rights of others and lack empathy; strong sense of entitlement, very poor treatment outcomes, (i.e., "the dreaded patient")
Substance-Abuse Disorder		Pain used to obtain narcotics	Need rigid treatment contracts
Malingering	Symptoms intentionally produced for a specific goal	Goal is compensation or avoidance of work	
Factitious Disorder	Symptoms intentionally produced	Goal is "winning," secondary goal not obvious	Munchausen syndrome
Psychosis (Schizophrenia or Psychotic Depression)	Pain as a fixed somatic delusion is uncommon	Bizarre distribution and quality	Treat underlying psychosis

From American Psychiatric Association. Diagnostic and Statistical Manual of Mental Disorders, 4th ed, text revision. Washington DC, American Psychiatric Association, 2000.

faulty perception and assessment of somatosensory input. Distress and interpersonal problems are common. These people are often anxious and depressed, and suicide attempts are not infrequent. There may be a family history of marital discord, abuse, alcoholism, and sociopathy in parents and spouses. The interview is difficult because the medical history and review of systems are vague, circumstantial, and disorganized. Patients often describe their symptoms in colorful, exaggerated terms but may lack specific factual information. The patients frequently report that their prior physicians were incompetent and often have a long history of poor compliance with medical recommendations and "doctor shopping." This disorder is much more common in women. Somatization disorder has a fluctuating course but seldom remits completely. Treatment is directed at assisting the patient to cope and preventing unnecessary workups and surgeries. These patients need frequent clinic visits for reassurance that the pain is not due to physical illness, and supportive psychotherapy is beneficial, if they will participate.

Hypochondriasis (hysteria) is a preoccupation with fears about having a serious disease based on a misinterpretation of normal body sensations or everyday aches and pains. The unwarranted fears persist despite medical reassurance. Concern about the feared illness becomes the focus of the individual's self image. The medical history is presented in great detail and at length, with multiple unsatisfactory doctor–patient relationships, and the conviction he or she is not receiving the proper care. Family history reveals illness was a prominent focus of attention. In the medical history it becomes apparent the patient is as concerned about the meaning and diagnosis of the symptom as with its relief. Hypochondriacs are preoccupied with their bodies and physiologic functioning and are obsessed with their health. Family and social relationships deteriorate because of the self-centered focus on "the condition" and demands for special treatment and consideration.[8] Doctor visits become a way of life, and these patients carry out elaborate self-treatment regimens. Treatment should be by a primary care physician who conceptualizes that the symptoms are a communication, not a disease to be eradicated. Group psychotherapy is also helpful as it provides the social interaction and support these patients need. Drug therapy should be avoided because hypochondriacs tend to develop side effects or simply replace a cured symptom with a new one. Hypochondriasis may begin at any age and is equally common in men and women. It has a waxing and waning course with occasional complete recovery. The individual is not delusional and may become able to consider that the feared disease is not present.

Conversion disorder is the presence of symptoms or deficits affecting voluntary motor or sensory function, suggesting a neurologic or medical condition. Pain may be one of the symptoms but not the only symptom. Deficits are not feigned and do not conform to anatomic pathways or physiologic mechanisms. Interestingly, the individual may show surprising indifference to the deficits or be overly dramatic. Conversion disorder usually begins before age 35, is more common in women, and symptoms more often involve the left side of the body. Deficit symptoms usually do not last more than 2 weeks but are often recurrent.[8]

The pain disorder (formerly somatoform pain disorder or psychogenic pain) is diagnosed in those patients with a predominant focus of pain and in whom psychologic factors are judged to have a significant role in the onset, severity, exacerbation, and maintenance of the pain.[8] There is substantial impairment of functioning and frequent health care use, with substantial use of medications and disruption of family and social relationships. Psychodynamic theories have focused on the unconscious meaning of the pain, such as childhood means of obtaining love and affection or as a punishment for real or imagined wrongdoing. The pain is constant, does not vary, and is not consistent with the innervation of the painful area. There is a long history of invalidism and frequent requests for surgery. Patients are preoccupied with the pain and claim all other areas of their lives are fine.

In some patients, psychophysiologic pain refers to a chronic pain syndrome that has recurred after a structural lesion was treated or healed and is accompanied by pain behavior (sometimes also referred to as somatoform pain disorder as described previously). Examples include postoperative return of pain following herniated disk surgery or pain after a musculoskeletal injury has healed. The pain is not related to progressive structural disease and is not life threatening, but it is associated with changes in personality and lifestyle that can be severely disabling (pain behaviors). Pain can be respondent (response to a nociceptive stimulus) or operant (response to the environment and the rewards for expressing pain in that environment). Moaning and grimacing increase attention or sympathy from a spouse and also gives the patient the ability to control his or her mileu and roles. Patients with personality disorders are vulnerable to these secondary gains. Patients often fear reinjury or jeopardizing disability payments by becoming active again or returning to work. The patients have strong but unconscious motivations to retain the pain. Emotional stress is a major factor in recurrences or exacerbations of the pain, but the patient has not made that connection. Treatment of chronic pain behaviors depends on controlling and changing these reinforcers (operant mechanisms).

Psychotic disorders such as schizophrenia, delusional disorder, and bipolar affective disorder do not commonly present with pain. However the finding of fixed, intense, somatic delusion (bizarre descriptions of body sensations) in a chronic-pain patient would suggest severe psychiatric disease such as schizophrenia or psychotic depression. The pain descriptors in these cases are typically nonanatomic.

Comorbidities between chronic pain disorder and Axis II personality disorders are common. The prevalence of personality disorders in chronic pain–disorder patients has ranged from 31 to 49 percent in different studies.[47] These patients present a great challenge to a successful doctor–patient relationship and are very difficult to manage in a primary care or rheumatology clinic. Personality disorders are defined by enduring maladaptive patterns of perceiving, relating to, and thinking about the environment and the self.[48] Patients with personality disorders use pain to manipulate others, obtain narcotics (substance-abuse disorder), avoid responsibilities, develop pathologic relationships with health care providers, and obtain nurturing attention (antisocial personality disorder).

Two other groups of patients present particular difficulties for assessment and successful treatment. Patients who are malingering or those with factitious disorder. Malingering is volitional fabrication of false symptoms or physical findings to attain some recognizable external gain, such as avoiding work or prosecution and obtaining drugs or financial compensation. Submaximal effort on muscle-strength testing often leads to the suspicion that the patient is lying. Be cautious when the patient was referred by an attorney for evaluation. Factitious disorder is presentation of false symptoms or self-inflicted abnormal findings with the poorly understood goal of "winning" or a psychologic need to assume the sick role (i.e., no obvious secondary economic gain or external incentives). Examples include the Munchausen syndrome, a chronic factitious disorder with self-induced physical abnormalities. The history is often dramatic but extremely vague and inconsistent. Complaints of pain and requests for analgesics are common. Some patients with chronic pain will not be categorizable. It is important to reinvestigate whether litigation is involved with the pain. Pain treatment is typically unsuccessful until litigation is settled.

The Pain-Sleep Connection

Dudley Hart suggested that "persistent and repeated recurrence of discomfort produces physical and mental fatigue and depression."[49] It is doubtful that clinician or patient would disagree, but objective data from sleep studies are lacking or insufficiently studied in the rheumatic diseases.[50-52] Interestingly, auditory perception remains active during sleep; however, responses to thermal and muscle pain stimuli during sleep appear to be attenuated.[53] At least 75 percent of patients with chronic pain report poor sleep,[54] and it is generally assumed that the complaint of poor sleep is directly attributable to the underlying pain. Regrettably, rigorous systematic, objective studies of sleep in either acute or chronic pain are lacking. It appears that chronic pain plays a lesser role in insomnia than might be thought.[55] In one small series of patients complaining of low back pain and poor sleep, the objective sleep parameters displayed wide variability.[56] Another objective study indicated that the sleep of patients complaining of pain was less disturbed than that of patients suffering from psychiatric disease unassociated with pain.[57] A recent objective study found no differences in sleep architecture between patients with chronic low back pain with subjective reports of sleep disturbance and normal controls. EEG power spectral analyses suggested some difference among groups, but the significance of these findings is unknown and they remain to be replicated.[58] Furthermore, there is some evidence that the degree of subjective sleep impairment correlates better with depressed mood than pain intensity, duration, or anxiety.[59] Another study of patients with chronic pain indicated that presleep cognitive arousal, rather than pain severity, was the primary predictor of sleep quality.[54] Other factors correlating with poor sleep include physical health, physical functioning, and psychosocial functioning.[60] The intuitively attractive assumption that chronic pain per se causes insomnia remains to be demonstrated. What is clear is that the severity of the chronic pain is not the primary predictor of the degree of subjective sleep disturbance. Identification of the precise nature of the sleep complaints associated with chronic pain has important therapeutic implications.

Standardized Approach to Assessment of Patients with Chronic Pain

Caring for a patient with chronic pain requires a thorough investigation of the medical, psychologic, and socioeconomic complexities of chronic pain (Table 64–6). Because acute pain and chronic pain are distinctly different clinical entities, the duration of the pain must be clearly identified first. With short-term acute pain, the patient can describe the onset precisely and the proximate circumstances such as injury or other illness. Acute pain usually has an identifiable noxious stimulus of limited duration (e.g., surgical incision, burn, fracture), responds to analgesics and rest of the affected area, and diminishes as the tissue heals. When pain has been persistent for more than 6 months, it is much more difficult for the patient to describe the onset, timing, and character precisely, and psychobehavior symptoms may have become disproportionate to the physical abnormalities evident. A multinational World Health Organization (WHO) study of more than 3000 primary care patients in 14 countries[61] demonstrated that only 51 percent of those with persistent pain at baseline had recovered 12 months later, and 8.8 percent of those without persistent pain had developed it 12 months later. The presence of persistent pain at baseline predicted the development of anxiety or depression and vice versa. Occupational disability was actually the strongest predictor for both pain and psychologic disorder. These findings underscore the need for detailed investigation of medical, psychiatric, and functional status in the evaluation of the patient with chronic pain.

Initial evaluation of the patient with chronic pain must contain essential elements to formulate a diagnostic impression of the most likely pathogenic mechanism causing the pain (Table 64–6). Pathogenic mechanisms causing chronic pain can be broadly divided into those related to (1) an active or progressive underlying structural disease (somatogenic) of the musculoskeletal system or nervous system, or (2) a psychiatric disorder producing pain as a somatic delusion or as a result of chronic pain or various combinations of these mechanisms (Fig. 64–1). The workup must include a standard medical history with focus on specific dimensions described in the following paragraphs, a thorough general physical exami-

TABLE 64–6 • STANDARDIZED ASSESSMENT OF THE PATIENT WITH CHRONIC PAIN

Pain History		**Physical Examination**	
Location	Onset	Vital signs, weight	
Intensity	Duration	General physical examination	
Descriptors	Frequency	Detailed neurological examination	
Aggravating Factors	Alleviating Factors	Mental state asessment	
Past Treatments	Injury/Litigation	Full musculoskeletal examination	
Current Treatments		Health Status/Diagnostic Screens	
		SF-36	PRIME-MD
Medical History	**Surgical History**	Timed Stands × 10	
Psychiatric history	**Trauma history**	Pain VAS	Qualitative Pain Relief
Review of Systems			
		Laboratory tests	
Psychosocial Function		Hematologic abnormality	Immune abnormalities
Mood	Depression	Hepatitis screens	Indicators of inflammation
Sleep	Energy level	Renal function	Liver function
Relationships	Cognition	Urinalysis	Urine Tox Screen
Activity Status			
Walk	Work at home	**Radiographic imaging**	
Sit	Work at job	Take image of part that hurts	Bone scan if radiographs negative
Stand	Self cares	CT scans	MRI scans
Lift/carry objects	Recreational activities	Angiograms	
Substance Use		**Additional Tests**	
Alcohol (CAGE)	Tobacco	EMG	
Illicit drugs	Caffeine	Biopsy rashes	
Misuse prescription meds	Misuse OTC meds	Nerve conduction study	
		Biopsy masses	
		Working Diagnosis	
		Probable cause of pain	Medical comorbidity impact
Family History		Pathophysiologic mechanism	Psychiatric comorbidity
Chronic pain	Medical illnesses		
Substance abuse	Psychiatric disease	**Treatment Plan**	
Physical/sexual abuse	Family dysfunction	Additional consults	Indicators to monitor
		Analgesics	Adjuvant meds
Concurrent Medications		Exercise recommendation	Benchmark of improvement
		Opioid rules	Opioid contract

Abbreviations: CAGE, Alcohol abuse screen; OTC, over the counter; PRIME-MD, Primary Care Evalution of Mental Disorders; SF-36, short from quality-of-life scale.

nation, and a meticulous neurologic and musculoskeletal examination.

The medical interview is focused on the history and character of the pain; medical, surgical, and psychiatric comorbidities; prior treatments, surgeries, and injuries; family history; current social history; education and vocational history; functional status; current medications; and current legal or disability issues. The pain history should define the cardinal features of the pain at its onset, progression since onset, and current condition. The clinician should attempt to determine the precise location and time of onset of the pain. He or she should ask the patient to describe the tempo of onset and progression, whether abrupt and fulminant, insidious and progressive, or waxing and waning. The patient should be asked to demonstrate the position or motion when the pain started. Was the onset of the pain immediate or delayed after an injury? The patient should characterize the current pain by indicating with a single digit the precise location of the pain. Is the pain spontaneous or produced by movement (incident pain), pressure, touch, or temperature? The patient should describe the character of the pain (i.e., burning, lancinating, sharp, dull, aching) (see Table 64–3). If the pain radiates, the patient should describe the radiation pattern and whether the current pain is persistent or intermittent. The clinician should determine what factors worsen the pain and what tends to relieve the pain. The patient should quantify the pain severity on a 0 to 10 scale, with 0 being no pain and 10 the worst possible pain.

The clinician should obtain a detailed general medical history to formulate a life profile of coexistent medical, surgical, and psychologic problems. A thorough review of systems should be undertaken to identify symptoms of systemic or localized disorders that might be associated with the pain. A detailed psychiatric history with attention to early family dynamics, history of abuse, alcoholism, and psychiatric disorders in the immediate family and spouse, and interpersonal problems with boss, friends, family, peers, and previous physicians may reveal indicators suggestive of significant psychopathology. It is often very informative to ask patients if the pain has influenced how a boss, friends, or family members perceive and treat them. It is essential to have the spouse or most significant peer present for the interview. Observation of the patient in the presence of a family member and interviewing the family member will help establish the accuracy of the history and self report of functional status, medication use, substance abuse, and vocational situation. Clues for identification of patients with primary psychopathology include prior psychiatric treatment; dysfunction in family, interpersonal, work roles, relationships, or some combination of these; polypharmacy, substance abuse, or both; and a history of multiple medical evaluations and treatments with little or no improvement. These patients have dissatisfied and hostile attitudes and are often manipulative and uncooperative. The clinician should define as concisely as possible the patient's prepain personality, family dynamics, and functional status.

An assessment of current overall functional status with a determination of how much the pain is affecting self-care, family, sexual, occupational, social, and recreational function status should be made. The clinician should have the patient identify several activities he or she is no longer able to do because of the pain and describe the impact of this functional loss. The amount of current monthly income should be determined, as well as how it changed because of the pain. The patient should articulate how coworkers, family, and friends treat him or her and whether this has changed since the pain began. The clinician should also inquire about worker's compensation or litigation issues.

A detailed inventory of all the patient's prior and current medications, both prescription and over-the-counter, as well as nutriceuticals and treatments, should be generated, including their effects and adverse side effects to avoid the mistake of recommending a prior failed treatment. The patient should describe the effects of previous treatments, including benefits, costs, and side effects. The clinician should emphasize the need to know all medications being taken because drug interactions and side effects could put the patient at risk.

Review of prior medical records is a tedious task, but it may be very time saving in the long run and permit more accurate interpretations of a patient's account of the complex medical and surgical history. For patients with chronic disease, recollection of prior events may be inaccurate or distorted and cause hostility about their prior treatments. Old medical records often reveal forgotten adverse effects, substance-abuse problems, and important psychosocial or legal issues. Spending sufficient time at the first interview, permittings patients to vent about their doubts and distrust, and reviewing old records creates a stronger basis for the therapeutic relationship.

IDENTIFICATION OF PSYCHIATRIC COMORBIDITIES

Identification of personality disorders is crucial for the clinician who must rely on the accuracy of history and behavioral observations during the interview. Expression of rage toward family members, employers, insurance adjusters, and every physician seen is a "red flag" for a personality disorder diagnosis (see Table 64–5). These patients are not appropriate for multidisciplinary treatment programs and will have to be managed medically using rigid opioid contracts because compliance is likely to become a serious issue. Detection of malingering and deception in chronic-pain patients is very problematic because assessment and treatment depends on accurate patient self-reporting for the clinician to reach valid conclusions. It is crucial for the clinician to understand the factors that may affect patient self-report accuracy. To trust the patient's complaints, the clinician must consider the possibility of deliberate distortion or deception because it is so common. The critical issue is that a clinician's ability to make an accurate diagnosis and effective treatment decisions depends totally on the completeness, honesty, and overall accuracy of the patient's self report. Nondeliberate and deliberate distortion by the patient can seriously jeopardize patient care and safety. Clinicians should have a strategy for deception analysis that is implemented in all patient assessments.[62] There are basically five patient-response styles, which refer to how patients report symptoms; these are honesty, maximization, minimization, mixed, and irrelevant (when the patient is not engaged with the interview so responses are not relevant to the question). Distortion refers to using a maximized, minimized, or mixed response style. Deception refers to intentional distortion of symptoms to achieve some desired target goal (i.e., the behavior seen in malingering). An observed lack of cooperation during the interview and examination should be viewed as a "red flag" for possible distortion or deception. The patient who reports numerous neurologic, pain, and musculoskeletal symptoms with little objective abnormality is likely demonstrating a maximizing response style. A fluctuating response style with little change in objective abnormalities suggests distortion. Nonintentional distortion is seen with distraught patients who are fearful the physician will not understand his or her pain and magnifies the symptoms as a cry for help. Complaints of unusual nonsensical symptoms likely represents intentional distortion. Patients who report no benefit from any treatment may be intentionally distorting the history, because most patients experience at least a small benefit from some treatments. Observation that symptoms worsened while the patient was being observed and lessened when distracted suggests deliberate distortion. Most patients who have disability have some degree of emotional distress and depression. Cases in which patients deny emotional stress or depression yet have significant disability suggest deliberate distortion. Refusal to permit access to old medical records and a history of multiple hospitalizations and compensation claims are also "red flags" for deception.

Several health status instruments are useful for the individual clinician evaluating a chronic pain patient and are recommended because they are self administered or can be administered by an assistant, are easy to score, and have been validated in populations with medical illnesses. The Primary Care Evalution of Mental Disorders (PRIME-MD)[63] is an excellent screen for depression, anxiety, somatoform disorders, eating disorders, and alcohol abuse. Pain severity is best quantified on a 0 to 10 scale, with 0 being no pain and 10 the most severe pain, and pain relief is best quantified with qualitative answers of none, some, a little, and a lot to monitor response to treatment. The short form quality-of-life scale (SF-36) is a standardized health-related quality of life functional test as is the HAQ, and both are useful in ongoing assessments (see Chapter 29).

The clinician and patient should establish the patient's goals. The clinician should ask the patient what he or she expects from evaluation and recommendations. The patient may be seeking a second opinion to validate another physician's evaluation and treatment recommendations, seeking a different diagnosis and treatment plan, applying for disability and needing a medical statement, or looking for a physician willing to prescribe opioids for chronic nonmalignant pain. It is important to establish at the outset that it is unlikely the pain will be eliminated completely, but some improvement can be anticipated.

The physical examination process serves to identify objective abnormalities associated with musculoskeletal and neurologic disorders that reasonably explain the patient's pain, find important coexistant abnormalities, and define functional status. During the examination, the decision-making process will "rule in" and "rule out" the items in the differential diagnosis generated during the interview and review of medical records. The musculoskeletal and neurologic examination must be meticulous. For the patient, it is the opportunity to observe the examiner's technical competence and to develop confidence in the quality of the assessment and recommendations. For the primary care physician or rheumatologist, the finding of a gross neurologic abnormality requires a prompt evaluation.

Initially, the clinician should observe the patient as he or she walks 20 feet away to observe spine deformities, pelvic tilt, knee and hip contractures, or instability. The patient should then turn and walk back, first on the heels, then up on the toes, and then walking heel to toe. The patient should hop first on one foot then the other to assess leg strength, balance, and coordination. As a test of lower extremity function, the patient should squat and stand up from a squat or stand up and down from a seated position in the chair, without using arms, 10 times (normal time for this is 11 to 14 seconds). The clinician should observe the patient as he or she undresses, puts on an examination gown, and climbs onto the examination table, noting imbalance, weakness, and pain behaviors. The clinician should enumerate pain behaviors such as moaning, groaning, grimacing, writhing, crying, or shouting. Unobtrusive observations of gait as the patient walks into the examination room and climbs onto the table are important to understand the effects of the patient's pain. Neurologic and musculoskeletal examination should be focused to identify abnormalities associated with the pain and to analyze maneuvers that reproduce, worsen, or alleviate the pain. The examiner should critically consider the different possible pathogenic mechanisms and tissue sources of the pain while performing the physical examination. Mental status examination provides clues to a central nervous system lesion and will reveal cognitive deficits that can influence a patient's description of and response to painful stimuli. Cognitive abilites will also influence treatment recommendations. The clinician should assess global mental status by asking name, place, year, date, location of examination, and inquiring about a current event or the president or governor, having the patient subtract serial sevens, testing the ability to interpret a proverb, naming a pen, and identifying a coin with eyes closed. Symptoms of a thought disorder should be sought by directly asking if the patient hears or sees things that are not there, if people are after or trying to hurt him or her, if he or she has trouble controlling thoughts, and by asking what the patient thinks is causing the pain. Detailed examination of all cranial nerves may provide evidence of unsuspected lesions in the brain stem or higher. Check for facial asymmetry, pupil diameter and light responses, extraocular eye muscles, facial sensation and gag reflex, as well as for snout and glabellar reflexes.The patient should flex the head (put chin to chest), extend the head (look at the ceiling), laterally extend right and left (put ear on shoulder), and rotate the head (put chin on each shoulder); the clinician should note increase in pain with these maneuvers, palpate for paracervical muscle tenderness, and check muscle strength of neck flexors and extensors.

The musculoskeletal examination (see Chapter 33) should assess redness, warmth, swelling, and tenderness or lack thereof at synovial reflections, joint capsule insertions, and tendon muscle insertions. Upper-extremity examination of joints, bursae, and tendons should be accompanied by muscle-strength testing of shoulder shrug, flexion, and abduction, with special attention to production of pain with resisted motion. Evaluation of resisted motion tests muscle strength and also puts tension on tendons and ligaments, which will reproduce pain if these structures are the site of pathology. Muscle-strength testing may be difficult in a patient with pain, because the pain may limit maximal effort. With manual muscle-strength testing and coaching, it is possible to distinguish true muscle weakness from "giving way" due to pain or lack of cooperation. The clinician should note whether the testing effort reproduces the pain or behaviors such as grimacing and moaning and carefully distinguish whether active versus passive motion reproduces or accentuates the pain. With synovial inflammation, synovial tissue is swollen and tender to palpation and both active and passive motion increase pain. With tendinitis, the joint itself is not tender but the area of tendon insertion will be focally tender, and active, but not passive, motion reproduces the pain. The clinician should note crepitance, joint instability, and the presence of trigger points or tender points around the joints. Unobtrusive observation of the patient's responses to range of motion (ROM) testing maneuvers and palpation during the joint examination can provide insight into pain severity and the patient's reaction to the pain. Elbow flexion and extension, wrist flexion and extension, grip strength, and finger abduction should be evaluated. The patient should make fists, flex elbows 90 degrees, and hold them at the torso. Instruct the patient to resist the examiner's attempts to bring the fists together at the midline (this checks infraspinatus, teres minor and deltoid muscles). Instruct the patient to resist the examiner's attempts to separate the fists (this resisted external rotation, checks the deltoid, pectoralis, subscapularis, teres major, and latissimus dorsi strength). Resisting attempts to extend the elbow checks biceps and brachioradialis strength, and resistance of attempts to flex the elbow checks triceps strength. The clinician should note whether changes in deep tendon reflexes (DTRs) correspond to changes in strength. DTRs at the triceps (C7 and C8), biceps, and brachioradialis (C6 and C7) tendons should be checked, as well as cutaneous sensation to light touch, pinprick, and Hoffman's reflex. The patient should perform rapid alternating movements of the hand and finger by touching the nose bilaterally. Sensory examination in upper and lower extremities should include testing of superficial (pinprick) and deep (tendon squeeze) pain, light touch, heat, cold, vibration, and position sense. The clinician should note whether changes conform to dermatome distribution (loss of pain, touch, and temperature sense), nerve root distribution (sensory loss, hyperesthesia, and radicular pain), or distribution of a peripheral nerve.

Examine the back with the patient sitting, standing, and prone to evaluate spinal tenderness, paravertebral muscle spasm, and ROM (flexion, extension, and rotation with pelvis fixed to eliminate hip-joint motion). Straight-leg raising test should be performed in the supine and sitting position, as both should reproduce pain from a radiculopathy.

Lower extremity examination of the joints, tendons, and bursae should be accompanied by muscle-strength testing of hip flexors, extensors, abductors, and adductors, with attention to production of pain with resisted motion in the four planes. Knee flexion and extension strength should be tested with patellar reflex testing (L3 and L4). Ankle plantar flexion, dorsiflexion, and great toe extension strength should be tested with Achilles tendon reflex (S1 and S2) testing and sensory testing to light touch and pinprick; vibration. Heel to chin coordination and Babinski's reflex should be assessed.

FORMULATING THE DIAGNOSTIC IMPRESSION

The clinician should decide whether the pain is primarily somatogenic or nonsomatogenic. If somatogenic, the clinician should decide whether the source of pathology is nociceptive, neuropathic, or both, and if neuropathic, whether peripheral or central. If arthritis is the most likely underlying cause, an appropriate laboratory and radiologic workup should be undertaken. If prior radiographs are more than 2 or 3 months old, they should be repeated and, if normal, bone scans, magnetic resonance imaging (MRI), or computed tomography (CT) scan should be obtained. If the underlying cause is most likely neuropathic, electromyography, nerve conduction studies provide immediate diagnostic information about neuromuscular disorders, as well as prognostic indicators for traumatic injuries. If central pain is likely, MRI of the spinal cord, brain, or both should be obtained. If weakness is found nerve or muscle biopsy should be considered. If a neurologic deficit is evident on the physical examination, a neurology consultation may be helpful. For patients with predominantly somatogenic pain, treatment strategies should be mechanism-based as described in the following paragraphs.

If the pain is predominantly psychologic, the clinician should determine whether there is primary or secondary psychopathology. Primary psychopathology predates the chronic pain problem (i.e., hypochondriasis, somatization and somatoform pain disorder, major depression, and substance abuse). These patients usually have had multiple medical problems, surgeries, and treatments and are dissatisfied and hostile toward doctors. They are often manipulative and uncooperative. They may appear overly depressed or surprisingly indifferent. Subjective pain report and pain behaviors are out of proportion to objective physical abnormalities, and physical signs may fluctuate from one examination to another. Secondary psychopathology occurs in those with healthy personality and functioning before the pain but who have developed significant psychologic dysfunction secondary to the pain, physical changes due to illness, or impaired socioeconomic function and vocational losses. These patients often have a negative attitude, are anxious, depressed, and angry, and they feel isolated and helpless. For patients with predominantly nonsomatogenic psychologic pain, additional psychiatric evaluation is often needed, and treatment of these factors should be the initial treatment strategy. When the decision has been made confidently that there is no significant somatogenic component to the chronic pain that requires specific medical or surgical treatment, requests from the patient for more workup should be declined. Most patients will not be diagnosable as having exclusively nociceptive, neuropathic, or psychogenic pain, but they will have components of all three in the total clinical picture.

Mechanism-Based Approach to Treatment of Chronic Musculoskeletal Pain

Inflammatory joint disease as cause for chronic pain should be treated as specifically as possible to reduce inflammation and prevent further joint damage (see Chapter 67). Most patients with chronic musculoskeletal pain have become physically deconditioned and will need a directed rehabilitation program when pain has been decreased enough to permit an increase in physical activity (see Chapter 55).

Analgesic selection, route, dosage, and scheduling should be individualized. If pain is present for most of the day, treatment should be scheduled regularly, rather than on an as-needed basis. The majority of patients with defined musculoskeletal disease will have pain incident to movement and should be taught how to schedule analgesic doses to permit as high a level of physical activity as possible. Adjuvant therapies can decrease pain by modifying pain pathways, mitigate analgesic side effects, and treat concomitant problems such as depression, which may aggravate pain. Alternatvie methods of analgesic administration, such as patient-controlled analgesic pumps, intrathecal administration of medications, or spinal cord stimulators, may be needed in a minority of patients.

How much reduction in pain is clincally meaningful? The most widely used scale to quantify pain severity in clinical trials, and now in clinical practice as the "fifth vital sign" is the pain-intensity numeric rating scale (PI-NRS) of 0 to 10, with 0 being no pain and 10 the worst possible pain. The patient's global impression of change (PGIC) is a qualitative measure of pain relief with a 7-point categorical scale (1 = very much worse, to 7 = very much improved).[65] Farrar and colleagues[65] examined the changes in the data from 10 different studies with more than 2700 subjects and demonstrated that both a 30-percent change and two-point raw change in score on the PI-NRS was associated with the PGIC of "much improved or better." A 50-percent reduction in pain-intensity score was associated with PGIC of "very much improved." It is advisable to use both scales when monitoring a patient's disease activity and response to treatment, rather than relying only on the pain-intensity scale.

ANALGESICS

Nonopioid analgesics are useful for mild to moderate pain, regardless of the underlying joint disease. Selection of acetaminophen, a salicylate, or one of the many available NSAIDs is determined by the patient's prior treatment history, age, and comorbid conditions that impact the risk profile for side effects (see Chapter ***). Acetaminophen has less gastrointestinal toxicity and nephrotoxicity and no antiplatelet activity. There may be an increased risk of hepatotoxicity in those with underlying liver disease. NSAIDs inhibit cyclooxygenase (COX) production of prostaglandins, which are known to directly sensitize peripheral nociceptors and may also have some central analgesic effects. There is a ceiling effect to NSAID-induced analgesia, such that above a certain dose there is no further increase in relief. There is patient variability in analgesic response and the occurrence of side effects. Therefore, if analgesic response is inadequate, several different NSAIDs should be tried. Elderly patients and those with renal disease, hypertension, and congestive heart failure should be given NSAIDs with caution. Increased risk of serious adverse gastrointestinal events (hemorrhage, perforation, or obstruction) is seen in those over age 65; who are taking prednisone, Coumadin, or both; who have a history of peptic ulcer disease or prior NSAID gastropathy; and who have poor health status. These individuals should be treated with a selective COX-2 inhibitor or opioid rather than NSAIDs. Nonopioid analgesics are usually not effective for moderate to severe pain.

Until recently, many physicians were reluctant to prescribe opioids for nonmalignant pain because of concerns about long-term opioid efficacy, side effects, tolerance requiring ever-increasing doses, and dependence, abuse, or addiction. Evidence is accumulating that opioids are safe without major organ toxicity, and side effects are manageable when anticipated and treated expectantly.[66-70] A survey of opioid use in a rheumatology clinic cohort found 45 percent of 644 patients had been prescribed opioids in the preceding 3 years: 153 of them for less than 3 months and 137 for 3 months or more. Opioids were highly effective in these patients with well-defined rheumatologic diseases.[71] Figure 64–6 illustrates the important observation that opioids have been just as effective in those treated with long-term opioids as in those treated with short-term opioids, suggesting that tolerance did not develop in these patients. Analysis of the causes for increases in daily opioid dose indicated that a progression of the underlying disease, a complication, or a new painful problem had developed in all but four patients. In the four patients with unexplained increases in opioid dose, problems with abuse behavior, addiction, or both became evident and required the assistance of a liaison psychiatrist for management. The cohort has been followed prospectively for another 5.5 years.[72] Opioid efficacy has been sustained, and no opioid tolerance has been seen in these patients. Side effects were common but easily managed in most patients. As in the initial 3-year study period, increases in opioid dose were related to worsening or complication of the underlying rheumatic disease or development of a new disease in all but three patients. There three patients also displayed abuse or addiction behaviors and were difficult to manage. The 8.5-year surveillance of this cohort of patients treated with long-term opioids for defined rheumatic disease pain supports the concepts that opioids are effective long term, tolerance is not inevitable, no serious organ toxicity is observed, side effects are manageable, and the incidence of substance-abuse behaviors is no greater than the general population.

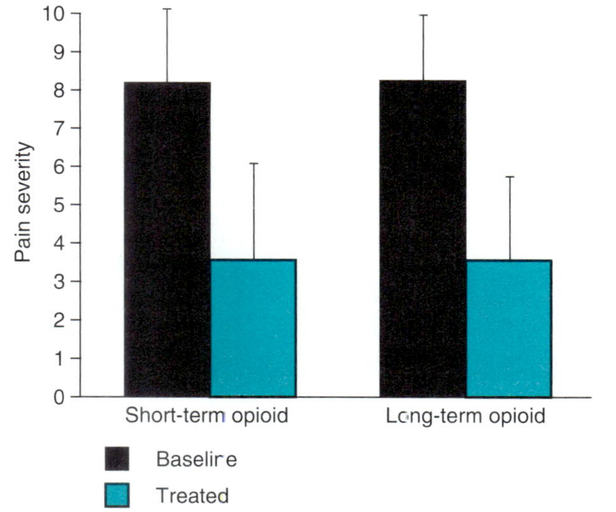

FIGURE 64–6 · Patient Contract for Chronic Opioid Therapy. Ratings of pain severity for short-term (n = 111) and long-term (n = 116) opioid users before and after a dose of an opioid analgesic. Error bars show ISD = $P < 0.001$. (From Ytterberg SR, Mahowald M, Woods SR: codeine and oxycodone use in patients with chronic rheumatic disease pain. Arthritis Rheum 41:1603, 1998.

Management of a large number of patients on opioids in a busy clinic with multiple physicians and trainees requires a controlled system for patient monitoring and prescription refills. The first step is the decision for an opioid trial. If the nonopioid analgesics are not sufficient to reduce pain below 4.5 rating, a weak opioid, such as codeine or hydrocodone with acetaminophen, should be tried next (Table 64–7). At this point it is important to discuss with the patient a plan of 2 to 3 months for gradual titration of the opioid. Opioids do not have a ceiling effect for analgesia, but if compounded with acetaminophen, the daily dose of acetaminophen should be less than 4 grams. It is important to anticipate opioid side

TABLE 64-7 • OPIOIDS FOR LONG-TERM TREATMENT OF CHRONIC MUSCULOSKELETAL PAIN

	Oral Dose	Dosing Intervals	Comments
Codeine	30-60 mg	4-6 hr	For moderate pain
Hydrocodone (Lortab, Vicodin)	5-10 mg	3-4 hr	For moderate pain
Morphine	7.5-15 mg	Q 4hr	For severe pain, titrate to pain relief, morphine-6-glucuronide can accumulate in renal insufficiency
Morphine (controlled release)	15-30 mg	Q 8-12 hr	Titrate slowly
Oxycodone	5-10 mg	3-4 hr	Monitor amount of acetaminophen given per day
Oxycodone (controlled release)	10-20 mg	Q 12 hr	Titrate slowly
Hydromorphone (Dilaudid)	1.5-3 mg	3-4 hr	Titrate to pain relief
Methadone	15-20 mg	6-8 hr	Slow titration
Fentanyl	25 µg	Q 72 hr	Titrate very slowly, variable responses
Propoxyphene	100 mg	4 hr	Caution in elderly
Tramadol	50-100 mg	6 hr	Binds mu receptor, inhibits uptake of serotonin and NE

Abbreviation: Q, Every.

effects and warn the patient to take a gut stimulant, rather than stool softener, to prevent constipation. When starting a new opioid medication, patients should be advised to take the first dose at home to determine whether sedation, dizziness, or confusion occurs. Caution patients about taking an opioid with other sedating medications or after drinking alcohol. If the patient has a history of substance abuse, more frequent monitoring may be necessary.

At the end of the 3-month opioid titration trial, a decision should be made as to whether the opioid reduced the pain, whether side effects were manageable, and whether the patient is now ready to begin an exercise program to increase function or is able to perform some activity he or she was unable to do before the opioids. If pain relief was only minimally improved, further dose titration or a trial of a stronger opioid is recommended. When the decision for long-term opioid treatment has been made, the rules for opioids must be clearly explained to the patient, preferably with an opioid contract signed by both the patient and the physician (Fig. 64–7). The patient must agree to keep all scheduled appointments, have random urine toxicology screens, seek opioid prescriptions only from a single provider, and not to go to the emergency room or come into the clinic unscheduled for an early prescription refill. With rare exceptions, there should be no excuses for early refills or "lost" medications. When the opioid dose has been selected, a trained nurse can take over the monthly monitoring for efficacy, side effects, signs of abuse or drug diversion, and the timely refilling of prescriptions (see Fig. 64–8). It is important to get all physicians in the clinic to agree to write only prescriptions prepared by the nurse managing opioid administration in the clinic. It is desirable to obtain cooperation from the local emergency room physicians not to refill opioid prescriptions at night or on the weekends.

How do opioids work? Opioids either block the release of neurotransmitter by preventing calcium influx into the presynaptic terminal, or they take the pain-transmission neuron out of the circuit by hyperpolarizing it through opening a potassium channel. Selection of opioid preparation should begin with the weaker opioids first (codeine or hydro-codone with acetaminophen), because the prescription can be written with five refills. It is important to remember that codeine and hydrocodone must be metabolized to their active metabolite, morphine, to exert an analgesic effect. There will be no analgesic effect in individuals who are poor metabolizers or if the enzyme CYP2D6 is inhibited by concomitant medications such as amiodarone, fluoxetine, haloperidol, paroxetine, and terbinafine.

Conversion among opioid preparations is straightforward. Long-acting morphine is converted to long-acting oxycodone at an equianalgesic ratio of 2:1 (60 mg controlled release Morphine = 30 mg controlled release Oxycodase every 12 hours). When converting morphine to transdermal fentanyl, use a 1:2:3 rule that says 1 mg parenteral morphine per day is equivalent to 2 µg per hour via fentanyl patch, which is also equivalent to 3 mg per day of oral morphine. Conversion ratios in the fentanyl package insert are recommended for opioid naïve patients and may not be high enough for those already taking regular opioids. Although there is no ceiling dose for opioid analgesia, side effects increase with increasing opioid dose and can produce confusion, agitation, myoclonus, dry mouth, itching, and sedation.

Methadone is an opioid that also blocks N-methyl-D-aspartate (NMDA) receptors in the brain and spinal cord. NMDA is an excitatory neurotransmitter responsible for pain amplification via "wind up" by releasing nitric oxide. When used to treat opioid addiction, the dose of methadone selected is 1:1 with morphine dose and administered every 24 hours. When using methadone to treat pain, the equianalgesic dose is 1 mg oral methadone for 3 mg morphine, and it must be dosed at 6-hour intervals.

TROUBLESHOOTING PROBLEMS WITH LONG-TERM OPIOID THERAPY

Problems do arise when managing patients with long-term opioids for chronic musculoskeletal pain. It is important to document opioid efficacy, increased function, side effects, and the lack of signs suggesting abuse (Fig. 64–8). The most common problem is patient report of loss of analgesia. This complaint has a differ-

Contract for Long-Term Chronic Opioid Therapy Between:

Patient Name **and Dr.** **At the Minneapolis VAMC**
Chronic Opioid Therapy for Intractable Pain Will Be Prescribed Under the Following Conditions:
1. If (drug prescribed) is effective for adequate pain control with tolerable side effects
2. If Scheduled appointments are kept: if appointment is failed the prescription will not be renewed
3. If the Patient agrees to obtain pain medications only from Dr: And NOT to go to the ER or Urgent Care for more meds
4. If the patient agrees NOT to request "early" or "partial" prescription refills from the MVAMC Pharmacy
5. If the patient agrees NOT to come to the Rheumatology clinic without an appointment to request more Pain Medications
6. There will be no acceptable excuses for "lost medications"
7. If the Patient agrees to be responsible for taking medications as directed. If the Pain medication supply is used up before the end of the prescription period, the patient has the option of admission for opioid withdrawal under supervision or will "tough it out" at home. NO additional pain medications will be prescribed.
8. Pain Severity and function will be re-evaluated after ________months of an Opioid Trial to determine whether continued use of chronic opiods is justified by clinical improvement
9. I understand that urine samples will be randomly tested for drugs
PATIENT AND PHYSICIAN ARE TO SIGN BELOW:
PATIENT SIGNATURE: **PHYSICIAN SIGNATURE:**

DATE			NAME SSN

MEDICINE SERVICE **RHEUMATOLOGY CLINIC**

FIGURE 64–7 · Opioid Contract.

3D Narcotic Telephone Renewal Clinic

Renewal For: **Last Filled on:** **# Pills Dispensed** **DATE STARTED**

How many pills are you using per day? LEAST MOST

Are you using any other Pain Medications? NO YES If yes what? ?OTC from another MD?

Does the medication help? A LOT SOME A LITTLE NOT AT ALL

Rate your pain from **0 to 10** BEFORE you take the pain medication ________ and AFTER taking it________

Have you had any side effects from the pain medications such as: FEEL SLEEPY OR SEDATED CONFUSION

DIZZINESS CONSTIPATION NAUSEA OTHER:

How do you feel your pain control is? Residual Pain Amount of Time with No Pain

How many days per week do you take the Pain Medications: How many pills per day do you take on those days?

Do you feel the Pain Medication has lost its effectiveness? NO YES If Yes have you increased the dose? NO YES

COMMENTS:

Do you receive pain medication from doctors not at the MVAMC NO YES If yes what medication

Reason it was prescribed by whom:

Have you become addicted to the opioid NO YES If yes describe

Are you afraid of becoming addicted? NO YES If yes comment:

Do you have a history of addiction to alcohol or other drugs? NO YES If YES describe

PRESCRIPTION WRITTEN FOR **# PILLS/MO** **RENEWED** **MD**

SCHEDULE ED NARCOTIC TELEPHONE RENEWAL CLINIC ON (DATE)________________

DATE	NAME: ssn

MEDICINE SERVICE **3D RHEUMATOLOGY CLINIC**

FIGURE 64–8 · Opioid Monitoring Form.

ential diagnosis that includes: (1) increased peripheral nociception from the original or a new problem with increased inflammation, tumor, neuropathic process, or osteoporotic fracture; (2) development of anxiety or depression; (3) cognitive change altering pain perception or reporting, such as delirium; or (4) opioid tolerance (rare). There are certain aberrant behaviors that raise the question of abuse or addiction behaviors. Highly suggestive behaviors include selling prescription drugs; prescription forgery; stealing drugs from others; injecting oral formulations; obtaining drugs from nonmedical sources; concurrent abuse of alcohol or illicit drugs; multiple dose escalations; multiple episodes of "lost medications"; aggressive complaining about the need for more medications; seeking medications from multiple prescribers or the emergency room; deterioration in work, family, or social functioning because of the drugs; and resistance to changing therapy despite adverse effects. These behaviors should prompt urine toxicology screens and request for addiction-disorder evaluation.

Side effects may be troublesome in some patients. Sedation is usually transient. Nausea usually abates within 2 to 3 weeks but can be treated with hydroxyzine or compazine suppositories. Constipation should be prevented by prophylactic gut stimulants, such as bisacodyl or senna, or an osmotic laxative, such as lactulose. Bulk-forming laxatives, such as psyllium and methyl cellulose, should be avoided because they can cause obstruction in an opioid-treated patient.[74] Opioid-induced confusion, disorientation, and hallucinations can occur in those with underlying encephalopathy or dementia and are more common with long-acting preparations. The patient should be switched to a short-acting preparation and the dose lowered if necessary. Urinary retention is usually transient, but the dose should be decreased or another opioid used. Pruritus may be secondary to histamine release from mast cells and may require switch to another opioid. Multifocal myoclonus is uncommon, usually transient, and may respond to a benzodiazepine such as lorazepam.

ADJUNCTIVE MEDICATIONS FOR CHRONIC PAIN

Tricyclic anti-depressant (TCA) and antiepileptic drugs are useful adjuncts to analgesic therapy in patients with low back pain, radiculopathy, PHN, and neuropathic pain.[75] The antiepileptic drugs may decrease ectopic discharges from injured nerves and decrease the lancinating pains. There are three basic mechanism-based approaches to treatment of a neuropathic pain component (Table 64–8).

1. Drugs to enhance the descending inhibitory pathways by interacting with biogenic amines
2. Drugs that modulate peripheral sensitization by interacting with voltage-sensitive sodium channels
3. Drugs that modulate central sensitization by interacting with calcium channels, NK1, or NMDA receptors (norepinephrine and serotonin)

There is strong evidence that TCA decrease neuropathic pain and weaker evidence that anticonvulsants, antiarrhythmics, and topical agents are effective.[76,77] Antidepressants inhibit reuptake of the biogenic amines serotonin and norepinephrine, modulate sodium channels, and inhibit excitatory neurotransmitters. The tertiary amines block uptake of both norepinephrine and serotonin (i.e., amitryptiline, imipramine, clomipramine, and doxepin) and the secondary amines block only norepinephrine uptake (i.e., nortriptyline and desipramine). TCAs have adverse effects of sedation, weight gain, and orthostatic hypotension and anticholinergic symptoms of dry mouth, urinary retention, and constipation, which are worse in the elderly. TCAs must be used with caution in those with heart disease, glaucoma, and prostatism. serotonin-norepinephrine reuptake inhibitors (SNRIs), such as venlafaxine, have little anticholinergic effects, fewer side effects than TCAs, and are effective in diabetic neuropathy pain. The selective serotonin reuptake inhibitors (SSRIs) are generally not very effective for pain but are better tolerated than the TCAs. Fluoxetine is not effective; paroxetine and citalopram have modest effects.[77] Narcotics have long been considered ineffective in neuropathic pain; however, recent studies have demonstrated that controlled-release oxycodone (20 to 99 mg/day),[78,79] morphine and methadone,[75] and tramadol[77] were effective for neuropathic pain.

Drugs that inhibit sodium channel activation can modulate peripheral sensitization by decreasing action potential propagation, membrane depolarization, and neurotransmitter release. Anticonvulsants tend to inhibit repetitive firing of action potentials under conditions of sustained neuronal depolarization.[34] First-generation antiepileptic drugs are carbamezepine and dilantin. Carbamazepine is structurally similar to the TCAs and can enhance sodium channel inactivation, reduce excitatory neurotransmitter release, and modulate L-type calcium channels. It has been shown to be effective in diabetic neuropathy and PHN pain.[34] Phenytoin has had variable efficacy in neuropathic pain. The side effects of these two drugs often limit their usefulness. The second-generation antiepileptic drugs (gabapentin, lamotrigine, topiramate) act via multiple mechanisms and show promise in clinical trials of painful neuropathy. Oxcarbazepine acts on sodium channels and N-type calcium channels and may modulate both peripheral and central sensitization. Lamotrigine acts on sodium channels, inhibits release of excitatory neurotransmitters, and modulates N-type calcium channels. It has had variable efficacy for peripheral neuropathic pain and is associated with common side effects, including rash. In one trial, 44 percent of patients with central post-stroke pain experienced a decrease with 200 mg/day of lamotrigine.[34] Topiramate has multiple mechanisms of action, inhibits voltage-gated sodium and calcium channels, has GABAergic and glutaminergic effects, and has shown modest effects in diabetic neuropathy.

Modulators of central sensitization such as gabapentin[34,76] and pregabalin, which are GABA analogues, may act on calcium channels within the spinal cord, modulate GABA release, inhibit sodium channels, and alter monoamine neurotransmitter release. Levetiracetam, a novel antiepileptic drug, binds to synaptic plasma membranes in the central nervous system and

TABLE 64–8 • ADJUVANT THERAPEUTIC MEDICATIONS

	Trade Name	Dose Ranges	Comments
Antidepressants			All effective in painful neuropathy independent of antidepressant properties; risk of arrhythmias in cardiac disease
Amitriptyline	Elavil	25-150 mg/day	S and NE reuptake inhibitor
Imipramine	Tofranil	25-150 mg/day	
Desipramine	Norpramin	25-150 mg/day	NE reuptake inhibitor
Nortriptyline	Pamelor	25-150 mg/day	NE reuptake inhibitor
Clomipramine	Anafranil	25-150 mg/day	S and NE reuptake inhibitor
SNRIs venlafaxine	Effexor	25-150 mg/day Titrate slowly	Not analgesic at low dose, S and NE reuptake inhibitor, AEs, nausea, dizziness, insomnia, anorexia, somnolence, and fatigue; fluoxetine not effective;
SSRIs			
paroxetine	Paxil	20 mg	AEs, less than TCAs; asthenia, sweating, GI disturbances,
citalopram	Celexa	20 mg	somnolence, dizziness, sexual dysfunction
Antiepileptic Drugs			**Enhance sodium channel inactivation**
Phenytoin	Dilantin	200-50 mg/day	Variable results, inhibits insulin release; AEs, dizziness, unsteadiness, drowsiness, rash
Gabapentin	Neurontin	300 mg at bedtime, slow increase up to 3600 mg/day on a tid schedule	Variable results in clinical trials; AEs, drowsiness, somnolence, fatigue are transient; no interaction with warfarin or birth control pills; accumulates in renal failure
Pregabalin	In trials	300-600 mg/day	Dizziness, somnolence, edema
Carbamezepine	Tegretol	200 mg bid to start up to 400-1200 mg/day	Effective for trigeminal neuralgia, diabetic neuropathy less effective in PHN; relative contraindication in heart disease, contraindicated with heart block, AEs, dizziness, drowsiness, diplopia, rash in 7-10%; risk of cytopenias is rare
Oxcarbazepine		75 mg bid up to 600-2400 mg/day	Fewer AEs than carbamazepine; hyponatremia drowsiness, dizziness, headache, GI sx
Lamotrigine	Lamictal	25 mg/day to start, slow increases up to 400 mg/day	AEs, dizziness, unsteadiness, drowsiness, rashes, ataxia
Topiramate	Topamax	25-50 mg/d up to 400 mg/day	Sulfonamide derivative, variable benefit in trials; AEs, somnolence, anorexia, weight loss, fatigue, behavioral problems and cognitive difficulties, confusion
Levetiracetam	Keppra	250 mg/day up to 1500-6000 mg	Few studies in painful neuropathy, some added benefit with gabapentin, few side effects
Valproic acid	Depakote		AEs drowsiness, nausea, vomiting, tremor, weight gain, rare hepatotoxicity, pancreatitis
Zonisamide		100 mg	Blocks sodium and T type calcium channels and increases GABA release
Topicals			
Lidocaine patch		Up to 3 patches at once for 12 hr	Must use on intact skin, modest benefit
Capsaicin		.025% to .075% applied 3-5 times/day	Adjunctive treatment, depletes substance P from C fibers, transient burning may be intolerable, lasts a few weeks
Miscellaneous			
Mexilitene		450-675 mg/day on tid schedule	An antiarrythmic, sodium channel blocker; equivocal efficacy, AEs, GI sx, dizziness, tremor, palpitations, chest pain, headache
Baclofen		10 mg tid up to 60 mg/day	Effective in trigeminal neuralgia
Carbidopa-levodopa		25:100 tid	Increases CNS dopamine
Ketamine		IV or subcutaneous injections	Blocks NMDA receptors; AEs dysphoria, sedation, dissociative episodes
Dextromethorphan		Up to 960 mg/day	Low-affinity NMDA receptor blocker

Abbreviations: AE, Adverse events; GI, gastrointestinal; NE, norepinephrine; S, serotonin.

inhibits burst firing. It is used primarily as adjunctive therapy with gabapentin in patients with seizures. In one small trial it showed some additional pain relief when added to gabapentin for painful neuropathy. Zonisamide, a sodium and T-type calcium channel blocker, increases GABA release and had marginal benefit and a high occurrence of adverse events[34]; however, some patients who had failed multiple prior medications did obtain pain relief. Mexiletine is a sodium channel blocker structurally similar to lidocaine. It improved nighttime pain relief and sleep in patients with diabetic neuropathy but had minimal daytime benefit, and its use is limited by side effects of tremors, confusion, agitation, nausea, and vomiting.

Blocking NMDA (an excitatory neurotransmitter) channels to decrease central sensitization has been limited by drug side effects.[80] Intravenous and subcutaneous ketamine at subanesthetic doses was effective but caused severe dysphoria, sedation, and dissociative episodes. Dextromethorphan, an over-the-counter cough suppressant, is a low-affinity NMDA channel blocker, an isomer of the codeine analog levorphanol, and is metabolized to dextrorphan, which also has NMDA-antagonist activity. The antitussive dose of 120 mg/day is not sufficient for neuropathic analgesia. In an NIH clinical trial of up to 960 mg/day, seven of 13 patients with diabetic neuropathy reported moderate or greater relief; however, the drug was ineffective in PHN.[80] Side effects were substantial, including sedation, dizziness, and ataxia. In the future, NMDA antagonists will likely be combined with other agents to decrease central sensitization because neuropathic pain is partially responsive to multiple agents.

Lidocaine patches may give local pain relief. Topical capsaicin, an alkaloid in hot chili peppers that binds to the vanilloid receptor on C and A-delta fibers, depletes SP from sensory nerve endings and may actually cause degeneration of nerve endings.

WHEN TO REFER TO A PAIN SPECIALIST OR A MULTIDISCIPLINARY PAIN PROGRAM

General internists and rheumatologists may become frustrated caring for patients with chronic pain disorders when elimination of the presumptive cause of the pain does not eliminate the pain. The medical, psychologic, and socioeconomic complexity of these patients often creates an intense demand on the clinician. Patients who have predominantly psychologic and socioeconomic or occupational features to their chronic-pain experience are best cared for by a multidisciplinary pain team, rather than an office-based single practitioner who would not have the breadth of skills and experience required to identify multiple layers of sensory and emotional components of the pain behaviors. Physicians who are unaware of the psychosocial dimensions of chronic psychophysiologic pain syndromes will fail to identify such patients and may become frustrated and suspicious of the lack of response to "standard" treatments. These patients have often had repeated attempts to identify and eliminate the cause of the pain; yet the pain persisted, and they have become depressed, angry, and hopeless.

Interestingly, the patients behave similarly. Regardless of the underlying pathophysiology, the debility is out of proportion to the tissue injury, and these patients have atypical nonanatomic sensory abnormalities. They seem intolerant to stress, sensory stimuli, and physical activity. The patient's response to the pain experience and coping style results in a "functional overlay" as an attempt to handle the fear and anxiety he or she is experiencing. The individual clinician usually does not possess the multiple skills and specialized knowledge to fully assess all the dimensions of the pain experience in patients with the chronic pain disorder. This chronic pain syndrome is the physical, psychologic, and social degeneration of the patient with chronic pain. Therefore, these patients need physical, psychologic, and social rehabilitation in concert with medical management. Such a biopsychosocial model of chronic pain syndrome requires a multidisciplinary pain-management program in which pain reduction has lower priority than pain acceptance and restoration of function. In specialty pain-treatment programs, behavior not focused on pain is rewarded and pain-focused behavior is ignored. This redirects the patient's efforts away from seeking pain relief toward changing behavior and reducing disability. Families are taught not to be solicitous and sympathethic to grimaces and complaints of pain. The program includes intensive exercise therapy, management of depression and anxiety, supportive psychotherapy, and patient education. Cognitive and behavioral therapy includes stress management, relaxation, and biofeedback techniques to gain control over factors that exacerbate the pain. Physical modalities are used to reduce pain and permit a progressive exercise program with a timetable to attain self care at a level consistent with objective physical abnormalities. Three to 6 weeks are required to initiate physical and emotional changes and an aftercare program to reinforce these changes. The primary criteria for selection of a patient for a multidisciplinary pain program is the definitive diagnosis of nonreversible pain (no planned surgery) and readiness to change (i.e., motivated toward rehabilitation goals). The patients must not have active substance abuse, suicidal ideation, cognitive impairment, or a personality or thought disorder that would interfere with the group milieu, learning, and communication. They may need additional specialized diagnostic testing (e.g., nerve blocks, electromyography, psychometric testing) or need detoxification from drugs. Chronic-pain programs vary in quality and should be carefully evaluated before referring patients. A pain specialty center should have multidisciplinary groups of medical specialists for intensive medical, neurologic, psychologic and physical therapy, not simply personnel to perform nerve blocks.

List of Website Pain Management Resources

American Academy of Pain Medicine
http://www.painmed.org
American Pain Foundation
http://painfoundation.org
American Pain Society
http://ampainsoc.org
International Association for the Study of Pain
http://halcyon.com/iasp
World Health Organization
http://www5.who.int/cancer/main.cfm

REFERENCES

1. American Pain Society. Guideline for the Management of Pain in Osteoarthritis, Rheumatoid Arthritis, and Juvenile Chronic Arthritis, 2nd ed. Glenview, IL, American Pain Society, 2002.
2. Katz WA: Musculoskeletal pain and its socioeconomic implications. Clin Rheumatol 21(Suppl 1):S2-S4, 2002.
3. Cassell EJ: Diagnosing suffering: a perspective. Ann Int Med 131:531-534, 1999.

4. Merskey HM: Classification of chronic pain syndromes: Description of chronic pain syndromes. Pain 3(Suppl):S217, 1986.
5. Russo CM, Brose WG: Chronic pain. Ann Rev Med 49:123-133, 1998.
6. Arner S: Opioids and long-lasting pain conditions: 25-year perspective on mechanisms-based treatment strategies. Pain Reviews 7:81-96, 2000.
7. Bolay H, Moskowitz MA: Mechanisms of pain moculation in chronic syndromes. Neurology 59(Suppl 2):S2-S7, 2002.
8. American Psychiatric Association. Diagnostic and Statistical Manual of Mental Disorders, 4th ed, text revision. Washington DC, American Psychiatric Association, 2000.
9. Becker N, Bondegaard Thomsen A, Olsen AK, et al: Pain epidemiology and health related quality of life in chronic nonmalignant pain patients referred to a Danish multidisciplinary pain center. Pain 73(3):393-400, 1997.
10. Sokka T, Kankainen A, Hannonen P: Scores for functional disability in patients with rheumatoid arthritis are correlated at higher levels with pain scores than with radiographic scores. Arthritis Rheum 43:386-389, 2000.
11. Picavet HSJ, Schouten JSAG: Musculoskeletal pain in the Netherlands: Prevalences, consequences and risk groups the DMC3-study. Pain 102:167-178,s 2003.
12. Bergman S, Herrstrom P, Hogstrom K, et al: Chronic musculoskeletal pain, prevalence rates, and sociodemographic associations in a Swedish population study. J Rheumatol 28:1369-1377, 2001.
13. Sternbach RA: Survey of pain in the United States: The Nuprin Pain Report. Clin J Pain 2:49-53, 1986.
14. American Geriatrics Society: The Management of chronic pain in older persons. J Amer Geriatrics Soc 46:635-651, 1998.
15. Ferrell BA, Ferrell BR, Osterweil D: Pain in the nursing home. J Am Geriatrics Soc 38:409-414, 1990.
16. Hunt SP, Mantyh PW: The molecular dynamics of pain control. Nat Rev Neurosci 2:83-91, 2001.
17. Willis WD, Westlund KN: Neuroanatomy of the pain system and of the pathways that modulate pain. J Clin Neurophysiol 14:2-31, 1997.
18. Schaible HG, Schmidt RF: Effects of an experimental arthritis on the sensory properties of fine articular afferent units. J Neurophysiol 54:1109-1122, 1985.
19. Sachs D, Cunha FQ, Poole S, et al: Tumour necrosis factor-alpha, interleiukin 1 beta and interleukin-8 induce persistent mechanical nociceptro hypersensitivity. Pain 96:89-97, 2002.
20. Stein C: The control of pain in peripheral tissues by opioids. N Eng J Med 332:1685-1690, 1995.
21. Honore P, Rogers SD, Schwei MJ, et al: Murine models of inflammatory, neuropathic and cancer pain each generates a unique set of neurochemical changes in the spinal cord and sensory neurons. Neuroscience 98:585-598, 2000.
22. Melzack R, Wall PD: Pain mechanisms: a new theory. Science 150:971-979, 1965.
23. LeBars D, Dickenson AH, Besson JM: Diffuse noxious inhibitory controls (DNIC). I. Effects on dorsal horn convergent neurons in the rat. Pain 6:283-304, 1979.
24. Schaible HG, Grubb BD: Afferent and spinal mechanisms of joint pain. Pain 55:5-54, 1993.
25. Mapp P, Kidd BL: The role of substance P in rheumatic disease. Semin Arthritis Rheum 23:3-9, 1994.
26. Schaible HG: Why does an inflammation in the joint hurt? Br J Rheum 35:405-406, 1996.
27. Matucci-Cerinic M, Konttinen YT, Generini S, Cutolo M: Neuropeptides and steroid hormones in arthritis. Curr Opin Rheumatol 10:220-235, 1998.
28. Garrett N, Cruwys SC, Kidd BL, Tomlison DR: Effect of capsaicin on substance P and nerve growth factor in adjuvant arthritic rat. Neuroscience Letter 230:5-8, 1997.
29. Buma P, Elmans L, van den Berg WB, Schrama LH: Neurovascular plasticity in the knee joint of an arthritic mouse model. Anatom Rec 260:51-61, 2000.
30. Konttinen YT, Sorsa T, Santavirta SS, Russel A: Via dolorosa: From the first to the second station. J Rheumatol 21:783-787, 1994.
31. Lotz M: Experimental models of arthritis: identification of substance P as a therapeutic target and use of capsaicin to manage joint pain and inflammation. Semin Arthritis Rheum 23:10-17, 1994.
32. Boyle DL, Moore J, Yang L, et al: Spinal adenosine receptor activation inhibits inflammation and joint destruction in rat adjuvant arthritis. Arthritis Rheum 46:3076-3082, 2002.
33. Honore P, Luger NM, Sabino MC, et al: Osteoprotegerin blocks bone cancer-induced skeletal destruction, skeletal pain and pain-related neurochemical reorganization of the spinal cord. Nat Med 6:521-528, 2000.
34. Backonja M: Use of anticonvulsants for treatment of neuropathic pain. Neurology 59(Suppl 2):S14-S17, 2002.
35. Jensen TS, Baron R: Translation of symptoms and signs into mechanisms in neuropathic pain. Pain 102:1-8, 2003.
36. Kost RG, Straus SE: Postherpetic neuralgia-pathogenesis, treatment, prevention. New Engl J Med 335:32-42, 1996.
37. Rice ASC: Gabapentin in postherpetic neuralgia: A randomized, double blind, placebo controlled study. Pain 94:215-224, 2001.
38. Alper BS, Lewis PR: Review: tricyclic antidepressants, capsaicin, gabapentin, and oxycodone are effective for postherpetic neuralgia. J Fam Pract 51:121-128, 2002.
39. Attal N, Brasseur L, Dupuy M, et al: Invravenous lidocaine in central pain: A double blind placebo controlled psychophysical study. Neurology 54:564-574, 2000.
40. Attal N, Guirimand F, Brasseur L, et al: Effects of IV morphine in central pain, a randomized placebo controlled study. Neurology 58:554-563, 2002.
41. Merskey HM, Bogduk N: Descriptions of Chronic Pain Syndromes and Definitions of Pain Terms. Seattle, International Association for the Study of Pain Press, 1994.
42. Kemler MA, Barendse GAM, van Kleef M, et al: Spinal cord stimulation in patients with chronic reflex sympathetic dystrophy. New Engl J Med 343:618-624, 2000.
43. Berklein F, Schmelz M, Schifter S, Weber M: The important role of neuropeptides in complex regional pain syndrome. Neurology 57:2179-2184, 2001.
44. van Hilten BJ, van de Beek WJT, Hoff JI, et al: Intrathecal baclofen for the treatment of dystonia in patients with reflex sympathetic dystrophy. New Engl J Med 343:625-630, 2000.
45. Koenig TW, Clark MR: Advances in comprehensive pain management. Psych Clin N Am 19:589-611, 1996.
46. Staab JP, Datto CJ, Weinrieb RM, et al: Detection and diagnosis of psychiatric disorders in primary medical care settings. Med Clin North Am 85:579-596, 2001.
47. Fishbain DA: Approaches to treatment decisions for psychiatric comorbidity in the management of the chronic pain patient. Med Clin North Am 83:737-760, 1999.
48. Miller MC: Personality disorders. Med Clin North Am 85:819-837, 2001.
49. Hart FD, Taylor RT, Huskisson EC: Pain at night. Lancet I:881-884, 1970.
50. Mahowald MW, Mahowald ML, Bundlie S, Ytterberg SR: Sleep fragmentation in rheumatoid arthritis. Arthritis Rheum 32:974-983, 1989.
51. Mahowald ML, Mahowald MW: Nighttime sleep and daytime functioning (sleepiness and fatigue) in well-defined chronic rheumatic diseases. Sleep Med 1:179-193, 2000.
52. Mahowald ML, Mahowald MW: Nighttime sleep and daytime functioning (sleepiness and fatigue) in less well defined rheumatic diseases. Sleep Med 1:195-207, 2000.
53. Lavigne G, Zucconi M, Castronovo C, et al: Sleep arousal response to experimental thermal stimulation during sleep in human subjects free of pain and sleep problems. Pain 84:283-290, 2000.
54. Smith MT, Perlis ML, Smith MS, et al: Sleep quality and presleep arousal in chronic pain. Int J Behav Med 23:1-13, 2000.
55. Wooten V: Medical causes of insomnia. *In* Dement WC (ed): Principles and Practice of Sleep Medicine. Philadelphia, W. B. Saunders, 1994, p 509-522.
56. Atkinson H, Ancoli-Israel S, Slater MA, et al: Subjective sleep disturbance in chronic back pain. Clin J Pain 4:225-232, 1988.
57. Wittig RM, Zorick FJ, Blumer D, et al: Disturbed sleep in patients complaining of chronic pain. J Nerv Ment Dis 170:429-431, 1982.
58. Harman K, Pivik RT, D'Eon JL, et al: Sleep in depressed and nondepressed participants with chronic low back pain: Electroencephalographic and behaviour findings. Sleep 25:775-783, 2002.
59. Sayar K, Arikan M, Yontem T: Sleep quality in chronic pain patients. Can J Psych 47:844-848, 2002.
60. Wilcox S, Brenes GA, Levine D, et al: Factors related to sleep disturbance in older adults experiencing knee pain or knee pain

with radiographic evidence of knee osteoarthritis. J Am Geriatr Soc 48:1241-1251, 2000.
61. Gureje O, Simon GE, Von Korff M: A cross national study of the course of persistent pain in primary care. Pain 92:195-200, 2001.
62. Eckman P, O'Sullivan M: Who can catch a liar? Am Psychol 46:913-920, 1991.
63. Spitzer RL, Williams JB, Kroenke K, et al: Validity and utility of the PRIME-MD patient health questionnaire in assessment of 3000 obstetric-gynecologic patients: The PRIME-MD Patient Health Questionnaire Obstetrics Gynecology Study. Am J Obstet Gynecol 183:759-769, 2000.
64. Brena SF, Koch DF: The pain estimate model for quantification and classification of chronic pain states. Anesth Rev 2:8-13, 1975.
65. Farrar JT, Young JP, LaMoreaux L, et al: Clinical importance of changes in chronic pain intensity measured on an 11-point numerical pain rating scale. Pain 94:149-158, 2001.
66. Papagallo M: Aggressive pharmacologic treatment of pain. Rheum Dis Clin North Am 25:193-212, 1999.
67. Peloso PM, Bellamy N, Bensen W, et al: Double blind randomized placebo control trial of controlled release codeine in the treatment of osteoarthritis of the hip or knee. J Rheumatol 27(3):764-771, 2000.
68. Portenoy RK: Opioid therapy for chronic nonmalignant pain: current status. *In* Fields HL, Liebeskind JC (eds): Progress in Pain Research and Management. Seattle, International Association for the Study of Pain Press, 1994, pp 247-287.
69. Portenoy RK (ed): Opioid tolerance and responsiveness: Research findings and clinical observations. *In* Proceedings of 7th World Congress on Pain. Seattle, International Association for the Study of Pain Press, 1994.
70. Portenoy RK, Dole F, Joseph H, et al: Pain management and chemical dependency: Evolving perspectives. JAMA 278:592-593, 1997.
71. Ytterberg SR, Mahowald ML, Woods SR: Codeine and oxycodone use in patients with chronic rheumatic disease pain. Arthritis Rheum 41(9):1603-1612, 1998.
72. Lazovskis J, Mahowald ML, Singh J: Lack of evidence for opioid tolerance in patients with rheumatic disease. Arthritis Rheum 46:S102, 2003.
73. Fields HL: Pain modulation and the action of analgesic medications. Ann Neurol 35:S42-S45, 1994.
74. Papagallo M, JN C: The pharmacologic management of chronic back pain. *In* JW F (ed) The Adult Spine: Principles and Practice. Philadelphia, Lippincott-Raven, 1997, pp 275-285.
75. Raja SN, Haythornthwaite JA, Papagallo M, et al: Opioids versus antidepressants in postherpetic neuralgia, a randomized, placebo-controlled trial. Neurology 59:1015-1021, 2001.
76. Backonja M, Beydoun A, Edwards KR, et al: Gabapentin for the symptomatic treatment of painful neuropathy in patients with diabetes mellitus: A randomized controlled trial. JAMA 280:1831-1836, 1998.
77. Sindrup SH, Jensen TS: Pharmacologic treatment of pain in polyneuropathy. Neurology 55:915-920, 2000.
78. Watson CP, Babul N: Efficacy of oxycodone in neuropathic pain. A randomized trial in postherpetic neuralgia. Neurology 50:1837-1841, 1998.
79. Gimbel JS, Richards P, Portenoy RK: Controlled-release oxycodone for pain in diabeti neuropathy: A randomized controlled trial. Neurology 60:927-934, 2003.
80. Nelson KA, Park KM, Robinovitz E, et al: High dose oral dextromethorphan versus placebo in painful diabetic neuropathy and postherpetic neuralgia. Neurology 48:1212-1218, 1997.

Index

Page numbers followed by "f" denote figures and "t" denote tables

D

F

G

K

N

P

Q

R

S

W

X

Y

Z